Y0-AQO-156

LATEST APPROVED METHODS OF TREATMENT
FOR THE PRACTICING PHYSICIAN

Edited by

ROBERT E. RAKEL, M.D.

Professor and Chairman, Department of Family Medicine
Associate Dean for Academic and Clinical Affairs
Baylor College of Medicine, Houston, Texas

W.B. SAUNDERS COMPANY
A Division of Harcourt Brace & Company
Philadelphia London Toronto Montreal Sydney Tokyo

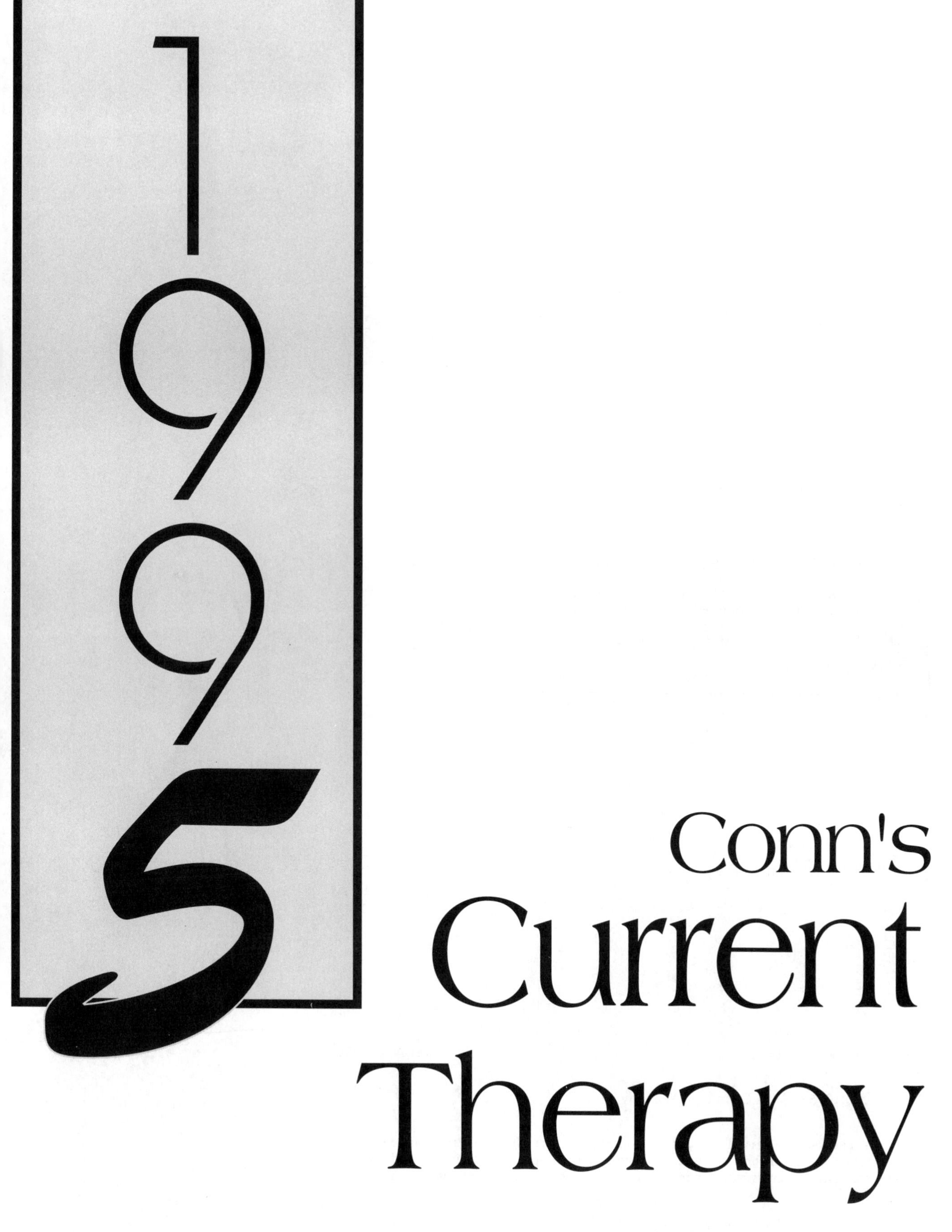

Conn's Current Therapy

W.B. SAUNDERS COMPANY
A Division of
Harcourt Brace & Company

The Curtis Center
Independence Square West
Philadelphia, Pennsylvania 19106

Library of Congress Cataloging-in-Publication Data

Current therapy; latest approved methods of treatment for the practicing physician. 1949–

v. 28 cm. annual.

Editors: 1949– H. F. Conn and others.

1. Therapeutics. 2. Therapeutics, Surgical. 3. Medicine—Practice. I. Conn, Howard Franklin, 1908–1982 ed.

RM101.C87 616.058 49–8328 rev*

ISBN 0–7216–4052–4

Conn's Current Therapy 1995 ISBN 0–7216–4052–4

Printed in the United States of America

Last digit is the print number: 9 8 7 6 5 4 3 2 1

Contributors

GEORGE AHTARIDIS, M.D.

Assistant Professor of Medicine, University of Pennsylvania; Graduate Hospital, Philadelphia, Pennsylvania
Diverticula of the Alimentary Tract

JAZILA AL-ATTAR, M.D.

Fellow in Infectious Diseases, Cornell University Medical College, New York, New York; Fellow, North Shore University Hospital, Manhasset, New York
Infectious Mononucleosis

C. KNIGHT ALDRICH, M.D.

Emeritus Professor of Psychiatry and Family Medicine, University of Virginia School of Medicine; Visiting Psychiatrist, University of Virginia Hospitals, Charlottesville, Virginia
Anxiety Disorders

CARL M. ALLEN, D.D.S., M.S.D.

Associate Professor and Director, Oral Pathology Section, Oral and Maxillofacial Surgery and Pathology, The Ohio State University, College of Dentistry, Columbus, Ohio
Diseases of the Mouth

MARK S. ALLEN, M.D.

Consultant in General Thoracic Surgery, Mayo Clinic; Assistant Professor of Surgery, Mayo Medical School; Consultant and Sur- Saint Mary's Hospital; Consultant and Surgeon, Rochester Methodist Hospital, Rochester, Minnesota
Pleural Effusion and Empyema Thoracis

CHARLES C. ALLING III, D.D.S., M.S., D.Sc. (Hon.)

Adjunct Professor, University of Iowa School of Dentistry, Iowa City, Iowa; Consultant Staff, Brookwood Medical Center, Birmingham, Alabama
Temporomandibular Disorders

CARRIE D. ALSPAUGH, M.D.

Resident in Dermatology, Vanderbilt University Medical Center Hospital, Nashville, Tennessee
Papulosquamous Eruptions

ARNOLD E. ANDERSEN, M.D.

Professor of Psychiatry, University of Iowa College of Medicine; Attending Psychiatrist and Director, Eating Disorders Program, University of Iowa Hospitals and Clinics, Iowa City, Iowa
Bulimia Nervosa

NANCY J. ANDERSON, M.D.

Associate Professor, Loma Linda University and Jerry L. Pettis VA Hospital; Consultant Staff, San Bernardino County Medical Center, San Bernardino, California; Riverside County Hospital, Riverside, California; and Loma Linda Community Hospital, Loma Linda, California
Granuloma Inguinale (Donovanosis); Lymphogranuloma Venereum

PHILIP C. ANDERSON, M.D.

Professor and Director, Division of Dermatology, University of Missouri—Columbia, Columbia, Missouri
Spider Bites and Scorpion Stings

GRANT J. ANHALT, M.D.

Professor, Johns Hopkins University School of Medicine and Johns Hopkins Hospital, Baltimore, Maryland
Bullous Diseases

DONALD ARMSTRONG, M.D.

Professor of Medicine, Cornell University Medical College; Chief, Infectious Disease Service; Director, Microbiology Laboratories, Memorial Sloan-Kettering Cancer Center, New York, New York
Acquired Immune Deficiency Syndrome (AIDS)

JAMES M. ATKINS, M.D.

Director, Emergency Medicine Education and Professor of Internal Medicine, University of Texas Southwestern Medical School, Dallas, Texas
Cardiac Arrest

PAUL AUERBACH, M.D., M.S.

Professor of Surgery and Emergency Medicine, Stanford University School of Medicine; Chief, Division of Emergency Medicine, Department of Surgery, Stanford University Hospital, Stanford, California
Disturbances Due to Cold

MILES AUSLANDER, M.D.

Assistant Professor, Division of Gastroenterology, Valley Presbyterian Hospital, Van Nuys, California
Gaseousness and Indigestion

BRUCE AVERBOOK, M.D.

Assistant Professor of Surgery and Assistant Professor of General Medical Sciences (Oncology), Case Western Reserve University and MetroHealth Medical Center, Cleveland, Ohio
Gastric Tumors

ROBERT L. BAEHNER, M.D.

Professor of Pediatrics, Department of Pediatrics, University of Southern California School of Medicine; LAC plus USC Medical Center, Women's and Children's Hospital, Los Angeles, California
Neutropenia

SAMIR K. BALLAS, M.D.

Professor of Medicine, Cardeza Foundation, Department of Medicine, Jefferson Medical College of Thomas Jefferson University; Director, Sickle Cell Center, Thomas Jefferson University Hospital, Philadelphia, Pennsylvania
Sickle Cell Disease

ROBERT W. BALOH, M.D.

Professor of Neurology, UCLA Medical School, Attending Staff, UCLA Hospital, Los Angeles, California
Episodic Vertigo

NICHOLAS M. BARBARO, M.D.

Associate Professor, University of California, San Francisco; Medical Director, Neurointensive Care Unit and Attending Neurosurgeon, University of California, San Francisco Hospitals, San Francisco, California
Trigeminal Neuralgia

BART BARLOGIE, M.D., Ph.D.
Professor of Medicine and Pathology and Director, Division of Hematology/Oncology, University of Arkansas for Medical Sciences; Director of Research, Arkansas Cancer Research Center, Little Rock, Arkansas
Multiple Myeloma

JOHN B. BARLOW, M.D.
Emeritus Professor and Honorary Research Fellow, University of Witwatersrand; Acting Head, Department of Cardiology, Johannesburg Hospital, Johannesburg, South Africa
Mitral Valve Prolapse

LEWIS A. BARNESS, M.D.
Professor of Pediatrics, University of South Florida College of Medicine; Staff Pediatrician, Tampa General Hospital, Tampa, Florida
Normal Infant Feeding

KURT T. BARNHART, M.D.
Clinical Instructor, Department of Obstetrics and Gynecology, University of Pennsylvania; Clinical Fellow in Reproductive Endocrinology, Hospital of the University of Pennsylvania, Philadelphia, Pennsylvania
Dysmenorrhea

RONALD J. BARR, M.D.
Professor of Dermatology and Pathology and Director, Dermatopathology Laboratory, University of California, Irvine, and University of California Medical Center, Irvine, California
Nevi

JOHN R. BARTHOLOMEW, M.D.
Staff, Department of Vascular Medicine, Cleveland Clinic Foundation, Cleveland, Ohio
Deep Venous Thrombosis of the Extremities; Stasis Ulcers

CHRISTOPHER J. BARTOLONE, M.D.
Associate in Medicine, University of Illinois Medical Center, Chicago, Illinois
Constipation

MORRISA BASKIN, M.D.
Clinical Instructor in Medicine, University of Washington, Seattle, Washington; Central Washington Hospital, Wenatchee, Washington
Warts (Verruca Vulgaris)

JOHN B. BASS, Jr., M.D.
Professor of Medicine, University of South Alabama; Director, Division of Pulmonary and Critical Care Medicine, University of South Alabama, Mobile, Alabama
Bacterial Pneumonia

ROY D. BAYNES, M.D., Ph.D.
Professor of Medicine, Division of Hematology, Department of Medicine, University of Kansas Medical Center, Kansas City, Kansas
Iron Deficiency Anemia

ANDREW BERCHUCK, M.D.
Associate Professor, Duke University Medical School; Associate Professor, Department of Gynecologic Oncology/Obstetrics and Gynecology, Duke University Medical Center, Durham, North Carolina
Cancer of the Endometrium

JEFFREY D. BERNHARD, M.D.
Professor of Medicine and Director, Division of Dermatology, University of Massachusetts Medical School, Worcester, Massachusetts
Pruritus (Itching)

SCOTT M. BERRY, M.D.
Nutrition Support Fellow and Senior Surgical Resident, Department of Surgery, University of Cincinnati, Cincinnati, Ohio
Acute Pancreatitis

PELAYO C. BESA, M.D.
Junior Faculty Associate, The University of Texas M.D. Anderson Cancer Center, Houston, Texas
Hodgkin's Disease: Radiation Therapy

JOHN P. BILEZIKIAN, M.D.
Professor of Medicine and Pharmacology, College of Physicians and Surgeons, Columbia University; Attending Physician, Columbia Presbyterian Medical Center, New York, New York
Hyperparathyroidism and Hypoparathyroidism

M. M. BLACK, M.D.
Chairman and Consultant Dermatologist, Department of Dermatopathology, St. John's Institute of Dermatology, St. Thomas' Hospital, London, England
The Specific Dermatoses of Pregnancy

MICHAEL S. BLAISS, M.D.
Associate Professor of Pediatrics, Assistant Professor of Medicine, and Director, Pediatric Allergy/Immunology Training Program, University of Tennessee; Division Consultant for Allergy, LeBonheur Children's Medical Center, Memphis, Tennessee
Anaphylaxis and Serum Sickness

CONRAD B. BLUM, M.D.
Associate Professor of Clinical Medicine, Columbia University College of Physicians and Surgeons; Associate Attending Physician, Presbyterian Hospital, New York, New York
Hyperlipoproteinemias

JOSEPH V. BONVENTRE, M.D., Ph.D.
Associate Professor of Medicine, Harvard Medical School; Associate Professor of Health Sciences and Technology, Massachusetts Institute of Technology; Associate Physician, Massachusetts General Hospital, Boston, Massachusetts
Acute Renal Failure

WILLIAM Z. BORER, M.D.
Associate Professor, Department of Pathology and Cell Biology, Thomas Jefferson University; Director, Department of Clinical Chemistry, Thomas Jefferson University Hospital, Philadelphia, Pennsylvania
Reference Intervals for the Interpretation of Laboratory Tests

STEVEN BORZAK, M.D.
Director, Cardiac Intensive Care Unit, Henry Ford Hospital, Detroit, Michigan
Acute Myocardial Infarction

JOHN M. BOWMAN, M.D.
Professor, Department of Pediatrics and Child Health; Professor, Department of Obstetrics, Gynecology and Reproductive Sciences, University of Manitoba; Medical Director, Rh Laboratory, Women's Hospital, Health Sciences Centre, Winnipeg, Manitoba, Canada
Hemolytic Disease of the Fetus and Newborn

OLGA BRAWMAN-MINTZER, M.D.
Assistant Professor of Psychiatry, Department of Psychiatry and Behavioral Sciences, Medical University of South Carolina, Charleston, South Carolina
Panic Disorder and Agoraphobia

MARTIN L. BRECHER, M.D.
Chairman, Department of Pediatrics, Roswell Park Cancer Institute; Associate Professor of Pediatrics, SUNY at Buffalo; Chief,

Division of Hematology-Oncology, Department of Pediatrics, Children's Hospital of Buffalo, Buffalo, New York
Acute Leukemia in Children

DOREEN B. BRETTLER, M.D.

Professor of Medicine, University of Massachusetts Medical School; Director, New England Hemophilia Center, Medical Center of Central Massachusetts, Worcester, Massachusetts
Platelet-Mediated Bleeding Disorders

SYLVIA L. BRICE, M.D.

Associate Professor of Dermatology, University of Colorado School of Medicine; University of Colorado Health Sciences Center, Denver, Colorado
Erythema Multiforme

MICHAEL S. BRONZE, M.D.

Associate Professor of Medicine, University of Tennessee; University of Tennessee Teaching Hospitals, Veterans Administration Medical Center, Memphis, Tennessee
Rheumatic Fever

WILLIAM A. BROUGHTON, M.D.

Associate Professor of Medicine, Division of Pulmonary Diseases/Critical Care/Sleep Medicine, University of South Alabama College of Medicine; Medical Director, Intensive Care Units, University of South Alabama Medical Center; Medical Director, University of South Alabama Knollwood Park Hospital Sleep Disorders Center; Medical Director, Cardiopulmonary Services, University of South Alabama Knollwood Park Hospital, Mobile, Alabama
Bacterial Pneumonia

THOMAS R. BROWNE, M.D.

Professor and Vice Chairman, Department of Neurology, Boston University School of Medicine; Associate Chief, Neurology Service, Veterans Administration Medical Center, Boston, Massachusetts
Epilepsy in Adolescents and Adults

GERARD N. BURROW, M.D.

Dean and Professor of Internal Medicine, Yale University School of Medicine; Yale-New Haven Hospital, New Haven, Connecticut; Veterans Administration Medical Center, West Haven, Connecticut
Goiter

WILLIAM J. BURTIS, M.D., PH.D.

Associate Professor of Medicine, Yale University School of Medicine, New Haven, Connecticut; Attending Physician, Endocrinology Section, Yale–New Haven Hospital, New Haven, Connecticut; Medical Director, Eastern Blind Rehabilitation Center, Veterans Administration Medical Center, West Haven, Connecticut
Paget's Disease of Bone

ROBERT K. BUSH, M.D.

Professor of Medicine (CHS), University of Wisconsin; Chief of Allergy, William S. Middleton Veterans Hospital, Madison, Wisconsin
Asthma in Adults and Adolescents

THOMAS BUTLER, M.D.

Professor of Internal Medicine, Texas Tech University Health Sciences Center; Attending Physician, University Medical Center, Lubbock, Texas
Plague

BLAKE CADY, M.D.

Professor of Surgery, Harvard Medical School; Chief of Surgical Oncology, New England Deaconess Hospital, Boston, Massachusetts
Diseases of the Breast

LEIGH A. CALLAHAN, M.D.

Assistant Professor of Medicine, Section of Pulmonary Diseases, Medical College of Georgia; Medical Director, Pulmonary Outpatient Clinics, Medical College of Georgia Hospital, Augusta, Georgia
Acute Respiratory Failure

D. W. CAMERON, M.D.

Assistant Professor of Medicine, Microbiology and Immunology, University of Ottawa; Ottawa General Hospital, Division of Infectious Diseases, Ottawa, Ontario, Canada
Chancroid

ELLIS S. CAPLAN, M.D.

Associate Professor of Medicine, University of Maryland School of Medicine and RA Cowley Shock Trauma Center; Chief, Department of Infectious Diseases, RA Cowley Shock Trauma Center, Baltimore, Maryland
Necrotizing Skin and Soft Tissue Infections

LOUIS R. CAPLAN, M.D.

Professor and Chairman, Department of Neurology, Tufts University; Neurologist-in-Chief, New England Medical Center, Boston, Massachusetts
Parenchymatous Brain Hemorrhage

THOMAS R. CARACCIO, PHARM.D.

Assistant Professor of Emergency Medicine, SUNY Stony Brook, New York; Assistant Professor of Pharmacology/Toxicology, New York College of Osteopathic Medicine, Old Westbury, New York; Assistant Professor of Clinical Pharmacy, St. John's University College Pharmacy, Jamaica, New York; Assistant Director of Long Island Regional Poison Control Center, East Meadow, New York; Winthrop University Hospital, Mineola, New York
Acute Poisonings

RALPH CARMEL, M.D.

Professor of Medicine and Pathology, University of Southern California School of Medicine; Attending Physician, LAC-USC Medical Center; Consultant, Kenneth J. Norris Cancer Center; Attending Physician, University Hospital, University of Southern California, Los Angeles, California
Pernicious Anemia and Other Megaloblastic Anemias

PAUL C. CARPENTER, M.D.

Assistant Professor of Medicine, Mayo Medical School; Consulting Staff, Rochester St. Mary's Hospital and Rochester Methodist Hospital, Rochester, Minnesota
Cushing's Syndrome

ANTHONY J. CASALE, M.D.

Associate Professor of Surgery (Urology), University of Louisville School of Medicine; Chief of Urology, Kosair Children's Hospital, Louisville, Kentucky
Bacterial Infections of the Urinary Tract in Girls

ALEXANDER S. CASS, M.D.

Staff Urologic Surgeon, Hennepin County Medical Center, Minneapolis, Minnesota
Genitourinary Trauma

PETER A. CATALDO, M.D.

Assistant Clinical Professor of Surgery, Wright State School of Medicine and Uniformed Services University of the Health Sciences; Staff Colon and Rectal Surgeon, Director of Surgical Research, Director of the Anal Physiology Laboratory, Wright-Patterson Medical Center, Wright-Patterson Air Force Base, Ohio
Hemorrhoids, Anal Fissure, and Anorectal Abscess and Fistula

LAURA A. CATTANEO, B.S.
Medical Student, Vanderbilt University Medical School, Nashville, Tennessee
Whooping Cough (Pertussis)

WILLIAM T. CEFALU, M.D.
Associate Professor of Medicine, Section of Endocrinology and Metabolism, The Bowman Gray School of Medicine of Wake Forest University; Bowman Gray/Baptist Hospital Medical Center, Winston-Salem, North Carolina
Diabetic Ketoacidosis

MICHAEL B. CHANCELLOR, M.D.
Assistant Professor of Urology, Thomas Jefferson University and Thomas Jefferson University Hospital, Philadelphia, Pennsylvania
Benign Prostatic Hyperplasia

STANLEY W. CHAPMAN, M.D.
Professor of Medicine, Associate Professor of Microbiology, and Director, Department of Infectious Diseases, University of Mississippi Medical Center and Veterans Administration Medical Center, Jackson, Mississippi
Histoplasmosis

LAURA W. CHEEVER, M.D.
Fellow, Division of Infectious Disease, Johns Hopkins School of Medicine, Baltimore, Maryland
Otitis Externa

CHIN-SANG CHUNG, M.D.
Fellow, Department of Neurology, New England Medical Center, Boston, Massachusetts; Associate Professor and Chair, Department of Neurology, Chungnam National University Medical College, Taejon, Korea
Parenchymatous Brain Hemorrhage

C. JAMES CHUONG, M.D., M.P.H.
Assistant Professor and Director, Premenstrual Syndrome Program, Division of Reproductive Endocrinology, Department of Obstetrics and Gynecology, Baylor College of Medicine; Active Medical Staff, St. Luke's Episcopal Hospital, The Methodist Hospital, and The Woman's Hospital of Texas, Houston, Texas
Premenstrual Syndrome (PMS)

RICHARD F. CLARK, M.D.
Assistant Adjunct Professor of Medicine, University of California at San Diego; Medical Director, San Diego Regional Poison Center; Assistant Director, Department of Emergency Medicine; Director, Medical Toxicology Services, University of California, San Diego Medical Center, San Diego, California
Venomous Snakebite

MARC D. COHEN, M.D.
Assistant Professor of Medicine, Mayo Medical School; Attending Staff Physician, St. Luke's Hospital, Jacksonville, Florida
Rheumatoid Arthritis

ANTHONY J. COMEROTA, M.D.
Professor of Surgery, Temple University School of Medicine; Chief of Vascular Surgery, Temple University Hospital, Philadelphia, Pennsylvania
Thrombophlebitis in Obstetrics and Gynecology

EDWARD M. CONWAY, M.D.
Assistant Professor of Medicine, University of Toronto; The Toronto Hospital, Toronto, Ontario, Canada
Disseminated Intravascular Coagulation; Thrombotic Thrombocytopenic Purpura

DAVID S. COOPER, M.D.
Associate Professor of Medicine and Co-Director, Thyroid Clinic, The Johns Hopkins University School of Medicine; Director, Division of Endocrinology, and Associate Physician-in-Chief, Sinai Hospital of Baltimore, Baltimore, Maryland
Hypothyroidism

JONATHAN CORREN, M.D.
Assistant Clinical Professor of Medicine and Director, Allergy-Immunology Clinic; Assistant Director, Allergy Fellowship Program, UCLA School of Medicine; Attending Physician, UCLA Center for Health Sciences, Los Angeles, California
Allergic Rhinitis Caused by Inhalant Factors

GEORGE J. CUCHURAL, JR., M.D.
Assistant Professor of Medicine, Pathology, and Community Medicine, New England Medical Center, Tufts University School of Medicine; Consultant in Infectious Diseases, Faulkner Hospital, Boston, Massachusetts
Tularemia

MARIANNE DALGAS, M.D.
Chief Physician, Department of Rheumatology, Holbaek Hospital, Holbaek, Denmark
Low Back Pain

MARY JANE DALTON, M.D.
Viral and Rickettsial Zoonoses Branch, National Center for Infectious Diseases, Centers for Disease Control and Prevention, Atlanta, Georgia
The Typhus Fevers

GILBERT H. DANIELS, M.D.
Associate Professor of Medicine, Harvard Medical School; Co-Director, Thyroid Associates; Physician, Massachusetts General Hospital, Boston, Massachusetts
Hyperthyroidism

JAMES H. DAUBER, M.D.
Professor of Medicine and Anesthesiology (Critical Care), University of Pittsburgh School of Medicine; Pulmonary Service, Veterans Administration Medical Center; Staff Physician, University of Pittsburgh Medical Center, Pittsburgh, Pennsylvania
Silicosis

SCOTT F. DAVIES, M.D.
Associate Professor, Department of Medicine, University of Minnesota; Director, Pulmonary Medicine Division, Department of Internal Medicine, Hennepin County Medical Center, Minneapolis, Minnesota
Blastomycosis

TERRY F. DAVIES, M.D.
Baumritte Professor of Medicine and Director, Division of Endocrinology and Metabolism, Mount Sinai Medical Center; Attending Physician, Mount Sinai Hospital, New York, New York
Thyroiditis

IRA C. DAVIS, M.D.
Instructor, Wake Forest University Medical Center, Winston-Salem, North Carolina
Cancer of the Skin

CHARLES S. DAYTON, R.PH., B.S.PHARM.
Adjunct Clinical Instructor, University of Iowa College of Pharmacy; Clinical Projects Coordinator, Interstitial Lung Disease SCOR Grant, College of Medicine, University of Iowa; Clinical Pharmacy Specialist, Pharmacy Department, University of Iowa Hospitals and Clinics, Iowa City, Iowa
Tuberculosis and Other Mycobacterial Infections

LISA M. DeANGELIS, M.D.
Assistant Professor of Neurology, Cornell University Medical College; Chief of Neurology Service, Memorial Sloan-Kettering Cancer Center, New York, New York
Brain Tumors

ARTHUR J. DeCROSS, M.D.
Senior Gastroenterology Fellow, University of Virginia, Charlottesville, Virginia; Gastroenterology Attending Clinical Faculty, Highland Hospital; Affiliate of the University of Rochester, Rochester, New York
Peptic Ulcer Disease

PRAKASH C. DEEDWANIA, M.D.
Clinical Professor of Medicine, UCSF School of Medicine; Chief of Cardiology Division and Director, Cardiovascular Research, Veterans Administration Medical Center, Fresno, California
Premature Beats

JAMES D. DOUKETIS, M.D.
Clinical Research Fellow, Department of Thromboembolic Diseases, McMaster University Medical Centre, Hamilton, Ontario, Canada
Acute Pulmonary Embolism

LAURA L. DOWNEY, M.D.
Resident, Department of Otolaryngology, New York University Medical Center, New York, New York
Tinnitus

STEPHEN C. DUCK, M.D.
Associate Professor of Pediatrics, Northwestern University Medical School, Chicago, Illinois; Attending Physician, The Evanston Hospital, Evanston, Illinois
Type I Diabetes Mellitus in Children and Adolescents

WILLIAM C. DUCKWORTH, M.D.
Degan Professor of Internal Medicine; Professor of Biochemistry; Chief, Section of Diabetes, Endocrinology and Metabolism, and Director, University Center for Diabetes and Metabolic Diseases, University of Nebraska Medical Center, University Hospital, Omaha, Nebraska
Diabetes Mellitus in Adults

MICHAEL J. DUNN, M.D.
Professor of Medicine and Physiology and Biophysics, Case Western Reserve University School of Medicine; Director, Division of Nephrology, Department of Medicine, University Hospitals of Cleveland, Cleveland, Ohio
Chronic Renal Failure

RICHARD F. EDLICH, M.D., PH.D.
Distinguished Professor of Plastic Surgery and Biomedical Engineering, University of Virginia School of Medicine, Charlottesville, Virginia
Bacterial Diseases of the Skin

KATHRYN M. EDWARDS, M.D.
Professor of Pediatrics, Vanderbilt University Medical School; Attending Physician, Vanderbilt Children's Hospital, Nashville, Tennessee
Whooping Cough (Pertussis)

N. LAWRENCE EDWARDS, M.D.
Associate Professor of Medicine, University of Florida; Chief, Section of Rheumatology, Veterans Administration Medical Center; Associate Professor of Shands Hospital and all University of Florida Affiliated Hospitals, Gainesville, Florida
Hyperuricemia and Gout

M. PATRICE EIFF, M.D.
Assistant Professor, Department of Family Medicine, Oregon Health Sciences University, Portland, Oregon
Common Sports Injuries

AL ELBENDARY, M.D.
Fellow, Gynecology Oncology, Duke University Medical School, Durham, North Carolina
Cancer of the Endometrium

DARREL L. ELLIS, M.D.
Assistant Professor, Department of Medicine, Division of Dermatology, Vanderbilt University Medical Center; Vanderbilt University Medical Center Hospital; Veterans Administration Medical Center, Nashville, Tennessee
Papulosquamous Eruptions

GERALD ERENBERG, M.D.
Staff Physician, Cleveland Clinic Foundation; Director, Learning Assessment Clinic, Cleveland Clinic Foundation, Cleveland, Ohio
Gilles De La Tourette Syndrome

BARRY FARR, M.D., M.SC.
William S. Jordan, Jr., Associate Professor of Medicine, University of Virginia; Hospital Epidemiologist, University of Virginia Health Sciences Center, Charlottesville, Virginia
Viral Respiratory Infections

MAKONNEN FEKADU, D.V.M., PH.D.
Medical Officer for Research, Rabies Division, Viral and Rickettsial Zoonoses Branch, Centers for Disease Control and Prevention, Atlanta, Georgia
Rabies

FRANCIS N. FERNANDES, M.D.
Senior Staff Physician, Henry Ford Hospital, Detroit, Michigan
Acute Myocardial Infarction

JOHN F. FIESELMANN, M.D.
Associate Professor, University of Iowa College of Medicine; Staff Physician and Director, Joint Office for Clinical Outreach Services and Contracting for Patient Care, University of Iowa Hospitals and Clinics, Iowa City, Iowa
Tuberculosis and Other Mycobacterial Infections

AARON S. FINK, M.D.
Associate Professor, Department of Surgery, Emory University School of Medicine, Atlanta, Georgia; Chief, Surgical Service, Atlanta Veterans Administration Medical Center, Decatur, Georgia
Acute Pancreatitis

BRUCE FLAREAU, M.D.
Assistant Director, Family Practice Residency, Bay Front Medical Center, St. Petersburg, Florida; Clinical Assistant Professor, Department of Family Medicine, University of South Florida, Tampa, Florida
Hazardous Marine Animals

W. P. FLEMING, M.D.
Private practice; Attending Physician, Memorial Medical Center, Las Cruces, New Mexico
Pelvic Inflammatory Disease

GERALD F. FLETCHER, M.D.
Professor and Chairman, Department of Rehabilitation Medicine; Professor in Medicine (Cardiology), Emory University School of Medicine; Medical Director, Center for Rehabilitation Medicine, Emory University Hospital; Medical Director, Emory Health Enhancement Program, Emory University Hospital, Atlanta, Georgia
Cardiac Rehabilitation

BARBARA J. FONER, M.D.
Pulmonary and Critical Care Fellow, University of South Alabama Medical Center, Mobile, Alabama
Bacterial Pneumonia

CARMEN FONSECA, M.D.
Clinical Associate, Cleveland Clinic Foundation, Cleveland, Ohio
Stasis Ulcers

CAROL A. FOSTER, M.D.
Fellow, Neurotology, UCLA School of Medicine, University of California, Los Angeles, California
Episodic Vertigo

JACKSON E. FOWLER, Jr., M.D.
Professor of Surgery, University of Mississippi School of Medicine; Chief of Urology, University of Mississippi Medical Center; Chief of Urology, Veterans Affairs Medical Center, Jackson, Mississippi
Prostatitis

JOHN P. FRANGIE, M.D.
Assistant Professor of Ophthalmology, Boston University School of Medicine; Ophthalmologist-in-Chief, Boston City Hospital, Boston, Massachusetts
Conjunctivitis

LAWRENCE S. FRIEDMAN, M.D.
Associate Professor of Medicine, Harvard Medical School; Associate Physician, Gastrointestinal Unit, Massachusetts General Hospital, Boston, Massachusetts
Acute and Chronic Viral Hepatitis

KAREN FRYE, M.D.
Assistant Professor of Surgery, University of South Alabama, Mobile, Alabama
Burns

DEREK A. FYFE, M.D., Ph.D.
Director of Imaging, The Children's Heart Center at Emory University, Atlanta, Georgia
Congenital Heart Disease

RON GALL, B.M.R.(P.T.)
Sports Physiotherapy Center and Pan Am Sports Medical Center, Winnipeg, Manitoba, Canada
Ankylosing Spondylitis

K. GAMBLE, M.D.
Lecturer, University of Toronto; Staff Physician, Tropical Disease Unit, The Toronto Hospital, Toronto, Ontario, Canada
Amebiasis

BRUCE J. GANTZ, M.D.
Professor and Interim Head, Department of Otolaryngology—Head and Neck Surgery, The University of Iowa Hospitals and Clinics, Iowa City, Iowa
Idiopathic Facial Paralysis (Bell's Palsy)

SUSAN J. GARRISON, M.D.
Associate Professor of Physical Medicine and Rehabilitation, Baylor College of Medicine; Medical Director, Rehabilitation Center, The Methodist Hospital, Houston, Texas
Rehabilitation of Hemiplegia

RONALD B. GEORGE, M.D.
Professor and Chairman, Department of Medicine, Louisiana State University School of Medicine; Chief, Medical Service, Louisiana State University Medical Center; Consultant, Shreveport VA Medical Center, Shreveport, Louisiana
Chronic Obstructive Pulmonary Disease

ALFRED L. GEST, M.D.
Assistant Professor of Pediatrics, Baylor College of Medicine, Houston, Texas
Resuscitation of the Newborn

RALPH A. GIANNELLA, M.D.
Mark Brown Professor of Medicine and Director, Division of Digestive Diseases, University of Cincinnati College of Medicine; Staff Physician, Veterans Administration Medical Center; Attending Physician, University of Cincinnati Medical Center; Attending Physician, Veterans Administration Medical Center, Cincinnati, Ohio
Malabsorption

JEFFREY S. GINSBERG, M.D.
Associate Professor, Department of Medicine, Faculty of Health Sciences, McMaster University, Hamilton, Ontario, Canada
Acute Pulmonary Embolism

DAN I. N. GIURGIU, M.D.
Research Fellow, Department of Surgery, The Medical College of Pennsylvania, Philadelphia, Pennsylvania
Cholelithiasis and Cholecystitis

RICHARD GLECKMAN, M.D.
Professor of Medicine, Boston University School of Medicine; Director of Medicine, Carney Hospital, Boston, Massachusetts
Infectious Bronchitis

PETER GLOVICZKI, M.D.
Professor of Surgery, Mayo Medical School; Consultant, Division of Vascular Surgery, Mayo Clinic and Foundation, Rochester, Minnesota
Acquired Diseases of the Aorta

MICHAEL R. GOLD, M.D., Ph.D.
Assistant Professor of Medicine, University of Maryland School of Medicine; Director, Cardiac Electrophysiology Service, University of Maryland Hospital, Baltimore, Maryland
Tachycardias

JAY L. GOLDSTEIN, M.D.
Associate Professor of Medicine, Section of Digestive and Liver Diseases, University of Illinois Medical Center, Chicago, Illinois
Constipation

EDMOND T. GONZALES, Jr., M.D.
Professor of Urology, Scott Department of Urology, Baylor College of Medicine; Head, Department of Surgery; Chief, Urology Service, Texas Children's Hospital, Houston, Texas
Childhood Enuresis

W. M. GOOCH III, M.D.
Professor of Pediatrics, University of Utah School of Medicine; Attending Physician, Primary Children's Medical Center, Salt Lake City, Utah
Streptococcal Pharyngitis

R. GOPINATH, M.D.
Infectious Disease Fellow, University of Toronto and The Toronto Hospital, Toronto, Ontario, Canada
Trichinosis

RALPH C. GORDON, M.D., M.A.
Professor of Pediatrics, Department of Infectious Diseases, Michigan State University, Kalamazoo Center for Medical Studies; Attending Physician, Pediatric Section and Consultant in Pediatric Infectious Diseases, Bronson Methodist Hospital and Borgess Medical Center, Kalamazoo, Michigan
Mumps

C. W. GOWEN, Jr., M.D.
Associate Professor of Pediatrics and Director of Pediatric Medical Education, Eastern Virginia Medical School, Children's Hospital of the King's Daughters, Norfolk, Virginia
Care of the High-Risk Neonate

NORMAN D. GRACE, M.D.
Professor of Medicine, Tufts University School of Medicine; Chief of Gastroenterology, Faulkner Hospital, Boston, Massachusetts
Hemochromatosis

J. ANDREW GRANT, M.D.
Professor, Departments of Medicine and Microbiology and Immunology, University of Texas Medical Branch at Galveston; Director,

Adult Allergy, University of Texas Medical Branch Hospital, Galveston, Texas
Stinging Insect Allergy

RICHARD N. GREENBERG, M.D.
Associate Professor of Medicine, Division of Infectious Diseases, University of Kentucky; Attending Physician, University of Kentucky Medical Center and Lexington Veterans Administration Medical Center, Lexington, Kentucky
Osteomyelitis

JOSEPH GREENSHER, M.D.
Professor of Pediatrics, SUNY at Stony Brook, Stony Brook, New York; Medical Director and Associate Chairman, Department of Pediatrics, Winthrop University Hospital; Associate Director, Long Island Regional Poison Control Center, East Meadow, New York; Winthrop University Hospital, Mineola, New York
Acute Poisonings

GABRIEL GREGORATOS, M.D.
Professor of Medicine, University of California, Davis; Director, Department of Clinical Cardiology, University of California, Davis Medical Center, Davis, California
Infective Endocarditis

DIETER H. M. GRÖESCHEL, M.D., PH.D.
Professor of Pathology and Medicine and Director of Microbiology, University of Virginia School of Medicine, Charlottesville, Virginia
Bacterial Diseases of the Skin

MARKO R. GUDZIAK, M.D.
Fellow in Neurourology, University of Texas Medical School; Hermann Hospital; Lyndon B. Johnson Hospital, Houston, Texas
Urinary Incontinence

RICHARD L. GUERRANT, M.D.
Thomas H. Hunter Professor of International Medicine and Chief, Division of Geographic International Medicine; Attending Physician, University of Virginia Hospital, Charlottesville, Virginia
Acute Infectious Diarrhea

JERE D. GUIN, M.D.
Professor and Chairman, Department of Dermatology, University of Arkansas for Medical Sciences, Little Rock, Arkansas
Urticaria

RICHARD H. HAAS, M.B., B.CHIR.
Associate Professor of Neurosciences and Pediatrics, University of California; Attending Physician, University of California San Diego Medical Center, Children's Hospital and Health Center, Mercy Hospital, San Diego, California
Reye's Syndrome

LEILA R. HAJJAR, M.D.
Senior Staff Physician, OB/GYN Department, Henry Ford Medical Center, Detroit, Michigan
Uterine Leiomyoma

PAUL E. HAMMERSCHLAG, M.D.
Resident in Otolaryngology and Associate Professor of Otolaryngology, New York University School of Medicine; Associate Attending Physician and Resident, Tisch Hospital, Bellevue Hospital, New York University Medical Center, New York, New York
Tinnitus

BRUCE H. HAMORY, M.D.
Professor of Medicine, Associate Dean for Clinical Affairs, Milton S. Hershey College of Medicine, Penn State University; Attending Physician, University Hospital, Hershey Medical Center, Hershey, Pennsylvania
Viral and Mycoplasmal Pneumonias

PETER HANSON, M.S., M.D.
Professor of Medicine, Cardiology Section, University of Wisconsin; Co-Director, Department of Preventive Cardiology, University of Wisconsin, Clinical Science Center, Madison, Wisconsin
Disturbances Due to Heat

RUSSELL N. HARADA, M.D.
Instructor of Surgery, Temple University School of Medicine; Fellow in Vascular Surgery, Temple University Hospital, Philadelphia, Pennsylvania
Thrombophlebitis in Obstetrics and Gynecology

KEN HASHIMOTO, M.D.
Professor and Chairman, Department of Dermatology, Wayne State University School of Medicine; Attending Physician and Chief of Department of Dermatology, Harper Hospital, Detroit, Michigan
Parasitic Infections of the Skin

CHRISTINE M. HAYES, M.D.
Associate Professor of Dermatology, University of Iowa Hospitals University, Iowa City, Iowa; Assistant Professor of Dermatology, Tufts University, New England Medical Center, Boston, Massachusetts
Premalignant Lesions

JOHN A. HEANEY, M.B., B.CHIR.
Professor of Surgery (Urology), Dartmouth Medical School, and Chief, Section of Urology, Dartmouth-Hitchcock Medical Center, Lebanon, New Hampshire
Epididymitis

LEE A. HEBERT, M.D.
Professor of Medicine and Director, Division of Nephrology, Department of Internal Medicine, The Ohio State University Medical Center, Columbus, Ohio
The Primary Glomerulopathies

PETER HEDERA, M.D.
Research Fellow, Alzheimer Center, Department of Neurology, Division of Behavioral Neurology, University Hospitals of Cleveland and Case Western Reserve University, Cleveland, Ohio
Alzheimer's Disease

DAVID HEIMBACH, M.D.
Professor of Surgery, Department of Surgery, University of Washington School of Medicine; Director, University of Washington Burn Center, Harborview Medical Center, Seattle, Washington
Burns

ROBERT M. HERNDON, M.D.
Professor of Neurology, Oregon Health Sciences University, Legacy Good Samaritan Hospital; Chairman, Neuroservices Department, Portland, Oregon
Multiple Sclerosis

DEIRDRE A. HERRINGTON, M.D.
Assistant Professor of Medicine, Bowman Gray School of Medicine, Wake Forest University; North Carolina Baptist Hospital, Winston-Salem, North Carolina
Typhoid Fever

STEVEN B. HEYMSFIELD, M.D.
Professor of Medicine, Columbia University College of Physicians and Surgeons; Deputy Director, Obesity Research Center, St. Luke's-Roosevelt Hospital, New York, New York
Obesity

CHARLES B. HICKS, M.D.
Assistant Professor, Division of Infectious Diseases, Duke University Medical Center, Durham, North Carolina
Gonorrhea

AKIRA HIRONO, M.D.

Research Associate, Okinaka Memorial Institute for Medical Research, Tokyo, Japan
Nonimmune Hemolytic Anemia

DANIEL J. HOGAN, M.D.

Professor of Medicine (Dermatology and Cutaneous Surgery), Professor of Pediatrics, Professor of Environmental and Occupational Health, College of Public Health, University of South Florida; Chief of Dermatology, Bay Pines Veterans Administration Medical Center; Staff Physician, Tampa General Hospital, Tampa, Florida
Contact Dermatitis

THOMAS M. HOOTON, M.D.

Associate Professor, Department of Medicine, University of Washington School of Medicine; Medical Director, Harborview Medical Center, Madison Clinic, Seattle, Washington
Nongonococcal Urethritis

DOUGLAS B. HORNICK, M.D.

Assistant Professor, University of Iowa College of Medicine; Staff Physician, University of Iowa Hospitals and Clinics; Director, TB Chest Clinic, University of Iowa Hospitals and Clinics, Iowa City, Iowa
Tuberculosis and Other Mycobacterial Infections

HAROLD W. HOROWITZ, M.D.

Assistant Professor of Medicine, New York Medical College; Attending Physician, Westchester County Medical Center, Valhalla, New York
Bacteremia

SHANNON HOWE, M.D.

Clinical Fellow, Department of Medicine, Division of Rheumatology and Clinical Immunology, University of Florida, Gainesville, Florida
Hyperuricemia and Gout

KATHY HOY, M.ED., R.D.

Research Coordinator, Obesity Research Center; St. Luke's-Roosevelt Hospital, New York, New York
Obesity

GORDON B. HUGHES, M.D.

Program Director, Clinical Staff, Department of Otolaryngology and Communicative Disorders, Cleveland Clinic Foundation, Cleveland, Ohio
Otitis Media

VICTOR IDROVO, M.D.

Research Fellow, Division of Hepatology, University of Miami School of Medicine, Miami, Florida
Cirrhosis

MOSHE IPP, M.B.B.CH.(RAND)

Associate Professor, University of Toronto; Hospital For Sick Children, Toronto, Ontario, Canada
Fever

ROBIN D. ISAACS, M.D.

Assistant Professor of Medicine, University of Mississippi Medical Center; Staff Physician in Infectious Diseases, Department of Veterans Affairs Medical Center, Jackson, Mississippi
Syphilis

TAKATERU IZUMI, M.D.

Professor of Environmental Respiratory Disease, Chest Disease Research Institute, Kyoto University; Professor and Chief, 2nd Department of Medicine, Chest Disease Research Institute Hospital, Kyoto University, Kyoto, Japan
Sarcoidosis

ROBERT R. JACOBSON, M.D., PH.D.

Director, Gillis W. Long Hansen's Disease Center, Carville, Louisiana
Leprosy (Hansen's Disease)

SUNDAR JAGANNATH, M.D.

Professor of Medicine and Pathology and Chief, Bone Marrow Transplantation, University of Arkansas for Medical Sciences, Little Rock, Arkansas
Multiple Myeloma

MICHAEL P. JOHNSON, M.D., M.P.H.

Assistant Professor, Department of International Health, Johns Hopkins School of Hygiene and Public Health, Johns Hopkins Medical Institutions, Baltimore, Maryland
Otitis Externa

SCOTT A. JOHNSON, M.D.

Postdoctoral Fellow in Neonatal/Perinatal Medicine, Baylor College of Medicine, Houston, Texas
Resuscitation of the Newborn

GERALD H. JORDAN, M.D.

Professor of Urology, Eastern Virginia Medical School; Attending Physician, Sentara Hospitals and Children's Hospital of the King's Daughters, Norfolk, Virginia
Urethral Stricture

JOSEPH L. JORIZZO, M.D.

Professor and Chairman, Department of Dermatology, The Bowman Gray School of Medicine, Wake Forest University, Winston-Salem, North Carolina
Pruritus (Itching)

STEPHEN JURD, M.B., B.S.

Clinical Lecturer, Department of Psychiatry, Sydney University; Visiting Medical Officer, Manly District Hospital and Royal North Shore Hospital, Artarmon, New South Wales, Australia
Alcohol-Related Problems

MARILYN A. KACICA, M.D.

Assistant Professor of Pediatrics, Albany Medical College; Attending Physician, Albany Medical Center Hospital, Albany, New York
Varicella (Chickenpox)

HARRIET KANG, M.D.

Montefiore Medical Center, Albert Einstein College of Medicine, Bronx, New York
Epilepsy in Infants and Children

HAROLD S. KAPLAN, M.D.

Professor, Department of Pathology, University of Texas Southwestern Medical Center; Medical Director, Transfusion Services, Parkland Memorial Hospital; Consultant, Blood Bank, Veterans Administration Medical Center; Consultant in Pathology, Children's Medical Center; Pathology Staff, Zale Lipshy University Hospital, Dallas, Texas
Adverse Reactions to Blood Transfusions

FREDERICK J. KASKEL, M.D., PH.D.

Associate Professor of Pediatrics, Physiology, and Biophysics and Director, Division of Pediatric Nephrology, University Medical Center at Stony Brook; Attending Physician, University Hospital, Stony Brook, New York
Parenteral Fluid Therapy for Infants and Children

ADRIAN I. KATZ, M.D.

Professor of Medicine, University of Chicago Pritzker School of Medicine; Attending Physician, University of Chicago Hospitals and Clinics, Chicago, Illinois
Hypertensive Disorders of Pregnancy

EUGENE KATZ, M.D.

Clinical Assistant Professor, The University of Maryland; Attending Physician, Women's Hospital Fertility Center, Greater Baltimore Medical Center, Baltimore, Maryland
Hyperprolactinemia

RAYMOND H. KAUFMAN, M.D.

Professor, Department of Obstetrics and Gynecology, and Professor, Department of Pathology, Baylor College of Medicine, Houston, Texas
Tumors of the Vulva

MARTIN B. KELLER, M.D.

Professor and Chairman, Department of Psychiatry, Brown University; Executive Psychiatrist-in-Chief, Butler Hospital, Emma Pendleton Bradley Hospital, Memorial Hospital, Miriam Hospital, Rhode Island Hospital, Roger Williams General Hospital, Providence Veterans Administration Medical Center, Women and Infants Hospital, Providence, Rhode Island
Mood Disorders

LARISA C. KELLEY, M.D.

Resident in Dermatology, Harvard Medical School; Massachusetts General Hospital, Boston, Massachusetts
Acne Vulgaris and Rosacea

CLARK M. KERR, M.D.

Chairman, Infection Control, St. Mary of the Plains Hospital; Chairman, Infection Control, Methodist Hospital, Lubbock, Texas
Psittacosis (Ornithosis)

RANDOLPH KESSLER, M.D.

Assistant Professor of Surgery and Pediatrics, University of New Mexico; Staff Surgeon, University of New Mexico Hospital, Lovelace Medical Center, Albuquerque Veterans Administration Hospital, Albuquerque, New Mexico
Atelectasis

J. S. KEYSTONE, M.D., M.Sc.(C.T.M.)

Professor of Medicine, University of Toronto; Director, Tropical Disease Unit, The Toronto Hospital, Toronto, Ontario, Canada
Amebiasis; Trichinosis

M. YOUSUF KHAN, M.D.

Head, Infectious Diseases, King Fahad National Guard Hospital, Riyadh, Saudi Arabia
Brucellosis

JEFFREY C. KING, M.D.

Associate Professor, Georgetown University School of Medicine; Director, Maternal-Transport Service, Georgetown University Hospital, Washington, District of Columbia
Vaginal Bleeding in Late Pregnancy

ROBERT L. KNOBLER, M.D., Ph.D.

Professor, Division of Neuroimmunology, Department of Neurology, Jefferson Medical College, Thomas Jefferson University; Attending Physician, Thomas Jefferson University Hospital, Philadelphia, Pennsylvania
Viral Meningitis and Encephalitis

MAHENDR S. KOCHAR, M.D.

Professor of Medicine, Medical College of Wisconsin; Attending Physician, Clement J. Zablocki Veterans Administration Medical Center, Froedtert Memorial Lutheran Hospital, John L. Doyne Hospital, St. Joseph's Hospital, St. Michael's Hospital, Milwaukee, Wisconsin
Primary Aldosteronism

BRIAN S. KOLL, M.D.

Attending Physician, Infectious Disease Service; Assistant Hospital Epidemiologist, Beth Israel Medical Center, New York, New York
Acquired Immune Deficiency Syndrome (AIDS)

ASHER KORNBLUTH, M.D.

Assistant Clinical Professor of Medicine, Mount Sinai School of Medicine; Assistant Attending Physician, The Mount Sinai Hospital, New York, New York
Crohn's Disease

ROBERT A. KOZOL, M.D.

Associate Professor of Surgery, Wayne State University School of Medicine, Detroit, Michigan; Chief of Surgery, Veterans Affairs Medical Center, Allen Park, Michigan; Staff Surgeon, Harper Hospital and Detroit Receiving Hospital, Detroit, Michigan
Gastritis

BERNICE R. KRAFCHIK, M.B., Ch.B.

Associate Professor, Departments of Pediatrics and Medicine, Division of Dermatology, University of Toronto; Staff Physician, Hospital for Sick Children, Toronto, Ontario, Canada
Atopic Dermatitis

SUMNER C. KRAFT, M.D.

Professor of Medicine, University of Chicago; Attending Physician, University of Chicago Medical Center, Chicago, Illinois
Ulcerative Colitis

BRUCE P. KRIEGER, M.D.

Associate Professor of Medicine, University of Miami, Miami, Florida; Chief, Pulmonary Intensive Care, Mount Sinai Medical Center, Miami Beach, Florida
Primary Lung Abscess

MARK G. KRIS, M.D.

Associate Professor, Cornell University Medical College; Associate Attending, Memorial Sloan-Kettering Cancer Center, New York, New York
Nausea and Vomiting

TIMOTHY M. KUZEL, M.D.

Assistant Professor of Medicine, Northwestern University Medical School and Robert H. Lurie Cancer Center; Attending Physician, Northwestern Memorial Hospital, Veterans Affairs Lakeside Medical Center, Chicago, Illinois
T Cell Lymphoma (Mycosis Fungoides and Sézary's Syndrome)

ROBERT G. LAHITA, M.D., Ph.D.

Associate Professor, Columbia University College of Physicians and Surgeons; Senior Attending Physician, St. Luke's-Roosevelt Hospital Center; Consulting Physician, The Rockefeller University Hospital, New York, New York
Connective Tissue Disorders: Systemic Lupus Erythematosus, Dermatomyositis and Other Myopathies, and Scleroderma

CHARLES R. LAMBERT, M.D., Ph.D.

Abraham Mitchell Professor of Medicine, University of South Alabama College of Medicine; Director, Cardiac Catheterization Laboratories, University of South Alabama Medical Center, Mobile, Alabama
Angina Pectoris

ROGER LARSON, M.D.

Clinical Professor of Medicine, University of California, San Francisco, California; Attending Physician, Valley Medical Center of Fresno, Fresno, California
Coccidioidomycosis

STEVEN A. LAUTER, M.D.

Assistant Professor of Clinical Medicine, Washington University School of Medicine; Attending Physician, Barnes Hospital, Jewish Hospital, Missouri Baptist Hospital, St. Louis, Missouri
Polymyalgia Rheumatica and Giant Cell Arteritis

JOE Y. LEE, M.D.

Staff Urologic Surgeon, Hennepin County Medical Center, Minneapolis, Minnesota
Genitourinary Trauma

STEPHANIE J. LEE, M.D.

Fellow in Medicine, Harvard Medical School; Fellow in Hematology-Oncology, Brigham and Women's Hospital, Boston, Massachusetts
Acute Leukemia in Adults

HOWARD M. LEIBOWITZ, M.D.

Professor of Ophthalmology, Boston University School of Medicine, Boston, Massachusetts; Ophthalmologist-In-Chief, Boston University Medical Center, Boston, Massachusetts
Conjunctivitis

BRUCE B. LERMAN, M.D.

Director, Cardiac Electrophysiology Laboratory, and Professor of Medicine, Cornell University Medical College; Attending Physician, The New York Hospital-Cornell University Medical Center, New York, New York
Heart Block

ALAN LERNER, M.D.

Assistant Professor of Neurology, Case Western Reserve University School of Medicine; Director, Division of Neurology, Saint Luke's Medical Center, Cleveland, Ohio
Alzheimer's Disease

BARRY LESHIN, M.D.

Associate Professor of Dermatology and Otolaryngology, Wake Forest University Medical Center; Staff, North Carolina Baptist Hospital, Winston-Salem, North Carolina
Cancer of the Skin

DAVID A. LEVY, M.D.

Chief Resident, Department of Urology, University Hospitals of Cleveland, Cleveland, Ohio
Renal Calculi

LUKE LEWIS, M.D.

Assistant Instructor, Texas Tech University Health Sciences Center, Lubbock, Texas
Viral Diseases of the Skin

MATTHEW H. LIANG, M.D., M.P.H.

Associate Professor of Medicine, Harvard Medical School; Director, Robert Brigham Multipurpose Arthritis and Musculoskeletal Diseases Center, Brigham and Women's Hospital, Boston, Massachusetts
Low Back Pain

ROBERT LIBKE, M.D.

Assistant Clinical Professor, University of California, San Francisco, California; Chief of Infectious Diseases, Valley Medical Center of Fresno, Fresno, California
Coccidioidomycosis

HENRY W. LIM, M.D.

Professor of Dermatology, New York University School of Medicine; Chief of Staff, New York Veterans Affairs Medical Center, New York, New York
Sunburn and Other Dermatoses Induced by Sunlight

MARSHALL D. LINDHEIMER, M.D.

Professor of Medicine, Obstetrics, and Gynecology and Clinical Pharmacology, University of Chicago, Division of Biological Sciences, Pritzker School of Medicine; Attending Physician, University of Chicago Hospital; Director, Medical High-Risk Clinic, Chicago Lying-in Hospital, Chicago, Illinois
Hypertensive Disorders of Pregnancy

BRUCE A. LOWE, M.D.

Associate Professor of Urology, Oregon Health Sciences University, Portland, Oregon
Genitourinary Cancer

FRANKLIN D. LOWY, M.D.

Professor of Medicine, Albert Einstein College of Medicine; Attending Physician, Montefiore Medical Center, Bronx, New York
Rat-Bite Fever

R. BRUCE LYDIARD, PH.D., M.D.

Professor of Psychiatry, Department of Psychiatry and Behavioral Sciences; Director, Anxiety Disorders Research; Director, Psychopharmacology Unit; Medical University of South Carolina, Charleston, South Carolina
Panic Disorder and Agoraphobia

DIANA L. MAAS, M.D.

Assistant Professor of Medicine, Medical College of Wisconsin; Staff Physician, Clement J. Zablocki Veterans Administration Medical Center, Froedtert Memorial Lutheran Hospital, John L. Doyne Hospital, Milwaukee, Wisconsin
Primary Aldosteronism

MAURIZIO MACCATO, M.D.

Clinical Assistant Professor, Baylor College of Medicine, Houston, Texas
Vulvovaginitis

ALAN J. MAGILL, M.D.

Infectious Disease Officer, Department of Immunology, Walter Reed Army Institute of Research; Attending Physician, Walter Reed Army Medical Center, Washington, District of Columbia
Leishmaniasis

DILIP MAHALANABIS, M.B., B.S.

Director, Clinical Sciences Division, International Centre for Diarrhoea Disease Research, Dhaka, Bangladesh
Cholera

SHARON B. MANNHEIMER, M.D.

Fellow, Division of Infectious Diseases, New York Hospital–Cornell University Medical Center, New York, New York
Toxoplasmosis

HARISH MARISIDDAIAH, M.D.

Fellow, Division of Infectious Diseases, New York Medical College, Valhalla, New York
Bacteremia

STEVEN M. MARKOWITZ, M.D.

Instructor in Medicine, Cornell University Medical College; Assistant Attending Physician, New York Hospital, New York, New York
Heart Block

THOMAS J. MARRIE, M.D.

Professor of Medicine, Department of Medicine, Dalhousie University; Associate Professor, Department of Microbiology, Dalhousie University; Active Staff, Victoria General Hospital; Consultant Staff, Camp Hill Medical Centre, Consultant Staff, Nova Scotia Rehabilitation Centre; Consultant Staff, Grare Maternity Hospital, Halifax, Nova Scotia, Canada
Legionellosis (Legionnaire's Disease and Pontiac Fever)

MARK G. MARTENS, M.D.
Associate Professor and Director of Gynecology; Head, Infectious Diseases, Department of Gynecology, and Obstetrics, Emory University; Emory University Hospital, Crawford W. Long Hospital, Veterans Affairs Medical Center, Grady Memorial Hospital, Atlanta, Georgia
Pyelonephritis

RONALD E. MASON, M.D.
Clinical Research Fellow and Instructor of Medicine, Division of Digestive Diseases, University of Cincinnati Medical Center; Attending Physician, University of Cincinnati Medical Center, Veterans Administration Medical Center, Cincinnati, Ohio
Malabsorption

BRUCE MATHERN, M.D.
Resident, Division of Neurosurgery, Medicial College of Virginia, Richmond, Virginia
Acute Head Injuries in Children

GLENN E. MATHISEN, M.D.
Associate Clinical Professor of Medicine, UCLA School of Medicine; Chief, Infectious Disease Service, Olive View Medical Center, Los Angeles, California
Brain Abscess

ALEXANDER MAUSKOP, M.D.
Assistant Professor of Neurology, State University of New York, Health Science Center at Brooklyn; Director, New York Headache Center, New York; Associate Attending Neurologist, Long Island College Hospital, Brooklyn, New York
Pain

JAMES R. McCORMICK, M.D.
Professor of Medicine, University of Massachusetts, Worcester, Massachusetts; Chairman, Department of Medicine, and Director, Internal Medicine Residency, Berkshire Medical Center, Pittsfield, Massachusetts
Cough

DAVID W. McFADDEN, M.D.
Associate Professor of Surgery, University of California, Los Angeles, UCLA Department of Surgery, School of Medicine; Chief of General Surgery, Sepulveda Veterans Administration Medical Center, Los Angeles, California
Chronic Pancreatitis

CARMEN M. McINTYRE, M.D.
Clinical Instructor, Medical College of Pennsylvania; Medical Director, Resource Day Treatment Center, Philadelphia, Pennsylvania
Schizophrenic Disorders

MARILYNNE McKAY, M.D.
Associate Professor of Dermatology and Gynecology, Emory University School of Medicine; Chief, Dermatology Service, Grady Memorial Hospital, Atlanta, Georgia
Pruritus Ani and Vulvae

WALLACE B. MENDELSON, M.D.
Director, Sleep Disorders Center, Cleveland Clinic Foundation, Cleveland, Ohio
Insomnia

DEBORAH A. METZGER, PH.D., M.D.
Associate Professor, Division of Reproductive Endocrinology and Infertility, Department of Obstetrics and Gynecology, University of Connecticut Health Center, Farmington, Connecticut
Endometriosis

MICHAEL M. MILLER, M.D.
Associate Professor and Director, Division of Reproductive Endocrinology and Infertility, Department of Obstetrics and Gynecology, University of Arkansas for Medical Sciences; Director of Reproductive Endocrinology/Infertility, University Hospital, University of Arkansas for Medical Sciences, Little Rock, Arkansas
Dysfunctional Uterine Bleeding

DANIEL R. MISHELL, JR., M.D.
Lyle G. McNeill Professor and Chairman, Department of Obstetrics and Gynecology, University of Southern California School of Medicine; Chief of Professional Services, LAC University of Southern California Medical Center Women's Hospital, and Children's Hospital, Los Angeles, California
Menopause

HOWARD C. MOFENSON, M.D.
Professor of Pediatrics and Emergency Medicine, SUNY at Stony Brook, Stony Brook, New York; Professor of Pharmacology/ Toxicology, New York College of Osteopathy, Old Westbury, New York; Professor of Clinical Pharmacy, St. John's University, Jamaica, New York; Attending Physician, Department of Pediatrics, and Medical Director, Long Island Regional Poison Control Center, East Meadow, New York; Winthrop University Hospital, Mineola, New York
Acute Poisonings

MARK E. MOLITCH, M.D.
Professor of Medicine, Center for Endocrinology, Metabolism and Molecular Medicine, Northwestern University Medical School; Attending Physician, Northwestern Memorial Hospital; Consulting Physician, Veterans Administration Lakeside Hospital, Chicago, Illinois
Acromegaly

F. J. MONTZ, M.D.
Associate Professor, University of California at Los Angeles School of Medicine; Consulting Surgeon, University of California at Los Angeles Center for Health Sciences, Los Angeles, California
Cancer of the Uterine Cervix

CASSANDRA MOORE, M.A., M.P.H.
Ph.D. Candidate, Columbia University, Department of Psychology, New York, New York
Contraception

PETER MORGAN-CAPNER, F.R.C.PATH.
Consultant Virologist, Department of Virology, Royal Preston Hospital, Preston, United Kingdom
Rubella and Congenital Rubella

MARVIN MOSER, M.D.
Clinical Professor of Medicine, Yale University School of Medicine; Senior Medical Consultant, National High Blood Pressure Education Program, National Heart Lung and Blood Institute; Emeritus Chief of Cardiology and Attending Physician, Cardiology, White Plains Hospital Medical Centre, White Plains, New York
Hypertension

ALISON A. MOY, M.D.
Postdoctoral Fellow in Endocrinology and Metabolism, Yale University and Yale-New Haven Hospital, New Haven, Connecticut
Paget's Disease of Bone

J. PAUL MUIZELAAR, M.D., PH.D.
Lind Lawrence Professor of Neurosurgery, Medical College of Virginia School of Medicine, Virginia Commonwealth University, Richmond, Virginia
Acute Head Injuries in Adults

KENRIC M. MURAYAMA, M.D.
Assistant Professor of General Surgery, University of Nebraska Medical Center, and Omaha Veterans Administration Hospital, Omaha, Nebraska
Bleeding Esophageal Varices

HENRY W. MURRAY, M.D.
Professor of Medicine, Cornell University Medical College; Chief, Division of Infectious Diseases, New York Hospital, New York, New York
Toxoplasmosis

JOHN C. MURRAY, M.D.
Assistant Professor of Medicine, Division of Dermatology, Duke University Medical Center, Durham, North Carolina
Keloids

GERALD V. NACCARELLI, M.D.
Professor of Medicine and Director, Department of Clinical Electrophysiology; Department of Cardiology, University of Texas Medical School at Houston; Medical Director, Hermann Hospital Arrhythmia Center; Courtesy Staff, West Houston Medical Center; Courtesy Staff, St. Luke's Episcopal Hospital, Houston, Texas
Atrial Fibrillation

SONOKO NAGAI, M.D.
Associate Professor, Department of Clinical Immunology, Chest Disease Research Institute,. Kyoto University; Associate Professor 2nd Department of Medicine, Chest Disease Research Institute Hospital, Kyoto University, Kyoto, Japan
Sarcoidosis

STEPHEN R. NEWMARK, M.D.
Chairman, Department of Internal Medicine, University of Nevada School of Medicine, Las Vegas, Nevada
Water-Soluble Vitamin Deficiency States

JUAN J. NOGUERAS, M.D.
Staff Colorectal Surgeon, Cleveland Clinic Florida, Fort Lauderdale, Florida
Malignant Diseases of the Colon and Rectum

GEORGE H. NOLAN, M.D., M.P.H.
Division Head, Maternal-Fetal Medicine, OB/GYN Department, Henry Ford Medical Center, Detroit, Michigan
Uterine Leiomyoma

MARGARET A. NOYES, PHARM.D.
Assistant Professor, University of Houston College of Pharmacy; Clinical Pharmacist, Houston Veterans Affairs Medical Center, Houston, Texas
Drugs Approved in 1993

DAVID L. OLIVE, M.D.
Associate Professor and Chief of Reproductive Endocrinology and Infertility, Yale University School of Medicine; Director of Reproductive Endocrinology and Infertility, Yale-New Haven Hospital, New Haven, Connecticut
Amenorrhea

JAMES G. OLSON, PH.D.
Chief, Viral and Rickettsial Zoonoses Branch, National Center for Infectious Diseases, Centers for Disease Control and Prevention, Atlanta, Georgia
The Typhus Fevers

ROBERT E. OLSON, M.D., PH.D.
Professor of Medicine Emeritus, School of Medicine, State University of New York at Stony Brook; Consultant in Medicine, University Hospital, State University of New York at Stony Brook, Stony Brook, New York
Vitamin K Deficiency

JOHN J. ORLOFF, M.D.
Assistant Professor of Medicine, Yale University School of Medicine; Yale-New Haven Hospital, New Haven, Connecticut; Staff Physician, Veterans Affairs Medical Center, West Haven, Connecticut
Goiter

DEBORAH ORTEGA-CARR, M.D.
Clinical Instructor, University of Wisconsin, Madison, Wisconsin
Asthma in Adults and Adolescents

SCOTT OSLUND, M.D.
Resident Physician, Division of Emergency Medicine, Stanford University Hospital, Stanford, California; Kaiser Permanente Medical Center, Santa Clara, California
Disturbances Due to Cold

JAMES R. OSTER, M.D.
Professor of Medicine, University of Miami School of Medicine; Associate Chief of Medical Service, Department of Veterans Affairs Medical Center, Miami, Florida
Diabetes Insipidus

GARY D. OVERTURF, M.D.
Professor of Pediatrics, University of New Mexico School of Medicine; Director, Pediatric Infectious Disease, University of New Mexico Hospital, Albuquerque, New Mexico
Diphtheria; Salmonellosis

MICHAEL W. OWENS, M.D.
Associate Professor of Medicine, Louisiana State University School of Medicine; Chief, Section of Pulmonary and Critical Care Medicine, Department of Veterans Affairs Medical Center, Shreveport, Louisiana
Chronic Obstructive Pulmonary Disease

CHARLES H. PACKMAN, M.D.
Professor of Medicine, University of Rochester School of Medicine and Dentistry; Attending Physician, Strong Memorial Hospital, Rochester, New York
Autoimmune Hemolytic Anemia

DARWIN L. PALMER, M.D.
Professor and Chief, Division of Infectious Disease, University of New Mexico School of Medicine; Chief, Infectious Disease Section, Veterans Administration Medical Center, Albuquerque, New Mexico
Q Fever

MICHAEL M. PAPARELLA, M.D.
Clinical Professor and Chairman Emeritus, Department of Otolaryngology, University of Minnesota; Staff Physician, Fairview Riverside Medical Center, Minneapolis, Minnesota
Menière's Disease

LAWRENCE C. PARISH, M.D.
Clinical Professor of Dermatology and Director of Jefferson Center for International Dermatology, Jefferson Medical College, Thomas Jefferson University, Philadelphia, Pennsylvania
Pressure Ulcer

DAVID O. PARRISH, M.S., M.D.
Assistant Director, Bayfront Family Practice Residency, St. Petersburg, Florida; Clinical Assistant Professor, Department of Family Practice, University of South Florida, Tampa, Florida; Chairman, Research Review and IRB Bayfront Medical Center; Executive Council, All Children's Hospital; Standards and Credentials, Bayfront Medical Center, St. Petersburg, Florida; Family Practice Faculty (Part time), U.S. Naval Hospital, Jacksonville, Florida
Hazardous Marine Animals

BEN PATAROQUE, M.D.
Resident in Medicine, Sinai Hospital of Baltimore, Baltimore, Maryland
Hypothyroidism

RICHARD D. PEARSON, M.D.
Professor of Medicine and Pathology, Division of Geographic and International Medicine, University of Virginia School of Medicine, Charlottesville, Virginia
Intestinal Parasites

ANNA MARIA PELUSO, M.D.
Doctor in Research, Department of Dermatology, University of Bologna, Bologna, Italy
Diseases of the Nails

ROBERT W. PETERS, M.D.
Professor of Medicine, University of Maryland School of Medicine; Chief, Division of Cardiology, Veterans Administration Medical Center, Baltimore, Maryland
Tachycardias

DAVID A. PEURA, M.D.
Associate Professor of Medicine, University of Virginia; Acting Chief of Gastroenterology, University of Virginia, Charlottesville, Virginia
Peptic Ulcer Disease

KATHERINE M. W. PISTERS, M.D.
Instructor, Cornell University Medical College; Clinical Assistant Attending, Memorial Sloan-Kettering Cancer Center, New York, New York
Nausea and Vomiting

BARBARA A. POCKAJ, M.D.
Surgery Resident, Case Western Reserve University, Cleveland, Ohio
Gastric Tumors

MICHAEL A. POLIS, M.D., M.P.H.
Senior Investigator, National Institute of Allergy and Infectious Diseases; Associate Clinical Professor of Emergency Medicine, The George Washington University Medical Center, Washington, D. C.
Food-Borne Illness

AMY E. POLLACK, M.D., M.P.H.
Assistant Clinical Professor, Columbia University, New York, New York
Contraception

ROBERT S. PURVIS, M.D.
Assistant Instructor, Texas Tech University Health Sciences Center, Lubbock, Texas
Viral Diseases of the Skin

PETER V. RABINS, M.D., M.P.H.
Professor of Psychiatry, Johns Hopkins University School of Medicine, Baltimore, Maryland
Delirium

REBECCA B. RABY, M.D.
Fellow, Division of Clinical Immunology, Department of Pediatrics, University of Tennessee, Memphis, Tennessee
Anaphylaxis and Serum Sickness

GARY S. RACHELEFSKY, M.D.
Clinical Professor, Department of Pediatrics, Associate Director of Allergy-Immunology Training Program, University of California at Los Angeles; Director, Allergy Research Foundation, Los Angeles, California
Allergic Rhinitis Caused by Inhalant Factors

DANIEL W. RAHN, M.D.
Professor and Vice Chairman, Department of Medicine, Medical College of Georgia, Augusta, Georgia
Lyme Disease

MARVIN RAPAPORT, M.D.
Clinical Professor, University of California at Los Angeles Medical Center; Attending Physician, University of California at Los Angeles and Cedars-Sinai Medical Center, Los Angeles, California
Pigmentary Disorders

L. ANDREW RAUSCHER, M.D.
Associate Clinical Professor, Columbia University, New York, New York; Clinical Chief, Department of Anesthesiology, Mary Imogen Bassett Hospital, Cooperstown, New York
Tetanus

HOWARD A. REBER, M.D.
Professor of Surgery, Vice Chairman, Department of Surgery, UCLA School of Medicine; Chief, Surgical Services, Sepulveda Veterans Administration Medical Center, Los Angeles, California
Chronic Pancreatitis

K. RAJENDER REDDY, M.D.
Associate Professor of Medicine, Division of Hepatology, Department of Medicine, University of Miami School of Medicine; Attending Physician, Jackson Memorial Hospital and Veterans Administration Medical Center, Miami, Florida
Cirrhosis

ALEXANDER REITER, M.D.
Assistant Professor, Department of Obstetrics and Gynecology, Baylor College of Medicine; Attending Physician, The Methodist Hospital, St. Luke's Episcopal Hospital, Texas Woman's Hospital, Houston, Texas
Postpartum Care

MARTIN I. RESNICK, M.D.
Lester Persky Professor and Chairman, Department of Urology, Case Western Reserve University School of Medicine; Director, Department of Urology, University Hospitals of Cleveland, Cleveland, Ohio
Renal Calculi

KAREN RHEW, M.D.
Special Expert, Voice and Speech Section, National Institute on Deafness and Other Communication Disorders, National Institutes of Health, Bethesda, Maryland
Hoarseness and Laryngitis

DALE H. RICE, M.D.
Tiber/Alpert Professor and Chairman, Department of Otolaryngology–Head and Neck Surgery, University of Southern California School of Medicine, Los Angeles, California
Sinusitis

MARILYN R. RICHARDSON, M.D.
Chief of Obstetrics and Gynecology, Permanente Medical Association of Texas; Clinical Associate Professor, University of Texas Health Science Center at Dallas, Dallas, Texas
Ectopic Pregnancy

LAYTON F. RIKKERS, M.D.
M. M. Musselman Professor and Chairman, Department of Surgery, University of Nebraska Medical Center, Omaha, Nebraska
Bleeding Esophageal Varices

DAVID A. RIVAS, M.D.
Instructor of Urology, Jefferson Medical College; Staff Physician, Thomas Jefferson University Hospital; Consulting Staff, Magee Rehabilitation Hospital, Philadelphia, Pennsylvania
Benign Prostatic Hyperplasia

DAVID J. ROBERTS, M.D.
Clinical Associate Professor, University of Minnesota Medical School, Minneapolis, Minnesota; Staff Emergency Physician and Toxicologist, North Memorial Medical Center, Robbinsdale, Minnesota
Drug Abuse

EDWARD J. ROCKWOOD, M.D.
Staff Ophthalmologist, Glaucoma Section, Division of Ophthalmology, Cleveland Clinic Foundation, Cleveland, Ohio
Glaucoma

STEVEN A. ROGERS, M.D.
Clinical and Research Fellow, Harvard Medical School; Clinical and Research Fellow, Massachusetts General Hospital, Boston, Massachusetts
Acute and Chronic Viral Hepatitis

ROLANDO H. ROLANDELLI, M.D.
Assistant Professor of Surgery, UCLA School of Medicine; Staff Surgeon, UCLA Medical Center, Los Angeles, California
Parenteral Nutrition in Adults

A. R. RONALD, O.C., M.D.
Associate Dean of Research Faculty of Medicine, University of Manitoba; Head, Infectious Disease, St. Boniface Hospital, Winnipeg, Manitoba, Canada
Bacterial Infections of the Urinary Tract in Women

STEVEN T. ROSEN, M.D.
Genevieve Teuton Professor of Medicine and Director, Robert H. Lurie Cancer Center, Northwestern University; Attending Physician, Northwestern Memorial Hospital, Chicago, Illinois
T Cell Lymphoma (Mycosis Fungoides and Sézary's Syndrome)

JOEL J. ROSLYN, M.D.
Professor and Chairman, Department of Surgery, The Medical College of Pennsylvania and Hahnemann University School of Medicine, Philadelphia, Pennsylvania
Cholelithiasis and Cholecystitis

JOHN C. RUCKDESCHEL, M.D.
Professor of Medicine, University of South Florida; Center Director and Chief Executive Officer, H. Lee Moffitt Cancer Center and Research Institute, Tampa, Florida
Carcinoma of the Lung

DELBERT C. RUDY, M.D., M.Sc.
Associate Professor of Surgery (Urology) and Director of Urology, The Institute for Rehabilitation and Research, Houston, Texas
Urinary Incontinence

CHARLES E. RUPPRECHT, V.M.D., Ph.D.
Associate Professor, Centre for Neurovirology, Thomas Jefferson University, Philadelphia, Pennsylvania; Chief, Rabies Section, Viral and Rickettsial Zoonoses Branch, National Center for Infectious Diseases, Centers for Disease Control and Prevention, Atlanta, Georgia
Rabies

ELISA B. RUSH, M.D.
Resident in Surgery, Cedars-Sinai Medical Center, Los Angeles, California
Malignant Melanoma

DAVID B. SACHAR, M.D.
The Dr. Burrill B. Crohn Professor of Medicine, Mount Sinai School of Medicine of the City University of New York; Director of the Dr. Henry D. Janowitz Division of Gastroenterology, The Mount Sinai Hospital, New York, New York
Crohn's Disease

HAMED SAJJADI, M.D.
Neurotology Fellowship Director, Minnesota Ear, Head and Neck Clinic, Minneapolis, Minnesota; Staff Physician, Fairview Riverside Hospital, Minneapolis, Minnesota; Mercy Health One Hospital, Coon Rapids, Minnesota
Meniere's Disease

JOSE H. SALGADO, M.D., M.P.H.
Fellow, Infectious Disease Division, University of Kentucky College of Medicine, Lexington, Kentucky
Osteomyelitis

DONALD B. SANDERS, M.D.
Professor of Medicine, Duke University Medical School; Neurologist, Duke University Hospital and Veterans Administration Medical Center; Director, Electromyography Laboratory, Duke University Medical Center, Durham, North Carolina
Myasthenia Gravis

GUILLERMO R. SAURINA, M.D.
Clinical Assistant Instructor, Harvard Medical School, Renal Fellow, Massachusetts General Hospital, Boston, Massachusetts
Acute Renal Failure

HARTZELL SCHAFF, M.D.
Professor of Surgery, Mayo Medical School; Consultant, Division of Thoracic and Cardiovascular Surgery, Mayo Clinic and Foundation, Rochester, Minnesota
Acquired Diseases of the Aorta

W. MICHAEL SCHELD, M.D.
Professor of Internal Medicine and Neurosurgery, Division of Infectious Diseases, University of Virginia School of Medicine, Charlottesville, Viriginia
Bacterial Meningitis

STEVEN SCHLOSSBERG, M.D.
Associate Professor of Urology and Anatomy, Eastern Virginia Medical School; Attending Physician, Sentara Norfolk General Hospital and Children's Hospital of the King's Daughters, Norfolk, Virginia
Urethral Stricture

DOUGLAS K. SCHREIBER, M.D.
Assistant Clinical Instructor, University of Texas Medical Branch, Galveston, Texas
Stinging Insect Allergy

MARK SCHUYLER, M.D.
Professor of Medicine, University of New Mexico School of Medicine; Associate Chief of Staff for Education, Veterans Administration Medical Center, Albuquerque, New Mexico
Hypersensitivity Pneumonitis

ERNEST SCHWARTZ, M.D.
Clinical Associate Professor of Medicine, Cornell University Medical College; Chief, Metabolic Bone Unit, Bronx Veterans Administration Medical Center, Bronx, New York; Associate Attending Physician, Hospital for Special Surgery, New York, New York
Osteoporosis

GARY R. SCHWARTZ, M.D.
Assistant Professor of Emergency Medicine, Vanderbilt University; Attending Physician, Vanderbilt University Hospital, Nashville, Tennessee
Toxic Shock Syndrome

DANIEL J. SEXTON, M.D.
Associate Professor, Department of Medicine, Duke University Medical Center; Staff Physician, Duke University Medical Center; Director, Infection Control Unit, Duke University Medical Center, Durham, North Carolina
Rocky Mountain Spotted Fever

REZA SHAKER, M.D.
Associate Professor of Medicine and Radiology, Medical College of Wisconsin; Senior Attending Staff, Froedtert Memorial Lutheran Hospital and John L. Doyne Hospital; Attending Staff, Veterans Administration Medical Center; Director, MCW Dysphagia Institute, Milwaukee, Wisconsin
Dysphagia and Esophageal Obstruction

GAIL G. SHAPIRO, M.D.
Clinical Professor of Pediatrics, University of Washington School of Medicine; Attending Physician, Children's Hospital and Medical Center, Seattle, Washington
Asthma in Children

HARRY H. SHARATA, M.D., PH.D.
Assistant Professor, Division of Dermatology, University of Wisconsin; Attending Dermatologist, University of Wisconsin Hospital and Clinics and Veterans Hospital, Madison, Wisconsin
Parasitic Infections of the Skin

PHILIP D. SHENEFELT, M.D.
Assistant Professor, Section of Dermatology and Cutaneous Surgery, Department of Internal Medicine, University of South Florida; Assistant Chief of Dermatology, James A. Haley Veterans Hospital; Staff Dermatologist, Tampa General Hospital, Moffitt Cancer Center, Tampa, Florida
Contact Dermatitis

GILLIAN M. SHEPHERD, M.D.
Associate Professor of Clinical Medicine, Cornell University Medical College; Associate Attending Physician, The New York Hospital; Consultant, Memorial Sloan-Kettering Cancer Center, New York, New York
Allergic Drug Reactions

DAVID H. SHEPP, M.D.
Associate Professor of Medicine, Cornell University Medical College, New York, New York; Attending Physician, North Shore University Hospital, Manhasset, New York
Infectious Mononucleosis

ELIZABETH F. SHERERTZ, M.D.
Professor and Vice Chairman, Department of Dermatology, Bowman Gray School of Medicine, Wake Forest University, Winston-Salem, North Carolina
Pruritus (Itching)

DAVID G. SHERMAN, M.D.
Professor and Chief, Division of Neurology, Department of Medicine, University of Texas Health Science Center at San Antonio; Staff Neurologist, University Hospital; Audie L. Murphy Memorial Veterans Hospital, San Antonio, Texas
Ischemic Cerebrovascular Disease

LAWRENCE N. SHULMAN, M.D.
Assistant Professor of Medicine, Harvard Medical School; Clinical Director, Hematology-Oncology Division, Brigham and Women's Hospital, Boston, Massachusetts
Acute Leukemia in Adults

LISA M. SHULMAN, M.D.
Assistant Professor of Clinical Neurology, University of Miami School of Medicine; Attending Physician, University of Miami Jackson Memorial Medical Center, Miami, Florida
Parkinson's Disease

JONATHAN SHUTER, M.D.
Fellow, Division of Infectious Diseases, Albert Einstein College of Medicine; I. D. Consultant, Montefiore Medical Center and The Albert Einstein College of Medicine, Bronx, New York
Rat-Bite Fever

AXEL SIGURDSSON, M.D., PH.D.
Associate Director, Division of Cardiology, Department of Medicine, Östra Hospital, Göteborg, Sweden
Congestive Heart Failure

ALLAN W. SILBERMAN, M.D., PH.D.
Associate Clinical Professor of Surgery, University of Southern California School of Medicine; Attending Surgeon, Cedars-Sinai Medical Center, Los Angeles, California
Malignant Melanoma

RICHARD T. SILVER, M.D.
Clinical Professor of Medicine, Cornell University Medical College; Director, Section of Clinical Oncology Chemotherapy Research, New York, New York
Polycythemia Vera

FREDRIC J. SILVERBLATT, M.D.
Professor of Medicine, Brown University; Chief, Medical Service, Veterans Affairs Medical Center, Providence, Rhode Island
Bacterial Infections of the Urinary Tract in Males

GEORGE M. SIMPSON, M.D.
Professor of Psychiatry and Pharmacology and Director of Clinical Psychopharmacology, Hospital of the Medical College of Pennsylvania/Eastern Pennsylvania Psychiatric Institute, Philadelphia, Pennsylvania
Schizophrenic Disorders

IRWIN SINGER, M.D.
Clinical Professor of Medicine, University of Miami School of Medicine; Staff Physician, Nephrology Section, Medical Service, Department of Veterans Affairs Medical Center, Miami, Florida
Diabetes Insipidus

LAURENCE SLUTSKER, M.D., M.P.H.
Medical Epidemiologist, Division of Parasitic Diseases, National Center for Infectious Diseases, Centers for Disease Control and Prevention, Atlanta, Georgia
Malaria

BENJAMIN N. SMITH, M.D.
Assistant Professor of Medicine, Tufts University School of Medicine; Staff Physician, Department of Gastroenterology, Faulkner Hospital and Lemuel Shattuck Hospital, Boston, Massachusetts
Hemochromatosis

BRADLEY E. SMITH, M.D.
Professor of Anesthesiology, Vanderbilt University School of Medicine; Attending Physician, Vanderbilt University Medical Center, Nashville, Tennessee
Obstetric Anesthesia

CARL V. SMITH, M.D.
Associate Professor and Vice-Chairman, Department of Obstetrics and Gynecology; Director, Maternal-Fetal Medicine, University of Nebraska Medical Center, Omaha, Nebraska
Antepartum Care

DAVID S. SMITH, M.D.
Professor Emeritus of Pediatrics, Temple University School of Medicine; Attending Pediatrician, St. Christopher's Hospital for Children, Philadelphia, Pennsylvania
Measles

EDGAR B. SMITH, M.D.
Professor and Chairman of Dermatology, University of Texas Medical Branch; Staff Physician, University of Texas Medical Branch Hospitals, Galveston, Texas
Superficial Fungal Infections of the Skin

MICHAEL C. SMITH, M.D.
Associate Professor of Medicine, Division of Nephrology, University Hospitals and Case Western Reserve University, Cleveland, Ohio
Chronic Renal Failure

PETER S. SMITH, M.D.
Associate Professor of Pediatrics, Brown University School of Medicine, and Associate Director, Department of Pediatric Hematology-Oncology, Rhode Island Hospital, Providence, Rhode Island
Hemophilia and Related Disorders

REBECCA SMITH-COGGINS, M.D.

Assistant Professor of Surgery/Emergency Medicine, Stanford University School of Medicine; Emergency Medicine Residency Director, Stanford University Hospital, Stanford, California
Disturbances Due to Cold

DAVID A. SOLOMON, M.D.

Clinical Assistant Professor of Psychiatry and Human Behavior, Brown University; Director, Outpatient Mood Disorders Program, Butler Hospital, Providence, Rhode Island
Mood Disorders

DIANE H. SOLOMON, M.D.

Assistant Professor, Division of Department of Medicine, Neurology, University of Texas Health Science Center at San Antonio; Staff Neurologist, University Hospital and Audie Murphy Veterans Administration Hospital, San Antonio, Texas
Ischemic Cerebrovascular Disease

STEVEN J. SONDHEIMER, M.D.

Professor of Obstetrics and Gynecology, University of Pennsylvania Medical Center; Staff Physician, Hospital of the University of Pennsylvania, Philadelphia, Pennsylvania
Dysmenorrhea

WILLIAM A. SPEIR, M.D.

Professor of Medicine, Section of Pulmonary Diseases, Medical College of Georgia; Medical Director, Medical Intensive Care Unit, Medical College of Georgia Hospital, Augusta, Georgia
Acute Respiratory Failure

CHARLES H. SPENCER, M.D.

Assistant Professor of Pediatrics, Department of Pediatrics, University of Chicago Medical Center; Acting Section Head of Rheumatology, La Rabida Children's Hospital and Research Center; Attending Staff in Rheumatology, Wyler Children's Hospital, Chicago, Illinois
Juvenile Rheumatoid Arthritis

EGILIUS L. H. SPIERINGS, M.D., PH.D.

Lecturer in Neurology, Harvard Medical School; Assistant Professor of Neurology, Tufts University School of Medicine; Physician, Brigham and Women's Hospital, Boston, Massachusetts
Headache

DAVID H. SPODICK, M.D., D.SC.

Professor of Medicine, University of Massachusetts Medical School; Director of Clinical Cardiology and Director of Cardiology Fellowship Training, St. Vincent Hospital, Worcester, Massachusetts
Pericarditis

KATHERINE M. SPOONER, M.D.

Medical Staff Fellow, National Institutes of Allergy and Infectious Diseases, Bethesda, Maryland
Food-Borne Illness

MARCUS D. STANBRO, D.O.

Adjunct Faculty Member, Kirksville College of Osteopathic Medicine, Kirksville, Missouri; Active Staff, Oakhill Hospital and Freeman Hospital; Associate Staff, St. John's Regional Medical Center, Joplin, Missouri
Deep Venous Thrombosis of the Extremities

MARTIN H. STEINBERG, M.D.

Professor of Medicine, University of Mississippi; Associate Chief of Staff for Research, Jackson Veterans Affairs Medical Center, Jackson, Mississippi
Thalassemia

SAMUEL M. STEINFELD, B.SC., B.M.R.(P.T.)

Sports Physiotherapy Center, Pan Am Sports Medicine Center, Winnipeg, Manitoba, Canada
Ankylosing Spondylitis

ROBERT S. STERN, M.D.

Associate Professor of Dermatology, Harvard Medical School; Dermatologist, Beth Israel Hospital, Boston, Massachusetts
Acne Vulgaris and Rosacea

CHARLES L. STEWART, M.D.

Assistant Professor, University Medical Center at Stony Brook; Attending Physician, Department of Pediatric Nephrology, University Hospital at Stony Brook, Stony Brook, New York
Parenteral Fluid Therapy for Infants and Children

S. H. SUBRAMONY, M.D.

Professor and Vice Chairman of Neurology, Department of Neurology, University of Mississippi School of Medicine; Attending Physician, University of Mississippi Medical Center; Consultant in Neurology, Veterans Administration Medical Center, Jackson, Mississippi
Peripheral Neuropathies

SIMON SUTCLIFFE, B.SC., M.D.

Professor, Department of Radiation Oncology, University of Toronto; President and Chief Executive Officer, Princess Margaret Hospital, Ontario Cancer Institute; Radiation Oncologist, Department of Radiation Oncology, Princess Margaret Hospital, Toronto, Ontario, Canada
Hodgkin's Disease: Chemotherapy

LAURIE J. SUTOR, M.D.

Assistant Professor, Department of Pathology, University of Texas Southwestern Medical Center; Associate Medical Director, Transfusion Services, Parkland Memorial Hospital; Scientific Director, Blood Bank, Veterans Administration Medical Center; Consultant in Pathology, Children's Medical Center; Pathology Staff, Zale Lipshy University Hospital, Dallas, Texas
Adverse Reactions to Blood Transfusions

SHERRY T. SUTTON, PHARM.D.

Clinical Specialist, Department of Pharmacy, University of Virginia Hospital, Charlottesville, Virginia
Bacterial Diseases of the Skin

KARL SWEDBERG, M.D., PH.D.

Associate Professor of Medicine, Göteborg University; Chief, Department of Medicine, Östra Hospital, Göteborg, Sweden
Congestive Heart Failure

ROBERT A. SWERLICK, M.D.

Associate Professor, Department of Dermatology, Emory University School of Medicine; Emory University Hospital and Grady Memorial Hospital, Atlanta, Georgia
Cutaneous Vasculitis

TED P. SZATROWSKI, M.D.

Assistant Professor of Medicine, Cornell University Medical College; Assistant Attending Physician, The New York Hospital, New York, New York
Chronic Leukemias

GARY B. TALPOS, M.D.

Attending Surgeon, Henry Ford Hospital, Detroit, Michigan
Thyroid Cancer

JAMES S. TAYLOR, M.D.

Head, Section of Industrial Dermatology, Cleveland Clinic Foundation, Cleveland, Ohio
Occupational Dermatoses

NATHAN M. THIELMAN, M.D., M.P.H.

Fellow in Infectious Diseases, University of Virginia School of Medicine, Charlottesville, Virginia
Acute Infectious Diarrhea

JEFFREY M. THOMPSON, M.D.
Assistant Professor of Physical Medicine and Rehabilitation, Mayo Medical School; Consultant, Department of Physical Medicine and Rehabilitation, Mayo Clinic and Mayo Foundation, Rochester, Minnesota
Fibromyalgia, Tendinitis, and Bursitis

W. GRANT THOMPSON, M.D.
Professor of Medicine, University of Ottawa; Chief, Division of Gastroenterology, Ottawa Civic Hospital, Ottawa, Ontario, Canada
The Irritable Bowel

GLEN T. D. THOMSON, M.D.
Assistant Professor, University of Manitoba; Director of Rheumatology Services, St. Boniface Hospital, Winnipeg, Manitoba, Canada
Ankylosing Spondylitis

PETER V. TISHLER, M.D.
Associate Professor of Medicine, Harvard Medical School, Boston, Massachusetts; Attending Physician, Brockton-West Roxbury Veterans Administration Medical Center, Brockton, Massachusetts
The Porphyrias

WILLIAM L. TOFFLER, M.D.
Associate Professor, Department of Family Medicine, Oregon Health Sciences University, Portland, Oregon
Common Sports Injuries

RICHARD B. TOMPKINS, M.D.
Consultant in Rheumatology and Internal Medicine, Mayo Clinic, Mayo Foundation, Rochester, Minnesota
Osteoarthritis

ANTONELLA TOSTI, M.D.
Associate Professor, Department of Dermatology, University of Bologna, Bologna, Italy
Diseases of the Nails

GREGORY C. TOWNSEND, M.D.
Clinical Instructor, Department of Internal Medicine (Infectious Diseases), University of Virginia, Charlottesville, Virginia
Bacterial Meningitis

JOHN TREANOR, M.D.
Assistant Professor of Medicine, University of Rochester School of Medicine, Attending Physician, Strong Memorial Hospital, Rochester, New York
Epidemic Influenza

JOAN R. ULLRICH, R.D.
Coordinator, Home Parenteral Nutrition Program, UCLA Medical Center, Los Angeles, California
Parenteral Nutrition in Adults

MARY LEE VANCE, M.D.
Associate Professor of Medicine, Department of Internal Medicine, Division of Endocrinology and Metabolism, University of Virginia Medical School; Attending Physician, University of Virginia Hospital, Charlottesville, Virginia
Hypopituitarism

ALEXANDER G. VANDEVELDE, M.D.
Associate Professor, University of Florida Health Science Center; Hospital Epidemiologist, University Medical Center, Jacksonville, Florida
Relapsing Fevers

S. A. VAUGHAN JONES, M.D.
Research Registrar, St. John's Institute of Dermatology, St. Thomas' Hospital, London, England
The Specific Dermatoses of Pregnancy

V. VEDANARAYANAN, M.D.
Assistant Professor of Pediatrics and Neurology, University of Mississippi Medical School; Attending Physician, University of Mississippi Medical Center, Jackson, Mississippi
Peripheral Neuropathies

DAVID VESOLE, M.D., PH.D.
Assistant Professor, Department of Medicine, University of Arkansas for Medical Sciences, Little Rock, Arkansas
Multiple Myeloma

JULIE M. VOSE, M.D.
Associate Professor, University of Nebraska Medical Center, Omaha, Nebraska
Non-Hodgkin's Lymphoma

MICHAEL WALL, M.D.
Associate Professor of Neurology and Ophthalmology, Department of Neurology, University of Iowa College of Medicine; Attending Physician, University of Iowa Hospitals and Clinics and Veterans Administration Hospital, Iowa City, Iowa
Optic Neuritis

JOHN D. WARD, M.D.
Director, Neurosciences Center, Professor and Executive Vice Chairman; Chief, Pediatric Neurosurgery, Division of Neurosurgery, Medical College of Virginia, Richmond, Virginia
Acute Head Injuries in Children

PETER C. WEBER, M.D.
Assistant Professor and Director, Department of Otolaryngology, Center for Hearing and Balance Disorders, Medical University of South Carolina, Charleston, South Carolina
Idiopathic Facial Paralysis (Bell's Palsy)

WILLIAM J. WEINER, M.D.
Director, Movement Disorders Center; Professor of Neurology, University of Miami School of Medicine, Miami, Florida
Parkinson's Disease

STEVEN D. WEXNER, M.D.
Chairman, Department of Colorectal Surgery, Cleveland Clinic Florida, Ft. Lauderdale, Florida
Malignant Diseases of the Colon and Rectum

DUANE C. WHITAKER, M.D.
Professor of Dermatology, University of Iowa College of Medicine; Director of Dermatologic Surgery and Cutaneous Laser Surgery, University of Iowa Hospitals and Clinics, Iowa City, Iowa
Premalignant Lesions

PETER WHITEHOUSE, M.D., PH.D.
Professor of Neurology, Case Western Reserve University; Director, Alzheimer Center, University Hospitals of Cleveland, Cleveland, Ohio
Alzheimer's Disease

DAVID A. WHITING, M.D.
Clinical Professor of Dermatology and Pediatrics, University of Texas, Southwestern Medical Center; Attending Dermatologist, Baylor University Medical Center, Children's Medical Center, and Parkland Hospital, Dallas, Texas
Hair Disorders

CAROLYN F. WHITSETT, M.D.
Associate Professor of Pathology, Emory University School of Medicine; Director, Blood Bank, Crawford W. Long Hospital of Emory University, Atlanta, Georgia
Therapeutic Use of Blood Components

PAUL V. WILLIAMS, M.D.
Clinical Professor of Pediatrics, University of Washington School of Medicine; Attending Physician, Children's Hospital and Medical Center, Seattle, Washington
Asthma in Children

JOSEPH A. WITKOWSKI, M.D.

Clinical Professor of Dermatology, University of Pennsylvania School of Medicine; Professor of Medicine (Dermatology), Pennsylvania College of Podiatric Medicine, Philadelphia, Pennsylvania
Pressure Ulcer

KIMBERLY A. WORKOWSKI, M.D.

Assistant Professor of Medicine, Division of Infectious Diseases, Emory University; Attending Physician, Crawford Long Hospital, Grady Hospital, and Emory Hospital, Atlanta, Georgia
Chlamydia Trachomatis

SETH W. WRIGHT, M.D.

Assistant Professor of Emergency Medicine, Vanderbilt University School of Medicine; Attending Physician, Vanderbilt University Hospital, Nashville, Tennessee
Toxic Shock Syndrome

JAMES S. T. YAO, M.D., PH.D.

Magerstadt Professor of Surgery, Northwestern University Medical School; Attending Surgeon and Chief, Division of Vascular Surgery, Northwestern Memorial Hospital, Chicago, Illinois
Peripheral Arterial Disease

ERIK Y. YEO, M.D.

Assistant Professor of Medicine, University of Toronto; Attending Physician, The Toronto Hospital, Toronto, Ontario, Canada
Disseminated Intravascular Coagulation; Thrombotic Thrombocytopenic Purpura

NEAL S. YOUNG, M.D.

Chief, Hematology Branch, National Heart, Lung and Blood Institute, Bethesda, Maryland
Aplastic Anemia

WILLIAM F. YOUNG, JR., M.D.

Associate Professor of Medicine, Mayo Medical School; Consultant, Division of Endocrinology, Metabolism, and Internal Medicine, and Consultant, Division of Hypertension and Internal Medicine, Mayo Clinic and Mayo Foundation, Rochester, Minnesota
Adrenocortical Insufficiency; Pheochromocytoma

TONY ZREIK, M.D.

Postdoctoral Fellow, Yale University School of Medicine; Staff Member, Yale-New Haven Hospital, New Haven, Connecticut
Amenorrhea

JANE ZUCKER, M.D., M.SC.

Medical Epidemiologist, Division of Parasitic Diseases, National Center for Infectious Diseases, Centers for Disease Control and Prevention, Atlanta, Georgia
Malaria

Preface

This 47th edition of *Current Therapy* is somewhat unique in that it has the highest percentage of completely new authors of any edition. Although each year we invite new authors to write on each topic in order to provide a new edition that is fresh and up to date, our tight deadlines make it difficult for some authors to submit their manuscripts on time and we end up asking several of the previous authors to update their material. In this manner, the information is always current but not as fresh. This year 95% of the authors are new, a considerable increase over the usual 80%. This is largely due to the excellent organizational skills and persistence of Jeanne Ullian, my editorial assistant, without whom this book would never have made it to press on time.

A new feature added to the Appendices in this edition is a list of drugs approved by the U.S. Food and Drug Administration during the year. This is a quick reference for new drugs that may not have made it into the usual texts and the only reference source for the busy physician is a journal advertisement that may not be easy to locate during office hours. This emphasizes that our primary objective is to assist the practicing physician by providing current information in a compact format to assist in easy retrieval for the patient in the office at that moment. The staff at W.B. Saunders are experts at editing the material so that it is concise and easy to read.

Articles on low back pain and otitis externa have been added this year, continuing the trend to focus on problems frequently encountered in primary care. In the article on otitis externa, the table showing the preferred drug for each of the most likely pathogens is an excellent example of how tables can aid the busy physician in quickly identifying the drug of choice.

The authors of each topic are experts in that area and see many more patients with these problems than the average physician is likely to encounter in practice. They are also familiar with ongoing research and frequently use drugs that have not yet been approved by the U.S. Food and Drug Administration for that indication. Although we add a footnote indicating that lack of approval, this does not mean the drug is not useful in that disease; it just means that the drug has not yet made it through the bureaucracy. I have also maintained Howard Conn's practice of indicating that the material presented is the "method of" the author to emphasize that this expert has found this technique or this drug combination the most successful way to manage the problem. This method may vary from previous authors, and the reader is encouraged to compare the methods of more than one author.

This book is intended to serve primary care physicians, but it may be even more useful to those physicians trained in subspecialties who find themselves called on to deliver more and more primary care. I would appreciate hearing whether it serves this purpose and welcome suggestions.

ROBERT E. RAKEL, M.D.

NOTICE

Medicine is an ever-changing field. Standard safety precautions must be followed, but as new research and clinical experience broaden our knowledge, changes in treatment and drug therapy become necessary or appropriate. The editors of this work have carefully checked the generic and trade drug names and verified drug dosages to ensure that the dosage information in this work is accurate and in accord with the standards accepted at the time of publication. Readers are advised, however, to check the product information currently provided by the manufacturer of each drug to be administered to be certain that changes have not been made in the recommended dose or in the contraindications for administration. This is of particular importance in regard to new or infrequently used drugs. It is the responsibility of the treating physician, relying on experience and knowledge of the patient, to determine dosages and the best treatment for the patient. The editors cannot be responsible for misuse or misapplication of the material in this work.

THE PUBLISHER

Contents

SECTION 1. SYMPTOMATIC CARE PENDING DIAGNOSIS

Pain 1
Alexander Mauskop

Nausea and Vomiting 4
Katherine M. W. Pisters
Mark G. Kris

Gaseousness and Indigestion 8
Miles Auslander

Acute Infectious Diarrhea 9
Nathan M. Thielman
Richard L. Guerrant

Constipation 16
Christopher J. Bartolone
Jay L. Goldstein

Fever 19
Moshe Ipp

Cough 21
James R. McCormick

Hoarseness and Laryngitis 25
Karen Rhew

Insomnia 33
Wallace B. Mendelson

Pruritus (Itching) 35
Jeffrey D. Bernhard
Elizabeth F. Sherertz
Joseph L. Jorizzo

Tinnitus 38
Laura L. Downey
Paul E. Hammerschlag

Low Back Pain 39
Marianne Dalgas
Matthew H. Liang

SECTION 2. THE INFECTIOUS DISEASES

Acquired Immune Deficiency Syndrome (AIDS) 42
Brian S. Koll
Donald Armstrong

Amebiasis 53
K. Gamble
J. S. Keystone

Bacteremia 55
Harold W. Horowitz
Harish Marisiddaiah

Brucellosis 62
M. Yousuf Khan

Conjunctivitis 63
John P. Frangie
Howard M. Leibowitz

Varicella (Chickenpox) 66
Marilyn A. Kacica

Cholera 69
Dilip Mahalanabis

Diphtheria 72
Gary D. Overturf

Food-Borne Illness 74
Katherine M. Spooner
Michael A. Polis

Necrotizing Skin and Soft Tissue Infections 78
Ellis S. Caplan

Epidemic Influenza 80
John Treanor

Leishmaniasis 83
Alan J. Magill

Leprosy (Hansen's Disease) 87
Robert R. Jacobson

Malaria 91
Laurence Slutsker
Jane Zucker

Bacterial Meningitis 98
Gregory C. Townsend
W. Michael Scheld

Infectious Mononucleosis 103
Jazila Al-Attar
David H. Shepp

Mumps 104
Ralph C. Gordon

Otitis Externa 105
Laura W. Cheever
Michael P. Johnson

Plague 107
Thomas Butler

Psittacosis (Ornithosis) 108
Clark M. Kerr

Q Fever 109
Darwin L. Palmer

Rabies 110
Charles E. Rupprecht
Makonnen Fekadu

Rat-Bite Fever 113
Jonathan Shuter
Franklin D. Lowy

Relapsing Fevers 114
Alexander G. Vandevelde

Rheumatic Fever 117
Michael S. Bronze

Lyme Disease 119
Daniel W. Rahn

Rocky Mountain Spotted Fever 124
Daniel J. Sexton

Rubella and Congenital Rubella 125
Peter Morgan-Capner

Measles 127
David S. Smith

Tetanus 128
L. Andrew Rauscher

Toxoplasmosis 131
Sharon B. Mannheimer
Henry W. Murray

Trichinosis 133
R. Gopinath
J. S. Keystone

Tularemia 134
George J. Cuchural, Jr.

Salmonellosis 136
Gary D. Overturf

Typhoid Fever 140
Deirdre A. Herrington

The Typhus Fevers 142
James G. Olson
Mary Jane Dalton

Whooping Cough (Pertussis) 144
Kathryn M. Edwards
Laura A. Cattaneo

SECTION 3. THE RESPIRATORY SYSTEM

Acute Respiratory Failure 147
William A. Speir
Leigh A. Callahan

Atelectasis 151
Randolph Kessler

Chronic Obstructive Pulmonary Disease 152
Ronald B. George
Michael W. Owens

Carcinoma of the Lung 156
John C. Ruckdeschel

Coccidioidomycosis 163
Roger Larson
Robert Libke

Histoplasmosis 166
Stanley W. Chapman

Blastomycosis 168
Scott F. Davies

Pleural Effusion and Empyema Thoracis 170
Mark S. Allen

Primary Lung Abscess 171
Bruce P. Krieger

Otitis Media 172
Gordon B. Hughes

Infectious Bronchitis 174
Richard Gleckman

Bacterial Pneumonia 176
Barbara J. Foner
William A. Broughton
John B. Bass, Jr.

Viral Respiratory Infections 187
Barry Farr

Viral and Mycoplasmal Pneumonias 189
Bruce H. Hamory

Legionellosis (Legionnaire's Disease and Pontiac Fever) 190
Thomas J. Marrie

Acute Pulmonary Embolism 192
James D. Douketis
Jeffrey S. Ginsberg

Sarcoidosis 195
Sonoko Nagai
Takateru Izumi

Silicosis 199
James H. Dauber

Hypersensitivity Pneumonitis 201
Mark Schuyler

Sinusitis 202
Dale H. Rice

Streptococcal Pharyngitis 204
W. M. Gooch III

Tuberculosis and Other Mycobacterial Infections 207
John F. Fieselmann
Charles S. Dayton
Douglas B. Hornick

SECTION 4. THE CARDIOVASCULAR SYSTEM

Acquired Diseases of the Aorta 213
Peter Gloviczki
Hartzell Schaff

Angina Pectoris 217
Charles R. Lambert

Cardiac Arrest 222
James M. Atkins

Atrial Fibrillation 227
Gerald V. Naccarelli

Premature Beats 230
Prakash C. Deedwania

Heart Block 233
Steven M. Markowitz
Bruce B. Lerman

Tachycardias 236
Michael R. Gold
Robert W. Peters

Congenital Heart Disease 241
Derek A. Fyfe

Mitral Valve Prolapse 249
John B. Barlow

Congestive Heart Failure 252
Axel Sigurdsson
Karl Swedberg

Infective Endocarditis 257
Gabriel Gregoratos

Hypertension 263
Marvin Moser

Acute Myocardial Infarction 280
Francis N. Fernandes
Steven Borzak

Cardiac Rehabilitation 285
Gerald F. Fletcher

Pericarditis 289
David H. Spodick

Peripheral Arterial Disease 292
James S. T. Yao

Deep Venous Thrombosis of the Extremities 296
Marcus D. Stanbro
John R. Bartholomew

SECTION 5. THE BLOOD AND SPLEEN

Aplastic Anemia 299
Neal S. Young

Iron Deficiency Anemia 302
Roy D. Baynes

Autoimmune Hemolytic Anemia 305
Charles H. Packman

Nonimmune Hemolytic Anemia 308
Akira Hirono

Pernicious Anemia and Other Megaloblastic Anemias 311
Ralph Carmel

Thalassemia 314
Martin H. Steinberg

Sickle Cell Disease 318
Samir K. Ballas

Neutropenia 327
Robert L. Baehner

Hemolytic Disease of the Fetus and Newborn 329
John M. Bowman

Hemophilia and Related Disorders 334
Peter S. Smith

Platelet-Mediated Bleeding Disorders 338
Doreen B. Brettler

Disseminated Intravascular Coagulation 342
Erik Y. Yeo
Edward M. Conway

Thrombotic Thrombocytopenic Purpura 344
Edward M. Conway
Erik Y. Yeo

Hemochromatosis 345
Benjamin N. Smith
Norman D. Grace

Hodgkin's Disease: Chemotherapy 348
Simon Sutcliffe

Hodgkin's Disease: Radiation Therapy 354
Pelayo C. Besa

Acute Leukemia in Adults 359
Stephanie J. Lee
Lawrence N. Shulman

Acute Leukemia in Children 365
Martin L. Brecher

Chronic Leukemias 369
Ted P. Szatrowski

Non-Hodgkin's Lymphoma 374
Julie M. Vose

T Cell Lymphoma (Mycosis Fungoides and Sézary's Syndrome) 377
Timothy M. Kuzel
Steven T. Rosen

Multiple Myeloma 382
Bart Barlogie
David Vesole
Sundar Jagannath

Polycythemia Vera 387
Richard T. Silver

The Porphyrias 389
Peter V. Tishler

Therapeutic Use of Blood Components 393
Carolyn F. Whitsett

Adverse Reactions to Blood Transfusions 398
Laurie J. Sutor
Harold S. Kaplan

SECTION 6. THE DIGESTIVE SYSTEM

Cholelithiasis and Cholecystitis 402
Dan I. N. Giurgiu
Joel J. Roslyn

Cirrhosis 405
Victor Idrovo
K. Rajender Reddy

Bleeding Esophageal Varices 413
Kenric M. Murayama
Layton F. Rikkers

Dysphagia and Esophageal Obstruction 417
Reza Shaker

Diverticula of the Alimentary Tract 422
George Ahtaridis

Ulcerative Colitis 426
Sumner C. Kraft

Crohn's Disease 433
Asher Kornbluth
David B. Sachar

The Irritable Bowel 435
W. Grant Thompson

Hemorrhoids, Anal Fissure, and Anorectal Abscess and Fistula 438
Peter A. Cataldo

Gastritis 441
Robert A. Kozol

Acute and Chronic Viral Hepatitis 443
Steven A. Rogers
Lawrence S. Friedman

Malabsorption 450
Ronald E. Mason
Ralph A. Giannella

Acute Pancreatitis 458
Scott M. Berry
Aaron S. Fink

Chronic Pancreatitis 463
Howard A. Reber
David W. McFadden

Peptic Ulcer Disease 469
Arthur J. DeCross
David A. Peura

Gastric Tumors 472
Barbara A. Pockaj
Bruce Averbook

Malignant Diseases of the Colon and Rectum 476
Steven D. Wexner
Juan J. Nogueras

Intestinal Parasites 479
Richard D. Pearson

SECTION 7. METABOLIC DISORDERS

Diabetes Mellitus in Adults 487
William C. Duckworth

Type I Diabetes Mellitus in Children and Adolescents 493
Stephen C. Duck

Diabetic Ketoacidosis 499
William T. Cefalu

Hyperuricemia and Gout 502
Shannon Howe
N. Lawrence Edwards

Hyperlipoproteinemias 505
Conrad B. Blum

Obesity 510
Steven B. Heymsfield
Kathy Hoy

Water-Soluble Vitamin Deficiency States 517
Stephen R. Newmark

Vitamin K Deficiency 520
Robert E. Olson

Osteoporosis 521
Ernest Schwartz

Paget's Disease of Bone 527
Alison A. Moy
William J. Burtis

Parenteral Nutrition in Adults 530
Rolando H. Rolandelli
Joan R. Ullrich

Parenteral Fluid Therapy for Infants and Children 538
Charles L. Stewart
Frederick J. Kaskel

SECTION 8. THE ENDOCRINE SYSTEM

Acromegaly 548
Mark E. Molitch

Adrenocortical Insufficiency 550
William F. Young, Jr.

Cushing's Syndrome 554
Paul C. Carpenter

Diabetes Insipidus 559
Irwin Singer
James R. Oster

Goiter 563
John J. Orloff
Gerard N. Burrow

Hyperparathyroidism and Hypoparathyroidism 565
John P. Bilezikian

Primary Aldosteronism 569
Diana L. Maas
Mahendr S. Kochar

Hypopituitarism 572
Mary Lee Vance

Hyperprolactinemia 575
Eugene Katz

Hypothyroidism 577
Ben Pataroque
David S. Cooper

Hyperthyroidism 580
Gilbert H. Daniels

Thyroid Cancer 584
Gary B. Talpos

Pheochromocytoma 588
William F. Young, Jr.

Thyroiditis 592
Terry F. Davies

SECTION 9. THE UROGENITAL TRACT

Bacterial Infections of the Urinary Tract in Males 595
Fredric J. Silverblatt

Bacterial Infections of the Urinary Tract in Women 596
A. R. Ronald

Bacterial Infections of the Urinary Tract in Girls 599
Anthony J. Casale

Childhood Enuresis 601
Edmond T. Gonzales, Jr.

Urinary Incontinence 604
Marko R. Gudziak
Delbert C. Rudy

Epididymitis 608
John A. Heaney

The Primary Glomerulopathies 609
Lee A. Hebert

Pyelonephritis 620
Mark G. Martens

Genitourinary Trauma 623
Joe Y. Lee
Alexander S. Cass

Benign Prostatic Hyperplasia 627
David A. Rivas
Michael B. Chancellor

Prostatitis 633
Jackson E. Fowler, Jr.

Acute Renal Failure 635
Guillermo R. Saurina
Joseph V. Bonventre

Chronic Renal Failure 642
Michael C. Smith
Michael J. Dunn

Genitourinary Cancer 648
Bruce A. Lowe

Urethral Stricture 658
Steven Schlossberg
Gerald H. Jordan

Renal Calculi 661
David A. Levy
Martin I. Resnick

SECTION 10. THE SEXUALLY TRANSMITTED DISEASES

Chancroid 666
D. W. Cameron

Gonorrhea 666
Charles B. Hicks

Nongonococcal Urethritis 669
Thomas M. Hooton

Granuloma Inguinale (Donovanosis) 670
Nancy J. Anderson

Lymphogranuloma Venereum 671
Nancy J. Anderson

Syphilis 671
Robin D. Isaacs

SECTION 11. DISEASES OF ALLERGY

Anaphylaxis and Serum Sickness 675
Rebecca B. Raby
Michael S. Blaiss

Asthma in Adults and Adolescents 678
Deborah Ortega-Carr
Robert K. Bush

Asthma in Children 682
Paul V. Williams
Gail G. Shapiro

Allergic Rhinitis Caused by Inhalant Factors 691
Jonathan Corren
Gary S. Rachelefsky

Allergic Drug Reactions 695
Gillian M. Shepherd

Stinging Insect Allergy 700
Douglas K. Schreiber
J. Andrew Grant

SECTION 12. DISEASES OF THE SKIN

Acne Vulgaris and Rosacea 703
Larisa C. Kelley
Robert S. Stern

Hair Disorders 706
David A. Whiting

Cancer of the Skin 709
Ira C. Davis
Barry Leshin

Papulosquamous Eruptions 711
Carrie D. Alspaugh
Darrel L. Ellis

Connective Tissue Disorders: Systemic Lupus Erythematosus, Dermatomyositis and Other Myopathies, and Scleroderma 715
Robert G. Lahita

Cutaneous Vasculitis 719
Robert A. Swerlick

Diseases of the Nails 721
Antonella Tosti
Anna Maria Peluso

Keloids 725
John C. Murray

Warts (Verruca Vulgaris) 727
Morrisa Baskin

Nevi 729
Ronald J. Barr

Malignant Melanoma 731
Elisa B. Rush
Allan W. Silberman

Premalignant Lesions 733
Christine M. Hayes
Duane C. Whitaker

Bacterial Diseases of the Skin 736
Richard F. Edlich
Sherry T. Sutton
Dieter H. M. Gröeschel

Viral Diseases of the Skin 740
Robert S. Purvis
Luke Lewis

Parasitic Infections of the Skin 745
Ken Hashimoto
Harry H. Sharata

Superficial Fungal Infections of the Skin 749
Edgar B. Smith

Diseases of the Mouth 750
Carl M. Allen

Stasis Ulcers 758
John R. Bartholomew
Carmen Fonseca

Pressure Ulcer 759
Joseph A. Witkowski
Lawrence C. Parish

Atopic Dermatitis 762
Bernice R. Krafchik

Erythema Multiforme 764
Sylvia L. Brice

Bullous Diseases 766
Grant J. Anhalt

Contact Dermatitis 772
Daniel J. Hogan
Philip D. Shenefelt

The Specific Dermatoses of Pregnancy 773
S. A. Vaughan Jones
M. M. Black

Pruritus Ani and Vulvae 775
Marilynne McKay

Urticaria 776
Jere D. Guin

Pigmentary Disorders 779
Marvin Rapaport

Occupational Dermatoses 781
James S. Taylor

Sunburn and Other Dermatoses Induced by Sunlight 784
Henry W. Lim

SECTION 13. THE NERVOUS SYSTEM

Brain Abscess 788
Glenn E. Mathisen

Alzheimer's Disease 790
Alan Lerner
Peter Hedera
Peter Whitehouse

Parenchymatous Brain Hemorrhage 794
Chin-Sang Chung
Louis R. Caplan

Ischemic Cerebrovascular Disease 798
Diane H. Solomon
David G. Sherman

Rehabilitation of Hemiplegia 801
Susan J. Garrison

Epilepsy in Adolescents and Adults 806
Thomas R. Browne

Epilepsy in Infants and Children 819
Harriet Kang

Gilles De La Tourette Syndrome 823
Gerald Erenberg

Headache 828
Egilius L. H. Spierings

Episodic Vertigo 837
Carol A. Foster
Robert W. Baloh

Meniere's Disease 841
Hamed Sajjadi
Michael M. Paparella

Viral Meningitis and Encephalitis 843
Robert L. Knobler

Reye's Syndrome 845
Richard H. Haas

Multiple Sclerosis 848
Robert M. Herndon

Myasthenia Gravis 856
Donald B. Sanders

Trigeminal Neuralgia 862
Nicholas M. Barbaro

Optic Neuritis 864
Michael Wall

Glaucoma 866
Edward J. Rockwood

Idiopathic Facial Paralysis (Bell's Palsy) 869
Bruce J. Gantz
Peter C. Weber

Parkinson's Disease 871
William J. Weiner
Lisa M. Shulman

Peripheral Neuropathies 879
S. H. Subramony
V. Vedanarayanan

Acute Head Injuries in Adults 889
J. Paul Muizelaar

Acute Head Injuries in Children 892
Burce Mathern
John D. Ward

Brain Tumors 895
Lisa M. DeAngelis

SECTION 14. THE LOCOMOTOR SYSTEM

Rheumatoid Arthritis 901
Marc D. Cohen

Juvenile Rheumatoid Arthritis 907
Charles H. Spencer

Ankylosing Spondylitis 911
Glen T. D. Thomson
Samuel M. Steinfeld
Ron Gall

Temporomandibular Disorders 914
Charles C. Alling III

Fibromyalgia, Tendinitis, and Bursitis 919
Jeffrey M. Thompson

Osteoarthritis 922
Richard B. Tompkins

Polymyalgia Rheumatica and Giant Cell Arteritis 922
Steven A. Lauter

Osteomyelitis 923
Jose H. Salgado
Richard N. Greenberg

Common Sports Injuries 929
M. Patrice Eiff
William L. Toffler

SECTION 15. OBSTETRICS AND GYNECOLOGY

Antepartum Care 933
Carl V. Smith

Ectopic Pregnancy 940
Marilyn R. Richardson

Vaginal Bleeding in Late Pregnancy 941
Jeffrey C. King

Hypertensive Disorders of Pregnancy 944
Marshall D. Lindheimer
Adrian I. Katz

Obstetric Anesthesia 948
Bradley E. Smith

Postpartum Care 955
Alexander Reiter

Resuscitation of the Newborn 957
Scott A. Johnson
Alfred L. Gest

Care of the High-Risk Neonate 962
C. W. Gowen, Jr.

Normal Infant Feeding 977
Lewis A. Barness

Diseases of the Breast 979
Blake Cady

Endometriosis 989
Deborah A. Metzger

Dysfunctional Uterine Bleeding 993
Michael M. Miller

Amenorrhea 994
Tony Zreik
David L. Olive

Dysmenorrhea 998
Kurt T. Barnhart
Steven J. Sondheimer

Premenstrual Syndrome (PMS) 1000
C. James Chuong

Menopause 1003
Daniel R. Mishell, Jr.

Vulvovaginitis 1006
Maurizio Maccato

Toxic Shock Syndrome 1008
Gary R. Schwartz
Seth W. Wright

***Chlamydia Trachomatis* Infection** 1010
Kimberly A. Workowski

Pelvic Inflammatory Disease 1012
W. P. Fleming

Uterine Leiomyoma 1014
Leila R. Hajjar
George H. Nolan

Cancer of the Endometrium 1015
Al Elbendary
Andrew Berchuck

Cancer of the Uterine Cervix 1018
F. J. Montz

Tumors of the Vulva 1021
Raymond H. Kaufman

Thrombophlebitis in Obstetrics and Gynecology 1026
Anthony J. Comerota
Russell N. Harada

Contraception 1031
Amy E. Pollack
Cassandra Moore

SECTION 16. PSYCHIATRIC DISORDERS

Alcohol-Related Problems 1037
Stephen Jurd

Drug Abuse 1040
David J. Roberts

Anxiety Disorders 1046
C. Knight Aldrich

Bulimia Nervosa 1048
Arnold E. Andersen

Delirium 1053
Peter V. Rabins

Mood Disorders 1054
David A. Solomon
Martin B. Keller

Schizophrenic Disorders 1061
Carmen M. McIntyre
George M. Simpson

Panic Disorder and Agoraphobia 1064
Olga Brawman-Mintzer
R. Bruce Lydiard

SECTION 17. PHYSICAL AND CHEMICAL INJURIES

Burns 1067
Karen Frye
David Heimbach

Disturbances Due to Cold 1073
Scott Oslund
Rebecca Smith-Coggins
Paul Auerbach

Disturbances Due to Heat 1077
Peter Hanson

Spider Bites and Scorpion Stings 1078
Philip C. Anderson

Venomous Snakebite 1080
Richard F. Clark

Hazardous Marine Animals 1082
Bruce Flareau
David O. Parrish

Acute Poisonings 1086
Howard C. Mofenson
Thomas R. Caraccio
Joseph Greensher

SECTION 18. APPENDICES AND INDEX

Reference Intervals for the Interpretation of Laboratory Tests 1133
William Z. Borer

Drugs Approved in 1993 1142
Margaret A. Noyes

Index 1145

Section 1

Symptomatic Care Pending Diagnosis

PAIN

method of
ALEXANDER MAUSKOP, M.D.
New York Headache Center
New York, New York

PHARMACOTHERAPY

Pharmacologic management has been the mainstay of treatment for many pain syndromes; however, nonpharmacologic therapies can at times be more effective and should not be used as methods of last resort. Examples include biofeedback for patients with headaches and physical therapy for patients with many forms of chronic low back pain.

The three major groups of drugs used in pain management are nonsteroidal anti-inflammatory drugs (NSAIDs), opiates, and adjuvant medications.

Nonsteroidal Anti-Inflammatory Drugs

Aspirin and ibuprofen (Advil, Motrin) are sold over the counter, and many patients try them before seeking medical care. It is necessary for the physician to establish that the dosage and the frequency of self-administration were sufficient before giving up on this group of medications. Failure of one NSAID to relieve pain does not mean that another one is not effective. Side effects can also be idiosyncratic. For example, naproxen (Naprosyn) and indomethacin (Indocin) can produce gastrointestinal side effects in a particular patient, whereas naproxen sodium (Anaprox) and diclofenac sodium (Voltaren) do not.

NSAIDs can be surprisingly effective in the relief of pain from metastatic bone disease. Opiates and NSAIDs have different mechanisms of action and together can have a synergistic effect. This combination may reduce the dose requirement of an opiate and consequently reduce its side effects. Longer acting NSAIDs, such as piroxicam (Feldene) given at 20 mg once a day, diflunisal (Dolobid), given at 500 mg twice a day, choline magnesium trisalicylate (Trilisate) given at 1500 mg twice a day, nabumetone (Relafen) given at 1000 mg once a day, and sustained-release indomethacin (Indocin SR) given at 75 mg once a day, are preferred in patients who have continuous pain. Short-acting NSAIDs include ibuprofen (Motrin, Advil) given at 400 to 600 mg every 4 hours, aspirin given at 650 to 1000 mg every 3 to 4 hours, and ketoprofen (Orudis) given at 50 mg four times a day. Ketorolac tromethamine (Toradol) is the first NSAID to be available in a parenteral form; the efficacy of a 30-mg intramuscular injection is comparable with that of an injection of 10 mg of morphine. Until the recent introduction of sumatriptan (Imitrex), ketorolac* (60 mg IM) and dihydroergotamine (DHE-45) were drugs of first choice for office management of a patient with an acute migraine attack. Sometimes the author injects ketorolac in the office to relieve acute low back or neck pain.

Opiates

Important characteristics of opiate drugs and their relative potencies are shown in Table 1. Unlike NSAIDs, opiate drugs do not have a ceiling effect. This means that with the development of tolerance, in order to regain pain relief the dose of an opiate can be escalated indefinitely. Usually, the development of side effects limits such escalation, although some patients can tolerate an equivalent of up to several grams of morphine a day, given parenterally. These patients remain functional because gradual escalation of the dose leads to the development of tolerance not only to pain relief but also to side effects. The development of tolerance to an opiate is usually manifested by a shorter duration of action. Because cross-tolerance between different opiates is incomplete, switching to a different opiate may forestall escalation of the dose. Combinations of NSAIDs and adjuvant analgesics with opiates constitute another useful approach. Development of tolerance and physical dependence is often mistakenly equated with addiction. In a tolerant patient receiving a high dose of an opiate drug, symptoms of withdrawal can appear within 6 hours of the last dose. Addiction, in contrast, is characterized by craving for the drug, efforts to secure a supply of the drug, and not following a physician's directions regarding usage.

Both physicians and patients have an instinctive fear of opiates because of the potential for addiction. Sometimes the use of an opiate in a cancer patient is equated with imminent death. A large amount of data indicates that the risk of iatrogenic opiate addic-

*Not FDA approved for this indication.

TABLE 1. **Dosing Data for Opioid Analgesics**

Drug	Approximate Equianalgesic Oral Dose	Approximate Equianalgesic Parenteral Dose
Opioid Agonist		
Morphine	30 mg q 3–4 h (around-the-clock dosing) 60 mg q 3–4 (single dose or intermittent dosing)	10 mg q 3–4 h
Codeine	130 mg q 3–4 h	75 mg q 3–4 h
Hydromorphone (Dilaudid)	7.5 mg q 3–4 h	1.5 mg q 3–4 h
Hydrocodone (in Lorcet, Lortab, Vicodin, others)	30 mg q 3–4	Not available
Levorphanol (Levo-Dromoran)	4 mg q 6–8 h	2 mg q 6–8 h
Meperidine (Demerol)	300 mg q 2–3 h	100 mg q 3 h
Methadone (Dolophine, others)	20 mg q 6–8 h	10 mg q 6–8 h
Oxycodone (Roxicodone, also in Percocet, Percodan, Tylox, others)	30 mg q 3–4 h	Not available
Oxymorphone (Numorphan)	Not available	1 mg q 3–4 h
Opioid Agonist-Antagonist and Partial Agonist		
Buprenorphine (Buprenex)	Not available	0.3–0.4 mg q 6–8 h
Butorphanol (Stadol)	Not available	2 mg q 3–4 h
Nalbuphine (Nubain)	Not available	10 mg q 3–4 h
Pentazocine (Talwin, others)	150 mg q 3–4 h	60 mg q 3–4 h

Adapted from Agency for Health Care Policy and Research: Acute Pain Management in Adults: Operative Procedures (Pub. No. 92-0032). Washington, DC, Public Health Service, U.S. Department of Health and Human Services, 1992.

tion is extremely small and can be predicted in the majority of cases by the patient's history of prior addictions. The author always brings up this topic because many patients do not verbalize their fears and, if not reassured, are reluctant to take sufficient amounts, if any, of the drug. Another obstacle to the proper use of opiates is an exaggerated concern about respiratory and central nervous system (CNS) depression. Tolerance to these side effects of opiates develops quickly. Patients do not become oversedated or stop breathing while in pain. When a patient receiving a steady dose of an opiate suddenly becomes drowsy or demonstrates respiratory depression, the most likely cause is a new systemic problem, such as an infection or liver or kidney failure. When pain can be controlled only with some degree of sedation, a stimulant, such as dextroamphetamine (Dexedrine), given at 5 mg twice a day, may not only improve the patient's alertness but may provide analgesia as well. Dextroamphetamine has mild analgesic properties synergistic with opioid analgesics.

The major side effect of opiates that must be anticipated is constipation. Senna concentrate (Senokot) is an anecdotal favorite used to combat this problem. Transdermal fentanyl (Duragesic) tends to produce less constipation than do oral opiates.

Meperidine (Demerol) is a popular drug, but it is the only opiate that should not be used continuously for more than a few days. Meperidine is metabolized into normeperidine, which is a CNS stimulant. With chronic administration, meperidine can cause irritability, tremor, and generalized seizures.

Until recently, the preferred route of administration of medications has been oral. With the introduction of transdermal fentanyl (Duragesic), the author has found that many patients do better with a fentanyl patch. This product provides a steady level of an opiate drug with practical and psychological benefits. The patches last for about 3 days and come in four strengths. Because of the long half-life of the drug, the process of determining the optimal dose of the patch may take up to a few weeks. While this adjustment is being made, patients should be given a short-acting opiate such as oxycodone (Percocet, Percodan), morphine sulfate (Roxanol), or hydromorphone (Dilaudid) for breakthrough pain. This also applies to the titration phase of other long-acting oral opiates, including sustained-release morphine (MS Contin, Oramorph SR), methadone (Dolophine), and levorphanol (Levo-Dromoran). Methadone is an excellent analgesic with good absorption and, in the author's experience, fewer side effects than other opiates. It is also one of the most inexpensive opiates, although it can be difficult to obtain from some pharmacies.

Rectal suppositories of morphine, hydromorphone, and oxymorphone (Numorphan) are useful for patients who cannot take oral preparations. The rectal route is not practical for long-term management and when high doses are needed.

Intranasal administration of butorphanol (Stadol NS) produces a rapid onset of action. The limitation of this drug in current formulation is that the dose contained in each spray is excessive for many patients. This results in a high incidence of CNS side effects. Reformulation at a low dose may improve the utility of this drug. Butorphanol is not a controlled substance because it is a partial agonist-antagonist drug with a lower potential for addiction. It should not be given to patients who are maintained on opiates that are pure agonists (see Table 1) because the antagonist properties can lead to a withdrawal reaction. Patients on chronic opiate maintenance become very sensitive to all opiate antagonists. Should a need arise to reverse the effect of an opiate in such a patient, naloxone (Narcan) must be diluted with saline and infused very gradually.

When a patient with continuous pain cannot take

oral medications, subcutaneous (SC) infusion of opiates is an alternative to the transdermal route and has many advantages over intravenous infusion. The fentanyl patch should be tried first, but when it is ineffective at a high dose (e.g., two Duragesic-100 patches) or causes side effects, SC infusion is the method of choice. SC infusion is administered with the use of a programmable, portable pump that can be filled with a solution of any opiate, including morphine, hydromorphone, methadone, and levorphanol. The pump is connected to a 25-gauge butterfly needle that can be inserted subcutaneously by the patient or a family member. An intravenous infusion of an opiate may be necessary only if a patient requires a very large volume of an opiate or if other routes are not tolerated.

The use of opiate analgesics has been limited mostly to cancer patients. Their prolonged use in non-cancer patients with pain remains controversial. Many anecdotal reports and the author's personal experience suggest that under strict supervision, selected non-cancer patients with pain can derive great benefits from chronic opiate therapy. Such patients are usually those who do not develop significant tolerance and can remain on a steady dose for long periods of time with few side effects. The author obtains an informed consent from such patients, sees them at least once a month, and tries to make opiates only a part of the pain management program.

Adjuvant Analgesics

This is a diverse group of medications that were not known to have analgesic properties when they were first introduced. The most useful drugs for chronic pain and headache management are tricyclic antidepressants (TCAs). Among the TCAs, amitriptyline (Elavil) has been studied most extensively but nortriptyline (Pamelor), imipramine (Tofranil), and desipramine (Norpramin) are also effective and may produce fewer anticholinergic side effects. If one TCA is ineffective or produces unacceptable side effects, another TCA should be tried.

The starting doses for any TCA are 25 mg in young or middle-aged patients and 10 mg in elderly persons. The average effective dose is 50 to 75 mg taken once a day in the evening. Some patients may require and tolerate antidepressant doses of up to 300 mg or more a day in order to achieve pain or headache relief. Patients must be told that these medications are antidepressants but that they are also used for chronic painful conditions, even if there is no associated depression. If patients discover from other sources that TCAs are antidepressant drugs, they may become angry and noncompliant; they may think that their reports of pain were interpreted as depressive symptoms and not real pain. Warning patients about possible side effects such as dryness of the mouth, drowsiness, and constipation also improves compliance. Some of the contraindications for the use of TCAs include concomitant use of monoamine oxidase inhibitors, recent myocardial infarction, cardiac arrhythmias, glaucoma, and urinary retention. An electrocardiogram should be obtained before the initiation of treatment in all elderly patients.

Other antidepressants including fluoxetine (Prozac), bupropion (Wellbutrin), sertraline (Zoloft), paroxetine (Paxil), and phenelzine (Nardil) may have some utility in pain management. No large trials of these drugs have been conducted in pain patients to show any benefits beyond their antidepressant effect.

Anticonvulsants that are commonly used for pain relief are carbamazepine (Tegretol) and phenytoin (Dilantin). It has been suggested that anticonvulsants are more effective for sharp, lancinating pain, whereas TCAs are better for burning, dysesthetic pain. Divalproex sodium (Depakote)* has been reported to be effective in the prevention of migraines.

Hydroxyzine (Vistaril, Atarax) has mild analgesic properties, but what makes it a useful adjuvant analgesic is its reduction of anxiety and nausea.

Caffeine has been shown to enhance the effect of other analgesics and to have mild analgesic properties of its own. It is useful in a variety of pain syndromes, but it is most commonly used for headaches. Overuse of caffeine in drinks (coffee, tea, colas) and medications (Excedrin, Anacin, Fiorinal, Esgic, Norgesic) can lead to severe withdrawal headaches and other symptoms, such as anxiety, depression, and insomnia. As little as three cups of coffee a day can lead to a withdrawal syndrome.

Corticosteroids can be effective in relieving pain from various causes. Long-term side effects and loss of efficacy limits their use in treatment of acute pain syndromes, such as those involving the spinal cord, a plexus, or nerve compression.

PSYCHOLOGICAL METHODS

These methods are indispensable in the management of patients with chronic pain. Chronic pain affects all aspects of patients' lives and the lives of people who live and work with them. For this reason, the psychologist is a crucial member of the pain management team. Chronic pain of long duration is very unlikely to respond to a single treatment modality. Patients should not be allowed to pick and choose their treatment. The author explains to such patients that pain control can be achieved only by attacking the problem with several methods at the same time. Psychological methods may include behavior modification, cognitive psychotherapy, biofeedback, and relaxation training. On occasion, in an anxious patient with acute or cancer pain, simple reassurance may reduce the need for opiate analgesics. In some patients, music therapy can have beneficial effects. Benzodiazepines usually have little utility in pain management, except for acute pain of muscle spasm. However, in an anxious patient with cancer pain, a short course of diazepam (Valium) or clonazepam (Klonopin) may help.

---

*Not FDA approved for this indication.

ANESTHETIC APPROACHES

Muscle spasm is a common primary cause of pain, and it often accompanies pain of other types. Trigger point injections are very effective in the management of acute pain caused by muscle spasm. They usually involve the use of a long-acting local anesthetic, bupivacaine (Marcaine).

Nerve blocks can provide temporary relief of pain in patients with local pain. Some physicians use them to predict possible efficacy of a nerve ablation. The author much more commonly injects a corticosteroid such as betamethasone (Celestone Soluspan) or methylprednisolone (Depo-Medrol) into an area surrounding the nerve. Although such an injection cannot be considered a nerve block, a similar technique is used. Examples of conditions that benefit from corticosteroid injections include carpal tunnel syndrome, meralgia paresthetica, and occipital neuralgia.

Sympathetic block is the most effective procedure for the treatment of reflex sympathetic dystrophy, especially when blocks are combined with vigorous physical therapy and, if necessary, pharmacotherapy and psychological methods. This combined treatment works best if it is started early in the course of the disease.

Epidural and spinal infusions of opiates and local anesthetics are useful in some cancer patients and in a few selected patients with a so-called failed back syndrome.

NEUROSURGICAL METHODS

In attempting to stop transmission of pain signals along the nervous system, neurosurgeons have tried placing lesions anywhere from the peripheral nerves all the way up to the frontal cortex. Nerve section can be effective in patients with meralgia paresthetica, occipital neuralgia, and some other focal neuropathic pains. It is not effective, however, in patients with postherpetic neuralgia. Some patients with trigeminal neuralgia find temporary relief when the nerve leading to the trigger area is sectioned. A lesion in the dorsal root entry zone can sometimes relieve pain caused by brachial plexus avulsion and anesthesia dolorosa. Section of half of the spinal cord (cordotomy) is effective in patients with cancer who have unilateral pain below the waist. Bilateral cordotomy usually leads to loss of sphincter control and should be reserved for cancer patients who have already lost such control. Hypophysectomy should be considered in women whose pain is resistant to other modalities and who have hormonal (breast or ovarian) cancers.

PHYSICAL METHODS

Physical therapy is the main treatment modality for most patients with low back and neck pain. It is also essential in the management of reflex sympathetic dystrophy. Patients with almost any pain syndrome benefit from regular exercise. Improved cardiovascular and pulmonary function from aerobic exercise is of significant benefit in itself, but it also provides important psychological benefits. Patients believe that they are regaining some control over their bodies and feel less helpless and hopeless. Regular exercise helps to alleviate stress, which is a major contributing factor in chronic headaches, back pain, and other pain syndromes.

Other physical methods include transcutaneous electrical nerve stimulation and acupuncture. Neither method has been scientifically proved to be effective; however, a large body of anecdotal evidence indicates that they can be very helpful in some patients. Results of experiments detailing opiate and nonopiate mechanisms of acupuncture analgesia in animals, as well as the successful use of acupuncture in veterinary medicine, suggest that the effect of acupuncture is superior to placebo. The author usually uses acupuncture in elderly patients, patients who do not tolerate any medications, and patients who have tried a variety of treatments without relief. In patients with chronic pain, acupuncture should be used as a part of a multidisciplinary approach.

NAUSEA AND VOMITING

method of
KATHERINE M. W. PISTERS, M.D., and
MARK G. KRIS, M.D.
Memorial Sloan-Kettering Cancer Center
New York, New York

Even though nausea and vomiting are among the most basic neural reflexes, they remain poorly understood. The functional area known as the “emetic center” in the brain stem controls the complex act of vomiting. This central emetic circuitry is related to respiratory centers and located near the floor of the fourth ventricle. It receives and processes input from the gastrointestinal tract and other areas of the brain. The chemoreceptor trigger zone (a bloodstream chemosensor located in the medulla), the vestibular complex, the labyrinth, and the diencephalon also provide input. Impulses from the emetic center are transmitted to the striated and smooth muscles of the thorax, abdomen, and gastrointestinal tract to initiate the vomiting reflex. The areas of the brain controlling nausea and vomiting, as well as the gastrointestinal tract, contain many different neurotransmitters including serotonin, dopamine, histamine, acetylcholine, and endorphins. The pharmacologic control of nausea and vomiting centers on the blockade of one or more neurotransmitter receptors in either the central nervous system or gastrointestinal tract.

APPROACH TO THE PATIENT WITH NAUSEA AND VOMITING

Nausea and vomiting are associated with many disorders as outlined in Table 1. In addition to occurring as a manifestation of an underlying illness, nausea and vomiting can develop iatrogenically as a result of drug administration, radiation, or surgery. Evaluation of the patient experiencing nausea and vomiting should include a thorough history including information on the presence of pain, change in bowel habits, fever, relationship to meals, prior history of

TABLE 1. **Causes of Nausea and Vomiting**

Gastrointestinal Causes
- Infectious gastroenteritis
- Peptic ulcer disease
- Intestinal tract obstruction or perforation
- Biliary tract disease
- Constipation/impaction
- Pancreatitis
- Peritonitis
- Hepatitis
- Adhesions
- Motility disorders
- Appendicitis
- Malignancy

Central Nervous System Disorders
- Malignancy
- Abscess
- Meningitis
- Migraine
- Motion sickness
- Labyrinthitis
- Meniere's disease

Iatrogenic Causes
- Chemotherapy
- Radiation
- Surgery
- Medication, e.g., theophylline, analgesics, digoxin

Endocrinologic Disorders
- Diabetic acidosis
- Adrenal insufficiency
- Pregnancy
- Uremia
- Hypercalcemia

Psychogenic

surgery, gallstones, kidney stones, liver disease, weight loss, medications, or other illnesses. A physical examination should be conducted. Screening laboratory tests should be performed to assess acid-base and electrolyte status, glucose, calcium, amylase, and beta human chorionic gonadotropin hCG-beta (if pregnancy is suspected). Evaluation of renal and liver functions are often helpful as well. Simple radiologic testing including a plain chest x-ray study and flat and upright films of the abdomen may also help in the initial assessment. If the precise etiology of the nausea and vomiting can be discovered, the best approach is to treat the underlying cause. During the initial evaluation of the patient with nausea and vomiting, supportive measures, including hydration, correction of any electrolyte abnormalities, and treatment of symptoms with medications, should be taken.

Nausea and Vomiting in the Cancer Patient

Patients with malignancies require special consideration. Bowel obstruction, either mechanical or nonmechanical, may occur secondary to prior surgery, intra-abdominal disease, metabolic effects, or abnormal bowel motility secondary to narcotic analgesics. Constipation and even fecal impaction may occur following the use of moderate to strong analgesics if prophylactic laxatives have not been used. In addition, central nervous system metastases may initially be exhibited as nausea or unexplained emesis.

In general, chemotherapy-related nausea and vomiting occur within 1 week of the administration of chemotherapy. Other causes of nausea and vomiting should be considered more likely in a patient who presents with these symptoms and who has not recently received chemotherapy.

TREATMENT

The optimal management of nausea and vomiting is to identify and treat the underlying cause. Once the patient has undergone an initial assessment, a differential diagnosis should be generated. In addition, patients should receive symptomatic care and intravenous fluids, if necessary. Patients presenting with abdominal pain may require evaluation by a surgeon.

Both pharmacologic and nonpharmacologic interventions may alleviate nausea and vomiting. Controlled clinical studies have identified many safe and effective antiemetic agents. The selection of specific antiemetic drugs or combinations should be based on the clinical setting. Nonpharmacologic interventions should be aimed specifically at the cause of the nausea and vomiting. Examples of nonpharmacologic therapy include dietary restrictions, surgery for bowel obstruction, radiation for symptomatic brain metastases, and behavioral therapy for conditioned nausea and vomiting. In addition to the use of specific antiemetic agents, other medications such as the H_2 antagonists, insulin, antibiotics or laxatives as indicated for treatment of specific diseases may alleviate the symptoms of nausea and vomiting.

Antiemetic Drugs (Table 2)

Serotonin Antagonists

Ondansetron (Zofran) and granisetron (Kytril) are members of the newly developed specific 5-HT_3 receptor antagonists. They are highly effective in controlling chemotherapy-induced nausea and vomiting, and they have few side effects. Headache, transient elevations of serum aspartate aminotransferase (AST) and alanine aminotransferase (ALT), and lightheadedness or dizziness may occur. Although effective for acute chemotherapy-induced nausea and vomiting (within 24 hours of chemotherapy administration), this class of agent has not been found to be as helpful for delayed nausea and vomiting (see later).

Substituted Benzamides

Metoclopramide (Reglan), a substituted benzamide, has been found to block both dopamine receptors and 5-HT_3 receptors when given in high doses. It is an effective and widely studied antiemetic. Studies have identified doses of 1 to 3 mg/kg, intravenously, every 2 hours for two doses beginning 30 minutes prior to chemotherapy as the optimal dose for use with highly emetogenic chemotherapy. In controlled trials, its efficacy is similar to that of ondansetron. Common side effects include mild sedation, akathisia, diarrhea, and acute dystonic reactions. Extrapyramidal symptoms may occur following treatment with any dopamine antagonist and occur more frequently in patients under the age of 30. In addition, these symptoms occur more frequently in patients receiving antiemetics on successive days. Extrapyramidal symptoms can be quickly controlled by 50

TABLE 2. **Antiemetic Agents: Doses and Administration Schedules**

Specific Serotonin Antagonists	
Ondansetron (Zofran)	0.15 mg/kg every 2–4 hours 3 doses, intravenously; 32 mg, once, intravenously; 8 mg, 3 times daily, orally, beginning 30 minutes before chemotherapy
Granisetron (Kytril)	10 μg/kg (or 1 mg) intravenously, once
Substituted Benzamides	
Metoclopramide (Reglan)‡	1–3 mg/kg every 2 hours, 2–5 doses, intravenously, beginning 30 minutes before chemotherapy*
Butyrophenones	
Haloperidol (Haldol)†	1–3 mg, every 2–6 hours, intravenously for cancer chemotherapy*
Droperidol (Inapsine)†, ‖	1–2 mg, orally or intramuscularly, 3 times daily; 0.5–2.5 mg intravenously, every 4 hours
Corticosteroids	
Dexamethasone (Decadron)†	4–20 mg orally or intravenously, once or every 4–6 hours*
Methylprednisolone (Solu-Medrol)†	250–500 mg intravenously, once or every 4–6 hours*
Cannabinoids	
Dronabinol (Marinol)	5–10 mg/m^2, orally, every 3–4 hours
Phenothiazines	
Prochlorperazine (Compazine)‡	5–10 mg, orally, 3–4 times daily; 5–10 mg, intramuscularly, every 3–4 hours; 25 mg per rectum, every 5 hours; 10–40 mg, intravenously, every 3 hours, 3 doses, beginning 30 minutes before chemotherapy*
Chlorpromazine (Thorazine)	10–25 mg, orally, every 4–6 hours; 25 mg, intravenously, every 3–4 hours; 100 mg, per rectum, every 6–8 hours
Thiethylperazine (Torecan)†	10 mg, orally, rectally, or intramuscularly, 1–3 times daily
Perphenazine (Trilafon)	8–16 mg, orally, in divided doses; 5 mg intravenously
Promethazine (Phenergan)‡	25 mg, orally, rectally, or intramuscularly, every 4–6 hours
Antihistamines	
Dimenhydrinate (Dramamine)	50 mg, orally or intravenously, every 4–6 hours
Meclizine (Antivert)	20–50 mg, orally, every 24 hours
Hydroxyzine (Vistaril)	25–100 mg, orally or intravenously, 3–4 times daily
Anticholinergics	
Scopolamine (Transderm-Scōp)	1 patch behind ear 4 hours before travel, change every 3 days
Adjunctive Agents	
Lorazepam (Ativan)†	1–1.5 mg/m^2, intravenously, 30 minutes before chemotherapy
Diphenhydramine (Benadryl)	25–50 mg, orally or intravenously, every 3–4 hours

*Investigational use, dose, or schedule.
†Not FDA approved for this indication.
‡Exceeds dosage recommended by the manufacturer.
§Oral form.

mg of diphenhydramine (Benadryl) given orally or intravenously.

Butyrophenones

Haloperidol (Haldol) and droperidol (Inapsine) block dopamine receptors and can control cisplatin-induced emesis when used intravenously. Side effects include sedation, extrapyramidal reactions, and hypotension.

Corticosteroids

Dexamethasone* and methylprednisolone* are effective, inexpensive, and safe. However, their mechanism of action is unknown. They prevent vomiting caused by all types of chemotherapeutic agents. Common side effects include insomnia, epigastric burning, and perineal sensations when given by rapid intravenous infusion.

Cannabinoids

Dronabinol (Marinol) is recommended for patients who have failed to respond adequately to conventional antiemetic treatments. In controlled trials, it has been found to be superior or equivalent to placebo and prochlorperazine in patients receiving chemotherapy of mild to moderate emetic potential. Side effects that limit its use include drowsiness, ataxia, dizziness, hypotension, and dysphoria, particularly in older adults.

Phenothiazines

Randomized trials have found prochlorperazine (Compazine) to be inferior to metoclopramide or dexamethasone. In general, prochlorperazine and other phenothiazines such as thiethylperazine (Torecan), chlorpromazine (Thorazine), perphenazine (Trilafon) or promethazine (Phenergan) should be restricted to those patients receiving mildly emetogenic chemotherapy or to those patients who have vomited despite prophylactic antiemetics with prior courses. Dose escalation in this class of drugs is associated with increased toxicity and side effects, particularly hypotension. Extrapyramidal effects, sedation, and anticholinergic effects may occur.

Anticholinergics/Antihistamines

These agents are used primarily for motion sickness. Scopolamine (Transderm-Scōp) is used in the form of a patch placed behind the ear. The patch should be changed every 3 days. This class of agent has not been extensively studied for the control of chemotherapy-induced nausea and vomiting. Dimenhydrinate (Dramamine), meclizine (Antivert), diphenhydramine (Benadryl), and hydroxyzine (Vis-

*Not FDA approved for this indication.

TABLE 3. **Recommendations for Prevention of Acute Chemotherapy–Related Vomiting**

Chemotherapy—Emetic Potential	Management
Rare Bleomycin, chlorambucil, etoposide, hydroxyurea, methotrexate, plicamycin, tamoxifen, vinblastine, vincristine	Patient education No prophylactic antiemetics required
Mild Fluorouracil, ifosfamide, mitomycin, paclitaxel	Patient education Dexamethasone (Decadron*) 20 mg, intravenously, 30 minutes prior to chemotherapy
Moderate to Severe Carboplatin, carmustine, cisplatin, cyclophosphamide, cytarabine, dacarbazine, dactinomycin, daunorubicin, doxorubicin, idarubicin, lomustine, mechlorethamine, procarbazine, combination chemotherapy	Patient education *Beginning 30 minutes prior to chemotherapy* Dexamethasone (Decadron) 20 mg, intravenously plus Ondansetron (Zofran), 0.15 mg/kg, every 2–4 hours, 3 doses, intravenously or 32 mg, once, intravenously or Metoclopramide (Reglan), 1–3 mg/kg, every 2 hours, 2–5 doses, intravenously with or without Lorazepam* (Ativan), 1–1.5 mg/m^2, intravenously, once or Diphenhydramine (Benadryl), 50 mg, intravenously, once

*Not FDA approved for this indication.
†Exceeds dosage recommended by the manufacturer.

taril) are examples of antihistamines that may be useful for motion sickness.

Benzodiazepines

Lorazepam (Ativan) has limited antiemetic effectiveness but is a useful adjunct to combination antiemetic therapies as described later. This agent controls extrapyramidal effects of dopamine antagonists and reduces anxiety.

Antiemetic Combinations

Controlled trials have demonstrated that the combination of dexamethasone and high-dose metoclopramide or ondansetron provide antiemetic control that is superior to these agents used alone for the control of cisplatin-induced emesis. Combination antiemetic therapy also reduces both disease- and treatment-related side effects. Prophylactic combination antiemetics should be prescribed for all patients receiving combination chemotherapy.

TABLE 4. **Medications for Prevention of Delayed Emesis After Chemotherapy**

Medication	Dosage
Dexamethasone (Decadron)*	8 mg, orally, two times daily for 2 days, then 4 mg, orally, two times daily for 2 days
plus	
Metoclopramide (Reglan)*,†	0.5 mg/kg, orally, four times daily, for 4 days
or	
Prochlorperazine spansules (Compazine)*,†	30 mg, orally, three times daily, for 2 days, then 15 mg, orally, three times daily for 2 days

*Not FDA approved for this indication.
†Exceeds dosage recommended by the manufacturer.

MANAGEMENT OF CHEMOTHERAPY-RELATED EMESIS

Acute Chemotherapy-Induced Emesis. The emetic potential of the prescribed chemotherapeutic agents should be assessed prior to administration. Patients should be educated as to the expected course following the chemotherapy. For patients receiving medication that rarely causes emesis (e.g., vinblastine, or tamoxifen), prophylactic antiemetics are not required. For patients receiving chemotherapy of mild emetic potential, education and dexamethasone given intravenously before chemotherapy should be employed. Any patient receiving chemotherapy of moderate to severe emetic potential or combination chemotherapy, should receive prophylactic combination antiemetics. Specific chemotherapeutic agents, their emetogenic potential, and recommended antiemetic management are presented in Table 3.

Delayed Emesis. This is vomiting that begins or persists 24 or more hours following chemotherapy. Delayed emesis occurs to some degree in the vast majority of patients treated with high-dose cisplatin. In general, delayed emesis is less severe than the vomiting seen in the initial 24 hours following chemotherapy. Oral antiemetic combinations such as dexamethasone plus metoclopramide or prochlorperazine spanules given routinely beginning the day after cisplatin are safe and effective for the control of this problem. Recommended regimens for delayed emesis are outlined in Table 4.

Anticipatory Emesis. Although this conditioned response is becoming less frequent with the use of prophylactic antiemetics, anticipatory emesis may develop in those patients who have poor control of emesis with chemotherapy. Anticipatory emesis can be triggered by the sights, sounds, or smells of the hospital or the appearance of the chemotherapy nurse or oncologist. At present, prevention is the best strategy. Behavioral modification or treatment with benzodiazepines may reduce symptoms in patients with this problem.

NAUSEA AND VOMITING ACCOMPANYING PREGNANCY

Nausea and vomiting are frequently reported during the first trimester of pregnancy. Surveys have found that at least 85% of pregnant women experience nausea and over 50% experience emesis. In general, these symptoms abate after the first trimester. It is generally assumed that pregnancy hormones cause this syndrome; however, there is no conclusive evidence to support this assumption.

Some patients may experience severe or protracted symptoms collectively known as hyperemesis gravidarum. In these instances, hospitalization and intravenous fluids may be required. There are no approved drugs for the control of nausea and vomiting in pregnancy. In general, reassurance, rest, frequent small meals, and dietary restrictions may be helpful.

POSTOPERATIVE NAUSEA AND VOMITING

Approximately 80% of patients undergoing surgery experience nausea and vomiting in the preoperative or postoperative period. Predisposing factors include the type of anesthetic agents used, the duration of anesthesia and the patient's age, sex, and type of operation. Women undergoing laparoscopic gynecologic procedures appear particularly prone to this complication. Randomized trials have found single 4-mg intravenous doses of ondansetron (Zofran) to be superior to placebo for the control of postoperative vomiting. Supportive measures including intravenous hydration and nasogastric suction may be helpful.

MOTION SICKNESS

The etiology of motion sickness is not completely understood. Anticholinergics and antihistamines are most commonly used to treat this disorder. These agents include scopolamine, especially in the transdermal dosage form; dimenhydrinate; cyclizine and meclizine. Medication should be started 1 to 4 hours prior to travel. Anxiolytic agents may also be helpful. Symptoms of motion sickness always abate with the cessation of motion.

GASEOUSNESS AND INDIGESTION

method of
MILES AUSLANDER, M.D.
Valley Presbyterian Hospital
Van Nuys, California

Gaseousness and indigestion are among the most common of gastrointestinal symptoms. Although they often coexist, they may have very different etiologies and significances.

GASEOUSNESS

The nonspecific complaints of eructation, flatus, bloating, and distention may be evidence of serious bowel obstruction or simple dietary indiscretion. Increased abdominal gas may be caused by excessive air swallowing, such as occurs in patients with chronic obstructive pulmonary disease or in anxious patients with aerophagia. In other patients, the excessive gas is hydrogen, methane, and carbon dioxide produced by the fermentation of nondigestible carbohydrates. High-fiber foods, especially vegetables such as broccoli and cauliflower, tend to produce gas. Many people maldigest the lactose of milk, ice cream, and soft cheeses. Blacks and Asians are particularly prone to lactase deficiency and experience gaseousness (as well as diarrhea) with excessive intake of dairy products. Other carbohydrates such as fructose and sorbitol that are found in certain fruits, apple juice, and dietetic sweeteners produce similar symptoms. Excessive gas from these mechanisms is also increased in patients with prolonged intestinal transit times. The spastic colon with chronic constipation causes gas retention and increased fermentation time within the colon.

Many patients with the irritable bowel syndrome feel gassy and bloated but do not actually have more gas than do normal people. Part of the functional disease of the gut is a heightened sensitivity to distention with resultant discomfort. Obstruction of the intestinal tract also causes gaseous distention. Gastric outlet obstruction distends the stomach, and adhesions may block the small bowel. Tumor, ischemia, inflammation, and ileus can all result in intestinal distention.

The evaluation of patients with gas should include a careful history and physical examination with special attention to diet and bowel movement patterns. The need for diagnostic tests is increased if the patient reports rectal bleeding, weight loss, localized pain, nausea, or vomiting. Physical findings of a mass, localized tenderness, and occult gastrointestinal blood loss also mandate evaluation.

For patients with acute symptoms or in whom the degree of gaseousness is in question, abdominal flat and upright radiographs can diagnose gastric outlet or bowel obstruction. The finding of a normal gas pattern but considerable retained fecal matter suggests constipation with a functional bowel. If dietary carbohydrate maldigestion is suspected on the basis of the history, breath tests for hydrogen and intestinal gas analysis can be performed. A simple elimination diet, however, is effective for diagnosis as well as for therapy. When more significant disease is suspected, the intestinal tract should be evaluated by means of barium contrast radiographs or endoscopic examination.

The therapy of gaseousness depends on the etiology. Aerophagia can be reduced by teaching the patient to recognize and avoid air swallowing and to limit the use of chewing gum and drinking straws. Because irritable bowel is a common cause of gaseousness, the restriction of gas-forming foods, antispasmodic medications such as dicyclomine (Bentyl) 20 mg before meals and bedtime), and stool softening and laxative combinations such as docusate sodium with casanthranol (Peri-Colace) (one at bedtime) are effective. Bulk-acting laxatives such as psyllium (Metamucil) and methylcellulose (Citrucel) may actually produce gas or a feeling of fullness, in which case they should be avoided. Dietary gaseousness resulting from lactose maldigestion can be improved by using lactase-pretreated milk (LactAid milk) or supplemental lactase enzyme (LactAid Tablets). The maldigested carbohydrates of beans and certain vegetables can be reduced by pretreatment with alpha-d-galactosidase (Beano liquid). Various antigas agents such as simethicone (Mylicon) and charcoal have limited use only for stomach gas resulting from swallowed air.

INDIGESTION

The sense of upper abdominal discomfort ranging from burning to mild nausea to a full, dull aching sensation may be termed "indigestion." In patients with the acute onset of symptoms, often with related fever and diarrhea, an infectious or toxic etiology may be suspected, and the illness is often self-limited. If the symptoms are recent but persistent, with burning pain in the epigastrium or lower chest and related to food, peptic disease is likely. The current recommendations for suspected, uncomplicated peptic disease is to treat the patient with one of the following H_2 blocking agents: cimetidine (Tagamet), 800 mg at bedtime; ranitidine (Zantac) or nizatidine (Axid), 150 mg twice per day; or famotidine (Pepcid), 20 mg twice per day. If the patient responds to the therapy within 10 days, the diagnosis is considered confirmed, and therapy is continued for 6 to 8 weeks. If symptoms persist, diagnostic evaluation, preferably by upper gastrointestinal endoscopy, is suggested. For resistant peptic disease, especially symptomatic esophageal reflux, omeprazole (Prilosec), 20 mg each morning for 6 to 8 weeks, is more effective.

Indigestion can be caused by gallbladder or biliary disease, suspected on the basis of the pattern of illness (occurring during the night, sometimes after a heavy or fatty meal, and associated with nausea and sometimes fever). Diagnostic ultrasonography can confirm gallstones, whereas nuclear biliary imaging can demonstrate the cystic duct obstruction of acute cholecystitis. Although gallbladder disease may be treated expectantly or by stone-dissolving medication, most confirmed cases are best managed by laparoscopic cholecystectomy. Early pancreatitis, bowel obstruction, hepatitis, or any abdominal catastrophe may be exhibited as indigestion, but the clinical picture soon points toward the correct diagnosis and therapy.

An increasingly recognized cause of indigestion is nonulcer dyspepsia. This functional disease of the upper intestinal tract causes upper abdominal discomfort, nausea, a feeling of fullness, early satiety, and general malaise, but it does not cause systemic features such as fever, weight loss, or gastrointestinal bleeding. Many patients also complain of fatigue, insomnia, and general anxiety. The diagnosis of nonulcer dyspepsia is made by exclusion. Upper gastrointestinal endoscopy is negative. *Helicobactor pylori* gastritis is sometimes detected; however, therapy does not improve symptoms. Solid-phase nuclear medicine gastric emptying is sometimes prolonged, and as in diabetics with gastric paresis, cisapride (Propulsid), 10 mg before meals and bedtime, may help. For many patients with indigestion, emotional support, low-fat diets, and nonspecific measures, including acid reduction, antispasmodics, and tranquilizers, may control symptoms while newer diagnostic and therapeutic options are awaited.

ACUTE INFECTIOUS DIARRHEA

method of
NATHAN M. THIELMAN, M.D., M.P.H., and
RICHARD L. GUERRANT, M.D.
University of Virginia School of Medicine
Charlottesville, Virignia

Diarrheal diseases, the majority of which are infectious, rank second only to cardiovascular disease as a cause of death worldwide. In developing countries, where poor sanitary conditions facilitate transmission, diarrheal illnesses lead to 5 to 10 million deaths per year, while in the United States an estimated annual 25 to 100 million cases lead to 8 million outpatient visits, 250,000 hospitalizations, and 10,000 deaths—cumulatively resulting in a projected cost of $23 billion dollars per year based on estimated medical costs and lost productivity.

EVALUATION

Because of the varied bowel habits of individual patients, it is useful to attempt to objectively define diarrhea. Although the medical literature puts forth a number of highly quantitative definitions of diarrhea based on stool weight and other factors, a practical clinical definition should include estimates of stool consistency and frequency. In general, if stool is liquid or semisolid and intestinal evacuations occur three or more times within a 24-hour period, the patient is said to have diarrhea. When an infectious etiology is suspected, a screening history and physical examination should help distinguish between four diarrheal syndromes, each of which requires a different management strategy (Fig. 1). Additional directed questioning and examination and the judicious use of laboratory tests help distinguish among the various potential pathogens and provide guidance for empiric or specific treatment. Table 1 lists other noninfectious considerations in the differential diagnosis of acute diarrhea.

Inflammatory Diarrhea

Although the majority of sporadic diarrheal illnesses are self-limited and short-lived, in patients with fever, severe

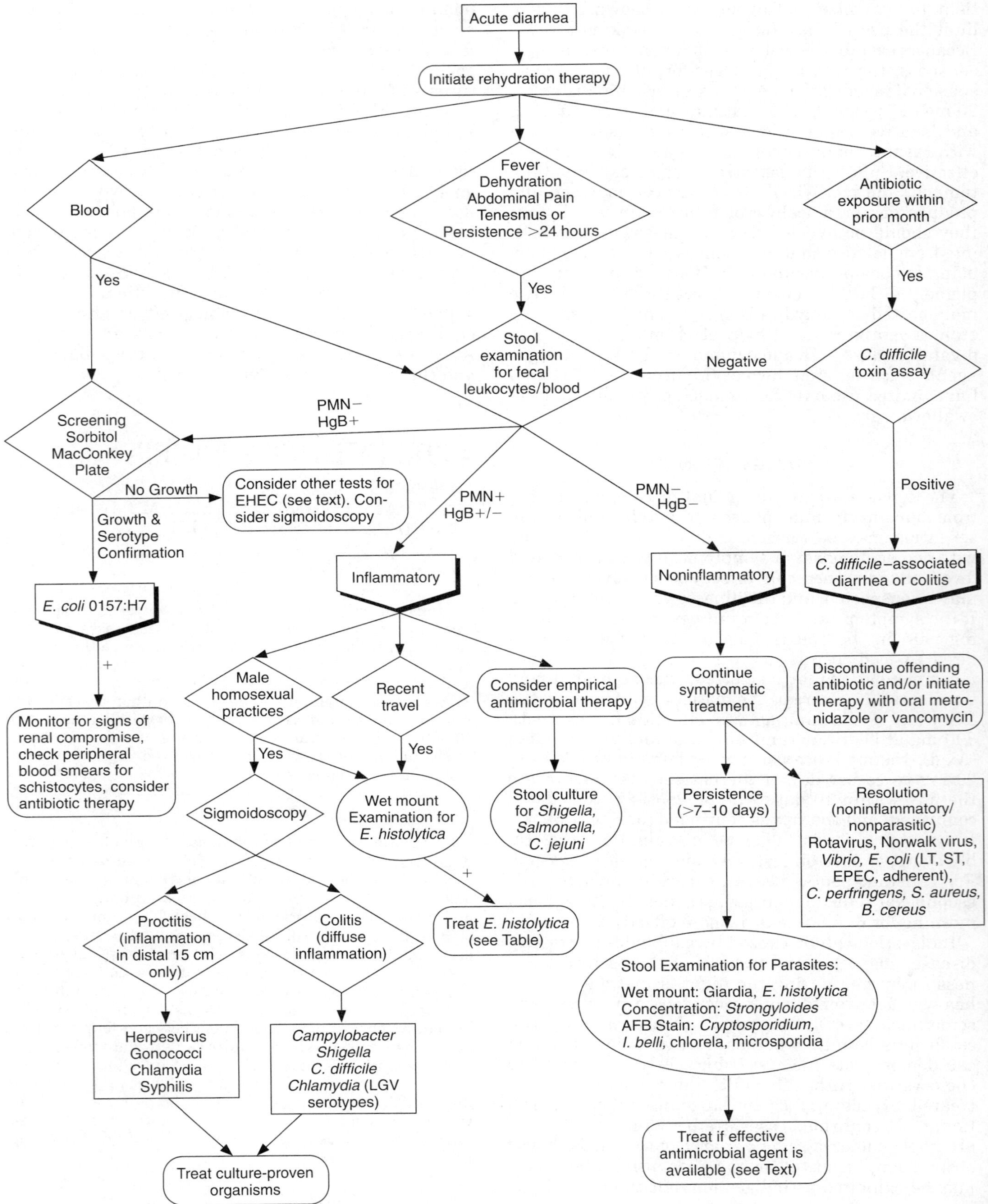

Figure 1. An approach to the diagnosis and management of acute infectious diarrhea.

TABLE 1. **Noninfectious Causes of Acute Diarrhea**

Gastrointestinal/Mechanical	Drug	Dietary Products
Fecal impaction	Laxatives	Sorbitol
Foreign body	Diuretics	Mannitol
Intussusception	Quinidine	Xylitol
Extraluminal compression	Colchicine	**Toxins (Nonbacterial)**
Villous adenoma	Theophylline	Organophosphates
Strangulation	Misoprostol	Insecticides
Bile salt diarrhea	Gold	Mercury
Lactose intolerance	Magnesium-containing antacids	Arsenic
Tropical sprue	Mesalamine	Cadmium
Celiac sprue	Anticholinesterase inhibitors	Mushrooms
Inflammatory bowel disease	Hydralazine	Ciguatoxin
Intestinal ischemia	Guanethidine	Brainerd agent?
Diverticulitis	Iron	**Others**
Appendicitis	Digitalis	Excessive alcohol ingestion
Endocrine	**Diet**	Uremia
Thyrotoxicosis	Prunes, unripe fruit, and others	Food allergy
Carcinoid syndrome	Diet colas	
VIPoma	Caffeine and other methylxanthines	
Gastrin-producing tumor		
Diabetes mellitus		
Addisonian crisis		

dehydration, abdominal pain, tenesmus, mucoid stools, or persistence for longer than 24 hours, a specimen of fresh stool should be examined for fecal leukocytes (or a leukocyte marker such as lactoferrin) and blood. The presence of leukocytes or surrogate leukocyte markers suggests colonic mucosal inflammation usually caused by infections with *Salmonella, Shigella,* or *Campylobacter,* but enteroinvasive *Escherichia coli, Clostridium difficile,* and *Entamoeba histolytica* should also be considered. Empiric antimicrobial therapy with coverage directed toward *Salmonella, Shigella,* and *Campylobacter* is reasonable, and culture of a fresh stool specimen for these organisms could guide future therapy. Male homosexual patients and those recently exposed to tropical regions should have stool examined for parasites, particularly *Giardia lamblia* (noninflammatory) and *E. histolytica* (although amoebic infections in this setting may be predominantly with the nonpathogenic strain *Entamoeba dispar*). Moreover, practicing male homosexual patients are at increased risk for acute colitis and proctitis primarily because of direct inoculation of organisms during receptive anal intercourse. In such men, sigmoidoscopy is useful to distinguish proctitis in the distal 15 cm of colon (usually caused by herpetic, gonococcal, chlamydial, or syphilitic infections) from colitis (*Campylobacter, Shigella, C. difficile,* or chlamydial serotypes causing lymphogranuloma venerum infections). In addition, noninflammatory diarrhea caused by *Giardia* is also seen with increased frequency in homosexual men.

Bloody Diarrhea

Enterohemorrhagic *E. coli* (EHEC), especially *E. coli* O157:H7, *Shigella,* and enteroinvasive *E. coli* are the most common causes of hemorrhagic diarrhea and colitis; and EHEC and *Shigella dysenteriae* have been associated with a potentially devastating sequela, the hemolytic uremic syndrome (HUS). When fecal blood is detected either by gross examination or by hemoccult testing, stool should also be examined for fecal leukocytes and cultures obtained for *E. coli* O157:H7. In general, when the illness is more consistent with an inflammatory process (i.e., fever, fecal leukocytes, tenesmus), *Shigella* and invasive *E. coli* are more likely causes.

In classic EHEC infections, patients with hemorrhagic colitis are often afebrile, and fecal leukocytes are detected in fewer than 30% of cases. Outbreaks have been linked to the ingestion of rare hamburgers, unpasteurized dairy products, fresh-pressed apple cider, and contaminated water usually 72 to 120 hours prior to the onset of symptoms. The development of fever and leukocytosis as the illness progresses may herald HUS (a constellation of microangiopathic hemolytic anemia, thrombocytopenia, and acute renal failure), which occurs most frequently in children between 1 and 4 years of age and in the elderly. Whereas in sporadic cases of hemorrhagic colitis, HUS occurs in approximately 10% of patients, following outbreaks of *E. coli* O157:H7, the attack rate of HUS may increase to as much as 24 to 40% in certain high-risk groups such as the mentally retarded.

Because *E. coli* O157, the most common serogroup of EHEC isolated from humans, and other shiga-like toxin-producing strains generally do not ferment sorbitol, sorbitol-MacConkey (SMAC) medium is widely used to screen for EHEC in fecal specimens. A recently described indirect hemagglutination assay shows promise as a specific test for the serologic diagnosis of *E. coli* O157 infections in children with HUS 1 week after onset of diarrhea. In addition to O:157, more than 30 *E. coli* serotypes have been associated with clinically significant EHEC disease, and they can be identified with more sophisticated testing in special laboratories.

Noninfectious causes of bloody diarrhea include inflammatory bowel disease, intestinal ischemia, bowel strangulation, and rarely, drug induced (gold and methyldopa) diarrhea.

Noninflammatory Diarrhea

The majority of noninflammatory diarrhea illnesses (those without fecal leukocytes) respond to simple oral rehydration therapy, are self-limited, and require no specific diagnostic work-up. If the noninflammatory illness lasts less than 10 days the etiology is likely to be viral (rotavirus, small round viruses such as Norwalk agent, caliciviruses, and astroviruses) or bacterial (*B. cereus, C. perfringens, S. aureus, Vibrio,* enterotoxigenic *E. coli,* enteropathogenic *E. coli,* and adherent *E. coli*).

When an illness persists for longer than 10 days, parasitic infection should be sought, employing a wet mount examination (*Giardia, E. histolytica, Trichurus trichuria* >5000 eggs/gm feces, rarely *Balantidium coli, Schistosoma mansoni* and *japonicum, Capillaria philippenensis*); stool concentration (Strongyloides); acid-fast staining *(Cryptosporidium, Isospora belli, Cyclospora),* and modified trichrome staining (microsporidia). In addition, if a pattern of chronic diarrhea emerges, noninfectious etiologies of diarrhea should be considered, including inflammatory bowel disease, irritable bowel syndrome, malabsorptive diseases (such as sprue and pancreatic insufficiency), diverticular disease, lactose intolerance, and laxative abuse (also see Table 1).

Antibiotic-Associated Diarrhea

The most commonly identified etiologic agent of antibiotic-associated diarrhea and colitis is *C. difficile.* Although almost all antibiotics have been implicated in *C. difficile*–associated disease, reports of large clinical experiences most frequently implicate the broad-spectrum and beta-lactamase–stable penicillins, cephalosporins, and clindamycin (Cleocin). In addition, antineoplastic agents with antimicrobial activity may also lead to *C. difficile*–mediated diarrhea or colitis.

Symptoms usually occur 5 to 10 days after the initiation of the antibiotic, but disease has been reported as late as 10 weeks after the cessation of therapy. The intestinal manifestations of toxigenic *C. difficile* may range from a brief self-limited illness to cholera-like voluminous stools to the classic inflammatory presentation of pseudomembranous colitis. Findings suggestive of pseudomembranous colitis include cramping abdominal pain, leukocytosis, fever, hypoalbuminemia, and the presence of fecal leukocytes or blood. Rarely, *C. difficile* colitis presents as an acute abdomen or toxic megacolon without diarrhea.

C. difficile may be implicated in antibiotic-associated diarrhea by a tissue culture assay for the cytotoxin (toxin B), by enzyme-linked immunoassay (ELISA) for toxin A, or by detecting pseudomembranes on endoscopy. The latex particle agglutination test does not detect a protein specific to toxigenic *C. difficile,* and it should not be used alone to establish the diagnosis of *C. difficile*–associated diarrhea.

Diarrhea in AIDS Patients

Most patients with AIDS will have some diarrheal illness in the course of their disease, and for many, especially in Africa, diarrhea of 1 month's duration or longer is the presenting complaint of HIV infection. Up to two-thirds of these patients will have identifiable pathogens. In addition to the usual pathogens discussed earlier, this group is particularly prone to symptomatic infections with cytomegalovirus, *Mycobacterium avium* complex, *Cryptosporidium,* microsporidia, *Isospora, Strongyloides* and *E. histolytica.* Thus, beyond the routine stool cultures, thorough examinations for ova and parasites, and special stains for acid fast organisms, endoscopic evaluation may be useful in establishing a diagnosis.

Traveler's Diarrhea

Around one-third of travelers acquire acute diarrhea, often in the first week of the trip or soon after returning home. Host factors for developing diarrhea include age less than 30 years, impaired gastric-acid barrier, achlorhydria, immunosuppression, and a previous history of severe travelers' diarrhea. Travel to tropical regions places the patient at particular risk for infection with enterotoxigenic *E. coli* (Latin America [42%] >Africa [36%] >Asia [16%]), *Shigella, Salmonella, Campylobacter,* and parasites *(Giardia, E. histolytica, Strongyloides, Cryptosporidium).* Travelers with diarrhea often respond to conservative measures or antimicrobial agents aimed at enterotoxigenic *E. coli,* and do not (or cannot) seek further medical attention. When such patients do present, stool cultures (with sensitivity patterns) in addition to ova and parasite examination should be obtained in patients with signs of systemic illness or intestinal inflammation.

Foodborne and Waterborne Outbreaks

Of reported outbreaks of foodborne illnesses, the majority are due to bacteria, but parasites (such as *G. lamblia, E. histolytica, Diphylabothrium latum, Anisakis,* and *Trichinella*), viruses (especially Norwalk-like viruses and rotavirus), and noninfectious or toxic agents (including heavy metals, fish and shellfish, mushrooms, solanine, rapeseed oil, and pesticides) also cause outbreaks.

TREATMENT

Supportive Measures

Rehydration. The focal point of therapy for any diarrheal disease is the replacement of lost fluid and electrolytes. Simple and inexpensive, the oral rehydration formula recommended by the World Health Organization (WHO) replaces the extracellular fluid deficit and prevents dehydration in patients with all types of diarrhea who are able to take fluids by mouth. The formula is based on the principle that sodium absorption, which is coupled with glucose transport in the small intestine, remains largely intact even in severe diarrhea. Conventional oral rehydration solution contains 3.5 g NaCl(or ¾ teaspoon of table salt), 2.5 grams $NaHCO_3$ (or 2.9 grams sodium citrate or 1 teaspoon of baking soda), 1.5 grams KCl (or one cup of orange juice or two bananas), and 20 grams of glucose (or 40 grams of sucrose, 50 to 60 grams of rice or other starch, or 4 tablespoons of sugar) in 1 liter (1.05 quarts) of clean water. Prompt therapy should aim to replace the existing fluid deficit in addition to replacing losses from continuing diarrhea and basal metabolism. Oral therapy is preferred not only because it is more physiologic (with an intact thirst mechanism overhydration is avoided) than intravenous rehydration but it is also less costly, less painful, safer (no risk of catheter-related infections), and much easier to administer in developing regions. The only contraindications to oral rehydration therapy are uncontrolled vomiting, ileus, severe fluid deficit with toxicity, or monosaccharide malabsorption. Food-based oral-rehydration therapy, prepared by replacing glucose in the above formula with 50 to 60 grams of cereal flour or 200 grams of mashed boiled potato, may help to reduce fluid output.

Refeeding. Food intake, starting as soon as dehydration has been corrected, is generally well tolerated, enhances the efficacy of glucose-based oral rehydration therapy, and provides intraluminal nutrition necessary to repair and maintain the gastrointestinal mucosa. Rice-based cereal has clearly documented efficacy in the refeeding diet; bananas, potatoes or other nonlactose carbohydrates may also be useful. The smaller meals low in fat content and without residues (such as seeds or peels), fiber, or spices traditionally recommended for patients seem to be better tolerated (or at least preferred) by patients recovering from a diarrheal illness. Children who usually drink milk or modified milk formulas should have them diluted to one-half to three-quarters of normal strength for several days to avoid lactose overloads. In infants with severe persisting diarrhea, fresh stool with pH less than 6, and/or reducing substances present in the stool, lactose-free formulas should be considered, if available, for 10 to 15 days.

Specific Antimicrobial Therapy

Antibacterial Agents. Appropriate antibiotics may be lifesaving in patients with shigellosis or severe *C. difficile*–associated pseudomembranous colitis; can reduce the duration and severity of diarrhea caused by enterotoxigenic *E. coli* (in travelers' diarrhea), *Vibrio cholerae,* enteroinvasive *E. coli,* and enteropathogenic *E. coli;* and are useful in preventing and treating complications of gastrointestinal salmonellosis. The use of empiric antibiotic therapy is often warranted in patients presenting with acute inflammatory diarrheal illness. Table 2 lists preferred and alternative antibacterial agents for specific bacterial pathogens. It is important to note that among these pathogens, emerging resistance patterns exhibit regional differences and that in vitro drug susceptibility may not always predict the clinical response. Thus careful follow-up and continued maintenance hydration of patients on antibacterial therapy is necessary.

SHIGELLOSIS. In the United States, approximately 60% of cases of shigellosis are caused by *Shigella sonnei,* and the majority of the remainder are caused by *Shigella flexneri.* The latter have remained relatively susceptible to ampicillin, while of the former strains, nearly half are resistant. Among foreign travelers returning to the United States, high rates of trimethoprim-sulfamethoxazole (TMP-SMX) (Bactrim, Septra) resistance have been documented in isolates of *Shigella* spp. Hence, ciprofloxacin has become the favored choice for treating *Shigella* infections in adults, and, when the bacteria are susceptible, TMP-SMX should be used in children. Nalidixic acid (NegGram) is also widely used in developing regions, but like the quinolones, chondral toxicity has been reported in young animals and resistance among *Shigella dysenteriae* type 1 isolates is increasing. Not unexpectedly, fluoroquinolone-resistant *Shigella* strains (which also demonstrate high-level nalidixic acid resistance) have now been reported in Japan. Thus, susceptibility data for *Shigella* strains are particularly useful for guiding treatment, especially if the organism was acquired during travel to developing regions where resistance is more common.

VIBRIO CHOLERAE. Although *Vibrio cholerae* infection is uncommon in the United States, the recent migration of the seventh pandemic into Latin America, the emergence of a new serotype (O139) on the Indian subcontinent, and the persistence of an endemic focus of *Vibrio cholerae* along the Gulf Coast all lend global relevance to this previously "Asiatic" disease. While oral fluid and electrolyte therapy remains the cornerstone of treatment for acute cholera and has saved thousands in developing regions, concomitant antimicrobial therapy further reduces fluid losses and the duration of diarrhea. Tetracycline, the drug of choice for most patients, can be given as 500 mg qid or 2 grams qd for two days, and because therapy is short, it is generally considered safe for use in children* (125 mg qid for 2 to 4 days). In addition, ampicillin, choloramphenicol, trimethoprim-sulfamethoxazole, doxycycline, and furazolidone are also effective. The latter has been suggested as an alternative treatment for children and pregnant women.

TRAVELER'S DIARRHEA. Early treatment of traveler's diarrhea with ciprofloxacin (Cipro), norfloxacin (Noroxin), or TMP-SMX typically shortens the duration of illness from 59 to 63 hours to 15 to 30 hours. Because of increasing resistance to doxycycline and more recently to TMP-SMX around the world, fluoroquinolones such as ciprofloxacin, norfloxacin, and ofloxacin (Floxin) are generally the preferred antimicrobial agents for traveler's diarrhea. Although possibly not as effective as TMP-SMZ, furazolidone presents a reasonable therapeutic option for children with traveler's diarrhea in areas of high TMP-SMZ resistance. The cautious use of an antimotility agent in adults with noninflammatory diarrhea may also help to reduce the duration and severity of symptoms in adults (see later).

ENTEROHEMORRHAGIC *E. COLI.* The use of antibiotics in enterohemorrhagic *E. coli* (EHEC) disease is controversial. In addition to potentially biased epidemiologic data suggesting that use of TMP-SMX may predispose some patients to HUS, there are reports of this drug and others increasing in vitro toxin production in clinical isolates of EHEC. However, additional epidemiologic data have suggested that prolonged appropriate antibiotic therapy either has no effect on or decreases the incidence of progression to HUS. Thus, the role of antibiotics in hemorrhagic colitis associated with EHEC remains unsettled at present, and their use in a given patient should be preceded by broad consultation and informed consent from the patient.

CLOSTRIDIUM DIFFICILE. Although nearly all antibiotics have been linked with *C. difficile*–associated diarrhea, ampicillin, clindamycin, and the cephalosporins are the agents most commonly implicated in *C. difficile* overgrowth and diarrhea. If possible, offending antibiotics such as these should be discontinued while the patient is observed closely and fluids and electrolyte losses are replaced. If symptoms persist or worsen, or if the offending antibiotic cannot be

*Not FDA approved for this indication in children younger than 8 years old.

TABLE 2. **Antibacterial Therapy for Acute Infectious Diarrhea***

Pathogen	Drug	Usual Adult Dosage	Notes
Shigella	**Ciprofloxacin†**	500 mg PO bid × 3–5 days	A single 1 gm dose of ciprofloxacin may be as effective as a 5-day/10-dose course in patients with *Shigella* other than *S. dysenteriae* Type 1
	Norfloxacin†	400 mg PO bid × 3–5 days	
	TMP-SMX	1 DS PO bid × 3–5 days	Increasingly resistant strains are reported in many developing regions
	Ampicillin	500 mg PO or 1 gm IV q 6 hours × 3–5 days	Increasingly resistant strains are noted in many developing regions
	Nalidixic acid	1 g q 6 hours × 3–7 days	Like 4-fluoroquinolones, causes arthropathy when given in high doses to immature animals
Non-typhoid *Salmonella*‡	**Ciprofloxacin†**	500 mg PO bid until patient is free of fever for at least 24 hours	Antimicrobial therapy may prolong intestinal shedding of *Salmonella* spp.
	TMP-SMX	1 DS PO bid	
	Amoxicillin/Ampicillin	500 mg PO tid/1–2 g IV q 4–6 hours	
	Cefoperazone	1 g IV q 12 hours	
	Ceftriaxone	1 g IV q 12 hours	
C. jejuni§	**Erythromycin**	250–500 mg PO qid × 5–7 days	Increased rates of resistance reported in Thailand
	Ciprofloxacin†	500 mg PO bid × 7 days	Rarely resistance and associated clinical relapse has developed during therapy
	Tetracycline‖	500 mg PO qid × 7 days	Higher resistance rates (~30%)
Traveler's diarrhea¶	**TMP-SMX**	2 DS once or 1 DS PO bid × 3–5 days	Loading dose regimen followed by standard doses for 3 days may be more effective
	Ciprofloxacin†	1 gm once or 500 mg PO bid × 3–5 days	
	Norfloxacin†	800 mg once or 400 mg PO bid × 3–5 days	
	Ofloxacin†	600 mg once or 300 mg PO bid × 3–5 days	
	Furazolidone	100 mg PO qid × 7 days	
*Clostridium difficile***	**Metronidazole**	250 mg PO qid × 10–14 days	Contraindicated in pregnant and nursing mothers
	Vancomycin	125–250 mg PO q 6 h × 10–14 days	Not absorbed systemically
	Bacitracin	25,000 units PO qid × 10–14 days	
Vibrio cholerae††	**Tetracycline‖**	500 mg qid × 2 days	Tetracycline-resistant outbreaks have been reported in Africa and Asia
	Doxycycline‖	300 mg PO × 1	
	TMP-SMX	1 DS PO bid × 3 days	
	Furazolidone	100 mg PO qid × 3 days	Alternative for treatment of children and pregnant women

*Preferred antibiotics are listed in bold; directed antibiotic therapy should also take into account local sensitivity patterns, if available.

†Quinolones in immature animals can cause arthropathy, and their safety and efficacy has not been established in persons <18 years of age, pregnant women and nursing mothers.

‡Treatment is particularly recommended for bacteremia prophylaxis in patients at extremes of age, with prosthetic material(s) present, or immunocompromised hosts (see text).

§Studies in which antibiotic treatment is initiated early in the course of illness (≤4 days) demonstrate clinical benefit.

‖Should not be used in children younger than 8 years of age.

¶Most common bacterial enteropathogens include enterotoxigenic, enteroadherent, and enteroinvasive *E. coli* as well as *Shigella, C. jejuni,* and *Salmonella.*

**The offending antibiotic should be discontinued, if possible.

††Although the mainstay of therapy should be volume replacement, antibiotics diminish volume and duration of diarrhea and volume replacement requirements.

withdrawn, anticlostridial therapy should be initiated with oral metronidazole (Flagyl) or oral vancomycin. Oral metronidazole is a much less expensive alternative to vancomycin and is equally effective.

CAMPYLOBACTER JEJUNI. Most *C. jejuni* strains are susceptible to erythromycin, the quinolones, aminoglycosides, tetracycline, chloramphenicol, and clindamycin but are relatively resistant to ampicillin, penicillin, and the cephalosporins. In well-designed studies, erythromycin eradicated *Campylobacter* from the feces but did not alter the natural course of disease when initiated 4 days or longer after the onset of symptoms. Ciprofloxacin has also been shown to effectively cure *C. jejuni* diarrhea, although occasional clinical relapse and ciprofloxacin resistance have been reported. Thus, the decision to treat *Campylobacter* enteritis must be made on clinical grounds. If the patient presents early in the course of the illness, appears toxic, or is immunocompromised, antibiotic therapy is reasonable; however, those with relatively mild disease presenting more than 4 days into their illness may not benefit directly from antibiotic therapy. Tetracycline is also effective in adults; in children, clindamycin or amoxicillin with clavulanic acid are reasonable alternatives.

SALMONELLA. Recent studies show that quinolones

TABLE 3. **Therapeutic Regimens for Parasites Causing Diarrhea***

Clinical Syndrome	Drug	Adult Dose	Notes
Amebiasis *(Entamoeba histolytica)*			
Asymptomatic cyst excretor	**Iodoquinol** or	650 mg tid × 20 days	At doses higher than those listed, risk of optic neuritis
	Paromomycin	25–30 mg/kg/day in 3 doses × 7 days	
	Diloxanide furoate (Furamide)	500 mg tid × 10 days	Available from CDC (404-639-3670 or 404-639-2888)
Mild to moderate intestinal disease	**#1 Metronidazole** or	750 mg tid × 10 days	Not recommended for pregnant women
	Tinidazole	2 grams/day × 3 days	Not available in the United States Appears to be as effective as metronidazole, but better tolerated
	#2 Intraluminal agent as listed above.	May also be given IV	
Severe intestinal disease	**#1 Metronidazole** or	750 mg tid × 10 days	
	Tinidazole	600 mg bid × 5 days	Available from CDC (404-639-3670 or 404-639-2888)
	Dehydroemetine	1 to 1.5 mg/kg/day (max 90 mg/day) IM for up to 5 days	
	#2 Intraluminal agent as listed above.		
Hepatic abscess	**#1 Metronidazole** or	750 mg tid × 10 days	
	Tinidazole	800 mg tid × 5 days	
	Dehydroemetine *followed by*	1 to 1.5 mg/kg/day (max. 90 mg/day) IM for up to 5 days	
	Chloroquine phosphate	600 mg base (1 gm)/day × 2 days, then 300 mg base (500 mg)/day × 2–3 weeks	
	#2 Intraluminal agent as listed above.		
Cryptosporidiosis† *(Cryptosporidium)*	Paromomycin	500 mg PO qid	An aminoglycoside similar to neomycin
Cyclospora infection†,‡	TMP-SMZ	1 DS PO bid × 3 days	Limited efficacy data
Giardiasis *(Giardia lamblia)*	**Metronidazole**	250 mg tid × 5 days	Considered investigational for this purpose by FDA
	Quinacrine HCl§	100 mg tid after meals × 5 days	Better cure rate than metronidazole, but more side effects
	Tinidazole	2 g once	Not marketed in United States
	Furazolidone	100 mg qid × 7–10 days	Drug of choice in children
	Paromomycin	25–30 mg/kg/d in 3 doses × 7 days	Not absorbed; may be used in pregnancy, although less effective.
Intestinal Microsporidiosis *(Enterocytozoon bieneusi, Septata intestinalis)*	Albendazole§	400 mg bid	May help treat *E. bieneusi;* can cure *S. intestinalis.*
Strongyloidiasis *(Strongyloides stercoralis)*	**Thiabendazole**	50 mg/kd/d in 2 doses (maximum 3 g/day) × 2 days	Prolonged therapy (which may be toxic) may be required in immunocompromised patients
	Ivermectin§	200 μg/kg/d × 1–2 days	
Isosporiasis *(Isospora belli)*	**TMP-SMX**	1 DS qid × 10 days, then bid × 3 weeks	Considered investigational for this purpose by FDA; in immunocompromised patients, may need to continue indefinitely; if sulfonamide-sensitive, pyrimethamine 50–75 mg qd may be effective.

*Dosing recommendations primarily derived from Med. Lett 35:111, 1993; all dosages are for PO administration except where indicated; drug of choice in bold.

†No antimicrobial agent has established efficacy.

‡Also referred to as cyanobacterium-like bodies.

§Not available in the United States.

Abbreviation: CDC, Centers for Disease Control

alone reduce the duration of symptoms in *Salmonella* gastroenteritis; however, they also appear to prolong the intestinal carriage state and may be associated with clinical relapse. Whereas the routine use of ciprofloxacin is open to question, antibiotic treatment to prevent metastatic seeding is clearly warranted in patients at risk for secondary complications. Patients with *Salmonella* gastroenteritis who are younger than 12 weeks of age or older than 50 years; those with lymphoproliferative disorders, malignancies, hemoglobinopathies, or AIDS; transplant recipients; those with vascular grafts, artificial joints, marked degenerative joint disease, valvular heart disease; and those on steroids should receive antibiotics until they are free of fever for at least 24 hours. If *Salmonella* is isolated from the bloodstream, treatment for 7 to 14 days (longer if a metastatic focus is present) is indicated. Although choramphenicol resistance has been recognized virtually worldwide, ciprofloxacin, ampicillin, and TMP-SMX are usually effective as are third generation cephalosporins such as cefotaxime, ceftriaxone, and cefoperazone. Second-generation cephalosporins have been less effective than third-generation agents and should not be used in the treatment of *Salmonella* disease.

Yersinia enterocolitica. The acute diarrhea caused by *Y. enterocolitica,* primarily occurring in children younger than 5 years of age and associated with food contamination (particularly raw pork), is generally self-limited. The organism is usually susceptible to aminoglycosides, tetracycline, TMP-SMX, choramphenicol, tetracyclines, third-generation cephalosporins, and quinolones in vitro, but there are no data to support the use of antibiotics in uncomplicated *Y. enterocolitica* diarrhea. If extraintestinal complications occur, treatment should be guided by in vitro susceptibly data of the causative isolate.

Antiparasitic Therapy. With the possible exception of some patients with acute amebiasis, diarrheal illnesses associated with parasites are generally more indolent and present as chronic or subacute infections. The most severe manifestations of these agents are in the AIDS population and other immunocompromised hosts. Table 3 summarizes the major parasitic pathogens that cause diarrhea and the current treatment options available.

Symptomatic Therapy

Antimotility Agents. Of the more than 100 antidiarrheal products on the market said to have antidiarrheal properties, few have proved to be both safe and effective in controlled trials for the management of acute nonspecific diarrhea and nondysenteric traveler's diarrhea. Loperamide (Imodium) acts directly to inhibit intestinal peristaltic contractions, thereby delaying transit of intestinal contents. Because it has minimal penetration into the central nervous system, unlike other opiates (e.g., diphenoxylate, codeine, and paregoric), loperamide does not cause nausea, vomiting or drowsiness, nor does it have significant addiction potential. Because patients with inflammatory colitides may worsen when given antiperistaltic agents, they should be avoided in *C. difficile* disease and other inflammatory diarrheas. Their use in shigellosis, in some studies, has been associated with prolonged fever and toxic megacolon and with progression to HUS in EHEC infection. Thus, if fecal leukocytes or blood are present or if the patient has a fever, antimotility agents should probably be avoided. In a recent small study, however, no adverse effects were noted when loperamide was administered along with ciprofloxacin to patients with dysentery caused by *Shigella* or enteroinvasive *E. coli.* Loperamide dosing should not exceed 16 mg/day or be continued for >48 hours.

Bismuth Preparations. Bismuth subsalicylate (Pepto-Bismol) has been used to treat diarrheal illnesses for nearly a century and is found in 60% of American homes. It is has demonstrated efficacy in preventing traveler's diarrhea and has shown modest efficacy in treating traveler's diarrhea as well as acute and chronic diarrhea in children. However, because small amounts of bismuth are absorbed and sequestered in multiple tissue sites even at conventional doses, and because of concerns of salicylate toxicity, treatment with any bismuth-containing compound should be restricted to 6 to 8 weeks.

Adsorbents. Although it is widely used, the adsorbent kaolin-pectin has not been shown to reduce the duration of diarrhea or the loss of fluid and electrolytes in patients with diarrhea. Attapulgite, a clay capable of adsorbing eight times its weight in water, has been shown to be more adsorbent than kaolin and may be as effective as loperamide in decreasing the frequency and increasing the consistency of stools in patients with nonspecific acute diarrhea. It is inert, not absorbed systemically, and has few side effects. In oral suspension, 1200 mg is usually given initially, and repeated after each subsequent bowel movement, not exceeding 8400 mg per day. Children 6 to 12 years of age should receive half the adult dose, and children 3 to 6 years of age should receive one-fourth of the adult dose.

CONSTIPATION

method of
CHRISTOPHER J. BARTOLONE, M.D., and
JAY L. GOLDSTEIN, M.D.
University of Illinois at Chicago
Chicago, Illinois

Constipation is the most common digestive complaint in the United States, affecting on average four million people annually. It is important to recognize that constipation is only a symptom and that when the term constipation is used, it often means different things to different people. Although there is no singularly accepted definition for constipation, individuals may describe stools that are perceived to be too hard or too small, the need to strain with defecation, infrequent defecation, and bloating or a sense of incomplete evacuation. Although these symptoms may reflect a temporary variant of normal physiology, they may also be a manifestation of an underlying medical problem (Table 1). The focus of the guidelines presented in this chapter is directed at the symptomatic treatment of acute and chronic constipation. It is assumed that an appropriate work-up for reversible and treatable medical problems has been conducted prior to or concurrent with the initiation of such therapy.

EVALUATION

Initially we obtain a detailed history of the patient's bowel habits, including the onset and duration of the symptoms. We especially focus on recent changes in bowel habits and fully investigate symptoms suggestive of acute or subacute mechanical bowel obstruction. It is equally important to evaluate the medications the patient has been using, including over-the-counter laxatives, which are often tried prior to seeking medical advice. Special attention is given to medications that alter bowel motility (e.g., nonsteroidal anti-inflammatory agents, anticholinergics, narcotics, and others). Because changes in diet can often influence bowel function, a careful dietary history highlighting recent changes should be obtained. Most important, this dietary history should include an estimate on the amount of daily fiber intake. Although symptoms of constipation are commonly seen in the geriatric population, they should not be attributed to aging alone. Instead, metabolic or endocrinologic disorders, colonic obstruction such as colon cancer or diverticular disease (stricture or abscess), and medications should strongly be considered as causing the patient's symptoms. Once patients have been evaluated and treatment has started, it is often necessary to periodically reevaluate these historical points especially in patients who do not respond to simple medical interventions. Although the physical examination often does not contribute significant information, signs of intestinal obstruction or localized perianal disease (e.g., anal fissures, fistulas) should be excluded. The physical examination may also be useful when findings suggest an underlying primary systemic medical problem that is associated with altered gut motility (Table 1).

Baseline laboratory studies should be obtained commensurate with the acuity or chronicity of the patient's complaints. We commonly obtain a complete blood count, thyroid function tests, and serum calcium and serum electrolyte measurements. As a minimum to exclude primary colonic disease (e.g., colitis) or colon cancer, stool testing for occult blood and proctoscopy or flexible sigmoidoscopy is performed. Depending on the patient's age, duration of symptoms, the presence or absence of occult or frank rectal bleeding, family history, and the physical examination, an obstructive series, barium enema or colonoscopy may also be indicated. Further studies of colonic and anorectal function are generally reserved for patients who do not respond to basic therapeutic measures and after an exhaustive medical work-up has failed to identify a primary medical problem. For these patients with presumed idiopathic constipation, colonic transit studies, anorectal manometry, and defecography should be considered.

MANAGEMENT

Before beginning any medical interventions, it is first important to dispel any preconceived ideas the patient might have as to what is considered a pattern of "(ab)normal bowel movements." In the absence of mechanical bowel obstruction, realistic goals of medical treatment must then be established between the physician and patient. After addressing primary medical problems and discontinuing medications that cause constipation, initial therapy should be directed at behavioral patterns the patient might have that may influence the frequency and pattern of bowel movements. For example, patients should be instructed not to suppress their urge to defecate when it is sensed. Increased mobility in the elderly and regular exercise in younger individuals is also encouraged because this facilitates the development of a regular pattern of defecation.

Dietary intervention is the next step in treating constipation. In the United States, the average intake of dietary fiber has been declining from about 40 grams per day 100 years ago, to the average current

TABLE 1. **Causes of Constipation**

Colorectal	Drugs	Metabolic/Endocrine	Neurogenic	Miscellaneous
Malignancy	Analgesics	Diabetes mellitus	Autonomic neuropathy	Idiopathic
Diverticular disease	Antacids (containing calcium and aluminum)	Hypothyroidism	Aganglionosis (Hirschsprung's disease)	Irritable bowel
Chronic volvulus	Anticholinergics	Panhypopituitarism	Cerebrovascular accidents	Inadequate dietary fiber
Hernias	Antidepressants	Hypercalcemia	Cerebral tumors	Inadequate fluid intake
Ulcerative proctitis/colitis	Anticonvulsants	Pheochromocytoma	Chagas disease	Lack of physical activity
Rectocele	Anesthetic agents	Glucagonoma	Neurofibromatosis	
Strictures	Antiparkinsonian agents	Porphyria	Multiple sclerosis	
Pelvic floor dysfunction	Barium sulfate	Pregnancy	Parkinson's disease	
Amyloidosis	Bismuth	Uremia	Spinal cord tumors or trauma	
Scleroderma	Diuretics		Shy-Drager syndrome	
Anal fissure	Heavy metal intoxication (arsenic, lead and mercury)		Tabes dorsalis	
	Iron			
	Laxative abuse			
	Nonsteroidal anti-inflammatory agents			
	Opiates			
	Psychotherapeutic agents			

intake of only 15 grams per day. This has contributed significantly to the increased prevalence of constipation. Whether or not additional stool softeners or laxatives will eventually be required, patients should initially be instructed to eat a diet high in natural fiber (> 30 grams per day). These instructions should stress the use of bran cereals, fresh fruits, root vegetables and legumes as well as an adequate intake of water (at least six 8-ounce glasses per day). Fiber retains luminal water in the colon and acts as a substrate for the colonic microflora. In patients with normal colonic function, it also reduces intracolonic pressure, decreases transit time, and produces softer stools.

Bulk-Forming Agents. For many patients with mild symptoms, dietary changes may be an adequate intervention. We believe that in patients with more significant complaints, any additional interventions will be more successful after initial dietary changes have already been made. For those who cannot incorporate adequate fiber into their diet, bulk-forming agents such as psyllium (Metamucil), methylcellulose (Citrucel), and polycarbophil (FiberCon) may be used in addition to dietary manipulation. These agents increase stool water content and stool bulk, and are available in a variety of forms including powders, wafers, candies and tablets. In the absence of significant mechanical obstruction, delayed gastric emptying or other gastrointestinal motility disorders, their margin of safety is high and they can safely be used over the long term. Patients should be instructed that adequate fluid intake (at least 1.5 liters per day) should be used daily to avoid obstruction and impaction. The desired effect of bulk-forming agents is usually seen after several days. It should be stressed to the patient that long-term success with these agents is predicated on their continuous and daily use. Although many patients initially experience bloating, cramping, and gas, these symptoms are generally minor and dissipate within a few weeks. These symptoms tend to occur less frequently with methylcellulose products. To avoid the early rejection and noncompliance with any of these agents, we start all bulk-forming agents at a lower dose than anticipated for maintenance (½ tablespoon daily) and increase the dose gradually (over 1 to 2 weeks) to 2 to 3 tablespoons daily. The final dose is generally titrated to the patient's response and the desired goal of therapy.

Lubricating Agents and Stool Softeners. If these initial measures with increasing oral fiber intake fail, there are a number of laxatives that are available for use, mainly on a short term basis. Emollients that include mineral oils and surfactants such as sodium docusate (Colace) or calcium docusate (Surfak) soften the stool. They are useful in situations when straining is to be avoided such as after myocardial infarction, during pregnancy, after rectal or abdominal surgery, and in patients with perianal disease. Mineral oils, if aspirated, can lead to lipid pneumonia and therefore are contraindicated in patients with dysphagia, esophageal dysmotility and in elderly or debilitated patients. Long term use of mineral oil can also decrease the absorption of fat-soluble vitamins A, D and K and, therefore, should be given between meals.

Saline Laxatives. Saline laxatives include magnesium hydroxide (Milk of Magnesia), sodium phosphate (Phospho-soda, Fleet enema), and magnesium citrate and magnesium sulfate. These agents exert an osmotic effect, thereby increasing intraluminal water. If given orally, their effects are seen within 3 hours; if given rectally, their effects are seen within 15 minutes. These agents are not recommended for patients with renal insufficiency because of the potential for magnesium toxicity. Other side effects mainly seen with long-term use may include hypocalcemia, hypophosphatemia, electrolyte imbalance, and volume depletion. These agents should only be used acutely for bowel preparation prior to radiographic or endoscopic procedures of the large bowel or when it is necessary to cleanse the gastrointestinal tract.

Hyperosmotic Agents. Hyperosmolar laxatives include the nonabsorbable sugars lactulose (Chronulac 15 to 60 mL per day) and sorbitol (70% solution:sorbitol to water, 15 to 60 mL per day) or the mixed electrolyte solutions containing polyethylene glycol (GoLYTELY, CoLyte and others). Lactulose and sorbitol are metabolized by colonic bacteria to lower molecular weight short chain fatty acids, subsequently lowering colonic pH and increasing colonic peristalsis. In a dose-dependent fashion, lactulose and sorbitol may cause abdominal cramping, diarrhea, gas and electrolyte imbalance. However, we find that these agents are usually well accepted by patients who require their long-term use. When adjusted to produce one or two soft stools a day, these two agents can be used safely on a long-term basis. Sorbitol has been shown to be as effective as lactulose and is much less expensive.

The polyethylene glycol solutions* are primarily used for bowel preparation prior to colonoscopy or surgery. Large volumes (1 gallon) need to be taken in a relatively short period of time (2 hours), and compliance is often an issue dictating their success. Recently, these solutions have also been used in chronically obstipated patients. The typical amount used is 8 to 16 ounces per day for these patients. Side effects include cramping, gas, nausea, and the unpleasant taste of the solution.

Stimulant Agents. The anthraquinones (cascara sagrada, senna, danthron, and casanthranol) and the diphenylmethanes (bisacodyl and phenolphthalein) are stimulant agents and include some of the most commonly used brand name over-the-counter laxatives such as Dulcolax, Peri-Colace, Correctol, Ex-lax, and Senokot. Some of these medications, when used on a long-term basis, can produce a benign pigmentation of the colonic mucosa known as melanosis coli. More importantly, long-term stimulant laxative use (or abuse) may lead to laxative dependence and, in later stages, recalcitrance to their action. This is referred to as the cathartic colon syndrome, which may,

*Not FDA approved for this indication.

in some individuals, reverse itself with slow tapering and finally withdrawal of the use of these agents. As such, regular use of stimulant laxatives should be avoided. Other potential problems associated with their use include electrolyte and fluid imbalance and cramping. Phenolphthalein (Correctol, Ex-lax) can cause erythema multiforme, hyperaldosteronism, and vitamin D malabsorption. Although they are quite popular, these agents should only be used intermittently for short-term management and should not be used on a long-term basis.

Prokinetic Agents. Cisapride (Propulsid), 10 mg, 4 times daily is a prokinetic drug that has recently become available in the United States. Although it is currently only approved for gastroesophogeal reflux disease, it has been shown to be effective in patients with constipation secondary to delayed colonic transit time.

Surgery for the management of constipation remains a controversial issue except in the patient with Hirschsprung's disease, in which it is the treatment of choice.

FEVER

method of
MOSHE IPP, M.B.B.CH.(RAND)
The Hospital for Sick Children
Toronto, Ontario, Canada

Fever is one of the most common clinical manifestations of disease. However, despite significant recent advances in our understanding of it, misconceptions still prevail. Many patients have an unrealistic fear of fever, which is compounded by the exaggerated concern expressed by many physicians. This phobia of fever often results in unnecessary phone calls and visits to the doctor's office, as well as the inappropriate use of medications and excessive use of laboratory investigations.

Fever does not cause much harm to the individual except in certain rare circumstances and in cases in which the fever is excessively high. Both physicians and patients need to be reassured that fever is merely a marker for an underlying condition, and in itself, it is essentially benign and not dangerous.

PATHOPHYSIOLOGY OF FEVER

Several mechanisms may cause an elevation of body temperature above normal. The most common mechanism seen in clinical medicine results from an elevation of the hypothalamic set point, an area in the anterior hypothalamus that functions like a thermostat. Infection is the most common condition responsible for raising the set point and initiates this process by triggering the release of a circulating polypeptide known as interleukin-1. This polypeptide is produced when pyrogens such as viruses and bacteria are engulfed by phagocytes and leukocytes. These cells release interleukin-1 into the blood, where it acts on the arachidonic acid pathway to stimulate the production of prostaglandin E_2 in the hypothalamus. The prostaglandin E_2 elevates the set point and causes fever by allowing the body to conserve heat through vasoconstriction and by increasing heat, generally through shivering. Among other effects of interleukin-1 are the proliferation of helper T cells and enhanced interferon production, although a decrease of certain immunologic functions has also been shown at high temperatures.

Other mechanisms of fever production do not affect the usual daily clinical practice of most physicians but should be borne in mind because they call for different treatment. Fever may result from excessive heat production in which the hypothalamic set point remains normal. The causes of such heat production include salicylate overdose, hyperthyroidism, and malignant hyperthermia. There are also clinical situations in which there is an impairment of heat loss (also with a normal hypothalamic set point) that may result in fever. This occurs in patients with ectodermal dysplasia, heat stroke, and anticholinergic drug poisoning. In terms of treatment, antipyretic agents are only useful for managing high set-point fevers. All other fevers require removal of the heat source.

WHAT DEFINES A FEVER?

Normal body temperatures fluctuate during the day in the range of 36° C to 37.8° C (96.8° F to 100° F), the lowest occurring in the morning and the highest in the evening. Fever is defined as a temperature above the normal range, and the reading is determined by the anatomic site of measurement. In adults and children over 5 years of age, an oral temperature above 37.5° C (99.5° F) constitutes a fever. In children under 5 years of age, in whom oral measurement is not practical, most authorities would accept a rectal temperature above 38° C (100.4° F) or an axillary temperature above 37.2° C (99° F) as constituting a fever. Axillary temperatures are generally less accurate but serve as a suitable screening site for measuring fever, whereas oral and rectal measurements are more accurate and reliable. With the recent introduction of tympanic membrane thermometers calibrated to measure core temperatures, the ear may be used in addition to the current standard oral, rectal, and axillary sites.

IS FEVER HARMFUL OR BENEFICIAL?

There is an evolutionary argument as well as scientific data to support the view that fever is beneficial (although contrary opinions still prevail). Many components of nonspecific and specific host immune responses to infection are enhanced by some elevation in temperature, and studies of bacterial and viral infections in animals have shown that, in general, moderate fevers decrease morbidity and increase the survival rate. Interleukin-1 is considered to be responsible for stimulating the host's defenses against infection and for providing the optimal temperature at which these beneficial effects occur. In other studies, suppression of fever using antipyretic drugs has been shown to lead to increased morbidity and mortality in laboratory animals.

Although fever is considered beneficial to the host in most circumstances, in certain clinical situations it may be maladaptive and harmful, such as in patients with impaired coronary perfusion in whom the hypermetabolic state resulting from the fever may aggravate the condition. During pregnancy, high temperatures may be teratogenic and cause birth defects.

Certainly, the types of fever that children usually experience are not harmful and do not cause brain damage or death. Fever may cause convulsions in fewer than 5% of children but these convulsions have no long-term sequelae. Death or any damage that may occur is usually caused by the underlying condition, such as meningitis, rather than by the fever itself. On the other hand, elevated set-point fevers that result from the host's neurologic response to a pyrogenic stimulus must be distinguished from externally imposed hyperthermia, as seen in heat stroke, in which set point remains normal. Under the latter circumstances, the body's normal defenses are overwhelmed: The temperature may rise above 41.7° C (107° F) and may cause central nervous system damage.

CLINICAL ASPECTS OF FEVER

When approaching the management of fever, the physician must determine both its underlying cause and its effects on the comfort of the patient. Although most fevers are viral in origin and require no specific treatment, fever has many other causes. If a focus for the fever is found, it should be treated specifically while appropriate symptomatic relief is provided for the patient to counteract both the effects of the underlying cause and those of the fever. If no focus for the fever is found, the physician must decide whether further investigations are necessary or whether it would be more prudent to wait for the fever to resolve spontaneously. These decisions depend on how ill the patient appears, the age of the patient, the duration of the fever, and other particular circumstances of both patient and illness. Generally speaking, the height of the fever is less important than how ill the patient appears. Most patients require symptomatic relief only because fevers are generally viral in origin, but caution must be exercised in the very young and the very old, in whom infection may be present without the clinical signs one might normally expect. For example, in the infant under 1 month of age, symptomatic treatment alone is not advised. Many recommend that these infants have a full sepsis evaluation and, if necessary, be admitted to hospital for administration of antibiotics and observation pending the outcome of laboratory investigations.

TREATMENT

Supportive Treatment

The one compelling reason to treat fever is to make the patient feel more comfortable: In essence, the patient should be treated, not the thermometer. Patients can be made to feel more comfortable with extra fluids to prevent dehydration, less clothing, and reduced activity. If the patient feels cold and is shivering with chills, a light blanket may give symptomatic relief.

Children should not be bundled up when they have a fever because this practice may not allow for adequate dispersion of heat and could, thus, be harmful. The room must not be overheated but rather kept at a comfortable 20° C (68° F). Children should not be covered with towels or wet sheets, which make them feel uncomfortable, and alcohol sponging is contraindicated because the alcohol can be absorbed through the skin. Lukewarm sponge baths for infants and children, although controversial, are recommended by some physicians, especially for a high fever that is unresponsive to acetaminophen. Although some doubt their efficacy, it may be worth sponging an uncomfortable and feverish child—not immersing him or her completely but leaving most of the body exposed to help speed evaporation. If the sponging makes the child feel chilled, shivery, or unhappy, it should be stopped. For safety reasons, children should never be left alone in the bathtub.

Pharmacotherapy

In addition to these supportive measures, antipyretic drugs may be useful in providing further symptomatic relief. However, they should not be given automatically and are necessary only if the patient is feeling uncomfortable. It must be emphasized that the purpose of antipyretic treatment is to make the patient feel more comfortable, not to keep the fever from rising any higher or to prevent convulsions, brain damage, or death. The objective should not be to reduce the temperature to normal but to a level at which the patient feels more comfortable. Patients do not need to be awakened for antipyretic treatment.

There are essentially three main choices of antipyretics currently available: acetaminophen, ibuprofen, and salicylates. Ibuprofen and salicylates are classic nonsteroidal anti-inflammatory drugs (NSAIDs) in that they inhibit prostaglandin synthesis. Acetaminophen differs pharmacologically from the other two and probably exerts its effect by central prostaglandin inhibition. The clinician must base the choice of antipyretic on the clinical situation, the age of the patient, the cost/benefit ratio, and the safety and efficacy of the different agents.

Acetaminophen

Despite being synthesized at Johns Hopkins Hospital in 1877, acetaminophen (Tylenol) has been marketed in the United States only since 1950. Acetaminophen is rapidly and completely absorbed after ingestion. It begins to act in approximately 30 minutes after dosing, achieves peak effects at 1 to 3 hours, and lasts from 3 to 6 hours. Its antipyretic efficacy is good, and it is an effective analgesic but a weak anti-inflammatory drug. The maximum antipyretic effect in terms of decrease in temperature appears to be equal among all the available antipyretics. The safety of acetaminophen for routine short-term treatment is excellent: It has the lowest incidence of adverse effects, causing less gastrointestinal upset, renal toxicity, and allergic reactions than the alternative antipyretics. Clinically significant toxicity (mainly hepatotoxicity) is seen only in massive overdose, which is less common in children than in adults. If treated early, the hepatotoxicity can be minimized by the use of *N*-acetylcysteine (Mucomyst).

From a clinical standpoint, it should be recognized that acetaminophen is available at relatively low cost, without a prescription, and in many easy-to-swallow forms, such as flavored chewable tablets, elixir, and drops. It is also available in the form of suppositories, tablets, capsules, and caplets. The recommended dose for children is 10 to 15 mg per kg given every 4 to 6 hours. The pharmacodynamics and safety data indicate that the higher dosage of 15 mg per kg is easily justified. The adult dose is 325 to 650 mg every 4 to 6 hours.

Ibuprofen

Ibuprofen (Motrin, Advil) has been used for many years, primarily for the treatment of inflammatory conditions such as rheumatoid arthritis as well as for pain and antipyresis. It has been used in the United States only within the past few years. Ibuprofen is a classic NSAID, inhibiting prostaglandin synthesis. Its absorption is rapid but not necessarily complete and is delayed and decreased by the presence of food. It has a longer duration of action than salicylates and acetaminophen, usually at least 5 to 6 hours and sometimes up to 8 hours.

The toxic effects of ibuprofen in adults are well recognized and are similar to those caused by aspirin. Because its use has been restricted in children, its safety needs to be confirmed with more widespread use. Most ibuprofen toxicity is minor or uncommon, but serious adverse renal, gastrointestinal, or pulmonary effects can occur. Ibuprofen interferes with platelet aggregation and, thus, may cause gastrointestinal hemorrhage both from its direct effect on the gastrointestinal tract and from dose-dependent platelet dysfunction. However, recent evidence in adults suggests that the rates of serious gastrointestinal complications during chronic use are lower for ibuprofen than for other clinically available NSAIDs (e.g., naproxen, aspirin). Bronchospasm, headaches, rashes, bone-marrow suppression, and aseptic meningitis have all been reported. A major advantage of ibuprofen is that it appears to be very safe in cases of overdose. The risk of Reye's syndrome remains unknown.

Ibuprofen is available over the counter for adults and children older than 12 years. In the United States, it has recently been made available in suspension form for children younger than 12 by prescription only, but at present, it is not available in this form in Canada. As a prescription drug it is more expensive than other available antipyretic agents. The recommended adult dosage is 200 to 400 mg given every 4 to 6 hours, that for children 5 to 10 mg per kg every 4 to 6 hours.

Salicylates

Aspirin and other salicylates represent the classic NSAID and antipyretic agents, but are now less commonly used than either acetaminophen or ibuprofen, largely because of safety concerns. In particular, the epidemiologic data associating aspirin usage with Reye's syndrome has dramatically affected its use in children.

All salicylates are rapidly and completely absorbed, with a duration of antipyretic effect of 3 to 4 hours. The major problem with aspirin is its narrow margin of safety. Adverse effects are common and include gastrointestinal irritation and hemorrhage, impairment of coagulation due to both irreversible and reversible platelet effects, renal injury, hypersensitivity and allergic reactions, and exacerbation of asthma. Therapeutic, accidental, and suicidal overdose is serious and not infrequent. Because of the availability of other less toxic alternatives, it is difficult to justify the use of salicylates for antipyresis, particularly in children.

COUGH

method of
JAMES R. McCORMICK, M.D.
Berkshire Medical Center
Pittsfield, Massachusetts

A cough, like a sneeze, is a protective reflex, designed to clear the upper or lower airways of foreign material or to warn of noxious stimuli in the environment. All of us cough from time to time, often after misswallowing with minor aspiration or during the course of an upper respiratory tract infection. In this latter circumstance, cough seems to serve no useful purpose; it results from the hypersecretion of mucus and inflammation, which must be endured until natural healing takes place. Persistent cough can be annoying to the afflicted individual because it may interfere with work, recreation, or sleep. It may also be socially challenging if the cough interrupts an audience's concentration at concerts, in the theater, classroom, or place of worship. Cough may also be a cardinal symptom of serious illness, requiring investigation for upper airway, cardiac, or pulmonary disorders. Some of the more common causes of cough are listed in Table 1.

When considering therapy for a patient with cough, it is appropriate to first determine whether the symptom is acute or chronic. A chronic cough has been defined arbitrarily by investigators as one lasting 3 weeks or more in order to distinguish its causes from common upper respiratory tract infections. Sometimes, a patient with a chronic cough develops an acute problem that alters its character, as in patients with chronic bronchitis who develop an acute exacerbation of their symptoms or bronchitic patients whose cough often changes in frequency and who experience persistent hemoptysis when a lung cancer has developed. Generally, a targeted history and physical examination enable the health care provider to identify a probable etiology and an approach to therapy (Table 2).

MANAGING ACUTE COUGH

For patients with acute upper respiratory tract infections, simple demulcents often suffice to suppress the urge to cough for a few minutes. Often, a viral cough is episodic anyway, an intrusive symptom heralded by a posterior pharyngeal tickle or substernal irritation that cannot be ignored. If tea with honey, licorice, or other candies are not sufficient to control the cough, some patients have used candied flavors combined with menthol, which may last a little longer. For those with nasal congestion and postnasal drip, a decongestant administered nasally or orally may diminish the cough and relieve the annoying fullness in the nose and over the sinuses. The author uses an oral decongestant, such as pseudoephedrine (Sudafed), 60 mg every 4 to 6 hours or 120 mg every 12 hours in adults, because of the local irritation of nasal sympathomimetics and their tendency to produce rebound edema after a few days of use. For persistent cough, the oral local anesthetic benzonatate (Tessalon, Forest Pharmaceuticals) has been effective for some individuals. Because it is structurally similar to tetracaine, this drug should not be used in individuals hypersensitive to that agent and should not be chewed because it might cause sufficient local anesthesia to impair swallowing (and it has a bitter taste). In overdosage, it can cause serious central nervous system side effects including seizures. For some annoying viral coughs, dextromethorphan, hydrocodone, or codeine may effectively suppress the symptom so that the patient can rest. The author sometimes uses dextromethorphan-containing lozenges for limited periods or oral codeine (10–30 mg every 4 to 6 hours for adults) for patients with particularly persistent cough. Note that liquid cough suppressants containing these agents are combinations of drugs. There is no convincing evidence that antihistamines or expectorants (such as guaifenesin) are effective in treating any of the symptoms related to an upper respiratory tract infection. Therefore, the author does not use cough and cold formulations that contain antihistamines or the phenothiazine promethazine to treat virally induced cough, in general. Any perceived benefit these drugs provide is probably mediated through their sedative effect. Guaifenesin is neither a cough suppressant nor even an expectorant, at least at the dose recommended by most manufacturers of cough and cold medications. Similarly, terpin hydrate has not been shown to be an effective expectorant, and it is not a cough suppressant. Therefore, for patients with symptoms due to an upper respiratory tract infection, the author recommends rest, fluids, and simple analgesics for the generalized aches, pains, and fever; humidified air, saline nose drops, or just standing in a warm shower for the congestion; and simple demulcents as necessary. For persistent cough and nasal congestion and, especially, postnasal drip, the author recommends a decongestant–cough suppressant combination for brief therapy. Table 3 lists some of these drugs and includes brands that also contain guaifenesin because this agent appears to be safe, if not effective.

TABLE 1. **Some Common Causes of Cough**

Inflammatory Disorders of the Upper and Lower Airways or Lung Parenchyma
Viral upper respiratory tract infections
Allergic rhinitis
Sinusitis
Acute and chronic bronchitis
Asthma
Pneumonia (bacterial, viral)
Bronchiectasis (associated with common variable hypogammaglobulinemia, cystic fibrosis, dyskinetic or immotile cilia syndrome)
Aspiration (of gastric contents, from esophageal diverticulum, or in patients with achalasia)
Diffuse pulmonary interstitial fibrosis
Neoplasms
Primary malignant or benign tumors of the upper airway or bronchi
Metastatic malignancy to the lung parenchyma or pleura
Mediastinal tumors (thymoma, germ cell tumors, lymphomas, metastatic malignancy)
Chemical Irritants
Tobacco smoke, other smokey products of combustion
SO_2, NO_2
Capsaicin (from all capsicum peppers)
Metabisulfites
Gastroesophageal reflux (reflex bronchoconstriction or aspiration)
Mechanical Stimulants (Inflammation May also Play Some Role in Cough Production)
Foreign body aspiration
Substernal thyroid
Mediastinal fibrosis
Irritation of external auditory canal
Congestive cardiac failure (interstitial edema leading to reduced lung volumes which may trigger cough receptors, also pleural effusions)
Drugs
Angiotensin-converting enzyme inhibitors (may act indirectly through bradykinin which stimulates prostanoid synthesis)
β-blockers (via bronchospasm or precipitation of congestive heart failure)
L-Dopa (? promoting disordered swallowing)
Drug-induced hypersensitivity pneumonitis or pleuritis (nonsteroidal anti-inflammatory agents, nitrofurantoin, others)

TABLE 2. **Evaluating the Patient with Cough**

History
Onset, duration, frequency
Factors causing exacerbation or remission
Associated symptoms (e.g., feverishness, upper respiratory tract symptoms, sinus pain, wheezing, shortness of breath)
Sputum
Volume, color, odor, consistency; if blood is present, how much? how often?
Chest pain
Hoarseness
History of allergies, seasonal changes in symptoms, atopy
Gastroesophageal reflux symptoms
Environmental causes (e.g., tobacco smoke, air conditioning or humidifying units, dry air, common allergens, inhalation of fumes or particulates associated with occupation or hobbies)
Medications; other drugs
Physical
Respiratory rate, check for abnormal degree of pulsus paradoxicus
Thorough upper respiratory tract evaluation, including indirect (or direct) laryngoscopy when appropriate
Complete chest examination (inspection, palpation, percussion, auscultation). Note whether trachea is in the midline.
Careful cardiac examination. (Do not forget that occult mitral stenosis may be associated with cough!)
Other
Simple, bedside swallowing assessment
Radiologic assessment of swallowing and esophageal anatomy and function
Radiologic evaluation of the sinuses when sinusitis seems likely
Chest roentgenogram if an intrathoracic cause is a possibility
Prolonged esophageal pH monitoring
Pulmonary function studies (with methacholine challenge testing if spirometry is normal and asthma is suspected).
Bronchoscopy when a lower respiratory tract lesion is suspected

Sinusitis or bronchitis should be considered in selected patients who have purulent nasal discharge or sputum and cough lasting longer than a week or two. Although a viral etiology may still be operative, one must consider primary or superinfection with bacterial organisms such as *Streptococcus pneumoniae, Haemophilus influenzae,* or *Moraxella catarrhalis* in the sinuses and *S. pneumoniae, H. influenzae, Chla-*

TABLE 3. **Decongestants–Cough Suppressants**

Drug	Antitussive	Expectorant	Other Agents
Isoclor (Fisons)	Codeine (10 mg)	Pseudoephedrine (30 mg)	Guaifenesin
Naldecon CX (Bristol)	Codeine (10 mg)	Phenylpropanolamine (12.5 mg)	Guaifenesin (200 mg)
Novahistine (Marion)	Codeine (10 mg)	Pseudoephedrine (30 mg)	Guaifenesin (100 mg)
Nucofed (SmithKline Beecham)	Codeine (20 mg)	Pseudoephedrine (60 mg)	Guaifenesin (200 mg)
Nucofed Pediatric (SmithKline Beecham)	Codeine (10 mg)	Pseudoephedrine (30 mg)	Guaifenesin (200 mg)
Robitussin-DAC (Robins)	Codeine (10 mg)	Pseudoephedrine (30 mg)	Guaifenesin (100 mg)
Ryna CX (Wallace)	Codeine (10 mg)	Pseudoephedrine (30 mg)	Guaifenesin (100 mg)
Triaminic (Sandoz)	Codeine (10 mg)	Phenylpropanolamine (12.5 mg)	Guaifenesin (100 mg)
Hycomine (Dupont)	Hydrocodone (5 mg)	Phenylpropanolamine (25 mg)	
Tussend (Lakeside)*	Hydrocodone (5 mg)	Pseudoephedrine (60 mg)	
Anatuss (Mayrand)	Dextromethorphan (15 mg)	Phenylpropanolamine (25 mg)	Guaifenesin (100 mg)
Conar (SmithKline Beecham)*	Dextromethorphan (15 mg)	Phenylephrine (10 mg)	
Conar Expectorant (SmithKline Beecham)*	Dextromethorphan (15 mg)	Phenylephrine (10 mg)	Guaifenesin (100 mg)
Dimacol (Robins)	Dextromethorphan (10 mg)	Pseudoephedrine (30 mg)	Guaifenesin (100 mg)
Dorcol Children's Cough Syrup (Sandoz)	Dextromethorphan (5 mg)	Pseudoephedrine (15 mg)	Guaifenesin (100 mg)
Naldecon-DX (Bristol)	Dextromethorphan (10 mg)	Phenylpropanolamine (12.5 mg)	Guaifenesin (200 mg)
Novahistine DMX (Lakeside)	Dextromethorphan (10 mg)	Pseudoephedrine (30 mg)	Guaifenesin (100 mg)
Robitussin-CF (Robins)	Dextromethorphan (10 mg)	Phenylpropanolamine (12.5 mg)	Guaifenesin (100 mg)
Ru-Tuss Expectorant (Boots)	Dextromethorphan (10 mg)	Pseudoephedrine (30 mg)	Guaifenesin (100 mg)
Sudafed Cough Syrup (Burroughs Wellcome)	Dextromethorphan (10 mg)	Pseudoephedrine (15 mg)	Guaifenesin (100 mg)
Triaminic-DM (Sandoz)	Dextromethorphan (10 mg)	Phenylpropanolamine (12.5 mg)	
Vicks Formula 44D	Dextromethorphan	Pseudoephedrine (20 mg)	
Tuss-Ornade	Caramiphen	Phenylpropanolamine (75 mg)	

*Not available in the United States
Content given per capsule or 5 mL.

mydia pneumoniae or *Mycoplasma* as causes of bronchitis. *Chlamydia* is emerging as a frequent cause of upper and lower respiratory tract infection (especially sinusitis and bronchitis), especially in individuals who have no prior pulmonary disease.

Sinusitis should be suspected clinically in patients who report or are observed to have purulent nasal discharge, who report a maxillary toothache, and who have had a poor response to nasal decongestants. If there is also abnormal transillumination of the sinuses and sinus tenderness, it is likely that acute sinusitis is present. Purulent sinusitis can contribute to the perpetuation of cough and should be treated empirically with an appropriate antibacterial agent. Failure of the patient to respond or progression of symptoms despite decongestant and antimicrobial therapy should lead to further investigation.

Patients with chronic obstructive pulmonary disease who develop acute bronchitis, manifested by an increase in sputum volume and purulence, generally respond to a 2- to 3-week course of antibiotics. The author generally uses doxycycline (100 mg twice daily), amoxicillin (250–500 mg three times daily) or trimethoprim-sulfamethoxazole (160 mg/800 mg twice daily). In previously normal patients with a viral-like syndrome heralded by a slight sore throat and complicated by hoarseness, purulent nasal discharge and bronchitis, the author is suspicious of chlamydial infection, particularly, and often begins with doxycycline (100 mg twice daily). This drug also treats infection with *Mycoplasma pneumoniae.* In parts of the country where as many as 50% of pneumococcal isolates are resistant to penicillin (and nearly as many to other commonly used oral antibiotics), culture of the purulent material should be performed and antibiotic therapy should be guided by sensitivity testing. Empirical antibiotic therapy should always be guided by the physician's clinical judgment in assessing the severity of the infection and by a knowledge of the drug sensitivity of the prevailing flora in your community.

EVALUATING THE PATIENT WITH CHRONIC COUGH

Generally, a thorough initial history and physical examination will disclose which patients have a serious underlying illness as the cause of their cough. In others, the cause may not be so readily apparent until laboratory data, such as pulmonary function studies or chest x-ray studies, are obtained. In a few patients, the reason for the cough will not be apparent even after these tests and a trial of antihistamines, cough suppressants and even antibiotics may be of little benefit. It is this group of patients with cough who are most difficult to treat and who present a great source of frustration to the primary care practitioner and to the patient. When the cause of the cough cannot be determined, specific therapy cannot be administered and the side effects of strong measures to suppress the cough seem difficult to justify. These are the patients who are most often referred to the pulmonary specialist or allergist for some help or at least for reassurance that nothing else can be done. Take heart! There is hope for these individuals and for the practitioner, who is searching for a means of treating them. A small group of investigators have evaluated large numbers of these patients, individuals with cough of more than 3 weeks' duration for which no cause can be found in the patient's history, physical examination, or selected routine laboratory studies. The patients studied did not have any obvious allergies (although skin testing may not have been performed upon most of them) and have had none of the usual symptoms or signs of asthma. Pulmonary function studies in this group have generally been normal. There was no consistent history suggesting gastroesophageal reflux, and some have undergone simple antireflux measures for brief periods of time without benefit. The investigators' work has suggested an approach that we may follow in evaluating patients with chronic cough for which no obvious cause can be found. Initial therapy should consist of the administration of a decongestant-antihistamine preparation such as Trinalin (azatadine, 1 mg, and pseudoephedrine, 120 mg; Key Pharmaceuticals) to be taken twice daily for at least 1 week, and the patient should be observed for improvement of symptoms. Combinations containing pseudoephedrine with chlorpheniramine, brompheniramine, terfenadine, or other antihistamines may be reasonable alternatives. The supposition is that most of these cases of chronic cough are due to a postnasal drip syndrome related to allergic rhinitis. Patients who improve should generally be continued on the medication for a month or more, and if symptoms resolve completely, the medication can be tapered gradually. Persistence of symptoms after the first week of therapy and the presence of edematous nasal mucosa suggest the need for topical corticosteroid therapy in addition to the decongestant-antihistamine agent. Topical cromolyn sodium may benefit some patients with obvious allergic rhinitis. Patients with symptoms of chronic sinusitis should have sinus roentgenograms and appropriate therapy if that diagnosis is confirmed. Patients with sinusitis who do not respond to the decongestants, antihistamines, nasal corticosteroids, and antibiotics should be referred to an otorhinolaryngologist.

Patients who do not receive much benefit from the initial therapy should be evaluated for the presence of occult asthma. Methacholine challenge testing should be performed on those patients who have normal pulmonary function studies. If asthma is present, an inhaled bronchodilator (e.g., metaproteranol, albuterol, or terbutaline) should be used initially because it may immediately benefit the cough. The author recommends the administration of inhaled corticosteroids twice daily as well in order to diminish the airway inflammation that is currently believed to be the root cause of the asthmatic response. Several agents are available, all of which are probably equivalent in anti-inflammatory potency at the doses recommended. The author generally uses triamcinolone acetonide (Azmacort), 200 μg, at an initial dose of four puffs twice daily. If this dose does not control symptoms, the author either increases the number of inhalations twice daily or the frequency *and* the number of inhalations. Cough may be the only manifestation of hyperreactive airways and, perhaps, frank asthma in some patients. This approach generally results in prompt resolution of symptoms so that the inhaled adrenergic bronchodilator may be discontinued after a couple of weeks of corticosteroids. The author generally continues the corticosteroids for several months before tapering in order to determine how the patient fares.

Patients who do not respond to either or both of the above-mentioned regimens may have occult gastroesophageal reflux disease, which may cause cough by poorly understood mechanisms. If gastroesophageal reflux is suspected, a trial of antireflux measures such as raising the head of the bed, avoiding food and alcohol before going to bed and a few weeks trial of an H_2 blocker such as ranitidine (Zantac), 150 mg at bedtime should be initiated. Patients who do not respond to these measures or have no obvious symptoms of reflux should be considered for prolonged (24-hour) esophageal pH-probe monitoring. Individuals found to have significant reflux should be managed appropriately.

Most patients with chronic cough have one of these entities or some combination of these three entities as the cause for their persistent symptom. The aforementioned therapies should result in dramatic improvement or complete resolution shortly after their institution. Patients in whom allergic rhinitis is suspected and who require constant therapy should be considered for allergy testing in order to attempt to remove the offending antigen or to desensitize the individual to its effects. Before referring a patient whose cough is refractory to the pulmonary or allergy specialist, however, keep in mind that angiotensin-converting enzyme inhibitors produce cough in 5 to 20% of patients, generally women, and do so without affecting pulmonary function tests. The cough may appear shortly after initiating therapy or months later and ceases within a few days after stopping the drug. It may occur with all of the available agents and generally precludes further use of any of them. You will be a heroine or a hero if you can deduce this cause of a chronic cough and cure it without expensive diagnostic investigation or referral.

If chronic cough is a difficult symptom to diagnose and to treat, it is at least as difficult to endure. The frustrated health care provider who finds no cause and no response to empiric therapy may wish to ascribe the cough to psychogenic origin. In my experience, chronic, troubling psychogenic cough is often associated with persistent throat clearing and other tics. Before considering that the cough may be psychogenic in origin, the author tries using benzonatate or an opiate cough suppressant like codeine (15 to 30 mg every 4 to 6 hours), or both, as needed for a week or two. Sometimes the cough will resolve completely and the drugs can be discontinued.

Patients who have irreversible pulmonary fibrosis, untreatable malignancy, or other unresolvable causes of cough may also benefit from this therapy. Individuals who suffer from bronchiectasis and who have difficulty raising sputum should be treated with antibiotics appropriate for the infecting organism, aerosolized saline and bronchodilators, and postural drainage with or without chest percussion. Some patients respond to aerosolized acetylcysteine (Mucomyst, diluted 1:1 in saline), which may act as a mucolytic expectorant. Aerosolized human recombinant deoxyribonuclease has been demonstrated to be an effective mucolytic agent in patients with cystic fibrosis and has recently become available in the United States.

SUMMARY

There are more than 200 nonprescription and prescription cough and cold preparations, reflecting the vast market for symptomatic relief of cough and associated symptoms. The author's approach has been to try to relieve symptoms by treating the specific etiology of the cough first, if possible. If a viral cause is likely, then a limited course of a decongestant and cough suppressant may be helpful. Antihistamines and expectorants are not useful cough suppressants or facilitators. Sinusitis or an acute bronchitis should respond to an appropriate antibiotic. For chronic cough of unknown cause, the algorithm provided by the author should cure the symptom in most individuals. Patients whose cough persists despite this approach may need to undergo further testing or referral to a specialist. Patients whose cough is due to an untreatable illness may find some relief with benzonatate or oral codeine (or an analogue), or both.

HOARSENESS AND LARYNGITIS

method of
KAREN RHEW, M.D.
National Institute on Deafness and Other Communication Disorders
National Institutes of Health
Bethesda, Maryland

Hoarseness and laryngitis are general terms commonly used to indicate an abnormal voice. A hoarse voice may be further described as raspy, scratchy, breathy, rough, gravelly, strained, or harsh. The term laryngitis is used more often when the voice change occurs in conjunction with a respiratory infection. Virtually any of the diseases or disorders that affect the larynx can affect the voice. Dysphonia, a more inclusive term, is used to indicate the various types of abnormal voice qualities regardless of exact laryngeal etiology.

Speech pathologists, laryngologists, and other professionals specializing in voice disorders are skilled in recognizing voice qualities that characterize specific laryngeal pathologies. They often suspect the correct diagnosis just by listening to the patient speak for a few minutes. However, in addition to a thorough history and examination of the head and neck, accurate diagnosis requires a laryngeal examination. This may be difficult because the larynx is relatively inaccessible without using special techniques and instruments. The traditional indirect laryngeal mirror examination is useful for initial identification of most problems. Flexible fiberoptic nasolaryngoscopes have become standard equipment in many offices and clinics because they are less likely to elicit a gag reflex and seem more easily tolerated by children and many adults. The enhanced visualization and video documentation made possible with fiberoptic laryngoscopes often eliminate the need for direct laryngoscopy in the operating room if benign lesions that do not require surgery are identified.

INITIAL EVALUATION

When consulted by a patient exhibiting symptoms of a laryngeal or voice disorder, the primary care physician must decide whether or not a laryngeal examination is necessary at that point and, if so, whether it is urgent or likely to require referral to a specialist. Decisions regarding the necessity, urgency, and extent of the laryngeal examination are based on several factors, such as the severity of the symptoms, whether the symptoms are acute or chronic, whether the patient is a child or an adult, or if the person uses his or her voice professionally.

Severity of Symptoms

Airway Obstruction. Hoarseness accompanied by evidence of upper airway compromise constitutes the most urgent reason for expert laryngeal examination. Stridor, in particular, is diagnostic of obstruction at the level of the larynx. Some conditions causing hoarseness are more likely to produce concomitant stridor than others (see Table 4).

The severity of symptoms determines the necessity of performing the examination in a hospital setting, perhaps in the operating room. Even in an office situation, emergency equipment for intubation, tracheotomy, and resuscitation must be available when a patient with such a condition is examined.

Dysphagia. The hoarse patient who also has significant

swallowing problems needs prompt evaluation. Aspiration, drooling, and odynophagia are especially worrisome symptoms (see Table 4).

Acute versus Chronic Symptoms

Acute Symptoms. If a patient with symptoms of upper respiratory infection and no previous voice problems presents with hoarseness of 48 hours' duration or less, acute infectious laryngitis is the most likely diagnosis. The causative organism is usually viral, but evidence of bacterial infection in the upper or lower airway, such as purulent sputum or sinus drainage, warrants appropriate antibiotic therapy. However, if no other serious symptoms exist, limitation of voice use (Table 1) and supportive measures (Tables 2 and 3) may be all that is needed. This same course can be taken for hoarseness that occurs after a bout of vocal abuse such as with shouting, cheering, and loud continuous talking. If the vocal symptoms do not lessen significantly after a week, laryngeal examination should be undertaken. Most patients presenting in this manner will experience resolution of their acute voice symptoms before laryngoscopy is needed.

Chronic Symptoms. Hoarseness that has been present for 3 weeks or longer requires a thorough inspection of the larynx. Examination should not be delayed if there is suspected cancer, worsening of the voice, or interference with work or daily functioning.

Pediatric versus Adult Patients

Hoarseness in infants, children, and adults has very different diagnostic and therapeutic implications. Infants and children can become hoarse from excessive vocal use such as yelling or prolonged crying or from self-limited viral upper respiratory infections just as adults can. However, the newborn or infant with a hoarse, weak, or absent cry most likely has a congenital anomaly of the larynx. Because laryngeal malformations are often accompanied by other anomalies of the head and neck, it is imperative that an infant with these symptoms have a complete examination of the respiratory tract, including nose, oral cavity, pharynx, larynx, trachea, and bronchi. Direct laryngoscopy in the operating room is the safest way to adequately examine the larynx of an infant or young child. Whether or not the child is in distress determines how urgently the procedure is performed, but a diagnosis should be made in a timely fashion. The opening of an infant's laryngeal glottis can be reduced to 35% of normal by a mere 1 mm of mucosal edema, which could be induced by the coughing and choking associated with gastroesophageal reflux or aspiration. The infant also may be more susceptible to a sudden fatal episode of laryngospasm under these circumstances. Although the airway enlarges with growth, young children are still at greater risk from laryngeal edema than older children and adults. Hospitalization is often advisable for even early symptoms of airway compromise associated with infections such as laryngotracheobronchitis and is mandatory for patients with epiglottitis.

Professional Voice Users

Performers such as singers, actors, and public speakers who present with complaints about their singing or speaking voices require a high level of clinical sophistication from the physician evaluating them. The extreme endurance and quality these patients demand from their voices can be affected by even slight alterations in the tissues or fine motor control of the larynx and other voice mechanisms. Any voice complaint from a performing artist should be taken seriously even if an abnormality cannot be heard or seen by the examiner. Often, the performer's career need to "go on with the show" must be weighed against the potential for vocal fold injury. A decision to perform based on the physician's assessment can have serious consequences. Suboptimal medical care in professional voice users can devastate their means of livelihood and possibly result in litigation. For these reasons, it is advisable to give professional voice users the option of seeing a laryngologist with expertise in treating such patients.

TABLE 1. **Voice Care: Avoiding Vocal Abuse**

Hoarseness and similar vocal problems have many causes, one of the most important being improper use of the voice. Here are some guidelines for avoiding vocal abuse:

- No yelling or shouting
  - Move closer to the listener
  - To attract attention from a distance, use clapping, a whistle, a bell, a noisemaker
- No loud continuous talking
  - Avoid talking in noisy places. (It is frequently very noisy inside many vehicles—cars, buses, trains, planes. Trying to talk above the noise causes wear and tear on the voice)
  - Use amplification for public speaking. Be sure you have a system that allows you to monitor your own voice to avoid speaking unnecessarily loud
- Talk less; shorten even the amount of quiet talking you do
- No unnatural vocal sounds (e.g., imitating animals, motors, explosions)
- No throat clearing. Try swallowing or taking a sip of water instead
- Suppress coughing
  - To get rid of mucus, use a quiet or silent cough in which a blast of air is forced from the lungs with the vocal folds apart or gently brought together so little sound is produced
  - Gentle rubbing of the anterior neck creates a counter stimulus and inhibits coughing
  - For a cough precipitated by a dry, tickling throat, try humidification, sipping fluids, and sucking on lubricating lozenges

Additional measures may be necessary during times when you have laryngitis or the voice sounds abnormal:

- Use voice rest—relative voice rest means speaking only when absolutely necessary; no casual conversations. Try to put off any meetings or other situations that will force you to use your voice. Have someone else explain to others ahead of time that you are on voice rest. Strict voice rest or complete silence may be necessary if speaking is painful or you have been told that there are hemorrhages on the vocal folds. Use a writing pad to communicate
- No whispering. Loud whispering strains the voice. When talking is absolutely necesary, use a soft voice with as little volume as possible
- No singing

GENERAL THERAPEUTIC MEASURES

The most common causes of hoarseness are acute infectious laryngitis and various forms of chronic laryngitis. Many of the supportive measures recommended for these problems are also appropriate for maintenance of a healthy vocal tract. In keeping with current health care trends emphasizing wellness and prevention, information in principles of self-care of the respiratory tract may have long-term benefits even for patients with self-limited forms of hoarseness. Patients prone to recurrent or chronic upper airway congestion and infection may wish to continue environmental controls and increased hydration even after their hoarseness has resolved. Patients whose occupations require a good deal of talking, such as teachers, lawyers, and telephone operators, often find some of these practices useful for preventing voice problems.

Recommendations involve avoiding vocal misuse and abuse and taking care of the tissues of the larynx and respiratory tract with hydration and elimination of irritants and infection. Many of the methods are old fashioned remedies that were used before antibiotics and modern pharmaceuticals were available. This information is presented in the form of patient handouts in Tables 1 to 3.

Modification of Vocal Behavior

Voice Rest. Any patient with hoarseness should be cautioned that attempting to continue the usual amount of daily talking may cause further irritation to the vocal folds. Using the voice for only essential communication is known as relative voice rest. Most patients are able to comply with this recommendation for the several days when an acute laryngitis is affecting their voice quality most severely. Infrequently, the laryngeal examination reveals vocal fold hemorrhages or severe inflammation, which requires complete silence or strict voice rest.

Avoiding Vocal Abuse. Certain vocal behaviors such as shouting, loud continuous talking, frequent coughing, and throat clearing traumatize the vocal folds and may even be the primary cause of hoarseness. Such vocal abuse should certainly be avoided by the hoarse patient whose vocal folds are in a state that is more vulnerable to injury.

Vocal Tract Hygiene

Measures used to restore and maintain healthy laryngeal tissues should be directed at the entire respiratory tract. When the mucosa of the nose and sinuses is in an unhealthy state, inhaled air is not properly humidified and filtered prior to contact with the more vulnerable tissues of the larynx, tracheobronchial tree, and lungs. In addition, infected or irritating secretions from the paranasal sinuses above or the lower airway below can involve the larynx. Irritated mucosa in the tracheobronchial tree and larynx may stimulate a persistent cough that traumatizes the delicate vocal folds. Even a small amount of edema can disrupt the fine vibratory function of the vocal fold mucosa, and hoarseness results.

The key defense mechanism of the upper and lower airways is the thin layer of mucus produced by mu-

TABLE 2. **Voice Care: General Measures**

Taking care of the tissues of the throat and voice box (larynx) is an important part of voice care. Here are some guidelines:

1. No smoking
2. Avoid inhaling irritants such as dust, smoke, and fumes (e.g., gasoline, ammonia, paint thinner, disinfectants)
3. Limit intake of alcohol and caffeine-containing beverages. Alcohol is an irritant to the mucous membranes that line the mouth and throat. It also causes acid to reflux from the stomach. Both alcohol and caffeine have a diuretic effect that causes water loss from the body
4. Avoid mouthwashes and gargles that contain alcohol or irritating chemicals. If gargling is necessary, use a salt water solution.* If you believe that you have bad breath, it is better to diagnose the cause and treat that condition. Halitosis can come from low-grade infections in the nose, sinuses, tonsils, gums, and lungs, as well as gastric acid reflux from the stomach.
5. Drink plenty of fluids—a minimum of 1½ to 2 quarts per day
6. Put moisture in the air indoors, especially in winter. (30% humidity is the proper amount. A higher percentage may be necessary if the vocal folds are swollen and inflamed.)
7. Treat acid reflux (stomach acid that regurgitates into the throat). Consult your doctor as to treatment
8. Maintain a well-balanced diet with plenty of whole grains, fruits, and vegetables. Foods containing vitamins A, E, and C are especially important in maintaining healthy mucous membranes
9. Seek treatment for any conditions that cause inflammation, infection, or swelling of tissues in the nose, sinuses, tonsils, or bronchial tubes. Bacteria or irritating secretions from these tissues can affect the voice box because they share common drainage pathways. Also, swollen tissues in the nose and throat can cause snoring and mouth breathing, which dry out the vocal folds and make them more susceptible to injury
10. Get adequate exercise. Proper speaking depends on maintenance of good posture and proper breathing. This requires a certain amount of stamina and general muscle tone. Just 30 minutes or so of aerobic exercise (walking counts), coupled with stretching before and afterward, performed 3 times a week is adequate. Keep the muscles of the neck, shoulders, and upper torso limber and stretched
11. Get adequate rest. General physical fatigue affects the voice
12. Reduce stress. Recognize unproductive tension and develop strategies for dealing with it, including obtaining professional advice if needed
13. Consider voice therapy. Getting rid of some harmful speaking habits such as excessive neck tension, improper breath support, or a vocal pitch that is too low or too high may require voice therapy from a speech pathologist experienced in treating voice problems

*Saline solution: Add ½ teaspoon of noniodized salt or sea salt to 1 cup (8 oz) of body temperature water.

TABLE 3. **Medications for Laryngitis and Upper Respiratory Infections**

The respiratory tract includes the sinuses, nose, throat, larynx (voice box), trachea (windpipe), and bronchial tubes. In order to be healthy and function normally, the tissues (mucous membranes) that line the respiratory airway must be moist and covered with a thin layer of clear mucus. This mucous blanket enables the nose and the sinuses to humidify and filter inspired air before it reaches the more delicate tissues in the larynx and lungs. These mucous secretions become scant and too thick when the body is dehydrated or the tissues become damaged by inhaled irritants or infected by viruses or bacteria. The dry, swollen vocal folds do not vibrate normally, causing hoarseness. The irritation may also cause a cough.

Most of the medications described here are designed to relieve dryness and swelling in the tissues of the entire airway, as well as the larynx, so that the normal mucous secretions and other natural defense mechanisms are able to work. This will help relieve symptoms during upper respiratory infections. Also, chronic hoarseness, cough, or sinusitis is less likely to develop.

The specific brands named below are used only as examples of a particular type of medication. There are usually several name brands and generic brands available for each of the medications recommended. Follow the instructions on the package carefully.

Moisturizers

Saline nasal spray (NāSal, SalineX)—Spray 3 to 4 squirts into each nostril every 2 to 4 hours. Buy several bottles so a new one can be used every day

Guaifenesin (Robitussin)—An expectorant that thins mucous secretions so that the respiratory tract can handle them in a more normal manner

Petroleum jelly—If the inside of the nose feels dry, apply petroleum jelly inside of each nostril. Gently insert a small glob of ointment on the end of a cotton-tipped swab or little finger into each nostril and then pinch the nostrils together to coat the inside of the nose. You may use antibiotic ointment (Polysporin ointment) if there are sore places or minor bleeding inside the nose. Ointments should be used in the nose for only a week unless your doctor advises you to do otherwise. If the problem does not resolve or becomes worse, stop applying the ointments and see your doctor

Humidifier—Either cool or warm mist is acceptable. The humidifier must be kept clean to avoid mold and bacterial contamination

Increased fluid intake—Drink at least 2 quarts of noncaffeinated liquids a day

Decongestants

Oxymetazoline (Afrin)—Use 1 to 2 sprays to each nostril twice a day for 3 days only. This 12-hour decongestant nasal spray is an effective immediate treatment for nasal, sinus, and some ear congestion. It can be used for only 2 to 3 days at a time because rebound congestion occurs, in which the nose stays stuffed up unless the spray continues to be used. If air travel is necessary when you are congested, using the nasal spray 20 minutes before take-off and landing may help avoid blocked sinuses and ears

Pseudoephedrine (Sudafed); phenylpropanolamine (Propagest)—Decongestants shrink swollen mucous membranes. They can cause a caffeine-like jitteriness, sleeplessness, heart palpitations, and increased blood pressure. These side effects may be increased in the long-acting forms, so start with the smallest dose (Sudafed 30 mg, or Propagest 25 mg) of the short-acting tablet to determine how it affects you

Antihistamines—It is best to avoid antihistamines unless you are treating an allergic condition. They can cause dryness as well as decrease and thicken mucous secretions, thereby reducing throat lubrication to the point of causing a dry cough

Cough Medications

Lozenges (NICE)—The most important function of cough drops is to stimulate saliva production, which lubricates the throat. Lozenges that numb the throat or have an antiseptic action may contain ingredients that are irritating to the tissues. A piece of hard candy can also be used to keep the mouth and throat moist

Dextromethorphan—This non-narcotic cough suppressant is as effective as codeine in depressing the cough reflex. It comes in many forms including syrup (Vicks Formula 44) and in a capsule with guaifenesin (Robitussin Cold and Cough Liqui-Gels)

Pain Medications

Acetaminophen (Tylenol)—If you have laryngitis, this nonprescription medication is preferable to aspirin and other anti-inflammatory drugs such as ibuprofen (Motrin, Advil, Nuprin), which may interfere with the clotting mechanism and increase the risk of vocal fold hemorrhages. Your doctor may believe narcotic cough medicines (e.g., codeine) are indicated even though they contribute to thicker mucous secretions

Hot packs, cold packs, heating pads, hot/cold water bottles—Use devices for applying heat or cold, whichever may be appropriate, to sore muscles, sore throat, strained tendons, bruises, headaches. Besides being therapeutic, thermal treatment can help make strong pain killers unnecessary

Treatment for a painful throat infection:

- Warm saline irrigations using a bulb syringe while leaning over the sink. Gargling may be painful and difficult
  Avoid mouthwashes and gargles that contain alcohol or irritating chemicals that temporarily numb or anesthetize the throat
- Warm packs to the neck
- Inhale mist or steam
- Sip warm drinks
- Pain medications

Note: If a bacterial infection such as a strep throat is suspected or if the severe pain persists longer than 24 hours, see your doctor promptly. You may need antibiotics

cous and serous glands in the respiratory mucosa and transported by cilia of the respiratory epithelium. Microbes, dust, pollen, and other foreign elements are caught up in the mucus produced in the sinuses and nose, moved posteriorly down the throat, and swallowed. The gastric acid and the excretory function of the digestive tract dispose of the foreign elements. Cilia of the tracheobronchial tree similarly move mucus up and out of the trachea and larynx and into the hypopharynx, where the secretions are swallowed. The airways are constantly cleaned, thus limiting the opportunity for inhaled irritants to elicit an inflammatory reaction and for microorganisms to multiply and infect the mucosal cells. The secretions can also contain substances such as lysosyme or IgG and IgA antibodies that block microbial invasion. Eustachian tube function also depends on the mucociliary flow mechanism.

The mucociliary flow system is disrupted by inflammation and edema caused by excessive dryness, allergic reaction, infection, and toxic or irritating inhalants. Many of the hygienic and therapeutic measures are directed at maintaining or restoring this normal protective mechanism.

Hydration. Daily intake of 1½ to 2 quarts of water and noncaffeinated liquids is ordinarily adequate to replenish bodily fluid losses. Conditions such as heat, exercise, or illness may increase the fluid requirements. Hot tea and warm broths stimulate normal mucociliary action besides adding to fluid intake. Patients should be instructed to monitor their state of hydration by observing oral and nasal mucous membranes as well as the quantity and color of urine output.

Humidification. Environmental dryness, especially when it is due to air cooling or heating, can be lessened with the use of either warm or cool humidifiers. Travelers can run a steamy shower or hang wet towels to humidify a hotel room. Thirty percent humidity is adequate for maintenance, but a higher amount may be desirable for therapeutic purposes during respiratory infections. If there is rawness or slight bleeding in the nose, a coating of antibiotic ointment (Polysporin) or petroleum jelly inside each nostril for a few days should promote healing.

Saline nasal irrigation is helpful in relieving dry or congested nasal mucous membranes. This may be accomplished with multiple squirts of saline nasal spray (NāSal, SalineX, Ayr Saline) every 2 hours or more. Also, saline solution can be introduced into the nose using a regular 20-mL syringe or an infant's nasal bulb syringe, or can be simply snuffed from the cupped hand.

Avoidance of Irritants. The direct damage of inhaled irritants such as dust, smoke, and chemical fumes (gasoline, ammonia, disinfectants, and paint thinner) makes the airway more susceptible to infection and the vocal folds more likely to develop mucosal changes such as chronic edema and polyps. Severe inflammation and cellulitis of the larynx can sometimes be traced to inhalation of fumes from household cleaners such as ammonia and sodium hypochlorite. All types of tobacco use should be discouraged. If contact with such inhalants is unavoidable, patients should be instructed as to proper precautions for ventilation, use of masks, and careful monitoring. Vitamins A, E, and C appear to have protective properties for the mucous membranes of the aerodigestive tract.

Medical Management

Allergy Management. Allergies to foods and inhalants such as dust, pollens, and molds can cause swelling and irritation of tissues throughout the airway. Nasal and sinus congestion are the most common symptoms associated with allergy, but cough and varying degrees of hoarseness occur as well. Hoarseness secondary to vocal fold edema and vocal nodules is more common in allergic children. Antihistamines may be helpful for relieving some symptoms of allergy but the mucosal dryness and the slowing of mucociliary action they cause is counterproductive in the larynx. They should be prescribed with instructions for increased oral hydration and nasal moisturization. Topical corticosteroid nasal spray such as beclomethasone (Beconase AQ), 1 spray to each nostril two to three times daily, is an effective alternative treatment for nasal symptoms of allergy. Orally inhaled aerosol medications are not recommended for allergic hoarseness or cough. Indeed, when such aerosols are used for bronchitis and asthma, laryngeal irritation develops from the propellants and the aerosolized steroid. Hyposensitization therapy should be considered for perennial or severe allergies.

Treatment of Upper Respiratory Infection. Many patients with chronic hoarseness report that the problem began during or immediately after an upper respiratory infection. Since the laryngeal tissues are vulnerable to injury during this time, it is important to choose medications which do not exacerbate the dryness and inflammation caused by infection. Patients should be advised as to the most appropriate non-prescription medications and the rationale for using them (Table 3).

Nasal and sinus decongestion can be accomplished with minimal drying and thickening of secretions using a long-acting decongestant nasal spray such as oxymetazoline (Afrin), 1 to 2 sprays to each nostril every 10 to 12 hours for 2 to 3 days only, and a systemic decongestant such as pseudoephedrine (Sudafed, Novafed) or phenylpropanolamine (Propagest). The slight drying effect can be ameliorated by taking an expectorant and increasing oral intake of liquids. Preparations that combine decongestants and expectorants, such as phenylephrine, phenylpropanolamine, and guaifenesin (Entex), are available. Before decongestants are recommended, consideration should be given to their side effects of increased blood pressure, sleeplessness, agitation, and urinary retention.

A key concept in treating a cough that stems from laryngeal irritation is delivering adequate moisture and lubrication to the throat. Breathing steam or nebulized moist air is effective. Dissolving lozenges or hard candy in the mouth will stimulate saliva production and lubricate the throat. Lozenges and gargles containing irritating antiseptic or topical anesthetic ingredients should be avoided. Dextromethorphan (Robitussin DM, Vicks Formula 44) is as potent for cough suppression as codeine but does not have the disadvantage of slowing mucociliary flow.

Acetaminophen (Tylenol) for analgesia is preferable to aspirin and other anti-inflammatory drugs such as ibuprofen, which may interfere with the clotting mechanism, increasing the risk of hemorrhages from the superficial dilated vessels on the inflamed vocal folds. Narcotics contribute to sluggish clearing of secretions. Devices for applying heat or cold, whichever may be appropriate for sore muscles, sore throat, and headache, may decrease the need for stronger analgesics as well as being therapeutic.

Warm saline gargles help when infection is the cause of inflammation, whereas chilled, not frozen, drinks may be more soothing for edema caused by overuse of the voice.

Related Infections. Acute infections in the nose, sinuses, tonsils, lungs, or bronchi generate irritating and infectious secretions that drain to the vicinity of the larynx. If they are not treated with appropriate antibiotics and measures to protect the respiratory mucosa, sequestered pockets of mucous secretions may stagnate, resulting in chronic sinusitis, tonsillitis, or bronchitis. Halitosis is more often caused by infection of this type than by dental sources.

Systemic Steroids. Although rapid relief from hoarseness caused by acute inflammatory laryngitis can be sometimes obtained by taking oral corticosteroids, their use is not usually warranted. Exceptions can be made in the case of a patient who has an important professional obligation to perform or communicate verbally. Some expertise is required in making this decision. The physician must be confident that the condition of the vocal folds is stable enough that fulfilling the speaking or singing commitment will not cause injury. Generally, dexamethasone (Decadron), 6 to 8 mg taken once and then in tapering doses over the next 3 to 5 days, is sufficient. If a bacterial infection is suspected, empirical antibiotic coverage is indicated. Diuretics are not useful for decreasing inflammatory vocal fold edema. The excess fluid that is sequestered in the superficial lamina propria is bound, not free, water and will not be mobilized by diuretics.

COMMON CAUSES OF HOARSENESS

As is evident from Table 4, the larynx is affected by many disease processes that result in hoarseness. Some of the more common causes of hoarseness are described briefly.

Infectious Laryngitis

Acute Infectious Laryngitis

Over 85% of cases of acute infectious laryngitis are of viral etiology; the pathogen typically is a rhinovirus. The onset is commonly associated with symptoms of upper respiratory infection such as rhinorrhea, pharyngitis, sneezing, and cough. The hoarseness that rapidly develops may be accompanied by throat pain, especially with speaking. The illness is usually self-limited but can progress to secondary bacterial infection, the most common pathogens being *Moraxella catarrhalis* and *Haemophilus influenzae.*

Treatment. General therapeutic measures such as described earlier can ease the symptoms of the laryngitis and the concomitant respiratory infection, as well as making residual chronic laryngitis or secondary bacterial infection less likely. If the hoarseness persists longer than a week, a laryngeal examination should be performed and antibiotic therapy considered.

Chronic Laryngitis

Continual exposure of the larynx to any number of irritants, such as smoking, irritative inhalants, gastroesophageal reflux, allergens, respiratory tract infection, alcohol abuse, vocal abuse, and coughing, may lead to a variety of chronic mucosal changes in the vocal folds and cause hoarseness. These changes range from generalized thickening of the vocal fold epithelium to discrete lesions or even atrophy.

Chronic Laryngitis. The vocal fold mucosa has diffuse inflammatory changes, usually with some edema. However, if heat and dryness are contributing factors, the mucosa may appear atrophic. Exposure to caustic and carcinogenic irritants may produce whitish patches of hyperkeratosis. Diffuse polypoid changes can result from fluid accumulation in the superficial lamina propria of the mucosa. Polyposis may be patchy or may be so extensive that one or both vocal folds appear to be one large polyp (Reinke's edema).

TREATMENT. The causative agents must be identified and eliminated. Measures to restore the mucous membranes of the respiratory and vocal tracts to a healthy state should be instituted. Lesions that do not subside may be removed with microsurgery, particularly if cancer must be ruled out. Faulty vocal habits that contribute to the problem should be corrected with voice therapy.

Gastroesophageal Reflux Laryngitis. Gastric secretions refluxing into the hypopharynx is a common cause of laryngeal irritation which can produce cough, throat clearing, and hoarseness. The patient may or may not complain of typical symptoms such as heartburn, gastritis, and a burning or lump-like sensation in the throat. On laryngoscopy, the mucosa of the arytenoids and posterior larynx is inflamed, sometimes with ulcerative granuloma formation.

TREATMENT. Once identified, reflux laryngitis can be effectively managed by the primary care physician with antacids, elevation of the upper body at night, dietary habits, and histamine H_2-receptor antagonists such as ranitidine HCl (Zantac) 150 mg twice daily or antisecretory agents such as omeprazole (Prilosec) 20 mg daily for 4–8 weeks. Repeated vomiting such as is seen in bulimia nervosa can produce changes in the larynx similar to those seen with reflux.

Vocal Nodules. Nodules are discrete, usually bilateral swellings which typically form just anterior to the midportion of the vocal fold. They are caused by improper use of the voice; in children, they are called screamer's nodes, and in singers, singer's nodes.

TREATMENT. Most nodules in compliant patients will resolve with voice therapy. A trial of therapy is indicated in all cases, even when surgical removal is necessary, as the nodules may form again if the voice misuse is not corrected.

Vocal Misuse. This term refers to the habitual use of phonation patterns that are inappropriate for the vocal mechanism of the particular speaker. Examples are speaking or singing in a pitch range that is too

TABLE 4. **Causes of Hoarseness**

Infectious Laryngitis
Viral
- Acute viral laryngitis
- · Laryngotracheobronchitis (croup)

Bacterial
- +· Epiglottitis
- +· Diphtheria
- + Infectious mononucleosis
- Tuberculosis
- Actinomycosis *(Actinomyces israeli)*
- + Syphilis
- · Rhinoscleroma *(Klebsiella rhinoscleromatis)*
- +· Deep space neck abscesses

Fungal
- Candidiasis
- Histoplasmosis
- Blastomycosis
- Coccidioidomycosis

Granulomatous Diseases
- · Sarcoidosis
- · Wegener's granulomatosis

Immune Diseases
- +· Rheumatoid arthritis
- Systemic lupus erythematosus
- Polymyositis
- · Relapsing polychondritis
- Pemphigus vulgaris

Systemic Disorders
- Hypothyroidism (myxedema)
- Amyloidosis
- +· Scleroderma

Neurologic Disorders
- +· Vocal fold paralysis or paresis
- Spasmodic dysphonia
- Essential tremor
- + Stroke
- + Supranuclear palsy
- + Pseudobulbar palsy
- + Cerebellar disorders
- + Multiple sclerosis
- + Parkinson's disease
- +· Multiple systems atrophy
- +· Amyotrophic lateral sclerosis
- Myasthenia gravis

Allergy
- Chronic allergic edema
- +· Angioneurotic edema
- · Spasmodic croup

Neoplasia
- · Papilloma
- Keratosis
- Malignancy

Congenital Malformations
- · Laryngomalacia
- · Vocal fold paralysis
- · Subglottic hemangioma
- · Subglottic stenosis
- · Laryngeal cysts/laryngoceles
- · Laryngeal web
- +· Laryngeal cleft

Laryngeal Trauma
- Endotracheal intubation
- After laryngeal surgery
- +· Upper aerodigestive tract foreign bodies
- +· Blunt and penetrating injuries
- · Toxic inhalation
- +· Caustic ingestion

Chronic Laryngitis
- Smoking
- Irritative inhalants
- Gastroesophageal reflux
  - Ulcers/granulomas
- Chronic vomiting (bulimia nervosa)
- Vocal abuse and misuse
  - Vocal nodules
- Reinke's edema
- · Polyps
- Muscle tension dysphonia

Presbylaryngis

Psychogenic Dysphonia

Other
- · Idiopathic midline destructive disease

· Patient may present with hoarseness and stridor.
+Patient may present with hoarseness and dysphagia.

high or too low, using inadequate breath support, or using excessive tension in the neck and laryngeal muscles. Vocal abuse, the exuberant overuse of the larynx for shouting, loud talking, or coughing, is more acutely traumatizing to the vocal cords.

Although vocal misuse is the main cause of some vocal fold lesions that result in hoarseness, it is also contributory to many others. For example, vocal abuse and misuse may not be present at the onset of hoarseness secondary to a chronic irritative laryngitis. However, in an effort to compensate for vocal impairment, the patient will often develop harmful speech patterns, such as increased tension in the jaw and neck muscles. A vicious circle develops in which the pathologic changes in the vocal fold mucosa, the abnormal voice quality, and the compensatory speaking techniques perpetuate, even exacerbate, each other. For this reason, elimination of the faulty vocal habits is always warranted even when they are believed to be secondary.

Muscle Tension Dysphonia. This term refers to hoarseness in a larynx that appears to be structurally and functionally normal. Usually, subtle patterns of excessive tension in the laryngeal and neck muscles can be identified. This is basically a condition due to a form of vocal misuse that may eventually result in mucosal changes if it is left untreated.

TREATMENT. Identification and elimination of vocal misuse habits usually require consultation with a speech pathologist who has had extensive experience in managing voice disorders.

Neurogenic Disorders

Vocal Fold Paralysis

Unilateral vocal fold paralysis is the most common neurogenic voice disorder in adults. The voice is characterized by weakness and breathiness that ranges from complete aphonia to an essentially normal voice that tends to fatigue at the end of the day. Any mass lesion, injury, or destructive process along the course of the recurrent laryngeal nerve can cause paralysis. Briefly, the nerve travels as part of the 10th cranial nerve (vagus) from the brain stem and base of skull into the neck, where it separates, goes into the mediastinum, and curves around the subclavian on the right and the aortic arch on the left before returning to the neck and the larynx. The primary care physician may want to initiate the evaluation of a vocal fold paralysis, which entails ruling out thyroid masses and obtaining a magnetic resonance image of the head, base of the skull, neck, and mediastinum. Locating the level of the nerve disruption is simplified if there is a history of recent trauma, endotracheal intubation, or surgery of the base of the skull, neck, or chest. At least 30% of vocal fold paralysis is idiopathic; virus-induced neuropathy is often suspected but has not yet been proved in such cases. Many neurodegenerative disorders produce characteristic alterations in the voice, usually as a result of vocal fold paralysis or paresis.

Bilateral vocal fold paralysis suggests a central lesion such as Arnold-Chiari malformation and usually is exhibited as airway obstruction with a fairly normal voice. An infant with unilateral vocal fold paralysis may present with significant airway compromise as a result of the small size of the larynx.

Treatment. At least half of idiopathic vocal fold paralysis and most crush injuries from trauma or surgery recover spontaneously with full movement of the affected side. It is also common for varying amounts of recovery to take place even when the vocal fold remains paralyzed, probably because of increased tone in the laryngeal muscles as a result of random reinnervation. Voice therapy is helpful in facilitating recovery. Voice changes secondary to neurodegenerative disorders will show little spontaneous improvement but may receive some benefit from voice therapy. For the patients who continue to have problems, a surgical procedure may be indicated. The available techniques all result in medializing the paralyzed vocal fold to improve contact with the mobile opposite fold during speech. Augmentation of the paralyzed fold with injected Gelfoam, collagen, or Teflon is the simplest method. Thyroplasty involves medialization by external placement of a laryngeal implant. Reinnervation by selective nerve graft to the damaged recurrent laryngeal nerve is also performed.

Spasmodic Dysphonia

Spasmodic dysphonia (SD) is believed to be a type of focal dystonia that affects the laryngeal muscles during phonated speech. This classification is reinforced by the occurrence of associated dystonias such as blepharospasm or torticollis in some SD patients. In spasmodic dysphonia, the voice is abnormal and effortful but the larynx has no lesions or structural abnormalities. However, there are characteristic laryngeal movements that correlate with the abnormal voice quality. In adductor spasmodic dysphonia, the vocal folds are adducted with abnormal force and duration, resulting in harsh, strained, choppy speech. The voice in the less common abductor spasmodic dysphonia is perceived as weak and breathy, even sobbing. During abductor voice breaks, the vocal folds are observed to remain apart for an abnormally long pause, allowing excessive air escape before vocal fold adduction and speech are resumed. Both the tightness of adductor SD and the breathiness of abductor SD are often described as hoarseness.

Treatment. Voice therapy may be all that is needed in mild cases of spasmodic dysphonia. However, for most cases of adductor SD, botulinum toxin injections* into the laryngeal muscles is the treatment of choice. Usually, 5 to 15 units is injected into one vocal fold or 1 to 3 units into each fold. This form of chemical denervation is usually effective for 3 to 5 months, at which time the symptoms return and reinjection is necessary. Botulinum toxin injections have limited success in abductor SD.

Neoplastic Lesions

Papilloma

Squamous cell papilloma is the most common benign tumor of the larynx at any age. There is a higher incidence in children, although the incidence appears to be rising in adults. Papilloma growth in adults is not as aggressive, with less spread and less recurrence after removal.

Juvenile Laryngeal Papillomatosis. Squamous cell papilloma occurring laryngeally in children usually appears with marked hoarseness as an early sign. The growths first appear between 6 months and 6 years of age. The papillomas tend to recur, requiring multiple removal procedures until their recurrence rate dramatically subsides or disappears at puberty. Although the condition is occasionally self-limited, usually the wartlike tumors spread aggressively from the vocal folds to the rest of the larynx and even to the respiratory mucosa in the airway above and below. Prevention of airway obstruction is the primary concern.

Treatment. Meticulous microscopic ablation with the CO_2 laser is the mainstay of therapy. The papillomas tend to recur, requiring multiple removal procedures until their recurrence rate dramatically subsides or disappears at puberty. Biopsies should be taken routinely during laser surgery because there is a low incidence of malignant transformation. Interferon given intramuscularly for a period of 6 to 12 months is used in cases that cannot be controlled with laser excision alone.

Squamous Cell Carcinoma

By far the most common malignant tumor of the larynx is squamous cell carcinoma. Invariably the patient is a long-term smoker, usually a male. Lesions most often occur first on the vocalis or glottic portion of the vocal fold.

---

*Not FDA approved for this indication.

Treatment. In most cases, hoarseness is an early sign in cancer of the larynx, allowing detection while the tumor is still confined to the glottic vocal fold and is curable with radiation or limited surgery. More advanced tumors require extensive surgery, which may require total removal of the larynx, radical neck dissection, and radiation.

The Aging Voice

The voice of the elderly person is often weak, breathy, and slightly tremulous. These qualities are a result of normal degenerative changes in the neurologic and soft tissues of the aging larynx. The decrease in muscle tone, tissue bulk, and elasticity of the vocal folds results in a bowed appearance of the vocal folds as they fail to tense properly during phonation. The persistent gap, or at best, a weak closure between the lax vocal folds allows an excessive escape of air during speech, producing a breathy, weak quality. The same neurodegenerative changes that produce tremor in other parts of the body also affect the larynx.

Treatment. Therapy for age-associated voice changes is usually sought only when the symptoms are severe or when the patient has a continuing need for vigorous verbal communication. Voice therapy is always indicated in these cases. Also, collagen injection of the vocal folds and thyroplasty have been reported as beneficial.

INSOMNIA

method of
WALLACE B. MENDELSON, M.D.
The Cleveland Clinic Foundation
Cleveland, Ohio

In many ways, insomnia is a symptom that is analogous to pain. If a patient were to enter the office complaining of chest pain, one would formulate a differential diagnosis to discover the etiology of this uncomfortable subjective experience. If a patient describes long-standing difficulty sleeping, similar reasoning applies. If one uses a "decision tree" approach to consider a differential diagnosis, a specific etiology and treatment can usually be derived.

ETIOLOGY

Our focus here is on chronic insomnia, a complaint of inadequate quantity or quality of sleep that has persisted for at least 1 month. Acute insomnias, those that have lasted for only a few days or weeks, generally are caused by obvious stresses, medical illnesses, or changes in sleep schedule. In most cases, these are self-limiting conditions, and the appropriate response is counseling patience, addressing the cause if feasible (e.g., responding to a medical illness causing poor sleep), and possibly temporarily administering sedative or hypnotic medication. A similar logic applies to intermittent insomnia, which is usually due to recurring stresses, changes in sleeping location, or illness. Chronic insomnia presents a much more complex situation.

TABLE 1. **Causes of Chronic Insomnia, Divided by Type of Complaint**

Difficulty Staying Asleep
Medication
Drug or alcohol abuse
Psychiatric disorders
Medical disorders
Primary sleep disorders: sleep apnea, nocturnal myoclonus
Difficulty Falling Asleep
Phase lag syndrome
Restless legs syndrome
Conditioned insomnia
Poor sleep hygiene

One useful approach is to formulate a differential diagnosis that begins with a description of the type of sleep complaint (Table 1). Let us first consider patients who complain of difficulties with sleep maintenance (e.g., frequent awakenings during the night). Among the first things to check is the possibility that sleep is disturbed by a medication the patient is receiving. Among common offenders are beta blockers, thyroid preparations, steroids including birth control pills, fluoxetine (Prozac), MAO inhibitors, desipramine (Norpramin), methyldopa (Aldomet), phenytoin (Dilantin), cancer chemotherapy, buspirone (BuSpar), and stimulants. (Conversely, acute withdrawal from a variety of sedatives and hypnotics may disturb sleep, but this is generally a self-limited process that lasts only a few days.) If any of these drugs are being taken, the best treatment is generally to decrease dosage or change medications, if feasible. Sometimes, this cannot be done, and all one can do is explain the situation to the patient and assure him or her that sleep will return to normal when the medication is discontinued. In the case of fluoxetine and MAO inhibitors, some papers have indicated that adding a low dose of trazodone (Desyrel)* at bedtime improves sleep. This is often useful, but one should be aware of the possibility of marked sedation or (rarely) confusional states, which can occur.

Another cause of chronic poor sleep can be alcohol or other drug abuse. Although it is common clinical experience that alcoholics have difficulty sleeping while they are drinking, it is also important to remember that very fragmented sleep may continue to occur for up to 2 years or so after these patients have stopped drinking. Abuse of a variety of agents, including cocaine, stimulants, and marijuana, may be associated with either poor sleep or alternating periods of hypersomnolence and insomnia. Rarely, cocaine use may cause inflammation of the nostrils sufficient to result in sleep apnea syndrome in susceptible individuals.

It is important to consider psychiatric disorders, particularly depression, as a cause of poor sleep. Indeed, a major epidemiologic study conducted by the National Institute of Mental Health has indicated that individuals who complain of poor sleep, and continue to do so after one year, are almost 40 times more likely to have a diagnosable psychiatric condition than those with no sleep complaints. Certainly, the most important among these complaints is major depression, both because it is so common and because giving a hypnotic to a patient with unrecognized depression may be unwittingly providing him or her with a method for suicide. Questions that are useful in looking for depression include those directed at uncovering affective and somatic symptoms (Table 2). If depression is thought to be the cause

*Not FDA approved for this indication.

TABLE 2. **Symptoms Suggestive of Major Depression in a Patient Complaining of Poor Sleep**

Affective Complaints
Depressed mood for at least several weeks
Irritability or suspiciousness
Feelings of hopelessness or helplessness
Loss of interest in sports, hobbies
Suicidal ideation or history of suicidal attempts

Somatic Symptoms
Change in appetite or weight
Decreased energy
Decreased libido
Poor sleep, especially early morning awakening

of the poor sleep, one should give the specific treatment, such as one of the tricyclic antidepressants. If sleep continues to be a difficulty, one can give a particularly sedating tricyclic such as amitriptyline (Elavil) or trimipramine (Surmontil) in a bedtime dose, either as the main treatment or in addition to a less sedating agent. Usually, this therapy will improve sleep rapidly, although it is unlikely to change the rapidity of the overall antidepressant response; just an improvement in sleep, however, is often taken by the patient as an encouraging sign that gives hope. Of course, it is also important to remember that tricyclics can be lethal in an overdose, and that they must be administered cautiously in potentially suicidal patients. Other psychiatric conditions that may be associated with poor sleep include generalized anxiety disorder, panic disorder, mania, and acute psychotic episodes.

The cause of poor sleep is often the same medical disorder that led to the primary care consultation. Examples might range from an elderly patient kept awake by pain from arthritis to a congestive heart failure patient receiving diuretics who needs to get up frequently to urinate. In these cases, the best strategy is to address the underlying medical illness itself. Thus, in the case of the arthritic patient, the best pharmacologic aid to sleep may be an analgesic rather than a hypnotic; in the congestive failure patient, readjustment of the diuretic schedule may be the most important intervention. The principle is the same for medical or psychiatric conditions: Treat the underlying disorder, and the sleep difficulty will usually resolve itself.

CLINICAL EVALUATION

Primary disorders of sleep are often found in patients with chronic insomnia. Sleep apnea is often divided into obstructive and central types. Although there is a great deal of overlap of symptoms, the general finding is that the obstructive form is more often associated with sleepiness, whereas the central form is more likely to result in insomnia. Central sleep apnea can occur at any age, but tends to be a disorder of the elderly. It is more difficult to diagnose in the office, because it is less often associated with snoring or obesity. In these cases, it is important to ask the spouse whether he or she has observed the patient to stop breathing during sleep. If sleep apnea is suspected, a visit to the sleep laboratory may be warranted. Regardless of whether a formal work-up is performed, if sleep apnea seems to be the likely diagnosis, it is important not to give medications that are respiratory suppressants, such as the commonly used hypnotics. Treatments that are sometimes useful in mixed or central apnea include protriptyline (Vivactil),* low doses of medroxyprogesterone acetate (Provera),* and acetazolamide (Diamox).* Although it is not yet well established in the literature, some clinicians have found that continuous positive airway pressure (CPAP), a major treatment for obstructive apnea, is effective in central apnea as well.

*Not FDA approved for this indication.

Periodic leg movement disorder (nocturnal myoclonus) is characterized by rhythmic kicking movements of the legs during sleep. The patient whose daytime neurologic examination is normal and whose waking electroencephalogram usually does not show seizure activity is generally unaware of these events. Clues from the office interview may come from asking the spouse about the patient's leg movements and enquiring whether the covers stay neatly on the bed at night or whether they end up being rumpled or on the floor. The treatment of choice for nocturnal myoclonus is usually the benzodiazepines. Perhaps the best well-known one used for this purpose is clonazepam (Klonopin).* Because of difficulties with daytime sleepiness, however, many clinicians prefer to use shorter-acting agents such as triazolam (Halcion)* or temazepam (Restoril).*

Difficulty with sleep onset may result from a variety of causes. Phase lag syndrome is a condition in which the body clock that regulates sleep and wakefulness runs in a stable but delayed relationship to the environment. A patient has trouble going to sleep because, although in the external world it may be midnight, the nervous system reacts as if it were 9:00 or 10:00 P.M. Thus, the complaint is both inability to fall asleep at conventional bedtimes and difficulty getting up in the morning. Some clues in the history are that once the patient does fall asleep, the sleep is usually sound, and that the patient believes that if he or she could go to bed at 2:00 or 3:00 A.M. every night and get up mid-morning that everything would be okay. Among the treatments for phase lag syndrome is exposure of the patient to bright light at conventional wake-up times in the morning. Another approach is to have the patient go to bed 2 hours later each night progressively until he or she has in effect moved around the clock to a more conventional bedtime.

Restless legs syndrome usually occurs in conjunction with nocturnal myoclonus (although many patients have myoclonus without having restless legs syndrome). In this condition, patients describe an uncomfortable feeling (which they often decline to characterize as pain) that appears at rest and is relieved by moving about. It is difficult to go to sleep because of the frequent need to get up and walk around to relieve this uncomfortable feeling. Restless legs syndrome often occurs in conjunction with anemia (either iron or B_{12} deficiency) or renal failure, and can transiently occur in patients after surgery. Treatment (aside from dealing with the related medical condition) may include baclofen (Lioresal),* carbamazepine (Tegretol),* levodopa (Laradopa),* and in very severe cases, the narcotic analgesics.

Conditioned insomnia, also known as psychophysiologic insomnia, results from a situation in which the act of going to bed triggers anxiety and other responses that are incompatible with sleep. The cues that trigger this response may be internal (disturbing thoughts such as "Oh boy, now I'm in for it") or external (the bedroom environment, which the patient associates with poor sleep). In summary, the worry about not sleeping has become a major contributor to the inability to sleep. Clues in the history are that the patient

*Not FDA approved for this indication.

TABLE 3. **Sleep Hygiene**

Try going to bed at about the same time every night
Reduce the total time in bed slightly
Reduce or stop consumption of nicotine, caffeine, and alcohol
Exercise, preferably in the late afternoon or evening
Worry about your troubles before going to bed, not in bed
For most (but not all persons), it is better not to take naps
Try a light snack at bedtime
Remember that not all of these rules work for all people; try them and pick the ones that seem best for you

is able to sleep when he or she is not trying to (e.g., when watching television in the living room) and that he or she sleeps better away from the bedroom, such as when on a trip. Training in sleep hygiene, which is discussed in the following section, can be useful, as can teaching the patient the principles of stimulus control therapy. In summary, this involves stripping the bedroom of all activities except sleep and sex, and instructing the patient that if he or she is ever lying in bed unable to sleep, to get up and go into another room. The principle is to avoid the association in the patient's mind of the bedroom being a place where one lies in bed unable to sleep.

TREATMENT

Psychological Treatment

Poor sleep hygiene is often a major contributor to poor sleep, either by itself or as a complication of some of the difficulties we have already described. Some of the principles involved appear in Table 3. Usually, it is difficult to implement all of these measures at once, and many clinicians prefer to concentrate on the one or two that seem most relevant to the particular patient. Many patients spend their time in bed worrying about the events of the day and planning tomorrow's battles. Some suggestions for avoiding this are to ask the patient to schedule a "worry time" during the evening and encourage him or her to worry then but not later when in bed. Another technique is to ask the patient to write out a list of worries, put it on the dresser, and to promise to look at it first thing in the morning in exchange for not thinking about it at night.

For patients who do not respond to sleep hygiene, one can also make a referral to a sleep center or a behaviorally oriented therapist for behavioral treatment of insomnia. There are many techniques available, which are listed in Table 4. Different therapists vary in their approach, but in general, this is a form of short-term therapy. In our clinic, for instance, most patients would come once a week for 2 or 3 months.

TABLE 4. **A Sampling of Behavioral Techniques**

Jacobsonian relaxation therapy
Sleep restriction
Stimulus control
Biofeedback
Imagery techniques
Desensitization by reciprocal inhibition
Paradoxical intention

During that time, we expose them to a variety of techniques and then ask them to help choose a package that seems right for them. As in all behavioral therapy, the emphasis is on empowering the patient to help himself or herself.

Medical Treatment

Finally, one must consider the role of hypnotic medications. As we mentioned earlier, the short-term use of these drugs can be very helpful in the acute insomnias. In the chronic insomnias, their use is more limited. Although guidelines are still being developed, most people in the field agree that long-term nightly use is probably not a good strategy. Short-term administration, while the patient is developing skills at sleeping using sleep hygiene and other behavioral interventions, can be helpful. One strategy is to give medication intermittently. When a patient is working on behavioral strategies in ongoing therapy for instance, we will often give a prescription for perhaps two nights a week. In effect we make a contract with the patient, which might be expressed something like this: "I know you are skeptical about learning to help yourself sleep by behavioral techniques. Work with me this way, and while you do, with an intermittent supply of pills you will never need to go more than two nights without a good night's sleep." The medication can also be useful as a benchmark; one can ask the patient how the relaxation or improved sleep from a behavioral method compares to that induced by a drug. Generally, the short-acting agents (benzodiazepines or new nonbenzodiazepines, such as zolpidem [Ambien]) are preferable because they minimize unwanted daytime sedation. In summary, the use of medication does not seem to be contradictory to nonpharmacologic approaches, and indeed, there is some suggestion that the two methods may be complementary.

PRURITUS
(Itching)

method of
JEFFREY D. BERNHARD, M.D.
University of Massachusetts Medical School
Worcester, Massachusetts

and

ELIZABETH F. SHERERTZ, M.D., and
JOSEPH L. JORIZZO, M.D.
Bowman Gray School of Medicine of Wake Forest University
Winston-Salem, North Carolina

Pruritus (itching) may be defined as an unpleasant sensation that evokes the inclination to scratch. Itching is the most common symptom of skin diseases and may also be troublesome in a patient without any visible signs of a primary skin problem. The pathophysiology of pruritus is incompletely understood: Depending on the disease or triggering factors, different mediators may be involved in the itch sensation. Histamine is an important mediator that can cause itching (e.g., in urticaria), but prostaglandins, leukotrienes, vasoactive and neuroactive peptides, kinins, and opioid peptides (e.g., itching after epidural morphine) may cause itching in different disease states. This explains why antihistamines are ineffective for many patients with pruritus, depending on the underlying diagnosis. The more clear the patient's diagnosis, the easier the choice of therapy to help control the itching.

DIAGNOSIS

Before symptomatic therapy for pruritus is initiated, a systematic approach to diagnosis should be undertaken. This can be conducted in a stepwise fashion. If skin disease is present, look for primary lesions that have not been scratched: Are there papules or vesicles? Is there dermatographism (a wheal and flare or linear "hive" at the site of scratching)? Is there dry, scaling skin? In a patient who has an acute onset of itching, the skin diseases most commonly associated are urticaria, contact dermatitis, scabies, insect bites, and dry skin. The list of skin disorders that can cause pruritus is extensive and is summarized in Table 1. Many of these disorders have diagnostic clinical appearances. For the common disorders, historical points, such as exposure to outside agents (e.g., poison ivy, fiberglass), and affected family members (e.g., scabies), drug ingestion, or flea-infested pets, may be very helpful in establishing the correct diagnosis. Overbathing and low ambient humidity (as in heated air in winter) may point to xerosis (dry skin). If the skin eruption is not recognizable, dermatologic consultation should be sought to help confirm a specific diagnosis.

TABLE 1. **Selected Skin Disorders Associated with Pruritus**

Common (Often Acute)
Asteatosis (xerosis, dry skin)
Contact dermatitis (irritant and allergic)
Scabies, pediculosis
Insect bites, flea bites
Urticaria, dermatographism
Varicella
Pityriasis rosea
Sunburn
Miliaria rubra (prickly heat)
Drug hypersensitivity
Common (Often Subacute or Chronic)
Atopic dermatitis (eczema)
Psoriasis
Dermatophytosis (ringworm)
Folliculitis
Lichen planus
Lichen simplex chronicus
Other physical urticarias (e.g., cold, solar, pressure)
Diminutive variants of urticaria (e.g., aquagenic pruritus)
Uncommon or Rare
Dermatitis herpetiformis
Bullous pemphigoid
Polymorphous light eruption
Mycosis fungoides (cutaneous T cell lymphoma)
Mastocytosis
Exfoliative dermatitis
Prurigo nodularis

TABLE 2. **Selected Systemic Conditions That May Be Associated with Generalized Pruritus**

Condition	Suggested Laboratory Tests
Chronic renal failure	Urine analysis, blood urea nitrogen (BUN), creatinine
Cholestatic liver disease	Bilirubin, alkaline phosphatase, aspartate amino-transferase (AST)
Hematologic disease	Complete blood count, differential
Hyperthyroidism	Thyroid panel
Occult malignancy (e.g., Hodgkin's disease)	Chest x-ray study (other work-up as indicated by history/physical examination)
Drug reaction	
Infestations/parasitosis	
Pregnancy	
Psychiatric illness	

When diagnostic primary skin lesions are not present or if only nonspecific or secondary changes such as scratch marks (excoriations) are seen, a different approach should be taken to evaluate the symptom of itching. Consideration needs to be given to the possibility that a systemic condition could be causing the pruritus, particularly chronic renal failure, cholestatic liver disease, hematologic disease, malignancy (especially Hodgkin's disease), and hyperthyroidism. The patient's history and general physical examination are critically important. Pay special attention to adenopathy and organomegaly. Table 2 lists some of the associated systemic illnesses and an approach to screening laboratory studies. Such a work-up may be indicated in a patient without a diagnosed skin disease who has generalized pruritus occurring daily for more than 2 weeks (PUO, pruritus of undetermined origin). Tests should be tailored to the individual patient's presentation to realize a more cost-effective yield. Since HIV infection and AIDS may lead to itching or to exacerbation of pruritic skin diseases, HIV testing may be indicated in some cases.

The possibility of drug-induced itching should not be overlooked. Opiate analgesic agents (e.g., epidural morphine) may cause severe itching without skin lesions. Other drugs that may cause itching include aspirin, quinidine, B complex vitamins, and drugs that can cause hepatic cholestasis such as phenothiazines, systemic hormonal therapy, and erythromycin estolate (Ilosone). The most common forms of localized pruritus—pruritus ani and pruritus vulvae—are discussed in another article.

SYMPTOMATIC TREATMENT OF ITCHING

General Patient Education and Topical Therapy

Some environmental factors can make itching worse, no matter what the underlying cause. Skin that is dry is more prone to itching, so that the frequency of bathing should be decreased, deodorant soaps should be discontinued, and milder products such as Dove or Cetaphil cleanser should be substituted. The temperature of the bath should not be too hot, because it may temporarily bring relief only to cause the itch to worsen afterward. The addition of baking soda, up to 1 cup per tub bath, or oilated oatmeal bath products (Aveeno) can also be soothing to the patient who itches. Older patients should be cautioned about getting into or out of a slippery tub.

Towel-drying should be done by patting rather than vigorous rubbing. Use of a bath oil or moisturizer applied immediately after bathing to help replenish moisture in the skin may also help. Fragrance-free products such as Eucerin cream, DML lotion, fragrance-free Lubriderm, Lacticare, or Vaseline are useful examples. Increasing humidity in the patient's environment through the use of a humidifier or open pans of water may help. Irritating fabrics such as wool and some textured synthetics should be avoided. The use of anti-static fabric softeners that are added to the dryer cycle should be discontinued because use of these products has been anecdotally associated with itching.

Heat triggers itching, so the patient with pruritus should avoid excessively warm environments by lowering the thermostat, using fewer bedcovers, or reducing exercise temporarily. Reduced intake of hot, spicy foods, alcohol, and caffeine may be helpful. Emotional stress may also worsen itching of any cause, and patients should be made aware of that fact.

Availability of specific topical treatment for pruritus is limited. Over-the-counter treatments containing anesthetic (such as benzocaine) or antihistamines (diphenhydramine [Benadryl]) should be avoided, because these products can cause contact dermatitis in some individuals. Preparations containing pramoxine (PrameGel, Prax) or those containing combinations of menthol and camphor (Sarna), applied several times daily, may give symptomatic relief. When inflammation accompanies xerosis, the addition of 1% hydrocortisone cream twice daily for 5 or 6 days is often helpful. Otherwise, the use of topical corticosteroids should be reserved for patients with diagnosed steroid-responsive inflammatory dermatoses, such as acute contact dermatitis. (See specific articles on skin disease.) Topical corticosteroids are usually not helpful for patients with urticaria. Be aware of the specific products a patient is using on his or her skin, so as not to overlook a subtle contact dermatitis due to the topical treatment as a cause of the pruritus.

TABLE 3. **Selected Antihistamines for Use in Symptomatic Treatment of Pruritus (Itching)**

Antihistamine	Adult Dose (mg)	Dosing Interval (h)	Sedation
Diphenhydramine (Benadryl)	25–50	6–8	+ + +
Hydroxyzine (Atarax, Vistaril)	10–25	6–8	+ + +
Chlorpheniramine (Chlor-Trimeton)	4	4–6	+ +
Clemastine (Tavist)	2.68	12	+ +
Trimeprazine (Temaril)	2.5	8	+ +
Cyproheptadine (Periactin)	4	8	+
Terfenadine (Seldane)	60	12	–
Astemizole (Hismanal)	10	24	–
Loratadine (Claritin)	10	24	–

Systemic Therapy

Oral antihistamines, such as diphenhydramine (Benadryl), hydroxyzine (Atarax, Vistaril), clemastine (Tavist) and trimeprazine (Temaril), are the agents most often used first to control itching. Suggested doses of antihistamines are given in Table 3. These agents are most helpful in histamine-mediated pruritic conditions, such as urticaria, but may also alleviate itching through their sedative effects. The antihistamines are more helpful if they are taken in adequate dosage at regular intervals, rather than taken on a PRN, or as-needed, basis. Bedtime dosing is useful, because itching is often worse at bedtime, and dosages may be increased to tolerance (sedation, dry mouth) under supervision. If no relief is obtained, switching to another type of antihistamine or combining agents of different chemical classes may be helpful. Nonsedating antihistamines such as terfenadine (Seldane, 60 mg every 12 hours), astemizole (Hismanal, 10 mg at bedtime), and loratadine (Claritin, 10 mg once daily) are useful in chronic urticaria. It takes 6 days for astemizole to reach steady-state plasma concentrations, and thus it is not useful for acute pruritus. Terfenadine may be suggested for a patient for whom there is great concern about sedating side effects of other antihistamines, but it is of limited efficacy for acute itching in our experience. Loratadine has a rapid onset of action, usually within 2 hours.

Other systemic agents for the treatment of itching should be reserved until a specific diagnosis has been made. Systemic corticosteroids should not be used because they are ineffective, have side effects, and may mask the underlying diagnosis. Tricyclic antidepressant agents, such as doxepin (Sinequan),* have antihistamine properties that may be useful at times and are used in oral dosages of 10 to 25 mg up to three times daily. H_2 histamine antagonists such as cimetidine (Tagamet)* may be useful in treating the itching associated with Hodgkin's disease. Oral cholestyramine (Questran, 5 mg twice daily) is helpful in controlling itching due to hepatic and sometimes renal disease. Ultraviolet B phototherapy is the treatment of choice for the itching experienced by some hemodialysis-dependent patients with chronic renal failure and has been helpful in controlling pruritus in some other situations. PUVA (oral methoxsalen photochemotherapy) may be indicated in others. It is often in the patient's interest for the physician to consult with a dermatologist prior to initiating systemic therapy other than antihistamines for the treatment of pruritus. (For further detailed information, see Bernhard JD: Itch: Mechanisms and Management of Pruritus. New York, McGraw-Hill, 1994.)

*Not FDA approved for this indication.

TINNITUS

method of
LAURA L. DOWNEY, M.D., and
PAUL E. HAMMERSCHLAG, M.D.
New York University Medical Center
New York, New York

Tinnitus is an abnormal perception of sound that is unrelated to an external stimulus. It is estimated that approximately 36 million Americans suffer from this disorder even though a minority of patients describe it as severe and disabling. Thus, tinnitus continues to receive clinical interest in its diagnosis and treatment.

CLASSIFICATION

Tinnitus is often divided in two categories—objective and subjective. Though this division can offer some aid in diagnosis, overlap of symptoms prohibits this classification from accurately identifying a cause.

Objective tinnitus classically refers to sound that can be heard both by the patient and by the examiner (with the aid of a stethoscope or ear tube, or both). This symptom often suggests a vascular or mechanical origin (Table 1). Vascular causes include arteriovenous malformations, carotid and other arterial bruits, and venous hums. In these instances, the patient may report pulsatile tinnitus or increasing symptoms with increased blood flow. On examination, the patient may have audible bruits of the neck or mastoid or have a lesion in the middle ear visible with otoscopy. Compression of neck vascular structures may suppress pulsatile tinnitus. Mechanical causes of tinnitus include a patulous eustachian tube and spasms of palate and stapedius muscles.

In contrast, subjective tinnitus can be heard only by the patient. It is thought to represent an electrophysiologic pathology. Underlying causes include otologic, metabolic, pharmacologic, infectious, and neoplastic disorders.

WORKUP

The evaluation of tinnitus begins with the patient's history. Description of the sound should include frequency, location, pitch, and pulsations. Tinnitus that varies in severity may indicate a fluctuating hearing loss, which is characteristic of endolymphatic hydrops or syphilis. Unilateral tinnitus may be associated with retrocochlear pathology, such as acoustic neuroma. High-pitched tinnitus often occurs with high-frequency sensorineural hearing loss. Associated symptoms such as ear pain may suggest acute infection, neoplasm, or temporomandibular joint syndrome as a cause.

TABLE 1. **Causes of Tinnitus**

Vascular	**Metabolic**
AV malformations	Diabetes
Bruits	Thyroid disease
Venous hums	Hyperlipidemia
Aneurysms	Demyelinating disease (MS)
Mechanical	**Pharmacologic**
Eustachian tube dysfunction	Aspirin; Aminoglycosides
Temporomandibular joint disease	Caffeine; NSAIDs
	Nicotine; Quinine
Otologic	Propranolol; Antidepressants
SNHL	**Infectious/Neoplastic**
CHL	Syphilis
Meniere's disease	Acoustic neuroma
Chronic otitis media	AIDS
Middle ear effusions	Autoimmune diseases

Abbreviations: AIDS, acquired immune deficiency syndrome; AV, arteriovenous; MS, multiple sclerosis; SNHL, sensorineural hearing loss; CHL, conductive hearing loss; NSAIDs, nonsteroidal anti-inflammatory drugs.

The patient's medical history should include inquiries about metabolic disease (diabetes and hyperlipidemia may cause capillary obstruction, possibly contributing to sensorineural hearing loss and tinnitus; hyperthyroidism may cause increased cardiac output resulting in pulsatile tinnitus), infectious disease (e.g., syphilis, acquired immune deficiency syndrome [AIDS], Lyme disease), autoimmune disease (e.g., systemic lupus erythematosus [SLE], rheumatoid arthritis), hypertension (which may increase blood flow and cause otherwise asymptomatic pulsatile tinnitus to become symptomatic), renal abnormalities (which alter renal clearance of drugs, rendering patients more sensitive to ototoxic medications), and psychiatric illness (anxiety and depression can make a patient less adaptable to the tinnitus). Medications, such as aspirin, can cause reversible tinnitus. Ototoxic medications, including aminoglycosides, cisplatin, and furosemide, may cause permanent hearing loss, or tinnitus, or both. A family history of hearing loss may suggest a genetic sensorineural hearing loss or otosclerosis, both of which are associated with tinnitus.

A complete head and neck examination should be performed. Pertinent otologic findings include perforations and infections (acute or chronic); these can render the ear more sensitive to labyrinthitis, leading to high-frequency sensorineural hearing loss and tinnitus. The nasopharynx should be examined to determine the patency of the eustachian tube orifice, which may be affected by enlarged adenoids or an occult carcinoma. A cranial nerve examination should concentrate on the function of the trigeminal nerve, because it is located at the apex of the temporal bone, and the facial nerve, because it transverses the temporal bone and the lower cranial nerves, which may be involved with a disorder of the skull base. Neck auscultation to identify bruits and blood pressure measurement to evaluate hypertension completes the examination.

All patients should receive an audiogram, which includes air and bone thresholds and speech discrimination. In those patients with unilateral tinnitus, a brain stem–evoked response (BSER) or magnetic resonance imaging (MRI) with gadolinium should be obtained to screen for retrocochlear pathology. Patients with symmetric hearing loss and a normal neurologic examination usually do not require a BSER or MRI.

Routine laboratory values should include hematocrit, glucose, erythrocyte sedimentation rate (ESR) and fluorescent treponemal antibody (FTA) (the Venereal Disease Research Laboratories [VDRL] test is not sufficient because it has a 20% false-negative rate). If no obvious cause is found at this point, other laboratory tests include thyroid function tests (TFTs) (to evaluate hyperthyroidism), lipid profile (looking for hypercholesterolemia), and antinuclear antibody (ANA) titers (autoimmune diseases that cause tinnitus may be difficult to diagnose if no other symptoms of disease can be found).

TREATMENT

Specific medical problems and etiologies should be addressed. For the remainder of patients, several treatment options exist including (1) reassurance, (2) masking, (3) biofeedback, (4) electrical stimulation, (5) surgery, and (6) medications.

Reassurance

For most patients, the tinnitus is neither severe nor debilitating. Approximately 25% of patients have complete resolution of the problem; 50% will have a gradual decrease. As the patient adapts, the tinnitus may become less symptomatic. For these patients reassurance of no underlying disease (cerebrovascular accident, tumor) suffices. This group, however, should be made aware of possible exacerbating factors including noise exposure, caffeine, nicotine, anxiety, and aspirin-containing medications.

Masking

For the remaining 25% of patients, tinnitus persists or increases in intensity and further therapy is required. Masking is the most common form of therapy. It is based on the premise that externally generated sound can cover the internally produced noise. Hearing aids are the simplest devices because they amplify the outside sound. This is particularly helpful for patients with tinnitus associated with hearing loss. If a hearing aid is not appropriate, a tinnitus masker may be tried. Evaluation for this therapy first determines the pitch and loudness of the perceived tone. The device then produces a matched tone. Vernon and Meikle report that 91% of their patients had significant improvement with the use of such a tinnitus synthesizer.

Biofeedback

Biofeedback is not a specific therapy for the relief of tinnitus but is a system for managing stress. In this modality, relaxation techniques are used to decrease the patient's attention to the tinnitus. This treatment is successful when the patient and the therapist are carefully selected. Hypnosis has also been employed; however, success has been infrequent.

Electric Stimulation

The basis of this modality was House's study of 53% of cochlear implant patients, which reported a decrease in their tinnitus. Still in its infancy, electric stimulation is introduced via a single channel electrode at the tympanic membrane, round window, or mastoid. Results to date are inconclusive.

Surgery

The role of surgery solely for the relief of tinnitus is inconsistent.

Medication

Because the exact causes of tinnitus are unknown, development of effective medications has been limited. It has long been known, however, that intravenous administration of lidocaine* can suppress tinnitus. Unfortunately, this drug had several disadvantages including (1) intravenous administration, (2) a short half-life, and (3) requirement of near anesthetic doses. An oral form of lidocaine, tocainide (Tonocard),* has also been tried with varying reports of minimal success.

At present, anxiolytics and antidepressants such as alprazolam (Xanax)* and amitriptyline (Elavil)* are the mainstays of therapy. Some drugs in these classes produce a paradoxic increase in tinnitus.

The American Tinnitus Association (ATA) (P.O. Box 5, Portland, OR, 67207) is an organization whose goal is to fund research and provide information for patients and clinicians.

*Not FDA approved for this indication.

LOW BACK PAIN

method of
MARIANNE DALGAS, M.D., and
MATTHEW H. LIANG, M.D., M.P.H.
Brigham and Women's Hospital
Boston, Massachusetts

Acute low back pain is the most common musculoskeletal complaint seen in an ambulatory care setting and usually has a benign cause. Atypical clinical features (Table 1) suggest more serious diagnoses. If the patient's history and physical examination are typical, further diagnostic tests are not needed in the initial evaluation.

Imaging studies by x-ray, computed tomography (CT), and nuclear magnetic resonance imaging (MRI) in acute back pain with typical clinical features have limited usefulness. Findings such as osteophytes, narrowed disk space, lumbarization, sacralization, mild scoliosis, facet arthrosis, subluxation, and spina bifida occulta are found in the same frequency in symptomatic and asymptomatic individuals and do not necessary indicate a specific causative disorder. Degenerative changes of the disk and disk bulging (seen by CT scanning and MRI) increase with age and correlate imperfectly with symptoms. In elderly subjects, multiple findings are the rule.

Imaging studies are indicated in (1) pain not significantly relieved by bed rest, (2) new onset of back pain without antecedent trauma in a patient younger than age 15 or older than 50 years of age, (3) back pain after major trauma, (4) history or physical examination suggestive of sacroiliitis, (5) unimproved or worsening symptoms, (6) pre-

TABLE 1. **Atypical Clinical Features Associated with Low Back Pain**

Back pain not relieved by supine or Fowler's position
Constitutional symptoms
Severe back pain
Bilateral back or leg pain, or both
Neuromotor deficit
Midline point tenderness
Morning symptoms more severe than evening symptoms

vious vertebral fracture or spine surgery, (7) spinal deformity, (8) known malignancy (kidney, breast, prostate), and (9) constitutional symptoms (fever and weight loss).

TREATMENT OF LOW BACK PAIN

Of patients with acute low back pain seen in the community, 44% are better within 1 week and 92% within 1 month; only 8% have pain persisting more than 2 months. Patients with physical findings of nerve root compression from a herniated disk have a 50% chance of recovering within 1 month.

The key to treating low back pain is unloading the spine. Bed rest should be individualized, ranging from an as-needed basis for mild symptoms to nearly complete bed rest for moderate to severe symptoms. Two days of rest seems to be as effective as seven. More back rest may be needed in a patient with evidence of nerve root compression, the patient with acute muscle spasm with compensatory scoliosis, and the person who has not responded to conservative therapy and for whom surgery is being considered.

A spinal support, either a brace or a corset, limits spinal motion, corrects posture, reduces mechanical stress on the lumbosacral spine, and reminds a patient to avoid extension stress on the back. A brace and corset are alike, except that a brace has rigid horizontal elements. In general, a brace limits all motion to a greater degree, and a corset is lighter and better tolerated. During lifting, trunk muscles contract proportionally to the load being lifted. When a corset is applied, the normal activity of the muscle is diminished. Therefore, corset use begets disuse muscle atrophy. Corsets and abdominal binders should be used only as temporary measures. They may reduce time lost in the workplace, especially in people who lift as part of their work.

Medications

The administration of non-narcotic analgesics such as acetaminophen, or acetaminophen with codeine, for a limited time on an as-needed basis is usually sufficient and should be presented to the patient as an adjunct to unloading the back. Nonsteroidal anti-inflammatory drugs (NSAIDs) can be used in patients without contraindications to their use and who experience back stiffness after prolonged inactivity or who do not respond completely to analgesics. No data support the theory that any NSAID is superior to any other.

Muscle relaxants are widely promoted to treat back pain. Although they are active agents, they are no more effective than NSAIDs in treating people with acute low back pain and cause drowsiness in patients.

There are no data to support the routine use of antidepressants, oral steroids, or colchicine in managing acute back pain.

Physical Treatment

A number of spinal manipulation techniques are used to move the spine to its end range of voluntary motion followed by an impulse load. Used in the first month of acute low back pain without radiculopathy, manipulation is effective. Beyond that time, it might be tried, but there are no data to indicate that it is effective.

Hot and cold are applied with a variety of techniques such as ultrasound, laser, and diathermy. These procedures can do little harm, but there is no evidence that hot is better than cold or that the way of applying these elements matters. Patients can try these procedures if they desire but should avoid heating pads, which occasionally can lead to first-degree burns.

Therapies that have not proved effective in treating acute low back pain in controlled trials include biofeedback, traction, acupuncture, and trigger-point and facet injections with a local anesthetic.

PATIENT EDUCATION FOR PREVENTION

An important task in managing back pain of any origin is to provide instructions on how to minimize stress on the lumbosacral spine. In the erect position, the weight of the body is transmitted to the intervertebral disks in the back, particularly L4–5—the focus of most low back pathology. With normal lordosis of the spine, the major stress is on the posterior edges of the disks. Minimizing the lordosis reduces these forces. The essential lesson for individuals with low back pain is to sit, stand, walk, and lie in positions that minimize this lordosis.

These recommendations regarding activities is derived from data on intradiskal pressure correlated with surface electrodes, which provide the most reliable estimates of mechanical stress for the lumbar spine. These studies suggest that back symptoms can be minimized if individuals avoid prolonged standing, bending forward, and sitting. The patient should try to change sitting positions and have a good lumbar support. Slouching in a chair with the knees above the waist can reduce back stress. Lifting should be done with the leg muscles. The object to be lifted should be faced and brought toward the body. Twisting, bending, and reaching while lifting increase stress on the back.

Factors that contribute to extension of the spine, such as weak abdominal muscles, tight hamstrings, obesity, and wearing high heels, should be eliminated or corrected.

Low-impact exercises such as walking, biking, and swimming improve endurance, muscle strength, and flexibility and probably lead to reduced symptoms, improved function, and fewer or less severe recurrences and engage a patient in a more active role. Exercises can be started during the first 2 weeks after onset for most patients with acute low back pain. Exercise should be advised and gradually increased. Patients improve faster when given specific quotas of exercises, rather than being told to stop exercise when it produces pain. Commonly used exercises focus on back flexion, back extension, strengthening hamstrings, strengthening abdominal muscles, generalized strengthening, or some combination, but no exercise type has proved more effective than any other.

Addressing a patient's concerns and giving prognostic information establish a therapeutic relationship, allay anxiety, and engage the patient in the program. Patients with acute low back pain should be reassured that no serious signs are present and no special investigation should be conducted. Ninety percent of patients recover within 1 month. However, 65% of patients who have one significant episode will have recurrent episodes within the next few years. There is evidence that printed and audiovisual material may reduce use of medical resources, decrease patient apprehension, and increase compliance with treatment.

"Back school" is a term applied to a variety of structured programs of education about low back problems, which are usually conducted in a group setting. The results of these programs are contradictory. In the occupational setting, such a program usually includes a work-site visit, which reduces the amount of total work time lost and, possibly, recurrences.

WORK RECOMMENDATIONS

Work restrictions need to be individualized. Physical tasks of a job may require a formal work assessment by an ergonomist, physical therapist, or occupational therapist. When possible, a return to a less physically demanding job should be encouraged.

Low job satisfaction, stressful life events, and substance abuse are poor prognostic features. If symptoms continue after 1 month of conservative treatment and the evaluation is unchanged, psychosocial factors should be considered. By 3 months, referral for psychosocial management might be considered.

EPIDURAL INJECTIONS

Epidural injections of local anesthetic with or without steroids are a valuable adjunct to the management of disk disease. A few patients respond dramatically, some are partially helped, and many others get transient relief.

SURGERY

The only absolute indication for lumbar disk surgery is a midline disk herniation and progressive neurologic deficit. Surgery for low back pain should be considered in the patient with pain and functional impairment with spinal stenosis, or the patient with a herniated disk who has not responded to conservative treatment. For most patients with low back pain from a degenerated disk, surgery is not necessary.

Section 2

The Infectious Diseases

ACQUIRED IMMUNE DEFICIENCY SYNDROME (AIDS)

method of
BRIAN S. KOLL, M.D., and
DONALD ARMSTRONG, M.D.
Beth Israel Medical Center
New York, New York

Since the appearance of *Pneumocystis carinii* pneumonia (PCP) and Kaposi's sarcoma in previously healthy homosexual and bisexual young men in 1981, the acquired immune deficiency syndrome (AIDS) has evolved from a deadly medical curiosity of unknown cause into a major pandemic of a new viral disease. At the end of 1991, over 200,000 cases of AIDS in the United States have been reported to the Centers for Disease Control and Prevention (CDC). More than 60% of patients with AIDS have died. The estimated prevalence of the human immunodeficiency virus (HIV), the etiologic agent of AIDS, ranges between 1 and 2 million people infected in the United States, and between 8 and 10 million people worldwide. Because AIDS is still a fatal disease, the social and economic impact has been substantial in high-incidence areas.

EPIDEMIOLOGY

HIV is not spread by casual contact, through the use of shared household facilities, or via aerosolization. It is spread through intimate sexual contact or by parenteral contact with blood or body fluids infected with the virus (Table 1). Incidental transmission through saliva, tears, minor bites, scratches, or insect bites has no solid scientific support. HIV infection is lifelong illness. Measures used to prevent transmission include the practice of safer sex, avoidance of sharing needles and syringes, and the adoption by health care workers of precautions similar to those used for hepatitis B infection.

In the United States, AIDS still affects homosexual men more than any other risk group. Curtailment of some high-risk behaviors has resulted in a relative decline in new-case rates among homosexual men. The risk of infection from contaminated blood products has also been reduced over the past decade. However, the epidemic is expanding in large urban areas in the United States, Western Europe, Asia, and South America, with a high prevalence associated with intravenous drug abuse. Equally disturbing is the pandemic spread of AIDS in Africa, Asia, and South America, where it is primarily a heterosexual disease.

TABLE 1. **Risk Factors for Transmission of HIV**

Sexual:	Heterosexual, homosexual intercourse (use of condoms reduces the risk)
Parenteral:	Intravenous drug abuse, transfusion of blood products (rare), needle stick (rare), invasive medical/dental procedure (very rare)
Maternal to child:	Perinatal, breast-feeding
Cutaneous (very rare):	Defects in mucous membranes or skin

PATHOPHYSIOLOGY

HIV-1 was shown to be the etiologic agent of AIDS in 1984. Since then, another retrovirus, HIV-2, has also been found to infect humans and cause AIDS. HIV is an RNA virus that has an affinity for cells expressing the CD4 receptor. CD4 T helper lymphocytes, a key component of cell-mediated immunity, are depleted by HIV infection, leading to the profound immunologic defects which are the hallmark of AIDS.

Other key cells of the immune system such as macrophages are also infected by HIV. Once within the macrophage, HIV remains undetected by the body's immune surveillance system and replicates freely. Thus, the macrophage can serve as both a haven and a reservoir for HIV. It also appears that macrophage function is impaired. Macrophages can introduce HIV to the brain and contribute to the AIDS dementia complex. HIV also infects myeloid monocyte precursor cells in the bone marrow. This is believed to contribute to the pancytopenia seen in patients with AIDS. B cell impairment, as well as functional impairment of neutrophils, is also seen in patients infected with HIV. Poor antibody responses are apparently due to a breakdown in CD4 T helper lymphocytes informing B cells to produce specific antibody. The reason for the functional impairment of neutrophils is not clear.

THERAPY

The opportunistic infections seen in AIDS occur because of the spectrum of immune defects that result from infection with HIV. Infection with HIV should be considered a process that evolves from asymptomatic carriage of the virus to full-blown AIDS, as defined by the CDC (Table 2), with a number of intermediate stages referred to as AIDS-related complex (ARC). The clinical approach to infection with HIV includes prevention of infection, which was discussed in the epidemiology section, management of asymptomatic infection and ARC, and management of AIDS-associated opportunistic infections and neoplasms.

When HIV infection is suspected, an enzyme-linked immunosorbent assay (ELISA) should be used to screen for HIV antibody. If a positive test is obtained, it should be confirmed with a Western blot test. Once infection with the virus has been documented, evaluation of the patient's immune system

TABLE 2. **Summary of CDC Surveillance Criteria for the Diagnosis of AIDS**

Without Laboratory Evidence of HIV Infection and with Definitive Evidence of:
Candidiasis of the esophagus, trachea, bronchi, or lungs
Cryptococcosis, extrapulmonary
Cryptosporidiosis with diarrhea lasting > 1 month
Herpes simplex esophagitis, bronchitis, pneumonitis; or mucocutaneous disease > 1 month
Cytomegalovirus disease of an organ other than liver, spleen, or lymph nodes in a patient > 1 month of age
Kaposi's sarcoma in a patient < 60 years of age
Primary brain lymphoma in a patient < 60 years of age
Lymphoid interstitial pneumonia in a patient < 13 years of age
Disseminated *Mycobacterium-avium* complex or *M. kansasii* disease
Pneumocystis carinii pneumonia
Progressive multifocal leukoencephalopathy
Toxoplasmosis of the brain in a patient > 1 month of age

With Laboratory Evidence of HIV Infection and:
A CD4 T lymphocyte count < 200 cells per cubic millimeter
Pulmonary or extrapulmonary tuberculosis
Any mycobacterial disease caused by mycobacteria other than *M. tuberculosis* disseminated at a site other than or in addition to lungs, skin, or cervical or hilar lymph nodes
Recurrent pneumonia within a 12-month period
Recurrent Salmonella spp. septicemia
Multiple infections with encapsulated or pyogenic bacteria in a child < 13 years of age
Invasive cervical cancer
Kaposi's sarcoma
Lymphoma of the brain
Other lymphomas of B cell or unknown phenotype
Coccidioidomycosis disseminated at a site other than, or in addition to, the lungs or cervical or hilar lymph nodes
Histoplasmosis disseminated at a site other than, or in addition to, the lungs or cervical or hilar lymph nodes
HIV encephalopathy
HIV wasting syndrome
Isosporiasis with diarrhea persisting > 1 month
Recurrent salpingitis

Presumptive Diagnosis of:
Esophageal candidiasis
Cytomegalovirus retinitis with loss of vision
Pneumocystis carinii pneumonia
Toxoplasmosis of the brain in a patient > 1 month of age
Disseminated mycobacterial disease (no culture)
Lymphoid interstitial pneumonia in a child < 13 years of age
Kaposi's sarcoma

should be undertaken with serial assays of T lymphocyte subsets and anergy testing.

Recently, individuals with profound and progressive CD4 T lymphocyte depletion and opportunistic infections, alone or with Kaposi's sarcoma, and with AIDS risk factors but without evidence for HIV-1 or HIV-2 by serology or culture have been reported. These individuals should be referred to the CDC for further evaluation.

Testing for exposure to potentially opportunistic pathogens should also be performed. Screening tests should include a tuberculin test and serology for toxoplasmosis, cytomegalovirus (CMV), and syphilis. If the patient's CD4 T lymphocyte count is less than or equal to 200 cells per cubic millimeter, and symptoms of fever, fatigue, weight loss, night sweats, or malaise are present, an aggressive evaluation to rule out an opportunistic infection should be undertaken.

Antiretroviral Therapy

Antiretroviral therapy has been shown to retard HIV replication, but it does not kill the virus. Since 1985, several clinical trials of antiretroviral agents have demonstrated benefits for patients infected with HIV. These benefits include (1) improved short-term survival in patients with CD4 T lymphocyte counts less than 200 cells per cubic millimeter, (2) improvement in neurologic function for some patients treated with zidovudine, (3) modest and transient increases in CD4 T lymphocyte counts in some patients, (4) a decrease in viral titers in the blood for a period of time, and (5) increased energy and weight gain in some patients.

There are presently three licensed antiretroviral agents approved for therapy of HIV infection: zidovudine (ZDV), dideoxyinosine (didanosine) (DDI), and dideoxycytidine (DDC). Studies to date have shown only small and somewhat conflicting differences between these three agents. At the present time, areas of uncertainty regarding therapy with ZDV, DDI, and DDC include (1) comparative drug efficacy, (2) effects of these agents on long-term survival, (3) when antiretroviral therapy should be initiated for patients infected with HIV, (4) optimal drug doses as well as minimum effective drug doses, (5) the importance of drug resistance of the virus, (6) efficacy of monotherapy versus combination therapy, and (7) when to change antiretroviral therapy during the course of a patient's illness.

Before antiretroviral therapy is begun, CD4 T lymphocyte counts should be determined by two separate assays performed at least 1 week apart. If CD4 T lymphocyte counts are greater than 500 cells per cubic millimeter, the patient should not be started on antiretroviral therapy. T cell subset counts should be followed every 4 to 6 months.

There has been some controversy as when to begin antiretroviral therapy. Several U.S. studies suggest benefit for patients with CD4 T lymphocyte counts between 200 and 500 cells per cubic millimeter, whereas a recent European study did not. Benefit for patients with CD4 T lymphocyte counts less than 200 cells per cubic millimeter is generally agreed on. Because of the different conclusions from these studies, a patient may be observed without therapy if the patient is asymptomatic, has CD4 T lymphocyte counts between 200 and 500 cells per cubic millimeter, and is stable over time. Antiretroviral therapy should be started if clinical or laboratory deterioration occurs. If a patient is symptomatic with CD4 T lymphocyte counts between 200 and 500 cells per cubic millimeter or has a history of an opportunistic infection regardless of CD4 T lymphocyte counts, antiretroviral therapy should be started.

ZDV has been the cornerstone of antiretroviral therapy and is usually used as the initial agent. It is a thymidine analogue that inhibits the in vitro replication of HIV by blocking the viral enzyme reverse transcriptase. The suggested dose is 500 to 600 mg a day (100 mg orally every 4 hours while awake or 200 mg orally every 8 hours). Complete blood counts should be monitored for the first 3 months. If no toxicity is discovered, the frequency of complete blood counts can be decreased to every 3 months thereafter. Higher doses may be indicated for HIV-associated idiopathic thrombocytopenia purpura (ITP) or HIV-related encephalopathy. The lowest dose that has been found to have antiretroviral activity is 300 mg a day.

Early toxicities of ZDV include nausea, vomiting, dyspepsia, malaise, and headaches. Symptoms usually occur during the first few weeks of therapy and tend to be self-limited. Elevations of liver transaminases, alkaline phosphatase, and bilirubin have also been reported. These elevations generally are not severe and do not require dose modification.

Bone marrow suppression is seen later with therapy and is the primary dose-limiting factor of ZDV therapy. Bone marrow suppression is thought to occur by suppression of cellular thymidine metabolism, DNA polymerase, and DNA synthesis. Some patients with AIDS- and ZDV-induced anemia have a suboptimal compensatory erythropoietin level response. Controlled trials have demonstrated a benefit from exogenous recombinant erythropoietin for those persons with serum erythropoietin levels less than 500 IU per liter. Granulocyte-macrophage colony-stimulating factor (GM-CSF) (Leukine, Prokine)* and granulocyte colony-stimulating factor (G-CSF)* (Neupogen)* are being studied as adjuvant agents for patients with ZDV-induced neutropenia.

Long-term ZDV use (over 1-year duration) has been associated with the development of myocyte mitochondrial toxicity resulting in clinical myopathy. The use of ZDV for more than 6 months in patients with advanced AIDS has led to the recovery of virus isolates resistant in vitro to ZDV. Resistance develops less often in patients with fewer HIV-related symptoms and higher CD4 T lymphocyte counts. The clinical significance of resistant isolates is unclear, but it is believed that patients with resistant isolates may have a more rapid clinical deterioration. These isolates remain sensitive to other antiretroviral agents.

Despite the proven benefits of ZDV, the disease still progresses over time in patients who take the drug. These patients should be evaluated for other antiretroviral therapy. DDI and DDC are two other nucleoside analogues used for HIV disease.

DDI has a mechanism of action similar to ZDV but a different toxicity profile. The two primary toxicities associated with DDI are peripheral neuropathy and acute pancreatitis. The peripheral neuropathy seen with DDI therapy is common but usually not severe. Persons who develop this complication complain of numbness, tingling, or painful extremities. Symptoms generally improve with discontinuation of the medicine, and some patients tolerate lower doses of the agent. Pancreatitis occurs less often and can be subclinical. A prior history of pancreatitis or excessive alcohol use should be considered a relative contraindication to therapy with DDI. DDI therapy should also be withheld during treatment with pentamidine to minimize the development of pancreatitis. Neurologic examinations and laboratory evaluations of amylase and lipase should be performed monthly to monitor for the development of these two toxicities.

At present, DDI is approved for adults who have advanced AIDS and who are intolerant to or fail to respond to therapy with ZDV. Therapeutic failure is considered to be the development of significant clinical or immunologic deterioration while receiving treatment with ZDV. DDI may also benefit patients who have received ZDV for 4 months or longer and have CD4 T lymphocyte counts less than 300 cells per cubic millimeter. Doses are based on weights in adults and are presented in Table 3. To date, no data exist to guide use of DDI in asymptomatic patients or those persons with CD4 T lymphocyte counts greater than 200 cells per cubic millimeter. Further studies with DDI alone and in combination with ZDV therapy are ongoing. Resistant HIV isolates have been recovered after 6 months of therapy with DDI. As with ZDV-resistant isolates, the clinical significance is unknown, but patients may have a more rapid clinical deterioration.

DDC is the third nucleoside analogue used for the treatment of patients infected with HIV. At present, it is approved for combination therapy with ZDV. Studies have shown that monotherapy with DDC provides beneficial effects that are equal to or more than those provided by monotherapy with ZDV. The side effects seen with DDC are similar to those seen with DDI but occur less often. Other adverse effects seen with DDC include transient aphthous mouth ulcers, skin eruptions, arthralgias, and fever. These early side effects are usually self-limited.

DDC should be considered as monotherapy or combination therapy with ZDV in adults with advanced HIV infection (CD4 T lymphocytes less than 300 cells per cubic millimeter) who have developed significant clinical or immunologic deterioration while receiving ZDV monotherapy. The dosage of DDC is 0.75 mg orally every 8 hours; with ZDV, the dosage is 200 mg orally every 8 hours. If side effects develop with DDC, 0.375 mg orally every 8 hours may be used. As with the other antiretroviral agents, resistant viral isolates have been recovered.

TABLE 3. **Recommended Dosages of Dideoxyinosine (DDI, Didanosine [Videx]) and Dideoxycytidine (DDC, Zalcitabine [Hivid])**

DDI	
Weight (kg)	*Tablets*
75	300 mg bid
50–74	200 mg bid
35–49	125 mg bid
DDI may be given as monotherapy or with zidovudine (Retrovir), 200 mg tid	
DDC	
0.75 mg tid as monotherapy or, with zidovudine (Retrovir), 200 mg tid	

*Not FDA approved for this indication.

TABLE 4. **Guidelines for Antiretroviral Treatment**

Regimens must be individualized, depending on allergies, compliance, and the need for other medications

CD4 T lymphocytes > 500 cells per cubic millimeter:
No antiretroviral therapy
Follow CD4 counts every 4 to 6 months

CD4T lymphocytes 200 to 500 cells per cubic millimeter:
If the patient is asymptomatic and stable over time, observe while off therapy. Begin antiretroviral therapy if clinical or laboratory deterioration.
If the patient is symptomatic or has a history of an opportunistic infection, begin antiretroviral therapy.

Initial antiretroviral therapy:
ZDV monotherapy or combination therapy with DDI or DDC

If the patient does well on ZDV monotherapy for 4 or more months and has a CD4 T lymphocyte count < 300 cells per cubic millimeter, change to DDI.

If clinical or immunologic deterioration on ZDV monotherapy:
Begin combination therapy with DDC or
Switch to DDI or DDC monotherapy or
Begin combination therapy with DDI

The newer nucleoside analogue reverse transcriptase inhibitors stavudine (d4T)* and 3TC* will enter efficacy trials as monotherapy and in combination with other antiretroviral agents. Preliminary results regarding the efficacy of the Tat-antagonist Ro24-7429* and several protease inhibitors (drugs that, contrary to the reverse transcriptase inhibitors, affect HIV replication in chronically infected cells) will be available soon. Present antiretroviral treatment recommendations are presented in Table 4. The use of combination therapy with two dideoxynucloside analogues that have differing toxicity profiles or with two agents of different classes and mechanisms of action or of three agents all inhibiting reverse transcriptase is presently being evaluated. Combination therapy likely provides the next major advancement in the treatment of HIV infection.

OPPORTUNISTIC INFECTIONS

Opportunistic infections are the major cause of morbidity and mortality in patients infected with HIV. The physician should have a low threshold for obtaining a diagnosis to explain the relatively nonspecific signs and symptoms that can herald the onset of a new infection. Empirical therapy, when possible, is discouraged because of the high incidence of multiple infections and diverse etiologies of various syndromes, and the toxicities that can occur with treatment. Although most infections are responsive to therapy, there is a high relapse rate, so chronic suppressive therapy and prophylaxis are important in the management of HIV-infected patients. Table 5 illustrates the common opportunistic pathogens seen in AIDS.

*Investigational drug in the United States.

Bacterial Infections

Mycobacteria. The mycobacteria have been a prominent part of the AIDS pandemic since it was first discovered. Two species predominate, *Mycobacterium tuberculosis* and *Mycobacterium avium* complex (MAC), the latter comprising those organisms previously identified as either *Mycobacterium avium* or *Mycobacterium intracellulare* but now are recognized as so similar as to be classified together. Recently, infection with *Mycobacterium haemophilum* has also been associated with AIDS. A remarkable cluster of cases has occurred in the New York City area. Other mycobacterial infections only rarely recognized until now include *Mycobacterium genavense* and *Mycobacterium malmoense.*

Infection with *Mycobacterium tuberculosis* has been seen in 2% to 10% of patients infected with HIV. Tuberculosis is often the first manifestation of HIV infection. It can be reactivated disease or primary infection. When tuberculosis occurs early in HIV infection, its features are indistinguishable from tuberculosis occurring in non–HIV-infected persons. The clinical features include night sweats, fever, weight loss, and productive coughs with typical chest x-ray findings. In the later stages of HIV infection, tuberculosis is more likely to present in an atypical manner with nonspecific constitutional symptoms and nonproductive coughs. Pulmonary disease is often atypical on chest film, lacking cavitation, and may involve the mediastinal lymph nodes, the lower lobes, or appear as a diffuse interstitial infiltrate. Histopathology may show poorly formed granulomas without caseation necrosis.

Furthermore, up to 70% of patients have extrapulmonary disease, often involving the adrenal glands. Lymphadenopathy is the most common manifestation of extrapulmonary tuberculosis and can be an unsuspected cause of lymphadenopathy in HIV-infected persons. Extrapulmonary tuberculosis also manifests itself in patients with AIDS as pericarditis, peritonitis, meningitis, brain lesions, bone and joint involvement, or disseminated tuberculosis.

The diagnosis of tuberculosis in HIV-infected patients can be difficult and is often missed because of its atypical presentation, the high frequency of extrapulmonary manifestations, occurrence of other mycobacterial diseases, and frequent poor delayed hypersensitivity response. Because anergy is seen in about 50% of HIV-infected persons and over 90% of people in the later stages of AIDS, many will have negative findings on a skin test, even when the classic test response criterion is relaxed and induration of <5 mm is considered positive.

Patients with pulmonary tuberculosis in the later stages of AIDS produce scanty sputum that may be nondiagnostic by direct microscopic examination. A positive sputum smear can be helpful, and at least three sputum smears should be tested; if they do not contain acid fast bacilli, other specimens should be obtained through induced sputums, bronchial washing and lavage, gastric lavage, pleural fluid, blood or

TABLE 5. **Common Opportunistic Infections in AIDS**

Pathogen	Usual Clinical Presentation
Bacteria	
Mycobacterium avium complex	Dissemination
Mycobacterium tuberculosis	Pulmonary or extrapulmonary disease
Mycobacterium haemophilum	Skin or joint lesions, pneumonia
Streptococcus pneumoniae	Pneumonia, sinusitis
Haemophilus influenzae	Pneumonia, sinusitis
Staphylococcus aureus	Pneumonia
Salmonella typhimurium	Enteritis or dissemination
Treponema pallidum	Central nervous system infection
Rochalimea sp.	Skin or hepatic lesions
Fungi	
Candida albicans	Oral thrush or esophagitis
Cryptococcus neoformans	Dissemination
Histoplasma capsulatum	Dissemination
Coccidioides immitis	Dissemination
Aspergillus sp.	Pneumonia
Pneumocystis carinii	Pneumonia or dissemination
Protozoa	
Toxoplasma gondii	Brain mass lesion or encephalitis; or chorioretinitis
Cryptosporidium	Chronic diarrhea
Isospora belli	Recurrent diarrhea
Viruses	
Cytomegalovirus	Chorioretinitis or pneumonitis or colitis or esophagitis; dissemination
Herpes simplex	Mucocutaneous ulcers or stomatitis
Varicella-zoster	Dissemination
Epstein-Barr	Lymphoma or oral hairy leukoplakia or lymphocytic interstitial pneumonitis
Papovavirus	Progressive multifocal leukoencephalopathy
Pox virus	Molluscum contagiosum

urine samples, and lymph node, bone marrow, or liver biopsy if indicated. A culture with complete identification of mycobacterial species and drug-susceptibility tests should be performed. Serologic tests are still limited and polymerase chain reactions are being developed.

When inactive infection is identified, prophylaxis with oral isoniazid (INH), 300 mg per day, for 1 year, is recommended (Table 6). Treatment for active tuberculosis should include oral INH, 300 mg per day, oral rifampin (RIF), 600 mg per day, and oral pyrazinamide (PZA), 20 to 30 mg per kg per day for 2 months, followed by INH and RIF at the same dosages for the remainder of the treatment. Therapy should continue for a minimum of 9 months. Oral ethambutol (EMB), 15 mg per kg per day, should be added if disseminated or central nervous system (CNS) infection is suspected. HIV-infected persons have a similar response rate to therapy when compared with uninfected patients. However, HIV-infected patients have a higher relapse rate.

HIV-infected patients are at a higher risk for developing drug-resistant tuberculosis. The initial treatment regimen should take into consideration the knowledge regarding the incidence of drug-resistant isolates from a given community. If drug-resistant tuberculosis is suspected, therapy may require starting with more than four drugs, including INH, RIF, PZA, EMB, streptomycin (STM) or amikacin, and one or more other drugs, which include ethionamide, cycloserine, kanamycin, capreomycin, *para*-aminosalicylic acid, ciprofloxacin, and ofloxacin.

Some studies have shown a higher frequency of side effects with drug therapy in HIV-infected patients with tuberculosis, whereas others have shown no significant difference. The most frequent adverse reactions included skin rashes; some cases of hepatitis have been reported. Treatment should be adjusted in cases of severe drug toxicity. There appears to be no drug interaction with zidovudine, but rifampin can increase the hepatic metabolism of fluconazole.

MAC is found antemortem in 20% of patients with AIDS, and has been found in more than 50% at autopsy. MAC usually presents as a disseminated infection in patients with far-advanced AIDS. Diffuse involvement of bone marrow and structures of the reticuloendothelial system in the spleen, liver, lymph nodes, lungs, and gastrointestinal tract with massive mycobacterial loads and poorly formed granulomas is

TABLE 6. **Guidelines for Tuberculosis Testing and Prophylaxis for HIV-infected Persons**

1. All HIV-infected persons should receive a PPD-tuberculin (5 TU) skin test by Mantoux method.
2. All HIV-infected persons should be tested for anergy at the time of PPD testing using at least two delayed-type hypersensitivity antigens by the Mantoux method.
3. Any induration measured at 48 to 72 hours is considered a positive PPD response; failure to elicit an induration with other antigens is evidence of anergy.
4. Persons with a positive PPD reaction are considered to be infected with *M. tuberculosis* and should be evaluated for active tuberculosis.
5. Preventive therapy should be given if PPD-positive and active TB has been ruled out, or if the patient is PPD negative, anergic, and at increased risk for tuberculosis infection.

often seen along with a continuous high-grade bacillemia.

Symptoms include persistent fevers, weight loss, and night sweats. Signs of end-organ involvement include diarrhea, anemia, an elevated alkaline phosphatase level, hypoalbuminemia, and progressive debilitation. Disseminated disease is associated with a relentlessly deteriorating clinical course and an extremely poor prognosis. It is rarely the only direct cause of death.

Diagnosis depends on culturing possible sites of involvement, including blood, lymph nodes, liver, stool, and bone marrow for mycobacteria. The finding of acid-fast bacilli in direct smears of stool with positive cultures often correlates with disseminated disease and should prompt consideration of treatment or intensive further evaluation. In contrast, the finding of MAC in sputum or bronchoalveolar lavage specimens does not necessarily imply systemic infection, because, unlike *M. tuberculosis,* MAC seldom causes invasive pulmonary disease.

Patients who are symptomatic usually benefit from a trial of therapy. However, no consistently effective or curative therapy has been found for MAC. Four and five drug regimens, using rifabutin (Mycobutin), clofazimine (Lamprene), rifampin, ethionamide, cycloserine, ciprofloxacin (Cipro), amikacin (Amikin), imipenem (Primaxin), clarithromycin (Biaxin), and azithromycin (Zithromax), have been used and have produced some improvement in symptoms, and often at least a temporary reduction in bacillemia. Rifabutin, 300 mg orally per day, is recommended to prevent the development of disseminated MAC infection in patients infected with HIV who do not have evidence of disseminated infection as determined by a negative culture for MAC from a sterile body site, are not infected with *M. tuberculosis,* and have CD4 T lymphocyte counts less than 100 cells per cubic millimeter.

Recently, *Mycobacterium haemophilum* has been found to infect the skin and underlying tissues of HIV-infected patients. Skin lesions begin as painful, erythematous, or violaceous nodules that can progress to form an abscess. They are often exudative and can form ulcers. The synovium of joints such as the knee, ankle, digits, and wrist, as well as tendon sheaths, can also be infected. Isolation from bronchoalveolar lavage, blood, skin ulcers, joint effusion, eye, or lymph nodes requires special culturing techniques. At present, the optimal treatment regimen and duration of therapy is unclear, but four drug regimens using rifampin or rifabutin, ciprofloxacin, clarithromycin, amikacin, or clofazimine may be effective. Infection with this organism should be included in the differential diagnosis of any HIV-infected patient who presents with cutaneous lesions, joint effusion, osteomyelitis, or unexplained pneumonia. The microbiology laboratory must be notified so that special culture conditions using hemin and room temperature incubation can be used.

Other Bacterial Infections

Other bacterial infections that HIV-infected persons are predisposed to develop secondary to defects in cell-mediated immunity include salmonellosis, listeriosis, legionellosis, and nocardial infections. Recurrent Salmonella bacteremia, usually with *Salmonella typhimurium,* is the most important, often requiring chronic suppressive therapy with amoxicillin, trimethoprim-sulfamethoxazole, or ciprofloxacin. The remaining organisms respond well to conventional treatment.

Syphilis is increasingly being recognized as a cause of CNS disease in patients with AIDS. Patients may be asymptomatic or have an array of signs and symptoms. Patients infected with HIV and with a history of treated primary or secondary syphilis may develop CNS infection months or years after therapy. The diagnosis is difficult. Cerebrospinal fluid (CSF) may show a pleocytosis and an elevated protein or may be normal, including a nonreactive Venereal Disease Research Laboratory (VDRL) test. Therapy with intravenous penicillin G, 12 to 24 million units per day, is given for a minimum of 2 weeks. Total length of treatment may be guided by serial CSF findings, but the duration of therapy and the need for suppressive therapy is unclear.

HIV-infected persons are also predisposed to infections with encapsulated organisms secondary to their impaired humoral immune system. Bacterial pneumonia occurs frequently in AIDS patients, and may be seen concurrently with PCP. *Streptococcus pneumonia* and *Haemophilus influenzae* pneumonia often occur in this patient population. Pneumococcal pneumonia is typically lobar and responds to conventional therapy. Pneumococcal vaccine is recommended for HIV-infected adults. Pneumonia due to *H. influenzae* can have a variety of radiographic presentations and may be indistinguishable from PCP. It is, therefore, recommended that treatment for *H. influenzae* be added to pentamidine when allergy to trimethoprim-sulfamethoxazole precludes its use in the early empirical therapy of presumed PCP.

Pyogenic infections with *Staphylococcus aureus* and *Pseudomonas aeruginosa* occur with increased frequency in HIV-infected patients, especially in those persons with neutropenia. The most common presentations are bronchitis, sinusitis, and pneumonia. These infections respond to conventional therapy, but relapse is common.

Campylobacter jejuni, Campylobacter fetus, and *Shigella flexneri* are also seen with increased frequency in patients with AIDS. These organisms are usually associated with chronic diarrhea, but bacteremia can occur. Conventional therapy is indicated.

Rochalimea henselae, the causative agents of cat-scratch disease, has been shown to cause small hemangioma-like lesions of the skin and liver in HIV-infected persons. Symptoms may be rare, absent, or mild. Disseminated disease has been reported. Therapy with macrolides may be effective.

Fungal Infections

Candida Albicans. Mucocutaneous candidiasis is often the first sign of infection with HIV. Although candida infections are common clinically, candidal organisms are infrequent causes of major morbidity or mortality in patients with AIDS. Oropharyngeal disease occurs most often, but cutaneous, vaginal, and esophageal involvement is not unusual in the absence of invasive disease. Hematogenous candidiasis can occur but is usually associated with intravascular catheters.

Diagnosis is made by wet mount with potassium hydroxide or Gram's stain of accessible lesions. Esophagitis clinically is associated with gradually progressive burning dysphagia, which can occur without oropharyngeal disease. When the clinical suspicion of esophageal candidiasis is strong, symptomatic improvement with therapy is presumptive support for the diagnosis. If improvement does not occur, endoscopy should be considered.

Topical therapy of cutaneous and vaginal disease is usually effective. Oropharyngeal disease often clears with oral preparations of nystatin (Mycostatin) or clotrimazole (Lotrimin). Suspensions, suppositories, and the troche forms of these medications are equally efficacious, although patients usually express preference for the troche form.

Systemic therapy with ketoconazole or fluconazole is indicated for candidal esophagitis. Ketoconazole (Nizoral), 100 to 200 mg twice daily, or fluconazole (Diflucan), 200 mg orally on the first day, followed by 100 mg daily, is usually well tolerated. Itraconazole (Sporanox), the newest oral azole, has no clear advantages over the other agents for candidal infections. It is unknown whether candidal infections refractory to other treatment regimens will respond to therapy with this agent. Patients may develop mild gastrointestinal side effects, and cross-reactivity with other medications can occur with either azole. Ketoconazole, unlike fluconazole, requires a normally low gastric pH to be absorbed. Recent studies have shown that fluconazole may be more beneficial than ketoconazole in the treatment of esophageal candidiasis. Refractory disease may require treatment with 0.5 mg per kg per day of amphotericin B (Fungizone). Following response to systemic therapy, suppressive use of topical preparations can be employed as needed. Recurrence is common, and more severe disease is seen with progression of infection with HIV.

Cryptococcus Neoformans. The spectrum of disease caused by *C. neoformans* ranges from asymptomatic pulmonary lesions to meningoencephalitis to fungemia with disseminated infection. Cryptococcal infections occur in approximately 5% of all patients with AIDS. It is the second most common fungal infection, the most common cause of fungal meningitis, and the fourth most common opportunistic infection in patients infected with HIV.

The CNS is the most frequent site of extrapulmonary involvement. Minimal inflammation is seen, and the symptoms can be subtle, often including fever, headache, and mental status changes lasting days to weeks. A presumptive diagnosis is made by a positive cryptococcal antigen in blood and in CSF. *C. neoformans* cultured from the blood and CSF establishes the presence the infection. The CSF should also be examined with an India ink preparation in the search for budding yeasts. The India ink preparation has a 15% false-negative rate. CSF pleocytosis may or may not be evident. CSF glucose and protein levels can also be normal.

Pulmonary infection can also occur, with or without cryptococcal meningitis. It can present as lobar pneumonia, interstitial pneumonia, or pleural effusion. Other manifestations of cryptococcal disease include adenopathy, mediastinitis, chorioretinitis, sinusitis, CNS cryptococcoma, arthritis, prostatitis, pustules, and molluscum-like skin lesions. Because of the protean manifestations of cryptococcal disease, it is recommended that a serum test for cryptococcal antigen be routinely performed in the evaluation of unexplained symptoms in persons infected with HIV, although the test result is usually negative with localized disease. Once the diagnosis is established, the patient should be treated with amphotericin B.

Amphotericin B is initially given as a 1-mg test dose. If this amount is tolerated, the dose is escalated to 1.0 mg per kg per day within the first 24 hours. Oral 5-flucytosine (5FC) (Ancobon), 50 to 100 mg per kg per day in divided doses every 6 hours, is given with amphotericin B. Treatment of acute reactions to amphotericin B infusion such as rigors and fevers can be managed as needed with acetaminophen, diphenhydramine, and meperidine. Both amphotericin B and 5FC are nephrotoxic, requiring frequent evaluations of renal function. The use of 5FC may be limited by myelosuppression or gastrointestinal intolerance. To minimize side effects, 5FC peak and trough levels should be measured and maintained between 25 and 50 μg per mL. Therapy with high-dose fluconazole regimens are presently being compared with therapy with amphotericin B and 5FC. Itraconazole may be inferior to fluconazole for the therapy of cryptococcal disease. It may be considered if the patient cannot receive any other therapy due to drug allergy or intolerance.

Therapeutic efficacy should be monitored by serial sampling of blood and CSF for culture and cryptococcal antigen. The amount of cryptococcal antigen is not predictive of response to treatment, but serial titers are useful in assessing a response to therapy. Although a positive response to treatment is expected, up to 33% of patients with cryptococcal disease succumb to their initial infection, 50% to 90% of patients experience a relapse, and most patients expire 5 months after their presentation with cryptococcal disease.

Cryptococcal infection is rarely, if ever, cured. Patients infected with HIV require chronic maintenance therapy to prevent relapse. Oral fluconazole maintenance therapy of 100 mg per day is believed to be more effective than treatment with amphotericin B once to 3 times weekly.

***Histoplasma capsulatum* and *Coccidioides immitis*.** Although cryptococci are ubiquitous, certain mycotic diseases such as coccidioidomycosis and histoplasmosis are epidemic in certain regions of North America. Disease with either organism should be considered in a person with AIDS who lives in or who has traveled to an endemic area and has an unexplained fever. Pulmonary involvement is most common, but disseminated disease has been noted with increased frequency in patients infected with HIV. Symptoms are often nonspecific, with complaints of cough, fever, malaise, and weight loss often reported.

Radiologic studies may reveal perihilar calcification or splenic calcifications, or both, with histoplasmosis. Serologic tests are valuable in the diagnosis of infection with either yeast. A positive test for histoplasma antigen in urine, serum, or CSF correlates with active disease. Positive cultures or demonstration of the organism by fungal stains in peripheral blood buffy coat, bone marrow, bronchoalveolar lavage, or in biopsy specimens of lung, skin, liver, or lymph nodes establishes the diagnosis of infection with these fungi.

Treatment with amphotericin B (Fungizone), 1.0 mg per kg per day up to a total dose of 2 to 2.5 grams, is recommended. As with cryptococcosis, chronic suppressive therapy is required. The azoles ketoconazole, fluconazole, or itraconazole can be used to prevent relapse, as can amphotericin B. At present, itraconazole is not recommended for coccidioidomycosis but is recommended for histoplasmosis.

***Aspergillus* spp.** Invasive aspergillosis is an uncommon infectious complication in patients with AIDS despite the frequent recovery of Aspergillus spp. from sputum. Risk factors associated with invasive aspergillosis include neutropenia, hematologic malignancy, and corticosteroid use. As more aggressive chemotherapy protocols are developed for Kaposi's sarcoma, lymphoma, and other malignancies that occur in patients infected with HIV, the predisposing factors for invasive aspergillosis will occur with increased frequency. Treatment with amphotericin B must be considered for the neutropenic patient with AIDS who has a pneumonia of uncertain etiology and from whom Aspergillus spp. has been isolated from a respiratory specimen. Itraconazole is also an effective agent for the treatment of aspergillosis. Every effort should be made to establish a definitive microbial diagnosis before therapy is initiated.

***Pneumocystis carinii*.** *P. carinii,* frequently thought of as a protozoan, has been recently reclassified as a fungus. PCP is the most common opportunistic infection in patients with AIDS. It is the initial manifestation of AIDS in 64% of patients. PCP is the leading cause of morbidity and mortality in patients infected with HIV and is the cause of death in 25% of patients. In the United States, 80% of patients with AIDS have had at least one episode of PCP. The onset of PCP can be insidious and prolonged, or acute. Cough and fever are the most common presenting symptoms. Other signs and symptoms include dyspnea, tachypnea, exercise intolerance, chest tightness, and spontaneous pneumothorax.

Because the signs and symptoms of PCP are nonspecific, additional studies are necessary to document this infection. *P. carinii* cannot be cultured, and at the present time, there are no reliable serologic tests. Therefore, to clearly establish the diagnosis of PCP, *P. carinii* must be identified in pulmonary secretions or in lung tissue. All specimens should be examined with toluidine blue and Giemsa stains, and examined cytologically with Gram-Weigert stain. Direct fluorescent antibody studies have been successful in some laboratories.

Sputum induction should be the first test performed when PCP is strongly suspected because it is the least invasive method. Depending on the institution, *P. carinii* can be detected in 52% to 92% of cases of PCP. With the increased use of aerosol pentamidine prophylaxis and ZDV, this percentage may have decreased. The diagnostic yield of bronchoscopy and bronchoalveolar lavage (BAL) has been reported to approach 100% However, the sensitivity of BAL may also have decreased with the use of aerosol pentamidine prophylaxis. The sensitivity increases to 100% when a transbronchial biopsy is performed. However, many patients cannot undergo transbronchial biopsy secondary to thrombocytopenia or an underlying coagulation disorder. An open lung biopsy is the diagnostic procedure of last resort to determine the diagnosis.

Because many patients cannot tolerate a bronchoscopy, several indirect tests to diagnose PCP are useful. The chest film is the best screening test for PCP. PCP can appear as diffuse interstitial infiltrates, cavities, or pneumothorax, or the lung may appear normal on a chest film. If a patient is receiving aerosol pentamidine, PCP can present as biapical disease. Gallium scanning is 100% sensitive but only 50% specific. It may be useful if PCP is strongly suspected and the patient has a normal chest film. An arterial blood gas (ABG) may reveal hypoxia and an increased arterial-alveolar (A − a) gradient. The ABG may be normal with early PCP. Paired rest and exercise ABGs, however, usually show a pronounced A − a gradient (>10 mmHg) with early PCP and is suggestive of an interstitial process. A decreased diffusing capacity is also suggestive of an interstitial disease and can indicate early PCP. The lactate dehydrogenase level is often elevated in PCP but is nonspecific.

Agents used for the treatment of PCP are presented in Table 7. Adverse reactions develop in 50% to 100% of patients receiving anti-PCP therapy. Side effects with trimethoprim-sulfamethoxazole include rash, leukopenia, thrombocytopenia, fever, nausea, and vomiting. Pentamidine can induce hypoglycemia, pancreatitis, nephrotoxicity, hepatic dysfunction, neutropenia, and hypotension. Corticosteroids are recommended when the presenting PO_2 is less than 70 mmHg. The dosage of prednisone as adjunctive therapy for PCP is also given in Table 7. Atovaquone (Mepron) is a new nonsulfonamide that has been recently approved as therapy for PCP in patients with

TABLE 7. **Recommended Regimens for PCP Therapy**

Drug	Dosage	Route
Trimethoprim-sulfamethoxazole (Bactrim, Septra)	Trimethoprim, 20 mg/kg/d, and sulfamethoxazole, 100 mg/kg/d, in four divided doses, for 21 days	Oral* or intravenous
Pentamidine (Pentam 300)	4 mg/kg in a single daily dose, for 21 days	Intravenous
Dapsone-Trimethoprim* (Trimpex)	Dapsone, 100 mg, in a single daily dose, and trimethoprim, 20 mg/kg/d, in q 8 hr intervals, for 21 days	Oral
Atovaquone* (Mepron)	750 mg in q 8 h intervals, for 21 days	Oral
Prednisone†	40 mg twice a day for 5 days, 20 mg twice a day for 5 days, 20 mg once a day for 5 days	Oral

*Not recommended by us for mild to moderate PCP. Would start with IV therapy and switch to oral therapy when disease is obviously under control.
†Adjunctive therapy to antibiotics as defined in the text

mild PCP and who are intolerant to trimethoprim-sulfamethoxazole. Notable failures have occurred along with early recurrence. With early diagnosis, treatment with trimethoprim-sulfamethoxazole or intravenous pentamidine should result in 90% response rates.

Alternative but less effective agents that can be used as treatment for PCP include dapsone, dapsone with trimethoprim, clindamycin with primaquine, trimatrexate, and eflornithine (DFMO). These agents are associated with a variety of toxicities and should be considered only if a patient is failing to respond to primary therapy.

Prophylaxis against PCP is indicated when the person infected with HIV has a CD4 T lymphocyte count less than 200 cells per cubic milliliter, a rapid decline in CD4 T lymphocyte counts, thrush, or any opportunistic infection. Agents used for prophylaxis are given in Table 8. Trimethoprim-sulfamethoxazole is the most effective agent.

P. carinii may disseminate. The organisms may be found in bone marrow, lymph nodes, thyroid, liver, or the retina. Aerosol pentamidine prophylaxis may predispose the patient to disseminated infection with *P. carinii*. Therapy with trimethoprim-sulfamethoxazole or intravenous pentamidine may be effective.

Parasitic Infections

Toxoplasma gondii. Neurologic disease occurs in up to 40% of patients with AIDS. *T. gondii* is the most common cause of focal encephalitis in individuals infected with HIV, and in 99% of cases, it is due to reactivation of latent infection. The neurologic manifestations of toxoplasmosis include encephalitis, meningoencephalitis, and mass lesions that can be exhibited as headache, fever, altered mental status, seizures, focal motor and sensory deficits, and coma. Pneumonia, pericarditis, chorioretinitis, and disseminated infection with *T. gondii* have also been reported.

Patients at risk of developing toxoplasmosis have elevated IgG titers representing past exposure to the parasite. The absence of IgG for toxoplasmosis makes the diagnosis unlikely. Because most patients will not mount a rising titer of IgG antibody as a result of defects in humoral immunity, serologic diagnosis of reactivated infection is difficult. CSF is also often negative for antibody against *T. gondii*.

Computed tomography or magnetic resonance imaging of the brain usually demonstrates multiple bilateral contrast-enhancing lesions in the cerebral hemispheres at the junction of the gray and white matter. Edema may or may not be present. Brain biopsy, used in the search for the tachyzoites of *T. gondii*, is the only certain way to make a definite diagnosis.

Empirical therapy may be required if the brain lesions are inaccessible or a brain biopsy is contraindicated. In practice, empirical therapy is now the rule. Improvement with empirical therapy for a presumptive diagnosis of cerebral toxoplasmosis should be expected within 14 days of treatment. If there is no improvement or if the patient deteriorates, further attempts at making a tissue diagnosis should be reconsidered.

The standard therapy for toxoplasmosis includes pyrimethamine (Daraprim), 100 mg orally a day, for 3 days, followed by 25 mg to 75 mg orally a day, and sulfadiazine, 4 gm orally as a loading dose, followed by 6 gm to 8 gm in four divided doses every day. Folinic acid (Wellcovorin), 5 mg orally a day, is usually given to minimize bone marrow suppression from these agents. Other side effects include rash, fever, and gastrointestinal intolerance. Most reactions are due to sulfadiazine. Response rates are in the 90% range with this regimen in patients diagnosed early.

Alternatives to sulfadiazine include clindamycin, 900 mg orally three times daily, or dapsone, 100 mg

TABLE 8. **Recommended Regimens for PCP Prophylaxis**

1. Trimethoprim-sufamethoxazole: 1 double-strength tablet daily, 7 days per week or two double-strength tablets bid 3 days per week

or

2. Aerosol pentamidine (Nebupent): 300 mg, once monthly via Respirgard II nebulizer or 60 mg 5 times over 2 weeks; then 60 mg every 2 weeks via Fisoneb nebulizer

or

3. Dapsone: 50–100 mg once or twice daily +/− trimethoprim 10 mg/kg/day (given bid). Pyrimethamine 25 mg/day or twice weekly can be substituted for trimethoprim if the patient is allergic to trimethoprim.

or

4. Fansidar (sulfadoxine 500 mg plus pyrimethamine 25 mg) one or two times orally weekly

orally a day. Pyrimethamine should be given with either agent. Alternative agents that may be effective include oral azithromycin, oral atovaquone, or intravenous trimetrexate.

Lifelong maintenance therapy is required to prevent relapse of infection as up to 80% of patients will relapse after treatment is discontinued. Maintenance therapy is usually begun after 4 to 6 weeks of initial therapy and clinical and radiographic improvement is observed. Most clinicians use decreased doses of pyrimethamine, 50 mg daily, and sulfadiazine, 4 gm divided in four doses. The efficacy of other agents has not been established. Pyrimethamine alone at doses of 50 mg/day and higher has been successful as a maintenance dose.

Cryptosporidium. Patients with AIDS with cryptosporidiosis may have protracted, voluminous, and watery diarrhea; profound malabsorption with electrolyte disturbances; and weight loss. Biliary tract involvement, seen in up to 10% of patients, can be associated with severe right upper quadrant abdominal pain, nausea, and vomiting. Laboratory studies reveal an elevated alkaline phosphatase, gallbladder wall thickening, and dilated bile ducts. It is seen mostly in Africa and Haiti, where 50% of patients with AIDS have cryptosporidiosis, although only 5% of patients with AIDS in the United States have this disease. Occasionally, patients have only mild diarrhea and spontaneous remissions occur.

The diagnosis is established by the detection of acid-fast cryptosporidial oocysts in the stool or by a sucrose gradient technique. No effective therapy for cryptosporidial infections has been established. Treatment with the oral aminoglycoside spiramycin (Rovamycine),* oral diclazuril,† oral azithromycin (Zithromax), or subcutaneous somatostatin has yielded inconsistent results. Recently, albendazole (Zentel),† has been tried as a therapeutic agent. Further clinical trials are ongoing.

Isospora belli. *Isospora belli* is also an acid-fast parasite mostly seen in patients of Haitian origin. It can also produce watery diarrhea, but unlike Cryptosporidium, it can cause disseminated disease and responds to treatment with oral trimethoprim-sulfamethoxazole, 1 double-strength tablet, four times daily for 10 to 14 days. Metronidazole and pyrimethamine-sulfadiazine are also effective. Recurrence is common, and chronic suppressive therapy may be required.

Microsporidia. Microsporidia, a tiny coccidian organism responsible for diarrhea in some patients with AIDS, is difficult to diagnose. A trichrome stain of the stool is now available through the CDC, and bowel biopsies have been diagnostic. There is no proven effective therapy, but metronidazole may be effective.

Other Parasitic Infections. *Entamoeba histolytica, Giardia lamblia,* and amebae are frequently implicated in acute enteritis in patients infected with HIV and often respond to standard treatment regimens. Disseminated *Strongyloides stercoralis* and severe visceral leishmaniasis has been reported in HIV-infected persons who have lived in or traveled to endemic areas.

*Investigational drug in the United States.
†Not available in the United States.

Viral Infections

Cytomegalovirus Infection. CMV infections are among the most common in persons with AIDS. CMV is transmitted sexually, by saliva, or by exposure to blood products. Approximately 100% of homosexual men infected with HIV are seropositive for CMV. Therefore, in this population, CMV disease is believed to be due to reactivation of latent infection. CMV itself may contribute to immunosuppression or to development of Kaposi's sarcoma. Retinitis is the major manifestation of infection with CMV, but encephalitis, polyradiculopathy, pneumonitis, esophagitis, hepatitis, and colitis are being found with increasing frequency. Adrenalitis with adrenal insufficiency may occur. Ventriculitis with pathognomonic CT scan results has also been seen.

Diagnosis of infection with CMV is not easy. Serologic testing is seldom helpful, owing to the high prevalence of seropositivity in the HIV-infected population. Positive cultures of CMV are difficult to interpret because it is difficult to distinguish between active disease due to CMV and intermittent viral shedding or even viremia with CMV.

Two clinical syndromes that may be accepted as presumptive evidence of invasive CMV disease include (1) a characteristic chorioretinitis with hemorrhages, exudates, and vascular sheathing and (2) adrenalitis in the presence of CMV infection viremia or uremia and without another explanation. Organ system involvement such as pneumonia, colitis, esophagitis, and hepatitis must be accompanied by histopathologic evidence of pathognomonic so-called owl's-eye inclusions before a diagnosis can be made. Papanicolaou smears of cells may also show the typical inclusions.

Presenting signs and symptoms of CMV infection depend on the organ system infected. Between 5% and 10% of patients with AIDS will develop CMV retinitis. Retinitis usually develops during the later stages of AIDS. Patients may complain of floaters, a change in acuity, or a unilateral visual field defect. Blindness will result if therapy is not instituted. Findings on blood and urine cultures are often positive for CMV at the time of diagnosis but can be negative.

Ganciclovir (DHPG) is an effective therapeutic agent in 80% of patients with CMV retinitis. Treatment is intravenous and is given initially as 10 mg per kg per day in two divided doses for 2 weeks, and then maintenance therapy 5 mg per kg per day indefinitely to prevent relapse. Patients may need to discontinue ZDV while receiving DHPG secondary to both drugs' myelosuppressive effects. The use of GM-CSF or G-CSF with DHPG may ameliorate the myelosuppression seen with therapy.

Intravenous foscarnet (Foscavir), is a broad-spectrum antiviral agent with good activity against CMV. It is effective in ganciclovir-resistant strains of CMV. The induction dose is 180 mg per kg per day in three divided doses for 2 weeks, then 90 to 120 mg per kg per day in a single dose indefinitely. Foscarnet does not cause myelosuppression, but a rise in serum creatinine is often seen and may require dose adjustments.

Because both DHPG and foscarnet are given intravenously, persons with CMV retinitis require indwelling vascular access devices for indefinite treatment. Patients should have frequent ophthalmologic examinations to assess the response to therapy and to monitor for recurrence of disease. Both drugs are equally effective but an apparent 4-month survival advantage has been seen with those patients receiving foscarnet.

Signs and symptoms of CMV pneumonitis resemble those of PCP or any interstitial pneumonitis. Patients with biopsy-proven disease and no other demonstrable pathogen to explain an interstitial pneumonia may benefit from treatment. Intravenous therapy with DHPG, 5 mg per kg given twice daily, is effective in 50% of patients. Optimal duration of therapy is not established. Some patients respond after 2 to 4 weeks of treatment, but many relapse. Chronic suppressive therapy may be necessary. Intravenous foscarnet, 60 mg per kg three times daily given for 14 to 21 days, has had promising results. The effective maintenance dose has not been determined.

CMV esophagitis is clinically indistinguishable from esophagitis due to *C. albicans* or herpes simplex virus. Endoscopy reveals erythema, submucosal hemorrhages, and diffuse ulcerations. Vasculitis, neutrophilic invasion, and destructive changes are seen at biopsy. Diagnosis is made by finding the pathognomonic inclusions seen with CMV. CMV colitis occurs in at least 5% to 10% of patients with AIDS. Findings at sigmoidoscopy are similar to the findings seen on endoscopy. Treatment with DHPG, 5 mg per kg twice daily, is effective in at least 75% of patients. Chronic suppressive therapy may not be required. All patients with CMV colitis should undergo an ophthalmologic examination to rule out retinitis.

Herpes Simplex Virus. Infections with herpes simplex virus (HSV) are common and unusually severe in HIV-infected patients. Manifestations of HSV infection include large persistent perianal erosions that may lack typical vesicle formation, stomatitis, and esophagitis. Diagnosis of perianal, oral, and genital HSV infection is made by culture of swabs of the lesions. Endoscopy is required to diagnose HSV esophagitis because it is clinically indistinguishable from esophagitis due to *C. albicans* or CMV.

Treatment with oral acyclovir, 200 mg 5 times daily, is usually effective for mild infections. More severe disease requires intravenous therapy with acyclovir (Zovirax), 5 mg per kg three times daily. DHPG is also effective for HSV esophagitis. Foscarnet is the drug of choice for acyclovir-resistant HSV. Recurrence is common and may require suppressive medication.

Varicella-Zoster Virus. Reactivation of varicella-zoster virus (VZV) infection is common in HIV-infected persons and can be the first sign of clinically significant immunosuppression. VZV can be severe and chronic, and although it is usually dermatomal, it may disseminate. Therapy with intravenous acyclovir, 10 mg per kg three times daily is usually effective. Intravenous foscarnet is required for resistant VZV infections.

Epstein-Barr Virus. High titers of antibody to Epstein-Barr virus (EBV) are found in many AIDS patients but have not been clearly associated with disease. There is evidence that B cell lymphomas and lymphoid interstitial pneumonitis seen in HIV-infected persons, especially children, are caused by EBV. EBV has also been associated with oral hairy leukoplakia. Patients may present with hypertrophy of the lateral tongue or painless white plaques anywhere on their tongue or posterior oropharynx. There is no known treatment, and the lesions usually do not progress. Regression of oral hairy leukoplakia has been seen with ZDV therapy.

Papovavirus. The JC and SV-40 papovaviruses are the most common causes of progressive multifocal leukoencephalopathy seen in patients with AIDS. Presentation depends on the area of the brain involved, ranging from a diffuse encephalopathy to focal deficits. Symptoms progress rapidly over several months, although some patients may have a waxing and waning clinical course. Brain imaging studies reveal multiple nonenhancing lesions scattered throughout the white matter. MRI is more specific than computed tomographic images. Diagnosis is made at brain biopsy, which shows focal myelin loss with abnormal astrocytes. There is no known therapy at present but ara-C may be useful and is currently being evaluated for treatment. The prognosis for patients with progressive multifocal leukoencephalopathy is poor.

Pox Viruses. Molluscum contagiosum occurs as an opportunistic infection in patients with AIDS. The presentation is clinically the same as in non–HIV-infected persons except that the lesions may not resolve spontaneously but instead continue to increase in size, number, and severity. Patients should be referred to a dermatologist for cryotherapy with liquid nitrogen.

Human Immunodeficiency Virus. HIV can cause a variety of clinical syndromes on its own. It has been associated with a mononucleosis-like syndrome, acute aseptic meningitis, immune thrombocytopenic purpura, progressive generalized lymphadenopathy, subacute encephalitis, spinal vacuolar myopathy, and peripheral neuropathies. Some of these syndromes respond to antiretroviral therapy.

AMEBIASIS

method of
K. GAMBLE, M.D., and
J. S. KEYSTONE, M.D., M.Sc. (C.T.M.)
The Toronto Hospital
Toronto, Ontario, Canada

Amebiasis is infection by the protozoan parasite *Entamoeba histolytica.* It has been estimated that the organism infects approximately 500,000,000 people, resulting in 50,000,000 cases of diarrhea and 40,000 deaths yearly. Although the species is found worldwide, it is most prevalent in countries having the lowest level of sanitation. In the developed world, amebiasis is concentrated in certain high-risk groups, including immigrants from endemic regions, travelers returning from developing countries, migrant workers, inhabitants of mental institutions, and sexually active homosexual men. The disease is most commonly acquired by ingestion of food or water contaminated with the cyst form of the parasite; person-to-person transmission through fecal-oral contact also occurs.

Relatively few of those infected with the parasite develop invasive disease. Recent studies suggest that less than 10% of strains have the potential to invade tissue. Although morphologically indistinguishable from the pathogenic variety, analysis of isoenzyme patterns (zymodemes) and studies using molecular genetic probes have shown the non-invasive strains of *E. histolytica* are genetically distinct species, now called *Entamoeba dispar.* Moreover, only about 10% of those infected with the potential pathogen *E. histolytica* eventually develop clinical disease. The pathogenic strain will continue to be known as *E. histolytica.*

The main clinical manifestations of amebiasis involve the large bowel and liver. Intestinal amebiasis occurs when pathogenic amebae invade the colonic epithelium and lyse mucosal cells, resulting in mucosal damage. In approximately 10% of cases, amebae enter the mesenteric circulation and reach the liver to form an abscess, the most common extraintestinal manifestation of amebiasis.

INTESTINAL AMEBIASIS

As noted earlier, approximately 90% of those infected with *E. histolytica* harbor nonpathogenic strains *(E. dispar)* and are asymptomatic. When a pathogenic strain produces intestinal disease, the spectrum ranges from mild diarrhea to fulminant dysentery and death. Patients with amebic colitis most often complain of crampy abdominal pain, diarrhea, bloody stools, tenesmus, and abdominal tenderness. Only 30% present with a fever, which is usually low grade. Fulminant colitis, associated with high fever, profuse bloody diarrhea, peritoneal signs, intestinal perforation, and a high mortality rate, is rare and most likely seen in immunosuppressed patients, pregnant women, very young children, and the malnourished. Chronic nondysenteric amebiasis, consisting of diarrhea, abdominal pain, and weight loss, may persist for years. Because these symptoms may resemble those of inflammatory bowel disease, amebiasis should be excluded by examination of stools and amebic serology before a diagnosis of inflammatory bowel disease is made and especially before corticosteroid therapy is begun.

Diagnosis

The diagnosis of intestinal amebiasis is made by detecting *E. histolytica* trophozoites or cysts, or both, in stool samples using light microscopy. Prior administration of bismuth, laxatives, antacids, hypertonic enemas, or antibiotics such as tetracycline and erythromycin may interfere with the detection of the organism in stools and should be avoided. Unfortunately, light microscopy cannot differentiate between *E. histolytica* (pathogenic) and *E. dispar* (nonpathogenic).

Virtually 100% of patients with amebic colitis test positive for occult blood; this is a cheap and effective screening test for the disease. Amebic serology is a useful adjunct because antibodies develop only during infection with pathogenic strains, even in those who are asymptomatic. For the most part, negative amebic serology excludes the presence of an invasive strain. However, in newly infected individuals, antibody levels may not be detectable during the first week of infection or symptoms. Moreover, in endemic areas, the presence of amebic antibodies may not reflect active disease because they may persist for years following infection.

Treatment of Intestinal Amebiasis

The treatment of amebiasis can generally be reduced to two basic tenets: (1) eradication of cysts or lumen-dwelling trophozoites with a lumen-active agent and (2) treatment of invasive disease with a tissue-active agent.

Treatment of Asymptomatic Cyst and Trophozoite Passers

Although most asymptomatic individuals with amebiasis are infected with a nonpathogenic strain *(E. dispar),* we favor treating these patients with a lumen-active agent alone in non-endemic areas until these strains can be readily differentiated from *E. histolytica.* From a therapeutic perspective, cyst passers and asymptomatic excreters of red blood cell–free trophozoites should be considered alike. Diloxanide furoate (Furamide), the preferred agent for eradicating intraluminal infection, is not readily available. A 10-day course has an 85% success rate in eliminating the organism. The advantage of this drug compared with other agents lies in its relative lack of toxicity. Occasional mild gastrointestinal symptoms and increased flatulence are the most frequent side effects. In the United States, the drug is available only from the Centers for Disease Control and, in Canada, only with the authorization of the

TABLE 1. **Treatment of the Asymptomatic Cyst Passer**

Drug	Adult Dosage (PO)	Pediatric Dosage (PO)
Diloxanide furoate* (Furamide)	500 mg tid × 10 days	20 mg/kg/day† × 10 days (maximum 1500 mg/day)
Paromomycin (Humatin)	30 mg/kg/day × 7 days	25 mg/kg/day† × 7 days (maximum 2 g/day)
Iodoquinol (Yodoxin)	650 mg tid × 20 days	30–40 mg/kg/day† × 20 days (maximum 2 g/day)

*In the United States, available only through the Centers for Disease Control: telephone 404-639-3670 or 404-639-3356; nights and emergencies, 404-639-2888. In Canada, authorized through the Bureau of Drugs, Health Protection Branch, Ottawa.

†Administered in three divided doses.

Bureau of Drugs, Health Protection Branch, Ottawa (Table 1). Paromomycin (Humatin), an aminoglycoside which is not absorbed from the gut, is safe in pregnancy. Diarrhea is the only significant side effect. Iodoquinol (diiodohydroxyquin [Yodoxin]), is marketed in North America and is equally effective to diloxanide furoate but needs to be administered in a 20-day course. In addition to gastrointestinal side effects, it may interfere with thyroid function tests because of its high iodine content. Rare dose-related neurotoxicity has been reported with prolonged drug use or inappropriate high doses. Metronidazole (Flagyl) should not be used to treat asymptomatic cyst or trophozoite passers because it often fails to eradicate these organisms from the lumen of the bowel (Table 1). It should be reserved for treatment of documented or suspected invasive disease.

Treatment of Invasive Disease (Amebic Colitis)

Metronidazole is the drug of choice for patients with invasive intestinal disease and amebic liver abscess (Tables 2 and 3). It is highly efficacious (90% cure rate in many studies) and is relatively well tolerated. Despite widespread use of this drug, *E. histolytica* resistance to metronidazole has not been a problem. Although most authorities recommend that amebic colitis be treated for 7 to 10 days, recent studies indicate that 2.4 grams of metronidazole given once daily orally for 3 days is equally effective. Metronidazole is not recommended for use in pregnancy even though it has not been shown to be teratogenic in humans. In one study, over 200 patients received the drug in the third trimester of pregnancy without adverse effects to the fetus. Therapy during pregnancy is warranted for invasive amebic disease because of the risk of severe complications if therapy were withheld.

Common side effects of metronidazole therapy include nausea, headache, metallic taste, abdominal discomfort, and dark-colored urine. Ataxia, confusion, insomnia, and paresthesias may occur occasionally.

TABLE 2. **Treatment of Invasive Disease***

Drug	Adult Dosage	Pediatric Dosage
Metronidazole (Flagyl)†	750 mg tid × 5–10 days **Alternative** 2.5 gm once daily × 3 days	30–50 mg/kg/day‡ × 10 days (maximum 2250 mg/day)
Tinidazole (Fasigyn)‖	2 gm once daily × 3 days	50 mg/kg/day × 3 days
Alternative		
Dehydroemetine§ (Mebadin)	1–1.5 mg/kg/day IM × 5 days (maximum 90 mg/day)	1–1.5 mg/kg/day IM × 5 days (maximum 90 mg/day)

*Treatment of intestinal disease is followed by a complete course of a luminal agent (e.g., diloxanide furoate) to eliminate intestinal colonization using the regimen in Table 1.

†May be administered intravenously if patient unable to take by mouth.

‡Administered in three divided doses.

§In the United States, available only through the Centers for Disease Control: telephone 404-639-3670 or 404-639-3356; nights and emergencies, 404-639-2888. In Canada, authorized through the Bureau of Drugs, Health Protection Branch, Ottawa.

‖Marketed outside of the United States and Canada.

Patients should avoid alcoholic beverages due to metronidazole's disulfiram-like properties. The drug is available for intravenous administration in patients unable to take medications by the oral route. Because metronidazole usually fails to eliminate intestinal carriage, a lumen-active agent should always be given in conjunction with metronidazole therapy for any form of invasive disease (colitis or amebic abscess) whether or not parasites are detected on stool examination. To reduce the likelihood of additive side effects, we recommend that these drugs be given sequentially (see Table 1).

Outside of the United States and Canada, tinidazole (Fasigyn),* a metronidazole derivative, is the preferred drug for the treatment of invasive disease because it is generally associated with fewer gas-

*Not available in the United States.

TABLE 3. **Treatment of Amebic Liver Abscess***

Drug of Choice	Adult Dosage	Pediatric Dosage
Metronidazole†	750 mg tid × 5–10 days or 2.5 gm orally stat	30–50 mg/kg/day‡ × 5–10 days
Alternative		
Dehydroemetine§ (Mebadin)	1–1.5 mg/kg/day IM × 5 days (maximum 90 mg/day)	1–1.5 mg/kg/day IM × 5 days (maximum 90 mg/day)

*Treatment of amebic liver abscess is followed by a complete course of a luminal agent (e.g., diloxanide furoate) to eliminate intestinal colonization using the regimen in Table 1.

†May be administered intravenously if patient unable to take by mouth.

‡Administered in three divided doses.

§In the United States, available only through the Centers for Disease Control: telephone 404-639-3670 or 404-639-3356; nights and emergencies, 404-639-2888. In Canada, authorized through the Bureau of Drugs, Health Protection Branch, Ottawa.

trointestinal side effects. The dose is 2 grams or 50 mg per kg orally once per day for 3 days. It, too, should be followed by a lumen-active agent.

Tetracycline and erythromycin followed by a luminal agent are effective alternatives for patients with mild amebic colitis who are unable to tolerate metronidazole. However, these regimens do not eradicate parasites in the liver. Although dehydroemetine (Mebadin)* is rapidly amebicidal, it has significant toxicity. At least 50% of patients experience gastrointestinal side effects; cardiotoxicity and myotoxicity are not uncommon. The drug has little activity against lumen-dwelling forms. In the United States, the drug is available only from the Centers for Disease Control and, in Canada, only with the authorization of the Bureau of Drugs, Health Protection Branch, Ottawa (see Table 2). Follow-up stool examinations 2 weeks after the completion of therapy should be carried out to screen for treatment failures. Amebic antibodies may take up to 2 years to disappear after successful treatment.

AMEBIC LIVER ABSCESS

Patients with amebic liver abscess generally present with fever, weight loss, abdominal pain, and hepatic tenderness. The diagnosis is established by demonstrating a space-occupying lesion in the liver radiographically (e.g., ultrasound, CT scan). Amebic serology is positive in 99% of patients but may be negative during the first week of symptoms.

Treatment of Amebic Liver Abscess

Amebic liver abscess can usually be managed by medical therapy alone (see Table 3). The drug of choice is metronidazole followed by an agent to eradicate intraluminal infection. In uncomplicated mild to moderate disease, single-dose therapy with 2.5 grams of metronidazole† has been shown to be effective and provides welcome relief to those patients who cannot tolerate the longer traditional 5-to-10 day regimen. Although some authors recommend the addition of chloroquine phosphate (Aralen) to metronidazole when treating critically ill patients, there are no data to support an improved outcome with this combination. Chloroquine was recommended because it is an amebicide that reaches extremely high levels in hepatic tissue (but not in bowel mucosa). Percutaneous drainage of liver abscesses should be reserved for patients who are not responding to medical therapy or who have large abscesses that are at risk for rupture. Open surgical drainage has been the standard approach in patients whose liver abscesses have ruptured into the peritoneal space, but some of these patients have now been managed with percutaneous drainage. All patients treated surgically still require a full course of antiamebic therapy. Patients should be followed up for at least 6 months. The abscess cavity often resolves slowly over several months, as determined by ultrasonography; up to 20% of patients will have a permanent hepatic cyst after the completion of therapy. Amebic antibodies may take 2 years or more to disappear after successful treatment.

*Investigational drug in the United States.
†Exceeds dosage recommended by the manufacturer.

BACTEREMIA

method of
HAROLD W. HOROWITZ, M.D., and
HARISH MARISIDDAIAH, M.D.
New York Medical College
Valhalla, New York

Bacteremia is defined as the presence of viable bacteria in the bloodstream. It is a frequent event, even in healthy individuals, and may occur transiently after brushing teeth, bowel movements, sexual intercourse in women, and endoscopic procedures such as cystoscopy or endoscopy (3 to 13% upper endoscopy and 0 to 27% colonoscopy). The bacteria that enter the bloodstream trigger a rapid systemic response generally leading to phagocytosis by polymorphonuclear cells, and active infection is aborted. However, when the immune system falters, a persistent or overwhelming infection of the bloodstream may lead to a series of physiologic responses that initiate sepsis. The incidence of primary bloodstream infections increased yearly from 1980 to 1989 in the United States, with increases ranging from 279% in small nonteaching hospitals to 70% in large teaching hospitals during that period.

Since nearly 25% of positive blood cultures are caused by contaminants, it is important clinically to attempt to determine whether a positive blood culture represents a true infection or simply contamination that may have occurred by drawing blood through colonized skin or intravascular devices. The specific organism that is cultured frequently gives an indication of whether contamination has occurred. For instance, 94% of *Staphylococcus epidermidis* and diphtheroid blood isolates are considered contaminants, as are nearly 80% of *Bacillus* sp. When blood cultures become positive after 48 to 72 hours of incubation (particularly from broth culture only), when multiple skin organisms are cultured simultaneously, or when cultures are positive from only one of several cultures drawn simultaneously, contamination should be suspected. Colonization is a particularly difficult problem to evaluate when cultures are taken from indwelling catheters of hospitalized patients owing to the frequent colonization of these catheters by skin organisms or secondary seeding of the catheter from distant sites of infection. Peripheral blood cultures generally remain negative when only central catheters are colonized. When foreign bodies such as Ommaya reservoirs or prosthetic devices are in place, bacteremia due to organisms generally considered contaminants must be considered seriously owing to the possible seeding of these devices. *Clostridium* sp., Enterococci, and *Streptococcus viridans* frequently represent contaminants when cultured from the blood. The treatment provided depends on the clinical setting in which these organisms are isolated. *Staphylococcus aureus, Streptococcus pyogenes,* Enterobacteriaceae, *Pseudomonas aeruginosa,* or gram-negative anaerobes must be considered significant pathogens when isolated from the blood. The frequency of the isolation of coagulase-negative staphylococci, *Enterococci,* and *S. aureus* has increased dramatically in the past 20 years compared with Enterobacteriaceae. These changes in the bacterial flora isolated from the blood probably reflect the advent of long-lasting central venous access devices and the availability and use of antibiotics with broad-spectrum, gram-negative coverage.

Bacteremia may be transient, intermittent, or continuous. Transient bacteremia occurs early in the course of localized infections such as pneumonia or urinary tract infections, or after the manipulation of colonized surfaces such as occurs during endoscopy or even after removal of a Foley catheter. Intermittent bacteremia generally occurs in the clinical setting of an undrained abscess, whereas continuous bacteremia occurs in the presence of endovascular infection such as endocarditis. A single blood culture has a sensitivity of 80 to 90%. However, the sensitivity of three blood cultures approaches 100%. Rarely are more than three blood cultures required in a 24-hour period to diagnose bacteremia except perhaps in instances in which patients have been treated with antibiotics within 1 to 2 weeks of culturing. Blood cultures become positive within 24 hours nearly 66% of the time and, within 72 hours, nearly 90% of the time. The sensitivity of blood cultures depends on the amount of blood that is cultured. The recommended volume is 10 mL per culture. The timing of drawing blood cultures is less important than traditionally thought owing to the unpredictability of bacteremia in relationship to fever in patients with transient and intermittent bacteremia and the fact that bacteremia is continuous with endovascular infection.

TREATMENT

Antibiotic Choice

Frequently, antibiotics are initiated before blood culture results are available in the febrile or otherwise clinically deteriorating patient, based on a suspected site of infection and the severity of the illness. Although multiple models have been developed to predict bacteremia, none have sufficient sensitivity and specificity to be of clinical utility. Fever higher than 38.3° C (100.92° F), the presence of a rapidly (<1 month) or ultimately fatal (<5 years) disease, shaking chills, intravenous drug abuse, findings of acute abdomen on physical examination, major comorbidity, low systolic blood pressure, and low platelet counts have been found to be independent predictors of bacteremia in patients who have had blood cultures for a multitude of reasons. In the patient with bacteremia, the appropriate empiric choice of antibiotics may be lifesaving.

The importance of a detailed history and physical examination cannot be overestimated in the choice of empiric antibiotic therapy, because the suspected site of infection determines the spectrum of antibiotic activity required for treatment (Table 1). Because the signs and symptoms of bacteremia are not specific and may be subtle, the treating physician must have a strong clinical suspicion of bacteremia, particularly in the elderly, neutropenic, or hospitalized patient with clinical status changes. When a primary site of infection can be found, the bacteremia is considered secondary bacteremia, in contrast to primary bacteremia, in which no localizing source of infection can be identified.

Specific epidemiologic information regarding the patient's age, travel history, recent surgical or other invasive procedures, occupation, intravenous drug use, risk factors for HIV infection, and recent antibiotic use (or treatment for infection) should be ascertained. Recent medication changes should also be determined to uncover possible drug fever. Moreover, any underlying disorders of the immune system must be determined because specific immune function abnormalities predispose individuals to specific infections (Table 2). A knowledge of the patient's prior antibiotic allergy and the nature of these sensitivities helps determine whether certain antibiotics are relatively or absolutely contraindicated. For instance, a history of a rash to penicillin would rarely deter the use of a cephalosporin, whereas a history of an anaphylactic reaction to penicillin would be a contraindication to cephalosporin use without prior desensitization. Nephrotoxic or hepatotoxic antibiotics, or both, should be used with caution in patients with a history of renal or hepatic disease respectively. System-specific information obtained from the review of systems is critical in helping localize the primary site of infection.

A detailed physical examination should also provide clues regarding the underlying site of infection. A wealth of information may be found in the dermatologic examination. For instance, peripheral signs of endocarditis such as splinter hemorrhages, Janeway lesions, Roth spots, disseminated purpura in meningococcemia, ecthyma gangrenosum generally caused by gram-negative bacteremia, or signs of sepsis such as petechiae or peripheral vasoconstriction may be found. Costovertebral angle tenderness in the presence of urinary frequency or dysuria may signify pyelonephritis. When a specific site of infection cannot be determined by the information gathered by historical or physical examination, the abdomen or lungs should be suspected as potential sources of primary infection.

Prior to initiating antibiotic therapy, appropriate laboratory studies should be performed, including complete blood count, urinalysis, chest roentgenogram, and cultures of blood, urine, sputum, and cerebrospinal fluid (when clinically indicated). When a single culture has been reported to be positive for an organism frequently considered a contaminant, two sets of blood cultures should be acquired prior to initiating antibiotics. If the second set of cultures is negative, frequently antibiotic therapy can be stopped. Drainage of abscesses for material to culture should be performed prior to antibiotic therapy, if possible. A Gram's stain of potentially infected material is a simple and very useful tool on which to base empiric therapy. Although obtaining material for culture prior to antibiotic therapy is optimal, antibiotic therapy should not be withheld in the face of severe infection while awaiting a diagnostic procedure.

The choice of antibiotics for initial therapy depends mostly on the spectrum of activity desired to treat

TABLE 1. **Empiric Antibiotic Therapy for Bacteremia Based on Suspected Site of Primary Infection***

Meningitis†		
Adult	*Streptococcus pneumoniae, Neisseria meningitidis*	Ceftriaxone, cefotaxime
Postneurosurgical	Enterobacteriaceae, *Pseudomonas aeruginosa, Staphylococcus aureus, Staphylococcus epidermidis*	Ceftazidime or antipseudomonal penicillin‡ plus aminoglycoside§ plus vancomycin
Pneumonia†		
Community acquired	*Streptococcus pneumoniae, Haemophilus influenzae*, mouth anaerobes, *Legionella* and other atypical bacteria	Cefuroxime or cefotaxime plus erythromycin if atypical pneumonia is suspected
Hospital acquired	Enterobacteriaceae, *Pseudomonas aeruginosa, Staphylococcus aureus*‖	Ceftazidime or antipseudomonal penicillin plus aminoglycoside
Endocarditis		
Native valve (acute)	*Enterococcus, Staphylococcus aureus, Streptococcus pneumoniae*	Vancomycin or penicillin plus nafcillin‖ plus gentamicin
Native valve (subacute)	*Enterococcus, Streptococcus bovis, Streptococcus viridans*	Penicillin G or ampicillin‖ plus gentamicin
Prosthetic valve (early)	Enterobacteriaceae, *Staphylococcus aureus, Staphylococcus epidermidis*	Vancomycin plus gentamicin plus third-generation cephalosporin¶
Intravenous drug user	Enterobacteriaciae, *Staphylococcus aureus*	Nafcillin‖ plus gentamicin plus anti-pseudomonal third-generation cephalosporin**
Urinary Tract†		
Community acquired	Enterobacteriacae, *Enterococcus*	Ampicillin plus gentamicin (trimethoprim/sulfamethoxazole or third-generation cephalosporin or quinolone†† if no gram-positive cocci on Gram's stain)
Hospital acquired or recurrent	Enterobacteriaceae, *Pseudomonas aeruginosa, Enterococcus*	Third-generation cephalosporin or anti-pseudomonal penicillin plus aminoglycoside
Gastrointestinal Tract		
Bowel or hepatobiliary	Enterobacteriaceae, anaerobes, *Enterococcus*	Clindamycin or metronidazole plus aminoglycoside
Primary peritonitis	Enterobacteriaceae, *Streptococcus pneumoniae*, group A streptococci	Aminoglycoside plus ampicillin; or cefoxitin or ampicillin/sulbactam alone
Skin and Soft Tissue		
Wound infection	*Staphylococcus aureus*, Enterobacteriaceae, *Staphylococcus epidermidis*	Vancomycin plus aminoglycoside or third-generation cephalosporin
Primary cellulitis	*Staphylococcus aureus, Streptococci*	Nafcillin or first-generation cephalosporin
Gynecologic Infection		
Endometritis	Enterobacteriaceae, Groups A and B streptococci, *Bacteroides* sp., esp. *Bacteroides bivivus*	Clindamycin or metronidazole plus aminoglycoside or third-generation cephalosporin
Pelvic inflammatory disease	*Neisseria gonorrhoeae, Chlamydia trachomatis, Bacteroides* sp., Enterobacteriaceae, streptococci	Cefoxitin or ampicillin/sulbactam plus doxycycline
Neutropenic Host	Enterobacteriaceae, *Pseudomonas aeruginosa*	Antipseudomonal third-generation cephalosporin or antipseudomonal penicillin plus aminoglycoside
Catheter-Related Sepsis	*Staphylococcus epidermidis, Staphylococcus aureus*, Enterobacteriaceae, *Pseudomonas aeruginosa*	Vancomycin plus antipseudomonal third-generation cephalosporin
Unidentified Site	Enterobacteriaceae, *Staphylococcus aureus*, streptococci	Aminoglycoside plus third-generation cephalosporin

*Initial therapy should be modified and simplified if possible when culture results are known.
†Base therapy on Gram's stain when possible.
‡Anti-pseudomonal penicillins and related compounds include ticarcillin, pipericillin, mezlocillin, imipenem/cilastatin, ticarcillin/clavulanate, and piperacillin/tazobactam.
§Aminoglycosides include gentamicin, tobramycin, amikacin.
‖Use vancomycin if high risk for methicillin-resistant *S. aureus* or penicillin allergic.
¶Third-generation cephalosporins and related compounds include ceftazidime, cefoperazone, ceftriaxone, ceftizoxime, and cefotaxime.
**Antipseudomonal third-generation cephalosporins and equivalents include ceftazidime, cefoperazone, aztreonam, quinolones.
††Parenteral quinolones include ciprofloxacin and ofloxacin.

TABLE 2. **Epidemiologic and Immunologic Risks for Specific Organisms Causing Bacteremia**

Bites	
Human	*Eikenella corrodens*
Cat	*Pasteurella multocida*
Dog	*Capnocytophagia canimorus*
After splenectomy	*Streptococcus pneumoniae, Neisseria meningitidis, Haemophilus influenzae*
Sickle cell anemia	*Haemophilus influenzae, Salmonella* sp., *Streptococcus pneumoniae*
Neutropenia	*Corynebacterium jekeium, Clostridium tertium, Clostridium septicum*
Late component complement deficiency	*Neisseria meningitidis*
Chronic granulomatous disease	*Staphylococcus aureus*
Multiple myeloma and other humoral immune deficiencies	*Streptococcus pneumoniae, Haemophilus influenzae, Neisseria meningitidis, Escherichia coli*
Cellular immune deficiencies	*Listeria monocytogenes, Salmonella* sp.
AIDS	*Salmonella* sp., *Staphylococcus aureus, Haemophilus influenzae, Streptococcus pneumoniae, Pseudomonas aeruginosa*
Rheumatoid arthritis	*Staphylococcus aureus*
Burn	*Pseudomonas aeruginosa, Staphylococcus aureus,* Enterobacteriaceae
Toxic shock	*Staphylococcus aureus*, Group A streptococcus
Pregnancy	Group B streptococci, *Listeria monocytogenes*
Achlorhydria/postgastrectomy	*Salmonella* sp.
Exposure to raw shellfish or brackish water	*Vibrio* sp.
Flea bite or contaminated meat ingestion	*Yersinia pestis*
Contact with body fluid or tissue of infected mammal or bite by infected arthropod (tick)	*Francisella tularensis*
Ingestion of unpasteurized milk or cheese, direct contact with contaminated tissues of cattle or swine	*Brucella*
Ingestion of unpasteurized milk or cheese	*Listeria monocytogenes, Salmonella*

Abbreviation: AIDS, acquired immune deficiency syndrome.

the suspected site of infection. Table 1 lists choices for empiric treatment based on a suspected site of infection. In patients without an obvious site of primary infection, empiric broad-spectrum coverage of both gram-negative and gram-positive bacteria should be started because clinical presentation alone cannot distinguish between these two broad groups of infecting organisms. Usually, more than a single antibiotic is given in order to provide broad coverage and treat potentially antibiotic-resistant organisms. This is particularly true in hospital-acquired infections, suspected intraabdominal sepsis, and when treating the immunocompromised host. However, in the patient who is not critically ill, therapy with extremely broad-spectrum antibiotics such as the carbapenem imipenem–cilastatin (Primaxin) or an antipseudomonal penicillin/B-lactamase inhibitor combination are appropriate choices for empiric therapy. For the hospitalized patient, the initial choice of antibiotics must take into account antibiotic susceptibilities of bacteria previously isolated from specimens such as sputum and urine that had been considered colonizing organisms.

In order to rapidly reach desired blood levels of antibiotics and because of potential problems with drug absorption, intravenous rather than oral therapy is generally initiated. When culture results and bacterial susceptibility patterns are completed, antibiotic regimens can often be simplified to less toxic, less costly, and narrower spectrum therapy. However, it is also important to recognize that the organism isolated from the bloodstream may be one of several organisms present at the primary site of infection. For example, *E. coli* may be the only bacterium cultured from the blood when the primary site of infection is a polymicrobial intra-abdominal abscess. In this instance, it would be inappropriate to treat the patient only with ampicillin, to which the *E. coli* is sensitive. There is no single way to initiate and subsequently complete antibiotic therapy. The treating physician should be aware that, owing to the proliferation of many antibiotics with similar spectra of activity, several different treatment options are available and acceptable.

Other factors that must be evaluated in choosing therapy include

1. Do the infecting organism(s) require synergistic therapy? Synergy between antibiotics represents the enhanced killing of bacteria that occurs when the antimicrobial activity of two or more agents is greater than that of the individual agents, either alone or when their modes of effectiveness are combined. Generally, synergy is achieved when antibiotics have different mechanisms of action. For instance, the treatment of serious enterococcal, group C streptococcal, or *P. aeruginosa* infections is improved with the use of a cell wall–active agent (ampicillin, penicillin, or vancomycin in the case of enterococcus or group C streptococcal infection and an antipseudomonal pen-

icillin for *P. aeruginosa*) that weakens the cell wall, thereby allowing penetration of the synergizing agent, and an aminoglycoside such as gentamicin, that acts at the ribosomal level.

2. Is single drug therapy likely to induce or promote a drug-resistant population? This most commonly occurs in the setting of *Enterobacter, Serratia,* and *P. aeruginosa* infections. Two antibiotics with different mechanisms of action may be preferred to a single antibiotic in treating these specific organisms.

3. What is the susceptibility pattern of specific bacteria at the treating institution? For instance, patterns of resistance to methicillin among *S. aureus;* to ampicillin and aminoglycosides among *Enterococci;* and extended spectrum cephalosporins, penicillins, and aminoglycosides among *P. aeruginosa* vary widely between institutions, even those located within the same geographic region.

4. Is the infection hospital acquired (nosocomial) or community acquired? In general, nosocomial infections, particularly pneumonias and urinary tract infections, have greater resistance to antibiotics than community-acquired infections. Prior to the availability of antibiotic sensitivity patterns, two antibiotics may be preferred for initial treatment to provide broad coverage. Moreover, in certain geographic regions, specific bacteria may be found as nosocomial but not community-acquired pathogens, such as *Legionella* species.

5. Are there specific requirements for antibiotic penetration or site-specific activity? For example, first-generation cephalosporins, second-generation cephalosporins with the exception of cefuroxime (Ceftin), and cefoperazone (Cefobid) and the third-generation cephalosporins do not penetrate the blood-brain barrier well and should not be used for the treatment of meningitis. Although concerns have been raised regarding inactivation of antibiotics in abscesses, such as the deacetylation of chloramphenicol or the reduced activity of aminoglycosides in the face of the anaerobic environment of an abscess, few clinical data suggest that this factor is of clinical importance. Moreover, multiple in vitro studies have reported wide variations of antibiotic penetration into bone or valvular vegetations that might influence the choice of antibiotic for the treatment of osteomyelitis and bacterial endocarditis, respectively. However, correlation of these factors with clinical outcome has been difficult to establish.

6. Can combination therapy be used to shorten the course of therapy? For instance, endocarditis caused by *Streptococcus viridans* with minimal inhibitory concentrations of penicillin G (less than or equal to 0.1 μg per mL) can be treated for 2 weeks with the combination of penicillin G plus gentamicin, compared with 4 weeks using single-agent therapy with penicillin G or ceftriaxone (Rocephin). Although the combination of an anti-staphylococcal penicillin plus an aminoglycoside is synergistic against *S. aureus* and decreases the duration of *S. aureus* bacteremia, clinical studies have not shown superiority of the combination compared with anti-staphylococcal penicillin therapy alone.

After antibiotic therapy has been initiated, the patient must be monitored closely for signs of treatment failure. Failure may represent a hidden focus of infection that must be drained or removed, antibiotics that are inactive against the infecting organism(s), inadequate serum or tissue antibiotic levels, and rarely, antibiotic antagonism. Fungal superinfection also must suspected when broad antibacterial therapy is failing. When appropriate, antibiotic peak and trough levels should be monitored and adjusted as needed. Vancomycin and aminoglycosides are the most commonly used antibiotics that require monitoring. A combined surgical-medical approach is required for many infections. Infected tissue may need to be debrided; abscesses, empyema or joints drained; prosthetic devices removed; or infected heart valves replaced. In some situations, simply removing an infected catheter may be enough to clear bacteremia. Re-evaluation of the patient should occur frequently, and blood and other cultures should be repeated if fever persists or signs of clinical deterioration occur. Toxicities that may be due to antibiotics, such as rashes, interstitial nephritis, diarrhea (*Clostridium difficile* and others), and cytopenias, must be monitored so that antibiotics can be switched or stopped as necessary.

The length of therapy for primary bacteremia is typically 1 to 2 weeks. *S. aureus* bacteremia, with or without an indwelling intravascular device, has traditionally been treated for a more prolonged (4-week) period of time owing to the high frequency of endocarditis with short courses of treatment. However, in uncomplicated *S. aureus* catheter-associated bacteremia, if the catheter is removed and defervescence occurs within 3 days, 10 to 14 days of intravenous therapy is sufficient. When secondary bacteremia occurs, the length of the treatment period may be prolonged owing to the requirement to treat the primary source of infection, such as endocarditis or osteomyelitis. In the neutropenic host, antibiotic therapy is generally continued until the resolution of neutropenia or until a specific infection has been treated, whichever is longer. Although it is possible to discontinue antibiotic therapy in a subset of neutropenic patients who are afebrile yet remain neutropenic, sepsis has been reported in up to 50% of cases in which this approach is taken. Until studies better define which neutropenic patients can safely have antibiotic therapy stopped, the aforementioned recommendations should probably be followed. With the enhanced gastrointestinal absorption and broader spectrum of antimicrobial activity of some of the newer oral agents such as the quinolones, oral therapy can be considered after defervescence using intravenous therapy. This has been best studied in patients with urosepsis, in whom after as few as 3 days of intravenous therapy, oral therapy has been used successfully.

SEPSIS

Approximately 300,000 to 500,000 cases of sepsis occur in the United States annually. The mortality rate ranges from 30 to 50% even with the appropriate use of antibiotics, making this the thirteenth leading cause of death in the United States. In an effort to control bacterial infection, macrophages, lymphocytes, neutrophils, and endothelial cells release a myriad of endogenous inflammatory mediators that initiate physiologic responses that are both beneficial and detrimental to the host (Fig. 1). Myocardial depression and dilatation, peripheral vasodilatation followed by vasoconstriction, leukocyte aggregation, and endothelial cell dysfunction will ensue if the systemic inflammatory response goes unmitigated, ultimately leading to refractory hypotension and multiple organ system failure.

Sepsis is actually but one of several inciting events including pancreatitis, burns, trauma, transplant rejection, hemorrhage, and even therapeutic cytokine administration that initiate the sepsis syndrome, which recently has been defined as the systemic inflammatory response syndrome. Sepsis implies that the primary cause for systemic inflammatory response syndrome is the release of bacterial products such as teichoic acid antigen, endotoxin, or exotoxins. If the clinical situation worsens, the patient may develop severe sepsis with the onset of hypotension (a systolic blood pressure less than 90 mmHg or a 40 mmHg decrease from baseline), hypoperfusion, and organ dysfunction reflected by lactic acidosis, oliguria, and altered mental status. Septic shock signifies a further deterioration of clinical status and represents the failure of fluid resuscitation to ameliorate hypotension and the presence of perfusion abnormalities as noted earlier. Septic shock develops in approximately 50% of septic patients and is a major cause of the adult respiratory distress syndrome. As physiologic status deteriorates the patient may develop the multiple organ dysfunction syndrome, signifying that homeostatsis cannot be maintained without supportive therapy. As the patient moves through the continuum from sepsis to multiple organ dysfunction syndrome, the chance for survival decreases.

Although antibiotics may prevent the development of sepsis in the bacteremic patient nearly 50% of the time and remain a mainstay of therapy, other supportive measures have major roles to play in patient survival. Management of the septic patient depends on the specific physiologic abnormalities that are present at any given point in time, and these abnormalities are apt to change rapidly in the critically ill patient. For the purposes of close physiologic monitoring, patient care of the septic patient is generally best achieved in an intensive care unit setting. Frequently, pulmonary artery catheters are required in order to accurately determine left-sided heart filling pressures.

During the early phases of the septic syndrome when systemic vascular resistance falls and cardiac output is elevated, early and rapid fluid resuscitation with potentially large volumes of fluid should be initiated. If hypotension persists despite fluid replacement and maintenance of pulmonary artery wedge pressures of 15 to 18 mmHg, then a vasopressor agent such as dopamine should be employed at doses from 2 to 20 μg per kg per minute (titrating upward from lower doses). If doses higher than this are needed to maintain the patient's blood pressure in the normal range, then a second agent such as dobutamine or isoproterenol should be added. The aim is to keep the systolic blood pressure high enough (usually >90 mmHg) to perfuse vital organs such as the brain, heart, and kidneys in order to prevent cerebral anoxia, myocardial ischemia, and acute tubular necrosis. Metabolic acidosis commonly develops due to tissue hypoperfusion, and if it is severe enough, it will impair the response to sympathomimetic agents and may cause myocardial depression. However, bicarbonate administration generally is not necessary and should be employed only when the arterial pH is less than 7.1. Ventilatory assistance with positive end-expiratory pressure is frequently required when supplemental oxygen cannot maintain the PaO_2 higher than 50 to 60 mmHg. The requirement for mechanical ventilation generally signifies the development of adult respiratory distress syndrome.

Multiple adjunctive therapies have been attempted to lower the rates of morbidity and mortality of the septic patient including corticosteroids, naloxone, and more recently, adoptive immunotherapy using monoclonal anti-endotoxin antibodies, as well as genetically engineered products that interfere with the cytokine network (Fig. 1). Although the use of corticosteroids as adjunctive therapy in shock was debated for many years, several recent controlled studies have demonstrated no significant survival advantage related to their use. They are presently not recommended for the treatment of shock. Naloxone* has provided transient improvement of hypotension in patients with sepsis without significantly altering the mortality rate. Several monoclonal antibodies directed against endotoxin have been tested in large human clinical trials. Using a mouse-derived antiendotoxin monoclonal antibody (E5), a subgroup of patients with gram-negative sepsis without refractory shock appeared to benefit from such therapy. However, the overall rate of mortality was not significantly different between treatment and placebo groups. Moreover, a second study could not verify the results of the first trial. A single trial testing HA-1A, a human-derived monoclonal anti-endotoxin antibody, demonstrated effectiveness of the antibody only in a subgroup of patients with gram-negative bacteremia without sepsis. Because of the difficulty in predicting which patients actually had gram-negative sepsis, approximately three patients without gram-negative sepsis received the monoclonal antibodies to every patient with gram-negative sepsis. This is problematic in light of the high costs of these products.

*Not FDA approved for this indication.

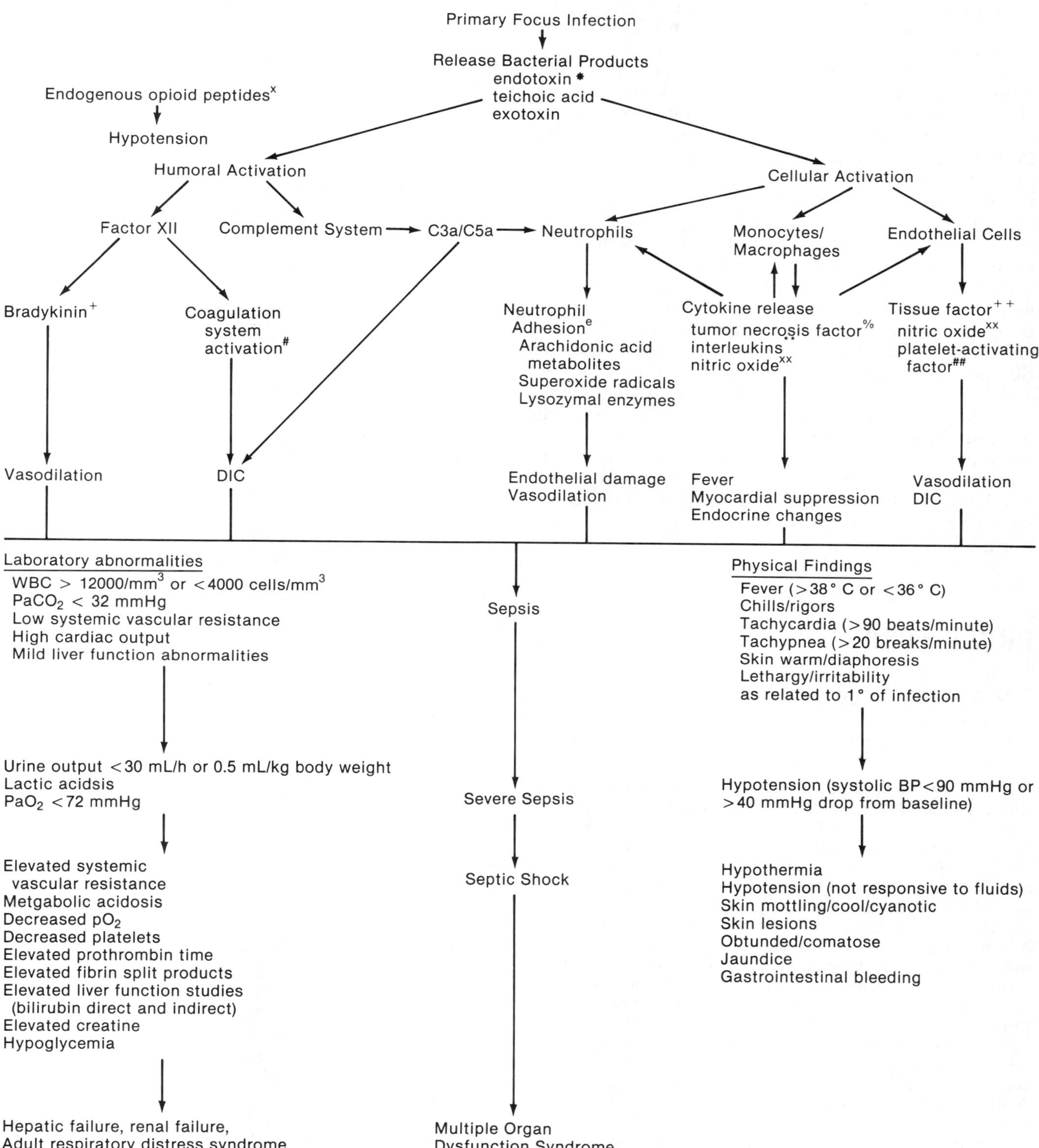

Figure 1. Pathogenesis of sepsis: Symbols represent specific therapeutic interventions in trial: *, antiendotoxin antibodies; ×, naloxone; +, bradykinin antagonists; #, antithrombin 3; e, cyclooxygenase inhibitors, antiphospholipase antibodies; %, tumor necrosis factor antibodies or receptor infusion; **, interleukin-1 receptor antagonist, anti-interleukin-6 antibodies, interleukin 10 infusion; ××, nitric oxide inhibitors; ++, tissue factor inhibitor; ##, platelet-activating factor antagonist, platelet-activating factor receptors, thromboxane synthetase inhibitors, thromboxane receptor blockers

Although infusion of anti-tumor necrosis factor antibodies, soluble tumor necrosis factor receptors, interleukin-1 receptor antibody (IL-1Rab), antithrombin III, inhibitors of nitric oxide, platelet-activating factor antagonists, and interleukin 10 have all shown some beneficial effects in altering various parameters of endotoxin-mediated sepsis in animal models, to date only limited data are available in human trials. Preliminary human trials of IL-1Rab and anti-tumor necrosis factor monoclonal antibodies have not demonstrated significant reduction in the mortality rate to date. Further studies aimed at interrupting the sepsis syndrome, possibly using combinations of agents, are in developmental or early stages.

Attempts to reduce the incidence of nosocomial infection in the intensive care unit (where such infection occurs in up to 10% of patients) through the use of bowel decolonization regimens (nonabsorbable antibiotics or nonabsorbable antibiotics plus systemic agents) have been extensively explored. Although the incidence of nosocomial pneumonia may be reduced, most studies have not demonstrated a shortening of hospital stay, total antibiotic administration, or decreased morbidity rate. Moreover, concerns about the development of bacterial resistance and overall costs have been raised. At present, such prophylaxis is not routinely recommended.

BRUCELLOSIS

method of
M. YOUSUF KHAN, M.D.
King Fahad Hospital
Riyadh, Saudi Arabia

Brucellosis is a microbial infection of domestic animals that is transmissible to humans. This infection is caused by gram-negative bacteria belonging to the genus *Brucella*. *Brucella* species commonly involved in human infections are *Brucella melitensis* (goats, sheep), *Brucella suis* (hogs), *Brucella abortus* (cattle), and *Brucella canis* (dogs). Human infection most frequently results from ingestion of unpasteurized milk or milk products, or by direct contact with infected animal tissues. Workers in certain occupations, especially those working in meat-packing plants or on dairy farms or those performing veterinary surgery or laboratory bacteriologic tests, can be at risk for acquiring brucellosis. This infection is frequently reported from the Middle East, Africa, Russia, India, Europe (Spain, France, and Italy), South America, and Mexico. In the United States, the number of cases of brucellosis has decreased from a peak of 6000 in 1947 to approximately 200 annually in recent years.

In humans, the acute infection is associated with fever, chills, weakness, sweats, malaise, headache, backache, and arthralgia. Acute arthritis, especially of the sacroiliac and hip joints, is a common finding. Various complications may occur in 5 to 10% of patients with brucellosis. These complications include osteomyelitis of the spine, epididymo-orchitis, granulomatous hepatitis, meningoencephalitis, and infective endocarditis. This infection, because of its varied manifestations, may be easily misdiagnosed.

Brucellosis should be suspected in patients with a febrile illness, arthralgia or arthritis, and a history of exposure. Routine laboratory tests are not diagnostic. Diagnosis depends on serologic test results, with or without culture of *Brucella* from body fluids. Cultures are not always positive, and even if they are, results may be available in 7 to 21 days; therefore, serologic tests are most helpful for early diagnosis. Nearly all cases of acute brucellosis show an agglutinin titer of 1:160 or higher. Cultures of body fluids should be attempted before antimicrobial therapy is begun. Blood cultures are most useful in acute disease and may be positive in 50 to 75% of patients. Cultures of infected tissues and biopsies of bone marrow and abscesses may also be helpful. Bone marrow cultures may be positive even when blood cultures are negative and may remain positive after antibiotic therapy.

TREATMENT

Most patients with acute brucellosis require a few days of hospitalization for bed rest, rehydration, and nutritional support. Patients may be treated in an outpatient setting provided that they are not very ill. A combination of tetracycline and streptomycin is the current treatment of choice and results in the lowest relapse rates. The adult dose of tetracycline is 0.5 gram orally four times daily for 6 weeks. Streptomycin is given at a dose of 1 gram intramuscularly once daily for 2 weeks. Doxycycline (Vibramycin), 100 mg orally twice daily, may be substituted for tetracycline. Although doxycycline is expensive, it is easier to administer and results in better patient compliance. Rifampin (Rifadin) is generally active against *B. melitensis* but not always against *B. abortus*. To avoid emergence of resistant strains, rifampin should not be used as a single agent. It has been effective as a companion to tetracycline or doxycycline. Rifampin is used at a single daily dose of 900 mg orally. The combination of doxycycline and rifampin has shown satisfactory results and is suitable for outpatient use.

Relapses are rarely caused by resistant *Brucella* strains. They are due mainly to the intracellular nature of the infection because organisms may remain protected from antibodies and certain antimicrobial agents for long periods. Relapses may be treated successfully with a second course of treatment.

Brucellosis commonly causes abortion in the first and second trimesters of pregnancy. Early treatment may prevent this complication. Tetracycline should not be used in pregnant women because of the dangers of staining the developing teeth of the fetus and inducing skeletal deformities. Streptomycin is also considered to be unsafe in pregnancy. We have treated pregnant women with trimethoprim-sulfamethoxazole (Bactrim, Septra).* The treatment course consists of one double-strength tablet (160 mg of trimethoprim plus 800 mg of sulfamethoxazole) given twice daily by mouth for 6 weeks. This treatment prevents abortion when given early in the course of illness in pregnant women. In areas where prevalence of strains resistant to trimethoprim-sul-

*Not FDA approved for this indication.

famethoxazole is high, rifampin* may be used in combination with trimethoprim-sulfamethoxazole.* We have used this regimen in a few patients with a satisfactory outcome of pregnancy. Complete blood counts and liver function tests should be monitored during therapy to screen for any untoward reactions.

Children younger than 8 years of age should not be treated with tetracycline. Treatment consisting of trimethoprim-sulfamethoxazole and rifampin has been successful in eradicating infection in children. The dose of trimethoprim is 10 mg per kg per day and that of sulfamethoxazole is 50 mg per kg per day orally as two equal portions given every 12 hours. The dose of rifampin is 10 mg per kg per day once daily orally. In complicated cases, streptomycin, 15 mg per kg as a single intramuscular injection, may be added to this combination for the first 2 to 3 weeks of the total course of 6 weeks.

Neurobrucellosis is difficult to diagnose and treat. A regimen combining tetracycline, rifampin, and trimethoprim-sulfamethoxazole has generally been found to be effective. A longer course of therapy from 2 to 4 months is required in these patients. The actual duration of therapy depends on clinical improvement and favorable response of pleocytosis in the cerebrospinal fluid. Streptomycin may have to be added to this regimen in patients who are extremely ill. Streptomycin given intramuscularly and trimethoprim-sulfamethoxazole given intravenously should be used, together with rifampin and tetracycline by nasogastric tube, in unconscious patients who cannot take medications orally. Use of streptomycin is limited to 2 to 4 weeks, to avoid toxicity. Corticosteroids appear to be beneficial in neurobrucellosis. Patients with increased intracranial pressure and cranial nerve involvement should receive dexamethasone,* 4 mg intravenously or orally four times daily. Prednisone,* 40-80 mg orally daily, may be used in place of dexamethasone. The dose of corticosteroids is tapered over a few days, and discontinued after a period of up to 4 weeks. The doses given are for adults and should be adjusted for pediatric patients.

Brucella osteomyelitis (spondylitis) also requires a longer course of therapy. A combination of doxycycline or tetracycline with rifampin* for 6 to 9 months gives satisfactory results. *Brucella* spondylitis can mimic tuberculous spondylitis. If tuberculosis cannot be excluded, isoniazid,* 300 mg per day orally, should be added to this combination. If possible, abscesses should be drained surgically. Abscesses of the spleen or of one kidney are cured by the removal of the organ.

Infective endocarditis is the most serious complication of brucellosis. Once established, *Brucella* endocarditis is difficult to treat and may result in death. Surgical replacement of the damaged valve with a prosthetic valve, together with treatment with bactericidal drugs, may be curative. We have used ceftriaxone (Rocephin),* 1.0 gram intravenously twice daily, together with tetracycline and rifampin orally, and

*Not FDA approved for this indication.

have had an excellent clinical response and sterilization of blood cultures. However, surgical replacement of the diseased aortic valve (with ring abscess) was necessary because of relapse of bacteremia 1 year later.

New antimicrobial agents such as third-generation cephalosporins (e.g., ceftriaxone*) and quinolones have shown in vitro activity against *Brucella* species. In the past, cephalosporins have been ineffective in brucellosis. A recent study has reported an unacceptable failure rate when ceftriaxone was used alone for the treatment of brucellosis. Similarly, treatment with ciprofloxacin* alone has not been as successful as the standard combination therapy. Another quinolone, ofloxacin,* along with rifampin* when given for 6 weeks was found to be as effective as doxycycline plus rifampin. However, quinolones have not been approved for use in children and pregnant women.

*Not FDA approved for this indication.

CONJUNCTIVITIS

method of
JOHN P. FRANGIE, M.D.
Boston City Hospital

and

HOWARD M. LEIBOWITZ, M.D.
Boston University School of Medicine
Boston, Massachusetts

The conjunctiva is a mucous membrane that lines the posterior aspect of the lids and then sweeps around the anterior surface of the globe, ultimately fusing with the corneal epithelium at the limbus. Conjunctivitis connotes an inflammatory process of the conjunctiva that may be infectious or noninfectious. Noninfectious causes of conjunctivitis include exposure, allergy, and toxicity. Infectious conjunctivitis may result from bacterial, viral, or chlamydial agents. Although any age group may be affected by conjunctivitis, the implications of possible systemic sequelae in the neonatal population dictates that conjunctivitis in this age group be discussed separately.

NEONATAL CONJUNCTIVITIS

Neonatal conjunctivitis, or ophthalmia neonatorum, is conjunctival inflammation that occurs during the first 30 days postpartum. A complete work-up of neonatal conjunctivitis requires a clinical examination including fluorescein staining, Gram's and Giemsa stains, culture and sensitivity, and conjunctival scrapings. The physical signs of neonatal conjunctivitis tend to be nonspecific and include lid edema, discharge, conjunctival injection, and edema. Additionally, determination of an etiologic agent on the basis of onset with relation to birth has been proved to be an unreliable index. Meticulous work-up is critical because isolation of an infectious agent(s) may provide the clinician with information that has relevance on a systemic level. Although the pathogens in the neonatal population are not very different from those seen in adults, the immature neonatal immune system is more susceptible to systemic dissemination, occasionally with catastrophic results. Almost without exception, microbes responsible for ophthalmia neonatorum are encountered in the birth canal (unless premature membrane rupture allows in utero infection).

Buffered 1% silver nitrate solution is the most common ophthalmic agent instilled at birth. This agent tends to destroy *Neisseria* organisms with little effect on other pathogens, notably *Chlamydia* and viruses. It is interesting to note that the silver nitrate compound is intrinsically toxic and has the potential to cause chemical conjunctivitis. Indeed, the most common form of neonatal conjunctivitis is secondary to the prophylactic agent. Chemical conjunctivitis from silver nitrate is characterized by the signs of conjunctivitis listed earlier; however, this entity is self-limited and typically resolves within 36 hours.

A wide spectrum of bacteria may cause ophthalmia neonatorum (Table 1). Staphylococci and streptococci represent the majority of gram-positive isolates. Gram-positive infections may be treated with topical erythromycin (0.5% ointment, 4 to 6 times per day) for two weeks. Gram-negative infections may be caused by a number of coliform bacteria including *Escherichia coli, Enterobacter* spp., *Proteus* spp., and *Serratia marcescens.* Additionally, *Klebsiella pneumoniae* and *Haemophilus* species have been isolated. Tobramycin (Tobrex), 0.3% ointment, 4 to 6 times per day for 2 weeks, is the drug of choice. With few exceptions, we recommend the use of ointments rather

TABLE 1. **Neonatal Conjunctivitis**

Organism	Topical Therapy	Systemic Therapy
Gram positive	Erythromycin 0.5% 4–6 times daily	Not indicated
Gram negative (except *Haemophilus* sp. and *Neisseria* sp.)	Tobramycin 0.3% 4–6 times daily*	Not indicated
Haemophilus sp.	Polymyxin B compound (Polytrim) 10,000 U per ml 4–6 times daily	May be indicated if associated with cellulitis
Neisseria sp.	Penicillin G 20,000 U per ml every half hour	Penicillin G 50,000 U/kg/day in 4 divided doses
Neisseria sp. (resistant to penicillin)	Bacitracin 500 μg/gm 8 times daily	Ceftriaxone 50 mg/kg per day
Chlamydia	Erythromycin 0.5% 4–6 times daily	Erythromycin 40 mg/kg per day orally
Herpes simplex virus	Trifluorothymidine 1.0% every 2 hours	If associated with signs of systemic dissemination

*Hourly instillation should be used for *Pseudomonas* sp.

than solutions; instillation of solutions in crying neonates may result in a dilution or total wash-out of the antimicrobial agents. The one exception is *Haemophilus* spp., which tend to be resistant to tobramycin. The use of a polymyxin B/trimethoprim compound (Polytrim), 4 to 6 times per day, is indicated. If *Pseudomonas* spp. are isolated, one should instill tobramycin hourly.

Prior to the introduction of Credé's prophylaxis (2% silver nitrate) in 1881, *Neisseria gonorrhoeae* was a major source of ophthalmic morbidity in the neonatal population. Although the occurrence of neonatal gonococcal conjunctivitis has decreased considerably, the significant morbidity associated with this condition mandates that this infection be diagnosed and treated promptly. *Neisseria gonorrhoeae* has the ability to penetrate an intact corneal epithelium, and, therefore, is capable of causing corneal perforation. Gonococci appear as gram-negative diplococci. Thayer-Martin medium provides the best medium for growth of this agent. Isolation of gonococci should prompt the physician to rule out other associated venereal pathogens including *Chlamydia,* syphilis, herpes simplex virus (HSV), and human immunodeficiency virus (HIV). Appropriate treatment of the mother and her sexual partner(s) should also be undertaken. It should be noted that owing to the chelating properties of tetracycline, this drug should not be used systemically in pediatric patients (up to age 8 years) or nursing or pregnant mothers. Lifelong discoloration of deciduous teeth has been reported in children following the administration of tetracycline.

Initial therapy of gonococcal conjunctivitis should include ceftriaxone (Rocephin), 50 mg per kg every 24 hours for 1 week. Should culture sensitivity to penicillin G exist, the suggested regimen is 50,000 U per kg per day intravenously, divided into four doses. Gonococcal conjunctivitis also requires simultaneous topical therapy. Penicillin G mixed in a concentration of 20,000 U per milliliter may be applied every 30 minutes when the pathogen is susceptible. Alternative agents include bacitracin 500 micrograms per gram or gentamicin 0.3%. Frequent lavage is also indicated to remove the typically copious exudate.

Chlamydia is the most frequent cause of infectious neonatal conjunctivitis, reflecting the prominence of this agent as a venereal pathogen. Chlamydia also is responsible for infectious neonatal pneumonitis, and this condition may be present in up to 20% of neonates with conjunctivitis. Chlamydial conjunctivitis has a spectrum of effects; although the condition is typically mild, corneal opacification and conjunctival scarring have been reported. The use of Giemsa's stain may demonstrate chlamydial inclusion bodies in involved epithelial cells. The development of an enzyme-linked immunoassay permits rapid and accurate diagnosis. Systemic therapy is indicated in chlamydial conjunctivitis and consists of oral erythromycin, 40 mg per kg per day in four divided doses for 2 to 4 weeks. In addition, topical erythromycin ointment 0.5% may be used four times daily. Again, the clinician should suspect and rule out the presence of concurrent venereal pathogens.

VIRAL NEONATAL CONJUNCTIVITIS

HSV conjunctivitis in the neonatal period typically is caused by Type II virus encountered in the birth canal period. HSV conjunctivitis may present unilaterally or bilaterally and has no defining characteristics unless there is coexistent HSV keratitis. Disseminated disease with significant morbidity may occur in up to two thirds of cases of HSV conjunctivitis and keratoconjunctivitis.

Ocular diagnosis has been aided by the development of monoclonal antibody immunologic techniques. Additionally, cell cultures from associated skin lesions may be diagnostic. Ocular treatment consists of topical trifluorothymidine 1% (Viroptic) given every 2 hours while the patient is awake. Follow-up of HSV conjunctivitis should be undertaken by an ophthalmologist, while the pediatrician must monitor the patient for possible dissemination of the HSV agent, including encephalitis. Because HSV conjunctivitis in the neonate has a nonspecific presentation, among the most important preventive tools is a high degree of clinical suspicion, a detailed maternal history of genital HSV infection, and close follow-up of these mothers. The presence of active genital lesions in these patients has been used as a criterion for proceeding with cesarean section. As in other cases in which a sexually transmitted disease is detected, work-up for other agents in both the patient and mother is appropriate.

ADULT CONJUNCTIVITIS

Conjunctivitis in the adult also can be caused by infectious or noninfectious agents. Physical findings include lid edema, conjunctival edema and injection, and an associated discharge. The patient may complain of minimal irritation or foreign body sensation and, possibly, mild photophobia. Severe pain or photophobia suggests corneal involvement and/or anterior uveitis. Referral to an ophthalmologist is indicated.

Common noninfectious causes of conjunctivitis include toxicity and allergy. Toxic conjunctivitis typically is exhibited with conjunctival injection, mild to moderate ocular discomfort, and occasionally a serous discharge. The diagnosis is made on the basis of the patient's history of exposure to an inciting agent. The treatment of toxic conjunctivitis is primarily supportive; artificial tears may be used for comfort, and avoidance of exposure to the agent is curative.

The prominent component of allergic conjunctivitis is a subjective complaint of bilateral (or, less frequently, unilateral) ocular itching. If a discharge is present, it may be serous, or in advanced cases, tenuous ropelike deposits of matter may be removed from the eyes. It is not unusual for the patient to give a history of hay fever or similar atopic phenomena with associated seasonal occurrence. Treatment modalities include supportive therapy using cold compresses and artificial tears four to six times daily (Table 2). Topical antihistamine agents such as pheniramine combined with decongestants such as naphazoline (Naphcon A) may afford symptomatic relief. Topical corticosteroid preparations (fluorometholone, prednisolone, and dexamethasone) tend to provide the greatest relief from allergic conditions. Unfortunately, steroid-induced adverse effects including elevation of intraocular pressure, potentiation of microbial proliferation, and cataractogenesis provide a significant risk factor given the usually self-limited course of allergic conjunctivitis. Because of the potential for sight-threatening complications, topical ophthalmic steroid use should be instituted and monitored by an ophthalmologist.

Another group of drugs that may be used in allergic disease are the mast cell–stabilizing agents. At present, only one member of this group of drugs, lodoxamide 0.1% (Alomide), is available for ophthalmic use in the United States. Although lodoxamide prevents the symptoms associated with allergy by preventing mast cell degranulation, this drug has no intrinsic anti-inflammatory capabilities and does not relieve symptoms if mast cell degranulation has already occurred. A time period of 1 to 3 weeks may be necessary before the effect of these agents is appreciated by the patient.

Infectious conjunctivitis may be caused by bacteria, viruses, or chlamydial agents. Unlike in the neonatal population, there are no data supporting the necessity to perform extensive laboratory work in the vast majority of cases. Obtaining a complete history generally gives a clinician insight about the etiologic agent. Viral conjunctivitis often causes symptoms of tearing and mild to moderate itching accompanying a serous discharge. The process typically starts in one eye with subsequent bilateral involvement within a matter of days. Viral conjunctivitis may be caused by a number of agents including picornavirus and adenovirus. Adenovirus subtypes are responsible for the highly contagious epidemic keratoconjunctivitis known as pink eye, which may be spread by fomites or person-to-person contact. An adenovirus subtype is also responsible for a symptom complex known as pharyngoconjunctival fever, in which the patient with conjunctivitis also is febrile and exhibits upper respiratory infection symptoms. The physical findings in viral conjunctivitis also may include a prominent ipsilateral preauricular node.

HSV conjunctivitis in the adult is often a nonspecific conjunctival inflammation in the absence of associated corneal lesions. HSV conjunctivitis typically represents primary ocular infection and is difficult to differentiate from other forms of viral conjunctivitis. The primary importance of HSV infection in the eye is the subsequent recurrence with corneal involvement.

At present, there are no specific cures for viral conjunctivitis. Treatment is primarily supportive with cold compresses and artificial tears. Occasionally, topical antibiotic preparations are prescribed as prophy-

TABLE 2. **Conjunctivitis in Other Age Groups**

Etiology	Signs/Symptoms*	Treatment
Bacterial	Discharge with lids sealed shut in A.M., conjunctival injection	Erythromycin 0.5% or polymyxin B/trimethoprim compound (Polytrim) four times daily
Gonococcal	Hyperpurulent conjunctivitis Beefy-red conjunctival injection	Topical bacitracin 500 U/gm 8 times daily PLUS Ceftriaxone 1 gm intramuscularly every 24 hours for 5 days
Chlamydial	Chronic unilateral or bilateral mucopurulent conjunctivitis	Tetracycline 500 mg or erythromycin stearate 500 mg orally four times daily for 3 weeks
Viral	Serous discharge starting unilaterally, then spreading bilaterally, mild itching, conjunctival injection	Artificial tears Cold compresses Fomite precautions
Allergy	Bilateral itching, increased lacrimation, conjunctival injection, associated systemic allergy	Topical antihistamine four times daily Consider prophylactic treatment with lodoxamide 0.1% 4 times daily in patients with documented seasonal allergic conjunctivitis Artificial tears four to six times daily Cold compresses prn
Toxic	Unilateral/bilateral irritation with associated conjunctival injection	Artificial tears Removal of inciting agent

*Corneal fluorescein staining and/or severe foreign body sensation suggest corneal involvement and should be managed with an ophthalmologist.

laxis against secondary bacterial infections. Although steroids are known to provide symptomatic improvement for some types of viral conjunctivitis, HSV replication is potentiated by these drugs. Therefore, administration of corticosteroids for the treatment of viral conjunctivitis should be under the direction of an ophthalmologist.

The patient with bacterial conjunctivitis typically reports a unilateral, red, irritated eye, associated with a mucopurulent discharge that causes the eyelids to be sealed shut on waking. Culture and sensitivity testing of these cases has not been cost efficient. Indeed, sensitivity testing is somewhat useless because drug sensitivity is reported for drug levels obtained in the blood and soft tissues. These levels are easily surpassed on the ocular surface by topical application of antibiotics. Typically, conjunctivitis may be treated effectively with a polymyxin B/trimethoprim compound (Polytrim) or, in the more severe cases, a 0.3% aminoglycoside drop (gentamicin, tobramycin) four times daily for a 7 to 10 day course.

The presence of a hyperpurulent conjunctivitis with a beefy red appearance to the conjunctiva in a sexually active adult should cause the clinician to consider gonococcal conjunctivitis. Unlike most other forms of adult conjunctivitis, gonococcal conjunctivitis requires concurrent parenteral therapy with ceftriaxone, 1 gm intramuscularly every 24 hours for 5 days, in addition to topical ophthalmic application of bacitracin 500 U per gram, eight times daily. Inadequate treatment may lead to rapid corneal perforation resulting in loss of the eye. Because of the virulent nature of this condition, gonococcal conjunctivitis should be managed with the aid of an ophthalmologist. Gonococcal conjunctivitis is typically an oculogenital condition; appropriate work-up of the patient and his or her sexual partner(s) is indicated.

Adult inclusion conjunctivitis is another oculogenital process. This mucopurulent conjunctivitis is caused by *Chlamydia,* and tends to have a chronic, remittent course. Adult chlamydial conjunctivitis typically results from sexual encounter with an infected partner. The infection is most commonly diagnosed in young (15 to 30 years of age) adults who have recently acquired a new sexual partner. Because this disease has a urogenital component, systemic therapy is indicated. Oral tetracycline, 500 mg, or erythromycin stearate, 500 mg orally four times daily for 3 weeks is recommended.

Conjunctivitis that persists following the recommended treatment schedules or worsens significantly during the course of treatment should be evaluated promptly by an ophthalmologist.

VARICELLA
(Chickenpox)

method of
MARILYN A. KACICA, M.D.
Albany Medical College
Albany, New York

Varicella (chickenpox) and zoster (shingles) are different manifestations of infections caused by the herpesvirus, varicella-zoster virus (VZV). Varicella is very common and highly communicable, and in normal children, does not cause a serious illness and is characterized by a generalized vesicular eruption. After primary infection, the virus produces latent infection of neuronal cells in the dorsal root ganglia. Zoster is a reactivation of the latent virus and consists of grouped vesicular lesions appearing in a dermatome distribution that are often painful. A variety of complications may occur as a consequence of chickenpox, and these may pose a serious problem in the immunocompromised person. Morbidity may be reduced by immunoprophylaxis or antiviral therapy in patients when indicated.

EPIDEMIOLOGY

Humans are the only known reservoir for VZV. Varicella is transmitted to a susceptible individual by direct contact with another person with varicella or zoster lesions, or by airborne droplet spread. Airborne droplet spread from patients with zoster is very rare but has been reported. Varicella is seasonal and epidemic, occurring most commonly during late winter and early spring. Patients are infectious for approximately 48 hours before the onset of rash and until all vesicles are crusted without the appearance of new lesions. The incubation period of chickenpox is generally regarded as being 14 to 15 days, but disease can appear within a range of 10 to 21 days. The incubation period may be prolonged to 28 days after the administration of varicella-zoster immune globulin (VZIG). Secondary attack rates in susceptible individuals within a household range between 70 and 90%.

VARICELLA IN THE NORMAL HOST

Diagnosis

Varicella is characterized by a generalized, pruritic vesicular rash with fever elevated to 37.7° C to 38.9° C (100° F to 102° F) and mild systemic symptoms. Varicella rash can be preceded by 24 to 48 hours of malaise and mild fever. The lesions begin as an erythematous papule, which progresses to a superficial vesicle with an erythematous base. The fluid in the vesicles is initially clear but then turns cloudy. Crops of vesicles continue to appear for 1 to 6 days. The first crop usually involves the head and trunk and progresses from vesicle to crusted lesion in about 3 days. The extremities are also involved but less so and lesions on mucosal surfaces are commonly seen. The total number of lesions varies but ranges from 200 to 500 in various stages of eruption and healing simultaneously. Secondary cases tend to be more severe than the index case in the same household and this may be due to a more intense exposure to a greater inoculum of virus.

In infants younger than 1 year of age, varicella may be mild depending on the degree of immunity conferred by maternal antibodies. Older adolescents and adults usually have a more severe illness than children. The incidence of pneumonitis in adults may be as high as 15%, with 10% being severe. The typical adult course of varicella lasts 10 to 14 days. The mortality rate of varicella is approximately 25 times higher in adults than in children.

If documentation of VZV is needed, the virus can be isolated from vesicular lesions for 3 to 4 days following eruption but may take as long as 1 to 2 weeks for culture results to be complete. Immunofluorescent staining of cells scraped from the base of a vesicle can confirm VZV in 1 to 2 hours. If the Tzanck smear using scrapings from the base of a lesion demonstrates multinucleated giant cells containing intranuclear inclusions, the presence of VZV or another herpesvirus is indicated. The serologic ELISA or FAMA antibody test can also be used to determine immune status.

Treatment

Varicella in the normal child is usually a self-limited illness. Therefore, management is supportive. Daily bathing is recommended to decrease the risk of secondary bacterial infection of the lesions, and the addition of baking soda or oatmeal to the bath water helps alleviate pruritus and discomfort associated with vaginitis or urethritis. The use of cool compresses as well as calamine lotion may also help relieve discomfort. Oral antihistamines may be helpful in the early stages if pruritus interferes with sleep, but these drugs must be used with caution so as not to mask neurologic symptoms. Fever can be treated with acetaminophen; salicylates are contraindicated because of the association with Reye's syndrome.

The use of oral acyclovir (Zovirax) for the treatment of varicella in the normal child remains controversial. The clinical reduction in illness—reducing the number and duration of vesicles, duration of fever, and constitutional symptoms—is modest. In order to have any effect, acyclovir must be begun within 24 hours of onset of rash. The high cost of acyclovir must also be considered. Generally, acyclovir therapy is not recommended for normal children under 12 years of age. However, acyclovir therapy is recommended for the adolescent and adult, and it is highly recommended for secondary household cases in older children.

Complications

Complications of varicella infection are uncommon. The most common problem seen is secondary bacterial infection of the skin lesions with *Staphylococcus aureus* and Group A beta-hemolytic streptococci. Pyoderma or cellulitis occurs in less than 5% of patients, but staphylococcal scalded skin syndrome and scarlet fever do occur. The lesions initially appear as impetigo and continue to have advancing margins, and the patient may have persistent or secondary fever. Bacteremia is rare, but if it is present, it may lead to other sites of infection, which include septic arthritis, osteomyelitis, pneumonia, and meningitis. After the lesions and any secondary sites are cultured, a beta-lactamase–resistant penicillin, a cephalosporin, or amoxicillin/clavulanate (Augmentin) should be initiated depending on the severity of illness.

Vesicular lesions of the conjunctivae can occur but usually resolve without residua. However, if ocular involvement is extensive, ophthalmologic evaluation for uveitis or keratitis is recommended. Topical antiviral therapy may be indicated at this point.

Central nervous system manifestations of varicella are well recognized. Manifestations range from aseptic meningitis to encephalitis. The most common complication is cerebellar ataxia, which usually occurs at the end of the first week or the beginning of the second week after the onset of varicella. However, it may occur as late as 3 weeks after the exanthem. This is a self-limited syndrome that resolves without treatment in 1 to 4 weeks without sequelae. Encephalitis may begin with symptoms of personality change, confusion, and dizziness, which is often associated with brain swelling. This may rapidly progress to seizures and coma, which can occur within a week of onset of rash. Increased intracranial pressure may require intensive care management with attention to maintaining the airway, fluid restriction, and possibly, the use of mannitol, steroids and hyperventilation. Encephalitis is estimated to occur in 1 per 1000 cases of varicella. The CSF obtained usually shows a moderate increase in white blood cells, predominantly lymphocytes, with a normal glucose and slight elevation of protein. Death is usually attributed to increased intracranial pressure, and the mortality rate is estimated at 10%. However, if intracranial pressure can be controlled, full recovery without sequelae is seen. Pathogenesis in healthy children is thought to be demyelination rather than viral infection of brain tissue. Antiviral therapy is of unproven benefit, although many physicians would use intravenous acyclovir for encephalitis.

Other neurologic complications, including transverse myelitis, Guillain-Barré syndrome, cranial nerve palsies, and optic neuritis with transient blindness have been described. Reye's syndrome may occur in association with varicella and, early on, may be confused with encephalitis. Children often present with persistent vomiting and elevation of serum transaminase, blood ammonia levels and prothrombin time, with minimal alteration in serum bilirubin. Hypoglycemia is often seen, especially in children younger than 2 years of age. Epidemiologic studies suggest a strong statistical association between intake of salicylates (aspirin) during the prodromal illness and the development of the syndrome. Therefore, the use of aspirin is contraindicated in children with varicella. Management of Reye's syndrome is supportive, and antiviral drugs are not likely to be helpful.

Pneumonia due to varicella is usually seen in adults and immunocompromised individuals. The onset is insidious, beginning with tachypnea and cough, progressing to dyspnea with occasional hemoptysis. Pneumonitis may also be asymptomatic with an abnormal chest x-ray study. Pulmonary involvement usually begins 3 to 5 days into the course of the illness. The chest radiograph usually reveals nodular or interstitial pneumonitis. Because pulmonary involvement occurs in approximately 15% of healthy adults, oral acyclovir is recommended for the treatment of varicella in adults and adolescents.

Hematologic and hemorrhagic complications of varicella may occur during the acute illness. Thrombocytopenia may occur as a postinfectious complication of varicella and rarely requires platelet support and corticosteroid therapy. Purpura fulminans is rare, but may require intensive care management and a full evaluation to rule out bacterial etiology. Henoch-Schönlein purpura, as well as transient thrombocytopenic purpura, have been reported following varicella.

Arthritis or acute glomerulonephritis that occurs following varicella may be of viral etiology. However, a coincident Group A *Streptococcus* infection must be considered. In addition, *Staphylococcus aureus* may cause arthritis or osteomyelitis.

Various uncommon manifestations of varicella have been reported. These include myocarditis, pancarditis, ulcerative gastritis, gastrointestinal bleeding, nephritis, and orchitis.

VARICELLA IN HIGH-RISK POPULATIONS

Pregnancy and Varicella

Pregnant women who are susceptible to varicella may be predisposed to a more severe illness with varicella secondary to the immunosuppression of pregnancy. For this reason, it is recommended that varicella-susceptible pregnant women who are exposed to varicella receive passive immunoprophylaxis with VZIG.* This approach may modify maternal illness, but protection of the fetus is unknown. Treatment of the pregnant woman who develops symptoms of chickenpox with acyclovir must be considered individually. However, the illness including pneumonia may be more severe.

A congenital varicella syndrome has been reported in about 5% of cases in which the mother developed varicella during the first trimester of gestation. Common manifestations of congenital varicella include cicatricial skin lesions, hydrocephalus, chorioretinitis, limb paresis, limb hypoplasia, and intrauterine growth retardation.

When the onset of maternal varicella occurs near the time of delivery, it places the infant at extreme risk for severe, disseminated infection. If the varicella rash develops in the mother from 5 days before delivery to 2 days after delivery, infants at risk should be given VZIG. If the infant progresses to active varicella infection, intravenous acyclovir should be begun. Left untreated, infected infants have a mortality rate of 31%, perhaps secondary to a large transplacental viral inoculum and the immature neonatal immune system.

Varicella in the Neonate

Neonates exposed to varicella later than 48 hours postpartum are not thought to be at risk for severe disease. However, case reports do reflect severe and fatal infections in infants exposed up to 3 weeks of age. The numbers reported are small so it is difficult to assess the true incidence of severe varicella in this setting. For this reason, consideration should be

*Not FDA approved for this indication.

given to the administration of VZIG to neonates younger than 2 to 3 weeks of age exposed to varicella. Premature infants and infants whose mothers have a negative history for chickenpox and are exposed to varicella should be considered for immunoprophylaxis in the first 2 months of life.

Varicella in the Immunocompromised Host

Varicella in immunocompromised hosts can lead to disseminated, progressive varicella involving multiple organ systems with persistent crops of vesicles and a high mortality rate. If exposure is recognized prior to development of infection, VZIG should be administered. However, often exposures are unknown, and when VZV develops, early therapy with intravenous acyclovir should be initiated. Individuals considered at high risk are those with a defect in cellular immune function. This includes patients with congenital immunodeficiencies, diseases such as leukemia, lymphoma, and human immunodeficiency virus infection; those receiving chemotherapy or radiation therapy; and transplant recipients.

For certain other groups considered at increased risk of severe varicella or its complications, oral acyclovir should be considered if initiated within the first 24 hours after the onset of rash. These groups include healthy nonpregnant individuals who are 13 years of age or older, children older than 12 months with a chronic cutaneous or pulmonary disorder, those receiving long-term salicylate therapy, and those receiving short, intermittent, or aerosolized courses of corticosteroids. If possible, corticosteroids should be discontinued after known varicella exposure. If an individual is immunocompromised because of the administration of high-dose steroids and develops varicella, intravenous acyclovir therapy is indicated. Oral acyclovir therapy should not be used prophylactically.

Immunoprophylaxis and Antiviral Therapy

Passive immunization, when indicated, is accomplished by the intramuscular injection of VZIG. One vial, with an approximate volume of 1.25 milliliters, contains 125 units. One hundred and twenty-five units are given for each 10 kg of body weight (and is the minimum dose), with a maximum dose of 625 units or five vials. For maximal effectiveness, VZIG should be given within 48 hours of exposure and, preferably, not more than 96 hours after exposure.

Both acyclovir and vidarabine are effective in treating varicella or zoster, but acyclovir is considered the drug of choice. Acyclovir is less toxic and easily administered. The recommended dose of acyclovir for treatment of varicella is 500 mg per M^2 per dose given every 8 hours. The medication should be given over 1 hour, and the patient should be kept well hydrated to prevent crystallization of the drug in the kidneys. Antiviral therapy should be begun early in the course of disease for best results.

Oral acyclovir is available in both tablets and suspension. The dose is 20 mg per kg to a maximum of 800 mg per dose four times daily for 5 days. This should be initiated within 24 hours of onset of rash to be effective. Therapy for zoster in normal adults, especially those older than 60 years of age, is oral acyclovir 800 mg per dose 5 times daily. In the immunocompromised host, intravenous acyclovir is indicated.

INFECTION CONTROL IN THE HOSPITAL SETTING

Because VZV is highly contagious and VZV infection may be life-threatening in certain populations, VZV is carefully screened for in hospitals, especially in the pediatric setting. If possible, patients with active infections should not be admitted to the hospital. If they must be hospitalized, normal patients with localized zoster should be placed on drainage and secretion precautions until lesions are crusted. Immunocompromised patients with zoster or chickenpox and normal patients with disseminated zoster or chickenpox should be kept in strict isolation for the duration of the illness.

Exposed susceptible patients, if not able to be discharged, should be placed in strict isolation from day 10 until 21 days after the onset of the rash in the index patient. Those who receive VZIG should be kept in isolation until 28 days after exposure.

VARICELLA VACCINE

The effectiveness of the live-attenuated varicella vaccine, developed in Japan in the early 1970s, has been documented in many clinical trials, but the vaccine is still investigational in the United States. The vaccine has been studied extensively in children with normal and compromised immune systems, as well as in healthy adults, affording protection with few reactions in the normal child and adult. Approximately one third of leukemic children develop papulovesicular skin lesions after immunization, but otherwise they tolerate it well. Breakthrough cases of chickenpox after exposure to VZV have been reported in both adults and children, although the cases are reported to be mild. Varicella vaccine is currently being evaluated for simultaneous administration with measles-mumps-rubella vaccine, either as a separate injection or as a mixture of the four vaccine viruses. However, the routine use of this vaccine in healthy children remains controversial.

CHOLERA

method of
DILIP MAHALANABIS, M.B., B.S.
International Centre for Diarrhoeal Disease Research
Dhaka, Bangladesh

Although cholera carries a case fatality rate of 50% or more when it is left untreated, almost all patients recover fully and rapidly when they are treated adequately. With rapid rehydration, a seriously ill patient in profound shock with no detectable pulse or blood pressure is able to sit, talk, and eat within a few hours and can return to work or school within 2 to 3 days. This lifesaving and dramatic treatment can be rendered at a very low cost; this is important because cholera affects mainly poor people in the least developed countries.

Cholera is caused by the bacterium *Vibrio cholerae,* which colonizes the mucosal lining of the small intestinal lumen. The toxin released is an 84-kilodalton protein consisting of an active A subunit (with A_1 and A_2 peptides) and a cluster of five B subunits. The B subunits bind the toxin molecule to the mucosal receptor GM_1 ganglioside; the active A subunit enters the cell and stimulates the secretion of water and electrolytes, resulting in secretory diarrhea.

TREATMENT

On examination, a typical cholera patient is extremely weak and thirsty, has a hoarse voice, and often complains of muscle cramps. Signs of dehydration include decreased skin turgor, sunken eyes, dry mucous membranes, and a weak or undetectable radial pulse. Patients often have severe metabolic acidosis. A remarkable aspect of the disease is how a healthy person can become so sick after only a few hours of diarrhea and vomiting. However, much less severe episodes of cholera are common, and mild cases cannot be distinguished clinically from other acute watery diarrheal diseases. Such an acute dehydrating diarrhea syndrome is sometimes caused by other etiologic agents, most notably the enterotoxigenic *Escherichia coli.*

Patients are assessed for signs of dehydration to estimate severity and fluid requirements. Rapid assessment is important because a severely dehydrated patient may literally be within minutes of death unless fluid therapy is started immediately. Clinical assessment is adequate for formulating a treatment plan for individual patients; laboratory tests (e.g., hematocrit, plasma specific gravity, total serum proteins) are used in research studies to compare groups of patients but are superfluous for clinical management. Clinical manifestations of severe cholera are mostly due to the loss of salts and water in the stool and vomitus. Complications arise only when appropriate rehydration is not accomplished rapidly.

Objectives of treatment are (1) rapid replacement of water and salts already lost; (2) maintenance of normal hydration until diarrhea stops, by replacing fluid losses as they occur; (3) reduction of the magnitude and duration of diarrhea with suitable antimicrobials; and (4) introduction of a normal diet as soon as the patient is able to eat without waiting for diarrhea to stop.

Until the early 1970s, fluid losses in cholera could be replaced only by intravenous therapy. Treatment has been revolutionized by the introduction of oral rehydration therapy (ORT), in which a solution containing glucose and three salts is used (Table 1). It has made cholera therapy practical, simple, inexpensive, and highly effective, particularly under field conditions. ORT is based on the fact that glucose-linked enhanced absorption of sodium and water from the small intestine remains largely intact during the massive secretory state of cholera. ORT is optimally employed by starting administration of the solution at the first sign of diarrhea in an amount equal to the losses that occur and continuing it until diarrhea stops. This may reduce the number of severe cases requiring intravenous therapy, conserving scarce medical resources. Research in the 1980s has shown that replacing 20 grams of glucose with 50 grams of rice flour (which requires cooking; see Table 1) for 1 liter of oral rehydration salt solution increases absorption and reduces fluid stool losses by 35% to 40% in comparison with glucose oral rehydration salt (ORS) solution.

Intravenous rehydration still plays a critical role in the treatment of cholera: In patients who present with severe dehydration and shock, infusion of appropriate intravenous fluids can be lifesaving. Intravenous fluids should replace the electrolyte losses via cholera stool, which in the severely affected patient range from 100 to 140 mmol per liter of sodium, 30 to 50 mmol per liter of bicarbonate, and 15 to 30 mmol per liter of potassium with an osmolality close to that of plasma (Table 2). Lactated Ringer's (Hartmann's) solution is commercially available and has a suitable composition (see Table 2). In cholera-endemic areas, special polyelectrolyte fluids can be prepared especially for diarrhea treatment (e.g., Dhaka's solution). Normal saline with or without glucose should be used only if a more suitable polyelectrolyte solution is not available. In such a situation, a complete ORS solution should be given as early as possible to provide the base and potassium.

Patients with severe dehydration and signs of hypovolemia should be rehydrated intravenously to

TABLE 1. **Oral Rehydration Salt Solution***

Amount of Oral Rehydration Salts Needed to Prepare 1 Liter of Solution	
Sodium chloride	3.5 gm
Trisodium citrate dihydrate	2.9 gm
OR	
Sodium hydrogen carbonate (sodium bicarbonate)	2.5 gm
Potassium chloride	1.5 gm
Glucose anhydrous†	20.0 gm

Molar Concentration of Solution (mmol/L)

	Citrate Solution	*Bicarbonate Solution*
Sodium	90	90
Potassium	20	20
Chloride	80	80
Citrate	10	—
Bicarbonate	—	30
Glucose	111	111

*Formula recommended by the World Health Organization was first used in 1971.

†50 gm rice powder can replace 20 gm glucose. To prepare a rice-ORS solution, put 50 gm rice flour in 1100 mL water and bring to a boil. Continue boiling for about 7–10 min. When the mixture is opalescent, cool, add the three salts. Serve warm and discard after 8 h. Rice-ORS can reduce purging by 30–40% in comparison with glucose-ORS.

TABLE 2. **Electrolyte Composition of Cholera Stool and Some Intravenous Solutions***

Concentration (mmol/L)	Cholera Stool		Ringer's Lactate†	Dhaka's Solution‡	Normal Saline§
	Adults	*Children*			
Na^+	135	105	131	133	154
K^+	15	25	4	13	0
Cl^-	100	90	111	98	154
HCO_3^-	45	30	26	48	0

*Do not use 5% dextrose in water to treat dehydrating diarrheal diseases.

†The best commercially available solution. Lactate yields bicarbonate; low potassium concentration is made up by optimum use of oral rehydration therapy.

‡In use for many years to treat cholera at the International Centre for Diarrhoeal Disease Research, Bangladesh. It is not commercially available but serves as a good example of a polyelectrolyte solution for cholera.

§Sodium concentration is high for children and solution does not contain a base or potassium. Prompt introduction of oral rehydration therapy may prevent potential problems.

achieve complete rehydration in 2 to 4 hours. After initial complete rehydration, most patients can be maintained with ORT, although about 10% to 15% of hospitalized patients may need an additional short course of intravenous therapy because of high purging rates and recurrence of signs of dehydration. A single solution is adequate for all age groups in cholera.

Rehydration and Maintenance Therapy

The severity of dehydration must be assessed and the fluid requirement estimated quickly. A severely dehydrated patient with a deficit of about 10% of body weight is very weak with very poor skin turgor, sunken eyes, and a barely perceptible or absent radial pulse. As an example, the estimated deficit in a 50-kg adult with severe dehydration is 5 liters. A moderately dehydrated patient whose deficit is estimated at about 7.5% has obvious signs of dehydration with dry mucous membranes, sunken eyes, and poor skin turgor; the radial pulse is palpable but soft and rapid. In severely dehydrated patients, intravenous fluids are infused rapidly to quickly restore circulating volume. As a guide, half of the estimated volume of fluid required in a severely dehydrated patient should be given over the first hour, initially as fast as possible until the radial pulse is palpable. The patient should be fully hydrated in 2 to 4 hours, at which time intravenous therapy may be discontinued and oral rehydration therapy started and continued until diarrhea stops.

For most patients with mild and moderate dehydration, ORT can be given both for initial rehydration and for replacement of ongoing fecal losses (see Table 2). ORT can continue in spite of some vomiting, which is common; with persistence and with small frequent feedings, most patients retain enough fluid to become rehydrated.

Adequate replacement is signaled by the return of the radial pulse to normal strength and rate (the pulse rates in an adult are usually below 90 beats per minute), return of skin turgor to normal, and a feeling of well-being. Children who are drowsy or stuporous may not become fully alert for 12 to 18 hours despite adequate rehydration. In addition, weight gain of about 8% to 10% in a severely dehydrated patient is observed. Return of urine output usually occurs within 12 to 20 hours of initial rehydration.

Patients are most conveniently treated with a cholera cot, which allows efficient collection and measurement of stool. In its simplest configuration, a cholera cot consists of a foldable canvas camp cot covered by a plastic sheet with a suitable hole in the center. A sleeve fits into the hole and guides the diarrheal stool into a plastic bucket underneath the cot so that it can be measured periodically. A vomit basin should also be available. A simple input-output chart at the patient's bedside shows the amounts of intravenous and ORS solutions and the volume of stool. A few hospitalized cholera patients may show signs of dehydration while on ORT. If dehydration occurs, additional intravenous fluids are given rapidly as for initial rehydration, after which oral maintenance should be resumed.

Antimicrobial Therapy

The goal of antimicrobial therapy is to drastically reduce or eliminate *V. cholerae* from the intestinal lumen so that no more cholera toxin is produced and only the residual toxin already bound to the gut mucosa remains. The use of a suitable antibiotic such as tetracycline reduces the duration of diarrhea by about 50%, to an average of 2 days; reduces the volume of diarrhea after start of treatment by about 50%; and reduces the duration of *Vibrio* excretion to an average of 1 to 2 days. Therefore, the use of an appropriate antibiotic has a profound effect on the cost and convenience of treatment.

Antibiotics are usually given after completion of initial rehydration, i.e., about 4 to 6 hours after starting treatment. Tetracycline, the antibiotic of choice, is given to adults at 500 mg every 6 hours for 48 to 72 hours and to children at 50 mg per kg per day in four divided doses for 48 to 72 hours (tetracycline should be avoided in children under 8 years of age). Doxycycline can also be used in a single dose of 300 mg in adults and 6 mg per kg body weight for children younger than 15 years of age; doxycycline may cause nausea and should be given after the patient eats some food. Alternative antibiotics are furazolidone, 100 mg every 6 hours (for children, 5 mg per kg per day in four divided doses) for 72 hours; erythromycin, 250 mg every 6 hours (for children, 30 mg per kg per day in three divided doses) for 72 hours; or trimethoprim-sulfamethoxazole (8 mg of trimethoprim and 40 mg of sulfamethoxazole per kg per day in two divided doses for 72 hours). Chloramphenicol is also effective in the same dosage as tetracycline but is usually not used because of potential serious side effects. Prophylactic antibiotics are not recommended because of the risk of the emergence of antibiotic-resistant strains.

Diet

Patients should be offered normal food as soon as the dehydration and acidosis are corrected and they feel able to eat.

COMPLICATIONS

Complications of cholera are rare if correct treatment is provided quickly because most result from delay in therapy or provision of inappropriate fluid therapy. Risks of pyrogen reaction, excessive hydration, or too-rapid correction of hypernatremia or hyponatremia or acidosis are minimized by optimal use of ORT and early resumption of a normal diet. Pneumonia, a not uncommon problem, may be due to aspiration of vomitus or altered tissue resistance secondary to shock and acidosis.

PREVENTION

The only effective means of preventing cholera is to ensure that healthy individuals are not infected with *V. cholerae* through food and drink. Therefore, washing hands with soap and water, using clean water for drinking and washing utensils and other activities, and appropriate excreta disposal are useful preventive measures. The injectable killed bacterial vaccines are not recommended because protection is inadequate, short lived, and ineffective in children. Oral killed whole-cell vaccines with or without added B subunit* are more effective and their usefulness in the public health field is being evaluated.

*Not available in the United States.

DIPHTHERIA

method of
GARY D. OVERTURF, M.D.
University of New Mexico—School of Medicine
Albuquerque, New Mexico

Diphtheria, an acute infection caused by *Corynebacterium diphtheriae,* is characterized by symptoms localized to the respiratory tract and toxin-induced neurologic, renal, and cardiac damage. The toxin is an extracellular phage-mediated protein elaborated solely by toxigenic strains. The infection is acquired by contact with a human carrier or person with active disease. The bacteria may be transmitted via droplets or contact with infected skin lesions. The period of communicability in untreated individuals ranges from 2 to 6 weeks, and the mean incubation period is 2 to 3 days but may be as long as 1 week. The usual portal of entry is the nose or mouth, or occasionally, the eyes, skin, or genital mucosa. The organism remains localized to mucosal or cutaneous surfaces. A localized inflammatory response results in tissue necrosis with formation of the characteristic diphtheritic pseudomembrane in the upper respiratory tract. Toxin produced and absorbed at the local site of infection is distributed via the blood causing potential damage to the heart, nervous system, or kidneys. Thus, the severity of disease and resultant symptoms depend on the site of the primary infection (e.g., nasopharynx, larynx, or trachea), immunization status of the infected individual, and the degree of toxin-induced damage. To avoid continuing toxigenic damage, the diagnosis of diphtheria and the decision to administer antitoxin should be made on the basis of clinical history and findings and not await cultural confirmation, which may take several days. Confirmation of the diagnosis requires the isolation of *C. diphtheriae* on culture with selective media and the subsequent demonstration of toxigenicity.

TREATMENT

Antitoxin Administration

Successful treatment of diphtheria is predicated both on neutralization of free toxin and elimination of further toxin production by eradication of the toxigenic organism. The only specific treatment available is antitoxin of equine origin (diphtheria equine antitoxin).

The antitoxin is delivered preferably by the intravenous route in a single dose. A history of prior sensitization or exposure to horses or horse serum should be sought. If the history is positive, testing for horse serum hypersensitivity should be first performed with either a scratch test or intracutaneous injection of dilute antitoxin. The scratch test is performed with application of one drop of a 1:100 saline dilution of serum to the site of a superficial scratch, prick, or puncture on the volar aspect of the forearm. A positive test response is indicated by a wheal with surrounding erythema of at least 3 mm larger than a control test with normal saline (at 15 to 20 minutes after application). Alternatively, for those patients with a positive history of possible horse serum hypersensitivity, a smaller intracutaneous injection of 0.02 mL of a 1:1000 saline dilution of antitoxin may be administered. Erythema greater than 10 mm or a wheal within 20 minutes is considered a positive reaction. For those patients with a negative history or for those with an initially negative intradermal test with dilute material, the intracutaneous injection should be performed or repeated, respectively, by injection of 0.02 mL of a 1:100 dilution.

If the patient is deemed hypersensitive to horse serum, then desensitization is required. All desensitization regimens require adequate preparation for the event of anaphylaxis (e.g., bedside resuscitative and monitoring equipment, and the availability of aqueous epinephrine 1:1000), and thus are optimally

TABLE 1. **Suggested Dosage Schedule of Diphtheria Equine Antitoxin for Desensitization**

Dose	Amount (mL)	Dilution	Preferred Route*	Alternate Route
1	0.10	1:1000	Intravenous	Intradermal
2	0.30	1:1000	Intravenous	Intradermal
3	0.60	1:1000	Intravenous	Subcutaneous
4	0.10	1:100	Intravenous	Subcutaneous
5	0.30	1:100	Intravenous	Subcutaneous
6	0.60	1:100	Intravenous	Subcutaneous
7	0.10	1:10	Intravenous	Subcutaneous
8	0.30	1:10	Intravenous	Subcutaneous
9	0.60	1:10	Intravenous	Subcutaneous
10	0.10	undiluted	Intravenous	Subcutaneous
11	0.20	undiluted	Intravenous	Subcutaneous
12	0.60	undiluted	Intravenous	Intramuscular
13	1.0	undiluted	Intravenous	Intramuscular

*Intravenous is the preferred route because of better control.

performed in an intensive care unit. The American Academy of Pediatrics Infectious Disease committee recommends a regimen employing increasing intravenous doses administered at 15-minute intervals as shown in Table 1. If no reaction occurs, the remaining dose is given by slow intravenous infusion. Patients may benefit from premedication with antihistamines, with or without the addition of hydrocortisone or methylprednisolone. Intravenous administration results in higher levels in saliva and presumptively more rapid neutralization of toxin, and subsequent detoxification of horse serum products.

The choice of the therapeutic dosage of equine antitoxin is empiric (Table 2) and is dependent largely on the site and duration of infection and degree of toxicity but not by the age or size of the patient.

Antitoxin is available in the United States from the Centers for Disease Control (CDC), Atlanta, Georgia. An immediate reaction may be seen in up to 16% of patients including a variety of rashes, fever, and anaphylaxis, whereas more commonly, a delayed reaction of serum sickness (rash, urticaria, fever, and arthralgia or arthritis) may occur in 10 to 20% of children or adults. Serum sickness characteristically occurs at 5 to 21 days after infusion and may be treated symptomatically with acetaminophen, aspirin or ibuprofen, or corticosteroids in severe cases.

Antibiotic Therapy

Antibiotics are important to eradicate the organism and prevent further toxin production. Both erythromycin and penicillin are effective. Erythromycin may be given orally or intravenously at a dosage of 40 to 50 mg per kg per day in four divided doses (maximum 2.0 grams per day). Penicillin may be given as aqueous penicillin, 100,000 to 150,000 U per kg per day divided in four doses (maximum, 10 mU), or procaine penicillin G 25,000 to 50,000 U per kg per day, intramuscularly in two divided doses (maximum, 1.2 mU per dose). All regimens of penicillin or erythromycin should be given for a total of 14 days. All these antibiotic regimens eliminate co-infecting group A streptococci. Elimination of the organism should be documented by three consecutive (daily) negative cultures after cessation of therapy.

TABLE 2. **Dosage of Diphtheria Antitoxin**

Clinical Indication	Antitoxin Dose
Pharyngeal or laryngeal disease of 48 hours duration or less	40,000 units
Nasopharyngeal lesions	40,000–60,000 units
Extensive disease of more than three days duration or brawny neck swelling	80,000–120,000 units

In cutaneous diphtheria, lesions should be cleaned vigorously with soap and water. Either oral erythromycin or penicillin V should be administered for 10 days. Antitoxin therapy is of unproven value for this form of diphtheria, but some authorities recommend the administration of 20,000 to 40,000 units of antitoxin. Because of its uncertain value, the material should not be given to patients who are sensitive to horse serum by history or by skin testing.

Supportive Therapy

Patients with diphtheria should be hospitalized for horse serum and antibiotic administration, as well as careful monitoring. Isolation of the patient with measures to prevent airborne spread is necessary for the duration of hospitalization or until the completion of antibiotic therapy. Isolation should continue until two cultures obtained 24 hours apart after cessation of therapy from both the nasopharynx and throat are negative for *C. diphtheriae.*

Continuous cardiac monitoring should be employed during acute hospitalization, and thereafter, serial electrocardiograms or echocardiography, or both, should be performed 2 to 3 times per week to assess for cardiac arrhythmias and myocardial function and for up to 4 to 6 weeks to detect myocarditis. Patients with diphtheria may be digitalized carefully if congestive heart failure develops. In severe cases, prednisone 1 to 1.5 mg per kg for up to 2 weeks has been employed, but its therapeutic efficacy is unknown. Serial urinalysis and renal functional screens should also be employed to detect renal damage. Similarly, serial neurologic examinations should be carefully performed to detect any evidence of neurologic toxicity. Maintenance of adequate hydration and nutrition, including parenteral nutrition, if necessary, should be provided because palatal paralysis may complicate oral hydration or alimentation. Patients with laryngeal disease may require diagnostic or therapeutic bronchoscopy with intubation in order to provide an unobstructed airway. A section of necrotic membrane in nasal or throat locations may dislodge and obstruct the airway.

Treatment of Contacts

A history of symptoms and immunization status should be sought in all contacts. Cultures should be performed in contacts irrespective of immunization status. Persons with positive cultures should be treated with either oral erythromycin or penicillin V for 7 days or a single intramuscular dose of benzathine penicillin G* (600,000 U for those weighing less than 30 kg and 1.2 mU for those greater than 30 kg). Asymptomatic, previously immunized close contacts should receive a booster dose of diphtheria toxoid (dT) (adults, and children more than 7 years) or pediatric diphtheria toxoid (DPT or DT) (children less than 7 years). Asymptomatic close contacts who are unimmunized or who are not fully immunized, or whose immunization status is unknown, should have cultures performed and should be started immediately on any of those antibiotic regimens used in carriers. Cultures should be repeated after treatment. Active immunization with DPT, DT, or dT should be initiated or boosted appropriate for the age of the contact. A close contact who cannot be kept under close surveillance should be given benzathine penicillin G* as noted earlier and a dose of an appropriate immunizing agent, depending on the person's age and immunization status.

PREVENTION

Universal immunization with the diphtheria toxoid is the only effective control measure. Children up to their seventh birthday should receive DPT (or DT for those in whom pertussis immunization is contraindicated) according to the currently approved schedule at 2, 4, 6, and 15 to 18 months, repeated at 4 to 6 years. After age 7 years, booster immunization with dT toxoid is recommended at 10-year intervals and/or with administration of tetanus prophylaxis for wounds. Childhood preparations of diphtheria toxin (DT or DPT) contain 7 to 25 flocculating units (Lf) of diphtheria toxoid per dose, as compared with preparations of vaccine for older children and adults (dT), which contain no more than 2 Lf per dose. A primary series of immunization for older children and adults who have not previously been immunized is two doses given at a 2-month interval and a booster dose at 6 to 12 months.

*Not FDA approved for this indication.

FOOD-BORNE ILLNESS

method of
KATHERINE M. SPOONER, M.D., and
MICHAEL A. POLIS, M.D., M.P.H.
National Institutes of Allergy and Infectious Diseases
Bethesda, Maryland

Food-borne disease syndromes are common and are the result of bacterial, viral, parasitic, chemical, or toxic agents found in a wide variety of foods. These syndromes are usually manifested by the acute onset of gastrointestinal symptoms with or without systemic complications. The true incidence of food-borne syndromes is not known, because reported outbreaks greatly underestimate the actual impact of the problem. From 1983 to 1987, the Centers for Disease Control and Prevention (CDC) received reports of 2393 outbreaks of food-borne illness (with an outbreak involving 2 or more cases from one food source), and these outbreaks represented 91,678 individual cases.

In the evaluation of suspected food-borne illness, the following general guidelines should be used to establish an etiologic diagnosis and treatment plan: (1) Define the clinical features of the illness, including the incubation time, type of symptoms, and severity of disease. (2) Define the epidemiology of the disease, including recent travel, the type of food ingested (including origin and method of preparation), time of year, and the presence of similar symptoms in the patient's recent contacts. (3) Attempt, when possible, to document the etiology by laboratory confirmation. This can be accomplished by collecting appropriate specimens and performing cultures as well as assays for the presence of toxins.

PATHOGENESIS AND CLINICAL PRESENTATION

Microbial Agents and Their Toxins

The diagnosis of food-related illness should be entertained when a patient develops an acute gastrointestinal or neurologic illness, and it should be strongly suspected when two or more persons develop an acute illness after ingesting food from the same source within the previous 72 hours. The presentation and time course of the illness provide important clues about the pathogenesis and cause of the syndrome. A summary of the common microbial agents causing food poisoning and their sources can be found in Table 1, and a summary of common chemical agents causing food poisoning can be found in Table 2.

In a patient who develops nausea and vomiting within 1 to 6 hours of ingestion of a food item, the major etiologic considerations are *Staphylococcus aureus* and *Bacillus cereus.* These are enterotoxigenic organisms, and the short incubation time is a reflection of a preformed toxin present in the food. *S. aureus* contamination is usually due to improper handling of the food during preparation, whereas *B. cereus* is most often associated with reheating fried rice. Both toxins cause an acute, self-limited illness lasting generally less than 12 hours. Therapy is supportive and includes fluid and electrolyte replacement.

In a patient who develops abdominal cramps and diarrhea within 8 to 16 hours after ingestion of food, the likely agent is also a toxin-producing organism. In this setting, the toxin is likely formed in vivo, as opposed to the preformed toxins produced by *S. aureus* and *B. cereus.* The most common pathogens are *Clostridium perfringens* and *B. cereus* (which produces both types of toxins), causing illness that tends to last longer than preformed toxin–related illness.

TABLE 1. **Microbial Agents and Their Sources**

Agent	Common Sources
Toxin-Producing Microbial Agents	
S. aureus	Dairy products, egg salad, pastry, human handling of cold foods
B. cereus	Dried food, fried rice, cereals, meat and dairy products
C. perfringens	Meats, poultry, dried foods, vegetables
C. botulinum	Canned vegetables, fruits, home-processed foods, honey (infant botulism)
Enterotoxigenic *E. coli*	Raw or undercooked food, milk
V. cholerae (01 and non-01)	Shellfish
Verotoxigenic *E. coli*	Beef, milk
Toxin Production and/or Tissue Invasion	
V. parahaemolyticus	Crabs
Y. enterocolitica	Milk, tofu, pork
Tissue Invasion	
C. jejuni	Poultry, raw milk
Salmonella	Beef, dairy products, eggs, poultry
Shigella	Egg salad, lettuce
Invasive *E. coli*	Handled food, dairy products
Aeromonas sp.	Contaminated water
Parasitic	
Giardia	Contaminated water
Amoeba	Contaminated water
Cryptosporidium	Contaminated water
Trichinella	Pork
Viral	
Norwalk agent	Shellfish, salads
Hepatitis A	Handled foods (salads, fruits), shellfish

The ailment is occasionally associated with nausea, vomiting, and rarely, fever. The illness is self-limited, resolving within 24 hours, and treatment is solely supportive.

In a patient who presents with fever, abdominal cramps, and diarrhea 16 to 48 hours after ingestion of contaminated food, the likely cause is microbial infection with tissue invasion. The major organisms to be considered are salmonellae, shigellae, *Campylobacter jejuni, Vibrio parahaemolyticus,* and invasive *Escherichia coli.* Fever and fecal leukocytes are evidence of tissue invasion; bloody diarrhea is common with *Shigella* and verotoxigenic *E. coli* O157:H7, and may occur as well with *Salmonella, V. parahaemolyticus,* and *Yersinia enterocolitica. C. perfringens* type C has been associated with a severe hemorrhagic jejunitis and ileitis, a syndrome known as enteritis necroticans, or pig bel. Recent outbreaks of *E. coli* O157:H7 have been associated with hamburger meat from a fast-food chain, as well as apple cider from a cider mill that used improperly processed apples. Symptoms from these invasive diarrheal illnesses generally last less than 1 week, but severe complications may occasionally occur such as the hemolytic-uremic syndrome with *E. coli* O157:H7, and rarely, seizures and meningism associated with shigellosis.

The presentation of abdominal cramps and watery diarrhea within 16 to 72 hours after exposure to contaminated food suggests an enterotoxin-producing agent. Typical strains include *E. coli, V. parahaemolyticus, V. cholerae* (either non-01, or 01 in endemic locales), and occasionally, *C. jejuni,* salmonellae, and shigellae. Occasionally, vomiting and fever may occur, and in the majority of cases, these illnesses resolve within 72 to 96 hours. Cholera has been described in outbreaks from contaminated Gulf Coast waters and, recently, in an isolated outbreak in Maryland due to contaminated imported coconut milk. Cholera needs to be treated with aggressive fluid replacement. Antibiotics have been shown to shorten the duration of disease, and tetracycline, 250 mg orally every 6 hours, is the drug most often used with alternatives including the fluroquinolones (e.g., Cipro), and trimethoprim-sulfamethoxazole (Bactrim, Septra). Doxycycline (Vibramycin),* 300 mg orally in a single dose, is recommended by many experts.

Nausea, vomiting, diarrhea, and progressive paralysis within 18 to 36 hours of food ingestion strongly suggests the diagnosis of food-borne botulism. Botulism is a syndrome that is caused by a neurotoxin produced by *Clostridium botulinum,* and it is manifested by progressive neurologic symptoms of dry mouth, diplopia, dysphagia, and progressive weakness, with respiratory failure in severe cases. Nausea, vomiting, and diarrhea can occur in the inital stages of the illness, but once the neurologic symptoms predominate, constipation is a common feature. The incubation period of this illness usually ranges from 12 to 36 hours but can be as long as 8 days. Typically, the disease results from the ingestion of

*Not FDA approved for this indication.

TABLE 2. **Chemical Agents**

Agent	Common Sources
Ciguatera	Barracuda, snapper, grouper, amberjack, parrotfish, sturgeon
Scombroid poisoning (histamine fish poisoning)	Tuna, mackerel, bonito, skipjack, mahi-mahi
Paralytic shellfish poisoning	Molluscs, oysters, clams
Neurotoxic shellfish poisoning	Molluscs, oysters, clams
Mushroom poisoning (short incubation)	*Amanita, Inocybe, Clitocybe, Coprinus, Psilocybe, Panaeolus* spp.
Mushroom poisoning (long incubation)	*Amanita, Galerina, Gyromitra* spp.
Monosodium-L-glutamate	Chinese food
Heavy metals	Acidic beverages

any of three distinct neurotoxins (A, B, and E) produced by *C. botulinum* spores. The source is usually inadequately prepared home-processed or canned foods. In Alaska, for example, home-processed fish prepared in oils and spices and allowed to ferment in plastic bags has been associated with botulism. Infant botulism is a similar illness, but in these cases, the toxin is produced in vivo after ingestion of the spores, with honey being the usual source. Botulism is a potentially deadly illness, with fatality rates estimated as high as 25%. Death is usually due to rapidly progressive neuromuscular paralysis. All patients with suspected cases of botulism should be hospitalized and should be considered for treatment with a trivalent antiserum available from the CDC. The CDC should be contacted immediately regarding the management of these patients, and the offices can be reached during days at 1-404-639-3753, and during nights and weekends at 1-404-639-2888. Apart from the antiserum, treatment is primarily supportive, including mechanical ventilation, as indicated. Penicillin has been used to eradicate *C. botulinum* in the gastrointestinal tract, but the clinical benefit is not known.

Several infectious diseases are transmitted by foods and present with symptoms other than those localized to the gastrointestinal or neurologic systems. Listeriosis, although rare in the United States, is potentially fatal and can be caused by ingestion of improperly pasteurized milk and cheese products, undercooked chicken, and non-reheated hot dogs containing *Listeria monocytogenes*. Other illnesses include brucellosis (from *Brucella abortus* found in goat's milk cheese), anthrax (from *Bacillus anthracis* found in contaminated, undercooked meat), a sepsis-like syndrome due to *Vibrio vulnificus* (from raw oysters), hepatitis A (from seafood and improperly prepared salads), trichinosis (from *Trichinella spiralis* found in contaminated pork), tularemia (from *Francisella tularensis* found in contaminated water from streams and wells and from contaminated meat), and Q fever (from *Coxiella burnetii* found in contaminated raw milk).

Seafood-Related Toxins

Although it is associated with many real and imagined pleasures, seafood ingestion is also associated with several types of food poisoning, usually related to toxin ingestion. Ciguatera poisoning has a worldwide incidence reported to be as high as 50,000 cases per year, and is believed to be due to a neurotoxin, produced by marine dinoflagellates and algae. This neurotoxin is transmitted through the food chain in grouper, snapper, barracuda, jack, surgeonfish, and sea bass. The largest concentrations of contaminated fish can be found in the Pacific and Indian Oceans and the Caribbean Sea during the spring and summer months. The onset of illness is usually a few hours after the consumption of the implicated fish, and the patient presents with nausea, vomiting, abdominal pain, pruritus, perioral paresthesias, dizziness, and blurred vision. Rarely, it can lead to temporary blindness, paralysis, and death. The toxin can be present in affected fish without any apparent indication of contamination. The heat-stable toxins are unaffected by cooking and processing methods, and can persist for weeks. Treatment is supportive, although one can consider cholinesterase-reactivating drugs because the toxin appears to inhibit cholinesterase activity in red blood cells. Pralidoxime chloride (Protopam), 1 to 2 grams in 100 mL saline, may be given intravenously over 15 to 30 minutes in severe cases by persons familiar with its use.

Scombroid poisoning is also toxin mediated and is frequently misdiagnosed as a seafood allergy. Although it is recognized worldwide, most incidents are reported from the United States, Japan, and Great Britain. The illness is caused by eating fish that contain high levels of histamine, produced as a result of the decarboxylation of histidine. Initially reported in association with fish of the Scombridae and Scombresocidae families (tuna, mackerel, and bonito), other species such as mahi-mahi have been implicated. Flushing, pruritus, urticaria, headache, nausea, and rarely, bronchospasm develop within 10 minutes to 2 hours of ingestion of contaminated fish. This self-limited process typically resolves within 4 hours, although antihistamines and bronchodilators may be used for symptomatic relief.

Other seafood-related, toxin-mediated illnesses include paralytic and neurotoxic shellfish poisoning and puffer fish poisoning. Paralytic shellfish poisoning is caused by the ingestion of shellfish contaminated with marine dinoflagellates (the cause of red tide), which contain saxitoxin. Molluscs feed on dinoflagellates, and contaminated species can be found in ambient waters at latitudes higher than 30 degrees. Most patients present with the onset of symptoms within 1 hour of food ingestion and develop paresthesias of the mouth, lips and face, and extremities. Rarely, patients develop severe complications, including dyspnea, dysphagia, weakness or paralysis, and respiratory failure. Treatment involves removal of the remaining toxin from the gastrointestinal tract (by use of cathartics, enemas), supportive care, and rarely, mechanical ventilation.

Neurotoxic shellfish poisoning is similar to paralytic shellfish poisoning, but paralysis does not occur. Outbreaks in North America have been reported in association with ingestion of oysters, clams, and other molluscs. Puffer fish poisoning is seen primarily in Japan and is caused by tetrodotoxin. This toxin is found in puffer fish, porcupine fish, ocean sunfish, as well as some newts and salamanders, and it is associated with improper cleaning of the fish. Tetrodotoxin is similar to saxitoxin; can cause a severe neuromuscular paralysis, including respiratory failure; and is associated with a mortality rate of up to 60%.

Mushroom Poisoning

Ingestion of toxic mushrooms may lead to clinically distinct syndromes depending on the type of mushroom ingested. At least six species of toxic mushrooms lead to illness within 2 hours of ingestion, whereas three species of mushrooms lead to an illness of longer incubation of up to 24 hours (see Table 2). Types of symptoms seen in the early presentations of poisoning include confusion, delirium (similar to alcohol intoxication), parasympathetic hyperactivity, acute psychotic behavior and hallucinations, a disulfiram-like reaction if alcohol is ingested, and gastrointestinal manifestations (nausea, vomiting, and abdominal cramps). With the exception of the illness associated with parasympathetic hypersensitivity, the symptoms are self-limited and require only supportive treatment. Mushrooms of the muscarine-containing varieties (*Clitocybe* and *Inocybe* species) produce an anticholinergic syndrome, which presents as sweating, salivation, bradycardia, as well as other indications of parasympathetic hyperactivity. Rarely, this syndrome is fatal and, thus, should be treated with parenteral atropine sulfate, 1 to 2 mg every 2 to 6 hours until the symptoms resolve (typically within 24 hours).

A patient developing abdominal cramps and diarrhea within 6 to 24 hours of mushroom ingestion suggests a more serious mushroom intoxication that can lead to hepatorenal failure. The cause is most commonly ingestion of amatoxin or phallotoxin, which produces a biphasic illness accounting for 95% of fatal mushroom poisoning. Initially, the patient presents with gastrointestinal symptoms (nausea, vomiting, abdominal cramps, and diarrhea) as well as fever in the first 6 to 12 hours after ingestion. These symptoms resolve within 24 hours, and then after remaining well for up to 2 days, the patient becomes severely ill with renal and hepatic failure. Treatment is with supportive intensive care, but the mortality rate approaches 50% even with this care.

A similar syndrome also develops with the ingestion of *Gyromitra* spp. of mushrooms containing gyromitrin that, after metabolism to methylhydrazine, inhibits pyridoxal phosphate. Initially, the patient experiences gastrointestinal symptoms, which are followed by hepatic failure, hemolysis, methemoglobinuria, convulsions, and coma. This syndrome is treated with pyridoxine hydrochloride,*† 25 mg per kg, given intravenously over 15 to 30 minutes. For assistance with the treatment of mushroom poisoning, the local poison control center should be contacted.

Miscellaneous Food-Related Illnesses

Ingestion of alkaloids found in fungi that contaminate wheat and rye may lead to ergotism, which is severe vasoconstriction that can progress to ischemic necrosis of muscle. Ingestion of the mycotoxin aflatoxin, found in peanut butter, can lead to gastrointestinal bleeding and hepatic complications. Other mycotoxins known as tricothecenes can be found as contaminants of grains, and can lead to gastrointestinal symptoms as well as anemia and leukopenia. Ingestion of the Italian fava bean can cause hemolytic anemia in patients with glucose-6-phosphate dehydrogenase deficiency. Ingestion of solanine, found in jimson weed and in the milk of cows ingesting this weed, can cause a syndrome similar to atropine poisoning with headache, confusion, abdominal pain, and diarrhea. Other toxin-related illnesses due to ingestion of food items include oxalic acid poisoning (rhubarb leaves, beets, spinach, houseplants), lathyrism (progressive spastic paraplegia due to ingestion of sweet peas of *Lathyrus* species), digitalis poisoning (home-brewed foxglove or oleander tea), and cyanide poisoning (rarely seen, after ingestion of large amounts of seeds from apples, cherries, pears, peaches, cassava, and lima beans).

The Chinese restaurant syndrome, due to the ingestion of monosodium L-glutamate (MSG), causes a flushing and burning sensation of the face and chest, headache, and diaphoresis. Most commonly, this condition occurs after eating wonton soup as a first course, because the MSG is more rapidly absorbed on an empty stomach. The syndrome is self-limited and rarely requires treatment.

DIAGNOSIS

Although the patient's history and clinical presentation can lead to a presumptive diagnosis of food-related illness, confirmation lies in laboratory evaluation. Appropriate specimens to evaluate include blood, stool, vomitus, and the suspected contaminated food. Most often, however, no diagnosis is made due to the rapid resolution of symptoms with appropriate supportive care.

Stool cultures are helpful for diagnosis of *Salmonella, Shigella, Campylobacter, Yersinia, V. cholerae* (types 01 and non-01), and *V. parahaemolyticus.* Gram's stain of the stool is rarely helpful, but the presence of fecal leukocytes on stool examination is useful in establishing the diagnosis of an invasive organism (e.g., salmonellae, shigellae, and invasive *E. coli*). In outbreaks of staphylococcal poisoning, the organism can be isolated from stool and vomitus, as well as the suspected food item. *B. cereus* can also be isolated from feces; however, this organism has been reported on occasion as flora in healthy patients, so confirmation by serotyping may be useful. *C. perfringens* is frequently seen in the normal flora of healthy patients, so stool culture is only helpful if a colony count of greater than 10^6 *C. perfringens* spores per gram of feces is found. Confirmation of this illness can be made by isolating the organism in the suspected food. Electron microscopy of the stool plays a role in identifying some viruses (e.g., Norwalk agent) but is not routinely available.

Toxin assays are important for identifying several causes of food poisoning. These are most helpful for *C. botulinum, E. coli* 015:H7, *S. aureus,* fish and shellfish poisoning, and mushroom poisoning. Most of these assays require the use of a reference laboratory.

*Not FDA approved for this indication.
†Exceeds dosage recommended by the manufacturer.

Scombroid poisoning can be documented by the presence of histamine in the suspected fish (100 mg of histamine in 100 grams of fish confirms the diagnosis). Ciguatera usually is diagnosed through the clinical picture alone. Assays demonstrating the toxin in suspected fish have been developed but are not commonly available. The clinician can contact local public health authorities for more specialized assays. Despite an extensive evaluation, one can only expect to find the cause of food-related illness in less than 50% of the cases.

TREATMENT

Although specific therapy is occasionally indicated, the mainstay of treatment of food-borne illness is supportive. The majority of the syndromes discussed are self-limited in nature but may require extensive fluid replacement. The patients should also be monitored closely for changes in vital signs and neurologic symptoms. When indicated, any remaining toxin should be removed, either by emetics, cathartics, or activated charcoal. This may be accomplished with the use of syrup of ipecac, 30 ml orally, or apomorphine, 6 mg subcutaneously. Gastric lavage and charcoal may also be useful, as are cathartics such as magnesium citrate (up to 300 ml). Emetics should not be used in patients with neurologic involvement, as the risk of aspiration is significant.

Fluid replacement can be either oral or parenteral, depending on the patient's clinical status. The degree of dehydration can be assessed by the patient's vital signs, as well as examination of mucous membranes and skin turgor. If oral hydration is chosen as the route of replacement, the patient must be advised to take a fluid with adequate sodium and carbohydrate content. Acceptable fluids include Rehydralyte, Ricelyte, or the WHO-oral rehydration formula or other replacement formula containing 3.5 grams NaCl, 1.5 grams KCl, 2.5 grams $NaHCO_3$ and 20 grams glucose in 1 liter of boiled water. Clear liquids, such as Gatorade, are less appropriate because the sodium content is lower. In severe cases, rapid infusion of intravenous fluids, such as normal saline, is necessary.

Symptomatically the patient can be treated for nausea and vomiting with antiemetics, such as prochlorperazine (Compazine), 5 to 10 mg orally, or 25 mg by rectal suppository. Agents offering symptomatic relief of diarrhea should be given to patients with mild, nondysentery gastroenteritis but should be avoided in those with toxin-related illness and severe invasive diarrhea. An appropriate agent is loperamide hydrochloride (Imodium), 4 mg followed by 2 mg after each episode of diarrhea, to a maximum of 16 mg daily.

The role of antibiotics has yet to be clarified in the treatment of most causes of invasive diarrhea, but these agents should be included in the treatment of shigellosis, cholera, and typhoid. Studies have been conducted showing that antibiotics may decrease the duration of microbial carriage but generally do not affect the clinical course of the illness. Antimicrobials are of no known benefit in the treatment of illness due to staphylococcal, *C. perfringens,* or *B. cereus* food poisoning and are likely to have minimal to no benefit in the treatment of food poisoning due to *V. parahaemolyticus, E. coli,* and *Y. enterocolitica.*

In cases of traveler's diarrhea, defined as more than 3 loose stools daily associated with at least one other gastrointestinal symptom, an appropriate treatment regimen would include a fluoroquinolone such as ciprofloxacin (Cipro), at a dose of 500 mg twice daily. Antidiarrheal agents, such as loperamide hydrochloride (Imodium), are useful in decreasing symptoms but are contraindicated in patients with evidence of invasive disease (e.g., fever and bloody stools). The issue of chemoprophylaxis for travelers has been debated over the last few years; the use of antimicrobial agents decreases the incidence of diarrhea but is associated with a significant incidence of side effects and potentially increased microbial resistance. The use of bismuth subsalicylate, two tablets chewed with meals and at bedtime, reduces the incidence of traveler's diarrhea with fewer side effects. This is more commonly recommended as chemoprophylaxis, and antimicrobials should generally be reserved for treatment of established illness.

NECROTIZING SKIN AND SOFT TISSUE INFECTIONS

method of
ELLIS S. CAPLAN, M.D.
University of Maryland School of Medicine
Baltimore, Maryland

Necrotizing infections of the skin encompass a variety of disorders that have been described individually in the past; monomicrobial necrotizing cellulitis, necrotizing fasciitis, gram-negative synergistic necrotizing cellulitis, and clostridial myonecrosis. For practical purposes, we consider them a single entity, necrotizing infection of the skin and soft tissue. Although this consolidation excludes infections of the muscles, in particular myonecrosis, much of this discussion applies to the presentations of muscle infections that the physician will encounter. Although necrotizing fasciitis is, in a sense, a more limited term, in general it is often used to include all necrotizing disorders of the skin and soft tissue.

The vast majority of these infections are secondary to trauma, although the trauma sometimes is minor. Most cases begin as a simple infection that, for reasons still unclear, quickly progresses into a fulminant, severe, life-threatening process. By far the most responsible organism is the group A beta-hemolytic streptococcus, either alone or frequently in combination with other organisms, particularly anaerobic organisms of the skin. Careful and skillful microbiologic techniques are frequently necessary to recover the anaerobic organisms, and in many reports, this has not been accomplished, thus giving a false impression as to their lack of a role in this disease. Occasionally, fungi have been implicated in these infections, particularly following natural disasters. For the most part, identifying the particular organism is not as important as recognizing the disease process itself, because antibiotic selection is based on the presentation and circumstances of the patient and not on which organism may be present.

The diagnosis of necrotizing infections is a clinical one. The patient presents with signs and symptoms of infection—usually fever, leukocytosis, and increasing pain. The infection may have started as a simple cellulitis that now has reached a crescendo as to pain and swelling. The skin rapidly changes color, and superficial blebs or small areas of necrosis may be the first sign of impeding deterioration. Biopsy has been advocated at this point to determine if deeper, more progressive infection is present. Histologic criteria are (1) necrosis of superficial fascia, (2) polymorphonuclear infiltration of the deep dermis and fascia, (3) fibrinous thrombi of arteries and veins passing through the fascia, (4) angiitis with fibrinoid necrosis of arterial and venous walls, (5) presence of microorganisms within the destroyed fascia, and (6) absence of muscle involvement. If muscle involvement is present, then we are dealing with myonecrosis and not fasciitis. Usually, however, a biopsy is not conducted, and treatment decisions are based on the clinical picture. With the onset of necrosis, toxicity ensues and the patient deteriorates rapidly. Without urgent intervention, multiple organ failure begins and death is a common outcome. The reported mortality rate is up to 75%, and 50% of these patients die within a week of admission.

At increased risk are patients with underlying diseases such as diabetes, alcoholism, congestive heart failure, and immune defects. Most lesions result from trauma sustained in a environment conducive to contamination with multiple organisms, such as farm injuries and hunting injuries. However, hospitalized, immobile, or poorly mobile patients are also at risk from pressure necrosis as the inciting event. Enlargement of the ischemic area leads to vascular occlusion and more ischemia. Skin changes herald the onset of extreme toxicity. Subcutaneous gas formation is frequently seen, even in the absence of clostridial infection. Unfortunately, gas formation is not very specific and many anaerobes, as well as *Escherichia coli*, are impressive gas producers. However, this does strongly suggest the diagnosis, if it has not already been made. X-ray films are helpful in that they can show subcutaneous gas, if present, as fine streaks or small bubbles along fascial, muscle or skin planes.

Once the diagnosis is made, the patient should be transferred to a facility that has experience in dealing with this type of infection. Because these infections are so uncommon, most physicians have not acquired sufficient experience to manage these patients.

A variety of classification schemes have been proposed to identify the various different syndromes that are included in necrotizing infections of the skin and soft tissues. Some depend on the particular organism (e.g., streptococcal gangrene, gram-negative synergistic necrotizing cellulitis), others on whether there are more than one organism present, and still others rely on the area involved (e.g., Fournier's gangrene). This classification is useful only if it helps the physician make treatment decisions. In fact, the only real decision to be made is the extent of surgery necessary. Only an experienced surgeon in the operating room can make this decision, and where the infection is located or what organism is involved does not influence this decision. Hence, we believe that if the patient is toxic and there is necrosis present, that that is the only information necessary to influence treatment.

TREATMENT

The cornerstone of treatment of all types of necrotizing infections is prompt and complete surgical debridement of all dead and compromised tissue. The debridement must be performed as soon as the patient is stabilized sufficiently to withstand the surgery. The most common mistake is that the initial surgery is inadequate because of the extent of debridement necessary; inexperienced physicians fail to remove all of the affected tissue. The initial operation is clearly the best time to undertake definitive surgery, so the patient should be stabilized as quickly as possible. Attention to fluid replacement and metabolic stabilization are imperative.

Antibiotic selection depends to some extent on the circumstances causing the necrotizing infection. By far, the most common organism involved is group A beta-hemolytic streptococcus, an organism that is still very sensitive to penicillin G. However, other organisms such as the staphylococci, a host of anaerobic organisms, and some gram-negative rods may be involved. We prefer ampicillin/sulbactam (Unasyn), 3 grams every 6 hours, as initial treatment for most patients while awaiting results of cultures. Doses must be adjusted if there is severe renal failure. Gram's stain frequently confirms a mixed infection and rarely is helpful at directing antibiotic selection. Ampicillin/sulbactam provide coverage for all streptococci including most enterococci, *Staphylococcus aureus, Clostridium,* other anaerobes, and many gram-negative rods. *Pseudomonas* species are not covered but are rarely associated with these types of infections, unless the patient has been on other antibiotics. Imipenem/cilastatin (Primaxin), ticarcillin/clavulanate (Timentin), piperacillin-tazobactam (Zosyn),* are also single agents that can be used if *Pseudomonas* is a possibility. This also allows aminoglycoside use to be avoided in patients with diabetes, a frequent underlying condition in these infections. For patients with penicillin sensitivity, a combination of clindamycin (Cleocin), 900 mg every 8 hours, and a quinolone or aztreonam (Azactam) offers coverage for most organisms. However, enterococci are not covered unless vancomycin is also added.

If the necrotizing infection is secondary to a water injury or to a water exposure, including rain water, then organisms such as *Aeromonas* and *Vibrio* must be considered, with *Vibrio* associated with salt water and *Aeromonas* with fresh water. In this case, trimethoprim-sulfamethoxazole (Bactrim, Septra), 15 mg per kg per day, or a quinolone in full doses, or an aminoglycoside must be added to the previous regimen pending identification and sensitivity results.

Because these necrotizing infections result in large open wounds, it is not uncommon to encounter both colonization and superinfection with more resistant organisms during the patient's hospital course. It is important to distinguish between the two. If the patient is improving and the wound is healing, isolation of a resistant organism is usually just a colonization and does not require additional antibiotics. On the other hand, if the patient is not improving in spite of adequate surgery and antibiotics, then isolation of a

*Not FDA approved for this indication.

resistant organism has to be considered as a possible superinfection, and changes in the antibiotic may be indicated.

Patients with fungal infections should be treated with amphotericin B, 0.6 to 1 mg per kg per day, to a total dose of 1500 to 2000 mg.

Hyperbaric oxygen is a controversial treatment for these infections. Although its value as an adjunct therapy has not been proved, it is often used, if available, for patients with these infections. Because the mortality rate associated with these necrotizing infections is so high and because most physicians have limited experience in treating them, we believe that patients with such infections should be transferred to centers with hyperbaric oxygen facilities, if at all possible. Physicians in those facilities tend to have the most experience in handling all aspects of these potentially life-threatening infections.

EPIDEMIC INFLUENZA

method of
JOHN TREANOR, M.D.
University of Rochester School of Medicine
Rochester, New York

Epidemic influenza refers to seasonal acute respiratory disease caused by influenza viruses. These enveloped viruses are divided into three types, based on antigenic and genetic differences, referred to as influenza virus types A, B, and C. Influenza A viruses are further characterized by hemagglutinin (HA or H) and neuraminidase (NA or N) subtypes. Standard nomenclature for these viruses includes the type, location of isolation, strain designation, year of isolation, and subtype for influenza A viruses, i.e., influenza A/Beijing/32/92 (H3N2) virus.

EPIDEMIOLOGY AND DISEASE IMPACT

Influenza A viruses possess a unique epidemiology that can best be understood in terms of the concepts of antigenic drift and shift. Antigenic drift refers to the gradual accumulation of point mutations in the HA or NA resulting in an antigenically variant virus able to successfully infect in the presence of immunity to the previous strain. Seasonal epidemics of influenza A occur each year, the severity of which is largely determined by the degree of antigenic drift between the epidemic virus and the virus immediately preceding it. Pandemics, or worldwide epidemics, of influenza are associated with new subtypes of HA and/or NA, referred to as antigenic shifts, so that the virus enters into a more or less completely susceptible population. Several pandemics have been recorded in recent history, notably in 1918 when the H1N1 viruses replaced previously circulating H3N8 viruses; in 1957, when H2N2 viruses replaced H1N1 viruses; and in 1968, when H3N2 viruses replaced H2N2 viruses. In contrast to influenza A virus, only single subtypes of the influenza B virus HA and NA are recognized, and antigenic shift and pandemics do not occur with influenza B virus. However, significant antigenic drift is seen, and yearly epidemics may be noted. Influenza C viruses also undergo antigenic drift but not antigenic shift.

Unlike other respiratory viruses, influenza epidemics are regularly associated with excess morbidity and mortality, usually seen in the form of excess rates of pneumonia and influenza-associated hospitalizations and death during epidemics. Both influenza A and B, but not influenza C, are associated with severe illness. Influenza affects all age groups, with the highest hospitalization rates in the very young and the very old. Excess morbidity and mortality are particularly high in those with certain medical conditions, including adults and children with cardiovascular and pulmonary conditions, or those requiring regular medical care because of chronic metabolic disease, renal dysfunction, hemoglobinopathies, or immunodeficiency. Recent reports also suggest that influenza may result in more severe disease and prolonged symptoms in individuals with human immunodeficiency virus infection.

CLINICAL FEATURES OF INFLUENZA VIRUS INFECTION

Influenza is characterized by a surprisingly sudden onset, and many patients can pinpoint the exact hour at which their symptoms began. Respiratory complaints include rhinitis, pharyngitis, cough, and hoarseness. Systemic symptoms, including high fever, myalgias, malaise, and prostration, are prominent and may overshadow respiratory complaints early in the course of illness. Myalgias of the extraocular muscles, associated with severe pain on lateral gaze, are a common complaint. Complete recovery may take weeks. The clinical features of influenza A and B virus infection are similar.

COMPLICATIONS

Classically, four types of lower respiratory complications of acute influenza have been described and contribute significantly to virus-related morbidity and mortality. Primary viral pneumonia is seen predominantly in those with prior cardiac disease. The patient presents with typical features of acute influenza but experiences a rapid progression of dyspnea, cough, cyanosis, and development of adult respiratory distress syndrome. Chest roentgenographs reveal bilateral interstitial infiltrates, sputum production is scanty, and Gram's stain reveals few organisms. Secondary bacterial pneumonia often appears 1 to 2 weeks after apparent recovery from an acute influenza episode with recurrence of fever, as well as signs and symptoms of typical lobar pneumonia. Common respiratory bacterial pathogens, including *Streptococcus pneumoniae,* beta-hemolytic streptococci, and *Haemophilus influenzae* are often isolated. In addition, the incidence of *Staphylococcus aureus,* an uncommon pulmonary pathogen, is much increased. Mixed viral-bacterial pneumonia may also occur, with features common to both syndromes. Finally, dyspnea and lower respiratory signs, such as rales, rhonchi, and wheezes, may be seen without visible roentgenographic infiltrates. Other lower respiratory tract complications include croup and bronchiolitis in younger children, and exacerbations of chronic pulmonary disease and asthma. Bacterial sinusitis may also occur as a complication of influenza.

Extrapulmonary complications appear to be uncommon. Myositis, with myoglobinuria and elevated serum creatine phosphokinase, has been seen predominantly in children. Both myocarditis and pericarditis have also been associated with influenza. Toxic shock syndrome has been reported following influenza, presumably reflecting colonization of the damaged respiratory tract with toxin-producing *S. aureus.* Encephalitis has also been reported in acute influenza. Of note, Reye's syndrome, an illness of unknown cause characterized by mental status changes and hepatic failure, has been associated with influenza, particularly influenza B, as well as with other respiratory viral infections. The use of aspirin greatly increases the risk of Reye's syndrome, and aspirin should not be administered to children with acute respiratory disease. Acetaminophen is not associated with an increased risk of Reye's syndrome.

DIAGNOSIS

Presentation with an acute febrile respiratory illness with prominent systemic symptoms during a recognized influenza epidemic is strongly suggestive of acute influenza. Conversely, a clinical diagnosis of influenza outside of the influenza epidemic season should be made with caution. Because of the frequent co-circulation of several subtypes of influenza and other respiratory viruses, a specific viral diagnosis cannot be made on clinical grounds alone.

The most accurate method for specific diagnosis is virus culture. Nasopharyngeal swab or nasal aspirate samples should be collected at the time of acute illness and transported on wet ice to the diagnostic laboratory. Freezing of the sample at −20° C (−4° F) should be avoided. Influenza viruses can be isolated from clinical samples in a variety of mammalian epithelial cell lines, and specific identification usually takes 5 to 7 days. Several rapid viral diagnostic tests for influenza have been described. Generally, these tests detect viral antigens in clinical samples using monoclonal or polyclonal antibodies in immunofluoresence or enzyme immunoassay type formats. Rapid tests based on the polymerase chain reaction technique have also been described. Most of these tests are specific, but the sensitivity of these tests compared with virus culture has been variable. The sensitivity of these tests often depends on a use of a specific sample collection technique.

PREVENTION OF INFLUENZA

Influenza Vaccination

Inactivated influenza vaccines are generated by the treatment of partially purified influenza virions with an inactivating agent, such as formalin. Whole virus, split-product or subvirion vaccines generated by disruption of the virus envelope, and purified HA/NA subunit vaccines are available. Generally, the immunogenicity of each of these types of preparations is similar. Because of the current co-circulation of both influenza A H3N2 and H1N1 subtypes as well as influenza B virus, inactivated influenza vaccines are administered as a trivalent preparation. The formulation of the 1993 to 1994 inactivated influenza vaccine included the influenza A/Texas/36/91 (H1N1), A/Beijing/32/92 (H3N2), and B/Panama/45/90 viruses.

Randomized, placebo-controlled trials of modern influenza vaccines have demonstrated these vaccines to be well tolerated. Mild local reactions occur in a minority of subjects, and systemic symptoms, such as malaise, headache, or myalgias, occur at a low rate, similar to placebo. Inactivated influenza vaccines do not cause respiratory illness. Reactions to whole virus and split-product vaccines at current doses are similar in adults, but whole virus vaccines are unacceptably reactogenic in children, and they should not be used in those under 12 years of age. Inactivated influenza vaccines are immunogenic when they are administered at the currently recommended dose of approximately 15 μg of each HA antigen in healthy adults, and they result in increases in hemagglutination-inhibition (HI) antibody in about 90% of adult recipients. Only a single dose of influenza vaccine is needed in individuals who have experienced prior infection with a related subtype, but a two-dose schedule is required in unprimed individuals, including children. Dosage recommendations for inactivated influenza vaccines are shown in Table 1.

TABLE 1. **Recommended Doses of Influenza Vaccine by Age Group**

Age Group	Product	Dosage (mL)	No. of Doses
6–35 months	Split virus only	0.25	1 or 2*
3–8 years	Split virus only	0.50	1 or 2*
9–12 years	Split virus only	0.50	1
> 12 years	Whole or split virus	0.50	1

*Two doses 4 or more weeks apart are recommended for unprimed individuals, e.g., children under 9 years receiving vaccine for the first time.

Inactivated influenza vaccine has been shown to be effective in the prevention of influenza A in several randomized or semirandomized controlled studies conducted in young adults, with levels of protection of 70 to 90%. Randomized controlled trials have not been conducted in other populations, particularly in high-risk individuals. However, numerous retrospective case-control studies are available that have documented the effectiveness of inactivated influenza vaccines in this group. In general, the effectiveness of inactivated vaccine is greatest for the prevention of lower respiratory tract disease, such as pneumonia, while being relatively less effective at preventing infection or upper respiratory tract disease. The effectiveness of influenza vaccination is directly related to the degree of antigenic similarity between the circulating epidemic influenza virus and the virus used to generate the vaccine. The duration of protective immunity also appears to be limited, particularly in the elderly. Thus, inactivated influenza vaccine should be administered annually, usually in the late fall. Current recommendations for groups in which influenza vaccination should be considered are given in Table 2. Vaccine may be administered on the same visit as pneumococcal vaccine, but should be given at a different injection site.

Chemoprophylaxis

Two antiviral drugs, amantadine (Symmetrel), and the related drug rimantadine (Flumadine), are currently licensed for the prevention and treatment of influenza A. Both amantadine and rimantadine are active against all strains of influenza A virus in a variety of cell culture sys-

TABLE 2. **Target Groups for Influenza Vaccination**

Groups at Increased Risk for Influenza-Related Complications
Persons ≥ 65 years of age
Residents of nursing homes and other chronic care facilities
Adults and children with chronic disorders of the pulmonary and cardiovascular systems
Adults and children requiring regular medical follow-up or hospitalization for chronic metabolic diseases, renal dysfunction, hemoglobinopathies, or immunosuppression
Children and teenagers requiring long-term aspirin therapy
Groups That Can Transmit Influenza to High-Risk Persons
Physicians, nurses, and other personnel
Employees of nursing homes and chronic care facilities
Providers of home care
Household members

tems and animal models, with rimantadine slightly more active on a per weight basis. Both drugs are active only against influenza A virus at clinically achievable levels.

The dose of both amantadine and rimantadine in individuals with normal renal function is 100 mg given twice daily. Both drugs are well absorbed orally. Amantadine is excreted unchanged in the urine, and the plasma half-life is prolonged in patients with impaired renal function. Only a small amount of drug is removed by dialysis. Amantadine dosage should be adjusted in the presence of renal dysfunction (Table 3). In contrast, rimantadine is extensively metabolized, and the pharmacokinetics of the drug do not appear to be altered significantly in individuals with hepatic or renal diseases. However, a dosage reduction to 100 mg per day is recommended in patients with severe hepatic dysfunction or renal failure (creatinine clearance less than 10 mL per min). Both drugs should be administered at a maximum dose of 100 mg per day in individuals over the age of 65 regardless of renal function.

Minor central nervous system side effects, such as insomnia, nervousness, and difficulty concentrating, are seen in approximately 10% of individuals given amantadine, and at a significantly lower rate with rimantadine. Seizures have also been reported rarely with both drugs and are more common in individuals with pre-existing seizure disorders. These drugs should be used with caution in such individuals.

Amantadine and rimantadine are approximately 70 to 90% effective in the prophylaxis of influenza A in healthy adults. Relatively less is known about the effectiveness of these drugs in the prevention of influenza in high-risk subjects. However, preliminary data suggest that rimantadine is effective in the prevention of influenza A in the elderly and that the protective effect is additive to that provided by inactivated influenza vaccine. Antiviral prophylaxis is not a substitute for vaccination but should be considered in situations in which vaccine cannot be given in time or is contraindicated. Examples of such situations include high-risk adults or their caregivers who have not received vaccine at the beginning of an epidemic. In this case, vaccine should be administered, and amantadine or rimantadine given for 2 weeks until immune responses to vaccine develop. In high-risk persons or caregivers for whom influenza vaccine is contraindicated, amantadine or rimantadine should be administered for the duration of the influenza A virus epidemic.

Amantadine and rimantadine may also be useful to prevent further spread of infection during institutional outbreaks of influenza A. Although no controlled, randomized trials have been conducted to evaluate the use of these drugs under these circumstances, retrospective analyses of such outbreaks support this recommendation. In this situation, the drugs should be administered to both vaccinated and unvaccinated residents for the duration of the epidemic.

TABLE 3. **Amantadine Dosage in Renal Failure**

Creatinine Clearance (mL/min)	Recommended Dose of Amantadine
≥ 80	200 mg daily
60–79	200 mg/100 mg on alternate days
40–59	100 mg daily
30–39	200 mg twice weekly
20–29	100 mg thrice weekly
10–19	200 mg/100 mg alternating once weekly

TREATMENT

Commonsense measures, including provision of fluids and adequate rest, provide symptomatic relief in acute influenza. Antipyretics and decongestants are also useful, but aspirin and aspirin-containing products should be avoided in children. Bacterial superinfections should be treated with supportive measures and appropriate antibiotics based on results of Gram's stain and bacterial culture and sensitivity.

Both amantadine and rimantadine are effective in the treatment of influenza A when administered within 48 hours of onset of symptoms. Most studies have shown more rapid reductions in symptoms and fever, and reduced levels and duration of virus shedding when compared with placebo or aspirin in young adults. Rimantadine has also been shown to reduce the level of virus shedding and clinical symptoms early in infection when compared with acetaminophen in children.* These drugs should be administered during the period of acute illness but no longer than 5 to 7 days. Relatively less is known about the efficacy of these drugs in the treatment of influenza in high-risk individuals or in individuals with complicated influenza, such as in hospitalized patients or those with pneumonia. However, most authorities would support the use of amantadine or rimantadine in the treatment of complicated influenza A virus infection, even late in the course of illness.

Influenza A viruses that are resistant to the antiviral effects of amantadine and rimantadine emerge frequently in individuals treated with these drugs, and they can be transmitted to and cause disease in susceptible contacts. Because resistant viruses typically are found late in the course of therapy, short courses of drug therapy may reduce the rate of resistance, but this has not been proved. When possible, individuals being treated with drugs should not be in close contact with those receiving chemoprophylaxis, to reduce the selection and transmission of resistant viruses in the population.

The antiviral drug ribavirin (Virazole) is active against both influenza A and B virus in vitro and in human challenge models when administered by small-particle aerosol. However, the relatively poor efficacy of the drug and its cumbersome method of administration have limited its utility in this situation. Intravenous ribavirin was recently reported to be effective in treatment of a case of influenza virus associated acute myocarditis. However, no firm recommendations can be made currently regarding the use of ribavirin in influenza virus infection.*

*Not FDA approved for this indication.

LEISHMANIASIS

method of
ALAN J. MAGILL, M.D.
Walter Reed Army Institute of Research
Washington, D.C.

Leishmaniasis refers to a variety of clinical syndromes caused by infection with a protozoan parasite of the genus *Leishmania.* Traditionally, human disease has been divided into three syndromes: (1) cutaneous leishmaniasis (CL), characterized by chronic skin ulcers that slowly resolve with residual scarring; (2) mucocutaneous leishmaniasis (MCL), characterized by ulcerative lesions of the oral, nasal, and pharyngeal mucosa that occur months to years following a primary cutaneous ulcer; and (3) visceral leishmaniasis (VL), characterized by widespread systemic infection. However, from a pathophysiologic point of view, it may be more useful to view the clinical manifestations of leishmaniasis seen in individual patients as a single point along a spectrum of disease. This spectrum can be defined by the parasite burden (numbers of parasites) and the predominant immune response (humoral versus cell mediated). A schematic representation of this concept is shown in Figure 1.

Parasites are transmitted to mammals by the bite of an infected female sand fly. Host macrophages ingest the promastigote, the flagellated form found in the insect, where it transforms into the amastigote, the oval form found in host macrophages. Within the macrophages, amastigotes fuse with a phagosome, grow, and replicate. Therefore, *Leishmania* are obligate intracellular parasites of host cells from the monocyte-macrophage lineage. The life cycle is completed when a sandfly acquires parasites from an infected mammalian host while taking a blood meal.

In most areas of the world, leishmaniasis is a zoonosis and human disease is incidentally acquired when humans intrude into the natural cycle. However, human-fly-human cycles can be established. Epidemics of visceral disease leading to tens of thousands of deaths in India and parts of Africa and South America periodically occur. Likewise, thousands of cases of cutaneous disease occur in endemic areas.

CLINICAL SYNDROMES

Cutaneous manifestations of leishmaniasis include solitary or multiple papules, plaques, nodules, and ulcerative lesions. Patients may present with solitary, regional, or generalized adenopathy, with or without associated cutaneous findings. Mucosal lesions may appear on any surface of the oral, pharyngeal, or nasal mucosa. Classic mucocutaneous disease is usually a manifestation of infection with *L. braziliensis* acquired in the New World, although rare cases have been reported from the Old World associated with *L. major* and *L. ethiopica.* Diffuse cutaneous leishmaniasis (DCL) has been described in Venezuela and Ethiopia. Clinically, it looks like lepromatous leprosy, with nodules found all over the body. The soft, fleshy nodules are teeming with amastigotes. Other uncommon presentations of leishmaniasis include granulomas and nonhealing ulcers at the site of trauma, surgery, or accidental inoculation.

Classic visceral leishmaniasis, also known as kala-azar, is characterized by the pentad of chronic fever, wasting, massive hepatosplenomegaly, hyperglobulinemia, and pancytopenia. Less well recognized are a host of other visceral syndromes including asymptomatic infection, transient undifferentiated febrile illness, mononucleosis syndromes, chronic viscerotropic syndromes, and incomplete stages of kala-azar, in which one or more of the classic findings are not present.

Leishmaniasis is an opportunistic infection in immunosuppressed patients. There have been multiple reports of disease owing to reactivation following organ transplantation, chronic steroid use, malignancy and its associated therapies, and more recently, as a late-stage opportunistic infection in patients with AIDS. In some endemic areas such as the Mediterranean basin, leishmaniasis has emerged as a significant problem in human immunodeficiency virus (HIV)–infected individuals. Response to traditional therapy with pentavalent antimony has been disappointing. Leishmaniasis may prove to be a leading acquired

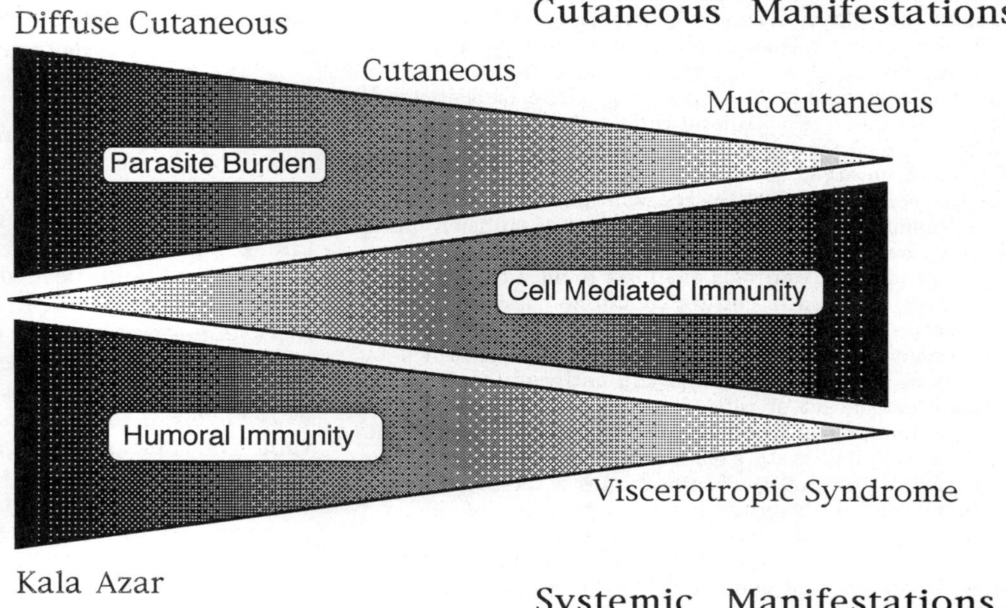

Figure 1. Bipolar spectrum of leishmaniasis. Cell-mediated immunity is defined by a delayed-type hypersensitivity reaction. Humoral response is defined by detecting antibody to whole promastigotes in an immunofluorescence assay.

immune deficiency syndrome (AIDS)–associated opportunistic infection in some areas of South America, Africa, and the Indian subcontinent.

Some parasite species are commonly associated with one clinical syndrome, such as kala-azar caused by *L. donovani* or cutaneous ulcers caused by *L. major;* however, it is clear that any species can be associated with more than one clinical syndrome. In addition, animal models have shown that even in classic cutaneous disease, there is widespread visceral dissemination of parasites. This suggests transient parasitemia or lymphatic spread in the majority, if not all, cases of leishmanial infection.

DIAGNOSIS

A definitive diagnosis is the demonstration of parasites (parasitologic diagnosis) in patient tissues, either by visualizing amastigotes or obtaining promastigotes from in vitro cultures. Therefore, an invasive procedure is required for the diagnosis of all forms of leishmaniasis. Also, the ease of diagnosis in visceral syndromes is proportional to the patient's parasite burden; the more organisms that are present, the easier it is to make a parasitologic diagnosis. Tissue samples are obtained from the margin of an active cutaneous ulcer, bone marrow, liver, spleen, or lymph nodes. Skin ulcers can be aspirated using a 23-gauge needle attached to a syringe with 0.1 mL of sterile saline. The bloody aspirate is placed directly onto glass slides and is smeared as with a peripheral blood smear. Smears of bone marrow aspirate are likewise prepared. Tissue obtained by biopsy is used to prepare touch preparations. Smears prepared from aspirates and touch preparations are fixed and then stained with Giemsa stain. Stains using monoclonal antibodies tagged to immunofluorescent markers are more sensitive, but require experienced observers. In addition, histopathologic sections of tissue should be stained with hematoxylin, eosin, and Giemsa. Review of sections requires a careful systematic search under oil by an experienced observer. The diagnosis is confirmed when an amastigote is identified as a 2- to 5-micron oval structure with a plasma membrane surrounding the nucleus and a dense rodlike structure, called the kinetoplast, next to the nucleus. The presence of the kinetoplast distinguishes the leishmanial amastigote from other intracellular organisms causing histoplasmosis or toxoplasmosis.

Aspirates and tissue should also be directly inoculated into an appropriate culture media such as Nicolle's modification of Novy and McNeal's medium (NNN) or Schneider's drosophila medium with fetal calf serum. Cultures should be maintained for 30 to 40 days at 22° to 25°C (71.6° to 77°F) and observed daily for evidence of promastigotes. A positive culture requires the transformation of amastigotes into promastigotes and their expansion to a sufficient number for visualization. In vitro culture is as much an art as a science and is not routinely available to most clinicians.

Isolates obtained in culture should be characterized, as the species of *Leishmania* may affect therapeutic decisions and prognosis. Characterization is usually performed by isoenzyme electrophoresis and the patterns obtained are compared to a set of reference standards. Thus, species designations reflect where arbitrarily defined enzymes migrate on cellulose acetate electrophoresis.

A bewildering variety of serologic tests, including immunofluorescent antibody tests, direct agglutination, indirect hemagglutinin, and enzyme-linked immunosorbent assays, have been used to detect antibodies to leishmanial parasites. Unfortunately, none have been standardized, so sensitivity and specificity are variable between laboratories and tests. Also, none are easily available to clinicians in North America. In general, a high titer is useful but low titers do not exclude infection. Detection of delayed-type hypersensitivity with a skin test, as with the PPD reaction in tuberculosis, would be a great aid to diagnosis in cutaneous syndromes and as an epidemiologic tool. Although skin test preparations are widely used in endemic areas of the world, no skin test is approved by the Food and Drug Administration (FDA) for human use in the United States. In summary, measures of the immune response to leishmanial infection are poorly characterized and are not readily available.

Partly because of the difficulty in measuring the immune response to an intracellular pathogen like *Leishmania,* techniques increasing the sensitivity of parasitologic diagnosis, such as the polymerase chain reaction (PCR) to amplify parasite DNA, have recently been introduced. Use of a sensitive parasitologic test such as the PCR promises to make diagnosis of all forms of leishmaniasis easier and may more fully define the spectrum of disease, especially the oligoparasitic spectrum of illness.

TREATMENT

There are no drugs for the treatment of leishmaniasis approved for use in the United States by the FDA. Pentavalent antimony, the drug of choice for all forms of leishmaniasis, is available to physicians in the United States only under investigational new drug (IND) protocols as the manufacturers have not sought a new drug application (NDA) with the FDA.

Worldwide, there are two preparations of pentavalent antimony available. Sodium stibogluconate* (SSG) (Pentostam, Burroughs Wellcome, UK)† is provided in 100-mL bottles at a concentration of 100 mg of antimony per mL. Meglumine antimoniate (Glucantime, Rhone Poulenc, France)† is provided in 15-mL ampules containing 85 mg of antimony per mL. SSG is traditionally used in the English-speaking countries of the world, whereas meglumine antimoniate is used in French-, Spanish-, and Portuguese-speaking countries. Although most consider the two drugs to be equivalent, there has been little comparative study of efficacy and toxicity.

In the United States, virtually all cases of leishmaniasis are treated with intravenous SSG (Pentostam). SSG is available for civilian use from the Centers for Disease Control and Prevention (telephone: 404-639-3670) and for military use (all branches) from the Walter Reed Army Medical Center (telephone: 202-576-1740).

Bottles should be stored in the dark at 4° C (46.4° F) until use. It can be given intramuscularly or intravenously, although the intramuscular route is painful owing to the large volume that must be given. We give the drug in a 1:10 dilution of 5% dextrose in water over 10 to 15 minutes through an antecubital vein. The solution to be given is prepared each morning and given to the patient via a butterfly needle, thus saving the patient from a prolonged indwelling catheter. Undiluted drug, given as an intravenous

---

*Investigational drug in the United States.
†Not available in the United States.

push, has been reported to cause thrombophlebitis. We have never seen this complication using the 1:10 dilution.

The decision to treat an individual patient is based on a number of factors. The drug rarely causes death or irreversible morbidity when it is used as recommended, so its therapeutic index is high. However, the drug is poorly tolerated by many patients, has a broad side effect profile, and requires daily intravenous infusions. We routinely offer treatment to all individuals who have acquired cutaneous leishmaniasis in the New World, especially those in whom we have demonstrated the presence of *L. braziliensis,* because of the possibility of late presentations of mucocutaneous leishmaniasis. Cutaneous lesions acquired in the Old World are usually self-healing (although the time required for complete healing may be many months) and do not always require therapy. Individuals who have cosmetically unacceptable lesions, functionally disabling lesions, painful lesions, or persistent lesions should be offered treatment. SSG is a lifesaving intervention for patients with kala-azar, and it is an effective treatment for patients with prolonged, febrile illness. Recognized cases of imported VL are uncommon in the United States.

We treat all forms of simple CL from both the Old World and the New World with SSG at 20 mg per kg per day for 20 days. We treat all forms of visceral disease and mucosal disease with SSG at 20 mg per kg per day for 30 days. There is no upper limit on the dose due to body weight, gender, or percentage of body fat. Prior to Operation Desert Storm, the majority of patients treated at WRAMC acquired simple CL due to *L. panamensis* at the Army jungle training center in Panama. Using 10 mg per kg per day for 20 days, 75% (15 of 20) patients were cured, whereas 100% (20 of 20) were cured using 20 mg per kg per day for 20 days. Despite successful treatment using the 20 mg per kg per day for 20 days regimen for dozens of cases over the last few years, we have had a few cases of clinical and parasitologic failure. These patients may require more treatment with SSG or the use of second-line agents. SSG was used successfully in treating several cases of VL caused by *L. tropica* in veterans of Operation Desert Storm. These patients all had a variety of systemic symptoms and few objective signs of disease. It is unclear whether these patients improved because of SSG therapy or whether it was the result of the natural history of their infections.

The side effects and toxicity of SSG are listed in Table 1. The cardiac toxicity associated with earlier trivalent preparations is not seen with the current pentavalent preparations. However, sudden cardiac death, which is presumed to be caused by a dysrhythmia associated with a prolonged QTc interval, has been documented in one Kenyan patient receiving 30 mg per kg per day. Therefore, we monitor our patients with a weekly electrocardiogram. T wave flattening and nonspecific ST segment changes are commonly seen but are not cause for discontinuing therapy. Therapy should be discontinued, or at least interrupted, if the QTc is prolonged to greater than 0.5 second.

TABLE 1. **Side Effects and Toxicity of Sodium Stibogluconate (Pentostam)**

Symptoms
Headache, somnolence, fatigue
Anorexia, nausea, vomiting, abdominal pain
Large joint arthralgias, joint stiffness, myalgias
Signs
Abdominal tenderness
Special Tests
Increased AST/ALT
Increased serum lipase and amylase
T wave flattening, nonspecific ST segment changes on ECG
Prolonged QTc interval on ECG
Anemia
Thrombocytopenia
Granulocytopenia

Abbreviations: AST = aspartate aminotransferase; ALT = alanine aminotransferase; ECG = electrocardiogram.

SSG will cause up to 10-fold elevations in serum liver enzymes in a majority of patients. These reversible abnormalities usually occur in the second to third week of therapy but can occur at any time. Enzyme levels tend to return toward normal before therapy is completed.

Recently, we have identified elevations in pancreatic enzymes in virtually all patients treated with SSG. Serum lipase tends to be much higher than serum amylase. This complication of SSG therapy had previously been noted in case reports but appears to be a very common if not universal complication of SSG therapy. Like hepatic enzymes, elevations in pancreatic enzymes are reversible. Most elevations tend to return to normal by the third or fourth week without interrupting therapy. About half of treated patients are asymptomatic, with only chemical pancreatitis, but the remainder have varying degrees of anorexia, nausea, vomiting, and mid-epigastric pain. For most patients, therapy can be continued despite mild symptoms, but in some individuals, we have elected to discontinue or interrupt therapy because of prominent symptoms. Gastrointestinal symptoms resolve and pancreatic enzymes quickly decrease when the drug is stopped. In many of these patients, therapy can be continued after symptoms resolve and enzyme elevations decrease significantly. The decision to temporarily hold or discontinue therapy is primarily a clinical one, but dramatic increases in pancreatic enzymes (>15-fold elevation above the upper limits of normal for lipase and >5-fold elevation for amylase) or the presence of significant nausea, vomiting, or abdominal pain should lead to at least a brief drug holiday.

Rare reports of drug-induced anemia, granulocytopenia, and thrombocytopenia have been published. We have seen two cases of significant thrombocytopenia (<50,000 platelets per cubic milliliter) during treatment for visceralizing *L. tropica.* We suggest performing a complete blood count once weekly.

Patients frequently report moderately severe frontal headaches, which often start a few hours after an infusion. Progressive fatigue also appears after the first week. Patients may experience significant somnolence beginning early in the therapy and lasting until 2 to 3 weeks after therapy. Patients have slept 12 to 18 hours daily. From the perspective of the patient, one of the most troublesome side effects of SSG is the gradual onset of severe, symmetric, large joint arthralgias occurring on day 7 to day 10 of treatment. True joint inflammation is not seen except for occasional effusions. Shoulders and hips are most affected with elbows and knees also involved. Some patients are so symptomatic, they cannot walk without assistance and cannot abduct their arms more than 10–20 degrees from the midline without considerable pain. Toward the end of therapy and during the first week or so post therapy, patients may also complain of small joint (fingers and wrists) stiffness. Plain x-ray studies and technetium bone scans are normal. Fortunately, the arthralgias are reversible and usually resolve within 2 to 3 weeks following the last dose. Although nonsteroidal anti-inflammatory medications are routinely given for relief of pain, their efficacy is questionable.

We obtain a complete blood count, liver enzymes, serum lipase, serum amylase, and electrocardiogram (ECG) before treatment on all patients. These tests are repeated at weekly intervals and at the end of therapy. If the patient develops any gastrointestinal symptoms, then more frequent monitoring of serum lipase and amylase is indicated.

In determining the patient's response to therapy, one must define objective end points. The most common definitions are clinical cure, which is defined as the resolution of signs and symptoms of disease, and parasitologic cure, which is defined as the eradication of parasites. It is unlikely that any drug therapy results in frequent parasitologic cure. For simple cutaneous ulcers with an inflammatory response, signs of inflammation often start to resolve with the first few doses. In many cases, the ulcer will be completely epithelialized by the end of a 20 day treatment period. Patients should routinely be seen 6 weeks following their last dose. A clinical cure must have at least a 75% reduction in the surface area of the ulcer. If an area remains ulcerated or there is an active nonhealing border, then attempts at isolating parasites by smear or culture are indicated. The ulcer site will be hyperpigmented and pruritic for many weeks. Pigmentation slowly returns to normal over many months.

Response to therapy in visceral syndromes is complicated by the lack of uniformity in the definition of VL. A staging system is needed to accurately stratify patients according to their parasite burden, immune response, nutritional status, infecting species of parasite, and intercurrent diseases. However, patients with the pentad of chronic fever, cachexia, marked hepatosplenomegaly, hypergammaglobulinemia, and pancytopenia that defines kala-azar do respond to SSG. Fever usually resolves in 3 to 4 days, the patient begins to feel better, and the organomegaly and pancytopenia also usually improve by the end of therapy. Patients' responses to therapy in milder forms of disease is less well documented.

There are two established second-line drugs for the treatment of leishmaniasis—amphotericin B (Fungizone), for visceral disease and pentamidine (Pentam 300), for visceral and cutaneous disease. Both are used primarily in antimony-resistant cases of VL, diffuse cutaneous leishmaniasis, and mucocutaneous leishmaniasis. However, they are both parenteral agents with their own significant side effect profiles. Other agents with demonstrated activity against some forms of leishmaniasis are allopurinol (Zyloprim), ketoconazole (Nizoral), and dapsone. These agents are attractive because they are orally administered and have little or tolerable side effect profiles. Allopurinol has been reported to be effective in VL in India and CL in Colombia, but other reports from Kenya and the Americas fail to support this promise. Allopurinol should not be used outside of an endemic area where efficacy has been demonstrated or in a controlled trial. Ketoconazole was shown to be effective in CL caused by *L. panamensis* when used at 600 mg per day for 28 days. Dapsone was shown to cure 82% of 60 patients with Indian CL treated with 100 mg every 12 hours for 6 weeks.

Several drugs are currently being tested worldwide and appear promising. Topical preparations containing paromomycin,* an aminoglycoside analogue, have proved effective in both Old and New World CL. Parenteral paromomycin (aminosidine),* used as a single agent and in combination with antimonials, has likewise been shown to be effective in Indian and Kenyan VL. Liposomal formulations of amphotericin B,† by selectively targeting amphotericin B to the host macrophage, theoretically will allow higher doses of the drug with less toxicity. Animal models and limited human data support this concept, and larger clinical trials are under way.

The clinical resolution of all forms of leishmaniasis is dependent on stimulating an appropriate cell-mediated immune response. Therefore, immunomodulating therapies such as interferon-gamma, a potent stimulator of macrophages, in combination with SSG have been used with some success in drug resistant kala-azar in Brazil. Bacille Calmette-Guérin (BCG) vaccine plus killed promastigotes of *L. mexicana* have also been shown to be as effective as drug therapy in curing CL caused by *L. braziliensis* in Venezuela. Indeed, the effectiveness of SSG, the primary agent for treating leishmaniasis, has been shown in animal models to be dependent on the presence of an intact immune system and the activation of CD4(+) lymphocytes to be effective. In the absence of host CD4(+) lymphocytes, SSG is ineffective.

Leishmaniasis is one of the exotic tropical infections that most North American clinicians only hear about in a medical school lecture. All forms of leishmaniasis are uncommonly seen in the United States, and so few clinicians develop the experience in clini-

*Not available in the United States.

†Investigational drug in the United States.

cal recognition, diagnosis, and treatment that are needed to optimally manage these patients. It is strongly recommended that any clinician who suspects one of the many clinical syndromes associated with leishmaniasis seek consultation with individuals experienced in this field.

LEPROSY
(Hansen's Disease)

method of
ROBERT R. JACOBSON, M.D., PH.D.
Gillis W. Long Hansen's Disease Center
Carville, Louisiana

Leprosy is a chronic infectious disease caused by *Mycobacterium leprae.* Because of the mobility of modern peoples, it is seen at least occasionally in nearly every country but is common only in a number of Third World countries in tropical or semitropical areas. The World Health Organization (WHO) estimates that there are now about 3.1 million cases worldwide. The United States has over 6000 cases, and the number of new cases detected annually in the United States is currently about 200. These new cases are found mostly among aliens, particularly those from Southeast Asia, Mexico, and the Philippines. Cases among native-born Americans currently constitute about 15% of the total.

Leprosy is best viewed as a spectrum of diseases, and the problems encountered in treatment vary considerably from one end of the spectrum to the other. Although most people (>95%) are not susceptible, those who are initially develop indeterminate leprosy. This condition may be self-healing, but it is always treated if it is diagnosed. When self-healing or treatment does not intervene, the disease eventually progresses to one of the advanced forms. Those with the most intact immune response, relatively speaking, keep the infection localized, manifesting tuberculoid leprosy, which is referred to as polar tuberculoid disease, or TT in the Ridley-Jopling classification. On the other hand, in those with a poor immune response to the infection, it becomes generalized, exhibiting polar lepromatous (LL) disease. Between the two extremes is a broad borderline (dimorphous) region where the disease may be classified borderline tuberculoid (BT), midborderline (BB), or borderline lepromatous (BL).

Classification is based on findings of physical examination, skin biopsy, and skin scrapings. Bacteria in biopsy sections and skin scrapings are evaluated to determine the morphologic index (MI), and their numbers are quantified using the bacterial index (BI). The MI is the percentage that appear fully intact and presumably viable, and is usually 5% or less in patients with newly diagnosed disease. The BI is a semilogarithmic scale ranging from 0, which indicates none found in 100 oil immersion fields, to 6+ (>1000 per oil immersion field). Indeterminate, TT, and most BT cases have a BI of 0 on skin scrapings at diagnosis, and only rare bacilli are detected on biopsy specimens. The BI on biopsy specimens and skin scrapings in BB, BL, and LL cases usually ranges from 2 to 3+, 3 to 5+, and 4 to 6+, respectively. The WHO classifies those with a BI of 0 on skin scrapings at all sites at the time of diagnosis (indeterminate, TT, and most BT) as paucibacillary (PB) and those with a BI of 1+ or above at any site as multibacillary (MB).

GENERAL TREATMENT

Antileprosy Drugs

At present, five drugs are widely used to treat leprosy: dapsone, clofazimine (Lamprene), rifampin (Rifadin),* and ethionamide (Trecator-SC),* and prothionamide.† Dapsone and clofazimine are weakly bactericidal against *M. leprae,* rifampin has potent bactericidal activity, and ethionamide and prothionamide are intermediate in activity. Ofloxacin, minocycline, and clarithromycin are also highly bactericidal against *M. leprae* but somewhat less than rifampin. Various combinations of these agents with the standard antileprosy drugs are now being evaluated in clinical trials for the treatment of this disease. Technically, only dapsone and clofazimine are approved by the U.S. Food and Drug Administration for the treatment of leprosy. However, rifampin is routinely used, both in the United States and throughout the world, for this purpose. Ethionamide and prothionamide are used to a lesser extent because there is no question as to the effectiveness of any of these drugs against *M. leprae.* Because *M. leprae* cannot be grown in artificial media, drug sensitivity testing is usually performed using the mouse footpad technique. Sensitivity to dapsone, rifampin, clofazimine, and ethionamide is routinely tested at the Gillis W. Long Hansen's Disease Center (GWLHDC).

Dapsone

Dapsone is available as 25- and 100-mg tablets, and the usual dosage is 100 mg daily for adults and 0.9 to 1.4 mg per kg for children. Because of its safety, low cost, and effectiveness, it is included in all treatment regimens, unless the patient is infected with fully dapsone-resistant bacilli or has had a serious adverse reaction to dapsone. Its most common side effect is anemia; however, except for occasional patients, the glucose-6-phosphate dehydrogenase (G6PD) deficiency is rarely severe enough to require discontinuation of the drug. Gastrointestinal complaints also rarely necessitate its discontinuation with the dosages used to treat leprosy. The most serious complications of dapsone therapy are agranulocytosis and the so-called dapsone syndrome (infectious mononucleosis-like syndrome). Fortunately, both are relatively rare. Other reported side effects are uncommon and include various rashes, peripheral neuropathies, hepatitis, cholestatic jaundice, hypoalbuminemia, the nephrotic syndrome, psychoses, and fever. Methemoglobinemia occurs but is rarely a problem in patients receiving the standard antileprosy dosage of dapsone. It may be severe, however,

*Not FDA approved for this indication.
†Not available in the United States.

if an overdose is taken and may require the use of supportive measures and the use of methylene blue.

Rifampin

Rifampin (Rifadin, Rimactane), is available as 150- and 300-mg capsules, and the usual adult dose is 600 mg daily, although it has been given intermittently at intervals of up to 1 month in doses ranging from 600 to 1500 mg.* Strains of *M. leprae* that are resistant to it can appear in as few as 3 to 4 years if it is given as monotherapy. Rifampin should, therefore, be used only in combination drug regimens. Its major side effect has been hepatotoxicity, but this has usually not been a major problem, except in patients receiving the drug in combination with ethionamide, which is also hepatotoxic. In general, it is discontinued only if the alanine aminotransferase (ALT) level rises to 2½ times the upper limit of normal. Thrombocytopenia is occasionally observed in patients taking the drug, but the platelet count rarely drops below 100,000 per mm^3, which would require discontinuation of rifampin therapy. The drug may also produce a reddish-orange to reddish-brown discoloration of urine, feces, saliva, sputum, sweat, and tears. Other reported side effects include an influenza-like syndrome, fatigue, drowsiness, headaches, dizziness, pruritus, various rashes, eosinophilia, and rarely, kidney damage. The drug also affects the metabolism of other medications. Those treating patients with leprosy should be aware that it decreases plasma levels of corticosteroids and reduces the effectiveness of oral contraceptives. Thus, higher dosages of corticosteroids may be necessary for the management of leprous reactions, and alternate methods of contraception may be required.

Clofazimine

Clofazimine (Lamprene), is available as 50- and 100-mg capsules. It is extremely useful in the management of leprosy. It not only treats the disease, but in higher dosages also suppresses reactive episodes. The usual adult dosage for treatment is 50 to 100 mg daily, but dosages as high as 300 mg daily may be used to suppress reactive episodes.* Although clofazimine-resistant *M. leprae* are rarely reported with monotherapy, clofazimine should be given only in combination with other antileprosy drugs.

The most obvious side effect is pigmentation of the skin. The severity of this complication is proportional to the dosage being given and the extent of infiltration of the skin by the disease process. The color can range from a reddish hue to purplish-black. It tends to be blotchy, being most pronounced in areas where skin lesions are present. The pigmentation occurs in essentially all patients with active disease, and its absence may indicate that the patient is not taking the drug. As the disease process clears from the skin, the coloration slowly diminishes and nearly disappears in patients with inactive disease. Discontinuation of the drug also leads to clearance of most of the pigmentation within 6 to 12 months, although traces of it may remain for several years.

The most serious toxic effect is on the gastrointestinal tract. Patients receiving 50 to 100 mg daily may have mild crampy or burning midabdominal to epigastric pain, which is sometimes associated with mild nausea or diarrhea, or both. Patients receiving greater than 100 mg daily for control of reactions, however, may develop severe crampy abdominal pain, diarrhea, nausea, vomiting, and weight loss, which with continued treatment may progress to symptoms suggesting partial or complete bowel obstruction. This problem usually clears rapidly if the drug is temporarily discontinued.

Other side effects include an anticholinergic activity, resulting in diminished sweating and tearing, and phototoxicity reactions, which are uncommon.

Ethionamide (Trecator-SC)

Ethionamide is available only as 250-mg tablets, and the usual dosage is 250 to 500 mg daily. Resistance to the drug develops rapidly if it is given as monotherapy, and it should, therefore, be used only as part of a combination drug regimen. Its most common side effects are various gastrointestinal complaints, such as metallic taste in the mouth, nausea, vomiting, abdominal pain, diarrhea, anorexia, and hepatotoxicity. These problems usually clear rapidly if the drug is discontinued. Giving ethionamide and rifampin together increases the chance of hepatotoxicity considerably, and patients taking this combination must be followed closely for evidence of such toxicity, particularly during the first year of therapy. The drug is normally discontinued if the ALT level rises to 2½ times the upper limit of normal. Other side effects include postural hypotension, mental depression, drowsiness, peripheral neuropathies, and asthenia.

TREATMENT REGIMENS

Standard United States Treatment Regimens

Patients with newly diagnosed disease in the United States are generally infected with fully sulfone-sensitive *M. leprae* (no growth in mice treated with 0.0001% dietary dapsone). Bacilli from occasional patients show varying degrees of primary resistance to dapsone in mouse footpad testing. Clinically, however, those treated with dapsone monotherapy in the past have shown a normal initial response to standard dosages, unless their bacilli were fully resistant to dapsone (there was growth in mice treated with 0.01% dietary dapsone). Such resistance is rare in new cases. Thus, dapsone probably remains useful in essentially all newly diagnosed disease. Standard therapy for paucibacillary adult patients seen at the GWLHDC is 100 mg of dapsone plus 600 mg of rifampin daily for 6 months, followed by dap-

*Exceeds dosage recommended by the manufacturer.

sone monotherapy for 3 years in indeterminate and TT cases and for 5 years in BT patients. Multibacillary patients receive dapsone plus rifampin for 3 years, followed by dapsone monotherapy for 10 years after inactivity (no bacilli found on skin scrapings or biopsy specimens) in BB patients, and indefinitely for BL and LL cases as a prophylactic measure to prevent reactivation. Because the BI generally falls at the rate of 0.5 to 1 per year, it usually requires 2 to 6 years for BB patients, and 5 to 10 years for BL and LL patients, to reach an inactive status.

There is a remote possibility that a new case may be infected with fully dapsone-resistant *M. leprae* and thus would, in effect, be receiving rifampin monotherapy. Performing mouse footpad studies on bacilli from all new cases, as conducted at the GWLHDC would avoid this risk, but this test is expensive and is not available to most of those treating this disease. Fortunately, this danger has so far proved more theoretical than real.

Patients infected with dapsone-resistant *M. leprae* are usually those who were treated for prolonged periods of time with dapsone monotherapy and who ultimately relapsed with fully dapsone resistant bacilli. Rarely, as noted earlier, patients with newly diagnosed disease may also be infected with dapsone-resistant bacilli. The treatment of choice for adults infected with dapsone-resistant bacilli is 50 to 100 mg of clofazimine daily, given for the same time intervals as dapsone for newly diagnosed disease, plus 600 mg of rifampin daily for the first 6 months in paucibacillary cases and for the first 3 years in multibacillary cases. If the patient does not accept the pigmentation produced by clofazimine, 600 mg of rifampin with 250 mg of ethionamide daily may be substituted, but he or she should be warned of the considerable risk of hepatotoxicity with this combination. Both rifampin and ethionamide are then continued for the same interval as the dapsone in individuals with newly diagnosed leprosy.

Although they are still investigational, consideration should be given to using the short-term WHO-like regimens now under trial in the United States rather than the standard therapy just described. They are effective whether or not the patient is infected with dapsone-resistant bacilli and only 2 years of treatment is required even for lepromatous cases as opposed to committing the patient to lifelong therapy. These regimens are described in the section that follows.

World Health Organization Treatment Regimens

Leprosy control has long been a major problem in many Third World countries because of the size of the problem and the often limited resources available to manage it. Most control programs were formerly based on long-term dapsone monotherapy, which was often taken irregularly, leading to the emergence of secondary dapsone resistance and the later primary dapsone resistance. Because of this problem, in 1981, the WHO organized a study group to make recommendations for the "chemotherapy of leprosy for control programs" (WHO Technical Report Series No. 675-1982). They proposed two regimens. Adult patients with paucibacillary disease would be given 100 mg of dapsone daily, unsupervised, and 600 mg of rifampin, once monthly, supervised, both for a total of 6 months; therapy is then discontinued. Multibacillary cases should receive 100 mg of dapsone daily, plus 50 mg of clofazimine daily, unsupervised, plus 600 mg of rifampin with 300 mg of clofazimine once monthly, supervised. Therapy is continued for at least 2 years, and preferably to a BI of 0, and then discontinued.

The WHO regimens clearly have certain advantages. Cost is relatively low and compliance should improve because of the shorter length of treatment. These regimens have thus far proved highly successful even when given for only 2 years in MB cases, and follow-up for up to 9 years has generally demonstrated a relapse rate of only about 1% over all. They are, therefore, now accepted as standard antileprosy therapy nearly everywhere. Although data are limited, as noted they appear to be effective even if the patient is infected with dapsone-resistant *M. leprae*. Furthermore, bacilli from patients who have relapsed have remained fully sensitive to the drugs used in mouse footpad studies performed thus far.

These regimens are now under investigation in the United States. However, the PB regimen is given for 1 year rather than 6 months, and the MB regimen is being used both as described and in a second version, with the rifampin given daily rather than monthly. Therapy of MB patients is also limited to only 2 years.

FOLLOW-UP OF PATIENTS ON TREATMENT

Patients are followed at varying intervals, depending on the severity of their disease, complications, and the drugs they are receiving. For example, patients receiving only dapsone with no complications may need to be seen only every 3 months, whereas those with severe reactions may require weekly or more frequent follow-up. It is generally useful to see the patient relatively frequently at first because complications are most likely to occur during the first 1 to 2 years. Later, as the danger of reaction diminishes and the patient has gained an understanding of his or her disease, the follow-up visits can be less frequent. Isolation of patients is not necessary because therapy rapidly renders them noninfectious, thus providing chemical isolation, and close contacts have already generally received maximal exposure prior to the time the diagnosis was established. Pregnancy has little effect on the disease process, except for increasing the likelihood for reaction.

Clinically, there is a gradual clearance of skin lesions. Within 3 to 4 months of the start of appropriate therapy, the MI should fall to 0, but as noted earlier, the BI on skin scrapings or biopsy specimens falls slowly. Routine follow-up laboratory studies would include a complete blood count, urinalysis, creatinine determination, and liver function tests. Drug toxicity, however, is uncommon after the first year of treatment, and serious toxicity may be exhibited clinically before it is detected in the laboratory. If possible, skin scrapings should be performed from several of the most active sites at least yearly. Routine follow-up biopsies are not performed unless skin scrapings are unavailable.

REACTIONS

About half the patients with leprosy have reactive episodes of varying degrees of severity during the course of their disease, although they appear to be less common in those treated with the WHO regimens. Some have them before treatment is started, but most occur during therapy, particularly during the first year. The occurrence of a reaction should not be regarded as a side effect of any drug; rather, it is apparently due to destruction of bacilli by whatever cause and the immune response to bacterial antigens released. Chemotherapy should be continued in spite of reactive episodes, and the episodes themselves should be suppressed as needed by other therapy.

Reactions can be broadly divided into two main categories: erythema nodosum leprosum (ENL, or type 2 reactions), occurring almost exclusively in BL and LL patients, and reversal (type 1) reactions, occurring throughout the leprosy spectrum, except for the lepromatous (LL) pole. A third type of reaction known as the Lucio phenomenon may only be an extreme variation of ENL, and it occurs in patients with diffuse lepromatous leprosy who are from Mexico and some other areas. It is occasionally seen in the United States and is managed with corticosteroids. A fourth type, known as downgrading reaction, is also uncommon. It represents inflammation associated with progression of the disease process in untreated patients and is usually managed by the initiation of antileprosy therapy.

Erythema Nodosum Leprosum

ENL usually is exhibited with fever and painful erythematous nodules, but peripheral neuritis, orchitis, lymphadenitis, iridocyclitis, nephritis, periostitis, and arthralgias may also occur. Mild episodes may require no therapy, or symptomatic measures, such as aspirin administration, may suffice. Several drugs are useful for the management of severe episodes.

Corticosteroids are effective in all patients and should always be used if an acute neuritis is present to prevent permanent nerve injury. Usually, 60 mg of prednisone daily is sufficient. When the initial episode has been completely controlled for several days, an attempt may be made to taper the drug dosage, over a period of 2 to 4 weeks. The reaction often recurs, however, and the dosage has to be increased again. If, as often happens, the process becomes chronic and recurs whenever attempts to reduce or discontinue the prednisone are made, prolonged therapy may be needed. In these patients, I try to taper the prednisone to alternate-day therapy. When an alternate-day schedule is reached, the dosage is reduced still more slowly until either the drug is eliminated or the lowest possible maintenance level is reached. However, because steroid-associated side effects are often a problem, other forms of therapy should be considered in chronic cases.

Thalidomide, which is investigational in the United States, is effective in most patients. The initial regimen is 100 mg four times daily, and the reaction is usually controlled within 48 to 72 hours. The dosage is then tapered over 2 weeks to a maintenance level, usually 100 mg daily. Regular attempts are made to discontinue it, but patients may need to continue taking thalidomide for months to years before it can be discontinued without recurrence of the reaction. Side effects are few, drowsiness being the most common. It cannot, of course, be given to fertile females because of its well-known teratogenicity. Information regarding procurement of the drug may be obtained from the GWLHDC in Carville, LA.

Clofazimine is also effective for the control of ENL. A dose of 100 mg two or three times daily usually is necessary, and the reaction should come under control during a period ranging from a few weeks to a few months, depending on its severity. Normally, reaction control is maintained with prednisone in these patients, and the dosage of prednisone is gradually diminished as the clofazimine begins to take effect. Because gastrointestinal symptoms may develop with high doses, the dosage should be reduced to 100 mg daily within a year, if possible. Pigmentation from the clofazimine is usually marked in these patients, and they should be fully cognizant of this problem before therapy is started.

Reversal Reactions

Clinically, these reactions usually are evidenced by fever, edema, and erythema of pre-existing lesions, which may progress to ulceration. Neuritis and adenopathy may also occur. If there is danger of a motor or sensory deficit or ulceration, high dosages of corticosteroids must always be used, such as 60 to 120 mg of prednisone daily. The reaction usually is controlled within 24 to 48 hours, and only a short course of therapy may be necessary if the patient has minimally active disease and no neuritis. Those with neuritis may require prolonged treatment (3 to 6 months), however, if neural damage is to be reversed. Patients with prolonged reaction may sometimes be managed with alternate-day steroids as noted for ENL, and some investigators have found clofazimine to be useful in these patients.

Other Complications

Neuritis may occur independently of any reactive episode. Immediate treatment with high dosages of corticosteroids is necessary to avoid permanent injury and recover lost function insofar as possible.

Iridocyclitis is a medical emergency and is probably best managed by an ophthalmologist. Atropine drops and corticosteroid drops must be started at once if permanent damage is to be avoided. Tear substitutes are used in patients with lagophthalmos or decreased lacrimation, or both.

Orchitis may occur with or independently of a reactive episode. It usually responds quickly to corticosteroids, but sterility may result.

Injuries are common in all patients with leprosy who have significant degrees of sensory or motor loss, or both. The patient must be taught how to avoid them by frequent inspections of involved skin and the use of protective measures, such as wearing gloves or special footwear. When an injury does occur in an insensitive area, it must be protected from further damage during healing.

CONTROL MEASURES

These include appropriate patient education and management, evaluation of contacts, and prophylaxis. Patient education is vital if treatment is to be successful. Prolonged compliance with any regimen is unlikely unless the patient fully understands the necessity for it. The family's cooperation is also important.

Evaluation of contacts in countries of low endemicity, such as the United States, is limited to the household. They should be checked for evidence of the disease annually for at least 5 years and know to seek immediate attention if suspicious changes occur at any time.

Three years of dapsone prophylaxis has been recommended by the Centers for Disease Control for household contacts younger than age 25 years of multibacillary patients. Compliance is often a serious problem, and it is uncertain whether such prophylaxis prevents or only delays the onset of the disease in those contacts destined to undergo development of multibacillary disease. The WHO does not recommend dapsone prophylaxis.

FUTURE PROSPECTS

Research emphasis has been placed on new drug development and improved use of existing drugs, cultivation of *M. leprae* in artificial media, antileprosy vaccine development, serodiagnostic and other tests for the early detection and follow-up of this disease, and the clarification of the immunopathology involved. For example, regimens as short as 1 month are under trial using a rifampin-ofloxacin combination. This duration of therapy may be too short, but it is possible that treatment can be shortened to intervals even less than those currently recommended by WHO, using one or more of the newer bactericidal drugs in combination with rifampin and dapsone and/or clofazimine.

MALARIA

method of
LAURENCE SLUTSKER, M.D., M.P.H., and
JANE ZUCKER, M.D., M.Sc.
National Center for Infectious Diseases
Centers for Disease Control and Prevention
Atlanta, Georgia

Malaria is one of the most prevalent infectious diseases in the world, with an estimated 120 million cases and over 1 million deaths occurring annually worldwide. Although most of the morbidity attributed to malaria occurs in young children and pregnant women living in endemic areas, travelers to malarious areas are also highly susceptible to this disease. *Plasmodium falciparum,* potentially the most lethal malaria species, has become increasingly resistant to many of the drugs used for prevention and treatment. Preventing severe or fatal malaria infections requires prompt evaluation for malaria as a possible source of fever in persons who have traveled to or resided in a malarious area. Treatment with appropriate antimalarial drugs can result in high cure rates when therapy is initiated before development of complications.

ETIOLOGY

Four species of *Plasmodium* cause malaria in humans: *P. falciparum, P. vivax, P. ovale,* and *P. malariae.* Infection occurs through the bite of an infected female anopheline mosquito. As the mosquito feeds, it releases malaria sporozoites from its salivary glands that enter the blood and rapidly gain entry to the human host's liver cells, where they multiply and release large numbers of merozoites into the bloodstream. Merozoites invade red blood cells (RBCs), where they mature to schizonts that contain a new generation of merozoites. The infected erythrocytes then rupture and release merozoites to repeat the cycle by invading other RBCs. The release of merozoites from erythrocytes initiates the paroxysms of fever and chills typical of malaria. In infections due to *P. falciparum* and *P. malariae,* no parasites remain in the liver after release; in infection with *P. vivax* and *P. ovale* some of the intrahepatic parasites undergo immediate development, while others may remain dormant in the liver (hypnozoites). Subsets of hypnozoites may mature after a dormant period lasting several months or even years.

Although it is unusual, malaria may also be transmitted by infected RBCs through blood transfusion, needle sharing, laboratory accidents, or transplacental infection.

EPIDEMIOLOGY

Distribution of the four *Plasmodium* species varies worldwide. Malaria occurs primarily in tropical and some subtropical regions of the world. *P. falciparum* occurs in almost all areas with malaria transmission and is responsible for the majority of illness in sub-Saharan Africa, Haiti, Dominican Republic, the Amazon region of South America, and parts of Asia and Oceania. *P. vivax* is the most common species in the Indian subcontinent, although *P. falciparum* malaria also occurs there. The intensity of *P. falciparum* transmission in sub-Saharan Africa is much greater than in other areas, resulting in over 80% of the estimated deaths worldwide. The epidemiology of malaria has changed in recent years with the spread of drug-resistant *P. falciparum,* the movement of nonimmune populations into disease-endemic areas (for example, refugees in Africa and Southeast Asia and prospectors in the Amazon basin), the increasing importance of urban malaria, and changes in short-term travel patterns.

The development of resistance to antimalarial drugs has complicated malaria therapy and chemoprophylaxis. The capacity of *P. falciparum* to develop resistance to a wide range of antimalarials has been particularly remarkable in the extension of resistance to the 4-aminoquinoline, chloroquine. First reported in Thailand and Colombia in 1961, chloroquine resistant *P. falciparum* has spread throughout the malarious areas of the world, leaving only Central America, Haiti, the Dominican Republic, Central America west of the Panama Canal, and some areas of the Middle East unaffected (Fig. 1). Resistance to the combination of pyrimethamine and sulfadoxine (Fansidar) is widely prevalent in some areas of Southeast Asia and the Amazon basin. Resistance to mefloquine has been reported from Thailand and Cambodia. In some areas of Southeast Asia, diminished responsiveness of *P. falciparum* to quinine has been reported.

Documented cases of chloroquine-resistant *P. vivax* have been reported from Papua New Guinea and Indonesia. However, because the frequency and geographic extent of chloroquine-resistant *P. vivax* remains unclear, no changes in therapy for *P. vivax* are recommended at present.

The vast majority of persons with malaria in the United States, Europe, and Canada are infected while visiting or residing in Africa, Asia, or Central America. In the United States, approximately 1000 cases of malaria are reported annually to the Centers for Disease Control and Prevention (CDC); half are in non-U.S. citizens, with the other half occurring in returning U.S. travelers. In 1992, 52% of reported cases were due to *P. vivax,* 32% to *P. falciparum,* 4% to *P. malariae,* and 3% to *P. ovale,* with the remainder undetermined. Although travel to Africa represents less than 2% of all travel to areas where *P. falciparum* is endemic, 83% of *P. falciparum* cases among U.S. citizens were acquired there. This disparity reflects the increased risk of exposure of travelers to Africa, who may generally stay overnight in rural areas with relatively high transmission. In contrast, travelers to other regions with *P. falciparum,* such as Central America or Southeast Asia, often stay in urban and resort areas, where transmission rates are much lower.

Death from malaria in the United States occurs at a rate of between 1% and 4% of all reported *P. falciparum* infections, and it is almost always due to infection with this species. The most important risk factors for death due to *P. falciparum* have been delay in seeking medical care, misdiagnosis, failure to take antimalarial prophylaxis, and older age. Most malaria fatalities in the United States, Canada, and Europe are preventable if appropriate diagnosis and therapy are initiated promptly.

Persons who have had malaria can develop short-lasting partial immunity that is insufficient to protect against subsequent infection with *Plasmodium* spp. but may increase the tolerance for low-density infections and limit the density of parasitemia. With repeated infections, the level of acquired immunity increases. With partial immunity the incubation period may be prolonged, and depending on the degree of immunity, the infection may be asymptomatic. In endemic areas, newborns are relatively protected by maternal antibody but become increasingly susceptible to malaria in later infancy and early childhood. Semi-immune adults who leave an endemic area lose their immunity after several years.

CLINICAL MANIFESTATIONS

The incubation period (interval from inoculation to the onset of malarial symptoms) varies, depending on the species involved, the immune status of the host, and whether or not antimalarial drugs for chemoprophylaxis have been taken previously. With *P. falciparum, P. ovale,* and *P. vivax,* the average incubation period is generally 10 to 14 days and rarely longer than 30 days. The incubation period for *P. malariae* may be as long as 30 to 45 days.

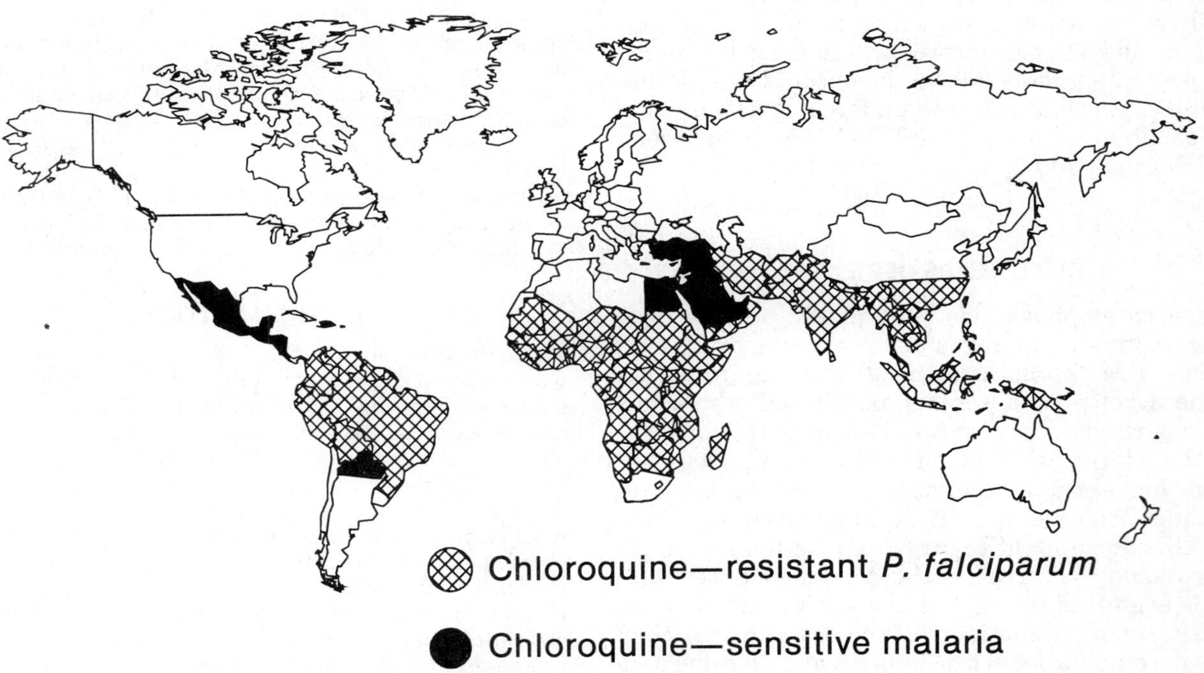

Figure 1. Distribution of malaria and chloroquine-resistant *P. falciparum,* 1993.

In synchronous infections, when a majority of parasites are undergoing erythrocytic development at the same time, fever paroxysms recur at approximately 48-hour intervals, except for *P. malariae,* which has a 72-hour erythrocytic cycle. The periodicity of the paroxysms is variable however, and most patients exhibit a more persistent, less periodic illness.

Typical symptoms include fever, chills, myalgias and arthralgias, headache, vomiting, diarrhea, and other nonspecific signs. Fever is the only consistent initial sign; temperatures higher than 41° C (105° F) are not unusual. Other findings may include an enlarged liver or spleen, anemia, and thrombocytopenia. In more severe disease, pulmonary or renal dysfunction and changes in mental status may be present. In infants, the initial signs may be less dramatic and can include poor appetite, restlessness, and lethargy.

Infections with *P. falciparum* may produce severe illness and death if not promptly diagnosed and treated. Recognized risk factors that predispose an individual to severe and complicated *P. falciparum* malaria include high-density parasitemia, pregnancy, age (either very young or elderly), and lack of immunity to malaria. A particularly grave complication of *P. falciparum* malaria is involvement of the central nervous system. Clinically, cerebral malaria may present as disorientation, stupor, seizures, psychosis, or coma with decerebrate posturing. Generalized seizures are frequently the initial manifestation of cerebral malaria, especially in children.

DIAGNOSIS

Malaria should be considered in any febrile patient with a history of travel to or residence in a malarious area, even when the patient gives a history of using chemoprophylaxis. A detailed travel history should be obtained to ascertain the patient's potential exposure to drug-resistant *P. falciparum.* Depending on the history of travel, other infections, and other illnesses, the differential diagnosis may include a variety of infectious agents. Infectious diseases co-indigenous with malaria include (but are not limited to) bacterial pneumonia, typhoid fever, viral hemorrhagic fevers, and meningococcal infection.

Infection with *Plasmodium* spp. is confirmed by finding the parasites on examination of the peripheral blood smear. Both thick and thin blood smears should be prepared on any patient suspected of having malaria. Initial blood smears may be negative on a patient who ultimately develops patent parasitemia. Therefore, a diagnosis of malaria cannot be dismissed on the basis of a single negative smear. Blood smears should be obtained when the diagnosis is considered and repeated every 6 to 12 hours until the diagnosis is confirmed or disproved. If parasitemia cannot be documented after 72 hours, the diagnosis of malaria can be considered unlikely. Blood smears may be collected at any time during the illness.

Non-immune persons may develop symptoms of malaria even with very low-density parasitemias; therefore, the examination of thick blood smears is required for maximal sensitivity. Thick blood smear examination is estimated to be 10 to 50 times more sensitive than thin blood smears alone. Thin blood smears permit assessment of the morphology of erythrocytes and parasites for accurate determination of infecting species. The optimal stain for thick and thin malaria smears is Giemsa; best results are obtained by using a 3% Giemsa solution (pH 7.2) for 30 to 45 minutes. Wright-Giemsa stain is an acceptable alternative; however, Wright stain alone will not reliably stain *Plasmodium* parasites.

In addition to species identification, the density of parasitemia should be determined because it is prognostic for severe or fatal *P. falciparum* infection. Parasite density can be estimated quickly from examination of the thin blood smear by counting the number of parasitized RBCs in a field of the smear where the red cells are evenly spread and assuming between 200 to 250 RBCs per oil immersion field and estimating the percentage of RBCs infected. A more accurate count can be obtained from a thick smear by counting the number of asexual forms per 300 white blood cells (WBCs) and multiplying by the WBC count to estimate the number of parasites per cubic millimeter of blood.

Standard laboratory tests do not confirm or exclude the diagnosis of malaria. The WBC count may be normal or decreased; similarly, the WBC differential is usually normal or has shifted toward the mononuclear series. Anemia is common. Thrombocytopenia is frequently seen in *P. falciparum* and *P. vivax* malaria.

TREATMENT

The following factors must be considered in choosing therapy for malaria: infecting species of *Plasmodium;* parasite density; presence of neurologic, renal, hematologic, or metabolic complications; geographic origin of infection that may suggest particular patterns of drug resistance; and the patient's ability to take oral medications. Of primary importance among medical complications is altered mental status, because cerebral complications can occur with any peripheral parasite density. Other potential complications include hypoglycemia, pulmonary edema, renal dysfunction, thrombocytopenia, severe anemia, and dehydration.

Because the risk of death and complications from *P. falciparum* increases with the density of infection and higher density infections require more aggressive therapy, different severity categories based on parasite density have been defined. *P. falciparum* infections with density below 1% and no complications are considered low density infections, 1 to 5% moderate, 5% to 10% severe, and >10% very severe infections. *P. vivax, P. ovale,* and *P. malariae* rarely cause infections with parasite densities greater than 1% of RBCs infected; therefore, infections due to these species may be treated as low-density infections. Appropriate therapy is best approached by a consideration of categories based on clinical and laboratory features (Table 1).

Uncomplicated *P. falciparum* Acquired in Areas Without Chloroquine Resistance, and *P. vivax, P. ovale,* and *P. malariae* Infections. Oral chloroquine is the drug of choice for treatment of *P. vivax, P. ovale, P. malariae,* and uncomplicated *P. falciparum* infections acquired in areas without chloroquine resistance. For adults, chloroquine is given at a dose of 600 mg (base) initially, followed in 6 to 8 hours with 300 mg (base), then 300 mg (base) daily for 2 days for a total dose of 1500 mg (base) (see Table 1 for pediatric dosages). Although usually well tolerated, chloroquine can cause gastrointestinal upset, pruritus, headaches, blurred vision, and dizziness. These side effects are generally mild and resolve after therapy is completed.

TABLE 1. **Treatment of Malaria**

Drug Susceptibility by Area of Acquisition, Species, Illness Severity, and Parasite Density	Drug of Choice	Adult Dosage	Pediatric Dosage
Areas with Chloroquine Resistance			
P. falciparum, uncomplicated, parasite density low (< 1%)	Quinine sulfate*	650 mg (salt) q 8 h orally for 3–7 days	10 mg/kg/salt q 8 h orally for 3–7 days
	PLUS		
	Tetracycline	250 mg qid orally for 7 days	5 mg/kg qid orally for 7 days†
	ALTERNATIVES		
	Quinine sulfate	As above	As above
	PLUS		
	Fansidar	3 tablets orally, single dose	< 1 year: 1/4 tablet single dose 1–3 years: 1/2 tablet 4–6 years: 1 tablet 9–14 years: 2 tablets > 14 years: 3 tablets
	OR		
	Mefloquine‡	15 mg/kg salt orally, single dose, up to a maximum of 1250 mg	15 mg/kg salt orally, single dose
	OR		
P. falciparum, uncomplicated, parasite density low (< 1%)	Halofantrine§	6 tablets (250 mg salt each) orally, given as 2 tablets 6 h apart for 3 doses; repeat the dose in 7 days	8 mg/kg salt orally given q 6 h for three doses; repeat the dose in 7 days
P. falciparum, uncomplicated, parasite density moderate (1 to 5%)	Quinine* PLUS tetracycline†	As above	As above
	OR ALTERNATIVE		
	Quinine* PLUS Fansidar	As above	As above
P. falciparum, complicated or parasite density high (> 5%)	Quinidine gluconate‖	10 mg (salt)/kg IV loading dose over 1–2 hours, then constant infusion of 0.02 mg/kg/minute; keep quinidine levels between 3–7 mg/L until density < 1%; then as above for moderate parasite density for a total of 3–7 days quinidine/quinine	Same
P. falciparum, parasite density very high (> 10%) or altered mental status at any parasite density	Exchange transfusion and Quinidine gluconate‖	See text As above for high density	Same Same
Areas without Chloroquine Resistance			
P. falciparum, uncomplicated, parasite density low or moderate (< 5%)	Chloroquine phosphate	600 mg (base) orally, then 300 mg (base) in 6 h, then 300 mg (base) daily for 2 days (total of 1500 mg base)	10 mg (base)/kg orally, then 5 mg (base)/kg in 6 h, then 5 mg (base)/kg daily for 2 days (total of 25 mg base/kg)
P. falciparum, complicated or high density (> 5%)	Quinidine gluconate‖ and, if indicated, exchange transfusion	As above As above	As above As above
P. vivax, P. ovale	Chloroquine phosphate	As above	As above
	Primaquine phosphate¶	15 mg (base) orally daily for 14 days	0.3 mg (base)/kg orally daily for 14 days
P. malariae	Chloroquine phosphate	As above	As above

*Quinine treatment should be given for 3 days with a second drug. *P. falciparum* infections acquired in Thailand should be treated with 7 days of quinine and tetracycline.

†The benefits of using tetracycline must be weighed against the known risks in children under 8 years of age.

‡Mefloquine at treatment doses is associated with an increased incidence of neuropsychiatric side effects that appear to be dose dependent. See text for contraindications.

§Halofantrine is licensed in the United States but is not yet available commercially. Persons should receive a second dose 7 days after the initial treatment to prevent recrudescence.

‖Patients receiving intravenous quinidine require cardiac monitoring.

¶Primaquine may cause hemolytic anemia in patients with G6PD deficiency. Primaquine should not be administered during pregnancy.

In order to decrease the likelihood of relapse, patients with either *P. vivax* or *P. ovale* infections require therapy with primaquine in addition to chloroquine. Primaquine is administered at a dose of 15 mg (base) once daily for 14 days for adults. Some *P. vivax* infections (especially those acquired in Oceania) frequently relapse after primaquine therapy. If this occurs, the standard course of therapy (15 mg per day for 14 days) should be repeated.

Because of the risk of hemolysis, all patients requiring primaquine should be tested for glucose-6-phosphate dehydrogenase (G6PD) deficiency prior to therapy. G6PD deficiency has been categorized into groups based on the level of enzyme activity in red cells. In adult patients with mild deficiencies (10 to 60% residual enzyme activity), primaquine may be better tolerated in a once-weekly dose of 45 mg (base) for 8 weeks; more severely deficient patients (<10% residual enzyme activity) and pregnant women should not be given primaquine.

Uncomplicated *P. falciparum* Acquired in Areas of Chloroquine Resistance in Patients Able to Tolerate Oral Therapy. Patients with low-density parasitemias (<1% of RBCs infected) should be treated with 650 mg quinine sulfate (salt) for adults given orally three times daily for 3 days, in addition to 250 mg tetracycline four times daily for 7 days. The use of tetracycline as an adjunct drug permits a shorter period of quinine dosing, thus decreasing the potential for quinine-associated side effects, which include tinnitus, nausea, blurred vision, and headache. These symptoms, collectively known as cinchonism, are typically transient and resolve after the drug is discontinued. Because of the reduced efficacy of quinine for the treatment of *P. falciparum* acquired in Thailand, quinine should be given for 7 consecutive days along with tetracycline. Pyrimethamine-sulfadoxine (Fansidar) as a single oral dose may be substituted for tetracycline; however, because of Fansidar resistance, this antimalarial should not be used for *P. falciparum* infections acquired in Southeast Asia or the Amazon basin.

Intermediate parasite densities (1 to 5%) should be treated with a combination of quinine sulfate and tetracycline, as described earlier. Fluid balance, blood glucose concentration, mental status, and renal function should be monitored closely in patients with parasite densities greater than 1%. Therapeutic efficacy should be monitored by repeating blood smears every 6 to 12 hours; a rapid decrease in parasite density should occur within 24 to 48 hours after therapy is initiated. Blood smears should be repeated until asexual parasites are undetectable and symptoms have abated.

High-density (>5%) *P. falciparum* or Infections in Patients Unable to Tolerate Oral Therapy. Patients with parasite densities higher than 5% are at significant risk of life-threatening complications and death. Because so few malaria-endemic areas have chloroquine-sensitive *P. falciparum* and because of the efficacy and wide availability in the United States of intravenous quinidine gluconate, high-density *P. falciparum* infections or those occurring in patients unable to tolerate oral therapy should be treated with quinidine regardless of area of acquisition.

In the United States, after a base line electrocardiogram (ECG) has been obtained, parenteral quinidine gluconate should be initiated using a loading dosage of 10 mg (salt) per kg given over 1 to 2 hours, followed by a constant infusion of 0.02 mg (salt) per kg per minute. Quinidine administration should be temporarily slowed or discontinued if the QT interval exceeds 0.6 seconds, the QRS complex widens beyond 50% of baseline, or significant hypotension develops. Quinidine blood levels of 3 to 7 mg per liter should be maintained until the parasite density falls below 1% of RBCs infected. At this time, if the patient is able to tolerate oral medications, quinine sulfate may be given orally for a total of 3 days of combined quinidine/quinine therapy (or 7 days for *P. falciparum* infections acquired in southeast Asia). A second drug should then be used, as described earlier.

Complicated or Very High-density (>10%) *P. falciparum* Acquired in Areas of Chloroquine Resistance. Patients with very high parasite densities (>10%) and patients with neurologic complications at any parasite density should be considered candidates for RBC exchange transfusion in addition to parenteral malaria drug therapy. Exchange transfusion is capable of rapidly removing infected RBCs and stabilizing vascular volume and perfusion, and can be life-saving. The exchange should continue until parasite density falls below 1% of RBCs infected (generally ½ to 1 full volume exchange). Drug therapy should be instituted promptly and intravenous infusion of quinidine continued during exchange transfusion.

Other Antimalarial Drugs

Mefloquine (Lariam). Mefloquine is an effective schizonticidal drug for the four species of human *Plasmodium* and can be used for treatment of multidrug–resistant *P. falciparum.* However, mefloquine at treatment dosage has been associated with a relatively high rate (approximately 1%) of severe adverse neuropsychiatric effects, including vertigo, convulsions, and psychosis; consequently, quinine plus tetracycline is the preferred treatment for uncomplicated *P. falciparum* infections acquired in areas with chloroquine resistance. The adult dosage of mefloquine for therapy for uncomplicated *P. falciparum* is 15 mg per kg orally as a single dose, up to a maximum of 1250 mg. Resistance of *P. falciparum* to mefloquine has been reported in southeast Asia.

Quinidine Sulfate. Oral quinidine sulfate* may be substituted for oral quinine sulfate. It is given at an adult dosage of 300 mg salt (or 10 mg salt per kg) three times daily for 3 to 7 days depending on where the infection was acquired, in addition to tetracycline, as described previously.

Hydroxychloroquine Sulfate (Plaquenil). This drug may be substituted at an adult dose of 400 mg (equivalent to 300 mg base) for 500 mg of chloroquine phosphate.

Halofantrine (Halfan). Halofantrine was licensed by the FDA in 1992, but at the time of this writing, it was not commercially available in the United States. Although effective against multidrug–resistant *P. falciparum,* halofantrine is absorbed at unpredictable rates, which may lead to low bioavailability; consequently, it should not be used for patients with

*Not FDA approved for this indication.

severe infections. In addition, recent evidence suggests that halofantrine therapy may be associated with a dose-related lengthening of the PR and QT interval in adult patients with uncomplicated *P. falciparum* malaria. Although the implications of these findings remain uncertain, until additional data are available, halofantrine use should most likely be avoided in patients with underlying cardiac conduction abnormalities.

Artemisinin Derivatives. These compounds are derived from the Chinese herb qinghaosu (*Artemisia annua*) and have been shown to have potent antimalarial properties. Recent trials with these drugs have demonstrated more rapid parasite clearance times than those achieved with chloroquine, quinine, or mefloquine. These findings suggest that the artemisinin* derivatives may ultimately prove to be superior to quinine for the initial treatment of severe malaria. Although further research is needed before recommendations for the use of these compounds for malaria treatment can be made, they promise to be a valuable addition to the drugs available for treatment of *P. falciparum* infections.

COMPLICATIONS

In *P. falciparum* infections, RBCs infected with schizonts develop altered surface characteristics, which may result in their adherence to the endothelial linings of post-capillary venules in deep organs, including the brain, lungs, liver, gut, and bone marrow. This sequestration may protect parasites from splenic destruction and may contribute to organ dysfunction mediated through a variety of potential mechanisms. These mechanisms may include obstruction of local blood flow, resulting in tissue hypoxia or the production of cytokines (such as tumor necrosis factor and interleukin-6 [IL-6]), or both. In malaria due to the other three species of *Plasmodium,* sequestration does not occur and organ failure is rare. High plasma concentrations of cytokines, such as tumor necrosis factor and IL-6, are found in severe malaria. Excessive production of these cytokines may contribute to the development of severe disease.

The likelihood of severe and complicated illness due to *P. falciparum* infection is generally related to parasite density on presentation; individuals with more than 5% of RBCs infected may frequently suffer complications involving multiple organ systems. Complications may be present at the time of presentation, or they may occur during the course of treatment. Most complications seen with severe malaria, such as hyperpyrexia or vomiting, are treated as for other medical illnesses; a few complications, however, deserve special comment.

Cerebral Malaria. Cerebral malaria is characterized by an alteration in mental status, ranging from disorientation to profound coma. Seizures are common, and may be focal or generalized. Coma may be accompanied by a variety of abnormal physical findings, including abnormalities of conjugate gaze, limb posturing, muscular hypertonicity, and opisthotonos. The prognosis in cerebral malaria is poor; case fatality rates range from 10 to 40%. The mechanisms responsible for cerebral dysfunction remain unknown. Intracranial pressure may be elevated, but there is no evidence to suggest that therapy directed against raised intracranial pressure (such as treatment with corticosteroids) is beneficial. In fact, treatment with dexamethasone has been demonstrated to prolong coma and increase the incidence of complications such as pulmonary edema and gastrointestinal bleeding. All the features of cerebral malaria may be found in hypoglycemia. The blood glucose level must be measured at presentation and monitored carefully thereafter. Principles of care for the unconscious patient must be carefully administered. Fluid status should be monitored closely to avoid dehydration or pulmonary edema.

Hypoglycemia. Hypoglycemia may be found in any patient with severe malaria, and it is especially common in children. Hypoglycemia may also develop in patients receiving quinidine or quinine, as a result of drug-induced hyperinsulinemia. Hypoglycemia must be recognized rapidly and treated with intravenous 50% dextrose to restore and maintain normoglycemia.

Pulmonary Disease. Pulmonary edema may occur secondary to fluid overload; respiratory distress syndrome can occur with normal volume status and must be distinguished from volume-overload pulmonary edema by measurement of central venous and pulmonary wedge pressures. Respiratory distress syndrome may occur after several days of therapy. Both conditions are characterized by tachypnea and hypoxemia. Intubation and mechanical ventilation may be necessary.

Renal Dysfunction. Early recognition of renal insufficiency may allow for restoration of renal function through judicious use of fluids and diuretics. Renal failure usually results from acute tubular necrosis secondary to hypotension or shock. Once renal failure is established, management is the same for acute tubular necrosis of any cause and may include diuretics, dialysis, and dietary restrictions.

Bleeding Disorders. Spontaneous bleeding may occur infrequently as a result of disseminated intravascular coagulation, most commonly in patients with hyperparasitemia and multiple organ system involvement. Thrombocytopenia is relatively common at all parasite densities. Platelet counts may drop as low as 10,000 to 20,000 per cubic millimeter. Thrombocytopenia is rarely accompanied by clinically significant bleeding and usually resolves after antimalarial treatment is initiated.

Pregnancy. In nonimmune pregnant women, *P. falciparum* infection is associated with an increased risk of adverse outcomes including prematurity, abortion, stillbirth, and maternal death. Chloroquine may be used safely during pregnancy. Quinine or quinidine may be used for treatment of severe malaria

*Not available in the United States.

TABLE 2. **Prophylaxis of Malaria**

Drug of Choice	Adult Dosage	Pediatric Dosage
Areas with Chloroquine-Resistant P. falciparum		
Mefloquine*	250 mg (salt) once weekly beginning 1 week before, during, and 4 weeks after exposure	15 to 19 kg: ¼ tablet / week 20 to 30 kg: ½ tablet / week 31 to 45 kg: ¾ tablet / week On return: continue dosage 4 weeks after exposure
ALTERNATIVES:		
Doxycycline alone	100 mg daily, 1 to 2 days before, during, and for 4 weeks after exposure	> 8 years: 2 mg/kg daily up to adult dose of 100 mg/day
OR		
Chloroquine	As below for areas without chloroquine resistance	As below for areas without chloroquine resistance
PLUS		
Fansidar	Carry a single dose (3 tablets) for self-treatment of febrile illness when medical care is not immediately available	< 1 year: ¼ tablet single dose 1–3 years: ½ tablet 4–8 years: 1 tablet 9–14 years: 2 tablets > 14 years: 3 tablets
Proguanil†	200 mg once/day in combination with weekly chloroquine	Used as for adults < 2 years: 50 mg/day 2–6 years: 100 mg/day 7–10 years: 150 mg/day > 10 years: 200 mg/day
Areas with Chloroquine-Sensitive P. falciparum		
Chloroquine	300 mg (base) once/week, 1 week before, during, and for 4 weeks after exposure	5 mg/kg (base) once/week up to 300 mg base; frequency as for adults
Prevention of Relapses of P. vivax *and* P. ovale		
Primaquine‡	15 mg base once/day for 14 days	0.3 mg/kg base once/day for 14 days

*See text for contraindications for use of mefloquine.
†Proguanil is not available in the United States.
‡Primaquine may cause hemolytic anemia in patients with G6PD deficiency. Primaquine should not be administered during pregnancy.

during pregnancy; there are conflicting reports on whether these drugs may be oxytocic, but the risk of malaria to the mother and fetus far outweighs any concern about their use. Although there is a theoretical concern about induction of hyperbilirubinemia and subsequent kernicterus in the newborn with the use of sulfonamides late in the third trimester, Fansidar has been used safely in pregnancy. Tetracycline and primaquine are not recommended for use during pregnancy. Patients with *P. vivax* or *P. ovale* infections should be given chloroquine prophylaxis for the duration of pregnancy to prevent relapses and can be treated with primaquine after delivery.

PREVENTION

Prevention modalities for travelers to malarious areas include both personal protection measures and chemoprophylaxis. Personal protection includes all measures designed to minimize contact with mosquitoes during evening and nighttime hours such as use of insect repellents, wearing protective clothing, sleeping in screened areas, using insecticide-impregnated bednets, and indoor spraying with pyrethrum-containing insecticides. Mosquito repellents containing *N,N*-diethylmetatoluamide (deet) are most effective, but skin contact with formulations containing high concentrations should be avoided, particularly in children, because of toxicity.

The choice of chemoprophylaxis depends on several factors including the exact travel itinerary, the risk of acquiring malaria in those areas, and whether those areas have chloroquine or multidrug-resistant *P. falciparum* (Table 2). Detailed information on the risk of malaria in various regions of the world can be obtained by calling the CDC Malaria Hotline 1-404-332-4555. In addition, the traveler's age, allergies, and any concurrent medications or medical conditions must be considered in the selection of chemoprophylactic regimens.

For travel to areas of risk where chloroquine-resistant *P. falciparum* exists, the drug of choice is mefloquine (Lariam), 250 mg once weekly, starting 1 week before entering the malarious area, and continuing during exposure and for 4 weeks after leaving the area. Recent studies indicate that weekly administration of mefloquine is significantly more effective than other antimalarial prophylactic regimens (such as the combination of chloroquine and proguanil*) in prevention of malaria in Peace Corps volunteers and European travelers in sub-Saharan Africa. The frequency and types of side effects observed with weekly

*Not available in the United States.

administration of mefloquine did not differ significantly from those seen with other regimens. Mefloquine has rarely been associated with serious adverse reactions at prophylactic dosage. Minor side effects observed at prophylactic dosage, such as gastrointestinal disturbance and dizziness, tend to be transient and self-limited. Mefloquine is contraindicated for use in persons with a known hypersensitivity to mefloquine, and it is not recommended for travelers with a history of epilepsy or psychiatric disorders, children less than 15 kg (30 lbs), and pregnant women. Mefloquine may be used in persons concurrently on beta blockers if they have no underlying cardiac arrhythmia. However, mefloquine is not recommended for persons with cardiac conduction abnormalities. It has not been established that mefloquine is contraindicated for persons involved in tasks requiring fine motor skills (e.g., pilots, drivers, and machine operators).

Travelers to areas with chloroquine-resistant *P. falciparum* in whom mefloquine is contraindicated or poorly tolerated may substitute 100 mg doxycycline (Vibramycin) daily (alone), beginning 1 to 2 days before entering the malarious area, continuing during exposure, and for 4 weeks after leaving the area. Adverse effects include gastrointestinal upset, photosensitivity (usually manifested as an exaggerated sunburn reaction), and an increased frequency of monilial vaginitis. Tetracyclines should not be taken by pregnant women and children younger than 8 years of age.

For travelers to areas where *P. falciparum* has not developed chloroquine resistance, or for those in whom mefloquine or doxycycline is contraindicated or poorly tolerated, chloroquine (300 mg base per week for adults, 5 mg per kg per week for children) beginning 1 week before, during, and for 4 weeks after exposure may be used. Travelers using this regimen should understand that it may be of limited efficacy.

All travelers should be counseled that the use of chemoprophylaxis and personal protection measures may reduce but may not eliminate the risk of malaria. Travelers should be counseled to seek medical evaluation promptly in the event of a febrile illness. For most travelers, adequate medical care is readily available. However, those taking chloroquine prophylaxis who are travelling in remote areas with chloroquine resistance where medical care may not be readily available should be advised to carry a treatment dose of sulfadoxine and pyrimethamine (Fansidar) with them. If febrile illness develops, and professional medical care cannot be obtained within 24 hours, self-treatment with Fansidar should be administered. Self-treatment with Fansidar for febrile illness is a temporary measure and does not obviate the need to seek medical care as soon as possible. Chloroquine prophylaxis should be continued after presumptive self-treatment. The utility of this measure is obviously limited to areas without Fansidar resistance. Persons with known sulfa intolerance should not be given Fansidar.

Chlorguanide (proguanil, Paludrine),* a dihydrofolate reductase inhibitor, has been recommended by some authorities for use in areas where *P. falciparum* has developed chloroquine resistance. Because resistance to proguanil occurs in many malarious areas, its efficacy is unpredictable. Limited data suggest that the combination of weekly chloroquine with daily proguanil is more effective than chloroquine alone in Africa. For travelers unable to take mefloquine or doxycycline, proguanil may be taken at a dose of 200 mg daily (adult dose) in addition to the weekly dose of chloroquine. Proguanil has few side effects (gastrointestinal upset and mouth ulcers are the most common) and can be used safely in pregnancy. At the time of this writing, proguanil is not available commercially in the United States but can be obtained in Canada, Europe, and many African countries.

Pregnant women traveling to malarious areas should be advised about the increased severity of malaria infection in pregnancy and the increased risk of adverse reproductive outcomes. In addition, the prophylactic drugs most effective in areas of chloroquine resistance (mefloquine and doxycycline) are contraindicated in pregnancy. Consequently, pregnant women should be advised to defer travel to malarious areas until after delivery. The indications for prophylaxis for children are identical to those for adults. Pediatric antimalarial dosages must be calculated carefully according to body weight (see Table 2).

*Not available in the United States.

BACTERIAL MENINGITIS

method of
GREGORY C. TOWNSEND, M.D., and
W. MICHAEL SCHELD, M.D.
University of Virginia Health Sciences Center
Charlottesville, Virginia

According to two recently published large studies of the epidemiology and outcome of bacterial meningitis in the United States, the attack rate for this disease is approximately 7 to 10 cases per 100,000 population per year; this suggests an annual incidence of approximately 18,000 to 25,000 cases of bacterial meningitis in the United States. Fortunately, the introduction of *Haemophilus influenzae* polysaccharide capsule-protein conjugate vaccines that are immunogenic in young infants has resulted in a rapid decline in the incidence of meningitis in children in recent years.

Despite significant advances in diagnosis and antimicrobial therapy, however, bacterial meningitis is still accompanied by significant morbidity and mortality rates. In the United States, case fatality rates are approximately 10% overall and approach 30% in the neonatal and elderly adult populations. The incidence of long-term neurologic sequelae, most notably hearing loss and seizures, and in chil-

Supported in part by a grant from the National Institute of Allergy and Infectious Diseases (RO1-AI17904). W. Michael Scheld is an Established Investigator of the American Heart Association.

dren, mental retardation and developmental delays, is 10 to 30% among long-term survivors. Unfortunately, the incidence of adverse outcomes has not decreased significantly over the last 15 years. This factor suggests that current management strategies that rely on the introduction of newer antimicrobial agents alone may not be entirely adequate for minimizing complications. Recent clinical and experimental studies have suggested newer promising adjunctive treatment options.

Meningitis is characterized by abnormally high numbers of white blood cells in the cerebrospinal fluid. Aseptic meningitis is meningitis that occurs in the absence of a readily identifiable bacterial pathogen. The most commonly identified causes of this syndrome are viruses, although a number of entities (including unusual bacteria, fungi, protozoa, neoplasms, and drugs) may be responsible. In the majority of cases, however, no cause is identified, and a benign self-limited course is usually followed. Because of the relative frequency with which bacterial meningitis and its potentially devastating consequences occur, this article focuses on acute bacterial meningitis.

INITIAL MANAGEMENT

The first step in the management of the patient with suspected bacterial meningitis is stabilization, which may include support of blood pressure and ventilatory assistance. Elevation of the patient's head to 30 degrees may help to combat increased intracranial pressure; other measures that may be effective include hyperventilation to maintain arterial carbon dioxide tension at 27 to 30 mmHg and the administration of hyperosmolar agents. Fluid restriction is often employed to prevent or to treat the syndrome of inappropriate antidiuretic hormone secretion.

The mainstays of therapy for bacterial meningitis are specific antimicrobial agents. The choice of antimicrobial therapy depends not only on the antimicrobial activity of an agent against certain pathogens but also on the ability of the drug to penetrate the blood-brain barrier in sufficient concentrations to achieve a bactericidal effect at the site of infection in the central nervous system. In general, animal studies have demonstrated that for optimal results, the drug must achieve mean peak cerebrospinal fluid concentrations at least 10 to 20 times greater than the in vitro minimum bactericidal concentration for a given pathogen early in the disease.

Empiric therapy should be instituted as soon as appropriate cultures have been obtained. If intracranial pressure elevation is suspected and an imaging procedure (e.g., head computed tomography scan) is to be performed to evaluate this possibility, therapy should not be delayed for the completion of radiologic evaluation. Empiric therapy should be based on the pathogens most commonly encountered in the patient's age group (Table 1), with other risk factors taken into account; once Gram's stain or culture results are available, therapy should be amended appropriately.

The pathogens most commonly isolated in cases of meningitis in neonates (<1 month old) are group B streptococci (*Streptococcus agalactiae*), *Escherichia coli,* and *Listeria monocytogenes.* Ampicillin combined with either an aminoglycoside or a third-generation cephalosporin (cefotaxime or ceftizoxime) is recommended as empiric therapy for this age group; ceftriaxone should not be administered during the neonatal period because of risk of kernicterus.

In the older child (3 months to 8 years old), *Haemophilus influenzae* is by far the most common pathogen, followed by *Streptococcus pneumoniae* and *Neisseria meningitidis.* The decline in the incidence of meningitis due to *H. influenzae* associated with the widespread use of the *H. influenzae* conjugate vaccine during infancy, however, is likely to lead to a change in the relative frequencies of infection caused by these organisms. Ampicillin and chloramphenicol have been the standard therapy for many years in this age group, but a third-generation cephalosporin alone is an acceptable alternative; cefuroxime (Zinacet), which is less active against *H. influenzae,* has been associated with a relatively high incidence of residual hearing loss in the treatment of children with bacterial meningitis and is not recommended.

In the young infant (1 to 3 months) all of the previously mentioned pathogens have been isolated in a significant percentage of cases of bacterial meningitis. A combination of ampicillin and a third-generation cephalosporin is recommended for empiric therapy in children in this age group.

S. pneumoniae and *N. meningitidis* are the organisms most commonly identified in cases of bacterial meningitis in older children (>8 years old) and young adults. In these individuals, ampicillin or penicillin alone are often employed because these agents are usually active against these bacteria. However, the increasing proportion of pneumococcal and meningococcal strains that are relatively penicillin resistant favor the use of a third-generation cephalosporin initially.

In addition to *S. pneumoniae,* gram-negative enteric bacteria and *L. monocytogenes* assume a greater role in the elderly patient, necessitating the use of a third-generation cephalosporin with the addition of ampicillin. Penicillin-allergic patients in this age group should receive high doses of trimethoprim-sulfamethoxazole, although experience with this regimen is limited.

Certain underlying or predisposing conditions may be associated with specific pathogens, some of which may be otherwise uncommon causes of bacterial meningitis and may necessitate alterations in antimicrobial therapy. For example, meningitis following open skull fracture or craniotomy, or that is associated with communications between the subarachnoid space (SAS) and the skin, is often caused by *Staphylococcus aureus,* coagulase-negative staphylococci, or aerobic gram-negative bacilli (including *Pseudomonas aeruginosa*). Bacterial meningitis associated with ventriculoperitoneal or ventriculoatrial shunts may also be caused by diphtheroids (e.g., *Propionibacterium acnes*) and enterococci. Empiric therapy for bacterial meningitis in these cases should include vancomycin and an antipseudomonal cephalosporin (e.g., ceftazidime), with the possible addition of an

TABLE 1. **Empiric Antimicrobial Therapy for Bacterial Meningitis Based on Age or Other Predisposing Condition**

Predisposing Condition	Common Pathogens	Suggested Regimen*
Age		
< 1 month	Group B streptococci *Escherichia coli* *Listeria monocytogenes*	Ampicillin + Gentamicin or cephalosporin 3†‡
1 month to 3 months	*Haemophilus influenzae* *Escherichia coli* Group B streptococci *Neisseria meningitidis* *Streptococcus pneumoniae* *Listeria monocytogenes*	Ampicillin + cephalosporin 3†
3 months to 8 years	*Haemophilus influenzae* *Streptococcus pneumoniae* *Neisseria meningitidis*	Ampicillin + chloramphenicol or Cephalosporin 3†
8 years to 60 years	*Streptococcus pneumoniae* *Neisseria meningitidis*	Cephalosporin 3†
> 60 years	*Streptococcus pneumoniae* Gram-negative enteric bacilli *Listeria monocytogenes*	Ampicillin + cephalosporin 3†
Post-craniotomy, open skull fracture, communication between skin and SAS	*Staphylococcus aureus* Coagulase-negative staphylococci Gram-negative enteric bacilli Diphtheroids§ Enterococci§	Vancomycin + ceftazidime‖ ± Rifampin¶

Abbreviations: Cephalosporin 3 = third-generation cephalosporin; SAS = subarachnoid space.

*Clinical efficacy for some regimens has not been evaluated, but is suggested by in vitro or in vivo data, or both. Consider adjunctive therapy with dexamethasone 0.15 mg/kg q 6 h intravenously for 4 days, beginning prior to or concomitant with initial dose of antimicrobial(s), in treatment of bacterial meningitis in children older than 2 months.

†Cefotaxime, ceftizoxime, or ceftriaxone.

‡Ceftriaxone and rifampin may displace bilirubin from serum albumin sufficiently to cause kernicterus, and thus should not be used in the neonatal period.

§Most commonly isolated in shunt-associated infections.

‖Cefoperazone, which also has excellent activity against *Pseudomonas aeruginosa* and other gram-negative bacilli, penetrates poorly across the blood-brain barrier and should not be used in the treatment of bacterial meningitis.

¶Consider adding an aminoglycoside given systemically, particularly if infection with *P. aeruginosa* is suspected. Shunt-associated infections may require shunt removal or intraventricular administration of antibiotics.

aminoglycoside given systemically. Shunt-associated infections may require, in addition to systemic antimicrobial therapy, removal of the shunt or intraventricular antimicrobials; systemic administration of rifampin should also be considered.

SPECIFIC THERAPY

Once an organism is identified by Gram's stain, culture, or rapid bacterial antigen detection assay, antimicrobial therapy should be modified to provide optimal activity against that organism (Table 2). Doses of specific agents for particular age groups are presented in Table 3.

Penicillin G remains the drug of choice for infections due to *S. pneumoniae;* alternatives for the penicillin-allergic patient include a third-generation cephalosporin, chloramphenicol, and vancomycin. Although isolates were formerly uniformly susceptible to penicillin, there have been recent reports in the United States and in other countries of isolation of strains that are penicillin tolerant (in vitro minimum inhibitory concentration [MIC] 0.1 to 1 μg/mL) or penicillin resistant (MIC >1 μg/mL). Because of this factor, it is important to perform susceptibility testing for all strains of pneumococci isolated from CSF specimens. Infections due to penicillin-tolerant strains of *S. pneumoniae* should be treated with a third-generation cephalosporin, and vancomycin (with or without rifampin) should be used to treat infections due to penicillin-resistant strains. In vitro and in vivo data from animal models of meningitis suggest that a third-generation cephalosporin in combination with either vancomycin or ampicillin may be effective in the treatment of infection caused by penicillin-resistant pneumococcal strains.

Infections due to *N. meningitidis* should also be treated with penicillin G. A third-generation cephalosporin or chloramphenicol may be used as an alternative to treat infections in penicillin-allergic patients or to treat those rare infections due to meningococcal strains that are beta-lactamase producers or display intermediate resistance to penicillin G, or both.

Since 25 to 35% of community-acquired strains of *H. influenzae* are now beta-lactamase producers, ampicillin is no longer acceptable as therapy for meningitis caused by this organism, unless the strain is known to be beta-lactamase negative. For treatment of strains that are not known to be beta-lactamase negative, a third-generation cephalosporin should be used and is usually employed in children. Chloramphenicol is an alternative treatment for those who are allergic to beta-lactams. Again, although cefuroxime possesses antimicrobial activity against most strains of *H. influenzae,* this agent has been associ-

TABLE 2. **Recommended Antimicrobial Regimens for Treatment of Bacterial Meningitis Due to Specific Bacteria**

Organism	Recommended Therapy*	Alternatives*
Streptococcus pneumoniae, penicillin-susceptible	Penicillin G	Cephalosporin 3†‡ Chloramphenicol Vancomycin
Streptococcus pneumoniae, penicillin-tolerant (MIC 0.1–1 μg/mL)	Cephalosporin 3†‡	Vancomycin
Streptococcus pneumoniae, penicillin-resistant (MIC > 1 μg/mL)	Vancomycin ± rifampin‡	Vancomycin + cephalosporin 3†‡ Ampicillin + cephalosporin 3†‡
Haemophilus influenzae, beta-lactamase negative	Ampicillin	Cephalosporin 3†‡ Chloramphenicol
Haemophilus influenzae, beta-lactamase positive	Cephalosporin 3†‡	Chloramphenicol
Neisseria meningitidis	Penicillin G	Cephalosporin 3†‡ Chloramphenicol
Enteric gram-negative bacilli	Cephalosporin 3†‡§	Aztreonam§ Extended-spectrum penicillin§‖ Ciprofloxacin§¶
Listeria monocytogenes	Ampicillin**	Trimethoprim-sulfamethoxazole‡ Vancomycin**
Group B streptococci (*S. agalactiae*)	Ampicillin**	Cephalosporin 3†‡** Vancomycin**
Staphylococci,†† methicillin-susceptible	Antistaphylococcal penicillin‡‡	Vancomycin Trimethoprim-sulfamethoxazole‡
Staphylococci,‡‡ methicillin-resistant	Vancomycin ± rifampin‡	Trimethoprim-sulfamethoxazole‡

Abbreviations: MIC = in vitro minimum inhibitory concentration; cephalosporin 3 = third-generation cephalosporin.

*Clinical efficacy for some regimens has not been evaluated, but is suggested by in vitro or in vivo data, or both. Regimens should be based ultimately upon antimicrobial susceptibility patterns for each isolate. Consider adjunctive therapy with dexamethasone 0.15 mg/kg q 6 h intravenously for 4 days, beginning prior to or concomitant with initial dose of antimicrobial(s), in treatment of bacterial meningitis in children ≥ 2 months.

†Cefotaxime, ceftriaxone, ceftizoxime, or ceftazidime. Ceftazidime should be selected if a third-generation cephalosporin is used to treat infections with *Pseudomonas aeruginosa*.

‡Ceftriaxone, rifampin, and trimethoprim-sulfamethoxazole may displace bilirubin from serum albumin sufficiently to cause kernicterus, and thus should not be used in the neonatal period.

§Consider addition of an aminoglycoside if infection with *P. aeruginosa* is known or suspected.

‖Piperacillin, ticarcillin, or mezlocillin.

¶Should not be administered to patients younger than 21 years unless no other alternative exists.

**Consider addition of an aminoglycoside.

††*Staphylococcus aureus* or coagulase-negative staphylococci.

‡‡Nafcillin or oxacillin.

ated with delays in cerebrospinal fluid sterilization and with an increased incidence of long-term neurologic sequelae in the treatment of *H. influenzae* meningitis when compared with a third-generation cephalosporin and, therefore, should not be used.

Infections due to enteric gram-negative bacilli, which may be particularly seen at the extremes of age, may be treated with a third-generation cephalosporin. This class of drugs has been associated with substantially improved mortality rates in the treatment of gram-negative bacillary meningitis since their introduction. If infection with *P. aeruginosa* is known or suspected, an anti-pseudomonal cephalosporin should be employed, and the addition of an aminoglycoside antibiotic administered systemically should be considered. Although little clinical data exist on the use of extended-spectrum penicillins (piperacillin, ticarcillin, and mezlocillin), aztreonam, or ciprofloxacin in the treatment of bacterial meningitis, data from in vitro or in vivo animal studies suggest that these agents may be acceptable as alternatives.

L. monocytogenes meningitis, which is also particularly common at the extremes of age and in patients with defects in cell-mediated immunity, should be treated with ampicillin; again, an aminoglycoside should be considered for synergy. Trimethoprim-sulfamethoxazole or vancomycin may be used as alternative agents.

Ampicillin is also the drug of choice for infections due to group B streptococci (*S. agalactiae*). Alternative agents include a third-generation cephalosporin or vancomycin. The addition of an aminoglycoside should be considered for all of these regimens.

Strains of *S. aureus* and coagulase-negative staphylococci which are methicillin-susceptible may be treated with an anti-staphylococcal penicillin (oxacillin or nafcillin); vancomycin (or possibly trimethoprim-sulfamethoxazole) may be substituted in the penicillin-allergic patient. However, until antimicrobial susceptibility is known, these organisms should be considered to be potentially methicillin resistant, and these infections should be treated with vancomycin; the addition of rifampin should also be considered.

The duration of therapy should be based at least in part on the clinical response but is often empiric. In general, 7 days of treatment are often recommended for meningitis due to *N. meningitidis,* 10 days for infection caused by *H. influenzae,* about 14 days for pneumococcal meningitis or disease caused by *L.*

TABLE 3. **Recommended Dosing Regimens of Antimicrobial Agents for the Treatment of Bacterial Meningitis**

	Individual Doses and Schedule by Age Group*					
	≤ 7 days†		*8 to 30 days*†			
Antimicrobial Agent (Trade Name)	≤ 2 kg‡	> 2 kg‡	≤ 2 kg‡	> 2 kg‡	*Children > 1 month*†	*Adults*
Aminoglycosides						
Amikacin§	7.5 mg	7.5–10 mg	7.5–10 mg	10 mg	5–10 mg	5 mg‖
(Amikin)	q 12 h	q 12 h	q 8 h	q 8 h	q 8 h	q 8 h
Gentamicin§	2.5 mg	2.5 mg	2.5 mg	2.5 mg	2.5 mg	2.5 mg‖
(Garamycin)	q 12 h	q 12 h	q 8 h	q 8 h	q 8 h	q 8 h
Tobramycin§	2 mg	2 mg	2 mg	2 mg	2–2.5 mg	1–1.5 mg‖
(Nebcin)	q 12 h	q 12 h	q 8 h	q 8 h	q 8 h	q 8 h
Penicillins						
Penicillin G	50,000 U	50,000 U	50,000 U	50,000 U	50,000 U	4,000,000 U
	q 12 h	q 8 h	q 8 h	q 6 h	q 4 h	q 4 h
Ampicillin	50 mg	50 mg	50 mg	50 mg	50 mg	2 gm
	q 12 h	q 8 h	q 8 h	q 6 h	q 4 h	q 4 h
AS penicillins						
Nafcillin	50 mg	50 mg	50 mg	50 mg	50 mg	1.5–2 gm
(Unipen)	q 12 h	q 8 h	q 8 h	q 6 h	q 6 h	q 4 h
Oxacillin	50 mg	50 mg	50 mg	50 mg	50 mg	1.5–2 gm
(Bactocill)	q 12 h	q 8 h	q 8 h	q 6 h	q 6 h	q 4 h
E-S penicillins						
Piperacillin¶	—	—	—	—	50–75 mg	3–4 gm
(Pipracil)					q 4 h	q 4 h
Ticarcillin	75 mg	75 mg	75 mg	75 mg	50–75 mg	3–4 gm
(Ticar)	q 12 h	q 8 h	q 8 h	q 6 h	q 4 h	q 4 h
Mezlocillin	75 mg	75 mg	75 mg	75 mg	50–75 mg	3 gm
(Mezlin)	q 12 h	q 8 h	q 8 h	q 6 h	q 4 h	q 4 h
Cephalosporin 3						
Cefotaxime	50 mg	50 mg	50 mg	50 mg	50 mg	2 gm
(Claforan)	q 12 h	q 12 h	q 8 h	q 6–8 h	q 6 h	q 4–6 h
Ceftriaxone**	—	—	—	—	40–50 mg	1–2 gm
(Rocephin)					q 12 h	q 12 h
Ceftizoxime	50 mg	50 mg	50 mg	50 mg	50 mg	3 gm
(Cefizox)	q 12 h	q 12 h	q 8 h	q 8 h	q 6 h	q 6–8 h
Ceftazidime	50 mg	30 mg	30 mg	30 mg	50 mg	2 gm
(Fortaz)	q 12 h	q 8 h	q 8 h	q 8 h	q 6–8 h	q 8 h
Aztreonam	30 mg	30 mg	30 mg	30 mg	30 mg	2 gm
(Azactam)	q 12 h	q 8 h	q 8 h	q 6 h	q 6 h	q 6 h
Chloramphenicol§	25 mg	25 mg	25 mg	25 mg	25 mg	1 gm
	q 24 h	q 24 h	q 24 h	q 12 h	q 6 h	q 6 h
Ciprofloxacin††	—	—	—	—	—	400 mg
(Cipro)						q 12 h
Rifampin**	—	—	—	—	10–20 mg	600 mg
(Rifadin)					q 24 h	q 24 h
TMP/SMX**	—	—	—	—	5 mg‡‡	5 mg‡‡
(Bactrim)					q 6 h	q 6 h
Vancomycin§	10 mg	10 mg	10 mg	10 mg	10–15 mg	500 mg
(Vancocin)	q 12 h	q 12 h	q 8 h	q 8 h	q 6 h	q 6 h

Abbreviations: AS = anti-staphylococcal; E-S = extended-spectrum; cephalosporin 3 = third-generation cephalosporins; TMP/SMX = trimethoprim-sulfamethoxazole.

*All doses given intravenously, based on normal renal and hepatic function.

†All pediatric doses are per kg body weight. Total daily dose should not exceed maximum daily dose for adults.

‡Birth weight.

§Monitoring of serum concentrations is recommended and may require change in dosing.

‖Doses are per kg body weight.

¶Insufficient data exist to recommend doses in the neonatal period.

**May displace bilirubin from serum albumin sufficiently to cause kernicterus and, thus, should not be used in the neonatal period.

††Should not be administered to patients younger than 21 years old unless no other alternative exists.

‡‡Doses are per kg body weight based on trimethoprim component.

monocytogenes or group B streptococci, and 21 days or longer are usually allowed for gram-negative bacillary meningitis.

ADJUNCTIVE THERAPY

As noted earlier, the rates of morbidity and mortality due to bacterial meningitis have not changed substantially over the last 15 years, the period in which the third-generation cephalosporins were introduced. Experimental studies have suggested several reasons for this relative lack of success. Clinical studies and studies of animals with experimental meningitis have demonstrated that the presence of bacteria and bacterial cell products within the SAS elicits an inflammatory response characterized by the presence of leukocytes within the SAS and by elevated cerebrospinal fluid concentrations of numerous host-derived inflammatory mediators such as the cytokines interleukin-1 and tumor necrosis factor, prostaglandins, and platelet-activating factor. The administration of bactericidal antibiotics may exacerbate this process by causing bacterial cell lysis and, thus, the release of bacterial cell surface components such as endotoxin and teichoic acid, which may provoke the release of endogenous mediators of inflammation. Antagonists to some of these mediators have been demonstrated to ameliorate indices of SAS inflammation, such as increases in blood-brain barrier permeability and brain edema. Thus, there has been a great deal of interest in the potential role of adjunctive therapies directed at the inflammatory response itself. Corticosteroids, which have potent anti-inflammatory effects, have been the subjects of several clinical and experimental studies and appear to be promising, at least in the management of bacterial meningitis in children.

Several studies have shown improved outcomes of patients with bacterial meningitis treated with concurrent dexamethasone and antibiotics. Improvements in the incidence of hearing loss and other neurologic sequelae and in mortality (in one trial) have been noted. However, these results have not been consistently noted across all of these studies. Also, it must be noted that most of the patients enrolled have been children and that most of the infections have been due to *H. influenzae;* the results of these studies, therefore, may not be generalizable to the management of meningitis in other age groups or due to other bacteria.

However, the data support the use of adjunctive dexamethasone, at a dose of 0.15 mg per kg intravenously every 6 hours for 4 days, in the treatment of bacterial meningitis in infants and children at least 2 months old. Dexamethasone should also be considered in the treatment of bacterial meningitis in adults in whom organisms are visible on Gram's stain; these individuals may have a large bacterial burden in the SAS and, thus, may be at increased risk for an exaggerated inflammatory response following the administration of bactericidal antibiotics. It is important that the first dose of dexamethasone be given prior to or simultaneously with the first dose of antibiotics, if at all possible, in order to abrogate the inflammatory response in the SAS. Although there were a small number of cases of gastrointestinal hemorrhage associated with the administration of dexamethasone among children in one study, other trials have not corroborated this finding. Dexamethasone use also did not adversely affect the outcome of children with aseptic meningitis in one study and has not resulted in clinically significant reduction in entry of antibiotics into the cerebrospinal fluid.

INFECTIOUS MONONUCLEOSIS

method of
JAZILA AL-ATTAR, M.D., and
DAVID H. SHEPP, M.D.
North Shore University Hospital—Cornell University Medical College
Manhasset, New York

THE CLINICAL SYNDROME

The hallmark of infectious mononucleosis (IM) is an excess of mononuclear leukocytes in the peripheral blood. Included among these cells is an increased number of activated atypical lymphocytes. Clinical features commonly associated with the syndrome are fever, pharyngitis, lymphadenopathy, fatigue, headache, and splenomegaly. The incidence of IM is highest in individuals 15 to 24 years of age. The acute illness usually lasts from 1 to several weeks and severity ranges from extremely mild to incapacitating.

ETIOLOGY

IM is caused by primary infection with Epstein-Barr virus (EBV), a ubiquitous member of the herpesvirus family. More than 95% of older adults have evidence of prior infection. Infection with EBV is common in childhood and usually subclinical. IM occurs most frequently when primary EBV infection is delayed until adolescence or adulthood.

EBV is excreted in oropharyngeal secretions for up to 18 months after the primary infection resolves and intermittently thereafter for life. Transmission occurs largely through intimate contact and exchange of saliva.

DIAGNOSIS

Polyclonal B cell activation during EBV-IM results in hypergammaglobulinemia. Abnormal antibodies reactive with horse, sheep, or ox red blood cells are present in 90% of patients. Detection of such heterophile antibodies forms the basis of common commercial rapid diagnostic tests. Heterophile antibodies are not common in IM-like syndromes due to agents other than EBV. A typical clinical syndrome combined with a positive heterophile test is sufficient to diagnose EBV-IM. However, heterophile antibody production is less common in children under 5 years of age and is occasionally detected in other disorders. In young children, when the typical syndrome is heterophile negative, or when the syndrome is atypical, EBV-specific antibodies should be measured.

Antibodies to EBV viral capsid antigen (VCA) develop early in IM. Both IgM and IgG antibodies to VCA usually are detected at presentation. IgM reverts to negative within 1 to 6 months, whereas IgG to EBV-VCA remains positive for life. Antibodies to the EBV nuclear antigen (EBNA) do not appear until convalescence. As with antibodies to VCA, IgM to EBNA remains positive for only 1 to 6 months, whereas IgG antibodies remain detectable for life. Thus, a typical patient with acute, symptomatic EBV-IM has antibodies to VCA (IgM or IgG, or both) and antibodies to EBNA are absent. A positive VCA IgG, a negative VCA IgM, and a positive EBNA IgG suggests remote infection.

IM must be differentiated from other causes of fever, pharyngitis, and lymphadenopathy, such as streptococcal or adenovirus infection, and from other primary infections that may resemble EBV-IM, including cytomegalovirus, human herpesvirus 6, human immunodeficiency virus, and *Toxoplasma gondii.*

COMPLICATIONS

Most cases of IM are mild and uncomplicated. Severe pharyngitis, fever, and anorexia may combine to produce significant dehydration. Occasionally, upper airway obstruction due to massive enlargement of tonsils and other oropharyngeal lymphoid tissues may occur. Splenic enlargement predisposes the spleen to rupture. The incidence of splenic rupture is highest in the second and third week of illness. Hepatic transaminase elevation is extremely common, but jaundice is uncommon and signs of liver dysfunction are very rare. Other rare complications of EBV-IM include meningoencephalitis, Guillain-Barré syndrome, transverse myelitis, Bell's palsy, optic neuritis, myocarditis, pericarditis, hemolytic anemia, aplastic anemia, and interstitial pneumonia.

Duncan's syndrome is a rare X-linked lacunar immunodeficiency associated with EBV. Affected males develop normally until primary EBV infection occurs. Overwhelming and invariably fatal infection results, often terminating with transformation to an aggressive lymphoma. A similar syndrome occurs in organ transplant recipients, usually after aggressive immunosuppressive therapy including T lymphocyte–depleting antibodies.

Convalescence after IM may be dominated by fatigue, which persists for several weeks to months. Gradual but complete resolution is the rule. There is no convincing evidence linking IM or EBV infection to the chronic fatigue syndrome.

TREATMENT

Treatment of IM is largely supportive. Antipyretics, analgesics, and hydration are the basics of care. When there is evidence of impending obstruction, oropharyngeal lymphoid swelling is rapidly reduced by a short course of intravenous corticosteroids, such as methylprednisolone, 1 mg per kg per day, given in divided doses. Corticosteroids also may be of benefit in the treatment of myocarditis, pericarditis, meningoencephalitis, hemolytic anemia, or marrow aplasia. Throat culture to identify streptococcal pharyngitis is advisable, but antibiotics should not be given unless a concurrent bacterial infection is proven. Ampicillin should be avoided because rash develops following administration in more than 90% of IM patients. To reduce the risk of splenic rupture, patients should avoid heavy exertion or contact sports for 1 to 2 months after onset of illness, or longer if splenomegaly persists. Splenic rupture requires urgent splenectomy or splenorraphy.

Antiviral therapy is not indicated. Acyclovir (Zovirax), does not modify the clinical course of IM. Ganciclovir (Cytovene), zidovudine (Retrovir), and interferons alpha-2b (Intron A), and gamma-1b (Actimmune), are active against EBV in vitro but are potentially toxic and have not been adequately evaluated for treatment of IM or its complications.

MUMPS

method of
RALPH C. GORDON, M.D., M.A.
Michigan State University
Kalamazoo, Michigan

Mumps is clinically recognized as acute parotitis and is caused by a single paramyxovirus, with infection usually occurring in late winter or early spring. Both parotid glands are generally involved in the infection, which may produce with pain and swelling of the salivary glands, fever, and other systemic signs and symptoms. A major resurgence during the last decade in older children, adolescents, and college students was attributed to a failure to adequately immunize a large number of individuals in infancy. This has been followed by return to an relatively low annual baseline of 4000 cases in the United States beginning in 1991, and the incidence appears to be remaining in that range for the present.

DIAGNOSIS

Parotid and submaxillary gland infection with mumps virus is differentiated from bacterial lymphadenitis based on a more diffuse pattern of inflammation and the prominence and erythema of Stensen's and Wharton's ducts in parotoid and submaxillary gland infection, whereas there is a much more discrete outline of the nodes with lymphadenitis. Bacterial parotitis is associated with inflammation over the gland and the ability to express pus from the ducts. The incubation period for mumps is 18 to 21 days, and inapparent infection may occur in 30% of individuals. The diagnosis can be confirmed by viral culture of secretions in the throat or by serologic studies, such as the demonstration of a fourfold increase in antibody titers between acute and chronic specimens. The serum amylase determination can also be a useful adjunctive test. A number of other viruses may infect the salivary glands as well, and the consideration of other causes of symptoms related to the parotid glands, including the ingestion of starch, iodine, and thiazides, and the development of tumors as noted in the literature, should not be omitted.

TREATMENT

The treatment of mumps is supportive because the special hyperimmune serum globulin preparation is no longer available because it was shown to be ineffective. An imperative aspect of the management of mumps is the recognition of a variety of potential complications of the infection.

COMPLICATIONS

Mumps virus has a predilection for glandular and nervous tissue. Approximately 20% of postpubertal men may develop orchitis, yet sterility is rare because testicular involvement is usually unilateral. Oophoritis may occur in women, resulting in severe complaints of pain. Other, more rare complications may include nephritis, pancreatitis, arthritis, thyroiditis, mastitis, transverse myelitis, myocarditis, and deafness. Deafness is usually unilateral and can have a sudden onset. The most common neurologic problem is mumps meningitis, which occurs in about 10% of cases and usually ends with a good outcome.

PREVENTION

The live attenuated mumps vaccine is usually administered as part of the measles, mumps, and rubella combination (MMR) and is effective in inducing antibody formation in over 95% of recipients. Uncommon complications of the vaccine include rashes, itching, and purpura, which are described as mild and self-limited. The vaccine is well tolerated when second doses are given, as is currently the case when the recommendation for routinely giving two doses of MMR, which consists of administration of one in early and one in late childhood or in adolescence is carried out. Mumps vaccine is well tolerated and should be given to all individuals without clinical or laboratory proof of immunity with the exception of pregnant women. The MMR vaccine has caused no problem when given to individuals infected with human immunodeficiency virus.

OTITIS EXTERNA

method of
LAURA W. CHEEVER, M.D.
Johns Hopkins School of Medicine
Baltimore, Maryland

and

MICHAEL P. JOHNSON, M.D., M.P.H.
Johns Hopkins School of Hygiene and Public Health
Baltimore, Maryland

The external auditory canal is a common site of infection. The canal usually contains skin flora, such as *Staphylococcus epidermidis,* diphtheroids, *Propionibacterium acnes,* and *Staphylococcus aureus,* but it is sterile in roughly one-third of individuals. Fungi, such as *Candida albicans* and *Aspergillus niger,* may also be present in one-third of normal hosts. Cerumen, with an acid pH, and hair follicles along the outer third of the canal combine with the normal skin flora to protect against infection. Factors that disrupt this ecology predispose the individual to infection. These factors include swimming, repeated ear cleansing, cotton swabs, and other foreign bodies.

Infection of the skin in the canal may be localized, diffuse, or invasive. These syndromes may be distinguished by the patient's history, physical examination, and in cases of suspected invasive disease (malignant external otitis), radiologic testing. Treatment may be local, systemic, or a combination of these approaches, depending on the severity and chronicity of the otitis externa. These are summarized in Table 1.

Localized otitis externa results from infection of the hair follicles. This is most often due to *Staphylococcus aureus* but may also be caused by group A streptococcus. The predominant clinical complaint is acute pain. Examination may show a localized area of erythema, sometimes with pustules or furuncles. Lymphadenopathy may be an associated clinical finding in severe cases. Treatment is with local and/or systemic antibiotics (depending on the severity of the infection), analgesics, and local heat. Occasionally, incision and drainage are necessary.

Diffuse otitis externa is nonlocalized inflammation of the external canal that is usually related to infection. Commonly associated with swimming and with hot, humid climates, *Pseudomonas aeruginosa* is the most frequent pathogen. *Staphylococcus aureus* is also a common pathogen. Infections of the external canal may also be polymicrobial, and rarely, they are due to fungi. Diffuse otitis externa is sometimes caused by noninfectious dermatologic conditions, such as contact dermatitis (sometimes due to treatment with topical neomycin), seborrheic dermatitis, or psoriasis. Infection of the external canal often follows precipitating dermatitis.

Itching and pain are the prominent symptoms. In severe cases, pain is exacerbated by chewing and movement of the tragus. The canal appears erythematous and edematous, and may contain seropurulent debris in the lumen. Hearing is usually intact, unless there is significant luminal occlusion, leading to conductive hearing loss. The tympanic membrane appears normal. When itching with dry, scaly skin is the predominant clinical picture, dermatitis without infection may be present.

Chronic forms of otitis externa may result from recurrent or incompletely treated disease, untreated underlying dermatologic conditions, or associated chronic draining otitis media. It is important to rule out underlying chronic otitis media with drainage, which leads to chronic irritation and inflammation of the external auditory canal. Unusual causes of otitis externa and otitis media, such as tuberculosis, syphilis, and leprosy, should be considered in the differential diagnosis of refractory cases.

Treatment of mild disease is with local antibiotics and steroids (which are combined in some preparations), and local treatment to cleanse the canal of debris (Burow's solution or 3% hypertonic saline*) and restore the acidic pH (acetic acid). Local débridement to allow maximal effect of topical therapy may be indicated if there is significant debris (e.g., pus, desquamated epithelium, and cerumen). Systemic antibiotics are required to treat severe disease. In cases of otitis externa due to draining otitis media, therapy should be directed at the underlying otitis media.

Invasive otitis externa (also called malignant external otitis) is a potentially life-threatening infection of the external auditory canal that occurs primarily in elderly diabetics. Although it was first described in 1959, the majority of cases have been reported since 1980, due to increased recognition of this clinical en-

*Neither agent is approved by the FDA for this indication.

TABLE 1. **Treatment of Otitis Media**

Otitis Externa	Clinical Manifestations	Likely Pathogens	Treatment
Localized	Acute pain Furuncle or pustule	*Staphylococcus aureus,* Group A streptococcus	*Local* polymyxin, neomycin, hydrocortisone (Cortisporin)—4 drops, four times daily incision and drainage occasionally necessary *Systemic* Dicloxacillin (Cloxacin)—500 mg orally, four times daily Amoxicillin/clavulanate (Augmentin)—500 mg orally, three times daily† Cefuroxime axetil (Ceftin)—250–500 mg orally, twice daily† Ciprofloxacin (Cipro)—500 mg orally, twice daily
Diffuse	Pain and itching Diffuse erythema, edema If chronic, luminal debris	*Pseudomonas aeruginosa, Staphylococcus aureus*	*Local* polymyxin, neomycin, hydrocortisone (Cortisporin) Burow's solution—2 tablets in pint of water, irrigate three to four times daily† Acetic acid (VoSol), with hydrocortisone (VoSol HC)—5 drops, four times daily *Systemic* Ciprofloxacin (Cipro)—500 mg orally, twice daily Cefuroxime axetil (Ceftin)—250–500 mg orally, two times daily Cefixime (Suprax)—400 mg once daily† Amoxicillin/clavulanate (Augmentin)—500 mg, three times daily
Invasive (malignant external otitis)	Pain, otorrhea Often in elderly diabetics	*Pseudomonas aeruginosa*	*Systemic* Ceftazidime (Fortaz)—2 grams intravenously, every 8–12 hours Ciprofloxacin (Cipro)—750 mg orally, twice daily Tobramycin*—1–1.5 mg per kg intravenously, every 8 hours Plus ticarcillin (Ticar)—3 grams intravenously, every 4 hours *Surgical* Local débridement Rarely, extensive surgical débridement

*Tobramycin dosage is adjusted through monitoring of serum levels and renal function
†Not FDA approved for this indication

tity and increased incidence related to the expanding population of elderly individuals.

Pseudomonas aeruginosa, which is not part of the normal flora in the external canal, is the pathogen in the overwhelming majority of cases. The specific factors that lead to deep invasion remain unclear, but the decreased polymorphonuclear leukocyte function and microvascular disease of diabetes may predispose the individual to tissue invasion. Early in the course of the disease, there is involvement of the soft tissues surrounding the external auditory canal. As the disease progresses, osteomyelitis of the base of the skull and cranial nerve impingement may develop. The infection rarely spreads to the central nervous system and surrounding blood vessels.

Clinical features include a history of multiple courses of topical or systemic treatment, or both, for diffuse, noninvasive otitis externa. Patients report severe otalgia and purulent otorrhea that have persisted for weeks to months. The pain is often worse at night and wakes the patient from sleep. Patients may report hearing loss, and fever is typically absent. Cranial nerve palsies occur in 20 to 30% of patients. Cranial nerve VII is involved most commonly, but the infection may affect cranial nerves IX, X, XI, and XII if the disease is progressive.

On physical examination, the external canal is usually edematous, and granulation tissue is present. The tympanic membrane may remain uninvolved. Often, there is tenderness at the temporomandibular joint. Laboratory abnormalities are unimpressive, with white blood cell counts of less than 14,000/mm^3. The erythrocyte sedimentation rate has not been systematically studied but is usually elevated. Cultures of the external canal reveal *Pseudomonas aeruginosa* as the pathogen in over 99% of cases, with occasional cases caused by *Aspergillus* and *Staphylococcus aureus.* Biopsy of the granulation tissue should be performed to rule out carcinoma.

Plain films may show bony erosions in advanced disease, but they lack both sensitivity and specificity. Technetium 99 bone scans and gallium scans are both highly sensitive but not specific. At present, computed tomography (CT) and magnetic resonance imaging (MRI) are the two principal imaging studies employed in diagnosis. Both methods delineate the extent of soft tissue and bony involvement.

Prior to the advent of effective anti-pseudomonal antibiotics, the treatment of this disease was primarily surgical and the mortality rate was 30%. Today, a majority of patients are treated with prolonged systemic antibiotics and local débridement of the involved area to drain abscesses and remove sequestered collagen. Radical surgery is rarely indicated.

Antibiotics employed include anti-pseudomonal penicillins with aminoglycosides, anti-pseudomonal cephalosporins, and quinolines. Topical antibiotics used alone are not appropriate. Anti-pseudomonal penicillins plus aminoglycosides have been used since the 1970s, with current cure rates of 86 to 90%. Ticarcillin (Ticar) with tobramycin (Nebcin) for 6 to 8 weeks is commonly used but carries significant risk of nephrotoxicity, ototoxicity, and bleeding complications. Monotherapy with anti-pseudomonal cephalosporins is now accepted therapy. Ceftazidime (Fortaz) has been used, either alone or in combination with aminoglycosides, with a similar cure rate but fewer complications. The quinolines offer an attractive alternative. High blood and tissue levels are achieved with oral administration of many of these agents. In over 100 patients given ciprofloxacin (Cipro), the cure rate was 90%. The quinolines are generally very well tolerated with minimal toxicities and obviate the need for long-term intravascular access.

Outpatient management, with local débridement and oral ciprofloxacin or home intravenous antibiotics for 6 weeks leads to cure rates of greater than 90%. Otorrhea resolves in most patients within 2 weeks of treatment. Cranial nerve palsies may improve with treatment but are not a sensitive indicator of response to therapy. If the ESR is initially elevated, it should fall within 2 weeks of effective therapy.

After discontinuation of antibiotics, 1 year of follow-up is recommended. The role of imaging studies in routine follow-up is unclear. CT scans and MRI scans remain abnormal for many months after clinical cure. Serial nuclear medicine scans may be helpful in evaluating the response to therapy.

Recurrence is reported in approximately 10% of cases, usually within 6 months of terminating antibiotics. Recurrence is indicated by recurrent otalgia and headache, often without otorrhea. Treatment of recurrence should be approached on a case-by-case basis. Some patients have responded to a repeated course of monotherapy with ceftazidime. There are also case reports of refractory cases that have been cured with prolonged oral quinoline therapy. It is at this stage that some patients require more aggressive surgical débridement of infected bone.

PLAGUE

method of
THOMAS BUTLER, M.D.
Texas Tech University
Lubbock, Texas

Plague is an acute bacterial infection of humans and animals caused by *Yersinia pestis.* The disease has a worldwide distribution, with the countries of Brazil, Burma, Madagascar, Peru, Tanzania, Uganda, Vietnam, and Zaire reporting several hundred cases in recent years. In the United States, about 15 cases occur annually in Arizona, California, Colorado, New Mexico, and Utah. The natural reservoirs of the organism are urban and wild rodents (including rats, squirrels, and prairie dogs), and it is transmitted among animals and occasionally to humans by bites of infected fleas. *Y. pestis* has caused devastating pandemics, in which pneumonic human-to-human transmission has occurred in addition to the usual flea-to-human spread. In the United States, a significant proportion of plague cases occurs as a result of hunters handling infected animal tissues, especially that of rabbits.

The most common clinical form of *Y. pestis* infection is an acute lymphadenitis called bubonic plague. Typically, the patient exhibits a sudden onset of fever and chills with headache and prostration. The development of the bubo is heralded by painful swelling in the femoral, inguinal, axillary, or cervical region. The buboes are tender, oval swellings, ranging from about 1 to 10 centimeters in length, which may produce elevation and erythema of the overlying skin. Most patients have a single bubo, which is commonly located in the femoral area, but some patients may have them in multiple sites.

Less common clinical presentations of plague include the septicemic, pneumonic, and meningeal forms. Septicemic plague is a rare variant, in which there is no obvious bubo while bacteria are in the bloodstream. Primary pneumonic plague is an inhalation pneumonia resulting from close contact with a sick cat or from human-to-human transmission by coughing. It presents as cough productive of purulent or bloody sputum and can be highly contagious and rapidly fatal. Meningeal plague is rare and usually occurs a week or more after inadequately treated bubonic plague.

A bacteriologic diagnosis is readily made in most patients by smear and culture of bubo aspirate. For definitive identification, cultures should be mailed in double containers to the Centers for Disease Control and Prevention, Plague Branch, P. O. Box 2087, Fort Collins, CO 80522 (1-303-221-6450). At this same laboratory, a serologic test, the passive hemagglutination test using Fraction I of *Y. pestis,* can be performed on acute and convalescent serum.

TREATMENT

Antibiotics

Untreated plague has an estimated mortality rate of greater than 50% and can evolve into a fulminant course of septic shock. Therefore, the early institution of effective antibiotic therapy is mandatory immediately after appropriate cultures have been taken. In 1948, streptomycin was shown to be the drug of choice for the treatment of plague by reducing the mortality rate to less than 5%. No other drug has been demonstrated to be better or less toxic. Streptomycin should be administered intramuscularly in two divided doses daily, totaling 30 mg per kg of body weight per day for 10 days. Most patients show improvement rapidly and become afebrile in about 3 days. The 10-day course of streptomycin is recommended to prevent relapses because viable bacteria have been isolated from buboes of patients during convalescence. The risk of vestibular damage and hearing loss caused by streptomycin is minimal during a 10-day course. However, it should be used cautiously in pregnancy, in older patients who would have trouble adapting to vestibular damage, and in patients who already have hearing difficulty. In these patients, the course of streptomycin can be reasonably shortened to 3 days after the patient becomes afebrile. Renal injury as a result of streptomycin therapy is rare with the usual clinical dosages, but renal function should be monitored. If the serum creatinine rises significantly, the dose of streptomycin should be reduced. In mild renal failure the recommended dose is 1.5 grams a day and, in advanced renal failure, 0.5 gram every 3 days.

For patients allergic to streptomycin or in whom an oral drug is strongly preferred, tetracycline is a satisfactory alternative to streptomycin. Tetracycline is administered orally in a dose of 2 to 4 grams a day in four divided doses for 10 days. Tetracycline is contraindicated in children younger than 7 years and pregnant women in order to avoid staining of developing teeth. It is also contraindicated in patients with renal failure.

For patients with meningitis, who require a drug that penetrates well into the cerebrospinal fluid, and for patients with profound hypotension, in whom an intramuscular injection may not be well absorbed, chloramphenicol should be administered intravenously, with a loading dose of 25 mg per kg of body weight, followed by 60 mg per kg per day in four divided doses. After clinical improvement, chloramphenicol should be continued orally to complete a total course of 10 days and the dosage may be reduced to 30 mg per kg per day to reduce the magnitude of bone marrow suppression, which is reversible after completion of therapy. The irreversible bone marrow aplasia associated with chloramphenicol is so rare (estimated as 1 in 40,000 patients) that its consideration should not deter the use of chloramphenicol for patients who are seriously ill with plague infection.

Other antimicrobial drugs have been used against plague with varying success. These include sulfonamides, trimethoprim-sulfamethoxazole, kanamycin, and ampicillin. Gentamicin, tobramycin, cephalosporins, and fluoroquinolones show good in vitro activity against *Y. pestis* but have not been tested in human infection.

Antibiotic resistance in human isolates of *Y. pestis* has never been reported, nor has resistance emerged during antibiotic therapy. The three antibiotics streptomycin, tetracycline, and chloramphenicol given alone are clinically very effective, and relapses are exceedingly rare. Therefore, there is no rationale for using more than one antibiotic to treat plague.

Supportive Therapy

Most patients with plague are febrile, with constitutional symptoms including nausea and vomiting. Hypotension and dehydration are common. Therefore, intravenous 0.9% saline solution should be given to most patients for the first few days and until clinical improvement occurs. Patients in shock require additional quantities of fluid and hemodynamic monitoring in an intensive care setting. There is no evidence that corticosteroids are beneficial.

The buboes usually recede without need of local therapy. Occasionally, they enlarge or become fluctuant during the first week of treatment, requiring incision and drainage. The fluid should be cultured to determine the presence of superinfection with other bacteria, but this material is usually sterile.

PREVENTION

All patients who are suspected of having plague must be reported to the Health Department. Patients with uncomplicated bubonic plague who are promptly treated present no health hazards to other persons. Those with cough or other signs of pneumonia, however, must be placed on strict respiratory isolation for at least 48 hours after the start of antibiotic therapy or until the sputum culture is negative. The handling of the bubo aspirate and blood must be performed with gloves and with care to avoid aerosolization of these infected fluids. Laboratory workers who process the cultures should be alerted to exercise precautions; however, standard bacteriologic techniques that safeguard against skin contact with and aerosolization of cultures should be adequate to protect the workers.

A formalin killed vaccine, Plague Vaccine U.S.P. (Cutter Laboratories, Berkeley, CA 94710), is available for travelers to epidemic or hyperendemic areas who must live and work in close contact with rodents. A primary series of two injections is recommended with a 1- to 3-month interval between them. Booster injections are given every 6 months for as long as exposure continues.

The control of plague requires knowledge of the epidemiology of infected rodents, fleas, and the contact of humans with these rodents in any particular area. In the United States, the Plague Branch of the Centers for Disease Control and Prevention in Fort Collins, Colorado, has a field team of entomologists, mammalogists, and epidemiologists to investigate cases. A specific approach to each patient should be chosen and usually consists of insecticide use around homes, trapping of animals, and educating people to avoid contact with certain animals.

PSITTACOSIS
(Ornithosis)

method of
CLARK M. KERR, M.D.
St. Mary of the Plains Hospital
Lubbock, Texas

Psittacosis is a chlamydial infection transmissible to humans usually via inhalation of dried bird excreta, in which the agent can survive for long periods. On rare occasions, albeit frequently causing more severe disease, infection may be transmitted from one human to another. Psittacosis must be considered an occupational hazard of pet shop employees, pigeon fanciers, zoo workers, veterinarians, and others who work with birds. In recent years, outbreaks have occurred in turkey processing plants, and duck farms and processing plants. Serologic testing on employees clearly indicated a strong association between years of employment and exposure to infection.

Three factors have contributed to the striking decline in cases over the past 1 to 2 decades: (1) use of tetracycline-medicated poultry feed, (2) prior medication of imported psittacine birds before entry to the United States, and (3) the growth of the domestic parakeet-breeding industry. The disease is more common in Great Britain, where import regulations are more lenient.

CLINICAL MANIFESTATION

The incubation period may range from 7 to 15 days or longer, with disease occurring suddenly with chills and high fever (38° to 40.5° C [100.4° to 104.9° F]), or the disease may start gradually over a period of 2 to 4 days with a gradual increase of fever and malaise. As with infection with other obligate intracellular bacteria (e.g., brucellosis, typhoid) the pulse rate may be disproportionately slow compared with the temperature elevation. Headache may be severe and is frequently a chief complaint. Malaise, anorexia, myalgias (especially of the back and neck), and arthralgias are common. Horder spots, a pale macular rash, may be confused with the rose spots of typhoid fever.

A persistent, dry, hacking cough frequently productive of small amounts of mucoid sputum is a hallmark feature of the disease. Splenomegaly is noted in 10 to 70% of patients, and when associated with a community-acquired undiagnosed pneumonitis, the diagnosis of psittacosis should be considered.

In the last several years, reports of associated reactive arthritis and psittacosis have been reported. *Chlamydia psittaci* is in the differential diagnosis of culture-negative endocarditis, along with *Mycoplasma pneumoniae* and Q fever. In a recent report, family members presented with icteric hepatitis as the cardinal manifestation of proven *Chlamydia psittaci* infection.

Key diseases in the differential diagnosis include *Mycoplasma pneumoniae, Chlamydia pneumoniae*, (TWAR) *Coxiella burnetii,* (Q fever), and *Francisella tularensis* tularemia. The diagnosis of psittacosis is arrived at primarily by clinical acumen through recognition that presenting features both on history and examination are consistent with the disease coupled with an exposure history. The laboratory is dominantly used for confirmation of diagnosis. Diagnosis may be confirmed by the isolation of *Chlamydia psittaci*. However, isolation is hazardous to laboratory personnel, and this study is available only in specialized laboratories. The diagnosis may also be confirmed by serologic studies, demonstrated by a fourfold rise in complement-fixing antibodies in acute and convalescent serum specimens. However, a single titer of 1:32 in a patient with compatible disease is regarded as presumptive evidence of psittacosis. Detection of *Chlamydia pneumoniae* and *Chlamydia psittaci* in sputum samples by polymerase chain reaction has been reported and may be commercially available for rapid diagnosis in the future.

TREATMENT

Tetracyclines are the most effective antimicrobial agent. Therapy with 2 to 3 grams of tetracycline daily usually results in improvement within 48 to 72 hours, although the response may be slower. Treatment should be continued for a period of 10 days to 2 weeks after defervescence to minimize recurrence. Doxycycline, 100 mg twice daily given orally, has also been used with excellent results. Erythromycin* is the drug of choice in the treatment of pregnant women and children. Rifampin,* 600 mg daily, has been reported to be of value in the treatment of disease unresponsive to tetracycline therapy. However, this is not a use of rifampin listed in the manufacturer's official directive.

PREVENTION

All clinical cases of psittacosis should be reported to public health officials, and any infected avian source should be identified and appropriately treated or quarantined, or both.

The prognosis for treatment of psittacosis is good. The prior case fatality rate of 20 to 40% of the pre-antibiotic era no longer prevails. With appropriate antimicrobial therapy available, the mortality rate is less than 1%.

*Not FDA approved for this indication.

Q FEVER

method of
DARWIN L. PALMER, M.D.
University of New Mexico School of Medicine and Veterans Affairs Medical Center
Albuquerque, New Mexico

A disease of protean manifestations, Q (Query) fever is found worldwide but with marked differences in regional prevalence. Although it is carried by many animals, the primary reservoirs of the rickettsial pathogen *Coxiella burnetii* are sheep, goats, cattle, cats and ticks, in whom it causes minimal illness. The organism is both extremely contagious and causes serious disease in humans, who are infected predominantly by aerosolized particles. Parturient livestock shed large numbers of organisms, which may remain viable in soil for weeks to months despite heat and drying. Sporadic infection (and occasional outbreaks) thus may occur in farmers, herders, veterinarians, abattoir workers, and laboratory workers dealing with sheep or goats or in others in contact with contaminated straw, manure, or dust.

CLINICAL AND LABORATORY FEATURES

After an average incubation period of 20 days, the most common form of Q fever (other than asymptomatic seroconversion in 50%) is an acute, self-limited febrile illness. Although patients suffer from severe headache, malaise, and myalgia, they may feel well between fever bouts. Of patients with acute illness who are sufficiently ill to be hospitalized, one-half have pneumonia, one-third have clinical hepatitis, 20% have skin rash, and 10% have neurologic symptoms. Pneumonia is atypical, with patchy pulmonary infiltrates, occasional round segmental opacities, and a small pleural effusion in 25% but with only modest cough and minimal sputum production. Although the condition is mild, resolution may take from 10 to 70 days. Hepatitis may occur alone or accompany the other clinical presentations and is characterized by mild liver dysfunction, tender hepatomegaly, and rarely, jaundice. Splenomegaly may also be found in 20% and hepatic biopsy may show a characteristic lesion, the so-called doughnut granuloma. The severe headache of Q fever may prompt a lumbar tap, but the cerebrospinal fluid is usually normal. Occasionally, encephalitis and aseptic meningitis may be seen. These forms of acute illness generally resolve without treatment; however, chronic Q fever, exhibited as endocarditis, is a rare but severe and often fatal disease. Prior valvular heart disease or valve replacement is a common antecedent. Endocarditis is slowly progressive from 1 to 20 years after acute infection and generally involves the aortic and less commonly the mitral valves. It is accompanied by fever, purpuric rash, hepatosplenomegaly, clubbing, arterial emboli, anemia, microscopic hematuria, hypergammaglobulinemia, and negative blood cultures.

Diagnosis of Q fever is reliant on a high degree of clinical suspicion in the correct epidemiologic setting and is confirmed by serologic test. *C. burnetii* culture is both risky and not available except in research settings. Commonly employed tests are the indirect fluorescent antibody and the complement fixation tests. The indirect fluorescent antibody test peaks earlier (4 to 8 weeks) than the complement fixation test (12 weeks), but with both, a fourfold rise is diagnostic. Phase variation of *C. burnetii* during illness reflects a gradual shift in carbohydrate surface antigens from phase II (acute infection) to phase I (chronic infection). Antibody titers should decline with recovery from acute disease over weeks to months; both tests may decline gradually over years. A very high phase I indirect fluorescent antibody or complement fixation titer (>1:800 or >1:200, respectively) or a ratio of phase I to II of greater than 1 suggests chronic Q fever endocarditis.

TREATMENT

Although acute Q fever in the patient with either pneumonia, hepatitis, or severe fever may be self-limited, the concern for development of chronic infection makes treatment advisable. Tetracycline (or doxycycline) has been standard for many years; however animal studies demonstrate that the addition of rifampin (Rifadin)* or trimethoprim (Trimpex)* is bactericidal rather than bacteriostatic. Therefore, recommendations are for tetracycline, 500 mg every 6 hours (or doxycycline, 100 mg every 12 hours) alone in acute infection; rifampin, 300 mg every 12 hours, should be added for patients who are immunosuppressed, severely ill, or elderly. Treatment should be continued for 5 days after resolution of fever. Erythromycin,* aminoglycosides, and beta lactams (penicillins, cephalosporins) are not effective against *C. burnetii,* but the quinolines and chloramphenicol have been useful for acute illness. In Q fever endocarditis, tetracycline or doxycycline, in combination with trimethoprim-sulfamethoxazole (Bactrim, Septra)* or rifampin, for 2 years has been successful although some recommend therapy for life. Indirect fluorescent antibody or complement fixation titers should be determined every 6 months during therapy. Even after optimum or prolonged therapy, relapse or clinical progression may occur and valvular surgery may be necessary. If the hemodynamic state permits, surgery should be deferred until treatment is well under way.

*Not FDA approved for this indication.

PREVENTION

Q fever is among the most infectious of human agents. Efforts should be made to prevent infection in abattoirs and research facilities conducting experiments on sheep. These efforts should include maintaining facility sterility, keeping pregnant sheep in isolation, and restricting employment of immunosuppressed or acquired heart-valve diseased individuals. Vaccines are of proven efficacy, but they are not yet licensed or commercially available. Their use in animals is not economically feasible because domestic livestock have no apparent illness. Inactivated vaccines in humans (obtained under investigational new drug protocol) may be helpful in veterinarians and for new employees in slaughter houses or laboratories using sheep.

RABIES

method of
CHARLES E. RUPPRECHT, V.M.D., Ph.D., and
MAKONNEN FEKADU, D.V.M., Ph.D.
Centers for Disease Control and Prevention
Atlanta, Georgia

Rabies is one of the oldest recognized zoonoses. Ancient Egyptian and Mesopotamian writings relate a syndrome akin to rabies that existed thousands of years ago. Later civilizations were not spared; the glory of Greece and the grandeur of Rome also had to contend with the horrible specter of rabies. Today, although many developed countries have successfully controlled domestic animal rabies, the disease remains a major health risk for people in many of the globe's developing countries. Although there is no effective treatment for clinical rabies, early consideration and prophylaxis of rabies exposure almost always completely prevents the development of the disease.

The worldwide magnitude of actual human rabies fatalities is essentially unknown. Annually, approximately 100,000 cases of human rabies may occur worldwide, some 5 to 10 times the number of reported cases. Under-reporting is due in part to inadequate resources for epidemiologic surveillance and laboratory diagnosis, the social stigma attached to persons with rabies, and the lack of any effective medical therapy, resulting in reluctance to seek medical care. In the developed world, the economic and emotional impact of evaluating exposure for rabies prophylaxis, stray animal destruction, quarantine, and domestic animal vaccination exacts a much greater toll than the overt mortality of the disease itself. Only a fraction of all the reported cases of human rabies occur outside the tropic and subtropic regions.

EPIDEMIOLOGY

Some geographic regions, particularly islands, including Antarctica, Australia, New Zealand, Hawaii, and Pacific Oceania, are free of indigenous rabies. Other areas, including the United Kingdom, Scandinavia, Japan, Malaysia, and a few areas of the Americas, have had a history of rabies but have achieved secondary eradication. Aggressive control measures, focused on both domestic animals and wildlife, have successfully eliminated rabies, and strict international importation/quarantine regulations have prevented its return.

Rabies infects a broad range of mammals; all are susceptible, but in greatly varying degrees. Most infected mammalian reservoirs belong to Carnivora or Chiroptera, but rabies may spill over into other mammalian species, such as hooved stock, usually as a dead-end infection. Animals in a specific geographic area are usually infected by a similar strain of virus, as documented by monoclonal antibody and genetic sequencing studies. In the United States, rabies is enzootic regionally among raccoons, skunks, foxes, and bats. Epizootic rabies has also involved raccoons in the northeastern states and coyotes in Texas. Domestic free-ranging dogs are among those animals with the greatest risk for transmission in developing parts of the world, along with wolves, jackals, mongooses, and raccoon dogs. Cats can transmit rabies but do not appear to maintain the disease in lieu of other primary hosts; feline rabies often outnumbers canine rabies cases, especially in areas where canine rabies has been largely controlled via induced herd immunity. Rodents, rabbits, and opossums rarely, if ever, transmit rabies to humans. Knowledge of the cause of rabies in local reservoirs is important in risk assessment for the probability of disease in humans following an animal bite.

With the exception of six human-to-human transmission cases due to corneal transplantation, infected animals are the ultimate sources of all known human rabies cases. From 1980 through 1993, there have been 18 cases of human rabies diagnosed in the United States; at least eight acquired the rabies abroad in canine enzootic rabies areas. There was no definite history of an animal bite in 10 of the 18 recent cases, raising the possibility that the event may have occurred at a time remote from the onset of symptoms and was forgotten or went unrecognized as an exposure.

MOLECULAR VIROLOGY

The etiologic agents of the acute encephalitis termed rabies are bullet-shaped, membrane-bound, single-stranded, negative-sense RNA viruses that belong to the Rhabdoviridae family, genus *Lyssavirus*. Monoclonal antibody and genetic sequence studies have demonstrated significant variation between strains of lyssaviruses. Besides rabies virus, at least three other lyssavirus strains (Mokola, Duvenhage, and European bat virus), all Old World in distribution, are known to cause human disease. It is unclear whether or not different lyssavirus strains produce distinct clinical manifestations. Despite considerable antigenic variation among lyssavirus strains of major public health significance, there appears to be adequate cross-protection resulting from vaccination. Analysis of the molecular structure of the virus has revealed an inner nucleocapsid core of ribonucleoprotein and an outer surface glycoprotein. These exterior glycoprotein spikes are involved in attachment and fusion to nerve cells. This glycoprotein is also the target of virus-neutralizing antibodies and cytotoxic T lymphocytes, but the contributory role of internal proteins to induced immunity cannot be discounted. Putative receptor molecules on nerve and muscle cells appear to be gangliosides, although the acetylcholine receptor is also implicated.

PATHOGENESIS

The virus usually enters the host via contaminated saliva through breaks in the skin caused by a bite or a scratch. Extremely uncommon routes of infection may also include contamination of mucous membranes, aerosols (laboratory accidents and bat cave aerosols), and corneal transplants. Following transdermal inoculation, the virus undergoes a so-called eclipse phase lasting several hours to days, during which time it may replicate in muscle cells at the site of entry. The virus is vulnerable to host immune defenses and neutralization by specific antibodies during this period. Viremia does not occur to any significant extent.

Infection of peripheral nerve tissue at the portal of entry initiates a sequence of events that may inexorably lead to the death of the patient. If clearence does not occur, the virus may bind to specific receptors in the vicinity of peripheral nerves and ascend centripetally by retrograde axoplasmic flow to the ganglia into the central nuclei in the brain. Infection of the parenchyma is progressive, with the virus spreading to most parts of the brain. There appears to be a predilection for the limbic system, the reticular formation, the pontine tegmentum, and the nuclei of the cranial nerves at the floor of the fourth ventricle. Nonspecific microscopic lesions include perivascular infiltrates, neuronophagia, and gliosis. Eosinophilic, intracytoplasmic inclusion bodies (Negri bodies) are identifiable in nerve cells at this stage of infection and are pathognomonic of rabies. Histology may demonstrate spongiform encephalopathy, but there may be little inflammatory response and minimal necrosis. The relative lack of structural neuronal damage in contrast to the profound encephalitic manifestations raises the issue of functional interference with neurotransmission as one pathogenic mechanism.

At the height of cerebral infection, the virus moves to the peripheral nerves and centrifugally invades highly innervated areas such as the cornea, the skin (especially of the head and neck), the salivary glands, and the buccal mucous membranes. There is heavy secretion of the virus into saliva at a time when agitation and aggressive biting behavior are present, increasing the risk of viral transmission.

CLINICAL HUMAN RABIES

The differential diagnosis of any rapidly progressive viral encephalitis should include rabies, especially with a history of animal bite. The disease typically progresses through a nonspecific prodromal stage to encephalopathy and death within 10 to 30 days. The prodromal period of rabies usually follows the bite by 4 to 8 weeks; however, incubation periods of less than 10 days or more than a year are well documented. Bites to the head and neck and to highly innervated areas may result in a shorter incubation period. Local cutaneous symptoms include paresthesia, pain, and itching at the site of the exposure, probably due to viral excitation of the sensory ganglia. Nonspecific symptoms include lassitude, sore throat, anorexia, dysphagia, insomnia, headache, fever, cough, nausea, vomiting, and diarrhea. Patients who developed rabies following corneal transplant from an infected donor also reported retro-ocular pain.

The acute period (furious or agitated rabies) follows the prodromal stage by 2 to 10 days. A generalized increase in neurologic activity is observed that is associated with agitation and aggressive behavior. The most profound and characteristic clinical manifestations of human rabies are hydrophobia and aerophobia, exaggerated respiratory protective reflexes that result in violent but painless contractions of the diaphragm and inspiratory accessory muscles triggered by attempts to swallow, the sight or sound of water, or air currents. Other cranial nerve manifestations include choking, drooling, and diplopia. Along with aerophobia and hydrophobia, there may be central nervous system excitation with anxiety, confusion, hallucinations, disorientation, photophobia, ataxia, and seizures. Autonomic excitation may result in labile hypertension, hyperventilation, priapism, panic attacks, palpitations, hypothermia, and hyperthermia.

A paralytic phase (dumb rabies) may follow the agitated phase, or the patient may progress directly to the paralytic phase from the prodromal stage. There is ascending symmetrical or asymmetrical paralysis leading to respiratory arrest and the need for mechanical ventilatory support. Hypothalamic and hypophyseal dysfunction may contribute to wasting, and cardiomyopathy has been described. Ultimately, rabies culminates in coma and generalized multiorgan failure that inevitably leads to death.

LABORATORY DIAGNOSIS

Routine clinical laboratory tests are nonspecific. Computed tomography and magnetic resonance imaging scans are not diagnostic, often because of the lack of inflammation and edema. The electroencephalographic patterns may reveal diffuse encephalitic and encephalopathic changes, but these findings are also nonspecific of rabies.

Direct histologic and immunohistologic examinations of infected tissue are the only tests that may produce a definitive diagnosis of rabies. Biopsy specimens of brain or of skin from the neck area can be submitted for rabies antigen detection by the immunofluorescent technique. Saliva (not sputum) can also be collected for virus isolation attempts. A positive result on a test for rabies antigen in brain, skin, or saliva has a high predictive value for rabies and may be positive before serum antibody can be detected. The presence of Negri bodies in brain biopsy specimens is also pathognomonic. Serum neutralizing antibodies may develop within 1 to 2 weeks of the onset of the prodromal phase. Positive serum antibodies are diagnostic in patients who have not received rabies immune globulin (RIG) or previous vaccination. Cerebrospinal fluid antirabies antibody at any titer, however, is highly predictive of rabies.

CLINICAL MANAGEMENT

Pre-exposure rabies prophylaxis is appropriate for high-risk groups, such as veterinarians, animal control officers, animal handlers, and rabies research, production, and diagnostic laboratory workers. In addition, any person who is likely to come into contact with potentially infected domestic animals or wildlife, such as spelunkers who explore caves, where there are bat colonies, and persons spending extended periods (>30 days) in contact with animals in Africa, Asia, or Latin America, should have pre-exposure vaccination. Pre-exposure prophylaxis consists of 1.0 mL of human diploid cell vaccine (HDCV) (Imovax) or Rabies Vaccine Adsorbed (RVA), given intramuscularly (deltoid area), or 0.1 mL intradermally (HDCV), on days 0, 7, and 21 or 28. Booster doses are recommended depending on the results of serologic testing and the relative risk of continued exposure. For example, if the risk category is deemed continuous, such as those who work with rabies virus, serological tests should be conducted every 6 months and a booster dose administered when the virus-neutralizing titer falls below an acceptable level. This period between serologic testing and booster administration becomes every 2 years for individuals in a frequent or common category of exposure. No serologic testing or vaccine administration beyond the primary course is needed for those with an infrequent risk, such as workers in an area of low rabies enzooticity. Pre-exposure vaccination may provide protection from nonapparent contact and simplifies the postexposure management of high-risk groups, without the necessity of costly human rabies immunoglobulin (HRIG).

Animal bites raise the issue of postexposure rabies treatment (prophylaxis). When confronted with a patient who has been bitten by an animal, the first step in the medical management is to determine if the exposure is rabies prone. If the exposure was due to an animal species that is essentially free of rabies in the wild (birds, cold-blooded vertebrates, invertebrates), then the patient should have appropriate local wound care with reassurance that no rabies prophylaxis is required.

If the bite or injury was caused by a rabies-prone animal that is available, the postexposure protocol is initiated if the animal (domestic dog or cat) has been observed and demonstrates signs of infection or if the animal has been euthanized and the brain is positive for rabies infection. Rather than delay for observation, treatment should begin immediately for any bites or scratches by dogs or cats, if rabies is strongly suspected by a veterinarian on the basis of presenting clinical signs. No treatment is necessary if the domestic animal remains healthy over a 10-day observation period or if the brain material produces negative test results, regardless of species. Wildlife rabies suspects should be humanely killed, because there is no recommended observation period. Additionally, if the exposure occurred from a wild carnivore or bat that escapes capture and diagnostic evaluation, the postexposure immunotherapy protocol should be initiated immediately. Consultation with local public health officials who are knowledgeable about regional rabies epidemiology is highly encouraged before treatment initiation. For example, bites by rodents and lagomorphs (rabbits and hares) almost never require anti-rabies treatment.

Postexposure treatment (prophylaxis), when performed promptly according to the following protocol, is remarkably successful in preventing human rabies:

1. While wearing gloves, one must wash the wound thoroughly with soap and water to remove any residual saliva that might contain rabies virus and to remove devitalized tissue.
2. Administer HRIG (Hyperab or Imogam), 20 IU per kg, up to 50% around the wound itself and 50% in the gluteal area.
3. Administer HDCV (Imovax) or RVA in the deltoid muscle. The dose is 1.0 mL on days 0, 3, 7, 14, and 28 following the exposure.
4. Start empiric antibiotics, inasmuch as bacterial infections are common following animal bites. For the previously vaccinated person, administer 1.0 mL of HDCV or RVA in the deltoid muscle on days 0 and 3, but HRIG is unnecessary.

Outside the United States, several different schedules and routes for use of alternative biologic agents (e.g., purified chick or duck embryo cell vaccine [PCEC, PDEV],* purified Vero cell rabies vaccine [PVRV]* and purified equine rabies sera [ERIG])* are available and may be more economical than the expensive strategies used in developed countries. Vaccines prepared from nerve tissue should not be used unless absolutely necessary because of the risk of neuroparalytic complications.

Without postexposure prophylaxis, the chance of developing rabies following the bite of a rabid animal depends in part on the dose of inoculated material and the severity and location of the injury. Only four people have survived documented rabies. Each of these patients required prolonged supportive therapy, including mechanical ventilation, and at least two suffered significant neurologic sequelae. There is no effective antiviral therapy for rabies once the neurologic infection has been established. Limited trials with interferon-alpha have been unsuccessful. The intraneuronal site of the infection is a barrier to the penetration of therapeutic agents. Avoid administering corticosteroid therapy because there is a risk of more rapid progression of infection and higher viral titers in the saliva. Supportive and symptomatic therapy may include antiseizure medications, sedatives, analgesics, and neuroleptics.

INFECTION CONTROL

Rabies virus may enter through breaks in the skin, intact mucous membrane, inhalation as an aerosol, or in an infected corneal graft. Blood products do not transmit rabies. Six cases of corneal transplant–associated rabies are the only documented examples of human-to-human rabies transmission. Human rabies has not been documented following the bite of an infected person. There has never been a reported case of rabies transmission from a patient to a health care worker. Strict adherence to universal biohazard precautions minimizes the fear of infection on the part of health care providers and markedly reduces the need for postexposure rabies prophylaxis.

The control and prevention of animal and human rabies is a great public health challenge for many areas of the world. Cost-effective prophylaxis must be made available for those who have suffered animal bites. Strict animal control measures and pre-exposure domestic animal vaccination need to be implemented. Oral rabies vaccines for free-ranging animals may provide an additional tool in the quest for worldwide rabies elimination.

*Not available in the United States.

RAT-BITE FEVER

method of
JONATHAN SHUTER, M.D., and
FRANKLIN D. LOWY, M.D.
Montefiore Medical Center and the Albert Einstein College of Medicine
Bronx, New York

Rat-bite fever (RBF) is a systemic febrile illness caused by either of two bacterial species—*Streptobacillus moniliformis* (streptobacillary illness) and *Spirillum minus* (spirillary illness). The disease and its association with rodent bites have been recognized in India since ancient times. In Japan, where spirillary infection predominates, RBF is termed sodoku (so: rat; doku: poison). RBF was first reported in the United States in 1839. The causative organisms of both forms of illness were isolated approximately 75 years thereafter. An outbreak of streptobacillary disease in 1926 secondary to consumption of contaminated milk in Haverhill, Massachusetts led to the designation Haverhill fever. More recently, in 1983, over three hundred children in England were infected from a rat-infested water supply. RBF is not a reportable illness in the United States, so its true incidence is unknown. Recognized cases of *S. moniliformis* infection in this country are rare and are largely limited to laboratory workers, farmers, and children in crowded urban centers. Proven cases of spirillary disease in the United States are exceptional.

Both *S. moniliformis* and *S. minus* are common members of the oropharyngeal flora of rats worldwide. In addition to rat bites and scratches, the disease may be transmitted by the bites of mice, squirrels, gerbils, and guinea pigs, as well as rodent-devouring carnivores, such as cats, dogs, and ferrets. *S. moniliformis* infection may also be acquired through ingestion of organisms via contaminated food or water, leading to Haverhill fever. This route of infection has not been described with *S. minus*.

BACTERIOLOGY

S. moniliformis is a nonmotile, unencapsulated, microaerophilic, pleomorphic gram-negative bacillus. It grows in branching filaments, which may appear beaded. Growth is optimized by the use of trypticase soy agar with 20% horse or rabbit serum, incubated in the presence of 8 to 10% CO_2. Sodium polyanetholesulfonate (Liquoid, or SPS), a common additive to blood culture broths, is inhibitory to the growth of *S. moniliformis*. Standard blood culture systems, therefore, frequently fail to detect the organism, particularly at low inocula. Resin-containing bottles may increase the yield by lowering the SPS concentration. Liquid cultures develop typical puffball-like colonies in 2 to 3 days, and culture on solid media is notable for tiny L-phase variants that lack cell walls and, as a consequence, are penicillin resistant.

S. minus is a short, thick, gram-negative spiral organism that exhibits darting motility. It does not grow on artificial media and can be cultured only via inoculation into mice or guinea pigs. If animal inoculation is undertaken, the laboratory must take care to ensure that pre-existing infection with *S. minus* is not present in the recipient animals.

CLINICAL MANIFESTATIONS

The diseases caused by these organisms are similar. However, they are distinct enough to warrant separate dis-

TABLE 1. **Distinguishing Features of Rat-Bite Fever Syndromes**

Feature	*Streptobacillus moniliformis*	*Spirillum minus*
Incubation period	~ 1 week	1–4 weeks
Reaction at site of bite	Healed by the time symptoms develop	Inflammation at the onset of symptoms
Lymphadenopathy	Rare	Regional
Rash	Maculopapular, morbilliform or petechial	Maculopapular
Joint involvement	Arthralgia and arthritis common	Rare
Laboratory diagnosis	Culture in specialized media. Gas-liquid chromatography	Animal inoculation. Dark-field microscopy
False-positive test for syphilis	≤ 25%	≤ 50%

cussions. The streptobacillary form of RBF tends to have a shorter incubation period, with most patients developing symptoms within 7 to 10 days of exposure. The illness is characterized by the abrupt onset of fever, chills, headache, myalgias, and severe migratory arthralgias. The site of the rat bite may be healed at the time of presentation. Within a few days after the onset of fever, most patients develop a pink-red maculopapular or petechial rash, or both, which frequently involves the palms and soles. Monoarticular or polyarticular arthritis develops in approximately 50% of patients. Joint effusions may be present, and in rare cases, culture of synovial fluid may yield the organism. Symptoms gradually resolve over 2 weeks, but in untreated patients, recurrent episodes of fever and arthritis are common. Haverhill fever follows a similar course but is notable for the prominence of pharyngitis and vomiting. Unusual complications of *S. moniliformis* infection include endocarditis, pneumonia, and abscesses. In the postantibiotic era, fatalities have been rare.

S. minus infection has an incubation period of 1 to 4 weeks. The site of the bite wound, which has often already healed, becomes indurated at the onset of symptoms. The illness is characterized by fever, chills, headache, myalgias, and lymphadenopathy in the region of the wound site. A rash consisting of large red-brown maculopapular lesions is common. Without treatment, a prolonged relapsing illness may ensue. Joint manifestations are unusual. Similar to streptobacillary disease, uncommon complications, including endocarditis, may occur. The clinical features of both diseases are summarized in Table 1.

DIAGNOSIS

In both infections, routine laboratory findings are nonspecific. Leukocytosis is common, as is a biologic false-positive test result for syphilis. The differential diagnosis of RBF includes disseminated neisserial infection, enteric fever, subacute bacterial endocarditis, leptospirosis, borreliosis, rheumatic fever, Rocky Mountain spotted fever, viral exanthem, Kawasaki disease, and collagen-vascular diseases.

S. moniliformis is definitively diagnosed by culturing blood, joint fluid, or pus. Typical bacterial forms may be seen on Gram's or Giemsa stain of these fluids. Gas-liquid chromatography may provide a means of rapid identification in the event of positive cultures. Specific agglutinin titers, of uncertain utility in streptobacillary illness, are no longer readily available. Although in rare cases *S. minus* may be visualized by dark-field microscopy in blood or body fluids, animal inoculation (as described in the section on bacteriology) is generally required. There is no available serologic test for spirillary disease.

TREATMENT AND PREVENTION

Procaine penicillin G, 600,000 units administered intramuscularly every 12 hours for 7 to 14 days, is the treatment of choice for both organisms. Accepted alternatives include tetracycline, 500 mg orally every 6 hours; erythromycin, 500 mg orally every 6 hours; and streptomycin, 15 mg per kg per day given intramuscularly in two divided doses. These alternative regimens are not of proven efficacy in spirillary disease. Treatment of endocarditis consists of 12 to 24 million units of penicillin G daily, administered intravenously for 4 to 6 weeks. In streptobacillary endocarditis, streptomycin may be added to treat resistant L forms.

To prevent illness, individuals who work with rodents should wear gloves. Wounds should be cleansed with soap and water, and tetanus vaccination should be administered if indicated. Although no data exist regarding the efficacy of prophylactic antibiotics, many experts recommend a 3-day course of oral penicillin, 500 mg every 6 hours, after any rat bite. This recommendation assumes particular importance in patients with pre-existing valvular heart disease.

RELAPSING FEVERS

method of
ALEXANDER G. VANDEVELDE, M.D.
University of Florida Health Science Center
Jacksonville, Florida

Relapsing fevers are a group of diseases in humans and animals that are characterized by recurrent fevers that last from 2 to 7 days, end by crisis, and alternate with a few days of relief before the next febrile episode.

ETIOLOGY, EPIDEMIOLOGY, AND PATHOPHYSIOLOGY

The diseases are caused by *Borrelia recurrentis* and other *Borrelia* spp, bacteria that belong to the spirochete group (Table 1).

Borrelia are spiral and thin (0.3 μm) but elongated (8 to 30 μm), microaerophilic organisms with three to ten coils. Borrelia have several flagella implanted along the long axis of their bodies, allowing them to swim with a screwlike movement. Surface proteins are programmed to change at regular intervals through DNA rearrangement. These antigenically different proteins, called variable major proteins, are the reason for the recurrence of fevers. During the progress of the same infection, several distinct serotypes appear in a sequential fashion. One serotype is predominant during the first febrile episode, but disappears after the build-up of antibodies. Another serotype emerges

TABLE 1. ***Borrelia* Species Identified as Causing Relapsing Fevers in Man**

Borrelia Species	Disease	Arthropod Vector	Vertebrate Carrier	Geographic Location
	Worldwide Disease			
B. recurrentis	Louse-borne relapsing fever	*Pediculus humanus* (body louse)	Humans	Epidemics worldwide in refugee camps; endemic pockets in and around Ethiopia and Bolivia
	New World Diseases			
B. hermsii	Tick-borne relapsing fever	*Ornithodoros hermsi* (an argasid, soft tick)	Wild rodents	Northwestern United States and western Canada
B. turicatae	Tick-borne relapsing fever	*O. turicata*	Wild rodents	Southwestern United States and Northern Mexico
B. parkeri	Tick-borne relapsing fever	*O. parkeri*	Wild rodents	Arizona, California, and Baja California
B. mazzottii	Tick-borne relapsing fever	*O. talaje*	Wild rodents	Mexico, adjacent Central America, and Caribbean islands
B. dugesii	Tick-borne relapsing fever	? An argasid tick	Wild rodents	Mexico, adjacent Central America, and Caribbean islands
B. venezuelensis	Tick-borne relapsing fever	*O. rudis*	Wild rodents	Northern South America, Central America, and Caribbean islands
	Old World Diseases			
B. hispanica	Tick-borne relapsing fever	*O. marocanus*	Wild rodents	Spain and northwestern Africa
B. duttonii	Tick-borne relapsing fever	*O. moubata*	Wild rodents	Sub-Saharan Africa
B. crocidurae	Tick-borne relapsing fever	*Alectorobius sonrai*	Wild rodents	West Africa, East Africa, and the Middle East
B. persica	Tick-borne relapsing fever	*Ornithodoros tholozani*	Wild rodents	Greece and the Middle East
B. caucasica	Tick-borne relapsing fever	*O. asperus*	Wild rodents	Southwestern Russia, the Caucasian republics, and Iraq
B. latyschewii	Tick-borne relapsing fever	*O. tartakowskyi*	Wild rodents	South-Central Russia, the steppe republics, Iran, and Afghanistan

during the second occurrence of fever until a new set of antibodies appears, and so on until as many as 25 different variable major protein genes have produced their surface protein. Thus, borrelia go through pulsating growth phases, and all relapsing fevers are multiphasic diseases.

B. recurrentis is transmitted from person to person by the body louse. The other *Borrelia* spp reside in rodents but are sometimes transmitted to humans by biting ticks, which fall off their usual hosts or depart from a dying host. These argasid (soft) ticks can outlive their rodent hosts and also pass the borrelia to their offspring through transovarian transmission. As such, the tick itself can also be considered as a definite host.

Endemic louse-borne relapsing fever (LBRF) still exists in certain regions of the world, such as Ethiopia and Bolivia and surrounding countries. The disease, however, has a propensity to break out in epidemics during times of disaster, when masses of people gather in refugee camps without adequate hygiene and laundering facilities. Tick-borne relapsing fevers (TBRFs) have been reported in many parts of the world where circumstances are right for the spread of these zoonoses to outdoorsmen (Table 1).

The body louse becomes infected during its blood meal on a spirochetemic patient. The suctioned organisms penetrate the gut of the louse and disperse into the tissues of the louse but not into the biting organs or the salivary glands. Therefore, the bite of the louse does not transmit the infectious agent per se, but crushing and scratching the lousy tissues into the abraded skin allows penetration of the microbe into the victim's bloodstream.

The ticks connected with TBRFs are evasive in the sense that their bites do not hurt, and they fall off the host after the 20 to 30 minutes that it takes to gather a blood meal. This is in contrast to Lyme disease, in which the ticks stay attached for days. The *Borrelia* spp in ticks are injected into the host during biting, not through the saliva but via the tick's coxal organ, which is located near the mouth of the tick and exudes excess fluid.

In animals, the borrelia reside in the liver, spleen, lymph nodes, and brain during the afebrile periods. In pregnant women, the fetus can become infected during the latter part of the gestation.

A smaller number of febrile episodes is seen in LBRF (2 to 3), but the disease is more dangerous because of the high number of bacteria in the bloodstream. The disease lasts about 2 weeks. If left untreated, the case fatality can be 10% and even higher during epidemics. Up to 10 relapses can be expected from TBRFs. Thus, TBRFs last much longer than 2 weeks.

SYMPTOMS, SIGNS, PROGNOSIS, AND DIAGNOSIS

Clinically, the patient runs high fevers (above 39.5° C [103° F]), starting with shaking chills, prostration, severe headaches, fatigue, and depressed mentation. The develop-

TABLE 2. **Treatment Guidelines for Relapsing Fevers**

Drug	Adult Dosage	Pediatric Dosage (Stay at or Below Adult Dosage)	Days of Treatment
Doxycycline*	100 mg q 12 h IV/PO	2 mg/kg q 12 h IV/PO	10–14
Erythromycin	500 mg q 6 hr IV/PO	10 mg/kg q 6 h IV/PO	10–14
Chloramphenicol†	500 mg q 6 h IV/PO	15 mg/kg q 6 h IV/PO	10–14
Penicillin V	500 mg q 6h PO	10 mg/kg q 6 h PO	10–14
Penicillin G	5 million units q 6 h IV	35,000 units/kg q 4 h IV	10–14
Ceftriaxone (Rocephin)	2 gm once daily IV	50 mg/kg once daily	10–14

*Contraindicated in pregnant women and children less than 8 years old.
†Incidence of aplastic anemia is reported at approximately 1 in 30,000 patients.

ment of splenomegaly, petechial rashes, and jaundice connotes a poor prognosis. Some patients will suffer from a true meningitis with nuchal rigidity and cerebrospinal fluid pleiocytosis. The fever will drop in lysis, and the patient will feel better, although exhausted, until the next bacterial breakthrough in the blood. The disease is milder in children than in adults. Relapsing fevers, even TBRFs, can be devastating to the point of a septic shock syndrome in patients with underlying diseases, as well as during pregnancy and malnutrition.

Differential diagnosis depends on the region where it is diagnosed and other circumstances. Malaria, viral hemorrhagic fevers, and epidemic typhus should be considered in refugee camps, especially in the tropics. In outdoorsmen and missionaries, one should consider other zoonoses such as leptospirosis, Lyme disease, sylvatic plague, Rocky Mountain spotted fever, and ehrlichiosis.

Diagnosis is easiest with a dark-field preparation, or a thick and thin blood smear, stained with Giemsa or Wright's stains, taken during the bacteremic phase. Serologic tests are available but are not in widespread use, and they are performed only in reference laboratories where animals can also be inoculated.

TREATMENT

Antimicrobial Therapy

The time at which the diagnosis is easiest to make may be the worst moment to treat. Indeed, the Jarisch-Herxheimer reaction (intensification of symptoms and signs of the disease after initiation of antimicrobial therapy) can be extremely violent and can even push the patient into a systemic inflammatory response syndrome with shock. Although the reaction has many traits in common with endotoxin infusion, it is not due to endotoxin. Inflammatory cytokines (tumor necrosis factor, interleukin-6, and interleukin-8) transiently increase to eight-fold above the pretreatment levels. Corticosteroids do not alter the course. The Jarisch-Herxheimer reaction in LBRF is seen in more than 80% of the patients, is more violent than in TBRFs, and is worse when a patient is treated at the end of the first febrile episode. One should anticipate that the patient will have a rough time for 12 to 24 hours.

The treatment of relapsing fevers should be initiated and monitored carefully in the hospital. The later stages of the treatment can be given on an outpatient basis with close follow-up. Clinicians in Africa believe that it is best to treat the patient with a small dose of penicillin* 1 day prior to the anticipated recurrence or at the very beginning of such recurrence, followed by a full dose of doxycycline (Vibramycin), the drug of first choice. In addition to the ones mentioned, antibiotics effective against the *Borrelia* spp in relapsing fevers include erythromycin,* chloramphenicol,* and ceftriaxone* (Rocephin) (Table 2). *Borrelia* spp are resistant to the sulfonamides and rifampin.

Relapses of TBRFs can occur following treatment with doxycycline and penicillin. Therefore, it is recommended to treat TBRFs for a full 2 weeks. If a relapse still occurs, the patient should be treated with a second course of the same antibiotics. In patients with meningitis, a regimen should be chosen with antimicrobials that penetrate the blood-brain barrier, such as double doses of doxycycline, high doses of intravenous penicillin,* ceftriaxone (Rocephin),* or chloramphenicol.*

Supportive Care

Patients with relapsing fevers need symptomatic and supportive care. The postperspiration dehydration and electrolyte imbalances need to be corrected, especially in malnourished refugees. High fevers above 40° C (104° F) can safely be controlled with tepid water soaks. Pain (especially headaches) is treated orally with acetaminophen (Tylenol and others), 500 mg every 4 to 6 hours. Narcotics may be necessary. Avoid aspirin because many patients develop bleeding abnormalities. Nausea and vomiting are treated with promethazine (Phenergan), 25 mg every 4 to 6 hours administered intramuscularly or rectally.

A few petechiae underneath the skin should not be regarded as dangerous but should be watched. However, severe diffuse intravascular coagulation with bleeding from the nose and other mucous membranes can be a devastating complication and may cause death. Disseminated intravascular coagulation should be treated in its own right. Treat with low doses of heparin 400 to 600 units per hour intravenously (total daily dose is 10,000 units), cryoprecipitates intravenously (one unit per 10 kg of weight),

*Not FDA approved for this indication.

and fresh frozen plasma. Monitor the fibrinogen level every four to six hours and give cryoprecipitates to keep the level of fibrinogen above 100 mg per dL. If the prothrombin time is prolonged, replace the prothrombin with fresh frozen plasma. Injection of phytonadione or vitamin K_1 (AquaMEPHYTON) is the preferred treatment for a prolonged prothrombin time without disseminated intravascular coagulation. Replace the platelets to keep the count above 20,000 cells per μL and even above 50,000 cells per μL if life-threatening bleeding has occurred.

The respiratory distress syndrome can be treated only with ventilatory support. If an acute abdomen develops, consider possible splenic rupture and the patient in need of an urgent splenectomy.

PREVENTION AND PUBLIC HEALTH

Prevention of LBRF is best established by preventing overcrowding in refugee camps, setting up adequate showering and laundering facilities, and delousing of the camps with malathion-type insecticides. TBRFs are prevented by eliminating rodents nesting in rafters and floors in the lodging cabins and through the use of DEET-containing insect repellents on skin and permethrin on clothing while outdoors in infected regions. LBRF is a disease under surveillance by the World Health Organization, and all relapsing fevers should be reported.

RHEUMATIC FEVER

method of
MICHAEL S. BRONZE, M.D.
University of Tennessee and Department of Veterans Affairs Medical Center
Memphis, Tennessee

For many years it has been known that pharyngeal infection with group A, beta-hemolytic streptococci (GABHS) may give rise to acute rheumatic fever (ARF) and rheumatic carditis. Although the putative agent is well known, the exact mechanisms by which streptococcal pharyngitis leads to rheumatic fever are still unknown. Studies from several laboratories suggest that the manifestations of ARF are the results of a host autoimmune response to streptococcal antigens, such as the surface M protein, which is a major virulence factor of the organism.

After decades of decline, there has been a significant resurgence in the incidence of ARF in the United States. Worldwide rheumatic heart disease is the leading cause of cardiac morbidity in children. The reasons for this resurgence are not fully understood, but studies suggest that it is not the result of inadequate access to health care. Additionally, only a minority of patients reported symptomatic sore throat, making primary prevention with antibiotic therapy difficult.

Prevention of ARF depends on the accurate diagnosis and treatment of group A streptococcal pharyngitis, which has been facilitated by rapid streptococcal antigen detection kits and simple culture techniques. The diagnosis of ARF is based on criteria established by Jones and modified by the American Heart Association (Table 1). These criteria apply to the initial attack and do not predict disease activity or clinical course or diagnose inactive or chronic rheumatic heart disease. The major manifestations include (1) carditis, which may be clinically manifested as an asymptomatic mitral or aortic insufficiency murmur or overt congestive heart failure or pericarditis; (2) polyarthritis, which is typically migratory, affecting the larger joints; (3) chorea, which often is a late manifestation presenting as involuntary, purposeless movements often associated with muscle weakness and behavioral changes; (4) subcutaneous nodules, which present as firm, painless nodules over extensor surfaces; and (5) erythema marginatum characterized as an evanescent, migratory rash of the trunk and proximal extremities. The minor manifestations are protean and by themselves offer limited diagnostic utility. These manifestations include arthralgias, fever, elevated erythrocyte sedimentation rate or C-reactive protein, and prolongation of the PR interval. Recent revisions of the Jones criteria no longer include previous rheumatic fever as a minor manifestation.

The diagnosis of ARF is based on the presence of two or more major criteria or one major criterion occurring with two minor criteria. In either case, there must be supporting evidence of a recent streptococcal infection unless the patient presents with isolated chorea or indolent rheumatic carditis. In these patients, evidence of positive streptococcal culture or antibody response (e.g., antistreptolysin O) may be lacking. A history of recent scarlet fever or bacteriologically or serologically confirmed GABHS pharyngitis is the best indication of recent infection. The most commonly used streptococcal antibody tests are the antistreptolysin O, antihyaluronidase, and antideoxyribonuclease B assays.

TREATMENT

The treatment of patients with ARF is directed at the elimination of GABHS from the throat, suppression of inflammation, treatment of congestive heart failure, and prevention of recurrences. Although treatment influences the course and severity of the illness, it has no proven influence on the subsequent development of chronic rheumatic heart disease.

TABLE 1. **Jones Criteria (Revised) for the Diagnosis of Acute Rheumatic Fever**

Major Manifestations	Minor Manifestations
Polyarthritis	*Clinical*
Carditis	Arthralgias
Arthritis	Fever ≥ 39° C (102.2° F)
Chorea	*Laboratory*
Subcutaneous nodules	Elevated ESR, CRP
Erythema marginatum	Prolonged PR interval (EKG)

plus

Supporting evidence of preceding streptococcal infection:
1. History of recent scarlet fever
2. Throat culture or rapid streptococcal antigen positive for group A streptococci
3. Increased antistreptolysin O* or other streptococcal antibodies

Abbreviations: ESR = erythrocyte sedimentation rate; CRP = C-reactive protein; EKG = electrocardiogram.

*ASO titer is usually reported in Todd units. Results may vary among laboratories, but significant Todd units may include those greater than 250 in adults and greater than 333 in children.

Adapted from JAMA *268*:2069, 1992. Copyright 1992, American Medical Association.

Eradication of Streptococci

Although the throat culture in patients with ARF may be negative at presentation, the concern for the possibility of residual GABHS in the pharynx has led to the recommendation that patients be treated with antibiotics. The recommended antibiotic regimens include a single intramuscular injection of benzathine penicillin G (600,000 units in children weighing less than 60 pounds and 1.2 million units for all others) or penicillin V, 125 to 250 mg orally four times a day for 10 days. For penicillin-allergic patients, erythromycin estolate, 20 to 40 mg per kg in two to four divided doses, may be used. Tetracyclines and sulfa-containing antibiotics should not be used for primary eradication. There is no direct evidence that antibiotic treatment has an effect on the clinical manifestations of established ARF.

Treatment of the Manifestations of ARF

The mainstay of treatment for patients with ARF is the use of anti-inflammatory drugs, namely salicylates and prednisone. Both agents suppress fever and the acute phase reactants, but neither prevents the development of rheumatic heart disease. Supportive measures include bed rest and restriction of physical activities, as well as the use of digoxin and diuretics in patients with congestive heart failure.

In general, salicylates are recommended as the anti-inflammatory agent when arthritis is the major manifestation (Table 2). This therapy results in prompt resolution of the arthritic symptoms. Failure of the patient to respond to salicylates should raise the concern about the accuracy of the diagnosis.

Corticosteroids have not been proved to be superior to aspirin except in cases of severe carditis. In the absence of overt moderate to severe congestive heart failure, carditis may be treated with salicylates (Table 2). For severe carditis, prednisone is given orally in four divided doses for 2 to 3 weeks, followed by initiation of aspirin with a concomitant steroid taper. Aspirin is continued as the sole agent for 6 to 8 weeks or longer. This approach is used to prevent rebound phenomena when steroids are tapered.

TABLE 2. **Treatment of the Manifestations of Acute Rheumatic Fever**

Manifestation	Recommended Treatment
Arthralgias	Aspirin not necessary, analgesics as needed
Arthritis	Aspirin, 75 to 100 mg/kg/day in four divided doses × 2 weeks, then reduce dose by one-half for next 2 to 3 weeks
Carditis	
Mild to moderate	Aspirin, 75 to 100 mg/kg/day in four divided doses for 2 weeks, then reduce by one-half for next 3 to 4 weeks
Severe	Prednisone 2 mg/kg/day (maximum 80 mg) in four divided doses for 2–3 weeks, then taper, adding aspirin 75–100 mg/kg/day for 6–8 weeks; then taper
Chorea	Bed rest; avoidance of stress; sedatives as necessary; role of steroids and aspirin unclear

Adapted from J. Rheumatol (Suppl 29) *18*:2, 1991.

TABLE 3. **Antibiotic Strategies for Secondary Prevention of ARF**

Drug		Dosage
Benzathine penicillin G		1.2 million units IM every 3 to 4 weeks
	or	
Penicillin V		250 mg orally twice daily
	or	
Sulfadiazine		1 gm orally daily (500 mg if < 60 lb)
	or	
Erythromycin		250 mg orally twice daily (primarily if allergic to penicillin)

The treatment of patients with chorea is less certain. The patient should be placed in a quiet environment. Controlled studies showing the efficacy of salicylates or steroids in patients with chorea are lacking. Because the manifestations of chorea often occur after arthritis and carditis have subsided, there appears to be a limited role for treatment with anti-inflammatory agents. Sedatives, especially phenobarbital* (3 to 6 mg per kg daily in three divided doses for children,and 60 to 200 mg per day in two or three divided doses for adults) have been effective in controlling the choreic movement. If it is ineffectual, haloperidol (Haldol)* (0.5 mg twice daily for children and 0.5 to 2.0 mg twice daily for adults) may be tried. Anecdotal evidence suggests that steroids in large doses may be effective, but controlled studies are again lacking.

Prevention of Recurrences

Patients with a history of ARF are at increased risk for recurrent attacks. These recurrences are often manifested by symptoms observed in the initial attack, and the incidence of recurrences declines with time. The mainstay of secondary prevention is the routine use of antibiotics to prevent recurrent infection by group A streptococci. Patients who present with only isolated chorea will require lifelong antibiotic prophylaxis.

The recommended regimen is parenteral or oral penicillin (Table 3). Intramuscular penicillin may be the most effective agent and is usually given every 3 to 4 weeks. Some studies advocate a 3-week interval because breakthrough cases have been reported with the 4-week schedule. Erythromycin is usually reserved for those patients who are allergic to penicillin or sulfadiazine.

The duration of antibiotic prophylaxis for secondary prevention is controversial and should be viewed in light of the patient's potential exposure to streptococcal infection. Some specialists recommend

*Not FDA approved for this indication.

TABLE 4. **Recommended Bacterial Endocarditis Prophylaxis Regimens***

Dental, Oral or Upper Respiratory Tract Procedures

Standard Regimen	*Penicillin-Allergic*
Amoxicillin <15 kg—750 mg 15–30 kg—1500 mg >30 kg—3000 mg	Erythromycin stearate <30 kg—20 mg/kg >30 kg—1000 mg *or* Clindamycin <30 kg—10 mg/kg >30 kg—300 mg

Dosing: Give full dose orally 1 hour prior to the procedure. Repeat one-half of the initial dose orally 6 hours later.

Genitourinary and Gastrointestinal Procedures

Standard Regimen	*Penicillin-Allergic*
Ampicillin (IM or IV) <30 kg—50 mg/kg >30 kg—2.0 gm *plus* Gentamicin (IM or IV) 2.0 mg/kg (up to 80 mg) *plus* Amoxicillin (PO) <30 kg—750 mg >30 kg—1500 mg	Vancomycin (IV) <50 kg—20 mg/kg >50 kg—1.0 gm *plus* Gentamicin (IM or IV) 2.0 mg/kg (up to 80 mg)

Dosing: For the standard regimen, give the ampicillin and gentamicin IM or IV 30 minutes prior to the procedure, followed by oral amoxicillin 6 hours after the initial dose. Alternatively, the ampicillin and gentamicin may be repeated 8 hours after the initial dose. For penicillin-allergic patients, vancomycin and gentamicin are given parenterally 1 hour prior to the procedure and are repeated in 8 hours.

Adapted from Committee on Rheumatic Fever, Endocarditis, and Kawasaki Disease of the Council on Cardiovascular Disease in the Young, American Heart Association. JAMA *264*:2919, 1990. Copyright 1990, American Medical Association.

that prophylaxis be continued indefinitely. Yet, the risk of streptococcal infection declines with advancing age, becoming low in older adults without heart disease who are not exposed to school-age children. The decision to discontinue antibiotic prophylaxis must be individualized.

Generally, it is recommended that prophylaxis of patients without carditis be continued until the patient is older than 18 years of age or 5 years have elapsed since the acute attack (whichever is longer). This recommendation probably should be prolonged to the greater of age 25 years or 10 years from the acute attack in patients with mild carditis as manifested by mild mitral regurgitation. For those patients with significant carditis, overt rheumatic heart disease, or chorea, prophylaxis should probably be lifelong.

In addition to rheumatic fever prophylaxis, patients with cardiac valvular abnormalities due to rheumatic heart disease should receive antibiotic prophylaxis to prevent bacterial endocarditis. The need to provide endocarditis prophylaxis should take into consideration the nature of the patient's underlying cardiac condition and the risk of bacteremia following certain dental and invasive procedures. The recommendations concerning prophylaxis have recently been updated by the American Heart Association (Table 4). Because daily oral penicillin prophylaxis may lead to the development of oral streptococci that may be resistant to amoxicillin, endocarditis prophylaxis for dental, oral, or upper respiratory tract procedures should use erythromycin or clindamycin.

Prevention of acute rheumatic fever depends on the treatment and prevention of streptococcal pharyngitis. This is problematic in that only one-third of the patients described in recent outbreaks of ARF reported symptomatic pharyngitis. Hence, the ultimate prevention may well depend on the development of safe and effective streptococcal vaccines. Recent studies from several laboratories have shown the protective efficacy of defined streptococcal vaccine preparations in laboratory animals. Future research efforts are being directed at the development of vaccines for humans that will prevent the pharyngeal infections that may give rise to acute rheumatic fever and rheumatic carditis.

LYME DISEASE

method of
DANIEL W. RAHN, M.D.
Medical College of Georgia
Augusta, Georgia

Lyme disease is a multisystem infectious disease caused by the spirochete *Borrelia burgdorferi.* This organism is transmitted to humans by *Ixodid* (hard-bodied) tick vectors. The rate of infection in the tick population (and hence the risk of acquiring Lyme disease when bitten) shows wide geographic variation. The primary vectors in the United States are *Ixodes dammini* (which may be a northern subspecies of *I. scapularis*) in the northeast from Maryland to Massachusetts and northcentral region primarily in parts of Minnesota and Wisconsin and *I. pacificus* along coastal regions of Northern California. The rate of infection in *I. scapularis* in the southeast United States is very low even though this is a suitable vector. Other species including *I. dentatus* and *Amblyomma americanum* may become infected but do not appear to be important in the ecology and epidemiology of Lyme disease.

The clinical spectrum of the disease is very broad, with manifestations varying dramatically among patients and over time in individual patients as the infection and inflammatory response evolve. The factors that determine geographic spread of *B. burgdorferi* are poorly understood at present but include the availability of reservoir hosts for the tick vectors and a means of transporting infected ticks. Further study of these important epidemiologic issues may provide guidance in designing environmental control measures in the future. Because of the wide geographic dispersion and varied clinical manifestations, patients with Lyme disease may present to physicians outside known endemic regions and in practice in most clinical specialties.

Lyme disease was originally recognized to be a distinct clinical entity in 1975 through the study of an epidemic of oligoarticular, inflammatory arthritis in a tight geographic cluster in three rural towns in Connecticut centering around the town of Lyme, from which the disease draws its name. Study of this epidemic led to the elucidation of the multisystem nature of the illness, the typical evolution of signs and symptoms, the response of individuals with all stages of disease to antibiotic therapy, the tick vector and eventually, in 1982, the spirochetal etiology. It is now known that Lyme disease is a clinical syndrome caused by *B. burgdorferi*. Infection begins in the skin at the site of a bite by an infected tick vector. The infection may disseminate to involve many organs. The heart, the nervous system, and the joints are favored targets.

The illness typically waxes and wanes over time, with symptoms resulting from persistence of infection or the inflammatory response engendered by the infecting organisms, or both. It is not known whether or not viable spirochetes persist in all patients throughout the course of the illness. In practice, it is often difficult to determine whether symptoms in individuals with a history of documented Lyme disease result from *B. burgdorferi* infection or postinfectious sequelae, an important distinction to make in planning therapy. Lyme disease is over-diagnosed in the United States at present, leading to unnecessary administration of potentially hazardous antibiotics for possible Lyme disease and failure to diagnose other underlying disorders. The leading reason for a patient's failure to respond to antibiotic therapy for Lyme disease is an incorrect diagnosis.

Lyme disease is generally divided into clinical stages. The staging system in common use is evolving as our understanding of the pathophysiology of signs and symptoms of the illness changes. In general, the disease begins with localized infection at the site of a bite by an infected tick (localized Stage I disease) and progresses through a phase of generalized signs and symptoms caused by dissemination of infecting organisms (disseminated Stage I). The illness typically spontaneously remits and some individuals subsequently develop acute inflammation in certain target organs, namely heart and nervous system (Stage II). Joint inflammation occurs months later beginning with episodic inflammation in one to three joints, and a minority of individuals eventually develop chronic inflammation in joints or nervous system characterized by persistent inflammation for more than 1 year (Stage III). Patients may present with any stage of disease, however, and stages may overlap, merge, or be skipped entirely. This staging system is somewhat arbitrary, but it has served a useful purpose in designing clinical trials and guiding therapy. Although all stages respond to appropriately chosen antibiotics, the illness is most responsive early in its course and response is less certain in chronic disease. Early detection and prompt institution of therapy is important in protecting against progression to later stages of illness. Antibiotic therapy for the various stages of Lyme disease must be individualized because it is often not possible to determine for certain the extent of the infection. In this chapter, therapy is discussed according to the staging system in common use and is distinguished by organ system for ease of reference. Antibiotic recommendations are summarized in Table 1.

TABLE 1. **Treatment Recommendations**

Early Lyme disease*
- Amoxicillin, 500 mg tid for 21 days†
- Doxycycline, 100 mg bid for 21 days
- Cefuroxime axetil, 500 mg bid for 21 days
- Azithromycin, 500 mg q d for 7 days‡ (less effective than other regimens)

Neurologic manifestations
- Bell's palsy (no other neurologic abnormalities)
  - Oral regimens for early disease suffice

Meningitis (with or without radiculoneuropathy or encephalitis)§
- Ceftriaxone, 2 gm q d for 14–28 days
- Penicillin G, 20 million U in divided doses daily for 14–28 days
- Doxycycline, 100 mg (PO or IV) for 14–28 days‖
- Chloramphenicol, 1 gm qid for 14–28 days

Arthritis¶
- Amoxicillin and probenecid, 500 mg each PO qid for 30 days**
- Doxycycline, 100 mg bid for 30 days
- Ceftriaxone, 2 gm q d for 14–28 days
- Penicillin G, 20 million U in divided doses daily for 14–28 days

Carditis
- Ceftriaxone, 2 gm in divided doses daily for 14 days
- Penicillin G, 20 million U in divided doses daily for 14 days
- Doxycycline, 100 mg PO bid for 21 days††
- Amoxicillin, 500 mg PO tid for 21 days

Pregnancy
- Localized early disease
  - Amoxicillin, 500 mg tid for 21 days
- Any manifestation of disseminated disease
  - Penicillin G, 20 million U in divided doses daily for 14–28 days
- Asymptomatic seropositivity
  - No treatment necessary

*Without neurologic, cardiac, or joint involvement. For early Lyme disease limited to single ECM lesion, 10 days are sufficient.

†Some experts advise addition of probenecid, 500 mg three times daily.

‡Experience with this agent is limited; optimal duration of therapy is unclear.

§Optimal duration of therapy has not been established. There are no controlled trials of therapy lasting longer than four weeks for any manifestation of Lyme disease.

‖No published experience in the United States.

¶An oral regimen should be selected only if there is no neurologic involvement.

**Amoxicillin is generally administered three times daily, but the only trial of this agent for Lyme arthritis employed a regimen that required the drug to be taken four times daily.

††Oral regimens have been reserved for mild carditis limited to first-degree heart block with PR ≤ 0.30 sec and normal ventricular function.

Adapted from Malawista SE and Rahn DW: Treatment of early Lyme disease. In Rogers D, Bone R, Cline M, et al (eds): 1994 Yearbook of Medicine. Chicago, Mosby–Year Book, 1994.

STAGE I (EARLY): LYME DISEASE

Clinical Features

The clinical hallmark of early Lyme disease is erythema chronicum migrans (ECM), the distinctive skin lesion that results from localized infection with *B. burgdorferi*. The only known means of acquiring infection in skin is through the bite of an infected tick. In mice, ticks must be imbedded in skin for more than 24 hours in order to transmit infection; the same likely holds true in humans. This largely asymptomatic skin lesion begins as an erythematous macule or papule. The lesion begins to expand a few days to as long as a month after the tick bite and expands at a rate of ½ to 1 centimeter per day, ultimately achieving a diameter of anywhere from five to 20 or more centimeters. This gradual expansion reflects local spread of spirochetes in the skin and is characteristic of ECM. These minimally symptomatic lesions are erythematous, warm to the touch, and flat with a sharply demarcated outer border and annular shape. Common skin sites include popliteal fossa, groin, axilla, and other skin folds. Spirochetes are relatively easily grown from ECM lesions if skin biopsy samples are cultured in appropriate media. Unfortunately, conditions for growth of *B. burgdorferi* are stringent, so culture is not available routinely in clinical laboratories. Diagnosis rests on clinical recognition of this highly characteristic skin lesion.

Approximately two-thirds of patients with Lyme disease present with ECM but most do not recall being bitten. If infection is localized to the skin, there are few accompanying systemic symptoms and laboratory results, including Lyme serologies, are also typically normal. More than 50% of untreated patients, however, develop disseminated infection after a variable period of local spread in skin (disseminated Stage I). Spirochetes enter the bloodstream and spread throughout the body.

Common symptoms at this stage of illness include fever, chills, arthralgias, myalgias, headache, stiff neck, multiple secondary skin lesions, and transient Bell's palsy. Symptoms wax and wane and often merge with Stage II disease, discussed later, in which central nervous system and cardiac manifestations predominate. Spirochetes have been recovered from blood and secondary skin lesions during this stage of infection. For the purpose of treatment decisions, patients have been considered to have early (Stage I) disease by the presence of ECM and the absence of central nervous system involvement, carditis, overt joint inflammation, or other major organ involvement.

Without antibiotic therapy, ECM and associated symptoms of early disease resolve within a month and patients become asymptomatic. This process may reflect spontaneous resolution of infection, but most patients (up to 80%) subsequently develop one or more manifestations of progressive Lyme disease. Antibiotic therapy, therefore, is indicated primarily to prevent the progression of infection.

Therapy

Imbedded ticks should be removed promptly, and the site of the tick bite should be watched for the appearance of a skin lesion. Controlled clinical trials have shown that prophylactic antibiotic therapy is not necessary following tick bites in routine clinical circumstances. Even in endemic areas, individuals with a definite ixodid tick bite should simply remove the tick and watch the bite site expectantly, reserving antibiotics for those individuals who develop ECM. An exception to this rule is the pregnant patient, in whom it may be advisable to administer antibiotics prophylactically to eliminate the risk of intrauterine infection.

A variety of antibiotic regimens have been proved effective in the treatment of early Lyme disease. Skin lesions fade promptly, and later manifestations of disease are prevented. Individuals with disseminated early disease seem to be at higher risk of failing antibiotic therapy than are those with disease limited to a single skin lesion and minor or no systemic symptoms. Although 10 days of therapy generally suffice to eradicate early disease, most experts currently recommend therapy of 3-weeks' duration because of the slow replication of *B. burgdorferi.* Amoxicillin (Amoxil), 500 mg three times daily, is preferred for most adults (30 mg/kg for children). Penicillin-allergic individuals can be treated with doxycycline (Vibramycin), 100 mg twice daily, which seems to be equally efficacious. Erythromycin and the related macrolide azithromycin (Zithromax) have been tested in clinical trials in the United States and were found to be less effective, particularly in individuals with disseminated early disease, resulting in a higher rate of progression or relapse, or both, after therapy. Azithromycin has been used in doses up to 500 mg daily for 7 days,* which should result in adequate tissue levels for at least 14 days; perhaps courses of longer duration (e.g., 14 days) would be equivalent to amoxicillin or doxycycline, but this is untested at present. Cefuroxime axetil (Ceftin), 500 mg twice daily, has been found equivalent to doxycycline and is an alternative for penicillin-allergic individuals. Reduced doses may be given to children under the age of 9 years for whom tetracyclines are contraindicated. Cefuroxime axetil is classified in pregnancy category B and is excreted in breast milk, so it should be used in pregnancy only when it is clearly indicated and consideration should be given to interrupting breast-feeding if it must be administered to women while nursing.

Several studies have shown that individuals with disseminated early infection have a different prognosis than those with localized early disease. These patients have a higher rate of antibiotic failure, with progression to subsequent development of central nervous system manifestations in particular. This factor probably indicates that spirochetes can spread to the central nervous system with minimal clinical symptoms early in the process of dissemination and that symptoms such as headache (even without meningismus) may reflect central nervous system infection. Therefore, it is advisable to search carefully for any evidence of carditis, actual arthritis, or central nervous system involvement in all individuals with dissemination of Lyme disease beyond a single skin lesion before deciding on short-course (3-week) oral antibiotic therapy. If clinical manifestations are limited to secondary skin lesions and non-neurologic systemic complaints, therapy should be the same as for early localized disease. Attention should be paid to compliance with a full 3-week course of antibiotics because symptoms are likely to resolve within 5 to 7 days and patients may tend to discontinue therapy once symptoms have resolved. The risk of progression is no doubt greater with a shorter course of therapy. Post-treatment sequelae, particularly a prolonged fatigue state and fibromyalgia, occur with some frequency after otherwise successful treatment of disseminated early Lyme disease. These symptoms do not reflect continued infection and should be treated supportively.

---

*Exceeds dosage recommended by the manufacturer.

STAGE II AND STAGE III (DISSEMINATED AND CHRONIC) LYME DISEASE

Clinical Features

As spirochetes spread throughout the body during the dissemination phase of early Lyme disease, they may seed a variety of target organs, resulting in organ-specific manifestations of infection. The natural history of Lyme disease and the likelihood of developing organ-specific manifestations of disseminated disease were determined through clinical observation of patients from Connecticut prior to the recognition of its spirochetal etiology and responsiveness to antibiotic therapy. In these patients, 10% developed carditis, 15% developed neurologic involvement, and 60% developed arthritis. Because carditis and acute neurologic abnormalities generally occur weeks after the onset of the disease and arthritis months later (mean of 6 months after the onset of the disease), carditis and neurologic abnormalities were dubbed Stage II and arthritis as Stage III disease. It is now known that there are both acute and chronic forms of neurologic and joint involvement, which leads to some breakdown in this classification scheme. The staging scheme is gradually being replaced by one in which, regardless of organ system involved, progressive disease of less than 1 year in duration is called disseminated Lyme disease, and disease lasting for more than 1 year in duration is called chronic Lyme disease. It is most helpful to think in terms of a spectrum of organ-specific involvement ranging from acute, intermittent, self-limited inflammation to progressive chronic involvement. Patients often have several organ systems affected simultaneously or in sequence. For the sake of discussion of treatment, it is useful to describe specific manifestations separately, particularly because the clinical literature is structured this way.

Carditis

Because the vast majority of patients presenting with erythema migrans are properly diagnosed, treated, and cured, most patients presenting to physicians with carditis do not recall preceding ECM. The clinical features of carditis include varying degrees of atrioventricular block, other rhythm disturbances, and less commonly, reversible impairment of cardiac contractility. Symptoms include palpitations, syncope, dyspnea on exertion, and other manifestations of disturbance of cardiac rhythm. Carditis results from spirochetal invasion of the myocardium and the attendant inflammatory response, which seems to affect specialized conduction system tissues preferentially. Electrophysiologic studies have demonstrated widespread disturbances of cardiac conduction, but predominant involvement is proximal to the atrioventricular node. Carditis generally occurs long enough after onset of infection that either IgM or IgG antibodies are present.

THERAPY

Carditis is generally self-limited. Even without treatment, rhythm disturbances revert to normal after days to weeks. The possible consequences of long-term persistence of spirochetes in the myocardium are unknown. Therapy must be focused on sustaining circulation, through electrical support of cardiac rhythm, if necessary, and antibiotic therapy to eradicate *B. burgdorferi.* There are no controlled studies of therapy for Lyme carditis. Recommendations are based on empirical observation of outcomes. Patients have been treated successfully with corticosteroids, nonsteroidal anti-inflammatory agents, oral tetracycline, and intravenous penicillin and ceftriaxone. Although conduction abnormalities result from an inflammatory reaction involving the conduction system, which responds acutely to anti-inflammatory therapy alone, it is prudent to treat all cases of Lyme carditis with antibiotics in sufficient doses and for sufficient duration to eliminate spirochetes from the heart or elsewhere in the body.

All individuals with carditis and significant conduction abnormalities (high-degree atrioventricular block or first-degree block with PR interval longer than 0.3 seconds) should be admitted to the hospital and placed on a cardiac monitor. If necessary, a temporary cardiac pacemaker should be inserted to support the circulation. We do not recommend the use of glucocorticoids, even though they have been shown to be effective in reversing high-degree atrioventricular block, because of the chance that immunosuppression might interfere with eradication of infection. Generally, patients should be treated with intravenous ceftriaxone (Rocephin) (2 grams daily) or penicillin (20 million units daily) for 14 days. Patients with first-degree heart block with PR equal to or less than 0.3 seconds seem to be at negligible risk of progressing on to high-degree block and have been treated successfully with oral antibiotics with frequent monitoring of cardiac rhythm. Generally, oral antibiotics are given for 1 month in this circumstance. Although carditis is usually self-limited, case reports have documented that conduction disturbances may persist long after therapy has been completed.

Neurologic Manifestations

The spectrum of neurologic abnormalities associated with disseminated Lyme disease is very broad. The disease may affect all levels of the neuraxis. Lesions have been described involving the brain, spinal cord, meninges, nerve roots and plexi, and cranial and peripheral nerves. Lesions may be acute as occurs with cranial neuropathy (particularly Bell's palsy), radiculoneuropathy, and meningitis or chronic lesions (e.g., encephalopathy and peripheral sensory neuropathy).

Approximately 15% of individuals with untreated Lyme disease in the United States develop acute neurologic abnormalities a few weeks to a few months after the onset of infection. Bell's palsy (which may be bilateral) is the most common lesion. Other cranial neuropathies are rare. Meningitis, characterized by headache, mental irritability, and stiff neck usually without frank meningismus, occurs alone or with an associated Bell's palsy or radiculoneuropathy (so-called Bannwarth's syndrome). Spinal fluid of patients with Lyme meningitis reveals a predominantly lymphocytic pleocytosis with a few to a few hundred cells and a modest elevation in protein. *B. burgdorferi* has been cultured from meningitic spinal fluid. In cases in which inflammation has persisted for many weeks, oligoclonal bands may be present, reflecting clonal expansion of B cells in the cerebrospinal fluid. Lyme serologies are usually positive with either IgM or IgG antibodies. In some cases, specific antibody levels in cerebrospinal fluid are elevated as well.

Chronic neurologic syndromes described to date include a subtle encephalopathy characterized principally by impairment of short-term memory and energy depletion, as well as a subtle sensory neuropathy causing distal paresthesias. Cerebrospinal fluid is usually abnormal in such patients with elevated protein and low-grade pleocytosis. Chronic fatigue alone is not an indication of persistent Lyme disease. These symptoms may evolve very gradually many years after onset of Lyme disease.

THERAPY

The acute neurologic manifestations of Lyme disease remit spontaneously but sometimes wax and wane for many months before finally resolving. In general, chronic lesions are less responsive to antibiotic therapy. The prognosis of Bell's palsy is excellent. Similar to Bell's palsy due to other causes, spontaneous complete recovery is the rule. If there is no associated abnormality of the central nervous system, Bell's palsy can be treated with oral antibiotics; 4 weeks of therapy are generally recommended. All other neurologic manifestations are treated with intravenous antibiotics. Excellent outcomes have been achieved with ceftriaxone or penicillin. Cefotaxime (Claforan) (2 grams three times daily) has also produced excellent results, particularly in Europe. Neurologic signs and symptoms may resolve slowly; it is not necessary to continue antibiotics until all abnormalities resolve. Optimal duration of therapy is unknown. The minimum length of therapy should be 2 weeks and the maximum should be 4 weeks. Within these limits, therapy should be individualized and all patients should be followed carefully for evidence of relapse.

Optimum therapy and expected response to treatment of chronic Lyme disease has not yet been defined. Some patients do not seem to respond to month-long courses of therapy; it is not clear whether this is due to persistence of infection or noninfectious, immunologic mechanisms. Such patients should be referred for expert evaluation. Courses of therapy longer than 1 month should not be administered except in a clinical research setting.

Arthritis

Months after the onset of Lyme disease, 60% of patients develop acute, intermittent oligoarticular arthritis. Attacks, typically asymmetrical and monoarticular, have a sudden onset, persist for days to a few weeks, and remit spontaneously. One or both knees are affected in most patients. Swelling may be massive, and popliteal cysts, which may dissect or rupture, are common. Knee effusions of 50 to 100 mL are common. Joint fluid is inflammatory in nature, resembling that of rheumatoid arthritis. At the time that attacks occur, most patients have strongly positive Lyme serologies, particularly of the IgG class. Studies with the polymerase chain reaction have recently demonstrated that *B. burgdorferi* is present in the joint space at the onset of arthritis. Without treatment, attacks peak in frequency and severity in the first 1 to 2 years of illness and then spontaneously decrease in intensity, ultimately ceasing. Some patients, particularly those with the HLA DR4 genotype, may develop chronic persistent synovitis, defined as lasting longer than 1 year. Recent evidence suggests that these individuals may not have persistent infection but rather persistent inflammatory arthritis triggered by previous infection.

THERAPY

The goals of treatment of Lyme arthritis are to eradicate acute inflammation and prevent joint damage thus preserving function. As is the case with other infectious arthritides, the attainment of these goals entails appropriate antibiotic therapy, joint protection during bouts of acute inflammation, and joint drainage to remove inflammatory mediators. Patients with Lyme arthritis respond, in most cases, to month-long courses of amoxicillin (probenecid has usually been added) or doxycycline given orally. Inflammation resolves gradually, however, often requiring up to 3 months after completion of antibiotics. Clinical experience has also been favorable with 2- to 4-week courses of intravenous penicillin or ceftriaxone. No studies have compared intravenous and oral therapy, but patients who have failed to respond to oral therapy generally do not respond to intravenous treatment either. Those who fail to respond to antibiotic therapy can be treated successfully with synovectomy. Because persistent arthritis generally involves large joints (especially the knees), this procedure can usually be performed through the arthroscope.

It is important to search for concomitant neurologic involvement when evaluating patients for Lyme arthritis. Oral therapy is inappropriate for individuals with concurrent neurologic Lyme disease. Arthralgias alone rarely occur as a mild form of Lyme arthritis. It has been difficult to demonstrate antibiotic responsiveness in such individuals, many of whom have been found to have fibromyalgia on closer examination. Joint complaints in an individual with a positive Lyme serology are not sufficient to conclude that the individual has Lyme disease; the Lyme serology may be falsely positive, or the joint complaints may be due to another cause even though there is a history of Lyme disease. The best course in evaluating individuals with subtle joint or neurologic complaints and a question of Lyme disease is to document the extent of their inflammatory lesion or deficit objectively prior to deciding on any course of therapy. Then, if an inflammatory lesion is found that is consistent with Lyme disease, a therapeutic trial may be undertaken with the knowledge of identifiable endpoints and objective measures by which to gauge the success or failure of therapy. The presence of unexplained symptoms alone does not provide a satisfactory justification for antibiotic therapy for suspected Lyme disease.

ROCKY MOUNTAIN SPOTTED FEVER

method of
DANIEL J. SEXTON, M.D.
Duke University Medical Center
Durham, North Carolina

Rocky Mountain spotted fever (RMSF) is an acute febrile vasculitic illness caused by *Rickettsia rickettsii.* The name RMSF is somewhat misleading because the illness often occurs in the eastern United States and not all patients exhibit a spotted rash. Indeed, documented cases of RMSF have been reported from almost every state in the continental United States. At present, the incidence of RMSF is highest in Oklahoma and the southeastern United States. Because of the ease and rapidity of modern travel facilities, physicians in areas not considered highly endemic for RMSF must be alert for cases of disease imported from endemic areas. Risk of infection is higher in rural dwellers and outdoor enthusiasts such as hikers and campers, but cases often occur in suburban settings and RMSF has even been reported in urban areas such as New York City. RMSF occurs predominantly during the spring and summer months; occasionally, cases occur in the autumn and even in winter in southern states. Both the vector and principal reservoir of RMSF are hard-shelled (ixodid) ticks. The two most important tick vectors in the United States are the Rocky Mountain wood tick (*Dermacentor andersoni*) and the American dog tick (*Dermacentor variabilis*).

CLINICAL MANIFESTATIONS

RMSF usually begins as a nonspecific illness characterized by fever, myalgia, malaise, and headache. The onset may be either gradual or abrupt. In its earliest stages, it may be impossible to distinguish RMSF from a nonspecific viral illness. A skin rash occurs in most but not all patients 3 to 7 days after onset. The rash is classically described as first appearing on the ankles and wrists, and then spreading centripetally; however, such an evolution has little diagnostic utility and is often not observed. The rash may be maculopapular or petechial and often involves the palms and soles. In severe cases, the rash can lead to superficial skin necrosis or even gangrene of the extremities.

Headache is often severe. A wide variety of neurologic symptoms and signs, including confusion, seizures, and focal neurologic deficits, may occur in severe cases. Gastrointestinal symptoms such as nausea, vomiting, abdominal pain, and diarrhea are common in the early phases of illness and may lead to diagnostic confusion. Because the basic pathophysiologic lesion of RMSF is a rickettsia-induced vasculitis, virtually any organ may be involved. Thus, RMSF may occasionally mimic the clinical features of meningoencephalitis, hepatitis, nephritis, and even interstitial pneumonitis.

DIAGNOSIS

It is axiomatic that the diagnosis of RMSF must be made solely on epidemiologic and clinical grounds. Antimicrobial therapy should never be withheld while awaiting laboratory results. An absence of a history of tick bite should not dissuade the physician from suspecting RMSF and instituting therapy, because many patients are unaware of having a tick bite prior to onset of illness. Furthermore, skin rash may not appear for 5 or more days after the onset of symptoms; thus, absence of a characteristic skin rash should not prevent initiation of therapy if the index of suspicion for RMSF is high. In some medical centers, skin biopsy can be useful in making an early diagnosis but proof of the correct diagnosis usually requires measuring anti-rickettsial antibodies in properly timed acute and convalescent serum samples.

TREATMENT

The only two drugs effective in the treatment of RMSF are chloramphenicol and tetracycline. Although all forms of tetracycline are effective against *R. rickettsii,* doxycycline (Vibramycin) is the recommended tetracycline. For adults and children who weigh more than 45 kg, the recommended loading dose is 200 mg, followed by 100 mg orally or intravenously every 12 hours. In children who weigh less than 45 kg, the recommended intravenous or oral dose of doxycycline is 2 mg per kg every 12 hours for the first 24 hours, then 1 mg per kg every 12 hours thereafter. Administration of doxycycline and other tetracycline derivatives are not recommended for pregnant women. Although tetracyclines may cause dental staining if given in repetitive courses to young children, the risk of such staining is minimal if the drug is used for a single short course of therapy for suspected RMSF.

Chloramphenicol may be administered to adults either orally or intravenously at 50 mg per kg per day in four divided doses. The recommended dose for children is 50 mg per kg orally or 100 mg per kg per day intravenously. Chloramphenicol should not be given intramuscularly because absorption is erratic and unpredictable by this route. Frequent checks of the platelet count, hematocrit, and white blood cell count are mandatory in patients receiving chloramphenicol. Two types of bone marrow toxicity can occur in chloramphenicol-treated patients: one is common, dose related, and reversible; the other is rare, idiosyncratic, and results in irreversible aplastic anemia. Because of its potential for hematopoietic toxicity, chloramphenicol is best reserved for patients with severe disease, in whom clinical differentiation between RMSF and meningococcemia is difficult. Total daily doses should not exceed 4 grams. Antimicrobial therapy for RMSF is usually effective within 48 to 96 hours of starting treatment and should be continued for 3 to 5 days after the patient has become afebrile.

R. rickettsii infection can produce illnesses ranging from mild to fatal; thus, the physician must individualize treatment accordingly. For instance, patients who are recognized and treated early often have a benign course and can be managed as outpatients. In more severe cases, hospitalization and intensive nursing care as well as oxygen, mechanical ventilation, intravenous fluids, and even pressors may be necessary.

Careful monitoring of vital signs and other parameters of intravascular volume as well as urine output are important factors in patients with severe or fulminant illness. Intravascular volume deficits should be corrected using either saline or colloid-containing solutions. Hyponatremia may be a prominent laboratory abnormality in patients with RMSF. If there is evidence of volume and salt depletion, such as postural hypotension, poor skin turgor, or dry mucous membranes, intravenous therapy with isotonic saline solution is indicated. Rickettsia-induced myocarditis may occur; thus, careful observation for signs and symptoms of congestive heart failure is required during administration of fluids.

Thrombocytopenia is common in hospitalized patients with RMSF, and disseminated intravascular coagulation may occur in some patients. When it is present, disseminated intravascular coagulation is best treated by combating its underlying cause (rickettsemia) with either tetracycline or chloramphenicol.

PREVENTION

Spotted fever group rickettsiae circulate in nature in a tick-animal cycle completely independent of infection in humans; therefore, traditional vector control methods are neither effective nor practical. Persons exposed to ticks and tick-infested areas should regularly inspect their bodies and remove attached ticks promptly and carefully.

RMSF vaccine is of only limited benefit and is not currently available for clinical use. Because a well-established cycle of rickettsial infection exists in nature, reduction in morbidity and mortality caused by RMSF is best accomplished by prompt recognition and treatment of human disease. Because even expert physicians in endemic areas often have difficulty distinguishing uncomplicated febrile illnesses from the early phases of RMSF, a high index of suspicion, a knowledge of the local and national epidemiology of this potentially fatal disease, and prompt institution of empirical anti-rickettsial therapy is the best way to prevent morbidity and mortality.

RUBELLA AND CONGENITAL RUBELLA

method of
PETER MORGAN-CAPNER, F.R.C.PATH.
Royal Preston Hospital
Preston, United Kingdom

Rubella (German measles) is now an uncommon infection in countries that have achieved a high uptake of measles, mumps, and rubella (MMR) vaccine in infants. It must still be considered, however, on all occasions when rashes or contact with rubelliform illness occur during pregnancy as recent clusters of congenital rubella in the United States demonstrate.

CLINICAL MANIFESTATIONS

Up to 50% of cases of rubella in children are subclinical, but with increasing age, the proportion of subclinical infection falls, and in a majority of adults, infection is symptomatic. Rubella usually presents as a maculopapular, pinkish red rash with an incubation period of 14 to 21 days (usually 15 to 17 days). The rash starts on the face and neck but rapidly spreads to involve the body and limbs. The individual spots may coalesce, but the rash usually clears within 3 to 4 days. Itching is uncommon. The rash is often preceded by a few days of nonspecific illness with fever and upper respiratory tract symptoms. Conjunctivitis can occur but is seldom as severe as that seen in measles. Lymphadenopathy is common, with the suboccipital nodes most often involved. It frequently precedes the rash and may persist for some days. Fever is usually mild and, particularly in children, may be absent. Children usually have only mild disease with little or no systemic upset and only a fleeting rash.

COMPLICATIONS

The major complication of rubella is the potential for adverse effects on the fetus when infection occurs early in pregnancy (see further on). Although arthralgia is rare in children, it occurs in up to 30% of adults. The small joints are most frequently involved, particularly the hands and wrists. Although the joint symptoms usually resolve within a month, they can persist for much longer. Thrombocytopenia and postinfectious encephalitis are rare complications, the latter occurring in about 1 in 10,000 cases. Infection in the immunocompromised patient is not unduly severe nor does it have an unusual presentation.

DIFFERENTIAL DIAGNOSIS

The clinical diagnosis of rubella is notoriously unreliable, even during epidemics. Infection with other viruses, such as enteroviruses, particularly echoviruses, parvovirus B19, and even measles, can be easily confused with rubella. Differentiating the rash of parvovirus B19 infection from rubella is particularly problematic in adults, with arthralgia of small joints a common complication of both, and the characteristic malar erythema of parvovirus B19 infection in children a rare manifestation in adults. Nonspecific pinkish red macular rashes are not uncommon, particularly in children, and may also be due to noninfective causes such as allergy. As rubella becomes increasingly rare, further difficulties arise because the infection may not even be considered in the differential diagnosis by medical practitioners unfamiliar with its manifestations.

CONGENITAL RUBELLA

Primary rubella in the first 16 weeks of pregnancy presents a major risk to the fetus. Although transplacental infection can occur throughout pregnancy, the risk of fetal damage varies with gestation. Infection in the first 8 weeks causes intrauterine death or major malformations in up to 85% of fetuses. The risk falls progressively with gestational age, so that at 12 to 16 weeks, the risk is 20% and the only damage likely is sensorineural deafness. Beyond 16 weeks, although occasional cases of deafness may be attributable to intrauterine infection, the risk to the fetus is very remote and is probably close to zero for infections past 24 weeks' gestation. Rubella prior to conception carries minimal, if any, risk to the fetus.

Infection in the first 12 weeks is associated with a wide range of congenital abnormalities. The classic triad of the congenital rubella syndrome consists of deformities of the eye (cataract, micro-ophthalmia, chorioretinitis), heart (patent ductus arteriosus, pulmonary artery stenosis), and ear (sensorineural deafness). Neurologic complications such as microencephaly and mental retardation also occur, and a wide range of other manifestations may be present (intrauterine growth retardation, purpura, hepatosplenomegaly). Further problems may develop after birth and include immune-mediated pneumonitis, progressive rubella panencephalitis, and diabetes mellitus.

EPIDEMIOLOGY

Patients are infectious for 7 days prior to and after onset of rash. Transmission is by direct nasopharyngeal droplet spread with no evidence for survival of infectious virus in the environment or spread by fomite. There is no animal reservoir. Infants with congenital rubella can remain infected for many years, although infectivity for susceptible contacts is negligible after 1 year of age, and failure to isolate virus may be demonstrated in even younger patients. Before widespread infant immunization, epidemics of rubella were seen every 7 to 10 years, but the current pattern is one of low-level endemic infection with localized outbreaks, infection being most common in the spring.

DIAGNOSIS

Primary Rubella

Because clinical diagnosis is so unreliable, laboratory investigation must be performed to make the specific diagnosis. As has been demonstrated in recent clusters, a history of past vaccination or positive antibody screening, even if documented, does not necessarily exclude recent rubella. Hence, it is essential to investigate all rubelliform rashes in pregnancy. Because subclinical primary rubella can occur and damage the fetus, it is wise to also investigate all pregnant contacts of patients with rubelliform illness. If possible, the source patient should also be tested to ascertain the validity of the diagnosis of rubella.

Virus isolation has no place in the diagnosis of postnatal primary rubella because it is unreliable and may take some weeks. Diagnosis is serologic, and serum should be obtained as soon as possible after contact or onset of illness. Procedures and tests vary by laboratory, but it is essential for correct testing and interpretation of results that full clinical details are given, including any past testing and immunization. Most laboratories will test either for total antibody by hemagglutination inhibition (HI) or for specific IgG by a wide variety of tests, and if the titer is high enough, for specific IgM. The detection of specific IgM is usually considered indicative of recent primary rubella, but all specific IgM assays may occasionally give false-positive results, and care is needed in their interpretation. False-positive specific IgM results can occur in infectious mononucleosis and parvovirus B19 infection, both of which may be clinically confused with rubella. Depending on the results obtained with the first serum, it will often be necessary to repeat tests 1 to 4 weeks later. The final interpretation will depend on the serologic results taken in conjunction with the clinical details and history of antibody testing and vaccination.

Reinfection

Reinfection is usually diagnosed in the laboratory by demonstrating a rise in antibody titer after recent contact with rubella by someone who has had natural rubella or successful immunization. The risk to the fetus posed by reinfection in early pregnancy is ill defined but likely to be less than 10%, substantially less than the risk with primary rubella. Reinfection is rarely symptomatic, but the differentiation of primary rubella from reinfection in the asymptomatic patient is critical in determining proper treatment. Routine rubella antibody tests may not be able to distinguish these conditions, however, because rubella-specific IgM can often be detected in reinfections, albeit usually at a lower concentration than in primary rubella.

If primary rubella or reinfection is diagnosed in pregnancy, further management will depend on patient counseling, including assessment of the degree and type of risk to the fetus and the possible prognosis for the baby.

Congenital Rubella

Isolation of virus from urine, throat swab, or tissue is of value in diagnosing congenital rubella, but sufficient virologic expertise for reliable isolation and identification is often not readily available. The detection of specific IgM in neonatal or infant serum is highly reliable, because almost all babies with congenital rubella are seropositive for the first 3 months of life, and most remain so for 6 months. At older ages, but before administration of MMR, persistence of specific IgG or total antibody is diagnostic, because maternal antibody will decline to negativity during the first year of life.

Rubella Antibody Screening

To determine whether a patient is susceptible to rubella, and hence should be immunized, testing for rubella-specific IgG or total antibody is required. There are many reliable assays, including HI, latex agglutination, radial hemolysis, and enzyme-linked immunosorbent assay (ELISA). Sensitivity of the assays varies, and debate continues about the protective efficacy of low concentrations of antibody. Although immunization may be advised for those with low concentrations of antibody (less than 15 IU), it may not boost their antibody levels. Protection against primary rubella can be assumed if two or more doses of vaccine have been given, even if the antibody concentration does not increase.

TREATMENT

There is no justification for the routine administration of gamma globulin to susceptible women after contact with rubella. Although there may be some attenuation of illness, no prophylactic effect or reduced transmission to the fetus has been demonstrated.

Antiviral drugs have not been used for the treatment of postnatal or congenital rubella.

RUBELLA VACCINE

Rubella vaccine (RA 27/3 strain) is available either as a component of MMR or as a single vaccine. It induces protection in more than 95% of recipients. Widespread administration of MMR vaccine to infants at age 15 months has had a major impact on the incidence of rubella. To ensure a continued low incidence, it is necessary to maintain high immunization levels by enforcing school entry laws and targeting socioeconomically deprived groups. Continued efforts must also be made to identify susceptible adolescent and adult women who would benefit from immunization. Screening in occupational health departments, prenatal clinics, family planning services, and college health services should continue.

Rubella vaccine is a live attenuated virus, and rarely a mild rubelliform illness will be seen 2 to 3 weeks after immunization. Arthralgia may occur, but an association with long-term arthritis is disputed and seems unlikely. Administration during pregnancy should be avoided, and an immunized female should not become pregnant for 3 months afterward. If inadvertent immunization in pregnancy does occur, the risk to the fetus is remote; no congenital abnormalities have been found in term infants (maximum risk is 2%, similar to that for nonexposed babies), although in occasional cases, the fetus may have been infected.

Vaccination in immunocompromised individuals, including those infected with human immunodeficiency virus, has not been associated with significant side effects, but further guidance should be sought if immunization of such individuals is considered.

Immunization should be postponed for 3 months after administration of intramuscular gamma globulin or blood transfusion. Anti-D antibody does not interfere with development of immunity, although follow-up serologic testing is advisable. Vaccine virus cannot be transmitted between the immunized individual and susceptible contacts.

MEASLES

method of
DAVID S. SMITH, M.D.
Temple University School of Medicine
Philadelphia, Pennsylvania

Measles is a highly contagious systemic disease caused by an RNA virus whose only natural hosts are humans. An incubation period of approximately 10 days is followed by fever, coryza, conjunctivitis, cough, and Koplik spots, which, in turn, are followed in 3 to 4 days by an erythematous, maculopapular rash that evolves in a cephalocaudad fashion. The cough often reflects an accompanying laryngotracheitis; abdominal pain is common, and diarrhea is frequent in small children. Koplik spots, which appear in the pre-eruptive phase on the buccal and labial mucosa, are bluish white specks on an erythematous base and are pathognomonic. Fever usually resolves after the sixth or seventh day of illness as the rash fades to a brownish tint, which may be followed by mild desquamation.

The distinctive pattern of symptoms and the troublesome cough usually make the diagnosis relatively easy, although confusion has occurred with Kawasaki disease, streptococcal and staphylococcal toxic shock syndromes, and drug eruptions. The clinical diagnosis of measles may be difficult in infants whose illness has been modified by transplacental passive protection or by previous immunization. Indeed, several recent studies have suggested that some secondary school students who had been previously immunized were susceptible to measles infection without rash.

Laboratory examinations that support the diagnosis of measles include virus isolation, serum IgM titers, and acute and convalescent sera for IgG titers. Leukopenia, lymphopenia, and thrombocytopenia are usual. An elevated erythrocyte sedimentation rate, an increase in platelet and leukocyte counts, and changes on echocardiogram may aid in the diagnosis of Kawasaki disease.

EPIDEMIOLOGY

Many physicians have seen measles for the first time in the past decade, which has added to the confusion in diagnosis. After a dramatic reduction in incidence in the United States following routine immunization, cases of measles increased annually from 1983 to 1993, when a decline was observed. Outbreaks of disease have occurred in urban areas involving unvaccinated children of preschool age and in young adults, most of whom had been previously immunized. It has also been apparent that the immunity provided to the fetus and newborn infant has been largely derived from a new generation of mothers whose own immunity has been vaccine derived. It has not been uncommon to observe measles in 6-month-old infants in contrast to the prevaccine era, when the diagnosis was rarely made in the first year of life and immunity of the mother was derived from the natural disease. Also missing from the immune experiences of a new generation has been the absence of periodic exposure to the wild virus from so-called subway contacts.

COMPLICATIONS

Measles remains a disease of significant morbidity and mortality; complications can be severe. Otitis media is common; pneumonia should be suspected in children with respiratory distress and persistent fever. Frequently, the presence of laryngotracheitis raises concerns of airway obstruction. Secondary bacterial pneumonia is the most common cause of death, although primary measles pneumonia may occur, particularly in immunocompromised children. Approximately one in a thousand children develops acute encephalomyelitis, most commonly between the second and sixth day after onset of rash. Drowsiness, seizures, and coma are seen, often with signs of meningeal irritation. Much clinical variation occurs, but death may ensue within 24 hours in approximately 15% of patients; 25% of patients survive with neurologic sequelae. The remaining 60% recover completely.

Subacute sclerosing panencephalitis as a complication of chronic infection of the central nervous system with the measles virus has virtually disappeared in the vaccination era.

Thrombocytopenia commonly is observed following the natural infection and the use of live attenuated measles vaccine. Infrequently, numbers of platelets are depressed enough to be complicated by capillary bleeding. No teratogenic effects have been noted when pregnancy is complicated by measles; however, fetal wastage and premature births are common. Activation of pulmonary tuberculosis has been noted; anergy to tuberculoprotein may persist for 6 weeks following clinical measles. Children with human immunodeficiency virus disease are at serious risk of pneumonia and death.

THERAPY

No specific therapy exists for the treatment of measles, although ribavirin (Virazole)* is effective in vitro. Limited data from Mexico, Brazil and the Philippines suggest reduction in severity and duration of disease when the drug is administered in the preeruptive phase. Although vitamin A deficiency is rarely recognized clinically in the United States, recent observations have led to recommendations by the American Academy of Pediatrics that vitamin A supplementation be considered for all hospitalized infants from 6 months to 2 years. Therapy recommended is a single dose of 200,000 units orally for children 1 year of age and older and 100,000 units for infants from 6 months to 1 year of age. The dose should be repeated in 24 hours and at 4 weeks for children with ophthalmologic evidence of vitamin A deficiency. It is important to recognize that these doses are 100 to 200 times the recommended dietary daily allowance and that patients should be monitored for toxicity.

Standard antibiotic therapy is recommended for otitis media and pneumonia. Cough suppressants are discouraged. Specific therapy for conjunctivitis is unnecessary, although corneal ulcerations occur rarely.

PREVENTION

Present recommendations provide for immunizing immunocompetent infants at 12 months of age with live attenuated measles vaccine routinely included in a trivalent preparation, measles-mumps-rubella (MMR). A second dose of MMR is recommended at 4 to 5 years of age (Advisory Committee on Immunization Practices) or at 12 years of age (American Academy of Pediatrics). Local or regional guidelines should be followed. In the presence of local epidemics, monovalent measles vaccine should be given at 6 months of age, followed by booster doses of MMR at 15 months and later in childhood, respectively.

Children with HIV infection who are asymptomatic should receive MMR. In addition, those children who are symptomatic with HIV should be considered for vaccination with live attenuated virus because of the severity of the disease in these children and the lack of reports of complications associated with vaccination.

Measles vaccine, however, is not to be given to persons (other than those with human immunodeficiency virus [HIV]) with impaired cell-mediated immunity, to pregnant women, and to individuals with a history of anaphylaxis due to egg or neomycin. Administration of vaccine should be deferred for 3 months after receipt of immunoglobulin or blood products and after immunosuppressive therapy has been discontinued.

POSTEXPOSURE PROPHYLAXIS

Measles vaccine can be given within 72 hours of exposure and likely provides protection against clinical measles as does the administration of standard intramuscular immunoglobulin when given within 6 days of exposure. The dose of immunoglobulin is 0.25 mL per kg for healthy children and 0.5 mL per kg for immunocompromised patients with a maximum dose of 15 mL. HIV-infected patients should receive immunoglobulin irrespective of vaccine status and even if they are being treated with immunoglobulin intravenously.

*Not FDA approved for this indication.

TETANUS

method of
L. ANDREW RAUSCHER, M.D.
The Mary Imogene Bassett Hospital
Cooperstown, New York

The clinical manifestations of tetanus are caused by an exotoxin, tetanospasmin, produced by the organism *Clostridium tetani,* which causes muscle rigidity, reflex spasms, and in some cases, autonomic dysreflexia.

ETIOLOGY

C. tetani is an anaerobic, gram-positive rod producing highly resistant spores that may survive for years. Vegetative forms produce two exotoxins: (1) tetanospasmin, a soluble, oxygen-resistant neurotoxin, second only to botulinum toxin in potency, and (2) tetanolysin, a clinically insignificant producer of hemolysis in vitro.

EPIDEMIOLOGY

Less than 50 cases of tetanus are reported in the United States each year, primarily in persons over 50 years of age. Approximately 5% of reported cases had received at least a primary immunization series. The disease is seen more frequently in rural, temperate, or tropical populations with poor immunization programs, poverty, and lack of adequate health care. Neonatal tetanus is an important cause of death in underdeveloped countries.

Spores of *C. tetani* are ubiquitous and are found in many locations, especially soil, clothing, household and hospital dust, animal and human skin, and the human intestinal tract.

PATHOGENESIS

Infection follows local injury, although no history of trauma or detectable wound is found in 20% of patients. The wound can be located anywhere but is more common on the hand or foot; many wounds are probably contaminated with the organism but do not present favorable conditions for vegetative growth.

In the presence of low oxygen tensions, infected or necrotic tissue, or low oxidation-reduction potentials, vegetative growth occurs locally, but exotoxin is disseminated by intra-axonal or blood-borne spread. Tetanospasmin produces dysfunction of motor end-plates, spinal cord internuncial neurons, and some cranial ganglia, resulting in reflex irritability, rigidity, dysinhibition of antagonistic muscles, and the early appearance of trismus and neck rigidity. Dysinhibition of the autonomic nervous system may produce sympathetic dysfunction as the disease progresses. There is no permanent effect of the toxin in patients who survive the disease.

CLINICAL COURSE

The incubation period for the development of symptoms is from 1 day to several months, with a median of 8 days. The shorter the incubation period, the more severe the disease is likely to be. Prodromal symptoms of malaise, irritability, and headache are unusual. Seventy-five percent of patients present with trismus, often to dentists. Others present with neck stiffness, dysphagia, or reflex spasm. As the disease progresses, muscle rigidity and reflex spasms increase in severity. The severity of the disease is indicated by the rate of onset from first symptoms to reflex spasms. Muscle rigidity and sustained contractions frequently begin in the facial and jaw muscles and progress to extensor movements in limbs and opisthotonos. Excruciatingly painful tonic/clonic spasms are present in 70% of patients and may be provoked by external stimuli such as noise, light, and handling; hypoxia and exhaustion are common. In the later stages, minimal stimuli may provoke severe and long-lasting spasms with increasing frequency. At any stage, gas exchange may be severely compromised by laryngospasm and respiratory muscle impairment. Hypoxia-associated brain, cardiac, or renal damage may occur, especially in older patients or those with other medical problems such as cardiovascular compromise. Although the overall mortality rate is 26%, the fatality rate in patients over 60 years of age at present is 52%.

Two rarer presentations have been described: (1) local tetanus is manifested by rigidity of muscle groups near the site of infection and (2) cephalic tetanus follows ear infections or head wounds and is characterized by cranial nerve dysfunction, especially of cranial nerves III, IV, VII, IX, X, and XII. Generalized tetanus may follow either of these rarer forms if left untreated.

Late in the course of the disease, signs of sympathetic overactivity may be associated with the more severe forms of tetanus, with labile hypertension or hypotension, tachycardia, and dysrhythmias. With treatment, the spasms gradually diminish in frequency and severity and end between 2 and 4 weeks after onset. During convalescence, residual stiffness may persist for some time. The development of tetanus does not confer immunity from future episodes, and formal immunization schedules must be implemented.

DIAGNOSIS

The diagnosis is clinical, with a history of injury followed by manifestations of the disease. Cultures are not reliable; white cell counts, creatine phosphokinase levels, cerebrospinal fluid examinations, and blood chemistries are frequently normal. Once the disease is clinically obvious, complicating cardiopulmonary, fluid, and electrolyte changes may become apparent. The absence of abnormal laboratory, radiologic, and other findings is itself diagnostic.

The differential diagnosis is one of exclusion of trismus due to localized conditions, phenothiazine toxicity, meningitis, tetany, strychnine poisoning, and subluxation of the mandible. Close observation of the patient and a high index of suspicion are usually confirmatory.

TREATMENT

All cases occurring in older persons and any other patient presenting with short incubation or onset periods should be managed aggressively given the high rates of morbidity and mortality in this group.

Human tetanus immune globulin (TIG) (Hyper-Tet), 3000 to 6000 units is given intramuscularly as soon as possible to neutralize free toxin. Only one dose is recommended, and hypersensitivity reactions are extremely rare. If human TIG is not available, horse-serum tetanus antitoxin is given after negative tests for hypersensitivity to equine serum, in doses of 50000 units intramuscularly and 50000 units intravenously. Immune globulin should be given in a different site from any previously administered tetanus toxoid.

Three to 4 hours after antitoxin administration, any identifiable wound is cultured and thoroughly debrided; the delay is necessary to ensure adequate antitoxin levels if tetanospasmin is liberated during débridement.

Antibiotics are given after débridement to destroy any remaining vegetative organisms. Metronidazole (Flagyl) may now be the drug of choice in doses of 7.5 mg per kg infused over 1 hour every 6 hours following a loading dose of 15 mg per kg over 1 hour; penicillin is the more traditional therapy in doses of 1.2 million units of procaine penicillin daily or penicillin G, 1 million units intravenously every 6 hours, although there is a potential for the development of nosocomial infections and potentiation of gamma-aminobutyric acid–induced hypertonia. Cephalosporins are also effective.

The mainstay of treatment is supportive while the toxin is slowly eliminated. Virtually all patients continue to deteriorate after initial admission and diagnosis. The high incidence of respiratory complications from the disease itself and the side effects of therapy designed to reduce oxygen consumption, spasms, and rigidity determine early and aggressive airway and ventilatory management. When there is any doubt about continued airway patency or difficulty with swallowing, or if there are any hypoxic episodes or drug-induced respiratory depression, tracheal intubation should be performed. Bedside continuous pulse oximetry is very helpful in assessment. Intubation is best accomplished by the careful induction of general anesthesia using short-acting barbiturates and muscle relaxants. Mivacurium (Mivacron), 0.15 mg per kg, or atracurium (Tracrium), 0.5 mg per kg, is preferable to succinylcholine (Anectine) to facilitate atraumatic intubation, as long as airway control can be established because hyperkalemia is less likely.

Initial nasotracheal intubation is desirable, pending assessment of progress of the disease over a number of days, and tracheostomy should not be considered until it is established that airway control will be required for more than 2 or 3 weeks. In mild cases managed by sedation alone, skilled staff and equipment for tracheal intubation must be immediately available until recovery is apparent.

Control of neuromuscular manifestations of tetanus is critical to reduce the pain, anxiety, and marked rise in oxygen consumption that accompany rigidity and skeletal muscle spasms. Diazepam (Valium) reduces oxygen consumption and rigidity and produces amnesia but does not prevent reflex spasms.

In mild cases, diazepam, up to 0.3 mg per kg, may be the only necessary treatment; in more severe cases, diazepam alone will only produce an oversedated patient with no guarantee of airway competency, while spasms will continue. Diazepam does not produce analgesia, and the addition of potent narcotics for pain control increases the potential for cardiorespiratory depression.

In moderate or severe cases, nondepolarizing neuromuscular blockers and ventilatory support should be used. Pancuronium bromide may be given in intermittent doses or by infusion, titrated to muscle tone or twitch response. Atracurium, 10 to 20 mg per hour, or vecuronium (Norcuron), 2 to 10 mg per hour, can be given by continuous infusion; infusion allows easier reassessment by temporary cessation of infusion without pharmacologic reversal of the neuromuscular block.

Sedation must be adequate in the paralyzed patient. Diazepam (Valium) (5 to 10 mg per hour, at least initially), lorazepam (Ativan), or midazolam (Versed), by continuous infusion ensures amnesia and sedation. Propofol (Diprivan), 3.5 to 4.5 mg per kg per hour, has also recently been found effective and has the advantage of rapid recovery of consciousness, unlike the benzodiazepines. A combination of diazepam or lorazepam and narcotics will produce sedation, amnesia, and pain relief. Morphine has been shown not only to function as an effective analgesic, but also to modify the severity of autonomic dysfunction.

Dantrolene sodium (Dantrium) has been used to inhibit excitation-contraction coupling in malignant hyperthermia, as well as in the control of several spastic complications of neurologic disease. There are isolated case reports of successful management of rigidity and spasm in tetanus by dantrolene in doses of 1.0 to 2.0 mg per kg, repeated every 4 to 6 hours.

General supportive measures include initial parenteral nutrition followed by tube feedings, and the prevention of pulmonary complications. Passive physiotherapy, frequent turning, and the use of a rocking bed minimize contractures, decubitus ulcers, and ventilation/perfusion mismatch problems. Risk of pulmonary embolus may be reduced by antiembolism stockings and low-dose heparin or aspirin. The administration of antacids or H2 antagonists minimizes the risk of peptic ulcer. All nursing and physical care should be performed during periods of maximum sedation in a quiet, semidark environment, and unnecessary stimulation should be avoided.

With a diminution in the frequency or severity of rigidity and muscle spasms, progressive withdrawal of muscle relaxants can be undertaken. Conventional criteria for extubation are used including lung mechanics, gas exchange criteria, normal chest x-ray study, and demonstrable airway control and swallowing, when muscle relaxants are no longer necessary.

Monitoring of moderate to severe disease includes direct arterial pressure and access for blood gas and chemistries, and pulse oximetry and capnography for continuous noninvasive vigilance and reduction of iatrogenic anemia by frequent sampling; nosocomial screening, fluid, electrolyte and nutritional assessments are made on a regular basis. Additional monitoring modalities are employed if complications develop.

COMPLICATIONS

In apparently mild cases, an important complication is a failure to recognize the actual severity of the disease. Loss of airway competence or cardiorespiratory depression may follow overzealous administration of sedatives.

General complications of moderate to severe cases are those of any long-term immobilized patient requiring mechanical ventilation, particularly malnutrition, stress ulcers, deep venous thrombosis, opportunistic infections, decubitus ulcers, and progressive ventilation-perfusion inequalities. General supportive measures have already been summarized.

Specific early respiratory complications are frequent; a restrictive ventilatory defect results from chest wall rigidity, with reduced chest wall compliance, shallow breathing, reduced ability to cough, and a fall in functional residual capacity; atelectasis and infection may follow. In addition, there is a decreased ventilatory response to carbon dioxide, which returns to normal after recovery from the disease.

Specific cardiac complications may follow hypoxemia (in older patients) or myocardial intoxication, with a histologic myocarditis similar to that sometimes seen in phaeochromocytoma. A direct intoxication of medullary cardiovascular centers has been postulated. Dysrhythmias are common and should be treated symptomatically. ST-T changes occur in about one-third of all patients but return to normal after recovery.

Sympathetic dysreflexia is the most serious of the specific complications and is not seen until late in the disease. An initial unexplained tachycardia is followed by labile hypertension and a high cardiac output, particularly in response to stimuli. Systemic vascular resistance becomes progressively elevated. Profuse sweating may occur in normothermic patients, and fever may develop in the absence of infection. Sodium and water retention, and increases in serum cortisol and urine catecholamines may occur. Bradycardia and hypotension appear late in the course of the disease and are ominous signs.

Recognition and aggressive management of circulatory instability are crucial to reduce late mortality. Monitoring should include direct arterial and pulmonary artery catheterization, reserved for the second or third week of the disease when circulatory instability occurs. The differential diagnosis of the circulatory changes requires filling pressure measurement but the usual calculated indices of cardiac function. The differential diagnosis includes pulmonary embolus, pneumonia, and septicemia, as well as other intercurrent illness, such as visceral perforation or gastrointestinal bleeding.

Management of sympathetic instability requires the use of alpha-blockade and beta-blockade and careful manipulation of filling pressures and cardiac output. Phentolamine (Regitine), pentolinium,* and guanethidine-like drugs are preferable to nitroprusside (Nipride), allowing smoother control of hypertension over a longer period without accumulation of cyanide. Propranolol (Inderal) is used to control tachycardia, either intravenously or intragastrically; labetolol (Normodyne) and, more recently, esmolol (Brevibloc) infusions titrated to effect have been used to control hypertensive and tachycardic episodes. Magnesium infusions have been used but require careful monitoring of magnesium and calcium levels and do not obviate the need for sedation. Continuous epidural block has also been used to modify the autonomic nervous system response and need for muscle relaxation.

Orthopedic complications include dislocation of the temporomandibular and shoulder joints. Thoracic vertebral fractures are often seen but usually do not result in neurologic sequelae. Urinary retention results when perineal muscles are affected.

Recurrent tetanus is a threat because survivors do not develop active immunity to the disease. A full course of passive tetanus immunization must be initiated during the rehabilitation phase of recovery.

*Not available in the United States.

TOXOPLASMOSIS

method of
SHARON B. MANNHEIMER, M.D., and
HENRY W. MURRAY, M.D.
Cornell University Medical College
New York, New York

Toxoplasmosis is a common and worldwide infection caused by the intracellular coccidian protozoan *Toxoplasma gondii.* After cysts or oocysts are ingested, liberated trophozoites spread hematogenously to virtually every organ. Intracellular replication commences following phagocytosis by tissue macrophages or invasion of parenchymal cells. With the development of an effective immune response, extracellular trophozoites are killed by specific serum antibodies, whereas intracellular *Toxoplasma* organisms are killed or inhibited by T cell–dependent mechanisms. Some organisms, however, survive and form tissue cysts. The brain, retina, myocardium, lung, and skeletal muscle are favored sites for encystment. During the acute stages of toxoplasmosis, most patients remain entirely asymptomatic; approximately 20% develop lymphadenitis or nonspecific flulike symptoms, or both. In addition, although all individuals probably remain infected with tissue cysts for life, clinical problems related to chronic toxoplasmosis (other than perhaps reactivated ocular disease) seldom, if ever, develop in the immunocompetent adult. Thus, in most infected individuals, treatment is never required. However,

TABLE 1. **Syndromes Caused by *Toxoplasma gondii* Infection**

Toxoplasma Infection	Treatment Appropriate?
Acute	
Asymptomatic	No
Lymphadenitis	Rarely
Laboratory acquired	Yes
Ocular (retinochoroiditis)	Yes
During pregnancy	Yes
Congenital	Yes
Chronic/reactivated	
Ocular	Yes
Disseminated/encephalitis	Yes

certain groups of patients do warrant specific therapy (Table 1).

ANTITOXOPLASMA THERAPY

The combination of pyrimethamine (Daraprim) plus sulfadiazine is the most effective regimen for the treatment of toxoplasmosis (see Table 2 for dosing and toxicity). These agents sequentially block folic acid metabolism and are synergistic against the proliferative trophozoite form of *T. gondii.* They have no activity, however, against tissue cysts. Folinic acid (leucovorin),* which is preferentially transported into mammalian but not protozoal cells, is used to minimize the bone marrow suppression associated with pyrimethamine. Complete blood and platelet counts should be followed closely in patients receiving pyrimethamine.

Among the sulfonamides, sulfadiazine, sulfapyrazine,† sulfamerazine, sulfamethazine, and sulfisoxazole all display activity against *T. gondii* and can act synergistically with pyrimethamine. Although sulfadiazine is most often used, trisulfapyrimidine (Triple sulfa)* which contains sulfadiazine, sulfamerazine, and sulfamethazine, can also be given along with pyrimethamine.

Clindamycin (Cleocin) in combination with pyrimethamine is an effective alternative regimen in sulfonamide-intolerant patients.

Spiramycin (Rovamycine)‡ is a macrolide antibiotic that appears to be useful in treating acute infection during pregnancy as well as congenital infection.

Other investigational agents with antitoxoplasma activity include atovaquone (Mepron),* azithromycin (Zithromax),* and clarithromycin (Biaxin). These three agents are also active against the tissue cyst form of *T. gondii* in experimental models.

INDICATIONS FOR THERAPY

Immunocompetent Individuals. Immunologically intact children and adults who develop acute symptomatic toxoplasmosis seldom require treatment.

*Not FDA approved for this indication.
†Not available in the United States.
‡Investigational drug in the United States.

TABLE 2. **Drugs Used in the Treatment of Toxoplasmosis**

Drug	Dosage		Adverse Effects
	Initial	*Maintenance*	
Pyrimethamine* (Daraprim)	50–75 mg daily†	50 mg daily	Thrombocytopenia, megaloblastic anemia, leukopenia, rash, vomiting, diarrhea
Sulfadiazine*	4–8 gm daily	2 grams daily	Hypersensitivity reactions (with rash and fever), nausea, vomiting, diarrhea
Clindamycin‡ (Cleocin)	450–600 mg qid (PO or IV)	300 mg qid	Diarrhea, pseudomembranous colitis, rash
Spiramycin‖ (Rovamycine)	3 grams daily		Nausea, abdominal pain
Atovaquone‡ (Mepron)	750 mg qid		Rash, fever
Azithromycin‡ (Zithromax)	500 mg q d		Diarrhea, nausea, abdominal pain
Clarithromycin‡ (Biaxin)	1000 mg bid		Diarrhea, nausea, abdominal pain

*Pyrimethamine is used in combination with either sulfadiazine or clindamycin. Folinic acid (leucovorin) (Wellcovorin) 10 mg per day is added to pyrimethamine-containing regimens to limit bone marrow suppression.
†After loading dose of 100 mg taken twice on day 1 of therapy.
‡Not FDA approved for this indication.
‖Investigational drug in the United States.
Spiramycin can be obtained from the U.S. Food and Drug Administration.

However, with either vital organ involvement or a particularly severe or protracted illness, pyrimethamine plus sulfadiazine can be given for 4 to 6 weeks. Infections acquired by blood transfusion or laboratory accident probably also should be treated. Acute infection during pregnancy also requires treatment because of the risk of congenital toxoplasmosis.

Retinochoroiditis. Active ocular toxoplasmosis most commonly follows congenital infection, with a peak incidence of reactivation in the second and third decades of life. Antitoxoplasma therapy may reduce the extent of disease and lead to less retinal scarring. Pyrimethamine plus sulfadiazine is the treatment of choice and is administered for 1 month. Clindamycin* alone or in combination with sulfadiazine and trimethoprim-sulfamethoxazole* alone have also been reported to be effective. With any regimen, retreatment may be required because of relapse. High-dose corticosteroids are added with sight-threatening lesions such as those involving the macula or optic nerve in order to reduce inflammation.

Acute Toxoplasmosis in Pregnancy. *T. gondii* can cross the placenta and infect the fetus during acute maternal infection. There is a lag time between maternal and fetal infection, and prompt maternal treatment can reduce fetal transmission. Spiramycin (Rovamycine),† a macrolide antibiotic with antitoxoplasma activity, concentrates in the placenta and can be used in pregnancy (see Table 2 for dosing and toxicity). When the prenatal diagnosis of fetal toxoplasmosis is established, women who wish to continue their pregnancies should be maintained on antitoxoplasma therapy for the duration of the pregnancy to try to minimize the sequelae of infection. Pyrimethamine (50 mg per day) plus sulfadiazine (3 grams per day) can be used after the sixteenth week of pregnancy in cases of documented fetal infection. This regimen is alternated with spiramycin every 3 weeks until delivery. Folinic acid* is added during the course of therapy with pyrimethamine and sulfadiazine.

Congenital Toxoplasmosis. Neonates who test positive for toxoplasma-specific IgM or who are strongly suspected of having congenital infection should be treated for 6 to 12 months to try to minimize the extent of tissue damage. Because the specific regimens are controversial and not necessarily based on firm clinical data, expert consultation should be enlisted to assist with management in such cases. Pyrimethamine plus sulfadiazine and folinic acid* are recommended for the first 6 months in infants with clinical infection. The pyrimethamine and sulfadiazine are then alternated with spiramycin for an additional 6 months. Prednisone (1 to 2 mg per kg per day) is added for infants with evidence of ongoing inflammation. Infants with subclinical infection should also be treated; spiramycin† alternating with pyrimethamine and sulfadiazine for 6 to 12 months has been suggested.

REACTIVATED TOXOPLASMOSIS

In immunocompetent individuals, *T. gondii* reactivation rarely occurs in areas other than the retina (see the section on Retinochoroiditis). In hosts with impaired cell-mediated immunity, however, quiescent cysts can reactivate and result in disseminated infection. Toxoplasmosis has become a major clinical problem in patients with the acquired immune deficiency syndrome (AIDS). Approximately one-third of human immunodeficiency virus (HIV)–infected individuals with evidence of prior exposure to *T. gondii* (positive IgG serology) will develop toxoplasma encephalitis.

Therapy. Empiric treatment is often initiated without a tissue diagnosis in HIV-infected persons with suspected toxoplasma encephalitis. Patients who do not respond clinically within 14 days are then considered for brain biopsy. Pyrimethamine (100 mg) twice on day 1, followed by 75 mg per day) combined

†Investigational drug in the United States.

*Not FDA approved for this indication.
†Investigational drug in the United States.

with sulfadiazine 100 mg per kg per day (4 to 8 grams) is the current treatment of choice for cerebral or disseminated toxoplasmosis in AIDS. Clindamycin* 450 mg three times a day orally or 600 mg four times a day intravenously is an effective alternative to sulfadiazine for sulfonamide-intolerant patients. Folinic acid (Leucovorin)* is added to these regimens to prevent bone marrow toxicity. Because relapse rates as high as 50% occur after the withdrawal of antitoxoplasma therapy, AIDS patients require lifelong maintenance therapy after responding to initial treatment. The maintenance regimens use the same agents at lower doses (Table 2). These regimens are all associated with significant toxicity, and alternative agents are under investigation.

Preliminary reports have demonstrated the efficacy of azithromycin* alone, atovaquone alone,* and clarithromycin* plus pyrimethamine in treating toxoplasmosis in AIDS patients who are intolerant of standard regimens. Trimetrexate† was not effective as monotherapy. At present, azithromycin plus pyrimethamine is being evaluated in the treatment of toxoplasma encephalitis in patients with AIDS.

Prophylaxis. HIV-infected persons with CD4 cell counts below 200 per mm^3 and evidence of previous *T. gondii* infection (positive IgG serology) are at obvious risk for reactivation of infection. This group has been targeted for primary prophylaxis. Unfortunately, many of the available data come from small retrospective studies of patients receiving primary or secondary prophylaxis for *Pneumocystis carinii* pneumonia. Both trimethoprim-sulfamethoxazole* alone (from 4 to 7 double-strength tablets per week) and dapsone* (50 mg per day) plus pyrimethamine (50 mg per week) appear to be effective in preventing reactivation of toxoplasmosis. Data from Europe suggest that roxithromycin‡ is also effective. Larger prospective comparative trials are needed. Pyrimethamine or trimethoprim-sulfamethoxazole monotherapy also appear to be effective as prophylaxis in preventing toxoplasmosis in organ transplant recipients.

---

*Not FDA approved for this indication.
†Investigational drug in the United States.
‡Not available in the United States.

TRICHINOSIS

method of
R. GOPINATH, M.D., and
J. S. KEYSTONE, M.D., M.Sc. (C.T.M.)
The Toronto Hospital
Toronto, Ontario, Canada

Trichinosis is a parasitic disease of humans characterized by fever, gastrointestinal symptoms, myositis, periorbital edema, and eosinophilia. The nematode is acquired by ingestion of meat containing infective encysted larvae of the genus *Trichinella*. Infection is widespread among wild mammals, particularly carnivores, wild pigs, and other animals that are cannibalistic or that eat carrion. Trichinosis remains a significant public health problem in several regions of the world—notably Europe, Southeast Asia, Africa, the United States, and the Canadian north. Garbage-fed pigs were considered the only important source of infection for humans, but in recent years, wild animal meat has accounted for an increasing number of cases. In 1986, infected boar meat accounted for 38% of traceable human infections in the United States, while in the former Soviet Union, 90% of cases were attributed to eating bear and wild boar meat. The consumption of raw pork in certain ethnic groups of central Europe and Southeast Asia is also important in the continuing transmission of this parasite.

When undercooked meat infected with *Trichinella* cysts is consumed by humans, the cysts are digested out of the muscle in the stomach and first-stage larvae, which are resistant to gastric juice, are released. These larvae burrow into the wall of the small intestine, develop into adults, and mate. Females begin to discharge newly formed larvae as early as 4 to 7 days after infection, and this process may continue for 4 to 16 weeks or more. The larvae are conveyed via the lymphatic system to the arterial circulation and are disseminated to all organs of the body. Although they can invade any tissue, they survive only in striated skeletal muscle. Once there, larvae begin to coil in nurse cells, around which a cyst forms in 17 to 21 days. Although calcification of the cysts may begin within 6 months, larvae remain viable within them for years.

The majority of individuals with trichinosis are asymptomatic; clinical manifestations attributable to the intestinal and systemic phases of the parasite's life cycle occur in heavy infections. In the intestinal phase of development, symptoms in the host include nausea, abdominal cramps, anorexia, vomiting, fever, and diarrhea or constipation, as well as headaches and dizziness. Some patients may experience severe diarrhea, which lasts for several weeks; this complication occurs particularly after consumption of undercooked Arctic mammals and seems to develop in those who have been infected previously. The muscle invasion phase begins about 7 to 9 days after exposure and is associated with a strong inflammatory response. Symptoms include periorbital and facial edema, myalgias, fever, urticaria, and splinter hemorrhages under the fingernails. In addition, conjunctivitis, anorexia, hoarseness, dysphagia and dyspnea may also occur. Pain can be prominent at this stage and can make talking, chewing, and swallowing difficult.

Complications of trichinosis may include intracerebral hemorrhage, meningeal irritation, seizures, dizziness, ataxia, monoparesis, and even coma. These manifestations result from larval migration through the central nervous system. Myocardial involvement occurring between the second and fifth week of infection can lead to sudden death from dysrhythmias, or a prolonged course with tachycardia, hypotension, elevated venous pressure, and peripheral edema. Myocarditis is a frequent complication and may lead to congestive heart failure 4 to 8 weeks after infection. The convalescent phase begins in the second month after infection and is associated with a decrease in symptoms. Although most patients who survive trichinosis recover completely, about 2% of cases in the United States end fatally and are usually associated with myocarditis, encephalitis, and pneumonitis.

The diagnosis of trichinosis is based on epidemiologic, clinical, and laboratory parameters. A definitive diagnosis of trichinosis usually depends on demonstration of the cysts on muscle biopsy, although this test may be negative due to sampling error. Circulating antibody is usually detected 3–4 weeks after infection, but may be in the circulation as early as 2 weeks after infection with a heavy parasite load. The bentonite flocculation test (BFT), and enzyme-linked immunosorbent assay (ELISA) are most useful. With the BFT, titers of 1:5 are positive and generally fall markedly after 1 to 2 years. The ELISA is more sensitive and can be used to detect a rise or fall in titer.

Anthelminthics are used in the treatment of trichinosis to stop the production of larvae by adult worms in the gut and to kill migrating and muscle-dwelling larvae. Anti-inflammatory drugs are used to alleviate systemic symptoms and may be lifesaving in severe disease. Although a variety of anthelminthics have been used, there are no good comparative data in the literature and little evidence to show that they shorten the course of the illness unless they are administered soon after the ingestion of infected meat. Thiabendazole (Mintezol), 50 mg per kg for 5 days; pyrantel pamoate (Antiminth), at a dose of 10 mg per kg for 4 days; or mebendazole (Vermox), 200 mg per kg for 4 days may be used. The use of thiabendazole has been associated with a systemic hypersensitivity response through the release of antigenic substances; mebendazole does not seem to provoke such severe reactions and may be more useful for that reason. Although it is not yet marketed in North America, albendazole (Zentel) is probably the drug of choice for the treatment of trichinosis. The drug is a well-tolerated benzimidazole derivative which, unlike mebendazole, is absorbed almost completely from the gastrointestinal tract. Experimental studies have shown that it kills both adult worms and migrating and encysted larvae in muscle. Albendazole is given in a dose of 400 mg twice daily for 2 weeks. In the United States, the drug may be obtained from SmithKline Beecham through the Centers for Disease Control in Atlanta, Georgia, and in Canada through the Health Protection Branch, Bureau of Human Prescription Drugs, Ottawa, Canada. Steroids are used in the acute stage at doses of 40 to 60 mg per day for their anti-inflammatory effect; they are recommended for severe disease complicated by central nervous system abnormalities, myocarditis, or severe systemic symptoms.

Trichinosis is prevented by avoiding infected meat or by cooking it adequately. The thermal death point for *T. spiralis* is 57.2° C (135° F); therefore, a temperature of 76.6° C (170° F) for 4 minutes will kill any encysted larvae in pork. Pork less than 6 inches thick is also safe if frozen at −15° C (5° F) for 20 days, −23.3° C (−10° F) for 10 days, or −28.8° C (−20° F) for 6 days. However, cysts in bear meat reportedly survive freezing for periods of over 1 year, and the meat must be properly cooked prior to consumption.

TULAREMIA

method of
GEORGE J. CUCHURAL, Jr., M.D.
Tufts University School of Medicine
Boston, Massachusetts

Tularemia is primarily a disease of wild animals caused by *Francisella tularensis.* Human infection is usually incidental and the result of contact with contaminated tissue or secondary to blood-sucking arthropod vectors. *F. tularensis* is a small pleomorphic, nonmotile, poorly staining, gram-negative rod. This organism is widely distributed in nature. Hundreds of wild mammals have been found to be infected with *F. tularensis,* including rabbits, hares, squirrels, voles, muskrats, beavers, and deer; domestic animals such as sheep, cattle, cats, birds, some amphibians, and fish; and arthropods, including ticks, deer flies, and mosquitos. Mud and water from streams and wells have also been shown to harbor this pathogen. The most important reservoirs in the United States are rabbits, hares, and ticks.

Tularemia is an uncommon infection in the United States, and its incidence has dropped from its peak in 1939 to levels of 0.6 to 1.3 per million population today. The disease occurs in all 50 states, but nearly 50% of all cases are reported from Arkansas, Missouri, Oklahoma, Texas, and Tennessee. Wild rabbits and ticks are the sources for most of the infection in this endemic area. Biting flies are the most common vectors in cases from Utah, Nevada, and California; whereas tick bites are the most common vector in the Rocky Mountain states. Seasonal distribution of cases varies with the mode of transmission. The incidence peaks in the spring and summer months in areas where tick-borne cases are prevalent and increases in winter where rabbit-associated cases are the principal mode of transmission. Humans are susceptible regardless of age, sex, or race. Attack rates are, however, highest in adult males and account for 60 to 75% of new cases. Individuals who are at increased risk include hunters, trappers, butchers, agricultural workers, campers, sheep herders, mink farmers, and laboratory technicians. The portals of entry include the skin and mucous membranes, gastrointestinal tract, and the respiratory tract. *F. tularensis* is capable of penetrating intact or broken skin. Direct inoculation occurs with tick or other blood-sucking insect bites and has occurred after the bite of a cat, a coyote or a squirrel. A skin papule usually develops within 3 to 5 days at the site of entry. Three to 4 days later, an ulcer forms and is usually accompanied by the abrupt onset of fever, chills, malaise, and fatigue. At this time, the organism has spread to regional lymph nodes. The nodes may enlarge, and a granulomatous reaction occurs with or without giant cells. Coalescence of granulomatous lesions may lead to abscess formation. Clinical manifestations depend on whether the disease is localized to the entry site, has reached the lymph nodes, or is more invasive and generalized. Clinical features of the disease syndromes associated with *F. tularensis* are highly dependent on the portal of entry. All forms of the disease are associated with fever, chills, and constitutional symptoms.

Ulceroglandular tularemia is the most common form of the disease and accounts for 80% of cases. This form is characterized by ulcerated skin lesions and painful regional lymphadenopathy. The ulcer develops in 3 to 5 days. It is erythematous and indurated and may look exudated at 2 weeks. Lymphangitis or nodular sporotrichosis-like lesion may rarely occur more proximally to the ulcer. This form of the disease represents entry of *F. tularensis* through penetration of the skin. Generalized lymphadenopathy may occur in 10 to 15% of patients with ulceroglandular disease as a result of bacteremia. Lymph nodes may suppurate and drain. The skin lesion is located in the fingers or hands in 90% of the rabbit-associated cases, and 20 to 90% of patients will have axillary or epitrochlear adenopathy. In tick-borne disease, the ulcer is usually located on the lower extremity or perineal area. In approximately 50% of the cases, multiple ulcers may occur in patients who have multiple inoculation sites. Sixty to seventy percent of those with tick-borne tularemia have inguinal or femoral adenopathy. The differential diagnosis of ulceroglandular tularemia includes bubonic plague, cat-scratch disease, sporotrichosis, ecthyma, rat-bite fever, and malignant anthrax pustule. Glandular tularemia is the term used when an ulcer is not found.

Oculoglandular tularemia is a rare variant of ulceroglandular disease. It results from the patient rubbing the eye with contaminated fingers. The organism penetrates the mucous membrane, and the eye rapidly becomes painful and congested. Severe conjunctivitis with photophobia, increased lacrimation, and purulent discharge occurs. The patient usually seeks medical attention rapidly, and adenopathy may not have developed at the time of first examination. A very painful preauricular adenopathy is unique to tularemia once it does develop. If left untreated, corneal ulceration and perforation may occur.

Gastrointestinal tularemia can vary in severity from mild to rapidly fatal. It is usually traced to the consumption of contaminated food or water. Patients develop fever, persistent diarrhea, nausea, vomiting, abdominal pain, and low back pain and may have gastrointestinal bleeding. Ulcerative intestinal lesions and large mesenteric adenopathy have been seen on autopsy of fatal cases suggesting a large inoculum.

Oropharyngeal tularemia is a result of penetration to the buccal or pharyngeal area by *F. tularensis.* A classic ulcer may be found there associated with an exudative pharyngitis. The tonsils become enlarged and covered with a yellow-white pseudomembrane similar to that described for diphtheria. The sore throat is described as more painful than it appears. Typhoid presentation of tularemia is an acute form of the infection with a mortality rate of 30 to 60% if it is left untreated with appropriate antibiotic therapy. The clinical appearance is similar to that of acute septicemia without an ulcer or lymphadenopathy. Toxemia, very severe headache, prostration, continuous high fever, and weight loss are common findings. Delirium and shock may develop. Typhoidal tularemia may be confused with typhoid fever, brucellosis, malaria, tuberculosis, mycotic infections, Q fever, sarcoidosis, and Legionnaire's disease.

Pulmonary tularemia occurs in 10 to 15% of ulceroglandular cases and 30 to 80% of typhoidal cases, and may be the result of direct bacteremic spread. Inhalation of aerosolized organisms is another potential route (running over a rabbit's nest with a lawn mower). The patient will usually complain of a nonproductive cough, shortness of breath, substernal chest discomfort, fever, chills, malaise, hemoptysis, and prostration. Chest x-ray studies reveal patchy infiltrates that may be bilateral and multilobar, and may be associated with hilar lymphadenopathy. Pleuritis, pleural effusion, and rarely, abscess formation occur. Pleural effusions are characterized by predominant mononuclear cellular response of the granulomatous tissue reaction that can be confused with tuberculous effusions. Some patients may develop hepatomegaly, abnormal liver function tests, renal failure, and rhabdomyolysis. Tularemia is rarely complicated by pericarditis, peritonitis, meningitis, and osteomyelitis. A rash may occur in up to 20% of patients, and may be macular, maculopapular, or blotchy. Rare cases have been associated with erythema nodosum or erythema multiforme.

LABORATORY FINDINGS

The usual laboratory tests are not helpful. Leukocytosis is unusual. The sedimentation rate is normal except in patients with severe disease. Gram's stain of infectious material is frequently negative because of the poor staining qualities of the bacteria. The organism is fastidious and usually requires rich media such as cystine glucose blood agar for growth. Most clinical microbiology laboratories do not attempt isolation because of the high infectivity of even small numbers of bacteria. At present, tularemia is listed as the third most common reported laboratory-associated bacterial infection. Technicians who may come into contact with the organism should be thoroughly trained and should wear protective gloves and a laboratory coat and work in an area of limited access. Procedures that may produce a high-aerosol concentration of the organism, such as centrifusion or grinding of tissues, should be performed in the biologic safety hood. All work areas should be thoroughly decontaminated. Inoculation of laboratory animals is very reliable for isolation of *F. tularensis* because less than 10 organisms can cause infection. These procedures must be performed in Bio-safety Level III. This is a dangerous procedure and, in general, is no longer used for routine diagnosis. Tularemia is most frequently confirmed by serology. Commercially available antigens can be used with standard tube agglutination tests. A four-fold increase during illness or single titer of 1:160 or greater is considered diagnostic. Titers into the thousands are common late in the progress of the infection and can persist for years at levels of 1:80. Agglutination titers are usually negative in the first week of illness and are positive in 60% of patients after 2 weeks of illness. Titers may reach a maximum in 4 to 8 weeks after the onset of illness. Cross-reacting antibodies occur with *Brucella* infection, and brucellosis titers should be obtained to rule out a false-positive serology for tularemia if it is appropriate to the clinical setting. The tularemia skin test becomes positive early in the illness, but unfortunately the skin test antigen is not commercially available.

TREATMENT

Because of the varied and protean manifestations of *F. tularensis* infection and the difficulty in isolation of the organism, a high index of clinical suspicion is critical in order to make a diagnosis and commence appropriate antibiotic therapy in a timely fashion. The mortality rate before the availability of antibiotics was 5 to 15% but has been maintained in the 1 to

3% range in recent years. The typhoidal form of tularemia carries a mortality rate two to three times higher than that of other forms of the disease. Streptomycin is considered the drug of choice for all forms of tularemia. Streptomycin, 15 to 20 mg per kilogram per day intramuscularly in divided doses for 7 to 14 days, is usually effective. Gentamicin at 3 to 5 mg per kilogram per day in divided doses is considered an appropriate alternative therapy. Adjustment of dosage is needed for patients with abnormal renal function. Relapse after this therapy is unusual, but if it does occur, it usually occurs within 2 weeks after the aminoglycoside has been discontinued. The patient usually responds to retreatment. Patients starting treatment after several weeks of illness have delayed resolution of fever and slower improvement in systemic complaints. Despite improvement of systemic signs, the natural history of the primary skin or mucosal lesion is not changed by therapy. Lymph nodes may continue to enlarge even after several days of therapy, and local nodes may occasionally develop suppuration requiring incision and drainage. Surgical manipulations of lymph nodes in untreated patients has resulted in spread of infection and severe complications. Drainage is best delayed until 2 days after the initiation of streptomycin therapy, when the nodes are generally sterile. The organism is also susceptible to tetracycline and chloramphenicol, but relapse rates with use of these antibiotics exceed 50%. If tetracycline or chloramphenicol are used, the duration of therapy should be 3 to 5 weeks to minimize relapse. All isolates have been found to be resistant to penicillin, cephalosporins, and polypeptide antibiotics. Third-generation cephalosporins and fluoroquinolones demonstrate good activity. There have been, however, disappointing clinical results with use of third-generation cephalosporins with tularemia. There are little clinical data on fluoroquinolone usage, and they should not be considered as adequate coverage at this time.

PREVENTION

Because there is no effective control of the disease in nature, the potential for human infections will continue, especially in the increased risk groups. In endemic areas, one should avoid handling dead or moribund animals (do not shoot slow-moving rabbits). Wearing of protective clothing and use of insect repellants help reduce the possibility of insect bites. Rapid removal of ticks is helpful. The tick should be removed by grasping its head and mouth and slowly extracting the biting parts. Avoid squeezing the body of the tick because its bodily fluids may be infectious. Hunters and trappers should wear gloves and proceed cautiously while skinning, dressing, or otherwise handling game, particularly rabbits. Wild game should not be undercooked. Laboratory workers should use caution when working with *F. tularensis*. Bio-safety Level II is recommended for clinical laboratory work of suspected material, and Bio-safety Level III is required for culturing or animal inoculation. Killed and live attenuated vaccines have been developed in an effort to prevent tularemia (contact Drug Service, Centers for Disease Control and Prevention, Atlanta, Georgia). However, the vaccines do not provide complete protection; they have been shown to reduce the severity of the disease in persons who develop clinical infections. Vaccination with live attenuated tularemia vaccine is suggested for persons working with *F. tularensis* or with infected animals, or for persons entering laboratory or animal facilities where *F. tularensis* cultures or infected animals are present. Prior infection with *F. tularensis* does not provide immunity to reinfection. Individuals with known exposure to *F. tularensis* should receive streptomycin treatment, which will prevent the development of clinical illness. Prophylactic treatment with tetracycline or chloramphenicol only results in prolongation of the incubation period.

SALMONELLOSIS

method of
GARY D. OVERTURF, M.D.
University of New Mexico–School of Medicine
Albuquerque, New Mexico

Salmonella spp. are gram-negative bacteria belonging to the family Enterobacteriaceae. Four major clinical syndromes with overlapping clinical features are caused by these bacteria: (1) acute self-limited enterocolitis caused chiefly by nontyphoidal *Salmonella* species; (2) bacteremia and/or focal extraintestinal infection (e.g., septic arthritis, intravascular infection, osteomyelitis, meningitis) complicating enterocolitis or other recognized or unrecognized primary infection; (3) enteric fever, caused primarily by *S. typhi,* with about 10 percent of cases caused by nontyphoidal species; and (4) chronic asymptomatic carriage, following asymptomatic or symptomatic infection.

Salmonella are identified chiefly by their lack of lactose fermentation on most primary stool media and production of hydrogen sulfide. The nomenclature of the genus *Salmonella* is currently under review; traditionally, these bacteria have been subgrouped by the Kauffman-White scheme using the relationship of O (somatic) lipopolysaccharide and H (flagellar) protein antigens. Within these subgroups, there are over 2000 serotypes. Molecular methods (e.g., plasmid analysis, ribotyping, DNA restriction polymorphisms) have been useful for epidemiologic tracking of strains. Except for *S. typhi* and *S. paratyphi,* for which humans are the only reservoir, *Salmonella* are widely distributed throughout vertebrate animals.

Human infection with *Salmonella* spp usually occurs after ingestion of more than 10^6 organisms in contaminated food or water. Impaired gastrointestinal defenses (e.g., in achlorhydria) may allow fewer organisms to cause disease. Other conditions predisposing to severe or invasive salmonella infection include (1) impairment of cellular immunity occurring with chemotherapy or malignancy, human immune deficiency viral (HIV) infection, Hodgkin's disease or other lymphoreticular malignancy, or malnutrition; (2) chronic hemolytic anemias such as sickle cell disease; (3) very young age (less than 6 months) or very old age; (4)

after functional or acquired splenectomy; and (5) the presence of intravascular devices or disease (e.g., aneurysms).

Most cases of salmonellosis occur sporadically; other cases occur in the context of an outbreak. During the past decade, 40,000 to 65,000 cases have been reported in the United States. Children younger than 5 years of age, particularly those younger than 1 year, and persons older than 60 years of age have the highest incidence of salmonellosis. Frequent contaminated food sources include poultry products (chicken, turkey), pork, beef, and unpasteurized dairy products. In the United States, contaminated eggshells have accounted for an increasing number of outbreaks, particularly associated with *S. enteritidis,* and unpasteurized milk has been a frequent source of infection with *S. dublin.* In order to prevent infection, foods should be thoroughly cooked and properly stored to avoid the multiplication of organisms that occurs at room temperature. Processed foods and dairy products should be appropriately heated or pasteurized. Direct person-to-person spread may occur in groups with poor fecal hygiene, such as young children in day care centers. *Salmonella* is an occasional bacterial cause (less than 5% of cases) of traveler's diarrhea.

Resistance to antibiotics is an increasing problem worldwide, with both typhoidal and nontyphoidal strains of *Salmonella.* This resistance may have been facilitated by the selective pressure of antibiotics in animal feeds and the indiscriminate use of over-the-counter antibiotics for the treatment of diarrheal illness. As much as 50% or greater of salmonella have become resistant to ampicillin in recent years. Susceptibility testing should be performed on all isolates and empiric therapy of severe disease should be initiated with broad antibiotic coverage. Only ampicillin or amoxicillin,* chloramphenicol, trimethoprim-sulfamethoxazole,* the quinoline antibiotics, and third-generation cephalosporins (e.g., cefotaxime* or ceftriaxone*) have been proved to be useful in invasive *Salmonella* infections; tetracyclines, aminoglycosides, and first-generation cephalosporins are not clinically efficacious, even when proved to be active in vitro.

ENTEROCOLITIS

Clinical Picture

Salmonella enteritis is the most common of the clinical syndromes, ranging from usually mild, self-limited diarrhea to dysentery. Twelve to 48 hours (range 6 to 96 hours) after ingestion of contaminated foods or liquids, symptoms develop including nausea, vomiting, abdominal cramps, and diarrhea; headache, myalgias, malaise, chills, and low-grade fever, with temperatures of 38° C (100.4° F), are common. Diagnosis is confirmed by stool or blood culture, or both. Stools may or may not contain polymorphonuclear leukocytes and occult or gross blood.

Most healthy adults have an uncomplicated course, and symptoms resolve without treatment within 48 to 72 hours. However, there are several groups for whom *Salmonella* can cause severe disease or infection is frequently complicated by bacteremia with localization to extraintestinal sites. These include those persons previously reviewed (see earlier); these patients may suffer disseminated infection during bacteremia, which may occur in 1 to 5% of cases of seemingly uncomplicated enterocolitis.

*Not FDA approved for this indication.

Treatment

Fluid and Electrolyte Therapy

The critical therapeutic modality in diarrhea is the replacement of fluids and electrolytes lost in diarrheal stools. Oral replacement with free water solutions, coupled with dietary modifications, is acceptable for most adults and children. However, commercial oral electrolyte solutions containing 40 to 110 mEq per liter of sodium with various simple sugar or polysaccharide sources are available for children and adults with more severe diarrhea; the World Health Organization recommends the use of an oral electrolyte solution with 90 millimoles per liter of sodium, 20 of potassium, 80 of chloride, 30 of base, and 111 of glucose (ideal ratio of sodium to carbohydrate of 1:1). In cases of enterocolitis in healthy adults and most children older than 12 months of age, this is usually the only treatment necessary. Rehydration fluids can be supplemented with caffeine-free liquids, lactose-free, bland soft foods (bananas, chicken, potatoes, and pasta) given in small frequent meals. When dehydration is severe or the patient is unable to take fluids orally, or when trials of these preparations have been unsuccessful, parenteral rehydration may be necessary with appropriate monitoring of blood pressure, body weight, urine specific gravity and stool and urine output, and serum electrolytes.

Antimotility and Antinausea Agents

The use of antimotility agents such as atropine-diphenoxylate (Lomotil) or loperamide (Imodium) in salmonellosis has generally been discouraged. Although they may slow the diarrhea, relieve cramping, and decrease nausea, they may prolong or worsen inflammatory enteritis. Thus, if there is gross blood or mucus in the stools, or fever greater than 38.5° C (101.3° F), these agents should not be used, and they should never be used in children younger than 5 years of age. Bismuth subsalicylate (Pepto-Bismol) is a preparation that is safe for both children and adults and may reduce the frequency of diarrhea; adults may be treated with 1 ounce of liquid (2 tablespoons) or two 262.5-mg tablets every 30 minutes for 8 doses, while children may be given 1.1 mL per kg at 4-hour intervals for up to 5 days.

Antinausea medications are generally not required. However, prochlorperazine (Compazine) may be administered orally to adults (5 to 10 mg, 3 or 4 times daily), via rectal suppository (25 mg twice daily), or by intramuscular injection (5 to 10 mg every 4 hours as needed). Promethazine hydrochloride (Phenergan) is preferable in children and may also be used orally (25 mg every 6 hours; 0.1 mg per kg every 6 hours in children), by suppository, or intramuscularly in the same doses.

Antibiotics

The use of antibiotics in uncomplicated enterocolitis in a healthy adult or child is not necessary. Prior trials using older classes of antibiotics demonstrated neither an improvement in symptoms nor shortened course. Antibiotics also contribute to the development of antimicrobial resistance and increase the risk of symptomatic and bacteriologic relapse. Young age and the presence of occult or overt gallbladder disease in addition to antibiotic therapy contributes to a more frequent long-term excretion or carriage of *Salmonella.* It is not known whether therapy with the newer, more active quinolines or cephalosporins will be associated with the same clinical problems. High-risk patients, as previously identified, should receive antibiotic treatment to prevent the potential complications of bacteremia. Additionally, treatment should be considered for patients with clinical illness lasting several days.

Depending on antimicrobial sensitivity, either trimethoprim-sulfamethoxazole (TMP/SMX, Bactrim or Septra)* (5 to 8 mg of TMP per kg two times daily for children; two single-strength tablets containing 80 mg TMP/400 mg SMX two times daily for adults) or ampicillin (50 mg per kg orally to 100 mg per kg per day intravenously, each in four divided doses for children; 2 to 4 grams per day in four doses for adults), or amoxicillin* in equivalent oral dosage, may be taken for 5 days. If bacteremia or systemic infections complicate enterocolitis, therapy should be appropriately prolonged for the clinical situation. Because of the high frequency of antibiotic resistance to ampicillin, TMP/SMX* has become the preferred initial regimen in the United States. Although they are more expensive, the fluoroquinone antibiotics, norfloxacin (Noroxin, 400 mg, twice daily)* and ciprofloxacin (Cipro 500 mg, twice daily)* for 5 to 7 days, are also effective and may be helpful in cases of resistant *Salmonella;* however, they are contraindicated in prepubertal children and pregnant women. In these patients, third-generation cephalosporins can be used in the regimens noted below.

BACTEREMIA AND FOCAL SUPPURATIVE INFECTION

Clinical Picture

Bacteremia in acute uncomplicated enterocolitis occurs frequently and may occur more often in persons in the high-risk categories. Therefore, blood cultures are not routinely necessary except in those patients with high-risk conditions or those with severe symptoms. Patients who have symptomatic bacteremia complicating enterocolitis usually present with fever and shaking chills in addition to diarrhea.

Localization of infection may occur at any site. *Salmonella* infrequently causes bronchopneumonia, empyema, infected aortic aneurysms, endocarditis (e.g., prosthetic heart valves), septic arthritis, and splenic or hepatic abscesses. When bacteremia occurs in persons older than 50 years of age, an infected vascular aneurysm should be suspected. Osteomyelitis can occur in areas of bone infarct in sickle cell disease, and overall, bone and joint infections are the most frequent sites of extraintestinal infection with *Salmonella.* Meningitis occurs primarily in infants younger than 5 months of age. Prolonged gastrointestinal infection with recurrent bacteremia has been a problem in AIDS patients.

*Not FDA approved for this indication.

Treatment

Both bacteremia and localized suppurative infection require adequate antibiotic therapy to prevent potentially life-threatening sequelae. Parenteral ampicillin (100 to 200 mg per kg per day, divided into six doses) or TMP/SMX* (8–10 mg per kg of TMP per day in three to four doses) is effective if the organism is sensitive. The minimal inhibitory concentration (MIC) of ceftriaxone (Rocephin)* or cefotaxime (Claforan)* is often 10-fold to 100-fold lower than the MIC of ampicillin or TMP/SMX. Ceftriaxone (Rochephin, 1 to 2 grams divided every 12 or 24 hours for adults; 50 to 75 mg per kg per day divided every 12 or 24 hours for children) or cefotaxime (Claforan, 1 to 2 grams every 6 hours for adults; 150 to 200 mg per kg per day divided every 6 to 8 hours for children)* has been found to be effective in meningitis, bone and joint infections, and a variety of other focal *Salmonella* infections. Because of the potential for bone marrow toxicity and the availability of excellent alternative agents, chloramphenicol is no longer preferred for invasive infections. In particular, it should not be used for patients with chronic hemolytic anemias.

Surgical drainage and débridement are often necessary for some localized infections. Vascular reconstruction is required for infected aneurysms, and most infected medical devices (e.g., heart valves, joint prostheses) require removal. Uncomplicated bacteremia should be treated for 10 to 14 days, meningitis for 2 to 3 weeks, and osteomyelitis and endovascular infection for 4 to 6 weeks or longer. Ciprofloxacin, 500 mg twice a day, may be helpful for prolonged therapy of osteomyelitis when an oral agent is desired. AIDS patients may require chronic, suppressive treatment to prevent relapses.

ENTERIC FEVER

Clinical Picture

Salmonella enteric fever is a systemic illness characterized by sustained fever; abdominal pain, tenderness, and distention; headache; profound malaise and a dry cough; and variable gastrointestinal signs and symptoms. There may be relative bradycardia, hepatosplenomegaly, and in 5 to 10% of patients, maculopapular lesions on the trunk called rose spots. The

*Not FDA approved for this indication.

toxicity of the illness when lasting more than 2 to 3 weeks can profoundly exhaust the patient, leading to multiple complications of pneumonia and gastrointestinal hemorrhage and perforation. Enteric fever is essentially a typhoid syndrome due to *Salmonella* spp. other than *S. typhi* or *S. paratyphi*.

Enteric fever is a disease primarily of the developing world, although several hundred cases occur each year in the United States. Approximately 10% of all enteric fevers are caused by nontyphoid *Salmonella* serotypes. Enteric fever is transmitted via food or water contaminated by the feces or urine of a symptomatic excretor or carrier. Enteric fever caused by nontyphoid serotypes may theoretically be caused by any *Salmonella* agent and may be acquired in the same fashion as for other enteric strains.

Treatment

If the disease is left untreated, the case fatality rate is 10 to 30% but has declined to less than 5% with modern treatment. Antimicrobial resistance of *S. typhi* has become increasingly common, particularly in areas of the Indian subcontinent, Southeast Asia, and Latin America, with increasing resistance to chloramphenicol, ampicillin, and TMP/SMX.* Thus, for many patients, therapy should be initiated with newer agents until susceptibility to the older agents has been established in vitro. Patients with infections caused by susceptible strains characteristically are afebrile in 5 to 7 days, and their bacteremia is cleared within 72 hours.

In patients infected with sensitive organisms, chloramphenicol remains an attractive agent because of its low cost, oral administration, and proven efficacy. It is given orally, except in severly ill persons for whom the intravenous route is used. The loading dose is 15 to 20 mg per kg, followed by 50 mg per kg per day in three to four divided doses (3 to 4 grams per day for adults). When the patient's temperature returns to normal, the dose may be decreased to 30 mg per kg per day, continued for at least 2 weeks minimum or 10 days following resolution of the fever. Relapses may occur in up to 10% of patients and usually respond to a second course of therapy with the same agent. Patients who are taking chloramphenicol should be observed for bone marrow toxicity, and the drug should not be used in neonates.

Ampicillin or amoxicillin* and TMP/SMX* are the most acceptable alternatives to chloramphenicol. The oral regimens of TMP/SMX or amoxicillin are often more acceptable for pediatric patients. Parenteral ampicillin, 8 to 12 grams per day in adults (150 to 200 mg per kg per day in children), in four divided doses, may be used; oral ampicillin is not reliable. Oral amoxicillin, 50 to 100 mg per kg per day in three divided doses, achieves high blood levels, is well tolerated, and is effective. TMP/SMX, two to four tablets (80 mg TMP/400 mg SMX per tablet) per dose two times per day for adults (5 to 8 mg TMP/25 mg SMX per kg per dose given twice daily in children), provides rates of response comparable to chloramphenicol; in patients unable to tolerate oral TMP/SMX, the same dose may be given intravenously.

*Not FDA approved for this indication.

There is increasing experience with expanded-spectrum cephalosporins such as ceftriaxone* and cefotaxime* given in the same dosages as for bacteremic salmonellosis. These agents have high efficacy rates (≥85%) and low relapse rates, and they may be particularly helpful in areas of known drug resistance; they provide the only alternative for prepubertal children with organisms resistant to ampicillin, chloramphenicol, and TMP/SMX.*

Recent comparative studies have shown rates of cure for ceftriaxone,* administered in a single daily dose (2 grams in adults; 50 mg per kg in children) for 3 days, comparable to those with the 10- to 14-day regimens of conventional antibiotics. Disadvantages include high cost, the need for intramuscular or intravenous injection, and the limited availability in most parts of the world. The quinoline antibiotics are effective in over 90% of patients, and are associated with rapid defervescence, low relapse rates, and infrequent development of the chronic carrier state following treatment. They are also effective against resistant *Salmonella*. The disadvantages are high cost and the concern about toxicity in children. Most clinical experience has been with ciprofloxacin* (500 to 750 mg) and ofloxacin* (Floxin, 200 to 400 mg) given twice daily for 14 days.

In addition to antimicrobial therapy, careful attention should be paid to fluid and electrolyte balance, nutrition, and prevention of complications. Fluids may be administered orally if tolerated. Otherwise, they should be administered parenterally. Control of fever is important, but salicylic acid should not be used because of occasional profound hypothermic reactions. High-dose corticosteroids (dexamethasone,† 3 mg per kg initially, followed by eight doses of 1 mg per kg every 6 hours) have been shown to be beneficial for *only* those patients who are delirious, obtunded, stuporous, comatose, or in shock. Some experts have questioned this high dose of dexamethasone; the use of corticosteroids may be associated with infectious complications and gastrointestinal bleeding. The treatment of occasional disseminated infections should follow those outlined earlier. Surgical exploration and treatment should be followed in patients who experience prolonged gastrointestinal bleeding or ileal perforation.

CARRIER STATE

Asymptomatic excretion of *Salmonella* after clinical nontyphoid enterocolitis occurs for greater than 2 months in 5 to 10% of patients. The chronic carrier state (persistence of asymptomatic fecal or urinary carriage of *Salmonella* for longer than 12 months) occurs in less than 1% of adults and in about 5% of

*Not FDA approved for this indication.
†Exceeds dosage recommended by the manufacturer.

children younger that 5 years of age. Chronic carriage occurs most often with *S. typhi* following typhoid fever (about 3% of cases). Carriers of nontyphoid *Salmonella* species are managed in the same fashion as carriers of *S. typhi.*

Convalescent carriers need only maintain strict personal hygiene so they will not transmit the agent to others. When treatment of chronic carriers with normal gallbladder function and no evidence of cholelithiasis is necessary, ampicillin or TMP/SMX has traditionally been used. Ampicillin is given in a dose of 100 mg per kg per day in four divided doses with probenecid (Benemid), 25 mg per kg per day in four divided doses, for 4 to 6 weeks. TMP/SMX* is given in doses used to treat enterocolitis; some authorities have combined this agent with rifampin* (600 mg per day in adults) for use in patients with cholelithiasis. High-dose ciprofloxacin* (750 mg twice daily) for 1 month has recently been shown to be effective, in some cases, in the presence of gallstones.

If medical attempts at eradication fail in the presence of gallbladder disease, cholecystectomy may be necessary. Even with all of these measures, permanent eradication may be difficult. Patients with intestinal schistosomiasis or urinary infection with *Schistosoma haematobium* may require treatment of their schistosomiasis before eradication of *Salmonella* carriage.

*Not FDA approved for this indication.

TYPHOID FEVER

method of
DEIRDRE A. HERRINGTON, M.D.
Bowman Gray School of Medicine, Wake Forest University
Winston-Salem, North Carolina

Typhoid fever is an acute, generalized infection of the reticuloendothelial system caused by *Salmonella typhi.* Typhoid fever and the related illness paratyphoid fever are also referred to as enteric fevers. In the United States, about 300 cases are reported each year, and the majority of these are imported. Occasional outbreaks occur, usually caused by a typhoid carrier involved in food preparation. However, in other parts of the world, typhoid fever is a significant public health problem because poor sanitation facilitates spread of the infection. Humans are both the only natural host and the only reservoir of *S. typhi,* which is spread by fecally contaminated food and water. Persons with human immunodeficiency virus (HIV) infection are at increased risk for infection with *S. typhi* as well as other salmonellae, and the worldwide spread of HIV infection may have an impact on the epidemiology of typhoid fever.

DIAGNOSIS

After an incubation period of 1 to 2 weeks, when the bacteria are multiplying in the organs of the reticuloendothelial system, sustained bacteremia develops and an insidious, flulike illness with fever, headache, malaise, sore throat, cough, myalgias, and arthralgias occurs. Symptoms progress over the next several days, and fevers rise in a stepwise fashion into the 40° C (104° F) range. Most patients have gastrointestinal symptoms, including abdominal pain and either constipation or diarrhea (constipation is more common in adults). Helpful physical signs to note are relative bradycardia, enlargement of the liver or spleen, lymphadenopathy, and erythematous, 2- to 4-mm maculopapular lesions on the thorax (rose spots). Typhoid fever should be suspected in toxic-appearing persons having undifferentiated fever and respiratory symptoms, especially if the illness is preceded by travel to a developing country. The diagnosis is confirmed by isolating *S. typhi,* usually from blood or stool. Culture of bone marrow is a more sensitive diagnostic tool, especially in persons previously receiving antibiotics. Serology (Widal test) lacks sensitivity and specificity, and may be misleading. Early diagnosis and treatment are imperative if complications are to be avoided. With appropriate management, the case fatality rate is less than 2%.

TREATMENT

Antimicrobial Agents

Chloramphenicol (Chloromycetin) has been used since 1948 to reduce mortality and morbidity in typhoid fever. In countries with a high prevalence of chloramphenicol-sensitive strains, it remains the drug of choice because of its low cost, practicality, and effectiveness. Dose-related bone marrow suppression is frequent but reversible. Rarely, chloramphenicol causes irreversible aplastic anemia (1 in 50,000 treatment courses). Unfortunately, chloramphenicol-resistant strains of *S. typhi* are now common in many parts of the world. If drug resistance is limited to chloramphenicol, furazolidone (Furoxone), amoxicillin (Amoxil), and trimethoprim-sulfamethoxazole (Bactrim, Septra) are inexpensive and effective alternative drugs. Each of these drugs can be given orally and has acceptable safety profiles in children and adults (see Table 1).

Since 1989, *S. typhi* strains resistant to multiple antibiotics have been prevalent on the Indian subcontinent and in the Arabian Gulf and have recently spread into northern Africa. These multiple drug–resistant strains are typically resistant to chloramphenicol, ampicillin (and amoxicillin), trimethoprim-sulfamethoxazole, and less commonly, furazolidone. The quinoline antibiotics and third-generation cephalosporins have been successfully used to treat typhoid fever due to multiple drug–resistant strains.

A number of quinoline drugs have been studied in controlled clinical trials and shown to be effective. The main advantage of the quinolines is that they can be given orally or parenterally to achieve high tissue concentrations and have been effective to date against drug-resistant strains. Their main disadvantage is their high cost and possible adverse effects on articular cartilage in children.

Among the third-generation cephalosporins, ceftriaxone (Rocephin), cefoperazone (Cefobid), and cefotaxime (Claforan) have all shown efficacy. Ceftriaxone has been studied the most because its long half-life permits once-daily dosing. The expense of these

TABLE 1. **Antimicrobial Therapy for Typhoid Fever**

S. typhi Strain	Drug	Adult Dose	Pediatric Dose	Duration (Days)
Chloramphenicol sensitive	Chloramphenicol (oral or intravenous)	750 mg q 6 h until fever resolves, then 500 mg q 6 h	15 mg per kg q 6 h until fever resolves, then 10 mg per kg q 6 h	14
Chloramphenicol resistant	Ciprofloxacin* (oral or intravenous)	500 to 750 mg every 12 hours	—not recommended—	10 to 14
	Ceftriaxone (intravenous)	3 to 4 gm q d	75 mg per kg q d	7 to 14
	Furazolidone† (oral)	200 mg q 6 h	3 mg per kg q 6 h	14
	Ampicillin† (intravenous)	2 gm q 6 h	50 mg per kg q 6 h	14
	Amoxicillin† (oral)	1 gm q 6 h	25 mg per kg q 6 h	14
	Trimethoprim-sulfamethoxazole† (oral or intravenous)	160 to 320 mg (trimethoprim) q 12 h	4 mg per kg (trimethoprim) q 12 h	14

*Other quinolines including ofloxacin, norfloxacin, pefloxacin, and fleroxacin have also been shown to be effective.
†Many chloramphenicol-resistant strains are also resistant to these drugs; check sensitivities before using.

drugs and the necessity to administer them intravenously limits their use in developing countries. Compared with chloramphenicol, ceftriaxone works more rapidly to clear bacteremia. Paradoxically, however, ceftriaxone-treated patients have a longer duration of fever, the explanation for which is unclear but may have to do with failure to kill intracellular bacteria. Ceftriaxone seems to be particularly useful in treatment of pediatric patients or pregnant women with chloramphenicol-resistant infection.

Aminoglycosides, despite good in vitro activity, are clinically ineffective, probably because they are less active in the low pH of the intracellular milieu where *S. typhi* reside. Similarly, tetracyclines are not effective in treatment even if they appear susceptible in vitro. Aztreonam (Azactam), a monobactam antibiotic for parenteral use, has also been found to be effective in the treatment of typhoid fever. However, experience with this drug is limited, and chloramphenicol was clinically superior in a controlled trial.

Data are insufficient to determine the optimal length of therapy with quinolones or third-generation cephalosporins or to determine whether relapse rates or the frequency of the chronic carrier state is lower with these drugs than with chloramphenicol. With this dearth of information in mind, suggested drugs and dosing schedules are given in Table 1. Because of the high prevalence of multiple drug–resistant strains of *S. typhi,* drug resistance should be presumed until culture and sensitivity data are available for persons who contract the disease on the Indian subcontinent, in the Arabian Gulf, or in northern Africa.

Supportive Measures

The clinical response in typhoid fever is not dramatic with any antibiotic regimen. Fevers typically do not abate for 3 to 4 days and may persist for longer than 1 week. High fevers may result in dehydration, and fluid and electrolyte losses should be replaced either orally or intravenously, as appropriate. Antipyretics should be avoided because they can cause wide temperature swings and hypotension. Sponging with tepid water is a preferred method to reduce high fevers.

Constipation may be treated with oral lactulose (Cephulac). This nonabsorbable disaccharide is a gentle physiologic stool softener, and the short-chain fatty acids produced as a result of its metabolism by normal enteric bacteria are probably inhibitory for salmonellae. Laxatives and enemas should be avoided because of the danger of precipitating intestinal hemorrhage or perforation.

Complications

The widespread dissemination of *S. typhi* early in the course of typhoid fever is evident in the wide array of complications that may be seen. These complications include intestinal perforation, intestinal hemorrhage, hemolytic anemia and disseminated intravascular coagulation, hepatitis, splenic abscess, empyema of the gallbladder, acalculous cholecystitis, meningitis, encephalopathy, pharyngitis, parotitis, myocarditis, bronchitis, pneumonia, osteomyelitis, septic arthritis, and orchitis. Although most of these complications are rare in antibiotic-treated patients, certain complications occur with some frequency and deserve separate mention.

A few patients with acute typhoid fever present with severe toxemia, accompanied by an altered state of consciousness or shock. In these cases, 2 days of dexamethasone therapy reduces mortality from 55% (with chloramphenicol alone) to 10%. An initial dexamethasone dose of 3 mg per kg should be given intravenously, followed by 1 mg per kg every 6 hours for a duration of 48 hours. Steroid usage should be reserved for this rare situation; otherwise, it plays no role in the therapy of typhoid fever.

Despite antibiotic therapy, up to 15% of patients undergo a relapse. The clinical syndrome is comparable to that seen initially, but all signs and symptoms are milder in nature. Treatment is the same as for the initial episode. Relapse is less common when therapy is begun late in the course of illness, perhaps because the cellular immune response has had time to fully develop.

Two serious complications of typhoid fever are still encountered in about 2 to 6 percent of cases: intestinal perforation and intestinal hemorrhage. Intestinal perforation remains an important cause of mortality in patients with typhoid fever. Perforation is most common in the second and third weeks of illness, is rare in children, and should be managed by both surgical and medical intervention. Most surgeons experienced in typhoid fever prefer wedge resection of the ulcer, although large or multiple ulcers may require resection of the affected bowel segment. Surgical treatment must be accompanied by additional antimicrobial agents to treat peritonitis caused by the normal enteric flora, including antibiotics with activity against anaerobes. Intestinal hemorrhage, which also occurs in the second or third week of illness, is managed by transfusion, unless there is evidence of perforation.

CARRIER STATE

Two to 5% of patients with typhoid fever develop chronic biliary carriage of *S. typhi* that persists for life. Most chronic carriers have cholecystitis with gallstones, and such individuals play a critical role in the transmission of disease. Fecal excretion of *S. typhi* in carriers may be intermittent, so multiple stool cultures may be necessary to identify a carrier. A serologic test for antibody to the *S. typhi* Vi capsular polysaccharide has proved a useful adjunct to identify chronic carriers.

Quinolone antibiotics are most effective in treatment of the carrier state, and response rates with norfloxacin (Noroxin) and ciprofloxacin (Cipro) have been around 80 to 90%. Cure of the chronic carrier state should be attempted with either ciprofloxacin (750 mg) or norfloxacin (400 mg) twice a day for 28 days. A less expensive alternative therapy is with 4 to 6 grams of ampicillin or amoxicillin together with 2 grams of probenecid given daily in four divided doses for 6 weeks. This regimen is about 90% effective but only in those without cholelithiasis. Patients who fail antibiotic therapy should be evaluated for the presence of gallstones, in which case cholecystectomy in combination with another course of antibiotics may be necessary for cure.

Vaccines

Two parenteral vaccines and one oral vaccine are available for immunization against typhoid fever. Typhoid vaccines afford reasonable protection in most circumstances but are poorly effective against heavily contaminated food or water. Whole cell heat-phenolized and acetone-killed *S. typhi* parenteral vaccines cause the most significant local and systemic reactions and, therefore, are generally less desirable than the typhoid Vi capsular polysaccharide (CPS) vaccine and oral attenuated Ty21a vaccines. Purified Vi CPS vaccine is not yet licensed in the United States. A single intramuscular injection is well tolerated and provides 60 to 80% protection to individuals living in endemic areas, similar to that conferred by the whole cell vaccines. The oral Ty21a vaccine (Vivotif) is given as 4 capsules taken over a period of 7 days and provides comparable protection to that provided by the parenteral vaccines. Ty21a is virtually free of side effects and is licensed for use in the United States for persons age 6 and older.

THE TYPHUS FEVERS

method of
JAMES G. OLSON, PH.D., and
MARY JANE DALTON, M.D.
National Center for Infectious Diseases
Centers for Disease Control and Prevention
Atlanta, GA

Typhus fevers, caused by obligate intracellular bacteria of the family Rickettsiaceae, are characterized by the sudden onset of nonspecific symptoms, including fever, chills, headache, myalgia, arthralgia, and rash. Anorexia, cough, and photophobia are less common. Malaise may progress to prostration, and in severe cases, shock and multisystem failure can ensue. Each species of *Rickettsia* is associated with a unique arthropod vector. Activities that bring humans in close contact with vectors and reservoirs increase the risk of acquiring a typhus fever. Table 1 lists the diseases and rickettsial species, vectors, and reservoirs and geographic distribution of each.

Rocky Mountain spotted fever, the most serious of the typhus fevers and the most commonly encountered one in the United States, is discussed in a separate section. Other rickettsial species within the spotted fever group cause boutonneuse fever (also called Mediterranean spotted fever, African tick typhus, or Kenya tick typhus), Israeli tick typhus, Astrakan fever, Siberian tick typhus, Queensland tick typhus, Oriental tick typhus, and rickettsialpox. Members of the typhus fever group cause louse-borne typhus (epidemic typhus), recrudescent typhus (Brill-Zinsser disease), and flea-borne typhus (murine or endemic typhus). Scrub typhus group rickettsiae cause mite-borne typhus (scrub typhus).

Humans are the primary reservoir of louse-borne typhus, which is transmitted from person to person by the human body louse. The disease is endemic among populations living at high altitudes or cold climates where pediculosis is common and bathing and laundering of clothing are infrequent. Disruption of community services such as electricity and water supplies during times of war provides the potential for epidemic (louse-borne) typhus. Brill-Zinsser disease, a milder recrudescence, occurs among persons who have been inadequately treated for acute louse-borne typhus, or who, after having recovered in the past, become immunocompromised.

Flea-borne typhus is maintained in rodent reservoirs. Human disease, which is mild, occurs among populations that live in close association with rodents and their fleas. Agricultural workers who enter fields to harvest cultivars can also be exposed. In the United States, 30 to 60 cases of flea-borne typhus are reported annually, primarily from Texas, California, and Hawaii.

TABLE 1. **Principal Vectors, Reservoirs, and Distribution of the Typhus Fevers**

Disease	Rickettsial Species	Vector	Reservoir	Distribution
Typhus Fever Group				
Epidemic (louse-borne) typhus	*R. prowazekii*	Body louse	Humans	Africa, Asia, Central America, South America, and Mexico
Flying squirrel typhus	*R. prowazekii*	Unknown	Flying squirrels	Eastern United States
Murine typhus	*R. typhi*	Rat flea	Rats, mice	Worldwide
Scrub typhus	*R. tsutsugamushi*	Mites	Mites, rats	Asia, Australia
Spotted Fever Group				
Rocky Mountain spotted fever	*R. rickettsii*	Ticks	Ticks, small mammals	North, Central, and South America
Boutonneuse fever	*R. conorii*	Ticks	Ticks, small mammals	Europe, Africa, Middle East
Queensland tick typhus	*R. australis*	Ticks	Ticks, small mammals	Australia
North Asia tick typhus	*R. sibirica*	Ticks	Ticks, small mammals	Central Asia
Rickettsialpox	*R. akari*	Mites	Mites, mice	Eastern United States, Russia, Africa, Korea

The spotted fever group rickettsiae, with the exception of *Rickettsia akari,* are tick-borne and can be found on every inhabited continent. Reservoirs are maintained both within tick populations (by transovarial passage) and in various wild animal hosts. Persons who venture into habitats infested with ticks seeking vertebrate hosts, such as campers, hikers, fishermen, and hunters, are at increased risk of acquiring a tick-borne rickettsiosis. Scrub typhus group rickettsiae cause mite-borne typhus, which is widespread throughout Asia and the Pacific Islands. Edge or scrub vegetation provides habitat for the rodent hosts of vector mites, and human populations, including military personnel and agricultural workers who frequent these areas, have increased risk of infection.

Infection occurs when rickettsiae are introduced through the skin by the bite of a tick or mite, or by rubbing infectious feces from lice or fleas into the skin. A necrotic skin lesion at the site of inoculation occurs commonly in patients with mite-borne typhus and occasionally in those with tick typhus or rickettsialpox. The rickettsiae proliferate in endothelial cells, causing vasculitis. Increased vascular permeability and leakage may result in electrolyte imbalance, azotemia, hypovolemia, and shock. Vessel thrombosis may cause gangrene of the skin and extremities. Cerebral dysfunction ranging from confusion to stupor, interstitial pneumonia, kidney failure, liver abnormalities, myocarditis, and disseminated intravascular coagulation can also occur with severe disease.

The diagnosis of typhus fevers depends on clinical judgment and careful gathering of the patient's medical history. Available serologic tests cannot confirm the diagnosis until the second or third week after onset of the disease. New techniques, including a polymerase chain reaction assay, detection of specific antigen in circulating endothelial cells, and detection of rickettsia-specific IgM antibody in serum, may have limited application in the future.

TREATMENT

Prompt antibiotic therapy decreases the risk of serious complications due to typhus fevers and must be begun empirically. Fulminant disease caused by Rocky Mountain spotted fever or louse-borne typhus may result in death before serologic confirmation can be made. If tolerated, oral therapy is adequate; otherwise, intravenous antibiotics should be used (Table 2). Tetracyclines and chloramphenicol are the drugs most suitable for treatment of typhus fevers. Both antibiotics are rickettsiostatic but are highly effective when administered in appropriate dosage early in the course of illness. Patients make spectacular improvements within 24 hours of initiation of therapy and frequently defervesce within 72 hours. Patients should be treated for 7 to 10 days; if the patient remains febrile, antibiotics should continue until at least 2 days following eradication of fever.

TABLE 2. **Drug Treatment of the Typhus Fevers**

Drug	Oral Therapy	Intravenous Therapy	Maximum Total Daily Dose
Tetracycline	25–50 mg per kg per day, in four divided doses q 6 h	(Tetracycline hydrochloride) 10–20 mg per kg per day, in four divided doses q 6 h	2 gm per day
Doxycycline	4.4 mg per kg per day, in two divided doses q 12 h	(Doxycycline hyclate) 4.4 mg per kg per day, in two divided doses q 12 h	200 mg per day
Chloramphenicol	50 mg per kg per day, in four divided doses q 6 h	(Chloramphenicol sodium succinate) 50–100 mg per kg per day, in four divided doses q 6 h	3 gm per day

WHOOPING COUGH
(Pertussis)

method of
KATHRYN M. EDWARDS, M.D., and
LAURA A. CATTANEO, B.S.
Vanderbilt University Medical School
Nashville, Tennessee

CLINICAL MANIFESTATIONS

Pertussis, also termed whooping cough, is a highly contagious, acute, infectious disease caused by the organism *Bordetella pertussis.* This fastidious, gram-negative, pleomorphic organism has a marked tropism for ciliated epithelial cells of the respiratory tract. The bacteria are not invasive, do not penetrate submucosal cells, and do not cause bacteremia. Infection with the organism produces a disease that is characterized by three phases as shown in Table 1. The symptoms of illness begin after an incubation period of 7 to 10 days. The initial symptoms noted in the first or catarrhal phase are rhinorrhea, conjunctival injection, mild cough, and low-grade or no fever. These symptoms do not lead the clinician to suspect pertussis. After several weeks, the second or paroxysmal phase begins. The paroxysmal phase generally lasts 2 to 4 weeks but may continue for an even longer period. This is the stage of illness in which the typical symptoms of paroxysmal cough with or without an inspiratory whoop, post-tussive vomiting, cyanosis, and apnea are present and is usually when the clinician first begins to entertain the diagnosis of pertussis. During this stage, a significant proportion of infants experience complications, such as apneic attacks, leading to cyanosis and occasionally respiratory arrest. Pneumonia is the most frequent complication of pertussis and is responsible for 90% of the deaths associated with disease. Seizures, encephalopathy, and coma have also been reported. The neurologic findings may be the result of hypoxia related to the coughing spells, subarachnoid or intraventricular hemorrhage associated with coughing, or direct effects of toxins released by the organisms. In children younger than 6 months, the current case fatality rate is 0.5%. The third or convalescent phase is characterized by less frequent coughing spells and a decreased severity of episodes. Coughing spells may last for many weeks and may recur with subsequent upper respiratory tract infections.

TABLE 1. ***Bordetella pertussis* Infection: Classic Clinical Stages and Diagnostic Tests***

Day: 1 - - - - - - - - - - 10 - - - - - - - - - 30 - - - - - - - - - 55			
	Catarrhal (1–2 wk)	Paroxysmal (2–4 wk)	Convalescent (3–4 wk)
Infectivity (# organisms)	+ + + + + +	+ + + −	None
Symptoms	Rhinorrhea Conjunctival injection Mild cough Low-grade fever	Paroxysmal cough Vomiting Cyanosis Apnea	Fewer paroxysms
Diagnostic tests	Culture	Serology (ELISA)	

Abbreviation: ELISA = enzyme-linked immunosorbent assay.
*Disease in older children and adults is more mild and atypical and tends to present as a prolonged bronchitis lasting several weeks.

DIAGNOSTIC STUDIES

As noted in Table 1, pertussis organisms can be detected in the nasopharynx of patients with pertussis early in the illness when the symptoms are similar to those of the common cold. However, by the time the symptoms of paroxysmal cough appear, the organisms have frequently decreased in number or have disappeared from the nasopharynx, making confirmation of the diagnosis by culture technique difficult. Techniques to optimize the rate of positive cultures include collecting the cultures within 21 days from the onset of symptoms; using nasal aspirates instead of nasal swabs; obtaining multiple cultures; using selective media (Bordet-Gengou or Regan-Lowe medium), which suppress the normal flora and allow the more fastidious *Bordetella* strains to grow; and using direct plating of the organisms at the bedside or clinic. Although absolute lymphocytosis is often present, it is a nonspecific finding and is rarely seen in partially immunized children or in adults. New serologic tests, such as the enzyme-linked immunosorbent assay (ELISA) antibody tests for individual pertussis antigens, are promising diagnostic methods but are not generally available for routine diagnostic use.

MANAGEMENT

Infants with pertussis frequently present with apnea and require hospitalization. Careful observation and the continuous monitoring of severely affected infants are of primary importance. Supportive care includes avoidance of stimuli that provoke coughing spells. The parents or caretakers need to be taught the natural history of the pertussis infection and the prolonged duration of illness, as well as methods to clear the airway of secretions and ensure adequate nutrition. Although the apneic episodes may persist for many days, the child should be free of life-threatening episodes for several days prior to hospital discharge. Secondary bacterial complications of otitis media and pneumonia also occur and require prompt antibiotic therapy. Although many pharmacologic agents have been used in patients with pertussis, no definite benefit of the use of corticosteroids, bronchodilators, or anticonvulsants has been confirmed in randomized clinical trials. Preliminary data from a recent controlled study have been presented, indicating that the administration of high titer antibody, prepared from adults immunized with acellular pertussis vaccine, remarkably reduces the severity and duration of the paroxysmal stage. This new hyperimmune product is not currently available for commercial use, but if initial studies are confirmed, it may be a promising new therapeutic agent.

Antibiotic Therapy

All patients with suspected pertussis should receive erythromycin therapy. Erythromycin, especially the estolate form (Ilosone), is the most active drug against pertussis. The dosage of erythromycin is 40 to 50 mg per kg per day (maximum of 2 grams/day) given every 6 hours for 14 days. For patients who cannot tolerate erythromycin, trimethoprim-sulfamethoxazole (Bactrim, Septra) (8 mg per kg per day

TABLE 2. **Components of *Bordetella pertussis* Infection**

Component	Biologic Activity	Role of Antibody to the Component
Pertussis toxin or lymphocytosis-promoting factor	A secreted exotoxin. Sensitizes to histamine, causes lymphocytosis, pancreatic islet cell activation, immune enhancement. Has been purified	Protects against respiratory and intracerebral challenge in mice; important for clinical protection in humans
Filamentous hemagglutinin	Involved in the attachment to ciliated respiratory epithelium. Has been purified	Protects against respiratory but not intracerebral challenge in mice
Agglutinogens	Surface antigens associated with fimbria involved in attachment. Types 2, 3 purified	Agglutinates organisms; correlated with protection in earlier studies in Great Britain
Pertactin or 69-kilodalton protein	Nonfimbrial agglutinogen associated with adenylate cyclase. Has been purified	Induces protection against respiratory challenge in mice

of trimethoprim and 40 mg per kg per day of sulfamethoxazole in two divided doses) has been recommended, although few data exist to confirm its efficacy. Although bacteria cannot be cultured after 5 days of therapy, treatment should be continued for 14 days because bacterial relapses have been reported with shorter courses of therapy. Early treatment in the catarrhal phase may modify the clinical course; however, once paroxysmal coughing spells have become established, antibiotics will have little effect on the clinical course of disease but will hasten clearance of the organism and limit spread of the disease to other susceptible contacts. Family members of patients with pertussis are at great risk of infection and should also be treated with antibiotics.

Isolation

Because pertussis is highly contagious, hospitalized patients and individuals in day care, school, or other settings with susceptible individuals should be isolated until they have received 5 days of erythromycin therapy. Exposed contacts should receive age-appropriate immunization and should be promptly treated with erythromycin as well. Prompt use of erythromycin chemoprophylaxis in households, schools, and day care centers is effective in limiting secondary spread.

BIOLOGY OF ORGANISM

Bordetella pertussis, first isolated in 1906 by Bordet and Gengou, produces many antigenic and biologically active factors (Table 2). Pertussis toxin, also termed lymphocytosis-promoting factor, appears to mediate many of the biologic activities of the organism, including attachment of the organism to ciliated respiratory epithelial cells, promotion of lymphocytosis, activation of pancreatic islet cells, and enhancement of immune responses. Antibody to pertussis toxin protects mice against lethal respiratory and intracerebral challenge with live organisms. *Filamentous hemagglutinin* (*FHA*) is crucial for the attachment of organisms to the respiratory epithelium. Mice immunized with filamentous hemagglutinin are also protected against lethal respiratory challenge with *B. pertussis* organisms. *Fimbriae* are surface structures that stimulate production of antibodies that agglutinate organisms. Studies in England in the 1950s suggested that the presence of agglutinins correlated with protection against disease. *Pertactin,* a 69-kilodalton (KDa) outer membrane protein, is produced by all virulent strains of *B. pertussis* and has been shown to be a protective antigen in mice and humans.

PREVENTION

Immunization of children with pertussis vaccine, composed of killed whole *B. pertussis* organisms, has remarkably decreased the incidence of disease. In the United States during the prevaccine era, there were 115,000 to 270,000 annual cases of pertussis, resulting in 5000 to 10,000 deaths per year. When standard pertussis vaccines prepared from killed whole cell *B. pertussis* organisms were introduced into the routine vaccination schedule for infants in the 1950s, the incidence of pertussis disease markedly declined. During the past 10 years, there have been 1200 to 4000 cases and five to 10 deaths per year. In spite of the success of the conventional pertussis vaccine, concern over reactions temporally associated with vaccine administration has limited its use in Europe, Japan, and the United States and has stimulated research efforts to produce a less reactogenic vaccine.

TABLE 3. **Adverse Reactions to Pertussis Vaccine**

Type of Reaction	Common Findings	Whole Cell (%)	Acellular Vaccine (%)*
Local	Redness	40.6	8.6–15.4
	Tenderness	52.4	5.1–7.3
	Swelling	37.8	5.3
	No reaction	27.8	UTD*
	Late local reactions	0	0–30
Systemic	Fever <37.7° C (100° F)	46.4	92.0–97.3
	Fever 37.7°–38.8° C (100°–102° F)	46.4	2.7–8
	Fever >37.7° C (102° F)	4.2	UTD*
	Crying	35.1	0.2–1.0
	Irritability	33.8	0–22
	None	18.2	UTD*
Uncommon	Persistent crying	3.1	0–0.7
	High-pitched, unusual cry	0.1	0–0.5
	Convulsions	0.06	0
	Hypotonic episodes	0.06	0–1

*Unable to determine from reports.

The identification of individual, purified pertussis antigens (pertussis toxin, filamentous hemagglutinin, fimbriae, and pertactin) has enabled the development of many new acellular vaccines using one or more of these antigens. Studies conducted in the United States have compared acellular vaccines with conventional whole cell vaccines and have demonstrated fewer reactions associated with the acellular products. The reaction rates seen in these studies are summarized in Table 3. In Japan, six different acellular vaccines are licensed and have been used routinely to immunize toddlers since 1981. Although two of the acellular vaccines are licensed for use as booster doses in the United States, the routine licensure of the acellular products for use in infants awaits further documentation of vaccine efficacy in this age group. These studies are in progress.

The prevention of pertussis in infants is a prime focus of vaccine research, yet it is becoming evident that adult pertussis disease is also a problem. Individuals older than 6 years of age do not routinely receive pertussis vaccination because the disease has not been perceived as having significant morbidity in older children and adults. In addition, adverse reactions to whole cell vaccine in adults have been considered to be significant. However, epidemiologic studies of infants with pertussis have repeatedly implicated adults in the transmission of pertussis to susceptible infants. Epidemics of pertussis have occurred among adult health care workers occupationally exposed to children with pertussis. Finally, data from adults with acute-onset cough of greater than 1 week's duration have shown that approximately 26% of these individuals are infected with *B. pertussis.* Preliminary studies of the acellular vaccines in adults have found them to be safe and immunogenic. Although more research is needed with the acellular vaccines in adults before they will be licensed for routine use, there is reason to believe that adults may be targeted for administration of the acellular vaccine within the next several years.

Section 3

The Respiratory System

ACUTE RESPIRATORY FAILURE

method of
WILLIAM A. SPEIR, M.D., and
LEIGH A. CALLAHAN, M.D.
Medical College of Georgia
Augusta, Georgia

Any process that interferes with the uptake of oxygen from the atmosphere and its transport to the tissues or impedes carbon dioxide elimination can lead to acute respiratory failure. Abnormalities of oxygenation and gas exchange as well as those of breathing mechanics, alone or together, can lead to acute respiratory failure. Clinically, analysis of arterial blood gases (ABGs) is required to determine the presence or absence of respiratory failure. In general, acute hypercarbic respiratory failure (ventilatory pump failure) is defined as a $PaCO_2$ of equal to or greater than 50 mmHg associated with respiratory acidemia (pH less than or equal to 7.35), and hypoxemic respiratory failure is defined as a PaO_2 of less than or equal to 55 to 60 mmHg. Arterial blood gas criteria for defining acute respiratory failure are arbitrary, and blood gases should be interpreted in light of the individual patient's baseline values. Often, trends in serial ABGs are more important than absolute values.

PHYSIOLOGIC BACKGROUND

Oxygenation and Gas Exchange. Normally, there is a balance between alveolar ventilation and pulmonary capillary blood flow, and the respiratory center regulates the rate and depth of breathing to maintain arterial blood gas values within narrow limits (PaO_2 80 mmHg or above, $PaCO_2$ 36 to 44 mmHg and pH 7.36 to 7.45). The minute ventilation rises and falls with increases or decreases in ventilatory demand. Increased ventilatory demand can result from factors such as agitation, exercise, fever, and increased carbohydrate intake. Changes in the respiratory rate and depth of breathing, as well as the balance between ventilation ($\dot{V}$) and blood flow ($\dot{Q}$), can profoundly alter arterial blood gas values.

There are two types of $\dot{V}/\dot{Q}$ abnormalities, high $\dot{V}/\dot{Q}$ and low $\dot{V}/\dot{Q}$. High $\dot{V}/\dot{Q}$ abnormalities occur when the ratio of blood flow is diminished in comparison with ventilation, leading to an increase in wasted ventilation or dead space. Large increases in physiologic dead space are closely related to elevated $PaCO_2$ (hypercapnia). Low $\dot{V}/\dot{Q}$ abnormalities result when the ratio of ventilation to pulmonary capillary blood flow is decreased, resulting in decreased oxygenation of the blood returning to the left atrium (shunt) and decreased PaO_2 (hypoxemia). Varying degrees of increased physiologic dead space (high $\dot{V}/\dot{Q}$) and physiologic shunting (low $\dot{V}/\dot{Q}$) may occur simultaneously in different regions of the lung.

The degree of impairment of oxygen transfer from the alveoli to the blood can be estimated by the alveolar air equation:

$$P_AO_2 = F_IO_2\,(P_B - P_{H_2O}) - (PaCO_2/R)$$

where P_AO_2 is the partial pressure of alveolar O_2, F_IO_2 is the fraction of O_2 in the inspired air, P_B is the barometric pressure, P_{H_2O} is the partial pressure of vapor, and R is the respiratory quotient. The F_IO_2 (P_B − P_{H_2O}) yields the P_IO_2, the partial pressure of inspired oxygen, and the $PaCO_2/R$ yields the respiratory exchange ratio. The $PaCO_2$ is approximately equal to the P_ACO_2. Using the usual values at sea level, $P_AO_2 = 0.21\,(760 - 47) - (40/0.8) = 100$; thus 100 mmHg is the normal P_AO_2. To calculate the alveolar-arterial oxygen difference, the $P(A - a)O_2$, the measured PaO_2 is subtracted from the P_AO_2 (if the patient's PaO_2 is 95 mmHg, at sea level the A − a difference is 100 − 95 = 5 mmHg). If the patient is receiving supplemental oxygen, the inspired oxygen concentration (%) multiplied by 7 may be used for P_IO_2. The normal $P(A - a)O_2$ increases with age. For individuals up to age 30, the $P(A - a)O_2$ should be less than 10 mmHg; between 30 and 50 years of age, a $P(A - a)O_2$ of less than 15 mmHg may be considered the upper limit of normal; and above age 50, a $P(A - a)O_2$ of less than 20 mmHg is accepted as normal.

Referring to the formula for estimating P_AO_2, it can be readily appreciated that when breathing room air, if the $PaCO_2$ is high, the P_AO_2 will be lower, and this will result in a lower PaO_2. Thus, in hypercapnic patients, hypoxemia can occur with a normal or near-normal alveolar-arterial O_2 difference. Such situations occur in patients with decreases in respiratory drive associated with respiratory center depression, in those who are unable to maintain adequate ventilation because of neuromuscular disease or chest wall deformities, and in those with widespread high $\dot{V}/\dot{Q}$ abnormalities, as in chronic obstructive pulmonary disease (COPD). In patients with widespread low $\dot{V}/\dot{Q}$ abnormalities, such as occur in adult respiratory distress syndrome (ARDS), the $P(A - a)O_2$ is high, indicating a substantial increase in the shunt fraction.

Mechanical Factors. Two mechanical factors play a major role in ventilation: resistance to air flow and compliance. Increased airway resistance, the hallmark of COPD and asthma, results in a pronounced slowing of expiratory flow rates, requiring an increase in expiratory time to empty the lungs. For this reason, patients with increased airway resistance have a high functional residual capacity (FRC), that is, the volume of air remaining in the lungs at the end of a tidal breath is increased. The resulting hyperinflation of the lungs flattens the normal curvature of the hemidiaphragms. Consequent to this flattening, the diaphragm is moved further from its ideal length-tension relationship, placing it at a distinct mechanical disadvantage.

Because of this mechanical impairment, the pressure required for generation by the diaphragm with each tidal breath is increased to nearly the maximum pressure the patient may be able to generate and approximates the transdiaphragmatic pressures produced by normal individuals during moderate exercise. In patients with obstructive airway diseases, increases in airway resistance require a lengthened expiratory time to fully empty the lungs. Increases in ventilatory demand, such as occur with exacerbations, cause an increased respiratory rate and a shortened expiratory time and result in inspiration beginning before the lungs are fully emptied. This leads to air trapping or dynamic hyperinflation, which is superimposed on an already elevated FRC. The consequences are far-reaching: the diaphragmatic muscle is put at a further mechanical disadvantage, and the patient's tidal breathing takes place at a higher lung volume, at which compliance (the pressure necessary to expand the lungs to the targeted volume) is decreased. For this reason, the mechanically impaired diaphragm is called on to generate even higher pressures, dramatically increasing the amount of work required to maintain adequate ventilation. Respiratory muscle fatigue often results from this increase in the work of breathing.

Decreased compliance is the defining mechanical factor of disease processes in which lung expansion is restricted. In patients with chest wall deformities, the compliance of the lungs is usually normal, and lung expansion is restricted because of the configuration of the chest and the resulting decrease in chest wall compliance. Although lung and chest wall compliance is usually normal, patients with neuromuscular weakness have difficulty in generating the breath-to-breath pressures required to maintain adequate ventilation. In this regard, their response to increased ventilatory demand is similar to that of patients with chest wall deformities. The respiratory muscles are unable to sustain the added workload of breathing for an appreciable length of time, and this results in respiratory muscle fatigue.

The decreases in lung compliance associated with conditions such as ARDS and multilobar pneumonias are due to alveolar filling and interstitial edema or inflammation. The increased pressures required to expand the resulting stiff lungs and maintain adequate ventilation result in a pronounced increase in the work of breathing and ultimately in respiratory muscle fatigue.

HYPERCAPNIC RESPIRATORY FAILURE

Acute hypercapnic respiratory failure occurs when the ventilatory pump fails and CO_2 elimination is impaired, resulting in acute respiratory acidemia (pH less than 7.36). There are two major types of hypercapnic respiratory failure: global hypoventilation and ineffective ventilation. Global hypoventilation is seen in patients with severe chest wall deformities (kyphoscoliosis), neuromuscular conditions (Guillain-Barré syndrome, myasthenia gravis, severe hypophosphatemia), and respiratory center depression (drug overdose, brain stem hemorrhage or infarction). Ineffective alveolar ventilation is the hallmark of COPD and asthma.

Global Hypoventilation. Acute respiratory failure occurs in patients with normal lungs when they can no longer sustain a ventilatory level adequate to maintain CO_2 elimination. The $PaCO_2$ rises, as does the P_ACO_2, causing a fall in P_AO_2 and PaO_2, the end result of which is hypercapnia, respiratory acidemia, and hypoxemia. An overdose of respiratory depressant drugs, such as narcotics, hypnotics, or sedatives, diminishes central drive. The decreased respiratory rate often results in global hypoventilation and acute respiratory failure. Patients with severe kyphoscoliosis or rotoscoliosis often have a fixed rib cage on the side of the curvature with a marked decrease in both lung volume and chest wall compliance. Because of this, the normal breathing pattern in these patients is a more rapid respiratory rate with a small tidal volume. As the chest wall deformity worsens, disease conditions requiring a sustained increase in ventilation result in respiratory muscle fatigue, global hypoventilation, and acute respiratory failure. Acute respiratory failure in patients with respiratory muscle weakness secondary to neuromuscular disease develops in a manner similar to that seen in patients with severe chest wall deformities. As respiratory muscle weakness and fatigue increase, tidal volume decreases, and the patient is unable to meet increased ventilatory demands.

Ineffective Alveolar Ventilation. The genesis of hypercapnic respiratory failure in patients with COPD and ineffective alveolar ventilation is decidedly more complex than that resulting from global hypoventilation. The pronounced slowing of expiratory flow rates and consequent chronic hyperinflation make these patients particularly susceptible to the development of dynamic hyperinflation with increases in ventilatory demand. This, in turn, leads to tidal breathing at higher lung volumes at which compliance is decreased, resulting in an increased work of breathing and diaphragmatic fatigue.

Patients with COPD have a combination of high and low $\dot{V}/\dot{Q}$ abnormalities. The cross-sectional area of the pulmonary capillary bed is reduced owing to emphysematous changes, and this hyperinflation compresses the pulmonary capillaries, thereby increasing areas of high $\dot{V}/\dot{Q}$ abnormalities. Additionally, increased resistance to air flow aggravates ventilation–blood flow mismatching, leading to more areas of low $\dot{V}/\dot{Q}$ abnormalities. For these reasons, many patients with advanced COPD have chronic elevation of the $PaCO_2$ in addition to chronic hypoxemia. Any condition that decreases respiratory rate and minute ventilation, such as the use of respiratory depressant drugs, or that increases ventilation demand, such as the presence of respiratory infections or fever, will magnify both high and low $\dot{V}/\dot{Q}$ abnormalities and result in acute respiratory failure.

Asthmatic patients usually have a much greater degree of reversibility of airway obstruction than do patients with COPD. Early in the course of status asthmaticus, hypoxemia with hypocapnia predominates owing to extensive mucous plugging and increased low $\dot{V}/\dot{Q}$ abnormalities. As the exacerbation worsens, airway resistance increases, hyperinflation progresses, and alveolar dead space (areas of high $\dot{V}/\dot{Q}$) increases, leading to worsening hypoxemia and hypercarbia.

HYPOXEMIC RESPIRATORY FAILURE

Acute hypoxemic respiratory failure is caused by diseases such as ARDS and diffuse pneumonia in which alveolar filling and interstitial edema or inflammation result in pronounced decreases in compliance and increases in shunt fraction (areas of low $\dot{V}/\dot{Q}$), with intrapulmonary shunting and absent ventilation. This situation severely impairs oxygen uptake by the blood. The shunt fraction is usually above 20%, and elevations to 50% or more are not uncommon. The increased work of breathing required to expand the stiff lungs, along with the increasing hypoxemia, results in fatigue of the respiratory muscles, worsening the severity of hypoxemic respiratory failure.

CONTRIBUTING FACTORS

Right ventricular dysfunction is present in a large percentage of patients with COPD. Cor pulmonale with impaired right ventricular function results from pulmonary arterial vasoconstriction (consequent to alveolar hypoxia) and a reduction in the cross-sectional area of the pulmonary vascular bed with compression of resistance vessels owing to parenchymal destruction and hyperinflation. Additionally, left ventricular dysfunction due to coronary artery disease is not uncommon in the age group of patients most likely to have advanced COPD. Hypoxemia and fluid overload resulting from retention and reabsorption of sodium and bicarbonate in response to respiratory acidemia may precipitate frank congestive heart failure, with increased lung water and decreased compliance, as well as decreased blood flow to already compromised respiratory muscles.

Cardiac dysfunction and failure is also a major cause of decreased oxygen transport and tissue oxygenation failure. For practical purposes, saturated hemoglobin is responsible for transport of oxygen to the tissues. Significant anemia greatly impairs oxygen delivery, even with normal cardiac function, and increases the risk of tissue hypoxia in patients with respiratory failure.

Patients with ARDS and sepsis usually have an increased cardiac output (in the absence of cardiac disease); however, the tremendously increased oxygen demands, in this extreme hypermetabolic state, may require a cardiac output of 15 liters per minute or more to meet the oxygen needs of vital organs and tissues. In sepsis, circulating myocardial depressant factor often prevents these increases. Additionally, tissue extraction of oxygen in sepsis decreases, rather than increases, in response to hypoxemia. Adequate tissue oxygenation depends on oxygen delivery, which mandates adequate increases in cardiac output.

Electrolyte disturbances such as hypokalemia, hypophosphatemia, and hypomagnesemia can seriously impair respiratory muscle function. Renal excretion of these electrolytes is enhanced by many of the drugs used in the treatment of acute respiratory failure, such as $beta_2$ agonists, theophylline, and corticosteroids. Many other important factors may contribute to the genesis and the severity of acute respiratory failure; however, limited space precludes an exhaustive discussion of this problem here.

MANAGEMENT OF ACUTE RESPIRATORY FAILURE

Hypercapnic Respiratory Failure. In patients with global hypoventilation and acute respiratory failure, the $P(A - a)O_2$ is low, and oxygenation is not a problem. Specific antagonists to reverse the respiratory depressant effects of opiates and benzodiazepines are available, and prompt administration with careful observation often obviates the need for intubation and mechanical ventilatory support. Unfortunately, specific antagonists for other respiratory depressant drugs are not available, and this can be problematic in patients with multiple drug overdose. Intubation and mechanical ventilatory support are usually necessary until the drug effects dissipate and the patient is able to sustain adequate spontaneous ventilation.

The major problems in patients with global hypoventilation and acute respiratory failure due to chest wall deformities and neuromuscular diseases are fatigue, weakness, and failure of the respiratory muscles. In some instances, intubation and mechanical ventilatory support can be avoided if the patient can be ventilated with bilevel continuous positive airway pressure (CPAP) using a nasal mask or specially adapted nasal prongs. High and low settings of the CPAP level create a gradient (the high level during inspiration, the low level during expiration) that noninvasively assists ventilation and provides partial rest for the respiratory muscles. Unfortunately, nasal masks or fitted prongs are often uncomfortable and are poorly tolerated.

In patients with obstructive airway disease and ineffective alveolar ventilation, regardless of the initial blood gas values, a trial of conservative therapy is warranted if the patient is conscious, responsive, hemodynamically stable, and able to cough and clear secretions. Conservative management consists of aggressive therapy with bronchodilators, inhaled $beta_2$ agonists, and usually intravenous theophylline, insistence on cough and sputum production (either spontaneously or aided by chest physiotherapy), prompt institution of antibiotics for respiratory infection, and controlled oxygen therapy. Controlled oxygen therapy consists of small, incremental increases in inspired oxygen concentration (usually 24 to 28% initially) and is used to minimize the decrease in respiratory drive that often occurs when oxygen is administered. In patients with severe $\dot{V}/\dot{Q}$ abnormalities, even very small decreases in respiratory rate result in large increases in $PaCO_2$ and worsening acidemia. The goals of conservative therapy are to relieve hypoxemia (PaO_2 55 to 60 mmHg within the first hours), decrease airway resistance, improve $\dot{V}/\dot{Q}$ relationships, and reduce hyperinflation (thus increasing compliance and decreasing the work of breathing). Conservative therapy for COPD is successful in approximately 75% of patients. If, despite maximum therapy, hypoxemia, hypercapnia, and acidemia do not improve or become worse, or if the patient becomes hemodynamically unstable or semiconscious or cannot cough up secretions, intubation and mechanical ventilatory support are indicated.

The nonventilator management of status asthmaticus is almost identical to that for acute respiratory failure due to COPD. Higher initial concentrations of supplemental O_2 may be required to achieve a PaO_2 of 60 mmHg quickly. In addition, a rising $PaCO_2$ (from hypocapnia to normal) is an ominous sign in asthmatics, indicating impending respiratory muscle failure.

Hypoxemic Respiratory Failure. The refractory hypoxemia and extremely low compliance associated with conditions that cause stiff lungs lead to rapid exhaustion of the respiratory muscles. The prudent course in any patient with ARDS or diffuse pneumonia who fails to achieve a PaO_2 of 60 mmHg with an inspired oxygen concentration of 60%, with or without CPAP, is intubation and mechanical ventilatory support.

Mechanical Ventilatory Support. Mechanical ventilatory support is just that—a supportive measure used to buy time so that the patient's underlying disease process can be identified and appropriately treated. It is important to take a physiologic, patient-oriented approach to mechanical ventilatory support.

Start with the patient, giving due consideration to the patient's psychological needs (for reassurance and empathy), physical needs (for as much comfort as possible), and physiologic needs (for mechanical ventilatory support). The overall goals of mechanical ventilation are simple: to provide adequate oxygenation (PaO_2 60 mmHg, SaO_2 90%) and adequate ventilation (pH 7.35 to 7.45, regardless of $PaCO_2$ level) and to protect the respiratory muscles.

Ventilator Modes and Settings. In patients with acute respiratory failure, the volume-assist (assist-control) or pressure-assist (pressure-support) modes should be used to allow the patient to trigger each breath and to vary the respiratory rate with changes in ventilatory demands and to rest the respiratory muscles.

When using the volume-assist mode, a ventilator that allows independent adjustment of the following parameters should be available: F_IO_2, tidal volume, rate, peak inspiratory flow rate, inspiratory flow pattern, sensitivity, and settings for the controlled backup mode. It is an absolute necessity to be able to vary these settings independently, particularly the inspiratory flow rate and the inspiratory flow pattern, to adapt the ventilator to the patient's needs rather than allowing the patient to be uncomfortable because of the limitations of the ventilator being used. The F_IO_2 is usually set at 1.0 and is then reduced to the lowest value that maintains a PaO_2 of 60 mmHg. Tidal volume should be set at 7 to 10 mL per kg of the estimated lean body weight. In the assist modes, the spontaneously breathing patient triggers each breath. The number of controlled backup breaths should be set at about 4 to 5 breaths lower than the patient's spontaneous rate so that if the patient hypoventilates or becomes apneic, an adequate minute ventilation will be delivered. Studies have shown that in almost all instances a decelerating inspiratory flow pattern results in better distribution of ventilation and improved gas exchange at lower peak inspiratory pressures than other inspiratory waveforms. Choosing a setting for the peak inspiratory flow rate is a bit more complicated. In patients with normal lungs, high inspiratory flow rates redistribute ventilation to areas with lower airway resistance and increase the dead space–tidal volume ratio as well as the $P(A - a)O_2$. For this reason, an initial inspiratory flow rate setting of 40 to 60 liters per minute is suggested in patients with normal lungs (those with hypercapnic respiratory failure due to drug overdose, chest wall deformities, neuromuscular disease, and so on). In patients with hypercapnic respiratory failure due to COPD or asthma, high-peak inspiratory flow rates of 70 to 100 liters per minute improve gas exchange and distribution of ventilation, increase expiratory time, and reduce end-expiratory volume. Recent evidence suggests that high-peak inspiratory flow rates combined with a decelerating inspiratory flow pattern improve gas exchange and decrease both dead space and dynamic compliance in patients with hypoxemic respiratory failure (ARDS).

The pressure-assist mode provides a high-peak inspiratory flow rate with a decelerating inspiratory flow pattern. The pressure limit should be set to maintain a tidal volume of 7 to 10 mL per kg of estimated lean body weight. The backup mode is the volume-controlled mode (settings as listed previously). For adequate backup ventilation, the apnea delay should be set at 10 seconds or less. If the patient makes no spontaneous inspiratory effort for the set length of time, the volume control mode takes over. Use of pressure-assist ventilation as a primary mode of mechanical ventilation has been hindered by lack of adequate backup systems in many of the currently used ventilators.

In patients with increased airway resistance, high ventilatory demand combined with an increased respiratory rate often results in the inspiratory cycle beginning before the FRC of the preceding breath has been reached. This results in air trapping or dynamic hyperinflation with measurable intrinsic end-expiratory pressure at the mouth. The intrinsic end-expiratory pressure increases the risk of circulatory depression with hypotension and of barotrauma to the lung. The determinants of dynamic hyperinflation with intrinsic positive end-expiratory pressure (PEEPi) are the airway resistance, the respiratory rate, the expiratory time, and the tidal volume. Appropriate ventilator settings almost invariably avoid this potentially dangerous complication.

Positive End-Expiratory Pressure. In patients with diffuse bilateral infiltrates and refractory hypoxemia, the addition of PEEP (beginning with 5 cm and increasing by 2- to 3-cm increments to 15 to 20 cm, if necessary) increases the FRC, keeps the alveoli open, and improves oxygenation. PEEP should not be used in patients with COPD and asthma because it often decreases PaO_2 and increases $PaCO_2$ by worsening the degree of hyperinflation, overdistending the alveoli, and further compressing the pulmonary capillaries.

Peak inspiratory pressures of 55 to 60 cmH_2O or more, with or without PEEP, can potentially increase acute lung injury in patients with ARDS. If the patient cannot be adequately oxygenated with peak inspiratory pressures (including PEEP) of less than 60 cmH_2O, a trial of pressure-controlled, inverted ratio ventilation should be considered. In this mode, the pressure limit is set to provide a tidal volume with an adequate minute ventilation at a respiratory rate of 25 to 30. Initially, the inspiratory-expiratory (I:E) ratio is set in the normal range, 1:3 or 1:2, and the inspiratory time is incrementally increased until adequate oxygenation is achieved whether the I:E ratio be 1:1, 1.5:1, or 2:1. Increasing the inspiratory time further (to an I:E ratio of 3:1 or 4:1) results in a sharp increase in the incidence of hypotension and barotrauma in adult patients. Inverting the I:E ratio, so that the inspiratory time exceeds the expiratory time, increases the FRC and may improve oxygenation in patients with hypoxemic respiratory failure who remain refractory to standard mechanical ventilatory approaches. A major drawback of this mode of ventilation is that the patient requires sedation and skeletal muscle paralysis.

ATELECTASIS

method of
RANDOLPH KESSLER, M.D.
University of New Mexico
Albuquerque, New Mexico

Atelectasis is collapse of the pulmonary parenchyma or incomplete alveolar inflation. It is of major clinical importance because of its high frequency of occurrence and the potential for associated morbidity. There remains ongoing controversy about the causes, incidence, diagnosis, and management of atelectasis. Perioperative atelectasis serves as an instructive model for all forms of atelectasis and is the focus of attention here.

CAUSES

Various theories have been proposed for the pathophysiologic mechanisms of atelectasis (Table 1). The most obvious cause is extrinsic compression of lung tissue from fluid, masses, or air. All of these are potential factors in patients who have undergone upper abdominal or thoracic operations. Airway obstruction results in atelectasis because the partial pressure of gases in the alveoli beyond the obstruction typically exceeds that in the alveolar capillaries; resorption of alveolar gases will lead to alveolar collapse unless fresh gas is periodically introduced. Retained mucous secretions, exuberant inflammatory exudates, foreign bodies, bronchospasm, and aspirated gastric contents are all potential factors contributing to perioperative airway obstruction. Regional hypoventilation leads to atelectasis because of reduced surfactant activity and premature airway closure with associated gas absorption. According to Laplace's law, alveolar surface tension increases as the alveolar radius decreases. Because of this, normal surfactant activity is required to prevent emptying of small alveoli into larger ones. Hypoventilation may also cause diminution in mucociliary function, which may lead to further alveolar collapse from mucus retention. Many perioperative factors may contribute to regional or global pulmonary hypoventilation. Anesthesia, abdominal distention, and the recumbent position all impair diaphragmatic function. Incisional pain and analgesic respiratory depression may markedly reduce chest wall and diaphragmatic excursion and therefore lung volumes. A high concentration of oxygen and the associated reduced nitrogen content in inspired gases may further serve to promote atelectasis from increased alveolar gas absorption.

CLINICAL CONSEQUENCES

The primary clinical consequences of atelectasis are impaired gas exchange, increased work of breathing, and formation of a substrate for infection. Hypoxemia resulting from a V/Q mismatch mechanism occurs as nonventilated alveoli continue to be perfused. Reflex hypoxic vasoconstriction only partially compensates for this. Reduced lung compliance is a primary factor in increasing the work of breathing and occurs in proportion to the extent of collapse and diaphragmatic dysfunction. Nonventilated alveoli provide a site for stagnation of secretions and fluid collections. This serves as a prime substrate for bacterial growth. Studies have demonstrated that the lower airway is commonly contaminated by oropharyngeal organisms during surgical operations, and blood-borne bacteria often infect atelectatic areas of lung.

TABLE 1. **Causes of Perioperative Atelectasis**

1. Extrinsic compression
2. Airway obstruction
3. Regional hypoventilation
4. Absorption

DIAGNOSIS

Diffuse microatelectasis or severe lobar collapse may cause symptoms of dyspnea, although important atelectasis can be unaccompanied by symptoms. Tachycardia and tachypnea may be present, and fever is common. Auscultatory findings may include tubular breath sounds, egophony, and crackles. Breath sounds may be reduced when there is major parenchymal collapse. Blood gas analysis and oximetry may demonstrate variable levels of hypoxemia. The chest radiograph may show one or more of a variety of patterns, including plate-like infiltrates, segmental or lobar collapse, and diffuse reticular or "miliary" densities. Other signs of volume loss, such as diaphragmatic elevation, displacement of fissures, mediastinal shift, and hilar displacement, may be present.

TREATMENT

Management should be directed at preventive measures, when possible, and should begin preoperatively in surgical patients. Cigarette use increases bronchopulmonary secretions and reduces mucociliary function and should be stopped at least 2 weeks before an operation. Patients with reactive airways, as demonstrated by history, examination, or spirometry, should receive preoperative bronchodilator therapy. Those with chronic bronchitis should be treated with antibiotics preoperatively based on sputum culture analysis.

Prevention and treatment perioperatively require (1) stretching of lung tissue to promote alveolar and airway expansion and (2) mobilization of secretions. In the anesthetized, obtunded, or otherwise neurologically impaired patient, lung stretch must be promoted by positive pressure mechanical ventilation at relatively high tidal volumes, for example 10 to 12 mL per kg. For the fully awake and cooperative patient deep inspirations are encouraged on a regular basis, for example ten times per hour, and may be promoted by an "incentive spirometry" program. In addition, early return to sitting and ambulatory activity is crucial in restoring normal respiratory mechanics. Clearing of secretions can occur only from tracheobronchial suctioning in the anesthetized or debilitated patient. In the cooperative patient purposeful and vigorous coughing is the preferred modality for management of secretions. In the awake but weakened or uncooperative patient, induced cough stimulation by nasotracheal suctioning, suctioning through a No. 4 French "minitracheostomy" tube, or instillation of saline through a small cricothyroid catheter, may all be effective. Chest percussion and postural drainage techniques may be helpful in the anesthetized, weakened, or uncooperative patient, more so in the pediatric population. They are of minor importance in the patient with an effective cough mechanism and should in no way substitute for coughing procedures. The effectiveness of active techniques for lung expansion and removal of secretions can be markedly enhanced by adequate pain control in patients with upper abdominal or thoracic incisions. These incisions have been shown to be associated with an important reduction in forced vital capacity. Narcotics are very effective but have the disadvantage of causing respiratory depression. Other measures such as regional anesthesia introduced through epidural or intrapleural catheters, use of nonsteroidal, non-narcotic analgesics such as ibuprofen (Motrin) or ketorolac (Toradol), or intrathecal narcotics introduced in the operating room, should be considered in the patient who is at high risk for atelectasis or the complications thereof.

CHRONIC OBSTRUCTIVE PULMONARY DISEASE

method of
RONALD B. GEORGE, M.D., and
MICHAEL W. OWENS, M.D.
Louisiana State University School of Medicine
Shreveport, Louisiana

Obstruction of air flow of a chronic or recurrent nature, which is seen most often in adults over the age of 40 who smoke, is commonly referred to as chronic obstructive pulmonary disease (COPD). The term usually refers to the presence of obstructive bronchitis associated with varying degrees of emphysema, bronchospasm (asthmatic bronchitis), and bronchiectasis. COPD results in over 10 million office visits, over 2 million hospitalizations, and over 25,000 deaths annually in the United States. COPD is one of only two of the 10 major causes of death in the United States that has increased in prevalence in recent years. The death rate from COPD is low in persons below age 45 years but rises progressively thereafter. The incidence and mortality are inversely related to socioeconomic status and are higher in males and in whites than in females and nonwhites.

The dominant physiologic abnormality, as the name implies, is chronic expiratory airflow obstruction that results from a variety of factors related to inflammation in the small peripheral airways. Mucus production is increased, and there is edema of the airway mucosa. Localized strictures and dilation of bronchi (bronchiectasis) occur, and mucus clearance is impaired. Variable degrees of bronchospasm and smooth muscle hypertrophy occur, the bronchial walls are thickened, and there is an increase in the numbers of inflammatory cells. The alterations of the peripheral airways result in mucus collection, and bacteria are present in areas where they are normally not found. An increase in lower respiratory infections, both bacterial and nonbacterial, is characteristic. Destruction of alveolar walls results in loss of elastic recoil and air trapping. Lung hyperinflation is the result of abnormalities of both the static and dynamic properties of the lungs.

PREVENTION

Cigarette smoking is by far the most important risk factor for the development of COPD. Approximately 15 to 20% of smokers suffer a rapid decline in the 1-second forced expiratory volume (FEV_1), two to three times the normal change with aging. This results in spirometric values that are below the expected range, which are first noted during the fifth decade of life prior to the onset of significant disability. It is at this time that smoking cessation is most successful in prolonging life and improving lifestyle. Thus, simple tests of air flow should be performed if possible in cigarette smokers in their forties and fifties who are seen in the office or clinic for any reason, whether or not they complain of cough or dyspnea.

A simple, office-based smoking cessation program can achieve quit rates of up to 50% in highly motivated patients. Simple, unequivocal advice ("you must stop smoking") has in itself been found to be successful in up to 10% of patients. It is helpful to pick a quitting date when outside pressures are low and to have the patient sign a simple contract ("I, John Smith, agree to quit smoking on the following date") written in the progress notes and witnessed by the physician. Most patients who quit smoking do so on their own, with advice and support from their physician and members of his or her office staff. The patient's efforts should be supported by a self-help program, available at minimal cost from a number of volunteer and government agencies, some of which are listed in Table 1. These programs usually assist the patient during the first critical weeks of withdrawal, and hot-line phone numbers are often available for emergency assistance. Commercial smoking cessation programs are available in most areas but tend to be relatively expensive. A choice of methods should be made available to the patient. Repeat office visits should be arranged for 2 weeks after cessation, again a month later, and thereafter as necessary.

Nicotine causes both psychological and physical addiction, and withdrawal symptoms occur as with alcohol or narcotics. The degree of addiction can be roughly assessed by a simple questionnaire such as the Fagerstrom test, available from suppliers of nicotine patches. The nicotine patch is an important advance in aiding smoking cessation

TABLE 1. **Some Recommended Sources for Self-help Guides for Smoking Cessation**

Title	Source
Smokers Self-Testing Kit	Office of Smoking and Health Department of Health and Human Services Atlanta, GA 30341 PHS Publication No. 1904
Freedom from Smoking in 20 Days A Lifetime of Freedom from Smoking	American Lung Association 1740 Broadway New York, NY 10019
Quit for Good	National Cancer Institute National Institutes of Health Bethesda, MD 20892
I Quit Kit	American Cancer Society 90 Park Avenue New York, NY 10016

in persons addicted to nicotine. It provides replacement blood levels during the early, severe withdrawal stages. Nicotine patches should be used only if the patient has quit smoking, and their use should be limited to the first 2 or 3 months of cessation. The highest dose is usually prescribed first, followed by the next lower dose, but patients are often able to eliminate the patches after 2 or 3 weeks at the high-dose level.

Immunization should be performed once with the pneumococcal vaccine and yearly with influenza vaccines. Some authorities are now recommending repeat pneumococcal vaccine after 5 years, especially if the patient's original vaccine did not contain all the currently available serotypes. The influenza vaccine should be given prior to expected outbreaks (October or November); if an unvaccinated patient with COPD is exposed during a known outbreak of influenza A, vaccine should be administered, and amantadine (Symmetrel), 200 mg daily (100 mg daily for adults 65 years of age or older), should be given for 14 days. Amantadine is effective only against the influenza A virus.

A general exercise program focused on improving exercise tolerance and quality of life can reduce respiratory symptoms and limitations and decrease hospitalizations. The exercise program should be simple, inexpensive, and task specific (walking, dressing, and so on). Emphysema clubs are present in larger communities, allowing patients to meet and walk together in air-conditioned malls, and to learn about their disease and its treatment. Nutritional status is important, and many advanced COPD patients are malnourished. A home monitoring program, in which the patient is asked to record the use of metered-dose inhalers (MDI) and symptoms, is useful; a home peak flowmeter will provide an objective record of the severity of obstruction.

Approximately 70,000 people in the United States have a severe hereditary deficiency of alpha$_1$-antitrypsin (α_1AT), demonstrating the phenotypes PiZZ, PiSZ, or Pi null. In the absence of α_1AT the target enzyme, neutrophil elastase, destroys lung tissue at the alveolar level, especially in the presence of cigarette smoking. Purified alpha$_1$-proteinase inhibitor (human) (Prolastin), concentrated from human plasma, is commercially available though rather expensive. It is approximately 80% pure and is infused weekly in carefully selected patients. Potential candidates for this therapy must have one of the previously listed phenotypes, plus moderate airway obstruction (FEV_1 <65% of normal) with documented progression of disease, and they must stop smoking. Patients with very severe COPD are not candidates for α_1AT replacement because therapy does not reverse damage that has already been done.

Recent reports from European clinical investigators indicate that a regular regimen of inhaled corticosteroid aerosol over a period of several years may alter the decline in FEV_1 in patients with COPD. The European group included patients with reversible airway obstruction in their study and found that long-term inhaled corticosteroids were most effective in subjects with the most variability in air flow. They found that an initial improvement in flow rates occurred following the addition of the corticosteroids, and although the decline in FEV_1 continued, it started from a new, higher level and appeared to occur at a slower rate than in controls. These reports have stimulated a number of trials of the usefulness of long-term inhaled corticosteroids in patients with COPD.

BRONCHODILATOR THERAPY

Bronchodilator therapy is indicated in most patients with COPD, even in those without significant improvement in air flow following bronchodilator administration in the laboratory. Subtle changes may not be measured at a given time, and bronchodilators may benefit patients by improving mucus clearance. The available bronchodilators include the anticholinergic agent ipratropium bromide (Atrovent), the beta-adrenergic agonists, and theophylline. Corticosteroids, although not classed as bronchodilators, may improve air flow by decreasing bronchial inflammation and edema and may increase the effectiveness of the bronchodilators.

Many authorities now agree that the anticholinergic agent ipratropium bromide, available now in metered-dose inhaler (MDI) form and as a nebulizer solution, should provide the basic bronchodilator therapy for patients with obstructive bronchitis. Ipratropium is a quaternary derivative of atropine sulfate, which produces bronchodilation in patients with COPD equal to that of the beta-adrenergic aerosols. Ipratropium has a relatively long duration of activity and has additive effects when combined with beta-adrenergic agonists. Its side effects are minimal because it is poorly absorbed from the bronchial mucosa. Ipratropium should be given three or four times daily on a regular basis. A convenient regimen is two puffs from an MDI three times during the day using a hand-held nebulizer (HHN) followed by postural drainage at bedtime.

The beta-adrenergic aerosols produce bronchodilation in COPD patients equivalent to that of ipratropium, but their onset of action is more rapid and their duration is shorter. A number of excellent beta-adrenergic agonists are available in various dosage forms, but they are most often prescribed for use with MDI. They provide similar bronchodilation in equivalent doses, and the choice of agent depends on such factors as patient preference, physician experience, and cost.

The beta-adrenergic MDI is best used on an as-needed basis by patients taking regular doses of ipratropium. Thus, the patient is instructed to carry the MDI with him or her and to take two puffs prior to exercise or whenever an attack of wheezing or dyspnea occurs. Used in this manner, the beta-adrenergic aerosol may be used as a monitoring device by asking the patient to record the amount and frequency of beta-adrenergic agonist use.

Theophylline is a relatively mild bronchodilator, and studies in patients with stable COPD indicate that the FEV_1 increases only slightly in the majority of cases at serum levels of 10 to 20 mg per liter. However, some studies show that theophylline improves functional status and decreases the sensation of dyspnea even without an improvement in air flow. This may relate to some of the nonrespiratory effects of theophylline, including improvement in oxygen delivery, diuresis, and a delay in diaphragmatic fatigue. Oral theophylline has one major advantage in its sustained-release form—that is, its long and relatively stable duration of action. Thus, it is best used as a bedtime therapy in doses of 200 to 400 mg based on measured peak serum levels. We see no rationale for the use of oral short-acting theophylline compounds.

The use of theophylline is complicated by its narrow therapeutic-toxic ratio, and it is one of the most common drugs associated with clinical toxicity. When prescribing oral theophylline for long-term therapy, the following three caveats should be carefully observed: (1) Measure a baseline serum theophylline level and then measure peak theophylline levels (4 to 6 hours after an oral dose) regularly when conditions or dosages change or when symptoms occur; (2) aim for a peak serum theophylline level of 8 to 12 mg per liter rather than the 10- to 20-mg-per-liter level recommended in some texts; and (3) carefully instruct patients and guardians about the wide variety of factors that may alter serum levels (Table 2). It is useful to prepare a handout of factors that raise or lower theophylline levels to give to patients for home use.

Alternative bedtime bronchodilator therapy for patients with nocturnal symptoms or hypoxemia includes use of the oral sustained-release beta-adrenergic agonist compounds. Albuterol (Ventolin, Proventil), metaproterenol (Alupent), and terbutaline (Brethine) are available in oral sustained-release form. These agents have not been very popular in the oral form owing to their side effects, which include tremor, anxiety, and sleep disturbances. The tremor is a beta-adrenergic effect and cannot be eliminated, although tolerance occurs over time. Another possibility for bedtime bronchodilation is now available with the very-long-acting beta-adrenergic aerosol salmeterol (Serevent). Salmeterol provides significant bronchodilation for up to 12 hours, making it an attractive alternative to oral beta-adrenergic agonists or theophylline, because it has very few reported side effects.

CORTICOSTEROIDS

The efficacy of corticosteroid therapy in patients with COPD has been a matter of controversy for some time, as noted earlier in the discussion of prophylactic inhaled corticosteroids. A recent meta-analysis of previous reports concluded that an improvement of 20% or more in flow rates occurs in about 10% of patients with well-documented COPD following the addition of corticosteroids to standard bronchodilator therapy. Steroid aerosols have minimal side effects, including hoarseness and oral moniliasis, which are easily prevented by using a spacer and rinsing and gargling with water after use of the MDI. Oropharyngeal candidiasis responds to topical therapy with nystatin (Mycostatin). Corticosteroid blood levels and alterations in pituitary-adrenal function are minimal when doses of up to 800 μg per day are used but may occur with higher doses, especially in children.

When initiating a trial of corticosteroids in a patient who is symptomatic after maximal bronchodilator therapy, measure a baseline FEV_1 or peak air flow rate, then prescribe oral prednisone, 40 mg once daily, or methylprednisolone, 32 mg daily, for 2 or 3 weeks. If, after this time, the FEV_1 or peak air flow has increased by 15% or more, the oral corticosteroid is tapered and an inhaled agent is begun. If possible, the improvement should be maintained with the inhaled agent; occasionally long-term alternate-day oral therapy is necessary, but this is associated with severe side effects, especially in older patients. The inhaled corticosteroid should be given initially in doses of 800 to 1000 μg per day, which are then tapered until a maintenance dose is found. An algorithm for optimum use of bronchodilator and corticosteroid therapy is shown in Figure 1.

TABLE 2. **Some Factors That May Affect Theophylline Clearance**

Decreased clearance
Liver disease
Congestive heart failure
Drug therapy: cimetidine (Tagamet), erythromycin, troleandomycin (Tao), allopurinol (Zyloprim), quinolones, oral contraceptives
Pneumonia, viral infections, vaccination
Fever; acute, severe illness
High-carbohydrate diet
Old age
Increased clearance
Smoking tobacco or marijuana
Drug therapy: rifampin (Rifadin), rifabutin (Mycobutin), phenobarbital, phenytoin, ethanol
High-protein, low-carbohydrate diet
Childhood

MANAGEMENT OF ACUTE EXACERBATIONS

The therapy of hypercapnic respiratory failure associated with severe COPD is discussed elsewhere; we will outline our approach to therapy of milder exacerbations of COPD, which are most often caused by an acute respiratory tract infection. Acute exacerbations are characterized by increases in cough and dyspnea and alterations in the type and amount of sputum produced. Common pathogens associated with these exacerbations include influenza and parainfluenza viruses, rhinovirus, coronavirus, *Mycoplasma pneumoniae, Chlamydia* (especially the TWAR strain), and bacteria including *Streptococcus pneumoniae Haemophilus influenzae, Moraxella catarrhalis, Legionella pneumophila,* and anaerobic organisms. Gross examination of the sputum is an important aspect of the work-up of COPD patients during acute exacerbations, and a change in its character is an important finding. A simple wet preparation of the sputum identifies the presence of neutrophils; Gram's stain and culture rarely add useful information because they generally show a variety of normal and pathogenic organisms.

Antibiotic therapy of acute exacerbations results in more rapid resolution of symptoms and an improvement in peak flow rate after 1 week of therapy. A variety of oral broad-spectrum agents are available, and the choice is dependent on physician preference and cost. Recommended antibiotics include ampicillin, amoxicillin, a tetracycline, co-trimoxazole, or a quinolone. Some bacterial strains from patients with COPD have been found to be beta-lactamase produc-

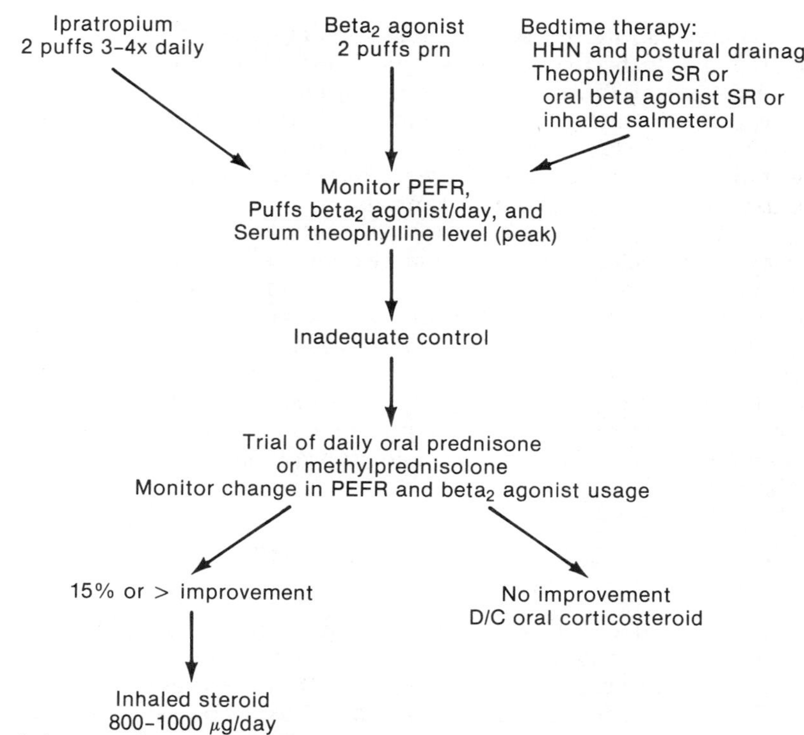

Figure 1. Bronchodilator therapy of COPD.

ers, so many authorities now recommend a beta-lactamase–resistant antibiotic. Because bronchial clearance is altered in COPD patients, we prefer to continue antibiotic therapy for at least 10 days to 2 weeks. The presence of fever and new chest radiographic infiltrates in patients with COPD is an indication for hospitalization and parenteral antibiotic therapy until symptoms subside.

In many cases, oral corticosteroid therapy is begun during an acute exacerbation of COPD, and is followed by long-term inhaled corticosteroid therapy. Patients should be encouraged to increase their oral fluid intake and bronchodilator therapy during acute exacerbations to improve mucus clearance. A course of chest physical therapy with modified postural drainage may be instituted at home by the patient and his or her associates. The patient should be instructed to lie flat in bed on the stomach, breathing deeply and coughing frequently until no more secretions are produced. An associate may assist by gently percussing the chest with a cupped hand while the patient rolls first to one side and then to the other. These treatments should be administered following HHN aerosol administration at least twice daily during exacerbations. If no HHN is available, the patient can inhale steam or vapor from a shower or facial sauna prior to the chest physical therapy sessions.

LONG-TERM OXYGEN THERAPY

A major manifestation of severe COPD is hypoxemia with pulmonary artery hypertension and cor pulmonale, manifested by fluid retention and peripheral edema. Hypoxemia also results in altered left ventricular function with symptoms of dyspnea, orthopnea, and paroxysmal nocturnal dyspnea. Several studies, including the NIH-sponsored Nocturnal Oxygen Therapy Trial (NOTT) and the British Medical Research Council study, have shown that long-term oxygen therapy improves symptoms and prolongs life in patients with severe COPD and hypoxemia. More recently, studies have shown that hypoxic COPD is associated with pulmonary artery hypertension and that prolonged oxygen therapy can significantly reduce mean pulmonary artery pressures and their effects on the right side of the heart.

Methods available to supply oxygen at home include oxygen concentrators, compressed oxygen cylinders, and liquid oxygen. The most cost-effective and reliable methods over time are oxygen concentrators because they require only an electrical source and

TABLE 3. **Criteria for Lung Transplantation in Patients with COPD**

Primary
Age <65 years
Expected survival <18 months
Adequate psychosocial status
Nonsmoking status
Relative
No extrapulmonary or systemic disease (renal, hepatic, malignant)
No previous thoracic surgery
Controversial
No recent steroid use
Weight within 10 to 15% ideal
Absence of ventilator dependency

occasional maintenance. A cylinder or liquid oxygen source should be available for emergency situations such as power failure. One disadvantage of oxygen concentrators is the lack of patient mobility required for their use; thus they are often used in conjunction with liquid or compressed oxygen containers. Oxygen is usually delivered by nasal cannula at a rate of 0.5 to 3.0 liters per minute continuously throughout the respiratory cycle. Newer cannula systems deliver oxygen only during inspiration. Alternative delivery devices used to improve the appearance and acceptance by patients include transtracheal oxygen catheters, which are inserted directly into the trachea through the cricothyroid membrane. Properly used, they are reported to decrease oxygen requirements, decrease dyspnea and hospitalizations, and improve exercise tolerance.

LUNG TRANSPLANTATION FOR PATIENTS WITH COPD

With the advent of improved methods of immunosuppression, lung transplantation has become a reasonable alternative for patients with end-stage COPD. At one time it was felt that double lung transplantation was necessary in these patients, but it is now known that single lung transplantation is successful, and at the present time severe COPD is the most common indication for single lung transplantation in the United States. Lung transplantation has been performed successfully for emphysema (including α_1AT deficiency), cystic fibrosis, obstructive bronchiectasis, and bronchiolitis obliterans. Patients without chronic infections are candidates for single lung transplantation, whereas those with chronic lower respiratory tract infections (cystic fibrosis and bronchiectasis) require double lung transplants. Selection criteria for transplantation in patients with COPD are shown in Table 3. In properly selected patients with COPD, the reported average 1-year survival rate is 78%, and most of those who survive 1 year are still alive after 2 or more years.

CARCINOMA OF THE LUNG

method of
JOHN C. RUCKDESCHEL, M.D.
H. Lee Moffitt Cancer and Research Institute and University of South Florida
Tampa, Florida

Carcinoma of the lung remains both the most common and the most lethal of the cancers affecting men and women, accounting for over 180,000 cases per year, with nearly 85% of those patients eventually succumbing to their disease. In most instances, the disease is caused by cigarette smoking, directly or indirectly, by the patient. Evidence is increasing that significant exposure to second-hand smoke is also associated with an increased risk of lung cancer. There is currently no agreed-upon method for screening for lung cancer, even in high-risk patients (e.g., heavy smokers). Consequently, I recommend a very low threshold of symptoms in a smoker before obtaining a chest x-ray study on the grounds that it is the fortuitously discovered lesion that is most often curable. Physicians who do not obtain chest x-ray studies in smokers with a new or changed cough (or other pulmonary symptoms) on the grounds that "there are no proven screening tests" are confusing screening and diagnosis.

For the primary physician, lung cancer often does not have a clear label that it is indeed cancer; many patients present with an array of symptoms that frequently are confused with less serious problems (Table 1). An upper respiratory infection that seems to hang on, an infiltrate on a chest film thought to be pneumonia, and hoarseness are frequently overlooked. All of these symptoms require a chest x-ray study in a current or former smoker. A substantial minority of patients present with signs or symptoms of metastatic disease on their first visit including bone pain, headaches, blurred vision, diplopia, progressive dyspnea with a heavy feeling in the chest, or significant weight loss (see Table 1). The first suggestion of lung cancer usually comes from an abnormal chest x-ray study, and it is from this point that our discussion of therapy will commence.

Therapy of cancer of the lung is based on three major factors: (1) the histology of the tumor, (2) the extent of disease, and (3) the condition of the patient. It is also based on the skill and knowledge of the therapist, be that a surgeon, radiation therapist, or medical oncologist.

A number of critical trials have come to fruition during the last 2 years that have indicated significant changes in what may be called "standard therapy." I

TABLE 1. **Signs and Symptoms of Lung Cancer That Determine the Initial Evaluation**

Sign or Symptom	Required Next Step
Possible metastatic disease	
Persistent headaches	Head CT or MRI
Blurred vision and diplopia	Head CT or MRI
Unexplained nausea	Head CT or MRI
Bone pain	Plain x-ray of area
Elevated alkaline phosphatase	Chest CT (liver) and bone scan
Elevated liver function tests	Chest CT (liver)
Low sodium or potassium value	Check medications, biopsy for SCLC
Likely locally extensive disease	
SVC syndrome	Mediastinoscopy or other accessible biopsy
Hoarseness	Chest CT, mediastinoscopy
Pleural effusion	Thoracentesis
Pulmonary symptoms only	
Persistent URI or infiltrate	Follow-up chest x-ray and then chest CT and bronchoscopy
Hemoptysis	Chest CT and bronchoscopy
Asymptomatic nodule	Chest CT

Abbreviations: SVC = superior vena cava; SCLC = small cell lung cancer; URI = upper respiratory infection.

will try to highlight those areas in which I think consultation with a multidisciplinary team is still required.

THE PRETHERAPEUTIC EVALUATION

The issues of histology, extent of disease or stage, and the patient's condition (performance status) are usually determined concurrently (Fig. 1). A patient with severe weight loss, bone pain, and an abnormal chest x-ray study does not need a computed tomography (CT) scan of the chest; he or she needs an x-ray study of the afflicted area and a biopsy of the most accessible tissue. On the other hand, patients with local symptoms or those whose lesion is found accidentally require a chest CT scan and a chemistry profile as the first procedures. The chemistry panel will suggest which patients may have unsuspected metastatic disease; an abnormal alkaline phosphatase level or evidence of liver dysfunction demands evaluation of the liver (usually accomplished adequately by the chest CT scan) and the osseous system, best assessed by a bone scan. Abnormal lesions on either of these studies need to be clarified before one embarks on tests intended to clarify cardiopulmonary reserve or otherwise assess local disease. A low sodium or potassium value, without the use of diuretics, is a strong suggestion that the patient may have a small cell carcinoma of the lung. The initial history and physical examination, chest x-ray study, chemistry profile, and chest CT scan define several groups of patients clinically who should be approached differently.

THE PATIENT WITH SYMPTOMS OF METASTASES

The classic symptoms of weight loss, headaches or visual changes, and bone pain will deflect the presurgical work-up but must not allow the diagnosis of the sites of metastases to be delayed owing to therapeutic nihilism. Suspected brain metastases can be detected on a CT scan or magnetic resonance imaging (MRI) scan of the head. Although an MRI scan is more sensitive and can suggest other diagnoses such as carcinomatous meningitis, it is not often needed to make the diagnosis in a symptomatic patient. The diagnosis should not be delayed to allow transport to a center performing MRI when CT is available. Steroids should be initiated immediately in symptomatic patients without waiting for the results of the CT scan because they can always be stopped promptly and rarely cause problems as a single dose. I give intravenous dexamethasone (Decadron) in doses of 10 to 100 mg depending on the severity of symptoms and follow this with dexamethasone 4 mg every 6 hours orally or intravenously while radiation is given (usually 3000 cGy in 10 to 14 fractions) (Table 2). I do not use anticonvulsants unless there has been evidence of grand mal or jacksonian seizure activity; phenytoin (Dilantin) 100 mg three times a day is usually sufficient when no active seizures are present. The most often overlooked symptom of brain metastases is persistent nausea, with or without vomiting and in the absence of another obvious cause.

Bone pain requires a prompt x-ray study of the afflicted area, especially if it is a weight-bearing area.

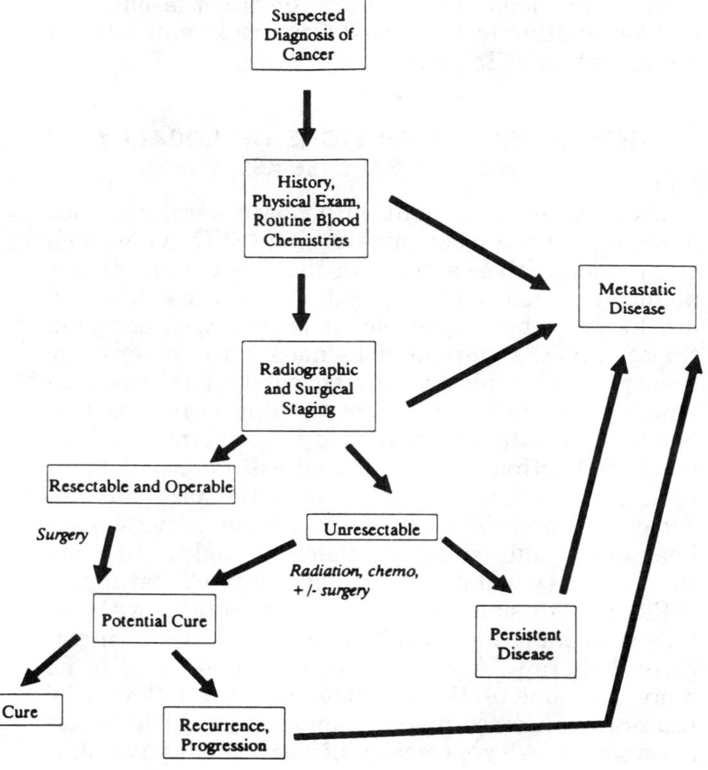

Figure 1. An algorithm for the diagnostic evaluation of non–small cell lung cancer in light of the various treatment options available. (From Ruckdeschel JC: Chemotherapy of metastatic non–small cell carcinoma of the lung. Hematol Oncol 10:25–30, 1992.)

TABLE 2. **Recommended Therapy for Brain Metastases and Spinal Cord Compression**

Clinical Setting	Therapeutic Approach
Spinal cord compression	
Impaired sphincter control, weakness, abnormal plantar reflexes	IV dexamethasone (Decadron) 100 mg and stat MRI
Radicular pain or severe back pain only (no neurologic deficit)	IV dexamethasome 10–100 mg depending on severity, then MRI
Brain metastases	
Seizures, grand mal or jacksonian	Control seizures with IV phenytoin (Dilantin) or diazepam (Valium), then IV dexamethasone 100 mg followed by CT or MRI
Headache, visual changes, persistent nausea	IV dexamethasone 10–100 mg depending on severity, then CT or MRI
Asymptomatic but suspicious findings on CT/MRI stabilization of above clinical situations	PO dexamethasone* 4 mg q 6 h (IV dexamethasone if PO not feasible)

*Prolonged use of Decadron leads to restlessness, gastric upset, and frequent candidal infections. Prophylactic sleeping medications, antacids, and antifungals can be very helpful.

Long bones can have significant lytic lesions that require pinning prior to the use of radiation. Back pain is a special category of pain that requires urgent care because of the presence of the spinal cord. All new or worsening back pain requires a plain film and usually an MRI scan of the area involved. If one lesion is found, the entire spine needs to be imaged. Signs of urinary or fecal incontinence, weakness, or upgoing plantar reflexes again require prompt use of high-dose intravenous and then oral dexamethasone in a fashion similar to that used for symptomatic brain metastases (see Table 2).

THE PATIENT WITH SIGNS OF LOCALLY ADVANCED DISEASE

These patients present with hoarseness, evidence of superior vena cava compression (SVC syndrome), or dyspnea with heaviness in the chest suggesting a pleural effusion. Patients with any of these findings are likely to be inoperable. It is now well accepted that the SVC syndrome does not require emergency therapy and a biopsy can be safely performed in nearly every instance before therapy is initiated. A biopsy is usually accomplished by performing a cervical mediastinoscopy or a mediastinotomy (Chamberlain procedure), which is also the procedure of choice for prompt assessment of the patient with hoarseness and bulky mediastinal nodes. In each case, a biopsy will direct the next steps in therapy.

Pleural effusions require a thoracentesis with cytologic evaluation; a positive sample leads to intrapleural therapy. A negative result should lead to no more than one additional diagnostic tap followed by thoracoscopy, since pleural biopsies add little to the assessment. A cytologically negative exudative effusion has the same poor prognosis as a cytologically positive one, but occasionally resection may be possible; this decision requires an experienced multidisciplinary consultation, however. Malignant effusions are most often treated with tube thoracostomy followed by use of a sclerosing agent. Several key points should be remembered in treating a malignant effusion: (1) excessive fluid should not be removed too quickly or rapid re-expansion pulmonary edema may occur, (2) the chest should not be drained dry at the first tap or loculations become more likely, and (3) the lung must re-expand to allow pleurodesis to occur. Alternative means of draining the fluid and treating the effusion include the use of soft small-bore catheters that can be used in the ambulatory setting, but no comparative trials across the full range of patients and effusions have been reported to date.

The intrapleural agent with the highest degree of effectiveness is talc given by insufflation, although this requires operative intervention and is therefore not optimal for many patients. Talc slurry given through a standard chest tube is currently under study, but intrapleural bleomycin (Blenoxane) is the current agent of choice despite its cost. The tetracycline substitutes require multiple instillations in 90% of patients and quickly price themselves out of competition when the cost of the entire treatment regimen is considered (Table 3).

THE PATIENT WITH PRIMARILY PULMONARY SYMPTOMS

The patient with primarily pulmonary symptoms most often presents with pneumonia in adulthood or with an upper respiratory infection that will not clear. These cases are underdiagnosed when the unsuspecting clinician does not follow the infiltrate to

TABLE 3. **Current Approaches to Management of Malignant Pleural Effusions**

Technique	Comments
Pleurectomy	100% effective but high morbidity, rarely indicated
Talc insufflation	Highly effective, requires operative exposure of pleura
Tube thoracostomy	
Alone	Effective perhaps 20% of the time
With sclerosing agent	
Bleomycin	Current agent of choice, but costly
Talc slurry	Effectiveness not fully assessed but promising
Doxycycline (minocycline)	Requires multiple injections
Other chemotherapy agents	No more effective than bleomycin, some absorption
With radioisotopes	Effective but requires special care and isolation, rarely used
Tube drainage by soft catheter	Can be done in ambulatory setting; unclear as to which patients it will help
Thoracentesis, repeated	Only used in terminal state
Pleuroperitoneal shunts	Tend to clog

complete resolution and are overdiagnosed when the presence of enlarged lymph nodes on CT scan is taken to mean that the lesion is unresectable. Particularly in the presence of an infection, the CT scan is sufficiently unreliable that surgical assessment of the mediastinum is required. Following initiation of a course of antibiotics, the patient needs both bronchoscopy and mediastinoscopy (see Fig. 1). Lobar or whole lung collapse may be due to an inauspiciously located tumor mass in the airway; if it is not accompanied by affected mediastinal nodes, the lesion may still be curable surgically. Hemoptysis is most often caused by bronchitis, but it usually scares the patient and physician sufficiently to be appropriately pursued by bronchoscopy and CT.

THE SOLITARY PULMONARY NODULE

These patients are usually discovered incidentally during evaluation for another problem and represent the group with the best chance of cure. The next step in evaluation is a CT scan, and if nodes of over 1 cm in greatest dimension are seen, mediastinoscopy is indicated. There is argument about the exact size of the node or nodes that should trigger mediastinal assessment (1 cm vs. 1.5 cm), but when surgery is the next approach it is wise to err on the conservative side because a patient with a small primary with multiple small, histologically positive nodes is not a candidate for surgery. When the nodes on CT scan are negative, the patient can be prepared for surgery without undergoing surgical assessment of the mediastinum. Fortunately, the technique of following the lesion for 3 to 6 months on chest x-ray has been all but abandoned in favor of fine-needle aspiration biopsy, which is now available in nearly every institution. However, confirmation that the lesion has been stable for at least a year, by comparing new films with earlier ones, can make biopsy unnecessary. Skin tests are almost useless in this situation because they can offer only suggestive advice.

WHICH PATIENTS WITH LOCALLY ADVANCED DISEASE ARE SURGICAL CANDIDATES?

The staging system for lung cancer was revised in 1986 to mirror the therapeutic options available, as seen in Table 4. Locally advanced tumors that are classified as T3 by virtue of extension into the chest wall, diaphragm, mediastinal pleura, or pericardium are resectable for cure (up to half the time) if they do not invade the heart, trachea, great vessels, or vertebral column. Deep invasion of the chest wall that can be resected en bloc is also curable. In each instance, the potential curability is determined by the absence of mediastinal lymph node invasion. T3 N0 lesions do unusually well, whereas T3 N2 lesions do not (see Table 4). This also holds true for superior sulcus tumors, the so-called Pancoast tumors. Direct invasion of the mediastinal fat is often a contraindication to surgery, but this is a difficult decision to make preoperatively. Mere abutment of the tumor against the mediastinum or other critical structures is not a reason to avoid surgery; consequently surgical expertise is critical. Most lesions within 2 cm of the main carina do not permit safe resection without specialized procedures. Some lesions that are classified as T4 by virtue of vessel or tracheal extension can be resected, but the procedures are heroic in nature; both of these situations require a specialized team. Patients with small adenocarcinomas who present with unsuspected mediastinal involvement at mediastinoscopy should undergo CT or MRI of the head before any surgical procedure is attempted because these tumors have an unusual propensity to metastasize to the brain.

THERAPEUTIC OPTIONS FOR THE PATIENT WITH LUNG CANCER: SURGERY AND THE PRESURGICAL ASSESSMENT

When it has been determined from the initial staging evaluation, including mediastinal assessment as indicated previously, that the lesion is resectable, the patient must also be assessed for "operability." The great majority of lung cancer sufferers have been chronic smokers and have significant cardiopulmonary compromise unrelated to the cancer. The clinical assessment, or "eyeball test," often suggests which patients will never be candidates for surgery. Before referring these patients for routine radiation therapy, however, it should be remembered that radiation will destroy the same lung volume as with surgery except that it will occur over a few months rather than hours. Therefore, the term inoperable must be clearly defined. Table 5 cites the traditional criteria for both cardiac and pulmonary ineligibility for surgery (or radiation). These must be interpreted in light of the stage, however; a patient with a T3 N2 or even a T2 N2 lesion is less likely to benefit from surgery, and slightly stricter criteria should therefore be applied. A T1 N0 lesion requires slightly looser criteria.

The cardiac assessment is rather easier: a myocardial infarct within the past 3 months, uncontrolled cardiac failure or arrhythmias, and severe coronary disease make surgery inadvisable or dangerous. When the decision about surgery is equivocal for reasons of potential cardiac insufficiency, there are several exercise-related procedures that can assess cardiac function more reliably, but again, this is a complex consultative process that is best left to experienced teams.

The pulmonary contraindications to surgery can be assessed more easily by the primary team. In general, it takes just under a liter of postoperative forced expiratory volume in 1 second (Fev_1) to leave an average-sized person comfortable with minor exertion. A value of much less than this indicates an increasing inability to get the patient through surgery or back to any kind of normal existence. Once again the likelihood of a curative procedure indicates the use of slightly looser restrictions. To assess the postoperative Fev_1 the total Fev_1 is reduced by subtracting the

TABLE 4. **International Staging System: TNM Classification**

TI A tumor that is 3.0 cm or less in its greatest dimension, surrounded by lung or visceral pleura, and without evidence of invasion proximal to a lobar bronchus at bronchoscopy.

A tumor more than 3.0 cm in its greatest diameter or a tumor of any size that invades the visceral pleura or has associated atelectasis or obstructive pneumonitis extending to the hilar region. At bronchoscopy, the proximal extent of demonstrable tumor must be within a lobar bronchus or at least 2.0 cm distal to the carcina. Any associated atelectasis or obstructive pneumonitis must involve less than an entire lung.

T2 A tumor of any size with direct extension into the chest wall (including superior sulcus tumors), diaphragm, or the mediastinal pleura or pericardium without involving the heart, great vessels, trachea, esophagus, or vertebral body, or a tumor in the main bronchus within 2.0 cm of the carina without involving the carina.

T3 A tumor of any size with invasion of the mediastinum or involving the heart, great vessels, trachea, esophagus, vertebral body or carina or the presence of malignant pleural effusion.

T4 A tumor of any size with invasion of the mediastinum or involving the heart, great vessels, trachea, esophagus, vertebral body or carina or the presence of malignant pleural effusion.

Nodal Involvement (N)

N0 No demonstrable metastasis to regional lymph nodes.

N1 Metastasis to lymph nodes in the peribronchial or the ipsilateral hilar region, or both, including direct extension.

N2 Metastasis to ipsilateral mediastinal lymph nodes or subcarinal lymph nodes

N3 Metastasis to contralateral mediastinal lymph nodes, contralateral hilar lymph nodes, and ipsilateral or contralateral scalene or supraclavicular lymph nodes.

Distant Metastasis (M)

M0 No (known) distant metastasis.

M1 Distant metastasis; specify site(s).

Stage Grouping

Stage I	T1–2, N0, M0
Stage II	T1–2, N1, M0
Stage IIIa	T3, N0–2, M0
	T1–3, N2, M0
Stage IIIb	T4, any N, M0
	Any T, N3, M0
Stage IV	Any T, any N, M1

Modified from Mountain CF: A new international staging system for lung cancer. Chest *89*:225S, 1986.

contribution of the part of the lung that will be removed on the basis of the quantitative lung scan. This is not merely an academic procedure; an obstructive lesion often leads to significant shunting through unaerated lung, so that pulmonary ventilation is actually improved by surgery rather than diminished.

TABLE 5. **Criteria for Assessing Operability***

Risk Factor	Comment
Age	Relative risk factor, based more on physiologic than chronologic age
Cardiac dysfunction	
Angina, stable	Minimal risk
Angina, unstable	Surgery contraindicated
Recent myocardial infarction	
<3 mo	37% reinfarction rate
3–6 mo	16% reinfarction rate
>6 mo	5% reinfarction rate
Poorly controlled PVC	Significant risk
Left ventricular dysfunction*	Variable risk, may need sophisticated study
Uncontrolled failure	Contraindication
Pulmonary dysfunction	
Continued smoking	Relative contraindication
Abnormal pulmonary function*	
Vital capacity <1.87/L, Fev$_1$ <1.2 L	
Predicted postoperative Fev$_1$ <35% or 0.8 L	Strong contraindication

*More sophisticated analysis of cardiac and pulmonary function can delineate a small group of otherwise inoperable patients who may survive a potentially curative resection, but an experienced team should be consulted.

If pulmonary function is borderline, the first task should be to attempt a "buffing" if the potential for cure is real with a surgical procedure. This entails first and foremost, an agreement to stop smoking by the patient because without this there will be little chance to improve the situation. A course of antibiotics, bronchodilators, and steroids often converts a marginally unacceptable into a marginally acceptable patient. More sophisticated measures of oxygen consumption can be employed, but again, the services of an experienced group are necessary. Up to this point the question of histology has not been relevant. In the remainder of this article I will discuss the therapy of non–small cell lung cancer (NSCLC) before returning to a discussion of the additional staging and therapeutic aspects of small cell lung cancer (SCLC).

SURGICAL PROCEDURES FOR PATIENTS WITH NSCLC

The intraoperative approach to patients should always include assessment of the mediastinal nodes. Often this is performed by mediastinoscopy during a procedure that immediately precedes the thoracotomy, but usually it occurs at the time of surgery. The various nodal stations are numbered, and both the surgical and pathologic reports should reflect this numbering system. Whether sampling of the various nodal stations or full resection of the nodes is required is unclear, but nodal sampling is a minimum. A lobectomy, sleeve lobectomy, or bi-lobectomy on the right is the procedure of choice if all tumor can be removed. Surgical mortality for this procedure should be under 3% (Table 6). A pneumonectomy is the procedure of choice only if the position and extent of the tumor or hilar nodes dictate such a step; mediastinal nodal involvement alone does not usually do so. Morbidity and mortality rates can rise precipitously for a pneumonectomy if proper patient selection is not carried out (see Table 6). Surgical experience with general thoracic procedures is also important because surgeons performing fewer than 10 operations per year experience a higher mortality rate. Good judgment in the operating room is paramount when the mediastinal nodes are found to be involved but resectable. Complex, extended operations to deal with locally invasive disease are contraindicated in the presence of N2 disease. On the other hand, upward of 30% of patients with N2 disease can be cured if the primary and nodes are completely resected and the extent of nodal involvement is minimal. When more than one nodal station is involved, or extracapsular spread occurs, there is a precipitous drop in the chance for cure. Lesions involving the chest wall should be resected en bloc. Superior sulcus tumors have often been treated surgically after a course of preoperative radiation, a technique that is of little benefit unless the patient has had a negative mediastinoscopy and the lesion is judged to be N0.

There has been an increasing interest in limited surgical procedures for patients who have marginal pulmonary function, and several reports have suggested that some lesser procedures such as segmentectomy or wedge resection are equivalent to lobectomy. A recent trial has demonstrated that survival is inferior when this is performed, but it is still a reasonable option in older patients with limited pulmonary reserve. Video-assisted thoracoscopic procedures have been introduced recently, extending the promise of shorter hospital stays and less morbidity; although this goal may be achievable, there has been a disturbing tendency to try to stage the disease this way when such staging cannot be adequately done by this method.

TABLE 6. **Postoperative Mortality Following Resection for Lung Cancer**

Type of Resection and Age of Patient	No. of Resections	30-Day Mortality (%)
All resections	2200	3.7
Pneumonectomy	569	6.2
Lobectomy	1508	2.9
Limited (wedge, segment)	143	1.4
≤60 years	847	1.3
60–69 years	920	4.1
≥70 years	443	7.2

Adapted from Ginsberg RJ, Hill LD, Eagen, RT, et al: Modern 30 day operative mortality for surgical resections in lung cancer. J Thorac Cardiovasc Surg *86*:654–657, 1983.

CAN PREOPERATIVE OR POSTOPERATIVE RADIATION OR CHEMOTHERAPY IMPROVE ON THE RESULTS OF SURGERY ALONE?

Most attempts to enhance the results of surgery, especially in groups in which recurrence rates are high, have involved the addition of radiation, chemotherapy, or immunotherapy in the postoperative setting. There has been no demonstrable benefit from immunotherapy, and the major randomized trial of postoperative radiation showed good local control but no improvement in survival—not unsurprising in light of the high incidence of systemic disease. These trials have been criticized as being not fully conclusive, leading to relatively routine use of postoperative radiation in the United States to "reduce local recurrences" and to near abandonment of the procedure in Canada. My own practice is to recommend postoperative radiation only when there is a question of an incomplete resection. Prophylactic cranial irradiation has likewise shown no benefit for patients with NSCLC.

Postoperative chemotherapy has been shown to lead to a slight to modest enhancement of survival in a few trials, and a major meta-analysis suggests a clearer benefit when modern cisplatin-based regimens are used. Because the benefit is modest at best, I usually use combined modality therapy (radiation plus chemotherapy) for young patients with a very high risk of recurrence but do not employ adjuvant therapy in older patients with a compromised performance status, but there is a lot of room for individualizing therapy. There are several large trials under way that are trying to resolve these issues, and referral to these trials should be a first choice for patients and physicians alike.

Preoperative chemotherapy and combined modality therapy have become increasingly popular for patients with disease that is at the border of resectability, usually Stage IIIA. A recent comparison suggests that combined-modality therapy is better than chemotherapy alone as preoperative therapy, but both approaches require specialized teams for management because the perioperative mortality can be significant. Patients in whom histologic clearing of the tumor occurs with preoperative therapy do strikingly well; these comprise about 10 to 15% of patients overall. A randomized trial of combined modality therapy plus surgery compared with combined modality therapy alone is currently under way.

THERAPY FOR PATIENTS WITH UNRESECTABLE BUT CLINICALLY NONMETASTATIC DISEASE

Patients in whom the tumor cannot be completely resected make up a sizable portion of patients with NSCLC, and previously the treatment of choice has been a continuous course of radiation therapy, usually to a dose of 6000 cGy over 6 weeks. Various attempts to enhance the activity and effectiveness of radiation by employing sensitizers and unconventional (hyper- or accelerated) fractionation schemes have met with mixed success. Several trials have suggested that chemotherapy given prior to radiation is superior to radiation alone, and a large randomized trial has demonstrated that two cycles of cisplatin-based chemotherapy (vinblastine and cisplatin) given prior to radiation is superior to the same amount of radiation given alone or to a similar dose of radiation given in a twice-daily (hyper-) fractionation. A large meta-analysis has confirmed the demonstration of a strong benefit in nearly all reported trials with chemotherapy plus radiation compared with radiation alone. The standard of therapy for Stage IIIB and unresectable Stage IIIA disease now appears to be combined-modality therapy.

CHEMOTHERAPY FOR PATIENTS WITH METASTATIC NSCLC

This form of therapy has been much maligned but has now been shown in several studies and in a large meta-analysis to be superior to supportive care alone; indeed, in the Canadian Multicenter Trial the employment of chemotherapy was less expensive than supportive care because patients stayed out of the hospital more often while on therapy than when off it. The arrival of the newer serotonin antagonist antiemetics has revolutionized the administration of cisplatin, and the development of carboplatin has further reduced the inconvenience of chemotherapy for less mobile patients. Most effective regimens (Table 7) employ cisplatin, with etoposide-cisplatin being the most common regimen. There are great variations in the dose of cisplatin employed, but there is little or no evidence that doses of 100 mg/m^2 are superior to the more standard dose of 60 mg/m^2. Mitomycin-containing regimens have a slightly higher initial response rate, but the drug cannot be used for more than two cycles because of significant toxicity and a diminished 1-year survival. Studies have demonstrated that patients with some symptoms will show improvement in their complaints, but patients who are severely symptomatic with a diminished performance status do not benefit from chemotherapy. A policy of waiting until symptoms appear before treatment is started is no longer warranted, and maximal quality and quantity of life are likely if patients with metastatic disease are treated before symptoms develop. For a group of patients with metastatic NSCLC the average survival is 4 to 6 months without therapy, and the 1-year survival is about 10%, although the presence of liver and bone metastases can shorten this time even further. With treatment with etoposide-cisplatin or several similar regimens the 1-year survival of the group climbs to 25% and is substantially higher for those responding to the therapy. This fact has led to a generally accepted policy of treating patients with a good performance status with one to two cycles of chemotherapy and then assessing the response, with responders going on to further therapy. Several new agents are coming into use, paclitaxel (Taxol) being the most exciting because it confers a 40% 1-year survival rate as a single agent. It is important when discussing therapy for the patient with metastatic disease not to fall into the trap of using median survival to give the patient an assessment of his or her outlook. To say that therapy leads to only 2 to 3 extra months of life based on such data is misleading. The chances of living to 1 or now 2 years is of far more interest to the patient.

WHAT IS DIFFERENT ABOUT THE PATIENT WITH SMALL CELL LUNG CANCER?

There has been an extraordinary increase in our knowledge of the fundamental biology of lung cancer based initially on our understanding of SCLC. These advances are now leading to studies of how to interfere in growth factor regulation of SCLC and to gene

TABLE 7. **Chemotherapy Regimens with Reported Efficacy in Metastatic NSCLC**

Regimen	Doses	Comments
EP: etoposide-cisplatin	E, 100–125 mg/m^2 days 1–3 P 60–90 mg/m^2 day 1	"Standard"
MVP: mitomycin, vinblastine, cisplatin	M, 8 mg/m^2 IV days 1, 29, 71 V, 4–5 mg/m^2 q wk × 5, then q 2 wk P, 100 mg/m^2 IV day 1	Mitomycin can be used for only a short period
VP: vinblastine-cisplatin	V, 4–5 mg/m^2 q wk × 4, IV P, 100 mg/m^2 day 1 q 4 wk IV	Demonstrated benefit with radiation therapy
VDS-P: vindesine*-cisplatin	VDS, 3 mg/m^2 q wk × 7, then qowk IV P, 60–120 mg/m^2 day 1 IV	Vindesine not available in United States
CAP: cyclophosphamide, doxorubicin, cisplatin	C, 400 mg/m^2 day 1 IV A, 40 mg/m^2 day 1 IV P, 40–60 mg/m^2 day 1 IV	Slightly less active
CAMP: cyclophosphamide, doxorubicin, methotrexate, procarbazine	C, 300 mg/m^2 days 1, 8 IV A, 20 mg/m^2 days 1, 8 IV M, 15 mg/m^2 days 1, 8 IV P, 100 mg/m^2 PO days 1–10	Slightly less active, but no toxicity
Taxol (paclitaxel)	T, 250 mg/m^2 day 1 q 4 wk IV† over 24 hours	40% 1-y survival as a single agent

*Investigational drug in the United States.
†Exceeds dosage recommended by the manufacturer.

transfection studies in NSCLC to overcome the effect of a mutated oncogene. The current therapy of SCLC has not changed as dramatically, however.

ADDITIONAL STAGING PROCEDURES FOR SCLC

This has been an area of increasing controversy, and there has been a significant drop in the number of studies required to stage the patient adequately. In a clinical trial it is often necessary to keep track of all known areas of disease, but in the community setting any evidence of metastatic disease should suffice to initiate therapy. Of course, the symptomatic areas in bone and brain, as described earlier, need to be pursued to prevent the development of catastrophic complications.

The staging system for SCLC is modestly illogical and comprises the concepts of local and extensive disease. The term local implies several variations of disease confined to the thorax, including supraclavicular nodes and pleural effusions. Different methods of labeling local disease make comparisons between studies difficult. My own preference is for the TNM system, but this is still a minority opinion. To declare that disease is localized, the bone scan, abdominal portion of the chest CT scan (liver and adrenals), and the brain need to be free from disease. The marrow was previously routinely sampled as well, but without other signs of spread, bone marrow as the sole site of metastasis is extremely rare. In the clinical trial setting, pre-therapy and post-therapy bronchoscopy is performed to assess for a complete response, but this is rarely required in the community setting.

THERAPY FOR PATIENTS WITH SCLC

The mainstay of therapy for SCLC is chemotherapy, etoposide-cisplatin being the usual choice or an alternating regimen consisting of etoposide-cisplatin and cisplatin, doxorubicin, and vincristine (CAV), although the benefits of the alternating scheme are modest at best. There are several other first-line regimens, but virtually no therapy is effective after initial chemotherapy has failed. For patients with localized disease, the use of consolidative chest irradiation, given as closely as possible to the chemotherapy, appears to be superior to other approaches. Surgery as a consolidation technique has not demonstrated superiority, but patients in whom an early SCLC lesion is found fortuitously should have it resected and receive postoperative chemotherapy. Prophylactic cranial irradiation remains controversial because it has produced no clear evidence that it improves survival, but it remains a commonly employed procedure that does seem to reduce the frequency with which the brain is the first site of recurrence. Several intense regimens are under development that should require referral to a medical center. There is an equally broad group of patients who are older, usually with a poorer performance status, who are being treated with less aggressive regimens, in particular oral etoposide. Results to date appear equivalent, but randomized trials are under way. In every instance the major threat to the 10 to 15% of patients who go into long-term remission appears to be the development of a second primary cancer, particularly NSCLC. This is strikingly true for those who continue to smoke.

UNUSUAL CLINICAL VARIATIONS OF SCLC

There is a subgroup of patients with atypical carcinoids who do poorly. Although these tumors are technically not true SCLC, they can behave with equal clinical viciousness. Molecular variations have been seen, but there is no reliable way histologically to differentiate those who will do poorly. I prefer to use the clinical behavior as a surrogate, treating those tumors that present with nodal metastases as SCLC. Similar reasoning is appropriate for patients with extrapulmonary SCLC, particularly those with the so-called "Merkel cell" tumors. There is also a series of mixed NSCLC and SCLC tumors as well as large cell neuroendocrine tumors that reflect the common stem cell heritage of NSCLC and SCLC. Outcome for all of these tumors is a function of the NSCLC component because the SCLC component responds well to chemotherapy. There does seem to be a degree of correlation between the extent of neuroendocrine differentiation in a NSCLC tumor and its responsiveness to chemotherapy.

The author gratefully acknowledges the expert secretarial assistance of Ms. Janet Moseley.

COCCIDIOIDOMYCOSIS

method of
ROGER LARSON, M.D., and
ROBERT LIBKE, M.D.
Valley Medical Center
Fresno, California

Coccidioidomycosis is an illness caused by the fungus *Coccidioides immitis.* This fungus grows well in soil in conditions found in the arid and semiarid regions of the southwestern United States and in a few places in Central and South America. Under proper conditions the fungus produces an abundance of arthroconidia, which are very light and are easily carried in the air. Infection occurs when the arthroconidia are inhaled and converted to spherules, which reproduce in the host by endosporulation. The primary infection is, therefore, almost always in the lung. In the great majority of cases the infection is quickly contained and remains confined to a limited area of the lung. In a few cases the organism is more aggressive and rapidly produces a diffuse pneumonia with an adult respiratory distress syndrome (ARDS)-like picture that may be fatal. In other cases the pulmonary lesions heal but the organism is successful in establishing an infection in other organs in the body through the blood or lymphatic channels. When this happens, the disease is considered to be disseminated and takes on a different character.

The pathology of infection with *Coccidioides immitis* is dimorphic like the fungus. The reaction of the body to the arthroconidia and to the endospores is an acute inflammatory reaction similar to that seen in acute bacterial infections. Reaction to the mature coccidioidal spherules is a granulomatous one similar to that seen in tuberculosis. Clinically, coccidioidomycosis reflects both of these processes—i.e., it can have features of both acute and chronic infection.

The primary infection in the lung is asymptomatic in the majority of instances. When symptomatic, it resembles many other acute lower respiratory tract infections. In some cases, however, clues are present that raise the suspicion of coccidioidomycosis. These are certain dermatoses (erythema nodosum, erythema multiforme, or a morbilliform maculopapular eruption), significant eosinophilia in the differential leukocyte count, a radiologic finding of hilar adenopathy on the side of the airspace consolidation, and a failure to produce a clinical response to conventional antibiotic therapy. Treatment has not been considered necessary in patients with uncomplicated primary infection. When the infection appears to be unusually severe and is progressing to an ARDS-like picture, however, it is prudent to undertake immediate diagnostic tests and initiate treatment with intravenous amphotericin B (Fungizone). Recovery from the primary pulmonary infection may be complete or may leave chronic residuals of either a cavity or a granuloma. Some cavities heal spontaneously within 2 years of the primary infection. Others are complicated by secondary infection, recurrent hemoptysis, or, rarely, rupture into the pleural space. Occasionally these complications are severe enough to warrant lobectomy, but this is the exception rather than the rule (except in cavitary rupture). Unlike tuberculosis, the chronic cavitary residuals of primary pulmonary coccidioidomycosis rarely progress. When they do, the progressive fibrocavitary disease may be indistinguishable from tuberculosis on radiographs.

The residual granuloma is only significant because of the difficulty of distinguishing it from a carcinoma of the lung when it is first discovered on a routine chest radiograph. If the patient is under 40 years of age or the lesion is calcified (coccidioidal granulomas calcify in less than 20% of cases), the lesion can be considered benign and merely followed with serial chest radiographs. Otherwise, enough tissue must be removed from the lesion to allow the pathologist to make a diagnosis. This may be obtained by transbronchial biopsy, thoracoscopic biopsy, or open biopsy, if necessary. (Occasionally organisms can be recovered from the lesion by fine-needle aspiration biopsy that will allow the pathologist to make the diagnosis without tissue biopsy.)

DIAGNOSIS

The diagnosis of coccidioidomycosis is established by finding the organism microscopically, by culture of tissue or body fluids, or by serology. Occasionally one is fortunate enough to be able to establish the diagnosis when a previously negative skin test converts to positive or by finding a positive skin test in a person who has only recently lived or traveled in an endemic area. Otherwise, the skin test is of no diagnostic value. In particular, a negative skin test should never be interpreted as excluding the possibility of a coccidioidal illness. Serologic reactions are the tests most frequently used for the diagnosis of coccidioidal infection. The best ones are both specific and sensitive. Some of the serologic tests are designed to detect IgM antibodies (the earliest and most evanescent); others detect IgG antibodies (which persist much longer and are quantitatively related to the severity of the infection), and others detect both. The most reliable techniques for detecting IgM antibodies are the tube precipitin test, the immunodiffusion technique, and an enzyme immunoassay. The most reliable tests for IgG antibodies are the complement fixation test and an immunodiffusion test. The former has the very great advantage of being quantitatively related to the severity of infection and therefore is useful in following the progression or resolution of the disease.

Dissemination is considered to occur when clinically apparent lesions are found outside the thoracic cavity. The most common sites of dissemination are the skin, lymph nodes, skeleton, synovia, and central nervous system. Almost any organ, however, can be involved. Dissemination may be focal, multifocal, or diffuse. The two most serious forms are diffuse dissemination and focal dissemination to the central nervous system. Prior to the advent of effective therapy, these two forms were almost always fatal. Even now, with effective antifungal agents, these two conditions carry a significant mortality. Dissemination usually occurs with the primary infection and only rarely as a late complication of a chronic pulmonary lesion. Cumulative clinical experience during the 9 decades since the first description of coccidioidomycosis now allows the clinician to predict with some accuracy the likelihood of dissemination. Coccidioidomycosis is unique among infectious illnesses in that humans have a genetically determined resistance to dissemination of the organism. This resistance is found most commonly in whites and least frequently in Filipinos. In between, in descending order of frequency of inherited resistance, are Asian, Native American, Hispanic, and African American. Infection in infancy and infection in the second or third trimester of pregnancy carry a high risk of dissemination, as does infection in persons with immunocompromised status. Clinical clues to the development of dissemination are a rapid rise in complement-fixing antibodies to a titer of 1:32 or greater, a prolonged primary illness (greater than 4 weeks), or development of mediastinal adenopathy on the chest radiograph. The risk of dissemination is so high in the latter two circumstances that treatment is advisable before actual evidence of dissemination occurs. The same can be said for infection in infants and in immunocompromised patients. Otherwise, the risk of dissemination is a matter of clinical judgment in weighing the number of unfavorable factors such as race, pregnancy, and complement-fixation titers.

TREATMENT

There is general agreement that disseminated disease is always an indication for treatment, but there is no consensus on the treatment of choice. Until recently, amphotericin B was the only effective medication. Now there are at least three other agents that have demonstrated some degree of effectiveness in both in vitro and clinical trials, namely, ketoconazole, fluconazole, and itraconazole. All three have the big advantage of being sufficiently absorbed from the gastrointestinal tract to achieve serum concentrations that are effective in in vitro studies. Fluconazole and itraconazole appear to have an advantage over ketoconazole in having considerably less toxicity and as good or better therapeutic effectiveness in initial clinical trials. Fluconazole is less dependent on gastric acidity for absorption and has the additional theoretical advantage of readily passing the blood-brain barrier to achieve good concentration in the cerebrospinal fluid. The only advantage of ketoconazole at present is its lower cost. So far, no direct comparative study has been done between itraconazole and fluconazole to determine any superiority in therapeutic effectiveness between the two drugs.

Considerably more cumulative experience exists with the use of amphotericin B than with the azole derivatives. Cure or control of focal and multifocal dissemination (exclusive of meningitis) with intravenous amphotericin B is the rule and therefore must be considered the gold standard against which all other drugs are measured. When dissemination is diffuse and rapid or an ARDS-like pulmonary picture develops, mortality is still significant regardless of the type of therapy used. The same may be said for coccidioidal meningitis, even when it is the only clinical site of dissemination. In view of the current uncertainty about the best therapeutic approach, we present the options to the patient (or the responsible person if the patient is not competent to make this decision), describing the routes of administration, the toxic effects, and the current knowledge about each drug's effectiveness. The patient is told in no uncertain terms that good results are presently most predictable with the use of amphotericin B because that is the drug that has the most experience behind it. Despite this weighing of the options, it is remarkable how seldom amphotericin B is selected by patients as primary therapy when the possibility of control with a much more convenient and pleasanter regimen exists.

Treatment with fluconazole (Diflucan) or itraconazole (Sporanox) should start with 200 mg per day and should be increased to tolerance to a maximum of 800 mg per day.* Because the half-life of both of these drugs is very long they can be administered in one dose or divided into a twice daily dosage schedule. The length of treatment is entirely dependent on the clinical course. Treatment should probably be continued for several months following complete clinical resolution. Relapse following cessation of therapy is common, and some patients may require lifelong treatment. When given for threatened rather than clinically evident dissemination, the course of treatment can often be shortened. From reports in the medical literature, toxicity appears to be greater with itraconazole than with fluconazole. The major unwanted side effects of the former are nausea and vomiting, edema, and hypertension.

Amphotericin B is the recommended treatment when the patient is desperately ill or when the clinical course is deteriorating rapidly. It is given intravenously in a concentration of 0.1 mg/mL over a period of 1 to 2 hours daily. It is customary to start with a small dose of 10 mg and increase it by 20-mg increments up to a daily dose of 50 mg. The dosage can be escalated more rapidly when demanded by the clinical situation. Toxic side effects are almost universal

*Exceeds dosage recommended by the manufacturer.

and should be anticipated by giving premedication of acetaminophen, 650 mg, and diphenhydramine (Benadryl), 50 mg, to lessen the rigors that frequently accompany the intravenous infusion. When this combination fails to control rigors, 25 mg of meperidine (Demerol) given as a slow intravenous bolus is often successful. Nausea and vomiting can frequently be ameliorated with antiemetics such as prochlorperazine (Compazine) or trimethobenzamide (Tigan). Renal tubular acidosis with hypokalemia, mild metabolic acidosis, and azotemia are also predictable results of continued amphotericin treatment. The metabolic acidosis is rarely significant enough to require attention, but the serum potassium and creatinine levels must be monitored daily until the response to treatment appears to be stable. Potassium can be replaced orally but sometimes requires very large doses. Amphotericin should be discontinued when the serum creatinine exceeds 3.0 and can be restarted when the creatinine drops below 2.5. After 0.5 gram of amphotericin has been given, administration can often be reduced to three times a week instead of daily. This makes outpatient administration quite practical for most patients. The total dosage of amphotericin should be determined by the clinical course and response to treatment. When given for threatened dissemination rather than clinically evident dissemination, 0.5 gram is often enough. For clinically apparent dissemination anywhere from 1 to 4 or more grams may be required.

In patients with coccidioidal meningitis it is customary to give only 0.5 to 1.0 gram of amphotericin intravenously but to give also intrathecal (cisternal or intraventricular)* amphotericin for an indefinite period of time as determined by the lumbar fluid parameters as well as the clinical response. It is desirable to continue intrathecal therapy until the lumbar fluid returns to normal and then for an additional 3 to 6 months. Cisternal injection is the preferred route of administration whenever possible. The starting dose is 0.05 mg, and this is increased daily to the largest dose tolerated or a maximum of 0.6 mg. After achieving a stable dose, the frequency of administration can be reduced to three times a week and, after lumbar fluid parameters have returned to normal, to once or twice a week.

Recent experience suggests that fluconazole is also effective in the treatment of coccidioidal meningitis. It has been used as sole therapy in doses of 400 to 1000 mg per day. Control of disease with improvement in cerebrospinal fluid parameters has occurred in the majority of patients, but relapse has been frequent when therapy has been stopped. It is now our policy, when treating patients with coccidioidal meningitis with fluconazole, to continue it indefinitely and possibly lifelong. When used in conjunction with intrathecal amphotericin, fluconazole may shorten the duration of intrathecal therapy.

*This therapy has not been approved by the Food and Drug Administration (FDA) for this indication.

HISTOPLASMOSIS

method of
STANLEY W. CHAPMAN, M.D.
University of Mississippi Medical Center
Jackson, Mississippi

Histoplasmosis is the systemic infection caused by the thermally dimorphic fungus *Histoplasma capsulatum.* At room temperature the organism grows as the mycelial form and produces both microconidia and tuberculated macroconidia. At 37° C the conidia convert to small (2 to 4 μm) nonencapsulated oval yeast cells that reproduce by polar budding. When seen in tissue specimens, the yeast cells are found almost exclusively within macrophages and neutrophils.

Histoplasmosis is the most common systemic fungal infection in the United States, and most cases occur in the Ohio and Mississippi River basins. Skin testing surveys indicate that greater than 80% of individuals in these endemic areas have been infected. Environmental surveys have shown that *H. capsulatum* grows in the soil as the saprophytic mycelial form. Although the factors that promote its growth in soil are incompletely understood, the organism flourishes in soil contaminated by bird and bat guano. Even within the endemic areas, however, the specific conditions that promote the growth of *H. capsulatum* are patchy, resulting in microfoci or point sources of infection (e.g., bird roosts, chicken houses, caves, attics, and old buildings.)

Infection occurs by inhalation of the conidia, which are small enough to reach the terminal bronchioles and alveoli. The conidia convert to the yeast form in 2 to 3 days and are efficiently phagocytized by macrophages. The organism continues to proliferate intracellularly, and other macrophages are recruited to the sites of infection, which results in focal infiltrates within the lungs. Infected macrophages then migrate to the regional lymph nodes of the lung hilum and mediastinum. Hematogenous spread of the organism may occur, especially to the liver and spleen, but in most cases infection is transient and is limited by the development of cellular immunity 1 to 3 weeks after infection. Healing of the primary infection occurs by a necrotizing granulomatous reaction with fibrosis and calcification. Cellular immunity diminishes over time and reinfection is common in the endemic areas. The illness seen with reinfection has a shorter incubation period, is generally less severe, and has a more rapid recovery time than primary disease. Exogenous reinfection is more common than reactivation of latent infection.

CLINICAL MANIFESTATIONS

The clinical manifestations of histoplasmosis vary from asymptomatic infection to widely disseminated disease. The specific clinical syndrome that results depends on the number of inhaled conidia and the patient's pulmonary anatomy and immune status. Three forms of infection are generally recognized. *Acute pulmonary histoplasmosis* refers to infection in the normal host. Most persons are infected with a low inoculum of conidia, and primary infection is usually subclinical or asymptomatic. The only evidence of infection in these cases is skin test conversion or calcifications in the lung or hilar lymph nodes. If a larger inoculum is inhaled, a flulike illness may develop approximately 2 weeks after infection. Fever, malaise, headache, myalgias, chest pain, and a nonproductive cough are frequently reported. Chest radiographs may show a patchy pneumonitis or diffuse nodular infiltrates. Enlargement of the hilar and mediastinal lymph nodes occurs frequently. Pleural effusions are uncommon. Findings on physical examination are minimal, but hepatomegaly and splenomegaly may be noted. Occasional patients may present with signs and symptoms of inflammatory complications, including erythema nodosum, arthritis, or pericarditis.

Chronic pulmonary histoplasmosis occurs primarily in patients with chronic obstructive pulmonary disease. Although cellular immunity is normal, the organism can colonize and proliferate in the abnormal airspaces that accompany centrilobular and bullous emphysema, resulting in a chronic cavitary pneumonia that clinically and radiologically mimics tuberculosis. Symptoms include low-grade fever, weight loss, anorexia, malaise, chest pain, productive cough, and hemoptysis. Segmental and subsegmental infiltrates are usually pleural based and are located in the apices of the lungs. Cavities and fibrosis develop with persistent infection and may progress to pulmonary insufficiency.

Disseminated histoplasmosis occurs in patients who do not develop cellular immunity against *H. capsulatum.* In these patients, the organism continues to proliferate, and progressive parasitization of the reticuloendothelial system results. Persons at greatest risk of disseminated disease are the very young and very old, those who are immunosuppressed, such as HIV-infected patients, transplant recipients, patients with lymphomas, and patients being treated with steroids or cytotoxic agents. The clinical presentation of disseminated disease is variable. In some patients, especially those with AIDS, the clinical course may be rapidly progressive with a sepsis-like syndrome, thrombocytopenia, coagulopathy, and multiple organ involvement. In other patients the clinical course is more chronic and is measured in months or even years. These patients have low-grade fevers, weight loss, hepatomegaly, splenomegaly, and mucosal ulcers. Pulmonary symptoms are minimal and may include cough or dyspnea. Chest radiographs are usually normal but may show diffuse, ill-defined interstitial infiltrates.

DIAGNOSIS

The diagnosis of histoplasmosis is often difficult. Definitive diagnosis requires culture of the organism from clinical material or visualization of the characteristic small yeast forms in histopathologic specimens. Sputum cultures are positive in fewer than 10% of patients with acute pulmonary histoplasmosis. Although sputum cultures are positive in up to 70% of patients with chronic pulmonary infection, multiple specimens are often required. In suspected cases of disseminated infection, blood, bone marrow aspirates, liver biopsy material, and scrapings of mucocutaneous ulcers should be examined microscopically and cultured. Bone marrow aspiration and biopsy are especially useful. The lysis-centrifugation method is more sensitive than other blood culture techniques. If granulomas are noted in the tissue specimens, methenamine silver staining should be performed to visualize the organism. AIDS patients with histoplasmosis may not form granulomas, and special stains should be performed routinely. The Wright and Giemsa stains are best for visualizing the organism in blood smears, buffy coat preparations, or bone marrow specimens.

Skin testing is of almost no diagnostic value because of the high incidence of skin test reactivity in the population in endemic areas and because skin tests are negative in most patients with disseminated disease. The detection of antibodies to antigens of *H. capsulatum* by serologic tests is most helpful when used in conjunction with a clinical syndrome compatible with active histoplasmosis. Complement fixation tests are suggestive of infection if a fourfold rise in titer is demonstrated, if a titer of 1:32 or higher is present, or if conversion from negative to positive is documented. The immunodiffusion test detects precipitating antibody to H and M antigens and is more specific for histoplasmosis but is less sensitive than complement fixation tests. The presence of an H band correlates best with recent or active disease. Because serologic tests for antibody are negative in about 50% of patients with disseminated disease, a negative test should never be used to rule out infection. Highly sensitive tests for antibody detection using enzyme immunoassay (EIA) and radioimmunoassay (RIA) have been described but are not yet commercially available. A radioimmunoassay for the detection of *Histoplasma* polysaccharide antigen in serum and urine has been developed. This test is both sensitive and specific for the detection of antigenuria and antigenemia in patients with disseminated disease. Antigen is usually not detected in patients with localized or self-limited infection. This assay should prove helpful in following a patient's response to therapy because antigen levels decrease with successful treatment and increase with relapse. Antigen testing is now available in a single commercial laboratory (Histoplasmosis Reference Laboratory, Indianapolis, IN).

ANTIFUNGAL THERAPY

General Principles

The treatment of histoplasmosis varies with the specific clinical syndrome, the severity of disease, and the immune status of the patient. Amphotericin B (Fungizone) was previously considered the treatment of choice for all clinical forms of histoplasmosis. Recent studies indicate, however, that either ketoconazole (Nizoral) or itraconazole (Sporanox) is an effective alternative in selected patients with mild to moderately severe disease. A third azole, fluconazole (Diflucan), is currently being investigated for the treatment of histoplasmosis. Amphotericin B remains the drug of choice in the presence of life-threatening disease, central nervous system infection, disease progression on an azole, or inability to tolerate an azole owing to toxicity.

Amphotericin B is a polyene macrolide that binds to ergosterol in the fungal cell membrane. Formation of pores in the membrane allows leakage of intracellular contents and cell death. Amphotericin is administered intravenously at a concentration of 0.1 mg per mL in dextrose and water. It does not need to be protected from light. Most patients tolerate a 1-hour infusion, but longer infusion times (4 to 6 hours) should be used in patients with renal failure because of the risk of cardiac arrhythmias. Unfortunately, amphotericin B also binds to the cholesterol in mammalian cells, and this probably accounts for many of its well-described toxic reactions. Infusion-related toxic reactions include chills, fever, and nausea and vomiting. Although these tend to diminish with subsequent doses, premedication with diphenhydramine (Benadryl) and aspirin or acetaminophen may be helpful. Rigors are best treated with intravenous meperidine (Demerol). If severe reactions persist, corticosteroids can be used as a premedication or added to the infusion. The patient should be carefully monitored for the appearance of dose-related toxicities including hypokalemia, hypomagnesemia, anemia, and renal failure. Hypokalemia and hypomagnesemia respond well to oral or intravenous replacement. Anemia occurs in almost all patients but usually does not require transfusion. If the serum creatinine rises above 2.5 mg/dL, I recommend that the dosage be reduced or, alternatively, if the drug is being given daily, that it be given only on alternate days or thrice weekly.

Both ketoconazole and itraconazole inhibit the synthesis of ergosterol, the major sterol in the fungal cell membrane. Both agents require gastric acid for absorption, and patients on antacids or H_2 blockers may have subtherapeutic levels. Rifampin (Rifadin), phenytoin (Dilantin), and carbamazepine (Tegretol) have been shown to increase the metabolism of both azoles, and the concurrent use of these drugs may result in treatment failures. Life-threatening ventricular arrhythmias have been reported when these azoles have been used simultaneously with terfenadine (Seldane) and astemizole (Hismanal). Neither drug should be used in patients with central nervous system histoplasmosis. Similar adverse effects have been reported with both azoles, although itraconazole appears to be better tolerated. Dose-related toxic reactions include nausea, vomiting, and endocrine dysfunction (e.g., impotence, gynecomastia, hypoadrenalism). Hepatitis has been reported with both agents, and hepatic transaminases should be monitored. Other reported toxicities include pruritus, skin rash, hypokalemia, edema, and hypertension. Regimens for both ketoconazole and itraconazole are presented for each clinical syndrome. However, it is my opinion that itraconazole is more effective and less toxic than ketoconazole and therefore is the oral agent of choice for patients with histoplasmosis.

Acute Pulmonary Histoplasmosis

Most patients with acute pulmonary histoplasmosis, even when symptomatic, have a self-limited illness and require no treatment. A few patients with very heavy exposure may develop a severe infection that is associated with respiratory compromise. Such patients appear to benefit from a brief course of amphotericin B, and I administer a total dose of 250 to 500 mg over 1 to 2 weeks. Some authors consider both ketoconazole (400 mg daily) and itraconazole (200 mg daily) administered for 2 or 3 months as alternatives to amphotericin B. Although some anecdotal reports have described rapid clinical improvement in patients treated with corticosteroids, I do not recommend their routine use in patients with acute pulmonary histoplasmosis.

Chronic Pulmonary Histoplasmosis

Spontaneous remission may occur in some patients with pneumonic disease or thin-walled cavities. Unless these patients are severely ill, they may be followed for 2 or 3 months and treated if their disease is progressive. Treatment of patients with thick-walled cavities and those with progressive fibrosis should be instituted at diagnosis. Recent studies indicate that either ketoconazole or itraconazole, when given for 6 months or longer, results in clinical response rates that compare favorably with previous reports on the use of amphotericin B. Thus, because of their ease of oral administration and greater safety compared with amphotericin, treatment with an oral azole should be the initial treatment for most patients with chronic pulmonary histoplasmosis.

Ketoconazole is initiated at a dose of 400 mg per day. If the clinical response is not satisfactory, the dose is escalated by 200-mg increments to a maximum daily dose of 800 mg. Itraconazole is usually started as a single daily 200-mg dose. When disease persists or progresses, the dose is increased in increments of 100 mg to a maximum daily dose of 400 mg. The optimal duration of therapy with azoles has not been determined with certainty, but a minimum of 6 months is recommended for both agents. I continue treatment for at least 6 months after sputum cultures have converted to negative. Treatment for a year or longer may be required in a few cases.

Amphotericin B should be used for patients on an azole whose disease progresses or who are unable to tolerate an azole owing to toxicity. In adults I begin at a daily dose of 10 mg and then increase it in 10-mg increments to a maximum daily dose of 0.6 mg per kg, not to exceed 50 mg per day. After a week of daily therapy, the treatment schedule is changed to thrice weekly. The best outcomes have been noted when total doses of 30 to 35 mg per kg (e.g., 2 to 2.5 grams in adults) are administered. Patients should be monitored carefully for renal failure, anemia, hypokalemia, and hypomagnesemia.

Disseminated Histoplasmosis

The treatment of disseminated disease must take into account the immune status of the patient, the severity of infection, and the presence or absence of central nervous system infection. All patients with central nervous system infection and those with life-threatening disease should be treated with amphotericin B. A total dose of 30 mg per kg has been reported to have the lowest relapse rates, and this dose should be administered over 10 to 12 weeks. In selected patients who do not have central nervous system infection, an oral azole may be successfully substituted for amphotericin B once clinical improvement ensues. Itraconazole is recommended in immunocompromised patients (see following paragraphs).

Both ketoconazole and itraconazole have proved effective in the treatment of patients with mild to moderately severe disease. Treatment failures are common when ketoconazole is used for immunocompromised patients, particularly AIDS patients. Itraconazole, in contrast, has proved effective in AIDS patients and also appears to be better tolerated than is ketoconazole. For these reasons, itraconazole is my oral agent of choice for disseminated histoplasmosis. The initial dose of itraconazole in non-AIDS patients is 200 mg daily, and this may be escalated in 100-mg daily increments to a maximum daily dose of 400 mg. Patients treated with an azole should receive a minimum of 6 months of therapy.

AIDS patients with severe disseminated disease should be treated initially with amphotericin B until the acute illness is controlled. Dose and duration of this induction phase vary from 15 to 30 mg per kg and 4 to 8 weeks, respectively. In AIDS patients with mild to moderately severe disease, itraconazole is begun at a dose of 300 mg twice daily for 3 days and then 200 mg twice daily for 12 weeks. Relapse after either induction therapy occurs frequently in AIDS patients, and maintenance therapy is recommended. Itraconazole, 200 to 400 mg daily, is the most effective maintenance regimen. Amphotericin B (1 mg per kg) administered weekly is a less effective alternative.

BLASTOMYCOSIS

method of
SCOTT F. DAVIES, M.D.
University of Minnesota Medical School and Hennepin County Medical Center
Minneapolis, Minnesota

Blastomycosis is an uncommon but important fungal infection. The infection is caused by the organism *Blastomyces dermatitidis,* which is endemic throughout most of the eastern half of the United States, excluding most of New England and the Florida peninsula. Disease activity is relatively high in the great river valleys of the central United States, where the disease is co-endemic with histoplasmosis. Many cases are reported from Arkansas, Illinois, Kentucky, and Tennessee. Compared with histoplasmosis, disease activity extends further north and west, across northern Wisconsin and Minnesota and far into the adjacent provinces of central Canada.

The disease is acquired by inhalation, and pulmonary illness is most frequent. Extrapulmonary spread may occur to any organ but is most common to the skin, bone, meninges, and male genitourinary tract, the first two sites being by far the most common.

Patients with pulmonary infection may present with an acute pneumonia with alveolar or even lobar infiltrates. The inflammatory response in blastomycosis is mixed with pyogenic and granulomatous components. Many patients have purulent secretions, which can be blood-streaked. The clinical syndrome closely resembles acute bacterial pneumonia.

More common is a chronic pulmonary disease with a mass lesion or multiple nodules. Symptoms are variable but less acute. Some patients are even asymptomatic. The illness can mimic lung cancer or a subacute pulmonary infection such as tuberculosis.

Symptoms may include productive cough, low-grade fever, night sweats, and weight loss and are present for weeks to months.

Rare patients have diffuse alveolar infiltrates and present in a highly toxic condition with severe hypoxemia, which is typical of the adult respiratory distress syndrome resulting from diffuse pulmonary infection.

Extrapulmonary blastomycosis includes skin lesions that are warty and crusted (resembling pyoderma gangrenosum) or ulcerative (resembling basal cell carcinoma). Bony lesions are destructive with granulomatous areas but also abscesses and necrosis. Extrapulmonary lesions may be found in patients with active pulmonary disease, or they may appear as isolated extrapulmonary lesions in patients whose symptomatic or even asymptomatic primary pulmonary infections have already cleared. Such patients have a normal chest roentgenogram when they present with extrapulmonary disease. Meningitis is a rare extrapulmonary complication of blastomycosis.

Diagnosis of blastomycosis is usually made by examining secretions or biopsy material directly (either after potassium hydroxide [KOH] digestion or after staining with special stains including Papanicolaou and Giemsa stains for cytologic material and periodic acid–Schiff [PAS] and silver stains for tissue biopsies) or by culturing the organism from these biologic materials. For pneumonia, the diagnostic progression is usually KOH preparation and fungal culture of sputum, followed by fiberoptic bronchoscopy with bronchoalveolar lavage and transbronchial biopsy. Specimens are examined directly after cytologic and histopathologic preparation and are also cultured. Occasional patients require needle biopsy, aspiration of pleural fluid, or thoracoscopic or traditional open lung biopsy for diagnosis. Skin and bone lesions are subjected to needle aspiration or biopsy, again with direct examination of the material using cytologic and histopathologic techniques as well as culture of these specimens. Cultures of lumbar spinal fluid have a relatively low yield in blastomycotic meningitis; sometimes cisternal or ventricular taps are necessary.

Treatment options include amphotericin B and the oral imidazoles—ketoconazole (Nizoral) and itraconazole (Sporanox). The oral agents, especially itraconazole, are potent, but they are not equal to amphotericin B. One important principle is that patients with life-threatening infections should always be treated with amphotericin B, the most powerful and really the only fungicidal agent available. Most patients do not present with life-threatening disease, however, but with mild to moderate acute or chronic pneumonias or with skin or bone lesions. Oral therapy is suitable and highly effective for all these patients. I prefer itraconazole over ketoconazole as the oral agent of choice because it is better absorbed, has fewer gastrointestinal side effects, has less effect on the synthesis of testosterone and other steroids, acts faster, and appears to be more potent based on many reports of successful therapy with itraconazole after failure with ketoconazole. However, ketoconazole has been proved effective in large trials and is much less expensive (about one-tenth the cost). Either oral agent is less costly and less toxic than a full course of intravenous amphotericin B.

The following recommendations are given for the treatment of the different clinical forms of blastomycosis.

1. Acute pulmonary blastomycosis resembling bacterial pneumonia, mild or moderately severe, can be treated with itraconazole, 200 to 400 mg orally given daily for 6 months.
2. Subacute or chronic pulmonary blastomycosis resembling lung cancer or tuberculosis can also be treated with a 6-month course of itraconazole (same dose).
3. Chronic skin, bone, or other nonmeningeal disseminated blastomycosis can also be treated with a 6-month course of itraconazole (same dose).
4. Severe acute pulmonary blastomycosis with severe toxicity or severe hypoxemia including all patients presenting with edematous lobar pneumonia, adult respiratory distress syndrome, or diffuse infiltrates should be treated with intravenous amphotericin B.

Intravenous amphotericin B is given daily over 1 to 2 hours. I give an initial dose of 10 mg and rapidly increase the daily dose to 40 to 50 mg. In severe cases a 10-mg dose can be followed later the same day with a 20-mg dose followed by a full 40- to 50-mg dose on the second day. In less urgent situations these three doses can be given over the first 3 days. The full daily doses are continued until there is objective improvement, including reduction of fever. Then the dosing interval is converted to three times weekly, usually on Monday, Wednesday, and Friday to facilitate outpatient administration. Serum creatinine and serum potassium levels should be monitored weekly. I usually use a 50-mg dose in adults of 70 kg or higher weight but decrease the individual doses to 40 mg if the serum creatinine increases to more than 2.5 mg per dL. All patients show some increase in serum creatinine, but permanent renal impairment is very rare. Renal tubular toxicity results in potassium wasting, and appropriate oral potassium supplementation is often necessary.

Acute amphotericin B reactions with fever and severe chilling can be troublesome. Pretreatment with acetaminophen (650 mg orally) and benadryl (50 mg orally) may produce minor benefit, but the most effective pretreatment to blunt these reactions is intravenous narcotic administration. Meperidine (50 to 75 mg) can be given intravenously 30 minutes before administration of amphotericin B). Other narcotics are also effective. Glucocorticoid preparations (hydrocortisone 50 to 100 mg) are sometimes added to the amphotericin B infusion, but the purpose is to reduce peripheral vein inflammation from the amphotericin B rather than to prevent the chilling reactions. The amphotericin B should be continued to a total cumulative dose of 2 grams. If a total of 120 to 150 mg is given each week (in three divided doses), the total duration of therapy will be 13 to 16 weeks. If the response to amphotericin is very good and the patient is clinically well fairly early in the treatment course, some clinicians stop the administration of amphotericin B after a cumulative dose of 500 mg and then complete a 6-month total treatment course with an oral agent, usually itraconazole, 200 mg orally each day. This approach seems to be effective, but there are no clinical studies comparing this approach with a full 2-gram course of amphotericin B.

Blastomycotic meningitis should always be treated with intravenous amphotericin B because the oral agents poorly penetrate the cerebrospinal fluid.

Blastomycosis is not a common problem in immunosuppressed patients. However, series of cases have been reported in renal transplant recipients and in patients with AIDS. The total experience is too small to make strong recommendations about therapy.

Renal transplant patients should be treated with amphotericin B if they are critically ill. Mild to moderate illness can be treated with itraconazole, 200 to 400 mg daily. The risk of relapse after a 6-month course of itraconazole has not been quantitated but is probably higher than after a full course of amphotericin B. However, the renal toxicity of amphotericin B in the presence of cyclosporine immunosuppression is so high that initial therapy with itraconazole is probably indicated in selected patients. Follow-up must be compulsive.

Blastomycosis in patients with AIDS is usually severe and widely disseminated. Amphotericin B should be used initially for critically ill patients. If there is clinical improvement, the patient can be switched to oral itraconazole, which should be continued for life because virtually all patients relapse if treatment is stopped. As for cryptococcal and histoplasma infections in AIDS patients, lifelong maintenance therapy is necessary. Milder infections can be treated with itraconazole from the onset.

PLEURAL EFFUSION AND EMPYEMA THORACIS

method of
MARK S. ALLEN, M.D.
Mayo Clinic and Mayo Foundation
Rochester, Minnesota

PLEURAL EFFUSION

Normally, only a few milliliters of fluid are present in the pleural space, although an estimated 5 to 10 liters of fluid move through the pleural space per day. When the rate of secretion exceeds the rate of reabsorption, an effusion occurs. Pleural effusions are classified as either transudates or exudates. If the fluid is protein poor, it is a transudate. Causes of transudates include congestive heart failure, cirrhosis, nephrotic syndrome, peritoneal dialysis, hypoalbuminemia, constrictive pericarditis, malignancy, atelectasis, and urinothorax. If the effusion is protein-rich, it is an exudate. Exudates result from changes in capillary permeability caused by inflammation or infiltration of the pleura. Causes of exudative effusions are more numerous and include infection, malignancy, and immunologic, inflammatory, iatrogenic, and subdiaphragmatic causes.

Symptoms of pleural effusion include dyspnea on exertion, pleuritic chest pain, fatigue, cough, weight loss, and fevers and chills. Physical examination usually reveals decreased breath sounds, dullness to percussion, and egophony over the affected area. A chest roentgenogram establishes the diagnosis; however, decubitus views, ultrasonography, or computed tomography (CT) may be necessary to localize and quantitate the effusion. Pleurocentesis should be the initial diagnostic test. The goal is to classify the effusion as a transudate or an exudate. Enough fluid should be removed for adequate analysis; however, if the patient is symptomatic, almost all of the fluid can be removed. The risk of re-expansion pulmonary edema is low as long as the pleural space is not connected to a high negative pressure and the volume removed is limited. The fluid need not be sent for every conceivable test but only those that will help to determine the cause of the effusion. It is helpful to save some of the fluid in a heparinized container in the refrigerator for future use as needed. Fluid obtained by thoracentesis should be examined for protein, lactate dehydrogenase (LD), cell count, culture, pH, and cytology. Table 1 shows the characteristics that differentiate an exudate from a transudate. The glucose level in pleural fluid is low in effusions caused by tuberculosis, rheumatoid arthritis, empyemas, or malignancies. The amylase concentration is elevated in effusions secondary to pancreatitis, pancreatic pseudocyst, esophageal perforation, or malignancy. In addition to chemical analysis, the color of the fluid can help to establish a diagnosis. Grossly

TABLE 1. **Differentiation of Transudates and Exudates**

	Transudate	Exudate
Protein	Low	>3 gm/dL
Pleural fluid protein/serum protein		>0.5
Lactate dehydrogenase (LD)	Low	>1000 IU
Pleural fluid LD/serum LD		>0.6
pH	Same as arterial	<7.20 implies empyema
Cytology	Negative	Can be positive in malignant effusion
Blood sugar	Same as serum	
White blood cell count	<1000/mm^3	>1000/mm^3
Color	Clear	Cloudy
Odor	Odorless	
Specific gravity	<1.016	>1.016
Culture	Negative	Can be positive in empyema
Red blood cell count	<10.000 mm^3	>10.000 mm^3

bloody effusions are associated with trauma, pulmonary infarctions, malignancy, traumatic pleurocentesis, and, rarely, thoracic endometriosis. Brown fluid may represent a ruptured amebic abscess, black fluid an *Aspergillus* infection, tube-feed–colored fluid a misplaced feeding tube, and white fluid a chylothorax. The smell of the fluid is also helpful; putrid-smelling fluid implies an anaerobic infection, and an ammonia smell indicates urinothorax.

Treatment of the effusion is usually directed toward the underlying cause. For symptomatic malignant effusions, video-assisted thoracic surgery (VATS) drainage with talc pleurodesis is the preferred method. Repeat thoracentesis or closed-tube thoracostomy and chemical pleurodesis are usually less effective. If the lung parenchyma is trapped from a malignant peel, placement of a pleuroperitoneal shunt can help to relieve symptoms.

EMPYEMA THORACIS

Pleural empyema is an accumulation of pus in the pleural space. Empyemas are classified into three phases based on the natural history of the disease. The first, or acute, phase is characterized by an expandable underlying lung surrounded by thin, purulent fluid. The second, or transitional, phase is characterized by turbid fluid that has an increased cellular content and by deposition of fibrin on the pleural surfaces. This forms a limiting peel that prevents extension of the empyema but also traps the underlying lung. The third, or chronic, phase is characterized by organization of the pleural peel and ingrowth of the fibrous tissue that entraps the lung.

Most empyemas are secondary to pneumonia. Other causes include lung abscess, chest trauma, subphrenic abscess, esophageal perforation, septic emboli, and postoperative factors. Empyemas occurring after a pulmonary resection can also be classified as pleural infections with or without a bronchopleural fistula.

The management of empyemas is related to etiology; however, adequate drainage of the empyema is important in all pleural space infections. As with any other collection of pus in the body, empyemas are seldom cured by antibiotic administration alone. Delay in treating an empyema, brought about by administering prolonged courses of antibiotics with inadequate drainage, significantly complicates the subsequent treatment of an infected pleural space.

Early empyemas, without bronchopleural fistulas, may be drained by thoracentesis. However, if there is a white blood cell count of more than 10,000 per mm^3, positive Gram's stain or culture results, a glucose level of less than 40, or a pH of less than 7.2, the effusion should be defined as an empyema and drained by tube thoracostomy. In addition, if the pleural fluid is thick or incompletely drained after thoracentesis, a chest tube should be placed. Chest roentgenograms or CT scans can be used to confirm adequate drainage of the pleural space. Appropriate antibiotics should be chosen to treat the acute phase of the pleural infection and the possible underlying pulmonary parenchymal infection.

With adequate drainage established, the patient's clinical course should improve, and after the underlying pneumonitis resolves, antibiotics can be stopped. Patients who have inadequate evacuation of the empyema with tube thoracostomy or loculated collections may require further drainage to resolve the infection. This may include additional chest tubes, VATS, or thoracotomy and decortication. VATS can debride an empyematous space but, when the empyema is large and well organized, it is tedious to perform decortication with VATS. After the pleural space has been adequately evacuated and the acute inflammation resolved, a CT scan should be performed to detect any residual space in the pleural cavity. If no residual space exists, the chest tube can be removed. If there is a small or moderate residual space, a chest tube can be left in place to provide adequate drainage and slowly advanced out over a period of weeks. Occasionally, it is necessary to resect a rib and place a larger tube, an empyema tube, in the dependent portion of the cavity. Another option for long-term open drainage is an Eloesser flap. However, for most patients with an entrapped lung, thoracotomy with decortication provides quicker resolution. If a large residual space is present, closure is accomplished by mobilizing a chest wall muscle or the omentum into the cavity. Alternatively, a Clagett procedure, whereby the space is filled with antibiotic solution and closed, can be performed. As a last resort, a thoracoplasty is used to eliminate the space.

Patients who have bronchopleural fistulas associated with empyema require special management. Drainage and the early administration of antibiotics are the key points of treatment. Immediate drainage removes the collection of pus and prevents the purulent material from infecting the contralateral lung through the bronchopleural fistula. The acute infection should be well controlled before repair of the bronchopleural fistula is undertaken. After drainage and resolution of the acute infection have been accomplished, plans for repair of the bronchopleural fistula can be made; such fistulas rarely close spontaneously. The fistula can be repaired by direct suture closure and reinforced with a muscle or omental flap. A transsternal, transpericardial approach has been used for postpneumonectomy bronchopleural fistulas with long bronchial stumps. After the bronchopleural fistula has healed, the residual space can be closed with a Clagett procedure.

PRIMARY LUNG ABSCESS

method of
BRUCE P. KRIEGER, M.D.
University of Miami School of Medicine
Miami, Florida

Primary lung abscess is a predominantly anaerobic pulmonary infection that destroys the lung parenchyma, resulting in one or more large cavities. The hallmark of the infection, lung necrosis, appears to be mediated by anaerobic bacterial production of volatile fatty acids, which produce a pH-dependent inhibition of phagocyte killing as well as an immunoregulatory T-cell "lymphokine." It is distinguished from necrotizing pneumonia by a larger cavity size (>2 cm), more frequent air-fluid levels, and a stronger association with other community-acquired anaerobic pleuropulmonary infections such as aspiration pneumonia and empyema. Knowledge of the pathophysiology of infection clarifies which populations are predisposed to the development of lung abscess and which organisms are most likely to be involved. The usual mechanism involves aspiration of an appropriate inoculum, usually from the upper airways, combined with an inability to clear the material or a condition characterized by abnormal bronchial drainage. Conditions that therefore predispose patients to lung abscess include (1) depressed mental status, (2) swallowing disorders, (3) immunocompromised hosts, (4) bronchial obstruction due to tumor, extrinsic compression, or foreign body, (5) bronchiectasis, (6) immotile ciliary syndromes, and (7) cystic fibrosis. When multiple abscesses occur, septic thrombophlebitis with hematogenous spread must be considered.

The causative organisms have been identified through transtracheal and transthoracic aspiration techniques. The infections are frequently polymicrobial, and anaerobes are involved in 90% of the specimens studied. The most common anaerobes are gram-positive cocci (*Peptostreptococcus* and *Peptococcus*) and gram-negative bacilli (*Fusobacterium* species and the *Bacteroides* genus). When the patient has been institutionalized (hospital or nursing home), mixed infections with aerobic gram-negative bacilli and gram-positive cocci (including staphylococci) can occur. Other infectious etiologies of lung abscess include *Mycobacterium,* fungi, *Nocardia,* and *Pneumocystis.*

DIAGNOSIS

Patients with lung abscess generally present with indolent (7 to 14 days) symptoms consisting of fever, weight loss (40%), night sweats, and putrid sputum (50%) along with moderate leukocytosis. The distinguishing radiographic finding is a solitary cavity with an air-fluid level in a dependent portion of the lung surrounded by an infiltrate. The differential diagnosis of this radiographic picture includes carcinoma, pulmonary infarction, infected bullae, and vasculitides (such as Wegener's granulomatosis); however, usually these cavitary lesions are not associated with infiltrates.

Diagnosis by culture is difficult because the specimen must be uncontaminated by the upper airway flora. Therefore, sputum and unprotected endotracheal aspirates are not adequate. Transtracheal and percutaneous transthoracic needle aspirates provide useful material but are generally considered excessively invasive and are rarely used today. Fiberoptic bronchoscopic techniques that provide useful microbiologic material include quantitative cultures of protected brush or bronchoalveolar lavage; of these, the latter tends to be more sensitive.

MANAGEMENT

The mainstay of treatment for primary lung abscess is empirical antibiotic therapy (based on the results of clinical trials) until the chest radiograph clears or shows a stable scar. For community-acquired lung abscess, clindamycin (Cleocin), 600 mg given intravenously every 6 to 8 hours, has supplanted penicillin G, 1 to 2 million units given intravenously every 4 hours, as the drug of choice. This change is based on the results of two clinical trials as well as in vitro detection of beta-lactamase in 30 to 65% of *Fusobacterium* and *Bacteroides* species. An alternative is to add metronidazole (Flagyl) to penicillin. Intravenous therapy is required for at least 1 week or until signs of objective and subjective improvement appear, at which time oral therapy with clindamycin, 300 mg four times daily, is continued for 2 to 3 months. In critically ill or immunocompromised patients, or when the lung abscess has occurred in a nosocomial setting, antibiotics with good activity against anaerobes as well as enteric gram-negative bacilli are appropriate. These include imipenem (Primaxin) or any combination of a beta-lactam–beta-lactamase inhibitor such as ampicillin plus sulbactam (Unasyn) or ticarcillin plus clavulanic acid (Timentin).

Treatment of any abscess includes appropriate drainage, which can usually be accomplished in these cases with an adequate cough mechanism. Adjunctive therapy in individual patients includes postural drainage and inhaled beta-adrenergic therapy to promote mucociliary clearance. Fiberoptic bronchoscopy, which can detect endobronchial obstruction due to tumor or foreign body, is reserved for patients with an atypical presentation (no predisposition to aspiration, low-grade fever and low white blood cell count, minimal systemic complaints) or those who remain acutely ill despite 7 to 10 days of appropriate antibiotic therapy. Surgical drainage is rarely necessary unless there is an associated empyema. Computed tomographic–guided drainage procedures may also help to decrease the need for thoracotomy. The reported mortality rate for lung abscess is less than 10%, and mortality is usually associated with bronchial obstruction or other debilitating medical conditions such as neoplasm or immunosuppression.

OTITIS MEDIA

method of
GORDON B. HUGHES, M.D.
Cleveland Clinic Foundation
Cleveland, Ohio

Otitis media is an inflammation of the middle ear cleft. Acute otitis media lasts 3 weeks, subacute disease lasts 3 weeks to 3 months, and chronic lesions last more than 3 months. Second only to viral upper respiratory infection (URI), acute otitis media is the most common disease of childhood; two-thirds of children have at least one infection by 12 months of age. In the United States otitis media is more common in white children, Native Americans and Eskimos; in those who have Down's syndrome, cleft palate, and craniofacial disorders; and in those who have immunodeficiency, immotile ciliary syndrome, and possibly allergy. Breast-feeding may confer some protection. Otitis media is much more common during the first 2 weeks after a viral URI.

The child usually tugs at the ear or complains of earache, is fussy and sleeps poorly, and may have fever. The tympanic membrane usually is hyperemic, and the middle ear contains fluid that may be pink or red. In the later stages, pus under pressure may produce a yellow-white eardrum that is distended under pressure, with indistinct landmarks and loss of the light reflex. The eardrum can rupture spontaneously. Complications such as meningitis are rare unless the child is immunocompromised.

On the other hand, examination of the ear can be remarkably benign. The drum may appear normal; middle ear fluid may be clear and colorless; body temperature may be normal. Nevertheless, the middle ear still may be infected. Thirty to 50% of children with subclinical (silent) otitis media with effusion have positive cultures on tympanocentesis. Therefore, if middle ear effusion is present during a URI, children should be treated for presumed otitis media.

TREATMENT

Presumably many cases of otitis media resolve spontaneously without ever being diagnosed. Those cases that are diagnosed should be treated with antibiotics. The most common bacterial species in acute otitis media are *Streptococcus pneumoniae* (pneumococcus), *Haemophilus influenzae,* and *Moraxella catarrhalis.* Group A streptococci and *Staphylococcus aureus,* by comparison, are rare. Gram-negative bacilli cause about 20% of cases of acute otitis media in infants under 6 weeks of age. Anaerobic bacteria and no growth results constitute the remainder of the culture reports. Some cases of *S. pneumoniae* infection are resistant to penicillin; most cases of *M. catarrhalis* and 30% of *H. influenzae* produce beta-lactamase and are resistant to ampicillin. Neither penicillin nor ampicillin should be given, therefore, unless the culture confirms that the organism is sensitive.

Tympanocentesis with culture is not required in routine cases if a beta-lactamase-stable antibiotic is selected unless the child is less than 6 weeks old, is immunocompromised, or does not improve clinically within 48 hours.

Antibiotic Treatment

Table 1 lists the various antibiotics that are approved for use in children and are available in oral suspension. Safety and efficacy have not been determined for loracarbef (Lorabid), cefixime (Suprax), and cefpodoxime (Vantin) in children below the age of 6 months; for sulfamethoxazole-trimethoprim (Septra) and erythromycin-sulfisoxazole (Pediazole) in children younger than 2 months; and for cefaclor (Ceclor) below the age of 1 month. Considering the spectrum of activity, tolerance, and cost, if the patient is not allergic to penicillin, my first choice is amoxicillin. If the patient is allergic to penicillin, I prescribe sulfamethoxazole-trimethoprim or erythromycin-sulfisoxazole. If there is no improvement in 48 hours, I select another antibiotic with a broader spectrum of activity. Physicians should note that cefaclor has limited activity against *H. influenzae* and cefixime has limited activity against pneumococci.

If there is still no improvement, or if the child is younger than 6 weeks old or is immunocompromised, I recommend tympanocentesis for definitive culture. If a complication of otitis media is suspected, the child should be hospitalized; myringotomy should be performed emergently to evacuate pus and obtain culture material; broad-spectrum intravenous antibiotics that will cross the blood-brain barrier should be started. Emergency CT scans (to rule out obstructive hydrocephalus from a possible brain abscess) followed by lumbar puncture should be performed if meningeal complications are suspected.

Antimicrobial prophylaxis can be given for recurrent acute otitis media if the middle ear effusion clears between episodes. Usually two-thirds of the total daily dose is given as a single dose each day. Because otitis media is more common during winter, I usually stop prophylaxis during the spring or summer.

In the future, vaccines for middle ear pathogens may prevent many cases of otitis media. Presently, *H. influenzae* vaccine for meningitis does not prevent (nontypable) *H. influenzae* otitis, and pneumococcal

TABLE 1. **Oral Suspension Antibiotics for Acute Otitis Media***

Antibiotic	Total Daily Dose	Divided Dose Frequency	Duration	Cost†
Amoxicillin (Amoxil)	40 mg/kg/d	q 8 h	10 days	$ 7.29
Amoxicillin/clavulanate (Augmentin)	40 mg/kg/d‡	q 8 h	10 days	$34.10
Cefaclor (Ceclor)	40 mg/kg/d	q 8 h	10 days	$34.50
Cefixime (Suprax)	8 mg/kg/d	qd or bid	10 days	$32.00
Cefpodoxime (Vantin)	10 mg/kg/d	q 12 h	10 days	$40.30
Erythromycin/sulfisoxazole (Pediazole)	50 mg/kg/d§	q 6 h	10 days	$23.70
Loracarbef (Lorabid)	30 mg/kg/d	q 12 h	10 days	$44.50
Sulfamethoxazole/trimethoprim (Septra)	40 mg/kg/d‖	q 12 h	10 days	$ 5.20

*See text for details.

†Approximate prices at the author's hospital in September, 1993 based on 10-kg body weight. Amoxicillin, erythromycin/sulfisoxasole, and sulfamethoxazole/trimethoprim are priced for generic equivalent; the others are brand-name drugs. Some costs are slightly higher because the concentrate or powder cannot be sold in smaller lots based on a 10-kg weight and 10 days' duration (e.g., Suprax).

‡Based on amoxicillin component.

§Based on erythromycin component.

‖Based on sulfamethoxazole component.

vaccine for respiratory disease does not prevent pneumococcal otitis.*

Surgical Treatment

I recommend myringotomy with placement of pressure equalization (PE) tubes if middle ear fluid persists for 3 months, if infections recur frequently (three episodes in 6 months or two episodes before the age of 6 months), if "breakthrough" infections occur despite antibiotic prophylaxis, or if craniofacial anomalies (e.g., cleft palate) predispose the patient to effusion. In my experience, short-term ventilating tubes last approximately 9 months; long-term tubes can last for years. I recommend short-term tubes unless cleft palate or another chronic condition is present. Most healthy children outgrow otitis media by the age of 6 or 7 years, if not earlier. Multiple short-term tubes are preferred to one long-term tube because disease prevalence decreases as the child grows older, and long-term tubes produce more chronic perforations of the tympanic membrane.

Adenoidectomy is performed if the child needs a second set of tubes and the adenoids are enlarged. Prospective studies have determined that adenoidectomy confers additional protection from recurrent middle ear disease. Generally, I do not perform adenoidectomy while the first set of tubes is in place unless the nasal airway is obstructed.

Tonsillectomy is performed for recurrent tonsillitis and may or may not help to prevent middle ear disease. Further studies on this relationship are needed.

Increased recognition of high-risk patients, early diagnosis, prompt treatment, appropriate follow-up, newer antibiotics, and timely placement of ventilation tubes produce significant control of otitis media in childhood and prevent many complications that may occur later in adolescence and adulthood.

INFECTIOUS BRONCHITIS

method of
RICHARD GLECKMAN, M.D.
Boston University School of Medicine
Wayland, Massachusetts

Patients with infectious bronchitis are usually classified into two broad categories: the previously well patient who develops an acute bronchitis syndrome, and patients with chronic bronchitis who experience an infectious "exacerbation."

ACUTE BRONCHITIS

Patients usually develop acute bronchitis in the winter months and have a cough preceded by a sore throat, coryza, and headache. Fever and sputum production are variable manifestations. Most episodes of acute bronchitis are caused by viruses (such as rhinovirus, coronavirus, adenovirus, influenza) and less frequently by *Mycoplasma pneumoniae, Chlamydia pneumoniae, Bordetella pertussis,* or *Legionella* sp. Experts disagree about whether or not *Streptococcus pneumoniae* and *Haemophilus influenzae* cause acute bronchitis syndrome in patients who are free of chronic bronchitis or emphysema.

The clinical findings and routine laboratory studies, such as the complete blood count and sputum analysis, offer no diagnostic assistance to the clinician who is attempting to define the responsible agent. Both viral and nonviral organisms can produce disease accompanied by leukocytosis. Patients can be adequately managed without analyzing the blood, processing sputum, or performing a chest x-ray study.

Patients with acute bronchitis syndrome experience spontaneous resolution, and progression to pneumonia occurs rarely, if ever (one potential exception is disease caused by influenza virus). Physicians should consider prescribing cough suppressants, codeine, or dextromethorphan for patients in whom the quality of life is significantly affected adversely by the illness. At least half of these patients experience cough for more than 2 weeks whether or not they receive any antibiotic.

Prescribing an antibiotic is controversial. A number of studies of this problem have been performed but have had deficiencies in their design. I do not recommend prescribing an antibiotic for the following reasons: The infection is usually caused by a virus and is self-limiting; there is no conclusive proof that an antibiotic accelerates resolution of the infection; and there are antibiotic-related costs and side effects. Most clinicians, however, elect to prescribe an agent such as erythromycin because of their patients' expectations and because of their own concern that the disorder could be caused by an organism such as *B. pertussis, M. pneumoniae,* or *C. pneumoniae* that could potentially be treated effectively. However, the data are not very convincing that acute bronchitis caused by these organisms is, in fact, improved by administration of this antibiotic. An alternative approach is to restrict antibiotic therapy to those patients who have had symptoms for longer than 1 week.

Amantadine (Symmetrel) or rimantadine (Flumadine) should be prescribed for patients with symptomatic influenza A–related acute bronchitis when the patient has had symptoms for less than 48 hours. Amantadine is not effective for disease caused by influenza B and should not be offered to patients who are pregnant or have a seizure disorder. Amantadine shortens the duration and severity of symptoms and accelerates resolution of altered airway function. When prescribed for a patient with renal insufficiency, the drug dose must be reduced. This medication should not be co-administered with chlorpheniramine. Adverse reactions attributed to amantadine include nervousness, lightheadedness, difficulty in concentrating, and insomnia.

*This vaccine has not been approved by the Food and Drug Administration (FDA) for these indications.

EXACERBATION OF CHRONIC BRONCHITIS

It has been estimated that approximately 7.5 million Americans have chronic bronchitis, a disorder attributed to chronic cigarette smoking, repeated childhood respiratory illnesses, and environmental pollutants. This disease is characterized by the chronic production of sputum and resembles other disorders, including cystic fibrosis, bronchiectasis, asthma, chronic sinusitis, and gastroesophageal reflux, that are also associated with prolonged cough and expectoration.

Exacerbation of this disease is usually recognized by a combination of abnormalities consisting of dyspnea on exertion, increased volume of sputum, and an alteration in the sputum appearance. Most exacerbations are not associated with fever. The exacerbation produces disabling symptoms, lost work time, significant financial costs, and, on occasion, a need for hospitalization. Pulmonary function worsens acutely during the exacerbation, and there is concern that infection can cause permanent alteration or an accelerated decline in pulmonary function.

Some, but certainly not all, exacerbations are precipitated by an infectious event. Those organisms most frequently associated with the exacerbation of chronic bronchitis include viruses, *M. pneumoniae, H. influenzae, S. pneumoniae,* and *M.* (*Branhamella*) *catarrhalis.* Limited data suggest a role for *Haemophilus parainfluenzae* and, rarely, *C. pneumoniae.*

As a general rule, there is no compelling need to analyze the blood or sputum or to obtain a chest x-ray study during the first encounter with a patient who does not appear seriously ill and is experiencing an exacerbation of chronic bronchitis. A blood gas determination would be appropriate for patients experiencing insomnia, agitation, or increasing dyspnea. If, however, a patient fails to respond to empirical treatment and compliance is ensured, there should be no hesitation about obtaining sputum for culture and susceptibility testing to exclude beta-lactamase–producing strains of *H. influenzae* and *M.* (*Branhamella*) *catarrhalis* and obtaining x-ray studies to help identify pneumonia, lung cancer, or congestive heart failure masquerading as an infectious exacerbation of chronic bronchitis.

It has been difficult to assess the value of prescribing an antibiotic for these patients because there is no precise definition of an exacerbation, not all exacerbations are initiated by bacterial infection, patients' symptoms are often relieved by co-medications, and meaningful end points of treatment are difficult to identify. One team of researchers noted the benefit of prescribing antibiotics for patients with a more severe exacerbation. In a randomized blinded study recipients of antibiotics experienced more complete resolution of symptoms, required additional medication or hospitalization less frequently, and experienced more rapid improvement in pulmonary function. Neither this study nor subsequent studies have identified the preferred antimicrobial agent, however. Each agent offers advantages and limitations. Tables 1 and 2 describe the characteristics of the traditional oral compounds (erythromycin, doxy-

TABLE 1. **Traditional Compounds for Exacerbations of Chronic Bronchitis**

	Advantages	Concerns
1. Erythromycin	Inexpensive Appropriate for *Mycoplasma, Chlamydia pneumoniae, Streptococcus pneumoniae,* and most *Moraxella (Branhamella) catarrhalis* species Safe for penicillin-allergic patients	GI adverse events (nausea, vomiting, or abdominal discomfort) Requires qid dosing Interacts with theophylline, warfarin, carbamazepine, cyclosporine, terfenadine Resistant *H. influenzae*
2. Doxycycline	Infrequent dosing Appropriate for *Mycoplasma, C. pneumoniae,* and most strains of *S. pneumoniae, Haemophilus influenzae* and *M. (Branhamella) catarrhalis* Inexpensive Safe for penicillin-allergic patients	Rare resistant pneumococci, *H. influenzae* GI adverse events (nausea, vomiting, or abdominal discomfort) Photosensitivity Absorption limited by milk, antacids, iron, food
3. Amoxicillin	Established track record Inexpensive	Contraindicated for penicillin-allergic patients Resistant *H. influenzae, M. catarrhalis*
4. Amoxicillin-potassium clavulanate (Augmentin)	Enhanced spectrum of activity compared to amoxicillin (includes beta-lactamase–producing *H. influenzae* and *M. (Branhamella) catarrhalis*	Contraindicated for penicillin-allergic patients Causes diarrhea Expensive
5. Cefaclor (Ceclor) Cefuroxime (Ceftin) Cefixime (Suprax)	Cefuroxime and cefixime require infrequent dosing	Contraindicated for penicillin-allergic patients Causes diarrhea Expensive
6. Trimethoprim-sulfamethoxazole (Bactrim, Septra)	Requires bid dosing Inexpensive Safe for pencillin-allergic patients	Some resistant pneumococci and *H. influenzae,* fever, rash, GI adverse events (nausea, vomiting, or abdominal discomfort), interaction with phenytoin, warfarin, methotrexate, oral hypoglycemic agents

TABLE 2. **Newer Compounds for Exacerbations of Chronic Bronchitis**

	Advantages	Concerns
1. Cefprozil (Cefzil) Cefpodoxime (Vantin)	Dosing bid	Contraindicated in penicillin-allergic patients Expensive Diarrhea from cefpodoxime Antacids and famotidine (Pepcid), inhibit the bioavailability of cefpodoxime
2. Loracarbef (Lorabid)	Dosing bid	Contraindicated in penicillin-allergic patients Expensive
3. Clarithromycin (Biaxin)	Can be taken with food Dosing bid Better tolerated than erythromycin Safe for pencillin-allergic patients Also appropriate for *Mycoplasma, Chlamydia pneumoniae*	Expensive Potential for drug interactions as with erythromycin
4. Azithromycin (Zithromax)	Once a day dosing Better tolerated than erythromycin Treatment course can be 3–5 days Also appropriate for *Mycoplasma, C. pneumoniae* Safe for penicillin-allergic patients	Expensive Cannot be taken with food
5. Ciprofloxacin (Cipro) Ofloxacin (Floxin) Lomefloxacin (Maxaquin)	Dosing bid (lomefloxacin prescribed once a day) Ofloxacin and lomefloxacin do not interact with theophylline Ofloxacin appropriate for *Mycoplasma, C. pneumoniae* Safe for penicillin-allergic patients Rarely cause pseudomembranous colitis	Expensive Ciprofloxacin interacts with theophylline Absorption in all three compounds is impeded by antacids, sucralfate (Carafate), iron, multivitamins with zinc Ciprofloxacin and lomefloxacin are not appropriate for infections caused by pneumococci

cycline, amoxicillin, amoxicillin-clavulanic acid, cefaclor, cefuroxime, cefixime, trimethoprim-sulfamethoxazole) and the newer agents (cefprozil [Cefzil], cefpodoxime [Vantin], loracarbef [Lorabid], clarithromycin [Biaxin], azithromycin [Zithromax], ciprofloxacin [Cipro], ofloxacin [Floxin], and lomefloxacin [Maxaquin]). The conventional antibiotic treatment duration is 7 to 10 days. Azithromycin treatment can be limited to 5 days, however.

It should be stressed that all the newer compounds are more expensive, require dose adjustment for patients with renal insufficiency, are not known to be safe for pregnant women, and have never been demonstrated to be more effective than the traditional and less expensive agents such as amoxicillin, doxycycline, and trimethoprim-sulfamethoxazole.

Ancillary treatment consists of instituting smoking cessation. The value of hydration and oral expectorants (quaifenesin, saturated iodide) remains undocumented. Evidence exists, however, that iodinated glycerol accelerates the rate of resolution of the exacerbation. As a general rule, patients improve within 3 to 4 days of the onset of treatment, and there is complete resolution of the exacerbation within 2 weeks.

Antibiotic prophylaxis with an agent such as tetracycline, ampicillin, amoxicillin, or trimethoprim-sulfamethoxazole,* prescribed once a day either four times a week or daily during the winter, has been recommended for patients who experience four or more exacerbations per year. Prophylaxis is designed to prevent the number of exacerbations; it is not offered to alter the rate of decline of pulmonary function.

Patients with chronic bronchitis are candidates for polyvalent inactivated influenza A and B vaccine. This vaccine is administered into the deltoid muscle. It is contraindicated for those rare patients known to have anaphylactic hypersensitivity to eggs. Unlike the 1976 swine influenza vaccine, contemporary vaccines prepared from other virus strains have not been associated with an increased frequency of Guillain-Barré syndrome.

Pneumococcal vaccination of patients with chronic bronchitis is recommended by the Immunization Practices Advisory Committee, Centers for Disease Control (CDC). The vaccine is not, however, administered to prevent exacerbation episodes. It is offered to prevent pneumococcal pneumonia and bacteremia.

BACTERIAL PNEUMONIA

method of
BARBARA J. FONER, M.D.,
WILLIAM A. BROUGHTON, M.D., and
JOHN B. BASS, JR., M.D.
University of South Alabama
Mobile, Alabama

Bacterial pneumonia remains a common and serious cause of morbidity and mortality in community

*None of these medications has been approved by the FDA for this indication.

and hospital settings. The specific etiologic agent in each case varies according to the host characteristics. These characteristics include the presence of underlying chronic disease, patient age, involvement in substance abuse, and living circumstances (i.e., whether the patient lives in the community or in a health care institution). Antibiotic treatment is almost always empirical owing to our inability to diagnose the infectious cause of pneumonia accurately. With the ever expanding selection of antimicrobial agents, the choice of a specific treatment must be based on a knowledge of the likely pathogen and usual resistance patterns. The identification of the organism should be sought using laboratory and radiographic data, but initial treatment is based on the host and the clinical situation.

METHODS OF DIAGNOSIS

In the attempt to ascertain the microbial cause of pneumonia the clinician often thinks of the sputum Gram's stain first. Authorities disagree on the utility of this exercise. The test is not reliably sensitive or specific. Those that recommend Gram's stains suggest that the smear is most useful if it is performed and examined by the treating physician at the time of initial evaluation. Criteria have been developed to ensure that a sputum specimen is adequate for evaluation. A smear is considered to be adequate when there are more than 25 polymorphonuclear cells (PMNs) per low-power field and fewer than 10 epithelial cells are present. The finding of typical lancet-shaped, gram-positive diplococci within the leukocytes is highly suggestive of pneumonia due to *Streptococcus pneumoniae.* Although this information can be very useful and can assist the physician in the choice of an appropriate antibiotic, the presence of other types of organisms is also helpful in that it suggests that a broader spectrum of antimicrobial coverage should be initiated. The Gram's stain will fail to show mycobacteria, fungi, and *Legionella.* In appropriate circumstances acid-fast, fungal, and direct-fluorescent antibody staining can be diagnostic and should be undertaken as indicated.

Most experts agree that cultures of expectorated sputum are of little use. Long ago Elizabeth Barrett-Conner showed that sputum cultures grew the pneumococcus in only about 50% of study patients with bacteremic pneumococcal pneumonia. It is also clear that the appearance of a potential pathogen in a sputum culture is no guarantee that the organism is the cause of the lower airway infection. Organisms like *Haemophilus influenzae* may colonize the upper and lower airways when no infection is present (e.g., in patients with chronic obstructive pulmonary disease [COPD]). The American Thoracic Society advised against the use of routine sputum cultures to determine the cause of pneumonia in their consensus statement on community-acquired pneumonia. They noted that sputum culture might be helpful in specific circumstances such as when resistant pneumococci are anticipated or in the presence of failing limited antibiotic therapy.

Because sputum cultures have such poor sensitivity and specificity, blood cultures are always recommended and should be performed before antimicrobial therapy is administered. The rate of bacteremia associated with pneumonia is only 5 to 10% (usually higher when lobar consolidation is present), but positive findings are specific and point to appropriate therapy.

Likewise, the presence of a pleural effusion represents another potential method of confirming a diagnosis. When large enough, any pleural effusion associated with pneumonia should be sampled. There are two reasons for this: empyema should be excluded, and cultures of the fluid may yield a pathogen. Although the sensitivity of pleural fluid is only approximately 30%, the findings are very specific. Pleural fluid should always undergo Gram's stain, culture and sensitivity testing, and determination of glucose, protein, and lactic dehydrogenase (LDH) levels. Simultaneously, serum specimens for protein and LDH concentrations should also be obtained.

A parapneumonic effusion should be drained if any of the following are present:

1. pH equal to or less than 7.2
2. Gross purulence
3. Bacteria on Gram's stain
4. Pleural fluid glucose of less than 40 mg per 100 mL

When deciding which parapneumonic effusions should be sampled, it is prudent to tap any fluid collection that layers out to a thickness of 10 mm or more on the lateral decubitus view of the chest roentgenogram. Fluid that is loculated will not layer on a lateral decubitus film. These collections can be sampled under ultrasound or CT guidance if necessary. If the character of a pleural fluid sample approaches the limits of the criteria for drainage listed previously, it should be resampled in 12 hours. Often the characteristics will change, indicating a need for chest tube drainage.

Other more invasive techniques are available for the diagnosis of pneumonia (see Table 1). These include transtracheal aspiration (TTA), percutaneous lung aspiration (PLA), bronchoscopy with protected specimen brush (BPSB), and bronchoalveolar lavage (BAL). Endotracheal aspiration (ETA) can be used to obtain a specimen in the intubated patient. The use of the ETA specimen in combination with quantitative cultures is currently being studied, and initial findings suggest that it may be a valid and economical technique.

TABLE 1. **Invasive Diagnostic Procedures**

Transtracheal aspiration (TTA)
Percutaneous lung aspiration (PLA)
Bronchoscopic protected specimen brush (BPSB)
Bronchoalveolar lavage (BAL)
Endotracheal aspiration (ETA)

Transtracheal Aspiration

TTA is an infrequently used method of obtaining lower airway microbiologic specimens. The main advantage of this procedure is that it bypasses the oral flora in the upper airway and provides an uncontaminated specimen that is particularly helpful in the diagnosis of aerobic and anaerobic lung infections. Bleeding diathesis, severe hypoxemia, and inability to cooperate with the procedure are the major contraindications. TTA is usually an unpleasant experience for the patient, mainly due to the sensation of a foreign body in the lower airway, which causes violent unsuppressible coughing. Patients tolerate the procedure best when it is performed very quickly.

The technique involves placing the patient in the supine position and hyperextending the neck. Supplemental oxygen is supplied. After preparing and anesthetizing the palpable notch between the lower border of the thyroid cartilage and cricoid cartilage, a 14-gauge needle with an internal catheter is inserted through the cricoid membrane with the open bevel facing anteriorly. The needle is cautiously advanced a few millimeters into the trachea, avoiding contact with the posterior trachea. The catheter is then directed inferiorly into the trachea. When it is fully advanced, the needle is withdrawn, leaving the catheter in place. An aspirated sample of lower airway secretions is obtained using a syringe or by suction aspiration into a Luken's trap with a Y connector. Saline wash should be avoided because it will dilute the specimen but can be used in the absence of return. A few drops of secretion are all that are necessary. These should be immediately processed in the laboratory. Serious complications of TTA include bleeding, subcutaneous emphysema, and death (which is thought to be vagally mediated). Pre-medication with atropine has been suggested. When performed correctly, however, it is relatively safe and of acceptable diagnostic accuracy.

Percutaneous Lung Aspiration

The basic idea behind PLA is to avoid lower airway specimen contamination by advancing a fine needle directly through the chest wall into the infected area of the pulmonary parenchyma. The technique produces reliable results but is not used widely because of the high incidence of complications. PLA is associated with a 20 to 30% incidence of pneumothorax and carries a theoretical risk of air embolus. Death is also a possible complication. TTA and PLA were once compared head to head. Both techniques seemed to be of comparable accuracy, but patients preferred PLA over TTA because of the great discomfort they experienced with tracheal puncture.

Bronchoscopic Protected Specimen Brush

In general, community-acquired lower respiratory tract infections are successfully treated using empirical antibiotics. However, there are certain circumstances in which a precise etiologic diagnosis of the infecting agent is critical. The BPSB is a sheathed microbiology brush with a distal plug that is introduced through a fiberoptic bronchoscope using a specialized technique to collect uncontaminated lower airway secretions. BPSB has an excellent safety profile and is highly sensitive and specific in the diagnosis of community-acquired pneumonia as well as hospital-acquired pneumonia in experienced hands. Special situations in which BPSB is useful include patients at risk for unusual infections, those with necrotizing pulmonary processes, those in whom there is a strong suggestion of a noninfectious cause of pulmonary infiltration, those in whom pneumonia progresses despite antibiotic therapy, and those who develop infiltrates while undergoing mechanical ventilation.

Reliable results from BPSB are highly dependent on technique. For the best results, BPSB should be performed exactly as originally described and before the administration of antibiotics. The bronchoscopic suction channel through which BPSB passes should not be used for injection or suctioning prior to sampling. For culture results to be meaningful, quantitative microbiologic methods *must* be employed. When the Gram's stain from BPSB smears reveals microorganisms, this almost always indicates later significant bacterial growth of an organism of a similar morphology from quantitative culture.

Bronchoalveolar Lavage

Concern about possible sampling errors from the small specimen obtained with BPSB led to development of a technique for the microbiologic analysis of BAL fluid. These specimens are obtained by injection and aspiration of a sterile physiologic solution through a fiberoptic bronchoscope wedged into a bronchial subsegmental orifice. The theoretical advantage is that BAL samples the alveolar space (approximately 1 million alveoli) rather than the possibly contaminated proximal airways sampled by BPSB.

Numerous studies have suggested that BAL is a valid technique, but so far there has been little standardization. Current recommendations are as follows: (1) Hand aspiration lessens the collapse of airways and improves fluid return. (2) The total injectate should be greater than or equal to 140 mL, and the first 20 mL is discarded. Aliquots of from 20 to 60 mL are suggested. (3) Quantitative cultures must be used to produce reliable results. The cut-off point for significant bacterial growth is not as clear as that used for BPSB. Bacterial growth greater than or equal to 10^4 colony-forming units per mL is considered significant. (4) A high number of cells from BAL fluid with intracellular organisms (ICO) has shown a high correlation with ongoing pneumonia; greater than 2% cells with ICO is suggestive of pneumonia. (5) BAL with quantitative culture is most useful prior to the administration of antimicrobial therapy.

Many of the aforementioned techniques are highly

specialized and require technical expertise and complex laboratory back-up. When such expertise and back-up are not available, all of the techniques described above are contraindicated.

TYPICAL VERSUS ATYPICAL COMMUNITY-ACQUIRED PNEUMONIA

Although the concept is somewhat artificial, it may be advantageous to think of community-acquired pneumonia (CAP) in the immunocompetent host as being divided into typical and atypical types. This allows one to categorize the suspected etiologic organisms and the empirical choice of antibiotic. The classic features, primary etiologic agents, and appropriate treatment are discussed in this section. A review of syndromes and therapy is found in Table 2.

Typical CAP

Typical CAP can occur in patients of all ages with normal immune status. The classic history involves an acute onset of fever, shaking chills, and productive cough with purulent sputum. Occasionally, sputum may be rust colored. Pleuritic chest pain may be present. The chest roentgenogram often shows lobar or multilobar involvement, although pneumonias caused by *Haemophilus influenzae* and pneumococcus may appear patchy. Pleural effusions may be present. Often there is a leukocytosis (often greater than 20,000 white blood cells/mL) with a left shift. These patients often appear toxic.

Traditionally, these infections have been called P pneumonias because they usually respond to penicillin or one of its derivatives. However, the rise of resistant strains of *Streptococcus pneumoniae* and the well-known resistant *H. influenzae* strains makes penicillin alone a risky choice. Penicillin resistance found in pneumococcus appears to be related to changes in the penicillin-binding protein. In general, resistance is either intermediate or high and is based on the minimum inhibitory concentration (MIC) (Intermediate MIC equals 0.1 to 1.0 and is treatable with higher-dose penicillin or cephalosporins. High-resistance MIC equals more than 1.0 and must be treated with vancomycin.) More specific drug therapy is addressed in a later section of this article, but perhaps these pneumonias might better be called C pneumonias (cephalosporin-responsive).

Specific Pathogens in Typical CAP

Streptococcus pneumoniae

Streptococcus pneumoniae (pneumococcus) is the leading cause of CAP in all age groups, with or without underlying co-morbidity. It is believed to account for up to 20% of pneumonias in otherwise healthy adults. The organism is a lancet-shaped, gram-positive facultative anaerobic diplococcus surrounded by a capsule. It is present as a commensal in the pharynx of roughly 20% of the population. Pneumonia due to this organism most often occurs in winter and early spring. Its incidence increases during influenza epidemics.

Pneumococcal pneumonia can be a mild illness or an overwhelming septic process proceeding rapidly to death. This "captain of the men of death" of years gone by should never be taken lightly. Patients with chronic underlying diseases such as heart failure, renal failure, sickle cell disease, diabetes mellitus, leukemia, or asplenia are more likely to have a complicated course.

TABLE 2. **Spectrum of Community-Acquired Pneumonia (CAP), Usual Pathogens and Therapy**

CAP Subgroup	Usual Pathogens	Therapy
Typical pneumonia	*Streptococcus pneumoniae* *Haemophilus influenzae* *Moraxella catarrhalis* *Staphylococcus aureus*	Cefazolin 1 gm IV q 8 h or cefuroxime 750 mg IV q 8 h (other cephalosporins are acceptable, or β-lactam in combination with β-lactamase inhibitors); also TMP-SMX
Atypical pneumonia	*Mycoplasma pneumoniae* *Chlamydia pneumoniae* (TWAR) *Legionella pneumophila* *Coxiella burnetti* (Q fever) Viruses	Erythromycin 500 mg PO or IV q 6 h or other macrolide. Tetracycline 500 mg PO qid or doxycycline 100 mg bid is also effective
Aspiration pneumonia	*Bacteroides* sp *Fusobacterium* sp Microaerophilic streptococci Peptococci and peptostreptococci *Viridans* streptococci *Eikenella corrodens*	Clindamycin 600–900 mg IV q 6 h or high-dose penicillin 3 to 4 million units IV q 4–6 h. (β-lactam and β-lactamase combinations are also effective but costly)
Aerobic gram-negative bacillary pneumonia	*Klebsiella* sp *Escherichia coli* *Enterobacter* sp *Proteus* sp *Pseudomonas* sp (rare and seldom resistant)	Third-generation cephalosporin such as ceftazidime 1–2 gm IV q 8 h or cefotaxime 2–3 gm IV q 6 h. In severe cases an aminoglycoside can be added (tobramycin may show higher levels in respiratory secretions)
Unsuspected immunocompromise	Typical (A) and atypical (B) pathogens *Pneumocystis carinii* *Mycobacterium tuberculosis* Fungi	Approriate coverage for AIDS-related pathogens, being sure that there is typical CAP +/− *Legionella* coverage as listed above

Complications are seen in fewer than 10% of cases and can include meningitis, empyema, septic arthritis, sinusitis, pericarditis, necrotizing pneumonia (rare), and a disseminated intravascular coagulation. With the advent of more effective antibiotics, the most common complication currently is superinfection with gram-negative organisms in patients receiving antibiotic therapy.

Blood culture or pleural fluid culture growing *S. pneumoniae* alone or the identification of pneumococcal polysaccharide antigen by counterimmunoelectrophoresis is diagnostic. Because the organism is a common commensal in the oropharynx, a positive sputum smear or culture from an expectorated sputum specimen is not confirmative. Invasive procedures, as mentioned earlier, can increase the sensitivity and specificity of the diagnosis, although they are usually not required. Mortality in severely ill hospitalized patients with bacteremic pneumococcal pneumonia can be as high as 20%. Early antibiotic administration improves outcome. When the organism is identified, its sensitivities should always be tested because there is an increasing tendency toward penicillin resistance. A pneumococcal vaccine is available, but the patients who need it, most including the elderly and debilitated, are the least likely to produce sufficient antibodies.

With the rising incidence of moderate penicillin resistance in pneumococcal strains, penicillin is no longer the empirical treatment of choice. At present, most strains exhibit only moderate resistance and remain sensitive to cephalosporins. Cefazolin (Ancef), 1 gram intravenously every 8 hours, and cefuroxime (Zinacef, Kefurox), 750 mg intravenously every 8 hours, are both effective therapies. Head-to-head comparisons have indicated little difference in outcome. Other cephalosporins can be considered if efficacy and cost considerations dictate. Sensitivity testing should always be performed on pneumococcal isolates to guide later modification of therapy. Penicillin alone is appropriate when the organism demonstrates sensitivity.

Haemophilus influenzae

Haemophilus influenzae is the second most frequent cause of CAP requiring hospitalization. It is often seen in patients with other illnesses such as underlying lung disease, diabetes, alcoholism, or some immune defect. Depending on the institution, up to 30% of isolates implicated in CAP may be beta-lactamase producers.

As a respiratory pathogen *H. influenzae* can cause pneumonia as well as other clinical manifestations including epiglottitis, bronchitis, and tracheitis. Pneumonia can occur in the lower lobes and may be bilateral or it can be a patchy process. Pleural effusion may be seen. Bacteremia is associated with a mortality rate of 25%, most likely related to the existence of an underlying disease.

Penicillin does not have a role in the treatment of *H. influenzae* infection. Acceptable treatments include cephalosporins and extended spectrum penicillins in combination with beta-lactamase inhibitors. Most isolates are susceptible to trimethoprim-sulfamethoxazole (TMP-SMX) as well. Ampicillin is appropriate if the organism is demonstrated to be sensitive. The newer macrolides, azithromycin (Zithromax) and clarithromycin (Biaxin), are reported to have activity against *H. influenzae* but are recommended only for mild cases at this time.

Moraxella catarrhalis

Moraxella catarrhalis has had several names over the years including *Neisseria catarrhalis* and *Branhamella catarrhalis.* It is a gram-negative diplococcus that often causes pulmonary infection in patients with underlying chronic lung disease or patients with immunoglobulin deficiency. Winter and early spring are associated with an increase in reported cases of tracheobronchitis or pneumonia due to this organism. Radiographically, an interstitial or mixed interstitial and alveolar filling type of pattern may be seen. The course is usually mild but is sometimes serious. Complications such as cavitation and empyema are not usually seen.

Treatment options include second- or third-generation cephalosporins and penicillins combined with beta-lactamase inhibitors. The newer macrolides, quinolones, TMP-SMX, and tetracycline are all considered effective alternative therapies.

Staphylococcus aureus

This gram-positive organism aerobe accounts for only 3 to 9% of cases of CAP, often striking the normal host who has recently had influenza and has diminished resistance owing to recovering denuded respiratory epithelium. Staphylococcal pneumonia is exceedingly rare in the totally normal host and therefore is more commonly seen in nosocomial settings, especially in patients who have undergone recent surgery or who have recently received multiple antibiotics. Other risk factors for the development of staphylococcal pneumonia include residence in a long-term care facility, diabetes mellitus, renal failure, hemodialysis, in-dwelling catheter, and intravenous drug abuse.

The presentation of staphylococcal pneumonia is similar to that of streptococcal pneumonia, with fever, chills, and chest pain. Gram's stain reveals clumps of gram-positive cocci. Other laboratory findings may include leukocytosis, anemia, and rarely, a positive blood culture. The roentgenogram shows parenchymal consolidation that is bilateral in 60% of cases. A pleural effusion or empyema may be present in as many as 50% of cases. Because the organism may gain access to the lung by hematogenous spread, multiple fluffy nodular infiltrates may be seen. There is a tendency toward bronchial wall necrosis, which can lead to pneumatoceles that occur when air passes into the interstitial spaces.

There are a number of treatment options. The semi-synthetic penicillins such as nafcillin and oxacillin are acceptable, as is cefazolin. Other choices include TMP-SMX and clindamycin (Cleocin). If methicillin-resistant *S. aureus* is suspected, vancomycin (Vancocin) must be used. Penicillin G, ampicillin, macrolides, and tetracycline are all unacceptable choices. The mortality from staphylococcal pneumonia is considerable, and appropriate therapy is imperative.

Atypical Pneumonia

Atypical CAP generally runs a more benign course, which may be shortened by using antibiotic therapy. The population at risk tends to be younger, but atypical CAP can occur in older patients. Flulike symptoms including fever, headache, arthralgia, and malaise are most often present. There is usually a cough that is nonproductive or minimally productive. Radiographically, it has been said that "the chest roentgenogram looks worse than the patient," meaning that diffuse bronchopneumonia or interstitial pulmonary involvement may be seen when the patient does not appear particularly toxic. The most common organisms causing atypical pneumonia are discussed subsequently.

It would be a great mistake to abandon the reader here thinking that the clinical distinction between typical and atypical pneumonia is reliable; it is not. Flulike symptoms occur in typical CAP. Purulent sputum and pleural effusions are seen in pneumonias due to *Mycoplasma* and *Legionella* spp. People can die from atypical pneumonia; retrospective French data suggest that survival from inappropriately treated *Legionella* pneumonia is less than 50%.

Whenever it is unclear whether pneumonia is typical or atypical it is acceptable for the clinician to "straddle the fence." Treatment with both a cephalosporin and a macrolide is a common occurrence in clinical practice. It is inappropriate, however, to "hedge" routinely with dual therapy. The typical-atypical diagnostic dichotomy is of some value. When a pneumonia looks obviously typical or atypical, it probably is.

Mycoplasma pneumoniae

The mycoplasmas have been called pleuropneumonia-like organisms. They are the smallest free-living microorganisms that can be cultured on media. *Mycoplasma pneumoniae* is generally considered the most common cause of clinical "nonbacterial" or atypical pneumonia. Infections can occur throughout the year with a rise in the fall and early winter. Although it is often thought to be a disease of children and young adults, patients of all ages are affected. Infection is acquired by droplet inhalation. The incubation period is usually 1 to 3 weeks. Upper respiratory symptoms develop initially, and only 3 to 10% of those infected develop pneumonia.

The clinical course is usually benign. A nonproductive cough and fever are the most common symptoms, although chills, myalgia, and headache can be seen. Bullous myringitis is traditionally a commonly associated occurrence but is rarely seen. Without treatment, the headache, fever, and malaise resolve within 3 to 10 days, and pulmonary symptoms clear more slowly. Rare pulmonary complications can include pulmonary infarction and cavitation, residual pleural scarring, and adult respiratory distress syndrome (ARDS).

Laboratory findings may not be impressive. The white cell count is usually normal with elevation seen in only 25% of cases. Occasionally, elevated transaminase levels may be seen. Electrocardiographic changes may result from pericarditis or myocarditis. The sputum Gram's stain may show a moderate number of white blood cells without a predominant organism. A routine sputum culture may yield normal throat flora.

The organism can be isolated from sputum or throat swabs. With a monoclonal antibody assay, diagnosis can be made in several hours. A DNA probe is also specific and sensitive in detecting *M. pneumoniae* in sputum. A fourfold rise in complement-fixing antibody titer can confirm the diagnosis, but the need for acute and convalescent samples limits its use. Elevated cold agglutinin titers are nonspecific and therefore not helpful because positive results are also seen with viral pneumonias, neoplastic disorders, and collagen vascular diseases.

The chest roentgenogram has two distinct patterns. One pattern involves segmental or lobar consolidation with or without atelectasis. Nineteen percent of these demonstrate a pleural effusion. The other pattern is a diffuse bilateral reticulonodular pattern, which at times shows Kerley B lines. The lobar pattern is more often associated with an acute respiratory syndrome that resolves rapidly, whereas the diffuse pattern implies a more protracted course of illness.

Several treatment options are acceptable. All of the macrolides, including erythromycin, 500 mg orally every 6 hours; clarithromycin (Biaxin), 500 mg orally every 12 hours for 10 days; and azithromycin (Zithromax), 500 mg orally, then 250 mg orally once daily for 5 days, in addition to tetracycline (250 to 500 mg orally every 6 hours) or doxycycline (Vibramycin, 100 mg orally every 12 hours) are effective. If gastric intolerance is an issue or if the patient is noncompliant, azithromycin may confer an advantage in both cases.

Chlamydia pneumoniae

Formerly known as the TWAR agent owing to its resemblance to two other *Chlamydia* serotypes (Taiwan 183 and Acute Respiratory 39), this obligate intracellular gram-negative bacterium has only recently been recognized as a separate species. Clinically, the disease resembles *Mycoplasma* pneumonia; however, it may be distinguished from *Mycoplasma* by the presence of severe pharyngitis associated with hoarseness that commonly precedes the onset of chlamydial pneumonia by 1 week. A nonproductive cough is often present. Physical examination of the chest is unimpressive except for crackles. There is often no fever. Sinusitis may be present.

The laboratory data are often not helpful because the white count, differential, and liver function test results are normal, and a sputum Gram's stain may show white blood cells without any predominant organism. The chest radiograph usually demonstrates a single segmental infiltrate but can be patchy.

The treatment of choice is tetracycline, doxycycline, or erythromycin at standard doses. The newer macrolides, azithromycin and clarithromycin, are reported to be effective and produce fewer gastrointestinal side effects, although the cost is significantly more.

Without treatment, the infection in most patients clears spontaneously, although there have been reports of respiratory failure requiring ventilatory assistance as well as deaths attributable to *C. pneumoniae*. Antibiotic therapy may abbreviate the course of illness. Without treatment, persistent cough, dyspnea, and a protracted infection are possible.

Legionnaire's Disease

See pages 190 to 192.

Q Fever

See pages 109 to 110.

ASPIRATION

The use of the term and the concept of aspiration creates confusion for many physicians. Three distinct syndromes exist, each with its unique pathogenesis and pathophysiology. The nature and size of the aspirate is the most significant factor in determining which aspiration syndrome is present. The first and most immediately lethal aspect is physical obstruction of the airway from aspiration of a large particulate load. This can be due to emesis or a foreign body such as occlusion of the airway with a bolus of food, commonly known as the "café coronary." Asphyxiation is the mechanism of death. The obvious treatment is clearing of the airway using the Heimlich maneuver, direct removal of the foreign body, or suctioning.

The remaining two entities of aspiration directly involve the pulmonary parenchyma: (1) aspiration syndrome involving aspiration of gastric fluid, resulting in chemical pneumonitis, and (2) aspiration pneumonia, which is the result of bolus or repetitive microaspiration from the oropharynx and resultant infection by its colonizing microorganisms.

The aspiration of small quantities of oropharyngeal fluid into the lungs is common and occurs in 50% of normal people while sleeping. In the same population the incidence of aspiration increases to 70% after intake of sedative substances. No untoward effects of this nightly aspiration are usually seen in the normal host. A change in the character of the aspirate occurs in debilitated patients and others who are colonized with gram-negative bacilli. An increase in the quantity of the aspirate and a decrease in its pH contribute to the pathogenicity associated with aspiration. Aspiration syndrome and aspiration pneumonia are discussed separately here with respect to risk factors, pathogens, and management, including the role of antibiotics.

Aspiration Syndrome

The aspiration of toxic fluids into the lower respiratory tract can lead to a primary inflammatory reaction. This is most commonly due to aspiration of a large volume of gastric acid. The syndrome was first described by Mendelson in 1946 in his series of 66 obstetric patients who aspirated gastric contents during anesthesia. Five of these patients had obstructive events from particulate matter. However, the majority of the patients developed what has been called Mendelson's syndrome—the acidic pH of the aspirant leads to a chemical pneumonitis with recruitment of inflammatory mediators at the alveolar level. Clinically, patients develop bronchospasm, respiratory distress, and hypoxemia with a normal or low PCO_2. This can progress to acute ARDS with decreasing lung compliance and a worsening physiologic shunt. Patients often have nonpurulent sputum and may become hypotensive owing to an immediate reflex reaction or volume depletion secondary to third spacing of fluid in the lung. Radiographically, the most common pattern is known as a "bat's wing" distribution, with infiltrates appearing in the posterior segments of the upper lobes and the superior segments of the lower lobes.

The most important element in treatment is the correction of hypoxemia with supplemental oxygen or mechanical ventilation if necessary. Tracheal suctioning may be necessary. Intravenous fluids may be administered if hypotension is present. Intravenous corticosteroids have not been demonstrated to be helpful after aspiration has occurred.

Antibiotics should not be routinely administered following macroaspiration with chemical pneumonitis. Antibiotic therapy should be reserved for patients who develop an obvious secondary bacterial pneumonia or those in whom it is deemed imprudent to wait. Clinical evidence of secondary pneumonia includes purulent sputum, significant increase in fever, and progression of leukocytosis and pulmonary infiltrates after 48 hours. Early use of antimicrobials following aspiration and before the clear-cut development of a secondary bacterial pneumonia has not been shown to prevent subsequent infection but has been shown to increase the incidence of resistant bacterial flora.

The microbiology of bacterial infection following macroaspiration has not been studied; however, the pathogens most likely include aerobic gram-negative rods mixed with oropharyngeal flora. Suspicion of this pathogenic flora is based on the assumption that these patients would have been in the hospital for 48 hours when secondary pneumonia develops and would essentially have nosocomial pneumonia.

Aspiration Pneumonia

Aspiration pneumonia develops in patients in whom there is a breakdown of the normal protective mechanisms that prevent the entry of oropharyngeal secretions, gastric secretions, or food and liquids into the tracheobronchial tree. Predisposing risk factors include debilitating disease, head injuries, cerebrovascular accidents, gastroesophageal reflux, achalasia, drug abuse, alcohol abuse, or decreased mental status for any reason. The presence of a nasoenteric tube also increases the risk of aspiration by disruption of the integrity of the lower esophageal sphincter. When poor dental hygiene is present it can lead to an increased gingival bacterial load, which may contain up to 10^8 anaerobes and 10^7 aerobes per mL of pharyngeal secretions. No single microorganism itself is implicated in the pathogenic process. Probably the repetitive microaspiration of oropharyngeal secretions heavily laden with mixed flora provides constant seeding of the dependent lung zones, overwhelming the normal mechanisms for removal. This leads to the reported indolent course of aspiration pneumonia in which there is slow onset of fatigue, weight loss, low-grade fever, and foul-smelling sputum.

Roentgenographically the dependent areas of the lungs are involved, most often the posterior subsegment of the upper lobe and the superior segments of the lower lobes. Cavitation is common. If an air-fluid level is seen, an abscess is present. Antibiotic treatment should be prolonged, extending for 3 to 4 months until roentgenographic resolution or stabilization is apparent.

The most frequently identified anaerobes include *Bacteroides* species, especially *B. fragilis, Fusobacterium* sp, peptostreptococci, microaerophilic streptococci, and peptococci. The aerobes most frequently found are enterobacteriaceae (encompassing *Klebsiella* sp, *Escherichia coli,* and *Enterobacter* sp), *Pseudomonas* sp, *viridans* streptococci, and *Eikenella corrodens.* In the past, high-dose penicillin was the therapy of choice; however, treatment failures have occurred that are believed to be due to anaerobic microbial resistance, especially in the cases of *B. fragilis* infection. A head-to-head comparison between penicillin and clindamycin revealed more treatment failures in the penicillin group. For this reason, clindamycin, 600 mg given intravenously every 6 hours, is the most conservative therapy for aspiration pneumonia. If the host is at increased risk for oropharyngeal colonization with aerobic gram-negative bacilli, empirical antibiotic treatment might also include a third-generation cephalosporin or antipseudomonal penicillin in conjunction with an aminoglycoside, encompassing both anaerobic and gram-negative coverage. The following section will describe the pathogenesis and treatment of aerobic gram-negative bacilli in further detail.

AEROBIC GRAM-NEGATIVE BACILLARY PNEUMONIA

In normal subjects gram-negative rods can transiently colonize the oropharynx in small numbers. Colonization is significantly increased in certain subgroups of patients including diabetics, alcoholics, and debilitated patients, especially those with urinary and fecal incontinence who for some reason cannot care for themselves. An otherwise able-bodied host who happens to live in a nursing home or other institution is not necessarily at risk for increased colonization with aerobic gram-negative rods.

The most common causes of community-acquired aerobic gram-negative bacillary pneumonia (AGNBP) are *Klebsiella* sp, *Enterobacter* sp, *E. coli,* and *Pseudomonas* sp. There is no characteristic clinical presentation or radiographic feature to assist in making this diagnosis. The clinician must assess the patient to determine whether he or she belongs in an appropriate host category at risk for this infection.

Empirical antibiotics for treatment of community-acquired AGNBP include a third-generation cephalosporin alone or in combination with an aminoglycoside. If aspiration is a concern, a third-generation cephalosporin with anaerobic coverage (e.g., cefotaxime [Claforan], cefotetan [Cefotan]) or extended-spectrum penicillins such as piperacillin-tazobactam (Zosyn) or ticarcillin-clavulanic acid (Timentin) may be used to cover potential anaerobic infection. Imipenem-cilastatin (Primaxin) should not be used routinely as a single agent because of the reported rapid induction of resistance when this drug is used as monotherapy.

In this subpopulation invasive diagnostic procedures such as BPSB and BAL with quantitative bacterial cultures may be helpful. Specific identification of pathogens helps to avoid the potential toxicity of empirical regimens and the unnecessary expense of prolonged therapy. Invasive procedures yield the most meaningful data if they are performed before the antimicrobial therapy is initiated. If a pathogen is identified, adjustment of the initial empirical antibiotic therapy can be tailored to the pathogen's sensitivity pattern.

In the event of negative cultures, many authorities recommend discontinuation of antimicrobial therapy. It is often difficult, however, to discontinue antibiotics in an extremely ill patient who has clinical signs of pneumonia. Also of note, when the radiographic pattern suggests a necrotizing process thought to be secondary to bacterial infection, oral antibiotics should be continued until the chest roentgenographic abnormality resolves or stabilizes.

COMMUNITY-ACQUIRED PNEUMONIA IN THE IMMUNOCOMPROMISED HOST

In the past it was possible to help to distinguish patients at risk for HIV infection and AIDS by standard questioning regarding intravenous drug use, unprotected sexual activity, prior transfusion, and a history of other opportunistic infections including dermatomal herpes zoster. At present, however, heterosexual spread of HIV is increasing. For this reason, it is possible that any patient evaluated for CAP may be immunocompromised. In fact, the attack rate of standard CAP in HIV-infected individuals is six to seven times that of the normal population.

The physical examination may be helpful in suggesting the presence of underlying immunocompromise. The findings of oral candidiasis, diffuse adenopathy, unusual skin lesions, or cachexia suggest the possibility of an immunocompromised state. Cachexia suggests a chronic underlying process as opposed to an acute infection. Oral candidiasis may be present in patients with HIV disease but can accompany other conditions that alter host defenses, such as the chronic administration of antibiotics or steroids.

When a patient is treated for suspected HIV-related pneumonia it should be remembered that TMP-SMX provides coverage for the standard community-acquired organisms as well as for *Pneumocystis carinii* pneumonia (PCP). When alternative therapies (such as aerosolized pentamidine, oral dapsone, and so on) are used for PCP the clinician should keep in mind that standard CAP pathogens are not covered by these regimens in patients who have an increased risk of same. If PCP is a consideration and the patient cannot tolerate TMP-SMX, pentamidine can be used in conjunction with another agent such as cefuroxime or erythromycin.

Tuberculosis can present an atypical appearance in HIV-infected patients. In fact, a healthy suspicion of tuberculosis in all cases of lung infection is worthwhile.

CRITERIA FOR HOSPITALIZATION OF PATIENTS WITH CAP

There are no specific guidelines for determining who should be admitted to the hospital with CAP. There are, however, certain risk factors that increase mortality or predict a complicated course for patients with CAP. In the presence of multiple risk factors, hospitalization should be more strongly considered. The following host factors portend greater mortality or a complicated course for CAP, as outlined by the American Thoracic Society Consensus Statement, Guidelines for the initial management of adults with CAP: diagnosis, assessment of severity, and initial antimicrobial therapy.

1. Age over 65 years
2. Chronic obstructive lung disease or other structural disease of the lung including bronchiectasis and cystic fibrosis
3. Diabetes mellitus
4. Congestive heart failure
5. Chronic liver disease
6. Chronic renal disease
7. Previous hospitalization within 1 year
8. Possibility of aspiration, either gastric or oropharyngeal
9. Altered mental status
10. Chronic alcohol abuse or malnutrition
11. Postsplenectomy state

The physical examination may also yield information that could predict a complicated course or increased mortality. These factors include

1. Respiratory rate greater than 30 breaths per minute
2. Temperature greater than 38.3° C (101° F)
3. Systolic blood pressure less than 90 mmHg or diastolic blood pressure less than or equal to 60 mmHg
4. Evidence of extrapulmonary sites of disease including septic arthritis, meningitis, sinusitis, and so on
5. Change in level of consciousness or confusion

Specific laboratory findings predict an adverse outcome:

1. PaO_2 of less than 60 mmHg or $PaCO_2$ of greater than 50 mmHg on room air
2. White blood cell count less than 4000/mL or greater than 30,000/mL or absolute neutrophil count below 1000
3. Abnormal renal function with creatinine greater than 1.2 mg/dL or blood urea nitrogen greater than 20 mg/dL
4. Hematocrit less than 30% or hemoglobin less than 9 grams per dL
5. Roentgenographic evidence of more than one lobe involvement, presence of a cavity, presence of a pleural effusion, or rapid radiographic progression
6. Need for mechanical ventilation
7. Other evidence of sepsis or multiorgan dysfunction as evidenced by metabolic acidosis, increased prothrombin time, increased partial thromboplastin time, low platelets, or fibrin split products greater than 1:40

Other factors must be considered as well. If the patient is unable to care for himself or herself or does not have a dependable caregiver in a stable home environment, hospital admission may be warranted. An appropriate antibiotic should be obtainable, and the patient should be able to tolerate its administration. Last, follow-up is critical. If a return appointment cannot be scheduled, admission should be strongly considered. Whenever there is doubt about any of these factors or the patient's medical stability, that patient should be admitted to the hospital.

NOSOCOMIAL PNEUMONIA

Nosocomial pneumonia (NP) is a serious and often fatal disease. It is defined as a pneumonia that was neither present nor incubating at the time of hospital admission and then becomes apparent at an interval greater than or equal to 48 hours after admission. Although hospital-acquired pneumonia follows urinary tract infection in frequency of occurrence, it has the highest mortality of all nosocomially acquired infections. Mortality is even higher for patients in intensive care units (ICU).

Situations conducive to the development of NP are (1) obtunded patients with ineffective cough or gag reflex, (2) patients with underlying pulmonary disease or congestive heart failure with impairment of the usual pulmonary defense mechanisms; and (3) patients requiring respiratory tract instrumentation or mechanically assisted ventilation.

Because NP is not a centrally reportable disease and is difficult to diagnose accurately, the true incidence is not known. One study of suspected NP in an intensive care unit found that only about a third of patients in whom NP was suspected actually had it (based on BPSB results). Accordingly, we believe that many patients are treated for NP when it is not present. Recent studies have indicated that prior treatment with antibiotics predisposes patients to NP with organisms associated with a higher mortality (*Pseudomonas* spp and *Acinetobacter*). Some invasive diagnostic techniques have been shown to improve our accuracy in diagnosing NP; however, these procedures are labor-intensive and expensive. Cost-efficacy for such techniques requires a willingness to discontinue antibiotics in the event of negative cultures. False-negative results have been reported; how low a false-negative rate is low enough? It is the absence of a widely available, accurate, and economical diagnostic test for NP that forces us into the host-based empirical schema outlined subsequently.

Tertiary care centers and municipal hospitals show an overall higher incidence of NP owing to the greater severity of underlying diseases in their patients as well as the more frequent use of invasive procedures and diagnostic tests. When bacteremia occurs, the mortality rate is increased to roughly 50%; however, certain organisms are more likely to be associated with mortality, as noted earlier. In NP due to *Pseudomonas aeruginosa,* mortality may approach 80% or higher.

Because NP is suspected more often than it actually occurs, it is imperative for the clinician always to consider other conditions that could mimic nosocomial pneumonia, including congestive heart failure, atelectasis, ARDS, pulmonary thromboembolus, and adverse drug reactions.

Pathogenesis

It is true that hospitalized patients are more often colonized with aerobic gram-negative bacteria than those in the community. However, not everyone in the hospital has the same risk of gram-negative colonization. Patients admitted for less serious illness and who are caring for themselves have a lower incidence of gram-negative carriage than the near-ubiquitous colonization seen in intubated patients in the ICU. Despite this difference, accurate lines of risk are difficult to draw.

Certain conditions predispose groups of patients to the nosocomial pathogens that will be defined later. These include diabetes mellitus, chronic renal failure, prolonged hospitalization, nasoenteric tube use, recent prior antibiotic use, admission to the ICU, prior surgery or trauma, or mechanical ventilation. The reasons for the increased risk are obvious in some of these conditions, whereas in many others the reasons for the predisposition to NP are unclear but have been verified by multivariate analysis.

We believe we understand part of the role played by mechanical ventilation in the occurrence of NP. Violation of the upper airway and the larynx provides a ready conduit for bacteria to gain access to the lower airway. As early as 48 hours, aerobic gram-negative rods have already established themselves as colonizers in a high percentage of patients receiving mechanical ventilation. It is thought that by this point receptors for gram-negative bacteria have been "revealed" on airway mucous membranes and that gram-negative organisms find no difficulty in adhering to them or to the inner surface of the endotracheal tube. Attempts have been made to decontaminate the bowel and pharynx or airway with topical, intravenous, and inhaled antibiotics. Results of several studies have shown a decline in NP due to gram-negative organisms after decontamination protocols but reveal an increased incidence of staphylococcal infections (in one study) and no change in overall mortality (in all studies).

Owing to the seriousness of NP, initial antimicrobial treatment must be timely and appropriate for the most probable pathogens. The patient's underlying risk factors should be assessed to guide therapy. In addition, the severity of the pneumonia is a consideration. A patient is considered to be seriously ill if any of the following are present: (1) PaO_2 of less than 60 mmHg on an FIO_2 of greater than 35% unless underlying chronic obstructive airway disease is present that accounts for the hypoxemia without pneumonia; (2) respiratory rate greater than 30 breaths per minute; (3) sepsis with evidence of end-organ dysfunction; (4) cavitation or involvement of more than one lobe on chest radiographs; (5) requirement for mechanical ventilation due to the infection or development of the pneumonia while on the ventilator.

Risk factors for the development of NP include: (1) prior antibiotic treatment (also increases risk of NP with an organism associated with higher mortality); (2) surgery, especially long preoperative stays and long operative procedures such as thoracoabdominal procedures; (3) hospitalization in an intensive care unit; (4) mechanical ventilatory support, especially if gastric pH has been elevated with H_2 antagonists, ventilatory support lasted longer than 3 days, or the patient underwent more than one intubation.

Host factors are of paramount importance in addressing the patient with NP. It may be helpful to think of patients with suspected NP in four general groups. These are Group 1: nonintubated patients who are not severely ill and have no risk factors; Group 2: patients with suspected NP with risk factors for specific pathogens; Group 3: previously healthy patients with ICU admission (less than 5 days) after trauma or after surgery; Group 4: patients with severe NP, ICU admission or mechanical ventilation, or combinations of risk factors noted earlier. Each of these groups has a spectrum of probable pathogens requiring specific adjustment in empirical therapy.

TABLE 3. **Treatment Groups for the Empirical Therapy of Nosocomial Pneumonia (NP)**

NP Group	Usual Pathogens	Therapy
Group 1 (patients with mild to moderate NP without risk factors)	Standard nosocomial organisms (SNO) (see Table 4)	Cefuroxime 750 mg IV q 8 h or Nonpseudomonal third-generation cephalosporin such as ceftriaxone, cefotaxime Ampicillin or sulbactam
Group 2 (NP with risk factors)		
Possible aspiration	SNO and anaerobes (as listed in text under Aspiration Pneumonia)	Same as Group 1 Fluoroquinolones and clindamycin
Diabetes mellitus Chronic renal failure IV drug abuse	SNO plus methicillin-resistant *S. aureus*	Group 1 drugs plus vancomycin when MRSA is suspected
Prolonged hospitalization Prior antibiotics Multiple risk factors	SNO plus resistant gram-negative rods and *Pseudomonas aeruginosa*	Refer to treatment for Group 4
Group 3 (NP in previously healthy patients < 5 days post-trauma or post-surgery)	SNO (without *P. aeruginosa*), plus *S. aureus, H. influenzae* and *S. pneumoniae*	Group 1 treatment plus staphylococcal coverage
Group 4 Severe NP ICU admission Mechanical ventilation Combined risk factors	SNO plus *P. aeruginosa, Acinetobacter calcoaceticus*	Antipseudomonal penicillin (plus or minus beta-lactamase inhibitor) and an aminoglycoside

Table 3 reviews these treatment groups and specific therapies.

Group 1 encompasses those patients who develop mild to moderate pneumonia after 48 hours of hospitalization. The pathogens usually encountered are essentially aerobic gram-negative rods, *S. aureus,* and *Streptococcus* spp. The gram-negative pathogens encountered include *Klebsiella* spp, *Enterobacter* spp, *E. coli, Proteus* spp, *Serratia marcescens, H. influenzae,* and do not normally include *Pseudomonas* spp (hereafter these organisms will be referred to as "standard nosocomial organisms" [SNO]—these are listed in Table 4). For this reason, broad-spectrum antibiotic monotherapy is acceptable. Appropriate antibiotic choices include third-generation cephalosporins with or without *Pseudomonas* activity (e.g., ceftazidime [Fortaz], ceftriaxone [Rocephin], cefotaxime [Claforan]), the second-generation cephalosporin cefuroxime (Zinacef), or ampicillin-sulbactam (Unasyn). For the patient with beta-lactam allergy, the fluoroquinolones, TMP-SMX, or a combination of clindamycin (Cleocin) and aztreonam (Azactam) would be appropriate. Quinolones alone do not have adequate coverage of gram-positive organisms. For this reason, if ciprofloxacin (Cipro) or ofloxacin (Floxin) is used, the addition of vancomycin or erythromycin may be beneficial.

Group 2 is that group of patients with suspected NP that are at risk for SNO (see earlier list) and have specific host risk factors that extend that spectrum as follows:

1. In the patient thought to have NP in whom aspiration is a consideration, therapeutic concern should include anaerobic organisms. Appropriate therapy includes ampicillin-sulbactam (Unasyn), cefuroxime (Zinacef), or third-generation cephalosporins with anaerobic activity such as ceftriaxone (Rocephin) and cefotaxime (Claforan). As noted earlier, fluoroquinolones are active against SNO, but these drugs have no antianaerobic activity. Thus, when fluoroquinolones are used they must be combined with an antibiotic with anaerobic activity such as clindamycin or metronidazole.

2. In patients with underlying diseases, specifically, chronic renal failure, diabetes mellitus, and a history of intravenous drug abuse; SNO and methicillin-resistant *S. aureus* (MRSA) should be pathogens of concern. Empirical treatment for this group of patients includes the same drugs used for therapy in Group 1 as well as vancomycin when *Staphylococcus* is suspected.

3. Patients who have a combination of these risks plus prolonged hospitalization, prior antibiotic use, or ICU admission should be considered to have severe NP. This topic is addressed in the discussion of Group 4.

Group 3 patients are those thought to have NP who were previously healthy and are less than 5 days post-surgery or post-trauma. These individuals are at risk for infection due to SNO and *S. aureus.* Studies have also indicated that these patients have an increased incidence of pneumonia due to *S. pneumoniae* and *H. influenzae.* Treatment options include cefuroxime, third-generation cephalosporins (such as ceftriaxone and cefotaxime), or ampicillin-sulbactam.

TABLE 4. **Standard Nosocomial Organisms Associated with Nosocomial Pneumonia**

Enterobacter sp
Escherichia coli
Klebsiella sp
Proteus sp
Serratia marcescens
Staphylococcus aureus (including methicillin-resistant strains)
Streptococcus sp (including pneumococcus)

The advantage of a single agent with SNO and staphylococcal coverage is that it obviates the need for a second agent to ensure gram-positive coverage. When these patients in Group 3 are severely ill, it is acceptable to cover SNO, *Pseudomonas aeruginosa,* and *Staphylococcus* spp.

Group 4 patients are those with severe NP or combinations of the risk factors noted previously. The major concern in this group of patients is the additional risk of *Pseudomonas aeruginosa* and *Acinetobacter calcoaceticus* as possible causes of NP. In one study of NP based on BPSB data, only 13% of patients with NP due to *P. aeruginosa* and *Acinetobacter* spp survived compared with 31% survival in those with SNO organisms. Therapy for this group of patients consists of an aminoglycoside plus an antipseudomonal penicillin. These drugs include piperacillin (Pipracil) and ticarcillin (Ticar) alone or with beta-lactamase inhibitors such as piperacillin-tazobactam and ticarcillin-clavulanate. It is possible that these combination drugs may be more effective against gram-negative organisms.

Other drugs that could be used in combination with aminoglycosides in Group 4 patients include imipenem-cilastatin and ciprofloxacin. Aztreonam (Azactam) could be substituted for an aminoglycoside in patients in whom marginal renal function is present and potential nephrotoxicity is a consideration.

Besides SNO and *Pseudomonas* or *Acinetobacter, S. aureus* is of significant concern as a cause of NP in these patients. When it is considered a possible pathogen, the major concern is that it will be methicillin resistant. Methicillin-resistant *S. aureus* (MRSA) has become a more common pathogen in hospital settings in recent years. It is thought to be possibly more virulent; however, the data come from nursing home patients and are not particularly convincing. Most would recommend initial therapy with vancomycin when MRSA is suspected and modification of therapy when sensitivities are available. The presence of renal failure in a patient in need of vancomycin therapy is not a contraindication. In fact, vancomycin can be administered at lower doses or at less frequent intervals, providing an additional cost advantage. In some institutions *Legionella* is also a significant nosocomial pathogen. The need for specific therapy must be based on local occurrence patterns. Specific therapy has been defined earlier in the CAP section.

Establishing the Diagnosis of Nosocomial Pneumonia

The diagnosis of NP is at least as difficult as that of CAP. As noted, the clinical evaluation can be misleading, sputum Gram's stain and culture are thought to be of little use, and blood and pleural fluid cultures are specific but infrequently positive. The invasive techniques described earlier may be helpful, although TTA cannot be performed in intubated patients, and PLA can be dangerous in the mechanically ventilated patients.

In intubated patients another type of specimen is available, the endotracheal aspirate (ETA). This specimen differs from sputum in that it is not mixed with saliva. Because tracheal colonization is common in intubated patients, positive results from qualitative cultures of ETA are not diagnostic of NP. Studies suggest that the underlying pathogen is usually present, but if multiple organisms are isolated it is not possible to know which is the true cause. For this reason, qualitative cultures of ETA can serve only to expand the spectrum of ongoing empirical therapy.

Recent studies involving quantitative cultures of ETA have been promising. Comparison of these results to BPSB as a gold standard suggests that this type of analysis is valid. At this time, the technique has not yet been standardized. In the future, this may prove to be an accurate and economical method of diagnosing ventilator-associated NP.

VIRAL RESPIRATORY INFECTIONS

method of
BARRY FARR, M.D., M.Sc.
University of Virginia
Charlottesville, Virginia

Viral respiratory infections are the most common acute illnesses of mankind and the leading reason for patient visits to physicians in the United States. They also account for a large proportion of industrial and scholastic absenteeism.

The majority of these viral respiratory infections result in the symptom complex known as the common cold. Cold symptoms include nasal obstruction and discharge, sore throat, sneezing, and coughing. Some cold sufferers develop laryngitis. Small children often have fever with a cold, but adults have fever in less than 1% of cases.

The common cold is caused by many antigenically distinct viruses, but the colds they produce cannot be distinguished from one another on clinical grounds. The rhinovirus group alone comprises more than 100 serotypes, for which only very limited cross-immunity is believed to occur. Other etiologic agents include coronavirus, parainfluenzavirus, respiratory syncytial virus, adenovirus, and even influenza virus, which does not always produce classic influenza. These cold viruses may cause other clinical syndromes in infants and young children such as bronchiolitis, croup, and pneumonia. These viruses account for about two-thirds of all colds, and the remaining third of cases are believed to be due to yet undiscovered viruses.

Influenza is a less common but more severe illness manifested by fever, malaise, myalgias, headache, cough, nasal discharge, chilliness, and occasionally rigors.

TREATMENT OF THE COMMON COLD

The common cold is easily diagnosed clinically, and virologic studies to determine the causative virus are unnecessary. The mainstays of therapy for this self-limited condition remain reassurance, rest, and fluids. Antiviral therapy is not yet available, and antibacterial treatment is not recommended because it does not shorten the duration of the cold and may lead to the development of antibiotic-resistant flora or potentially hazardous side effects.

Treatment is confined to relief of symptoms, but combination cold remedies containing compounds for all possible cold symptoms should be avoided because they expose the patient to a higher risk of unnecessary side effects. Instead, medications should be prescribed to relieve the specific symptoms of the individual patient.

The most frequently required medication is a nasal decongestant. Topical preparations such as 0.1% xylometazoline (Otrivin) or 0.05% oxymetazoline (Afrin) may be administered to adults as intranasal drops or sprays. A less concentrated solution of xylometazoline (0.05%) may be used for children. Sprays are administered with the patient upright (one or two sprays per nostril), whereas drops are administered with the patient in a recumbent position with the neck extended and the head rotated toward the side being treated (one or two drops per nostril). These preparations should be used regularly every 12 hours for 2 to 3 days until obstructive cold symptoms diminish. The patient should be warned about the hazard of rhinitis medicamentosa, which follows prolonged usage of nasal decongestants. Patients treated with monoamine oxidase (MAO) inhibitors should not use decongestants.

Oral preparations are available such as pseudoephedrine hydrochloride (Sudafed), which may be given three to four times daily at a dosage of 15 mg per dose for children aged 2 to 5 years, 30 mg per dose for those 6 to 11 years old, and 60 mg per dose for those over 11 years old. Oral preparations are probably less effective than topical preparations. Recent studies have suggested that one week's therapy with pseudoephedrine does not cause a significant rise in blood pressure in patients with prior controlled hypertension.

Antihistamines exert a drying effect on the nasal mucosa owing to an anticholinergic side effect, but used alone they do not relieve nasal congestion. The slight possible benefit afforded by adding an antihistamine to a decongestant must be weighed against the antihistamine's prominent side effect of drowsiness, which may impair work performance and automobile driving safety. Newer antihistamines lacking these anticholinergic side effects do not cause drowsiness, but they also do not dry the nasal mucosa because histamine is not involved in the pathogenesis of the common cold.

Sore throat is usually mild and may be relieved by saline gargles, but occasionally an analgesic is required. Aspirin may be given orally every 4 hours (adult dose 325 to 650 mg, pediatric dose 10 mg per kg of body weight to a maximum of 650 mg). Acetaminophen (Tylenol, Tempra) may be given orally every 4 hours to patients who are unable to take aspirin. Each dose of acetaminophen is 60 to 120 mg for children between 1 and 3 years old, 120 mg for those 3 to 6 years old, 240 mg for those 7 to 11 years old, and 325 to 650 mg for those over 11 years old. Severe sore throat, especially with exudate, cervical adenopathy, and fever, should suggest the possibility of streptococcal pharyngitis, which may be confirmed by throat culture or a streptococcal antigen test. Treatment for this condition is discussed in another article.

Cough does not usually require therapy in patients with the common cold, but moderate to severe coughing may require a suppressant after the possibility of pneumonia has been excluded by history, physical examination, and (if necessary) radiography. Effective cough suppressants include codeine and dextromethorphan hydrobromide (Romilar, Congesprin). Codeine may be given orally every 4 to 6 hours at the following doses: 2.5 to 5 mg per dose for a child 2 to 5 years old, 5 to 10 mg for a child 6 to 11 years old, and 10 to 30 mg for those over 11 years old. Dextromethorphan dosage is the same, not to exceed four doses in 24 hours. Patients taking MAO inhibitors should not receive these cough suppressants. Expectorants have not been proved to provide effective cough therapy.

Constitutional symptoms and headache are usually minimal with a cold but occasionally require treatment with one of the antipyretics or analgesics previously listed.

The most frequent bacterial complication of the common cold is otitis media, which occurs in approximately 2% of colds, involving mostly children. Otalgia, or diminished auditory acuity, indicates the need for pneumatic otoscopy.

Recent studies have shown that about 90% of patients with a common cold have fluid in their sinuses during the first few days of a cold, apparently because of obstruction of the nasal ostiomeatal complex by inflammation due to the viral infection. Acute bacterial sinusitis follows about 1 of 200 colds and tends to occur more frequently in adults. It cannot be distinguished from a cold on the basis of purulent nasal discharge, which may occur in the uncomplicated cold owing to the viral infection itself. Persistent nasal obstruction and facial pain suggest the need for sinus transillumination or radiography or both. These bacterial complications require antibiotic therapy as discussed in other articles in this book.

Patients and their families should be instructed that colds are caused by infectious viruses that spread from person to person. Although the mechanism of spread in the natural setting has not been definitively established, experimental evidence suggests that rhinoviruses are spread by hand contact and also by large-particle aerosols created by sneezing or coughing. Handwashing and conscious avoidance of finger-to-nose or finger-to-eye contact (which inoculates the virus) after exposure to a cold sufferer may reduce the risk of transmission. Staying more than 5 feet away from a sneezing or coughing patient may also reduce the risk of transmission because large-particle aerosols usually do not travel more than 5 feet. Covering the mouth tightly with a tissue during sneezing and coughing will reduce the number of particles aerosolized.

Ingestion of large doses of vitamin C has been shown to provide ineffective prophylaxis against or therapy for the common cold. Zinc lozenges have also been shown to be ineffective therapy in multiple randomized trials. Prospects for a vaccine are poor because of the multiplicity of viral agents. Interferon* has shown activity as a prophylactic agent but has prevented only a minority of colds and has not been considered cost effective.

TREATMENT OF INFLUENZA

The diagnosis of influenza is made on clinical and epidemiologic grounds. As with colds, diagnostic virology is usually unnecessary for management of the patient with influenza, but the practitioner should be aware of reports on influenza activity by the Centers for Disease Control and Prevention or the state health department. During winter these reports give evidence of the predominant type and frequency of influenza virus isolates in sentinel practices.

The systemic symptoms of influenza are the primary target of therapy. Bed rest and increased fluid intake are necessary. During an influenza A epidemic, amantadine (Symmetrel) has been considered the drug of choice because it is more effective than acetaminophen or aspirin and reduces illness duration by half. The oral dosage for adults is 200 mg initially followed by 100 mg twice daily and for a child 1 to 2 mg per pound of body weight twice daily (not over 150 mg per day). The dose for elderly adults is 100 mg once daily because higher doses are associated with a high rate of side effects. Treatment should continue for 3 to 4 days. Its use has been associated with minor and reversible side effects on the central nervous system such as insomnia, difficulty in concentrating, and dizziness. Rimantadine (Flumadine) is now available commercially and provides equivalent therapeutic efficacy for influenza A at the same dosage but has a lower incidence of side effects than amantadine. The cost of rimantidine is about twice that of amantadine, however.

When influenza B predominates in the area, acetaminophen may be prescribed (dosage given previously) because amantadine and rimantidine lack activity against this virus. Aspirin should not be prescribed for children in view of recent epidemiologic evidence relating Reye's syndrome to salicylate use for influenza or varicella. Although Reye's syndrome is rare in adults, case reports suggest that aspirin may play a role, and acetaminophen is thus preferred.

Cough is often moderate to severe, requiring prescription of a cough suppressant such as codeine or dextromethorphan (dosage given previously) after the possibility of pneumonia has been excluded. Nasal congestion may warrant a topical decongestant as previously described.

Prevention of influenza is possible by vaccination, which is recommended for those at risk for serious complications and death from influenza. This group includes principally the elderly (over 65 years of age) and those with a chronic disease, especially of the heart or lungs. Health care workers in contact with such high-risk patients should also be vaccinated to prevent transmission to their patients. Persons providing essential services to the community should be vaccinated as well. Egg allergy is one of the few contraindications to vaccination.

High-risk individuals who are unable to receive the vaccine may be treated prophylactically with amantadine (Symmetrel) (100 mg once daily for adults) during an epidemic of influenza A. If amantadine is begun prophylactically at the time of vaccination, it should be continued for 14 days to allow time for an effective vaccine response. Rimantidine (Flumadine) provides equal protective efficacy against influenza at the same daily dosage as for amantadine (100 mg per day for an adult).

*This drug has not been approved by the Food and Drug Administration for this indication.

VIRAL AND MYCOPLASMAL PNEUMONIAS

method of
BRUCE H. HAMORY, M.D.
Pennsylvania State University
Hershey, Pennsylvania

Viral and mycoplasmal pneumonias are the most frequent causes of lower respiratory infection in both children and adults. During the past 5 years, treatment regimens have become available for the most common viral causes of lower respiratory tract infection (influenza and respiratory syncytial virus [RSV]). However, successful treatment depends on a specific diagnosis and institution of appropriate therapy within the first 24 hours of clinical disease. With the exception of influenza A, antiviral therapy is expensive and is not necessary unless the patient is immunosuppressed or has severe heart or lung disease. Mycoplasmal pneumonias are frequent in young adults and are being recognized with increasing frequency among older adults and immunosuppressed patients.

The diagnosis of a viral or mycoplasmal infection should be suspected in the presence of a lower respiratory tract illness characterized by fever (usually not over 102° F), gradual onset without true rigors, and a prominent cough that is nonproductive. The chest radiograph shows an infiltrate out of proportion to the findings on physical examination. The specific etiologic agent must be suspected on the basis of the season, the epidemiologic setting, and the presence of confirmed cases of the disease in the community. In the absence of an epidemic, the specific agent should be demonstrated whenever possible by a rapid assay such as direct immunofluorescence on respiratory tract secretions.

VIRAL INFECTIONS

Influenza A

Both amantadine and rimantadine are effective in the treatment of influenza A virus infection if they are instituted within 24 hours of the first symptoms. They are also additive to vaccine in preventing disease. The dose of amantadine (Symmetrel) is 100 mg orally twice a day for 5 days. The dose of rimantadine (Flumadine) is 100 mg orally twice a day. Both drugs must be used with caution in the elderly and those with decreased renal function. Amantadine may be associated with increased irritability, loss of concentration, or other minor CNS side effects. Rimantadine should probably not be used in people with a history of seizure disorder who are not taking anticonvulsants.

Patients should also receive symptomatic treatment with oral fluids and analgesia. Because of the possibility of Reyes' syndrome, I prefer acetaminophen rather than aspirin for muscle aches and headache.

Respiratory Syncytial Virus

RSV causes the croup syndrome seen in young children during the winter and early spring. Ribavirin (Virazole) is specific therapy for this infection but is of proven benefit only in children with profound cardiac or respiratory impairment. Administration requires hospitalization and aerosolization of the drug using a tent or respirator. The drug may clog the nebulizer of the respirator, so care must be taken to check it frequently.

There is concern about the safety of pregnant women who are continuously exposed to the aerosol (ribavirin is mutagenic in rats), and respiratory irritation is common among both nursing and respiratory therapy staff. Because ribavirin has no effect on the other viruses that cause the croup syndrome (parainfluenza and influenza viruses), some attempt to demonstrate the presence of the virus in respiratory tract secretions should be made prior to or simultaneously with instituting this medication.

Viral Infections in the Impaired Host

Varicella-Zoster Virus Infection

Varicella-zoster virus (VZV) pneumonia is a complication of disseminated VZV infection in profoundly immunocompromised patients such as those with acute leukemia and certain organ transplants. In this situation, intravenous treatment with acyclovir (Zovirax), 5 mg per kg body weight every 8 hours for a total daily dose of 15 mg per kg per day, should be given for 7 days. If the infection is primary, some experts give intravenous varicella-zoster immune globulin (VZIG) as well. There is no evidence that either acyclovir or immunoglobulin ameliorates the course of the illness if it is given after onset of the rash. Supportive care and careful observation for secondary bacterial pneumonia are needed.

Cytomegalovirus Infection

Cytomegalovirus (CMV) pneumonia is rare except in patients with profound depression of cell-mediated immunity such as those with AIDS or organ transplants. Because of the plethora of other causes of pulmonary infiltrate in this population, bronchoscopy or lung biopsy for diagnosis is required. Once diagnosed, treatment with ganciclovir (Cytovene), 5 mg per kg given intravenously over 1 hour and repeated every 12 hours for 2 to 3 weeks, together with intravenous gamma globulin is warranted. If the patient cannot tolerate ganciclovir, foscarnet (Foscavir) is an acceptable alternative.

MYCOPLASMA PNEUMONIA

The young, previously healthy adult or teenager who develops prominent cough, usually without sputum, fever, and systemic illness during a period not epidemic for influenza may be presumed to have *Mycoplasma pneumoniae* pneumonia. Demonstration of high levels of "cold agglutinins" or of specific IgM antibody to *M. pneumoniae* are helpful. The treatment is supportive care and erythromycin, 500 mg orally every 8 hours for 10 to 14 days.

Every patient with suspected *M. pneumoniae* infection should be questioned about exposure to parrots, parakeets, and other birds because ornithosis (*Chlamydia psittaci* infection) presents in exactly the same manner but does not respond to erythromycin. Tetracycline or doxycycline (Vibramycin), 100 mg orally twice a day for 10 days, is required. Some studies of *M. pneumoniae* infection suggest a roughly equal response to therapy whether tetracycline or erythromycin is used.

In treating any presumptive lower respiratory tract infection, the first obligation of the physician is to make a reasonable effort to identify the causative agent. Each of the drugs available for treatment of viral or mycoplasmal infection has its own side effects and costs. Most healthy people handle influenza and RSV infections fairly well and require no treatment. Those patients for whom treatment would be required should they become ill should receive influenza vaccine yearly and pneumococcal vaccine as well.

LEGIONELLOSIS
(Legionnaire's Disease and Pontiac Fever)

method of
THOMAS J. MARRIE, M.D.
Dalhousie University and Victoria General Hospital
Halifax, Nova Scotia, Canada

Legionellosis refers to two clinical syndromes caused by bacteria from the family Legionellaceae. These two syndromes are pneumonia (legionnaires' disease) and a self-limited flulike illness (Pontiac fever).

The family Legionellaceae now includes 29 species and more than 49 serogroups. At least 17 members of this family have been implicated in pneumonia; however, *Legionella pneumophila* serogroup 1 accounts for 70 to 90% of these cases. *L. micdadei* (also known as Pittsburgh pneumonia agent) is the most common of the non-*pneumophila* species of Legionellaceae to cause pneumonia.

L. pneumophila is an aerobic gram-negative rod that is widely distributed in natural and artificial water systems. In these systems *Legionella* is amplified by growth in amebae and ciliated protozoa.

EPIDEMIOLOGY

Legionnaires' disease can be both community and hospital acquired and can occur in sporadic, endemic, and epidemic forms. Exposure to *L. pneumophila*–contaminated aerosols (showers, tap water faucets, cooling towers, evaporative condensers, whirlpool baths, decorative fountains, ultrasonic mist machines) is the prime mode of acquisition of epidemic legionnaires' disease. Legionnaires' disease accounts for about 2% of cases of community-acquired pneumonia in adults. The attack rate of nosocomial legionnaires' disease varies considerably, but outbreaks occur from time to time.

Domestic hot water heaters are frequently contaminated with *Legionella* organisms, and the importance of this contamination as a source of sporadic community-acquired legionnaires' disease is currently undergoing investigation.

CLINICAL MANIFESTATIONS

Legionnaires' disease appears as pneumonia that may range from mild to severe and overwhelming disease requiring ventilator support. Fever is present in 75% of patients. Contrary to initial descriptions, cough may be productive, especially in the elderly. Pleuritic chest pain, anorexia, and nausea and vomiting occur in one-third to one-half of the patients. Myalgia, chills, and confusion are found in about one-third. Headache or abdominal pain and diarrhea occur in 7 to 20% of patients. Hemoptysis is unusual but occasionally is present, and the clinical picture of legionnaires' disease in this situation may mimic that of pulmonary infarction. Almost half of the patients have the physical findings of consolidation. On occasion, extrapulmonary manifestations may dominate the clinical picture. These manifestations include encephalitis, cerebellar ataxia, fulminant diarrhea, hepatitis, rapidly progressive glomerulonephritis, myoglobinuria, myocarditis, pericarditis, prosthetic valve endocarditis, hemodialysis shunt infection, and erythema multiforme.

DIAGNOSIS

Knowledge of the local epidemiology and a high index of suspicion are the keys to the diagnosis of legionnaires' disease. This entity should be suspected in all cases of rapidly progressive, community-acquired pneumonia, which is defined as the presence of any two of the following—involvement of most of two or more lobes by the pneumonia; increase in extent of the opacity by 50% or more within 48 hours; a respiratory rate of greater than 32 per minute, or a state of shock due to the pneumonia. Cigarette smoking, chronic lung disease, immunosuppression, and chronic illness are risk factors for this infection. Corticosteroids are the most important immunosuppressive agents predisposing patients to legionnaires' disease. Onset of pneumonia following travel (exposure to contaminated air conditioning) also suggests legionnaires' disease. However, even a trip to the local grocery store (involving exposure to a contaminated ultrasonic mist machine) can be a clue to the source of the *Legionella.*

Despite these clues, the diagnosis cannot be made on clinical grounds alone and must be confirmed by the laboratory. The organism can be grown from sputum; however, this takes 3 to 5 days. The direct fluorescent antibody test for detecting the organism in sputum has a sensitivity of 25 to 75% and a specificity of 95 to 99%. A radioimmunoassay is available for detecting *L. pneumophila* antigen in urine. This test is 80 to 99% sensitive and 99% specific. The antigen may persist in the urine for days to weeks, even after initiation of specific therapy. The major drawback to this test is that it detects only disease due to *L. pneumophila.*

The diagnosis can also be confirmed by testing acute and 6- to 9-week convalescent serum samples for antibodies to *Legionella.*

TREATMENT

The choice and route of therapy depend on the severity of the illness. For patients who are seriously ill with confirmed or suspected legionnaires' disease, I start treatment with erythromycin, 1 gram intravenously every 6 hours. In addition, I add rifampin (Rifadin),* 300 mg orally every 12 hours. Once definite clinical improvement has occurred, the rifampin can be discontinued and the erythromycin given orally in a dose of 500 mg every 6 hours. The total duration of therapy should be at least 21 days because relapses occur when the duration is shorter than this. High-dose erythromycin can result in temporary hearing loss.

If erythromycin and rifampin cannot be given, my second choice is doxycycline (Vibramycin),* 100 mg every 12 hours for two doses, and then 100 mg once daily intravenously. Other options for therapy include ciprofloxacin (Cipro),* 400 mg every 12 hours intravenously or 750 mg every 12 hours orally. Trimethoprim-sulfamethoxazole, 5 mg of the trimethoprim* component per kg every 8 hours, has also been used, usually in conjunction with rifampin; however, there have been reports of failure of therapy with trimethoprim-sulfamethoxazole alone for legionnaires' disease in patients with AIDS.

A newer macrolide, clarithromycin (Biaxin),* at a dose of 500 mg every 12 hours orally, has also been effective in the treatment of legionnaires' disease.

PREVENTION

If nosocomial legionnaires' disease is identified, the hospital's water distribution should be cultured for *Legionella.* If *Legionella* is found, a variety of methods can be used to eliminate the organisms from the distribution system. These include heating the water to about 160° F (70° C) for several days and then flushing the hot water through all the outlets. The

*This drug has not been approved by the FDA for this indication.

water may be hyperchlorinated, or copper and silver ions can be added to the water supply. If the bacteria Legionellaceae cannot be eradicated from the water supply, all organ transplant recipients and all those who are receiving corticosteroids should not drink the water or shower in it.

ACUTE PULMONARY EMBOLISM

method of
JAMES D. DOUKETIS, M.D., and
JEFFREY S. GINSBERG, M.D.
McMaster University Medical Centre
Hamilton, Ontario, Canada

Venous thromboembolism, which includes pulmonary embolism (PE) and deep vein thrombosis (DVT), is the third most common disease involving the cardiovascular system, after coronary artery disease and stroke. DVT and PE can be considered part of a single disease entity given that the majority of pulmonary emboli originate from lower extremity venous thrombi and that approximately half of all patients with proximal DVT have evidence of PE. The true incidence of PE is not known because PE can be silent clinically. It is estimated that 276,000 new cases of PE are diagnosed in North America annually in acute care hospitals alone. In this clinical setting the mortality rate of untreated PE has been reported to be as high as 30%. PE may be the most common preventable cause of death among hospitalized patients because many cases of PE are preventable and effective therapy is available for patients with documented PE. In patients with suspected PE, the clinician's task is to confirm or exclude this diagnosis, so that effective anticoagulant therapy can be provided to patients with PE, and so that the potential risks of long-term anticoagulation can be avoided in patients without PE.

DIAGNOSIS OF PULMONARY EMBOLISM

The clinical features of acute PE are nonspecific, and objective diagnostic testing is required to diagnose this condition. A detailed history, physical examination, and an electrocardiogram and chest radiograph may be useful in identifying conditions that are included in the differential diagnosis of PE (Table 1). The clinical likelihood of PE depends on the clinical features and whether or not there are any coexisting risk factors for DVT (Table 2).

TABLE 1. **Differential Diagnosis for Acute Pulmonary Embolism**

Pulmonary disease
Viral or inflammatory pleurisy
Pneumonia
Acute bronchitis, exacerbation of chronic obstructive lung disease
Pneumothorax
Atelectasis
Cardiovascular disease
Acute pericarditis
Acute myocardial infarction
Dissecting aortic aneurysm
Miscellaneous disease
Musculoskeletal and chest wall pain
Esophageal spasm
Anxiety

In patients with clinically suspected PE, a ventilation/perfusion (V/Q) scan should be performed. The results of this test coupled with the pre-test likelihood of PE determine whether a diagnosis of PE can be made or excluded or whether further objective testing is required (Fig. 1). A normal perfusion scan excludes PE, whereas a high-probability V/Q scan represents PE in the large majority of cases. In patients with a nondiagnostic V/Q scan, duplex ultrasound (DU) or impedance plethysmography (IPG) can be performed to identify DVT as a source of PE from the lower extremities. If the IPG or DU is negative, PE cannot be excluded, and, therefore, pulmonary angiography can be considered. Alternatively, serial testing can be done with either IPG or DU over a 7- to 14-day period. Pulmonary angiography is strongly recommended in patients with a high clinical likelihood of PE, a nondiagnostic V/Q scan, and a normal IPG or DU. If serial IPG or DU is used, anticoagulant therapy can be started if the initial or a repeat IPG or DU is positive. Patients with serially negative IPG or DU tests do not require anticoagulant therapy.

TREATMENT OF PULMONARY EMBOLISM

Anticoagulant therapy has been shown to reduce mortality in patients with acute PE, probably by preventing recurrent thromboembolism and halting the growth of an existing thrombus. In patients with suspected PE, intravenous heparin can be started empirically if one anticipates a delay before objective testing can be performed to confirm or exclude PE. If there are no contraindications to anticoagulation, heparin should be given as an intravenous bolus of 5000 units followed by an infusion that will deliver approximately 31,000 units over 24 hours, or 1300 units per hour. Alternatively, heparin can be administered at a dose of 17,500 units subcutaneously twice daily. In either case, an activated partial thromboplastin time (aPTT) should be done 6 hours after the start of treatment; dosing adjustments can be made while targeting the aPTT to a therapeutic range. The therapeutic range varies among different laboratories and depends on the reagents used, but it usually corresponds to an aPTT of approximately two to three times the control aPTT value. A nomogram can be used to adjust the dose of intravenous heparin according to the aPTT result (Table 3). Patients with subtherapeutic aPTT results are at risk for recurrent thromboembolism, whereas an aPTT that is tempo-

TABLE 2. **Risk Factors for Venous Thromboembolism**

Previous venous thromboembolism
Prolonged immobilization (e.g., postoperative, leg paralysis)
Extensive surgery (especially for malignant disease), major orthopedic surgery
Fracture of tibia, femur, pelvis
Major medical illness (e.g., malignancy, sepsis, heart failure, stroke, myocardial infarction, inflammatory bowel disease)
Age over 60
Underlying prethrombotic disease stage (e.g., deficiency in protein S or C or antithrombin III)

From Hirsh J: Venous thromboembolism: Guide to management. Du Pont Pharmaceuticals, Mississauga, Ontario, 1993.

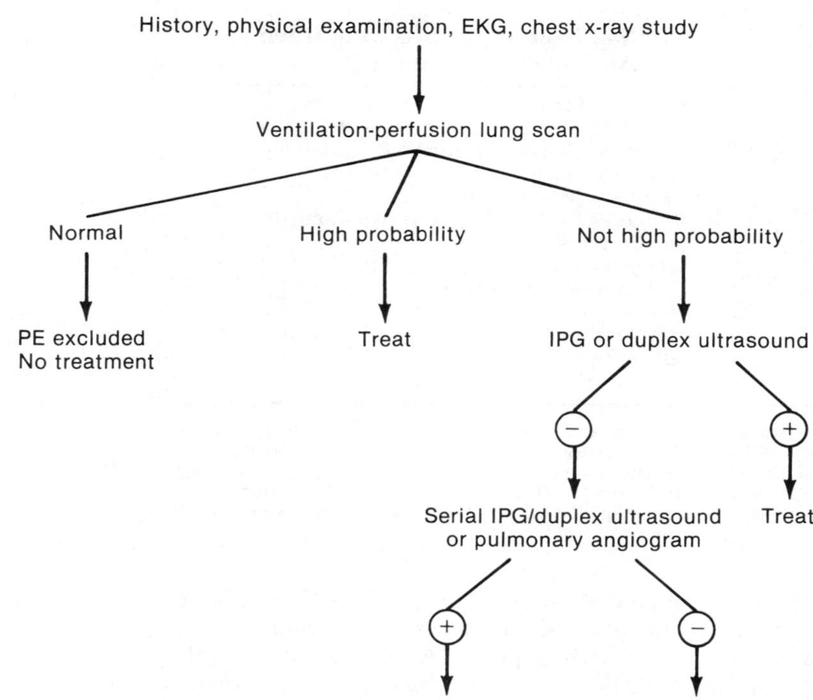

Figure 1. Diagnosis of clinically suspected pulmonary embolism.

rarily above the therapeutic range may not confer a substantially increased hemorrhagic risk. In patients with acute PE, heparin should be administered for a minimum of 4 to 5 days, and in patients with a large PE or hemodynamic instability, it is reasonable to continue heparin for 7 to 10 days.

The most frequent complication of heparin treatment is hemorrhage. Minor hemorrhage, which occurs in 5 to 20% of all patients receiving heparin, is usually self-limited and is often related to bleeding at venipuncture sites. Major hemorrhage requiring either a blood transfusion or the cessation of heparin occurs in only 2 to 5% of patients receiving heparin. The lack of a clear dose-response relationship between the aPTT level and the development of hemorrhage may reflect the variable effect of heparin on platelet and endothelial cell function. There are several risk factors that can increase the risk of bleeding in patients treated with heparin or warfarin (Table 4).

Heparin-induced thrombocytopenia (HIT) occurs in 2 to 4% of patients treated with heparin. The diagnosis of HIT should be considered if there is a greater than 50% drop in the platelet number or if there is an absolute decrease in the platelet count to less than 100,000/ml³. HIT usually occurs 6 to 12 days after the start of heparin therapy, although it can become manifest earlier, especially in a patient who has been exposed previously to heparin. In approximately 10% of cases, HIT may present paradoxically as venous or arterial thrombosis. A complete blood count should be done on the first day of heparin treatment and every 3 days thereafter to monitor for occult hemorrhage as well as for HIT. If HIT is suspected, heparin should be discontinued and replaced with ancrod*

*Ancrod is an investigational drug in the United States. It is not currently approved by the Food and Drug Administration (FDA) but may be supplied by the manufacturer, Knoll Pharmaceuticals, on a compassionate basis.

TABLE 3. **Intravenous Heparin Dose Titration Nomogram**

Starting dose: 5000 units bolus; 31,000 units per 24-hour infusion

aPPT (s)	Bolus Dose	Stop Infusion (min)	Rate Change		Repeat aPPT
			*mL/h**	*units/24 h*	
<50	5000 units	0	+3	2880	6 h
50–59	0	0	+3	2880	6 h
60–85	0	0	0	0	next A.M.
86–95	0	0	−2	1920	next A.M.
96–120	0	30	−2	1920	6 h
>120	0	60	−4	3840	6 h

*1 mL = 40 units/h.

From Cruickshank MK, et al: A standard heparin nomogram for the management of heparin therapy. Arch Intern Med *151*:333–337, 1991. Copyright 1991, American Medical Association.

TABLE 4. **Risk Factors for Bleeding During Anticoagulant Therapy**

Risk factors for bleeding with heparin
Recent (<2 wk) surgery or trauma
Concomitant aspirin or thrombolytic therapy
Renal insufficiency
Excessively prolonged aPPT*
Risk factors for bleeding with warfarin
Age >65 years
History of gastrointestinal bleeding
Stroke (present or previous)
Renal insufficiency
Atrial fibrillation
Acute myocardial infarction
Severe anemia

*The evidence that an excessively prolonged aPPT leads to an increased risk of bleeding is not strong, and significant bleeding can occur with an aPPT in the therapeutic range.

From Levine MN, Hirsh J, Landefeld S, and Raskob G: Hemorrhagic complications of anticoagulant therapy. Chest *102*(Suppl):352S–363S, 1992.

(Arvin), a fibrinolytic agent, or Organon 10172 (Lonoparin),* a heparinoid that does not appear to have cross-reactivity with heparin. Alternatively, an inferior vena cava (IVC) filter can be inserted to prevent PE, although the underlying thrombotic source of the PE will remain untreated and could cause significant morbidity owing to recurrent DVT or the post-phlebitic syndrome. Therefore, if an IVC filter is inserted, warfarin therapy should be considered in patients with coexisting symptomatic DVT to reduce morbidity from the post-phlebitic syndrome and to prevent recurrent thromboembolism.

In some patients with acute PE, heparin resistance may occur whereby a therapeutic aPTT is not attained despite high doses of intravenous heparin (i.e., >35,000 units in 24 hours). Heparin resistance can be caused by several factors. The rate of heparin clearance has been found to be increased in patients with PE compared to those with DVT alone. Heparin-binding proteins, which can be elevated in patients with acute PE, can bind with heparin to inactivate it. Both of these conditions cause true heparin resistance manifesting as a subtherapeutic aPTT and reduced plasma heparin levels. On the other hand "pseudo–heparin resistance" is manifested by a shortened aPTT combined with a therapeutic plasma heparin level. This can occur with an increase in factor VIII (acting as an acute phase reactant), which can shorten the aPTT without neutralizing the in vivo anticoagulant effects of heparin. If heparin resistance is suspected clinically, plasma heparin levels can be measured. Adequate heparin bioavailability is defined by a heparin level of more than 0.2 unit per milliliter measured by thrombin-protamine titration, or by an anti–factor Xa level of more than 0.35 unit per milliliter. If the heparin level reflects an adequate heparin effect, dose adjustments should be made according to heparin levels targeted to 0.2 to 0.4 unit per milliliter by thrombin-protamine titration, or 0.35 to 0.70 unit per milliliter by anti–factor Xa.

*Lonoparin is an investigational drug in the United States.

In patients with submassive PE, oral anticoagulant therapy should be started within 24 to 48 hours of the start of heparin. Heparin should be given for a minimum of 4 to 5 days and can be discontinued when the International Normalization Ratio (INR) has been in the therapeutic range of 2.0 to 3.0 for 2 consecutive days. A higher targeted INR range of 3.0 to 4.5 does not reduce the thromboembolic recurrence rate, but the rate of hemorrhagic complications increases fourfold. In patients with massive PE, heparin should be given for 7 to 10 days.

The optimal duration of long-term warfarin treatment has not been clearly defined, although it is generally accepted that oral anticoagulants, with a targeted INR of 2.0 to 3.0, should be given for at least 3 months, or until there are no ongoing risk factors for venous thromboembolism (VTE). In patients with idiopathic VTE, defined as VTE occurring in the absence of any known risk factors, a longer period of anticoagulant therapy can be considered, given the higher rate of recurrent VTE compared with VTE occurring in the presence of a transient risk factor (e.g., orthopedic surgery). In patients with a single previous episode of VTE and no coexisting risk factors for VTE, oral anticoagulants can be given empirically for 1 year. In patients with an ongoing irreversible risk factor for venous thrombosis (e.g., neoplastic disease, deficiency of protein C or S or antithrombin III), or in patients who have had more than two episodes of VTE, anticoagulants should be continued indefinitely. If anticoagulants are contraindicated or if treatment failure occurs despite adequate anticoagulant doses, the placement of an IVC filter should be considered. The Greenfield filter is an effective device for preventing lower extremity venous thrombi from reaching the lungs. It can be inserted percutaneously through the internal jugular or femoral vein.

Thrombolytic or surgical treatment for acute PE may be indicated in certain clinical situations. Thrombolytic therapy should be reserved for patients who are hemodynamically unstable or who have developed acute respiratory failure as a result of acute PE. In this subgroup of patients with PE, thrombolytic drugs may decrease mortality, and we recommend using a short infusion of tissue plasminogen activator (tPA), although other regimens can also be used (Table 5). In patients with less severe forms of acute PE, heparin therapy is probably as effective as thrombolysis in reducing mortality and long-term morbidity. Surgical embolectomy can be considered in patients who are persistently unstable hemodynamically despite thrombolytic therapy. Embolectomy should be performed by an experienced surgical team because the perioperative mortality is very high, ranging from 10 to 75%.

The use of low-molecular-weight heparins (LMWHs) has not yet been evaluated in large clinical trials for the treatment of patients with acute PE. However, because they are efficacious and safe for the treatment of patients with DVT, it is highly likely that they will prove to be effective for the treatment of patients with PE.

TABLE 5. **Thrombolytic Therapy for Acute Pulmonary Embolism***

Stop heparin infusion; when aPPT is <1.5 times control, thrombolytic therapy can be started	
Streptokinase (Streptase)	250,000 IU loading dose 100,000 IU/h infusion over 24 h
Urokinase (Abbokinase)	4400 IU/kg loading dose 4400 IU/kg/h infusion over 12 h
Tissue plasminogen activator (Activase)	100 mg (56 million IU) infusion over 2 h Alternatively, short infusion: 0.6 mg/kg intravenous bolus over 2 min*

*Heparin infusion can be continued during bolus of tPA.

From Hyers TM, et al: Antithrombotic therapy for venous thromboembolic disease. Chest *102*(suppl): 408S–425S, 1992; and Levine M, et al: A randomized trial of a single bolus dosage regimen of recombinant tissue plasminogen activator in patients with acute pulmonary embolism. Chest *98*:1473–1479, 1990.

TABLE 6. **Risk Categories for Venous Thromboembolism (in Hospitalized Patients Who Are Immobilized)**

High risk	Hip and major knee surgery Previous venous thromboembolism Extensive surgery for malignant disease
Moderate risk	General surgery in patients >40 years of age Leg fracture in a young (<40 years) patient Coexisting chronic medical illness Acute myocardial infarction
Low risk	Uncomplicated surgery Minimal immobility Young patient (<40 years of age)

From Hirsh J: Venous thromboembolism: Guide to management. Du Pont Pharmaceuticals, Mississauga, Ontario, 1993.

PREVENTION OF PULMONARY EMBOLISM

Hospitalized patients who are immobilized for 24 to 48 hours because of surgery, trauma, or medical illness should receive DVT prophylaxis. The importance of DVT prophylaxis is evident when one considers that among hospitalized patients DVT and PE are often asymptomatic and that the initial clinical manifestation may be hemodynamic collapse or sudden death. It has been estimated that if DVT prophylaxis were administered to all patients undergoing general surgery, 4000 deaths could be prevented in the United States annually. Furthermore, in patients undergoing general or orthopedic surgery, DVT prophylaxis with low-dose heparin has been found to be safe and more cost effective than placebo in the prevention of DVT.

In patients undergoing surgery the optimal method of DVT prophylaxis used depends on the patient's risk of developing DVT. This risk is determined by the type of surgery and whether the patient has other risk factors for DVT, such as a previous history of DVT or the coexistence of a hypercoagulable state (Table 6). Patients are considered at high risk for postoperative DVT if they are undergoing certain orthopedic procedures or if they have had previous DVT or PE. These patients should receive DVT prophylaxis with either moderate-dose warfarin, adjusted-dose heparin, or enoxaparin sodium (Lovenox). If warfarin is used, it can be started on the day of surgery or on the first postoperative day in patients undergoing hip or knee surgery. The dose of warfarin should be adjusted to target an INR to approximately 2.0 by the fourth to fifth postoperative day. This method of DVT prophylaxis is effective in reducing the frequency of postoperative DVT by 55% and of proximal postoperative DVT by 70%. Another effective approach for prophylaxis of DVT in high-risk patients is to start heparin 3500 units three times daily and adjust the dose to maintain the aPTT at the upper range of normal. Recently, LMWH has been approved for the prophylaxis of DVT in patients undergoing hip surgery. LMWH has been found to be more effective than standard heparin for the prophylaxis of DVT following hip or knee surgery without an increased risk of bleeding. In patients who have had hip surgery, the use of LMWH postoperatively results in a 70 to 80% risk reduction for DVT compared to placebo. The long half-life and the predictable bioavailability of LMWH obviate the need for monitoring with coagulation assays. Intermittent pneumatic compression is the method of choice for DVT prophylaxis for patients in whom anticoagulants are undesirable such as those undergoing neurosurgical, urologic, or certain ophthalmologic procedures.

In patients at moderate risk for DVT, the methods of prophylaxis include low-dose heparin (5000 units subcutaneously twice daily) or intermittent pneumatic compression. Both of these methods have been shown to reduce the risk of DVT by approximately 70% in general surgery patients. It is reasonable to supplement low-dose heparin or intermittent pneumatic compression with graduated compression stockings because they are effective, inexpensive, and free of serious side effects. Patients who are considered at low risk for postoperative DVT do not require active DVT prophylaxis, although early ambulation should be encouraged.

Overall, primary DVT prophylaxis using any of the aforementioned modalities has been found to be more cost effective than using surveillance screening tests to detect asymptomatic DVT. Moreover, noninvasive screening tests for DVT such as DU and IPG are relatively insensitive for detecting proximal DVT in asymptomatic postoperative patients compared with symptomatic patients, and these tests are insensitive in detecting calf DVT.

SARCOIDOSIS

method of
SONOKO NAGAI, M.D., and
TAKATERU IZUMI, M.D.
Kyoto University
Kyoto, Japan

Sarcoidosis is a systemic granulomatous disorder of unknown etiology. Although most organs of the body may be affected and the clinical findings often under-represent the incidence of pathologic organ involvement, overt clinical manifestations are usually found in the lung, eyes, skin, and superficial lymph nodes. Sarcoidosis most commonly affects adults of both sexes and almost all age groups. Disease in younger patients tends to be detected by abnormal findings on the chest radiograph with or without symptoms. Older patients tend to show clinical manifestations with various symptoms. Symptoms are induced by (1) mass effect of an epithelioid cell granuloma; (2) dysfunction due to metabolically active granulomas at the lesion sites; (3) nongranulomatous immune complex vasculitis, which produces acute symptoms; and (4) distortion due to fibrotic changes that remain even after the granulomatous lesions resolve.

Chest abnormalities occur in three stages: Stage I, bilateral hilar lymphadenopathy (BHL); Stage II, BHL and diffuse pulmonary infiltrate; and Stage III, only diffuse pulmonary infiltrate with or without fibrosis. The majority of patients have symmetrical BHL. Relatively few symptoms are referable to intrathoracic sarcoidosis compared with the findings obtained by radiographic examination.

The prevalence of sarcoidosis varies from less than 1 to 64 cases per 100,000 population, depending on the country, area, and race evaluated. Also, the involved organs and course of the disease differ greatly among countries, geographic areas, races, and individuals.

There are three requirements for diagnosis: (1) a clinical and radiographic picture that is consistent with sarcoidosis, (2) histologic findings of noncaseating epithelioid cell granulomas in an affected organ, and (3) exclusion of other causes of granulomatous inflammation. Elevated levels of serum angiotensin-converting enzyme (ACE) are highly suggestive of but not specific for sarcoidosis. A more atypical presentation requires more thorough diagnostic confirmation. The diagnosis is most commonly confirmed by transbronchial lung biopsy, endobronchial biopsy, or biopsy of the skin or lymph node. Currently, the Kveim-Siltzbach test is restricted because a validated antigen is usually not available and transmissible agents may be dangerous.

Initial evaluation of patients with suspected sarcoidosis includes a chest film (including a computed tomography [CT] scan), pulmonary function tests (spirometry, lung volumes, and diffusion capacity); complete blood count; serum calcium, glucose, liver enzymes, and serum ACE; total protein and gamma globulin, IgE, anti-human C-type hepatitis antibody, anti-human hepatitis B antigen and antibody, and cortisol; electrocardiogram; gallium-67 scan; and bronchoalveolar lavage (BAL).

For clinical management of patients with sarcoidosis, the routine tests needed at present to stage the activity of disease can be limited to the following: (1) clinical investigation, (2) chest radiography (facultatively CT scan), (3) lung function tests, (4) serum ACE, (5) gallium-67 scan, and (6) BAL. Although there are several markers of disease activity, there are no useful prognostic markers.

The course of the disease is often suggested by the mode of presentation. Asymptomatic BHL, with or without erythema nodosum, usually resolves spontaneously. Especially in patients younger than 30 years old, the shadows seen on the radiographic film usually diminish spontaneously or disappear within 2 years. In contrast, disease with an insidious onset and multiple organ involvement often has a chronic course. The prognosis of elderly patients, especially females, seems to be poor compared to that of younger patients. Unfortunately, it is difficult to foresee the prognosis in an individual patient.

IMMUNOPATHOGENESIS

Epithelioid cell granuloma, a hallmark of the lesion in sarcoidosis, resembles the histologic picture observed in tuberculous lesions. Because tuberculous lesions are known to result from a Type IV hyperimmune reaction (delayed hypersensitivity), the pathogenesis of sarcoidosis has been considered similar to that of tuberculosis. Studies of lung cells obtained by BAL have helped to elucidate the mechanisims that contribute to the formation of sarcoid lesions.

The basic pathologic process is the accumulation of macrophages and granulomas that form as a result of hyperfunction of T cells at the site of the lesion. The initial trigger of T cell activation is unknown. However, T cells can be activated as a result of antigen receptor stimulation of $CD3^+$ T cells by an antigen or autoantigen bound to histocompatibility leukocyte antigen (HLA) Class II molecules on mononuclear phagocytes. Activated T cells produce interleukin-2, which promotes the proliferation of T cells in an autocrine manner. Activated T cells also produce lymphokines such as monocyte chemotactic factor and interferon-gamma, which cause an accumulation of blood monocytes in the lesion and promote the differentiation of monocytes into macrophages and epithelioid cells. Activated macrophages and epithelioid cells produce various monokines or mediators, some of which enhance the inflammatory processes in an autostimulatory manner. ACE and active vitamin D are likely to play such a role.

Most sarcoid granulomas regress spontaneously, and only a few develop into fibrotic lesions in sarcoidosis. The question of whether sarcoid granulomas will develop into fibrotic lesions is the most important factor clinically. However, little is known yet about the progression of the fibrotic process. It is well known that patients with sarcoidosis fail to react to the intradermal tuberculin test and at the same time have an increased serum gamma globulin level. Negative conversion of the tuberculin test is explained by the lack of lymphocytes responding at the site of the tuberculin injection. This is due to an inability to accumulate cells at the site because of a diminished concentration gradient of local lymphokines caused in part by the systemically high concentration of lymphokines. It is probably not an actual disturbance of T cell function. The increase in the serum gamma globulin level results from the stimulation and activation of B cells by interleukin-4 or interleukin-6 produced by activated T cells.

ETIOLOGY

Extensive efforts have been made to identify the causative factor of sarcoidosis since Jonathan Hutchinson first described the disease in 1869. Mycobacteria, atypical mycobacteria, pine pollen, and viruses have been the center of attention. Recent studies have revealed a preferential usage of some T cell receptor subunits in sarcoidosis patients. Not only a preferential usage of the T cell receptor but also a high frequency of the presence of the HLA-DR3 subtype, which is strongly connected with the $V\alpha2.3$ TCR gene, was found in patients in Sweden. These results may indicate that sarcoidosis is not a disease caused by one agent but rather the result of the effects of various pathogenic materials that cause T cell activation.

Detection of mycobacterial DNA at the lesion site by molecular genetic approaches is fascinating but is still controversial as a method of confirmation of mycobacteria as an etiologic agent in sarcoidosis.

Considering the prevalence of sarcoidosis, some individuals may be susceptible to the causative agents and may have a tendency to develop sarcoidosis. Familial incidence and correlation with HLA subgroup (for example, HLA-DR52w has a high frequency in Japanese patients) have been studied.

TREATMENT

Because its etiology is unknown, sarcoidosis has been treated empirically with a wide variety of therapeutic modalities. Fundamentally, careful observation without treatment should be the initial approach by the clinician, especially when patients are asymptomatic. Patients who show symptoms and functional deterioration should be treated.

Corticosteroids

Corticosteroids are the mainstay of treatment of sarcoidosis. Theoretically, sarcoidosis is an antigen-driven disease, and if this process could be blocked there would be no need for a debate about the role of steroids. However, no causative antigen has been confirmed, so steroids are currently the best and most widely used therapy. They are the most effective drugs for the treatment of sarcoidosis and often produce dramatic resolution of the disease—that is, relief from symptoms and a clear improvement in chest radiographic findings. In addition, current understanding of events leading to the disease confirms that corticosteroids are a rational therapy. Corticosteroids are known to regulate the control and amplification of the synthesis of many cytokines including interleukin-1, interleukin-2, and tumor necrosis factor alpha. Thus, there is some logic for their use early in the inflammatory process because they may be expected to have an impact on the mechanisms operating at this time.

Some evidence of the disease-modulating effects of corticosteroids is obtainable from various sources. Nevertheless, corticosteroids are not used in all patients with sarcoidosis for the following reasons. (1) Spontaneous remission is observed frequently in patients with sarcoidosis. (2) For a short time corticosteroids are effective in stabilizing the patient's condition; they cause regression of the symptoms and chest radiographic findings. However, there are no data showing that administration of corticosteroids is beneficial for the long-term course and prognosis. (3) Corticosteroids have serious side effects such as osteoporosis.

Considering these conditions, with our current knowledge, the use of corticosteroids is justified and essential to promote symptomatic relief and control of disabling systemic involvement. But the administration schedules, including the time, dosage, and duration of treatment with corticosteroids, still need to be resolved. In addition, there are few reports of long-term observations of the effect of treatment with corticosteroids to clarify the point that corticosteroids can prevent the irreversible fibrotic process or the persistence of the inflammation, regardless of the presence or absence of symptoms. In our retrospective study of 185 patients with asymptomatic pulmonary sarcoidosis whose disease was mainly detected by health examinations and whose clinical symptoms, chest radiographic findings, and prognosis were followed for more than 10 years after the first detection of the disease, it was observed that administration of corticosteroids was not beneficial.

The goal of treatment is to resolve inflammatory lesions that interfere significantly with organ function. The variability of the clinical course and the potential hazards of therapy influence the decision of whether to begin corticosteroid treatment. It is important to use corticosteroids judiciously, avoiding unnecessarily large doses. There are two ways of approaching the problem—that of the early treaters and that of the late treaters. The early treaters think as follows: Treatment with corticosteroids can prevent irreversible fibrosis and should be applied early, preferably before the onset of pulmonary symptoms. Therefore, small doses and long-term treatment are desirable to restore normal structure and function. Furthermore, by using corticosteroids earlier, they may be withdrawn without causing relapse. On the other hand, late treaters reason that sarcoidosis is a benign self-limiting condition and often resolves spontaneously. In addition, corticosteroids have side effects, and if fibrosis is going to develop, it will do so despite the steroids. These clinicians hold the view that corticosteroids may alleviate pulmonary symptoms but do not interfere with the inexorable course of irreversible fibrosis. Therefore, they are not willing to use corticosteroids in the early stage.

Consequently, patients with sarcoidosis must be carefully monitored. The dose and duration of corticosteroid regimens must be tailored to the activity of the disease as monitored by one of a number of indices, such as clinical symptoms, chest radiographic changes, or pulmonary function. Furthermore, in select clinical settings, either serum ACE, BAL lymphocytes, or findings on gallium-67 citrate lung scan or high-resolution CT scan have been used as an index of disease activity. No treatment with corticosteroids is needed in patients with acute presentation and Stage I disease (BHL) because the majority of such patients will recover spontaneously despite showing a high initial inflammatory activity.

Practically, the administration of sufficient doses of corticosteroids will ensure that anti-inflammatory effects cause remission of symptoms and disease. Initially, a dose of 40 mg of prednisone is administered daily (or 60 mg on alternate days) for 4 to 8 weeks. If effective, the dosage can be reduced gradually over a 6-month period and maintained at 5 to 10 mg daily, which will produce few side effects. Just how long corticosteroids should be administered is unclear. Another strategy is to discontinue treatment when symptoms have disappeared and restart it promptly if there is a relapse. A dosage higher than the previous maintenance dosage will be needed at that point. Alternate-day treatment with corticosteroids is preferred if this approach will control the disease; certainly, this method will help to reduce the side effects and control adrenal suppression. When corticosteroid treatment is ineffective in terms of the previously mentioned indices of clinical symptoms, chest radiographic changes, and pulmonary function, the dosage should be reduced and stopped within a short time.

ALTERNATIVE THERAPY

Occasionally, corticosteroid treatment is absolutely contraindicated because of its side effects. In such cases, anti-inflammatory agents and immunosuppressive drugs such as cyclophosphamide, azathioprine, and cyclosporine* may be necessary. A recent report indicated that low-dose methotrexate* is effective in treating refractory sarcoidosis. However, the side effects of these alternative drugs are more common and severe than those associated with corticosteroids. From personal experience, we cannot recommend such agents as standard for the treatment of pulmonary sarcoidosis in advanced stages. There are few controlled trials relevant to the effect of these drugs on sarcoidosis.

Recent therapeutic approaches have focused on lung transplantation in patients with advanced pulmonary sarcoidosis with severe dysfunction. However, we have never performed such operations in our own patients, although several advanced cases have been reported in Japan.

SPECIFIC TREATMENT CONSIDERATIONS

Specific treatments should be considered depending on the specific manifestations of sarcoidosis.

Pulmonary Lesions. In advanced cases, supplemental oxygen is needed, including home oxygen therapy. When patients have an acute exacerbation, pulse therapy with methylprednisolone (1 gram for 3 days intravenously) can be tried.

Hemoptysis may complicate bronchiectasis due to endobronchial involvement, or aspergilloma may occur in fibrocystic sarcoidosis. Effective antibiotics or antifungal drugs are administered, and bed rest with antitussives may be necessary. Bronchoscopic embolization or surgical resection may be needed in severe cases.

In some cases, we have encountered bronchial hyperreactivity. For such patients, inhalation therapy with a corticosteroid with a bronchodilator may be effective.

Ocular Lesions. Patients with anterior uveitis complain of blurred vision, redness, or pain in the eyes. Ophthalmologic examinations should be done in every patient with sarcoidosis. Funduscopy is required to rule out other lesions. Some patients suffer from glaucoma, which causes eye pain. The effect of topical corticosteroids seems to diminish with progression of the disease. Some patients need systemic treatment with corticosteroids.

*These drugs have not been approved by the FDA for this indication.

Central Nervous System. Unilateral facial palsy, cerebellar signs, diabetes insipidus, or visual defects may be present owing to hypothalamic involvement. Hearing loss may be present because of neuropathy. CNS sarcoidosis usually requires prompt and prolonged therapy with corticosteroids.

Myocardial Involvement. Myocardial involvement is frequently detected by electrocardiography (ECG). Some patients experience tachycardiac or bradycardiac arrhythmias as anterior chest discomfort or palpitations. Patients who are over 40 years of age should be examined routinely by ECG in an outpatient clinic. A thallium scan may be useful, although abnormalities due to sarcoidosis resemble those due to ischemic heart disease. Endomyocardial biopsy is often nondiagnostic because of the patchy distribution of the granulomatous lesions in the myocardium. Corticosteroids should be administered to patients with myocardial involvement because this lesion often causes sudden death. In addition to corticosteroids, antiarrhythmic drugs are prescribed. Some patients need a pacemaker.

Muscle Involvement. Muscle involvement often causes gait disturbance or other complaints. The serum ACE level may be highly increased. Corticosteroids are administered to relieve the symptoms and disability.

Skin Lesions. Erythema nodosum is a self-limited nongranulomatous immune complex vasculitis, which is often found at the onset of sarcoidosis. Other skin lesions may persist longer. Their manifestations sometimes occur in parallel with other clinical manifestations. Because some patients want to take drugs to combat disfiguring lesions, corticosteroids are given orally. We have seen improvements even in chronic persisting lesions. But the majority of skin lesions tend to persist or relapse.

Joint Involvement. Joint involvement may occur acutely with erythema nodosum. Some patients may show a painful deformation of a joint that mimics rheumatoid arthritis. Corticosteroids are administered to symptomatic patients.

Bone Involvement. Bone lesions cause severe pain and disability. They should be treated with corticosteroids or other anti-inflammatory drugs.

Massive Enlargement of Lymph Nodes and Salivary Glands. Lymph node lesions are usually painless. Salivary gland enlargement may cause pain or a dry mouth. Corticosteroids may be effective, but the effects seem to be temporary.

General Symptoms. Some patients may complain of general malaise or a high fever. These symptoms respond to a short course of treatment with corticosteroids.

Liver Lesions. Liver biopsy frequently reveals the presence of granulomatous lesions. Patients may present with right quadrant discomfort, anorexia, and nausea, but jaundice is rare. Liver enzyme levels usually remain elevated with or without hepatomegaly. Symptoms lessen after treatment with corticosteroids, but liver enzyme levels may remain elevated for a prolonged period. If portal hypertension develops, surgical operation is needed.

Hypercalcemia and Renal Lesions. Activated macrophages or epithelioid cell granulomas produce an increased amount of 1,25-dihydroxycholecalciferol (calcitriol), so that some patients have excessive absorption of calcium from the gastrointestinal tract. These patients present with nausea, vomiting, and lethargy. Renal stones sometimes cause acute abdominal pain and severe back pain. The stones tend to be found bilaterally, but only a few patients develop chronic renal failure. Renal biopsy rarely demonstrates the presence of epithelioid cell granuloma. Most cases of nephropathy are due to hypercalcemia. Corticosteroids may be effective for both conditions. Exposure to sunlight, dietary calcium, and vitamin D should be restricted.

SILICOSIS

method of
JAMES H. DAUBER, M.D.
University of Pittsburgh School of Medicine
Pittsburgh, Pennsylvania

Silicosis was probably the first-recognized occupational lung disease. Accounts of chronic respiratory illness and disability in miners date back more than 6000 years. The Industrial Revolution created many more types of exposures and greatly expanded the number of individuals with clinically significant disease. The direct association between pulmonary fibrosis and the inhalation of siliceous dust, however, was not confirmed until the early twentieth century. Since then, considerable effort has gone into both limiting exposure to respirable-sized particles of free crystalline silica (<5.0 μm) and defining the pathogenesis of this still too common disease. Unfortunately, acceptable results have not yet been achieved in either arena.

DEFINITIONS AND EPIDEMIOLOGY

When the amount of free silica required to produce a clinically significant reaction in the lung accumulates from prolonged exposure (20 to 40 years) to low levels of respirable dust that exceed the threshold limit of 100 μg per M^3, the disease is called *chronic silicosis.* Levels of dust in the environment that are 10 to 50 times this amount produce clinically significant disease after only 5 to 10 years of exposure. This is called *accelerated silicosis.* Finally, a relatively uncommon condition called *acute silicosis* ensues after only 6 to 12 months of exposure to even higher levels of dust. Most exposures leading to silicosis occur in the work place, but there are a few instances of household exposure producing disease, most commonly in the form of scouring powder. Table 1 outlines the major forms of occupational exposure. Several of the exposures that have the potential to cause accelerated and even acute silicosis deserve mention here. The production of "silica flours" creates very high concentrations of particles, the vast majority of which are respirable. The same is true of abrasive blasting. In fact, recent improvements in the technology of sand blasting have led to even greater levels of respirable and highly reactive particles than were encountered in the past, a development that has not been fully appreciated by owners and operators of this equipment. Exposures are likely to be higher in workers employed by small companies that find it financially unrewarding or inconvenient to adhere to present standards of dust control and worker protection. Consequently, the examining physician must always keep in mind the possibility of silica exposure as the cause of unexplained fibrotic lung disease in young patients.

TABLE 1. **Occupations Associated with Exposure to Silica**

Category	Source of Free Silica
Mining	Drilling and cutting siliceous rock Sand for traction on rails
Manufacturing	
Stone dressing	Cutting, grinding, polishing
Abrasives	Crushing quartz
Foundries	Removing sand from castings
Pottery	Cleaning surfaces to be enameled
Refractory products	Crushed quartz in products (quartz was removed from "fire bricks" in 1950s)
Inert fillers	"Silica flours"
Filter materials	Heated diatomaceous earth
Construction	
Tunneling	Dust from drilled rock
Road building	Crushing rock for roadbeds
Renovation	Dust from drilling concrete
Steel fabrication	Sand blasting
Boiler scaling	Flue dust may contain silica

PATHOLOGY AND PATHOGENESIS

The hallmark of chronic and accelerated silicosis is the so-called silicotic nodule. These lesions, which consist of a core of concentrically arranged connective tissue surrounded by a halo of mononuclear inflammatory cells, typically contain abundant silica particles. They are distributed preferentially in the subpleural, paraseptal, and peribronchiolar interstitial spaces of the lung. Given such a distribution, they have the potential to invade the lymphatics, pulmonary arteries and veins, and small and medium-sized airways. Usually the density is greater in the upper lung zones than in the lower zones. This situation is known as *simple silicosis.* Nodules are present in draining lymph nodes as well and rarely may cause clinically significant adenitis in anatomically remote regions, which usually is mistaken for primary or metastatic cancer. These nodules coalesce in the lungs of up to 30% of afflicted individuals, forming much larger masses that consist primarily of amorphous hyaline material. Inflammatory cells and silica particles are much less conspicuous in such massive lesions compared to the nodules. Massive lesions occur more commonly in the upper lobes of individuals who have a high density of silicotic nodules. Infection with *Mycobacterium* also predisposes individuals to their formation. These massive lesions tend to grow inexorably, and as they enlarge they migrate toward the hila, destroying the lung parenchyma and compressing the nearby arteries and airways. These lesions may also cavitate owing to ischemic necrosis or superimposed tuberculosis. The contraction of large areas of severely involved lung leads to emphysematous changes in adjacent regions and less involved lobes. This situation is known as *complicated silicosis* or *progressive massive fibrosis.* When large amounts of dust accumulate in a matter of months to produce acute silicosis, the reaction is different. Inflammation is diffuse and involves both the alveolar wall and the alveolar space. Well-formed silicotic nodules in the interstitium are distinctly uncommon. There is usually an abundance of eosinophilic material in the alveolar space that takes up periodic acid–Schiff stain, suggesting that it contains lipoproteins. Such a reaction has been called silicoproteinosis.

In regard to pathogenesis, the macrophage has occupied center stage for the last 30 years. The observation that silica is toxic to these cells led to the hypothesis that dying cells release substances that stimulate the growth and synthetic activity of fibroblasts. Dying cells also release their burden of particles. The particles disgorged from dying macrophages are then taken up by fresh macrophages, which are destined to undergo the same fate as their predecessors. In the last 5 to 10 years this hypothesis has been recognized as being overly simplistic. Experimental studies have clearly demonstrated that prior to their demise, macrophages release a host of inflammatory mediators that influence the function not only of fibroblasts but also of a variety of inflammatory cells, including lymphocytes. This complex interaction leads not only to the formation of the typical silicotic nodule but also to a constellation of immunologic abnormalities seen with this disease. There is also a growing body of evidence of a genetic predisposition to silicosis. An unexpected proportion of individuals with advanced silicosis have the HLA-Bw54 phenotype and share similarities in genes for HLA-DP, the fourth component of complement, and the immunoglobulin lambda chain–variable region. These findings suggest that a gene predisposing to this disease is closely linked with the HLA-B locus.

CLINICAL FEATURES

Because individuals with simple silicosis are usually asymptomatic, the diagnosis is considered most often only after the incidental discovery of characteristic radiographic abnormalities (see Table 2 for a comparison of simple and complicated silicosis). The chest film reveals a profusion of fine nodules that are usually smaller than 0.5 cm and are most dense in the upper lung zones. Hilar and mediastinal nodes may also be enlarged and in more advanced situations show a peripheral rim of calcium. This pattern, often called eggshell calcification, is seen with other chronic granulomatous diseases but should always alert the physician to the possibility of silicosis. These individuals not infrequently admit to a chronic productive cough, but this symptom usually is related to chronic bronchitis resulting from smoking and exposure to nonsiliceous dusts. At this stage lung function is generally well preserved. Serologic abnormalities include polyclonal hypergammaglobulinemia and elevated titers of rheumatoid factor, antinuclear antibodies, and anticollagen antibodies. Angiotensin-converting enzyme activity in serum is greater than expected in 30% of individuals. Clinically evident autoimmune disease is uncommon but occurs at a greater than expected rate.

Dyspnea usually signifies the presence of massive fibrotic lesions in the lung. These individuals nearly always have a productive cough as well. The masses, which by definition are greater than 1 cm in diameter on the chest radiograph, have a predilection to grow in the upper lung zones and may eventually occupy a large part of the involved lobe. They always develop in association with a high density of small nodules on the radiograph, but as the massive lesions enlarge, the density of the small nodules may actually decrease owing to their inclusion in the growing mass and the rarefaction of the adjacent lung. Lung function studies typically reveal a combination of obstruction and restriction. The diffusing capacity is decreased, and the alveolar-arterial oxygen gradient is widened. Inhalation of a beta-agonist partially reverses the obstruction to air flow. In far-advanced situations cor pulmonale supervenes as a consequence of pulmonary hypertension. The latter condition reflects damage to the pulmonary vasculature from the advanced silicotic reaction and associated chronic hypoxemia. In these instances total disability ensues from progressive cardiopulmonary insufficiency.

Acute silicosis usually produces both systemic and respiratory symptoms. Dyspnea is accompanied by fever, fatigue, malaise, weakness, and even a full-blown lupus-like illness. The chest radiograph reveals an airspace-filling pattern with confluent infiltrates and air bronchograms. Superinfection with mycobacteria is frequent and must always be excluded. Death from respiratory failure or active tuberculosis usually ensues within 1 to 2 years of the onset of symptoms.

DIAGNOSIS

In most instances the diagnosis can be made by documenting sufficient exposure to silica in an individual with the characteristic radiographic abnormalities. A lung biopsy is not required unless there is a history of exposure to other fibrogenic dusts as well as silica and it is necessary to document that pulmonary disability is due to more than a single agent. Exposure to coal dust can produce an identical picture, but usually the diagnosis of coal workers' pneumoconiosis presents no difficulty for the experienced physician. Cavitation of a massive lesion strongly suggests co-existing infection with mycobacteria. A mass in the lung of an individual with a history of exposure to silica should not be attributed to complicated silicosis unless it can be confirmed that it arose in conjunction with a high profusion of small nodules (i.e., simple silicosis). Bronchogenic carcinoma must be excluded first in this situation. A series of

TABLE 2. **Comparison of Simple and Complicated Silicosis**

Feature	Simple Silicosis	Complicated Silicosis
Dyspnea	Uncommon	Common
Chronic cough	Depends on smoking history and degree of exposure to dust	Usual, regardless of smoking history and exposure to dust
Cor pulmonale	Rare	Common in later stages
Pulmonary function	Usually normal	Obstruction, restriction, and hypoxemia
Radiographic abnormalities	Small nodules (<0.5 cm), particularly in upper lung zones	Masses >1.0 cm usually in upper zones *along with* small nodules
Predisposition to tuberculosis	Strong	Strong; infection may also accelerate formation of massive lesions
Predisposition to lung cancer	Strongly suspected	Probable
Disability	Rare	Common

recent studies in populations of individuals with silicosis suggests that mortality due to lung cancer in silicotics is greater than expected regardless of the smoking history, suggesting that silica is carcinogenic. Until this situation is further clarified, monitoring subjects with silicosis for the development of lung cancer with annual chest radiographs seems reasonable. The appearance of a new mass on the film that does not demonstrate the usual findings of progressive massive fibrosis must be aggressively pursued.

TREATMENT

Young individuals with accelerated silicosis should cease exposure to silica, but whether older workers with asymptomatic simple silicosis who are near retirement need to do so is debatable. No specific therapy exists for the treatment of any form of silicosis, however. There may be a role for high doses of corticosteroids in patients with acute silicosis but certainly not in those with the chronic or accelerated form, in whom such therapy may create a further predisposition to tuberculous infection. Recent experimental evidence is beginning to confirm past anecdotal reports that inhalation of aluminum ameliorates the reaction to silica in the lung, but controlled studies using such an approach in humans have yet to be mounted. For these reasons, treatment should be directed toward complications such as airway obstruction and infection.

Inhaled beta-agonists and anticholinergics partially reverse obstruction to air flow. Low doses of oral corticosteroids or inhaled corticosteroids may augment the activity of bronchodilators. Acute exacerbations of chronic bronchitis deserve prompt therapy. Afflicted individuals should be vaccinated against influenza and pneumococcal pneumonia. The diagnosis and treatment of infection with mycobacteria must be aggressively pursued in all subjects with silicosis, particularly in light of the resurgence of this infection and the growing prevalence of drug-resistant organisms. Careful monitoring of the tuberculin skin test status of silicotics is warranted. Converters should be considered to have active tuberculosis. Appropriate cultures should be obtained and therapy with four drugs initiated and continued until the results of cultures and follow-up studies exclude the presence of active infection. In the absence of active infection, prophylaxis with isoniazid (INH), 300 mg daily, should be continued for 1 year. Recent evidence suggests, however, that after completion of what is presently considered adequate prophylaxis, a much greater than expected proportion of these subjects will develop active infection. Treatment of active infection should always employ agents to which the organism is sensitive. The duration of therapy is controversial. Relapse after completion of treatment regimens that are effective in the general population is all too common, leading some experts to propose lifelong therapy.

Chronic respiratory failure and cor pulmonale should be treated in the usual fashion. Continuous oxygen therapy and pulmonary rehabilitation should be employed when indicated. Young to middle-aged patients with acute silicosis or advanced accelerated silicosis are candidates for pulmonary transplantation. Although experience with recipients who have received a lung allograft for silicosis is limited, preliminary results have been encouraging. Realistically, this approach is presently the only hope for prolonged survival in such individuals. Because active tuberculosis is virtually an absolute contraindication to transplantation, control of this infection today has even greater significance than it had in the past. Given this state of affairs, efforts to limit exposure remain of paramount importance. Lowering the legal threshold limit of exposure may ultimately be successful, but instituting such regulatory actions does not ensure uniform compliance on the part of employers and employees.

HYPERSENSITIVITY PNEUMONITIS

method of
MARK SCHUYLER, M.D.
VA Medical Center
Albuquerque, New Mexico

Hypersensitivity pneumonitis (HP), or allergic alveolitis, is a group of immunologically mediated granulomatous pulmonary diseases caused by inhalation of finely dispersed antigenic material. Any environment that allows inhalation of large numbers of appropriate-sized antigenic particles can be associated with HP. Table 1 lists common examples of HP.

Unlike other granulomatous lung diseases (e.g., sarcoidosis), HP is limited to the lung. It occurs more frequently in adult men than in women and children but only as a reflection of their patterns of work and avocational exposure. Most patients with HP are nonsmokers.

CLINICAL PRESENTATION

Short-term, high-level exposure tends to cause acute disease, and the long-term, relatively low-level exposure tends to cause chronic disease.

Acute Hypersensitivity Pneumonitis. Four to 12 hours after exposure to the responsible agent, the subject develops fever (up to 40° C), chills, myalgias, nonproductive cough, and dyspnea and also may develop headache, anorexia, cyanosis, myalgias, and arthralgia. There is no wheezing, but bilateral basilar rales and often cyanosis occur. These symptoms abate spontaneously if exposure is discontinued, usually after several hours to several days. However, if exposure has been especially intense, symptoms may persist for 1 to 2 weeks. The chest roentgenogram typically displays miliary nodules 1 to 3 mm in diameter in the lower lung fields, but it may be normal or demonstrate larger nodules or the residuals of previous episodes of disease (interstitial fibrosis with upper lobe predominance). Pleural effusion and hilar adenopathy are rare. Peripheral blood leukocytosis with neutrophilia, but without eosinophilia, and arterial hypoxemia are usually present. Despite the terms hypersensitivity and allergic, these diseases are not allergic or atopic in nature. Levels of IgE and eosinophils are normal in peripheral blood both during an episode of disease and during remission.

TABLE 1. **Common Examples of Hypersensitivity Pneumonitis**

Disease	Source of Antigen	Type of Antigen	Probable Antigen
Farmer's lung disease	Moldy hay	Thermophilic actinomycetes, fungi	*Micropolyspora faeni* *Thermoactinomyces vulgaris* *Aspergillus*
Bird fancier's disease	Bird droppings	Animal proteins	Altered bird serum (probably IgA)
Humidifier lung	Contaminated humidifiers, dehumidifiers, air conditioners	Thermophilic actinomycetes, fungi	*Thermoactinomyces candidus* *Thermoactinomyces vulgaris* *Penicillium* *Cephalosporium*

Chronic Hypersensitivity Pneumonitis. This condition presents as interstitial pneumonitis with symptoms of dyspnea, weight loss, and cough. Radiologically, interstitial fibrosis due to HP tends to predominate in the upper lobes, whereas in most forms of pulmonary fibrosis the lower lobes are more heavily involved.

DIAGNOSIS

Serum antibody directed against the pertinent antigens is found in most patients with acute HP. Simple immunodiffusion (i.e., Ouchterlony technique) is as sensitive and specific as any other method used to detect antibody.

The presence of serum antibody demonstrates that a subject has been exposed to and has developed antibody to a particular antigen but does not always indicate that he or she has HP because many exposed subjects develop serum antibody without disease. Conversely, a negative antibody test in a patient with HP may occur if inappropriate antigen is used for testing or if sufficient time (years) has elapsed between the last exposure and the test. Immediate (allergy) type skin tests are not useful in evaluating a patient with suspected HP.

A biologic challenge may be very helpful in the diagnosis of HP. This consists of measuring simple physiologic parameters (temperature, respiratory rate, expiratory flow rates, and arterial oxygen saturation, with perhaps a chest roentgenogram) before and after an exposure that is suspected to cause HP. If the appropriate changes occur 4 to 12 hours after exposure and remit spontaneously, the diagnosis of HP is supported.

The symptoms and signs of acute and chronic HP are not specific and may mimic those of other diseases such as infectious pneumonia, sarcoidosis, and idiopathic pulmonary fibrosis. Often, only the history of repetitive, stereotypical episodes of disease occurring 4 to 12 hours after exposure to a particular environment, associated with serum precipitins, allows the diagnosis of HP to be considered. Obviously, the history is an extremely important diagnostic tool. This implies that one must inquire about previous illnesses and the occupational and avocational history in a detailed and complete manner in patients with "recurrent pneumonia," "sarcoidosis," and "idiopathic pulmonary fibrosis."

THERAPY

Avoidance of repeated exposure is the only established effective treatment. If exposure is stopped before permanent radiologic or pulmonary function test abnormalities occur, the prognosis is excellent. However, advanced abnormalities may not be completely reversible and can lead to disability (predominantly respiratory insufficiency and cor pulmonale) and death.

Systemic glucocorticosteroids are often used in both acute and chronic disease. A standard regimen is prednisone, 0.5 to 1 mg per kg per day, or the equivalent in divided doses after 2 weeks, tapered to zero over another 6 weeks. Antihistamines, bronchodilators, inhaled steroids, and immunotherapy are not useful.

SINUSITIS

method of
DALE H. RICE, M.D.
University of Southern California School of Medicine
Los Angeles, California

Sinusitis is an inflammatory process involving the mucosa of the paranasal sinuses and commonly the nasal cavity as well. A number of local and systemic factors may predispose to sinusitis (Table 1). These include decreased humidity, pollution, nasal medications, airborne antigens, and viruses and bacteria. Diseases such as cystic fibrosis and ciliary dyskinesia are also predisposing conditions. All may either impair ciliary motility or cause seconday edema. It is well known now that many of the initial events of sinusitis occur in the ostiomeatal complex. This is a particularly narrow area in the lateral nasal wall underlying the middle turbinate where the anterior ethmoid, frontal, and maxillary sinuses drain. This area is so narrow that minimal edema may cause mucus stasis or sinus obstruction. Other physical abnormalities may also cause obstruction, including foreign bodies, polyps, septal deviation, and middle tur-

TABLE 1. **Possible Predisposing Factors in Sinusitis**

Local	Systemic
Decreased humidity	Cystic fibrosis
Topical nasal medications	Ciliary dyskinesia
Air pollution	Immunosuppression
Foreign bodies	Nasal allergies
Lateralized middle turbinate	Immunodeficiencies
Deviated nasal septum	
Chronic adenoiditis	

binate expansion or lateral displacement. Other abnormalities in other locations may also lead to infection. An important one in children is adenoidal hypertrophy, in which the gland may serve as a bacterial reservoir. Pressure changes such as those occurring in diving may occasionally force bacteria under pressure into otherwise sterile sinuses. Immunosuppression from any cause may also predispose to infection and may lead to opportunistic infections. A wide variety of immune deficiencies may exist in childhood or adulthood and should be sought in the patient with recurrent bacterial sinusitis when there is no other obvious cause.

ACUTE SINUSITIS

An acute inflammatory reaction may be allergic, viral, or bacterial in origin. A careful history may distinguish between them, but either of the former two will predispose to the latter. Allergic reactions may be seasonal or perennial; the latter are much more difficult to distinguish from other causes. In allergic rhinitis, however, episodic sneezing, pruritus, and erythema of the conjunctiva are often associated. Allergic rhinosinusitis is best treated with antihistamines started before the attack if possible, with or without decongestants. Viral rhinosinusitis, on the other hand, typically is accompanied by systemic symptoms, unlike those of acute bacterial sinusitis. Commonly implicated viruses include a large number of rhinoviruses, influenza virus, parainfluenza virus, and adenoviruses. Treatment is supportive.

Acute bacterial sinusitis is usually associated with purulent discharge, nasal congestion, and facial pain or pressure. Fever is uncommon. The most common organisms are the same as those causing acute otitis media, including *Streptococcus pneumoniae, Haemophilis influenzae, Moraxella catarrhalis,* and *Streptococcus pyogenes.* In the absence of an accurate culture, which is difficult to obtain, a 2-week course of amoxicillin–clavulanic acid (Augmentin) is the recommended first line of therapy. Excellent second choices include trimethoprim-sulfamethoxazole (Bactrim, Septra),* cefaclor (Ceclor), cefuroxime (Ceftin),* and the newer antibiotics loracarbef (Lorabid), clarithromycin (Biaxin), and azithromycin (Zithromax).* Symptomatic response should occur within 48 to 72 hours, but therapy is continued for 10 to 14 days. Topical decongestants and nasal saline irrigation may improve drainage and mucociliary function. Topical nasal decongestants are not recommended for more than 1 to 2 days because of the inevitable rebound vasodilatation. Oral decongestants may also be beneficial. Antihistamines are generally not recommended because of their theoretical drying effect unless the infection has an allergic component. Acute frontal or sphenoidal sinusitis should be viewed with some suspicion and should be treated more aggressively because complications are more apt to occur in this situation.

*This drug has not been approved by the Food and Drug Administration (FDA) for this indication.

CHRONIC SINUSITIS

Chronic sinusitis is best defined operationally as a bacterial infection that continues beyond an initially good response to a therapeutic trial. In general, most of the symptoms of acute sinusitis persist but may be less severe. In addition, anaerobic organisms often are prominent at this point. The treatment is similar to that used for acute sinusitis, although care should be taken to cover anaerobic organisms well. A prolonged course of antibiotics is generally necessary, and even this may fail, necessitating operative intervention. Clearly, any underlying cause that can be corrected should be treated.

FUNGAL SINUSITIS

Fungal infections may occur in several varieties. Noninvasive fungal sinusitis, the so-called mycetoma, may occur in patients who have undergone prolonged administration of antibiotics or steroids. These infections are most commonly caused by *Aspergillus* or *Candida* and do not involve mucosal invasion by the fungus. Treatment generally requires drainage of the sinus, but the prognosis is excellent.

Allergic fungal sinusitis is a relatively recently described entity in which an exuberant eosinophilic response to the fungal hyphae leads to a dense expansile mass within one or more sinuses. Bone expansion and erosion are common in long-standing cases. Treatment requires drainage of all of the involved sinuses with thorough removal of the inspissated material within the sinus and a postoperative course of saline irrigation, systemic or topical steroids, and occasionally antibiotics. The fungi most commonly involved are *Aspergillus* and *Bipolaris,* with other occasional strains reported.

Invasive fungal sinusitis is a much more serious problem and generally occurs in uncontrolled diabetic or immunocompromised patients. *Aspergillus* and *Mucor* are the two most common fungi involved. There is rapid mucosal invasion and often rapid spread far beyond the sinus. Symptoms include proptosis, facial swelling, cranial neuropathies, and a bloody nasal discharge. Intranasal examination often reveals necrosis of the nasal and sinus mucosa. Treatment consists of systemic amphotericin B with aggressive débridement and attempts to correct the underlying problem. Unless diagnosed early and treated aggressively, these infections have a high mortality.

DIAGNOSIS

Several recent advances have improved our ability to diagnose bacterial sinusitis. However, in patients with routine uncomplicated acute sinusitis it is most cost effective to make a clinical diagnosis and treat accordingly. X-rays are unnecessary. In such patients, symptomatic response should occur within 24 to 48 hours. Full-course antibiotics should be continued for 10 to 14 days.

In any other situation, several additional steps

should be taken. The first is a fiberoptic intranasal examination, best performed with the rigid 2.7-mm sinus endoscope. The outstanding optics and illumination offered by this device allow a thorough examination of the entire nasal cavity.

A further important adjunct, especially if symptoms suggest a possible complication or in patients with chronic sinusitis, is coronal computed tomography (CT) scanning (usually performed without intravenous contrast unless one suspects an intraorbital or intracranial process). CT scanning has made plain sinus x-rays obsolete. Both the false-positive and false-negative rates are too high with plain x-rays to justify their use. If imaging information is needed, CT is the technique of choice for inflammatory disease.

COMPLICATIONS

Complications of sinusitis generally involve spread of the process beyond the confines of the sinus. The only exception to this is osteomyelitis, which generally involves the frontal bone. The other bones appear to be remarkably resistant to this complication. Osteomyelitis of the frontal bone requires aggressive treatment including drainage of the frontal sinus and prolonged high-dose antibiotic therapy following culture and sensitivity of the organism.

Orbital complications generally result from infection of the ethmoid sinus and are most common in children. The most common infection is the so-called periorbital or preseptal cellulitis, which is characterized by edema of the eyelids with associated erythema and fever. There is no proptosis or involvement of the extraocular muscles, and vision is normal. Treatment consists of high-dose antibiotics. It would be prudent to obtain a CT scan to rule out the possibility of a subperiosteal or orbital abscess. The presence of either abscess requires immediate drainage. Prior to this development, however, preseptal cellulitis generally progresses to orbital cellulitis. The latter is manifested by proptosis, chemosis, edema, orbital tenderness, and pain. Extraocular motion may be minimally impaired, but visual acuity is unaffected. Treatment in this instance requires high-dose intravenous antibiotics with careful observation. Should progression occur despite this treatment, in general a subperiosteal abscess will precede an orbital abscess. In either case, drainage is required in addition to high-dose antibiotics. CT scanning in this situation is invaluable in differentiating one from the other.

Other rare complications include the orbital apex syndrome (or superior orbital fissure syndrome), which is manifested by diminished vision and ophthalmoplegia. This may progress to cavernous sinus thrombophlebitis with symptoms of high fever and chills and signs of meningeal irritation. Other intracranial complications include epidural abscess, subdural abscess, brain abscess, and meningitis. Treatment for these includes high-dose intravenous antibiotics that cross the blood-brain barrier as well as the appropriate neurosurgical interventions.

STREPTOCOCCAL PHARYNGITIS

method of
W. M. GOOCH III, M.D.
University of Utah School of Medicine
Salt Lake City, Utah

Sore throat is the third most common cause of a visit to a physician. In spite of its common occurrence and the fact that acute, suppurative tonsillopharyngitis has been the subject of extensive study for centuries (the observation of the relationship with acute rheumatic fever is at least 200 years old), the proper approach to diagnosis and management of sore throat remains the subject of considerable discussion. Acute tonsillopharyngitis may present as only one element of the presentation in diverse clinical states, including influenza, diphtheria, yersiniosis, and even respiratory allergy. The following discussion focuses on the patient who presents with acute tonsillopharyngitis as the predominant complaint.

Many respiratory viruses as well as *Mycoplasma pneumoniae, Arcanobacterium haemolyticum, Neisseria gonorrhoeae,* groups C and G streptococci, and *Chlamydia pneumoniae* (TWAR agent) have been incriminated as causes of tonsillopharyngitis, but infections with these agents are usually associated with clinically mild disease in narrowly defined adult populations. Approximately one-third of cases of acute tonsillopharyngitis in children during the "strep season" (September through May in the United States) is due to group A beta-hemolytic streptococcus (GABHS), with fewer cases occurring in children during the summer months and in adults. Approximately one-third of sore throats have no detectable infectious cause.

CLINICAL PRESENTATION

The characteristic clinical appearance of group A beta-hemolytic tonsillopharyngitis consists of abrupt onset of throat or pharyngeal pain and dysphagia, tonsillopharyngeal erythema with yellow exudate, palatal petechiae, fever, headache, anterior cervical lymphadenopathy, nausea, and abdominal pain. The absence of conjunctivitis, rhinorrhea, hoarseness, and cough is also important in distinguishing viral from GABHS infection. Unfortunately, although this picture is characteristic, it is neither consistent nor specific, particularly in young infants and adults. Even the clinical scorecard devised by Breese to increase the accuracy of clinical diagnosis achieves a specificity of only about 70% with GABHS tonsillopharyngitis. Indeed, the use of clinical judgment alone may lead to as much as 85 to 90% overtreatment, depending on the population at risk and the season of the year. Complicating the bacteriologic diagnosis is the fact that children are commonly asymptomatic carriers of GABHS; the incidence of carriage varies with the season and geographic location, but the mean rate is about 15 to 20%, with much lower rates in adults.

LABORATORY DIAGNOSIS

The peripheral white blood cell count is commonly greater than 12,000 per microliter, although this test is not commonly employed for routine cases of tonsillopharyngitis. The gold standard of laboratory diagnosis of GABHS tonsillopharyngitis has been the sheep blood agar overnight culture, although many primary care physicians do not use it owing to its expense and inconvenience. Inhibition of growth about a differential bacitracin disk (not a susceptibility disk) provides practical differentiation from other hemolytic microflora. The need for pure culture can be obviated by placing a trimethoprim-sulfamethoxazole susceptibility disk against the bacitracin disk to inhibit the growth of most other oropharyngeal bacteria. Use of agar-containing trimethoprim-sulfamethoxazole has not proved practical owing to quality control problems.

More recently, the rapid antigen detection test for GABHS has replaced the culture in many offices. Published and product literature indicates that this test is a useful alternative to the culture. However, evaluation of published studies has revealed that although mean sensitivity-specificity results of the test in university and office-practice settings were 87 and 96% and 96 and 90%, respectively, sensitivity actually falls below 50% in some office settings. Consequently, the common recommendation today is to obtain duplicate throat swabs so that a negative test can be confirmed by culture of the second swab. Specificity is generally considered sufficient to justify treatment of positive reactors.

TREATMENT

The goal of antibacterial treatment of GABHS tonsillopharyngitis is relief of intensity and duration of febrile morbidity, rapid elimination of contagiosity, eradication of GABHS from the oropharyngeal tissues, and prevention of acute rheumatic fever and suppurative complications. As a general rule, patients may be considered noncontagious after 36 to 48 hours of a standard therapeutic regimen. Adequate treatment to prevent acute rheumatic fever has become a more compelling need in recent years owing to the reappearance of this historically significant, but until recently very uncommon, nonsuppurative complication of GABHS tonsillopharyngitis.

As noted previously, clinical judgment is not a reliable indicator for therapeutic intervention in patients with GABHS tonsillopharyngitis, and the issue is not only one of unnecessary expense. Additional concerns include the risk of penicillin hypersensitivity and alteration of the normal oropharyngeal microflora. Many clinicians dismiss the risk of penicillin hypersensitivity because of the usually mild nature of the adverse events that occur with a frequency of less than 5% and the fact that serious penicillin hypersensitivity reactions are very infrequent. However, in this era of growing numbers of immunocompromised patients, hypersensitivity resulting from an unnecessary exposure to penicillin or another beta-lactam antibiotic early in life may result in loss of access to a life-saving class of antibacterials later in life.

The gold standard for management of GABHS tonsillopharyngitis has long been a 10-day course of oral penicillin V. An alternative treatment, not often used today, is an injection of benzathine penicillin G. During the past decade, however, an alarming increase in the frequency of therapeutic failures (to as high as 38%) has been observed by many investigators. Therapeutic failure may be defined as bacteriologic failure (persistence of positive pharyngeal culture of GABHS after a course of therapy), symptomatic failure (persistence or recrudescence of symptoms), or both. The former is a common problem that occurs in community practice when a patient who is persistently culture-positive presents with viral pharyngitis. Some authorities also believe that the bacteriologic carrier is at risk for development of acute rheumatic fever. Several mechanisms have been suggested to explain therapeutic failure.

Patient Noncompliance. Patient noncompliance with the prescribed therapeutic regimen is probably the most common cause of therapeutic failure. The reasons patients or parents give for noncompliance include bad taste, excessive cost, undesirable side effects, and the need for frequent dosing. Bad taste is not limited to suspension formulations; newer beta-lactam preparations given as tablets may result in a bitter aftertaste. It has been demonstrated that approximately two-thirds of patients show therapeutic noncompliance when the prescribed regimen requires administration of a drug three times a day.

Early Treatment. Recent studies have demonstrated that when treatment is initiated within 24 to 36 hours of onset of symptoms, as may occur with sophisticated patients or with rapid antigen detection tests, the risk of recurrent disease is increased threefold compared with patients whose treatment is delayed for 2 to 3 days. This phenomenon presumably results from compromise of the normal host immune response owing to reduction of GABHS antigen exposure. Appropriate application of this knowledge is unclear. Although one may delay treatment up to 9 days without exposing the patient to the risk of acute rheumatic fever, postponement of symptomatic relief poses an ethical dilemma, and treatment should not be withheld from the severely ill patient or during an outbreak of rheumatic fever or invasive streptococcal infections. In addition, many patients or parents are reluctant to defer treatment.

Antibacterial Tolerance. This phenomenon is the simultaneous expression of considerable resistance to the bactericidal effect of a given antibacterial by a bacterium and susceptibility to the inhibitory effect of that agent. There is evidence that some strains of GABHS that have been isolated from cases of tonsillopharyngitis manifest tolerance, but the phenomenon is subject to considerable variation depending on the experimental design, and there is no evidence that this mechanism is a common cause of failure.

Bacterial Copathogenicity. This pathogenic mechanism is defined as the manifestation of enhanced virulence of one microorganism as the result of some biologic expression of another microorganism. In this context, beta-lactamases (penicillinases) elaborated by the bacterial microflora indigenous to the oropharynx hydrolyze penicillin before sufficient concentrations of penicillin have been present for a sufficiently long time to kill the pathogenic streptococci. Members of the microflora implicated in this mechanism include *Staphylococcus aureus, Hae-*

mophilus influenzae, Haemophilus parainfluenzae, Moraxella catarrhalis, and various enteric and anaerobic bacteria. Some published studies have proferred evidence supporting the clinical significance of this putative mechanism of therapeutic failure, while other investigators have published data refuting its significance, but flaws in experimental design have compromised the conclusions of the latter.

An approach to each of the listed mechanisms of therapeutic failure, except that of early treatment, that might be expected to increase therapeutic efficacy is to use an alternative antibacterial that is unaffected or less affected by beta-lactamases and penicillin tolerance and that possesses pharmacokinetic and formulation properties that result in increased compliance. Rational therapeutic alternatives include cephalosporins, beta-lactamase-blocking combination agents, and the newer macrolides. Because amoxicillin (Amoxil) and expanded spectrum penicillins may be hydrolyzed by oropharyngeal beta-lactamases, they offer no advantage, whereas the sulfonamides and tetracyclines are not sufficiently active against established GABHS infection, and their toxicity profile is not as advantageous as the other alternatives.

Many cephalosporins are attractive alternatives because they are active against GABHS, resist the hydrolytic effects of oropharyngeal beta-lactamases (although they may not kill the bacterium that elaborates the enzyme), require less frequent dosing, and possess a favorable adverse events profile; selected members of the class are palatable (even tasty) in suspension formulation. First-, second-, and third-generation oral cephalosporins have demonstrated superior efficacy compared with penicillin V in standard regimens (Table 1). There are, however, some members of this class that are not recommended alternatives to penicillin. For example, cefixime (Suprax), a third-generation cephalosporin, possesses broad resistance to the beta-lactamases produced by aerobic and facultative gram-negative bacteria of the oropharynx. However, it is insufficiently active against *Staphylococcus aureus* to justify its use to circumvent copathogenicity in the oropharynx owing to the potential role of this microorganism. Cefaclor (Ceclor), commonly considered a second-generation agent, is also an inappropriate choice owing to its lability in the presence of diverse oropharyngeal beta-lactamases.

The sole beta-lactamase–blocking product available for oral use in the United States is amoxicillin–clavulanic acid (Augmentin), and its extremely broad antibacterial coverage includes the oropharyngeal, beta-lactamase–producing microflora. This agent also has been demonstrated to be more successful than penicillin in eradicating GABHS from patients with recurrent tonsillopharyngitis.

The antimicrobial spectrum of the newer macrolide antibiotics includes *H. influenzae* while retaining the broad spectrum of activity of erythromycin against diverse other respiratory pathogens. These agents are not affected by either beta-lactamases or beta-lactam tolerance, and they achieve high concentrations in respiratory tissues, including the oropharynx. Erythromycin has been demonstrated to be less effective than penicillin or cephalosporins as therapy for GABHS pharyngitis, and it is also ineffective against nonstreptococcal pharyngitis. However, a 5-day course of azithromycin (Zithromax) has shown efficacy comparable to that of a 10-day course of penicillin.

Clindamycin (Cleocin), because it is also unaffected by beta-lactamases and beta-lactam tolerance and is quite active against anaerobes and facultative gram-positive cocci, might be considered an alternative to penicillin for treatment of GABHS tonsillopharyngitis. However, it remains the single agent most frequently implicated in the cause of antibacterial-associated pseudomembranous colitis due to *Clostridium difficile.*

TREATMENT OF RECURRENT DISEASE

When evaluating patients with apparent recurrence of GABHS tonsillopharyngitis, there is always the concern that one may be observing a viral infection in a patient who has become a carrier of a strain of GABHS. There are data to support this notion; however, longitudinal evaluation has demonstrated that recurrences do occur with the same strain. Spread within institutions and within family groups is common. Close contact is required for interpersonal transmission; neither respiratory spread by

TABLE 1. **Antibacterial Agents with Proved or Theoretical Advantages Over Penicillin V for Management of GABHS Tonsillopharyngitis**

Antibacterial Agent	Brand Name	Dose	Frequency	Duration
Cephalosporins				
Cefadroxil	Duricef, Ultracef	30 mg/kg/day	Twice daily	10 days
Cefuroxime axetil	Ceftin	250 mg*	Twice daily	10 days
Cefprozil	Cefzil	15 mg/kg/day	Twice daily	10 days
Cefpodoxime proxetil	Vantin	10 mg/kg/day	Twice daily	10 days
Beta-lactamase blockade				
Amoxicillin-potassium clavulanate	Augmentin	Amoxicillin: 40 mg/kg/day	Three times daily	10 days
Macrolides				
Clarithromycin	Biaxin	250 mg*	Twice daily	10 days
Azithromycin	Zithromax	500 mg* first day, then 250 mg	Once daily	5 days

*Not available in suspension formulation at this writing.

droplet nuclei nor exposure to contaminated fomites is a significant mode of transmission. In such circumstances, inadequate therapy (noncompliance, beta- [illegible] hogenicity) or early treatment [illegible]) may result in recrudescence [illegible] ction with the same strain. In [illegible] ment with penicillin is inap- [illegible] re rates with this approach [illegible] ad-spectrum alternative ther- [illegible] f other family members may [illegible] proaches fail, long-term pro- [illegible] similar to that used for acute [illegible] laxis and even tonsillectomy [illegible] ns.

[illegible] ND OTHER [illegible] INFECTIONS

[illegible] NN, M.D.,
[illegible] N, R.PH., B.S.PHARM.,
[illegible] CK, M.D.
[illegible] *als and Clinics*

[illegible] mbers of newly diagnosed cases [illegible] *sis* (MTB) infection declined an- [illegible] However, in 1985 a reversal in [illegible] l. From 1985 to 1991, the num- [illegible] s reported increased by 18%. It [illegible] cess" cases have been reported [illegible] at has caused the resurgence of [illegible] e emergence of HIV/AIDS has [illegible] s remarkable increase. TB is a [illegible] may be transmitted from the [illegible] with a normal immune system. [illegible] s highly susceptible to infection [illegible] his group are reported to be as [illegible] tients infected with TB are at [illegible] B at a rate of up to 10% per [illegible] e risk of about 10% in the non- [illegible] rge numbers of persons have [illegible] States from areas with a high [illegible] utheast Asia and Latin Amer- [illegible] ssness, and substance abuse [illegible] he spread of TB. Tuberculosis [illegible] ominant among the impover- [illegible] leterioration in some areas of [illegible] re has been a factor. Funding for state TB programs fell dramatically in the 1980s, and the ability to track tuberculosis patients through the many months needed for a complete drug therapy program was impaired owing to lack of personnel. A consequence of the move from inpatient drug treatment in TB sanatoriums to unsupervised outpatient therapy has been the development of drug-resistant TB. The haphazard way in which some patients self-administer TB medicines has aided the evolution of single-drug- and multidrug-resistant tuberculosis (MDRTB). MDRTB organisms are resistant to at least isoniazid (INH) and rifampin. Resistance rates across the nation have been rising during the last decade. Data from parts of New York City indicate alarming resistance rates among new isolates, which are close to 45% resistant to one or more drugs; 30% were MDRTB organisms. Nationally, for the first quarter of 1991, 3% of new TB cases were MDRTB, which is up from only 0.5% during the period 1982 to 1986. Unfortunately, HIV-infected patients are at highest risk for becoming infected by MDRTB.

TB does not fit the classic mold in the HIV-infected population, and diagnosis in these patients requires a higher index of suspicion. One cannot completely rely on sputum samples, the Mantoux skin test (5 tuberculin units [TU] of purified protein derivative [PPD]), or histologic demonstration of granulomas. Extrapulmonary involvement is more common in HIV-infected patients, and the search for active disease may require demonstration of acid-fast bacilli in extrapulmonary tissue. Despite the nonclassic presentation, HIV-infected patients infected with susceptible MTB strains do respond to classic antituberculosis prophylaxis and treatment.

The Centers for Disease Control and Prevention (CDC) have updated the guidelines for treatment of TB to face the prospect of increased numbers of TB cases, individuals coinfected with HIV and TB, and the increasing numbers of single- and multiply-resistant organisms. These guidelines form the basis of the treatment options that follow.

TREATMENT GUIDELINES

Immediate therapy and isolation of the patient should be initiated based on presumptive evidence of active pulmonary TB infection because of the risk to public health. Drug susceptibility studies should be performed when samples are cultured for MTB. To facilitate this aspect of diagnosis, many laboratories now have available a less cumbersome and more rapid system of culturing, identifying, and checking the drug susceptibility of MTB. For example, the Bactec system can detect growth in 7 to 10 days. Then, utilizing specific DNA probes, MTB, *M. avium* complex (MAC), and *M. gordonae* (common contaminant) can be identified from the culture medium in 1 day. The same rapid-growth detection method can then be used to determine MTB drug susceptibility to INH, rifampin, streptomycin, and ethambutol in approximately 1 additional week.

Daily Drug Therapy for 6 Months

Since the advent of early chemotherapy regimens for the treatment of TB, the use of multiple drugs to prevent the emergence of resistant organisms has been the cornerstone of therapy. A drug regimen consisting of INH, rifampin, pyrazinamide, and either streptomycin or ethambutol is the preferred initial treatment for disease caused by MTB (see Table 1 for doses). Four drugs are administered daily for 2 months, followed by therapy with INH and rifampin administered daily for 4 additional months. Supervised intermittent therapy, either two or three times weekly, is an option that may be used following the initial 2-month daily regimen. With either regimen, susceptibility to INH and rifampin determines whether ethambutol or streptomycin and pyrazinamide can be discontinued after 2 months. Although 6 months is the total recommended length of treat-

TABLE 1. **Recommended Adult Doses for Antituberculosis Medications***

Drug	Regimen		
	Daily	*Twice Weekly*†	*Three Times Weekly*
Isoniazid (INH)	300 mg	900 mg	900 mg
Rifampin	600 mg	600 mg	600 mg
Pyrazinamide	15–30 mg per kg (max. 2.0 gm)	50–70 mg per kg (max. 3.5 to 4 gm)	50–70 mg per kg (max. 2 to 3 gm)
Ethambutol	15 mg per kg (max. 2.5 gm)	50 mg per kg (max. 2.5 gm)	25–30 mg per kg (max. 2.5 gm)
Streptomycin	Up to 1 gm	Up to 1 gm	Up to 1 gm

*Pyridoxine in doses of 50 mg may be used with any of the regimens listed.
†For example, a 70-kg man would receive, on Monday and Thursdays, INH 900 mg, rifampin 600 mg, pyrazinamide 4.0 gm, and ethambutol 2.5 gm or streptomycin 1.0 gm.

ment, chemotherapy must be continued for at least 3 months after the last negative culture for MTB. In HIV-infected patients, INH and rifampin should be continued for at least 9 months, or 6 months beyond sputum conversion. Drug resistance necessitates a change in strategy. If single-drug resistance to INH is shown, INH may be discontinued. Rifampin, pyrazinamide, and ethambutol or streptomycin should be administered for the duration of the 6-month treatment period. This treatment regimen should be implemented only if directly observed therapy is being employed. The use of daily unsupervised therapy in patients with any drug-resistant TB strains is not advocated. In circumstances in which rates of resistance to INH and rifampin are high, a five- or six-drug regimen may need to be used as initial therapy. The four-drug regimen discussed earlier, plus additional agents to which the organism may be susceptible, should be employed. Additionally, if multiple drug resistance is demonstrated or suspected, advice from a TB consultant should be sought.

Directly Observed Therapy

Directly observed therapy (DOT) is a method by which patients are observed while ingesting antituberculosis medications. Since noncompliance is a major cause of the increase in drug-resistant strains of MTB, direct observation of therapy precludes patients' taking medications sporadically and inappropriately. Advocates for universal DOT point out that socioeconomic status is not necessarily an indicator of compliance, and to halt the development of more new strains of MDRTB, all TB medicines should be administered by DOT. There are two options for DOT that differ in whether it is initiated with or without a daily component.

When DOT is initiated with a daily component, INH, rifampin, pyrazinamide, and either ethambutol or streptomycin are given daily for 2 weeks in the doses described previously for daily therapy. Following the initial phase, these same drugs are given at increased doses twice weekly (intermittent therapy) under direct supervision for an additional 6 weeks (see doses listed in Table 1). The final 4 months of treatment consist of twice-weekly therapy with INH and rifampin.

A DOT program consisting of no initial daily therapy has been shown to provide satisfactory cure rates for TB. This regimen involves administration of four drugs three times weekly for the entire 6-month therapy program. Agents used are INH, rifampin, pyrazinamide, and ethambutol or streptomycin (doses are found in Table 1). It is important to note that all four drugs chosen need to be given for the entire 6 months and by DOT. If single-drug or multidrug resistance is demonstrated, the same guidelines apply as for the daily 6-month regimen. For HIV-infected patients with TB, the duration of therapy is increased to 9 months or 6 months after sputum conversion.

Note that in any of these options, if the patient is symptomatic or has a positive smear or culture after 3 months of antituberculosis chemotherapy, a reassessment of the drug regimen should be undertaken. The advice of a TB consultant is recommended.

Monitoring for Adverse Drug Reactions

Adverse drug reactions in patients receiving antituberculosis chemotherapy may include hepatotoxicity (INH, rifampin, pyrazinamide), ocular toxicity (ethambutol), ototoxicity and renal toxicity (streptomycin), peripheral neuropathy (INH), thrombocytopenia (rifampin), and increases in serum uric acid levels (pyrazinamide). In light of these potential toxic reactions, it has been recommended that baseline measurement of hepatic enzymes, bilirubin, and serum creatinine and a complete blood count, and a platelet count be performed in patients treated with the drug regimens outlined earlier. In addition, serum uric acid should be measured if pyrazinamide is included in the regimen. If ethambutol is selected as part of the treatment regimen, baseline tests for visual acuity and red-green color perception should be performed. If symptoms occur during treatment that suggest toxicity to one of the agents employed, further laboratory testing should be done to exclude possible adverse drug reactions.

Treatment of Tuberculosis in Special Situations

Extrapulmonary TB may be treated in much the same manner as described for pulmonary TB. Although drug therapy regimens may remain the same, some TB experts extend the length of treatment in some cases of extrapulmonary TB. The treatment of TB in children is essentially the same as that outlined for adults. Specific questions relating to pediatric cases, including drug dosages and length of treatment, are beyond the scope of this article. Pregnant patients with active TB may be given antituberculosis drug therapy. However, the use of streptomycin is not recommended because of concerns about fetal ototoxicity, and the routine use of pyrazinamide is not recommended because of the lack of teratogenicity studies. Therefore, the drugs commonly used while awaiting susceptibility data are INH, rifampin, and ethambutol.

Preventive Therapy for Tuberculosis

Preventive therapy with INH has been shown to be effective in reducing the incidence of tuberculous disease in those persons with latent tuberculosis. Controlled trials conducted by the U.S. Public Health Service have shown that INH reduces the incidence of active tuberculosis by 54 to 88% in this group. In fact, in persons known to be compliant with the prescribed regimen, INH is 93% effective.

Between 10 and 15 million persons in the United States are infected with MTB, and about 90% of new, currently active tuberculosis cases come from this pool. Therefore, identification and treatment of this segment of the population are very important for the control of tuberculosis.

The size of the induration of a PPD skin test (Mantoux test) indicates the presence of tuberculosis infection. Table 2 defines a positive skin test reaction to the intradermal administration of five test units of PPD by category of persons in the infected pool. These "cut points" for positivity are helpful in determining which people are at greatest risk for development of active tuberculosis. Particular attention should be paid to HIV-infected patients, especially those with $CD4^+$ T cell counts of lower than 100 per mm^3, because they may develop only a minimal reaction to PPD.

Certain groups within the pool of persons with latent tuberculosis have been categorized either as high-incidence or high-risk for the development of tuberculosis. Persons with any of the risk factors listed in Table 3 (high-risk category) should be considered for preventive therapy with INH, regardless of age, if they have not been previously treated. Persons in the high-incidence groups, also listed in Table 3, should be considered for preventive therapy with INH if they are less than 35 years of age. Figure 1 is a flow diagram intended to help the clinician determine who should be considered for preventive therapy.

TABLE 2. **Definition of Positive PPD Reaction**

≥ 5 mm Induration
HIV-positive persons
Close contacts of tuberculosis patients
Persons with old fibrotic lesions on chest radiograph
≥ 10 mm Induration
High-risk and high-incidence groups
Infants and children under 4 years of age
≥ 15 mm Induration
Persons with low tuberculosis risk

TABLE 3. **Indications for Tuberculosis Preventive Therapy**

High-Risk Groups (regardless of age)
Persons with HIV infection and persons with risk factors for HIV infection
Close contacts of persons with newly diagnosed infectious tuberculosis
Recent tuberculin skin test converters
Persons with old fibrotic lesions on chest radiographs
Intravenous drug users (HIV-negative)
Persons with medical conditions known to increase the risk of tuberculosis
High-Incidence Groups (younger than 35 years of age)
Foreign-born persons from areas of high tuberculosis prevalence
Medically underserved groups
Residents of facilities for long-term care
Staff of schools, correctional, health, and child care facilities

The drug of choice for preventive therapy for tuberculosis is INH, which is given in doses of 300 mg daily in adults and 10 mg per kg in children, up to 300 mg daily. Most adult patients should receive INH for 6 months, but those with HIV infection should receive the drug for 12 months. Nine months of therapy is recommended for children. For patients with known exposure to INH-resistant organisms, rifampin is used in standard daily therapeutic doses for the same length of time. Some clinicians add a second drug to this regimen, such as ethambutol. For persons exposed to multiply resistant organisms, the approach remains controversial. Some clinicians, however, recommend treatment for 6 months with ethambutol and pyrazinamide, or a quinolone (ofloxacin [Floxin] or ciprofloxacin [Cipro]) and pyrazinamide.

Persons being treated with INH should be monitored for signs and symptoms consistent with liver damage. Assessment should be performed monthly. For persons over the age of 35, monitoring with initial liver function tests is indicated, combined with tests done periodically during the course of therapy.

NONTUBERCULOUS MYCOBACTERIA

The role of the nontuberculous mycobacteria (NTM) in human disease was unclear until the 1950s although they were recognized soon after the identification of MTB in the late 1800s. Historically, NTM were classified by Runyon based upon the morphology, growth rates, biochemical differentiation, and pigmentation characteristics of the colonies. Today we rely on other criteria for clinical decision making and treatment.

Most NTM are found naturally in water sources and soil. In nonimmunosuppressed persons, patient-to-patient spread is not recognized. The mode of infection may be secondary to direct inoculation as in

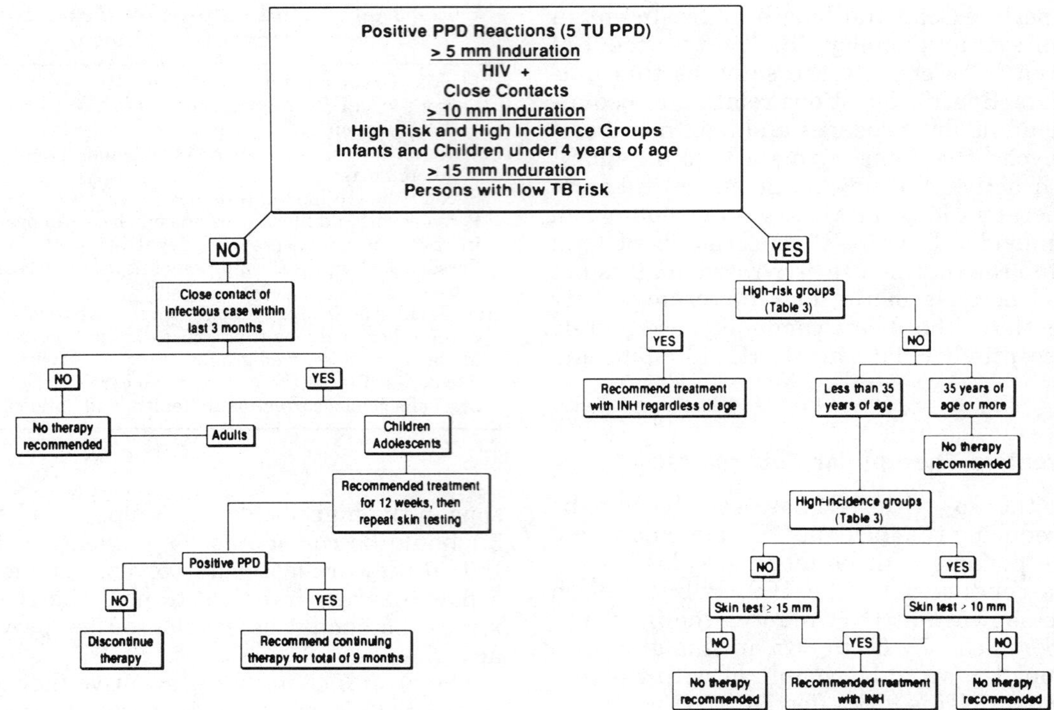

Figure 1. Isoniazid (INH) prophylaxis decision tree.

cases of trauma or aerosolization of the bacteria. Based on two CDC surveys prior to the existence of widespread HIV infection, the prevalence of NTM has been estimated at 1.8 cases per 100,000 population. The two studies varied somewhat in their findings of the frequency of individual organisms. MAC was most common, accounting for 61 to 72% of isolates, *M. kansasii* accounted for 10 to 19%, *M. fortuitum* for 6 to 19%, and others for 3 to 10%.

NTM strains commonly cause extrapulmonary disease in the HIV-infected patient and pulmonary disease in the nonimmunocompromised host. In the latter circumstance the clinical features are nonspecific and indistinct from those of classic tuberculosis. Immune response in these patients may cause weak cross-reactivity with the 5-TU PPD (range, 5- to 10-mm induration). Species-specific skin tests have not proved reliable owing to cross-reactivity between shared antigens. Chest x-ray findings are similar to those seen in patients with TB, although cavitary disease has less surrounding infiltrate and preferentially involves the apical and anterior segments.

The diagnosis of NTM infection relies partially on positive cultures. Unfortunately, a positive culture may represent either disease or colonization. The likelihood of disease is related to species, origin of culture, and clinical features. For example, MAC (including *M. intracellulare*), *M. scrofulaceum, M. kansasii, M. marinum, M. xenopi, M. szulgai, M. simiae, M. fortuitum, M. chelonei, M. malmoense, M. haemophilum,* and *M. asiaticum* are often associated with disease, whereas *M. gordonae, M. terrae, M. flavescens, M. gastri, M. triviale,* and *M. smegmatis* are often colonizers. Positive cultures taken from usually sterile tissue are more likely to represent a true pathogen. All species must be considered pathogens in the right clinical context. The recommended diagnostic criteria for pulmonary disease are findings on chest x-ray compatible with mycobacterial infection and the presence of two or more sputum cultures that result in moderate to heavy growth while excluding other causes of disease. Growth and identification in traditional culture techniques may take from 4 to 8 weeks. As mentioned earlier, rapid techniques that rely on the Bactec system and DNA probes have reduced the identification time to 10 to 20 days.

TREATMENT PRINCIPLES

The initial decision to treat is based on the separation of disease from colonization. This issue is complicated further by the age, underlying pulmonary disease, and immune status of the patient. However, the compelling reasons to treat patients aggressively are to stop progression of the disease, relieve symptoms, and ultimately, prevent death.

Specific treatment is based on the location and extent of the disease and the specific organism involved. Patient compliance and drug side effects also play a role in treatment decisions. Surgical removal of a confined area of infection, with or without combined chemotherapy, is a valid treatment for patients with cervical adenitis, isolated pulmonary infection, or localized cutaneous disease.

The following are treatment recommendations for the most common NTM infections. Drug susceptibility testing has minimal impact on treatment decisions. Treatment choice for NTM infections has been based on clinical experience and very limited susceptibility data. Lacking large multicenter controlled trials, recommendations for treatment are based on the results of several small published series. Agreement on a standard course of therapy has been difficult to achieve.

M. avium Complex Infection

MAC infection is a significant cause of morbidity in the nonimmunosuppressed host and most recently in the HIV-infected host. In contrast to the nonimmunocompromised host, in whom MAC most frequently causes pulmonary infection, MAC infection in HIV-infected individuals frequently presents as a nonpulmonary infection. The prevalence of MAC infection in HIV-infected individuals ranges from 15 to 40% and is highest in advanced HIV infection, in which $CD4^+$ T-cell counts are lowest. Localized extrapulmonary disease (cervical adenitis, skin lesions, endophthalmitis, hepatic dysfunction, abscesses) is a more common presentation of MAC infection when the $CD4^+$ T cell count is greater than 100 per mm^3. Disseminated disease with bacteremia predictably occurs when $CD4^+$ T cells measure 10 to 50 per mm^3. Symptoms, signs, and laboratory data for MAC infection often are nonspecific. Often the diagnosis is confounded by concurrent illness in these patients. Isolation of MAC in stool samples is a harbinger of MAC bacteremia. Generally, systemic symptoms such as fever, night sweats, diarrhea, and weight loss can be attributed to MAC infection when bacteremia is documented. One positive blood culture is sufficient for diagnosis. Disseminated MAC infection is associated with reduced survival in HIV patients. Specific and preventive therapies are believed to improve the survival and quality of life for HIV-infected patients.

Treatment of MAC infections is challenging because of the inherent resistance of these organisms to most antituberculosis agents. The treatment approach for HIV-infected patients is different from that for nonimmunosuppressed patients. The following approach for HIV-infected patients with disseminated disease is based on the 1993 recommendations of the Public Health Service Task Force on Prophylaxis and Therapy for MAC Infection. Physicians prescribing therapy for MAC infections in HIV patients should be aware that the FDA has not approved many of these agents for use in this situation.

HIV-infected patients with disseminated MAC infection should receive at least two drugs (and up to four), and therapy should continue for life. A reasonable core therapeutic regimen consists of a choice of macrolides (azithromycin [Zithromax], 500 mg per day, or clarithromycin, 1000 mg per day) plus ethambutol, 15 mg per kg per day. INH and pyrazinamide, drugs commonly used for MTB infections, have no role in therapy for this disease. The following drugs should be considered in the order listed: clofazamine (Lamprene), 100 to 200 mg per day; rifabutin (Mycobutin), 450 to 600 mg per day; ciprofloxacin (Cipro), 1500 mg per day; and last, amikacin (Amikin), 7.5 to 15 mg per kg per day, when a third or fourth drug is added.

Therapy aimed at delaying or preventing the onset of MAC dissemination is considered beneficial in HIV-infected patients with $CD4^+$ counts of less than 100 per mm^3. The physician should exclude active infection with MAC, MTB, or other NTM prior to initiating prophylactic therapy. Rifabutin (300 mg per day) for life may be used for prophylaxis unless active MAC infection develops. Rifabutin induces hepatic enzymes, which may result in lower drug levels for agents that are similarly metabolized, such as zidovudine. The clinical relevance of this effect is currently unknown. There is no evidence that the susceptibility pattern differs for MAC isolated from patients who develop disseminated infection while on rifabutin. However, this prophylactic regimen risks the development of rifampin-resistant MTB should the patient develop active TB.

MAC pulmonary infection in the nonimmunosuppressed host is also prolonged, and success rates vary from a low of 40% to a high of 90%. Pulmonary symptoms, a compatible chest x-ray, and at least two positive sputum cultures or a positive lung biopsy are required to initiate treatment. Four drugs are recommended for a minimum of 18 months and for at least 12 months after conversion of the sputum to culture negative. An initial regimen should include a combination of ethambutol, 15 mg per kg per day, and rifampin, 600 mg per day, which offer synergistic effects against MAC, and azithromycin, 500 mg per day, or clarithromycin, 1000 mg per day. Clinical studies have shown that inclusion of streptomycin, 1 gram two to three times per week up to 100 grams, results in an improved outcome. Other agents that might be effective include clofazamine, 100 to 200 mg per day, and ciprofloxacin, 1500 mg per day.

M. kansasii Infection

M. kansasii has proved to be one of the most eradicable of the NTM species, although only a moderate degree of drug susceptibility is demonstrated in vitro. Although no randomized controlled studies exist, a combination of INH, 300 mg per day, rifampin, 600 mg per day, and ethambutol, 15 mg per kg per day, given daily for 18 to 24 months (or 6 to 12 months

TABLE 4. **Less Common but Drug-Susceptible Nontuberculous Mycobacteria**

Species	Suggested Regimen
M. marinum	Rifampin and ethambutol; tetracycline, minocycline or doxycycline; trimethoprim-sulfamethoxazole; and newer macrolides
M. szulgai	INH, rifampin, streptomycin, and ethambutol
M. xenopi	INH, rifampin, and ethambutol with or without streptomycin. Other alternatives include amikacin, clofazimine, newer macrolides or quinolones

after sputum conversion) has been successful. The rate of failure to convert sputum is under 10%, and relapse is rare. Recently, short-course regimens have been instituted with some success, combining a standard regimen with the addition of streptomycin twice weekly during the first 3 months. This 12-month regimen appears to be a good alternative to the standard recommendations. Intermittent therapy for *M. kansasii* infection has not been adequately tested. Extrapulmonary disease may be treated in the same way as for pulmonary disease. Acquired resistance to standard drugs has been demonstrated. Other drugs with activity against *M. kansasii* include ethionamide, erythromycin, sulfamethoxazole, amikacin, and rifabutin.

Rapid Growers—*M. fortuitum* and *M. chelonei*

Infections due to the rapid growers may exhibit a wide spectrum of disease, ranging from skin and soft tissue diseases to pulmonary disease. In most cases of pulmonary disease, there is a history of underlying lung infection, making the differentiation between colonization and disease difficult. Treatment is based on the clinical symptoms, progression of disease, and extent of disease even though drug susceptibility panels may show universal resistance to standard antituberculosis drugs. The newer macrolide and quinolone antibiotics have shown some promise for treatment. Other antibiotics that may be effective include cefoxitin, amikacin, sulfonamides, doxycycline, erythromycin, and clofazimine. Surgical débridement or resection for localized disease should be strongly considered because of the difficulty of consummating a medical cure.

All other NTM species account for 3 to 6% of disease. Table 4 describes treatment for the more easily eradicable remaining organisms.

Section 4

The Cardiovascular System

ACQUIRED DISEASES OF THE AORTA

method of
PETER GLOVICZKI, M.D., and
HARTZELL SCHAFF, M.D.
Mayo Clinic and Foundation
Rochester, Minnesota

Results of elective operations for both aneurysmal and occlusive disease of the aorta have considerably improved during the last decade, and there is now a mortality of 3 to 10% following repair of thoracic aortic aneurysms and less than 3% following elective abdominal aortic reconstructions. Ruptured aortic aneurysms, however, continue to take a high toll, and mortality continues to be close to 50% even in tertiary referral centers.

PREOPERATIVE EVALUATION

Patients with aneurysmal or occlusive diseases of the aorta are frequently elderly and have several risk factors for atherosclerosis. These include a positive family history of atherosclerosis, male gender, hypertension, diabetes, history of smoking, or hypercholesterolemia. Atherosclerosis may involve the coronary, carotid, renal, and lower extremity arteries. Coronary disease is present in 60% of the patients, and preoperative assessment of cardiac disease is mandatory. Noninvasive cardiac testing is performed selectively based on the presence of angina, history of myocardial infarction or congestive heart failure, abnormal electrocardiogram (ECG) with Q waves, diabetes mellitus, or aortic aneurysms in patients in their fifties. Five percent of the patients with asymptomatic abdominal aortic aneurysm need preoperative cardiac revascularization.

Duplex scanning of the carotid artery may reveal significant disease, and a history of claudication or decreased pulses warrants noninvasive assessment of the lower extremity circulation. Patients with decreased renal function need hydration before aortography is performed. Chronic obstructive pulmonary disease is common, and pulmonary function tests should be done in symptomatic patients.

Careful preoperative assessment, combined with invasive intraoperative monitoring using ECG, an arterial line, a central intravenous line, and frequently a pulmonary artery catheter and selective transesophageal echocardiography have been essential in decreasing perioperative morbidity and mortality.

MANAGEMENT

Abdominal Aortic Aneurysm

The infrarenal aorta is the most frequent site of aortic aneurysm. Most aneurysms are fusiform and atherosclerotic. Rarely, the aneurysm is mycotic or inflammatory in type. Five percent of males over age 65 and 10 to 15% of those with symptomatic lower extremity arterial occlusive disease have an abdominal aortic aneurysm, half of which are 4 cm in size or larger. The usual growth rate of an aneurysm is 0.2 to 0.4 mm per year. Rupture is the most frequent complication. The rate of rupture correlates with the size of the aneurysm. Five-cm aneurysms have an annual rupture rate of 4%, and 7-cm aneurysms have an annual rupture rate of 19%. In good-risk patients, aneurysms between 4 and 5 cm can be repaired, but patients with a high surgical risk should be considered for repair only if the aneurysm is 5 cm or larger. Those with small aneurysms are followed at regular intervals with ultrasonography, which is first performed 6 months after diagnosis and then yearly if the size of the aneurysm is unchanged.

Infrarenal aortic aneurysm is repaired most frequently through a midline incision using the transperitoneal approach. The aorta is cross-clamped distal to the renal arteries, and the iliac arteries are clamped distal to the aneurysm. The sac is opened, thrombus is removed, and a Dacron graft, most frequently a knitted type coated with collagen or gelatin to prevent bleeding, is inserted in the aneurysm and sutured first proximally to the infrarenal aorta. A straight graft is sutured to the terminal aorta, and a bifurcated graft is sutured to the iliac arteries. The sac of the aneurysm is sutured around the graft to separate it from the duodenum to prevent graft-duodenal fistula. Cell-saver devices have substantially decreased transfusion of banked blood. Clinical studies with transfemoral placement of endovascular grafts have already begun.

Most patients with a ruptured abdominal aortic aneurysm present with sudden abdominal or back pain and hypotension, and about half have a pulsatile abdominal mass. Seventy percent of these patients did not know before rupture that they had an aneurysm. Timely referral and resuscitation, prompt operative management with rapid control of the proximal aorta, and expert postoperative care are needed for the patient to have a chance of survival. Those with preoperative shock and cardiac arrest have the worst prognosis. Because of the high mortality, screening of the high-risk population and early elective repair of abdominal aortic aneurysms are suggested.

Thoracic Aortic Aneurysms

Aneurysms of the thoracic aorta may be classified according to etiology (atherosclerotic, syphilitic, and so on), morphology (fusiform versus saccular), or location (ascending aorta, arch, descending aorta). Degenerative diseases including atherosclerosis account for the majority of thoracic aneurysms in North America. The following discussion is divided according to location of the aneurysm because of the special considerations required in surgical treatment in each area.

Ascending Aortic Aneurysms. The ascending aorta includes the sinus portion adjacent to the aortic valve, the sinotubular junction, and the aorta distal to the sinotubular junction but below the origin of the innominate artery. This area is intrapericardial, and leakage of blood from an aneurysm or traumatic injury often causes death due to cardiac tamponade rather than exsanguinating hemorrhage.

Patients with ascending aortic aneurysms may be asymptomatic, and the aneurysm is discovered on routine chest radiograph or during evaluation of a murmur of aortic valve insufficiency. Diagnosis can be made by echocardiography, computed tomography, or magnetic resonance imaging. Before operation most patients should undergo coronary arteriography.

Elective repair is usually indicated when the aortic aneurysm diameter is 5.5 cm or greater. Repair is performed using extracorporeal circulation, usually with systemic hypothermia. Cannulation for arterial inflow can be performed in the aortic arch or in the femoral or iliac artery. During bypass, an atraumatic clamp is used to occlude the aorta just beneath the innominate artery, and the heart is arrested with cardioplegia delivered through the coronary ostia or retrogradely through the coronary sinus, or through both routes. The ascending aorta is excised and replaced with a woven or knitted Dacron graft, impregnated with collagen or albumin.

When the aneurysm involves the sinotubular junction or the sinus portion of the aorta, aortic valve insufficiency is often associated. When the aortic valve also has to be replaced, a decision must be made about whether to perform separate or composite (integral valve and vascular graft) replacement. For annuloaortic ectasia, as is present in Marfan's syndrome, a composite replacement is usually indicated, with implantation of the coronary arteries into the graft.

Aneurysms of the Aortic Arch. Repair of arch aneurysms is hazardous because of the problems encountered in managing the cerebral circulation during graft insertion. There are two basic strategies for protecting the brain during repair. The first is perfusion of the brachiocephalic vessels, and the second is profound hypothermia and circulatory arrest. Clinical and laboratory data suggest that with hypothermia of 16° to 18° C, cerebral blood flow can be interrupted for 45 minutes with the expectation of full neurologic recovery. With longer periods of ischemia, the risk of cerebral damage increases. Profound hypothermia and circulatory arrest also provide ideal operating conditions with an operative field uncluttered by perfusion cannulas and clamps. This technique also has less risk of embolization.

Aneurysm repair is accomplished through a median sternotomy or left posterolateral thoracotomy. When a median sternotomy is used, cardiopulmonary bypass is established with a venous cannula in the right atrium and an arterial cannula in the femoral artery. Venous access through a lateral thoracotomy is obtained by cannulating both the femoral vein and the pulmonary artery. Patients are cooled by means of perfusion hypothermia to 16° to 18° C, and the operation is performed with the patient in a steep Trendelenburg position. Perfusion is then discontinued, and no effort is made to isolate or occlude the brachiocephalic arteries or the distal aorta. When additional cardiac procedures are planned, or when the period of cardiac arrest is anticipated to be longer than 45 minutes, intracoronary crystalloid or blood cardioplegia is administered for myocardial protection. Drugs used for cerebral protection include pentobarbital, dexamethasone, mannitol, and nimodipine. Graft replacement of the arch is facilitated by excising as a button or island the superior aspect of the aorta that gives rise to the innominate, carotid, and subclavian arteries. This aortic portion is then anastomosed to the superior aspect of the graft. The risk of perioperative death is 10 to 15%, and neurologic injury occurs in 5 to 10% of patients.

Descending Thoracic Aortic Aneurysms. The general indications and methods of repair of descending thoracic aortic aneurysms caused by atherosclerosis or chronic dissection are similar to those described for the abdominal aorta. The major area of controversy is whether circulatory support during aortic clamping is useful. We use left atrial-to-femoral artery bypass with a centrifugal pump because this system does not require systemic heparinization. Circulatory support during cross-clamping appears to improve renal function and prevent acidosis after release of the aortic cross-clamp.

Paraplegia or paraparesis occurs in approximately 5 to 10% of patients undergoing repair of descending thoracic aortic aneurysms. The risk is increased if the aortic segment to be replaced is extensive or if aortic cross-clamping is prolonged. The risk of this serious complication should be discussed thoroughly with patients and their families preoperatively.

Thoracoabdominal Aortic Aneurysms

Thoracoabdominal aneurysms involve varying segments of the thoracic and abdominal aorta. The cause is atherosclerosis or previous aortic dissection. Aneurysms of over 6 cm in diameter are considered for repair. The risk of surgical repair is high because critical arteries to the spinal cord and abdominal viscera originate from the aneurysmal portion of the aorta. Early mortality of elective repair is 14%. The rate of paraplegia is 2 to 29% depending on the extent of aortic involvement, cross-clamp time, the presence of dissection, and the age of the patient. Attempts to decrease paraplegia include expeditious operation, reimplantation of intercostal arteries, bypass or shunts, mild systemic hypothermia, deep hypothermic circulatory arrest with cardiopulmonary bypass, drainage of cerebrospinal fluid, and the use of drugs to decrease ischemic and reperfusion injuries. None of these techniques, however, have been fully successful.

Aortic Dissection

Aortic dissection is the most common aortic disease leading to sudden death. Autopsy studies estimate that fatal aortic dissections occur in 5.2 patients per 1 million population per year. Although connective tissue diseases and congenital cardiovascular malformations may predispose to dissection, aortic dissection is most often a complication of arterial hypertension. Dissecting aneurysm is an inaccurate term because there is little aortic dilatation during the early phase of the disease. Usually the intramedial hematoma involves one-half to two-thirds of the aortic circumference and is associated with an intimal tear. Typically, the intimal tear is transverse and is located in the right anterolateral aspect of the ascending aorta, in the medial aspect of the descending aorta close to the left subclavian artery, or, less frequently, in the posterior aspect of the aortic arch.

Various classifications exist. The simplest and most useful scheme divides dissections into *ascending* and *descending* types based on extension of the dissection into the ascending aorta. This classification is not related to the site of the intimal tear. Clinicians should also be familiar with the original DeBakey classification in which ascending aortic dissections are designated Type I if the intramural dissection extends into the descending aorta or Type II if the ascending dissection extends only to the level of the innominate artery. Type III dissections in this classification involve only the descending aorta.

Rapid downstream propagation of the intramedial hematoma produces the characteristic clinical findings, which are excruciating thoracic pain and sequelae of occlusion of major aortic branches. In the ascending aorta, proximal extension may lead to fatal intrapericardial rupture and cardiac tamponade. Death may also result from sudden aortic insufficiency or occlusion of the coronary arteries. Distal propagation of ascending aortic dissection may cause stroke, visceral ischemia, or spinal cord ischemia and flaccid lower extremity paralysis.

Chest pain, usually abrupt and excruciating, accompanies acute aortic dissection in approximately 90% of patients. Arterial hypertension is present in at least half of patients at presentation, and physical examination should include measurement of blood pressure in both arms and careful palpation and recording of peripheral pulses. A diastolic murmur along the right or left upper sternal border suggests aortic valve insufficiency due to dissection of the ascending aorta.

Typical findings on chest radiographs include progressive widening on the upper mediastinal shadow, prominence of the ascending aorta, and enlargement of the aortic knob with or without a double shadow. Computed tomography with intravenous contrast confirms the diagnosis. Transthoracic and transesophageal echocardiography with Doppler and magnetic resonance imaging are additional useful diagnostic tests.

The outlook for untreated patients with aortic dissections is poor; mortality is 37% within the first 48 hours, 74% within 2 weeks, and 90% within the first year. The 30-day survival of patients with dissections that involve the ascending aorta only is approximately 5%, much worse than the 63% 30-day survival for patients with dissections of the descending aorta. Death among patients with ascending aortic dissection is due to hemopericardium in 78% of patients.

Control of hypertension is the sine qua non of medical treatment, and antihypertensive therapy is crucial before and after surgical repair. All hypertensive patients with a presumptive diagnosis of acute aortic dissection should have prompt, aggressive antihypertensive therapy started *before* diagnostic studies are undertaken. An arterial line and urinary catheter are necessary for monitoring therapy. Patients with aortic dissection who have normal blood pressure at presentation should also have the systolic blood pressure lowered by 20 to 30 mmHg to prevent extension of the dissection and to alleviate chest pain.

The goals of surgical repair are to prevent early fatal complications (hemorrhage into the pericardium, aortic rupture), restore normal blood flow as nearly as possible through the true lumen of the aorta and its branches, and obliterate the false channel to prevent aneurysm formation.

For patients with dissection of the ascending aorta, operation should be undertaken as soon as possible. The aorta is approached through a median sternotomy and repaired during cardiopulmonary bypass. The dissection usually extends well beyond the limits of anterior exposure, and it is preferable to cannulate the femoral or external iliac artery for inflow. A single large cannula in the right atrium is sufficient for venous return. It is prudent to perform arterial cannulation before sternotomy, and in patients with hemodynamic distress, concomitant insertion of a femoral venous cannula will permit circulatory support during thoracotomy.

Systemic hypothermia (20° to 25° C) is useful in these patients because reduced whole-body perfusion or circulatory arrest or both may be required during distal anastomosis of the graft to the aorta. The aorta is cross-clamped just proximal to the innominate artery. A longitudinal aortotomy along the anterior or right anterior aspect of the aorta usually opens the false channel. The true lumen surrounded by intact intima is considerably narrower than the outer aortic diameter. An incision in the intima is extended proximally to allow exposure of the coronary ostia and infusion of cardioplegia.

Aortic insufficiency secondary to the dissection can usually be repaired, and valve replacement is reserved for patients who have combined intrinsic aortic valve disease, annuloaortic ectasia, or extensive dislocation of the valve. The aorta is divided proximal to the aortic clamp, and an interposition Dacron graft, as described in the section on repair of ascending aortic aneurysm, is implanted.

For repair of descending aortic dissections, we favor the use of left heart bypasses or partial cardiopulmonary bypass. Shunts or partial bypasses reduce (but do not eliminate) the risk of spinal cord injury. Paraplegia occurs in 14% of patients undergoing repair of acute descending thoracic aortic dissections and is significantly higher without than with shunt or bypass.

The descending aorta is exposed through a left posterolateral thoracotomy. Standard techniques are used for partial bypass from the femoral vessels. Intraoperative autotransfusion will reduce requirements for homologous blood use and the attendant risks of infectious disease transmission. The intimal tear initiating descending aortic dissections begins just below the origin of the left subclavian artery. The entry site should be excised or excluded with the graft repair. Often the dissection extends a few centimeters proximal to the initiating tear; proximal control of the aorta is best obtained between the left carotid and left subclavian arteries. Distally, the aorta is occluded so that a graft segment of approximately 6 cm can be inserted. If the posterior aortic wall is intact, patent intercostal vessels can be preserved including those into an oblique proximal or distal anastomosis.

Mortality following operation for acute aortic dissections remains high (20 to 30%). The risk is closely tied to preoperative variables including hemodynamic factors, medical condition of the patient, and the presence or absence of visceral artery occlusion, and to intraoperative factors such as the fragility of tissue, which is more difficult to quantify. Preoperative completed stroke or paraplegia rarely improves following operation.

Acute descending aortic dissections have a better natural history than ascending aortic dissections, and the early prognosis of uncomplicated descending dissections with medical treatment alone is reasonably good. Approximately 80% of patients with descending aortic dissections survive 3 years, but this figure may overestimate the prognosis of patients who present with acute dissections. We favor aggressive medical treatment in the early stages of descending aortic dissection, in an intensive care unit with parenteral medications and monitoring as previously described. This approach is almost always successful in relieving pain and halting progression of dissection. Elective repair is considered as early as 4 to 6 weeks after the initial presentation.

A high proportion of patients (75%) have a residual false lumen and distal dissection after initial successful repair. Late complications of aortic dissection necessitate careful follow-up with control of hypertension and serial CT scans. Progressive enlargement of the aorta has serious implications, and reoperation should be considered in appropriate candidates. Development and rupture of secondary aneurysms account for 29% of all late deaths among survivors following successful repair of aortic dissection.

AORTIC TRANSECTION FOLLOWING BLUNT TRAUMA

Acute aortic transection is, unfortunately, not uncommon after rapid deceleration injuries as often occur in motor vehicle accidents. The most common site of aortic disruption is the descending aorta below the origin of the subclavian artery and just above or adjacent to the ligamentum arteriosum. Expeditious diagnosis using aortography or computed tomography with intravenous contrast and immediate surgical repair is necessary. Without treatment, approximately 40% of patients who survive the initial accident will die during the first 2 days of hospitalization.

Repair of aortic transections is accomplished through a left posterolateral thoracotomy. We prefer, when possible, to insert a left atrial-to-femoral bypass circuit or a Gott shunt prior to clamping the aorta in order to minimize the risk of spinal cord injury. When the aorta is completely transected, a short interposition Dacron graft is used. If the posterior wall of the aorta is intact, the anterior wall can sometimes be repaired directly with interrupted felt-reinforced mattress sutures.

ABDOMINAL AORTIC OCCLUSIVE DISEASE

Chronic aortoiliac occlusive disease is the cause of claudication in more than half of patients less than 40 years of age. In those over 40 years, aortoiliac disease alone is responsible in 18% of claudication cases, and together with infrainguinal disease it is responsible in another 17%. Atherosclerosis is the most frequent cause, but nonspecific aortoarteritis in young patients should be considered as well.

Leriche's syndrome is caused by chronic aortoiliac occlusion and includes buttock and thigh claudication, impotence, and absence of pulses on the lower extremities. The presence of ischemic ulcer or gangrene usually indicates additional infrainguinal disease. The progress made in percutaneous endovascular procedures (transluminal angioplasty, thrombolytic treatment, stents) has changed the indications for surgical treatment. Iliac artery stenosis can effectively be treated with balloon angioplasty or sometimes with placement of stents. Stenosis of the infrarenal aorta, especially the so-called shaggy aorta with evidence of microembolism to the feet (blue toe syndrome), should be treated surgically, usually with bifurcated aortic graft replacement. Chronic occlusion of the infrarenal aorta is also a surgical disease. Because involvement of the iliac arteries is frequent, an aortobifemoral Dacron graft is the operation of choice. Pelvic flow to the sigmoid colon can be ensured either in a retrograde way, through a patent external iliac artery, or through a separate graft sutured to one of the internal iliac arteries. If the aortoiliac segment is patent but stenosed, an end-to-side proximal anastomosis can also be considered to preserve pre-existing pelvic flow. Concomitant renovascular hypertension or renal failure caused by renal artery disease can be treated by transaortic endarterectomy of the renal arteries or by aortorenal bypass, using reversed saphenous vein or a Dacron graft.

In patients who have had multiple previous operations on the abdominal aorta, thoracofemoral bypass is a good alternative. In high-risk patients or in those who need removal of an infected aortic graft, extra-anatomic revascularization using axillofemoral and femorofemoral bypass is performed. We use an extended polytetrafluoroethylene (ePTFE) graft with external ring support.

Five-year patency of aortobifemoral grafts is 85 to 90%. The patency of axillobifemoral grafts during the same interval is 50 to 70%, but revision or thrombectomy is frequently needed. Perioperative mortality has decreased to less than 3% in most series. However, one-third of these patients die within 5 years because of generalized atherosclerosis and underlying coronary artery disease.

NONSPECIFIC AORTITIS

Nonspecific aortoarteritis or Takayasu's arteritis is an autoimmune inflammatory vascular disease. Ninety percent of the patients are under 30 years of age. Signs and symptoms of the acute systemic illness are fatigue, low-grade fever, and tachycardia. The erythrocyte sedimentation rate is frequently elevated. Prednisone is the treatment of choice in this stage. The disease may cause stenosis of the low thoracic or upper abdominal aorta, although more frequently the primary branches of the aortic arch or the abdominal aorta are involved. Half of the patients have renovascular hypertension. Surgical treatment performed in the chronic phase of the disease includes prosthetic grafting from a proximal nonaffected site of the aorta to the more distal aortic segment or to an artery distal to the diseased segment. Endarterectomy of the visceral or renal arteries is rarely possible and should be avoided. Recurrence is frequent.

ANGINA PECTORIS

method of
CHARLES R. LAMBERT, M.D., PH.D.
University of South Alabama Medical Center
Mobile, Alabama

Angina pectoris is a symptom complex associated with myocardial ischemia. Classically, it consists of a pressure type of discomfort that is usually substernal, although it may originate from or radiate to the epigastrium, jaw, neck, back, or arm. Anginal "equivalents" may include dyspnea, palpitations, dizziness, or other cardiac symptoms. The differential diagnosis of angina pectoris includes pulmonary, pericardial, musculoskeletal, pleural, gastrointestinal, and great vessel pathology. Angina pectoris is generally classified as stable or unstable. Stable angina is usually exertional with a relatively constant threshold required for precipitation. Patients with stable angina have a relatively predictable symptom complex and are generally able to adjust their day-to-day activities and medication regimens to avoid its onset. Unstable angina represents a change in this stable pattern or the new onset of angina pectoris in a previously asymptomatic individual. Changes may include an increase in the frequency or intensity of angina, the occurrence of symptoms at rest, a lower exercise threshold for provocation of angina, or the onset of nocturnal symptoms. Most authorities include angina occurring after a myocardial infarction as unstable. Angina may occur in a similar pattern in patients with Prinzmetal's or variant angina. Stable angina, unstable angina, and Prinzmetal's angina all result from myocardial ischemia; however, the pathophysiologic mechanisms differ, and the approach to treatment of these clinical syndromes may differ as well.

PATHOPHYSIOLOGY OF STABLE ANGINA PECTORIS

Large coronary angiographic studies of patients presenting for evaluation of chronic stable angina consistently reveal severe epicardial coronary atherosclerosis as the major finding. In the Emory University database of 1586 patients catheterized for the first time for evaluation of stable angina pectoris, 9% had no disease, 3% had mild disease, 4% had moderate disease, and 84% had significant disease (>75% area reduction) in at least one major epicardial coronary artery. Furthermore, several investigators have shown that the morphology of coronary artery stenoses can be linked to the clinical syndrome present for a given patient. These findings suggest that stable angina pectoris is more often associated with a "stable coronary stenosis" characterized angiographically by smooth, usually concentric borders and not usually associated with plaque rupture, intramural hemorrhage, or thrombus. Thus, stable angina pectoris is most likely to be associated with severe epicardial coronary atherosclerotic obstruction; however, plaque morphology tends to be "stable" and is not associated with marked eccentricity, thrombus, or ulceration.

In the normal heart the epicardial coronary arteries offer little resistance to blood flow and serve largely as conductance vessels. In most patients with stable angina pectoris, as noted previously, major atherosclerotic lesions are present within these vessels and major limitations to coronary blood flow may occur, especially during periods of increased metabolic demand. If an increasingly severe stenosis is imposed on an epicardial coronary artery, resting blood flow is affected little until the luminal diameter has been severely reduced by around 90% or so. Peak hyperemic blood flow is limited much earlier at a diameter reduction of approximately 50%. Vasomotor tone and hydrodynamic factors may also affect the importance of a given coronary artery stenosis. With an appreciation of the dynamic nature of coronary stenoses, many pathophysiologic mediators have been proposed as instigators of ischemia in patients with coronary artery disease. Such potential mediators include the sympathetic nervous system, histamine, serotonin, thromboxane, leukotrienes, and a basic alteration in smooth muscle activational processes. Some vasodilators require intact endothelium to exert their effects on vascular smooth muscle. These substances are thought to cause the release of an endothelial-dependent relaxant factor (EDRF). In the absence of endothelium a substance that usually causes vasodilation when introduced through the luminal surface of a vessel may cause vasoconstriction owing to the lack of EDRF. Such observations have been made in atherosclerotic human coronary arteries studied in vitro as well as in patients studied in the cardiac catheterization laboratory. These observations suggest that an important pathophysiologic mechanism for the production of ischemia in coronary artery disease may be the loss of normal endothelial vasodilator function as a result of atherosclerotic injury.

Beside the obvious link between coronary atherosclerotic lesions and flow-related myocardial ischemia in patients with angina pectoris, several other pathophysiologic mechanisms may be important. One of these factors is the transmural distribution of resting myocardial blood flow from the epicardium to the endocardium. Because of greater systolic compressive forces and the resultant wall stress, the distribution of blood flow to the subendocardium is around 1.25 times greater than that to the epicardium. This preferential subendocardial flow is dependent upon the vasodilation of vessels in this region, and thus the subendocardium has less coronary flow reserve to respond to further stress. Because of this, factors such as lowering coronary perfusion pressure, elevation of left ventricular end-diastolic pressure, and tachycardia all tend to make the subendocardium ischemic before they affect the epicardial layers. In the presence of coronary artery obstruction the effective subendocardial perfusion pressure is determined by the gradient distal to the stenosis and the left ventricular end-diastolic pressure. If ischemia occurs and left ventricular end-diastolic pressure begins to rise, a vicious cycle may be set up whereby the effective subendocardial perfusion pressure is reduced, further intensifying ischemia, which further raises the end-diastolic pressure, and so on. Subendocardial ischemia also plays an important role in the genesis of certain forms of nonatheromatous angina such as that seen with severe left ventricular hypertrophy.

In patients with stable angina pectoris most significant pharmacologic interventions are targeted at the determinants of myocardial oxygen demand. At the bedside or in the office these determinants are approximated by heart rate, blood pressure, and volume status. With exercise, heart rate and blood pressure increase while peripheral vascular resistance falls and cardiac output increases. Precipitation of ischemia in this circumstance is usually a function of increased metabolic demand by the myocardium, although dynamic coronary mechanisms may also contribute, as noted in the previous section. Ischemia due to increased myocardial oxygen demand may also be a function of inadequate collateral development. A primary mediator of demand-side ischemia in many patients with stable angina is the sympathetic nervous system through its direct influence on heart rate, contractility, and afterload. Many investigations have established that the majority of ischemic episodes in patients with stable angina pectoris are not accompanied by angina but are asymptomatic or silent. Thus, clinical inquiries regarding symptoms may be inadequate in assessing the true ischemic burden in a given patient.

A discussion of the pathophysiology of myocardial ischemia would not be complete without mention of circadian patterns of ischemic events. Definite circadian variation has been described for myocardial infarction, sudden cardiac death, thrombotic stroke, Prinzmetal's angina, and transient myocardial ischemia in patients with stable angina. The majority of such events appear to cluster in the morning hours after awakening. Although ischemia tends to track the circadian variation in heart rate and blood pressure, patients are more likely to become ischemic in the morning than in the afternoon at the same heart rate and blood pressure. If the circadian variation in heart rate is abolished by beta-adrenergic blockade, most ischemia is abolished; however, that which remains has different frequency characteristics than the previously dominant circadian pattern. This latter observation suggests a heterogeneous etiology for the total ischemic burden in such patients. Although platelet activation may play a role in the circadian variation of ischemia in some patients, pharmacologic trials designed to alter this mechanism have had variable results. Detailed examination of ambulatory recordings shows episodes of ischemia followed by but not preceded by an increase in heart rate, suggesting a possible supply-side mechanism. Time-related variations in coronary artery tone may also play a role in modulating circadian variation of myocardial ischemia. Overall, currently available data suggest that such variation is mediated by a combination of factors that may include heart rate, blood pressure, platelet activation, coronary blood flow, mental activity, and dynamic alterations in coronary artery stenoses, among others.

PATHOPHYSIOLOGY OF UNSTABLE ANGINA PECTORIS

Coronary angiography in patients with unstable angina reveals lesions with eccentric geometry, irregular or scalloped borders, unstable plaque geometry, and a high incidence of thrombus. The mechanisms by which unstable

TABLE 1. **Commonly Used Nitrate Preparations**

Medication	Recommended Daily Dosage (mg)	Onset of Action (min)	Peak Action (min)	Duration
Sublingual NTG	0.3–0.8	2–5	4–8	10–30 min
Sublingual ISDN	2.5–10	5–20	15–60	45–120 min
Sublingual PETN	10–40	5–30	15–60	45 min
Sublingual ET	5–10	5	15–30	30–180 min
Oral NTG spray	0.4	2–5	4–8	10–30 min
Buccal NTG	1–3	2–5	4–10	30–300 min
Oral ISDN	10–160	15–45	45–120	2–6 h
Oral ISMN	40	60	60–240	7–12 h
Oral NTG	6.5–19.5	20–45	45–120	2–6 h
NTG ointment (2%)	0.5–2 inches	15–60	30–120	3–8 h
NTG discs (transdermal)	10–50	30–60	60–180	Up to 24 h

NTG = nitroglycerin (Nitrostat, Nitro-Bid, Nitro-Dur, Deponit, Minitran, Transderm-Nitro, Tridil, Nitrong, Nitrolingual Spray); ISDN = isosorbide dinitrate (Isordil, Sorbitrate); ISMN = isosorbide monotitrate (ISMO); PETN = pentaerythritol tetranitrate (Peritrate): ET = erythrityl tetranitrate (Cardilate).

TABLE 2. **Commonly Used Beta-Adrenergic Blockers**

Drug	Beta-Receptor Blocked (Cardiac Selectivity)	Membrane-Stabilizing Activity	Intrinsic Sympathomimetic Activity	Lipid Solubility	Serum Half-Life (h)	Duration of Action (h)	Protein Binding (%)	Usual Oral Dosage Range (mg/day)
Acebutolol (Sectral)	1[b]	+	+	Low	7–10	24	26	400–1800
Atenolol (Tenormin)	1[b]	−	−	Low	5–9	24	6–16	100–200
Betaxolol (Kerlone)	1[b]	−	−	Mod	12–22	23–25	50–60	10–40
Carteolol (Cartrol)	1 and 2	−	+	Low	5–7	72	23–30	15–30
Esmolol (Brevibloc)	1[b]	−	−	Low	9 (min)	10–20 (min)	55	None
Labetalol[a] (Normodyne, Trandate)	1 and 2	+	−	Mod	3–4	8–12	50	150–1200
Metoprolol (Lopressor, Toprol)	1[b]	±	−	Mod	2–6	10–12	13	150–400
Nadolol (Corgard)	1 and 2	−	−	Low	14–24	39	20	80–240
Penbutolol (Levatol)	1 and 2	+	+	High	12–20	>24	99	40–60
Pindolol (Visken)	1 and 2	±	+ + +	Low	3–4	8	57	10–20
Sotalol (Betapace)	1 and 2	−	−	Low	5–13	24	5	240–480
Timolol (Blocadren)	1 and 2	−	−	Mod	3–4	15	10	15–45

+ = Present; − = absent; ± = weak to variable response; Mod = moderate.
[a]Has postsynaptic $alpha_1$-adrenergic blocking ability.
[b]Blocks $beta_2$ receptors at higher doses of therapeutic range.

plaques become unstable are the object of intense investigation and appear to be multifactorial in origin. In any event, these coronary angiographic findings are associated clinically with worsening ischemia either at rest or with minimal exertion. Although all of the pathophysiologic mechanisms described earlier for stable angina also apply to unstable angina, limitation of blood flow due to the particular coronary lesions described previously appears to be of prime importance.

PATHOPHYSIOLOGY OF VARIANT ANGINA

Variant or Prinzmetal's angina is associated with coronary vasoconstriction or spasm that is usually focal and is manifested by rest pain with associated transient electrocardiographic (ECG) alterations. Although this type of angina may occur with angiographically normal coronary arteries, it is most often seen in conjunction with some degree of underlying coronary atherosclerosis. Variant angina may progress to an unstable ischemic syndrome such as unstable angina or myocardial infarction by the mechanisms discussed previously.

ANTIANGINAL MEDICAL THERAPY

Nitrates

Nitrates are among the oldest and most widely used antianginal drugs and are available in a variety of preparations (Table 1). Nitrates act principally as vasodilators affecting the venous capacitance vessels. Some effect may be demonstrated on the peripheral and coronary arterial systems, although the latter probably plays a minor role in antianginal clinical efficacy. When given acutely, nitrates reduce venous return and lower cardiac output and systemic arterial pressure, and they may have a variable effect on heart rate. Care must be taken during administration of nitrates to patients with diminished cardiac reserve or hypovolemia.

In acute cases nitrates are most commonly administered using the sublingual route, although a spray or intravenous administration may also be utilized, if available. The clinical effects of nitroglycerin and its metabolites with these three routes of administration are similar from a practical standpoint. Continuous nitroglycerin administration is usually done in acute cases using an intravenous infusion. Careful blood pressure monitoring must accompany this practice, and this therapy is most commonly used for patients with unstable ischemic syndromes in the intensive care unit. Topical or percutaneous nitroglycerin administration using paste may also be useful in these patients. Patch or transdermal administration is not generally useful in acute or subacute cases because of its slow onset of action and the difficulty in adjusting the dosage. In addition, tolerance commonly develops with continuous transdermal systems unless care is taken to provide a nitrate-free interval. Oral nitrate preparations such as isosorbide dinitrate, pentaerythritol tetranitrate, erythrityl tetranitrate, and isosorbide mononitrate offer convenient dosing intervals and are associated, in general, with fewer tolerance problems, although a nitrate-free interval is still needed. These agents are most often used for chronic therapy. Nitrates have side effects that include reflex tachycardia, headache, and flushing. Tolerance to most of these effects will develop in most patients, and careful dose titration can be used to minimize them.

Beta Blockers

Beta blockers are widely used in patients with ischemic heart disease because of their clinical efficacy in achieving symptomatic and objective control of ischemia as well as their documented value in secondary prevention. Beta blockers differ primarily with regard to $beta_1$-receptor (cardiac) selectivity, alpha-blocker activity, solubility, intrinsic sympathomimetic activity, and membrane-stabilizing activity. Beta blockers are available in various formulations and vary widely in pharmacologic properties as outlined in Table 2.

TABLE 3. **Side Effects and Adverse Reactions With Beta-Blocker Therapy**

Cardiovascular manifestations (beta$_1$ effects)
- Bradycardia
- Hypotension
- Ventricular dysfunction

Peripheral vascular manifestations (beta$_2$ effects)
- Increased total peripheral resistance
- Decreased blood supply to extremities
- Muscle fatigue

Respiratory dysfunction (beta$_2$ effects)
- Bronchospasm
- Dyspnea

Carbohydrate homeostasis (beta$_2$ effects)
- Inhibition of insulin release
- Inhibition of metabolic response to hypoglycemia
- Inhibition of hemodynamic response to hypoglycemia

Central nervous system effects
- Vivid or disturbing dreams
- Lethargy
- Depression
- Acute confusion
- Hallucinations

Gastrointestinal effects
- Mild indigestion
- Nausea
- Constipation

Skin reactions (uncommon)

Sexual dysfunction
- Impotence

Neuromuscular effects
- Myasthenic syndrome
- Worsening of myasthenia gravis or myotonia

Practolol syndrome*
- Psoriasis-like lesions
- Ocular disorders
- Sclerosing peritonitis

Overdosage
- Bradycardia
- Hypotension
- Low-output cardiac failure
- Cardiogenic shock
- Bronchospasm
- Grand mal seizures

Beta-blocker withdrawal
- Rebound hypertension
- Rebound angina

Use in pregnancy
- Low birth weight
- Neonatal bradycardia
- Neonatal hypoglycemia

Use in the elderly
- May require dosage reduction

*Practolol is not available in the United States.

Beta blockers reduce resting heart rate depending upon the degree of resting adrenergic tone present and the dose administered. They also produce a marked reduction in heart rate at any level of exercise and in the peak heart rate attainable. Drugs with and without beta$_1$ specificity appear to reduce heart rate equally during rest and exercise, whereas agents with intrinsic sympathomimetic activity may have a lesser effect on heart rate during periods of low adrenergic tone (e.g., sleep). Beta blockers generally produce a small reduction in resting cardiac output and a large reduction in exercise cardiac output. Similar changes are seen in blood pressure that are probably secondary to cardiac output because systemic vascular resistance is usually unchanged or slightly increased with beta blockade during exercise. Beta blockers have little direct effect on left ventricular diastolic function but do reduce contractile state and must be used with caution in patients with significant left ventricular dysfunction. Beta blockers may increase the ventricular fibrillation threshold, decrease automatic arrhythmias by reducing phase 4 depolarization, reduce afterdepolarizations, and alter refractoriness. Sotalol has unique Class III antiarrhythmic properties that are effective in controlling certain atrial and ventricular arrhythmias. Side effects and related problems with beta-blocker therapy are common (Table 3). Many of these may be avoided or minimized by trying alternate dosing or drugs with a different solubility or selectivity.

Calcium Channel Blockers

Calcium channel blockers all inhibit the entry of calcium into the cell; however, the receptors and subcellular mechanisms involved may differ for different compounds. From a clinical standpoint a classification scheme that includes verapamil (Calan, Isoptin), diltiazem (Cardizem), and the dihydropyridines (e.g., nifedipine [Procardia]) as three separate groups is useful. Calcium channel blockers all act as vasodilators, negative inotropic agents, and conduction-depressing agents. The in vivo dose-response relationships for these various effects are markedly different in the different classes, and thus the clinical effects may also be different. In clinical doses verapamil exerts the strongest depressant effect from the myocardial (negative inotropic) and conduction standpoints. The dihydropyridines produce little myocardial or conduction depression but are much more potent arterial vasodilators. Diltiazem is intermediate with respect to these effects. It follows, therefore, that verapamil must be avoided in patients with bradycardia and compromised left ventricular function. On the other hand, if myocardial depression is a desired characteristic, as in a patient with severe hypertension, left ventricular hypertrophy, and diastolic dysfunction, verapamil might be preferred. If a predominantly arterial vasodilator effect is desired, the dihydropyridines might be the agents of choice.

Calcium channel blockers are effective for treating hypertension as well as ischemic heart disease. During exercise they tend to prolong the time elapsed before ischemia occurs by prolonging the time needed to reach a given workload as defined by heart rate and blood pressure. Calcium channel blockers may or may not increase coronary blood flow, although the second-generation dihydropyridines display some coronary vascular selectivity. The dihydropyridines may provoke a reflex increase in heart rate owing to their potent vasodilator effects. This effect is generally not seen with chronic administration and may differ between agents. Dosing and pharmacokinetic information for these agents is outlined in Table 4. Diltiazem,

TABLE 4. **Commonly Used Calcium Channel Blockers**

Parameter	Diltiazem (Cardiazem, Dilacor)	Nifedipine (Adalat, Procardia)	Verapamil (Calan, Isoptin, Verelan)	Isradipine* (DynaCirc)	Nicardipine (Cardene)	Amlodipine (Norvasc)
T max (h)	1–4 6–11 (SR)	0.5–4 6 (SR)	0.5–1 7–9 (SR)	1–3	0.5–2 1–4 (SR)	6–12
Bioavailability (%)	24–74	43–65 29–85 (SR)	13–35	16–18	35	64–90
Protein binding (%)	77–93	92–98	83–92	97	>98	93
Half-life (h)	2–7	2–3 6 (SR)	2–7	5–11	0.75–2 8.6 (SR)	30–50
Excretion						
Renal	40	90	70	65	60	60
Fecal	60	10	16	30	35	40
Usual daily dose (mg)	180–360	30–90	120–360	5–10	60–120	5–10

Abbreviations: T max = time to maximal concentration; SR = sustained release.
*This drug is not approved by the FDA for this indication.

verapamil, and nicardipine are available in intravenous preparations. Dosing adjustments may be needed when calcium channel blockers are used in conjunction with digoxin, cimetidine, or quinidine. Side effects include headache, edema, bradycardia, worsening of ventricular function, flushing, palpitations, and hypotension. Severe cardiovascular side effects can be reversed by intravenous calcium administration. Nimodipine (Nimotop) is a dihydropyridine calcium channel-blocking drug approved for use in patients with subarachnoid hemorrhage.

APPROACH TO TREATMENT

General Principles

All patients with angina pectoris of any variety should be evaluated with respect to the underlying factors that may precipitate or exacerbate ischemia. These include hypertension, tachycardia, hyperthyroidism, anemia, smoking, hypoxia, drug use (sympathomimetics, cocaine), and hypotension. The initial evaluation generally includes stress testing of some variety unless the patient is acutely ill. The heart rate and blood pressure response to exercise may be very helpful in choosing which therapeutic agents to use.

Stable Angina

Initial monotherapy for stable angina may include agents of the nitrate, beta-blocker, or calcium-channel blocking class. The most innocuous side effects may be associated with calcium channel-blocking therapy, and many physicians use these agents as first-line therapy. Objective testing usually shows that beta blockers are more effective as monotherapy. Patients are also instructed about the use of nitroglycerin and are generally placed on aspirin unless a contraindication exists. If symptoms persist, pending other indicated tests, a second agent may be added to an adequate dose of the primary compound. Nitrates or a dihydropyridine calcium channel blocker is generally added to beta blockers, whereas nitrates are generally added to calcium channel blockers. Care must be used in adding calcium antagonists that have negative effects on conduction and ventricular function (verapamil more than diltiazem) to beta blockers. Triple therapy with nitrates, beta blockers, and calcium channel blockers may be needed in some patients. The principles of pathophysiology outlined previously are of primary importance when titrating such therapy. One can alter preload, afterload, and heart rate to produce a desired effect by making careful alterations in dosage and choice of compounds.

Unstable Angina

Patients with unstable angina require rigorous control of the determinants of myocardial oxygen demand as noted earlier. Beta blockers are a mainstay in this therapy, and rapid-acting agents such as esmolol (Brevibloc)* may be useful. Calcium channel blockers may also be useful, especially in patients who may develop a non–Q wave myocardial infarction without congestive heart failure. Intravenous nitroglycerin is considered standard therapy; however, attention must be paid to volume status because such patients are often dehydrated and may respond to small doses of nitroglycerin with a profound fall in systemic blood pressure. Intravenous heparin and aspirin are also considered standard therapy in patients with unstable ischemic syndromes. This makes sense given the pathophysiology noted earlier, and multiple clinical studies have supported the use of these agents in patients with unstable angina. With initial control of symptoms, oral therapy can generally be instituted early in such patients and must be individualized on the basis of the clinical presentation, pathophysiology, and coronary anatomy if known.

Cardiac Catheterization and Revascularization

Patients with stable angina are generally evaluated by stress testing, and the advisability of cardiac

*This drug has not been approved by the FDA for this indication.

catheterization should be based on these findings and the particular clinical situation. Published guidelines for selecting patients for invasive evaluation are available. Patients with high-risk anatomic conditions as shown by cardiac catheterization may require revascularization using either catheter technology (angioplasty, atherectomy) or coronary artery bypass surgery. The indications for these procedures are in constant evolution; however, they generally include severe ischemia during stress with or without normal left ventricular function.

Patients with unstable angina commonly undergo angiography in the United States, although noninvasive evaluation has been shown to be effective and safe if medical therapy is successful in converting unstable angina to a stable situation. Revascularization may be indicated in patients with unstable angina depending upon the clinical factors and coronary anatomy. Both angioplasty and bypass surgery have been shown to be effective in selected patient groups with unstable angina; however, the decision to proceed with revascularization must be made on an individual basis.

CARDIAC ARREST

method of
JAMES M. ATKINS, M.D.
The University of Texas Southwestern Medical School
Dallas, Texas

Sudden death is a frequent occurrence in the United States. Although trauma, suicide, and homicide make up a proportion of these incidents of sudden death, most of them are cardiac in nature. Thus, the term sudden cardiac death is used to describe this group of victims. Although cardiovascular disease has shown a dramatic decrease in mortality during the last 30 years, it still accounts for half of all deaths in the United States, or about 960,000 deaths per year. Of these deaths, about 525,000 are sudden in nature. Of these 525,000 sudden cardiac deaths, 75 to 80% occur in patients with known cardiovascular disease. Therefore, sudden cardiac death is the first symptom in 20 to 25% of patients.

ETIOLOGY AND RISK FACTORS

Whenever autopsy or resuscitated-patient series are examined, about two-thirds of patients suffering a cardiac arrest are found to have coronary artery disease. The distribution of coronary artery disease is similar to that seen in patients with stable angina, acute myocardial infarction, and unstable angina. About 40 to 50% of patients with any of these conditions have three-vessel coronary artery disease, 30% have two-vessel coronary artery disease, and 20 to 25% have one-vessel coronary artery disease. Thus, the distribution of coronary artery stenoses is the same in patients who suffer different coronary artery disease syndromes. The majority of patients who die suddenly from coronary artery disease do not have myocardial infarction. It appears that the most frequent cause of death is ischemia due to coronary artery disease in the presence of ventricular ectopy; the ischemia alters the fibrillation threshold, making the ventricular ectopy lethal. This mechanism may partially explain why control of ventricular ectopy does not reduce mortality. However, control of ischemia and platelet function will reduce mortality. The second most frequent mechanism inducing death is an acute myocardial infarction. The balance of sudden cardiac deaths is due to other forms of heart disease including cardiomyopathies (both hypertrophic and dilated), valvular heart disease, and hypertensive heart disease. Cardiac conduction abnormalities are associated with an increased incidence of sudden death, including the QT prolongation syndromes, the pre-excitation syndromes, and heart block. Many drugs can also cause sudden death by various mechanisms. Metabolic causes, including hypokalemia, hyperkalemia, and hypomagnesemia, also play a role. In some cases no cause can be found.

Because the majority of sudden cardiac death victims have coronary artery disease, it is not surprising that the risk factors for coronary artery disease are the same as those for sudden cardiac death. The major modifiable risk factors are smoking, hypercholesterolemia, hypertension, lack of exercise, and diabetes mellitus. However, the impact of treatment of diabetes on modification of cardiovascular risk is debatable. Equally important but not modifiable major risk factors include family history, increasing age, and the male sex. Stress and obesity are also risk factors, but they are not as important as the factors just mentioned. Besides the risk factors for atherosclerosis there are some additional risk factors for sudden cardiac death. The presence of ventricular ectopy correlates with sudden death. The more frequent and complex the ventricular ectopy, the greater the risk of sudden cardiac death. Poor ventricular function is also a predictor of sudden death. The worse the ventricular function, the greater the risk. The frequency and complexity of ventricular ectopy increases as ventricular function deteriorates. Suppression of ventricular ectopic activity with antiarrhythmic agents does not reduce mortality, but treatment of poor ventricular function with angiotensin-converting enzyme (ACE) inhibitors does reduce mortality and sudden death rates. This fact has led many practitioners to think that ventricular function is the independent variable associated with sudden cardiac death, whereas ventricular ectopic activity is a secondary marker of poor ventricular function, thereby correlating also with sudden cardiac death. Thus, many risk factors for sudden cardiac death can be recognized.

MECHANISMS AND RATES OF SURVIVAL

In patients with cardiovascular disease, the dominant mechanism of cardiac arrest is ventricular fibrillation or ventricular tachycardia. Although the exact incidence of ventricular fibrillation as the mechanism of cardiac arrest in patients with cardiovascular disease is not known, estimates have ranged from 60 to 90%. A second major mechanism is pulseless electrical activity (PEA) or electromechanical dissociation. PEA is a common occurrence in patients with hypovolemia or hypoxia; thus, it is frequently seen in patients who suffer traumatic arrest. PEA is also seen in cardiac patients with very severe cardiovascular disease. Asystole is usually a secondary arrhythmia. Primary asystole occurs particularly in patients with infra-His heart block (Mobitz II). However, the great majority of patients with asystole probably have ventricular fibrillation or PEA first, and then after 20 to 30 minutes or longer finally became asystolic.

Long-term survival following cardiac arrest occurs primarily in victims of ventricular fibrillation or ventricular tachycardia. Long-term survivals of 30 to 40% have been achieved by means of pre-hospital care by paramedic ambulance services. Coronary care unit long-term survivals of greater than 90% have been achieved when cardiac arrest is not associated with pre-existing shock. Long-term survival of patients with asystole and PEA has been very poor, less than 5%. In fact, 95 to 97% of survivors of cardiac arrest at hospital discharge have had ventricular fibrillation or ventricular tachycardia. Hence, ventricular fibrillation and ventricular tachycardia are the mechanisms of cardiac arrest associated with the greatest chance of survival.

TREATMENT

Resuscitation and the Chain of Survival

When studies of successful resuscitation from cardiac arrest are examined, four dominant factors that differentiate survivors from nonsurvivors are apparent. These factors are time, defibrillation, drugs (particularly epinephrine), and cardiopulmonary resuscitation (CPR). Time to defibrillation is the most important determinant of survival. Time to epinephrine and time to CPR are also important determinants. CPR only widens the window of time during which defibrillation or epinephrine can be effective. Thus, CPR should be looked on as a holding action, a losing holding action that merely prolongs the window of opportunity. Most long-term survivors of cardiac arrest are victims of a witnessed cardiac arrest due to ventricular fibrillation or ventricular tachycardia in whom CPR was begun within 4 minutes and defibrillation and advanced cardiac life support measures were instituted within 7 to 8 minutes. The American Heart Association has identified the chain of survival as four steps—early access, early CPR, early defibrillation, and early advanced cardiac life support (Fig. 1).

Early Access

Rapid recognition of the problem and activation of the emergency medical service (EMS) system is essential. Whenever unresponsiveness is recognized outside the hospital, EMS should be activated through the 911 system. Inside the hospital, the call for assistance should be made to the appropriate communication point for the hospital (code team, code blue, doctor heart, and so on). One problem outside the hospital is that the 911 number is not universal. It is present in many urban areas but not in rural areas or smaller towns. Only six states have universal 911 systems in place today; only seven more have laws establishing universal 911 systems by the year 2000. Despite this lack of universality, the 911 system is present in the majority of urban areas and large towns. Hence, the physician must instruct patients in the proper method of interacting with the EMS system in the area where the patient lives, recognizing that it may be different from the system that exists in the physician's location. Rapid recognition is also a problem. When a patient has a myocardial infarction, he frequently delays asking for help for more than 2 hours, but half of all deaths occur within the first hour of an acute myocardial infarction. To prevent sudden cardiac death, patient and family education is needed to allow rapid recognition and quick access to the EMS system. The physician must take the time to instruct the patient and family adequately about the proper time and mechanisms of activating the system. Dispatchers can be trained to assist lay rescuers over the telephone.

CHAIN *of* SURVIVAL

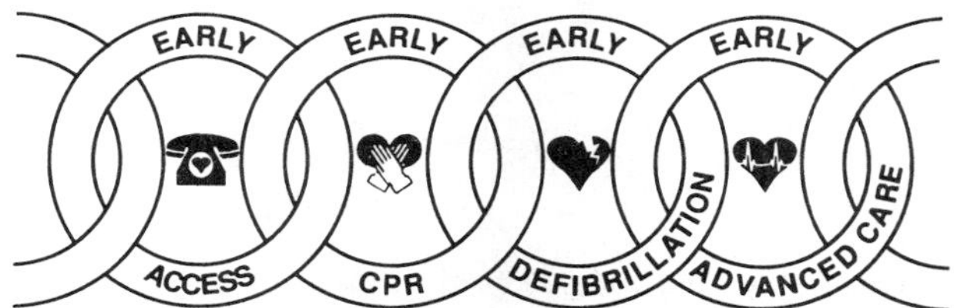

Figure 1. Sequence of events in emergency cardiac care is displayed schematically by the "chain of survival" metaphor. (From American Heart Association: Improving survival from sudden cardiac arrest: The "chain of survival" concept. Circulation *83:*1832–1847, 1991. By permission of the American Heart Association, Inc.)

Early Cardiopulmonary Resuscitation—Basic Life Support

Early initiation of CPR increases the victim's chances of survival by widening the window of opportunity for definitive therapy. CPR should be begun promptly and should continue until definitive therapy can be instituted. If a defibrillator is present and the patient is in ventricular fibrillation or ventricular tachycardia, immediate defibrillation should be accomplished; CPR should never delay defibrillation. Mass training in CPR increased the number of rescuers able to perform CPR during the 1970s and early 1980s. However, fear of AIDS and other communicable diseases has led to a decline in bystander or citizen CPR today. Recent studies have shown that bystanders performing CPR were related to the patient, friends of the patient, or health professionals. It has become rare for lay people to perform CPR on a person they do not know. Hence, training should emphasize family members and friends of patients who are at risk. CPR can be performed by untrained callers with the aid of a trained EMS dispatcher. EMS dispatchers have been able to talk untrained callers through the steps of CPR and have been successful in assisting in the resuscitation of victims. However, trained dispatchers who can give instructions over the telephone are present in only a minority of EMS systems. The method of CPR (basic life support) is outlined in Table 1. Newer methods of CPR such as vest CPR or active compression-decompression CPR (plumber's helper CPR) improve cardiac output during CPR. It remains to be proven whether they can significantly improve survival in large controlled trials.

TABLE 1. **Technique of Cardiopulmonary Resuscitation**

Establish unresponsiveness: Shake and shout
Rapid access: Call 911
Open the airway: Tilt the head back using a chin or jaw lift
Establish apnea: Place your ear over the patient's mouth and nose, listen and feel for breath, watch for rise and fall of the chest
Ventilate: Form a tight seal around the victim's mouth with a mask or your mouth (pinching off the nostrils if mouth-to-mouth) and deliver two breaths, allowing a brief time for exhalation
Establish pulselessness: Feel for the carotid pulse
Begin chest compressions: Place the heel of hands on the lower half of the sternum just cephalad of the sternal xiphoid junction and compress the sternum 1.5 to 2 inches at a rate of 80 to 100 compressions per minute
One-rescuer CPR: After 15 chest compressions, reopen the airway and give two breaths; alternate 15 compressions with two ventilations
Two-rescuer CPR: After five chest compressions, pause and allow second rescuer to give one ventilation; alternate five compressions with one ventilation

Early Defibrillation

Early defibrillation is also an important link in the chain of survival. Defibrillators should be quickly available wherever there is a risk of a cardiac arrest. Every ambulance should have a defibrillator, but it is estimated that less than 25% of American ambulances have one (a more realistic estimate is between 10 and 15%). Thus, there is a great need for defibrillators in all ambulances. Automated defibrillators can be used by first-responder units (fire engine, police cruiser, office building staff, stadium staff, and so on). Automated external defibrillators (AEDs) are attached to the patient with paste-on electrodes. They use a built-in computer that first recognizes that there is good electrode contact and then analyzes the rhythm for the presence of fibrillation waves and the absence of QRS complexes. The device charges the defibrillator and then either discharges the defibrillator or advises the rescuer to discharge it. These devices are very rapid. Some are totally automatic in that they shock the victim three times after an operator has pushed the "start" button. Other devices require a two-step interaction with the operator for each shock (one button activates the analysis, a second button delivers the shock). Manual defibrillators can also be used by trained individuals. Rapid defibrillation should be the goal for patients in ventricular fibrillation or pulseless ventricular tachycardia.

Early Advanced Cardiac Life Support

Protocols for the major actions to be taken during a cardiac arrest are shown step by step in Tables 2, 3, and 4. These protocols are adapted from the 1994 Textbook of Advanced Cardiac Life Support published by the American Heart Association. Drugs should be given intravenously, if possible, during a cardiac arrest. It is preferable to give drugs in the upper extremity or in a central line. Drugs instilled into a leg vein or the femoral vein may take many minutes to

TABLE 2. **Treatment for Ventricular Fibrillation, Pulseless Ventricular Tachycardia**

Perform CPR until defibrillator available
↓
Defibrillate 200 J
↓
Defibrillate 200 to 300 J
↓
Defibrillate 360 J
↓
CPR
↓
Intubate
↓
IV access
↓
Epinephrine 1 mg 1:10,000 intravenously every 3 to 5 min
↓
Defibrillate 360 J 30 to 60 s after each epinephrine dose
↓
Lidocaine 150 mg intravenously (1.5 mg per kg)
↓
Defibrillate 360 J 30 to 60 s after lidocaine
↓
Lidocaine 150 mg intravenously (1.5 mg per kg)
↓
Defibrillate 360 J 30 to 60 s after lidocaine
↓
Bretylium 500 mg intravenously (5 mg per kg)
↓
Defibrillate 360 J 30 to 60 s after bretylium
↓
See text

TABLE 3. **Treatment for Pulseless Electrical Activity (PEA)**

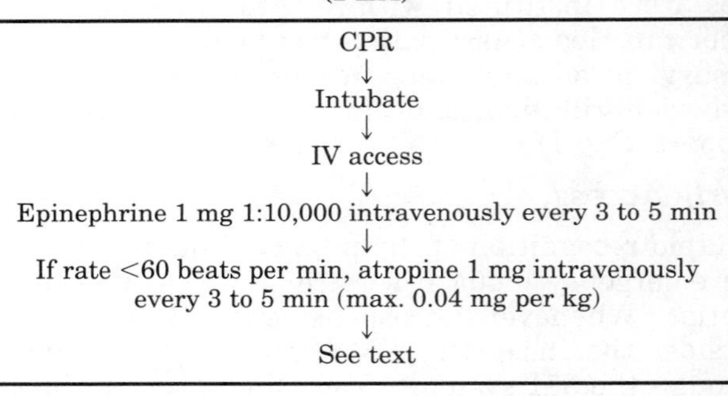
CPR
↓
Intubate
↓
IV access
↓
Epinephrine 1 mg 1:10,000 intravenously every 3 to 5 min
↓
If rate <60 beats per min, atropine 1 mg intravenously every 3 to 5 min (max. 0.04 mg per kg)
↓
See text

TABLE 4. **Treatment for Asystole**

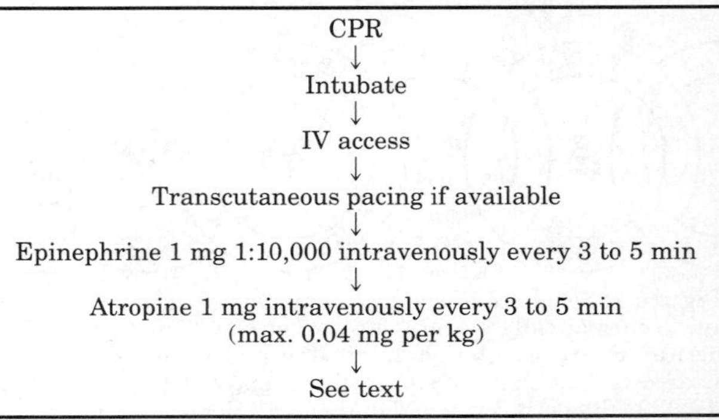
CPR
↓
Intubate
↓
IV access
↓
Transcutaneous pacing if available
↓
Epinephrine 1 mg 1:10,000 intravenously every 3 to 5 min
↓
Atropine 1 mg intravenously every 3 to 5 min (max. 0.04 mg per kg)
↓
See text

reach the central circulation because blood flow below the diaphragm during CPR is minimal. Blood flow during closed chest CPR occurs predominantly in the head and upper extremity.

It is generally recommended that intravenous lines contain no glucose. In certain models, glucose can increase brain injury. Although there is no direct evidence that glucose causes harm during cardiac arrest, the potential does exist. For these reasons, most authorities now recommend that the intravenous line contain either normal saline or Ringer's lactate in a keep-open flow.

Ventilation is also an essential component of CPR. Thus, early intubation is recommended because that is the best method of providing good oxygenation and hyperventilation to lower the PCO_2 in the patient's blood supply.

Ventricular Fibrillation (VF) and Pulseless Ventricular Tachycardia. The patient should be defibrillated as rapidly as possible, as shown in the algorithm given in Table 2. When a manual defibrillator is used, the rhythm should be checked after each defibrillation and after each drug has been added. A pulse check should be done if there is a change in rhythm or after each drug. When an automated defibrillator is used, the pulse is *not* checked after each shock; it is checked only after a group of three shocks. Whenever the rhythm changes or a pulse is present, change to the appropriate protocol.

Antiarrhythmic agents that can be used during the VF protocol include lidocaine, bretylium, and procainamide. There is no clear-cut advantage of any one of these drugs over another. If lidocaine is used, an initial dose of 150 mg or 1.5 mg per kg intravenously is recommended; repeat doses of 0.5 to 1.5 mg per kg (up to a maximum of 3 mg per kg) can be given. Bretylium, 5 mg per kg intravenously, can also be used, followed by repeat doses of 10 mg per kg every 5 minutes; no maximum dose is known, although most clinicians stop at 25 to 30 mg per kg total dose. Procainamide, 30 mg per minute up to 1000 mg intravenously, has also been used and is acceptable. My preference is to try lidocaine first because it is the least toxic and then go to bretylium if the lidocaine is not effective. One must always remember to shock the patient within 30 to 60 seconds after each dose of medication.

If this treatment is ineffective, higher doses of epinephrine may be considered (see later section, Epinephrine). Sodium bicarbonate may be beneficial in a few patients (see later section, Sodium Bicarbonate). Magnesium sulfate may also be beneficial in patients with torsades de pointes, suspected hypomagnesemic state, or refractory ventricular fibrillation. The recommended dose of magnesium sulfate is 1 to 2 grams intravenously given over 1 to 2 minutes. Routine administration of magnesium has not been shown to improve survival.

Pulseless Electrical Activity. The presence of organized electrical activity on the monitor with no palpable pulse is called pulseless electrical activity (PEA). This includes any rhythm without a palpable pulse—electromechanical dissociation (EMD), pseudo-EMD, idioventricular rhythms, ventricular escape rhythms, brady-asystolic rhythms, and post-defibrillation idioventricular rhythms. The treatment algorithm is shown in Table 3. In addition to the treatment shown in the algorithm, one must look for the cause and try to correct it. Table 5 shows the possible causes of PEA with the possible treatments. If one of these conditions is present, one should attempt to correct the cause. If the arrest remains refractory, higher doses of epinephrine may be considered (see Epinephrine section later). Sodium bicarbonate may be beneficial in a few patients (see later section, Sodium Bicarbonate).

Asystole. Asystole should be confirmed in two leads about 90 degrees apart (II and aVL) to make certain that the patient does not have ventricular fibrillation. The treatment algorithm is shown in Table 4. If the patient has asystole, some of the causes that can be treated should be considered—these include hypoxia, hyperkalemia, hypokalemia, pre-existing acidosis, drug overdose, and hypothermia. If the arrest remains refractory, higher doses of epinephrine may be considered (see following section, Epinephrine). Sodium bicarbonate may be beneficial in a few patients (see section on Sodium Bicarbonate, later).

Epinephrine. Epinephrine is the most important drug for treatment during a cardiac arrest. The mechanism of action of epinephrine is only partially understood. Epinephrine increases cerebral and cardiac blood flow during CPR, probably owing to its alpha effects. It appears that these effects on cerebral and cardiac blood flow are more important than any of the beta effects of epinephrine. The minimum dose of intravenous epinephrine is 1 mg for average-sized adults or 0.01 mg per kg for children or very large adults. The upper limit of epinephrine dosage is not known. Higher doses of epinephrine have been suggested from both human and animal studies because higher doses of epinephrine are associated with a higher return of spontaneous circulation (ROSC or pulse). However, in randomized trials higher doses of epinephrine failed to increase survival at 1 hour or at hospital discharge, or to improve neurologic status despite an increased ROSC. Higher doses of epineph-

TABLE 5. **Causes and Treatment of Pulseless Electrical Activity**

Possible Cause	Possible Therapy
Hypovolemia	Volume infusion
Hypoxia	Ventilation, supplemental oxygen
Cardiac tamponade	Pericardiocentesis
Tension pneumothorax	Needle decompression
Hypothermia	Rewarming
Massive pulmonary embolus	Surgery, thrombolytics
Hyperkalemia	Bicarbonate, calcium, dextrose
Acidosis	Bicarbonate
Drug overdoses	Specific antagonist
Massive myocardial infarction	Thrombolytics, angioplasty, surgery

rine did not cause any increase in side effects. Therefore, higher doses of epinephrine may be used. Alternative regimens include high-dose epinephrine, 0.1 mg per kg every 3 to 5 minutes, intermediate-dose epinephrine, 2 to 5 mg every 3 to 5 minutes, and escalating-dose epinephrine, 1 mg followed by 3 mg followed by 5 mg 3 minutes apart. If there is no intravenous access, epinephrine, 0.1 mg per kg of 1:1000 can be given through the endotracheal tube.

Sodium Bicarbonate. The use of sodium bicarbonate is controversial. Evidence about the benefits of bicarbonate has been contradictory. Sodium bicarbonate has been shown to be definitely effective and helpful in patients with known pre-existing hyperkalemia. On the other hand, it has been shown to be of no benefit and possibly harmful in patients with hypoxic lactic acidosis. In between are several situations in which bicarbonate might be helpful. It is probably helpful in patients with known pre-existing bicarbonate-responsive acidosis and overdose of tricyclic antidepressants. Sodium bicarbonate may be helpful in patients with prolonged cardiac arrests, in those who are intubated, or in those in whom a pulse returns after a prolonged arrest; however, the evidence of benefit is only possible and not proved. If a decision is made to give sodium bicarbonate, the recommended dose is 1 mEq per kg.

Beginning and Terminating Resuscitation

The decision to begin CPR and resuscitation is based on both medical and legal grounds. Resuscitation should be used in cases of sudden unexpected death that do not have a medical or legal contraindication for resuscitation. Medical contraindications to resuscitation include the presence of rigor mortis, decapitation, decomposition, and severe dependent lividity. Traumatic injuries, comprising visually recognizable injuries to the brain or cardiovascular system that are not compatible with life, are also used by some authorities. Legal contraindications include court orders, advance directives to physicians, and, in some states, living wills. Resuscitation should not be begun when there is no chance of reversing the primary illness. Patients with terminal illnesses who cannot be treated are not candidates for resuscitation in most circumstances. Terminal diseases may include certain end-stage cancers, end-stage AIDS, and cardiogenic shock that is refractory to therapy. In patients with terminal disease, the physician should discuss the situation with the patient and family and develop a mutually acceptable plan of action should a cardiac arrest occur.

Resuscitation should be terminated in two different situations. If after resuscitation has begun it is found that there was a reason not to begin resuscitation at all, it is reasonable to terminate it. Otherwise, resuscitation should be continued until it is obvious that the cardiovascular system is nonresponsive. Most successful resuscitations succeed in the first 10 minutes of advanced cardiac life support. A few more patients are resuscitated when a reversible cause is found and treated. Hence, a rule of thumb is to discontinue resuscitation after 20 to 25 minutes of advanced cardiac life support when any treatable cause has been treated. Rarely, a patient can be resuscitated after prolonged effort; however, in such cases neurologic impairment is frequent. One exception occurs in patients with hypothermia in whom prolonged cardiac arrest can be reversed after partial rewarming.

Prevention of Cardiac Arrest

Prevention of cardiac arrest is a laudable but difficult goal. Avoidance of certain precipitating factors may reduce the incidence of this situation. Common metabolic precipitating factors include hypokalemia, hyperkalemia, and hypomagnesemia. Although it makes good sense to treat and try to prevent these precipitating factors, prophylactic therapy may not be of benefit. The recent large studies of magnesium usage in patients with acute myocardial infarction showed no benefit from prophylactic administration of magnesium. Because certain drugs can be precipitating factors, excessive blood levels of these drugs should be avoided. Adequate blood levels of certain drugs such as digitalis and antiarrhythmic agents may reduce the incidence of arrhythmias. However, many drugs have idiosyncratic reactions that may not be predictable. Many antiarrhythmic agents can precipitate cardiac arrest in normal therapeutic doses in some patients. Other drugs such as terfenadine (Seldane) and astemizole (Hismanal) may cause sudden death by prolonging the QT interval. Many other drugs may also be precipitating causes in some patients, but because of their complexity and the presence of comorbid conditions, it is difficult to predict some of these interactions.

Treating and preventing some of the causes of PEA can also reduce the incidence of cardiac arrest. Treatment of conditions such as hypovolemia, hypoxia, hypoventilation, cardiac tamponade, pneumothorax, hypothermia, hyperthermia, sepsis, thrombophlebitis, and cardiogenic shock may prevent a secondary cardiac arrest. Hence, good and efficient medical therapy of patients with any serious illness may reduce the incidence of cardiac arrest in a particular population.

Treatment of certain conditions in a patient with acute cardiac disease may also reduce the incidence of cardiac arrest. Patients with an acute myocardial infarction have a lower incidence of sudden cardiac death when they are treated by therapies that cause reperfusion such as thrombolytic therapy, coronary angioplasty, or coronary bypass surgery in the first few hours after an acute myocardial infarction. The earlier patients are reperfused, the lower the incidence of sudden cardiac death. Beta-adrenergic blocking agents have also been shown to reduce the incidence of sudden cardiac death; these are metoprolol (Lopressor), propranolol (Inderal), and timolol (Blocadren). Other beta-blocking agents have not been as effective, have been ineffective (those with ISA [intrinsic sympathomimetic activity]), or have not been studied.

Prevention of asystole may also be beneficial. Some

patients with bradycardia, most frequently Mobitz II or complete heart block, may have a cardiac arrest. Thus, pacing either transcutaneously or transvenously may be beneficial in patients with Mobitz II or complete heart block. Sinus bradycardia and Wenckebach or Mobitz I block rarely lead to cardiac arrest; treatment of these bradycardias is usually given to treat symptoms related to the bradycardia.

Ventricular ectopic activity presents a difficult challenge in trying to prevent cardiac arrest. Although ventricular ectopic activity increases the likelihood of ventricular fibrillation in patients with acute myocardial infarction, prophylactic therapy of ventricular ectopy has not improved survival. Meta-analysis of prophylactic lidocaine therapy in victims of acute myocardial infarctions revealed a tendency to do harm by increasing the incidence of asystole and PEA more than reducing deaths from ventricular fibrillation. The only form of ventricular ectopy for which there is evidence of benefit is sustained ventricular tachycardia. Sustained ventricular tachycardia should be treated by cardioversion or antiarrhythmic therapy.

Aside from acute situations, there is some evidence that certain factors may reduce the incidence of cardiac arrest. Because most patients with sudden cardiac death have coronary artery disease, prevention of cardiac artery disease can also prevent sudden death. Hence, treating lipid abnormalities, ceasing smoking, treating hypertension, exercising routinely, reducing stress, and controlling diabetes and weight may help to reduce the incidence of sudden cardiac death by primarily or secondarily preventing coronary artery disease. Aspirin therapy may also reduce the incidence of events. Beta-blocking agents taken by patients who have had an acute myocardial infarction and possibly those with other coronary artery disease syndromes may also reduce the incidence of sudden cardiac death. Angiotensin-converting enzyme (ACE) inhibitors have also been shown to reduce the risk in persons with reduced ejection fractions or congestive heart failure.

Antiarrhythmic agents have not been shown to reduce the incidence of sudden cardiac death. In fact, antiarrhythmic agents may reduce ventricular ectopy only to increase the risk of sudden cardiac death. Patients who have sustained ventricular tachycardia or have been resuscitated from a cardiac arrest should be evaluated to see whether they may benefit from an automatic implantable cardioverter-defibrillator (AICD) with or without antiarrhythmic activity. Electrophysiologic testing may help in making this decision. Other high-risk patients may also benefit. However, there is no agreement on exactly what constitutes "high risk" other than the presence of sustained ventricular tachycardia or ventricular fibrillation occurring outside of the first 24 hours of an acute myocardial infarction.

ATRIAL FIBRILLATION

method of
GERALD V. NACCARELLI, M.D.
University of Texas Medical School at Houston
Houston, Texas

Atrial fibrillation is the most common pathologic cardiac tachyarrhythmia. Over 1 million persons are affected in the United States. The incidence of atrial fibrillation increases with age, rising from 0.05% at age 25 to 30 to more than 5% of patients over 69 years old. Atrial fibrillation may exist in either the chronic or paroxysmal form. Prognostically, the presence of atrial fibrillation is associated with a fivefold increased risk of morbidity, a twofold increase in mortality, and an increased incidence of embolic stroke. Although atrial fibrillation may be asymptomatic, it usually causes symptoms such as palpitations, dizziness, weakness or syncope. In patients with systolic or diastolic dysfunction, loss of atrioventricular (AV) synchrony may be associated with a decrease in cardiac output and a worsening of congestive heart failure.

ETIOLOGY

Hypertensive heart disease, coronary artery disease, rheumatic heart disease, cardiomyopathy, and sick sinus syndrome are the most common causes of associated conditions in patients with atrial fibrillation. Lone or idiopathic atrial fibrillation is one of the most common findings in patients presenting to an office-based clinician. Other common causes are listed in Table 1.

EVALUATION

A history and physical examination may help in diagnosing an associated condition that is responsible for the arrhythmia. The presence of an irregularly irregular pulse warrants an electrocardiogram to confirm the diagnosis of the arrhythmia. Echocardiography may be used to confirm the presence or absence of organic heart disease and assess left atrial size and left ventricular function. An electrocardiogram may aid in the diagnosis of the arrhythmia and screen for cardiac hypertrophy or old myocardial infarctions. A Holter monitor, stress test, and even recorders may be useful for documenting paroxysmal arrhythmias, assessing the ventricular response, and screening for other arrhythmias or conduction disturbances.

TABLE 1. **Causes of Atrial Fibrillation**

Hypertensive cardiovascular disease
Coronary artery disease
Rheumatic mitral valve disease (mitral stenosis or regurgitation)
Cardiomyopathy (dilated or hypertrophic)
Congestive heart failure
Tachycardia-bradycardia (sick sinus syndrome)
Post-thoracotomy
Hyperthyroidism
Pericarditis
Congential heart disease
Idiopathic (lone)
Wolff-Parkinson-White syndrome
Alcohol, toxins, caffeine
Pulmonary embolism

TREATMENT

In all patients an attempt should be made to treat the underlying cause (e.g., thyrotoxicosis) as part of the acute and chronic treatment for the arrhythmia. Treatment strategies for atrial fibrillation include (1) rate control, (2) prevention and maintenance of sinus rhythm, and (3) antiembolic therapy. In the acute situation, rate control can be achieved with intravenous digoxin, esmolol, propranolol, metoprolol, diltiazem, or verapamil (see Table 2 for doses). Although loading with intravenous digoxin may be the safest initial therapy, rate control may be delayed for several hours. During loading, signs of digitalis toxicity, such as a very slow ventricular response or regularization secondary to complete AV block and an accelerated junction rhythm, should be avoided. Intravenous diltiazem and verapamil have the advantage of slowing the ventricular response by 25% within 3 minutes of administration and may give partial rate control for up to several hours. However, because of their negative inotropic potential, the calcium channel and beta-blocking agents must be used with caution in patients with abnormal left ventricular function or hypotension. Esmolol, verapamil, and diltiazem can all be given as continuous intravenous infusions if continued subacute rate control is needed.

About 50% of patients who present with new-onset atrial fibrillation convert to sinus rhythm spontaneously within 12 to 24 hours even if no active therapy is given. However, therapy specifically aimed at medical conversion includes intravenous procainamide or oral quinidine, procainamide, disopyramide, flecainide, propafenone, sotalol, or amiodarone. Oral therapy may take days to reach steady state. Asymptomatic patients with long-standing atrial fibrillation (more than 1 year's duration) or a large left atrial size (greater than 5.0 cm) or those with acute processes such as thyrotoxicosis should be treated with rate control and antiembolic drugs because long-term successful maintenance of sinus rhythm by Type I or III antiarrhythmic agents is unlikely.

If chemical cardioversion is ineffective, direct current (DC) cardioversion should be attempted. Unless the patient has rapid rates and is hemodynamically unstable, this procedure should be performed with the help of an anesthesiologist. Common intravenous anesthetic drugs used for cardioversion include methohexital (Brevital), etomidate (Amidate), and propofol (Diptivan). We rarely apply shocks of less than 100 to 200 joules in this situation. If ineffective, we apply 300 to 400 joules before abandoning this approach. DC cardioversion should be performed carefully, synchronizing the shock to the QRS complex and using an intravenous line and adequate airway protection.

Fewer than 60% of patients remain in sinus rhythm after cardioversion. Therefore, chronic oral prophylactic therapy is often required, and antiarrhythmic doses or agents may need to be altered owing to inefficacy or adverse effects. Depending on the patient's history of organic heart disease, left ventricular function, or other concomitant conditions, we usually choose one of the following for chronic maintenance of sinus rhythm: quinidine, procainamide, disopyramide, flecainide, propafenone, or sotalol. In patients with refractory arrhythmia, low-dose amiodarone is commonly used. Amiodarone may be effective in treating up to 60% of patients in whom Type I antiarrhythmic agents have failed to control the arrhythmia. When using these drugs, a knowledge of drug interactions (e.g., digoxin-quinidine, digoxine-amiodarone) is helpful to achieve proper dose titration. Type I and III antiarrhythmic agents may be associated with subjective end-organ or proarrhythmic effects such as torsades de pointes. Several studies suggest that some of these agents may be

TABLE 2. **Pharmacologic Therapies of Atrial Arrhythmias**

Drug	Loading Dose	Maintenance Dose‡
Agents that Control Ventricular Response		
Digoxin	0.75–1.0 mg IV 0.75–1.5 mg PO	0.125–0.25 mg (PO or IV) qod–qd
Propranolol (Inderal)	0.15–0.20 mg/kg IV	40–160 mg PO qd
Esmolol (Brevibloc)	500 μg/kg/min IV	50–300 μg/kg/min IV
Metoprolol* (Lopressor)	5 mg IV	50–200 mg PO qd
Verapamil (Isoptin)	5–10 mg IV	120–360 mg PO qd
Diltiazem (Cardizem)	0.25 mg/kg IV	0.005 mg/kg/min IV§ 90–300 mg PO qd
Agents that Restore and Maintain Sinus Rhythm		
Propranolol†	0.15–20 mg/kg IV	40–160 mg PO qd
Procainamide*† (Pronestyl)	10–15 mg/kg IV	2000–4000 mg PO qd
Quinidine†		800–1600 mg PO qd
Disopyramide*† (Norpace)		400–800 mg PO qd
Flecainide (Tambocor)		100–300 mg PO qd
Propafenone* (Rythmol)		450–900 mg PO qd
Amiodarone* (Cordarone)	800–1600 mg PO qd	200–400 mg PO qd
Sotalol* (Betapace)		160–480 mg PO qd

*Not FDA approved for treatment of SVT.
†Sustained release formulations available.
‡Total daily maintenance doses taken one, two, three or four times a day, depending on formulation.
§Exceeds dosage recommended by the manufacturer.

associated with enhanced drug-induced mortality, especially if organic heart disease and left ventricular dysfunction are present. Dosing should usually be performed under telemetry control in the hospital, especially in sicker patients with significant organic heart disease. Based on the results of the Cardiac Arrhythmia Suppression Trial (CAST) trial, flecainide should be avoided in post–myocardial infarction patients. In patients not controlled with the drugs just listed, chronic rate control and antiembolic therapy should be considered.

Because atrial fibrillation often occurs paroxysmally, a patient who reverts spontaneously to sinus rhythm after only one attack can be treated only with antiembolic drugs as long as the presenting ventricular response is slow enough to be hemodynamically stable. If and when the patient develops frequent paroxysms, preventive therapy can be initiated.

NONPHARMACOLOGIC THERAPEUTIC APPROACHES

In some patients rate control or suppression of atrial fibrillation cannot be achieved. Rate control may be a problem in patients with congestive heart failure that limits the chronic use of large doses of oral beta-blocking and calcium channel agents. Some of these patients may need to be referred to an electrophysiologist, who can perform radiofrequency catheter ablation of the AV junction. With this procedure, radiofrequency current (electrocautery) is delivered through an electrode catheter tip to transect the AV junction electrically, thus causing complete heart block; the patient therefore remains in atrial fibrillation with a junctional escape rhythm. A ventricular-demand rate-responsive (VVIR) pacemaker is usually inserted in such patients to provide a reliable escape rhythm and chronotropic competence (the ability to increase heart rate with exertion).

Recently, the MAZE operation has been performed in several hundred patients with refractory atrial fibrillation. This procedure consists of multiple atrial incisions and suturing, which eliminate the atria's ability to allow micro-reentrant circuits and thus prevents atrial fibrillation. This procedure should be reserved for symptomatic patients with medically refractory arrhythmias. Research is currently ongoing to develop an implantable atrial defibrillator that can be used to terminate atrial fibrillation spells in refractory patients in the near future.

PREVENTION

Prevention of atrial fibrillation may be difficult. However, control of hypertension and risk factors for coronary artery disease as well as early thrombolytic therapy to minimize myocardial infarction size may be some practical methods of achieving this goal. Insertion of atrial-ventricular instead of ventricular pacemakers has lowered the incidence of atrial fibrillation in patients with sick sinus syndrome. Prophylactic use of beta blockers prior to open heart surgery has lowered the incidence of post-thoracotomy atrial fibrillation.

ANTIEMBOLIC THERAPY

Patients with atrial fibrillation have an increased risk of thromboembolic events and embolic strokes. The risk is highest in patients with organic heart disease, especially rheumatic heart disease and cardiomyopathy (hypertrophic, dilated, or ischemic). These patients should be chronically anticoagulated with warfarin to 1.3 to 1.6 times the control value. Even patients with nonvalvular atrial fibrillation have up to a 5% annual incidence of peripheral embolic events. Many recent trials have demonstrated that low-dose warfarin (1.3 to 1.6 times control) is effective in reducing this risk, although the results are less impressive in patients older than 75 years. In patients with nonvalvular disease, one aspirin a day also seems to reduce embolic events compared to placebo in controlled trials. However, aspirin appears to be less useful in patients older than 75 years. Low-risk patients who may not need chronic anticoagulation include young patients with nonvalvular, idiopathic atrial fibrillation, especially if there is no history of hypertension, cardiac chamber enlargement, or a previous embolic event.

The risk of thromboembolic events following cardioversion of atrial fibrillation ranges from 1 to 5% in nonanticoagulated patients compared to 1% in patients on warfarin. In patients who have a history of atrial fibrillation lasting more than several days to weeks, warfarin therapy for 4 weeks is recommended prior to medical or DC cardioversion. Recent studies suggest that transesophageal echocardiography (TEE) may be useful in screening patients at low risk for acute embolic events. Even if cardioversion is successful, antiembolic therapy should be continued for at least 1 month after cardioversion because atrial contractility may take days to recover, and atrial fibrillation may recur.

ATRIAL FIBRILLATION AND WOLFF-PARKINSON-WHITE SYNDROME

In patients who present acutely with rapid atrial fibrillation and intermittent pre-excited conduction along an accessory pathway, AV node–blocking agents such as verapamil, digoxin, and beta blockers should be avoided. These drugs may block induction to the AV node, thus preselecting accessory pathway conduction. In addition, drug-induced hypotension may accelerate the pre-excited ventricular response. If the patient is hemodynamically stable, intravenous procainamide can be carefully given at a loading dose of 10 to 15 mg per kg at a rate of 25 mg per minute. Acute administration of procainamide may slow conduction. If the arrhythmia is unstable, synchronized DC cardioversion is the acute method of choice. In the chronic setting, drugs such as quinidine, flecainide, and propafenone may be used to suppress atrial fibrillation and slow or block conduction down the accessory pathway. Pharmacologic and nonpharmacologic options are best prescribed with the help of an electrophysiologic study. Often intracardiac map-guided radiofrequency catheter ablation (which has replaced map-guided surgical resection) is performed to eliminate accessory pathway conduction and the need for chronic antiarrhythmic therapy.

PREMATURE BEATS

method of
PRAKASH C. DEEDWANIA, M.D.
Veterans Administration Medical Center
Fresno, California

Premature beats result from electrical depolarizations of myocardium that occur earlier than the sinus beat. Premature beats have been referred to by a variety of names, including premature contractions, premature complexes, ectopic beats, and early depolarizations. Although no single term is ideal, most electrophysiologists refer to them as premature complexes because although the term ectopic beat denotes the abnormal site of origin of the depolarization, it does not necessarily require it to be premature, and in some cases an ectopic rhythm may indeed occur as an escape phenomenon.

Premature beats are the most common form of cardiac arrhythmia encountered in clinical practice. Although most premature beats usually occur as a result of enhanced automaticity, other electrophysiologic mechanisms, including reentry and triggered activity, may also play a role. Based on the corresponding site of origin, premature electrical depolarizations are called premature atrial complexes (PACs), premature junctional complexes (PJCs), and premature ventricular complexes (PVCs).

PREMATURE ATRIAL COMPLEXES

PACs are the most common form of atrial arrhythmias and can originate at any site in the atria. The exact morphology of the atrial activation (P wave) varies depending on the site of origin of the PAC. A careful and systematic examination of the electrocardiographic features of PACs can usually distinguish them from PVCs.

Electrocardiographic Features

The cardinal features of PACs include their prematurity with reference to the sinus beats, an abnormal P wave morphology, and, in most cases, a QRS morphology similar to that of sinus beats. The P wave morphology of the PAC generally differs from the sinus P wave unless the premature complex is originating in the high right atrial area adjacent to the sinus node, in which case it might be difficult to distinguish a PAC from sinus arrhythmia. Although sinus arrhythmias are generally phasic in nature, being influenced by the respiratory cycle, this feature is helpful in differentiating sinus arrhythmia from a high right atrial PAC only when the PACs are frequent and repetitive. When the PAC occurs early in the diastolic phase, the P wave may not be obvious on the surface electrocardiogram (ECG) because it is often hidden in the preceding T wave and is evident only on careful observation for the notched or peaked T wave. In such cases, if the PAC is too premature, it may also fail to conduct to the ventricles if it reaches the atrioventricular (AV) node when it is refractory owing to conduction of the preceding sinus impulse. Such nonconducted PACs are called blocked PACs and are important because they may be thought to be instances of AV block. Such erroneous interpretations can, however, be avoided by simply remembering a common rule of thumb, which requires normal successive P-P intervals for all sinus beats, including the interval for blocked P waves, before considering a diagnosis of AV block. Although most PACs have a normal or prolonged PR interval, the relationship of the PAC to the subsequent QRS complex depends on the site of origin of the PAC and the prematurity index. For example, a PAC originating in the lower atrial area near the AV node generally has a shorter PR interval, whereas a PAC that is very premature and originates in the upper left atrial area may have a longer than usual PR interval. In general, the PR interval of a PAC is inversely related to its prematurity.

Because most PACs are able to depolarize the sinus node, they can usually reset the sinus automaticity, and therefore the subsequent pause following most PACs is generally less than compensatory because the sinus node fires earlier than expected. In this case, the measurement of the P-P interval between the sinus P wave preceding the PAC and the P wave following the PAC is generally less than twice the basic sinus cycle length. In contrast, a full compensatory pause is often observed in conjunction with PVCs. In some cases, the PAC may collide with the sinus impulse in the perinodal tissue and thus fails to reset the sinus node, thereby resulting in a full compensatory pause.

In general, the electrical depolarization below the AV node is normal with a PAC and results in a normal QRS complex. Aberrant conduction, however, may be encountered when the PAC reaches the infranodal tissue during the period when it is still refractory. Most commonly, the aberrant conduction usually occurs when a short-coupled PAC follows a long pause in patients with sinus bradycardia (long-short cycle). This is commonly referred to as the Ashman phenomenon and usually results in a right bundle branch block pattern.

Clinical Features

Although PACs can occur in normal individuals of all ages, they are quite infrequent. Their frequency increases with age, with as many as 50 to 70% of the elderly experiencing occasional PACs. Some elderly individuals without organic heart disease may have frequent PACs, occasional atrial bigeminy, or two to three PACs in a row. Whether the increased frequency of PACs in these individuals is secondary to senile amyloidosis or is due to diastolic dysfunction secondary to aging-related changes in the heart is not known. PACs are extremely common in patients with heart disease and in patients with acute as well as chronic respiratory failure. The frequency of PACs can increase markedly during periods of acute febrile illness, shock states, and metabolic disorders, especially hyperthyroidism or increased catecholamine levels. The use of excessive caffeine, alcohol, and tobacco can also increase the frequency of PACs. In patients with acute myocardial infarction (MI), frequent PACs are usually precursors of atrial fibrillation and result from decompensated left ventricular failure.

In general, PACs are usually benign except when they are a marker of an underlying cardiopulmonary disorder. The major clinical importance of PACs is related to the increased risk of atrial tachyarrhythmias in patients with a prior established history of such arrhythmias. As indicated earlier, in rare instances the blocked PACs may be confused as episodes of AV block; however, careful examination of the ECG features described easily establishes the correct diagnosis.

Treatment

Correction of the underlying structural cardiopulmonary disorder and other precipitating factors is usually all that is needed. No specific treatment is generally required in most patients because PACs are usually benign except in patients with a history of recurrent atrial tachyarrhythmias, e.g., atrial fibrillation. In such patients, specific treatment may be indicated and could include digoxin, a beta-blocker, or the calcium channel-blocking agent verapamil. Recent studies have shown that verapamil (Isoptin, Calan) is quite effective in patients with frequent PACs and multifocal atrial tachycardia in the setting of acute or chronic ventilatory insufficiency. In patients who are at risk of recurrent atrial fibrillation, treatment with type 1a antiarrhythmic agents may be required, but these should be used only when absolutely necessary because of the increased risk of proarrhythmia, especially in high-risk patients with recurrent ischemia or heart failure.

PREMATURE JUNCTIONAL COMPLEXES

PJCs are rarely seen in normal individuals and are infrequently encountered even in patients with organic heart disease.

Electrocardiographic Features

The ECG characteristics of PJCs are distinct from those of PACs in that the P wave is usually inverted in the inferior leads (II, III, and avf) because of retrograde conduction from the ectopic foci in the junctional area. The second feature of PJCs is that the PR interval is almost always shorter than the normal PR interval because of the proximity of ectopic foci to the AV node and bundle of His. In most cases, the P wave may not even be visible on surface ECGs because it lies hidden within the QRS complex. Rarely, the P wave may precede the QRS complex when the ectopic impulse traverses the atria before depolarizing the ventricle. In general, the infranodal conduction of PJCs is normal, and thus, the QRS morphology of the conducted PJCs is similar to that noted during sinus rhythm. When the PJC is closely coupled to the preceding sinus beat, aberrant conduction may occur if the impulse traverses the bundle branch during the refractory period. Because in many instances there is no obvious P wave accompanying a PJC, aberrantly conducted PJCs may be hard to differentiate from PVCs.

In some instances when PJCs occur when the AV node and the infranodal conduction system are both refractory, the PJC may encounter both retrograde and antegrade block for impulse propagation. In such situations, there will be no P wave or QRS complex related to the PJC. Although the ectopic impulse is invisible on the surface ECG, it may penetrate a portion of the conduction system and thus make it partially or completely refractory for conduction of the subsequent sinus impulse. This is manifest as a sudden prolongation of the subsequent PR interval in cases of partial refractoriness or as an episode of "pseudo AV block" due to the blocked sinus beat if the infranodal tissue is unable to conduct the sinus impulse. Thus, even though some PJCs might have no surface ECG complexes, their presence can be suspected by their influence on the conduction of the following sinus beat due to the electrophysiologic phenomenon of "concealed conduction."

Clinical Features

PJCs are usually not seen in normal persons and are rarely encountered in cardiac patients except in those with digitalis intoxication. In patients with digitalis toxicity, PJCs may lead to junctional tachycardia that occasionally results in palpitations, but they are rarely associated with hemodynamic compromise. Because in some cases concealed conduction of PJCs may result in periods of varying degrees of pseudo AV block, it is clinically important to recognize their presence to avoid undue concern and inappropriate pacemaker implantation.

PREMATURE VENTRICULAR COMPLEXES

PVCs are the most common form of arrhythmia and are encountered frequently in both healthy individuals and patients with a variety of cardiac disorders.

Electrocardiographic Features

PVCs occur as a result of premature depolarization of the ventricles due to ectopic foci in the ventricular myocardium or Purkinje fibers. In general, PVCs result in wide QRS complexes with the T wave axis usually opposite to that of the QRS. In the great majority of cases, PVCs do not conduct retrogradely and thus do not result in a distinct P wave. The sinus beats may, however, continue uninterrupted and thus manifest as an instance of AV dissociation in conjunction with PVCs. For the same reason, because PVCs usually do not conduct retrogradely and depolarize the atrium and the sinus node, there is usually a full compensatory pause that is clearly in contrast to the partial compensatory pause generally seen with PACs. In patients with slow sinus rates, however, interpolated PVCs may occur. If the ectopic foci for PVCs are located high in the His-Purkinje system, the resulting premature complexes may have a narrow QRS morphology similar to that seen during sinus rhythm. Additionally, if the PVCs occur rather late, in close proximity to the sinus impulse, there may also be a narrow complex QRS because of fusion between the normal depolarization due to the sinus impulse and the abnormal activation sequence due to ectopic foci. In the instance of fusion beats, there will be a normal P wave preceding the QRS; the PR interval will be shorter, and the QRS morphology may be only partially altered and in some cases may give an appearance of intermittent bundle branch block or pre-excitation (Wolff-Parkinson-White syndrome).

Based on the morphologic features of PVCs, they have been classified as uniform or multiform and also are referred to as unifocal or multifocal. It has also been recommended that PVCs be classified according to their coupling interval with the preceding sinus beat; PVCs with a short coupling interval near or on the previous T wave have been described as showing the R-on-T phenomenon or, alternatively, they may have long coupling intervals. Based on the underlying electrophysiologic mechanism responsible for PVCs, the coupling interval may be fixed as in reentrant beats or variable as seen with ventricular parasystole. PVCs may also have a repetitive pattern such as bigeminy, trigeminy, and so on, or they may occur in pairs. It is now believed that the repetitive pattern of PVCs, such as couplets or triplets, is prognostically more important than the frequency of PVCs.

Clinical Features

PVCs are recorded frequently in normal individuals and, like PACs, their frequency increases with age. In patients without organic heart disease or prior evidence of sustained ventricular tachyarrhythmias, the mere presence of frequent PVCs is not considered prognostically important. It should, however, be noted that individual exceptions do exist, and the clinician is advised to evaluate a given patient accordingly. In patients with organic heart disease, PVCs are the most common form of arrhythmia and carry significant prognostic importance, especially in survivors of acute MI and patients with recurrent ischemia and advanced heart failure. It has been well established during the past 2 decades that frequent PVCs during the acute phase of an MI are associated with an increased risk of sustained ventricular arrhythmias in the initial 48 hours, but they do not predict long-term outcome or risk of arrhythmic events in the post-infarction period. Although as many as 80 to 90% of patients with chronic heart failure have frequent PVCs, the results of several recent studies have shown that only the presence of nonsustained ventricular tachycardia (NSVT) at a rate greater than 100 beats per minute is strongly predictive of an increased risk of sudden cardiac death in these patients. This is clearly in contrast to the findings in post-MI patients, in whom several large clinical trials have previously shown that more than 10 PVCs per hour are predictive of a poor prognosis and an increased risk of death due to arrhythmia. More recently, it has been shown that in patients receiving thrombolytic therapy an increase in the frequency of PVCs, particularly runs of NSVT, is generally short lived and represents a sign of myocardial reperfusion.

Overall, the association between PVCs and an increased risk of ventricular tachyarrhythmias and sudden cardiac death appears to be related not only to the frequency and complexity of PVCs but also to the severity of the underlying structural heart disease. For example, a patient with mitral valve prolapse and frequent PVCs has a relatively lower risk of arrhythmic events than a patient with advanced heart failure who has repetitive PVCs and NSVT. Proper evaluation of the risk of PVCs has become more crucial now than ever before because most currently available therapeutic choices are not suitable and have the potential to cause serious adverse reactions in patients with advanced cardiac disorders.

Treatment

Traditionally, it has been a common practice to administer intravenous lidocaine routinely in an effort to suppress PVCs during the initial phase of acute MI; however, some recent data suggest that routine use of lidocaine is not necessary and should be avoided because of the risk of side effects, especially CNS side effects in the elderly. Based on accurate and early identification of ventricular tachyarrhythmias in monitored settings in coronary care units and an aggressive treatment strategy for patients with ventricular arrhythmias, it has been stated that the prophylactic use of lidocaine is generally not beneficial. It has also been demonstrated that routine use of prophylactic lidocaine during the acute or healing phase of an MI does not alter the overall mortality in patients with acute MI.

Although it is now well established that frequent PVCs (≥10 per hour) in survivors of acute MI predict an increased risk of arrhythmic death and overall cardiac mortality, recent studies have demonstrated that suppression of PVCs with most currently available antiarrhythmic drugs is not beneficial in reducing this risk. In the Cardiac Arrhythmia Suppression

Trials (CAST I and II), it was clearly demonstrated that, compared with placebo, treatment with class 1c antiarrhythmic drugs (which primarily work by slowing conduction) was associated with an increased risk of arrhythmic death despite adequate suppression of PVCs. These findings, as well as those from several other clinical trials, indicate that although frequent PVCs may be a marker for adverse events, suppression of PVCs does not favorably influence the associated increased risk of death. Whether newer antiarrhythmic drugs, class III agents, which work primarily by their effect on cardiac repolarization, would be useful remains a question for future clinical trials. For now, it is generally recommended that prophylactic suppression of PVCs with currently available antiarrhythmic drugs is not advisable for most patients primarily because of the increased risk of proarrhythmic effects associated with these drugs. In the occasional patient who is disabled by the annoying symptoms due to PVCs, an initial trial of beta-blocker therapy may be recommended and appears to be effective in some patients. Sotalol is a unique new antiarrhythmic agent that has combined beta-blocking (class II) as well as class III properties. Although not yet proved in clinical trials, the use of sotalol (Betapace), could be safe and effective in patients with symptomatic PVCs.

HEART BLOCK

method of
STEVEN M. MARKOWITZ, M.D., and
BRUCE B. LERMAN, M.D.
The New York Hospital–Cornell University Medical College
New York, New York

Heart block refers to an interruption of the orderly conduction of impulses from one part of the heart to another. Under normal circumstances, impulses originate in the sinus node and propagate through atrial myocardium to the atrioventricular (AV) node. Generally, conduction slows as impulses traverse the AV node, allowing for a delay between atrial and ventricular systole. Impulses exit the AV node through the bundle of His, which conducts rapidly and penetrates the fibrous skeleton of the heart. In the ventricular septum, the His bundle branches into a complex network that can be represented as three divisions: the right bundle, the left anterior fascicle, and the left posterior fascicle. The terminal portions of the bundle branches form the Purkinje network, which activates the endocardial surface of both ventricles.

Block in impulse propagation may occur at any point within this conduction system. The cellular mechanisms responsible for heart block and slowed conduction are the topics of active investigation. Simple cell death in the conduction system and replacement with fibrous tissue may account for conduction block. But most instances of heart block occur in viable cells that are unable to propagate impulses normally. In "tachycardia"-dependent heart block, for example, conduction block occurs in viable cells only *above* a critical heart rate. Under these circumstances, an impulse reaches cells when they are still refractory from the preceding beat. In "bradycardia"-dependent heart block, conduction block occurs *below* a critical heart rate. The mechanism of this form of heart block is more complex. For example, a group of cells in the region of the AV node or His-Purkinje system may undergo spontaneous phase 4 depolarization owing to a slow rate, and are therefore activated from a less negative membrane potential, resulting in impaired conduction.

SINOATRIAL BLOCK AND SINUS PAUSE

Sinoatrial block refers to an interruption of impulse propagation from the sinus node to the atrium. Sinus pause refers to the slowing or arrest of sinus node activity.

ECG Features. Both sinus exit block and sinus pause can be identified by the absence of a normal P wave. In sinus exit block, the length of the pause is a multiple of the P-P interval during sinus rhythm, reflecting the fact that automaticity in the sinus node is preserved but conduction to the atrium is blocked. In sinus pause, the length of the pause is not a multiple of the P-P interval in sinus rhythm.

Pathogenesis. Sinus node dysfunction may occur in patients with primary conduction system disease ("sick sinus syndrome"), myocardial infarction, myocarditis, drug toxicity, or hypervagotonia.

Clinical Features. Prolonged episodes of atrial asystole, in the absence of an adequate escape rhythm, may result in lightheadedness or syncope.

Treatment. In patients with symptomatic sinus pauses or sinus exit block not due to a reversible cause, permanent pacing is recommended. In cases of drug toxicity, withdrawal of the responsible agent is advised prior to determining the need for permanent pacing.

ATRIOVENTRICULAR BLOCK

AV block refers to interrupted conduction between the atria and the ventricles. The causes of AV block are listed in Table 1.

First-Degree AV Block

ECG Features. First-degree AV block is defined as a PR interval greater than 0.20 second in adults.

Pathogenesis. In this condition, conduction from the atria to the ventricles is slowed but not blocked. The site of slowing cannot be inferred from the surface electrocardiogram. With normal intraventricular conduction (a narrow QRS complex), the responsible site may be within the sinoatrial junction, the atria, the AV node, or the His bundle. With bundle branch block, the site of slowing may be in any of these

TABLE 1. **Causes of Atrioventricular Block**

Congenital
Hypervagotonia
Electrolyte disorder
Drugs
Digoxin
Beta blockers
Calcium channel blockers
Antiarrhythmics
Coronary artery disease
Ischemia
Infarction
Degenerative disease
Lev's disease
Lenegre's disease
Myocarditis
Valvular heart disease
Calcific aortic stenosis
Mitral annular calcification
Post-cardiac surgery
Congenital heart disease
Aortic valve replacement
Infiltrative heart disease
Sarcoidosis
Amyloidosis
Hemochromatosis
Infection
Endocarditis/valve ring abscess
Lyme disease
Chagas' disease
Myxedema
Collagen vascular disease
Polymyositis
Muscular dystrophy
Radiation exposure

structures as well as in a diseased bundle branch or fascicle.

Clinical Features. Isolated first-degree AV block does not cause symptoms. The clinical presentation is related to the underlying heart disease.

Treatment. No intervention is required for first-degree AV block. If first-degree AV block is secondary to a drug, withdrawal of the drug may be indicated if clinically appropriate. First-degree AV block in the setting of bundle branch block is discussed subsequently.

Second-Degree AV Block

In second-degree AV block, most atrial impulses are conducted to the ventricles, but occasional beats are blocked before the ventricles are depolarized. In electrocardiographic terms, most P waves are followed by QRS complexes, but occasional P waves are nonconducted and therefore are not followed by ventricular activation.

Second-Degree AV Block—Mobitz Type I

ECG Features. In second-degree AV block (Mobitz Type I), there is progressive prolongation of the PR interval terminating in a nonconducted P wave. Each sequence is called a Wenckebach cycle and may be characterized by the ratio of atrial beats to conducted beats (e.g., 3:2 or 4:3). This gives rise to the typical pattern of "grouped beating." Frequently, the R-R interval progressively shortens prior to the dropped beat. A clue in diagnosing Mobitz Type I block is comparison of the PR interval of the last conducted beat with the PR interval beginning the next cycle; in Mobitz Type I block, the last conducted beat has a longer PR interval than the first beat of a new cycle.

Pathogenesis. The Wenckebach phenomenon is a normal feature of the AV node. Thus Mobitz Type I block usually localizes the site of block to the AV node, above the bundle of His. Rarely, this type of block occurs within the His bundle or below.

Mobitz Type I AV block can occur with very rapid supraventricular rates. It is seen in the setting of hypervagotonia (e.g., inferior myocardial infarction). Drugs that slow conduction through the AV node, such as digoxin, beta blockers, and calcium channel blockers, may also provoke this type of AV block.

Clinical Features. Most episodes of Type I AV block carry no particular significance, especially in the absence of underlying heart disease. Clinical manifestations depend on the resulting heart rate. If severely bradycardic, patients may present with signs and symptoms of low cardiac output or congestive heart failure.

Treatment. Asymptomatic patients with Mobitz Type I block do not require treatment. For symptomatic episodes of Mobitz Type I block, atropine (1 to 2 mg intravenously) is useful as a first-line agent, particularly in the presence of inferior myocardial infarction. A temporary pacemaker may be required for short-term hemodynamic support. Usually these episodes are self-limited and require no long-term therapy. Occasionally, patients may manifest recurrent symptoms and require permanent pacing.

Second-Degree AV Block—Mobitz Type II

ECG Features. This form of AV block is characterized by abrupt failure of AV conduction. Occasional P waves are blocked, whereas conducted beats exhibit constant PR intervals. Typically, the QRS complexes of the conducted beats are wide, reflecting infranodal conduction system disease.

Pathogenesis. The site of block is typically within the bundle of His or below. Type II heart block may occur in the presence of anterior myocardial infarction and reflects extensive damage to the conduction system in the anterior septum. Type II block may also occur with Type Ia and Ic antiarrhythmic drugs, which slow conduction below the His bundle.

Clinical Features and Treatment. Type II block implies extensive disease of the infranodal conduction system and therefore confers a high risk of complete heart block. Symptomatic patients require permanent pacing. For asymptomatic patients with transient or permanent Type II block, permanent pacing is frequently advised.

Third-Degree (Complete) Heart Block

ECG Features. In complete AV block, the atria and ventricles exhibit independent electrical activity.

Thus, the P-P and R-R intervals are each regular, but the PR intervals vary, reflecting the loss of synchrony between the atria and ventricles. The escape focus determines the rate and characteristics of the ventricular rhythm. If the escape focus is within the AV junction, the ventricular complex is narrow with a rate of 50 to 60 beats per minute. If the escape rhythm originates below the His bundle in the Purkinje network or ventricular myocardium, the QRS complex is wide and slow. A key feature of complete heart block is that the atrial rate is *faster* than the ventricular rate. When the atrial rate is *slower* than the ventricular rate, heart block is not necessarily present. This latter situation is called AV dissociation without block. In this condition, an automatic infranodal focus drives the ventricles faster than the native atrial rhythm.

Pathogenesis. Complete AV block can occur in the AV node itself, in the His bundle, or below. When block occurs in the AV node or the His bundle, the escape rhythm is narrow and usually supports adequate cardiac output. When block occurs below the His bundle, the QRS complex is wide and the escape rhythm is slow.

Clinical Features. The presence of symptoms depends on the rate and stability of the escape rhythm. Patients with slow ventricular escape rhythms can present with fatigue, lightheadedness, syncope, altered mentation, congestive heart failure, or chest pain.

Treatment. The need for treatment depends on the presence of symptoms and the ventricular rate. In symptomatic patients, treatment with atropine (1 to 2 mg intravenously) may reverse complete heart block due to hypervagotonia. Isoproterenol (Isuprel) (2 to 6 μg/min) is utilized as a second-line agent but is contraindicated in patients with myocardial ischemia or infarction. Patients with unstable ventricular escape rhythms require permanent pacing.

Fascicular and Bundle Branch Block

Conduction may be blocked or slowed in any of the three fascicles that originate from the bundle of His. The 12-lead electrocardiogram is required to identify the sites of infra-Hisian block.

ECG Features. The electrocardiographic features of bundle branch and fascicular block are well described. The bundle branch blocks are characterized by wide QRS complexes (≥0.12 second). Right bundle branch block (RBBB) is distinguished by late activation of the right ventricle. In left bundle branch block (LBBB), the bulk of the left ventricle is depolarized late, and there is reversal of normal septal activation. In isolated left anterior fascicular block (LAFB) and left posterior fascicular block (LPFB), the QRS complex is narrow. Block in the left anterior fascicle results in late activation of the anterolateral wall of the left ventricle, whereas block in the left posterior fascicle results in late depolarization of the inferoposterior wall.

Bifascicular block refers to abnormal conduction in two fascicles. The most common combination is RBBB and LAFB. Less commonly, combined RBBB and LPFB are observed. The term trifascicular block refers to evidence of disease in all three fascicles. One example is alternating RBBB and LBBB. Another example is RBBB with alternating LAFB and LPFB. More commonly, trifascicular block is used to describe bifascicular block with first-degree AV block. Unfortunately, this last ECG pattern is not a good predictor of disease in all three fascicles because the prolonged PR interval may represent delay in the AV node or His bundle rather than the third fascicle.

Prognosis and Management. Most patients with bundle branch block have or develop underlying organic heart disease. The most common associated conditions are hypertension, coronary artery disease, and congestive heart failure. In addition, degenerative disease of the conduction system can cause this disturbance. Bundle branch block is associated with a higher incidence of syncope, sudden death, and cardiovascular mortality. Most of these deaths are related to the underlying cardiovascular disease and are secondary to myocardial infarction, congestive heart failure, and tachyarrhythmias. The incidence of high-grade heart block among patients with bifascicular block is increased compared to that in the general population, but the rate remains relatively low, approximately 1 to 1.5% per year. Rarely is complete heart block a cause of death in this population. When complete heart block does develop, the site of block is not necessarily below the His bundle; in half of patients, heart block occurs in the AV node. The role of invasive electrophysiologic studies has been investigated in identifying those patients with bundle branch block who are at high risk for future events. A prolonged HV (His to ventricular) interval is associated with a small increased risk of complete heart block and sudden cardiac death. But a prolonged HV interval also correlates with underlying organic heart disease; thus it is unclear whether the HV interval is indeed an independent predictor of future events. Pacing-induced block below the His bundle, a rare finding during electrophysiologic studies, also predicts future AV block.

In contrast to most patients with bundle branch block, there is a subset of young patients with RBBB who are free of underlying organic heart disease and have a favorable prognosis. Therefore, RBBB in young persons is generally not a sign of cardiovascular disease.

The patient with syncope and bundle branch block poses a difficult problem. In this population, syncope may be secondary to a tachyarrhythmia, and bradycardia cannot be assumed to be the cause of symptoms. In 20 to 40% of cases, ventricular tachycardia can be induced during electrophysiologic testing. In symptomatic patients with bundle branch block, a full electrophysiologic study is indicated, with measurement of sinus and AV nodal function as well as atrial and ventricular stimulation.

Prophylactic pacing of patients with chronic bifascicular block and prolonged HV intervals has not resulted in improved survival. Similarly, trifascicular block does not warrant prophylactic pacing. Permanent pacing is indicated for (1) bundle branch block complicated by symptomatic complete heart block and (2) bifascicular or trifascicular block with intermittent Type II second-degree AV block, even without symptoms. Relative but not universal indications for pacing include (1) bifascicular or trifascicular block with unexplained syncope and (2) bifascicular or trifascicular block with a markedly prolonged HV interval (>100 msec, normal 35 to 55 msec) or pacing-induced infra-Hisian block.

SPECIAL SITUATIONS

Myocardial Infarction and Heart Block

Blood Supply to the Conduction System. The blood supply of the AV node derives from the right coronary artery (RCA). The His bundle has a dual blood supply from the RCA and the left anterior descending (LAD). The right bundle and the left anterior fascicle, which both lie in the anterior septum, are supplied mainly by perforators from the LAD. The left posterior fascicle receives blood from the posterior descending artery and the LAD.

Inferior Myocardial Infarction. Inferior myocardial infarction (MI) may be complicated by block in the AV node, including first-degree AV block, second-degree AV block (Mobitz Type I), and complete heart block. In complete heart block, the escape rhythm is typically narrow, arising in the AV junction with a rate of 50 to 60 beats per minute. AV block occurring early after inferior infarction is often secondary to enhanced parasympathetic activity and is generally responsive to atropine. AV block that is atropine resistant is frequently due to the effects of adenosine (released during ischemia) on the AV node. Temporary pacing is rarely required in patients with inferior infarction because of stable escape rhythms that support adequate cardiac output. Complete heart block usually resolves within 1 to 2 weeks after inferior infarction. Infranodal block rarely occurs as a consequence of inferior MI.

Anterior Myocardial Infarction. Anterior infarction is associated with injury to the infranodal conduction system. Thus, anterior MI can be complicated by isolated fascicular block, bifascicular block, or trifascicular block, depending on the extent of myocardial damage. Complete heart block can develop abruptly without earlier stages of AV block; the escape rhythm may be unstable, and ventricular asystole may result. In anterior infarction, bundle branch block may be the only warning of impending complete heart block.

New bundle branch block complicating an acute anterior infarction carries a poor prognosis and is usually related to progressive pump failure. However, some patients with bundle branch block do not develop overt pump failure but instead develop high-grade AV block and death secondary to bradyarrhythmias. The most common bundle branch blocks complicating anterior infarction are LBBB and combined RBBB/LAFB. Combined RBBB/LPFB implies greater myocardial damage and a worse prognosis.

Several criteria have been identified that predict progression to high-grade or complete heart block. Patients with new bilateral bundle branch block (RBBB/LAFB, RBBB/LPFB, or alternating RBBB/LBBB), regardless of the PR interval, are at high risk for progressing to advanced AV block. Although no data have demonstrated improved survival, prophylactic temporary pacing is indicated for these subsets of patients. Prophylactic pacing has also been recommended for new LBBB and for new RBBB associated with first-degree AV block. Pacing for isolated RBBB remains controversial. As a rule, high-grade AV block (second- and third-degree AV block) also warrants temporary pacing.

Permanent pacing after myocardial infarction is indicated for patients with *persistent* high-grade AV block. Those patients who survive *transient* episodes of high-grade AV block and associated new bundle branch block also require long-term pacing. For patients with persistent bundle branch block in the *absence* of high-grade AV block, no survival benefit has been demonstrated with permanent pacing.

Bundle Branch Block and Noncardiac Surgery

In patients with chronic bifascicular or trifascicular block, the development of complete heart block with general anesthesia is very rare, and prophylactic pacing is not required for surgery.

TACHYCARDIAS

method of
MICHAEL R. GOLD, M.D., PH.D., and
ROBERT W. PETERS, M.D.
University of Maryland School of Medicine
Baltimore, Maryland

Tachycardia is broadly defined as any heart rhythm with a rate greater than 100 beats per minute. The specific rhythm disorders vary widely in their pathogenesis, mechanism, anatomic origin, and treatment. For instance, sinus tachycardia arises from the sinoatrial (SA) node and may be a normal physiologic response to exercise, whereas ventricular fibrillation is a life-threatening ventricular arrhythmia that requires immediate intervention. Yet both are examples of tachycardias.

The mechanisms underlying cardiac arrhythmias include reentry, enhanced automaticity, and triggered activity. Although these mechanisms are difficult to establish clinically, they have important implications for treatment. Reentrant arrhythmias such as ventricular tachycardia can be terminated by overdrive pacing or cardioversion, which has led to the frequent and successful use of the implantable defibrillator in the management of this disorder. Enhanced automaticity does not respond to pacing or cardioversion but usually requires pharmacologic suppression of the arrhythmic focus. Triggered activity is often due to drug effects such as digitalis toxicity and requires prompt discontinuation of the drug and possible reversal of its effects.

DIAGNOSIS

Before discussing specific tachycardias, a general approach to arrhythmias must be adopted. The diagnosis of an arrhythmia is often aided by a careful review of the electrocardiogram and the history and physical findings of the patient. Whenever possible a 12-lead electrocardiogram (ECG) should be obtained during the tachycardia and compared with previous ECGs. Often this will provide important clues to the origin of the arrhythmia. For instance, P waves preceding each QRS complex of the same morphology as in the basal state suggest sinus tachycardia. Atrioventricular (AV) dissociation during a wide-complex tachycardia strongly suggests ventricular tachycardia. Sometimes the diagnostic clues are present in only one or several leads, which is why a 12-lead ECG can be so important. This is often true of atrial flutter, in which flutter waves may be seen only in lead II or VI in many patients.

The previous medical history of the patient is often very useful in the evaluation of tachycardia. A history of myocardial infarction strongly predicts that a wide-complex tachycardia is ventricular tachycardia. An underlying pulmonary disorder is almost always present in patients with multifocal atrial tachycardia. Knowing that a patient has Wolff-Parkinson-White syndrome suggests that a regular tachycardia, whether narrow- or wide-complex, is an AV reciprocating tachycardia.

The treatment of all arrhythmias should begin by identifying any metabolic or pharmacologic causes or contributors to the tachycardia. Acidosis, hypoxia, hypokalemia, and hypomagnesemia can all lead to arrhythmias and should be promptly treated. The discontinuation of chronic beta-blocker therapy several days before initiation of a tachycardia suggests acute withdrawal as a contributing factor, whereas the development of torsades de pointes during treatment with a Type IA or III antiarrhythmic drug strongly suggests a proarrhythmic response to that agent.

The cornerstone of tachyarrhythmia treatment is the use of antiarrhythmic drugs. The most common grouping of these agents is the Vaughan-Williams classification. This classification, with examples and dosing ranges, is presented in Table 1. Missing from this classification scheme are several drugs commonly used in the treatment of supraventricular arrhythmias including digoxin (Lanoxin) and adenosine (Adenocard).

Nonpharmacologic therapy has become more important in the treatment of tachycardia because of the side effects, inefficacy, and proarrhythmias associated with drugs. Such therapies include catheter ablation, usually with radiofrequency energy, and implantable defibrillators.

Tachycardias are customarily divided into two main groups, ventricular and supraventricular, depending on the site of origin. Ventricular arrhythmias originate within the ventricular myocardium or ventricular specialized conduction system and are characterized by a prolonged (>120 msec) QRS complex, whereas supraventricular tachyarrhythmias originate within or above the AV junction and usually have a narrow QRS. The differentiation between ventricular tachycardia and supraventricular tachycardia with aberrantly conducted beats may be difficult, especially when the rate is rapid. Although there are a variety of morphologic criteria that can be used to differentiate these two types of arrhythmias, the presence of AV dissociation, sinus capture beats, or fusion beats most reliably identifies the rhythm as ventricular.

SUPRAVENTRICULAR TACHYCARDIA

There are a variety of supraventricular tachycardias that are due to several different mechanisms and are seen in diverse clinical settings (Table 2). Because the diagnostic and therapeutic approaches to these arrhythmias differ considerably, it is appropriate to consider each of them separately.

Sinus Tachycardia

Sinus tachycardia is usually considered a physiologic response to external stimuli, especially hyperadrenergic states such as fever or fright, rather than a true dysrhythmia. However, because it can occasionally create a diagnostic or therapeutic dilemma, it is worth considering separately. Sinus tachycardia is a regular rhythm characterized by a P wave morphology that is identical to the P wave seen in normal sinus rhythm and a rate that fluctuates gradually, as opposed to the sudden onset of rapid rate found in paroxysmal supraventricular tachycardia. In addition, the sinus rate should be appropriate for the clinical setting. For example, it might be expected that a patient who is hypotensive with a fever of 104° F would have a sinus rate of 120 to 130 beats per minute, whereas this rate would be inappropriate in an afebrile patient who is hemodynamically stable. Because sinus tachycardia is usually not a primary rhythm disorder, therapy is usually directed at the underlying condition (e.g., bronchodilator therapy in a patient with an acute exacerbation of chronic obstructive pulmonary disease, diuretics for those with congestive heart failure, and so on).

Paroxysmal Supraventricular Tachycardia

The term paroxysmal supraventricular tachycardia (PSVT) includes a variety of disorders of diverse mechanisms that, in general, are characterized by a

TABLE 1. **Antiarrhythmic Drugs**

Type	Mechanism	Drugs	Dose
1A	Blocks sodium channel	Quinidine sulfate	200–400 mg q 6 h
		Quinidine gluconate (Quinaglute)	324–648 mg q 8 h
		Procainamide (Pronestyl) oral	500–2000 mg q 6 h
		Procainamide IV	15 mg/kg load 1–5 mg/min main
		Disopyramide (Norpace)	50–200 mg q 6 h
1B	Blocks sodium channel	Lidocaine (Xylocaine) IV	50–200 mg load 1–4 mg/min main
		Mexiletine (Mexitil)	150–250 mg q 8 h
		Tocainide (Tonocard)	400–800 mg q 8 h
1C	Blocks sodium channel	Flecainide (Tambocor)	50–150 mg q 12 h
2	Blocks beta receptors	Metoprolol (Lopressor) oral	50–100 mg q 12 h
		IV	0.02 mg/kg load
		Esmolol (Brevibloc)	500 μg/kg/min load 50–200 μg/kg/min main
3	Blocks potassium channel	Bretylium (Bretylol) IV	5–10 mg/kg load 1–2 mg/min main
		Amiodarone (Cordarone)	10–20 gm load over 10 days, then 800 mg daily for 4 weeks 400 mg daily
		d,l-Sotalol (Betapace)	80–240 mg q 12 h

Abbreviations: IV = intravenous; main = maintenance; load = loading dose.

regular rhythm, a narrow QRS complex, and an abrupt onset and termination. A full discussion of the various types of PSVT is beyond the scope of this chapter. The majority of episodes of PSVT seen in clinical medicine are due to reentry within the AV node or reentry involving the retrograde use of an accessory pathway. The relationship of the P wave to the QRS complex during an episode of PSVT can provide important clues to the mechanism (Table 3). The initial therapeutic approach to an episode of PSVT often involves autonomic maneuvers such as carotid sinus massage or the Valsalva maneuver, which often terminate the arrhythmia. If these are unsuccessful, pharmacologic therapy should be considered (Table 4). Intravenous adenosine (Adenocard, 6- to 12-mg bolus) is probably the ideal drug for terminating an episode of PSVT because of its efficacy and extremely short duration of action, which gives it an excellent safety profile. Alternatively, intravenous administration of verapamil (Calan, Isoptin, up to 10 mg); a beta blocker, especially a very-short-acting one like esmolol (Brevibloc); edrophonium (Tensilon);* a vagomimetic agent; digoxin (Lanoxin); or procainamide (Pronestyl)* may be effective in terminating the acute episode. Nonpharmacologic therapy (Table 5) for an acute episode of PSVT includes overdrive pacing and direct current cardioversion, the treatment of choice when the episode is accompanied by severe hemodynamic compromise. Pharmacologic therapy for prevention of recurrent PSVT may include beta blockers, calcium channel blockers, digitalis, and Types 1A, 1C, and 3 antiarrhythmic drugs, either alone or in varying combinations. The specific drug regimen chosen for a particular patient depends on the precise mechanism of the tachycardia and the presence and severity of any underlying cardiac disease. However, recent developments suggest that these arrhythmias

*This drug has not been approved by the Food and Drug Administration (FDA) for this indication.

TABLE 2. **Types of Supraventricular Tachycardia**

Type	Atrial Rate (beats/min)	Ventricular Response	Relation of P to QRS	Response to Vagal Maneuver	P Wave Morphology	Mechanism	Comment
ST	>100	1:1, regular	Precedes	$\downarrow$ Rate	Sinus	Sinus	Rate change gradual
PSVT	120–240	1:1, regular	*	*	*	*	*
MAT	>100	irregular	Precedes	$\downarrow$ Rate	Multiple	Automaticity	Seen in COPD
A Fl	250–350	2:1, may vary	Precedes	$\downarrow$ Rate	Superior axis		
A Fib	>350	irregular	—	$\downarrow$ Rate	—	Multiple reentrant wavelets	

Abbreviations: ST = sinus tachycardia; PSVT = paroxysmal supraventricular tachycardia; MAT = multifocal atrial tachycardia; A Fl = atrial flutter; A Fib = atrial fibrillation.

*See Table 3.

TABLE 3. **Types of Paroxysmal Supraventricular Tachycardia**

Type	Relation of P to QRS	Response to Vagal Maneuver	P Wave Morphology	Comment
SA node reentry	Precedes	May terminate	Sinus	Uncommon
IA reentry	Precedes	Rate decreased	*	Relatively uncommon
AVNRT (typical)	P buried in or just after QRS	May terminate	Superior axis	Common; slow pathway is antegrade limb
AVNRT (atypical)	P closer to next QRS	May terminate	*	Uncommon
AVRT (orthodromic)	Follows	May terminate	*	Common
AVRT (antidromic)	Precedes or merges with QRS	May terminate	*	Uncommon; wide QRS may mimic VT

Abbreviations: AVNRT = AV nodal reentrant tachycardia; AVRT = AV reciprocating tachycardia; VT = ventricular tachycardia; IA = intra-atrial; SA = sinoatrial.
*P wave morphology depends on the pattern of atrial depolarization but is constant for a given episode of PSVT.

may be permanently eliminated by means of radiofrequency catheter ablation in a remarkably high percentage of cases. Although the risk-benefit ratio of this approach must be decided on an individual basis, the benefits of providing a "cure" and avoiding a lifetime of antiarrhythmic drug therapy with its attendant risks and inconveniences cannot be emphasized too strongly.

MULTIFOCAL ATRIAL TACHYCARDIA

Multifocal atrial tachycardia (MAT) is a rapid irregular rhythm characterized by several (>3) P wave morphologies and correspondingly varying PR intervals. It is most often due to competing atrial foci in the setting of acute or chronic pulmonary disease. MAT is best treated by correcting the underlying problem (hypoxia, acidosis, and so on) and tends to be relatively refractory to antiarrhythmic drugs. There is some evidence that beta blockers may be helpful, although they should be administered with caution in this clinical situation, especially if any component of bronchospasm is present.

ATRIAL FLUTTER

Atrial flutter is a relatively common dysrhythmia that is most easily identified by recognizing the characteristic "flutter waves" on the electrocardiogram. These consist of regular P waves occurring at a rate of between 250 and 350 beats per minute that typically form a "sawtooth" pattern in the inferior leads. The ventricular response is most frequently 2:1, but 3:1, 4:1, and a variable response pattern are not uncommon. Atrial flutter should be strongly suspected when sinus P waves are not clearly visible and the ventricular rate is around 150 beats per minute, especially if the rapid rate seems inappropriate for the

TABLE 4. **Pharmacologic Therapy of Supraventricular Tachycardia**

Medication Type	Drug Names	Mechanism of Action	Comment
Vagotonic	Edrophonium* (Tensilon)	May terminate reentry involving SA or AV nodes	Given by rapid IV push, short duration of action
Vasoconstrictors	Phenylephrine (Neo-Synephrine) Methoxamine (Vasoxyl)	May terminate reentry node	Given by continuous IV infusion
Nucleoside	Adenosine (Adenocard)	May terminate reentry involving AV node, slow the response in other SVT similar to adenosine	Similar to edrophonium
Digitalis	Digoxin (Lanoxin)		Given orally or IV, longer duration of action
Beta blockers	Metoprolol (Lopressor)* Esmolol (Brevibloc)	May terminate reentry involving AV or SA nodes, slow the response in other SVT	Given orally or IV, may slow sinus rate (esmolol can only be given IV)
Calcium channel blockers	Verapamil (Calan, Isoptin) Diltiazem* (Cardizem)	Similar to beta blockers	Similar to beta blockers
Antiarrhythmic drugs			
Type 1A	Quinidine Procainamide (Pronestyl) Disopyramide (Norpace)	Slows accessory pathway conduction, decreases automaticity	Have vagolytic action so should be used with AV nodal blocker
Type 1C	Flecainide (Tambocor)	Slows conduction in most cardiac tissues	Should not be used in setting of ASHD and LV dysfunction
Type 3	d,l-Sotalol (Betapace) Amiodarone (Cordarone)	Prolongs refractoriness in most cardiac tissues	Blocks conduction in AV node and accessory pathways

Abbreviations: IV = intravenous; ASHD = arteriosclerotic heart disease; LV = left ventricular; SA = sinoatrial; SVT = supraventricular tachycardia; AV = atrioventricular.
*Not approved by the FDA for this indication.

TABLE 5. **Nonpharmacologic Therapy of Supraventricular Tachycardia**

Procedure	Comment
Acute	
Vagal maneuvers	May terminate reentrant SVT involving SA or AV nodes
Overdrive pacing	May terminate atrial flutter, many types of PSVT
Cardioversion	Terminates most SVT except for sinus tachycardia and MAT
Recurrent or Chronic	
Overdrive pacing	Used for reentrant PSVT; can cause atrial fibrillation
Catheter ablation of accessory pathways	Procedure of choice for AVRT
Catheter AV nodal modification	Procedure of choice for AVNRT
Catheter AV nodal ablation	Used for SVT refractory to other therapy; has disadvantage of requiring permanent pacemaker

Abbreviations: PSVT = paroxysmal supraventricular tachycardia; MAT = multifocal atrial tachycardia; AVRT = AV reciprocating tachycardia; AVNRT = AV nodal reentrant tachycardia.

clinical situation. When the diagnosis is in doubt, vagal maneuvers may increase the degree of AV block, permitting visualization of the characteristic P waves. Atrial flutter is usually associated with significant cardiac or pulmonary disease. Because the ventricular rate is usually relatively rapid, prompt therapeutic intervention is often required. Overdrive atrial pacing and especially direct current cardioversion are effective means of restoring sinus rhythm. Medication alone can be expected to restore normal sinus rhythm in approximately 20 to 40% of cases, the success of this type of therapy depending partly on the severity and reversibility of the underlying disease. The initial aim of medication is usually to slow the ventricular response by means of a digitalis preparation, a beta blocker, or a calcium channel blocker (see Table 4). Subsequently, a Type 1A antiarrhythmic drug is initiated, and the dosage is carefully titrated upward until a therapeutic serum concentration is attained or sinus rhythm supervenes. If atrial flutter persists, pacing or cardioversion will be required. Currently, antiarrhythmic drugs are the mainstay of therapy for prevention of recurrent atrial flutter. Typically this involves the use of an AV nodal blocking agent plus a Type 1A or occasionally a Type 3 antiarrhythmic drug. In patients whose arrhythmia becomes resistant to medication, radiofrequency ablation of the flutter pathway may be attempted. If this is unsuccessful, radiofrequency ablation of the AV node with permanent pacemaker insertion may be performed as a last resort (see Table 5).

ATRIAL FIBRILLATION

Atrial fibrillation is a common arrhythmia that is observed most frequently in patients with underlying cardiac, pulmonary, or metabolic disorders. It is recognized electrocardiographically by the absence of clearly identifiable P waves and an irregularly irregular ventricular response. When the diagnosis is in doubt, vagal maneuvers may be helpful in eliciting the characteristic undulating baseline. Customarily, patients with atrial fibrillation are initially treated with medications because the arrhythmia is unaffected by overdrive pacing and may recur following direct current cardioversion, especially if the ventricular response is rapid. Initial therapy is directed at slowing the ventricular response with a drug that blocks at the AV node. If the arrhythmia is of unknown duration or is known to have existed for more than 48 hours, the patient should be anticoagulated (if there is no contraindication) for a period of 3 to 4 weeks, after which chemical or direct current cardioversion can be performed. Subsequently, Type 1 or Type 3 antiarrhythmic drugs may be employed to maintain sinus rhythm. Patients with atrial fibrillation with a rapid ventricular response should be considered candidates for catheter ablation of the AV node with permanent pacemaker insertion.

VENTRICULAR ARRHYTHMIAS

Nonsustained Ventricular Arrhythmias

In the presence of left ventricular dysfunction, ventricular arrhythmias (see Table 6) have been demonstrated to be a risk factor for cardiovascular mortality and sudden cardiac death. Yet in this population, ventricular arrhythmias, especially ventricular premature beats, are virtually ubiquitous. Attempts to reduce cardiovascular mortality by suppressing ventricular premature beats by means of antiarrhythmic drugs have generally been disappointing. In the recently completed Cardiac Arrhythmia Suppression Trial (CAST), suppression of ventricular ectopy with encainide (Enkaid), flecainide (Tambocor), or moricizine (Ethmozine) in patients with left ventricular dysfunction following myocardial infarction was associated with a significantly higher incidence of death due to arrhythmias. In contrast, beta blockers have been demonstrated to reduce mortality significantly following acute myocardial infarction despite their merely modest effects on ventricular arrhythmias. Currently, studies are under way to determine whether the Type 3 antiarrhythmic drug amiodarone (Cordarone) will improve survival in patients with recent acute myocardial infarction and in patients with congestive heart failure. Similar studies are being planned with the Type 3 drug sotalol (Betapace). Results of these studies will help to clarify the relationship between ventricular ectopy, arrhythmic drugs, and sudden cardiac death.

TABLE 6. **Types of Ventricular Arrhythmias**

1. Ventricular premature beats—single, complex, couplets
2. Nonsustained ventricular tachycardia
3. Sustained monomorphic ventricular tachycardia
4. Sustained polymorphic ventricular tachycardia, torsades de pointes
5. Ventricular fibrillation

Nonsustained ventricular tachycardia, variously defined as three or more consecutive ventricular premature beats at a rate of more than 100 or 120 beats per minute (for up to 15 to 30 seconds), is generally considered a somewhat more malignant variant of ventricular ectopy, especially in the presence of left ventricular dysfunction. Nonetheless, it is not yet clear that treatment of these patients, either with drugs or with nonpharmacologic means, will decrease cardiovascular mortality. This issue is currently being investigated in several large clinical trials. For the present, the decision to work up a patient with nonsustained ventricular tachycardia and subsequently to initiate therapy with antiarrhythmic drugs must be made on a case-by-case basis.

Sustained Ventricular Arrhythmias

Sustained ventricular tachyarrhythmias include sustained monomorphic and polymorphic ventricular tachycardia and ventricular fibrillation. All are associated with increased mortality and warrant prompt therapeutic intervention. As with all tachycardias, ventricular arrhythmias causing hemodynamic compromise should be treated with direct current cardioversion. In patients with monomorphic ventricular tachycardia that is well tolerated (this usually occurs at a rate below 150 beats per minute), a trial of pharmacologic therapy may be warranted. Pharmacologic therapy (see Table 1) is usually initiated either with intravenous lidocaine (Xylocaine), 50- to 100-mg boluses up to 200 mg, followed by a maintenance infusion of 1 to 4 mg per minute, or intravenous procainamide, 15 mg per kg administered at a rate of 50 mg per minute followed by a continuous infusion of 1 to 5 mg per minute. Subsequent oral therapy is aimed at preventing a recurrence of the arrhythmia and is generally guided by either electrophysiologic testing or serial ambulatory electrocardiographic (Holter) monitoring. Oral therapy is usually initiated with a Type 1A agent, a combination of a Type 1A and 1B agent, or a Type 3 antiarrhythmic drug. Because a successful drug or combination of drugs is found only 20 to 50% of the time (depending on the method of drug testing employed), nonpharmacologic therapy is often required (Table 7). Although surgical or catheter ablation may be performed in selected patients, the implantable cardioverter defibrillator (ICD) has become the mainstay of therapy because of its documented efficacy in preventing sudden cardiac death, its flexibility (newer generations of the device have incorporated antitachycardia pacing, programmable energy levels, back-up bradycardia pacing, and other desirable features) and its relative ease of implantation (most of these units are implanted transvenously).

The approach to patients with sustained polymorphic ventricular tachycardia is similar to that for those with monomorphic tachycardia except that reversible causes, such as drug effects and electrolyte abnormalities, should be carefully considered as possible causes. In particular, torsades de pointes ("twisting around a point"), a variant of polymorphic ventricular tachycardia characterized by shifting polarity of the QRS complexes, occurs in the setting of QT interval prolongation associated with a variety of conditions including congenital QT interval prolongation, several medications (especially Type 1A antiarrhythmic drugs), and low serum concentrations of potassium or magnesium.

Ventricular fibrillation (aborted sudden cardiac death) is also customarily evaluated by the same methods used for sustained ventricular tachycardia except that it is less frequently reproducible in the electrophysiology laboratory or on Holter monitoring, precluding serial drug testing. Accordingly, most survivors of ventricular fibrillation require implantable defibrillators.

TABLE 7. **Therapy of Recurrent Ventricular Tachycardia**

Therapy	Comment
1. Beta blockers	Reduces incidence of sudden cardiac death following myocardial infarction; not very effective for recurrent VT
2. Type IA drugs	First-line therapy for VT; effective in 10 to 30% of cases
3. Type III drugs	Effective in 30 to 40% of patients with recurrent VT
4. ICD	Very effective in preventing sudden cardiac death; addition of antitachycardia pacing adds flexibility
5. Catheter ablation	Technique still evolving
6. Surgical ablation	Usually performed with concomitant CABG, especially in patients with ventricular aneurysms

Abbreviations: VT = ventricular tachycardia; ICD = implantable cardioverter-defibrillator; CABG = coronary artery bypass graft.

CONGENITAL HEART DISEASE

method of
DEREK A. FYFE, M.D., PH.D.
Emory University
Atlanta, Georgia

Although congenital heart disease occurs with a frequency of only 8 per 1000 live births, the diagnosis and management of patients with congenital heart disease not only is the purview of the pediatric cardiologist but has also become the responsibility of the obstetrician, pediatrician, family physician, internist, and adult cardiologist. Although recognition of congenital heart disease in utero increases the likelihood of survival at birth, the now common practice of early discharge of newborns means that symptoms due to undiagnosed ductal-dependent heart defects may not occur during the initial hospitalization, and these infants may subsequently present in extremis after a brief period of wellness at home. When a neonatal diagnosis of serious congenital heart disease is made, surgical rescue is becoming increasingly more successful, even with previously uniformly lethal lesions such as hypoplastic left heart syndrome.

Because surgical treatment for many heart defects has been performed since the 1960s, there now exists a large cohort of children with surgically corrected congenital heart disease who, although they survived the operation, may yet have significant postoperative sequelae such as cardiac failure or life-threatening arrhythmias. As children with surgically treated and untreated congenital heart disease grow, they may desire to participate fully in school and sports activities; therefore, practitioners need to be familiar with the need for and appropriateness of any limitations or restrictions on activity. As they enter the work place, insurability becomes a significant issue. In young women with surgically corrected and uncorrected congenital heart disease, the risks and advisability of pregnancy and the recurrent risk of heart disease in their offspring become important questions.

THE FETUS

Nearly all forms of congenital heart disease and arrhythmias can be diagnosed before birth using fetal echocardiography. If all obstetrician ultrasonographers include a four-chamber view of the heart in routine ultrasound scans, the frequency of undiagnosed heart disease will decrease. A four-chamber view demonstrating the atria and ventricles can identify more than 90% of major congenital heart defects, and this can be accomplished by the eighteenth week of gestation. Specific indications for fetal echocardiography are congenital heart disease in the parents or in previous children, maternal illness such as diabetes or lupus erythematosus, the presence of somatic or genetic abnormalities in the fetus, maternal exposure to teratogens or drugs, and non-immune hydrops.

The severity of congenital heart defects detected in utero is worse than that found in term babies because fetal loss will occur in some cases. When a major cardiac defect is identified, amniocentesis should be considered because genetic and chromosomal abnormalities occur with increased frequency. Following identification of a fetus with congenital heart disease, elective transportation of the mother to a tertiary care center where pediatric cardiologists are available for delivery improves neonatal outcome and eliminates the need for emergency transportation of a critically ill child.

Recognition of a fetal arrhythmia in utero may prevent the development of hydrops fetalis and neonatal death. Maternal drug administration in patients with supraventricular tachycardia or atrial flutter may correct the arrhythmia; however, the fetal drug level cannot be monitored.

THE PREMATURE INFANT

The premature infant is vulnerable to heart failure usually caused by a patent ductus arteriosus (PDA) even when the left-to-right shunt is small. Neonatologists treating PDA with indomethacin should be aware that echocardiography can rule out ductal-dependent cardiac lesions, and therefore echocardiographic imaging of the aortic arch and the normal heart should be done before indomethacin is used. In premature babies, atypical clinical findings, such as a lower than expected arterial saturation for the degree of coexisting lung immaturity, may suggest cyanotic heart disease. When congenital heart diseases are identified in low-birthweight babies, the prognosis is often poor with or without surgery. Surgical success is improved if the operation can be delayed and the children are allowed to grow using hyperalimentation and high caloric density feeding. In many cases, a chronic continuous prostaglandin infusion is required to maintain ductal patency. Progression of pulmonary hypertension may, however, be accelerated in premature babies who have unrestricted pulmonary blood flow due to cardiac defects with intercirculatory communication.

THE NEWBORN WITH CONGESTIVE HEART FAILURE

Children born with hydrops fetalis or congestive heart failure from any cause have approximately a 90% neonatal mortality. Causes other than hemolytic anemia include sustained intrauterine supraventricular tachycardia, intrauterine asphyxia with myocardial dysfunction, congenital heart disease associated with mitral and tricuspid regurgitation, or complete heart block. Most commonly, however, the ravages of serious congenital heart disease are not expressed until after birth. The fetus has a biventricular circulation in which the systemic and pulmonary circuits communicate via the ductus arteriosus and the foramen ovale, allowing one side of the heart to compensate for deficiencies in the other. Within 2 to 72 hours following delivery, however, functional closure of the ductus arteriosus usually occurs. Pulmonary vascular resistance then falls, and the adult pattern of circulation through the heart and lungs is established. Obstruction to blood flow in any region of the heart will then be manifest, and signs and symptoms of congenital heart disease will appear rapidly.

THE CYANOTIC INFANT

The cyanotic infant in whom perinatal asphyxia has occurred is likely to have persistence of the fetal pattern of circulation (PFC) associated with sustained pulmonary hypertension. This results in right-to-left shunting at the foramen ovale and ductus arteriosus and desaturated venous blood entering the systemic arterial circulation. Arterial blood samples derived from the left ventricle and pumped to the ascending aorta and right radial (pre-ductal) artery are usually significantly more highly oxygenated than those obtained from the descending aorta, into which systemic venous blood is shunted through the ductus arteriosus. The crucial differential diagnosis in such babies is to demonstrate that no anomalies of the heart and especially of the pulmonary venous connection exist. Two-dimensional and color flow Doppler echocardiography readily identify the site of entry of each pulmonary vein into the left atrium.

Asphyxiated babies may have profound myocardial dysfunction sometimes associated with papillary muscle injury, which causes severe tricuspid regurgitation and poor right ventricular ejection into the pulmonary artery. This may result in severe cyanosis and "functional pulmonary atresia."

In the cyanotic infant in whom asphyxia has not occurred, complex congenital heart disease is *likely* to be present. Careful physical examination should determine the presence or absence of associated dysmorphic features, such as those associated with trisomy syndromes. Observation of the respiratory rate and effort may reveal profound tachypnea, particularly if pulmonary venous or left atrial obstruction or severe metabolic acidosis resulting from low cardiac output is present. Usually, however, no respiratory distress is apparent. Palpation of the arterial pulses with measurement of the arm and leg blood pressure and observation of peripheral capillary filling may identify discrepancies between the upper and lower extremities due to aortic arch interruption or severe coarctation. Palpation of the precordium may detect an overactive heart due to severe valvular regurgitation and enlargement, as occurs in Ebstein's malformation of the tricuspid valve. The presence of a palpable thrill and an easily audible long systolic murmur may be due to severe right or left ventricular outflow obstruction. Auscultation may also reveal a single second heart sound due to the absence of a semilunar valve in pulmonary atresia and truncus arteriosus or to the abnormal anterior position of the aorta in transposition of the great arteries. The presence of a systolic heart murmur in the left chest and back in a cyanotic patient is suggestive of right ventricular outflow tract obstruction, as is present in tetralogy of Fallot. A holosystolic murmur may be due to severe atrioventricular valve regurgitation such as Epstein's malformation. In this disorder, tricuspid regurgitation is often so severe that no forward flow occurs from the right ventricle to the pulmonary artery causing profound cyanosis. The presence of multiple clicks may accompany Ebstein's malformation and truncus arteriosus.

The absence of a heart murmur in a profoundly cyanotic patient is consistent with lesions such as transposition of the great arteries or total anomalous pulmonary venous connection in which no AV valve regurgitation is occurring.

Medical Therapy for Cyanotic Infants

During the resuscitation, stabilization, and diagnostic phases of care for cyanotic infants, a chest radiograph should be obtained to ascertain the presence of intrathoracic abnormalities such as hypoplastic lungs, diaphragmatic hernia, or pneumonia. The chest radiograph of the child with congenital heart disease associated with a right-to-left intracardiac shunt may show underperfused "black" lungs in which the pulmonary vascular markings are profoundly diminished. The heart itself may be of normal size and configuration; however, certain lesions have been associated with characteristic cardiac silhouettes. In tetralogy of Fallot and truncus arteriosus, the aortic arch may be to the right of the trachea in one-fourth of patients and the pulmonary artery silhouette is diminished owing to hypoplasia of the main pulmonary artery. Transposition of the great vessels produces the classic "egg on a string" appearance with a narrow superior mediastinum due to the abnormal position of the great vessels. The "basketball-size" heart of Ebstein's anomaly, due to massive right atrial enlargement, is almost unmistakable. It should be emphasized, however, that the presence of an enlarged thymus may confuse the interpretation of neonatal chest radiographs. In cyanotic patients in whom pulmonary plethora is present, transposition of the great vessels with ventricular septal defects and also pulmonary venous or left atrial obstruction must be considered.

Analysis of blood gases obtained during the resuscitative phase may show evidence of hypoxia with a low PO_2 and reduced PCO_2 due to hyperventilation. Carbon dioxide retention, however, may occur owing to low cardiac output or concurrent pulmonary insufficiency, especially in preterm infants. The cornerstone of therapy for a child with presumed cyanotic heart disease or heart disease in which aortic blood flow is impeded, such as hypoplastic left heart syndrome, is prostaglandin E_1 infusion (Table 1). This should be available in all hospitals and is carried by transport teams from tertiary pediatric cardiology centers. The decision to start prostaglandins is best made in conjunction with telephone consultation with the pediatric cardiology center to which the child is to be transported. If echocardiography is obtainable at the referring hospital, an attempt to image the heart may be useful while the child is awaiting transportation. It should be emphasized, however, that adult cardiologists are often uncomfortable in attempting to diagnose congenital heart defects and may make incorrect diagnoses owing to unfamiliarity with the lesions and technical limitations of equipment not designed for pediatric work. However, it may still be beneficial for the pediatric cardiologist to "talk through" an echocardiogram with the technologist or cardiologist to get an overall impression of the cardiac structure and function prior to transportation.

Following transportation, definitive diagnosis is made with echocardiography. Catheterization is usually reserved only for individuals in whom interventions, such as balloon atrial septostomy, are required to facilitate intracardiac circulatory admixture. Emergency preoperative catheterization may also be required for children who need systemic to pulmonary artery shunting when the arterial vessels involved are small or indistinct on echocardiography. Noninvasive magnetic resonance imaging is replacing catheterization for this purpose.

ACYANOTIC CONGENITAL HEART DISEASE IN INFANCY

The clinical presentation of acyanotic congenital heart disease in the neonatal period is varied. Certain babies should be screened by echocardiography for heart disease regardless of the absence of cardiac symptoms and signs. Down's syndrome children may have an electrocardiogram showing left axis deviation due to an atrioventricular canal defect. Because 40% of Down's syndrome infants have some type of cardiac lesion, echocardiography should be performed. Patients with other genetic syndromes that should be screened exhibit Turner's syndrome (coarctation of the aorta), trisomy 18 and 13 (ventricular septal defect [VSD]), Marfan's syndrome (mitral and aortic regurgitation and dysplasia), Williams syndrome (supravalvular aortic stenosis), Noonan's syndrome (supravalvular pulmonary stenosis), and some inborn errors of metabolism such as Pompe's disease (infiltrative cardiomyopathy). Although intermittent soft systolic murmurs due to the closing ductus arteriosus are common in asymptomatic infants on the first day of life, the presence of a persistent loud, long systolic murmur on the first and second days of life suggests an obstructive lesion such as aortic or pulmonary stenosis, left ventricular outflow tract obstruction with hypertrophic cardiomyopathy such as occurs in infants of a diabetic mother, or right ventricular outflow tract obstruction with pulmonary stenosis such as occurs in tetralogy of Fallot. In such patients, cardiac consultation with two-dimensional and Doppler echocardiography should be obtained. A soft systolic murmur may merely be mild branch pulmonary stenosis, particularly if it is audible well over the back.

CONGESTIVE HEART FAILURE DEVELOPING IN THE FIRST WEEK

In the child who develops symptoms of congestive heart failure within the first week of life after initially appearing well, the differential diagnosis of septicemia must be considered. Infants may be increasingly tachypneic and tachycardiac as the heart attempts to increase cardiac output. Feeding is accomplished only with difficulty because the increased work of breathing interferes with maintaining the nipple in the baby's mouth for any length of time. The child may appear pallid and may sweat. Perfusion eventually decreases with impending hemodynamic collapse. The

TABLE 1. **Frequently Used Cardiac Medications in Cyanotic Children**

Drug	Dose	Route	Desired Effects	Side Effects
Iron ($FeSO_4$)	1 mg Fe/kg/day	PO	↑ Hematocrit	GI irritation
Morphine	0.1 mg/kg/dose	IM or IV	Sedation, ↓ Hyperpnea	Apnea, hypotension
Phenylephrine (Neo-Synephrine)	0.1–0.5 μgm/kg/min	IV	Vasoconstriction (↑ afterload)	↓ Perfusion
Prostaglandin E_1 (Prostin VR Pediatric)	0.03–0.1 μg/kg/min	IV	Ductal patency	Apnea, seizures, ↑ temperature, ↓ Na^+, rash
$NaHCO_3$	1 mEq/kg/dose	IV	Correct acidosis	Alkalosis
Propranolol	0.1 mg/kg/dose IV 1–4 mg/kg/day divided qid	IV or PO	↓ Heart rate, ↑ pulmonary flow	Bradycardia, bronchospasm

development of heart failure associated with hyperactive precordium accompanied by diminished pulses or deteriorating perfusion suggests the presence of hypoplastic left-sided heart syndrome. Interruption of the aortic arch and severe coarctation of the aorta are similarly responsible for the rapid onset of congestive heart failure in the first few days of life. Prior to surgery, palliation with prostaglandin E_1 is lifesaving (see Table 1).

Sustained arrhythmias such as sustained supraventricular tachycardia or, more rarely, ventricular tachycardia or atrial flutter with rapid ventricular conduction may also occur with heart failure. Electrocardiography is invaluable in diagnosing supraventricular tachycardia and usually shows a heart rate of 220 to 300 beats per minute with an abnormal P wave axis. If dissociation of the P wave and QRS is present, this suggests a diagnosis of ventricular tachycardia. Fax transmission of electrocardiographic 12-lead and rhythm strips can provide diagnostic data instantaneously to the pediatric cardiology referral center, and telephone discussion can be initiated to guide therapy. The recent introduction of adenosine as an intravenous pharmacologic agent has revolutionized the acute termination of supraventricular tachycardia in children and may be used even when heart failure is present (Table 2). Direct current cardioversion is also reliable and is the immediate treatment of choice for the patient who is hypotensive. Verapamil is contraindicated in children under 1 year of age because its intravenous use in this age group has led to cardiovascular collapse. Digoxin is not useful for acute therapy and is useful as a maintenance therapy only when no pre-excitation suggestive of Wolff-Parkinson-White syndrome is present. Propranolol or tenormin is useful for chronic therapy for tachycardia (see Table 2).

Congestive heart failure in the newborn child or infant may be due to an arteriovenous malformation occurring in the vessels of the brain or the liver. These are often associated with a systolic ejection murmur due to the increased cardiac output, and an audible bruit is sometimes heard over the head or abdomen. Thrombocytopenia frequently ensues with disseminated intravascular coagulation as the turbulent flow in the fistula destroys cellular elements in the blood. Therapy for these conditions is treatment of the underlying malformation with surgical ligation if possible.

Congenital Heart Disease with Congestive Failure Presenting After the First Week of Life

Due to the initial high pulmonary vascular resistance of the newborn that may only gradually decrease during the first week of life, it is common for babies to be discharged from the newborn nursery with a congenital heart defect still undetected. Ventricular septal defects may be silent until pulmonary vascular resistance has diminished sufficiently to allow establishment of the left-to-right shunt through the ventricular septal defect. Only then is the murmur audible and, when fully established, the unmistakable holosystolic, harsh-quality murmur is often first noted at the first outpatient check-up. Similarly, a patent ductus arteriosus murmur may have the brief systolic ejection quality of the functional murmur during the newborn period and yet acquire machinery-like systolic and diastolic components at the follow-up examination owing to the

TABLE 2. **Frequently Used Cardiac Medications in Children—Arrhythmia Treatment**

Drug	Dose	Route	Desired Effects	Side Effects
Adenosine (Adenocard)	50–200 μgm/kg/dose IV	IV, rapid push	Transient AV block	Prolonged AV block
Propranolol (Inderal)	0.1 mg/kg/dose IV 1–4 mg/kg/dose PO	IV or PO	↓ HR	Bradycardia, bronchospasm
Phenytoin (Dilantin)	3–5 mg/kg IV (slow) 3–5 mg/kg/day divided bid	IV or PO	↓ PVC, ↓ VT	Hypotension (IV), allergic reaction
Lidocaine (Xylocaine)	1 mg/kg bolus then 20–50 μgm/kg/min IV	IV	↓ PVC, ↓ VT	Seizures
Procainamide (Pronestyl)	15 mg/kg bolus over 1 hr then 20–50 μgm/kg/min IV	IV	↓ PVC, ↓ VT, ↓ SVT	Hypotension
Atenolol (Tenormin)	1–1.5 mg/kg/day	PO	↓ SVT, ↓ VT	Depression, bradycardia
Direct current cardioversion	1–2 joules/kg	Transthoracic	↓ SVT, ↓ VT, ↓ VF	Myocardial injury at excessive voltages

Abbreviations: AV = atrioventricular; HR = heart rate; PVC = premature ventricular contraction; VT = ventricular tachycardia; SVT = supraventricular tachycardia; VF = ventricular fibrillation.

changes due to pulmonary resistance described earlier. Although blood flow through the ductus arteriosus usually stops within the first 24 hours of life, anatomic constriction of the ductus tissue itself may progress over a period of several weeks. If coarctation of the aorta is present in the juxtaductal region, the coarctation becomes more severe hemodynamically as the ductus arteriosus scars down. Often it takes 2 to 3 weeks after discharge from the newborn nursery before clinical findings of congestive heart failure become apparent. Coarctation, therefore, may result in heart failure at almost any time during the first 6 weeks of life. Often, coarctation of the aorta is associated with VSD and bicuspid aortic valve. The development of tachypnea in an infant with hypertension in the upper extremities and absent or diminished pulses in the lower extremities is diagnostic of coarctation. Prostaglandin E_1 infusion may reestablish patency of the juxtaductal region in young infants, thus ameliorating heart failure prior to surgery. Echocardiography and magnetic resonance imaging provide preoperative delineation of the important anatomic features, and these children may be operated on without catheterization.

Development of congestive heart failure in patients with lesions characterized by intercirculatory communications is facilitated by the physiologic changes in pulmonary resistance described earlier. VSD, single ventricle, truncus arteriosus, atrioventricular canal, and other lesions in which systemic arterial shunting occurs all begin to exert their detrimental effects after about 3 weeks of life. Clinical manifestations of congestive heart failure are often present by 6 to 8 weeks of age in patients with these defects. Failure to thrive is a prominent symptom owing to the high caloric requirements of the child who is tachypneic and is using the external muscles of respiration excessively. The cardiac examination may reveal a very overactive precordium with a systolic murmur. Often, a diastolic flow rumble is heard. This is due to the increased pulmonary venous return passing through the mitral valve, rendering it relatively restrictive. Hepatomegaly may indicate systemic vascular congestion. Chest radiographs usually have increased pulmonary vascular markings, and the electrocardiogram may now show hypertrophy as well as a sinus tachycardia. Serum electrolytes may demonstrate dilutional hyponatremia caused by excessive water retention. Yet despite fluid retention it is uncommon for infants to be edematous.

Therapy for Infants with Congestive Heart Failure

Therapy is usually initiated with specific agents directed toward the underlying physiologic abnormalities. In patients with atrioventricular valve regurgitation (e.g., those with atrioventricular canal defects and those with large left-to-right shunts due to VSD, single ventricle, and patent ductus arteriosus), afterload reduction with angiotensin-converting enzyme inhibitors such as captopril or enalapril (Table 3) is beneficial. Reduction of preload with diuretics such as furosemide is often sufficient to control heart failure and enable the child to grow and gain weight. The use of nutritional modification with formulas of increased caloric density up to 27 calories per ounce is beneficial. If heart failure is intractable despite medical therapy, surgery is indicated. Complete neonatal repair of intracardiac defects is now preferred. Pulmonary artery banding is still done in some cases to reduce pulmonary blood flow temporarily and facilitate growth prior to complete repair. Subsequent intracardiac repair with removal of the pulmonary artery band is best performed within 9 months because pulmonary bands cause distortion of the pulmonary arteries.

MANAGEMENT OF THE CHILD WITH CONGENITAL HEART DISEASE

The child with untreated congenital heart disease may decompensate clinically owing to congestive heart failure and may require intensive care therapy. Support of cardiac output is now possible with drugs such as amrinone (see Table 3), which has both an inotropic effect on the heart and dilator effects on the vascular bed. This action optimizes both contractility and afterload reduction and increases cardiac output. Amrinone is a noncatecholamine drug that has significantly improved our ability to deal with profound congestive heart failure due to congenital heart disease or cardiomyopathy. This drug, when combined with a catecholamine-based inotropic agent such as dobutamine and low doses of dopamine, may have synergistic beneficial effects. Side effects of such medications are serious and include ventricular arrhythmia, decreased renal perfusion, electrolyte abnormal-

TABLE 3. **Frequently Used Cardiac Medications in Children—Heart Failure**

Drug	Dose	Route	Desired Effects	Side Effects
Furosemide (Lasix)	0.5–2.0 mg/kg/dose up to q 8 h	PO, IM, IV	Diuresis	↓ K^+, ↓ Cl^-, ↑ HCO_3^-, dehydration
Captopril (Capoten)	1–5 mg/kg/day divided tid	PO	Vasodilation, ↓ BP	Hypotension, ↑ BUN, ↑ HR
Enalapril (Vasotec)	5 mg/day (adult dose)	PO, IV	Vasodilation (long-acting)	Hypotension, ↑ BUN (especially IV)
Spironolactone (Aldactone)	2–4 mg/kg/day divided bid	PO	Diuresis, potassium conservation	↑ K^+
Digoxin	8–10 μg/kg/day divided bid PO Decrease by ⅓ for neonates or IV	PO or IV	Inotropy	Nausea, toxicity with increased dose
Amrinone (Inocor)	0.75 μg bolus over 20 min; then 5–10 μgm/kg/min	IV	Inotropy, vasodilation, diuresis	Thrombocytopenia, arrhythmia
Dopamine (Intropin)	3–20 μgm/kg/min	*Central* IV	↑ Renal perfusion, ↑ inotropy, ↑ BP	Arrhythmia, ↑ vasoconstriction, tachycardia
Dobutamine (Dobutrex)	3–20 μgm/kg/min	*Central* IV	↑ Inotropy	Arrhythmia, tachycardia

Abbreviations: HR = heart rate; BUN = blood urea nitrogen.

ities, and thrombocytopenia. The thrombocytopenia due to amrinone is a reversible condition that improves 24 hours after discontinuation of the drug (see Table 3).

Hypercyanotic spells most commonly occur in infants with tetralogy of Fallot but can occur in infants with other defects that have a similar physiologic basis. These alarming episodes usually happen during the first year of life and may be precipitated on awakening in the morning or by prolonged crying. During spells, the otherwise loud pulmonary outflow murmur is markedly diminished or absent because little blood is flowing to the lungs, and desaturated blood floods through the VSD into the aorta. Initial treatment consists in placing the infant in a knee-chest position if squatting has not spontaneously occurred. Medications such as intramuscular morphine (see Table 1) calm the respiratory drive and may abort the spell. Intravenous fluids may expand the intravascular volume and enhance pulmonary blood flow. Neo-Synephrine infusion will cause systemic vasoconstriction, and propranolol will decrease heart rate and improve diastolic filling and pulmonary blood flow. Acidosis must be avoided because this stimulates the respiratory rate, and therefore bicarbonate may be given.

The occurrence of "tet" spells may be temporarily prevented by chronic administration of propranolol, but surgical treatment must be scheduled because the obstruction to right ventricular outflow becomes progressively worse. Dietary iron supplements should be given in all patients with cyanotic heart diseases because anemia causes significant worsening of hypoxemia.

SURGERY FOR CHILDREN WITH CONGENITAL HEART DISEASE

Neonatal correction of complex congenital heart disease is now offered in many cardiac centers and may be the optimal approach. Palliative surgery, however, may be preferred initially because surgical mortality may be less. In the cyanotic infant with reduced pulmonary blood flow, systemic to pulmonary shunts are established by inserting a synthetic tube from one or another subclavian artery to a pulmonary artery. This modified Blalock-Taussig shunt procedure provides palliation for 1 to 2 years. Intracardiac intercirculatory mixing is essential, and preoperative balloon atrial septostomy may be performed in patients with tricuspid or mitral atresia, transposition of the great vessels, and pulmonary atresia with an intact ventricular septum.

Definitive repair of transposition of the great arteries is accomplished with the arterial switch operation, which requires removal and retransposition of the arteries with relocation of the coronary arteries to the new aortic trunk. This operation is extraordinarily difficult technically, especially for patients with anomalous coronary artery origins, and cannot be done when pulmonary stenosis is present. In patients who do not undergo the arterial switch operation for transposition, the Senning operation is performed. Atrial channels are created to divert systemic venous blood to the left ventricle and pulmonary artery, and another channel is placed to divert blood from the left atrium to the right ventricle and aorta. Although arterial saturation is now normal, this maneuver does not correct the pressure overload to which the right ventricle is subjected because of its subaortic location. Long-term problems with atrial arrhythmias requiring permanent pacemakers, chronic pharmacologic therapy (see Table 2), and right-sided heart dysfunction may ensue many years after the Senning or Mustard operation.

Repair of tetralogy of Fallot with right ventricular outflow tract reconstruction and VSD closure may be performed either in the first months of life or as a staged operation following initial palliation with a modified Blalock-Taussig shunt with subsequent complete repair in the second and third years of life.

Patients with otherwise lethal critical left-sided heart disease such as hypoplastic left heart syndrome with aortic or mitral valve atresia have benefited from creative surgical approaches. The Norwood operation has revolutionized the treatment of hypoplastic left-sided heart disease in some surgeons' hands. In this operation, the aorta is joined to the pulmonary artery, and the pulmonary arteries are disconnected and then resupplied with blood through a small central shunt. This enables the right side of the heart to pump blood to both pulmonary and systemic circuits and provides palliation until a more definitive procedure, the Fontan operation, can be performed (see later discussion). Some cardiologists, however, have been dissatisfied with the results of this approach and have proceeded with infant heart transplantation. Currently, the early surgical results of transplantation and the Norwood operation are similar, with an approximately 30% perioperative mortality. Due to the very limited availability of infant heart donors, many infants die while awaiting transplantation, increasing the overall mortality of this procedure to approximately 50%. The late problems are multiple reoperations after the Norwood procedure and rejection, infection, and lymphoma following heart transplantation.

In patients with a single ventricle, limitation of pulmonary blood flow by pulmonary banding may be required in the first month of life. Subsequently, the Fontan-type operation can be performed. In this operation, the systemic venous or right atrial blood is surgically channelled to the pulmonary artery, leaving the single ventricle to be the pump for the aorta and systemic circulation. Owing to elevation of pulmonary vascular resistance, Fontan operations do not work well in children under 1 year of age; therefore, a partial "hemi"-Fontan procedure or a fenestrated Fontan operation may be performed. In these operations, only a partial isolation of the systemic venous circuit from the arterial circuit is made, such that some venous blood still enters the ventricle. Later reoperations close these communications and complete the Fontan operation when the child is older.

This staged approach has significantly improved the perioperative survival. The Fontan operation itself and the Norwood operation may also be used as a stage toward subsequent heart transplantation.

Operations for VSD closure are usually performed before age 2 to prevent the development of pulmonary vascular obstructive disease, and similarly, atrial septal defects are generally closed in children aged 2 to 3 years because the operation can be done with a high degree of safety and little impairment to the child's development.

EARLY COMPLICATIONS AFTER HEART SURGERY

With the increased numbers of survivors of surgery for congenital heart disease, the prevalence of postoperative patients has increased in the population. The practitioner is now confronted with many new clinical problems. After complex heart surgery, infants return home and may be taking formulas with a high caloric density as well as several cardiac medications. These all may have significant deleterious effects when a common childhood illness intervenes. Respiratory viral infections, pneumonia, and similar illnesses may severely compromise such patients, requiring rehospitalization. Diarrheal illness in patients taking diuretics may predispose them to electrolyte abnormalities and require temporary discontinuation of some medications.

In patients in whom cardiac arrhythmias have occurred following surgery, home monitoring or transtelephonic devices may be used during times of clinical symptoms of arrhythmia such as syncope, dizziness, and palpitations. These may be reported to the practitioner and may have profound significance. Good communication between the cardiologist and the practitioner will facilitate optimal management of these complex problems.

Fever occurring after the child has recently left the hospital is significant. Careful examination of the surgical sites for redness or exudation is necessary. It is advisable to obtain a complete blood count, blood cultures, and a urinalysis and urine culture because many of these children have had instrumentation of the urinary tract intraoperatively. One to 3 weeks after cardiac surgery, some individuals may develop fever and chest pain associated with pericardial and pleural effusions. Possible infection must be evaluated; negative studies suggest a diagnosis of the postpericardiotomy syndrome. This may be treated initially with nonsteroidal anti-inflammatory drugs such as aspirin but may be severe enough to require rehospitalization and aspiration of pericardial and pleural fluid with institution of steroids for their anti-inflammatory effect. The duration of this illness may be brief, or it may be prolonged for several weeks to months. Finally, bacterial endocarditis is a rare but devastating illness. Endocarditis is usually characterized by malaise and indolent fevers and may produce peripheral manifestations of systemic embolization such as hematuria, splinter hemorrhages, and retinal abnormalities.

Endocarditis prophylaxis is mandatory for patients with essentially all kinds of heart disease. Prophylaxis with the antibiotic regimens published by the American Heart Association should be employed prior to dental work and surgical procedures. These regimens usually recommend penicillin or amoxicillin unless the urogenital or gastrointestinal tract is invaded by instruments, and then an aminoglycoside is added.

LATE COMPLICATIONS AFTER HEART SURGERY

In patients who have undergone an operation for congenital heart disease, the repaired heart may function perfectly. There are, however, many patients who are left with sequelae from the heart defect or from the surgery itself. The most problematic sequela is the occurrence of abnormalities of heart rate and rhythm. Following repairs of atrial septal defects, the Senning or Mustard atrial baffle operations for transposition of the great vessels, and the Fontan operation, sinus node dysfunction may gradually evolve, causing decreased resting heart rates and an inability to respond to the physiologic demands of exercise. Additionally, serious life-threatening tachycardia or bradycardia may occur, and sudden deaths have been reported. All patients with atrial surgery should be documented to have normal sinus rhythm after surgery. Syncope, dizziness, and palpitations all suggest an arrhythmia and should be carefully evaluated. Some medications are hazardous for the treatment of arrhythmias in these patients because they may further depress sinus node function and lead to profound bradycardia and death. Permanent pacemakers have been implanted in many such patients and are required if more than digoxin is used for control of arrhythmia. Antiarrhythmic drugs themselves often have systemic side effects (see Table 2), and therapeutic drug levels may require monitoring; poor patient compliance is itself a problem.

Antiarrhythmic agents used in children differ considerably from those used in adults after myocardial infarction. Flecainide (Tambocor) is a safe and effective medication when monitored appropriately. Quinidine, however, has been associated with sudden death when used after atrial repair of transposition of the great vessels. Phenytoin (Dilantin) is most commonly used to prevent sudden death from ventricular arrhythmias after repair of tetralogy of Fallot (see Table 2).

Abnormalities of right or left ventricular function may persist or develop after surgery. When left ventriculotomy is required for closure of muscular defects, left ventricular contractility may be poor. Following repair of tetralogy of Fallot, in which the right ventricular outflow tract and pulmonary valve are incised, pulmonary insufficiency is severe and presents a chronic volume load to the right ventricle. In addition, the right ventricle itself has impaired function at the site of the incision. Not only does poor right ventricular function impair performance, it also predisposes to life-threatening ventricular arrhythmias. Postoperative catheterization with electrophysiologic studies may be indicated in many such patients to help define the risks of ventricular tachycardia and fibrillation.

Residual defects such as mild aortic stenosis and mild coarctation of the aorta or small residual VSDs are not uncommon and are well tolerated. Continued endocarditis prophylaxis, however, requires lifetime vigilance.

CARDIAC DEFECTS NOT REQUIRING INFANT SURGERY

Mild to moderate aortic and pulmonary valve stenosis may simply be followed over the years using serial Doppler echocardiographic assessment of the pressure gradient. Aortic stenosis may progress during the first years, whereas pulmonary stenosis gradients tend to remain the same. Stenotic gradients of 60 to 80 mmHg suggest the need for valvotomy or valvuloplasty.

Atrial septal defects that cause left-to-right shunting and right ventricular volume overload are usually asymptomatic and are best repaired before the child reaches school age because unrepaired defects lead to atrial arrhythmia and pulmonary hypertension in adulthood.

VSDs not causing heart failure in infancy are evaluated during the first 24 months of life. If the pulmonary-to-systemic flow ratio through the VSD exceeds 2:1, surgery is performed to prevent pulmonary hypertension developing in childhood. Small defects tend to decrease in size with age.

Each of these defects requires endocarditis prophylaxis for life even after repair.

SPORTS PARTICIPATION AND INSURANCE

Patients in whom congenital heart disease has essentially been cured by surgery should not be restricted in any activity. Patients with ventricular and atrial septal defects in whom no residual abnormalities or arrhythmias are present have essentially a normal prognosis for their lifetime. If these patients were operated on at an advanced age, however, pulmonary vascular obstructive disease or ventricular dysfunction may be present, and pulmonary hypertension may progress despite surgery. Insurability for health and life insurance should not be proscribed by many kinds of previous heart surgery; however, careful postoperative evaluation by a cardiologist may be necessary for patients to qualify.

SURGICALLY UNCORRECTED CONGENITAL HEART DISEASE

The practitioner may be confronted with patients with mild defects such as small VSDs, mild pulmonary stenosis, or bicuspid aortic valves, whose primary need is for endocarditis prophylaxis.

Lesions in which pulmonary blood flow is unrestricted and intracardiac communication occurs, such as large patent ductus arteriosus defects and VSDs that have not been operated on in childhood, will probably lead to pulmonary vascular obstructive disease and Eisenmenger's syndrome. These patients may have cyanosis with an elevated hemocrit that may cause significant fatigue, dyspnea, hemoptysis, and headaches. Such patients are at constant risk for development of brain abscess or stroke owing to the unfiltered blood passing into the systemic arterial circulation. Therapy with a heart-lung transplantation offers the only long-term hope for these individuals.

Patients with surgically untreated coarctation of the aorta as well as those in whom operation was delayed until their teens or late childhood years are likely to have hypertension. This is difficult to treat even using angiotensin-converting enzyme inhibitors and may lead to early vascular disease.

PROSTHETIC HEART DISEASE

New reconstructive surgical techniques are reducing the number of children who require artificial heart valves for severe regurgitant or stenotic valve defects. A number of children do, however, still have prosthetic valves. The use of cadaver-derived, preserved homograft valves has further reduced the use of metal valves in children. Homograft valves are unlikely to develop thrombi, and therefore anticoagulation is not required. They do, however, calcify and deteriorate with time, and constant observation for the development of new murmurs due to regurgitation through these valves is needed.

In patients who have implanted metal prosthetic valves, anticoagulation with either warfarin (Coumadin) or dipyridamole (Persantine) and aspirin is used to prevent thromboembolic events. Again, poor patient compliance is a major problem, particularly in the adolescent age group.

PREGNANCY

Birth control should be tailored to consideration of the cardiac defect present. Prevention of pregnancy may be mandatory to preserve the life of patients with severe ventricular dysfunction, cyanosis, or cardiomyopathy. A profound risk to both fetus and mother is present in such women in whom pregnancy occurs. In others, the risk of thrombosis is increased (e.g., after the Fontan operation), and therefore high-progesterone contraceptive pills are discouraged and barrier methods are preferred.

Pregnancy is a serious risk particularly to those individuals taking warfarin because it may lead to warfarin embryopathy as well as uncontrolled bleeding. Thromboembolic events are more likely to occur, and the management of anticoagulation in these patients is extraordinarily difficult and requires close collaboration between obstetrician and cardiologist.

The risk of pregnancy in patients who have had repair of congenital heart disease depends on the cardiac function at the time of the pregnancy. In individuals with VSD and tetralogy repair who have had a good surgical result, the risk of pregnancy is low. After repair of coarctation of the aorta, patients should be evaluated for aneurysm formation prior to pregnancy because aortic rupture has occurred at childbirth. In patients with poor ventricular function, the volume load imposed by pregnancy may lead to the development of congestive heart failure and arrhythmia. It is notable, however, that a few patients with complex heart disease that has been palliated by the Senning or Fontan operation have managed to go through pregnancy. The risk of congenital heart disease in these offspring is above that in the general population, and these patients should be examined by fetal echocardiography.

NEW TREATMENTS FOR CONGENITAL HEART DISEASE

Surgical pulmonary valvotomy is now seldom performed in patients with pulmonary stenosis because of the advent of balloon valvuloplasty performed in the catheterization laboratory. Similarly, the aortic valve may be dilated by balloon even in infants; however, recent microsurgical techniques may continue to make operation preferable. Reoperation for recurrent coarctation of the aorta is rarely performed because balloon angioplasty is efficacious. Treatment of native coarctation of the aorta by balloon angioplasty is, however, still controversial.

Coils and occluder devices that close atrial septal defects, patent ductus arteriosus, and VSDs are still experimental but will probably be available within the next 1 to 2 years.

Treatment for arrhythmias such as those associated with the Wolff-Parkinson-White syndrome can now be completed in the catheterization laboratory using radiofrequency ablative techniques. These avoid the need for open heart surgery or lifetime medical therapy by simply obliterating the focus of the electrophysiologic abnormality.

MITRAL VALVE PROLAPSE

method of
JOHN B. BARLOW, M.D.
University of Witwatersrand and Johannesburg Hospital
Johannesburg, South Africa

For more than 3 decades an "information explosion" relating to mitral valve prolapse (MVP) or billowing mitral leaflets (BML) resulted essentially from two principal observations. The first, made in 1963, confirmed the mitral valve origin of an apical late systolic murmur and mid (nonejection) systolic click. The second was the subsequent correlation of the symptoms, clinical signs, hereditary factors, and other features associated with the degenerative mitral valve anomaly that justify its designation as a specific syndrome. There are not many new diseases, however. In some instances, an individual doctor has neither read nor heard about a condition he has not previously encountered and believes has never been previously reported. Alternatively, earlier recognition and description may have been related to different aspects of the same disease. Patients with degenerative MVP, for example, are often anxious, and it has been suggested that observations of MVP by physicians in the nineteenth and early twentieth centuries were labeled neurocirculatory asthenia, soldier's heart, irritable heart, effort syndrome, functional heart disease, or Da Costa's syndrome. The widespread interest continues. An estimated 1545 articles during the decade prior to 1991 have addressed aspects of this subject.

TERMINOLOGY

Consequent on cineangiographic observations of abnormal bulging of the bodies of the mitral leaflets, the term prolapse of the mitral valve was introduced in 1966. After the advent of echocardiography, however, the evaluation of mitral valve prolapse, based on variable echocardiographic criteria and with ongoing use of that term, has caused much confusion. Webster's dictionary defines prolapse as "the slipping out of place or falling of some internal organ," and this state, whether intermittent or permanent, implies disease and thus abnormality, as exemplified by prolapse of hemorrhoids, the rectum, the uterus, an intervertebral disk, or the lens of the eye. It is regrettable that the term, which to some patients understandably has ominous connotations, is still widely used even when the anomaly is mild and clinically silent and the valve is functionally normal.

In accordance with observations and descriptions of functional anatomy by cardiac surgeons undertaking mitral valve repair procedures, MVP should be defined as failure of leaflet edge apposition resulting in displacement of the involved leaflet's edge toward the left atrium. Unless a leaflet is fibrosed, shortened, or retracted or has a cleft or hole in it, a mitral valve is competent throughout systole because sustained coaptation of leaflets occurs. When the leaflets are normal in size or larger, failure of sustained apposition must result in leaflet edge prolapse and hence mitral regurgitation. The terms billowing, floppy, and flail also require clarification in the context of correlating echocardiographic, cineangiocardiographic, and clinical evaluation with mitral valve functional anatomy. It is essentially the functional anatomy of the mitral valve mechanism that is evaluated by invasive or noninvasive investigations and that forms the principal basis for medical or surgical management. Immediately after leaflet edge apposition (and thus closure of the mitral valve), the bodies of normal leaflets bulge slightly into the left atrial cavity causing the C wave of that chamber's pressure tracing. The term billowing remains appropriate to describe this physiologic bulging when it becomes exaggerated. BML and its more advanced form, a floppy leaflet, are anatomic descriptions of the leaflet bodies; there is a gradation of mild billowing of part or all of near-normal leaflets to advanced displacement when the leaflet bodies are floppy and voluminous and the chordae tendineae are elongated. A floppy mitral valve, albeit anatomically pathologic, may still be functionally competent throughout systole.

MVP and its extreme form, a flail leaflet, reflect failure of sustained coaptation and therefore displacement of a leaflet's edge toward, or into, the left atrial cavity. The terms mainly describe abnormal valve function. Two-dimensional echocardiography contributes to the evaluation of both the rheumatic and degenerative processes that involve the complex mitral valve mechanism and may result in MVP, but the functional anatomy and hence the echocardiographic appearances are importantly different (Table 1).

RHEUMATIC MITRAL VALVE PROLAPSE

Active rheumatic carditis remains prevalent in developing countries and is the most common overall cause of pure severe mitral regurgitation. Patients are seldom older than 20 years, usually in their early teens, but they may be as young as 5 years. The primary defect in active rheumatic carditis causing pure mitral regurgitation is dilatation of the posterior anulus; the anterior anulus comprises dense fibrous tissue and is relatively fixed. Although chordal elongation is related in part to rheumatic inflammatory involvement, exposure of the chordae to enhanced tensile stresses during ventricular systole is the principal factor. Chordal tension in the normal mitral valve during ventricular systole is attenuated by the "keystone mechanism," whereby the left ventricular pressure generated during systole is applied against opposite sides of the apposing mitral leaflets, forming a competent seal. A normal leaflet-to-anular area ratio is essential for this mechanism to operate optimally. Following posterior anular dilatation, which is the initial and predominant manifestation of active rheumatic carditis, functional shortening of the stretched posterior leaflet occurs, the area of apposition of the leaflets is reduced, the keystone effect is diminished, and chordal tension rises. The chordae then stretch or rupture, the relatively normal anterior leaflet prolapses, and mitral regurgitation supervenes. Because of the mitral regurgitation, the left atrium enlarges causing further dilatation of the posterior anulus and perpetuation of the process. Important billowing, redundancy, or floppy leaflet bodies are not features of rheumatic mitral regurgitation, and thus two-dimensional echocardiography easily demonstrates the dilated anulus and prolapse of the anterior leaflet whose edge fails to achieve coaptation with the apparently shortened posterior leaflet. Scarring and true retraction of mitral leaflets or commissural fusion are infrequent or mild at this time.

TABLE 1. **Anatomic and Echocardiographic Features of Mitral Valve Prolapse**

	Degenerative	Rheumatic
Leaflets	Localized or diffuse billowing of bodies of leaflets Posterior leaflet primarily affected Failure of leaflet edge apposition (i.e., prolapse) seldom demonstrated on two-dimensional echocardiography unless mitral regurgitation is severe and leaflet "flail" exists	Posterior leaflet stretched and functionally shortened Anterior leaflet usually normal in size. Failure of coaptation with shortened posterior leaflet and displacement of edge (i.e., prolapse) toward left atrium is clearly detected on two-dimensional echocardiography
Chordae tendineae	Elongated and attenuated. Rupture of chordae to middle scallop of posterior leaflet common in middle-aged males	Elongation, seldom rupture, of strut and other chordae to anterior leaflet
Anulus	Moderate or severe dilatation in 20%	Primarily involved by rheumatic process. Severe dilatation invariable

MANAGEMENT OF RHEUMATIC ANTERIOR MITRAL LEAFLET PROLAPSE WITH HEART FAILURE

Rheumatic MVP causing mild, moderate, or even fairly severe mitral regurgitation is treated with the usual medical therapy as long as the patient remains well compensated. When rheumatic activity and carditis are detected, physical rest is mandatory. Left or right ventricular failure never results from active rheumatic carditis in the absence of a hemodynamically severe valvular lesion. Any possible role of a myocardial component, so-called toxic rheumatic myocarditis, remains uncertain, but that entity, unlike viral myocarditis, does not by itself cause ventricular dilatation or heart failure. The principal valve lesion causing heart failure in patients with active rheumatic carditis is mitral regurgitation. The hemodynamic overload seems to aggravate the rheumatic activity and may initiate virulent rheumatic carditis. A vicious cycle is then established, and the heart failure becomes intractable. The sole effective management of such patients is surgical treatment. Neither the rheumatic activity nor the cardiac failure responds satisfactorily to medical therapy. Contrary to misleading doctrine, steroids are neither a "lifesaving" nor beneficial measure in patients who have fulminant rheumatic carditis with heart failure. Surgery should not be delayed, and hospital mortality is less than 5%. We perform mitral repair rather than replacement in approximately 80% of patients and achieve a good immediate outcome. The surgical technique addresses essentially the anular dilatation and the prolapsed anterior leaflet by narrowing the anulus with a Carpentier-Edwards ring and shortening the anterior leaflet strut chordae. The rheumatic activity abates dramatically during the first few weeks of the postoperative period.

DEGENERATIVE BILLOWING MITRAL LEAFLETS AND PROLAPSE

Primary BML or MVP is a degenerative process of the leaflets and chordae that has been described as a "dyscollagenosis" and is associated with myxomatous degeneration. The redundancy of leaflet tissue may be mild and focal, involving only a portion of one scallop of the posterior leaflet, or it may be severe and diffuse, involving both leaflets. The valve is functionally abnormal only when mitral regurgitation, and therefore true MVP, supervenes. Clinical or echocardiographic features of BML alone are prevalent and have been detected in approximately 15% of the normal population. Primary MVP in its advanced form is the most common cause of pure mitral regurgitation requiring surgery in developed countries.

THE SYNDROME: DESCRIPTION AND MANAGEMENT

The syndrome associated with this anomaly is variously called primary MVP, floppy valve, myxomatous leaflet, click-murmur, or Barlow's syndrome, but the term BML syndrome is still favored by us. Idiopathic or primary MVP syndrome is a misnomer in the large number of patients who have no evidence, principally on auscultation, of mitral regurgitation. A distinction between BML syndrome alone and BML syndrome with MVP is crucial in formulating a management policy. The physician has to decide whether repeated auscultation for an apical late or pansystolic mitral murmur, vasoactive maneuvers, echocardiography, or Doppler ultrasound will contribute to determining whether regurgitation is present. Clinical auscultation for the appropriate apical regurgitant murmur, particularly if it is late, pansystolic, or whooping, remains a consistently reliable and practical method of evaluating mitral regurgitation. Clinical cardiology as practiced in the 1990s, especially in the developed countries, regrettably reflects a decline in the use, accuracy, and status of auscultation. Confirmation of mitral regurgitation, or indeed its detection, is now sought by Doppler techniques. Doppler ultrasonography also has pitfalls, however, and color Doppler, as well as the bi-plane transesophageal color Doppler criteria for mild mitral regurgitation that has pathologic significance, still requires clarification. Depending in important ways on the criteria used, two-dimensional echocardiography may indicate billowing of part or all of a leaflet body, primarily the posterior leaflet, on the left atrial side of the anulus. Such cases are prevalent and relatively mild, and an associated constant or intermittent nonejection systolic click may be heard on auscultation. Most of these cases should be regarded as variants of normal. A major contribution of two-dimensional echocardiography is to identify a subgroup of patients in whom the leaflet bodies show advanced billowing, sometimes confined to the posterior leaflet's middle scallop, and such leaflets may also be thickened. Although the failure of leaflet edge apposition is seldom discerned on echocardiography, a majority of patients in this subgroup do have true MVP with consequent mitral regurgitation. They are at increased risk for important complications such as spontaneous progression to significant mitral regurgitation, infective endocarditis, systemic emboli, and life-threatening ventricular arrhythmias.

In addition to the auscultatory, anatomic, and electrocardiographic features recognized as a syndrome in 1965, other components include skeletal abnormalities, arrhythmias, conduction defects, systemic emboli, hereditary factors, and possibly neurologic and autonomic disorders. The importance of making the diagnosis of primary BML syndrome, particularly in symptomatic patients, lies in the knowledge that in the large majority of cases, reassurance can be given that there is no serious heart disease and that the prognosis for life is excellent. Symptoms are bizarre and include chest pain, palpitations, lightheadedness, breathlessness, and fatigue. It may often be thought that these cannot be explained on an organic basis. Nonetheless, the patient seeks assistance, and the medical adviser should be wary before concluding that all symptoms are not causally related to the valve anomaly. Palpitations may be a reflection of the ventricular arrhythmias that occur when mitral leaflets are markedly billowing or floppy, and it has yet to be demonstrated that a BML does not indeed cause chest pain, albeit by an unexplained mechanism. Many symptomatic patients are anxious. Reasons for extreme anxiety are not always apparent, and the role of a causally related autonomic disorder remains arguable. Anxiety is aggravated in some patients by an incorrect diagnosis of occlusive coronary artery disease or when scant interpretation of the chest pain, sometimes allegedly severe, is provided. An explanation that there is "a very mild but also very common anomaly of a heart valve, which sometimes causes ill-understood symptoms of nuisance value only" is a comprehensible explanation from which many patients derive reassurance. Some fail to respond to reassurance alone but improve on a small dose of a beta-adrenergic blocking drug.

Although most patients with BML syndrome follow a benign course, complications in a few warrant attention.

Infective Endocarditis and Progression of Mitral Regurgitation

Whether symptomatic or not, patients with mitral regurgitation invariably have marked BML, which is easily demonstrated on echocardiography, and both prophylaxis against infective endocarditis and observation for progression of the MVP are indicated. Most nonpansystolic mitral murmurs, whether confined to early or late systole, remain unchanged for many years. Nonetheless, rapid progression of mitral regurgitation, even in the absence of infective endocarditis, may occur unpredictably. The overall incidence of such progression during a 10-year period is probably 10%, and this figure may be higher in middle-aged males. On the other hand, it is important to reiterate that unequivocal billowing on echocardiography or a loud nonejection systolic click on auscultation does not imply that MVP, let alone severe mitral regurgitation, will inevitably ensue.

Systemic Emboli

Bland emboli manifesting as transient ischemic attacks or partial strokes are a rare complication. Deposits of fibrin and platelet thrombi on the atrial surface of a floppy posterior leaflet may be the site of origin. Coronary emboli with coronary artery spasm have been suggested as the mechanism of otherwise unexplained myocardial infarction in a few instances. A purported association of BML and migraine requires confirmation, as does a common role of increased platelet aggregability in both conditions. Antithrombotic therapy is recommended in patients who have had emboli. We have had good results with aspirin (160 to 320 mg daily) plus dipyridamole (Persantine),* 100 mg three times daily. The effectiveness

*This drug has not been approved by the FDA for this indication.

of dipyridamole as an antithrombotic agent has been challenged, and aspirin alone may be adequate. If systemic emboli are large or if an underlying supraventricular tachyarrhythmia is suspected, warfarin (Coumadin) therapy is suggested.

Arrhythmias and Sudden Death

Palpitations, lightheadedness, or dizziness may reflect an underlying arrhythmia, but exercise electrocardiography or ambulatory monitoring are advisable for evaluation. Just as arrhythmias may occur without symptoms, dizziness and palpitations are sometimes prominent complaints when electrocardiographic monitoring and clinical examination provide no objective confirmation. Orthostatic hypotension should be excluded in all patients with these symptoms. Arrhythmias encountered in patients with the primary BML syndrome include supraventricular tachycardia, atrial fibrillation and flutter, atrial ectopic beats, ventricular tachycardia, and ventricular fibrillation. Ventricular extrasystoles are the most common rhythm disturbance; they may be unifocal or multifocal and may occur with or without an abnormal resting electrocardiogram. This arrhythmia is frequently precipitated or aggravated by emotion and exercise. When symptoms are troublesome, even if the arrhythmias are not potentially dangerous, patients should be treated with antiarrhythmic drugs, preferably verapamil (Isoptin) (if the rhythm is supraventricular) or beta-blocking agents. Although any beta-receptor blocking agent may contribute and will usually suffice, in more intractable cases we have had favorable experience with the unique beta-receptor-blocking agent sotalol (Betapace) (usual dose range 120 to 480 mg daily). Because of its important Class III activity, sotalol has the potential to precipitate ventricular tachycardias of the torsades de pointes variety and should be used with caution in high dosages, with concomitant diuretic therapy, or in the presence of hypokalemia. Amiodarone (Cordarone), 200 to 400 mg daily after a loading dose, is extremely effective for the treatment of refractory ventricular tachyarrhythmias, but serious side effects mitigate against its long-term use, especially in young subjects. In the absence of syncope and regardless of whether other symptoms are present or not, overall experience currently suggests that the prognosis for life is excellent despite the demonstration of multiple and multifocal ventricular ectopy.

A reliable history of syncope, provided that it occurs outside a context of probable vasovagal syncope, is cause for concern. It is estimated that at least 200 patients with the BML syndrome and causally related sudden death or "sudden death syndrome" have been reported or observed. Identification of patients at higher risk is crucial. In addition to a history of unexpected syncope and detection of multiform ventricular ectopy, other risk factors include a prominent BML that is demonstrable on M-mode or two-dimensional echocardiography, indisputable mitral regurgitation evaluated clinically or by color Doppler, abnormal T waves on the resting ECG, and a family history of unexpected sudden death. The important observation that BML patients with mitral regurgitation have more ventricular ectopy than those without mitral regurgitation almost certainly reflects the fact that the former have more advanced floppy and voluminous leaflets. Ventricular arrhythmias are not a feature of rheumatic anterior leaflet prolapse, in which the mitral leaflets are not voluminous regardless of the severity of the mitral regurgitation.

Optimal management of these high-risk patients, commonly relatively young women, with the BML syndrome but without hemodynamically important mitral regurgitation, remains a challenge. There are no data to justify treatment with Class IA antiarrhythmic drugs. Successful short-term results have been attained with implantable defibrillators, but this approach fails to address the basic cause of the life-threatening problem. The degenerative floppy mitral valve is particularly amenable to a surgical repair, and the durability of this repair over at least 10 years has been confirmed. Cardiac surgeons throughout the world are now gaining meaningful experience with valvuloplastic procedures. We recommend and practice surgical excision of excess leaflet tissue, appropriate shortening of the chordae tendineae, and insertion of a Carpentier ring for the management of high-risk MVP patients with potentially fatal arrhythmias despite the absence of a hemodynamic indication for surgery. Mitral valve repair in this context is justifiable, and it is now incumbent on surgeons experienced in valve repair to adopt this policy. Mitral valve replacement, with its need for anticoagulation and the attendant risk of thromboembolism or hemorrhage, is not recommended in these patients at this time.

CONGESTIVE HEART FAILURE

method of
AXEL SIGURDSSON, M.D., PH.D., and
KARL SWEDBERG, M.D., PH.D.
University of Göteborg,
Östra Hospital,
Göteborg, Sweden

Heart failure is a clinical syndrome caused by an abnormality of cardiac function that is responsible for the failure of the heart to pump adequate amounts of blood to meet the needs of the metabolizing tissues. Heart failure is furthermore characterized by a number of important adaptive and maladaptive responses involving the heart, kidneys, peripheral vasculature, and skeletal muscles. Each of these responses is variably modulated by complex neurohormonal mechanisms.

The primary event in heart failure is myocardial damage that leads to the loss of a critical quantity of contractile myocardial tissue. The initial injury is caused by different mechanisms such as acute myocardial infarction, prolonged volume or pressure overload (hypertension, valvular disorders), toxins (alcohol or cytotoxic drugs), or infections (viral myocarditis or Chagas' disease). The cause of the myocardial damage may sometimes be unknown, as for example in idiopathic dilated cardiomyopathy.

DIAGNOSIS

No single symptom or clinical finding is pathognomonic for the diagnosis of heart failure. Careful history and physical examination may reveal symptoms of dyspnea, orthopnea, paroxysmal nocturnal dyspnea, exertional fatigue, and signs such as pulmonary rales, third heart sound, distended neck veins, and peripheral edema. Further evaluation of patients with heart failure is aimed at identifying the underlying cause of the disorder. The electrocardiogram may show signs of a prior myocardial infarction and reveal arrhythmias. A chest radiograph is valuable to exclude obvious pulmonary diseases. Doppler echocardiography is indicated to clarify the degree of left ventricular dysfunction, segmental wall motion, size of the cardiac chambers, diastolic function, and valvular disorders. Cardiac performance may also be assessed with radionuclide techniques. If coronary artery disease is suspected, exercise testing and coronary arteriography are indicated. A normal echocardiographic evaluation and exercise test exclude heart failure.

PATHOPHYSIOLOGY

Heart failure may develop immediately after an acute myocardial injury or after a period of asymptomatic left ventricular dysfunction. Because of compensatory mechanisms, cardiac output and peripheral perfusion can be maintained in many patients without symptoms for some time. These adaptive responses are the result of a complex interplay between hemodynamic, neurohormonal, peripheral, and myocardial factors. Following a large myocardial infarction, the infarcted segment tends to dilate and become thinned, a process termed infarct expansion. Subsequently, hypertrophy and dilatation of the noninfarcted, contractile myocardium also occur. The overall result is an alteration in the geometry of the ventricle and an increase in left ventricular volume. The process, termed left ventricular remodeling, may precede a deterioration in left ventricular function.

Left ventricular dysfunction and clinical heart failure are also characterized by activation of the neuroendocrine systems (sympathetic nervous system and the renin-angiotensin-aldosterone system). Although supportive in hemodynamic terms, the modern concept of the pathophysiology of heart failure considers neuroendocrine activation to be maladaptive in the long run, causing further harm to the myocardium that leads to progression of heart failure. These effects may be temporarily opposed by activation of counterregulatory vasodilator mechanisms, such as increased secretion of natriuretic peptides from the atria and ventricles. However, over time, these vasodilator responses tend to become overwhelmed by activation of vasoconstrictor mechanisms such as the sympathetic nervous system and the renin-angiotensin system. Thus, at some point in time, compensatory mechanisms appear to become exhausted, and clinical heart failure emerges or progresses. At this stage cardiac filling pressures are usually elevated, cardiac output is reduced, and peripheral vasoconstriction exists. Reduced blood flow to the kidneys leads to retention of sodium and the occurrence of peripheral and pulmonary edema, the hallmarks of congestive heart failure. The exact role of neuroendocrine activation in the transition from left ventricular dysfunction to symptomatic heart failure is incompletely understood.

TREATMENT

Treatment of heart failure depends on the underlying etiology of myocardial dysfunction and on the clinical severity of the disorder. The pharmacologic treatment of chronic heart failure has traditionally been targeted toward reducing symptoms such as dyspnea and fluid retention. Because of their symptomatic effects, diuretic drugs are the cornerstone of therapy. In acute severe heart failure, intravenous treatment with vasodilators or inotropic drugs is often needed. Treatment is primarily aimed at achieving hemodynamic stability, preserving renal function, and alleviating pulmonary congestion and peripheral fluid retention. However, during the past few years physicians have become increasingly aware of the progressive nature and high mortality of this disorder. Several large-scale clinical trials have shown that the natural history of chronic heart failure may be influenced by pharmacologic interventions. Thus, treatment with angiotensin-converting enzyme inhibitors improves survival whereas treatment with inotropic drugs such as the phosphodiesterase inhibitors may actually increase mortality. Cardiac transplantations are now being successfully performed and provide improved survival and quality of life for many patients with end-stage heart failure, although the limited number of donor organs does not match the demand.

ACUTE HEART FAILURE

Acute heart failure is defined as moderately severe to severe heart failure of rapid onset or rapid worsening of previous chronic congestive heart failure. The condition is characterized by dyspnea, coughing, fatigue, anxiety, and an affected sensorium. The clinical findings include tachypnea and orthopnea, rales, a third heart sound, tachycardia, cold extremities, and sweating, with fulminant pulmonary edema in extreme cases. Clinical signs of bronchospasm may occur. The most severe form of acute heart failure is cardiogenic shock, which is characterized by the triad of hypotension, oliguria, and a clouded sensorium.

The underlying cause of acute heart failure should, when possible, be ascertained to allow choice of optimal treatment. Acute heart failure may be triggered by myocardial ischemia or infarction, an acute volume load caused by intraventricular septal rupture, papillary muscle dysfunction, acute aortic insufficiency, aortic stenosis, cardiac tamponade, rhythm disturbances, infections, and anemia. Emergency surgical correction of severe aortic stenosis may be lifesaving. Drugs with fluid-retaining properties such as the nonsteroidal anti-inflammatory drugs should be kept in mind as possible precipitating factors as well as compounds with negative inotropic properties, such as some of the calcium antagonists and large doses of beta blockers.

Initial treatment includes appropriate positioning of the patient propped up in bed, oxygen, nitroglycerin, and diuretics. Morphine is administered when pulmonary edema or anxiety is present. Theophylline may be given when there is bronchospasm. This treatment, or parts thereof, should be given as early as possible and is preferably started before the patient arrives at the hospital. The effects of treatment are assessed by repeated measurements of the patient's condition including blood pressure, heart rate, and urinary production.

The clinical signs of acute right ventricular failure include an increased jugular venous pressure with tricuspid insufficiency, hypotension, and a clouded sensorium. Despite a low blood pressure, initially these patients usually have warm extremities. The heart rate may be paradoxically low and the respiratory rate normal. Oliguria is common. When the underlying cause of right ventricular failure is an acute myocardial infarction, this is nearly always located in the inferior left ventricular wall, and an electrocardiogram may reveal evidence of right ventricular involvement in the right ventricular leads (V_{4R}). The prognosis is better for these patients than for those with severe left heart failure with hypotension or shock, and the treatment is somewhat different. It is therefore important to diagnose this condition, and this is an indication for a Swan-Ganz catheter to guide treatment with volume expansion, diuretics, and positive inotropic drugs. It is particularly important that high right ventricular pressures are maintained in these patients.

Raised Ventricular Filling Pressures

Breathlessness is the main symptom in acute heart failure. Treatment consists of administration of nitroglycerin, morphine when needed, and loop diuretics.

Nitroglycerin is given sublingually (0.4 mg), or by spray (0.4 mg). The dose may be repeated every 10 minutes until there is clinical improvement. Buccal nitroglycerin may also be used (2.5 to 5 mg). Administration may be limited by a fall in blood pressure. Nitroglycerin is preferably given as an intravenous infusion to hospitalized patients, starting at a dose of 0.25 μg per kg per minute and increasing it every 5 minutes until a fall in systolic blood pressure by 15 mmHg or to a level of 90 mmHg is observed.

Loop diuretics are given in the form of furosemide (Lasix) intravenously. Usually 20 to 40 mg is a sufficient dose, but repeated doses are often required. Large bolus doses may be hemodynamically unfavorable. High doses, preferably administered by intravenous infusion (doses of up to 4 mg per minute can be administered), are, however, often necessary in patients with reduced renal function.

Morphine, 2.5 to 10 mg, is given intravenously and may be repeated every 15 minutes. Apart from its beneficial effect on anxiety, it produces a favorable hemodynamic dilatory effect on the capacitance vessels.

Continuous positive airway pressure (CPAP) administered by face mask provides quick relief of symptoms in many patients with pulmonary edema. CPAP may decrease the work of breathing, relieve symptoms, and exert beneficial hemodynamic and respiratory effects. It should be used with caution in patients with hypovolemia, hypotension, or chronic obstructive pulmonary disease. Vomiting, pneumothorax, and a clouded sensorium are considered contraindications to CPAP. When administered, CPAP should be started with a regulator that provides a resistance of 7.5 cmH_2O, which may be increased to 10 cmH_2O if necessary. Close monitoring of PO_2 and PCO_2 is mandatory and should be assessed every 2 to 3 hours or more frequently if the patient is unstable. If the patient's condition improves, CPAP can often be discontinued after a stable period of 10 to 15 minutes.

Low Cardiac Output

If a low cardiac output is suspected, attempts should be made to lower the peripheral vascular resistance and give inotropic support. Heart rate and rhythm should be regulated to the optimal value. The beneficial effect of relatively low heart rates in the presence of valvular stenoses should be remembered. Dobutamine (Dobutrex), initial dose 2.5 μg per kg per minute, gradually increased by 2.5 μg per kg per minute after 5 to 10 minutes, is used primarily. The dose may be increased until the desired hemodynamic effect has been obtained. Blood pressure, heart rate, and urinary volumes are carefully monitored. Patients who remain oliguric may benefit from an additional low dose of dopamine (Intropin), 2.5 to 5 μg per kg per minute. Tachycardia is a common problem in this situation.

Phosphodiesterase inhibitors such as amrinone and milrinone may be administered intravenously. Amrinone (Inocor) may be an ideal agent for selected patients with heart failure that persists despite treatment with diuretics who are not hypotensive and who are likely to benefit from both an enhancement in contractility and afterload reduction. Amrinone is administered as an intravenous bolus dose of 0.75 mg per kg body weight followed by an intravenous infusion, starting with 5 μg per kg per minute and increasing the dose up to 10 μg per kg per minute.

The following combinations can be tried: dobutamine plus dopamine; dobutamine plus phosphodiesterase inhibitor (amrinone, milrinone); and dobutamine plus dopamine plus phosphodiesterase inhibitor. The choice of which combination to use is guided by the hemodynamic situation of each patient.

Digitalis may be given to patients with supraventricular tachycardia that is considered relevant to the heart failure situation at hand. Caution should be exercised in patients who are already taking digitalis. Nitroglycerin may be useful in the presence of markedly elevated filling pressures (see earlier). If peripheral resistance is low, norepinephrine may be administered temporarily at a dose of 0.025 to 0.4 μg per kg per minute to elevate the systolic blood pressure to 90 to 100 mmHg.

Drugs under investigation in this situation include

dopexamine with predominant beta$_2$-agonist activity and ibopamine with dopaminergic agonist activity.

Cardiogenic Shock

The importance of a correct diagnosis of cardiogenic shock cannot be overemphasized. Myocardial infarction is the most common cause, but other causes include aortic stenosis, cardiac tamponade, pulmonary embolism, and arrhythmias. The prognosis for patients with cardiogenic shock is very poor. Emergency percutaneous transluminal coronary angioplasty (PTCA) or revascularization may be lifesaving and should be considered at an early stage. Supportive treatment with a balloon pump may be useful to help the patient survive until such procedures can be started. Patients in cardiogenic shock can be assumed to be acidotic. Correction of the latter is essential because catecholamines have little effect in an acid medium. Ventilator support could be used to handle the acidosis.

CHRONIC HEART FAILURE

When a diagnosis of chronic heart failure has been established, patients should be offered advice and support about their lifestyle and psychosocial situation. Lifestyle changes include fluid and salt restriction, avoidance of large meals, mobility service, use of parking facilities for disabled persons, and an evaluation of the patient's working situation. Physical activity is to be encouraged if symptoms permit. Smoking should be stopped because it has hemodynamically unfavorable effects, impairs the oxygen-binding capacity of blood, and is thrombogenic. Attention should be paid to the negative effects on the myocardium caused by alcohol.

Asymptomatic Left Ventricular Dysfunction

Patients with reduced systolic left ventricular function (ejection fraction lower than 35 to 40%) but no overt heart failure are recommended for long-term treatment with an angiotensin-converting enzyme inhibitor. Data from large clinical trials performed in recent years have demonstrated that such treatment may delay the development of symptomatic heart failure and lower the incidence of myocardial infarction or unstable angina. Furthermore, such treatment appears to reduce mortality among patients with reduced systolic left ventricular function following myocardial infarction.

Mild Heart Failure

Symptoms caused by fluid retention are treated primarily with diuretic drugs. Thiazide diuretics may be preferable to loop diuretics because the former provide more constant diuresis. An angiotensin-converting enzyme inhibitor should be administered because it will slow the progression to more severe congestive heart failure and reduce mortality. In patients who show symptomatic improvement and when dose reductions seem indicated, dose reduction should begin with the diuretic. A potassium-sparing agent is prescribed to patients with normal renal function if the diuretic is not combined with an angiotensin-converting enzyme inhibitor. Amiloride (Midamor) is used primarily. Digitalis is prescribed to patients with atrial fibrillation or flutter.

Moderate to Severe Heart Failure

Diuretics and angiotensin-converting enzyme inhibitors are used for maintenance treatment. This combination decreases both morbidity and mortality in patients with moderate to severe heart failure. Though the value of digitalis has not yet been established, it is known to improve symptoms and exercise tolerance in patients in whom left ventricular function is markedly impaired.

Management of Pharmacologic Therapy

Treatment with loop diuretics is given intravenously to severely ill patients. Suitable doses are 20 to 40 mg of furosemide (Lasix) or, alternatively, 0.5 to 1.0 mg of bumetanide (Bumex). Rapid dehydration should be avoided. During maintenance treatment, daily doses of more than 120 mg of furosemide or 3 mg of bumetanide are rarely required in the absence of renal insufficiency. Spironolactone, 25 to 50 mg daily, may be added when the diuretic effect of thiazides or loop diuretics is insufficient. When these patients also receive an angiotensin-converting enzyme inhibitor there is, however, a risk of hyperkalemia. Metolazone (Zaroxolyn) may be added in patients who have marked fluid retention or fail to respond to loop diuretics. During such combination treatment, careful monitoring of fluid balance, electrolyte levels, and renal function is necessary. Potassium-sparing agents, primarily in the form of amiloride, are used to counteract the development of hypokalemia. Potassium chloride or other corresponding agents are second-line drugs for these purposes because they have no effect on losses of other electrolytes such as magnesium.

Treatment with angiotensin-converting enzyme inhibitors can often be initiated in an outpatient setting. Patients with severe heart failure, impaired renal function, and a tendency to develop electrolyte disturbances should, however, be monitored in the hospital when treatment is introduced. A reduction in the diuretic dose is recommended when treatment with a converting enzyme inhibitor is initiated. Potassium-sparing diuretics are withdrawn when treatment is started. Patients are preferably kept under observation for a few hours after receiving the first dose of a converting enzyme inhibitor when outpatient treatment is initiated. A suitable initial dose of enalapril (Vasotec), lisinopril (Zestril), or ramipril (Altace) is 2.5 mg with an observation time of about 3 to 4 hours. Treatment should be targeted at a maintenance dose of 20 mg daily (10 mg daily for ramipril). The starting dose of captopril (Capoten) is 6.25 to 12.5 mg, and the suitable outpatient observation time is 1 to 2 hours. The optimal maintenance dose is 100 to 150 mg daily, divided among two or three doses. Serum electrolytes and creatinine levels should be monitored 1 week after treatment with a converting enzyme inhibitor is initiated and whenever doses are increased. An increase in serum creatinine of 20 to 30% is acceptable, but it is important to exclude a further elevation of creatinine levels.

Digitalis is often added to the combination of a diuretic and an angiotensin-converting enzyme inhibitor. Digitalis treatment may positively influence symptoms, although the effect on mortality is unknown. Digitalization may be achieved with oral or intravenous administration of digoxin. Maintenance doses are adjusted according to age and renal function. Digitoxin is an alternative in patients with impaired renal function.

Combination treatment with hydralazine and isosorbide dinitrate may be considered in patients who fail to improve or in whom adequate treatment with an angiotensin-converting enzyme inhibitor cannot be given because of side effects. Hospitalization is often required for adjusting treatment in these patients.

Beta-adrenergic blockers appear to improve symptoms in patients with heart failure due to idiopathic dilated cardiomyopathy. Long-term treatment with positive inotropic agents such as beta-adrenergic agonists and phosphodiesterase inhibitors is not recommended and may have adverse effects on survival. Calcium channel blockers have not been demonstrated to be of value in patients with heart failure. Ongoing trials are evaluating whether the newer dihydropyridines (amlodipine [Norvasc], felodipine [Plendil]) are valuable.

Antiarrhythmic Treatment and Chronic Heart Failure

Ventricular arrhythmias are common in patients with chronic heart failure. About 50% of deaths are sudden. Antiarrhythmic drug therapy for asymptomatic ventricular arrhythmias in the presence of heart failure has not been shown to influence survival positively or reduce the risk of sudden death. Instead, some studies indicate an increased mortality in patients receiving Class I antiarrhythmic drugs after myocardial infarction. In patients with symptomatic ventricular arrhythmias there is a lack of well-designed trials assessing the possible value of antiarrhythmic drugs, and controversies exist about how to predict the efficacy of such therapy. In general, only gravely ill patients with symptomatic ventricular arrhythmias should be treated. Currently, the Class III antiarrhythmic agent amiodarone or sotalol (Betapace), which is a beta blocker with Class III properties, should be considered primarily. There are strong data indicating that beta-adrenergic blocking drugs may reduce the risk of sudden death among patients with heart failure following myocardial infarction. The use of an automatic implantable defibrillator should be considered in patients with life-threatening ventricular arrhythmias. The potential benefit of these devices is currently under evaluation in ongoing clinical trials.

Antiarrhythmic drug therapy may be needed in patients with paroxysmal atrial fibrillation or supraventricular tachycardia in the presence of heart failure. Amiodarone is often selected because of its lack of significant negative inotropic properties. Digitalis is the drug of choice in patients with chronic atrial fibrillation and concomitant heart failure. The addition of a beta blocker or a calcium channel blocker such as verapamil (Calan) may be required for optimal regulation of the heart rate. However, these drugs should be used with caution because of their negative inotropic effects. His bundle ablation may be considered when drug treatment fails or is not tolerated.

SURGERY FOR CONGESTIVE HEART FAILURE

Nonpharmacologic treatment of heart failure should be considered when symptomatic relief cannot be achieved with drugs or when the risk of death is considered too high, regardless of symptoms.

Coronary Revascularization

Patients with coronary artery disease and reduced left ventricular ejection fraction may benefit from coronary artery bypass surgery. Segmental myocardial dysfunction may be caused by ischemia and therefore may be potentially reversible. Although such myocardial areas may be detected by positron emission tomography (PET), there are no generally available methods for detection of myocardial viability. Because of the absence of clinical trials, coronary artery bypass surgery cannot be generally recommended to patients with heart failure who have no angina or detectable ischemia on positive exercise tests.

Cardiomyoplasty

Left ventricular performance may be improved when a skeletal muscle flap is wrapped around the ventricular wall and allowed to contract synchronously with it. Most commonly, the latissimus dorsi muscle is used for this purpose. Patients with end-stage heart failure who are considered for heart transplantation in areas with insufficient donor availability may be considered for cardiomyoplasty. It takes about 2 months to condition the skeletal muscle by electrical stimulation to become resistant to fatigue. Therefore, patients should be considered somewhat earlier for cardiomyoplasty than is normally recommended for heart transplantation. Data on both short-term and long-term results are limited. Although some centers have reported positive results, the initial enthusiasm for cardiomyoplasty has diminished because the beneficial effects seem to vanish during long-term therapy (>3 to 6 months).

Heart Transplantation

Heart transplantation is fairly well established as a treatment for end-stage heart failure. Careful selection of patients for this therapy is necessary because of the limited supply of donor organs. Patients with chronic heart failure, who are expected to live less than 12 months with conventional pharmacologic treatment, should be considered for heart transplantation. The upper age limit is usually considered to be about 60 years because of the limited availability of donor organs. Following the introduction of cyclosporine in 1980, a marked improvement in long-term survival was found with triple immunosuppressive therapy compared with earlier results when only azathioprine and steroids were used. According to international data, the operative mortality is about 10%. One-year survival is about 80%, and 5-year survival is about 70%.

DIASTOLIC HEART FAILURE

Heart failure is traditionally defined as a failure of systolic function in which an impaired inotropic state of the ventricle is the primary abnormality. Diastolic heart failure represents an abnormality of ventricular filling caused by abnormalities in ventricular relaxation or stiffness. Diastolic function is commonly assessed using pulsed Doppler echocardiography to study the velocity of transmitral blood flow, which reflects the left ventricular filling rate. The major consequences of diastolic failure are related to an elevation of ventricular filling pressures. Usually systolic and diastolic heart failure coexist. Hypertrophic cardiomyopathy or subendocardial fibrosis may be examples of pure diastolic heart failure. Diastolic failure is often claimed to be more important in heart failure among the elderly. Because pulmonary congestion is a common presentation in patients with diastolic heart failure, diuretics and venodilators such as nitrates may provide symptomatic relief in the acute situation. Maintenance therapy should, however, avoid excessive preload reduction. Therefore, when diastolic failure is supposed to be the dominant cause, diuretics and nitrates should be reduced or avoided. In patients with coexisting systolic and diastolic dysfunction, this balance may become difficult. Beta-adrenergic blockers and calcium antagonists may be of value in some patients with diastolic dysfunction.

INFECTIVE ENDOCARDITIS

method of
GABRIEL GREGORATOS, M.D.
University of California, Davis
Davis, California

Infective endocarditis is a microbial infection of the cardiac valves, the endocardium, or the endothelium adjacent to a cardiac or vascular malformation. It is caused by a large variety of microorganisms, and the infection may pursue either a prolonged (subacute) or a fulminant (acute) course. Although a great deal of overlap exists, it is clinically useful to classify endocarditis as acute (usually caused by invasive microorganisms such as *Staphylococcus aureus, Streptococcus pyogenes,* or *Neisseria* species) or subacute (caused by more indolent organisms such as *Streptococcus viridans* or *Staphylococcus epidermidis*). Prognosis and therapy differ considerably for these two forms.

Approximately 70% of patients with endocarditis have evidence of pre-existing structural cardiac abnormalities. Patients at high risk are those with prosthetic cardiac valves, aortic stenosis or insufficiency, mitral insufficiency, patent ductus arteriosus, or ventricular septal defect and those undergoing hyperalimentation through indwelling right heart catheters. On the other hand, patients with mitral stenosis, mitral valve prolapse, tricuspid valve disease, hypertrophic obstructive cardiomyopathy, calcific aortic sclerosis, or tetralogy of Fallot have an intermediate risk of infection. The presence of an atrial septal defect, luetic aortitis, transvenous pacemakers, or aortocoronary bypass grafts involves only a low or negligible risk. In the remaining 30% of patients who develop endocarditis, no pre-existing cardiac abnormality can be documented.

Infective endocarditis occurs frequently in intravenous drug abusers. The prognosis in this subgroup of patients is variable and has a reported mortality of 0 to 30%. By comparison, mortality for native valve endocarditis ranges from 20 to 40% in various series, and prosthetic valve endocarditis carries a mortality of 20 to 60%. Clinically, the tricuspid valve is most commonly involved in intravenous drug abusers, followed by the aortic and mitral valves, whereas in the general population infections of the mitral valve predominate, followed closely by aortic valve endocarditis. The causative agents in various patient subgroups are listed in Table 1.

DIAGNOSIS

When endocarditis is suspected, careful serial examinations are necessary to detect the development of a new *organic* murmur due to valvular destruction by the infectious process. A change in intensity or character of a pre-existing organic murmur is a much less reliable sign because alterations in cardiac output, body temperature, or hematocrit may produce impressive changes in the intensity and quality of a cardiac murmur completely independent of changes in valvular integrity. Peripheral cutaneous manifestations such as petechiae, splinter hemorrhages, Osler's nodes, Janeway's lesions, and so on are seen in 20 to 40% of cases, while clubbing of the fingers and splenomegaly are rare clinical manifestations today, seen in only 5 to 15% of all patients with endocarditis.

Blood Cultures. Definitive diagnosis of infective endocarditis is made by isolating the infecting microorganism from the circulation. Three sets of blood cultures, obtained a few hours apart during the first day of hospitalization, yield the causative organism in 98% of all cases unless the patient has been partially treated with antibiotics during the previous 2 weeks. Because the bacteremia of endocarditis is most often continuous, it is not necessary to obtain blood cultures at the time of high fever or chills. Blood cultures should be repeated 2 and 5 days after initiation of antibiotic therapy to document clearing of the bacteremia and should be repeated again 1 and 3 weeks after cessation of therapy because of the possibility of relapse. Once the causative organism has been isolated, it is essential to test

TABLE 1. **Microorganisms Commonly Responsible for Infective Endocarditis (Listed in Order of Decreasing Frequency)**

Native Valves	In IV Drug Abusers†	Prosthetic Valves
Streptococcus viridans	*Staphylococcus aureus*	*Staphylococcus epidermidis*
Enterococci or other streptococci	Streptococci	*Staphylococcus aureus*
Staphylococcus aureus	Enterococci	Gram-negative bacilli
Culture-negative	Gram-negative bacilli	*Streptococcus viridans*
Gram-negative bacilli	Fungi	Fungi
Fungi *(Candida, Aspergillus)*	Culture-negative	Enterococci
Diphtheroids	*Staphylococcus epidermidis*	Diphtheroids
Staphylococcus epidermidis	Diphtheroids	Culture-negative
Miscellaneous*	Miscellaneous*	Miscellaneous*

*Miscellaneous organisms: Gonococci, pneumococci, meningococci, rickettsiae, *Listeria, Haemophilus, Chlamydia, Clostridium, Eikenella*
†In 5% of IV drug abusers more than one organism is isolated

its sensitivity to antibiotics. In most cases when dealing with streptococci, routine disk (Kirby-Bauer) sensitivity studies are sufficient to select the appropriate antibiotic therapy. However, when dealing with penicillin-resistant streptococci, staphylococci, and other relatively resistant organisms, it is necessary to perform quantitative tube dilution sensitivity studies and determine both minimum inhibitory concentration (MIC) and minimum bactericidal concentration (MBC) to determine the appropriate antibiotic dosage. It is recommended that a peak serum sample obtained 30 minutes after the antibiotic has been administered be proved to be bactericidal in a dilution of 1:8 or greater (although an MBC of 1:8 or greater does not uniformly predict successful outcome). "Culture-negative" endocarditis is usually due either to administration of antibiotics before blood cultures are drawn or to poor bacteriologic technique with reference to microorganisms with special growth requirements. Prolonged culture incubation (3 weeks) with media supplemented with thiol may be necessary to identify slow-growing organisms.

Echocardiography. Echocardiography has become an indispensable tool in making the diagnosis and following the progress of treatment in patients with infective endocarditis. A combined M-mode and two-dimensional echocardiogram (with Doppler evaluation of the cardiac valves) should be performed immediately after hospitalization and again 2 to 3 weeks later unless the clinical course dictates an earlier study. Echocardiographic studies are useful in determining the valve or valves involved by the infectious process, the severity of valvular dysfunction, and ventricular function, and occasionally in documenting the extracardiac progression of the disease (e.g., development of an aortic ring abscess). Transesophageal echocardiography is a more sensitive technique for identifying valvular vegetations than M-mode or two-dimensional echocardiography studies and is especially useful in identifying extravalvular complications (ring abscesses, fistulas, and myocardial abscesses). The presence of very large valvular vegetations should suggest a fungal etiology and may be an indication for early surgical therapy.

TREATMENT

General Principles

It is important to categorize patients with infective endocarditis into complicated or uncomplicated groups. Patients with infection due to *S. viridans, S. bovis,* or *S. faecalis* may be placed in the uncomplicated group if there is no evidence of hemodynamically significant valve dysfunction, because these organisms are all relatively sensitive to penicillin. Prognosis in this group is generally good, and a 90 to 97% percent bacteriologic cure is achieved with 4 weeks of antibiotic therapy. These organisms do not become resistant during therapy, and the treatment regimens have been standardized for years and are well tested and accepted. Disk diffusion studies are adequate guides of therapy for this group of patients.

Patients should be classified in the complicated group if the causative organism is a staphyloccus, a fungus, or a gram-negative organism or if "culture-negative" endocarditis is present. Similarly, patients with intracardiac prosthetic devices, patients allergic to penicillin, intravenous drug users, and pregnant women also belong in the complicated group. Finally, patients presenting with heart failure, renal failure, extensive distal embolization, CNS complications, and extravalvular cardiac complications also must be considered to have complicated disease. Prognosis in this group is uncertain, with only a 20 to 80% bacteriologic cure being reported. Organisms involved in this group of patients frequently become resistant during therapy, and therapeutic regimens are not well standardized. Quantitative tube dilution sensitivity studies are necessary, and cardiovascular surgical support is often required to achieve cure and to treat complications. Whereas patients with uncomplicated endocarditis may be effectively treated in almost any well-staffed facility with an adequate microbiology laboratory, patients with complicated disease are best treated in a tertiary referral center where sophisticated microbiologic and surgical support services are available.

General Principles of Therapy

1. Microbiologic diagnosis and accurate studies of the sensitivity of the isolated organism to antibiotic agents must be established as early as possible.

2. Patients with acute fulminant infective endocarditis must be treated with an empirical antimicrobial regimen as soon as possible after three sets of blood cultures have been obtained at 15-minute intervals.

3. Early cardiovascular surgical consultation should be obtained in all patients with native aortic

valve endocarditis and patients with a valvular prosthesis even if they are hemodynamically stable.

4. Repeat blood cultures should be obtained after initiation of antibiotic therapy, as mentioned previously.

5. Careful serial physical examinations should be performed because subtle changes often precede abrupt hemodynamic catastrophes.

6. In the great majority of cases, antibiotic chemotherapy must be administered parenterally in a hospital setting because absorption of orally administered antibiotics may be unpredictable, and compliance is always in question.

7. Every patient should be examined to determine the portal of entry, especially the oral cavity. Necessary dental therapy should be performed under the umbrella of antibiotic treatment. Patients with endocarditis caused by *S. bovis* must undergo complete examination of the colon in search of neoplasia or other colonic pathology.

Specific Antibiotic Therapy (Table 2)

Streptococcal Endocarditis. *S. viridans* and *S. bovis* are usually highly sensitive to penicillin, as evidenced by a zone of inhibition of 30 mm or more surrounding a 10-μg penicillin disk or an MIC of less than 0.1 mg per milliliter. If streptomycin or gentamicin is added to the penicillin regimen, parenteral therapy may be limited in this group of patients to 2 weeks with an additional 2 weeks of oral penicillin or amoxicillin and probenecid therapy. Elderly patients and those with pre-existing renal dysfunction should not be given streptomycin or gentamicin, and penicillin therapy should be continued parenterally for a minimum of 4 weeks. Patients with prosthetic valve endocarditis due to these organisms should receive 6 weeks of penicillin therapy with the addition of streptomycin or gentamicin for the initial 2 weeks. Patients allergic to penicillin may be treated with vancomycin or a cephalosporin if the history of allergy does not indicate the presence of anaphylaxis or urticaria.

Enterococcal Endocarditis. *S. faecalis* organisms generally demonstrate an intermediate sensitivity to penicillin by disk testing. In general, the combination of penicillin and an aminoglycoside antibiotic is most effective in treating this organism because of its demonstrated synergism. If the organism is relatively resistant to streptomycin, gentamicin or tobramycin should be used. Ampicillin may be substituted for penicillin in this situation because enterococci are more sensitive in vitro to this antibiotic than to penicillin. However, ampicillin cannot be relied on to cure *S. faecalis* infection, and therefore an aminoglycoside is still necessary. A 6-week course of therapy may be necessary for these organisms. Patients allergic to penicillin should be treated with a combination of vancomycin and gentamicin.

Staphylococcal Endocarditis. Patients with *S. aureus* endocarditis are often acutely ill, and initiation of antibiotic therapy is urgent. The antibiotic agents of choice are the penicillinase-resistant penicillins (methicillin [Staphcillin], nafcillin [Unipen], or oxacillin [Bactocill]) unless the MIC to penicillin G is less than 0.1 μg per milliliter. Despite differences in in vitro activity, protein binding, and other pharmacodynamics, all three penicillins have proved equally effective in the treatment of staphylococcal endocarditis in both experimental animals and humans. I prefer nafcillin or oxacillin because of the occasional development of interstitial nephritis with methicillin therapy. Treatment is necessary for a minimum of 4 weeks, and in many instances 6 weeks are required. Relapses may occur, and the patient must be retreated. A relapse in a patient with staphylococcal endocarditis strongly suggests the presence of a myocardial abscess or other extravalvular extension of the infection. Vancomycin is the agent of second choice and should be used both in patients allergic to penicillin and in those with methicillin-resistant staphylococcal infections. The addition of an aminoglycoside antibiotic to these regimens is of unproved benefit.

S. epidermidis is the most common cause of *late* prosthetic valve endocarditis, and infection with this organism carries a 40 to 60% mortality rate. If the organism is sensitive to methicillin, a regimen similar to that used for *S. aureus* endocarditis should be employed. However, the majority of *S. epidermidis* isolates are methicillin resistant, and in these cases a combination of vancomycin and rifampin is recommended. *S. epidermidis* is often sensitive to cephalosporins, but these agents seem to be less effective, and vancomycin is preferred. The addition of gentamicin to the combined vancomycin and rifampin regimen has been recommended, but triple-drug therapy is not generally accepted.

Gram-Negative Microorganisms. Infective endocarditis may be caused by a variety of enteric and nonenteric gram-negative bacilli. Therapy must be guided by in vitro sensitivity studies, and two-drug regimens are generally necessary. *Pseudomonas aeruginosa* is a common infecting organism in intravenous drug abusers. This organism is frequently resistant to many antibiotic agents, and the use of multiple drug regimens is necessary. Most often, an antipseudomonal penicillin in combination with an aminoglycoside is indicated, as determined by in vitro bacteriologic studies. Because of the resistance of this organism to many agents and the persistent bacteremia despite optimal antibiotic therapy, surgical excision of the infected valve is often necessary. Infection by fastidious, slow-growing, nonenteric gram-negative bacilli, the so-called HACEK group (*Haemophilus, Actinobacillus, Cardiobacterium, Eikenella,* and *Kingella* species), is often characterized by large vegetations that frequently result in systemic embolization. Careful sensitivity studies are necessary, but most of these agents are susceptible to ampicillin, cephalosporins, and aminoglycosides. A combination regimen of ampicillin plus gentamicin for 4 weeks is the commonly recommended therapy. Cef-

TABLE 2. **Antimicrobial Treatment Regimens for Infective Endocarditis in Adults**

Responsible Organism	Therapy of Choice	Alternative Therapy	Duration of Therapy (Weeks)
Streptococcus			
1. Penicillin G-sensitive—e.g., *S. viridans, S. bovis, S. equinus,* anaerobic and microaerophilic streptococci (MIC $\leq$ 0.1 mg/mL)	Aqueous penicillin G 10–20 million U IV daily in divided q-4-hr doses	Vancomycin 1 gm IV q 12 hr	4
	OR Aqueous penicillin G as above *plus* streptomycin 0.5 gm IM q 12 hr OR gentamicin 1 mg/kg IV q 8 hr	OR Cephalothin 2 gm IV q 4 hr or cefazolin 1 gm IV q 6 hr *plus* streptomycin 0.5 gm IM q 12 hr or gentamicin 1 mg/kg IV q 8 hr for initial 2 weeks	4
	OR Procaine penicillin G 1.2 million U IM q 6 hr *plus* streptomycin or gentamicin as above	OR Amoxicillin 1 gm PO q 6 hr *plus* probenecid 0.5 gm PO q 6 hr (oral regimen, used when parenteral therapy is not feasible)	4
2. Penicillin G-resistant—e.g., enterococci, other streptococci (MIC $>$ 0.1 mg/mL)	Aqueous penicillin G 20–40 million U IV daily in divided q-4-hr doses *plus* streptomycin 0.5 gm IM q 12 hr or gentamicin 1 mg/kg IV or IM q 8 hr OR Ampicillin 12 gm daily IV in divided q-4-hr doses *plus* streptomycin or gentamicin as above	Vancomycin (for patients allergic to penicillin) 1 gm IV q 12 hr *plus* streptomycin or gentamicin as in regimen of choice	4–6
Staphylococcus aureus			
1. Penicillin-sensitive	Aqueous penicillin G 20–40 million U IV daily in divided q-4-hr doses	Vancomycin 1 gm IV q 12 hr	4–6
2. Penicillin-resistant (methicillin-sensitive)	Nafcillin or oxacillin 1.5–2.0 gm IV q 4 hr	Cephalothin 2 gm IV q 4 hr or cefazolin 2 gm IV q 8 hr *plus* gentamicin 1 mg/kg IV q 8 hr (optional) OR Vancomycin, as above	4–6
3. Methicillin-resistant	Vancomycin 1 gm IV q 12 hr		4–6
4. Methicillin-resistant in prosthetic valve endocarditis	Vancomycin 1 gm IV q 12 hr *plus* gentamicin 1 mg/kg IV q 8 hr *plus* rifampin* 300 mg q 8 hr PO (if initial response unsatisfactory)		
Staphylococcus epidermidis			
1. Methicillin-sensitive	Same as for methicillin-sensitive *S. aureus*		6
2. Methicillin-resistant	Vancomycin 1 gm IV q 12 hr *plus* rifampin 300 mg PO q 8 hr	Vancomycin and rifampin* *plus* gentamicin 1 mg/kg IV q 8 hr	6
Gram-Negative Organisms			
1. HACEK group (penicillin-sensitive)	Ampicillin 2 gm IV q 4 hr *plus* gentamicin 1 mg/kg IV q 8 hr		4
2. HACEK group (penicillin-resistant)	Cefotaxime 2 gm IV q 6 hr		4–6
	OR Imipenem 1 gm IV q 6 hr		4–6
	OR Aztreonam 2 gm IV q 6 hr *plus* gentamicin 1 mg/kg IV q 8 hr		4–6
3. Enterobacteriaceae (*E. coli, Klebsiella, Proteus, Serratia,* etc.)	Cefotaxime OR Imipenem OR aztreonam *plus* gentamicin as above		4–6
4. *Pseudomonas aeruginosa*	Piperacillin 3 gm IV q 6 hr		6
	OR Ceftazidime 2 gm IV q 8 hr		6
	OR Imipenem 1 gm IV q 6 hr		6
	OR Tobramycin 1.7 mg/kg IV q 8 hr		6
Fungi			
Candida spp.	Amphotericin B 1.0–1.5 mg/kg IV daily (start with 0.25 mg/kg and increase by 0.25 mg/kg/day)	Amphotericin B *plus* flucytosine 150 mg/kg daily in four divided PO doses	6–8
Aspergillus spp.	Amphotericin B as above		6–8

*This indication for rifampin has not been officially approved by the Food and Drug Administration (FDA).

triaxone (Rocephin) has been shown to be highly effective in vitro and may be a suitable alternative.

Fungal Endocarditis. The most common fungi responsible for endocarditis are various *Candida* and *Aspergillus* species. Fungal endocarditis is seen commonly in postoperative cardiosurgical patients, intravenous drug abusers, and patients receiving hyperalimentation or immunosuppressive therapy. Amphotericin B has been demonstrated to be effective in the treatment of fungal endocarditis; however, there has been a high incidence of primary drug failure in both native and prosthetic valve fungal infections. Current concepts suggest the need for surgical removal of the infected valve and continuation of amphotericin B for a period of 6 to 8 weeks. Valve resection without prosthetic replacement has been recommended for fungal tricuspid endocarditis but has not gained widespread acceptance owing to the frequently intolerable hemodynamic burden it places on the right heart. The role of flucytosine and ketoconazole (two new antifungal agents) remains to be determined.

Culture-Negative Endocarditis. The most common cause of failure to isolate the infective microorganism from blood is the use of antibiotic therapy in the 2 weeks preceding the culture. In the usual patient with infective endocarditis and negative blood cultures, my practice is to direct initial therapy against *S. faecalis* and use antibiotic regimens as outlined previously. Exceptions to this general rule include narcotic addicts, postoperative cardiosurgical patients, and patients with an acute fulminant septic course. In these circumstances, a regimen consisting of an aminoglycoside antibiotic and a semisynthetic penicillin must be used until the microorganism is positively identified. The clinical response to various antibiotic regimens should be followed carefully, and therapy should be continued for 4 to 6 weeks with a combination antibiotic regimen that produces symptomatic improvement and defervescence.

Prosthetic Valve Endocarditis. Treatment of infection of a prosthetic valve, regardless of the infective organism, requires prolonged large doses of antibiotic agents, frequently in combination regimens, as well as a combined team approach that includes specialists in infectious diseases, cardiology, nephrology, and cardiovascular surgery. Aggressive bactericidal antimicrobial therapy alone or in combination with early surgery can successfully cure a substantial number of patients. Surgical removal of the prothesis is necessary when the infective microorganism is a fungus, the infection relapses despite adequate antimicrobial therapy, or there is a major embolic event or evidence of prosthetic valve dysfunction.

Allergy to Penicillin. Because the penicillins are the antibiotic agents of choice in the treatment of many different types of endocarditis, the patient with documented allergy to penicillin presents a difficult therapeutic problem. However, history of penicillin allergy is often unsubstantiated, and the so-called allergy is either insignificant or nonexistent. To verify a significant history of penicillin allergy, a history of anaphylactic or anaphylactoid reaction to any penicillin in the past or a history of penicillin-induced urticarial skin reaction within the past 2 years is required. Skin testing may be undertaken, and if definite penicillin hypersensitivity exists, the clinician has the choice of either desensitizing the patient (a minimally risky procedure) or substituting another effective antimicrobial regimen. Concurrent administration of corticosteroids to suppress the hypersensitivity reaction in allergic patients cannot be recommended.

Antibiotic Administration. In general, antibiotics should be administered parenterally either intravenously or intramuscularly. Oral antibiotic therapy is thought to be too unpredictable to be used in treating potentially lethal infections. Penicillin and vancomycin must be administered intravenously as indicated in Table 2. Central venous lines are not recommended in patients with bacteremia because of the risk of colonization. The use of 23-gauge scalp vein needles in a peripheral vein with rotation of the intravenous infusion site every few days has been a satisfactory method in my experience in the great majority of cases. Some patients require the placement of a central line because of severe chemical phlebitis due to the sclerosing nature of some antibiotics (especially vancomycin). Antibiotic infusions should be given intermittently over a short period of time. Penicillin is administered as a bolus over a 30-minute period every 4 hours. Vancomycin is administered more slowly over a 1-hour period every 12 hours. Aminoglycosides are given intramuscularly but may also be given intravenously slowly over a period of 30 to 60 minutes to avoid their potential curare-like side effects. Aminoglycosides should not be mixed in solution with penicillin or cephalosporin. Rifampin is administered orally every 12 hours.

Patient Monitoring. Patients should be monitored carefully for the development of complications while undergoing parenteral antibiotic therapy. Congestive heart failure is a common complication of infective endocarditis, developing in approximately 50% of patients because of severe valvular regurgitation. Patients with congestive heart failure secondary to aortic or mitral regurgitation should be monitored carefully in a critical care unit, and placement of a Swan-Ganz balloon flotation catheter may be necessary to monitor the degree of congestive heart failure and the results of therapy. Medical therapy should be initiated promptly at the first sign of congestive heart failure and should include diuretics and digoxin. Vasodilator therapy is often necessary in the presence of severe mitral or aortic valve regurgitation. Even if medical therapy temporarily ameliorates the congestive heart failure, most patients with this complication will require valve replacement (see later section, Surgical Therapy). Patients should be monitored for the development of atrioventricular block, which indicates extravalvular extension of the infection to the conduction system and, if advanced, may require transvenous pacemaker insertion. The development of purulent pericarditis is most often associated with

TABLE 3. **Cardiac Conditions***

Endocarditis Prophylaxis Recommended
Prosthetic cardiac valves, including bioprosthetic and homograft valves
Previous bacterial endocarditis, even in the absence of heart disease
Most congenital cardiac malformations
Rheumatic and other acquired valvular dysfunction, even after valvular surgery
Hypertrophic cardiomyopathy
Mitral valve prolapse with valvular regurgitation
Endocarditis Prophylaxis Not Recommended
Isolated secundum atrial septal defect
Surgical repair without residua beyond 6 months of secundum atrial septal defect, ventricular septal defect, or patent ductus arteriosus
Previous coronary artery bypass graft surgery
Mitral valve prolapse without valvular regurgitation†
Physiologic, functional, or innocent heart murmurs
Previous Kawasaki disease without valvular dysfunction
Previous rheumatic fever without valvular dysfunction
Cardiac pacemakers and implanted defibrillators

*This table lists selected conditions but is not meant to be all inclusive.

†Individuals who have a mitral valve prolapse associated with thickening or redundancy of the valve leaflets may be at increased risk for bacterial endocarditis, particularly men who are 45 years of age or older.

From Dajani AS, Bisno AL, Chung KJ, et al: Prevention of bacterial endocarditis: Recommendations of the American Heart Association. JAMA *264*:2919, 1990. Reproduced with permission © 1990 American Medical Association.

S. aureus endocarditis of the aortic valve. It almost always requires prompt surgical management with drainage and frequently pericardiectomy. Additionally, patients should be monitored carefully for the development of complications from the antibiotic therapy. In patients receiving streptomycin, vestibular function should be followed carefully by means of audiography. Similarly, renal function should be monitored frequently in patients receiving gentamicin.

Surgical Therapy

Patients who develop pulmonary edema during the active phase of aortic or mitral valve endocarditis have a mortality ranging from 50 to 80% with medical therapy alone. Early operative treatment with replacement of the incompetent valve has significantly improved the outcome in this subgroup of patients, leading to reduced mortality ranging from 8 to 28%. Pulmonic and tricuspid valve resection without valve replacement has been used in patients with right-sided endocarditis caused by *P. aeruginosa* and fungal organisms that are relatively resistant to antimicrobial chemotherapy. However, right ventricular failure almost always results from this procedure, and current thinking suggests that maintaining tricuspid valve competence by insertion of a prosthesis is preferable. Other indications for early surgery in patients with infective endocarditis include recurrent embolization, uncontrolled sepsis despite adequate antimicrobial chemotherapy, fungal infection, development of extravalvular complications (conduction defects or pericarditis), development of prosthetic valve dysfunction, and recurrence of the infection despite adequate antimicrobial chemotherapy.

Despite the theoretical risk of inserting a foreign body in a potentially infected vascular bed, recurrence of the endocarditis following urgent valve replacement has been low even when blood cultures remain positive up to the time of surgery. A number of studies have clearly indicated that mortality is lower among patients undergoing valve replacement during the active phase of the infection than among those in whom needed surgery was delayed until the bacteremia had cleared. Current thinking indicates that timing of valve surgery should depend on the patient's hemodynamic needs rather than on the status of the infection.

PREVENTION OF INFECTIVE ENDOCARDITIS

Numerous studies have documented the occurrence of transient bacteremia after a variety of procedures,

TABLE 4. **Dental or Surgical Procedures***

Endocarditis Prophylaxis Recommended
Dental procedures known to induce gingival or mucosal bleeding, including professional cleaning
Tonsillectomy or adenoidectomy
Surgical operations that involve intestinal or respiratory mucosa
Bronchoscopy with a rigid bronchoscope
Sclerotherapy for esophageal varices
Esophageal dilation
Gallbladder surgery
Cystoscopy
Urethral dilation
Urethral catheterization if urinary tract infection is present†
Urinary tract surgery if urinary tract infection is present†
Prostatic surgery
Incision and drainage of infected tissue†
Vaginal hysterectomy
Vaginal delivery in the presence of infection†
Endocarditis Prophylaxis Not Recommended‡
Dental procedures not likely to induce gingival bleeding, such as simple adjustment of orthodontic appliances or fillings above the gum line
Injection of local intraoral anesthetic (except intraligamentary injections)
Shedding of primary teeth
Tympanostomy tube insertion
Endotracheal intubation
Bronchoscopy with a flexible bronchoscope, with or without biopsy
Cardiac catheterization
Endoscopy with or without gastrointestinal biopsy
Cesarean section
In the absence of infection for urethral catheterization, dilation and curettage, uncomplicated vaginal delivery, therapeutic abortion, sterilization procedures, or insertion or removal of intrauterine devices

*This table lists selected procedures but is not meant to be all inclusive.

†In addition to prophylactic regimen for genitourinary procedures, antibiotic therapy should be directed against the most likely bacterial pathogen.

‡In patients who have prosthetic heart valves, a previous history of endocarditis or surgically constructed systemic pulmonary shunts or conduits, physicians may choose to administer prophylactic antibiotics even for low-risk procedures that involve the lower respiratory, genitourinary, or gastrointestinal tract.

From Dajani AS, Bisno AL, Chung KJ, et al: Prevention of bacterial endocarditis: Recommendations of the American Heart Association. JAMA *264*:2919, 1990. Reproduced with permission © 1990 American Medical Association.

TABLE 5. **Antibiotic Regimens for Endocarditis Prophylaxis in Adults**

Dental, Oral, and Upper Respiratory Tract Procedures	
Standard regimen	Amoxicillin 3 gm PO 1 hr before procedure and 1.5 gm 6 hr after initial dose
Allergy to penicillin	Erythromycin ethylsuccinate 800 mg or erythromycin stearate 1 gm PO 2 hr before procedure; then half the dose 6 hr after initial dose *OR* clindamycin 300 mg PO 1 hr before procedure and 150 mg 6 hr after initial dose
For patients unable to take oral medications	Ampicillin 2 gm IV or IM 30 min before procedure; then 1 gm IV or IM 6 hr after initial dose (amoxicillin 1.5 gm PO may be substituted for second dose)
Patients at high risk (individuals with prosthetic valves, conduits, etc.)	Ampicillin 2 gm IV plus gentamicin 1.5 mg/kg IV (not to exceed 80 mg) 30 min before procedure; then amoxicillin 1.5 gm PO 6 hr after initial dose *OR* repeat initial regimen 8 hr after first dose
Patients at high risk *and* allergic to penicillin	Vancomycin 1 gm IV over 1 hr, starting 1 hr before procedure; no repeat dose necessary
Regimens for GU/GI Procedures	
Standard regimen	Ampicillin 2 gm IV or IM plus gentamicin 1.5 mg/kg (not to exceed 80 mg) 30 min before procedure; then amoxicillin 1.5 gm PO 6 hr after initial dose or repeat parenteral regimen 8 hr after initial dose
Alternate regimen for low-risk patients	Amoxicillin 3 gm PO 1 hr before procedure; then 1.5 gm PO 6 hr after initial dose
Allergy to penicillin	Vancomycin 1 gm IV over 1 hr *plus* gentamicin 1.5 mg/kg (not to exceed 80 mg) 1 hr before procedure; may be repeated once 8 hr after the initial dose

From Dajani AS, Bisno AL, Chung KJ, et al: Prevention of bacterial endocarditis: Recommendations of the American Heart Association. JAMA *264*:2919, 1990. Reproduced with permission © 1990 American Medical Association.

including dental manipulations and surgical procedures or instrumentation involving mucosal surfaces or contaminated tissue. Other studies have confirmed that pretreatment of patients with antimicrobial drugs markedly reduces the incidence and severity of postprocedure bacteremia. It has therefore become accepted medical practice to administer antibiotic chemoprophylaxis to susceptible patients (patients with valvular, endocardial, or endothelial structural abnormalities) prior to procedures carrying a potential for inducing transient bacteremia (Tables 3 and 4). These procedures include all dental manipulations (but not simple adjustment of orthodontic appliances or shedding of deciduous teeth), tonsillectomy and adenoidectomy, surgical procedures or biopsy involving the respiratory mucosa, bronchoscopy with a rigid bronchoscope, and incision and drainage of infected tissue, as well as genitourinary tract instrumentation in the presence of infection.

Although the effectiveness of antibiotic prophylaxis has not been absolutely documented, the potential consequences of endocarditis are so serious that the American Heart Association has proposed specific recommendations and antimicrobial chemotherapeutic regimens. All physicians should have available the booklet *Prevention of Bacterial Endocarditis* published by the American Heart Association for easy reference. A summary of current prophylactic antimicrobial chemotherapy recommendations is listed in Table 5.

Antibiotic prophylaxis must consist of the bactericidal drug most likely to be effective against the bacterial flora colonizing the anatomic area that is to be manipulated. The drug should be administered 1 to 1 and a ½ hours prior to the invasive procedure in an effort to obtain maximal blood levels at the time of the anticipated bacteremia. Beginning the antimicrobial chemotherapy 24 hours before the anticipated procedures is not required and may be detrimental. Continued antimicrobial chemotherapy beyond 6 to 8 hours after the invasive procedure is not necessary because the bacteremia associated with the procedure is self-limited and transient.

HYPERTENSION

method of
MARVIN MOSER, M.D.
Yale University School of Medicine
New Haven, Connecticut

Hypertension remains the most common reason for American adults to visit their physicians. More than 50 million people have blood pressures that are elevated enough to increase their risk of cardiovascular disease and stroke and warrant some type of treatment.

Data accumulated during the past several years have helped to clarify many of the controversial issues in the management of this common disease; these data have a direct bearing on decisions about the diagnostic evaluation and treatment of the hypertensive patient.

DIASTOLIC OR SYSTOLIC BLOOD PRESSURE—WHICH IS IMPORTANT?

For many years physicians were told that a diastolic blood pressure elevation was of more significance than the systolic in determining the risk of cardiovascular disease. One hundred mmHg plus age was considered a "normal" systolic blood pressure; a blood pressure of 170/90 mmHg was once considered normal in a 70-year old man or woman. Recent data have confirmed, however, what many investigators have known for years, that an elevated systolic blood pressure is of as great or greater importance in estimating cardiovascular risk as the diastolic pressure. These conclusions are based on a follow-up of more than 300,000 people in the Multiple Risk Factor Intervention Trial (MRFIT) as well as data from the Framingham, Massachusetts Study. Even borderline isolated systolic hypertension, defined as 140 to 160/<90 mmHg, increases risk at any age, not just in the elderly (Table 1). The Joint National Committee on Detection, Evaluation and Treatment of High Blood Pressure (JNC V) in 1993 considered

TABLE 1. **Significance of Borderline Isolated Systolic Hypertension (ISH) (140–159/<90 mmHg)**

	Normal BP*		Borderline ISH*	
	No.	*Percent*	*No.*	*Percent*
Progression to definite hypertension >160/>90 mmHg (20-year follow-up)	2416	45	351	80
Cardiovascular morbidity and mortality		**Percent Incidence**		
All cardiovascular disease, including coronary heart disease		57		89
Congestive heart failure		7		16
Stroke or transient ischemic attack		9		16
Cardiovascular mortality		13		29
All cause mortality		38		59

*At baseline.
From Sagie A, Levy D, and Larson M: The natural history of borderline isolated systolic hypertension. N Engl J Med *329*:1912, 1993.

these data and now includes systolic blood pressures in their new definitions. Hypertension is defined as a persistently elevated blood pressure above 140/90 mmHg, with levels of systolic pressures being used to define the various stages of hypertension (Table 2). Although the designation of a high-normal pressure as *130* to 139/85 to 89 mmHg rather than *135* to 139/85 to 89, as in previous years, may create unnecessary anxiety in a large number of people, this new designation at a lower level of systolic pressure is put forth to suggest follow-up, especially in those individuals with other risk factors for heart disease, i.e., smokers and patients with hyperlipidemia, obesity, diabetes, and so on.

WHITE COAT HYPERTENSION

Much has been written in the past several years about white coat hypertension, i.e., increased blood pressure in a physician's office with normal blood pressure at home. Some investigators believe that these patients should merely be followed and not treated. Recent data confirm, however, that patients with elevated blood pressure in a doctor's office and normal pressure at home or at work are different physiologically from people who do not demonstrate the white coat syndrome. Increased peripheral resistance is present in the high office–lower home blood pressure subjects, and they also have increased lipid levels and insulin resistance. Thus, patients who have white coat hypertension should not be ignored and probably should be treated. It is also important to remember that all of the data on which we base our estimates of risk are based on casual blood pressures taken in a physician's office or clinic—the higher the pressure, the greater the risk of cardiovascular disease. In addition, we base our treatment decisions on the results of the treatment trials. Blood pressures in these trials were taken in a physician's office or clinic; the lower the blood pressure, the fewer the complications. The importance, therefore, of casual blood pressures as a predictor of outcome should be maintained and not dismissed. There are some instances in which home blood pressure recordings are useful, e.g., some patients may insist on knowing what their pressures are, and sometimes unusual symptoms may be clarified by knowing what the pressure is at home. Finally, there are some patients who appear to be resistant to therapy; having home blood pressures recordings may be useful in treating these patients. It is our belief that these pressures can be obtained using an anaeroid or even a digital sphygmomanometer, avoiding the need for expensive ambulatory blood pressure monitoring. Pressures taken repeatedly over time provide more and better information than a 24- or even a 48-hour record.

TABLE 2. **Classification of Blood Pressure (BP) for Adults Aged 18 and Older***

Category†	Systolic BP (mmHg)	Diastolic BP (mmHg)
Normal	<130	<85
High normal	130–139	85–89
Hypertension‡		
Stage 1 (mild)	140–159	90–99
Stage 2 (moderate)	160–179	100–109
Stage 3 (severe)	180–209	110–119
Stage 4 (very severe)	≥210	≥120

*Not taking antihypertensive drugs.
†When systolic and diastolic BP fall into different categories, the higher category should be selected to classify the patient's BP status (e.g., 160/92 mmHg should be classified as Stage 2; 180/120 mmHg should be classified as Stage 4). Isolated systolic hypertension (ISH) is defined as systolic BP ≥140 mmHg and diastolic BP <90 mmHg.
‡Based on an average of two or more readings taken at each of two or more visits following an initial screening.

THE J CURVE

Another confusing issue that has a bearing on treatment decisions relates to the so-called J curve of response, i.e., the concept that (1) higher pressures (>90 mmHg) lead to an increase in deaths from congestive heart disease (CHD); (2) lowering the diastolic blood pressure to about 85 to 90 mmHg decreases this risk; but (3) decreasing the diastolic blood pressure to below 80 to 85 mmHg may actually increase the incidence of myocardial infarction, especially in patients with ischemic heart disease in whom a decrease in diastolic pressure may further compromise coronary flow during diastole. Most of the studies supporting this concept include small numbers of patients and are retrospective. More recent analyses show that although the J curve may exist as a statistical phenomenon, it is probably of little importance in clinical practice. In the recent Systolic Hypertension in the Elderly Program (SHEP) study, 60% of the patients had abnormal electrocardiograms at baseline and presumably had some degree of heart disease. A decrease in diastolic pressure to below 70 was achieved in many patients and was associated with a definite *decrease* in coronary heart disease events. There is little good evidence at present to warrant a specific recommendation in regard to lowering diastolic blood pressure too much (consistent with a lack of symptoms). Obviously, if blood pressure is lowered to 115 to 120/70 to 75 mmHg and the patient feels weak or dizzy, therapy should be altered.

TABLE 3. **Effect of Antihypertensive Drug Treatment on Coronary Heart Disease, Strokes, and Vascular Mortality in Seventeen 3- to 5-Year Clinical Trials**

	Active Treatment			Control			Risk Reduction (%)*	
	Fatal	*Total*	*No.*	*Fatal*	*Total*	*No.*	*Fatal*	*Total*
Coronary heart disease	470	934	23,847	560	1104	23,806	16	16
Strokes	140	525	23,847	234	835	23,806	40	38
Vascular mortality	768		23,847	964		23,806		21

*Highly statistically significant.

Adapted from Hebert PR, Moser M, Mayer J, Glynn RJ, and Hennekens CH: Recent evidence on drug therapy of mild to moderate hypertension and decreased risk of coronary heart disease. Arch Intern Med *153*:578, 1993. Copyright 1993, American Medical Association.

DOES LOWERING BLOOD PRESSURE REDUCE CORONARY HEART DISEASE? DOES IT REDUCE MORBIDITY AND MORTALITY IN THE ELDERLY?

These important questions have been answered to a great extent during the past few years, and the answers provide guidance in selecting appropriate therapy. More than 75,000 people have now been followed in 3- to 6-year controlled hypertension treatment trials. Effective treatment has (1) decreased progression to more severe disease (a factor not often considered when estimating the benefit of therapy), and (2) dramatically reduced the incidence of congestive heart failure, strokes, and stroke deaths, but the effectiveness of lowering the blood pressure in reducing coronary heart disease complications has been questioned. A recent meta-analysis, however, concluded that a statistically significant reduction of 16% in coronary heart disease events occurred in clinical trials when blood pressure was lowered by antihypertensive medication (Table 3). This reduction in incidence occurred despite the short duration of treatment (3 to 5 years) and with a reduction of only approximately 10 to 12/5 to 6 mmHg in blood pressure in treated compared with placebo or control subjects. In addition, approximately 25% of patients in the treated groups did not even achieve their goal blood pressures. It is interesting to speculate on the results of treatment over a longer period of time with better control of blood pressure. The same meta-analysis reported a 38 to 40% decrease in strokes and stroke deaths. Evidence, therefore, indicates that treatment of hypertension reduces the incidence not only of cerebrovascular but also of cardiovascular disease.

Three recent 3- to 5-year studies in the elderly—the Medical Research Council (MRC), the Swedish Trial in Older Patients with Hypertension (STOP-Hypertension), and SHEP—have all demonstrated a statistically significant decrease in strokes and stroke deaths (25 to 47%) and overall cardiovascular mortality (17 to 40%) in patients 65 years or older who were treated with a relatively simple regimen. In addition, CHD events were reduced by 13 to 27%. Therapy included a diuretic or a beta blocker, given singly or in combination (Table 4). These data confirm previous information from other trials in the elderly.

ARE THE METABOLIC CHANGES RESULTING FROM THE USE OF CERTAIN ANTIHYPERTENSIVE DRUGS OF SIGNIFICANCE?

Controversy has existed during the past 10 years about the metabolic changes noted with use of two of the more commonly used antihypertensive drugs, diuretics and beta-adrenergic inhibitors. All of the clinical trials to date have used one or the other of these agents as initial monotherapy. As noted, the trials reported a reduction in morbidity and mortality from cardiovascular disease.

Effects on Lipids

DIURETICS. A 5 to 7% short-term increase in total cholesterol levels results from the use of high-dose diuretics. After 1 year, however, this effect disappears to a great extent. None of the longer term trials report a more than minimal increase in cholesterol levels; most report a decrease (Table 5). The recent Treatment of Mild Hypertension Study (TOMHS) and a new study comparing different classes of drugs from the Veterans Administration have also failed to demonstrate an increase in cholesterol levels in diuretic-treated subjects after the first year of treatment. In addition, in the Hypertension Detection and Follow-up Program (HDFP), which was also diuretic based, cholesterol levels actually decreased in patients who had pre-treatment hyperlipidemia.

TABLE 4. **Effects of Therapy in Older Hypertensive Patients**

Clinical Trial	Australian	EWPHE	Coope and Warrender	STOP-Hypertension	MRC	SHEP	HDFP*
No. of patients	582	840	884	1,627	4,396	4,736	2,374
Age range (yr)	60–69	>60	60–79	70–84	65–74	60–>80	60–69
Mean BP (mmHg) at entry	165/101	182/101	179/100	195/102	185/91	170/77	170/101
% Reduction							
Stroke	33	36	42†	47†	25†	33†	44†
Coronary artery disease	18	20	—	13‡	19	27†	15†
Congestive heart failure	—	22	32	51†	—	55†	—
All cardiovascular disease	31	29†	24†	40†	17†	32†	16†

*Includes data calculated by the HDFP Coordinating Center.

†Statistically significant.

‡Myocardial infarction only; sudden deaths decreased from 13 to 4.

Abbreviations: MRC = Medical Research Council; STOP-Hypertension = Swedish Trial in Older Patients with Hypertension; SHEP = Systolic Hypertension in the Elderly Program; HDFP = Hypertension Detection and Follow-up Programs; EWPHE = European Working Party on Hypertension in the Elderly.

Many hypertensive individuals have increased insulin resistance *prior* to any treatment. The use of diuretics may increase insulin resistance still further. This suggests that a diuretic should not be used, especially in those patients with a strong family history of diabetes or with diabetes. The incidence of diabetes increased by only a minimal amount of about 1%, however, in diuretic-treated subjects in the clinical trials, which used dosages considerably higher than we use today (Table 6). In addition, a case control study of more than 11,000 hypertensive patients treated with various antihypertensive drugs reported that the number of individuals who became diabetic did not differ whether they took diuretics, beta-adrenergic inhibitors, calcium channel blockers, angiotensin-converting enzyme (ACE) inhibitors, or alpha blockers. Finally, recent studies from the SHEP group have shown that the reduction in mortality from coronary heart disease in subjects treated with low-dose diuretics is as great or greater in diabetics as in nondiabetics.

Thus, it appears that the importance of the adverse effects of diuretics on lipids and serum glucose levels has probably been overemphasized. Physicians should not be concerned about using these drugs in subjects with hyperlipidemia or diabetes. These chemical parameters should be monitored several times during the first year of treatment to detect the few people who might develop changes.

BETA-ADRENERGIC INHIBITORS. Beta blockers have a longer term effect on lipid levels; triglyceride levels may increase and high-density lipoprotein (HDL) levels may decrease to some extent with most beta blockers other than those with some agonist activity (intrinsic sympathomimetic activity [ISA]). Because of the nature of their action, beta-adrenergic inhibitors may decrease insulin release, mask some of the symptoms of hypoglycemia, such as tachycardia, and actually delay recovery from hypoglycemia (they should be used with care in patients with Type I insulin-dependent diabetes). These metabolic effects apparently do not reduce the ability of these agents to prevent second myocardial infarctions (MI) in patients with previous evidence of an MI (secondary prevention trials). In one of the recent hypertension treatment trials (MRC in the Elderly), a beta blocker did not prove as effective in reducing CHD events as a diuretic, but in an earlier MRC (primary prevention) trial, it appeared to be more effective in preventing them.

Other Effects. Other effects of diuretics that have concerned physicians include hypokalemia, which is clearly dose related. This is not a major problem with the dosages presently suggested, i.e., 25 mg per day or the equivalent of hydrochlorothiazide. Several recent studies involving 24- and 48-hour Holter monitoring have also demonstrated that even with diuretic-induced hypokalemia, ventricular

TABLE 5. **Effect of Relatively High-Dose Diuretic-Based Therapy on Serum Cholesterol in Long-Term Clinical Trials**

Trial	Duration	Total Cholesterol Level (mg/dL)		Difference
		Baseline	*Treatment*	
Berglund and Anderson	6 Yr	267	255	−12
MRC Trial	3+ Yr			
Men				
Active treatment		245	245	0
Placebo		244	239	−5
Women				
Active treatment		261	260	−1
Placebo		260	256	−4
MAPHY Study	6 Yr	244	243	−1
HDFP	5 Yr			
SC group		232	223	−9
Oslo	4 Yr			
Active treatment		272	273	+1
Control		278	280	+2
MRFIT	6 Yr			
SI group		254	236	−18
UC group		254	240	−14
HAPPHY Trial	4 Yr	242	242	0
EWPHE	3 Yr			
Active treatment		256	238	−18
Placebo		259	239	−20
MRC in Elderly	5 Yr			
Active treatment		228	232	+4
Placebo		228	232	+4
Jeunematre et al	20 Mo	228	232	+3.8
SHEP	5 Yr			2.2*
TOHMS	2 Yr			
Active treatment		231	226.5	−4.5
Placebo		225	219.9	−5.1
VA Multi Drug	2 Yr	†		

*2.2% more patients on diuretic versus placebo developed cholesterol level of >300 mg/dL at any time

†"No significant differences in any lipid fractions between 6 classes of drugs (including diuretics) and placebo at 1 and 2 years of treatment."

Abbreviations: MRC = Medical Research Council; MAPHY = Metoprolol Atherosclerosis Prevention in Hypertension; HDFP = Hypertension Detection and Follow-up Program; MRFIT = Multiple Risk Factor Intervention Trial; HAPPHY = Heart Attack Primary Prevention in Hypertension; EWPHE = European Working Party on Hypertension in the Elderly; SHEP = Systolic Hypertension in the Elderly Program; TOMHS = Treatment of Mild Hypertension Study; VA = Veterans Administration.

TABLE 6. **Effects of High-Dose Diuretic Therapy on Glucose Metabolism**

Study	Duration (Yr)	Serum Glucose (mg/dL)	Hyperglycemia or Diabetes
Oslo	5	No difference between diuretics and placebo	
EWPHE	3	Increase of 6.6—diuretics:placebo	Excess of 6/1000 patient years
MRC	3		Excess of 6/1000 patient years
HAPPHY	4		Excess of 6/1000 patient years
HDFP	5		1.6% (57/3563)
SHEP	1	Difference of 5—diuretics:placebo	1 of 483
	5	Not reported	More than 2.0% developed glucose levels of >200 mg/dL at any time in 5 yr compared to placebo
MRFIT	6		Excess of 7%* in SI group on diuretics vs. Excess of 2%* in UC group no diuretics
VA	2	Increase of 1.7—diuretics:placebo	
TOHMS	1	Decrease of 0.9—diuretics Decrease of 3.2—placebo	

*Fasting glucose >110 mg/dL.

Abbreviations: EWPHE = European Working Party on Hypertension in the Elderly; MRC = Medical Research Council; HAPPHY = Heart Attack Primary Prevention in Hypertension; HDFP = Hypertension Detection and Follow-up Program; SHEP = Systolic Hypertension in the Elderly Program; MRFIT = Multiple Risk Factor Intervention Trial; VA = Veterans Administration; TOHMS = Treatment of Mild Hypertension Study; SI = special intervention; UC = usual care.

ectopy is not increased. Concern about the risk of producing serious arrhythmias as a result of the use of diuretics has also probably been overemphasized.

These new data on the potential metabolic effects of medication have an important relationship with the choice of initial therapy. Based on the fact that diuretics and beta-blockers are the only two classes of drugs that have been tested and shown to reduce morbidity and mortality in hypertensive individuals, the JNC V considers these the preferred first-step therapy in a high percentage of hypertensive individuals. That decision takes into account the effects described earlier.

AN APPROACH TO TREATMENT

Clarification of the aforementioned issues makes it easier to make treatment decisions. Approximately 70 to 75% of the hypertensive population in the United States are patients with Stage 1 hypertension, that is, they have blood pressures of 140 to 160/90 to 100 mmHg. Because the immediate risk of a complication is not great, these patients can be followed for several weeks to as long as 6 months before specific antihypertensive medication is initiated. The 1993 JNC recommendations suggest that patients with Stage 1 or even the lower end of Stage 2 hypertension (i.e., 160 to 165/100 mmHg) with few additional risk factors can safely be evaluated on a second or third occasion within 3 to 6 months, but during this time they should be treated with lifestyle modifications—weight loss if appropriate, sodium restriction, exercise, and efforts at stress reduction. Weight loss has been shown to be the most effective nonpharmacologic intervention. Even a loss of 5 to 10 pounds may reduce systolic and diastolic blood pressure by 2 to 5/2 to 4 mmHg or more, changing a patient's status from Stage 1 to a high normal level. Even if this approach proves ineffective as monotherapy, it is one of the adjunctive treatments recommended if medication does become necessary. Sodium restriction may be important in some patients, but in others this may produce no change at all in blood pressure. A sodium intake of approximately 2 grams per day (salt intake of 5 grams) can be achieved by most people without significant deprivation. If this lifestyle modification combined with weight reduction is effective in reducing blood pressure to normotensive levels, the patient can be followed at 6-month intervals without other interventions (Table 7).

ALCOHOL INTAKE AND OTHER LIFESTYLE CHANGES

Excessive alcohol intake correlates with the presence of hypertension. There is a higher incidence of hypertension in people who drink more than three to four alcoholic beverages a day. Reducing this intake may lower blood pressure toward normal. The JNC V urges moderation, defined as no more than 1 ounce of ethanol (i.e., 2 ounces of whiskey, 8 ounces of wine, or 24 ounces of beer) daily. For some people, this may represent more than a moderate intake; certainly this recommendation should not be adhered to by those with a family history of alcoholism or a sensi-

TABLE 7. **Lifestyle Modifications for Hypertension Control and/or Overall Cardiovascular Risk**

Weight loss if overweight
Reduce sodium intake to less than 100 mM/day (2.3 gm of sodium or approximately <6 gm of sodium chloride)
Limit alcohol intake to <1 oz/day of ethanol (24 oz of beer, 8 oz of wine, or 2 oz of 100-proof whiskey)
Exercise (isotonic) regularly
Stop smoking and reduce dietary saturated fat and cholesterol intake for overall cardiovascular health; reducing fat intake also helps reduce caloric intake—important for control of weight and Type II diabetes
Maintain adequate dietary potassium, calcium, and magnesium intake

tivity to alcohol. A reduced incidence of CHD (compared with that in nondrinkers) has also been linked to a small daily intake of alcohol, presumably because of a favorable effect on HDL levels.

Other nonpharmacologic interventions, including smoking cessation, are recommended. This may not have any effect on blood pressure but will reduce the risk of pulmonary disease, cancer, coronary heart disease, and sudden death. Although stress reduction and relaxation efforts may transiently lower blood pressure, the long-term effects of these interventions are questionable; further data are necessary to conclude that this approach represents an effective treatment for hypertension.

Finally, isotonic exercises such as walking, bicycling, and swimming are good health measures; again, there is little definitive evidence in well-controlled studies that this approach by itself will lower blood pressure. Exercise burns up calories and aids in weight reduction.

In our experience, normotensive levels are achieved by lifestyle intervention in about 20 to 25% of patients with Stage I hypertension. It is a mistake to believe, however, that nonpharmacologic measures constitute definitive therapy in the majority of hypertensive individuals.

MORE SEVERE HYPERTENSION

In patients who present with Stage 2 or 3 hypertension, i.e., diastolic pressures higher than 100 mmHg (even without other risk factors), we institute pharmacologic therapy simultaneously with nonpharmacologic treatment. If, after 6 to 12 months blood pressures have been reduced to normal levels, it is a simple matter to reduce the medication gradually to see whether the nonpharmacologic measures will maintain normotensive levels. In those who present with Stage 3 or 4 hypertension, immediate pharmacologic therapy is necessary, most often with the use of multiple drugs.

PHARMACOLOGIC THERAPY

Therapy has evolved during the past 45 years from the era of the *Veratrum* derivatives, which had a narrow therapeutic range—a small dose might not be effective whereas a slightly larger dose might lower blood pressure but also produce severe and potentially life-threatening side effects—to the next era of reserpine, which is a moderately effective blood pressure-lowering agent by itself in only about 20% of patients but is more effective in a larger number of patients when combined with other drugs such as hydralazine (a vasodilator). In the 1950s ganglion blockers (e.g., hexamethonium,* macamylamine,* and so on) were introduced; these were potent antihypertensive drugs but were either poorly absorbed, producing erratic or extreme reductions in blood pressure, or caused numerous and often serious side effects. Both the sympathetic and parasympathetic nervous systems were blocked by these drugs. When diuretics became available in the middle 1950s, management was greatly simplified. When these agents were combined in the 1960s and 1970s with reserpine, beta-adrenergic inhibitors, or central agonists like methyldopa, a high percentage of patients responded with normotensive levels. In the 1970s and 1980s the armamentarium available to physicians increased dramatically with the introduction of the alpha antagonists, calcium channel blockers, and ACE inhibitors.

*Not available in the United States.

Today physicians have numerous medications to choose from when approaching the treatment of hypertension. I believe that many investigators have attempted to make the decision about initial therapy more complex than it needs to be. Therapy should be individualized to some extent, as outlined subsequently, but in the majority of patients a relatively straightforward approach can be followed. This was recognized by the 1993 JNC, which, although stressing individualization of therapy, suggested thiazide diuretics or beta blockers as the preferred medications for initial treatment. Other agents, such as the ACE inhibitors or calcium channel blockers, are useful and have a definite place in management, but because they have not been tested in long-term studies and found to reduce morbidity and mortality, they were suggested as alternative therapy by the JNC. We continue to institute therapy in a great majority of our patients with diuretics alone or in combination with other medications.

The Antihypertensive Agents

A brief review of the physiologic effects of the various antihypertensive medications is given, together with a discussion of when and how they should be used.

Diuretics

The *thiazide diuretics,* which include hydrochlorothiazide and chlorthalidone (Hygroton), the most commonly used agents, all have a similar action and produce a natriuresis, with an initial reduction in plasma volume and cardiac output along with a lowering of blood pressure. After approximately 4 to 6 weeks, the plasma volume returns almost to normal, cardiac output returns toward normal, peripheral resistance is decreased, and blood pressure lowering is maintained. In effect, diuretics produce vasodilation over the long term. With the continuing reduction in plasma volume, however, the renin-angiotensin system is stimulated; this physiologic effect attempts to correct volume changes and, in some instances, lessens the blood pressure–lowering effect of the diuretic. In most cases, the effect on the peripheral blood vessels is great enough to overcome the increased degree of renin activity.

Patients on diuretic therapy are less responsive to pressor substances, so that sympathetic nerve stimuli do not cause as much vasoconstriction in these patients as they usually do. No one has clearly defined the exact mechanism of the long-term blood pressure–lowering effectiveness of the thiazide diuretics.

Because thiazide diuretics increase the sodium load in the distal tubules, more sodium is exchanged for potassium, and some degree of hypokalemia may result in a high percentage of patients, especially when doses of more than 50 mg a day of hydrochlorothiazide or chlorthalidone are used. With the currently recommended doses (25 to 50 mg per day), hypokalemia (defined as levels of less than 3.5 mEq per liter) is not as common. Hypokalemia induced by high-dose thiazides may be counteracted by the simultaneous use of potassium-sparing agents; these agents are available in combinations such as hydrochlorothiazide-triamterene (Dyazide, Maxzide), hydrochlorothiazide-amiloride (Moduretic), or spironolactone (Aldactone), which is a more specific aldosterone inhibitor.

Tubular reabsorption of urate is also increased by thiazides, uric acid excretion is reduced, and plasma uric acid levels may increase. This is probably of little significance in most patients, but gout may occur in approximately 3 to 4% of patients. If uric acid levels rise above 11 mg per 100 mL even without symptoms, some physicians advocate the use of agents such as allopurinol (Zyloprim, 100 to 300 mg/day), which reduces excessive amounts of circulating uric acid. In these patients, especially those with recurrent gout, it may be wise to substitute another medication. As noted, thiazides may increase insulin resistance and may also produce transient elevations of serum lipid levels; the clinical significance of these findings is questionable.

Thiazide diuretics are as effective as or more effective than any of the other major classes of antihypertensive drugs. Some data suggest that they are more effective in lowering systolic blood pressure than the calcium channel blockers or ACE inhibitors. Two recent studies that compared all classes of drugs showed that the thiazides and calcium channel blockers were more effective in elderly and black patients than beta blockers or ACE inhibitors. Thiazides were, however, somewhat less effective than these latter agents in the treatment of young white patients. It should be noted that thiazide medications do produce normotensive levels in about 40% of young white patients when used as monotherapy.

The *loop* diuretics, furosemide (Lasix) and bumetanide (Bumex), are more potent because of their site of action, which is closer to the glomerulus in the ascending loop of Henle. These agents have not been shown, however, to be as useful as antihypertensive agents as the other diuretics, presumably because of their short duration of action and the dosages employed. However, loop diuretics are especially effective in patients with diminished renal function, in those in whom acute lowering of blood pressure is needed, or in patients with congestive heart failure.

In addition to the metabolic effects of diuretic therapy, some patients experience fatigue, frequent urination, which is especially annoying in patients with prostatic hypertrophy, and, in rare cases, a rash. If this occurs, it is presumably secondary to the sulfa-containing component of the thiazide. Substitution of ethacrynic acid (Edecrin), the only diuretic without a sulfa component, is suggested. Sexual dysfunction is an annoying symptom in about 10% of men and a small percentage of women. The mechanism causing this effect has not been clearly established. In our experience, it is one of the few symptoms that interferes with the quality of life of diuretic-treated subjects. Numerous quality of life studies have, however, demonstrated that there is little difference in quality of life when the four most frequently used classes of antihypertensive drugs are compared, i.e., diuretics, most beta blockers, ACE inhibitors, and calcium antagonists. Some measures of quality of life are adversely affected by the centrally acting and alpha-blocking drugs.

Diuretics have been used as initial therapy in all of the major clinical trials and as a comparative agent in several recent trials of beta-adrenergic inhibitors. Diuretics used as monotherapy lower the blood pressure in more than 50 to 60% of patients with Stage 1 hypertension, and, used in combination with a beta-adrenergic inhibitor, an ACE inhibitor, or a calcium channel blocker, they reduce blood pressure in approximately 75 to 80% of patients, including those with more severe disease. Table 8 lists the more commonly used diuretics along with their dosages and side effects.

Beta-Adrenergic Inhibiting Agents

These medications have been recommended as one of the two preferred initial therapies in the treatment of hypertension by the JNC V. Beta blockers inhibit the effects of stimulation of beta-adrenergic receptor sites by epinephrine and norepinephrine that are either circulating or released from postganglionic adrenergic nerve endings. This action blunts the effect of sympathetic nerve stimulation on the heart; heart rate, myocardial contractility, and myocardial oxygen demand are decreased following beta blockade. In addition, renin release is inhibited. Cardiac output is reduced by up to 20%; blood pressure is lowered; renal blood flow may be reduced to a slight extent or not at all. Calculated peripheral resistance may actually increase despite the reduction in blood pressure because of the decrease in cardiac output.

Beta-adrenergic inhibitors also have an effect on peripheral smooth muscle, blunting the usual sympathetic dilatory or agonist effect on the bronchi and peripheral arterioles. These agents tend to aggravate or precipitate asthma in susceptible individuals and may precipitate Renaud's phenomenon or increase symptoms of intermittent claudication.

Beta blockers are particularly indicated in hypertensive patients with angina pectoris or a history of myocardial infarction or cardiac dysrhythmias because they decrease myocardial oxygen demand and cardiac work. Migraine headaches may be prevented by the use of beta blockers; this constitutes a specific indication for their use in hypertensive patients with

TABLE 8. **Some Commonly Used Diuretics and Beta Blockers in the Treatment of Hypertension**

	Total Dosage (mg)	Times/ Day	Physiologic Effects	Comments
Thiazides and Related Agents				
Bendroflumethiazide (Naturetin)	2.5–5	1	Initial decrease in plasma volume, extracellular fluid volume, and cardiac output, followed by a decrease in total peripheral resistance with normalization of cardiac output	More effective than loop diuretics except in patients with serum creatinine >2.5 mg/dL. Hydrochlorothiazide or chlorthalidone was used in most clinical trials
Chlorthalidone (Hygroton)	12.5–50	1		
Hydrochlorothiazide (Esidrix, HydroDIURIL, Oretic)	12.5–50	1–2		
Indapamide (Lozol)	1.25–5	1		
Methyclothiazide (Enduron)	2.5–5	1		
Metolazone (Zaroxolyn, Diulo)	0.5–5	1		
Loop Diuretics				
Bumetanide (Bumex)	0.5–5	2		Higher doses may be needed for patients with renal impairment or congestive heart failure. Ethacrynic acid is alternative for patients with allergy to sulfur-containing diuretics
Ethacrynic acid (Edecrin)	25.0–100	2–3		
Furosemide (Lasix)	20.0–320	2–3		
Torsemide (Demadex)	5–10	1		
Potassium-Sparing Agents				
Amiloride (Midamor) as part of Moduretic	5–10	1–2	Increased potassium reabsorption	Weak diuretics; used mainly in combination with other diuretics to avoid or reverse hypokalemia. Avoid when serum creatinine >2.5 mg/dL
Triamterene (Dyrenium) as part of Dyazide or Maxzide	50–150	1–2		
Spironolactone (Aldactone)	25–100	2–3	Aldosterone antagonist	
Beta Blockers				
Atenolol (Tenormin)*	25–100	1	Decreased cardiac output; may increase total peripheral resistance; decreased plasma renin activity	In higher dosages the cardioselective agents also inhibit $beta_2$ receptors; all may aggravate asthma
Bisoprolol (Zebeta)*	5–10	1		
Metoprolol (Lopressor)*	50–200	1–2		
Metoprolol (Toprol XL)*	50–200	1		
Betaxolol (Kerlone)*	5–30	1		
Nadolol (Corgard)	20–240	1		
Propranolol (Inderide LA)	80–160	1		
Beta Blockers with ISA†				
Acebutolol (Sectral)*	200–1200	2	Less effect on heart rate and vascular and bronchial smooth muscle	Possible advantage in subjects with bradycardia who must receive beta blocker; they may produce fewer metabolic effects
Pindolol (Visken)	10–60	2		
Alpha + Beta Blocker				
Labetalol (Normodyne, Trandate)	200–1200	2	Same as beta blockers, plus $alpha_1$ blockade	Probably more effective in blacks than other beta blockers. May cause postural effects; titration should be based on standing BP.

*Cardioselective
†ISA = intrinsic sympathomimetic action (slight $beta_2$ receptor stimulation)

this type of headache. The drug should not be used in patients with second-degree heart block or worse or in most patients with congestive heart failure.

The beta-adrenergic inhibiting agents that are presently available are listed in Table 8. Some of these, specifically, acebutolol (Sectral), atenolol (Tenormin), bisoprolol (Zebeta), betaxolol (Kerlone), and metoprolol (Lopressor), are cardioselective; most of their activity is confined to receptors in the heart muscle ($beta_2$ blockade), and they have less effect on bronchial or peripheral smooth muscle ($beta_1$ receptors). However, in the dosages used to treat hypertension, some of the cardioselective properties are lost; these agents should, therefore, not be used in patients with asthma or chronic obstructive pulmonary disease (COPD). Some of the beta blockers (e.g., acebutolol [Sectral] and pindolol [Visken]) have some intrinsic sympathomimetic activity (ISA), that is, a tendency to increase vasodilation and bronchodilation and minimize the effects of beta blockade on heart rate and so on. These agents may be useful if a beta blocker is clearly indicated and a resting bradycardia is present; the degree of additional bradycardia will be significantly less than if a non-ISA blocker were used.

Beta-blocking agents may be specifically indicated for initial treatment in younger patients with faster resting heart rates, palpitations, or ectopy. They are less effective as monotherapy in many elderly patients and in blacks.

Combined Alpha and Beta Blockers

At present only one combined alpha plus beta blocker is available in the United States, i.e., labetalol (Normodyne or Trandate). This medication combines both $beta_1$- and $beta_2$-adrenergic blocking properties with some $alpha_1$-blocking activity. Several other combination medications are being developed. Carvedilol* (marketed as Kredex) is presently available in Europe. These agents possess a greater degree of beta- than of alpha-blocking activity. Blood pressure is reduced, mainly as a result of a decrease in peripheral resistance. There is less effect on heart rate and cardiac output than with the beta-adrenergic inhibitors alone. Heart rate decreases to only a slight degree. There is less fluid retention and orthostatic hypotension than occurs with simple alpha blockers. Changes in renin and catecholamine levels are minimal (Table 8). Labetalol and carvedilol are effective antihypertensive agents. One of the more common side effects of these drugs is postural hypotension and dizziness, which is noted in about 8 to 10% of patients. This occurs not only with the initial dose but also with increasing dose levels. Fatigue, headache, and tingling of the scalp may be noted in about 5% of patients. Titration to an effective dose may be time consuming, especially with labetalol. This drug has a short duration of action, and multiple daily doses may be necessary. For these reasons, labetalol has not been widely accepted in the United States as a suitable initial agent. The JNC V, however, has recommended it as a possible alternative for initial treatment. Carvedilol has a longer duration of action and is effective in a once-a-day dose, and titration is relatively simple.

Part of the problem with labetalol may have been the dosages that were originally advocated. If a dosage of only 100 mg twice a day is used initially, with an increase to a maximum of only 400 or 600 mg per day, side effects are less frequent. When the drug was first introduced, dosages of up to 1200 mg per day were commonly prescribed.

One adverse reaction noted with beta blockers is hair loss; this may not be as frequent with labetalol. As with other agents, if small doses of this drug do not work, combining it with a small dose of a diuretic increases the response rate significantly. Labetalol is effective in black patients to a greater degree than some of the beta blockers and lowers blood pressure to the same degree as a beta blocker and an $alpha_1$ blocker given separately. Intravenous labetalol is useful in the treatment of hypertensive crises or accelerated hypertension. This agent or carvedilol (if it is approved for use in the United States) can be used as alternative initial monotherapy but should be used with caution in older people; titration of blood pressure-lowering effects should be based on the levels of standing blood pressure.

Peripheral Adrenergic Inhibitors

The drugs in this class are rarely used. Two of them, guanethidine (Ismelin) and guanadrel (Hylorel), are potent medications and inhibit the activity of the sympathetic nervous system by blocking the exit of norepinephrine from storage granules. Guanethidine was widely used in the 1950s and 1960s. It is effective on a once-a-day basis even in severe hypertensives and, when combined with a diuretic, reduces blood pressure in a high percentage of patients. The occurrence of severe postural hypotension in some patients, diarrhea, and sexual dysfunction limits its usefulness. We still use guanethidine, however, in small doses of 10 to 20 mg per day in combination with a diuretic in a small number of patients who are resistant to other therapy. Unlike some other antihypertensive drugs, which may have a relatively flat dose-response curve, increasing the dose of guanethidine increases the degree of blood pressure response. Guanadrel (Hylorel) is similar to guanethidine but has a shorter duration of action. Because of this, it is somewhat less potent than guanethidine and may have fewer side effects.

Reserpine (Serpasil), a *Rauwolfia* derivative, acts on the central nervous system by decreasing the transport of norepinephrine into storage granules; eventually the amount of norepinephrine available when nerves are stimulated is reduced. This drug has been in use in the United States since the early 1950s but had been used as a sedative, tranquilizer, and blood pressure–lowering agent for many years before that in eastern European countries and India. As monotherapy, reserpine and its derivatives are only effective in approximately 20% of patients. However, when given in combination with a diuretic, blood pressure is reduced to goal levels of less than 140/90 mmHg in about 75 to 80% of patients. Unfortunately, when we used reserpine or its derivatives in the 1950s and early 1960s, dosages that were unnecessarily high (0.5 to 1.0 mg per day) were given. Side effects, which include nasal stuffiness, sedation, and, most importantly, depression, were not uncommon. But in those early days of antihypertensive drug treatment, many of us thought that the higher the dose, the better the response—with any of the blood pressure–lowering drugs; this included the beta blockers. Propranolol (Inderal) was given in doses of up to 3 grams a day; hydralazine (Apresoline) was often given in doses of up to 1200 mg per day, alpha methyldopa (Aldomet), up to 2.0 to 3.0 grams per day, and the diuretics were prescribed up to the equivalent of 200 mg per day of chlorthalidone (Hygroton). Today we know that most of these drugs are effective in much smaller dosages. When reserpine is given in doses of 0.05 to 0.1 mg per day, a blood pressure response may be obtained without many of the undesirable side effects. The reserpine (and whole root *Rauwolfia*) medications are still being used in small doses with a diuretic in some patients. Reserpine has the advantage of being inexpensive; most patients tolerate it well except for the occasional patient who develops symptoms of depression. These symptoms may include fatigue, insomnia, disturbing dreams, or just a general lack of interest in one's daily activities and job. Symptoms may persist for many weeks after the drug is stopped. Combinations of reserpine (Serpasil, 0.1 or 0.25 mg) or the whole root *Rauwolfia*

*Not available in the United States.

(Raudixin, 50 mg) and a diuretic are available as Salutensin, Rauzide, and other preparations. Table 9 lists the dosages and side effects of the peripheral adrenergic inhibitors. Maximum suggested doses are lower than those listed in the *Physicians' Desk Reference.* This modification is based on long experience and the fact that most of these drugs are used in combination with a diuretic.

The *ganglion blockers,* which block not only sympathetic but parasympathetic activity, are extremely potent arteriolar and venodilators. Their side effects limit their usefulness in the majority of patients. They are now used almost exclusivly as intravenous injections for control of blood pressure during operative procedures or in hypertensive emergencies. Table 10 summarizes our present indications for the use of these as well as other agents in treating hypertensive crises. Not all available medications are included, only those that we believe are most effective and easiest to use.

Central Agonists as Adrenergic Inhibitors

The central agonists have an unusual mechanism of action in the vasomotor centers of the brain. They stimulate inhibitory neurons and decrease sympathetic outflow from the central nervous system. Their hemodynamic effects include (1) a decrease in peripheral resistance; (2) a slight decrease in cardiac output; and (3) a decrease in blood pressure. Among the available central agonists are alpha methyldopa (Aldomet), clonidine (Catapres), guanabenz (Wytensin), and guanfacine (Tenex). These medications reduce blood pressure to normotensive levels in about 35 to 50% of patients and, in combination with small doses of a diuretic, are more effective. But side effects occur in a high percentage of patients, and dropout rates from therapy are as high as 20 to 30% in most series. The most common side effects include sedation, dry mouth, drowsiness, dizziness, fatigue, headaches, depression, and disturbing dreams. Symptoms of depression may be subtle, as they are with reserpine, and include a decrease in mental alertness, vivid dreams, and an inability to enjoy life. Quality of life measurements are decreased when the central agonists are used; diuretics, ACE inhibitors, most beta blockers, and calcium channel blockers do not adversely affect these measures. Table 9 lists these agents, their physiologic effects, and their duration of action.

In addition to the adverse effects just cited, which are shared by methyldopa, clonidine, guanabenz, and guanfacine, methyldopa may induce certain autoimmune disorders, as indicated by abnormal liver function tests, and fever may occur in about 5 to 10% and a positive Coombs' test in as many as 30% of patients. The incidence of hemolytic anemia, however, is uncommon.

There are many patients who have done well on methyldopa (usually in combination with a diuretic) through the years with normal blood pressures, few side effects, and no evidence of an autoimmune reaction. In these patients there is no reason to change therapy. Dosages of methyldopa (Aldomet) should probably not exceed 750 to 1000 mg per day. Doses closer to the starting range (i.e., 250 mg per day) should be used in combination with a diuretic when therapy is started.

Clonidine is similar in action to alpha methyldopa,

TABLE 9. **Peripheral Adrenergic Inhibitors, Central Agonists, and Alpha$_1$ Receptor Blockers**

	Total Dosage (mg)	Times/ Day	Physiologic Effects	Comments	Other Adverse Reactions
Peripheral Adrenergic Inhibitors					
Guanadrel (Hylorel)	10–50	2	Inhibit catecholamine release from neuronal storage sites	May cause orthostatic and exercise-induced hypotension	Sexual dysfunction
Guanethidine (Ismelin)	10–50	1			
Rauwolfia alkaloids					
Rauwolfia serpentina (Raudixin)	50–100	1	Depletion of tissue stores of catecholamines		Depression, nasal stuffiness, activation of peptic ulcer
Reserpine (Serpasil)*	0.05–0.25	1			
Central Agonists					
Clonidine (Catapres)	0.1–0.8	2	Stimulate central alpha$_2$ receptors that inhibit efferent sympathetic activity, leading to decreased BP, decreased peripheral resistance	Clonidine patch is replaced once a week. None of these agents should be withdrawn abruptly because of rebound hypertension	Dry mouth, drowsiness, headaches, fatigue, depression Possible immune reactions
Clonidine (patch)	0.1–0.2	1 wk			
Guanabenz (Wytensin)	4–16	2			
Guanfacine (Tenex)	1–3	1			
Methyldopa (Aldomet)	250–1000	2	No significant effect on heart rate, cardiac output, renal blood flow, or glomerular filtration rate		
Alpha$_1$ Receptor Blockers					
Doxazosin (Cardura)	1.0–12	1	Block postsynaptic alpha$_1$ receptors→vasodilatation, decreased peripheral resistance, decreased BP	All may cause postural effects; titration should be based on standing blood pressure	Dizziness, palpitations, GI disturbances
Prazosin (Minipress)	1.0–15	2–3			
Terazosin (Hytrin)	1.0–15	1–2			

*0.1-mg dose may be given every other day to achieve this dosage.

TABLE 10. **Management of the Hypertensive Crisis: Emergencies and Urgencies**

	Dose	Onset	Cautions
Parenteral Vasodilators			
Sodium nitroprusside (Nitropress)	0.25–10 μg/kg/min as IV infusion; maximal dose for 10 min only	Instantaneous	Nausea, vomiting, muscle twitching; with prolonged use may cause thiocyanate intoxication, methemoglobinemia, acidosis, cyanide poisoning. Bags, bottles, and delivery sets must be light resistant
Nitroglycerin	5–100 μg/min as IV infusion	2–5 min	Headache, tachycardia, vomiting, flushing, methemoglobinemia; requires special delivery system owing to drug binding to PVC tubing
Diazoxide (Hyperstat)	50–100 mg IV bolus, repeated, or 15–30 mg/min by IV infusion	1–2 min	Hypotension, tachycardia, aggravation of angina pectoris, nausea and vomiting, hyperglycemia with repeated injections
Parenteral Adrenergic Inhibitors			
Trimethaphan camsylate (Arfonad)	1–4 mg/min as IV infusion	1–5 min	Paresis of bowel and bladder, orthostatic hypotension, blurred vision, dry mouth
Labetalol (Normodyne, Trandate)	20–60 mg IV bolus every 10 min; 2 mg/min IV infusion	5–10 min	Bronchoconstriction, heart block; hypotension
Oral Agents			
Nifedipine (Procardia) (not extended release)	10–20 mg PO, repeat after 30 min	15–30 min	Rapid, occasionally uncontrolled reduction in blood pressure
Captopril (Capoten) or other ACE inhibitor	25 mg PO, repeat as needed	15–30 min	Hypotension, renal failure in bilateral renal artery stenosis
Clonidine (Catapress)	0.1–0.2 mg PO, repeat every hour as required to a total dose of 0.6 mg	30–60 min	Hypotension, drowsiness, dry mouth
Labetalol (Normodyne, Trandate)	200–400 mg PO, repeat every 2–3 hr	30 min–2 hr	Bronchoconstriction, heart block, orthostatic hypotension

It is often appropriate to administer a diuretic agent with any of the above.
Not all possible therapies are included.

although it has a somewhat shorter duration of action, but the advantage is that it is available as a transdermal patch. Use of the patch may result in fewer adverse reactions. The 0.1-mg starting dose patch can be used and changed every 7 days. Local skin reactions occur in as many as 30% of patients with the transdermal patch. The initial dose of clonidine given orally should be 0.1 mg twice a day, increasing to a maximum dose of 0.3 or 0.4 mg given twice a day. Clonidine should probably be used with small doses of a diuretic to increase its effectiveness and reduce side effects.

A deterrent to the widespread use of clonidine is the fact that if the drug is stopped, the sympathetic nervous system becomes overactive from a suppressed state; there can then be a marked overshoot in blood pressure with episodes of severe and often symptomatic hypertension. This diagnosis should be considered in any patient who abruptly stops clonidine therapy; restarting the drug will reduce blood pressure.

The clonidine patch has also been used in the treatment of nicotine addiction, with varying results.

Guanabenz (Wytensin) is similar to clonidine. Starting doses are 2 to 4 mg twice a day; the maximum dose should probably not exceed 16 mg per day. Guanfacine (Tenex) is also similar to clonidine, with a dosage range of 1 to 3 mg per day (Table 9).

The use of this class of drugs has decreased in recent years because of the availability of medications that are better tolerated. There are, however, some possible indications for their use as second- or third-step agents: (1) in insulin-dependent diabetics, patients with asthma, and those with peripheral arterial disease in whom a beta blocker should probably not be used, and (2) in patients who may have experienced annoying side effects from ACE inhibitors (angioedema, cough, loss of taste, and so on), or calcium channel blockers (palpitations, dizziness, persistent edema, constipation, and so on). Some patients respond well to a small bedtime dose of one of the central agonists when blood pressure has not been controlled by a diuretic alone. All of these medications have been found to be effective in reducing left ventricular hypertrophy. Methyldopa is still used in treating the hypertension of toxemia of pregnancy.

Alpha Blockers (Alpha-Adrenergic Inhibitors)

At present three $alpha_1$ blockers are available in the United States—prazosin (Minipress), terazosin (Hytrin), and doxazosin (Cardura). These drugs act by blocking or inhibiting the postsynaptic $alpha_1$ receptors on vascular smooth muscle. This inhibits the uptake of catecholamines by smooth muscle cells. Vasoconstriction is blunted, and peripheral vasodilatation occurs.

There are also several *non*selective alpha blockers

available—e.g., phentolamine (Regitine) and phenoxybenzamine (Dibenzyline). These agents block not only the postsynaptic $alpha_1$ receptors but also the presynaptic $alpha_2$ receptors located on the neuronal membrane itself. These latter drugs have not proved effective for the treatment of hypertension. Although they reduce blood pressure, often dramatically, their effect on the alpha receptors removes an inhibiting effect on norepinephrine release; more of this substance is released into the circulation, tachycardia occurs, and tachyphylaxis to blood pressure lowering occurs fairly quickly. In addition, postural hypotension and other adverse reactions militate against their use except in the therapy of pheochromocytoma, for which they are highly effective.

Although recent studies have shown that the $alpha_1$ receptor blockers (prazosin, terazosin, and doxazosin) reduce diastolic pressure to as great an extent as other classes of antihypertensive drugs, our experience suggests that their effect on systolic blood pressure is somewhat less. In addition, symptomatic side effects occur in a higher percentage of patients than with other drugs. For example, in one study of an $alpha_1$ receptor blocker, 18 of 42 patients dropped out of therapy because of adverse reactions; only three of 48 patients on hydrochlorothiazide discontinued therapy. Side effects include postural hypotension, tachycardia, dizziness, and occasional gastrointestinal distress. The postural hypotension and dizziness may occur with initiation of therapy or with any increase in dosage. These side effects are less common with the longer acting $alpha_1$ blocker doxazosin (Cardura). Dosage of this drug should be started at 1 mg per day at bedtime and gradually titrated to a maximum of 5 mg twice a day. We usually use an alpha blocker such as doxazosin (Cardura) as a second- or third-step drug in combination with a diuretic or a beta-adrenergic inhibitor. Dosages are kept at a minimum with fewer and tolerable side effects. These agents are particularly effective in reducing diastolic blood pressure if this has not been brought to normotensive levels with other medications. Table 9 reviews the actions, side effects, and dosages of the $alpha_1$ receptor blockers.

Several recent trials have demonstrated that the $alpha_1$ receptor blockers may have a favorable effect on lipid levels. Because of this possible advantage, it has been suggested that the $alpha_1$ blockers may be ideal antihypertensive agents. However, because of the more complicated titration and greater number of symptomatic adverse reactions, they have not been widely accepted by physicians as an initial step-one therapy. The addition of an $alpha_1$ blocker such as doxazosin to a beta-adrenergic inhibitor (which may raise serum triglycerides and in some instances reduce HDL levels) is a reasonable approach to therapy. The $alpha_1$ blockers reduce symptoms of prostatic hypertrophy and may be useful in the management of older hypertensive men with this problem.

Direct Vasodilators

Two vasodilators, hydralazine (Apresoline) and minoxidil (Loniten), have been available for the treatment of hypertension for many years. They act directly on vascular smooth muscle (possibly as potassium channel openers). Hydralazine was used for many years in combination with reserpine and a diuretic and later in the 1950s and 1960s as a third-step drug with a beta blocker and a diuretic. These combinations effectively lowered blood pressure in a high percentage of patients, even those with severe hypertension. Diastolic pressure is often specifically reduced when hydralazine is added to other drugs.

As a result of the dilatation of arterioles leading to a decrease in peripheral resistance and blood pressure, baroreceptors are stimulated; an increase in catecholamines and heart rate results. Renal retention of sodium with expansion of fluid volume may occur. Because of these effects, hydralazine and minoxidil by themselves may be only temporarily effective as blood pressure–lowering agents; tachyphylaxis to their effects develops rapidly. Side effects also limit their usefulness as monotherapeutic agents. Most prominent among these are tachycardia, fluid retention, flushing, headaches, and, in the case of minoxidil, excessive hair growth, not just on the face but on the body as well. This is especially troublesome in women. The compensatory mechanisms that prevent long-term blood pressure lowering and produce side effects may be mitigated by the concurrent use of an adrenergic inhibitor such as reserpine, clonidine, or a beta blocker. In patients taking minoxidil, large doses of a potent diuretic may have to be used to prevent the massive accumulation of fluid that may occur. In these cases, drugs such as furosemide (Lasix) may have to be used in doses of up to 200 mg per day or more or metolazone (Zaroxolyn or Diulo) in doses of up to 10 mg per day.

We currently use hydralazine infrequently and prefer the use of an $alpha_1$ blocker as a second- or third-step drug. However, in some patients who have not responded to a diuretic plus a beta blocker, hydralazine may be useful if it is used in appropriate doses of 25 mg twice a day to start, increasing to about 100 mg twice a day. We rarely use doses higher than this because of a lupus-like syndrome that may occur with higher doses. This is not common, but positive ANA (antinuclear antibodies) tests may occur in as many as 40% of patients. If a patient on hydralazine does develop a fever, rash, or arthralgias, the drug should be stopped and other drugs substituted. Minoxidil is rarely, if ever, used as initial therapy; its use is limited to patients with severe hypertension and renal insufficiency or patients who are resistant to or unable to tolerate other medications.

Although direct vasodilators are effective antihypertensive drugs, there is little or no place for them as initial monotherapy. Hydralazine is useful in some cases of accelerated or malignant hypertension or in toxemia of pregnancy.

Angiotensin-Converting Enzyme (ACE) Inhibitors

ACE inhibitors are among the most effective vasodilating antihypertensive drugs. These drugs prevent the conversion of angiotensin I, which is an inactive octapeptide, to angiotensin II, which is a potent vasoconstrictor and aldosterone stimulator. In addition, the ACE inhibitors prevent the degradation of bradykinin, a vasodilator substance, by inhibiting kininase II, an enzyme that inactivates bradykinin. Bradykinin levels are increased; this enhances the synthesis of various prostaglandins (which also act as vasodilators). Thus, ACE inhibitors have a combined action that decreases the generation of angiotensin II and increases the levels of bradykinin and various prostaglandins. In recent studies comparing five different classes of drugs, blood pressure reduction with an ACE inhibitor was essentially equivalent to that of the other medications except in black patients, who proved less responsive. A list of ACE inhibitors presently available in the United States is given in Table 11. Others are under investigation. Most of these have similar actions, although they differ chemically. Some contain a sulfhydryl group, for example, captopril (Capoten). This was believed to be a factor in causing some of the side effects, such as loss of taste. However, this concept has not been proved.

ACE inhibitors differ in their duration of action and mode of excretion and therefore in frequency of administration. They produce some degree of natriuresis and potassium retention as a result of decreasing aldosterone secretion. Blood pressure decreases as a result of vasodilatation and reduced peripheral resistance. Cardiac output remains the same and, despite the decrease in blood pressure, there is usually only a slight increase in heart rate. We have, however, seen some patients who develop a persistent tachycardia following the use of an ACE inhibitor.

ACE inhibitors are particularly effective as unloading agents in the treatment of heart failure because they reduce afterload. In heart failure, the levels of angiotensin II are high; reducing these levels is beneficial and may have a favorable effect on cardiac function over and above the effect on vascular resistance. In long-term studies, patients with heart failure have improved clinically with regard to exercise tolerance and other symptoms. Mortality due to CHD has also been reduced by the use of ACE inhibitors in subjects with ischemic heart disease and reduced left ventricular function (ejection fractions below 40%). ACE inhibitors are one of the groups of drugs suggested as an alternative first-step therapy by the JCN V. Long-term studies have not yet been done to demonstrate reductions in morbidity and mortality when these drugs are used. Several trials are under way. It is probable that they will demonstrate that ACE inhibitors are as effective as the drugs that have thus far been tested, that is, diuretics and beta blockers.

If an ACE inhibitor is used as a first-step monotherapy, small doses should be used initially; often these are effective. As noted in Table 11, the maximum suggested dose is less than that recommended in the *Physicians' Desk Reference.* Rather than increase the dosage to a maximum, we prefer to add a small dose of a diuretic if the blood pressure goal is not achieved with minimal or at most a moderate dose of an ACE inhibitor. This approach is similar to our approach to therapy with other medications. For example, if a patient is taking 10 mg per day of enalapril (Vasotec) or lisinopril (Zestril) or 50 mg per day of captopril (Capoten) and blood pressure has not become normal, a diuretic in doses equivalent to 25 mg per day or less of hydrochlorothiazide should probably be added. Numerous combinations of an ACE inhibitor and a diuretic are available.

Side Effects. Side effects of the ACE inhibitors are relatively uncommon except for cough. Most patients tolerate these medications well; quality of life is not compromised, and in fact, some people feel better on an ACE inhibitor. Several adverse reactions should be noted: (1) About 15 to 20% of patients develop a dry, hacking cough, which is persistent and annoying. If it is recognized early, patients can be saved the trouble of going through extensive diagnostic evaluations for various types of allergies, bronchitis, or pulmonary disease. The cough will disappear 3 to 5 days after the medication is stopped. The cough is reported to be more common in women, but in our experience, almost an equal number of men develop it. The cause is unknown but may be related to increased levels of bradykinin or substance P. (2) Postural hypotension

TABLE 11. **Some of the More Commonly Used ACE Inhibitors in the Treatment of Hypertension**

	Total Dosage (mg)*	Times/ Day	Physiologic Effects	Comments	Other Adverse Reactions
Benazepril (Lotensin)	10–20	1–2	Block formation of angiotensin II, promoting vasodilation and decreased aldosterone; also increase bradykinin and vasodilatory prostaglandins	Diuretic doses should be reduced before starting ACE inhibitor whenever possible to prevent hypotension. Reduce dose in patients with serum creatinine >2.5 mg/dL. May cause hyperkalemia in patients with renal impairment or in those receiving potassium-sparing agents. Can cause acute renal failure in patients with bilateral renal artery stenosis	Cough, rash, loss of taste, palpitations, angioedema
Captopril (Capoten)	12.5–150	2			
Enalapril (Vasotec)	2.5–20	1–2			
Fosinopril (Monopril)	5–20	1–2			
Lisinopril (Zestril, Prinivil)	5–20	1–2			
Perindopril (Aceon)	1–12	1–2			
Quinapril (Accupril)	5–20	1–2			
Ramipril (Altace)	1.25–15	1 or 2			

*Recommended dosages may differ from those suggested in the *Physicians' Desk Reference.*

and dizziness may occur, especially in patients who are already receiving a diuretic (this is actually an uncommon occurrence). (3) Angioedema is rare but can be serious; difficulty in breathing or swallowing may be noted. This reaction has occurred in three of our patients. It usually occurs within several days to 1 week of institution of therapy and usually clears quickly when the drug is stopped. Emergency care may be necessary. (4) A macular rash is occasionally seen (in about 3 to 5% of cases). (5) Loss of taste and appetite is also uncommon but does occur, especially in older people. Symptoms may be subtle, and weight loss can result if the medicine is not stopped within a short time. It may take more than several weeks for taste to return to normal.

Although the *Physicians' Desk Reference* suggests that diuretics be stopped prior to the addition of an ACE inhibitor as a second medication, we do not do this. We usually reduce the diuretic dosage to about one-half and start the ACE inhibitor in small doses. In some cases, measures of renal function (e.g., BUN or creatinine levels) rise following the institution of therapy with an ACE inhibitor, especially if a diuretic is being used concurrently. This occurs not only in patients with bilateral renal artery stenosis but also in others, especially older people who have nephrosclerotic changes. In patients with bilateral narrowing of the renal arteries and renovascular hypertension, blood pressures are often dependent on high levels of angiotensin II (a decrease in renal blood flow increases renin release, which leads to an increase in angiotensin II in an attempt to establish an adequate pressure and flow in the renal arteries). The decrease in blood pressure and intrarenal glomerular pressure brought about by ACE therapy may significantly reduce renal blood flow. BUN and creatinine levels should be checked within 1 to 2 months after beginning ACE inhibitor therapy; if a marked change occurs, therapy should be reevaluated.

Although it was originally believed that ACE inhibitors would be effective only in hypertensive patients with high renin levels, this has not proved to be true. Although these medications are more effective in patients with high renin hypertension (about 15 to 20% of all hypertensives), they also lower blood pressure in many patients with normal or low renin levels (we do not, however, determine renin levels as a diagnostic procedure and find it of little value in choosing an appropriate mode of therapy).

ACE inhibitors are effective as antihypertensive agents in young or middle-aged white persons. They are less effective in blacks and may, in some instances, be less effective in the elderly. The combination of an ACE inhibitor with small doses of a diuretic does, however, results in a significant decrease in blood pressures in young and old, black and white patients.

Normal blood pressure levels are achieved in 30 to 40% of patients with Stage 1 or Stage 2 hypertension when an ACE inhibitor is used as monotherapy. When a small dose of a diuretic is added, goal blood pressures of less than 140/90 mmHg are achieved in approximately 75 to 80%. The ACE inhibitors represent a major advance in the management of hypertension. Their availability has led to an increased rate of control and has simplified management of many patients.

Some investigators believe that ACE inhibitors should be the preferred therapy in patients with diabetes. This conclusion is based on the facts that (1) ACE inhibitors tend to decrease rather than increase insulin resistance; (2) these drugs lack even short-term or minor metabolic effects; (3) patients with diabetic nephropathy who are given ACE inhibitors experience a slowing of the decrease in glomerular filtration rate and a decrease in proteinuria. It should be noted, however, that in one recent study more than three-quarters of the patients on an ACE inhibitor also required a diuretic or a beta-adrenergic inhibitor to lower blood pressure to goal levels. Our approach to diabetic patients is somewhat similar to that used in nondiabetics, that is, we prescribe small doses of a diuretic along with an ACE inhibitor if the diuretic is ineffective. In our experience, blood pressure is not reduced to normal in many of these patients without the addition or use of a diuretic. Reduction of blood pressure may be the main factor in slowing the progression of diabetic nephropathy.

ACE inhibitors may also be considered preferentially in the subset of patients with obesity, elevated triglyceride levels, and low HDL levels, that is, individuals who are candidates for Type II diabetes.

NEWER MEDICATIONS IN RESEARCH

Numerous agents that block or inhibit the renin-angiotensin-aldosterone system at various sites are presently in development. Renin inhibitors as well as angiotensin II inhibitors are presently under investigation. The angiotensin II inhibitors, such as Losartan,* may have the advantage of achieving the same degree of blood pressure lowering as the ACE inhibitors without producing a cough.

Calcium Channel Blockers

In the past 10 to 15 years numerous calcium channel blockers have been introduced. A list of these appears in Table 12. The calcium channel blockers lower blood pressure by inhibiting the entry of calcium ions into vascular smooth muscle cells. This reduces vascular tone and contractility, vasodilatation occurs, peripheral resistance is reduced, and blood pressure is decreased. There are different types of calcium channel blockers. Diltiazem (Cardizem) and verapamil (Calan, Isoptin) act on heart muscle as well on peripheral arterioles. This results in partial blockade of the AV or sinoatrial (SA) node as well as a negative inotropic effect. Sinus rate may be slowed and the degree of heart block increased. These agents (especially verapamil) may be useful in the treatment of cardiac arrhythmias, especially supraventricular arrhythmias. Because of the negative inotropic effects, however, left ventricular function may

*Not available in the United States.

TABLE 12. **Some Commonly Used Calcium Antagonists**

	Total Dosage (mg)*	Times/ Day	Physiologic Effects	Comments and Possible Side Effects
Diltiazem (Cardizem)	90–240	3	Block inward movement of calcium ion across cell membranes and cause smooth muscle relaxation	Block slow channels in heart and may reduce sinus rate or produce heart block
Diltiazem (SR or CD) (Cardizem SR or CD)	120–240	2		
Diltiazem (ER) (Dilacor XR)	180–240	1		
Verapamil (Calan SR)	120–240	2		
(Isoptin SR)	120–360	1		
Verapamil (Verelan)	120–360	1		
Dihydropyridines				
Amlodipine (Norvasc)	2.5–10	1		Dihydropyridines are more potent peripheral vasodilators than diltiazem and verapamil and may cause more dizziness, headache, flushing, peripheral edema, and tachycardia
Felodipine (Plendil)	5–20	1		
Isradapine (DynaCirc)	2.5–10	2		
Nicardipine (Cardene)	60–90	3		
Nifedipine (Procardia)	30–60	3		
(Procardia XL) (Adalat)	30–60	1		

*Recommended dosages may differ from those suggested in the *Physicians' Desk Reference.*

be adversely affected, and congestive heart failure may result. This may be noted in patients with ischemic heart disease if this type of calcium blocker is given alone or in combination with a beta blocker. The long-acting formulations of diltiazem (Cardizem SR or CD) and verapamil (Calan SR or Isoptin SR) are probably effective on a once-a-day basis.

The dihydropyridine calcium channel blockers, such as nifedipine (Procardia), nicardipine (Cardene), amlodipine (Norvasc), felodipine (Plendil), and isradipine (DynaCirc), act primarily on the peripheral vascular beds and have no effect on cardiac muscle contraction or AV conduction. Nifedipine (Procardia XL), nicardipine (Cardene), amlodipine (Norvasc), and felodipine (Plendil) are probably effective on a once-a-day basis.

Calcium channel blockers may be more effective in the elderly and black patients than beta-adrenergic inhibitors or ACE inhibitors.

Adverse Reactions. Side effects differ considerably among the various calcium channel blockers. This is not unexpected in view of their different sites of action. The dihydropyridine derivatives, felodipine (Plendil), nicardipine (Cardene), nifedipine (Procardia XL), amlodipine (Norvasc), and isradipine (DynaCirc), may cause flushing, headaches, postural dizziness, palpitations or tachycardia, and ankle edema. Although some studies suggest that tachycardia is not common, this has not been our experience. Ankle edema is especially annoying to patients who are used to being warned about ankle swelling as a sign of congestive heart failure. Swelling may occur with small doses of any of these compounds and may not respond to the use of diuretics. Edema results from seepage of fluid from the capillary bed as a result of vasodilation. It usually clears with bed rest. *Verapamil* may cause severe constipation, postural hypotension, headache, and dizziness, and, as noted, it may have a negative inotropic effect on cardiac contraction. *Diltiazem* may cause headaches, tachycardias, and some gastrointestinal disturbances. Calcium channel blockers have not been shown to have any adverse effects on lipid metabolism or on insulin sensitivity. There is no evidence of any renal functional deterioration when these drugs are used.

Calcium channel blockers are effective as monotherapy in Stage 1 and 2 hypertension; approximately 35 to 40% of patients respond to such therapy. As with other drugs, about 75 to 80% of hypertensive patients become normotensive when a diuretic and calcium channel blocker are given together. A single combination pill is not yet available. The hypothesis that use of calcium channel blockers will reduce morbidity and mortality in hypertensive patients has not yet been tested. It is possible that when studies presently under way are finished, this will be shown to be true.

Studies with several calcium channel blockers have not shown a significant benefit in preventing a recurrence of myocardial infarction. Some data with the dihydropyridine derivatives suggest that the incidence of sudden death may actually be increased when these drugs are used. A recent 3-year study* failed to demonstrate a difference in carotid artery lesions between one of the dihydropyridine derivatives and a diuretic; cardiovascular events were more numerous in the calcium channel blocker group.

MANAGEMENT PLAN

The JNC V suggests initiation of therapy with a diuretic or beta-adrenergic inhibitor. We generally start most of our patients on a small dose of a diuretic, e.g., 25 mg or the equivalent of hydrochlorothiazide (HCTZ) with or without a potassium-sparing component. Many of our patients, especially those who are elderly and may be on a poor diet or are diabetics, are often started with a compound such as

*Grimm RH: Results of the Multicenter Isradipine/Diuretic Atherosclerosis Study (MIDAS), presented at the International Hypertension Society Meeting, Melbourne, Australia, March 20, 1994.

TABLE 13. **Modification of the JNC V Pharmacologic Treatment Algorithm***

If Inadequate→ Response	III.	Increase dosages or add medication from a different class ↑	Increase dosages or add medication from a different class ↑	Increase dosages or add medication from a different class ↑
If Inadequate→ Response	II.	Add ACE inhibitor, calcium channel blocker, beta blocker, $alpha_1$ blocker, or alpha and beta blockers ↑	Add diuretic ↑	Add diuretic ↑
Initial Therapy→	I.	Diuretic	Beta blocker	Alternative therapies: ACE inhibitors or calcium channel blockers. In some cases $alpha_1$ blockers or alpha and beta blockers

*Medication should be started at lowest recommended dosages.

Dyazide (HCTZ 25 mg, triamterene 50 mg) or Maxzide-25 MG (HCTZ 25, triamterene 37.5 mg). If a compound containing a larger quantity of HCTZ is used (e.g., Moduretic [HCTZ 50 mg, Amiloride 5 mg]), we start therapy with half of one tablet per day. If patients do not respond, we often increase the dosage to a maximum of 50 mg or the equivalent of HCTZ, but rarely, if ever, do we increase doses any further. If a beta-adrenergic inhibitor is used as initial therapy, the lower end of the dose range, given in Table 13, is used.

The JNC V suggests that if normotensive blood pressure levels are not achieved in a Stage 1 or early Stage 2 hypertensive patient after several months or in a Stage 2 or 3 hypertensive patient after several weeks, the physician can (1) proceed to a higher dose of the initial drug, (2) switch to an alternative class of drugs, or (3) add a second agent. We do not believe that sequential monotherapies (i.e., switching from one agent to another to another) is a useful method of treatment. It requires more frequent office visits and results in greater expense. We prefer instead to add a small dose of a second agent from a different class of medication. In our experience, this produces normotensive levels in a high percentage of patients without adding to side effects. The addition of a second agent often counteracts some of the physiologic responses to the first drug. For example, use of a diuretic results in an increase in the activity of the renin-angiotensin system. Adding an ACE inhibitor or a beta blocker will help to moderate this effect. In fact, an argument could be made for starting patients who have diastolic pressures greater than 100 mmHg on one of the various combinations that are available (Table 14). Two of these have been approved as initial monotherapy by the Food and Drug Administration: Capozide 25/15, which combines 25 mg of captopril and 15 mg of HCTZ, and Ziac, which contains small doses of a new cardioselective beta-adrenergic inhibitor, bisoprolol, 2.5, 5.0, or 10 mg, and HCTZ, 6.25 mg. Although this dosage of a thiazide is relatively ineffective when used as monotherapy, it augments the effectiveness of the beta-adrenergic inhibitor when combined with it. The addition of small doses of a diuretic often prolongs the action of the agent with which it is combined, and side effects are usually not increased.

Some physicians argue against using combination therapies initially; there is always a question as to which drug was effective. But if an agent combining two classes of medications with different actions can produce a higher percentage of responders without an increase in side effects or metabolic changes, this approach to therapy makes sense. If therapy with a diuretic plus a beta blocker, an ACE inhibitor, or calcium channel blocker in small and slightly increasing dosages is ineffective, we then add an alpha blocker such as prazosin (Minipress, 1 to 10 mg per day), terazosin (Hytrin, 1 to 10 mg per day), or doxazosin (Cardura, 1 to 10 mg per day), or, in a few instances, hydralazine (Apresoline, 50 to 150 mg per day). Another approach might include the addition of a cal-

TABLE 14. **Some Available Thiazide Combination Therapies (Other Than Diuretic and Potassium-Sparing Medications)**

Generic Name	Trade Name	Lowest Dosage Available (mg)
Atenolol + thiazide	Tenoretic	50/25
Propranolol + thiazide	Inderide	40/25
Nadolol + thiazide	Corzide	40/5
Bisoprolol + thiazide*	Ziac	2.5/6.25
Captopril + thiazide*	Capozide	25/15
Lisinopril + thiazide	Zestoretic	20/12.5
Enalapril + thiazide	Vaseretic	10/25
Rauwolfia + thiazide	Salutensin-Demi	0.125/25

*Approved as initial once-a-day therapy.

TABLE 15. **Specific Indications and Contraindications for Particular Antihypertensive Drugs**

Clinical Situation	Preferred Medications	Requires Careful Follow-up	May Be Contraindicated
Cardiovascular			
Angina pectoris	Beta blockers, calcium channel antagonists	—	Direct vasodilators
Bradycardia, heart block, sick sinus syndrome	—	—	Beta blockers, labetalol, verapamil, diltiazem
Cardiac failure	Diuretics, ACE inhibitors	—	Beta blockers, calcium channel antagonists, labetalol
Hypertrophic cardiomyopathy with severe diastolic dysfunction	Beta blockers, diltiazem, verapamil		ACE inhibitors, diuretics, $alpha_1$ blockers, hydralazine, minoxidil
Hyperdynamic circulation	Beta blockers	—	Direct vasodilators
Peripheral vascular occlusive disease	—	Beta blockers	—
After myocardial infarction	Non-ISA beta blockers	—	Direct vasodilators
Renal			
Bilateral renal arterial disease or severe stenosis in artery to solitary kidney	—	—	ACE inhibitors
Renal insufficiency			
Early (serum creatinine, 1.5–2.5 mg/dl)	—	—	Potassium-sparing agents, potassium supplements
Advanced (serum creatinine, ≥2.5 mg/dL)	Loop diuretics	ACE inhibitors, diuretics	
Other			
Asthma, chronic obstructive pulmonary disease	—	—	Beta blockers, labetalol
Cyclosporine-associated hypertension	Nifedipine, labelatol	Verapamil, nicardipine, diltiazem	—
Depression	—	$Alpha_2$ agonists	Reserpine
Diabetes mellitus Type 1 (insulin dependent)	—	Beta blockers	—
Liver disease	—	Labetalol	Methyldopa
Vascular headache	Beta blockers	—	—
Pregnancy			
Preeclampsia	Methyldopa, hydralazine	—	ACE inhibitors
Chronic hypertension	Same medications as used prior to pregnancy	—	ACE inhibitors

cium channel blocker if a patient has not responded to a diuretic and an ACE inhibitor, but cost may be a problem with this type of therapy. There are numerous combinations that can be used after initial monotherapy. Combinations of a beta blocker, diuretic, and vasodilator or alpha blocker may have to be used in resistant cases. Other than in patients with severe disease, a period of at least 1 to 3 months should be allowed before increasing or changing the medication. If blood pressure is controlled adequately for about 1 to 2 years, it is appropriate to step down therapy, removing small doses of each of the drugs or eliminating one of the drugs if more than two were necessary to control blood pressures.

SPECIAL POPULATIONS

Hypertension in the Elderly

There are now abundant data from numerous studies in the elderly showing that lowering blood pressure (not just systolic-diastolic but also isolated systolic hypertension) by appropriate therapy reduces morbidity and mortality not just from cerebrovascular disease but also from coronary heart disease. Table 4 summarizes the results of clinical trials in the elderly. In these studies small doses of diuretics or beta-adrenergic inhibitors were used as monotherapy with the addition of one of the other medications if blood pressures were not controlled. In general, elderly subjects tolerate medication well. There are some patients, however, who experience annoying side effects on even small doses of antihypertensive medications. All efforts should be made to lower blood pressure to normal (less than 140/90 mmHg) in the elderly, but this may not be achievable because of undesirable symptoms from side effects.

Antihypertensive Therapy in the Surgical Patient

Medications that have controlled blood pressure should be continued until the day of surgery and begun shortly thereafter. Blood pressure fluctuates less during anesthesia induction in patients who are well controlled. Serum potassium levels should be obtained and hypokalemia treated vigorously if the patient has been on a diuretic and is being prepared for surgery.

Patients with Renal Disease

It is important to maintain normotensive blood pressure levels in all patients with impaired renal function. This is especially true in those with diabetes mellitus. BUN and creatinine levels should be followed, and if these rise while the patient is taking agents such as diuretics or ACE inhibitors, the medication should be modified or changed. Some specific indications for medication are listed in Table 15.

CONCLUSION

We have made great progress in the treatment of hypertension during the past 20 years, achieving a dramatic decrease in stroke death rates of more than 57%. Some of this can be attributed to behavioral changes—people are smoking less, exercising more, and are less obese, but a great deal of the credit must be attributed to the better treatment of hypertension in a larger number of patients. Coronary heart disease deaths have also decreased by almost 50% during this same period of time. Some of this benefit can also be attributed to the better management of hypertension. Management can be undertaken without the use of expensive testing, and most patients can be treated with a simple regimen as outlined in the recent JNC V report.

ACUTE MYOCARDIAL INFARCTION

method of
FRANCIS N. FERNANDES, M.D., and
STEVEN BORZAK, M.D.
Henry Ford Hospital
Detroit, Michigan

Annually about 1,500,000 patients sustain an acute myocardial infarction (MI) in the United States. Despite a marked decrease in incidence and mortality during the past 3 decades, MI remains the leading cause of death, accounting for one-fourth of all fatalities.

PATHOPHYSIOLOGY

Abrupt coronary artery occlusion is the proximate cause of the great majority of MIs. Occlusion occurs through the interaction of disrupted atherosclerotic plaque, intracoronary thrombus formation, and arterial spasm. Clinically detectable MI develops when ischemia is prolonged, usually for more than 30 minutes.

The presence or absence of Q waves does not correlate completely with transmural or nontransmural MI. Q wave MIs are usually due to thrombotic occlusions on plaques. Non–Q wave MIs often occur with severe coronary stenoses and transient occlusions or states of increased myocardial demand. Non–Q wave MIs can also result from thrombolysis (spontaneous or induced) and in areas supplied by collaterals.

PRE-HOSPITAL PHASE

Most deaths in patients with acute MI occur during the first hour from ventricular fibrillation. This can be treated with prompt defibrillation. The maximum benefit from thrombolysis is also obtained during the first few hours. Therefore, it is important for patients to seek early medical attention. Delay is often due to the patient's nonrecognition or denial of the situation.

EMERGENCY ROOM MANAGEMENT

Patients suspected of having an acute MI should be evaluated without delay. This requires a coordinated effort from physicians, nurses, and other personnel. A protocol for a diagnostic work-up is useful to reduce the time needed for the initial evaluation. Table 1 lists the components of the initial assessment of the patient with a suspected MI.

DIAGNOSIS

An acute MI should be suspected if angina-like chest pain or discomfort persists for more than 30 minutes. The importance of the history is due to the limitations of objective tests.

An initial electrocardiogram (ECG) is diagnostic in approximately 60% of patients. In 25% of patients with acute MI it is abnormal but not diagnostic. It is normal in about 15% of patients. If clinical suspicion of an acute MI exists, serial ECGs should be obtained, and these may reveal evolving ST changes. The characteristic pattern includes an initial T wave abnormality followed later by ST elevation in the leads facing the infarcted segment. Reciprocal ST depression is often seen in the leads remote from the infarct zone. Q waves may be present on the initial ECG or may take hours to develop. With time, the QRS amplitude decreases and may be replaced by a QS complex except in patients with posterior MIs. Posterior MIs are associated with tall R waves in leads V_1 and V_2 with ST depression. In non–Q wave MIs persistent ST depression or nonspecific ECG changes may be seen. The appearance of a new bundle branch block with prolonged chest pain also suggests an acute MI. The initial ECG is important because only patients with ST segment elevation or bundle branch block derive benefit from thrombolysis. ST segment depression constitutes a high-risk marker, but thrombolysis in these patients has produced no benefit.

Creatine kinase (CK)-MB isoenzymes take 4 to 8 hours to rise and peak at around 24 hours. An earlier peak occurs with reperfusion. A normal initial CK concentration does not exclude the presence of MI. Serial CK measurements

TABLE 1. **Initial Assessment of Patients with Suspected MI**

Cardiac monitor
Rapid history
Directed physical examination
12-lead ECG; repeat if necessary
Aspirin, 160–325 mg, chewed or swallowed
Indications and contraindications to thrombolysis are checked
Intravenous thrombolytic infusion started if appropriate

should be obtained every 6 to 8 hours over a 24-hour period. The typical rise and fall is a characteristic pattern in an acute MI. If an acute MI has occurred more than 24 hours earlier, serum lactic dehydrogenase (LDH) levels should be obtained. Serum LDH rises in 24 hours and peaks in 3 to 6 days. An LDH1-to-LDH2 ratio of greater than 1 suggests an MI.

TREATMENT

Because many medications are available and valuable time may be lost in choosing among them, priority should be given to those that have proved effective in reducing mortality, as outlined in Table 2.

Pharmacologic Therapy

Aspirin

Aspirin (ASA) prevents platelet aggregation and has an additional beneficial effect on thrombolysis. Because of its high benefit-to-risk ratio, ASA should be given to all patients suspected of having an acute MI except those with known hypersensitivity to ASA. ASA in a dose of 160 to 325 mg should be chewed or swallowed as soon as possible. Enteric-coated ASA may delay its absorption.

The Second International Study of Infarct Survival (ISIS-2) demonstrated that streptokinase given intravenously reduced mortality after an acute MI by 25%. In addition, the administration of ASA orally at doses of 160 mg per day beginning within the first 24 hours of an MI independently reduced mortality by 23%. The combination of ASA and streptokinase was additive, reducing the 5-week mortality by 42%.

Thrombolytics

Systemic thrombolytics available include streptokinase (SK [Streptase]), anisoylated plasminogen–streptokinase activator complex (APSAC [Eminase]), and tissue plasminogen activator (tPA [Activase]). These agents activate plasminogen to form plasmin, which lyses the intracoronary thrombus. Table 3 lists the standard indications and dosages of these agents.

Maximal benefit of thrombolytic therapy is achieved in the first few hours. When used in the first hour there is a 50% reduction in mortality. Mortality reduction is 25% when thrombolytics are given within 6 hours. Results from pooled data also indicate a benefit from the use of thrombolytics in the 6- to 12-hour period, and for some patients in the 12- to 24-hour time frame.

The Third International Study of Infarct Survival (ISIS-3) and the second Gruppo Italiano per lo Studio della Streptochinasi nell'Infarto Miocardico (GISSI-2) showed that SK and tPA were equally effective in reducing mortality. The Global Utilization of tPA and Streptokinase for Occluded Coronary Arteries (GUSTO) trial showed a 14% reduction in mortality with front-loaded (accelerated) tPA compared with SK. Front-loaded tPA produces more rapid thrombolysis and earlier but no more effective artery patency. The stroke rate with tPA is greater by 2 to 3 per 1000 compared with SK, especially in the elderly. Front-loaded tPA has clinically important advantages compared with SK in patients under the age of 75 who present within 4 hours of onset of symptoms. In other patients SK is probably as good. The approximate 1993 costs of SK, APSAC, and tPA are $320, $1800, and $2300, respectively. However, regardless of the agent used, the most important factor is the need to reduce avoidable delays in starting treatment. Currently, thrombolysis is used in only one-third of all patients with MIs, and so earlier administration of thrombolytics to all eligible patients is more important than which agent is used. If the patient has received SK or APSAC in the last 12 months, tPA should be used to avoid neutralizing antibodies, which make the drug less effective. tPA should also be used in hypotensive patients in place of SK.

Elderly patients are frequently excluded from thrombolysis, although the absolute reduction in mortality from this therapy is greatest in this age group. ISIS-2 showed that patients over the age of 70 had the highest mortality (22%), which was reduced by 15 to 37% with thrombolytic therapy.

Contraindications to thrombolytic therapy are listed in Table 4. The risks of thrombolysis include a 1 to 5% risk of hemorrhage requiring transfusion and a 0.5 to 1.5% risk of intracranial bleeding. Invasive procedures should be limited during the first 24 hours after thrombolysis.

TABLE 2. **Initial Therapy with Proved Reduction in Mortality in Acute MI**

Drug	Mortality Reduction	Comments
Aspirin	23%*	Few exclusions
Thrombolytics	25%*	More benefit with earlier therapy
IV beta blockers	14%†	Impact greatest when started early
ACE inhibitors	5–25%‡	Limited early benefit, main effect is long-term

*Combined mortality reduction of 42%.
†Reduced mortality occurs in nonthrombolysed patients; in thrombolysed patients further mortality reduction is unknown.
‡Depending on duration of treatment and extent of left ventricular dysfunction.

TABLE 3. **Indications for Thrombolytic Therapy**

History of chest pain or pressure suggestive of an acute MI
ST elevation of 0.1 mV or more in two contiguous leads or bundle branch block (new or old) with a clinical diagnosis of acute MI
Presentation within 12 hr of symptoms or 12–24 hr with ongoing symptoms of a large infarct or a stuttering pattern
Lack of contraindications (see Table 4)

Dosage

Streptokinase (Streptase, Kabikinase), 1.5 million units infused over 1 hr
Tissue plasminogen activator (alteplase, Activase), accelerated dose 15 mg bolus, 0.75 mg/kg over 30 min (not to exceed 50 mg), followed by 0.5 mg/kg (up to 35 mg) over the next 60 minutes
Anisoylated plasminogen-streptokinase activator complex (anistreplase, Eminase), 30 units over 5 minutes

TABLE 4. **Contraindications to Thrombolytic Therapy***

History of intracranial bleed or surgery
History of nonhemorrhagic stroke within 6 mo
Active peptic ulcer disease within 3 mo
Surgery within 2 wk
Pericarditis or aortic dissection
Traumatic resuscitation or prolonged CPR
Active bleeding or bleeding diathesis
Pregnancy
Uncontrolled hypertension with persistent systolic blood pressure of >200 mm Hg or diastolic blood pressure of >110 mm Hg

*If SK or APSAC was used in the last 12 months, tPA should be given.

Beta Blockers

Beta blockers reduce myocardial oxygen demand by reducing heart rate, blood pressure, and contractility. The incidence of sudden death is reduced by the beneficial effects of these drugs against arrhythmias and possibly cardiac rupture. The ISIS-1 trial showed a 14% decrease in mortality when beta blockers were used before the advent of thrombolysis. The benefit of immediate intravenous beta blockers on mortality was independent of their long-term effect in the postinfarction period. In the Thrombolysis in Myocardial Infarction (TIMI-2) trial the addition of early intravenous beta blockade to thrombolytic therapy decreased the incidence of recurrent MIs and intracerebral hemorrhage. There was no reduction in mortality and no improvement in ejection fraction. Table 5 lists the beta-blocker regimens used for patients with acute MI. Contraindications include cardiogenic shock, second- and third-degree heart block, severe bradycardia, severe heart failure, hypotension, and obstructive airway disease.

Heparin

A study conducted by the Research Group on Instability in Coronary Artery Disease (RISC) examined the role of ASA, heparin,* and a combination of both agents in patients with unstable angina and non–Q wave MIs. ASA demonstrated a reduction in mortality, whereas heparin alone did not. The combination, however, was associated with the lowest event rate in the first 5 days. Patients who do not receive thrombolysis should be given both ASA and heparin if there are no contraindications.

Following thrombolysis the role of heparin was studied in the ISIS-3 and GUSTO trials. ISIS-3 showed that subcutaneous heparin added no further benefit to thrombolysis and ASA. The GUSTO trial found no difference between intravenous and subcutaneous heparin given after SK and ASA administration. Routine heparin use is therefore not recommended after SK and ASA. Smaller studies have examined the role of intravenous heparin after tPA and have shown a higher rate of coronary artery patency with excessive bleeding. Currently, intravenous heparin is used after tPA along with ASA. An intravenous bolus of 5000 units is followed by a heparin infusion during the first 24 to 48 hours. Certain subgroups of patients such as those with a large anterior wall MI, a low ejection fraction, or atrial fibrillation benefit from intravenous heparin and long-term anticoagulation.

*This drug has not been approved by the FDA for this indication.

Heparin binds thrombin indirectly after first binding antithrombin III. The role of direct-acting thrombin inhibitors such as hirudin is being studied.

Angiotensin-Converting Enzyme Inhibitors

The ISIS-4 trial showed a 5% reduction in mortality when captopril* was started within 24 hours of an acute MI. This benefit may be greater in patients with large anterior wall MIs and heart failure. The previous Cooperative New Scandinavian Enalapril Survival Study (CONSENSUS-2) had shown no benefit with early intravenous enalapril.* The long-term role of ACE inhibitors was examined by the Survival and Ventricular Enlargement (SAVE) trial. It showed a 19% reduction in mortality over 42 months when oral captopril was started 3 to 16 days after an acute MI in asymptomatic patients with ejection fractions of less than 40%. ACE inhibitors should be considered in all patients with symptomatic or asymptomatic left ventricular dysfunction. They may be started safely within 24 hours, but little is lost if initiation is postponed for several days.

Nitrates

Although intravenous nitroglycerin* (NTG) is frequently a first-line therapy in the emergency room, it has not been shown to reduce mortality. Hence, its priority should be lower than that of aspirin, thrombolytics, and beta blockers. In the pre-thrombolytic era, small studies with intravenous NTG showed that infarct size was reduced. However, ISIS-4 and GISSI-3 showed very little benefit from the addition of nitrates in patients with or without thrombolytics. Nitrates can be used for persistent chest pain or heart failure. NTG counteracts arterial spasm, dilates collaterals, and reduces preload. Intravenous NTG is started at a dose of 5 μg per minute and titrated to lower the mean arterial pressure by 10%. Possible adverse effects include hypotension, especially in patients with inferior wall MIs and right ventricular wall infarctions.

*This drug has not been approved by the FDA for this indication.

TABLE 5. **Beta-Blocker Regimens for Acute MI**

Metoprolol (Lopressor)
5 mg intravenously given over 2 min for three doses, 5 min apart, followed by 50 mg orally, q 6 hr for 2 days; then 100 mg bid
Atenolol (Tenormin)
5 mg intravenously given over 5 min for two doses, 5 min apart, followed by 50 mg orally, q 12 hr for 2 days; then 100 mg qd
Esmolol (Brevibloc)
500 μg/kg intravenously given over 1 min; then 50–250 μg/kg/min infusion

Lidocaine

In previous studies lidocaine was shown to reduce the incidence of primary ventricular fibrillation (VF) and ventricular tachycardia (VT), but overall mortality did not decrease owing to an increase in bradycardic and asystolic events. The incidence of primary VF and VT has decreased from 5% to less than 2% in the present decade; hence, routine prophylatic use of lidocaine is not recommended. It may be used in patients with primary VF or VT for 6 to 24 hours to prevent recurrences. The loading dose is 100 mg or 1.5 mg per kg given as an intravenous bolus. This is followed in 20 to 40 minutes by a second bolus of about half the initial dose. A lidocaine infusion is then continued at a dose of 1 to 4 mg per minute. Lower doses should be used in the elderly and in patients with liver and heart failure.

Magnesium

The Leicester Intravenous Magnesium Intervention Trial (LIMIT-2) suggested that lower mortality occurred with intravenous magnesium given after an MI. However, the larger ISIS-4 trial showed no benefit from the addition of magnesium to thrombolytic therapy or other standard treatment.

Calcium Channel Blockers

Despite their wide use, no reduction in mortality has been found with calcium channel blockers after MI. The dihydropyridine group (Nifedipine*) in fact was associated with an increased mortality. The rate-slowing calcium channel blockers such as diltiazem* (Cardizem) and verapamil* (Calan, Isoptin) may have a role in secondary prevention of MIs if beta blockers cannot be given. Verapamil and diltiazem should be avoided in patients with left ventricular dysfunction and should not be started for at least several days after an MI.

General Measures

Morphine sulfate can be given intravenously in doses of 2 to 4 mg every 5 to 15 minutes until the pain is relieved; the blood pressure and respiratory status are monitored during this time. The serum potassium level should be maintained above 4.0 mEq per liter because hypokalemia enhances ventricular arrhythmias. Nasal oxygen at 2 to 4 liters per minute is also administered. The diet should consist of clear, caffeine-free liquids during the first 4 to 12 hours. Heavy meals are avoided. Stool softening medications such as docusate sodium (Colace) may be used to prevent constipation. During the first 24 hours following an acute MI the patient is placed on bed rest with commode privileges. Stable patients with uncomplicated MIs may be permitted to sit in a chair within 24 to 48 hours and can undertake supervised ambulation after 48 to 72 hours. These patients may be transferred from the coronary care unit to the ward within 48 to 72 hours.

*This drug has not been approved by the FDA for this indication.

Cardiac Catheterization

Primary percutaneous transluminal coronary angioplasty (PTCA) is an acceptable alternative to thrombolysis, particularly when contraindications to thrombolysis exist. However, the majority of patients with an acute MI do not have prompt access to facilities in which this procedure can be performed.

Routine coronary angiography is not necessary in patients after an MI. Patients should be observed closely and cardiac catheterization performed if postinfarction angina, heart failure, or other complications develop or if positive results on a predischarge low-level stress test are found.

Urgent cardiac catheterization should be performed if there is evidence of a complication such as cardiogenic shock, acute ventricular septal defect, or severe acute mitral regurgitation.

COMPLICATIONS OF MYOCARDIAL INFARCTION

The mechanical complications of acute MI are associated with a high mortality and should be recognized early so that prompt treatment can be implemented. Table 6 lists the early complications and their management.

Late complications include left ventricular aneurysms, which are more common after large anterior wall MIs. They predispose to the formation of left ventricular thrombi. Intravenous heparin* followed by warfarin for 3 to 6 months lowers the embolic risk associated with these MIs.

Pericarditis may occur in the first week following an MI. It is associated with a pericardial rub, widespread ST elevation, and PR interval depression. Treatment includes aspirin and analgesics.

Arrhythmias associated with acute MI may include tachyarrhythmias or bradyarrhythmias. VF and hemodynamically significant VT should be treated with prompt defibrillation (200 to 360 joules). Electrolyte imbalances and hypoxemia should be corrected. Intravenous lidocaine (1 to 4 mg per kg per minute) may be used for 6 to 24 hours to prevent recurrences. VT and VF within the first 48 hours do not predict a poor long-term prognosis. However, patients with VT or VF after 48 hours should be considered for cardiac catheterization, revascularization, and possibly electrophysiologic (EP) testing or empirical Class III antiarrhythmic treatment.

Accelerated idioventricular rhythm is often associated with reperfusion and usually does not require treatment unless hemodynamic compromise is present.

Atrial fibrillation may indicate atrial infarction or pump failure. When associated with ischemia and hemodynamic instability, cardioversion should be performed. Intravenous digoxin or beta blockers may be used to control the heart rate.

Sinus bradycardia with hypotension and Mobitz

*This drug has not been approved by the FDA for this indication.

TABLE 6. **Mechanical Complications of Acute MI**

	Diagnosis	Management
Cardiogenic shock (60–80% mortality)	Hypotension or hypoperfusion Lung rales PA catheterization	Cardiac catheterization and early revascularization Dobutamine (Dobutrex), 5–15 μg/kg/min IABP until revascularization can be performed
Acute ventricular septal defect and acute MR	Heart failure Systolic murmur LLSB or at the apex (MR) Echocardiography PA catheterization	Emergency surgical repair Dobutamine (Dobutrex) and/or nitroprusside (Nipride) if tolerated IABP
Right ventricular infarction	Occurs with 50% of inferior MIs Hypotension and JVD Absent lung rales ECG, ST elevation, $V4_R$ PA catheterization	IV fluids Avoid nitroglycerin Dobutamine (Dobutrex) or dopamine IABP may be necessary
Cardiac rupture	Electromechanical dissociation	Emergency pericardiocentesis and surgery

Abbreviations: PA = pulmonary artery; IABP = intra-aortic balloon pump; LLSB = left lower sternal border; MR = mitral regurgitation; JVD = jugular venous distension.

Type I second-degree atrioventricular (AV) block are common with inferior wall MIs. When these conditions produce symptoms, they should be treated with atropine, 0.5 mg intravenously every 5 minutes, up to a total dose of 2 mg if necessary. The dosage of beta blockers, digoxin, or calcium channel blockers should be reduced or stopped. A temporary transvenous pacemaker should be used for asystole, third-degree AV block, Mobitz Type II second-degree AV block, bradyarrythmias not responsive to atropine, new bifascicular block, and new left bundle branch block.

RISK STRATIFICATION AFTER ACUTE MYOCARDIAL INFARCTION

Three major independent risk factors exist for mortality after an acute MI: left ventricular systolic dysfunction, recurrent myocardial ischemia, and ventricular arrhythmias after the initial 24 to 48 hours. The single most important prognostic indicator after an acute MI is the ejection fraction. Ventricular function can be estimated by echocardiography, radionuclide scanning, or left ventriculography.

Patients who develop recurrent angina following an infarction should be considered for early cardiac catheterization and revascularization. After an uncomplicated MI, asymptomatic patients should undergo a submaximal or low-level exercise stress test prior to discharge. Concomitant nuclear imaging or stress echocardiography may be required in patients with baseline ECG abnormalities. A positive low-level stress test indicates the need for coronary angiography, and consideration should be given to revascularization with either PTCA or CABG. Patients who have a negative low-level stress test usually can undergo a symptom-limited full stress test within 6 weeks of the infarction.

Ventricular arrhythmias are a risk factor for mortality; however, the Cardiac Arrhythmia Suppression Trial (CAST) revealed that Class I antiarrhythmic agents in patients with minimally symptomatic ventricular arrhythmias increased rather than decreased the incidence of subsequent sudden death. Hence, the use of antiarrhythmic agents is limited to patients with serious arrhythmias. All patients should be given a beta blocker barring the presence of contraindications after an infarction.

SECONDARY PREVENTION OF RECURRENT INFARCTION

Long-term beta blocker treatment reduces mortality by about 21% and decreases the incidence of nonfatal reinfarction by 22%. A dose should be chosen that produces a detectable effect on the resting or exercise heart rate.

Aspirin therapy following an infarction reduces the reinfarction rate by about 25%. Aspirin at 160 to 325 mg daily should be continued for a minimum of 2 years.

The role of ACE inhibitors has been shown by several large trials to be associated with important reductions in mortality over the long term. Candidates include patients with symptomatic or asymptomatic left ventricular dysfunction.

Diltiazem and verapamil reduce the rate of reinfarctions and are safe in patients with good ventricular function. Both are contraindicated in patients with heart failure. They are a weak alternative if lung disease prohibits beta blocker administration.

One particular subset of post-infarction patients that warrants particular attention is the group with non–Q wave MIs. Although these patients have a lower early mortality than their Q wave counterparts, the mortality in the two groups is equal by the end of the first year. Therefore, patients with non–Q wave MIs should have a lower threshold for a recommendation for catheterization and revascularization. No clear differences in the principles of medical management exist between patients with Q wave MIs and those with non–Q wave MIs.

Prior to discharge from the hospital the patient

should be counseled on the cessation of cigarette smoking and should meet with a dietitian to discuss a cholesterol-lowering diet. Patients should be considered for a cardiac rehabilitation program. Fasting cholesterol and triglyceride levels should be measured 6 weeks after infarction, and vigorous diet and pharmacologic therapy should be instituted if necessary.

SUMMARY

Major advances have been made in our understanding of the pathophysiology and treatment of MI, and there has been a corresponding decline in mortality during the past 2 decades. Further successes in treatment are less likely to result from new drugs than from a fuller understanding of the currently available therapy and its prompt and widespread application.

CARDIAC REHABILITATION

method of
GERALD F. FLETCHER, M.D.
Emory University School of Medicine
Atlanta, Georgia

The principle of cardiac rehabilitation evolved as early as 1772, when William Heberden described one of his patients with severe coronary artery disease who "became better" after chopping wood 45 minutes a day for 6 months. In more recent years, with increased recognition and successful management of cardiovascular disease, the true "father" of cardiac rehabilitation and preventive cardiology in the United States was Dr. Paul Dudley White. White believed in "safe exercise" for normal subjects and also for those with coronary artery disease. He believed that exercise was a good tranquilizer and benefited one spiritually, physically, and psychologically. In accord with his pioneering ideas, interest, and efforts in this field, many cardiac rehabilitation programs have evolved.

The *categories* of subjects seen in coronary rehabilitation programs include post-myocardial infarction subjects, those who have undergone coronary artery bypass surgery or coronary angioplasty, and many with stable coronary artery disease with clinical manifestations such as controlled angina pectoris and arrhythmias.

The *inpatient phase* of cardiac rehabilitation is usually quite limited in scope owing to the need for early discharge. In patients with stable coronary disease and angioplasty, hospitalization may be no longer than 1 to 2 days. Inpatient rehabilitation, therefore, predominantly entails education of the patient about the disease process. Special emphasis is placed on education about dietary control of cholesterol and saturated fat intake and on calorie control, when necessary, for the overweight patient. This education is best provided by a registered dietitian, who is both knowledgeable and experienced in this particular area of nutrition. In addition to the educational process, there is usually time for early ambulation activities and physical therapy exercise in certain patients. However, further exercise programming is usually scheduled in the outpatient setting.

Objective data are usually obtained by special tests carried out in the *outpatient* rehabilitation program, most often by use of the standard exercise test (to be discussed later) and, in addition, by the electrocardiographic (ECG) rate and rhythm recorded during the exercise sessions. Angiographic studies are frequently needed as part of the diagnostic evaluation, based on the exercise test data, and the nearness of such capabilities in a medical center is most valuable. Such medical back-up resources may not be available in independent cardiac rehabilitation programs, but this does not detract from the safety and efficacy of such programs if they are managed according to the standards set by health agencies such as the American Heart Association (AHA).

The *basic principles* of cardiac rehabilitation include several components in addition to prescribed physical activity. It is of great importance that subjects know the extent of their disease. This central nidus of knowledge by patients about the degree and type of their disease, the interventions and medications used, and the major coronary risk factors is an overall mission of cardiac rehabilitation. Nutrition guidelines for weight control as well as the normalization of abnormal blood lipids (with medication as needed) are essential and important components of cardiac rehabilitation. Of all coronary risk factors an elevated total blood cholesterol level correlates most closely with the development and progression of coronary artery atherosclerosis. This is evident at a level of 180 mg/dL or more, and the correlation becomes progressively stronger at levels above 180 mg/dL. Accordingly, the National Cholesterol Education Program and the AHA have strongly recommended that total blood cholesterol be maintained at 200 mg/dL or less in all subjects but especially in those with known coronary artery disease. Current guidelines dictate that optimal blood cholesterol levels be 180 mg/dL or less. Therefore, a most important component of all cardiac rehabilitation programs is control of blood cholesterol using dietary guidelines or medications.

Substance control in the form of cessation of cigarette smoking and control of high blood pressure (over and above the controlling effect produced by exercise and diet) is another important goal of cardiac rehabilitation. In certain people stress management on a one-to-one basis or in a group setting may be an important intervention.

There are two basic *types* of cardiac rehabilitation programs: group and home-based. The most popular is the *group* program; these sessions may be ECG monitored or nonmonitored, supervised or nonsupervised. In general, at least six or more monitored sessions are recommended for all subjects, including blood pressure monitoring (recording) and education of the patient about the modes and progression of exercise. Many programs, however, use as many as 36 sessions of ECG monitoring. Categorizing patients as low risk, moderate risk, or high risk usually indicates the appropriate number of monitored sessions.

The *prescribed activity* for cardiovascular exercise has five important components, all of which can be carefully monitored (with active patient education by staff) during ECG-monitored sessions. The basic components of activity addressed are intensity (how hard), frequency (how often), and duration (how long). Mode (or type) and progression of exercise are the other important components that are provided through specific protocols. It is most important that subjects learn to use different types of exercise equipment properly. Such equipment adds variety to the exercise program. Various devices (ergometers, cycles, and treadmills) have been made "prescriptively specific" for subjects so that they can progress safely through the various levels of exercise.

The basic fundamentals of the prescription are similar; however, the *monitored* phase is usually more structured and more closely supervised. For example, in the early monitored phase, maximal oxygen consumption ($\dot{V}O_2$ max) achieved at peak exercise level is converted to metabolic equivalents (METs; $\dot{V}O_2$ max divided by 3.5 equals maximal MET level), and the prescription is written for levels ranging from 30 to 75% of maximal MET level attained on exercise testing. These MET levels can then be individually adjusted so that each subject can achieve a 50 to 75% target heart rate (THR). This THR is arbitrarily selected based on previous observations and recommended established guidelines. If oxygen consumption studies are not available, THR end points derived from exercise testing can be quite safely and effectively used in writing the exercise prescription, and this is often done. Using the level of perceived exertion (PE) or how hard the subject is working is valuable as a subjective end point in prescribing the level of intensity.

Subjects then follow a progressive activity level protocol in sessions held three to four times weekly, in which the activities are individually prescribed based on available data in normal subjects. Such a program familiarizes patients with warm-up, flexibility, and light calisthenic exercises for the major muscle groups. In addition, patients are educated about the use of various types of exercise equipment, such as arm and arm-leg combination ergometers and motorized treadmills, in addition to walking. Usually patients complete this monitored phase in six to 12 sessions or more.

The *nonmonitored* exercise program is a continuation of the principles of the monitored protocol. In this medically supervised but nonmonitored training program, the patient continues the calisthenic and stationary exercises, usually adding more walk-jog activities. At this point, THR may be increased to 85% of the maximal level achieved with exercise testing. Water exercise and team activities such as volleyball may also be included as an additional recreational component. Subjects progress in the nonmonitored program until they achieve a maintenance program level. In many patients, repeat exercise testing may be needed 2 to 6 months after the initial test to evaluate symptoms further and to reassess $\dot{V}O_2$ max, THR, and PE.

The Emory University Health Enhancement Program in Atlanta uses a six-level protocol for the initial exercise phase of cardiac rehabilitation. This protocol is used not only for ECG monitoring but also for blood pressure recording, assessment of PE, and recording of specific symptoms. Education about the modes or types of exercise equipment and the rate of progression of exercise is also incorporated in this phase. With close monitoring by staff, accurate records can be made of responses such as angina and dyspnea as well as heart rate, rhythm, and blood pressure fluctuations. The subject may progress through all six levels in six sessions or may be delayed at any level for several sessions. The various modes in the six-level protocol include treadmill walking and leg, arm-leg, and arm ergometry. Precise prescriptions can be adapted for any category of subject for each of these modalities based on the initial exercise test results and use of methodology described elsewhere. After the six-level monitored protocol has been completed, subjects graduate to the nonmonitored phase through a 20- to 40-week period, during which time they acquire a fixed level of exercise prescription for long-term maintenance.

It is most important for the exercise prescription to be up to date. This is achieved by periodically evaluating the PE and heart rate response to exercise and making the appropriate changes in the prescription. However, regular use of repeat exercise testing at intervals is the most accurate and important means of updating the exercise prescription (see subsequent section on Exercise Testing).

Safety is a major factor in cardiovascular exercise programs. The instant ECG recorder may be used for heart rate and rhythm analysis. The defibrillator must be readily available for use with airway support and appropriate cardiac drugs in the event of an emergency; this equipment should be properly serviced at regular intervals. An emergency plan for patient transfer to a medical facility must be up to date and should be posted in the exercise room.

Supervision by a physician, nurse, or other trained professional has been an issue of concern and has been addressed in detail in recent guidelines published by the AHA. It is recommended that a physician be responsible and should be immediately available in the exercise facility. Well-trained cardiovascular nurses may, however, provide immediate supervision of the patients' exercise activities if a physician is not in the exercise room.

The other basic type of program used in cardiac rehabilitation is the *home-based* (or individual) program. Data are available from two centers on the safety and efficacy of such programs. These programs are convenient for subjects if they live far away, but of course they have no medical supervision. If exercise is done at home, heart rate and rhythm may be monitored by transtelephonic ECG transmission, and significant symptoms can be reported by voice transmission. A YMCA or exercise club may also be adequate if the subject chooses such a facility. In such settings there is usually an exercise leader or someone who can work closely with the subjects as a group. In such individual and home programs, the use of a lower intensity (perhaps 60 to 70% of maximum) exercise and regular interval exercise testing are of great importance.

EXERCISE TESTING

In cardiac rehabilitation programs, regular exercise testing is very important and should be carried out in adults of all ages. It should be performed initially in any coronary disease patient who enters a program and at least yearly thereafter. In the early phases of the program, exercise testing may be indicated in some subjects at the end of 3 or 4 months and then at least yearly afterward.

There are a number of end points to be considered in exercise testing. The development of angina pectoris, ST segment changes, and an abnormal blood pressure response are important predictors of cardiac function. Left ventricular function can be readily assessed during the exercise test by simply measuring the blood pressure by cuff sphygmomanometer and making particular note of the systolic response. Certain subjects who are taking beta-adrenergic blocking drugs may have only a modest blood pressure response initially; however, if there is good left ventricular function, the eventual response should be normal. Other specific end points to note in exercise testing are the duration of test time, the heart rate response, and the development of ventricular arrhythmias. The diastolic blood pressure response is important in subjects who are "potentially hypertensive" or who have hypertension that may not be well controlled by drug therapy.

There are good clinical prognostic correlations with exercise test results. Of great importance are the severity of ST segment displacement on ECG, the presence of angina pectoris, a fall in blood pressure, short exercise test time, and a low exercise heart rate.

Clinically, if a patient can produce a high-level performance on the treadmill, it is unlikely that he or she has significant coronary artery disease. If the blood pressure responds properly with an increasing systolic measurement and no rise in diastolic pressure, this is further confirmation of a normal cardiovascular response. On occasion, a normal individual may show a transient decrease in systolic blood pressure at the point of maximal exhaustion. However, an early drop in pressure (before the maximal exercise end-point) may reflect severe left ventricular dysfunction. Beta blockade may delay the increase in systolic blood pressure with exercise, but in the presence of good left ventricular function the pressure will eventually increase appropriately.

In summary, there are certain nonelectrocardiographic negative predictors in exercise testing that are quite useful: (1) a low achieved heart rate, less than 120 beats per minute in the absence of beta blockade; (2) hypotension greater than a 10-mmHg drop in systolic pressure below baseline; (3) a rise in diastolic blood pressure; (4) a low achieved rate-pressure product; and (5) a limited exercise test time.

Also of importance is the role of exercise testing in the evaluation of ventricular arrhythmias. With exercise, ventricular ectopy may develop, increase, or decrease in frequency, or, in some instances, disappear. Ventricular ectopy that increases in complexity, especially in the form of ventricular tachycardia, is of concern in subjects with cardiovascular disease and should be managed appropriately. Cardiac rehabilitation provides an excellent means of managing such patients. Physicians with trained nurses and health professionals in cardiac rehabilitation programs have an excellent opportunity to evaluate the subjects' symptoms and signs and refer them for other studies and possible interventions.

STUDIES AND TRIALS IN CARDIAC REHABILITATION

A number of studies support the benefit of cardiac rehabilitation programs. A meta-analysis of 22 trials of cardiac rehabilitation in various centers around the world is the most comprehensive of these reports. One of these trials was the National Exercise Heart Disease Project (NEHDP), in which Emory University of Atlanta participated. In the NEHDP, which was of 3 years' duration and involved post-infarction men, the exercise group had a significantly decreased percentage of cumulative mortality compared to the control or free activity group. Another well-controlled study from Finland revealed a lower cardiac death rate and lower overall mortality in exercising subjects compared to controls. The 22 trials, analyzed collectively, included 4500 subjects with an average 3-year follow-up. These trials included post-infarction subjects only, and no other category of coronary artery disease was considered. There was a total of only 3% women, and only 4 of the 22 studies included women. All patients participated in exercise programs of 2 to 6 months' duration. At 3 years, the results revealed that the odds ratio was significantly lower for the rehabilitation group in total mortality, cardiac mortality, and fatal reinfarction, and at 1 year it was lower for sudden cardiac death. There was no difference in the incidence of nonfatal reinfarction. There was an overall 20% reduction in mortality in the cardiac rehabilitation exercise group. Therefore, the data now reveal that these programs are beneficial, at least for 3 years after myocardial infarction. More recently, early results of a dual center study on high-level (85% $\dot{V}O_2$ max) versus low-level (50% $\dot{V}O_2$ max) intensity exercise training reveal that high-level exercise improves left ventricular ejection function as well as ventilatory threshold. Other studies in cost containment show that subjects in cardiac rehabilitation programs have fewer hospital readmissions and diagnostic tests than those not in such programs—a significant decrease in cost of care.

ONGOING CONCERNS IN CARDIAC REHABILITATION

Beta Blockade. Many patients are taking various types of beta-adrenergic blocking drugs. Once a subject begins such medication, it is often continued indefinitely. With regard to cardiac rehabilitation, there is more concern about the nonselective preparations such as propranolol (Inderal) and nadolol (Corgard) because they often produce other systemic side effects, such as fatigue and depression, in addition to heart rate depression. Because of the former, metoprolol (Lopressor) and atenolol (Tenormin) seem to be better tolerated as cardioselective drugs.

Disabled Individuals. Some subjects with coronary artery disease have had a stroke or an amputation with resultant hemiplegia, paraplegia, or other limb deficiency that allows them the use of fewer than all four extremities. Special modalities of exercise testing and training can be used effectively in this group of subjects. The more commonly used modalities are the leg or arm ergometer and the combined arm-leg ergometer. These subjects comprise a significant portion of the coronary artery disease population, a group that is now being referred for cardiac rehabilitation.

The Elderly. The average age of patients admitted to cardiac rehabilitation programs in the early 1970s was 52 years; currently, the average age is the mid-sixties, but some patients are in the 70- to 90-year age range. The aging process is associated with decreases in heart rate (at maximal exercise and at rest) and with increases in systolic blood pressure and systemic and pulmonary pressure. There is less fibrinolysis, and pulmonary function decreases. After the age of 30 years, there is also a decrease in maximal strength, which is greater in the legs than in the trunk. In the elderly, there is a decrease in cardiac output and stroke volume. All of these factors may affect the exercise prescription. In prescriptive exercise for the elderly, the heart rate and blood pressure response are important factors, and because of the changes occurring with aging, the use of metabolic studies to prescribe exercise is desirable. Another point of concern with elderly patients is the possibility of ventricular arrhythmias, which usually increase with age. The clinical significance of such arrhythmias must be assessed, particularly in the presence of clinically manifest coronary artery disease. This latter factor emphasizes the need for effective cardiovascular nursing and medical care to determine the indications for treatment intervention. Lastly, in the elderly, the musculoskeletal system may be affected by such conditions as degenerative arthritis, muscular soreness, and tendon laxity, which may discourage exercise training by these patients and lead to noncompliance.

Heart Failure. Currently, more subjects enter cardiac rehabilitation exercise programs with some degree of heart failure, defined as a decrease in cardiac output or ejection fraction, but without cardiac decompensation to the degree of pulmonary congestion or "congestive" heart failure. Patients who undergo careful exercise training may show modest improvements in oxygen consumption but usually have significant improvements in endurance and exercise capacity on retesting. This improvement is thought not to be due to improved cardiac function but rather to improved skeletal muscle recruitment, improved flexibility and strength, and general psychologic motivation. In prescribing exercise in subjects with heart failure, one must keep prescribed exercise to a low level. Even in subjects with marked left ventricular dysfunction (ejection fraction of <30%), musculoskeletal strength and endurance may be improved with a very low level prescription.

Several studies on the duration of exercise testing and maximal oxygen consumption after exercise training in subjects with heart failure are available. Regardless of the use of various drugs for treatment of heart failure, including placebo, most patients improve after training. This is probably due to improved musculoskeletal strength because improvement in maximal oxygen consumption is less marked. Several factors may cause the decrease in oxygen consumption in patients with heart failure: (1) increased body weight, (2) decreased heart rate, (3) anemia, (4) impaired vasodilatation, and (5) poor blood pressure control. All of these factors may be managed optimally in a cardiac rehabilitation program.

Ventricular Arrhythmias. Ventricular ectopy occurs frequently in subjects in cardiac rehabilitation programs and may increase, decrease, or develop for the first time with exercise. Development of increased ventricular ectopy or more complex ectopy in a cardiac rehabilitation population is of concern. There are data supporting the observation that ventricular ectopy increases with previous myocardial infarction. In addition, one must always consider the fact that ventricular ectopy in patients with coronary artery disease may reflect underlying left ventricular dysfunction and be a marker of poor prognosis. Such patients benefit from careful surveillance in a cardiac rehabilitation program.

Peripheral Vascular Disease. Atherosclerotic vascular disease is a diffuse process. Often patients with coronary disease who exercise present with intermittent claudication, suggesting the presence of occlusive disease of the lower extremities. This can usually be managed conservatively; however, when symptoms become severe, angiography and definitive intervention may be in order. In certain instances of claudication, long-term exercise has been found to be effective in alleviating and reducing symptoms. One study in subjects with atherosclerotic disease of the lower extremities showed that a 12-week period of treadmill walking for 1 hour per day, 3 days weekly, significantly improved exercise performance and decreased the severity of claudication pain. Concurrent with this, a 26% decrease was seen in the resting plasma short-chain acylcarnitine concentration (an index of ischemic skeletal muscle).

LONG-TERM CORONARY RISK FACTOR MODIFICATION

In long-term follow-up of patients in cardiac rehabilitation programs, the ever-present problems are those of resumption of cigarette smoking, inadequate blood pressure control, and poor adherence to dietary guidelines that provokes weight gain and abnormal blood lipid levels. The total program of cardiac rehabilitation must regularly address these issues on a long-term basis. By doing so, the patient will have the overall benefit of coronary risk factor modification as well as prescriptive exercise. This comprehensive approach provides the basis for retarding the progression and, in some instances, of provoking the regression of the atherosclerotic process.

PERICARDITIS

method of
DAVID H. SPODICK, M.D., D.Sc.
University of Massachusetts Medical School
Worcester, Massachusetts

Treatment of pericarditis is aimed at (1) suppressing symptoms, (2) relieving cardiac compression by pericardial effusion or constriction, and (3) controlling or destroying the etiologic agents and processes.

SUPPRESSION OF SYMPTOMS

Pain, Fever, and Discomfort

Pain is managed by using the lowest effective doses of individual or combined analgesic agents. Except in some patients with surgically induced pericarditis, escalation to maximal dosages and combined therapy with simpler medications should be attempted before resorting to corticosteroid treatment. Careful attention to contraindications and monitoring for side effects are mandatory, particularly for anti-inflammatory agents and especially for nonsteroidal agents. In any case, management of symptoms should be commensurate with the patient's distress. Frequently, in mild cases no symptomatic treatment is necessary.

Nonsteroidal anti-inflammatory drugs (NSAIDs) are the mainstay of treatment of both pain and inflammation (in patients with fever aspirin should be considered first—325 to 650 mg every 4 to 6 hours). The principal NSAID of value, ibuprofen, has the best side effect profile and the largest dose range among patients who can tolerate it, beginning with 800 mg every 8 hours and increasing the rate to every 6 hours with the option of raising the dose to 1000 mg.* Otherwise, any NSAID may be tried with the exception of indomethacin (Indocin), a drug that reduces coronary flow and increases the size of experimental myocardial infarcts. If pain is refractory or severe before the effects of these agents become manifest (usually a matter of a few hours at most), an icebag on the precordium occasionally suffices (not to be used in patients with ischemic heart disease). Otherwise, codeine, 60 mg every 4 hours, is particularly useful if there is a distressing cough, or morphine sulfate, 10 to 15 mg intramuscularly every 4 to 6 hours, or pentazocine (Talwin), 50 mg every 2 hours for up to 10 doses* a day may be tried. Tranquilizers may be needed for anxious patients who are not taking an opiate, notably those with heart disease, related or unrelated, who are often worried by any chest discomfort.

*Exceeds the dosage recommended by the manufacturer.

Occasional marked nausea or vomiting may require a 5- to 25-mg suppository of prochlorperazine (Compazine). Palpitations are uncommon and usually subside after suppression of pain. Important rhythm disturbances occur only in patients with underlying valve or myocardial disease (not in those with pure pericarditis without myocarditis); these patients require specific anti-arrhythmic agents if the arrhythmia causes hemodynamic impairment or is unusually distressing.

Large nontamponading effusions may cause thoracic or abdominal distress requiring a palliative pericardiocentesis.

Corticosteroid agents should be a last resort (unless pericarditis is produced by a syndrome for which such treatment is necessary) because of the growing number of individuals with chronic recurrent or incessant pericarditis who are "hooked" on an agent, usually prednisone, and cannot discontinue it without experiencing disabling discomfort.

RELIEF OF CARDIAC COMPRESSION

Acute Cardiac Tamponade

This is a major emergency requiring removal of pericardial fluid by paracentesis or surgical drainage. The technique of pericardiocentesis should be learned from an experienced mentor. In any case, needle drainage should always include a pericardial catheter to remain in situ for continuous drainage until the effusion ceases. The echocardiogram can demonstrate the optimal site for needle-catheter drainage, which is at the subxyphoid location in approximately 50% of patients. However, surgical drainage is safest. Until recently, most experience has been with a subxyphoid incision, which is extrapleural and extraperitoneal and permits resection of a large specimen of pericardium and inspection manually or by scope of the pericardial cavity and both layers of the pericardium. In any case, except in an emergency, needle paracentesis should be avoided if there is less than a 5-mm depth of anterior effusion fluid. Another option is thoracoscopic drainage, which also permits both

*Exceeds the dosage recommended by the manufacturer.

resection of large amounts of pericardium and creation of a window into the adjacent pleural cavity, usually the left. Pericardial windows can also be made with a double balloon technique via a pericardial catheter.

Medical therapy supporting the heart and circulation during cardiac tamponade remains controversial and has not been conclusively demonstrated to be effective except in patients who are dehydrated. In any case, administration of oxygen, blood volume expansion, and use of inotropic agents have increased the ejection fraction, especially when this treatment is combined with afterload reduction. Theoretically, dobutamine (Dobutrex) is the best agent; however, there is no substitute for drainage.

Under certain conditions, open thorocotomy with pericardial resection is necessary; these conditions are (1) recurrence of tamponade after partial (subxyphoid) pericardial resection, (2) recurrence of malignant pericardial effusion, (3) tamponade in dialyzed uremic patients who are unresponsive to increased dialysis and intrapericardial instillation of a corticosteroid, and (4) almost every patient with severe suppurative pericarditis (particularly children). If cardiac compression can be even partially relieved by needle drainage, this procedure is optimal before general anesthesia is induced. Anti-inotropic and anticoagulant treatments must be discontinued.

Chronic or Recurrent Acute Cardiac Tamponade

Although pericardiocentesis may be a temporary expedient, recurrent tamponade or epicardial constriction often makes pericardiectomy mandatory. Although very sick patients may undergo a window operation with fenestration of the pericardium into the adjacent pleural cavity, *all pericardial windows eventually close.* Therefore, the widest excision is best, preferably through a thoracoscope unless other conditions make thoracotomy necessary.

Constrictive Pericarditis (Chronic, Subacute, or Acute)

All patients recovering from any kind of acute pericarditis (excepting rheumatic) should be followed indefinitely because of the possibility of eventual constriction. Naturally, some causes, for example, tuberculosis, require a more intense follow-up. Patients with only asymptomatic pericardial thickening and calcification do not require treatment even if the calcification is extensive. On the other hand, they should be followed especially closely.

The definitive treatment is extensive (complete or quasi-complete) pericardiectomy. In occasional patients with mild acute constriction (and there is some evidence that this occurs frequently, although subclinically, after many instances of acute pericarditis), the syndrome resolves spontaneously or with anti-inflammatory management. In patients with definite constriction, the usual measures to relieve heart failure and systemic congestion may be tried, paying careful attention to avoid overdosing and side effects. In truly chronic cases (now quite rare in advanced countries) ascites may require abdominal paracentesis. The patient's clinical response is the best guide to optimal control. However, the presence of advanced liver involvement and atrial fibrillation, as seen in chronic cases, reduces the chances of surgery being successful in the long term.

Chronic Pericardial Effusion

Chronic, apparently nontamponading effusion may be present for very long periods, even many years, with no effect on the patient's quality of life, although in some cases reduction of lung volume induces a restrictive pulmonary defect. Recently, a number of cases have been observed in which progressive, rapid, or even sudden decompensation occurs, causing cardiac compression, so that there is a tendency to favor early surgery. Naturally, etiologic sources should be sought, particularly hypothyroidism, although most cases are idiopathic. A few cases are due to cholesterol pericarditis or chylopericardium that are for some reason asymptomatic or minimally symptomatic.

CONTROL OR DESTRUCTION OF ETIOLOGIC AGENTS AND PROCESSES

Table 1 shows the broad etiologic range of pericardial disease, which falls into 10 major categories, indicating the involvement of the pericardium in every kind of medical and surgical disorder. This list should be learned as a catechism because every new case of pericardial disease will fall into one of these categories, which may not be immediately apparent. Fortunately, the great majority of acute cases are idiopathic; when pericarditis is part of a generalized disorder, appropriate specific treatment, if available, is indicated. For example, drug-related "hypersensitivity" pericarditis calls for discontinuance of the drug. For infectious forms of pericarditis, most antibiotics tested produce effective levels in pericardial fluid when given orally or intravenously.

Idiopathic Pericarditis

Here the exact cause is never determined, although viral pericarditis probably accounts for most cases.

TABLE 1. **Etiologic Categories of Acute Pericarditis**

Idiopathic (syndrome; resembles viral pericarditis)
Infectious
Parasitic
Vasculitis–connective tissue disease group
Immunopathies; "hypersensitivity" (including drug-related) states
Diseases of contiguous structures
Metabolic
Neoplastic
Traumatic (direct and indirect)
Of uncertain origin or associated with syndromes of uncertain pathogenesis

The main therapeutic problems are pain, recurrences (sometimes for years), occasional tamponade, and constriction. Corticosteroid dependency occurs mainly in this group. All female patients with this syndrome should undergo screening tests and follow-up for systemic lupus erythematosus.

Pericarditis Caused by Living Agents

Viral pericarditis, usually diagnosed by inference from the epidemiologic and serologic findings, usually has no specific therapy. When a specific agent, such as Epstein-Barr virus, is involved, acyclovir (Zovirax) may be effective. Most cases are self-limiting, although occasionally pericarditis is combined with an element of myocarditis (myopericarditis).

Nontuberculous Bacterial Pericarditis. Mortality in patients with purulent pericarditis has been reduced from almost 100% to well under 50% by surgical drainage alone. Antibiotics have further cut the remainder drastically. Because this condition remains dangerous, particularly in children and in compromised hosts, rapid control is essential. Pus must be removed from the pericardium, preferably by surgery. Antimicrobial treatment should be matched to organisms found in the pericardial drainage or the bloodstream. While awaiting conclusive proof, treatment with oxacillin (Bactocill), 1 gram every 3 hours,* plus gentamicin (Garamycin), beginning with 6 mg per kg per day* may be attempted with subsequent dosages adjusted according to serum assay or creatinine level. For penicillin-sensitive patients, cephalothin sodium (Keflin) may be substituted for oxacillin. However, specific treatment should be instituted as soon as possible.

Fungal and parasitic pericarditis requires specific therapeutic agents plus surgical excision and drainage.

Tuberculous Pericarditis. Tuberculous pericarditis, whether seriously suspected or actually demonstrated, requires vigorous antituberculous therapy, usually with multiple drug regimens. Pericarditis in AIDS patients is becoming more and more common and is often produced by mycobacteria, particularly "atypical" organisms requiring special therapeutic protocols (bacterial and viral infections of the usual kinds also occur in AIDS patients).

Because of the tendency of tuberculous pericarditis to provoke constriction, early surgery is necessary if the symptomatic constitutional response is poor or if fluid reaccumulates despite multiple drainage procedures (painless cases seem to follow a more insidious chronic course). In any case, patients who are known to have had tuberculous pericarditis must be followed indefinitely for late complications.

Pericarditis in the Vasculitis–Connective Tissue Disease Group

Here the treatment is sometimes disease-specific, although anti-inflammatory treatment, notably with corticosteroid therapy in the most severe cases, usually is successful. In patients with rheumatic pericarditis, antistreptococcal therapy is added.

Drug-Related Pericarditis

An increasing number of drugs have been associated with acute pericarditis. The major ones are procainamide, hydralazine, certain antineoplastic agents, phenytoin, and some antibiotics. The offending agent must be discontinued.

Diseases of Contiguous Structures

Pericarditis in the course of pleural and pulmonary disease requires attacks on the originating process. The course of acute pericarditis is followed with frequent electrocardiograms, which should be examined for evidence of myocardial infarction. (Computer reports on electrocardiograms should always be read over by an experienced electrocardiographer because the computer frequently either misses the diagnosis or identifies acute pericarditis as "anterolateral infarct," and antithrombotic and anticoagulant therapies have been given, sometimes provoking a life-threatening hemopericardium with tamponade.)

Metabolic Pericarditis

Classic uremic pericarditis is usually well controlled by chronic dialysis, but tamponade requires aspiration, and the occasional constriction requires pericardiectomy. A pericardial effusion may be decompensated to frank tamponade by rapid hemorrhage or by dialysis if fluid is removed too rapidly from the intravascular compartment. The success with this form of treatment contrasts with *dialysis pericarditis,* in which continued dialysis does not suffice, and the patient may have to undergo drainage with instillation of a nonabsorbable corticosteroid or eventual pericardial resection. Occasionally switching from hemodialysis to peritoneal dialysis solves the problem (the latter for unknown reasons is associated much less often with induction of pericarditis).

Traumatic Pericarditis

Direct trauma, wounds of the heart and pericardium, requires emergency pericardiocentesis, treatment of shock, and early surgical drainage and repair. The surgical approach with careful inspection of the pericardium, heart, and adjacent structures is nearly always the safest and most successful because cardiac wounds can be temporarily stopped by clotting and later insidiously or suddenly result in hemopericardium. *Indirect trauma* caused by blunt blows to the chest should be observed and managed like idiopathic pericarditis. *Iatrogenic indirect trauma* is due to radiation therapy of lesions in the vicinity and produces all forms of pericarditis, the most dangerous being delayed tamponade and constriction, which should be treated as outlined previously.

---

*Exceeds the dosage recommended by the manufacturer.

Pericarditis of Uncertain Origin

There is a great variety of patients in this category, for example, cholesterol pericarditis, which occurs in association with rheumatoid arthritis, myxedema, or tuberculosis but is usually idiopathic. This is treated by drainage of effusions and resection of the pericardium. Another example is pericarditis associated with thalassemia major (relatively frequent in younger patients), which is treated like idiopathic pericarditis. Most patients in this group mainly require specific therapy of the associated condition.

PERIPHERAL ARTERIAL DISEASE

method of
JAMES S. T. YAO, M.D.
Northwestern University Medical School
Chicago, Illinois

OCCLUSIVE DISEASE OF LOWER EXTREMITY ARTERIES

In an elderly population, arterial occlusive disease of the lower extremity arteries is most likely due to atherosclerosis as part of the manifestation of the disease process affecting the coronary and carotid circulation. These patients share a common medical history such as a smoking habit, diabetes mellitus, lipid disorders, and hypertension. Arterial occlusion can also occur in younger patients less than 40 years old. In these patients, the cause is often entrapment of cystic degeneration of the popliteal artery, Buerger's disease, or arteritis. Table 1 lists the causes of chronic arterial occlusive disease of lower extremity arteries.

Clinical manifestations of chronic arterial occlusive disease include claudication, rest pain at the metatarsal head, and tissue loss such as ulceration or gangrene of the digits. Claudication is often the initial symptom, characterized by reproducible pain of the calf muscle after a fixed distance of walking followed by a brief period of relief by rest. Pain at rest, in particular at night when cardiac output is low, is a more severe form of ischemia. Some of these patients seek relief by dangling their feet by the bedside. In advanced ischemia, ulceration or gangrene of the digits is present.

TABLE 1. **Causes of Chronic Arterial Occlusion of the Lower Extremity**

Arteriosclerosis
Buerger's disease
Arteritis
Collagen disease
Rheumatoid arteritis
Takayasu's disease
Antiphospholipid syndrome
Popliteal artery entrapment
Adventitial cystic degeneration
Ergot poisoning
Antithrombin III deficiency

Diagnosis of arterial occlusion is not difficult. Palpation of the pedal pulses helps to establish the diagnosis and the site of occlusion. The availability of ankle pressure measurements and flow velocity waveform recordings from the pedal arteries by Doppler ultrasonography has greatly simplified the assessment of arterial occlusive disease. Comparison of the ankle systolic pressure with the brachial pressure to derive an ankle-brachial index (ABI) offers an instant determination of the diagnosis and the adequacy of the collateral circulation. In normal subjects, the ankle pressure is usually greater than or equal to the brachial pressure with an ABI of greater than 1.0. An ABI equal to or less than 0.97 almost always represents some degree of arterial occlusive disease. In patients with claudication, the ABI is often at the range of 0.50 to 0.80. An ABI of less than 0.25 or an absolute ankle systolic pressure of 50 mmHg or less indicates the presence of critical ischemia. In patients with diabetes, ankle pressure recording is less reliable because calcified arteries may give false-high readings. In such patients, the use of toe pressure is helpful to determine the degree of ischemia.

At present, arteriography is not needed to establish the diagnosis. If percutaneous transluminal balloon angioplasty or bypass graft is contemplated, arteriography helps to determine the type of therapeutic procedure to be used. Arteriography is also helpful to define the anatomic pattern of the disease process. In general, there are three patterns of arteriosclerotic occlusive disease: (1) aortoiliac, (2) femoropopliteal or tibial, and (3) combined aortoiliac and femoropopliteal occlusions.

Aortoiliac Disease

The classic occlusive disease is Leriche's syndrome, which produces an angiographic appearance of tapering of the terminal aorta and symptoms of lower extremity fatigue, muscle atrophy, and skin trophic changes, and an inability to sustain an erection. In females, the "small woman syndrome" is characterized by diffuse narrowing of a small aorta and hypoplastic iliac arteries. Most of these patients are in the younger age group (35 to 55 years). This pattern of arterial pathology in women appears to be similar to that of Leriche's syndrome in men with the exception of impotence. Other aortoiliac pathologic changes include juxtarenal aortic occlusion. This represents a late stage in the disease process. Although atherosclerosis tends to be diffuse, focal lesions such as solitary iliac artery stenosis, segmental stenosis of the aorta, and penetrating ulcer of the aorta are not infrequent disease patterns of the aortoiliac segment.

Femoropopliteal or Femorotibial Occlusive Disease

In patients with infrainguinal occlusive disease, claudication is often due to single segmental occlusion of the femoropopliteal artery, whereas severe ischemia such as rest pain or tissue loss is often a result of multiple occlusions affecting not only the femoropopliteal segment but also the tibial or pedal arteries. In diabetics, the atherosclerotic process often starts at the infrapopliteal artery and its trifurcation. Both anterior and posterior tibial arteries are often occluded. Fortunately, the peroneal artery is often spared the disease process and is suitable as a recipient artery for distal bypass. In young adults with symptoms of arterial occlusion, the possibility of nonatherosclerotic disease should be considered. Both entrapment and cystic degeneration tend to affect the popliteal artery. There are four main types of popliteal entrapment, the anomalous medial head of the gastrocnemius muscle being the most common form of compression. Adventitial cystic degeneration is an unusual but important cause of arterial occlusion. Accumulation of gelatinous fluid within the cyst can compress the popliteal artery, causing ischemic symptoms.

Combined Aortoiliac and Femoropopliteal or Tibial Occlusive Disease

This is the most severe form of atherosclerotic disease, affecting both inflow and outflow arteries. Because of the diffuse nature of the disease process, patients often present with severe claudication, rest pain, or tissue loss.

Treatment of arterial occlusive disease depends on the symptoms and not on the arteriographic appearance of the disease process. In most patients with claudication, nonoperative treatment should be offered. Patients should be instructed about risk reduction including cessation of smoking, control of hypertension, modification of diet if there is associated obesity, and correction of hyperlipidemia. Rehabilitation programs with standard forms of exercise are now readily available in many hospitals and should be offered to patients with claudicating symptoms. The pharmacologic management of intermittent claudication has been disappointing. Pentoxifylline (Trental), a drug that increases red blood cell deformability, has been advocated to increase perfusion to muscles but has not yet met clinical expectations. New drugs such as crantine and anti-platelet drugs are now undergoing multicenter trials to determine their effectiveness in the treatment of claudication. It is important to remember that claudication due to segmental occlusion of the femoropopliteal artery often runs a benign course. Only 5% of patients progress to limb-treatening ischemia during a 5-year period.

Several interventional procedures are now available for the treatment of arterial lesions. Laser ablation and atherectomy enjoyed a period of favor but have failed to sustain satisfactory long-term results. Recurrent stenosis is common with these two procedures. As a result, these two techniques are little used in clinical practice. In contrast, percutaneous transluminal angioplasty (PTLA) or balloon dilatation remains a very effective procedure, especially for short segmental stenosis of the iliac artery. The patency rate of PTLA for iliac stenosis is 75% at 1 year and 50% at 5 years. The combination of stent placement and balloon angioplasty offers an even better outlook for iliac artery stenosis, especially stenosis of the external iliac artery with diffuse atherosclerotic changes and also recurrent iliac stenosis. PTLA, however, is less durable in femoropopliteal segments, with a patency rate of about 50% at 1 year. At present PTLA is recommended only in patients with short segmental stenosis of the femoropopliteal artery. Recently, the use of intra-arterial infusion of urokinase has been reported to be effective in reopening a thrombosed artery of recent onset (less than 3 weeks). The role of urokinase* in the treatment of chronic occlusion awaits ongoing multicenter trials to determine its efficacy.

Surgical treatment of patients with claudication must adhere to strict criteria, especially in patients with femoropopliteal segmental occlusion. For severe aortoiliac disease such as Leriche's syndrome or juxta-aortic occlusion, aortobifemoral bypass using a Dacron or polytetrafluoroethylene (PTFE) graft is the preferred procedure. Aortic grafting is a durable procedure and has an expected patency rate of approximately 85 to 90% at 5 years, 75% at 10 years, 70% at 15 years, and 60% at 20 years. Mortality for aortic reconstruction is less than 3%. In young patients with unilateral iliac occlusion, a femorofemoral graft is the procedure of choice because the procedure avoids operative dissection of the iliac artery causing ejaculatory dysfunction. The results of femorofemoral grafts, however, are slightly inferior to those of aortofemoral grafts, with primary patency rates of 63%, 56%, and 40% at 5, 10, and 15 years, respectively.

Bypass grafting is needed in patients with limb-threatening ischemia. Prior to surgery, a complete evaluation of cardiac status is needed, especially for those who are candidates for aortic procedures. In general, a thallium scan is used as the initial guide for work-up in these patients. The type of surgical procedure used depends on the site of occlusion and the extent of the disease process. Because of the diffuse nature of the atherosclerotic process, a bypass graft is often the procedure of choice. Endarterectomy is reserved only for focal lesions. For aortoiliac artery occlusion, an aortobifemoral graft is an effective procedure. In patients with prohibitive cardiopulmonary risks, an alternative inflow procedure such as an axillofemoral graft should be considered. Severe ischemia is often due to combined inflow and outflow lesions. Correction of the inflow lesion by aortofemoral graft or axillofemoral graft is all that is needed to reverse the ischemia. Limb-threatening ischemia due to infrainguinal disease often requires the use of autogenous saphenous vein graft in either a reversed or in situ manner with the distal anastomosis placed on the tibial or peroneal arteries at the calf or on the pedal arteries at the ankle level. It is generally agreed that autogenous vein grafts fare much better

*Urokinase has not been approved by the Food and Drug Administration (FDA) for this indication.

than prosthetic grafts, especially when the distal anastomosis is placed on the tibial arteries (68% patency rate for vein vs. 38% for PTFE at 5 years). Whenever possible, an autogenous vein graft should be the conduit of choice. PTFE grafts are used only when autogenous vein is not available. Femorodistal bypass is now a safe procedure and has a mortality rate of less than 2%. The expected primary patency rate in autogenous vein graft is about 80% at 5 years and 43% at 10 years.

ACUTE ARTERIAL OCCLUSION

Unlike chronic occlusive disease, the onset of acute ischemia is often sudden and abrupt. The most common cause of acute ischemia of the lower extremity is embolic occlusion. Most emboli are cardiac in origin and have an incidence ranging from 90 to 94%. Another source of emboli is atheromatous ulcerating plaque or an aneurysm sac. These emboli are microemboli originating from cholesterol crystals or platelet debris of the ulcerating surface of the plaque. In these patients, the presenting symptoms include blue toe syndrome or livedo reticularis of the thigh or trunk of the body. In approximately 10% of patients with an embolic event, the source remains unknown despite an exhaustive search. Table 2 shows the sources of peripheral emboli. An acute embolic occlusion must be distinguished from acute thrombosis developed in an atherosclerotic artery. The latter often presents with a history of claudication with the clinical stigma of arterial occlusive disease in the contralateral limb. Another cause of acute occlusion is development of sudden thrombosis of a popliteal aneurysm.

The diagnosis is often not difficult. A history of cardiac fibrillation or myocardial infarction in the presence of sudden limb ischemia establishes the diagnosis of acute embolic occlusion. A cardiac embolism is commonly dislodged into the femoral artery. Diagnostic features of acute ischemia include loss of the pedal pulse, paresthesia, and motor function disturbance. Examination must include pulse palpation, test of nerve function, and palpation of the anterior and posterior compartments of the leg. Acute compartment syndrome can develop as a result of sudden arterial occlusion. The patient often complains of calf tenderness and inability to dorsiflex the forefoot or big toe. Acute saddle emboli at the bifurcation of the aorta can cause sensory and motor weakness of both extremities, and the diagnosis must be differentiated from acute dissection.

TABLE 2. **Sources of Peripheral Emboli**

Cardiac
- Left atrium
  - Atrial fibrillation
  - Atrial myxoma
  - Arrhythmia
- Chronic sinoatrial disorder
- Rheumatic mitral stenosis
- Endocardium: myocardial infarction
- Ventricular aneurysm
- Prosthetic heart valve

Peripheral artery
- Atheromatous ulcerating plaque
- Shaggy aortic syndrome (disseminated atherosclerosis)
- Aneurysm
- Prosthetic graft

Paradoxical emboli: Venous thrombosis with patent foramen ovale

Treatment of acute arterial occlusion requires immediate intravenous heparinization. Intra-arterial urokinase* infusion is now an effective therapeutic procedure and should be used following arteriographic examination if there is no contraindication to thrombolytic therapy. Most acute emboli respond to a 24- to 48-hour infusion of urokinase. In an acute thrombosed artery, urokinase may uncover the cause of occlusion (stenotic plaque or popliteal aneurysm), and the appropriate corrective procedure is instituted after the relief of acute ischemia.

Surgical treatment of acute embolic occlusion by catheter embolectomy remains the procedure of choice in patients with profound ischemia such as loss of motor sensory function or compartment syndrome, and in those for whom thrombolytic therapy is contraindicated. Treatment can be performed under local anesthesia to expose the femoral artery, pass a Fogarty balloon catheter beyond the embolic occlusion, and extract the obstructing embolus and the superimposed thrombi. All patients with cardiac emboli should be treated with heparin and subsequently should receive anticoagulation with long-term warfarin (Coumadin) therapy.

Atheromatous embolization is the second most common form of acute ischemia. This form of embolization is due to microembolization arising from cholesterol or platelet debris from an ulcerating plaque. Typically, it affects arteries of 50 to 200 μm in diameter. Unlike emboli of cardiac origin, treatment by heparin or urokinase is less effective. In these patients, the primary goal is to establish the source of the emboli. In the presence of palpable pedal pulses, the use of an infusion computed tomography (CT) scan may uncover an aneurysm of the aorta or of the iliac and popliteal arteries as the primary source of microembolization. The recent introduction of transesophageal echocardiography allows a complete evaluation of the thoracic aorta. Arteriography may also be needed, and occasionally a solitary ulcerating plaque of the aortoiliac segment or the common femoral artery is detected by this routine diagnostic technique. Treatment of atheromatous embolization is designed to eliminate the source of emboli either by placing a graft, excluding the aneurysm from the circulation, or by performing an endarterectomy to remove the ulcerating plaque.

ANEURYSMS OF THE AORTA AND PERIPHERAL ARTERIES

Aortic Aneurysm. Aneurysm formation of the aorta is a complex process, involving arteriosclerotic

*Not approved by the FDA for this indication.

change of the arterial wall and an alteration of the matrix protein metabolism of elastin and collagen. Enzymic destruction, gene mutation of Type III collagen, and participation of inflammatory cells have recently been implicated in the formation of aneurysms. Most aneurysms form in elderly people of more than 55 years of age and steadily increase in incidence up to 80 years of age. The infrarenal aorta is the most common site of aneurysm formation, followed by the iliac artery, the descending aorta, and the popliteal artery. Approximately 15% of patients with aortic aneurysm have a familial history of aneurysm. Men appear to be affected more often than women.

Aortic aneurysm is often asymptomatic and can be detected as a painless pulsatile mass during routine physical examination. In obese patients, however, palpation of the abdomen often fails to detect the aneurysm. Plain film radiographs of the abdomen, especially in the lateral projection, may show the aneurysm by its calcified wall. Unfortunately, in only 20% of cases is there enough calcification to allow clear depiction of the aneurysms on plain film radiographs. Aneurysms occur more often in patients with chronic arterial occlusive disease and in those with a family history of aneurysm. Screening of this population is best done by ultrasonography. Once a patient is thought to have an aneurysm, the most accurate diagnostic test is infusion CT scan of the abdominal aorta, which determines the extent of the aneurysm (above or below the renal artery), the wall characteristics (whether the aneurysm is an inflammatory aneurysm), and the relation of the aneurysm to the surrounding structures. Most abdominal aortic aneurysms are infrarenal, and only 5% have a proximal extension above the renal artery. Arteriography should not be used for diagnosis of an aortic aneurysm. In many instances, intramural thrombus may result in an angiographic appearance of a relatively normal aortic lumen. Arteriography, however, is needed in patients with hypertension, horseshoe kidney, or other visceral or peripheral artery occlusion. For a thoracoabdominal aneurysm, arteriography examination is mandatory prior to surgery.

The natural course of aneurysm is expansion leading to rupture, the development of acute thrombosis, and embolization. The growth rate of aneurysms is about 0.4 to 0.5 cm per year. Rupture of an aortic aneurysm appears to be related to size. Aneurysms 5 cm in diameter carry a 50% risk of rupture within 5 years. Rupture is less likely in aneurysms of 4.0 cm or less but still may occur. If surgery is not contemplated, small aneurysms must be followed by CT scans at 6-month intervals.

The mortality of patients with a ruptured aneurysm treated surgically is about 40 to 50%. This is in sharp contrast to the less than 5% mortality seen in elective surgery. Surgical intervention, therefore, is recommended for all aortic aneurysms greater than 5 cm in size or for small aneurysms that produce symptoms. Small aneurysms with recent expansion should also be considered for surgery. Prior to surgery, evaluation of the coronary artery status is mandatory. This can be accomplished with a thallium scan and, if indicated, a coronary arteriogram. For patients with thoracoabdominal aneurysms, coronary arteriography is desirable. Significant coronary disease must be corrected either by PTLA or surgery to maximize cardiac function prior to aortic surgery. The surgical procedures used depend on the extent of the aneurysm. For aneurysms confined to the aorta, a tube graft replacement is all that is needed. An aortoiliac or aortofemoral graft is used if there is an associated iliac artery aneurysm. For thoracoabdominal aneurysms, the technique advocated by E. S. Crawford using a Carrel patch for reimplantation of visceral arteries has greatly simplifed the procedure. At present, the 5-year survival rate is 70% after successful aortic aneurysm repair, with corresponding 10- and 15-year life expectancy rates of 40% and 18%, respectively.

Iliac Aneurysm. Iliac aneurysm is often associated with aortic aneurysm, and most aneurysms are located either at the common iliac artery or the internal iliac artery. For unknown reasons, the external iliac artery is often spared from aneurysm formation. Detection of isolated iliac aneurysm is often difficult unless a complication such as rupture or embolization has occurred. In patients with large iliac aneurysms, rectal examination often detects the pulsatile mass. Confirmation of an iliac aneurysm is best achieved by infusion CT scan.

Popliteal Aneurysm. One of the serious complications of popliteal aneurysm is distal embolization causing blue toe syndrome or digital gangrene. Diagnosis of a popliteal aneurysm can be difficult because the popliteal artery is hidden in the popliteal fossa, making palpation difficult. A prominent popliteal pulse raises the suspicion of aneurysm formation. Confirmation of the aneurysm can be achieved by duplex scan or infusion CT scan. Aneurysmal disease is systemic. A patient with one popliteal aneurysm has about a 50% chance of having one on the other side. He or she has a 30% chance of having an aortic aneurysm. In patients with an aortic aneurysm, a search for a popliteal aneurysm must be made. Although rupture is relatively uncommon, expansion of the aneurysm can cause compression of the adjacent nerve and venous structures. Not infrequently, sudden thrombosis may develop, causing limb-threatening ischemia. Surgical treatment is accomplished by proximal and distal ligation of the aneurysm to exclude it from the circulation, followed by a femoropopliteal bypass graft to restore distal perfusion.

Femoral Aneurysm. This is a less frequent aneurysm that is seen in the peripheral arteries, and in most instances it is commonly associated with popliteal or aortic aneurysm. Like all aneurysms, a femoral aneurysm can cause distal embolization or acute thrombosis causing severe limb ischemia. Treatment is rather simple and consists of resection of the aneurysm followed by an interposed prosthetic graft to restore continuity of the artery.

DEEP VENOUS THROMBOSIS OF THE EXTREMITIES

method of
MARCUS D. STANBRO, D.O., and
JOHN R. BARTHOLOMEW, M.D.
Kirksville College of Osteopathic Medicine
Kirksville, Missouri

Deep venous thrombosis (DVT) is a common yet underappreciated problem in hospitalized patients. It has two major complications: pulmonary embolism (PE) and chronic venous insufficiency (CVI). These constitute a significant source of morbidity and mortality in the United States.

It is estimated that venous thromboembolism results in 250,000 to 600,000 hospitalizations each year in the United States. Pulmonary embolism has been estimated to cause up to 100,000 deaths annually, making it one of the most common causes of sudden death in the United States. The actual number is undoubtedly higher because of the often "silent" nature of this disease. Many of these deaths are preventable.

The exact incidence of CVI following DVT is unknown but is believed to be low in cases of upper extremity and calf DVT but nearly 50% or greater in cases of iliofemoral DVT.

PATHOGENESIS

The pathogenesis of venous thromboembolism is based on vessel wall damage, venous stasis, and hypercoagulability, often referred to as Virchow's triad. Table 1 lists some of the common risk factors associated with DVT.

DIAGNOSIS

The diagnosis of DVT based on the history and physical examination is often unreliable. The physical examination may be normal or may demonstrate the classic signs: increased skin temperature, edema, erythrocyanotic discoloration, or dilated superficial veins. Pain or discomfort may or may not be present. The differential diagnosis of DVT includes a ruptured Baker's cyst, cellulitis, lymphedema, lymphangitis, muscle hematoma or tear, compartment syndrome, arthritis, arterial insufficiency, heart or liver failure, and iliac vein compression.

Duplex ultrasonography has emerged in recent years as the diagnostic test of choice for detecting upper and lower extremity DVT. In experienced hands, duplex scanning of the lower extremities has a sensitivity and specificity greater than 95% for proximal DVT. The sensitivity falls with examination of the calf veins; accuracy and reliability are often operator dependent.

Venography, still considered the gold standard by many, is usually reserved for inadequate or equivocal duplex examination results and for detecting calf vein thrombosis.

Impedance plethysmography (IPG) has been shown to have high sensitivity and specificity for proximal DVT; however, it is not useful for detecting calf thrombi, and it does not allow exact anatomic localization.

TABLE 1. **Deep Venous Thrombosis Risk Factors**

Advanced age	Previous DVT
Immobilization	Congestive heart failure
Malignancy	Myocardial infarction
Stroke	Pregnancy
Surgery	Varicose veins
Trauma	Long bone fractures
Lupus anticoagulant	Oral contraceptive use
Protein S or C deficiency	Inflammatory bowel disease
Antithrombin III deficiency	Antiphospholipid syndrome

PREVENTION

Every patient considered at risk for the development of venous thromboembolism should receive DVT prophylaxis. This constitutes the majority of hospitalized patients. Table 2 lists some currently recommended prophylaxis regimens.

TREATMENT

Once the diagnosis of DVT is suspected, the patient should receive immediate anticoagulation therapy unless there are contraindications. Treatment is aimed at preventing further thrombus formation and minimizing complications such as PE or CVI.

Heparin remains the drug of choice and is administered intravenously. Its primary action involves binding to antithrombin III and accelerating the inactivation of thrombin. This effectively and rapidly prevents further thrombus formation. Heparin is usually given as a 5000- to 10,000-unit intravenous bolus followed by an infusion rate of 500 units per kg per 24 hours. An activated partial thromboplastin time (APTT) should be checked every 4 to 6 hours until it achieves a therapeutic level and then once daily to maintain it between 1.5 and 2.5 times control. There are now substantial data indicating that recurrent venous thromboembolism is unlikely and that treatment is adequate for DVT if heparin is given for 5 days, assuming that warfarin (Coumadin) is also started on the first day of treatment.

A complete blood count (CBC) with platelets should be monitored at least every other day to guard against occult bleeding or heparin-induced thrombocytopenia.

Oral anticoagulation with warfarin is begun on the first day if possible. Warfarin is a vitamin K antagonist that depletes Factors II, VII, IX, and X. Factor VII has the shortest half-life: 8 to 12 hours compared with 60 to 70 hours for Factors II and X. Consequently, depletion of Factor VII occurs rapidly and may result in a prolongation of the prothrombin time (PT), often within 1 to 2 days. However, until the other remaining factors have been adequately depleted, there is a possible risk of new thrombus formation. Warfarin and heparin therapy should be overlapped by 4 to 5 days to prevent this possibility.

Warfarin is given as a 10-mg loading dose. Subsequent daily doses are adjusted to keep the International Normalized Ratio (INR) between 2.0 and 3.0 (PT should be 1.3 to 1.5 times control). After dose stabilization, the INR/PT should be monitored weekly. It is generally recommended that the initial episode of DVT be treated for 3 months. A second episode is treated for 6 to 12 months and a third episode, especially if unexplained, may necessitate lifelong anticoagulation.

TABLE 2. **Deep Venous Thrombosis Prophylaxis Regimens**

General medical patients (including those with MI, CHF, stroke)	LDH (SC q 12 hr) or IPC
Hemorrhagic stroke	IPC
Abdominal or thoracic surgery	LDH (SC administered 2 hr before surgery, then q 12 hr) or IPC
Orthopedic surgery	
Knee replacement	IPC, warfarin, or adjusted-dose heparin
Hip replacement	IPC, warfarin, LMWH, or adjusted-dose heparin
Eye or neurologic surgery	IPC
Indwelling CVP catheters	Warfarin, 1 mg/day

Abbreviations: LDH = Low-dose heparin (5000 units); SC = subcutaneous; IPC = intermittent pneumatic compression; LMWH = low-molecular-weight heparin; MI = myocardial infarction; CHF = congestive heart failure; CVP = central venous pressure.

Thrombolytic Therapy for DVT

Selected cases of DVT have been treated successfully with thrombolytic therapy* with the intent of preserving valvular function and thereby avoiding CVI. This approach appears to be most effective in patients with axillary-subclavian or iliofemoral DVT of less than 7 days' duration. Other indications may include preservation of catheter and vein function in patients with indwelling central venous catheters. Thrombolysis is the treatment of choice for phlegmasia cerulea dolens or venous gangrene.

Patients must be screened for absolute contraindications such as active bleeding or a recent stroke, or relative contraindications such as recent (<10 days) surgery, trauma, or organ biopsy. The risks and benefits of thrombolytic therapy must be weighed carefully.

Best results are obtained when the thrombolytic agent is delivered directly into the thrombus through a multiport catheter. The standard dosage for urokinase (Abbokinase) is a bolus of 4400 units per kg followed by a 4400-unit per kg per hour continuous intravenous infusion. If tissue plasminogen activator (tPA) (alteplace) is selected, the dosage is a 0.05- to 0.06-mg per kg per hour infusion. The dose for streptokinase (Kabikinase, Streptase) is a 250,000-unit bolus, followed by 100,000 units per hour. There is no set infusion time or maximal dosage because the goal is complete clot lysis; however, doses of tPA above 100 mg have been associated with higher bleeding rates. Most new DVTs are dissolved within 24 to 48 hours. Thrombolysis can also be given through a peripheral line, but it is associated with longer infusion times, which may lead to potentially higher bleeding complication rates.

Surgery

With the introduction of thrombolytic therapy, the need for venous thrombectomy has become uncommon. However, if thrombolysis is contraindicated, surgery can be used to treat phlegmasia cerulea dolens.

*Thrombolytic therapy is not approved by the FDA for this indication.

Vena Caval Interruption

The method of choice for vena caval interruption is now percutaneous placement of a caval filter. There are several indications for filter placement, including recurrent PE despite adequate anticoagulation, a contraindication to anticoagulation, chronic recurrent PE, and pulmonary thromboembolectomy. Although filters in the inferior vena cava (IVC) are 95% effective in preventing significant emboli from reaching the lungs and remain patent in 95% of patients, they do not prevent further thrombus propagation. Anticoagulation is recommended whenever possible for patients with newly placed filters or for patients who continue to be at high risk.

SPECIAL CONSIDERATIONS

Pregnancy

Studies have shown heparin to be safe and effective during all three trimesters of pregnancy. Gravid patients with acute DVT should be treated with intravenous heparin initially and then switched to full-dose subcutaneous heparin. The daily subcutaneous dose is usually higher than that of intravenous infusions and is adjusted to prolong the APTT at 1.5 to 2.5 times control. Anticoagulation should be maintained until 4 to 6 weeks postpartum. If the DVT occurred late in the pregnancy, the patient should be treated for 3 months after delivery. Unfortunately, one of the side effects of heparin is osteoporosis, which can occur with prolonged use as in pregnancy.

Axillary-Subclavian Venous Thrombosis

Although the clinical significance of axillary-subclavian venous thrombosis (ASVT) has been a source of controversy in the past, this entity is currently believed to be an important cause of morbidity and mortality. It appears that the incidence of ASVT is rising, possibly due to the increased use of central venous catheters. Risk factors for ASVT are similar to those for thrombosis of the lower extremities. Additional causes to consider include the thoracic outlet syndrome, effort-related thrombosis (Paget-Schrotter's syndrome), trauma, tumor, pacemakers, or intravenous drug abuse.

All patients with ASVT should undergo anticoagulation. Serious consideration should also be given to thrombolytic therapy, especially to preserve vein integrity and catheter function in patients requiring long-term central venous access.

Calf DVT

Isolated calf DVT constitutes an area of considerable controversy. There are two general approaches.

First, full anticoagulation can be recommended in the belief that proximal clot propagation will be prevented. This approach is reasonable if the clot is symptomatic or extensive or if the predisposing factors are still present. Treatment duration is typically limited to 6 to 8 weeks, and repeat objective testing is usually not needed. The second approach consists of observation with serial duplex scanning. This can be recommended in patients who are ambulatory or who have minimal risk factors for extension of DVT, or in whom the bleeding risk is deemed unacceptable. Duplex scanning two times a week for 2 to 3 weeks will ensure that any proximal propagation of thrombus will be detected and treated appropriately.

Low-Molecular-Weight Heparin

Low-molecular-weight heparins (LMWHs) are fragments of heparin with a molecular weight roughly one-third that of standard heparin. In addition to binding to antithrombin III, LMWHs also display an increased ability to catalyze the inactivation of Factor Xa. Currently, the only LMWH available in the United States is enoxaprin (Lovenox), which is approved by the FDA for prophylaxis in orthopedic surgery. In Europe, LMWHs are used not only for prophylaxis but also for treatment of acute DVT. LMWHs have predictable responses based on weight-adjusted dosing, making dose adjustments unnecessary. In the future, this mode of therapy may make outpatient treatment for acute DVT possible.

Section 5

The Blood and Spleen

APLASTIC ANEMIA

method of
NEAL S. YOUNG, M.D.
National Heart, Lung, and Blood Institute
Bethesda, Maryland

Aplastic anemia is pancytopenia with bone marrow hypocellularity. The disease, first described by Ehrlich just over a century ago, appears infrequently but is not rare: Formal epidemiologic studies in Europe found an incidence (annual new cases) of about 2 per million; the rate is higher in the Orient. Acquired aplastic anemia occurs predominantly in young adults (15 to 25 years old) and among older persons over the age of 60 years. Aplastic anemia can also be constitutional and is then described as Fanconi's anemia, or dyskeratosis congenita. Fanconi's anemia is often, but not always, associated with short stature and specific physical anomalies of the skeletal and urogenital systems. The diagnosis rests on the characteristic susceptibility of chromosomes to chemicals like mitomycin C and diepoxybutane, detected by cytogenetic analysis of blood cells. Inherited aplastic anemia may not become clinically manifest until adolescence or later, and therefore, these pediatric syndromes enter into the differential diagnosis of pancytopenia in the adult. Acquired aplastic anemia, especially when blood count suppression is incomplete or the marrow is only moderately hypocellular, must also be distinguished from myelodysplasia (hypocellular in about 20% of cases), aleukemic leukemia (especially in the very young and the very old), and myelofibrosis.

Aplastic anemia has many clinical associations. Direct toxicity to marrow clearly occurs in three circumstances: following acute irradiation, after treatment with myelosuppressive drugs (especially alkylators and nitrosoureas), and with benzene exposure. High doses of these agents are required to produce irreversible marrow failure; for example, the dose of radiation predicted to result in death from hematologic causes in 50% of an exposed population is probably in excess of 2.5 Gy. Except in cancer patients undergoing chemotherapy, direct toxicity is an infrequent etiology of acquired aplastic anemia. Pesticides, insecticides, and many drugs have also been associated with bone marrow failure, but here the relationship is idiosyncratic, meaning that despite their wide use, they only occasionally are linked to disease in an individual. In formal epidemiologic studies, nonsteroidal anti-inflammatory drugs, anticonvulsants, and sulfa drugs have been most strongly incriminated. Historically, chloramphenicol appeared to initiate an epidemic of aplastic anemia on its introduction in the 1950s, but this drug is now infrequently used in medical practice in the United States and Europe. Although a suggestive history of drug or chemical exposure may be obtained from a patient, establishing an etiologic relationship in an individual case is difficult, even with research laboratory studies.

Aplastic anemia also occurs in the setting of viral infections. In the hepatitis/aplasia syndrome, severe bone marrow failure follows an uncomplicated episode of hepatitis, which is non-A, non-B, non-C by serologic and molecular studies; the putative viral agent has not been identified for hepatitis/aplasia or non-A, non-B, non-C fulminant hepatitis alone. Rarely, aplastic anemia is a sequela of infectious mononucleosis, and Epstein-Barr virus can be demonstrated in the marrow in these cases. Cytopenias in patients with acquired immune deficiency syndrome (AIDS) are usually characterized by a cellular, dysplastic bone marrow.

Paroxysmal nocturnal hemoglobinuria (PNH) is strongly associated with aplastic anemia. In a high proportion of patients, especially young persons, PNH evolves into aplasia, and conversely, a significant proportion of aplastic anemia patients will develop a positive acidified serum lysis (Ham) test months to years after successful immunosuppressive therapy. PNH is now known to be secondary to a defect in the PIG-A gene, the protein product of which is responsible for the phosphatidylinositol (PI) linkage of a family of proteins to the cell membrane. Absence of certain cell-surface proteins leads to increased complement sensitivity of red cells, but the relationship of PI-linked proteins to hematopoietic failure is unknown. Detection of absent PI-linked proteins by flow cytometry is more sensitive than the Ham test for the diagnosis of PNH in aplastic anemia.

Rarely, aplastic anemia occurs in relation to pregnancy and may be resolved or improved by its termination. Aplastic anemia is associated with the collagen vascular disease eosinophilic fasciitis. Graft-versus-host disease, which develops after transfusion of blood products containing viable lymphocytes into an immunocompromised host, can produce fatal marrow aplasia.

Despite the large numbers of clinical associations, in most series, the majority of cases of aplastic anemia are labeled idiopathic.

Studies of marrow cells in vitro have shown that almost every patient has a severe defect of hematopoietic progenitors. Marrow stroma and hematopoietic growth factor production are usually normal, consistent with the success of marrow transplantation and the relative ineffectiveness of growth factor administration in this disease. In vitro assays of stem cells are more difficult to perform in humans, and stem cells have been reported as low to normal in a few studies. The basis for suppression of hematopoiesis in aplastic anemia is probably immunologic in most cases. Many laboratories have demonstrated inhibition of patient or normal progenitor cells by lymphocytes in colony culture. Activated cytotoxic lymphocytes may be present at high levels in blood and marrow, and overexpression of lymphokines that exert a negative effect on hematopoiesis, especially gamma-interferon and lymphotoxin, can be measured as protein in peripheral blood T cell cultures and by direct molecular analysis of marrow mRNA. Presumably, chemical and viral antigens incite an abnormal immune system response in some individuals that targets bone marrow stem cells. The high rate of clinical responses to immunosuppressive therapy (see further on) supports an immune hypothesis. However, no current assay of immune function can reliably predict response to therapy.

DIAGNOSIS AND LABORATORY FEATURES

Prompt diagnosis is important in order to avoid unnecessary complications and to provide the appropriate definitive therapy. In a classic case, there is abrupt onset of bleeding symptoms; blood counts show severe thrombocytopenia, neutropenia, and anemia, and the marrow is empty. However, distinguishing aplastic anemia with incomplete blood count suppression or moderate degrees of marrow cellularity from other hematologic diseases can be difficult.

In the typical severely affected patient, blood counts are uniformly low; lymphocytes are usually better preserved than neutrophils but are commonly also reduced in number. The absolute or corrected reticulocyte count is very low. Red cells on the blood smear appear normal, but macrocytosis is the rule on automated cell analysis. The differential diagnosis is more difficult in moderate aplastic anemia, in which blood counts and marrow cellularity are better preserved; these cases can be hard to distinguish from hypocellular myelodysplasia. Atypically, aplastic anemia may present with only two or even a single hematopoietic lineage affected and so resemble pure red cell aplasia, amegakaryocytic thrombocytopenia, or a chronic neutropenia. Fever, night sweats, weight loss, and other constitutional symptoms are unusual in aplastic anemia, and the presence of lymphadenopathy or hepatosplenomegaly should suggest alternative diagnoses. Patients with Fanconi's anemia may have short stature, café au lait spots, and abnormal formation of the hand; dyskeratosis congenita can be diagnosed from the peculiar nail changes.

The diagnosis of aplastic anemia rests on the bone marrow examination. At least a 1-cm biopsy specimen should be obtained from the iliac crest, and the sternum should be aspirated if no spicules are obtained from the hip site. In general, the bone marrow is aspirable but watery. The biopsy specimen may appear white rather than red. On microscopic examination, hematopoietic precursor cells of all types are markedly reduced or absent, and the aspirate smear shows only residual lymphocytes, plasma cells, and fibroblastoid stromal cells. There may be a few small "hot spots" of erythropoietic activity. The biopsy specimen is largely replaced by fat. Megakaryocytes are absent. A careful search should be made for blast cells, adjacent to the spicule, or infiltrating carcinoma, at the edge of the smear. Mild abnormalities of erythroid differentiation, "megaloblastoid" changes, occur commonly, but marked dysmyelopoiesis or aberrant megakaryocytes point to myelodysplasia.

Some other laboratory tests are important. In a young patient or an older individual with an unusual family history or physical findings, Fanconi's anemia should be excluded by chromosomal analysis of a peripheral blood specimen. Bone marrow cytogenetics are useful in the diagnosis of unusual marrow morphology, because they are usually normal in aplasia but abnormal in myelodysplasia. Magnetic resonance imaging of marrow has also been proposed to help in this differential diagnosis. A Ham test or, better, flow cytometric analysis of peripheral blood cells for PI-linked proteins makes the diagnosis of PNH. Elevated serum transaminases suggest a recent bout of hepatitis, and such a finding should be followed by specific serologic assays. Finally, tissue typing to determine HLA antigens should be performed as early as possible in patients who may require a bone marrow transplantation; this information is also useful for the selection of platelet donors (see later).

CLINICAL FEATURES

Most patients seek medical help because of bleeding from the gums or nose or in the skin rather than massive gastrointestinal or other blood loss. Patients also commonly complain of symptoms related to anemia: dizziness, fatigue, shortness of breath, and a pounding sensation in the ears. Infection is uncommon initially but becomes problematic as the disease progresses. The first physical examination in acquired aplastic anemia is often remarkably normal, with the exception of pallor, petechiae, and ecchymoses.

The course may be fulminant, and unfortunately death still occasionally occurs in a matter of days as a result of intracranial bleeding or overwhelming infection. During the course of aplastic anemia, the patient's symptoms and medical complications arise from the alterations in blood components. Thrombocytopenic bleeding rarely is massive or life threatening in the absence of concomitant infection. Platelet transfusions are effective in most patients (see later). Infection is the major cause of morbidity and mortality in aplastic anemia. Neutropenia predisposes the patient to bacterial infections, most commonly with organisms that originate in the patient's gut or enter via intravenous catheters. Many, perhaps most, febrile or septic episodes do not yield culture evidence of a specific organism. Local infections of skin, sinuses, and the perianal areas occur. As neutropenia persists, fatal fungal disease may develop, especially aspergillosis of the lungs and sinuses. Death usually results from invasive fungal disease or overwhelming bacterial sepsis.

The prognosis in aplastic anemia depends on the blood counts. Severe disease has been defined as the presence of two of the following three criteria: (1) absolute neutrophil count (ANC) below 500 per mm^3, (2) platelets below 20,000 per mm^3, and (3) corrected reticulocyte count of less than 1% (corresponding to an absolute reticulocyte count in automated blood counters of less than 90,000 mm^3). Extreme neutropenia (ANC $<200/\text{mm}^3$) carries an especially high mortality.

TREATMENT

Aplastic anemia is a hematologic emergency. The patient requires the most fastidious attention to the bleeding and infectious complications of the disease, and the correct, definitive therapy should be instituted quickly. Moderate aplastic anemia can be observed, but there is *no* place for "watchful waiting" or trials of low-dose corticosteroids or novel growth factors in severe aplastic anemia.

Supportive therapy consists of appropriate transfusions and aggressive treatment of infections. The patient should be warned to avoid aspirin and other nonsteroidal anti-inflammatory drugs that inhibit platelet function. Menses should be suppressed. Dental attention to gingivitis can alleviate much gum oozing. Active bleeding responds to platelet transfusions, and one to two transfusions weekly can alleviate all symptoms. All transfused products should be depleted of donor leukocytes, and family donors should never be employed for a patient who may need to undergo marrow transplantation. Massive hemorrhage is unusual and requires much more frequent transfusion for control. The effectiveness of platelet transfusion is most easily assessed by a 1-hour post-transfusion blood count. About one-third of patients become refractory to random donor platelet transfusions; refractoriness does not correlate with the number of units received and is probably genetically determined. Some refractory patients will show adequate increments using histocompatible donors. Inhibitors of fibrinolysis may be useful in controlling mucosal bleeding in some cases despite their ineffectiveness in controlled trials. Whether platelet transfusions in chronic thrombocytopenia are better administered prophylactically or solely on demand for symptoms remains unsettled. Mucosal hemorrhage increases at platelet counts below 5000 per mm^3, and about 10,000 per mm^3 is therefore a reasonable trigger value for preventive platelet infusions.

Red cell transfusions are given to maintain the hemoglobin at a level compatible with full activity, at least 7 grams per dL in general and 9 grams per dL in older persons with cardiopulmonary impairment. Transfusional hemosiderosis in chronic aplastic anemia should be treated with iron chelation therapy.

Fever, local areas of inflammation, and symptoms suggestive of sepsis in a severely neutropenic patient require careful clinical assessment. Treatment of infection, either documented or suspected, consists of broad-spectrum parenteral antibiotics administered for at least a week. The specific combination of antibiotics is less important than their prompt application. Persistent fever is addressed by modification of the regimen, as for example the addition of vancomycin for a suspected catheter infection or the empiric institution of the antifungal amphotericin B (Fungizone). The threshold for introduction of antibiotics should be low, because neglect or delay in the treatment of infection will likely be fatal in a granulocytopenic individual.

Bone Marrow Transplantation

Transplantation is curative therapy for aplastic anemia and should be the first consideration in every suitable candidate. The preferred donor is a histocompatible sibling, who unfortunately is available only in a minority of cases. In minimally transfused young patients, transplantation has a high success rate (probably >80% long-term survival). Among all young recipients, 5-year survival is 65 to 70%. The outcome of transplantation is affected by the recipient's age, prior transfusion history, and clinical condition. Age correlates with the major complication of graft-versus-host disease. Although aplastic patients to the age of 50 years have been successfully transplanted, morbidity and mortality increase over the age of 20 years. Transfusions lead to allosensitization and an increased risk of graft rejection. However, especially when leukocyte-depleted blood products are used, a few blood transfusions do not adversely affect outcome. A patient who is infected, is refractory to platelet transfusions, or has active liver disease has a poor prognosis after transplant. Transplantation from alternative donors, sometimes mismatched family members, and more often histocompatible nonfamily members has been successful, particularly in very young patients, but carries too high a risk at present to be routinely recommended. Although more expeditious arrangements of unrelated donor transplants may be helpful, ultimately the procedure may be limited by graft rejection and graft-versus-host disease due to minor antigen incompatibility.

Immunosuppression

Immunosuppression is effective in the majority of patients with aplastic anemia and is the first therapy in older patients and those without a sibling marrow donor. Antithymocyte globulin (ATG) (Atgam) is the commercial preparation of antilymphocyte sera available in the United States. Response rates to ATG vary depending on patient selection, but hematologic remission rates are about 50%. ATG is administered intravenously; a recommended schedule is 40 mg per kg per day for 4 days. Methylprednisolone (Solu-Medrol) at about 1 mg per kg per day is also given to alleviate symptoms of serum sickness but should be rapidly tapered beginning about 2 weeks after the first dose of ATG. Extremely high doses of corticosteroids are no more effective than ATG and have more associated complications, especially aseptic necrosis in major joints.

Cyclosporine (Sandimmune) is also effective in aplastic anemia. Cyclosporine can salvage about half of patients who have failed ATG therapy. When cyclosporine is added to ATG as first therapy, hematologic remission rates increase to about 75%, and both children and absolutely neutropenic patients respond to combined immunosuppression. Cyclosporine is administered orally at a dose of 12 mg per kg per day in adults and 15 mg per kg per day in children, with dose adjustments to blood drug levels or creatinine, for 3 to 6 months. Prophylaxis for *Pneumocystis pneumoniae* infection during cyclosporine therapy is advisable.

Patients who experience relapse often respond to a second course of immunosuppression. Occasionally, blood counts depend on continued cyclosporine treatment. Some patients who have responded to immunosuppression therapy will later develop clonal hematologic abnormalities, most frequently laboratory evidence of PNH but also marrow failure due to myelodysplasia and acute leukemia. Although immunosuppression cannot be considered curative therapy for most patients, it should be noted that long-term survival in patients receiving transplants and those treated by immunosuppression is equivalent.

Hematopoietic Growth Factors

Growth factors should be used as an adjunct to definitive treatment by marrow transplantation or immunosuppression. Both granulocyte colony stimulating factor (G-CSF) (Neupogen)* and granulocyte-macrophage colony stimulating factor (GM-CSF) (Leukine)* can increase neutrophil numbers and even marrow cellularity in some patients. Addition of G-CSF or GM-CSF to antibiotics is reasonable in an infected neutropenic patient; growth factors might also be useful as a regular part of an immunosuppressive regimen. The utility of growth factor therapy is limited: Severely neutropenic patients are less likely to respond than those with moderately depressed granulocyte numbers; continued therapy is required to sustain neutrophil numbers; and neither platelets nor reticulocytes are affected. Interleukin 1† and interleukin 3† have not been active in aplastic anemia. Stem cell factor† and combinations of growth factors will undergo testing in research protocols.

Androgens

Male hormones have not been proved to be generally effective in randomized trials. Nevertheless, occasional patients appear to improve or demonstrate dependence on androgen therapy. A trial of androgens is appropriate only in patients with moderate disease or in severely affected patients who have failed immunosuppression. We prefer nandralone decanoate (Deca-Durabolin), a formulation with little hepatotoxicity, administered intramuscularly at a dose of 5 mg per kg per week‡ for 3 months (prolonged pressure at the injection site will prevent local hemorrhage).

---

*Not FDA approved for this indication.
†Investigational drug in the United States.
‡Exceeds dosage recommended by the manufacturer.

IRON DEFICIENCY ANEMIA

method of
ROY D. BAYNES, M.D., PH.D.
University of Kansas Medical Center
Kansas City, Kansas

Although iron deficiency has been significantly reduced in the developed world, it continues to be a public health problem in certain high-risk subpopulations and is a major concern in many developing regions. Although this deficiency can be readily treated, therapeutic efficacy is often suboptimal on account of poor compliance. Attempts at improving therapeutic efficacy must include aggressive nutritional education, reduction of side effects, and active compliance surveillance.

IRON STATUS

As mentioned, although iron deficiency remains a public health problem of major significance on a global basis, in recent decades there has been marked improvement in the iron nutritional status of populations in developed nations. This, together with a greater appreciation that mild excess body iron may be deleterious, particularly in relation to cardiovascular events and cancer, dictates that iron status be carefully defined in individual subjects. In addition, unscreened supplementation of subpopulations deemed at risk appears to no longer be tenable in developed nations. It is important to note that major complications of iron deficiency, including reduced work capacity, impaired neurologic development in growing children, and an adverse outcome in pregnancy, correlate with functional iron depletion. Functional iron refers to the iron in hemoglobin in red blood cells, myoglobin in muscles, and small amounts in other iron proteins important to cellular metabolism. Iron present in stores serves only to replenish the functional compartment. Not surprisingly, therefore, storage iron depletion is not associated with any demonstrable clinical manifestations, but identification of this state, particularly in subjects who would normally have adequate stores, should raise concern about and mandate a search for pathologic blood loss.

Assessment of iron status in recent years has undergone progressive refinement. It is of importance to understand the significance and limitations of the various indices of iron status. These are outlined briefly in Table 1.

The most practical way of assessing the amount of iron in the storage compartment is to measure the serum ferritin concentration, which ranges in normal subjects from 12 to 300 μg per liter. Within this range, the serum ferritin is related to stores, with 1 μg per liter equivalent to 8 to 10 mg of storage iron. The measurement, however, is increased disproportionately to stores in infection, inflammation, neoplasia, and liver disease. Consequently, serum ferritin loses diagnostic utility in these settings. In these situations, stores are better assessed by a semiquantitative evaluation of macrophage iron observed on a bone marrow aspirate smear stained for iron. Serum ferritin has no value in the assessment of functional iron, but a level below 12 μg per liter establishes iron deficiency as the cause of anemia.

The best measure of functional iron is the serum transferrin receptor concentration, which shows an early and highly predictable increase with depletion. It is abnormal earlier, is more sensitive, and is more specific than other measures of functional deficiency including red cell distribution width, percentage saturation, mean cell volume, and free erythrocyte protoporphyrin. Because the serum receptor is unaffected by infection, inflammation, neoplasia, or pregnancy, it is useful in the diagnosis of iron deficiency in these settings.

The combination of serum ferritin concentration as a reflection of stores, serum receptor as a measure of functional iron deficit, and hemoglobin concentration as an index of anemia allows for comprehensive iron assessment in individual subjects and is ideally suited for population screening. Screening of subpopulations at risk for iron deficiency should include preschoolers, pregnant women, trained athletes, and people who habitually consume a calorie-restricted diet. Such screening will facilitate the safer, targeted use of iron supplements. The cost of this battery is not insignificant, however, and in certain settings there may still be a place for a therapeutic trial of iron as a diagnostic approach in patients with a high probability of iron deficiency. If this approach is used, it is imperative that the patient be reevaluated after 4 to 6 weeks. If the hemoglobin deficit has not decreased by 50% or more, a complete laboratory evaluation is indicated.

TREATMENT

Oral Iron Therapy

In a patient with significant iron deficiency anemia, oral iron therapy should be initiated to provide

TABLE 1. **Measurements Commonly Used to Evaluate Iron Status**

Test		Normal	Depleted Stores	Functional Deficiency	Anemia	Comments
Serum ferritin (μg/L)		>12	<12	<12	<12	Unreliable in infection, inflammation, neoplasia, and hepatic dysfunction
Bone marrow iron		+	–	–	–	Invasive
% Saturation		>16	>16	<16	<16	Lacks sensitivity and specificity
Red cell distribution width (RDW)		<15	<15	>15	>15	Insensitive and late
Mean cell volume (MCV) (fL)		>80	>80	<80	<80	Insensitive and late
Free erythrocyte protoporphyrin (FEP) (μg/dl RBC)		<70	<70	>70	>70	Insensitive and late, false positive in lead toxicity
Serum transferrin receptor* (mg/L)		<8.5	<8.5	>8.5	>8.5	Sensitive, early, unaffected by infection, inflammation, neoplasia and hepatic dysfunction
Hemoglobin (gm/L)	Male	>130	>130	>130	<130	
	Female	>120	>120	>120	<120	

*Kansas City monoclonal ELISA.

150 to 200 mg of elemental iron daily in divided doses. The form of iron is relatively unimportant, provided that it is in the reduced or ferrous state. The most important consideration is the amount of elemental iron contained in each tablet. Ferrous sulfate tablets generally contain 60 to 65 mg elemental iron, whereas ferrous gluconate tablets contain only about half this amount. Ferrous sulfate is the most widely prescribed oral iron supplement because of its high solubility and low cost, especially when calculated on the basis of its elemental iron content. There is little convincing evidence for the use of a number of other proprietary iron preparations on the basis of therapeutic advantage. Although the combination with ascorbic acid is employed in many pharmaceutical preparations, the higher amount of absorption realized can be achieved at lower cost and with no more side effects merely by increasing the amount of iron in each dose. Maximal absorption is obtained by taking the iron separately from meals. The most rapid erythropoietic reconstitution is observed when the iron is taken 1 to 2 hours before meals and is further enhanced by an additional dose at bedtime. Iron absorption from this intensive regimen will approach 50 mg daily, an amount that can compensate for daily blood losses in excess of 100 ml in chronically anemic patients. Maximal absorption, however, declines rapidly as iron deficiency is corrected.

The major limitation to oral iron therapy is the gastrointestinal side effects that affect a significant number of patients on maximal dosage. Lower gastrointestinal symptoms include constipation and diarrhea, but these appear to be unrelated to dosage and indeed are reported with almost equal frequency in patients receiving placebo. Such side effects can generally be managed symptomatically and are not an indication for dose modification or discontinuation. Upper gastrointestinal symptoms tend to be more significant and troublesome. When mild, these generally take the form of nausea, epigastric pain, and heartburn, but when profound can include vomiting and severe abdominal cramps. These symptoms usually appear within 1 hour of administration and are related to the concentration of ionized iron in the stomach and small intestine. The frequency and severity of these symptoms are closely associated with dosage.

In most patients, mild nausea or epigastric discomfort will be reduced by taking the therapeutic iron with or immediately after meals; food ligands complex significant amounts of the bioavailable elemental iron. Coadministration of iron with food also delays gastric emptying, thereby reducing the concentration of unbound iron in the duodenum. These influences lead to a 50 to 75% reduction in iron absorption, the extent of which depends on dietary composition, with the least effect noted in a diet rich in meat and ascorbic acid. Because there is rarely a need for urgent reversal of anemia, it is sometimes preferable to prescribe iron with meals and thereby avoid the development of gastrointestinal symptoms.

If scheduling doses with meals does not reduce the troublesome symptoms, then the amount of iron should be reduced. This is conveniently accomplished by using a preparation such as ferrous gluconate, which contains less elemental iron. Further reductions can be achieved by the use of a liquid preparation of ferrous sulfate. Such dosage reductions are usually more effective in limiting side effects than is decreasing the number of doses per day. An additional approach for patients with gastrointestinal side effects not alleviated by the aforementioned maneuvers is to employ sustained-release forms of iron, which are aggressively promoted by many pharmaceutical firms. These limit side effects by delaying the release of iron within the lumen until it is beyond the sites of maximal assimilation in the upper small intestine. Not surprisingly, this is paralleled by a reduction in iron absorption. Indeed with certain preparations, such as enteric coated tablets, the impairment of absorption may be profound. However, with other proprietary preparations, absorption in the presence of food may be comparable to that obtained with ferrous sulfate. Sustained-release preparations deserve a trial in patients with intractable, severe upper gastrointestinal symptoms. A major drawback to their use is their cost, which may be 20 to 30 times that of an iron-equivalent amount of ferrous sulfate. Sustained-release preparations should be reserved for patients who suffer intractable side effects with conventional forms of iron and should be used with the expressed understanding that absorption may be substantially less than with standard tablets of ferrous sulfate.

Response to Oral Iron

Because iron deficiency impairs erythroid marrow proliferation, it takes 7 to 10 days following commencement of iron therapy to achieve a maximal reticulocyte response. Although the increase in reticulocytosis is never dramatic, the reticulocyte count should rise to two to three times the basal level. In patients with an initial hemoglobin concentration below 100 grams per liter, full therapeutic doses of oral iron should produce an increase in the circulating hemoglobin level of about 2 grams per liter of whole blood daily after the first week of treatment. An increase of less than 1 gram per liter per day is a suboptimal response, although from a clinical perspective the slower rate of increase is acceptable.

Iron therapy should be continued until iron stores are replenished. A reasonable target is to increase iron reserves to 500 mg, or the amount of iron contained in 2 units of whole blood. In the past, this has usually been obtained empirically by continuing oral iron for 2 to 6 months beyond the point at which the hemoglobin deficit is fully corrected. However, the replenishment of iron stores can now be accurately monitored by the rise in serum ferritin concentrations. Employing this strategy, oral iron should be continued until serum ferritin concentration reaches 50 μg per liter. Ferritin determinations are useful in detecting recurrent storage compartment depletion.

Failure of Oral Iron Therapy

By far the most frequent cause of failure to obtain a complete response to oral iron is suboptimal patient compliance. Because of widespread fortification of dietary constituents and the ubiquitous presence of iron in multivitamin preparations, many patients regard medicinal iron as just another supplement. Treatment failures can be reduced if the physician takes time to explain the importance of optimal dosing and compliance. Compliance can be crudely monitored by prescribing only enough iron to last until the next visit; most patients will not request a prescription refill while they have an unused supply. Compliance can also be roughly assessed by inquiring as to stool color and directly evaluated by examining the stool.

Although a lack of response to oral iron therapy is commonly attributed to intestinal malabsorption, this is in fact an exceedingly rare cause of therapeutic failure. Patients with a prior partial gastrectomy absorb medicinal iron poorly when it is taken with food but absorb it well when it is taken between meals. Patients who have undergone total gastrectomy or extensive small bowel resections have a more profound defect in iron absorption and generally are nonresponsive to oral iron. Disorders of the small intestine such as celiac disease may, on occasion, present with iron deficiency on the basis of malabsorption. If there is any reason to suspect malabsorption, a convenient and simple test is to administer 100 mg of elemental iron while the patient is fasting and to measure the rise in the serum iron level 1 and 2 hours afterward. In iron-deficient patients with a basal serum iron level below 50 μg per dL, an increase to 200 to 300 μg per dL is commonly seen. A rise of less than 100 μg per dL warrants further small intestinal evaluation.

A common cause of so-called refractory iron deficiency anemia is the incorrect diagnosis of the anemia of inflammation as iron deficiency. This situation can be avoided by the careful application of the laboratory tests already outlined and by concomitantly obtaining an index of inflammation such as the erythrocyte sedimentation rate or serum C-reactive protein concentration.

In some patients, continued blood loss manifests as an incomplete response to oral iron. This is suggested by the finding of a sustained reticulocytosis, persistent mild thrombocytosis, or occult blood in the feces.

Parenteral Iron Therapy

Parenteral iron administration should not be undertaken lightly. It should not be employed to attain a more dramatic hematologic response nor as a matter of convenience to the physician or patient. Parenteral iron is no more efficacious at repairing iron deficiency than an optimal oral regimen. The indications for parenteral iron are malabsorption, severe recurrent iron deficiency due to uncontrollable blood loss, and intractable, severe gastrointestinal side effects of oral iron. Although the latter tends to be the most common indication, the number of patients in this category can be markedly reduced by attention to designing an oral regimen that minimizes side effects and by encouraging patients with minor side effects to persist with therapy. If iron requirements are not excessive, patients with a degree of malabsorption can absorb sufficient iron to correct iron deficiency or delay its recurrence. Repeated courses of parenteral iron may be required when there is large, uncontrollable blood loss, as in patients with hereditary telangiectasia. Whenever repeated parenteral iron is administered, serum ferritin should be carefully monitored to avoid inadvertent iron overload.

Iron dextran, a complex of ferric hydroxide and dextrans ranging in molecular mass between 5 and 8 kilodaltons, is now used exclusively for parenteral therapy in the United States. Intramuscular administration should be avoided on account of erratic absorption from the site, tissue staining, pain at the injection site, rare development of necrosis at the injection site, and the theoretic possibility of developing sarcomas in the region.

Intravenous administration is the route of choice, and the most convenient and safest approach is a single intravenous total dose infusion. The amount of iron required is calculated from the deficit in circulating hemoglobin, assuming that 1 gram hemoglobin per 100 mL whole blood corresponds to 150 mg iron in an average-sized adult. An additional 500 mg is given to replenish stores. This can be calculated by the formula.

Total iron required (mg) = [Hgb deficit (gm/dL)/ 100 × estimated blood volume × 3.4] + 500

This amount of iron dextran is diluted in normal saline to a concentration not exceeding 5% and administered slowly over 2 to 3 hours.

The major concern with total dose infusion is anaphylaxis, and patients should be warned of this risk. Iron dextran should be given intravenously only when resuscitation equipment is immediately available. To safeguard against severe anaphylaxis, the rate of intravenous infusion should be kept at less than 10 drops per minute during the first 10 to 15 minutes of administration. If no reaction occurs, the rate can be increased to several hundred milliliters per hour. A variety of less serious side effects, such as skin rash, fever, arthralgias, and lymphadenopathy have been documented. Although they are relatively uncommon, these side effects are important because they may herald the development of more serious reactions with subsequent therapy. Iron dextran administration is contraindicated in patients with rheumatoid arthritis because it is known to exacerbate synovitis.

Injected iron dextran cannot be used directly for erythropoiesis but requires initial reticuloendothelial processing before the iron can be released to bind to transferrin. The large amount of iron dextran passing through the reticuloendothelial system results in some of the iron being diverted into insoluble sequestered forms. These may be only slowly mobilized during recurrence of iron deficiency, leading to the seemingly anomalous situation of iron deficiency anemia in the presence of stainable macrophage iron in the marrow.

AUTOIMMUNE HEMOLYTIC ANEMIA

method of
CHARLES H. PACKMAN, M.D.
University of Rochester School of Medicine and Dentistry
Strong Memorial Hospital
Rochester, New York

Autoimmune hemolytic anemia (AIHA) is a collection of diseases in which shortened red cell survival is mediated by autoantibodies. The entities that comprise AIHA are classified primarily on the basis of the temperature at which the autoantibodies bind most efficiently to the patient's red cells. In adults, most cases (80 to 90%) are mediated by antibodies that react optimally with red cells at 37° C (98.6° F) (warm-reactive autoantibodies). Patients with cryopathic hemolytic syndromes exhibit autoantibodies that bind more avidly to red cells at temperatures below 37° C (98.6° F) (cold-reactive autoantibodies). The warm- and cold-antibody types are further classified by the presence or absence of underlying diseases. When no recognizable underlying disease is evident, the AIHA is designated *primary* or *idiopathic*. The term secondary is used when the AIHA is a manifestation or complication of an underlying disorder. Primary (idiopathic) AIHA and secondary AIHA occur with approximately equal frequency. Finally, certain drugs can cause immune destruction of red cells by three different mechanisms. True autoantibodies are involved in only one of these mechanisms. The hapten/drug adsorption mechanism and the ternary (immune) complex mechanism involve antibodies directed primarily against drugs or their metabolites rather than red cell antigens. The classification of the immune hemolytic anemias is shown in Table 1.

CLINICAL FEATURES AND DIAGNOSIS

The annual incidence of AIHA is approximately 1 to 2 cases per 100,000 population. It occurs in people of all ages with peak incidence in the seventh decade. No racial predisposition is known and familial occurrence is rare.

In warm-antibody AIHA, the presenting complaints are usually referable to the anemia itself. The onset of symptoms is typically insidious over months, but occasional patients may experience sudden symptoms of severe anemia and jaundice over a few days. In secondary cases, the symptoms and signs of the underlying disease may overshadow the hemolytic anemia. The physical examination is often normal. Modest splenomegaly may be noted in patients with relatively severe hemolytic anemia. Patients with acute hemolysis may exhibit fever, pallor, hyperpnea, angina, tachycardia, hepatosplenomegaly, heart failure, and jaundice. In secondary cases, other physical findings may be contributed by the associated disorder.

Patients with cold agglutinin disease usually exhibit

TABLE 1. **Diseases Characterized by Immune-Mediated Red Cell Destruction**

- Autoimmune hemolytic anemia due to warm-reactive autoantibodies
  - Primary (idiopathic)
  - Secondary
    - Lymphoproliferative disorders
    - Connective tissue disorders (especially systemic lupus erythematosus)
    - Nonlymphoid neoplasms (e.g., ovarian tumors)
    - Chronic inflammatory diseases (e.g., ulcerative colitis)
- Autoimmune hemolytic anemia due to cold-reactive autoantibodies (cryopathic hemolytic syndromes)
  - Primary (idiopathic) cold agglutinin disease
  - Secondary cold agglutinin disease
    - Lymphoproliferative disorders
    - Infections (*M. pneumoniae,* infectious mononucleosis)
  - Paroxysmal cold hemoglobinuria (primary or associated with syphilis)
  - Donath-Landsteiner hemolytic anemia (associated with viral syndromes)
- Drug-induced immune hemolytic anemia
  - Hapten/drug adsorption
  - Ternary (immune) complex
  - True autoantibody induction

chronic hemolytic anemia with or without jaundice, but some patients experience episodic acute hemolysis with hemoglobinuria induced by chilling. Acrocyanosis is sometimes seen, due to sludging of red cells in the cutaneous circulation. Hemolysis in patients with *Mycoplasma pneumoniae* infections is acute in onset, often appearing as the patient is recovering from pneumonia, and lasting 1 to 3 weeks. Hemolytic anemia in infectious mononucleosis can occur at any time within the first 3 weeks of illness. Splenomegaly, which is most characteristic of lymphoma and infectious mononucleosis, may also occur in idiopathic cold agglutinin disease.

Paroxysmal cold hemoglobinuria (PCH) is a chronic illness characterized by periodic episodes of massive hemolysis following cold exposure. It occurs in an idiopathic form and in patients with congenital or tertiary syphilis. Donath-Landsteiner hemolytic anemia is a related disorder that occurs more commonly in children and young adults; it presents as an acute, self-limited hemolytic anemia usually following a viral syndrome. In both diseases, paroxysms are characterized by prominent constitutional symptoms including aching pains in the back or legs, abdominal cramps, headaches, and chills and fever occurring a few minutes to several hours after cold exposure. The urine typically contains hemoglobin. The constitutional symptoms and hemoglobinuria generally last a few hours.

Drug-induced immune hemolytic anemias are usually slow in onset. However, those caused by the ternary (immune) complex mechanism are characterized by a rapid onset after only a few days of drug exposure, or after a single dose in patients who have taken the drug previously. Some common drugs implicated in immune red cell injury are shown in Table 2.

Laboratory Features

General. In both warm- and cold-antibody AIHA, the anemia can be mild or severe, with hemoglobin levels occasionally as low as 3 to 4 gm per dL. Patients with drug-induced immune hemolysis mediated by the hapten/drug adsorption mechanism or by true autoantibodies usually exhibit mildly depressed hemoglobin levels, whereas those with hemolysis mediated by the ternary (immune) complex mechanism may have severe, life-threatening anemia. Polychromasia on the blood smear indicates reticulocytosis, reflecting an increased rate of red cell production. Spherocytes are usually seen as well. Most patients exhibit mild leukocytosis and neutrophilia; occasionally leukopenia and neutropenia are noted. Platelet counts are usually normal. Although not usually indicated, bone marrow examination may reveal an underlying lymphoproliferative disorder.

TABLE 2. **Drug-Induced Immune Hemolytic Anemia**

Examples of causative drugs, by mechanism*
- Hapten/drug adsorption mechanism (penicillins, cephalosporins, tolbutamide)
- Ternary (immune) complex mechanism (quinine, quinidine, cephalosporins, chlorpropamide)
- True autoantibody induction (alpha-methyldopa, levodopa, cephalosporins, procainamide)
- Mechanisms uncertain (phenacetin, acetaminophen, thiazides, ibuprofen, erythromycin, omeprazole)

*These are examples of commonly used drugs that are well documented to cause immune hemolysis. The list is incomplete; many other drugs have been implicated. Generally speaking, in patients with immune hemolytic anemia, any recently ingested drug should be considered etiologically suspect until proven otherwise.

The reticulocyte count is usually elevated, but transient reticulocytopenia may be seen early in approximately one-third of patients with AIHA for unknown reasons. Usually, reticulocytes appear in the circulation of these patients in a few days. Reticulocytopenia may also be seen in patients with compromised marrow function related to infection, toxic chemicals, or nutritional deficiency. Such patients must be monitored carefully and transfused promptly (see further on), since life-threatening anemia can develop quickly in patients with hemolysis and decreased RBC production.

Total bilirubin is often mildly increased (up to 5 mg per dL) and is chiefly unconjugated (indirect). Bile is not detected in the urine unless serum conjugated (direct) bilirubin is increased. Serum haptoglobin levels are typically low, and lactate dehydrogenase (LDH) levels are usually elevated. In warm-antibody AIHA and in cold agglutinin disease, hemoglobinuria is encountered only in those uncommon patients who develop hyperacute hemolysis. In patients with PCH or Donath-Landsteiner hemolytic anemia, hemoglobinuria is characteristic, starting shortly after chilling. Hemoglobinuria may be a prominent feature of drug-induced hemolysis due to the ternary (immune) complex mechanism and may cause renal failure.

Serologic Features. The diagnosis of AIHA depends on the demonstration of an immune response directed against autologous red cells. The evidence for this usually comes in the form of a direct antiglobulin reaction (Coombs' test) or by demonstrating direct agglutinins or hemolysins in the patient's serum.

WARM-ANTIBODY AIHA AND THE DIRECT ANTIGLOBULIN TEST. Most patients with warm-antibody AIHA exhibit neither direct agglutinins nor hemolysins. Rather, their red cells are coated with nonagglutinating antibodies, almost always of the IgG class, and/or complement components. Antibodies and complement components on patient red cells are detected by antiglobulin serum (Coombs' reagent), which cross-links the red cells to produce visible agglutination. This procedure is called the direct antiglobulin (Coombs') test. The broad-spectrum antiglobulin (Coombs') reagent detects both immunoglobulin and complement components (principally C3). More specific reagents that detect *only* IgG or complement may be used to refine the pattern of red cell coating. Three *major* patterns of direct antiglobulin reaction have been noted in warm-antibody AIHA: red cells coated with IgG alone; red cells coated with IgG plus complement components; red cells coated with complement components alone.

In patients with warm-antibody AIHA, the autoantibody exists in a reversible, dynamic equilibrium between red cells and plasma. If sufficient free autoantibody is present in the plasma or serum of these patients, it may be detected by the *indirect* antiglobulin test. In general, the presence of plasma autoantibody may be viewed as "overflow" or excess above that bound to red cells. Thus, patients with a positive indirect antiglobulin test due to a warm-reactive autoantibody must also have a positive direct antiglobulin test. A patient who exhibits a serum anti–red cell antibody (positive indirect antiglobulin reaction) in the presence of a negative direct antiglobulin reaction probably does not have an autoimmune process but rather an alloantibody stimulated by prior transfusion or pregnancy.

CRYOPATHIC HEMOLYTIC SYNDROMES: DIRECT AGGLUTININS AND HEMOLYSINS. Direct agglutinins, as the name implies, directly agglutinate normal or autologous human red cells. These antibodies, largely of the IgM class, are present in patients with cold agglutinin disease. Cold agglutinins cause red cells to agglutinate maximally at 0 to 5° C (32° to

41° F). In patients with chronic cold agglutinin disease, the serum cold agglutinin titers are commonly 1:10,000 or higher, and may reach 1:1,000,000 or more. The direct antiglobulin test is positive only with anticomplement reagents. The antibody itself (i.e., the cold agglutinin) is not detected by the antiglobulin test because the antibody molecules readily dissociate from the red cells during the washing steps of the standard antiglobulin procedure. In contrast, complement components are covalently bound to target red cells and cannot be washed off.

In PCH and Donath-Landsteiner hemolytic anemia, patient serum contains hemolysins, antibodies that lyse red cells in the presence of complement. The direct antiglobulin reaction may be positive during or briefly following an acute attack, due to coating of surviving red cells with complement. The antibody is a nonagglutinating IgG that binds only in the cold. It is detected by the biphasic Donath-Landsteiner test in which the patient's fresh serum is incubated with red cells initially at 4° C (39.2° F) and then warmed to 37° C (98.6° F). Intense hemolysis follows.

Drug-Induced Immune Hemolytic Anemia. The serologic findings in drug-induced immune hemolytic anemia vary according to the mechanism. When hemolysis is mediated through the hapten/drug adsorption mechanism, the direct antiglobulin test is positive for IgG alone. The indirect antiglobulin test is positive only when the test red cells have been previously coated with the drug. In hemolysis mediated by the ternary (immune) complex mechanism, the direct antiglobulin test is positive only for complement components. The drug does not bind in measurable quantity to the red cell membrane, but if drug is included in the mixture with test red cells, patient serum as a source of antibody, and fresh serum as a source of complement, the cells become coated with complement components which can then be detected by the indirect antiglobulin test. In patients with drug immune hemolysis mediated by autoantibody induction, the direct antiglobulin reaction is generally positive for IgG alone. The direct antiglobulin test may be positive in as many as 25 to 30% of patients receiving alpha methyldopa (Aldomet), the most common drug to induce autoantibodies, but hemolysis occurs in fewer than 1% of these patients. The indirect antiglobulin reaction is almost always positive in those who experience hemolysis.

TREATMENT

Warm-Antibody Autoimmune Hemolytic Anemia

Transfusion. The clinical consequences of anemia are related to both the severity of the anemia and the rapidity with which it develops. Most patients with AIHA are in little danger of circulatory failure because the anemia usually develops over a sufficient period of time to allow cardiovascular compensation to occur. It is not usually necessary to transfuse these patients. The best guide to the need for blood transfusion is the patient's clinical condition rather than a predetermined hematocrit or hemoglobin level. In patients with significant comorbid diseases such as coronary artery disease with angina, or in patients who suddenly develop severe anemia and exhibit signs and symptoms of circulatory failure, transfusion is often required and may prove lifesaving. As noted previously, transfusion should be considered early in a patient with AIHA and reticulocytopenia, since the anemia may become severe very rapidly.

Transfusion of red cells in AIHA presents two issues: The need for crossmatching and the likelihood of rapid hemolysis of transfused cells. It is usually impossible to find truly serocompatible donor blood. The autoantibody in the patient's serum usually reacts with all potential donor red cells except in those unusual cases in which the autoantibody exhibits its specificity for a defined blood group antigen and binds only to cells exhibiting that antigen. Absent such specificity, candidate units of blood should be chosen on the basis of least incompatibility with the patient's serum in crossmatch testing. Furthermore, before transfusing such an incompatible unit, it is essential to assay patient serum for an alloantibody that could cause a severe hemolytic transfusion reaction directed toward the donor red cells. Alloantibodies are more likely to be found in patients with a history of pregnancy or prior transfusion. Once selected, packed red cells should be infused very slowly while the patient is monitored for evidence of a hemolytic transfusion reaction. The transfused cells are often destroyed as rapidly as the patient's own cells. Nonetheless, the temporarily increased hemoglobin level may maintain the patient's oxygen carrying capacity during the time required for more definitive therapy to become effective.

Corticosteroids. Corticosteroids cause cessation or slowing of hemolysis in about two-thirds of patients. About 20% of patients with warm-antibody AIHA achieve a complete remission with corticosteroids; about 10% show minimal or no response. Treatment is initiated with oral prednisone, 1 to 2 mg per kg daily. Critically ill patients with severe hemolysis should receive intravenous methylprednisolone, 2 to 4 mg per kg in divided doses over the first 24 to 48 hours. High doses of prednisone may be required for 10 to 14 days. When the hemoglobin level begins to increase, prednisone may be decreased in fairly large steps to approximately 30 mg per day. With continued response, prednisone is further decreased by 5 mg per day every week, to a dose of 15 to 20 mg daily. This dose should be continued for 8 to 12 weeks after the acute hemolytic episode has subsided. The patient may then be weaned from the drug over 4 to 8 weeks. If continued corticosteroid therapy is needed, treatment on an alternate-day schedule may be helpful; for example, 20 to 40 mg of prednisone every other day. Alternate-day therapy causes fewer corticosteroid side effects but should be attempted only after the patient maintains a stable hemoglobin level on daily prednisone in a dose range of 15 to 20 mg per day. Many patients achieve complete remission of hemolysis but relapses often occur after discontinuation of corticosteroids. Patients should be followed for several years after treatment. If relapse occurs, the patient may require further corticosteroid therapy and eventually splenectomy, or immunosuppression.

Splenectomy. About one-third of patients with warm-antibody AIHA require prednisone in doses greater than 15 mg daily to maintain an acceptable hemoglobin concentration. Such patients are candidates for splenectomy. It is usually reasonable to continue corticosteroids for 4 to 8 weeks while waiting for a response. However, if the patient's clinical condition deteriorates, the anemia is very severe, or there is no response to prednisone, splenectomy should be done sooner. Approximately two-thirds of splenectomized patients have a partial or complete remission, but relapses are disappointingly common. Postsplenectomy, some patients maintain acceptable hemoglobin levels only with further prednisone treatment, albeit at lower dosage than required prior to splenectomy.

After splenectomy, there is a slightly increased risk of pneumococcal sepsis, more likely in children than in adults. Pneumococcal vaccine is generally given prior to surgery. Prophylactic penicillin (250 to 500 mg daily) is also of value in children.

Immunosuppressive Drugs. Immunosuppressive therapy is not universally accepted, but responses to immunosuppressive drugs have been observed in some patients who do not to respond to corticosteroids. It is important to note that most patients with warm-antibody AIHA respond to corticosteroids and/or splenectomy. Immunosuppressive therapy is usually considered only for those patients who do not respond to glucocorticoids and splenectomy or for those who are poor surgical risks. The most commonly used drugs are cyclophosphamide (Cytoxan),* 1.5 to 2.0 mg per kg, or azathioprine (Imuran),* 1.5 to 2.0 mg per kg, given daily. If the patient tolerates the drug, treatment may be continued for up to 6 months while awaiting a response. When response occurs, the drug dose may be slowly decreased over 2 to 3 months. If there is no response, the alternative drug may be similarly tried. Because cyclophosphamide and azathioprine cause marrow suppression, blood counts must be monitored closely during therapy. Both agents increase the risk of subsequent neoplasia, and cyclophosphamide may cause severe hemorrhagic cystitis.

Other Therapies. Plasma exchange (plasmapheresis) has been used in warm-antibody AIHA. Improvement has been noted in a few cases, but its use remains controversial. The literature contains anecdotal reports of short-term successful treatment with high-dose intravenous gamma globulin, as well as reports of treatment failures. Danazol (Danocrine), a nonvirilizing androgen, was reported as useful in one uncontrolled study.

Cryopathic Hemolytic Syndromes

Keeping the patient warm, particularly the extremities, provides symptomatic relief. This may be the only measure required in patients with mild chronic hemolysis, who generally have a benign course and survive for many years. When a cold agglutinin is associated with a lymphoproliferative disorder, treatment of the underlying neoplasm often corrects the hemolysis. Interferon-alpha was remarkably successful in one patient with cold agglutinin disease, and this approach deserves further trials. Splenectomy and corticosteroids generally have been disappointing, although exceptions have been reported. As in warm-antibody AIHA, red cell transfusions are generally reserved for patients with severe anemia in danger of cardiorespiratory complications. The use of washed red cells may avoid replenishing depleted complement components that could reactivate the hemolytic process. Plasma exchange (with replacement by albumin-containing saline) has been tried in refractory cases. The procedure may temporarily slow the rate of hemolysis but does not provide long-term benefit. The postinfectious forms of cold agglutinin disease are usually self-limited, with recovery expected in a few weeks. When massive hemoglobinuria is complicated by acute renal failure, a period of hemodialysis may be required.

Acute attacks in both chronic and transient forms of PCH may be prevented by avoidance of cold. Corticosteroids and splenectomy have not been useful. PCH associated with syphilis often responds to effective treatment of the syphilis. Patients with chronic idiopathic PCH may survive for many years in spite of occasional paroxysms of hemolysis. Donath-Landsteiner hemolytic anemia following viral infections in children is usually self-limited.

Drug-Induced Immune Hemolytic Anemia

Discontinuation of the offending drug is usually all that is required. This measure is particularly important and potentially lifesaving in patients with severe hemolysis mediated by the ternary (immune) complex mechanism. In these patients, hemoglobinuria may lead to renal failure, requiring a period of dialysis. Corticosteroids are generally unnecessary and are of questionable efficacy. Transfusions should be reserved for the unusual circumstance of severe, life-threatening anemia. As in warm-antibody AIHA, crossmatching may present a problem in patients with a strongly positive indirect antiglobulin test. Patients with hemolytic anemia due to the hapten/drug adsorption mechanism should have a compatible crossmatch, since the serum antibody reacts only with drug-coated cells. In hemolysis due to ternary complex or hapten/drug adsorption mechanisms, the direct antiglobulin test becomes negative once the drug is cleared from the circulation, usually a few days after it is discontinued. Hemolysis due to autoantibodies induced by alpha-methyldopa ceases promptly after the drug is discontinued. However, the autoantibodies may remain in the patient, as evidenced by a positive direct antiglobulin test, for weeks or months.

NONIMMUNE HEMOLYTIC ANEMIA

method of
AKIRA HIRONO, M.D.
Okinaka Memorial Institute for Medical Research
Tokyo, Japan

Hemolytic anemia is defined as an anemia caused by shortening of the red cell life span. Although it is often

*Not FDA approved for this indication.

regarded as a syndrome with a triad of (1) reduction in red cell mass, (2) jaundice, and (3) splenomegaly, a considerable number of patients lack one or more of these signs. Hemolytic anemia may be classified into two categories from an immunologic point of view. One form is characterized by the presence of antibodies to antigens on the red cell membrane responsible for the red cell destruction (immunohemolytic anemia); in the other type, such antibodies are not involved (nonimmune hemolytic anemia). This classification is convenient from a therapeutic point of view, because the former usually responds to corticosteroids and the latter does not. Nonimmune hemolytic anemias are hereditary or acquired (Table 1). It has been suggested that environmental factors also play an important role in some hereditary hemolytic anemias.

DIAGNOSIS

Hemolytic Anemia or Not

When encountering a patient who is suspected of having hemolytic anemia, the physician should attempt to verify this diagnosis. The shortening of red cell life span usually causes a compensatory increase in erythropoiesis in bone marrow. In some cases of chronic hemolysis, the accelerated erythropoiesis compensates completely for the early destruction of red cells. Such patients have marked jaundice but no anemia and are sometimes misdiagnosed as having liver disease.

The most important routine laboratory findings indicating hemolysis are reticulocytosis and increased serum unconjugated bilirubin. Decreased serum haptoglobin level and increased activity of serum lactate dehydrogenase are often associated with hemolysis, but these are less specific findings. The direct determination of red cell life span using radioisotope-labeled erythrocytes is the most accurate way to prove the existence of hemolysis, but the procedure is rather complex and time consuming.

TABLE 1. **Classification of Nonimmune Hemolytic Anemia**

Hereditary
- Defects in the erythrocyte membrane
  - Hereditary spherocytosis
  - Hereditary elliptocytosis
  - Others
- Deficiencies of erythrocyte enzymes (erythroenzymopathies)
  - Pyruvate kinase deficiency
  - Glucose phosphate isomerase deficiency
  - Glucose-6-phosphate dehydrogenase deficiency
  - Pyrimidine 5′-nucleotidase deficiency
  - Others
- Defects in globin structure and synthesis
  - Unstable hemoglobin disease
  - Sickle cell disease
  - Thalassemia
- Etiology unknown

Acquired
- Intrinsic
  - Paroxysmal nocturnal hemoglobinuria
- Extrinsic
  - Mechanical trauma
    - Microangiopathic hemolytic anemia
    - Heart valve anemia
    - March hemoglobinuria
  - Infections
  - Chemicals

Differential Diagnosis

As is true in every disease, the first step in the differential diagnosis of hemolytic anemia is careful history taking, particularly the family history, the age of onset, and the existence of apparent precipitating factors.

History. A clear family history strongly suggests that the hemolytic anemia is hereditary, and in these cases, careful investigation of the pattern of inheritance may provide an important diagnostic clue. However, it should be noted that a negative family history does not always mean that the anemia is not hereditary. For example, hereditary spherocytosis is characterized by autosomal dominant inheritance, but one-fifth of the patients do not have a clear family history. Diseases with autosomal recessive inheritance, such as most of the erythroenzymopathies, are often found in siblings but not in the parents. This kind of hemolytic anemia is found more frequently in patients with consanguineous parents than in other populations. Glucose-6-phosphate dehydrogenase (G6PD) deficiency is a typical X-linked disorder, and hemizygous males are usually affected. Random inactivation of one of the two X chromosomes in early embryonic development may cause the deficiency of red cell G6PD in heterozygous females. G6PD deficiency is frequent in African blacks and Mediterranean peoples, but it is rare in northern Europeans. It is also common in southern China and Southeast Asia but rare in northern China, Korea, and Japan. Homozygous female patients with G6PD deficiency are not unusual in populations with high gene frequency of this disorder. Thalassemias and sickle cell disease show a similar distribution.

Onset. The onset of hereditary hemolytic anemia is generally early. Existence of anemia at birth, prolonged neonatal jaundice, or both are frequently observed in patients with hereditary hemolytic anemia. However, some patients with mild hereditary hemolytic anemia may be unaware of any symptom until reaching middle age. Pregnancy can be a precipitating factor for hereditary hemolytic anemias as well as for autoimmune hemolytic anemia. Paroxysmal nocturnal hemoglobinuria (PNH) is an acquired hemolytic anemia that is usually diagnosed after the third decade of life. Because the hemolysis usually occurs during sleep, patients with typical PNH frequently complain of dark-colored urine in the morning. A history of acute hemolysis after taking drugs is a very important clue to the diagnosis of G6PD deficiency. Viral or bacterial infections and exposure to chemicals, including insecticides or weed killers, or fava beans can also be precipitating factors in G6PD deficiency.

Laboratory Findings. The peripheral blood film provides important clues in the differential diagnosis of nonimmune hemolytic anemia. Microspherocytes in hereditary spherocytosis, elliptocytes in hereditary elliptocytosis, drepanocytes in sickle cell disease, and schistocytes in microangiopathic hemolytic anemia are strongly suggestive of each disease. Although less specific, target cells in thalassemia and basophilic stippling of red cells in pyrimidine 5′-nucleotidase deficiency or lead poisoning may be useful in the diagnosis.

A direct Coombs' antiglobulin test, osmotic fragility test, and Ham test should be performed in all suspected cases of hemolytic anemia. A negative direct Coombs' test suggests, but does not prove, that the hemolytic anemia is nonimmune in origin. Red cell osmotic fragility is markedly increased in many disorders with red cell membrane abnormalities, including hereditary spherocytosis and hereditary elliptocytosis. The Ham test is one of the most simple and specific screening tests for PNH, a disease that is often misdiagnosed or even overlooked. The final diagnosis of erythroenzymopathies or unstable hemoglobin diseases needs specific laboratory examinations such as a panel of red cell enzyme assays or hemoglobin electrophoresis. It is noteworthy that even after an extensive diagnostic work-up, the etiology of hereditary nonspherocytic hemolytic anemia remains unknown in about 70% of cases.

TREATMENT

In some nonimmune hemolytic anemias, hemolysis is caused and accelerated by specific extrinsic precipitating factors, and their identification and removal are the initial step in treatment. Hemolytic attack in G6PD deficiency is usually triggered by infection or by administration of certain drugs. Table 2 lists the drugs that can induce hemolysis at usual therapeutic doses. Although many other drugs, including acetaminophen and acetylsalicylic acid, have been reported to cause hemolysis in G6PD-deficient patients, they are generally considered to do so only when administered in extremely large doses or when coincident with other precipitating factors such as infections. Thus, only the drugs listed in Table 2 should be avoided by G6PD-deficient patients without chronic hemolysis. Hemolysis can also be caused by ingestion of fava beans or inhalation of the plant's pollen. The onset is sudden and the hemolysis is usually more severe than that caused by drug administration. Favism often affects patients of Mediterranean or Southeast Asian origin but is rare in African blacks.

Management of underlying disease is urgent in patients with hemolytic anemia caused by sepsis or microangiopathic hemolytic anemia associated with disseminated intravascular coagulation, thrombotic thrombocytopenic purpura, or hemolytic uremic syndrome. Patients with artificial heart valves may manifest various degrees of hemolytic anemia due to the mechanical destruction of red cells. Replacement of the artificial valves should be considered if marked anemia develops. Hemolysis caused by mechanical trauma to red cells associated with prolonged exercise (march hemoglobinuria) can be prevented by wearing thicker soled shoes or by changing training methods or intensity.

TABLE 2. **Drugs and Chemicals That Can Induce Hemolysis in G6PD Deficiency**

Analgesics
acetanilid*
Antimalarials
primaquine
Antimicrobials
nitrofurantoin (Furadantin)
furazolidone (Furoxone)
nalidixic acid (NegGram)
sulfamethoxazole (Gantanol)
phenazopyridine (Pyridium)
Anthelmintics
niridazole (Ambilhar)*
Antineoplastics
doxorubicin (Adriamycin)
Chemicals
methylene blue
naphthalene (mothballs)

*Not available in the United States.

Transfusion

Blood transfusions are sometimes required in patients with severe nonimmune hemolytic anemia. Physicians should bear in mind that blood transfusions can cause dangerous, and sometimes lethal, complications. Although hemoglobin levels of 7 to 8 grams per dL are generally adequate in patients with chronic hemolytic anemia, repeated transfusions are often mistakenly performed to maintain hemoglobin levels of 10 grams or even higher. When transfusion is necessary, leukocyte-poor packed red cells are the component of choice in most cases of nonimmune hemolytic anemia. In patients with PNH, washed red cells must be prepared to avoid hemolysis triggered by transfused complements in plasma. Although transfusion hemosiderosis due to repeated transfusions is a serious problem in other types of chronic anemia such as aplastic anemia, it is less common in nonthalassemic nonimmune hemolytic anemia.

Splenectomy

Because the spleen is responsible for the increased red cell destruction in nonimmune hemolytic anemia, splenectomy may result in significant correction of anemia. The most consistent response to splenectomy occurs in patients with hereditary spherocytosis or hereditary elliptocytosis. Patients with pyruvate kinase deficiency, glucose phosphate isomerase deficiency, pyrimidine 5′-nucleotidase deficiency, or unstable hemoglobin may be improved by splenectomy, but the response is usually partial. Splenectomy is indicated in patients with apparent splenomegaly, cholelithiasis, or consistent severe hemolytic anemia that requires repeated transfusions. Cholecystectomy should be performed during the same operation. Secondary spleens should be carefully searched for and if found, should be removed completely; otherwise relapse can occur. Although the operative risk of splenectomy is low and postoperative complications are rare in adults, it is well recognized that there is an increased susceptibility to infection after splenectomy in infancy, and splenectomy in children under the age of 4 should be avoided if possible.

Because the spleen plays an insignificant role in the hemolysis of G6PD deficiency, splenectomy is not considered to be of benefit to those patients. However, when G6PD deficiency is associated with severe chronic hemolytic anemia and splenomegaly, splenectomy may be worth trying. It may also be a practical approach to the treatment of severe hereditary nonspherocytic hemolytic anemia of unknown etiology associated with apparent splenomegaly. Splenectomy is not recommended in patients with PNH because of the poor response and the increasing risk of thrombosis after operation.

Drug Therapy

Unlike many other types of anemia, there are few drugs that can cause significant improvement in nonimmune hemolytic anemia. Glucocorticoids are used in patients with PNH. Thirty to 60 mg of prednisone daily should be given for 2 or 3 weeks followed by a slow taper over 2 months. Androgens such as fluoxymesterone* (Halotestin), 20 to 30 mg daily, are also used in the therapy of PNH. Some patients with PNH respond to these therapies and transfusion requirements are thereby reduced, but usually the effect is temporary. Anticoagulants such as heparin are indicated for preventing the thrombosis that is a fatal complication in PNH patients.

Iron deficiency due to the loss of iron in the urine is sometimes associated with PNH and heart valve anemia. In other types of nonimmune hemolytic anemia, iron is usually contraindicated. Although little beneficial effect is observed, folic acid is often administered to patients with hemolytic anemia to correct the folate deficiency caused by the marrow hyperactivity.

Bone Marrow Transplantation

Bone marrow transplantation is now recognized as a highly beneficial treatment for severe aplastic anemia and leukemias. Although marrow transplantation has the potential to cure any hemolytic anemia caused by an intrinsic red cell defect, the risk of marrow transplantation prevents its use in most types of nonimmune hemolytic anemia. Severe PNH that does not respond to any conventional therapy might be an indication for marrow transplantation if the patient is young enough and an appropriate donor is available.

*Not FDA approved for this indication.

PERNICIOUS ANEMIA AND OTHER MEGALOBLASTIC ANEMIAS

method of
RALPH CARMEL, M.D.
University of Southern California School of Medicine
Los Angeles, California

The optimal management of megaloblastic anemia requires one to be certain of the specific vitamin deficiency involved (folate versus cobalamin) and to establish as precisely as possible the specific disorder responsible for that deficiency. This ensures that the right vitamin is given, that the route and duration of therapy are appropriate, that the underlying process is managed properly and, if possible, reversed, that appropriate information is given to the patient, and that common complications are anticipated. Megaloblastic anemia can occur in disorders unrelated to cobalamin (vitamin B_{12}) or folate deficiency, but those are rare and are not considered here.

Changes in serum levels of cobalamin and folate usually identify the specific vitamin deficiency, although exceptions may occur. Measurement of serum levels of methylmalonic acid and homocysteine may be helpful in some cases; levels of both metabolites are elevated in cobalamin deficiency, while folate deficiency affects levels of homocysteine only.

Several general diagnostic principles apply (Table 1). First, atypical or mild expressions of deficiency, especially in the case of cobalamin, may be more common than we think. Megaloblastic anemia is often minimal or even absent. Thus, a patient can have pernicious anemia, which is defined gastroenterologically (cobalamin malabsorption due to inadequate gastric intrinsic factor secretion), and yet may not be anemic. Cobalamin deficiency can also produce serious neurologic symptoms with few or no hematologic abnormalities.

Second, cobalamin deficiency virtually always arises because of gastric or intestinal disease. It is rarely caused by poor diet and never by malnutrition of only a few weeks' or even a few months' duration. Therefore, tests of cobalamin absorption, such as the Schilling test, are central to the evaluation of all cases of cobalamin deficiency. Cobalamin deficiency should not be attributed to a dietary cause until malabsorption has been excluded.

On the other hand, folate deficiency frequently has a dietary basis. Alcohol contributes to many, if not most, cases of dietary folate deficiency. Therefore, alcoholism, often otherwise unsuspected, must be considered whenever dietary folate deficiency is diagnosed. Malabsorptive diseases and drug-induced disorders are the major nondietary causes of deficiency.

TABLE 1. **General Principles in the Diagnosis and Management of Megaloblastic Anemia**

Diagnosis

Remember that vitamin deficiency can be present without megaloblastic anemia.
Obtain both serum folic acid and cobalamin levels before treatment.
Pay attention to even mildly subnormal serum vitamin levels.
If the clinical picture is suggestive, do not let normal serum vitamin levels dissuade you.
Always establish why the patient became cobalamin or folate deficient.
Do not automatically equate cobalamin deficiency with pernicious anemia.
Cobalamin deficiency is malabsorptive in origin until proved otherwise; it is very rarely dietary in origin.
Consider the possibility of underlying alcoholism in the folate-deficient patient.

Therapy

Avoid shotgun therapy or preparations of multiple hematinics unless the patient is known to need all of them (a rare event).
Avoid treating with the wrong vitamin; if in doubt, restudy the patient completely.
The need for blood transfusion should be determined solely by symptoms and the clinical setting, not by the blood count.
A single injection without follow-up is never appropriate for treating cobalamin deficiency.
Discuss the disorder fully with the patient to make sure that its nature and the required duration of therapy are well understood.
Warn the patient with irreversible malabsorption (e.g., pernicious anemia) against discontinuing vitamin therapy when symptoms have abated or the blood count is normal.
Monitor the patient's response to therapy.

TREATMENT OF THE VITAMIN DEFICIENCY

General Principles

The initial goal is to determine whether the deficiency is of cobalamin or folate, or both, in order to avoid using the wrong vitamin in therapy. The chief danger arises from the fact that the hematologic abnormalities in cobalamin deficiency can respond to doses of folic acid as small as 0.2 mg. Neurologic abnormalities of cobalamin deficiency, however, do not respond to folate. As a result, neurologic dysfunction can progress, or may even appear for the first time, while the anemia becomes masked by the folate therapy. This danger underscores the twin necessities of making certain that the diagnosis is correct and of monitoring the patient's response to treatment.

Fortunately, emergency treatment of the deficiency state is rarely required. There is almost always ample time to obtain the necessary tests first, especially measurement of the vitamin levels. It is usually advisable (and safe) to defer therapy for a few days until the vitamin deficiency has been satisfactorily identified. Many of the diagnostic abnormalities become blurred once the patient is treated, and it is sometimes difficult to retrace one's diagnostic steps if treatment is given prematurely.

Only two situations generally call for urgent therapy. One is severe or deteriorating neurologic disease, for which cobalamin therapy should be started as soon as the appropriate tests have been obtained. The longer the neurologic abnormalities go untreated, the greater the risk of irreversibility or incomplete reversibility.

Emergency therapy is sometimes thought necessary when severe anemia exists. The urgency of this situation is tempered by two considerations, however. Because reticulocytosis takes several days to develop, vitamin therapy will not affect the blood count for some time. So-called shotgun therapy is therefore useless in extreme situations. If the clinical situation is so severe that the anemia truly requires immediate reversal, blood transfusion is needed. However, an even more important consideration is that the clinical picture rather than the blood count must determine the urgency of the situation and dictate the need for transfusion. Megaloblastic anemia is a chronic process that develops slowly, thus allowing compensatory adjustments to the low blood count. As a result, hemoglobin levels as low as 4 or 5 grams per dL (and sometimes lower) are usually well tolerated by the patient. Symptoms are often limited to fatigue and inability to tolerate exertion. Bed rest may be all that is needed while waiting for vitamin replacement to produce the desired effect.

Blood transfusion, with all its risks, should be avoided whenever possible. Only serious cardiopulmonary or cerebral symptoms or the risk of decompensation due to coexisting serious disease compromising those systems warrants transfusion. Because plasma volume is often increased, volume overload must be avoided and any transfusion should be given slowly, with re-evaluation after each unit of blood is administered.

Cobalamin Deficiency

There are three goals in treating cobalamin deficiency. The first is to reverse the sequelae of the deficiency. The megaloblastic anemia can be reversed with as little as 1 to 10 μg of cobalamin, but larger doses are usually used. Injections are given intramuscularly, although subcutaneous injection is preferable if the patient is thrombocytopenic. A single 100- or 1000-μg injection produces full, albeit temporary, hematologic remission, as long as no coexisting disorders blunt the therapeutic response. Whether larger doses are necessary to reverse neurologic deficits is unknown. Nevertheless, it is common practice to treat neurologic symptoms of cobalamin deficiency with more frequent injections, at least in the beginning, than are used to treat the hematologic abnormality.

With therapy, the patient quickly feels better even before the blood count rises. Other manifestations of deficiency, such as glossitis, also resolve quickly.

The second goal of treatment is to prevent relapse. Reversal of the disorder that produced the deficiency can accomplish that goal. However, most underlying causes of cobalamin deficiency are not reversible, and therefore regular, lifelong vitamin supplementation is usually necessary. The daily requirement seems to vary among individuals but usually approximates 1 to 2 μg per day. Adequate maintenance is best achieved with monthly intramuscular injections of 100 or 1000 μg. Variable fractions of these relatively large doses are retained. I prefer to use the 1000-μg dose; even though much more of it is immediately excreted than with the 100-μg injection, a larger absolute amount of cobalamin is retained. The larger dose thus provides a better margin, and it is not much more expensive than the 100-μg dose.

In unusual circumstances in which injections are refused or for some reason are impossible to administer, oral maintenance therapy can be used. Even if the specific intrinsic factor–mediated absorptive process for cobalamin is impaired, diffusion allows a tiny fraction of the oral dose (less than 1%) to be absorbed. Thus, daily oral ingestion of at least 100 μg may be adequate maintenance in malabsorption, although the patient's status will require regular monitoring. As a rule, however, oral therapy is advisable only in those rare patients whose deficiency is dietary in origin. Once adequate repletion has occurred, preferably with injections, such patients can take oral supplements of 10 μg daily if they choose not to discontinue their limited diet. A gel preparation of cyanocobalamin for nasal instillation and a preparation for sublingual use* provide no known advantage over the oral form and are expensive.

The third goal of treating cobalamin deficiency is to replenish the depleted body stores. Although par-

*Not available in the United States.

tially repleted patients do not seem to do worse than fully repleted ones as long as daily requirements are met, it seems prudent to provide a safety net both for unsuspected patients who have higher daily requirements and for those who fail to continue regular supplementation.

Although many regimens can achieve all three goals satisfactorily, and little evidence exists for recommending one over another, my approach is to begin with a series of about a dozen intramuscular injections of 1000 μg of cobalamin spread over a 2-month period. Thereafter, adequate maintenance can be achieved by monthly injections of 1000 μg of cobalamin. Infrequently, patients may complain of symptoms like fatigue before the end of the monthly interval. The reason for this is unclear, and it may even be psychological in origin, but it may represent a higher cobalamin requirement in some cases and warrants a trial of more frequent injections. Finally, many patients can be taught self-injection, thus saving the time and expense of office visits. However, self-injection does not obviate the need for periodic follow-up by the physician.

It bears repeating that the successful long-term management of cobalamin deficiency has less to do with doses, routes, and schedules than with patient education and compliance.

Several forms of cobalamin are available for replacement therapy. The most widely used form is cyanocobalamin, a stable but nonphysiologic form that is converted to metabolically active cobalamins in the body. A more physiologic form, and one that is better retained in the body after injection, is hydroxocobalamin. This preparation is preferred by many European physicians because less frequent injections are required, but it is not widely used in the United States and is somewhat more expensive than cyanocobalamin.

Cobalamin has no known toxicity even in very large doses. The excess is rapidly excreted in the urine, and body stores cannot become overloaded. Allergic reactions are infrequent and most often are due to the preservative in the parenteral solution; recurrences usually can be prevented by changing to a different preparation (e.g., from another manufacturer). Autoantibody to cobalamin-binding proteins may occasionally appear in patients who take depot preparations of cobalamin or hydroxocobalamin. Such autoantibodies can produce unusually high serum cobalamin levels, but there seem to be no adverse clinical effects.

Finally, the old report of frequent sudden death after cobalamin therapy of severe megaloblastic anemia has never been substantiated. As long as one avoids fluid overload, such as occurs with excessive blood transfusion, and manages any coexisting problems such as congestive heart failure appropriately, the prognosis is excellent. As mentioned earlier, most patients tolerate even severe anemia surprisingly well. My approach has been to simply provide standard, prudent medical care while waiting for cobalamin replacement to take effect.

Folate Deficiency

The therapeutic goals for folate deficiency and the responses obtained are very similar to those described for cobalamin deficiency.

As little as 0.1 mg of folic acid can ultimately reverse the megaloblastic anemia caused by folate deficiency. The widely available formulations usually contain 1 mg of folic acid, and such doses are optimal. Unless there is a drug-induced or hereditary metabolic block, folic acid is the preferred form, and the more expensive formyl tetrahydrofolic acid (folinic acid) should not be used.

Repletion can be, and usually is, achieved orally. Unlike cobalamin deficiency, which is almost always malabsorptive in origin, folate deficiency is most often produced by dietary insufficiency, with or without coexisting alcohol abuse. Parenteral therapy is needed only if oral doses cannot be absorbed. Indeed, even folate deficiency due to malabsorption can often be treated with oral folic acid. In such cases, higher doses (e.g., 2 to 5 mg twice daily) are advisable, and serum levels and the patient's response should be monitored.

Unlike cobalamin deficiency, whose underlying cause is usually irreversible, folate deficiency often need not be treated indefinitely. A 3- or 4-week course of 1 mg of folic acid daily generally suffices to reverse the megaloblastic anemia and replete tissue stores. If the underlying cause (e.g., inadequate diet or a malabsorptive disorder) has been corrected, it is sufficient simply to recheck the patient's folate status with a serum folate level determination and a blood count several months after folate replacement has been completed. If the underlying disorder is not reversible, therapy with 1 mg of folic acid daily can be maintained indefinitely.

Folic acid is nontoxic even in large doses. Rarely, children with seizure disorders, who may become folate deficient during hydantoin therapy, have been reported to suffer increased seizures if large doses of folate are given parenterally. The only truly serious toxicity of standard therapy, however, occurs when folic acid is given in error to a patient with cobalamin deficiency.

TREATMENT OF THE UNDERLYING DISORDER

Identifying the underlying disorder that produced the vitamin deficiency is almost as important as treating the deficiency itself. Such identification allows specific treatment of the disorder if it is reversible (e.g., antibiotics for the bacterial overgrowth in the small bowel that produced the cobalamin malabsorption or counseling for the alcoholism that contributed to the dietary folate insufficiency). If the underlying disorder is reversed, periodic monitoring is advisable because it may recur.

Even if the underlying defect is not treatable, its correct identification has important clinical benefits. Informed decisions can be made about the route of vitamin replacement and its duration. Identification of the underlying disorder allows reliable prognostic information to be given to the patient. Early recognition of known complications is also facilitated. For example, hypothyroidism, iron deficiency, gastric cancer, and gastric carcinoid all occur with increased frequency in patients with pernicious anemia and may develop at any time. Because of the increased risk of gastric neoplasms in pernicious anemia, the issue of preventive screening has long been debated. The consensus at this time is that annual endoscopy or barium studies are not worthwhile. However, it is my practice to perform endoscopy in all patients once, usually at the time of diagnosis of pernicious anemia. Whether or not this is done, part of the regular follow-up of patients with pernicious anemia must include stool testing for occult blood and questioning about dyspeptic symptoms.

FOLLOW-UP AND PATIENT EDUCATION

Many important benefits accrue from careful follow-up. Assessing whether a full clinical response occurred is the most obvious benefit and provides the ultimate proof of the correctness of the diagnosis of deficiency. It also permits the uncovering of coexisting disturbances that are often not diagnosable until the megaloblastic anemia has been reversed. The major example of the latter is iron deficiency, which occurs at some point in nearly 50% of patients with pernicious anemia but may be difficult to diagnose before the cobalamin deficiency has been treated.

Reticulocytosis does not begin until the second or third day, but the patient often feels better within 24 hours of beginning therapy, even before the blood count has risen. The best objective hallmarks of an adequate response to cobalamin or folate replacement are peak reticulocytosis after 7 days and full normalization of the blood count no later than 6 to 8 weeks after the start of therapy, no matter how severe the initial anemia. The failure of these events to occur indicates a suboptimal response, either because the diagnosis and therapy were incorrect or because coexisting disorders prevented a full response.

The neurologic symptoms of cobalamin deficiency usually respond to therapy, but may not always be fully reversible. Since it may take several months and sometimes as long as a year to obtain maximal recovery, some patience is required. However, even if neurologic dysfunction cannot be reversed by cobalamin therapy, it should cease to progress. Any evidence of progression during cobalamin therapy requires evaluation for coexisting neurologic disease.

During follow-up, appropriate testing to establish the underlying disorder can be completed (e.g., the various Schilling tests in cobalamin-deficient patients). Follow-up also permits a fuller explanation of the diagnosis and prognosis to the patient. For example, patients with pernicious anemia and other irreversible disorders often fail to appreciate the permanent nature of their malabsorption at first. All too often, as a result, they may discontinue cobalamin injections once they feel better. Follow-up provides the opportunity to explore more fully the patient's and family's understanding of the disease and to address any questions that they may have. It is particularly helpful to re-emphasize to the patient the gastrointestinal origin of many of the disorders, in contrast to the cured hematologic or neurologic expressions of the deficiency.

Follow-up should include dietary counseling for the folate-deficient patient. Emphasis must be given not only to the appropriate foods but also to their methods of preparation. Folate is a labile vitamin; storage, cooking, or canning often destroys much of its activity. Increased intake of fresh vegetables may be helpful. Finally, follow-up also permits exploration of delicate issues, such as alcoholism, that may initially be denied or deferred.

THALASSEMIA

method of
MARTIN H. STEINBERG, M.D.
VA Medical Center and University of Mississippi School of Medicine
Jackson, Mississippi

Inherited abnormalities of hemoglobin are of two general types: (1) abnormal hemoglobins that may have unusual properties, exemplified by sickle cell disease, and (2) insufficient synthesis of normal hemoglobins, which results in the constellation of diseases termed thalassemia. Thalassemias may be the most prevalent genetic disorder of humanity and extract a substantial medical and economic toll upon those afflicted.

The thalassemia phenotype is characterized by hypochromic and microcytic erythrocytes, hemolytic anemia, and splenomegaly. However, all these elements may not be present in every patient with thalassemia. When they are present, they may range from florid to insignificant. Consequently, thalassemias can be nearly undetectable and silent clinically or result in intrauterine death or anemia incompatible with life. These variations are well understood. Many different mutations can cause thalassemia. Different hemoglobin types can be involved in these mutations, patients can be heterozygous or homozygous for mutations, and mixtures of thalassemia mutations often exist in a single individual. The proclivity for variation seems almost endless.

To grasp the essential elements of the pathophysiology, diagnosis, and treatment of thalassemia, a brief summary of how hemoglobin (Hb) is made is warranted. Hb A is the predominant hemoglobin in humans and has two alpha-globin and two beta-globin chains interacting in a tetramer ($\alpha_2\beta_2$). Four genes control the synthesis of alpha-globin, and two direct beta-globin synthesis. The alpha- and beta-globin genes are present on different chromosomes and are regulated independently. Equal amounts of alpha and beta globin are normally made; that is, globin synthesis is balanced, and excessive amounts of neither chain are present. The clinically significant thalassemias occur when a mutation causes reduced synthesis of the alpha- or beta-globin chain. Thalassemia-causing mutations are many and, depending upon their nature, can totally abolish the synthesis

TABLE 1. **The Thalassemias**

*β-Thalassemia**
β^+ Thalassemia (suboptimal beta-globin synthesis)
β^0 Thalassemia (total absence of beta-globin synthesis)
α-Thalassemia
Silent carrier, heterozygous α-thalassemia-2 (3 alpha-globin genes present; -α/αα)†
α-Thalassemia trait, heterozygous α-thalassemia-1, homozygous α-thalassemia-2 (two alpha-globin genes present; -α/-α or --/αα)
Hb H disease (one alpha-globin gene present; -α/--)
Hydrops fetalis (no alpha-globin genes present; --/--)

*Within each broad category of β-thalassemia there is a considerable clinical and hematologic heterogeneity that can be accounted for by the numerous thalassemia-causing mutations, most of which involve just a single base change in the gene. Patients may be heterozygous, homozygous, or mixed heterozygous for these mutations.

†The usual cause of α-thalassemia is deletion of alpha-globin genes (indicated by a dash). Combinations of chromosomes with one or two alpha gene deletions cause the different α-thalassemias. Point mutations are a rare cause of α-thalassemia.

of a globin chain or cause merely slight suppression of globin production. When either the alpha- or the beta-globin chain fails to accumulate in sufficient quantities, the cell is damaged by the continued accumulation of the unaffected globin. Neither alpha nor beta globin alone can form stable hemoglobin molecules. Their presence within the developing and mature erythrocyte injures the cell membrane and its contents and causes early cell death in the bone marrow and hemolytic anemia. Table 1 provides a brief classification of the most prevalent types of thalassemia.

Different racial and ethnic groups have predominant mutations that determine the phenotype of thalassemia in the population. Italians and other ethnic groups of Mediterranean origin have β-thalassemias that severely interfere with beta-globin synthesis, and homozygotes have a relentless disease sometimes called Cooley's anemia, Mediterranean anemia, or thalassemia major. Blacks commonly have mild β-thalassemia mutations, and homozygotes usually have thalassemia intermedia, a milder phenotype. Heterozygous carriers of any β-thalassemia mutation are rarely ill.

α-Thalassemia is most prevalent in Asians and blacks. Asians often carry the chromosome that has two missing alpha-globin genes; blacks uncommonly have this chromosome. As a result, Asians have the two clinically significant types of α-thalassemia, Hb H disease and Hb Barts hydrops fetalis, while these entities are rare or absent in blacks.

Some laboratory diagnostic features of the thalassemias are shown in Table 2. Splenomegaly is present in the more severe thalassemias but is minimal or absent in thalassemia heterozygotes.

TREATMENT

Thalassemia treatment can be classified as preventive, symptomatic, or curative. These modalities are applied almost exclusively to the severe forms of homozygous α- and β-thalassemia. The specialized nature of the treatments employed makes management in thalassemia centers or by specially qualified hematologists most likely to result in a good outcome.

Heterozygous α- and β-Thalassemia

These conditions seldom require active treatment but are worthwhile recognizing for several reasons. First, their recognition raises the issue of population screening to detect carriers and to identify couples at risk for pregnancies with homozygous fetuses. Second, the presence of hypochromic and microcytic erythrocytes and perhaps mild anemia often leads to the confusion of heterozygous thalassemia with iron deficiency anemia. Thalassemias do not respond to iron replacement, and in fact such treatment may be harmful. Therefore, in evaluating patients with microcytic red cells, the distinction between iron deficiency and thalassemia, which is not difficult, must be clearly drawn to avoid injudicious treatment. Almost without exception, heterozygous thalassemias need no treatment.

Homozygous Thalassemia

Screening and Antenatal Diagnosis. Homozygotes for β-thalassemia are desperately ill, and in the α-thalassemias, in which all four alpha-globin genes are absent or defective, stillbirth is the rule. Population screening can identify heterozygous carriers of these thalassemias and, therefore, couples at risk for homozygous fetuses. Some countries have used government-supported programs for screening, prenatal diagnosis, and termination of affected pregnancies to markedly reduce the incidence of new cases of homozygous disease. Given the current expense of and imperfect methodology for managing severe thalassemia, these have been an effective means of reducing the medical and economic liability of disease. β-Thalassemia carrier detection, by measuring erythrocyte indices and Hb A_2 levels, is usually uncomplicated and inexpensive. Prenatal diagnosis of thalassemia is a feasible option in the United States and many parts

TABLE 2. **Laboratory Diagnosis of Thalassemia***

	PCV	MCV (fL)	Reticulocyte Count (%)	Hb A_2 (%)	Hb F (%)
Normal	38–55	80–90	1	2–3	1
Heterozygous β-thalassemia	35–45	60–75	1–3	4–6	1–3
Homozygous β-thalassemia	15–25	60–80	5–30	2–5	10–100
α-Thalassemia silent carrier	Normal	75–85	Normal	2–3	1
α-Thalassemia trait	35–45	65–80	1–2	2–3	1
Hb H disease	20–30	60–70	5–15	1–2	1

*The values given are approximate ranges and may vary among individuals according to the genotype and mutation.
PCV = packed cell volume; MCV = mean corpuscular volume.

of the world where these disorders are common. Prenatal diagnosis should be carried out within a program of screening and education of high-risk groups. The major goal of screening for heterozygotes is family counseling regarding the risks and potential outcomes of pregnancy. Comprehensible information about the medical problems of the heterozygote, although these are minor in thalassemia trait, should accompany the screening process.

Recombinant DNA technology has revolutionized prenatal diagnosis of thalassemias. Before this, antenatal diagnosis was not possible before 18 weeks' gestation, and the tests occasionally produced equivocal results. Prenatal diagnosis can now be done on fetal DNA from amniotic fluid cells at 14 weeks of gestation, and if chorionic villi are used, diagnosis can be made even earlier (at 10 weeks). The risk of miscarriage with the former method is about 1%, whereas for the latter it is near 5%. α-Thalassemia hydrops fetalis can be detected by the complete absence of alpha-globin genes when DNA is probed with alpha-globin gene–specific probes. β-Thalassemia–causing mutations cluster in different racial and ethnic groups. Direct mutation detection in fetal DNA, using gene amplification and groups of DNA probes specific for the mutations common in the patient's ethnic group, has become the standard means of detection.

Transfusion and Chelation in β-Thalassemia. Most homozygotes for β-thalassemia are dependent upon blood transfusion to sustain life. The magnitude of anemia and the body's attempt to compensate for the destruction of red cells in the marrow and the circulation lead to an exceptional metabolic burden. Skeletal deformation occurs as the marrow expands within the bone and elsewhere in a futile attempt to provide sufficient erythrocytes. In the absence of transfusion, the anemia is often incompatible with even a modest level of activity, and growth and normal development fail. Experience has shown that a program of continuous transfusion can ablate the worst features of the disease.

When transfusion is started very early in life and the hemoglobin levels are kept between 9 and 10 grams per dL, erythropoiesis is suppressed. Because of this, marrow expansion does not occur, severe hemolysis is not present, and growth and development approximate normal. It is customary to initiate transfusion when the hemoglobin concentration remains below 7 grams per dL, although some patients are symptomatic at higher hemoglobin levels. Before transfusion therapy is begun, vaccination for hepatitis B should be given to individuals who are antibody negative, and the red cell antigen phenotype should be ascertained to help detection of isoimmunization to minor blood group antigens. Washed or filtered packed red cells are given at the intervals needed to maintain the desired hemoglobin level. Recent studies have shown some advantage to using blood enriched in young red cells for transfusion as this may reduce blood requirements because of the longer life span of young cells. Transfusions are usually given at 3- to 4-week intervals. The amount of blood per transfusion required to maintain the desired hemoglobin level differs among patients and must be individualized.

The need for transfusion may change as time progresses. Splenectomy may be indicated when the red cell survival shortens; it reduces the excessive red cell destruction and the cytopenias of hypersplenism, and lengthens the interval between transfusions. Severe postsplenectomy infection is a risk to be confronted, and if possible the operation should be delayed until after age 5. Polyvalent *Streptococcus pneumoniae, Haemophilus influenzae,* and *Neisseria meningitidis* vaccine should be given before surgery and prophylactic penicillin V,* 250 mg orally twice daily, administered afterward.

In addition to the usual complications of transfusion (e.g., alloimmunization and transmission of retroviral infection), iron can be deposited in tissue owing to destruction of transfused blood. Transfusion-induced hemochromatosis then develops and ultimately causes death if iron is not removed by chelation. Serum ferritin levels, iron staining and measurement of the iron content of liver biopsy tissue, urinary iron excretion following a standard dose of deferoxamine, and magnetic resonance imaging of the liver can all be used to assess body iron stores. Deferoxamine (Desferal), currently the sole chelating agent available, is given by prolonged subcutaneous or intravenous infusion, 8 to 12 hours daily, 5 to 6 days weekly, at doses of 2 to 6 grams per day, using a portable infusion pump. The regimen must be individualized as the amount of iron excreted varies. While optimum chelation therapy can induce negative iron balance, the ultimate effects of this treatment are not yet known. When treatment is started after significant iron accumulation, iron-induced cardiomyopathy, a leading cause of death, may not always be reversible, although intense chelation may reduce the prevalence of arrhythmias and congestive failure.

Ideally, chelation should be started in young children before the acquisition of excessive iron stores and coincident with the onset of transfusions. However, reports of deferoxamine-associated growth retardation argue for delaying chelation until the iron stores begin to increase.

Low doses of vitamin C (100 mg daily) may increase the excretion of iron by deferoxamine and can be used in vitamin C–depleted individuals while they are receiving chelation treatment. A glass of fresh orange juice daily can accomplish the same result. Chelation is not easy for the patient, parents, or supervising medical professionals. The rate of compliance with optimal regimens, especially in adolescence, is low. The financial burden imposed by lifelong transfusion and chelation is considerable.

An effective oral chelating agent may soon be available, providing relief from the arduous regimen of subcutaneous infusion. If the promise of an effective

*Not FDA approved for this indication.

oral chelating drug is realized, the value of early transplantation (discussed in the next section) may have to be reconsidered.

Transplantation. Bone marrow transplantation has been employed in severe β-thalassemia and considerable experience has been gained, mainly in Italian thalassemia centers, which have been in the vanguard of this treatment. Successful transplantation can cure β-thalassemia: successfully treated individuals have either normal hemoglobin or the innocuous β-thalassemia trait, depending upon the genotype of the donor. The best candidates are the youngest children; older, more heavily transfused patients are less likely to become engrafted and have higher morbidity and mortality. Transfusion and chelation can allow normal development and a decent quality of life for many years. Because bone marrow transplantation still has appreciable short-term mortality, the decision to recommend this therapy has in the past been a difficult one. However, in children who have little or no liver disease because of efficient chelation, transplantation using haplo-identical donors has resulted in disease-free survival of 95% in experienced hands. As these results become achievable in all marrow transplant centers, early transplantation may become the most efficacious and cost-effective method of treatment, freeing the patient from the lifelong burden of transfusion and chelation therapy.

α-Thalassemia

Hb H disease is best managed by periodic observation so that any increase in the degree of anemia (e.g., from a supervening aplastic crisis or an enlarging spleen) can be properly treated. Hb H disease can be clinically heterogeneous depending on its molecular causes, and some patients may need blood transfusion.

In Asians, in whom chromosomes lacking both alpha-globin genes are common, screening can identify couples in jeopardy of bearing hydropic fetuses. Prenatal diagnosis should be made in pregnancies at risk for this fatal disorder. When a hydropic fetus is found, the pregnancy should be terminated, as stillbirth is almost universal and the course of pregnancy is accompanied by a high rate of maternal complications.

General Measures

Optimal nutrition is a general feature of the management of all chronic diseases and is especially important in severe thalassemias because of the high metabolic rate that results from hemolysis. The diet can be supplemented with 1 mg of folic acid daily by mouth. As with all types of chronic hemolytic anemia, gallstones develop early and should be suspected at any age when abdominal pain is present. Silent stones should probably be left alone; symptomatic stones should be removed, and laparoscopic surgery is the method of choice unless contraindicated.

The aplastic crisis of hemolytic anemia is caused most often by infection with the human B19 parvovirus. It can be recognized by a sudden fall in hemoglobin level without bleeding and the presence of reticulocytopenia. Depending upon the rapidity of its development and severity, it can be managed by observation or transfusion. If patients with homozygous β-thalassemia are properly transfused, the consequences of this cause of marrow aplasia are less dramatic and severe than in hemolytic anemias that are not treated with intensive transfusion.

Experimental and Future Therapies

Preliminary studies have suggested that hydroxyurea* may increase the level of Hb F and raise the hemoglobin level in some individuals with severe β-thalassemia. This therapy may be enhanced by the administration of erythropoietin. These are experimental observations, and further study is needed before their clinical application can be recommended. Also over the horizon may be other Hb F–inducing agents, such as butyrate analogues.

The most exciting possibilities for treatment involve alteration of the genetic defects of thalassemia by gene therapy. In this procedure, a viral vector that cannot replicate within a human cell, or even a nonviral vector, such as a liposome, is used to introduce a gene with therapeutic potential into a human cell. Along with the "therapeutic" gene, regulatory sequences for high-level, tissue-specific expression are needed. To fulfill the requirements for successful gene therapy of thalassemia, hematopoietic stem cells should be targeted for gene insertion, and sufficient numbers must be transduced with the therapeutic gene to be useful clinically. Transduced cells should have the selective advantage needed for proliferation, self-renewal, and differentiation in vivo, or else host bone marrow must be destroyed so that the transplanted cells containing the transferred gene can proliferate.

There are generic problems inherent in gene therapy that may appear only with time. Without site-specific recombination between the host and transgenome, the specter of insertional mutagenesis activating oncogenes or inactivating antioncogenes is present. Recombination might lead to production of deleterious fusion proteins. Theoretically, recombinant viral vectors might revert to competent virus particles. The coupling of therapeutically useful genes to powerful transcriptional activators may induce the expression of normally quiescent genes, disrupting the normal cell cycle or leading to the production of a normal protein in abnormal amounts. Even if some of these theoretical problems do occur, they may turn out to be sufficiently rare that the risk/benefit ratio for an effective gene therapy protocol is favorable. Work on gene therapy is rapidly progressing, and this treatment may be feasible within this decade.

*Not FDA approved for this indication.

SICKLE CELL DISEASE

method of
SAMIR K. BALLAS, M.D.
Cardeza Foundation for Hematological Research, Thomas Jefferson University
Philadelphia, Pennsylvania

BASIC CONSIDERATIONS

Sickle cell disease is a generic term for a group of chronic inherited disorders of hemoglobin structure in which the affected individual inherits two mutant globin genes (one from each parent), at least one of which is always the sickle mutation. The latter results from a single nucleotide change (GAT→GTT) in the sixth codon of exon 1 of the beta-globin gene responsible for the synthesis of the beta-globin chain. The resulting replacement of the normal glutamic acid by valine at position 6 in the beta-chain leads to the formation of sickle hemoglobin (Hb S). Sickle cell anemia (SS) is the homozygous state, in which the sickle gene is inherited from both parents. Other sickle cell syndromes result from the co-inheritance of the sickle gene and a nonsickle gene, such as Hb C, Hb O^{Arab}, Hb D, β^+-thalassemia, or β^0-thalassemia. Table 1 lists the common sickle cell syndromes arranged in order of decreasing prevalence among African-Americans. The deoxy form of Hb S is characterized by decreased intracellular solubility and a tendency to polymerize within red blood cells, causing the familiar sickle shape and forming long fibers visible by electron microscopy of red cells from patients with SS. The pathophysiologic findings are thought to be due to in situ sickling of red blood cells, leading to microvascular obstruction of blood flow associated with consequent microinfarcts in the affected tissue(s) and possible direct damage to local endothelium. The rate and extent of intracellular polymerization of Hb S, with consequent vascular occlusion, depend on the intracellular concentration of Hb, the intracellular hemoglobin composition, and the percentage of oxygen saturation. Accordingly, any factor that decreases the intracellular polymerization of Hb S may have a salutary outcome on the clinical manifestations of the disease. Moreover, α-thalassemia, characterized by the deletion of one or two alpha-globin genes, may be co-inherited with any of the sickle cell syndromes listed in Table 1. This association usually ameliorates the anemia and may have a bearing on certain clinical manifestations of the disease, as will be mentioned later.

TABLE 1. **Sickle Cell Syndromes Affecting African-Americans***

Disorder	Abbreviation
Sickle cell anemia	SS
Hemoglobin SC disease	Hb SC
Sickle-β^+-thalassemia	S-β^+-thal
Sickle-β^0-thalassemia	S-β^0-thal
Other hemoglobinopathies	
Hemoglobin SO^{Arab}	Hb SO^{Arab}
Hemoglobin SD	Hb SD
Other combinations	Hb SX

*Syndromes are listed in decreasing order of prevalence.

CLINICAL CONSIDERATIONS

The clinical manifestations of sickle cell disease vary considerably from patient to patient and in the same patient over time. Some patients with sickle cell anemia have very mild disease, while others suffer from severe disease and die at a relatively young age. In our experience the majority of patients with sickle cell disease (about 60%) treat themselves effectively at home and require management in the emergency department or hospital less than once a year. About 15 to 20% of the patients, on the other hand, have severe disease, seem to be in continuous pain, and require frequent hospitalizations.

Several factors have been proposed as modulators of certain aspects of the clinical expression of sickle cell disease. Most important among these is the Hb F level and the total hemoglobin (Hb) value. Recent studies have shown that (1) there is an inverse relation between Hb F level and the frequency of painful episodes; and (2) there is a direct relation between the hematocrit (or Hb) value and the frequency of painful episodes. The sickle cell gene seems to be pleiotropic in nature; i.e., it is a typical single gene inherited in a simple mendelian pattern but the resulting pathology has some of the clinical features of a polygenic disorder.

The comprehensive management of sickle cell disease, especially in adults, raises certain difficulties (Table 2). These stem from the fact that these patients are at a triple disadvantage as follows: (1) they suffer from an inherited chronic disease that involves frequent and unpredictable attacks of acute pain that may require relatively large and frequent doses of narcotic analgesics; (2) psychosocial factors may create barriers to effective management; and (3) they are often the target of negative attitudes by a subset of health care providers who have neither interest nor experience in sickle cell disease. Although there is, to date, no curative therapy for sickle cell disease in adults, the sociocultural aspects of the disease and the negative attitude of some health care providers are amenable to change through support groups, education, counseling, and enhanced communication. It is with this aim and hope that this article has been written.

TABLE 2. **Obstacles to Effective Management of Sickle Cell Disease**

Sickle cell disease is inherited, chronic, and incurable.
Disparity in the sociocultural backgrounds of patients and health care providers.
Heavy use of narcotic analgesics by some patients.
Overemphasis by some health care providers on the addictive side effects of narcotic analgesics.
Lack of affluent insurance coverage in the majority of patients.

CLINICAL MANIFESTATIONS OF SICKLE CELL DISEASE

The clinical picture of sickle cell disease is dominated by three sets of signs and symptoms (Table 3): (1) painful episodes; (2) hematologic manifestations; and (3) specific organ involvement. Pain management is the most practical aspect of treating sickle cell disease in adults. In infants and young children, prophylactic treatment with antibiotics and anti-pneumococcal vaccine as well as prompt treatment of intercurrent infectious episodes is essential in decreasing mortality and morbidity. One would expect that an illness like sickle cell disease with its protean clinical picture would be of great teaching value in urban medical institutions, since almost all subspecialties in internal medicine could find a model of pathophysiologic events that affect their organ of interest. Unfortunately, this is not the case in many institutions. The difficulties previously mentioned that surround the comprehensive management of patients with sickle cell disease may be responsible, in part, for this state of affairs. There may be other complex factors that are not addressed here.

Acute Pain Syndromes

Acute Painful Episodes (Painful Crises)

The acute painful sickle cell crisis is the hallmark of sickle cell anemia and is the most common complaint among patients with this disease. The majority of painful episodes are of mild to moderate severity and are usually treated at home with oral analgesics, bed rest, adequate oral hydration, and local measures such as application of heat to the painful area. Severe painful episodes necessitate treatment in the emergency room and/or the hospital. In our experience, over 90% of hospital admissions of adult patients with sickle cell disease are for the treatment of acute painful episodes. Typically about 125 patients are admitted about 500 times to our hospital per year, with an average length of stay of 9 to 11 days and a range from 1 day to several weeks.

The frequency and severity of these painful episodes vary considerably among patients and in the same patient from time to time. Infection, physical stress, and emotional upheaval may precede a painful crisis. In the majority of patients, however, there is no obvious precipitating factor. Objective signs of a painful crisis, such as fever, leukocytosis, joint effusions, and tenderness, occur in about 50% of patients at initial presentation. During the evolution of the painful crisis, objective laboratory signs become evident in the majority of patients, provided these parameters are determined serially. Thus, the percentage of irreversibly sickled cells or dense cells is high early in the painful crisis and decreases gradually as the crisis evolves. About 10% of patients with sickle cell anemia have very frequent severe crises (more than 20 per year). The factors that lead to this severe clinical picture are unknown. This subset of patients are almost always hospital and/or emergency room–bound and evoke considerable resentment among some health care providers who, in turn, develop stereotyped misconceptions about sickle cell disease in general. Pain usually involves the low back, legs, knees, arms, chest, and abdomen in decreasing order of frequency. Pain may be throbbing, sharp, dull, or stabbing in nature. Bone marrow infarcts are associated with the most severe pain, which is pounding-stabbing in nature and forces the patient to assume certain postures (e.g., crouching, raised legs) in an effort to find relief.

The sequence of pathophysiologic events that lead to the sensation of pain in sickle cell disease is not well understood. Available data in the literature suggest that tissue ischemia due to vascular occlusion consequent to in situ sickling causes infarctive tissue damage, which in turn initiates a secondary inflammatory response. The latter may enhance sympathetic activity via interactions with neuroendocrine pathways and trigger release of norepinephrine which, in the setting of tissue injury, causes more tissue ischemia, thus creating a vicious circle (Fig. 1). It is this combination of ischemic tissue damage and

TABLE 3. **Major Clinical Manifestations of Sickle Cell Disease**

- Pain syndromes
  - Acute pain syndromes
    - Painful crises
    - Acute chest syndrome
    - Right upper quadrant (RUQ) syndrome
    - Priapism
    - Hand-foot syndrome
    - Splenic sequestration
  - Chronic pain syndromes
    - Avascular (aseptic) necrosis
    - Vertebral body collapse
    - Leg ulcers
- Hematologic manifestations
- Organ failure

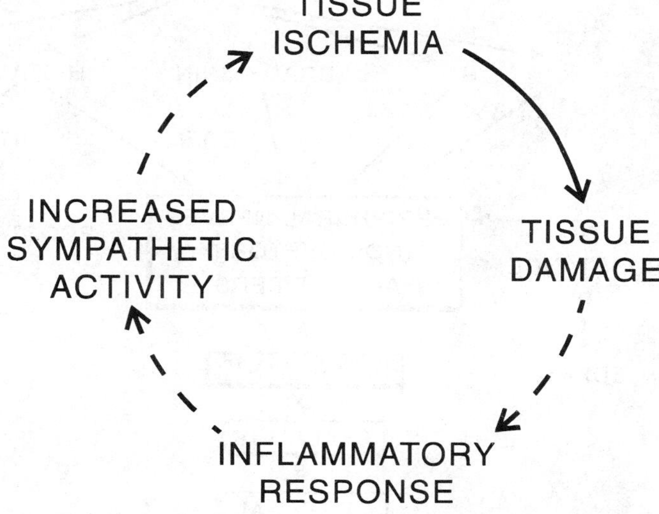

Figure 1. In situ sickling initiates a vicious circle of ischemic tissue damage and subsequent inflammatory response.

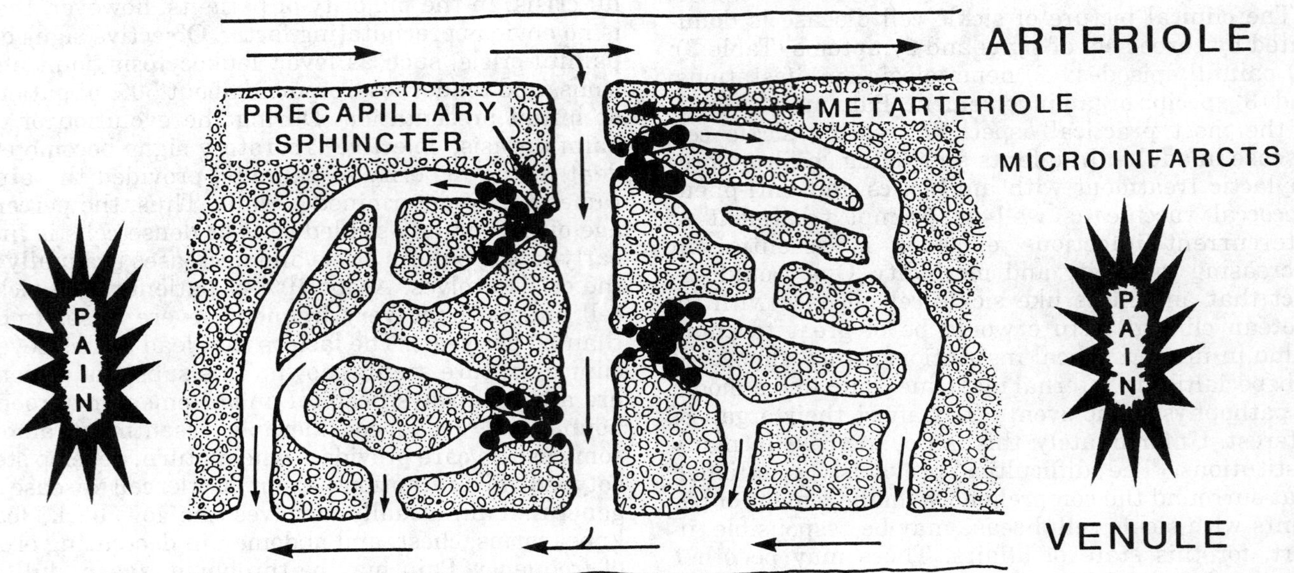

Figure 2. Impairment of microcirculation by sickle RBC. Adhesion of sickle RBC causes vascular occlusion with consequent hypoxic and tissue damage secondary to microinfarcts that initiate the acute painful episode. Arrows indicate the direction of blood flow.

secondary inflammatory response that makes the pain of sickle cell disease unique in its acuteness and severity. Figure 2 depicts vascular occlusion and its consequences. Figure 3 illustrates the major pain modulators that are generated by tissue injury. Interleukin-1 (IL-1) is an endogenous pyrogen and also activates the cyclooxygenase gene leading to synthesis of prostaglandins E_2 and I_2. Bradykinin, K^+, H^+, and histamine activate nociceptive afferent nerve fibers and evoke a pain response. Prostaglandins sensitize peripheral nerve endings and facilitate the transmission of painful stimuli that reach the cerebral cortex via the spinal cord and the thalamus. Moreover, activated nociceptors release stored substance P, which itself facilitates the transmission of painful stimuli. Bradykinin and substance P also cause vasodilation and extravasation of fluids that can lead to local swelling and tenderness. The pathway for painful stimuli is subject not only to activators, sensitizers, and facilitators but also to inhibitors

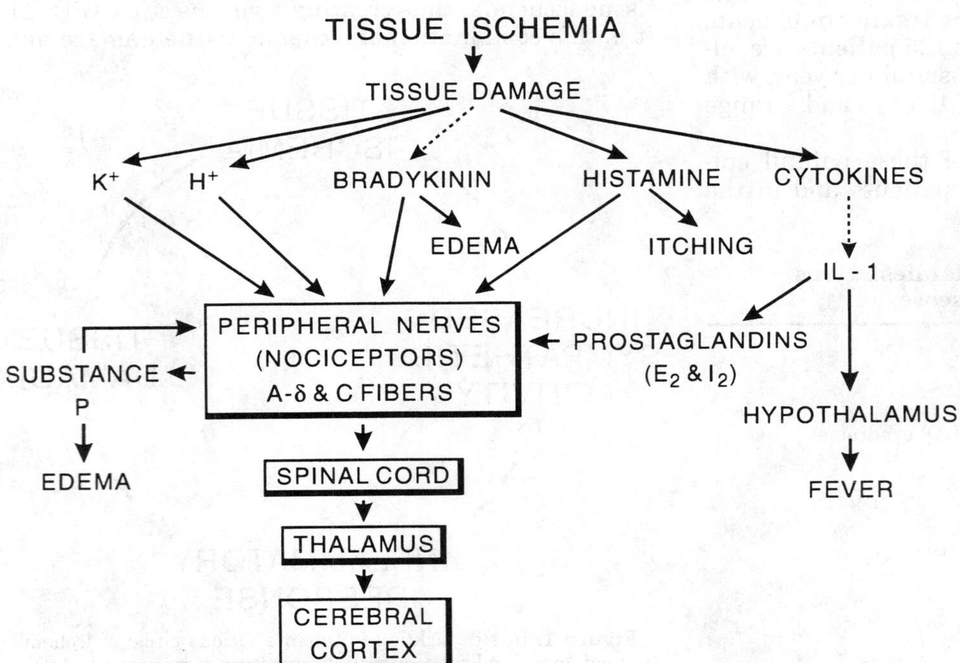

Figure 3. Pain pathway. Tissue damage results in the release of noxious stimuli, which activate peripheral nerves, which, in turn, transmit painful stimuli to the central nervous system.

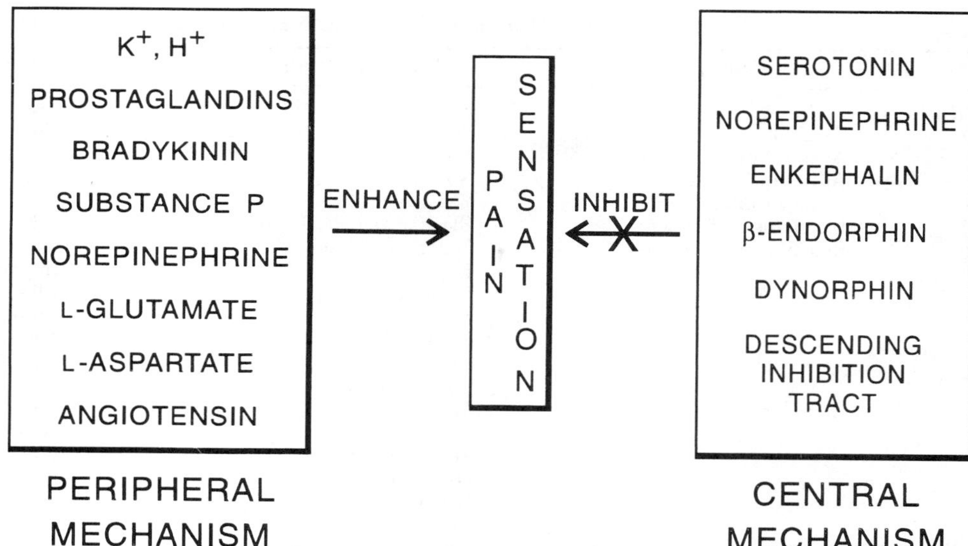

Figure 4. The severity of pain sensation following tissue damage depends on the net balance of pain stimulators versus pain inhibitors.

(Fig. 4). Serotonin, enkephalin, β-endorphin, and dynorphin are endogenous central pain inhibitors. Thus, in a given patient the net outcome of tissue ischemia may be severe or mild pain, depending on the extent of tissue damage and the net balance of pain stimulators versus pain inhibitors. This may explain, in part, the considerable variation in the frequency and severity of painful crises among patients and in the same patient over time.

Treatment of acute painful episodes is empiric and depends on the severity of pain and the presence or absence of other complications of the disease itself. Table 4 lists the three major principles of treatment of acute painful episodes. Modification of the source of pain should include a thorough search for an infectious process that might have precipitated the crisis. Specific organ involvement should be systematically evaluated. Patients are the best authority on their pain. If the pain they describe is not typical of their usual crises, then other causes should be sought. If the initial evaluation reveals an uncomplicated painful episode, proper assessment of the pain should ensue; categoric or visual analogue scales may be of value in this regard. The aim of treatment at this point should be interruption of the transmission of painful stimuli along peripheral fibers and alteration of the perception of pain in the central nervous system (CNS), as listed in Table 4.

TABLE 4. **Principles of Treatment of Acute Painful Episodes**

Principle	Method of Treatment
Modify the source of pain	Treat precipitating factors (e.g., infection) if identified Bed rest and local measures such as heating pad may be helpful
Interrupt the transmission of painful stimuli along nociceptors	Anti-inflammatory agents; salicylates, acetaminophen, and other NSAIDS
Alter the perception of pain at the CNS level	Narcotic analgesics Biofeedback Self-hypnosis

Non-narcotic analgesics exert their effect peripherally, whereas narcotic analgesics act centrally by blocking the μ and κ receptors. Major differences between narcotic and non-narcotic analgesics are listed in Table 5. Antagonists to bradykinin and substance P are not available for clinical use at present but are being used in animal experiments. Pain of mild severity may be treated with oral non-narcotic analgesics or weak narcotics such as oxycodone, codeine, or propoxyphene. Severe pain necessitates the administration of narcotic analgesics in an effective manner. Table 6 lists recommended guidelines for the treatment of severe acute painful episodes in hospitalized adult patients. The same format may be used in abbreviated form (i.e., treatment over 6 to 12 hours) to treat painful episodes in the emergency room. An example of a comprehensive regimen to manage severe episodes of pain in the hospital follows:

Maintenance Therapy

Narcotic Analgesic

Morphine sulfate, 0.1–0.2 mg/kg intravenously (IV), intramuscularly (IM), or subcutaneously (SC) q 2–3 h

or

Meperidine, 1.5 mg/kg IV or IM q 2–3 h

or

Hydromorphone, 0.02–0.04 mg/kg IV, IM, or SC q 2–3 h

Non-Narcotic Analgesic

Ibuprofen, 600 mg orally (PO) q 6 h

or

Ketorolac (Toradol), 60 mg IM initially followed by 30 mg IM q 6 h for a maximum of 5 days

Rescue Therapy for Breakthrough Pain

One-fourth to one-half the maintenance dose of the narcotic analgesic given parenterally 30–60 minutes after the maintenance dose

Adjuvant Therapy

Diphenhydramine (Benadryl),* 25–50 mg IM q 4–6 h

or

Hydroxyzine (Vistaril),* 25–50 mg IM q 4–6 h

*Not FDA approved for this indication.

TABLE 5. **Major Differences Between Narcotic and Non-Narcotic Analgesics**

Feature	Narcotic Analgesics	Non-Narcotic Analgesics
Ceiling effect	No	Yes
Sedation	Yes	No
Anti-inflammatory effect	No	Yes
Antipyretic effect	No	Yes
Habit forming	Yes	No
Mechanism of action	Block μ and κ CNS receptors	Inhibit prostaglandin synthesis
Side effects	Sedation	GI ulceration
	Euphoria	Impaired hepatic function
	Respiratory depression	Bleeding
	Myoclonus	Interstitial nephritis
	Seizures	Acute renal failure
	Emesis	Hypersensitivity reactions
	Constipation	
Commonly used agents	Meperidine	Ibuprofen
	Hydromorphone	Acetaminophen
	Morphine sulfate	Salicylates
	Oxycodone	Ketorolac
	Codeine	
	Propoxyphene	

Anxiolytics—Muscle Relaxants
Diazepam (Valium), 2–10 mg PO q 8 h prn
Antiemetics
Prochlorperazine (Compazine), 5–10 mg PO or IM q 6 h prn
Laxatives
Magnesium citrate 8 oz PO qd prn
Other Supportive Measures
Hydration (oral or intravenous)
Heating pads
Hydrotherapy
Biofeedback
Relaxation
Diversion

It should be emphasized that this scheme is only an example, and any of the drugs and dosages could be changed according to individual circumstances.

Decreased pain intensity and improvement in the patient's mood justify tapering of pain medications. This should be done gradually by decreasing the dose of the narcotic analgesic by 25% of the maintenance dose every 12 to 24 hours. Another possibility is to switch from parenteral to oral narcotic analgesics, in which case the oral/parenteral equianalgesic ratio should be taken into consideration (Table 7). Another approach to discharge planning is to start the patient on an oral long-acting narcotic analgesic such as controlled morphine sulfate (MS Contin) in divided doses without discontinuing the parenteral narcotic. The latter can be tapered rapidly after two to four doses of the oral long-acting narcotic. Such an approach may be contraindicated in patients with compromised pulmonary function. Patients are ready for discharge once they are pain free without medication or their pain is adequately controlled with oral medication.

Other approaches for the delivery of narcotic analgesics, such as patient-controlled analgesic (PCA) and fentanyl patches, have not been used widely in patients with sickle cell disease, and specific guidelines for these modalities are not available at the present time.

Acute Chest Syndrome

The full-blown clinical picture of acute chest syndrome includes chest pain, fever, dyspnea, hypoxia, pulmonary infiltrates on chest x-ray, and decreasing Hb level. These signs and symptoms vary from very mild to very severe and even life-threatening. The syndrome may be caused by rib or sternal infarction, pneumonia, pulmonary infarcts due to in situ sickling, fat embolism, or pulmonary embolism. The diagnostic work-up should include a chest x-ray, sputum and blood cultures, arterial blood gas monitoring, hemoglobin monitoring, ventilation and perfusion ($\dot{V}/\dot{Q}$) scans, examination for fat bodies in sputum and urine, and assessment for thrombophlebitis in the pelvis or lower extremities. Blister cells have been described in the peripheral smear of patients with pulmonary infarcts secondary to sickle cell disease. Treatment includes antibiotic therapy, oxygen, and in severe cases, exchange transfusion. Caution should be exercised in giving narcotics, especially the slow-release preparations, to the hypoxic

TABLE 6. **Guidelines for Effective Management of Adult Patients with Acute Severe Painful Episodes**

1. Believe the patient.
2. Conduct thorough clinical assessment periodically, including documentation of pain severity, pain relief, and mood.
3. Select the appropriate narcotic analgesic and its dose based on previous history.
4. Administer narcotic analgesics parenterally on a regular basis (maintenance dose).
5. Monitor vital signs with special attention to the respiratory rate (RR).
6. Titrate the maintenance dose of narcotic analgesic (taper or escalate).
7. Give rescue doses (¼–½ maintenance dose) for breakthrough pain.
8. Decrease or skip maintenance dose if RR $<$ 10/min.
9. Give non-narcotic analgesics and adjuvant analgesics in combination with narcotic analgesics.
10. Taper narcotic analgesics gradually once the pain severity score decreases and the patient's mood improves.
11. Consider discharge once pain relief is achieved without medication or if pain is adequately controlled with oral medications.
12. Design a discharge plan.

TABLE 7. **Oral Equianalgesic Doses of Commonly Used Narcotic Analgesics**

Analgesic	Parenteral Dose	Oral Dose	Oral/ Parenteral Ratio†
Meperidine	100 mg	400 mg*	4
Hydromorphone	2 mg	10 mg	5
Morphine sulfate	10 mg	60 mg	6

*It is not advisable to give meperidine in oral doses greater than 200 mg to avoid neurologic complications.

†The ratio may be smaller in patients taking narcotic analgesics regularly for several weeks.

patient. Heparin is usually reserved for patients with proven pulmonary embolism. Repeated attacks of acute chest syndrome with pulmonary infarcts predict the onset of pulmonary hypertension, pulmonary failure with cor pulmonale, and terminal adult respiratory distress syndrome. Moreover, the sudden death syndrome in adults may be related to chronic sickle cell lung disease via a sudden episode of pulmonary hypoxia.

Because acute chest syndrome is relatively frequent in sickle cell anemia and in view of the need for arterial blood gas monitoring, it is important to establish baseline values for blood gases and pulmonary function tests for all patients. These determinations will be of value in evaluating patients who present with acute onset of pulmonary signs and symptoms.

Right Upper Quadrant (RUQ) Syndrome

Sickle cell patients with this syndrome present with pain in the RUQ. The differential diagnosis includes painful crisis, cholecystitis, acute hepatic sequestration, and hepatic crisis. Acute hepatic sequestration is characterized by hepatic enlargement associated with significant fall in Hb level and no appreciable disturbance in liver function. The most likely mechanism seems to be sequestration of sickled erythrocytes in liver sinusoids. Hepatic crisis (also called sickle cell intrahepatic cholestasis) is characterized by the sudden onset of RUQ pain, progressive hepatomegaly, increasing bilirubin level (mainly indirect), and prolongation of the prothrombin time (PT) and partial thromboplastin time (PTT). Liver enzymes (GGT and AST) are also elevated, but not to the levels seen in acute viral hepatitis. It should be emphasized that hepatic crises, like acute splenic sequestration, vary in severity from minor episodes to severe life-threatening situations. Total blood exchange is a recommended form of therapy. In the author's experience blood exchange should be initiated when the total bilirubin level increases progressively to values greater than 50 mg/dL. At that level, the PT values are usually prolonged to greater than 20 seconds. Blood exchange should be total; i.e., whole blood is removed and replaced with red cells and fresh frozen plasma in order to correct the coagulation abnormality.

Priapism

Priapism occurs when sickle cells congest the corpora and prevent emptying of blood from the penis. It can result from tricorporal involvement (both the corpora cavernosa and the corpus spongiosum) or bicorporal involvement (both corpora cavernosa). The latter is more common in children and is not regularly associated with impotence. There are two major clinical presentations of priapism: acute and chronic. The acute presentation is characterized by a prolonged painful erection that persists beyond several hours, responds poorly to exchange transfusion, and frequently requires surgical intervention. Acute priapism may be followed by complete or partial impotence. The chronic form of priapism is characterized by repetitive, reversible, painful erections called *stuttering priapism.* It usually occurs after intercourse or it may awaken patients early in the morning. Stuttering priapism responds well to diazepam (Valium)* or pseudoephedrine hydrochloride (Sudafed).* Some patients report that exercise is helpful. Patients who become impotent may benefit from psychological counseling and the insertion of penile implants.

Hand-Foot Syndrome

This acute pain syndrome occurs most commonly in infants and young children between the ages of 6 months and 2 years with a few reported cases involving children up to age 7 years. The clinical picture is characterized by acute painful swelling of one or more extremities. Fever and leukocytosis may be present. The episode is usually self limited and resolves within 1 week, but recurrent attacks are common. Treatment is symptomatic, and if the attack persists, acute osteomyelitis should be ruled out.

Splenic Sequestration

The spleen is the first organ to suffer from the destructive effects of sickle microvasculopathy, which eventually leads to autosplenectomy. During infancy, the spleen is enlarged in about 75% of patients with sickle cell anemia. Children between the ages of 5 months and 2 years are most vulnerable to splenic sequestration, which varies in severity from mild to life-threatening. Splenic sequestration is characterized by an increase in the size of the spleen and a decrease in Hb. Minor episodes may resolve spontaneously, but severe episodes may be fatal and may be mistaken for sudden infant death syndrome. Because acute splenic sequestration tends to recur, splenectomy has been recommended for patients who survive the initial severe episode. By age 5 or 6 years, the spleen undergoes fibrosis and the risk of splenic sequestration decreases. It should be emphasized, however, that adults with certain sickle cell syndromes and splenomegaly (sickle cell anemia with two alphagene deletions, Hb SC disease, S-β-thalassemia) are at risk for acute splenic sequestration episodes. The onset of splenic sequestration correlates with the in-

*Not FDA approved for this indication.

creased risk of septicemia from *Streptococcus pneumoniae* and *Haemophilus influenzae*. For this reason, it is recommended that all patients with sickle cell syndromes receive anti-pneumococcal vaccine. Because the spleen is the major organ that produces IgM, patients with autosplenectomy typically have low levels of this immunoglobulin, as do patients with anatomic splenectomy.

TABLE 8. **Anemia in Sickle Cell Syndromes**

Sickle Cell Syndrome*	Typical Hemoglobin Level (gm/dL)
Sickle cell anemia	7.0–8.0
Sickle-β^0-thalassemia	7.0–10.0
Sickle-β^+-thalassemia	>10.0
Hb SC disease	>10.0

*Syndromes are listed in decreasing order of severity of the anemia.

Chronic Pain Syndromes

Avascular Necrosis and Vertebral Deformities

Chronic bone complications include avascular necrosis of the humeral and femoral heads as well as vertebral deformities. The limited terminal arterial blood supply and the paucity of collateral circulation make these areas vulnerable to sickling and consequent bone damage. Patients with sickle cell anemia and alpha-gene deletion have a greater incidence of avascular necrosis of the humeral and femoral heads because of the relatively high hematocrit level that increases blood viscosity and thus microvasculopathy in these areas. Treatment of avascular necrosis is symptomatic in its early stages, but advanced forms of the disease in the hips and shoulders require total bone replacement. The role of core decompression in the management of avascular necrosis remains controversial.

Leg Ulcers

Leg ulceration is a painful and sometimes disabling complication of sickle cell anemia that occurs in 5 to 10% of adult patients. Leg ulcers are more common in males and older patients and less common in patients with alpha-gene deletion, high total Hb level, and high levels of Hb F. Treatment includes the use of wet-to-dry dressings soaked in saline or Burow's solution. With good local care, many ulcers heal within a few months. Leg ulcers that persist beyond 6 months may require transfusion or skin grafting, although results of the latter treatment have been disappointing. Treatment with oral hydroxyurea* may be promising. The role of hyperbaric oxygen and zinc preparations in the treatment of leg ulcers remains controversial.

Hematologic Manifestations

Sickle cell anemia is characterized by normochromic normocytic anemia with a mean Hb of 7.8 ± 1.13 and a mean corpuscular volume (MCV) of 90 fL. It should be noted that the MCV is within normal limits despite an increased number of reticulocytes (mean 13.2 ± 6.93), cells with high MCV. This presence of normocytic indices despite high reticulocyte count is sometimes referred to as relative microcytosis. The presence or absence of alpha-gene deletion has an effect on the anemia, the indices, and the hemoglobin electrophoresis pattern. Thus, patients with sickle cell anemia and homozygous α-thalassemia-2 ($\beta^S\beta^S$; -α/-α) have milder anemia, lower reticulocyte count, low MCV, and high Hb A_2 level. Both the white blood cell count and the platelet count are increased in sickle cell anemia owing to increased marrow activity secondary to chronic hemolysis and, in the case of platelets, to autosplenectomy. Normally, about one-third of circulating platelets are stored in the spleen, and patients with splenectomy typically have high platelet counts. Patients with splenomegaly (S-β-thalassemia, Hb SC disease, and sickle cell anemia with α-thalassemia) typically have low or low normal platelet counts, depending on the degree of splenomegaly.

Patients with S-β^0-thalassemia have a hematologic picture that is characterized by microcytosis, hypochromia, high Hb A_2 level, and variable Hb F values. The anemia in Hb S-β^+-thalassemia is mild and the Hb level is usually greater than 10 gm/dL. Hb SC disease is typically characterized by microcytic and hyperchromic red cell indices. Table 8 lists the sickle cell syndromes in order of the severity of the anemia.

In addition to the chronic hemolytic anemia typical of sickle cell disease, patients with sickle cell anemia may develop other types of anemia (Table 9). Hyperhemolysis (hyperhemolytic crisis) is characterized by a decrease in Hb level and an increase in the reticulocyte count, indirect bilirubin, and lactate dehydrogenase. Hyperhemolysis can be caused by infection (e.g., *Mycoplasma* pneumonia), coexistent G6PD deficiency with exposure to oxidant stress, or delayed hemolytic transfusion reaction. Recently, a hyperhemolytic state has been described during the evolution of the sickle cell painful crisis. Aplastic crisis characterized by a decrease in both Hb and reticulocyte values is most commonly caused by infection, both bacterial and viral. Megaloblastic crisis is occasionally seen in patients who become folate deficient

TABLE 9. **Types of Anemia Associated with Sickle Cell Anemia**

- Chronic hemolytic anemia
- Hyperhemolytic anemia
  - Infection
  - G6PD deficiency
  - Delayed hemolytic transfusion reaction
  - Painful crises
- Aplastic crisis
  - Infection
- Megaloblastic crisis
- Iron deficiency

*Not FDA approved for this indication.

owing to poor dietary habits and who do not take folic acid supplements. Iron deficiency anemia may complicate sickle cell anemia, especially in young menstruating females who refuse blood transfusion. Whether iron deficiency anemia has a salutary effect on the phenotypic expression of sickle cell anemia because of impaired Hb S polymerization secondary to decreased mean corpuscular hemoglobin concentration has yet to be determined.

Blood Transfusion

The chronic anemia of sickle cell disease is well tolerated by most patients. Hb S has decreased oxygen affinity and is thus efficient in delivering oxygen to tissues. Moreover, recent studies have shown that there is a direct relation between the frequency of painful crisis and the hematocrit value. Thus, the frequency of painful episodes in patients with SS and relatively mild anemia is greater than in those with severe anemia. It seems that the higher blood viscosity in patients with milder anemia may accentuate the severity of vaso-occlusion and, hence, the frequency of painful crises.

The two main purposes of blood transfusion in sickle cell disease are (1) improvement of oxygen-carrying capacity and transport and (2) dilution of circulating sickled red cells in order to improve microvascular perfusion. Specific indications for blood transfusion in sickle cell disease are listed in Table 10.

Exchange transfusion may be considered in patients with cerebral infarcts, fat embolism, acute chest syndrome, unresponsive acute priapism, or leg ulcers. It may also be required before eye surgery, possibly surgery on the central nervous system, or injection of contrast material. It must be emphasized that there have been only a few properly controlled studies of blood transfusion in sickle cell disease. Uncontrolled data from one study in which the Hb S level was kept below 30% by exchange transfusion suggest a significant reduction in the risk of recurrence of neurologic complications. A well-controlled study showed that prophylactic transfusion during pregnancy had *no* effect on fetal morbidity and mortality but was associated with decreased frequency of painful episodes. The evidence for the beneficial effects of blood transfusion in other situations, such as acute chest syndrome, priapism, and leg ulcers, comes from anecdotal case reports and uncontrolled studies. Any prolonged hypertransfusion or exchange transfusion regimen will result in iron overload and the need for iron chelation therapy.

TABLE 10. **Indications for Blood Transfusion in Sickle Cell Disease**

Hb <5.0 gm/dL and significant signs and symptoms of anemia in association with erythroid aplasia or hypoplasia (aplastic crisis)
Angina or high-output failure
Acute hemorrhage
Acute cerebral infarction
Acute splenic sequestration
Acute chest syndrome with hypoxia (PO_2 <70 mm Hg on oxygen)
Preoperative preparation with general anesthesia

Organ Failure

Almost all organs are affected in sickle cell disease. Table 11 lists the major systems affected, the manifestations of organ damage, and recommended management. Some of the manifestations of organ failure such as acute chest syndrome have been discussed. Others are as follows.

Infection

Sickle cell anemia has an unusual relationship to certain infectious agents. Individuals with sickle trait are resistant to infection by *Plasmodium falciparum*, but patients with sickle cell anemia are susceptible. Individuals with Fy(a-b-) red cells are resistant to infection by other types of malarial parasites. Several acquired abnormalities render patients with sickle cell disease immunocompromised and hence susceptible to a number of infections that are a major cause of mortality and morbidity. The increased susceptibility of patients to infection with polysaccharide-encapsulated bacteria (*Streptococcus pneumoniae* and *H. influenzae*) is secondary to absence of splenic function. Cellular immunity may be compromised by transfusion-related iron overload, and abnormalities in B cell immunity may explain antigen processing defects. Infections due to *Escherichia coli* are usually associated with urinary tract infection in adult patients. Patients with sickle cell anemia are susceptible to osteomyelitis secondary to *S. typhimurium* in addition to the usual causes of bacterial osteomyelitis such as *S. aureus*. The susceptibility to infection by *Salmonella* may reflect the ability of this organism to flourish in partially necrotic bone.

Central Nervous System

Neurologic complications occur in 25% of patients with sickle cell disease and are more common in sickle cell anemia than in other sickle cell syndromes (Hb SC disease, S-β-thalassemia). Cerebral infarction is more frequent in children, whereas intracerebral hemorrhage is more prevalent in adults. Microaneurysms involving fragile dilated vessels that develop as compensatory collateral circulation around areas of infarction seem to be responsible for hemorrhage in adults. Unlike other vascular beds, large vessels rather than microvessels seem to be the site of occlusion with consequent infarction. About two-thirds of children with cerebral infarction (who are not transfused) may develop further ischemic events within 3 years.

The appropriate therapy for a child with cerebral infarction due to vaso-occlusion is exchange transfusion or hypertransfusion to maintain the Hb S level below 30%. Red cell transfusions are usually continued for a minimum of 5 years after which transfusion therapy is individualized. Whether chronic transfusion therapy for adults with cerebral infarction secondary to vaso-occlusion is indicated or not remains

TABLE 11. **Manifestations of the Major Organs Affected in Sickle Cell Disease and Recommended Management**

Manifestation	Management
Central Nervous System	
Cerebral infarction in childhood	Exchange transfusion for at least 5 years and possibly for life. Iron chelation therapy
Cerebral infarction in adults	Transfusion in acute episode. Role of transfusion on a long-term basis unknown
Cerebral aneurysm	Careful follow-up. Consider surgery
Cerebral hemorrhage	Possible surgery
Seizure disorder	Avoid meperidine. Antiepileptic therapy if focal lesion identified
Ocular Lesions	
Retinal neovascularization Retinitis proliferans Retinal hemorrhage	Photocoagulation with either xenon arc or argon laser vitrectomy
Cardiopulmonary System	
High-output failure	Transfusion. Symptomatic and supportive therapy
Mitral valve prolapse with mitral regurgitation	Symptomatic treatment Prophylactic antibiotics for dental work-up
Acute chest syndrome	
Rib or sternal infarct	Symptomatic treatment
Pneumonia	Antibiotics, oxygen, hydration; simple transfusion if needed
Pulmonary infarct	Symptomatic treatment if mild; exchange transfusion if severe Care with narcotic analgesics
Fat embolism	Exchange transfusion
Pulmonary embolism	Anticoagulation therapy
Reticuloendothelial System	
Splenic sequestration	Transfusion; splenectomy Polyvalent anti-pneumococcal vaccine
Autosplenectomy, functional asplenia, or hyposplenia	Prophylactic penicillin in infants and children for a minimum of 5 years Polyvalent antipneumococcal vaccine
Hepatobiliary System	
Cholelithiasis/calculous cholecystitis	Symptomatic treatment; antibiotics; cholecystectomy
Mild hepatic crisis (bilirubin <50 mg/dL, mostly indirect)	Symptomatic treatment
Severe hepatic crisis or intrahepatic cholestasis (bilirubin >50 mg/dL and prolonged PT)	Exchange transfusion
Genitourinary System	
Urinary tract infection	Antibiotics
Hematuria	Strict bed rest; ε-aminocaproic acid, desmopressin acetate* Transfusion if severe
Priapism	Symptomatic treatment Benzodiazepines, pseudoephedrine HCl,* exchange transfusion, irrigation with epinephrine, shunt surgery
Proteinuria	One study suggests angiotensin-converting enzyme inhibitors
Nephrotic syndrome	Kidney biopsy; treat according to results
Chronic renal failure	Hemodialysis; renal allograft
Pregnancy	Comprehensive prenatal care in a high-risk pregnancy clinic Transfuse if needed
Musculoskeletal System	
Avascular necrosis	Symptomatic treatment. Bone replacement. Possible core decompression
Leg ulcers	Symptomatic treatment. Topical management with wet-to-dry dressings, hypertransfusion, or exchange transfusion. Possible skin graft
Osteomyelitis	Bone biopsy to identify organism and antibiotic sensitivity. If positive, intravenous antibiotics for 6 weeks

*Not FDA approved for this indication.
PT = prothrombin time.

unknown. Similarly, the appropriate treatment for an adult patient with cerebral hemorrhage has yet to be determined. A thorough search for aneurysms should be made, and surgical intervention considered.

Seizures in sickle cell disease may be secondary to an epileptic focus due to infarction or treatment with large doses of meperidine, or they may be idiopathic. Antiepileptic therapy is recommended for patients with abnormal electroencephalograms.

Ophthalmic Complications

Sickle retinopathy results from occlusive arteriolar lesions in the retina that lead to microaneurysms and collateral neovascular proliferation (the so-called sea fans). This is followed by vitreous hemorrhage and retinal detachment. Sickle retinopathy seems to be more common in Hb SC disease than in other sickle cell syndromes. Regular follow-up by an ophthalmologist is highly recommended since photocoagulation therapy of early retinopathy may prevent progression to neovascularization, retinal detachment, and blindness. The frequency of retinopathy is time dependent and age specific, and the older patient is at a higher risk.

Cardiac Complications

High-output failure, right heart and/or congestive heart failure, cardiac hemosiderosis, and cardiomegaly are known manifestations of sickle cell anemia. Recent evidence suggests that myocardial ischemia can occur as well, and myocardial infarction has been reported. Mitral valve prolapse was reported to have a high prevalence (25%) in sickle cell disease in one study but was not confirmed by another group. The signs and symptoms of mitral valve prolapse (e.g., chest pain, dyspnea, fatigue, syncope, palpitations) overlap with those of sickle cell disease and may elucidate the protean manifestations of sickle cell disease in case there is an association between these two disorders.

Genitourinary Complications

Urinary tract infection is usually caused by *E. coli* and is more common in females than in males. Its increased frequency in sickle cell disease may relate to renal infarction or to immunodeficiency. The hypoxic, acidotic, and hypertonic microenvironment of the renal medulla causes sickling of red cells in the vasa recta, leading to infarction of the renal medulla, hyposthenuria, and hematuria (gross or microscopic). Patients may also be unable to acidify the urine after an acid load. These tubular defects of the kidney (hematuria, hyposthenuria) affect not only patients homozygous for the sickle gene but heterozygotes as well (e.g., AS, SC, SD, SO). Enuresis occurs in children. Potassium excretion is also impaired, and episodes of hyperchloremic acidosis have been reported. Papillary necrosis seems to be more common in Hb SC disease. Hyperuricemia in sickle cell anemia is due to increased marrow activity with consequent enhanced purine metabolism and to an acquired defect in the renal tubules. Gout has been described in a few patients.

Nephrotic syndrome occurs infrequently with or without hypertension. Microscopic hematuria, proteinuria, hypertension, and the nephrotic syndrome are markers of incipient end-stage renal failure. The pathologic lesion is usually glomerulosclerosis. Once chronic renal failure sets in, patients require chronic hemodialysis and are candidates for kidney transplantation.

NEUTROPENIA

method of
ROBERT L. BAEHNER, M.D.
University of Southern California School of Medicine
Los Angeles, California

Neutropenia is defined as an absolute granulocyte count (AGC) of less than 1500 granulocytes per mm^3. The AGC is calculated as follows:

AGC = neutrophils + bands × total white cell count

Depending on the AGC, neutropenia may be noted during evaluation for severe infection or may be an isolated laboratory finding. Neutropenia can occur alone or in combination with other hematologic abnormalities suggestive of more generalized marrow disease, such as aplastic anemia or leukemia. The family history, association with other disease or cancer therapy, degree and duration of neutropenia, and ability to handle infection should be considered in the evaluation and management of neutropenia.

CLINICAL PRESENTATION

In the absence of infection, there are no signs or symptoms associated with neutropenia itself. The degree of neutropenia determines the probability of infectious complications such as sepsis, periodontal disease, or skin, mouth, or gastrointestinal ulceration. A history of recurrence of fever every 19 to 30 days is suggestive of cyclic neutropenia.

DIFFERENTIAL DIAGNOSIS

Isolated neutropenia can be either acquired or congenital. Certain congenital neutropenias are due to marrow failure, but most are benign and immune in origin. Patients with the latter type do well despite very low absolute neutrophil counts. Acquired neutropenia can be due to marrow failure, as in the case of drug toxicity; increased margination of neutrophils to the microvasculature, as in complement activation or severe burns; or peripheral destruction, as in hypersplenism or immune neutropenia. An important correctable, although rare, cause of neutropenia is vitamin B_{12} or folate deficiency. In the newborn, neutropenia may be a sign of sepsis. Primary or metastatic marrow malignancy can present with neutropenia; however, other hematologic abnormalities are usually present as well. Transient neutropenia can follow viral infection or immunization.

EVALUATION

In the absence of any clinical findings or history, isolated mild neutropenia requires only observation. Medications known to be associated with neutropenia should be stopped. Most postviral neutropenias resolve within 4 to 8 weeks. The blood count should be followed weekly until recovery and with each subsequent febrile episode until it is clear that the neutropenia is not recurrent. If anemia or thrombocytopenia develops in conjunction with the neutropenia, bone marrow aspiration should be performed immediately. If the neutropenia is persistent, bone marrow aspiration and biopsy, determination of vitamin B_{12} and folate levels, collagen vascular evaluation, and a serum antineutrophil antibody assay should be performed. Twice-weekly blood counts for 6 weeks are required to rule out cyclic neutropenia. Epinephrine or steroid stimulation tests and serum lysozyme determinations are sometimes done but are of no help in establishing a diagnosis or selecting treatment.

TREATMENT

Supportive Management

Supportive management of the neutropenic patient depends on the degree of neutropenia, the cause, and the patient's past history of ability to handle infection. Because it is not possible to predict the duration or progression of neutropenia at first presentation, management must be much more aggressive than in the case of chronic neutropenias. The absolute granulocyte count can be used as a guide (Table 1). There is rarely room for clinical judgment in the management of patients with absolute neutrophil counts below 250 per mm.^{3} If these patients have significant fever (>38.5° C [101.3° F]), they must be admitted to the hospital and then, after appropriate cultures are obtained, should receive empiric broad-spectrum parenteral antibiotics. Common bacterial causes of febrile episodes in neutropenic patients include gram-negative bacilli and cocci (*Pseudomonas aeruginosa, Escherichia coli, Klebsiella* species) and gram-positive bacilli and cocci (*Staphylococcus aureus* and *epidermidis, Streptococcus pneumoniae, pyogenes,* and *viridans* group, *Enterococcus faecalis, Corynebacterium* species). In the clinical setting of prolonged periods of neutropenia, concomitant polymicrobial and sequential infections are not uncommon. Systemic fungal infections, especially candidiasis and aspergil-

TABLE 1. **Clinically Significant Absolute Neutrophil Counts**

Neutrophil Count (granulocytes/mm^3)	Significance
>1000	Normal host defenses against infection
500–1000	At some increased risk; will still show signs of infection; may have chronic periodontal disease
200–500	Some protection but at great risk for infection; may not show signs of infection; usually treated with antibiotics parenterally in the hospital
<200	At marked risk of overwhelming infection; few signs of inflammation; must be hospitalized and empirically treated with antibiotics

losis, often occur during the course of broad-spectrum antibiotic therapy. Such a large armamentarium of highly effective antibiotics is currently available that it is difficult to recommend a specific antibiotic or combination of antibiotics. Based on the *1990 Guidelines for the Use of Antimicrobial Agents in Neutropenia Patients with Unexplained Fever* by the Infectious Diseases Society of America, the following regimens are suggested.

In patients without renal impairment, combinations of an aminoglycoside (gentamicin, tobramycin, or amikacin, 2.5 mg per kg every 8 hours), and an antipseudomonal carboxy- or ureido-penicillin (piperacillin [Pipracil], ticarcillin with [Ticar] or without [Timentin] clavulanic acid, azlocillin [Azlin], or mezlocillin [Mezlin], 350 mg per kg per day divided every 4 hours), or an aminoglycoside with a third-generation antipseudomonal cephalosporin (ceftazidime [Fortaz, Tazidime], or cefoperazone [Cefobid]), 30 to 50 mg per kg every 8 hours, are effective. Serum levels of the aminoglycoside should be monitored and doses adjusted as needed to achieve the following therapeutic concentrations: peak, 5 to 8 μg per mL; trough, 2 μg per mL or less.

In patients with renal impairment, combinations of a third-generation cephalosporin, such as ceftazidime or cefoperazone, 30 to 50 mg per kg every 8 hours, and a ureido-penicillin, such as piperacillin or mezlocillin, 350 to 500 mg per kg every 4 hours, are effective.

In patients in whom coagulase-negative staphylococci, methicillin-resistant *Staphylococcus aureus, Corynebacterium* species, or alpha-hemolytic streptococci are suspected (e.g., those with indwelling central venous catheters), vancomycin can be added later if gram-positive bacteria are isolated in culture or if no response is obtained from the initial antibiotics after a few days. In the author's opinion, this limits the number of patients receiving the drug therapy, reduces the costs of treatment, and minimizes adverse drug reactions and the development of antimicrobial resistance. If the cultures are negative and the fever has resolved, antibiotics can be discontinued after 3 to 5 days. If a source of infection is documented, specific therapy should be instituted, and it may need to be continued longer than in the non-neutropenic patient. Granulocyte transfusions may be of limited use in patients who have blood culture–proved gram-negative sepsis. For patients who remain febrile and neutropenic for more than a week, a systemic fungal infection should be diligently sought: Common sites include the lower esophagus, chest, and sinuses. Amphotericin B infusions starting at 0.1 mg per kg per dose in 0.1 mg per ml 5% dextrose water to a maximum of 1 mg per kg per dose should be infused over 2 to 6 hours on a daily basis. If a systemic fungal infection is identified, the course of antifungal therapy will be determined by the extent and response of disease. It is suggested that if after 2 weeks of daily doses of amphotericin B no discernible lesions can be found by clinical evaluation, chest radiograph, endoscopy, and computed tomography (CT) of abdominal organs, the drug can be stopped.

In treating children with benign congenital neutropenia, it is not always necessary to be as aggressive as one would for neutropenias of equal degree due to other causes. The child should be hospitalized and treated with parenteral antibiotics during the first few episodes of fever. If the child responds well to therapy, hospitalization will not be mandatory for future episodes, even though the granulocyte count may be below 250 per mm^3. Because most of these patients have immune-mediated neutropenia, a trial of high-dose intravenous gamma globulin, 400 mg per kg per day for 3 days, may result in a transient increase in the neutrophil count and is indicated for more serious infections such as pneumonia, osteomyelitis, or cellulitis. Steroid therapy (prednisone, 2 mg per kg per day) could also be used to raise the neutrophil count, but it has obvious disadvantages in the case of acute infection.

Standard reverse isolation procedures are of no benefit in these patients and probably hinder good care. Rectal examination and rectal thermometers should be avoided. Insistence on excellent dental care with regular professional cleaning and good oral hygiene is important.

Specific Treatment

During the past several years, remarkable progress has been made in the use of recombinant human colony-stimulating factors. Granulocyte colony-stimulating factor (G-CSF) and granulocyte-macrophage colony-stimulating factor (GM-CSF) currently are approved for use in the treatment of neutropenia associated with cancer chemotherapy and bone marrow transplantation. Patients with a variety of malignancies who receive GM-CSF after standard doses of chemotherapy have demonstrated significant reductions in the duration of leukopenia. Use of GM-CSF after high-dose chemotherapy with or without bone marrow rescue appears to hasten recovery of a normal white blood count and reduce infective complications. Definitive data are not yet available to guide dosage for most potential indications, but dose ranges of 0.3 to 10 μg per kg per day of GM-CSF appear appropriate. Subcutaneous injection is convenient and generally tolerated except for local site inflammation. However, the intravenous route may be used and is preferred for bone marrow transplantation enhancement. In cases of severe neutropenia resulting in significant clinical morbidity, such as congenital neutropenia (Kostmann's syndrome), cyclic neutropenia, and acquired idiopathic neutropenias, G-CSF administration has resulted in a dose-dependent increase in the levels of circulating neutrophils and a significant reduction in the number of infections. Dose levels of G-CSF required to achieve clinical success vary from 1 μg per kg per day to 20 μg per kg per day given either intravenously or subcutaneously. Sequential combinations of other bone marrow growth factors such as interleukin-3 and GM-CSF appear to have synergistic action in some cases of bone marrow failure, reducing the risk of neutropenia, associated infections, and thrombocytopenic bleeding. Clinical trials employing other combinations of bone marrow growth factors are under way.

Side effects of G-CSF include bone pain, which can be controlled by analgesics, and rarely, vasculitis. G-CSF is contraindicated in patients with known hypersensitivity to *E. coli*–derived proteins. Caution should be exercised in using G-CSF in any malignancy with myeloid characteristics. In order to avoid potential complications of excessive leukocytosis, a complete blood count is recommended twice a week during therapy. Side effects of GM-CSF include fluid retention, pleural effusion, pericardial effusion, respiratory symptoms, cardiac arrhythmias, and renal and hepatic dysfunction. Although rare, these side effects are potentiated by pre-existing organ dysfunction. GM-CSFs are contraindicated in patients with excessive leukemic myeloid blasts in the bone marrow (≥10%) or peripheral blood and in those with known hypersensitivity to GM-CSF yeast-derived products or any component of the product. Transient rashes and local injection site reactions have occasionally been observed, but no serious allergic or anaphylactic reactions have been reported. If the absolute neutrophil count exceeds 20,000 per mm^3 or if the platelet count exceeds 500,000 per mm^3, GM-CSF administration should be stopped. Biweekly monitoring of the CBC with differential should be performed to preclude development of excessive counts.

G-CSF is marketed as filgrastim (Neupogen) by Amgen, Inc. GM-CSF is marketed as sargramostim (Prokine) by Immunex and distributed by Hoechst-Roussel Pharmaceuticals, Inc.

HEMOLYTIC DISEASE OF THE FETUS AND NEWBORN

method of
JOHN M. BOWMAN, M.D.
Women's Hospital and University of Manitoba
Winnipeg, Manitoba, Canada

Hemolytic disease of the fetus and newborn (erythroblastosis fetalis) is characterized by hemolytic anemia, extramedullary erythropoiesis, and hyperbilirubinemia. Anasarca (hydrops fetalis) with fetal or neonatal death occurs in 25% of cases. Severe neonatal jaundice (icterus gravis) with the risk of brain damage (kernicterus) occurs in another 25%.

Since 1940, the complexities of the Rh blood group system have been unraveled, and many other blood group systems have been discovered. Sensitive manual and automated methods of screening maternal blood for blood group antibodies and measuring their strength have been developed. The pathogenesis of icterus gravis, kernicterus, and hydrops fetalis has been determined. Methods of diagnosing hemolytic disease after birth (a direct antiglobulin or Coombs' test), of determining severity of hemolytic disease in utero (amniocentesis, fetal blood sampling) and of treating the affected fetus and newborn (early delivery, fetal transfusion, exchange transfusion) have been introduced. Finally, prevention of Rh immunization is now possible with administration of Rh antibody in the form of Rh immune globulin (RhIG).

THE Rh BLOOD GROUP SYSTEM

Although other blood group antigens may cause alloimmunization and hemolytic disease of the fetus and newborn, the D antigen in the Rh blood group system is still the most important. According to the CDE nomenclature, there are three pairs of genetically determined antigens: Cc, D(d), and Ee. The presence or absence of D indicates the Rh-positive or Rh-negative status of the individual, since no antibody with the specificity anti-d has ever been found. It is the production of anti-D in the Rh(D)-negative woman and the transplacental passage of anti-D into the circulation of the Rh-positive fetus that causes hemolytic disease of the fetus and newborn. Each parent transmits a set of the three antigens, CDe, c(d)e, and cDE, to the fetus, who may therefore be Rh(D) negative (dd), Rh positive heterozygous for D (Dd), or homozygous for D (DD). The zygosity for D of the Rh-positive husband of the Rh-negative woman is important. If he is homozygous, all of their children will be D positive; if heterozygous, in each pregnancy the chances are equal that the fetus will be D positive or D negative. Only the D-positive fetus can provoke Rh immunization, and only the D-positive fetus will be affected by the anti-D produced. About 15% of whites are D negative, and almost half of those who are D positive are homozygous for D. The incidence of D negativity in other races is much lower, ranging from about 8% in North American blacks to less than 1% in Asians.

IMMUNIZATION

Blood transfusion remains a common cause of atypical alloimmunization to other antigens of clinical importance, such as c, Kell, C, and E. Only when there is a hospital or laboratory error is transfusion a cause of Rh(D) immunization. It is through transplacental passage of fetal D-positive red cells that the Rh-negative mother becomes Rh immunized. Transplacental hemorrhage occurs in 75% of pregnancies, increasing in frequency and amount as pregnancy progresses and reaching a maximum at the time of delivery. In the majority of cases, transplacental hemorrhage involves less than 0.1 ml of red cells, but on occasion the amount can be greater than 12 to 15 ml.

Following exposure to D-positive red cells, the development of a primary immune response is slow, requiring weeks or even months, and initially may consist of IgM, which does not cross the placenta. Immunization occurs in 8 to 9% of women at risk within 6 months after delivery of an ABO-compatible fetus and in 1.5 to 2% after delivery of an ABO-incompatible fetus. An equal number demonstrate that they were immunized by mounting a secondary immune response in the next Rh-positive pregnancy. In addition, sensitive enzyme screening tests have shown that 1.8% of women at risk undergo primary immunization during pregnancy.

The amount of Rh antigen influences the risk of immunization. As little as 0.1 ml of ABO-compatible, D-positive cells can provoke a primary immune response; a dose in excess of 5 ml will provoke a response in 65% of women. The overall risk of immunization is 16 to 17% if the D-positive fetus is ABO compatible. Spontaneous or therapeutic abortion carries with it a 2 to 4% risk of Rh immunization. Preeclampsia and obstetric procedures such as amniocentesis, external version, cesarean section, and manual removal of the placenta increase the risk of transplacental hemorrhage of fetal red cells and the risk of Rh immunization. The secondary immune response, which can be evoked by a very small amount of fetal red cells, is rapid in onset, strong, and predominantly IgG in nature.

HEMOLYSIS

IgG anti-D traverses the placenta and coats fetal Rh-positive red cells, which form rosettes around macrophages, primarily in the spleen. Phagocyte pseudopodia invaginate the red cell membrane, causing membrane loss, sphering, erythrophagocytosis, and ultimately lysis. Hemolysis produces anemia, erythropoietin production, compensatory medullary and extramedullary erythropoiesis, and hepatosplenomegaly with an outpouring of immature nucleated red cells.

In the most severe cases, portal and umbilical venous pressures rise and ascites develops. Further anemia and intrahepatic circulatory obstruction cause hepatocellular damage, hypoalbuminemia, and generalized anasarca. The fetus, now hydropic, either dies in utero or, if born alive, frequently cannot be salvaged.

In utero, the toxic product of hemolysis, unconjugated bilirubin, is cleared across the placenta. It is conjugated by the maternal liver into bilirubin diglucuronide and is excreted. Despite placental clearance, total bilirubin levels in the severely affected fetus at birth may be as high as 135 to 170 μmol per liter (8 to 10 mg per dL), a significant portion of which may be direct acting conjugated bilirubin due to hepatocellular damage. After birth, the infant's immature hepatic Y-transport and glucuronyl transferase mechanism cannot conjugate the large amounts of bilirubin produced. In the absence of treatment, the bilirubin-binding capacity of albumin is exceeded. Free, lipid-soluble unconjugated bilirubin traverses the lipid cell membrane of the neuron, interferes with vital intracellular metabolic processes, and causes neuron cell death. At autopsy, cerebellar tonsils, hippocampal gyri, and midbrain and medullary nuclei are stained yellow (kernicterus).

CLINICAL SEVERITY (Table 1)

Mild Disease

About one-half of affected fetuses are mildly affected. They develop only mild to moderate hyperbilirubinemia and anemia and recover completely without treatment (just as they did when no treatment was available).

TABLE 1. **Degrees of Severity of Fetal-Neonatal Hemolytic Disease**

Severity	Clinical Manifestations	Prevalence
Mild	Only mild anemia and moderate hyperbilirubinemia No treatment required	50%
Moderate	In good condition at birth near term, but unless treated will develop significant anemia and severe hyperbilirubinemia ending in kernicterus	25%
Severe	Hydrops fetalis with fetal death in utero	
	After 34 weeks' gestation	12.5%
	17–34 weeks' gestation	12.5%

Kernicterus

Twenty-five percent of affected fetuses are born near term, in good condition, but with mild to moderate anemia. If left untreated they develop jaundice, which progresses rapidly (icterus gravis), and within 2 to 4 days of birth they show evidence of brain damage. Initially they become hypotonic and refuse to suck; then they lose their neurovegetative reflexes, become spastic, lie in a position of opisthotonus, and may have seizures. Respiratory failure supervenes, and most of these infants die. The 10% who survive have devastating brain damage, characterized by choreoathetosis, severe nerve deafness, and some degree of mental retardation. Prematurity and its complications, such as asphyxia and acidosis, which lower the blood-brain barrier and interfere with albumin binding, increase the risk of kernicterus at bilirubin levels that would not be hazardous in a full-term, nonasphyxiated, nonacidotic infant. Similarly, the presence of salicylate, benzoate, or sulfonamide radicals, which bind to albumin, reduce reserve albumin binding capacity and increase the risk of kernicterus.

Hydrops Fetalis

The most severely affected 25% of erythroblastotic fetuses are grossly hydropic. Half become so between 34 and 40 weeks' gestation, and the other half, between 17 and 34 weeks' gestation. The majority die in utero. The occasional hydropic infant born alive presents with extreme pallor, gross ascites, and generalized edema. Pleural effusion and pulmonary compression frequently thwart all resuscitative attempts. Moderate disease and hydrops grade one into the other. Intermediate, prehydropic, and early hydropic babies present with severe pallor, marked hepatosplenomegaly, petechiae, and moderate edema. Although heart failure is usually not present at birth, exchange transfusion and other ancillary treatment measures frequently precipitate heart failure.

Mothers carrying severely erythroblastotic fetuses often present with polyhydramnios and a preeclampsia-like syndrome (the mirror syndrome). If the disease is ameliorated by fetal transfusion, the maternal syndrome disappears.

ERYTHROBLASTOSIS DUE TO BLOOD GROUP ANTIBODIES OTHER THAN ANTI-D

Anti-c and anti-Kell erythroblastosis do not differ in clinical expression from anti-D erythroblastosis, nor does anti-k (Cellano) in the very few instances when it occurs. Only rarely do anti-C and anti-E produce hydrops. However, since on occasion they do, mothers with these antibodies should be managed in the same manner as mothers who are Rh immunized. Although anti-A and anti-B have been reported to produce severe anemia and even hydrops, in 40 years of experience encompassing over 180,000 pregnancies 35,000 of which produced ABO-incompatible babies, 12,000 having cord blood red cells that were weakly direct Coombs'-positive, not a single instance of hydrops or severe anemia (cord hemoglobin less than 10 gm/dL) was found. Jaundice and the risk of kernicterus are the only clinical problems in anti-A and anti-B and for the most part in anti-C and anti-E hemolytic disease.

LABORATORY MANAGEMENT

Maternal Evaluation

Maternal blood group antibody screening during pregnancy is essential. Only if alloimmunization is diagnosed early and followed carefully will optimal clinical management be possible. At the first prenatal visit, the Rh group of maternal blood should be determined and the plasma screened for alloantibodies. Testing of the unimmunized Rh-negative mother should be repeated at 20 weeks' gestation and thereafter every 6 weeks until delivery, and she is a candidate for Rh prophylaxis at 28 weeks' gestation and after delivery if she remains unimmunized. At the time of delivery, a test for fetomaternal hemorrhage should be carried out to determine the presence and size of transplacental hemorrhage, if any.

If the mother is found to be alloimmunized, the specificity of the antibody and its titer should be determined. Repeat antibody titration should be carried out at 17 to 18 weeks' gestation and every 2 to 4 weeks thereafter until delivery. Since hydrops can develop as early as 17 to 18 weeks' gestation and fetal transfusions may be successful as early as 18 to 20 weeks' gestation, the antibody titer upon which further laboratory tests will be based must be known by 17 to 18 weeks' gestation.

Fetal Evaluation

History and Antibody Titer. The determination of the risk of hydrops and fetal death is based partially upon history and antibody titer. The disease is usually, but not always, as severe or more severe than in previously affected siblings. The risk of hydrops develops at antibody titers of 1:16 to 1:32. History and antibody titer by themselves will predict severity of hemolytic disease accurately in only 62% of cases. They do, however, allow the identification of the woman at risk, who requires further investigation in order to define the severity of hemolytic disease.

The management of the highly immunized mother and her severely affected erythroblastotic fetus requires all of the resources of a tertiary antenatal-perinatal-neonatal center. The primary care family physician or family obstetrician rendering antenatal care must follow the laboratory screening procedures outlined. If a history of severely affected babies or an antibody titer of 1:16 or greater places the present conceptus at risk, prompt referral to such a center for appropriate further investigative and management measures is mandatory.

Amniotic Fluid Spectrophotometry. Serial spectrophotometric measurements of the optical density of amniotic fluid at 450 nm, available since 1961, provide information about the severity of hemolytic disease. Bilirubin absorbs light at 450 nm, and the degree of absorption (the Δ O.D. 450) is an accurate measurement of amniotic fluid bilirubin. The amount of amniotic fluid bilirubin (a fetal product), when measured serially, is an indicator of the severity of hemolytic disease. The Δ O.D. 450 measurement predicts the severity of hemolytic disease with 95% accuracy and should be started as early as 18 weeks' gestation. Although amniocentesis carries no risk to the mother, traversing the placenta can be hazardous to the fetus and, by causing fetomaternal transplacental hemorrhage (TPH), may increase the severity of alloimmunization. Amniocentesis should be carried out in a tertiary unit with careful ultrasound placental localization, which minimizes the risk of placental trauma. It should be performed only when the maternal history, antibody titer, or both indicate that the fetus is at significant risk.

Recently the accuracy of Δ O.D. 450 measurements in predicting the severity of hemolytic disease during the second trimester of pregnancy has been brought into question. There is no doubt that in early pregnancy, Δ O.D. 450 measurements are not as reliable, but nevertheless, if serial measurements are made and followed carefully they are of some value in determining the severity of disease.

A modification of the amniotic fluid zone boundaries, inclining the zone boundaries downward before 24 weeks' gestation (Fig. 1), has increased the accuracy of prediction of severity of hemolytic disease in early gestation.

Perinatal Ultrasonography. The development of ultrasound imaging techniques in the late 1970s was a major advance in the management of maternal blood group alloimmunization. Ultrasound allows an estimate of placental and hepatic size and shows the presence or absence of edema, ascites, and other effusions (hydrops fetalis). It is of great benefit in assessing fetal well-being. It has increased the accuracy of placental localization and has reduced the incidence of placental trauma at amniocentesis. Ultrasonographic guidance is essential in directing the transfusion needle in both intraperitoneal and intravascular fetal transfusions. Following intraperitoneal fetal transfusion, ultrasound confirms the presence of blood in the peritoneal cavity and serial examinations monitor its absorption. At the time of fetal intravascular transfusion, ultrasound observation of turbulence within the fetal umbilical vessel as the blood is injected confirms that it is being transfused into the fetal circulation. Unfortunately, although ultrasound allows the diagnosis of hydrops with great accuracy, it may not identify impending hydrops. However, after fetal transfusions, ultrasound biophysical profile scoring provides an accurate assessment of fetal well-being and indicates whether improvement or deterioration is occurring.

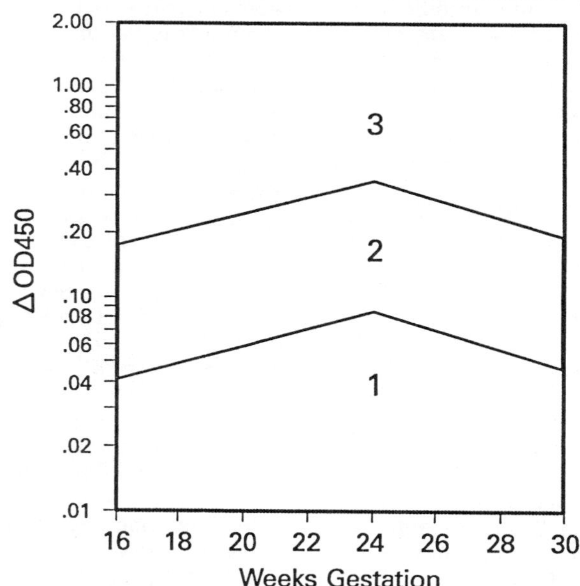

Figure 1. Modification of Liley △ O.D. 450 reading, zone boundaries before 24 weeks' gestation; zone boundary angle of declination before 24 weeks' gestation is the same as the zone boundary angle of inclination after 24 weeks' gestation. (From Bowman JM: Rhesus haemolytic disease. *In* Wald NR, [ed]: Antenatal and Neonatal Screening, 2nd ed. Oxford, England, Oxford University Press, 1994 [in press].)

Percutaneous Umbilical Blood Sampling (PUBS). Highly sophisticated real-time ultrasound equipment allows insertion of a 22- or 20-gauge spinal needle into a cord blood vessel (usually the vein) with surprisingly little risk. The fetal blood sample obtained thereby can be blood grouped and Coombs tested. Hemoglobin, hematocrit, serum bilirubin, serum protein, blood gas estimations, and erythropoietin levels can be measured and an accurate profile of severity of hemolytic disease can be obtained. If the cord insertion is accessible, PUBS should be carried out prior to any other form of fetal therapy.

Neonatal Evaluation

At the time of delivery, cord blood findings, taken in conjunction with the clinical appearance of the infant, will determine the need for and the type of treatment. A direct antiglobulin (Coombs') test should be done; it is positive in all forms of erythroblastosis with the exception of ABO hemolytic disease. However even in this condition, cord red cells are usually weakly positive if a sensitive Coombs' test is used. Cord blood hemoglobin and unconjugated bilirubin estimations reflect the severity of disease. Prompt treatment is indicated if the cord blood hemoglobin is less than 11.0 to 11.5 grams per dL or the indirect bilirubin level is greater than 75 to 85 μmol per liter (4.5 to 5.0 mg/dL). If the infant is premature or has been asphyxiated, prompt treatment should be carried out at hemoglobin levels of less than 12.5 grams per dL and bilirubin levels greater than 60 μmol per liter (3.5 mg/dL). Reticulocyte counts, although elevated, are not in themselves of much value in management; nucleated red cell counts are more helpful in assessing the degree of disease and the need for prompt treatment. The presence in cord blood of conjugated bilirubin of more than 45 μmol per liter (2.5 mg/dL) or heme (red/brown discoloration) is always indicative of severe hemolytic disease.

Whether treatment is required initially or not, serial hemoglobin and unconjugated bilirubin measurements at 8- to 12-hour intervals help to determine further management. Unconjugated bilirubin levels rising at greater than 7 to 8 μmol per liter (0.4 to 0.5 mg/dL) per hour or absolute levels of 170 μmol per liter (10 mg/dL) at 12 hours, 260 μmol per liter (15 mg/dL) at 24 hours, 300 μmol per liter (17.5 mg/dL) at 36 hours, 320 μmol per liter (19 mg/dL) at 48 hours, or 340 μmol per liter (20 mg/dL) or more thereafter are indications for prompt therapeutic intervention. These criteria may be modified somewhat if measurements of free bilirubin or reserve albumin-binding capacity are available. If the reserve albumin-binding capacity is greater than 50% and the infant is mature and not acidotic, there is little if any risk of kernicterus, and therapeutic intervention can be delayed until indirect bilirubin levels are 375 μmol per liter (22 mg/dL).

Thrombocytopenia is a common finding in severely affected infants. Platelet counts should be carried out at frequent intervals if thrombocytopenia is present. Levels below 30,000 per microliter carry a risk of cerebral, pulmonary, or gastrointestinal hemorrhage and should be treated with transfusion of platelet concentrate.

Persistent elevation of conjugated bilirubin to levels as high as 340 to 540 μmol per (20–30 mg/dL) is due to hepatocellular damage. Although it indicates severe disease that may have a poor outcome, conjugated hyperbilirubinemia in itself is benign. If the infant survives, the conjugated bilirubin levels subside over the first few weeks or months, leaving no residual hepatic damage.

Following recovery from the acute phase of hemolytic disease of the newborn, transient marrow inactivity with anemia is universal. Hemoglobin estimations should be carried out every 7 to 14 days until the infant is 6 to 10 weeks of age. The anemia is well tolerated and no treatment should be undertaken unless the hemoglobin drops below 7 grams per dL. After 6 to 10 weeks, marrow activity returns and the hemoglobin level rises without treatment.

DIFFERENTIAL DIAGNOSIS

Anasarca due to thalassemia or cardiac, renal, hepatic, placental, or idiopathic causes (so-called nonimmune hydrops) is differentiated from alloimmune hydrops fetalis by the lack of any blood group antibodies in the mother's blood and the failure of her serum to react with the father's red blood cells.

Other types of associated anemia and jaundice in the newborn (e.g., hereditary spherocytosis, enzyme-deficient hemolysis, extravasated blood) may also be differentiated by the absence of maternal antibodies and the negative direct Coombs' test of the infant's red cells. Other forms of indirect hyperbilirubinemia due to glucuronyl transferase inhibition or delayed development are not associated with anemia or a positive direct Coombs' test. The conjugated hyperbilirubinemia of hepatitis, biliary atresia, and galactosemia may also be differentiated from the conjugated hyperbilirubinemia of severe erythroblastosis by the absence of maternal alloantibodies and neonatal anemia and a negative direct Coombs' test.

On occasion, ABO erythroblastosis may be hard to differentiate from hereditary spherocytosis and enzymopathies if the direct Coombs' test is negative. Anti-A or anti-B red cell elution studies may be helpful, as may be studies of red cell enzymes and red cell morphology.

TREATMENT

Fetal Therapy

Management of a fetus who, according to amniotic fluid Δ O.D. 450 readings or fetal blood sampling measurements, has impending hydrops depends upon fetal maturity. If gestational age is beyond 33 to 34 weeks and the amniotic fluid lecithin/sphingomyelin ratio and phosphatidyl glycerol measurements indicate pulmonary maturity, prompt delivery is indicated, either vaginally or, in the presence of fetal distress, by immediate cesarean section.

If the fetus is immature (i.e., between 20 and 33 weeks' gestation) or is over 33 weeks' gestational age without evidence of pulmonary maturity, fetal blood sampling and intrauterine fetal transfusions, if necessary, should be carried out.

Fetal Transfusions

Fetal transfusion was initially done by the intraperitoneal route (IPT). IPT revolutionized the outcome for the 8 to 10% of affected fetuses doomed to become hydropic before 33 weeks' gestation. However, IPT is of little value for the moribund hydropic fetus who does not absorb blood from the peritoneal cavity and invariably dies despite IPT. Further, when an anterior placenta must be traversed by the IPT needle, the procedure carries a fetal mortality rate of 7%.

Following availability of highly sophisticated real-time ultrasound equipment and obstetric expertise in its use, not only could a fetal blood sample be obtained for laboratory tests, but also direct transfusion of compatible red cells into the fetal circulation could be carried out through insertion of a 22- or 20-gauge spinal needle into the umbilical vein. Direct intravascular transfusion (IVT) has improved the prognosis for those fetuses otherwise destined to become hydropic and die in utero; salvage rates varying from 75 to 90% have been reported. With this technique, moribund hydropic fetuses with hemoglobin levels as low as 1.0 gram per dL have been salvaged with reversal of their hydrops in utero. Direct IVT represents a major advance in the management of fetal hemolytic disease.

Neonatal Therapy

Exchange Transfusion

Exchange transfusion after delivery is the cornerstone of management. A two blood volume exchange transfusion removes about 85 to 90% of antibody-coated hemolyzing red cells, preventing anemia and further bilirubin production. However, it removes only 25 to 30% of preformed bilirubin. Bilirubin removal may be increased by the addition of 4 to 5 grams of human albumin to each unit of blood used. Prior to transfusion, a volume of plasma equivalent to the volume of citrate anticoagulant or anticoagulant plus added albumin should be removed from the blood unit to restore the hemoglobin concentration to normal.

The donor blood should be group O or group specific if the mother and baby are ABO compatible, and it must be negative for the red cell antigen to which the mother is immunized. It must be crossmatched against maternal serum for the initial exchange transfusion and against the previous postexchange transfusion blood sample for subsequent exchange transfusions. The blood should be not more than 96 hours old, or less if the infant is prehydropic, severely anemic, and/or thrombocytopenic. The exchange transfusion should be carried out in 10- to 20-ml aliquots. Careful attention should be paid to the venous pressure, with production of a suitable volume deficit if it is elevated, thereby reducing the likelihood of heart failure. Repeated exchange transfusions should be carried out for the indications outlined under laboratory management.

Phototherapy

Visual light in the blue spectrum bypasses the glucuronyl transferase mechanism, converting toxic unconjugated bilirubin into water-soluble nontoxic isomers, which are excreted in urine and bile. Phototherapy is a valuable adjunct in the management of all forms of neonatal hyperbilirubinemia, reducing the need for repeated exchange transfusions and sometimes obviating the need for exchange transfusion altogether. Since phototherapy does not prevent hemolysis, the hemoglobin level of the erythroblastotic infant must be followed carefully.

Albumin

Albumin administration (1 g per kg body weight per day) raises reserve albumin binding capacity. It decreases the risk of kernicterus and reduces the need for exchange transfusion. Albumin should not be given to the severely anemic infant who may be in borderline heart failure.

Phenobarbital

Phenobarbital* induces enzyme maturation and when given to the mother (30 mg three times daily) or to the infant (5 mg per kg per day) after birth, it enhances glucuronyl transferase formation and lowers peak bilirubin levels. Since there is a 48-hour latent interval, phenobarbital is not very effective once hyperbilirubinemia has developed.

Ancillary Measures

Optimal management of the very sick hydropic or prehydropic premature erythroblastotic infant will tax the resources of the neonatal intensive care unit. Abdominal and pleural paracentesis, mechanical ventilation, and treatment of congestive heart failure, thrombocytopenia, patent ductus arteriosus, and necrotizing enterocolitis may all be required. Every effort must be made to prevent hypoxia and acidosis, which can materially increase the risk of kernicterus, cerebral hemorrhage, and cardiac and renal failure.

Whether or not the affected infant has required intrauterine and/or exchange transfusion, progressive anemia in the first 6 to 10 weeks of life may require treatment. In the infant whose hemoglobin level drops below 7 grams per dL, 20 ml per kg of body weight of compatible packed red cells should be transfused by scalp vein.

Suppression of Rh Immunization

Only intensive plasma exchange and intravenous immune serum globulin (IGIV) have been shown to be of any value in reducing Rh antibody levels and ameliorating the severity of hemolytic disease.

Intensive plasma exchange is costly and its benefits are marginal. It will, however, reduce anti-D levels by about 75%. It should be reserved for the pregnant woman with a history of hydropic fetal death before 26 weeks' gestation and a homozygous husband. Ten to 20 liters of plasma should be exchanged weekly starting at 14 to 16 weeks' gestation in an effort to postpone the need for fetal transfusions until 23 to 26 weeks' gestation, when the hazards are less.

Large doses of IGIV* (400 mg per kg body weight daily for 5 days repeated every 3 weeks, or 1 gm per kg body weight daily each week), have been reported to reduce the severity of fetal hemolytic disease. IGIV may ameliorate hemolytic disease by reducing total (and anti-D) maternal IgG production by negative feedback. By saturating placental Fc receptors, it may also reduce transplacental maternofetal passage

*Not FDA approved for this indication.

of Rh antibody, and by saturating splenic reticuloendothelial receptors, interfere with macrophage rosetting and erythrophagocytosis of IgG-coated Rh-positive red cells. If IGIV therapy is elected, it should begin at 10 weeks' gestation, and it should not preclude other investigative measures such as amniocentesis and fetal blood sampling at the appropriate gestational age. Again, the only value of IGIV may be in delaying the need for fetal transfusions.

Prevention of Rh Immunization

Whether Rh immunization can be suppressed once it has developed is debatable, but there can be no question about its prevention. Von Dungern, in 1900, was the first to demonstrate that the administration of antibody to an antigen prevented active immunization to the antigen. This information was used 65 years later to develop a practical method of preventing Rh immunization. Experimental work and clinical trials have shown that Rh antibody administered in the form of Rh immune globulin (RhIG) (RhoGAM) to the Rh-negative, unimmunized woman carrying an Rh-positive fetus or delivered of an Rh-positive baby and therefore at risk of Rh immunization, prevents Rh immunization. To be effective it must be given prior to the beginning of the primary Rh immune response, and the dosage must be adequate.

Systematic administration of RhIG in doses of from 100 to 300 μg after delivery has reduced the incidence of Rh immunization by 85%. In order to reduce Rh immunization to the lowest possible level (95 to 97%), RhIG (300 μg) must be given in situations during pregnancy in which there is an increased risk of transplacental hemorrhage and Rh immunization, such as after amniocentesis, chorionic villus sampling, or obstetric procedures such as external version. It must also be given to the Rh-negative woman who threatens to abort or who aborts. If massive transplacental hemorrhage is diagnosed, or in the rare event of an Rh-incompatible blood transfusion, it should be given in doses in excess of 25 μg for every ml of Rh-positive red cells in the maternal circulation. It must also be administered routinely (300 μg dose) at 28 weeks' gestation if Rh immunization is to be prevented in the 1.8% of women at risk of becoming Rh immunized during pregnancy.

Conclusion

With modern management of hemolytic disease of the fetus and newborn, the perinatal mortality has been reduced from 13% in the mid 1960s to 3% in the early 1990s. With successful Rh prevention programs embodying antenatal, postnatal, and postabortion prophylaxis, the number of severely affected Rh erythroblastotic fetuses at risk of hydrops fetalis and neonatal death will continue to diminish but will never disappear entirely. The small number of severely affected anti-c, anti-Kell, and other antibody-related erythroblastotic fetuses will not change and will become of relatively greater importance as anti-D immunization becomes less frequent.

HEMOPHILIA AND RELATED DISORDERS

method of
PETER S. SMITH, M.D.
Brown University School of Medicine
Providence, Rhode Island

Hemophilia is one of the oldest described genetic diseases: its depredations were first depicted in the Babylonian Talmud (3rd–6th centuries). Four sisters, presumably carriers, had sons, three of whom died after ritual circumcision. For this reason the fourth was exempted from this rite by Rabbi Ben Galiel. But it was not until much later, in 1803, that the first medical description was published by Dr. John C. Otto, who described a Mrs. Smith from Plymouth, New Hampshire, all of whose sons bled excessively. The scientific approach by Wright in 1893 resulted in the recognition that the clotting time of hemophilic blood was prolonged. Addis realized that plasma was involved in clotting, since the time blood took to clot in hemophilia could be shortened by adding normal plasma. However, it was not until 1937 that it was established that the clotting property resided in the globulin fraction, the deficiency of which was noted in hemophilia.

As in many other diseases, treatment of hemophilia was predicated upon an understanding of its pathophysiology. Hence, it is understandable that until 1923, when Feissly reported the successful use of citrated plasma, treatment for hemophilia was crude and, at best, consisted of whole blood transfusions. Infusion of either whole blood or plasma, which contain 1 unit or less of coagulant protein per milliliter, easily caused fluid overload. In 1964, hemophilia treatment entered the modern era when Judith Pool discovered that the antihemophilic globulin contained within the plasma was enriched by cold precipitation of fresh-frozen plasma. This cryoprecipitate was some 20 times more effective in shortening the clotting time, and much less was required to stop hemorrhage. Shortly thereafter in the 1970s, chemical manipulation of cryoprecipitate resulted in a product several times more potent. This freeze-dried concentrate, which could be reconstituted quickly with water, was easily stored, had a long shelf life, and was portable. Concentrates ushered in the era of home care, which revolutionized the management of hemophilia while leading to almost complete normalization of the lives of people who, until then, were destined to be crippled, frequently hospitalized, and often died from hemorrhage at an early age.

Unfortunately, the euphoria brought on by these improvements was to be of short duration. The concentrates, each lot of which was derived from hundreds of donors, were contaminated in the late 1970s and early 1980s by a new pathogen. By the time the cause of acquired immunodeficiency syndrome (AIDS) was elucidated, the deadly human immunodeficiency virus (HIV) had infected half of the known hemophilia population, and more than 2000 persons with hemophilia have died.

The AIDS epidemic led to intensive efforts to develop ways to kill the virus in concentrates and to further purify them. A new generation of ultrapure products has reached the market, and as a result there have been no reports of seroconversion in previously untransfused hemophiliacs since 1985. There is now a wide array of products for treatment of hemophilia and related bleeding disorders, but before discussing their use, a review of the pathophysiology, manifestations, and complications of hemophilia is in order.

DEFINITION

Hemophilia is an X-linked recessive disorder resulting from a deficiency of factor VIII (hemophilia A, or classical hemophilia) or factor IX (hemophilia B, or Christmas disease). Hemophilia A is more common, accounting for approximately 85% of the cases. Although the term *hemophilia* has been applied to deficiencies of factors V, VII, and XI respectively, it is more properly reserved for more severe coagulation disorders in which there is spontaneous and profuse bleeding.

The prevalence of hemophilia is between 1 in 5000 and 1 in 7500 males. It is found in all countries and all races, although prevalences may vary. One-third of the cases are considered to result from spontaneous mutations, owing to the lack of a family history of abnormal bleeding. The factor VIII gene appears to be very mutagenic. The number of persons with hemophilia in the United States is estimated at between 17,000 and 20,000. There are women with hemophilia, but they are few.

PATHOPHYSIOLOGY

All patients with hemophilia A and some with hemophilia B have an aberrant clotting protein. When immunologic methods, such as rabbit anti-human factor VII, are used to measure factor VIII, the antigen is found to be present, whereas functional assays such as the activated prothrombin time detect decreased or no procoagulant activity. Therefore for factor VIII deficiency, the typical laboratory slip will show decreased VIII:C (factor VIII procoagulant activity, modified APTT assay) with normal VIIIR:Ag (factor VIII related antigen, an immunologic assay).

Factors VIII and IX are both involved in the activation of factor X via the intrinsic pathway of coagulation. In this pathway, several clotting proteins react upon each other to form the end product, fibrin, which holds together the definitive platelet plug.

Joints are thought to be the main location of bleeding because synovial vessels have thin walls and synovial fluid lacks tissue factor. With its iron and proteolytic enzymes, blood directly damages the cartilage cells and sets up an inflammatory response in the synovium. Ultimately, if bleeding is not stopped promptly by the intravenous infusion of clotting proteins, degenerative joint changes occur, ranging from the boggy chronically swollen, fully flexible, and painless joint seen in chronic proliferative synovitis to the fixed fibrous and bony fusion seen in ankylosis. More typical of hemophilia is the *acute bleeding episode,* often of spontaneous onset, involving the large joints of the knee, ankle, hip, and elbow. Initial discomfort leads to excruciating pain, swelling, and marked limitation of motion. A toddler may begin to limp and spare a limb before he cries inconsolably and parents, or the physician, notice joint swelling. Mucosal and cutaneous bleeding is less frequent because hemostasis is more platelet dependent in these tissues. Bleeding from the mouth, however, is common in toddlers, who often bite their tongue or cheek when falling and dislodge the clot with their tongue. By and large bleeding can involve any part of the body. Nerve damage may follow bleeding into a closed compartment such as the carpal tunnel or into the forearm or iliopsoas muscle sheaths. Intracranial bleeding usually follows trauma and is the most common cause of hemorrhagic death in hemophilia.

LABORATORY DETECTION OF HEMOPHILIA

The prothrombin time (PT) is normal, while the activated prothrombin time (APTT) is very prolonged, often over 100 seconds. The Ivy bleeding time is normal, but the template bleeding time is frequently prolonged. The platelet count is normal.

Hemophilia A and B are confirmed by specific assays using factor VIII– or factor IX–deficient plasma (modified APTT). Hemophilia A must be differentiated from von Willebrand's disease, in which VIII:C- and VIII-related antigens are often decreased and the bleeding time is prolonged.

CLINICAL SEVERITY

The clinical severity of hemophilia roughly matches the plasma level of the deficient clotting factors. In *severe hemophilia,* the factor VIII or IX levels are less than 1% of normal, and bleeding is generally spontaneous and frequent, often one or more times weekly. In hemophilia of moderate severity, the factor levels lie between 1 and 5%, and clinical manifestations usually follow trauma: a fall, a blow, a sprain or strain. The frequency of bleeding events depends largely upon how risky the patient's favored activities are and his level of training. Generally, such events occur at intervals of months. Persons with mild hemophilia often do not know they have a bleeding disorder, since it usually goes undetected until abnormal bleeding is noticed after major surgery or the diagnosis is established following presurgical screening. In such cases, the factor level is generally over 5%.

CLINICAL MANIFESTATIONS OF SEVERE HEMOPHILIA

Hemophilia may present in the neonate. Because of improved technology and techniques, bleeding from circumcision has become less frequent in developed countries. A thigh hematoma from the intramuscular administration of vitamin K is equally typical. Clinically, overt intracranial hemorrhage is rare. After a variable "honeymoon period" of months to a few years, clinical manifestations become evident as the hemophilic child becomes more active.

Common Bleeding Events. Hemarthrosis and Muscle Hemorrhage. The most common bleeding sites are the large joints and the limb muscles. The knees, ankles, and elbows are commonly involved. The episode may begin with discomfort or a limp and progress to agonizing pain, overt distension, and functional incapacity. With more experience, the patient learns to recognize the prodromal sensations. The physician is well advised not to ignore the early symptoms of bleeding, since delay in treatment can lead to both short- and long-term complications: contractures, subluxation, muscle atrophy, and progressive loss of cartilage and bone.

Some bleeding episodes are difficult to identify because they mimic other diseases. Bleeding into the iliopsoas muscle causes abdominal discomfort, which resembles appendicitis. The leg on the affected side is held in flexion at the hip, and there may be paresthesia on the anterior thigh because of femoral nerve compression. These manifestations promptly subside with factor infusions. Muscle bleeding is often acknowledged late by both patient and clinician, presumably because of the lack of pain receptors within the muscle. By the time of diagnosis there is usually much blood in the muscle compartment and discernible swelling. The affected part is held in flexion, the position of greatest comfort. The treatment of intramuscular hemorrhage consists of an infusion of 20 to 30 U per kg of factor VIII daily for at least 3 days. A shorter period of treatment is frequently followed by recurrence.

Occasional Bleeding Events. Hematomas, bleeding from the buccal mucosa, and bleeding from the urinary tract occur from time to time in both adults and children. Epistaxis in children can be a problem and can cause anemia. Hematomas tend to follow trauma or an intramuscular injection. Although they are rarely serious, they may become quite impressive in size. When located in the upper areas of the body, hematomas gravitate downward after a day or so, and discoloration is seen both at the primary site and below. Thus, a scalp hematoma can cause a raccoon's eye appearance suggestive of a basal skull fracture.

Rare Bleeding Events. Although skin lacerations rarely bleed excessively and require only an adhesive bandage, deeper lacerations with gaping borders will bleed excessively without both concentrates and suturing; suturing alone is not sufficient. Spontaneous hemorrhage into the central nervous system is fortunately rare but can be catastrophic. Trauma to the head is usually the triggering event. Headache that does not respond to minor analgesics suggests such an event and calls for immediate infusion. Bleeding into the retroperitoneum or the soft tissues of the neck is equally alarming and infrequent. The onset is typically preceded by trauma, such as a blow to the abdomen or the neck. This may eventually result in hypovolemic shock in the first instance and respiratory distress from airway compression in the second.

MANAGEMENT OF HEMOPHILIA AND RELATED DISORDERS (Table 1)

General Preventive Care

Routine immunizations may be given to children with hemophilia. To avoid hematoma formation, providers should either give a protective dose of factor VIII (about 10 units/kg) or apply pressure to the injection site for 15 minutes or more. Hepatitis B vaccine is recommended in all HBAb-negative patients.

Strong muscles function as shock absorbers to the large joints, protecting articular tissues from sudden compression. Thus physical fitness is effective in decreasing the frequency of bleeding events. Equally important following hemorrhage into a limb is physical therapy to restore muscle strength and joint range of motion.

Hemostatic Agents

The presence of pathogens in human blood has led to continuing efforts to purify blood derivatives by a variety of techniques on the one hand and to find alternatives to human blood on the other. There are an unprecedented number of products on the market, and the future holds the prospect of an unlimited supply of coagulation concentrates totally free from human pathogens, including those for hepatitis and as yet unknown microorganisms. Since early 1993, concentrates from nonhuman sources have been available through recombinant biotechnology for persons with factor VIII deficiency. All human-derived concentrates are either immunoaffinity purified to isolate the functional procoagulant or treated by a variety of physical and chemical methods to kill pathogens, or both.

Because of the rapid pace of developments, the Medical and Scientific Advisory Council (MASAC) of the National Hemophilia Foundation (NHF) periodically updates its recommendations on specific products for use in hemophilia. Copies are available from the NHF's Hemophilia and AIDS Network for Dissemination of Information (HANDI) at 1-800-424-2634. The therapeutic guidelines in Table 1 are based on these recommendations.

The following treatment guidelines are general and do not consider particular proprietary products. Treatment differs in hemophilia A and B and in patients who are seronegative or seropositive for HIV. *In all cases, recommended products have been virus inactivated by heat, pasteurization, solvent detergents, immunoaffinity purification, or a combination thereof.* No untreated products are currently available in the United States.

Severe Hemophilia. For persons with severe he-

TABLE 1. **Replacement Therapy for Bleeding Episodes**

Bleeding Event	Hemophilia A: Factor VIII Concentrates	Hemophilia B: Factor IX Concentrates or PCC	Von Willebrand's Disease
Joint–severe: tender, swollen, very painful	30 units/kg BW*	40 units/kg BW	Very rare: concentrates rich in vW factor such as Humate P† or Koate HP.† The dose is similar to that for hemarthroses in hemophilia A
Joint–moderate: slightly swollen, limitation of motion, moderate pain	20 units/kg BW	30 units/kg BW	
Joint–mild: mild discomfort	10 units/kg BW	20 units/kg BW	
Mucous membranes	10 units/kg BW	10 units/kg BW	DDAVP 0.3 μg/kg over ½ hour
Menorrhagia	10 units/kg BW	15 units/kg BW	As above, followed by OC
Life-threatening: intracranial, blunt trauma	50 units/kg BW	70 units/kg BW	Concentrates rich in vW factor as above

*The dose of concentrate is always rounded off to the closest vial.
†Not available in the United States.
DDAVP = desmopressin acetate; OC = oral contraceptives; BW = body weight; PCC = prothrombin complex concentrates; vW factor = von Willebrand factor.

mophilia A who are HIV seropositive, immunoaffinity-purified factor VIII products are recommended over those of intermediate purity because of data suggesting an association with preservation of helper lymphocyte levels. Inadequate studies preclude similar recommendations for recombinant products. For patients who are HIV seronegative, there is no evidence of superiority of one product over the other, although there is apprehension about transmission of viruses other than HIV that do not have a lipid envelope, such as the parvovirus and hepatitis viruses. Many clinicians, therefore, prefer to use the purest products available despite their greater cost.

Vials of concentrate are labeled in units and come in quantities of approximately 250 units, 500 units, and 1000 units. One always calculates the dose to the closest vial. High-purity products are now available for factor A and factor B deficiency, in addition to other virus-inactivated products of intermediate purity.

One unit per kg of factor VIII raises the plasma level by 2%, and the half-life is approximately 6 to 10 hours. One unit of factor IX per kg raises the plasma level by 1.5% and the half-life is approximately 24 hours.

Mild Hemophilia. There is constitutive secretion of endogenous sources of factor VIII in mild hemophilia that can be stimulated by certain drugs. Desmopressin acetate (DDAVP), a derivative of vasopressin, is effective at a dose of 0.3 μg per kg infused over ½ hour and generally triples the factor VIII level.

For all bleeding events *treat at the earliest onset of symptoms,* such as a limp or any other sensation recognizable by the patient as the beginning of a bleed. Waiting for paradigmatic symptoms too often results in significantly greater risk to life and limb.

For mucocutaneous bleeding (e.g., from the mouth or nose) aminocaproic acid (Amicar), an oral syrup, 200 mg per kg per dose followed by 100 mg per kg per dose q 6 h, or tranexamic acid (Cyklokapron) tablets, 25 mg per kg tid, are frequently effective without factor concentrate infusion. Both inhibit fibrinolysis and are generally given for 3 to 5 days.

Fresh frozen plasma and cryoprecipitate, even though harvested from fewer donors than concentrates, are used less and less frequently in hemophilia because they may still contain pathogens. The risk is reduced if cryoprecipitate is drawn from repeatedly tested single donors. A bag of cryoprecipitate contains about 100 units of factor VIII and a variable amount of fibrinogen. It lacks factor IX. Fresh-frozen plasma contains approximately 1 unit of any coagulation factor. There are better and safer products for treating hemophilia A and B, but fresh-frozen plasma retains its role in the replacement therapy of rare deficiencies of those factors for which there are no concentrates: VII, X, XI, and XIII. The standard loading dose is 10 to 15 mL per kg. If more is necessary, administration of a diuretic will decrease the risk of fluid overload. When fresh-frozen plasma is given repeatedly, prior administration of diphenhydramine and acetaminophen prevents minor transfusion reactions such as hives and fever.

Hemarthroses are classified for treatment purposes by severity. In *mild* cases there are no signs, simply recognizable sensations that herald the onset. It is wise to infuse 10 to 15 units of factor VIII or IX per kg body weight. Relief is almost immediate and the patient can resume his activities immediately. The signs of *moderate* joint hemorrhage include tenderness to touch, painful passive motion, and moderate swelling. The corresponding dose of concentrate is 20 to 25 units of factor concentrate per kg. For *severe hemarthrosis,* described previously, the dose is 30 to 40 units per kg.

The duration of treatment varies with severity: mild hemarthrosis requires only a single infusion, a moderate bleed, one to two infusions a day apart, and severe bleeding, several infusions once or twice daily. A hospital stay may be advisable in severe hemarthrosis for better pain control, limb immobilization, and even joint aspiration.

Muscle Hematomas. Inadequately treated large hematomas can cause nerve damage and contractures. Particularly vulnerable are muscles of the calf and forearm and the iliopsoas. Do not wait for swelling; pain is a sufficient indication for treatment. The dose is 20 units per kg repeated once or twice daily.

Superficial Skin Lacerations. These usually require only moderate pressure. Factor concentrate is rarely necessary.

Oral Bleeding. Children occasionally bite their tongue or cheek and may bleed when shedding teeth. Ten to 20 units per kg of factor VIII or IX followed by aminocaproic acid for a week is usually effective.

Gingival bleeding usually results from poor oral hygiene and can often be stopped temporarily with aminocaproic acid or tranexamic acid. A dental visit for plaque removal and restoration should be scheduled.

Life-Threatening Hemorrhage. A fall on the head, trauma to the neck, or a blow to the abdomen can cause serious hemorrhage. Give 40 to 50 units per kg of the missing factor (VIII or IX), admit, and observe closely.

Hematuria. Ten units per kg of factor VIII followed by increased oral hydration is often effective. Encourage the patient to drink frequently and not to remain supine for long periods lest clots form in and obstruct the ureters. Many clinicians empirically prescribe prednisone, 2 mg per kg for 1 week.

Major surgery. Surgery is safe if the factor level is above 80% for the procedure and the following two postoperative days. Usually a continuous infusion of 3 to 5 units per kg per hour of factor VIII and somewhat more for factor IX is sufficient. Precise factor levels should be monitored frequently in the perioperative period and daily thereafter and doses adjusted to achieve the recommended level. Maintain the level over 40% until the seventh to tenth postoperative day. Joint replacement surgery often requires longer periods of factor administration to allow for physical therapy. Daily boluses of 30 units per kg tapered to alternate days for up to 6 weeks postoperatively may be necessary.

Inhibitors

When there is a congenital absence of a protein, the body may recognize it as foreign when exposed to it, and such is the case in severe hemophilia. Studies show that from 10 to 15% of these people have inhibitors to the factor VIII coagulant protein. In factor IX deficiency, inhibitor formation is much less common. The appearance of inhibitors usually follows exposure to exogenous factor VIII, often within a year. There appears to be a genetic predisposition. Inhibitors are immunoglobulin G antibodies directed against specific regions of the factor VIII molecule. Disastrous consequences may develop when the titer is so high that the hemostatic effect of therapeutic infusions is totally suppressed. Clinically, individuals are said to be *high responders* when the titers rise rapidly to very high levels after infusion and *low responders* when titers rise slowly after exposure to factor VIII. In low responders it is often possible to achieve a therapeutic effect by simply infusing more factor VIII (e.g., 50 to 100 units per kg).

A number of options are available to treat patients with severe inhibitors, but because none is ideal, there is no best approach, although the first listed alternatives are currently favored.

Porcine factor VIII (Hyate C)* has the advantage of a slightly different molecular structure; this maintains its hemostatic properties while protecting it from inactivation by anti-human antibodies. Many people with high-titer inhibitors, however, quickly develop antibodies against porcine factor VIII, and if their titer is very high, porcine factor is usually not effective. Thus, Hyate C is best suited for persons with titers less than 50 Bethesda units.

Prothrombin complex concentrates (PCCs), of which there are several brands, are used for factor IX deficiency. They are deemed to be effective because they contain not only factor IX but also factors II, VII, and X along with small amounts of their activation products. They are said to have factor VIII inhibitor bypassing activity, which can be shown by the shortened activated partial thromboplastin time (aPTT).

Activated prothrombin complex concentrates contain the same factors as PCCs, but with a higher proportion of activated congeners; i.e., they are intentionally more thrombogenic. However it is still unsettled whether they are more effective than PCCs.

Although commercially not yet available in the United States, *activated factor VII,* which directly generates a clot through activation of the common pathway, has been at least as effective as aforementioned agents. It is likely to become available soon, owing to favorable clinical trials.

There are other options when none of the listed products is effective. Such very serious situations merit referral to a dedicated hemophilia center with expertise in experimental protocols. In these cases, the patient's antibodies are bound after passing his plasma through a column and infusing it with exogenous factor VIII.

*Not available in the United States.

Comprehensive Management

Hemophilia is a disease with protean manifestations and complications. Because it has an impact on every aspect of the patient's life, it is important that the patient be seen periodically in a center providing comprehensive hemophilia care. In this environment, the patient benefits from evaluation by a multidisciplinary team that assesses any long-term problems in a coordinated fashion. This approach has benefited a growing number of hemophiliacs in the Western Hemisphere. Several studies have conclusively demonstrated that comprehensive care not only results in better medical outcomes but is cost effective as well.

A representative center offers home care. After patients are acquainted with the theoretical and practical aspects of their condition, they or their parents are taught home infusion therapy so that bleeding can be arrested immediately. Many centers offer rehabilitative surgery: older hemophiliacs with advanced degenerative joint and muscle changes may undergo corrective surgical procedures to increase motility and decrease pain. Because of this, many have become self supporting. All centers offer psychosocial support and the services of a nurse specializing in hemophilia care, and many provide care for HIV infection, including access to national therapeutic trials.

The future bodes well for patients with severe hemophilia. Gene therapy trials in hemophilic animals have been successful, and hemophilia may be added to the very small but growing list of devastating diseases that can be cured by gene insertion.

PLATELET-MEDIATED BLEEDING DISORDERS

method of
DOREEN B. BRETTLER, M.D.
The Medical Center of Central Massachusetts
Worcester, Massachusetts

In primary hemostasis, platelets form a vascular plug after an initial injury and then provide a surface that promotes blood coagulation. Once a vessel is injured, the platelets adhere to subendothelial components and collagen in the vessel wall, a function that is enhanced by von Willebrand factor. Subsequently, aggregation between platelets occurs. This reaction is mediated by thrombin, released adenosine diphosphate (ADP), and thromboxane A_2, a product of arachidonic acid metabolism created when platelets are stimulated. Platelet secretion of serotonin, adenosine triphosphate, calcium from dense granules and fibrinogen, Factor V, and von Willebrand factor from alpha granules occurs in response to the same stimuli that cause aggregation and stimulates more aggregation. Platelet membranes contain multiple glycoprotein receptors that bind various proteins, such as von Willebrand factor, fibrinogen, ADP, and thrombin. Inherited bleeding disorders that are platelet mediated are most often due to qualitative defects involving membrane glycoprotein deficiencies or abnormalities of the granules. Acquired platelet-mediated disorders may be qualitative or quantitative.

CLINICAL PRESENTATION AND TESTING OF PLATELET-MEDIATED BLEEDING

Patients with platelet-mediated bleeding disorders most often present to their primary care physician with increased bruising, mucocutaneous bleeding, or both. Epistaxis, gingival bleeding, and menorrhagia may also be presenting complaints, and petechiae and ecchymoses may be found on examination. However, some patients are asymptomatic, with a decreased platelet count found only on a routine complete blood count. Before a work-up is instituted for thrombocytopenia, pseudothrombocytopenia must be ruled out. This is caused by platelet clumping secondary to the anticoagulant used in the tube, most often EDTA. If the smear shows platelet clumps, the test should be performed again using tubes that contain a different anticoagulant, such as citrate.

In addition to the platelet count, two clinical tests are performed routinely to evaluate platelet function: bleeding time (BT) and platelet aggregation. The bleeding time is dependent on platelet number as well as their ability to adhere and aggregate. There are various methods used to measure the BT, but most laboratories currently use a modified Ivy method, in which a commercial disposable spring-loaded blade is released when a trigger is pressed. A single incision 6 mm long and 1 mm deep is made on the forearm. At 30-second intervals, blood from the incision is absorbed on filter paper discs until bleeding stops. The BT almost always is prolonged if the platelet count is very low or the platelets are qualitatively abnormal. Up to 7 minutes is considered normal, but each laboratory has its own range. However, conditions unrelated to platelet number or function can also prolong the BT, such as collagen defects (Ehlers-Danlos syndrome), poor skin quality, and subcutaneous edema, and the BT should be interpreted accordingly.

Platelet aggregation tests are carried out to assess platelet function. They are most helpful when the BT is prolonged with a normal platelet count. The ability of platelets to aggregate with ADP, thrombin, epinephrine, and collagen or to adhere with ristocetin is assessed in an aggregometer.

TREATMENT

Inherited Disorders of Platelet Function

In these disorders, a specific membrane receptor on the platelet is absent or dysfunctional or the alpha or the dense granules may be absent. Several of these disorders may also have associated thrombocytopenia. Most of them are rare.

Bernard-Soulier syndrome, inherited as an autosomal recessive trait, usually presents in infancy or early childhood with ecchymosis or gingival bleeding. In adulthood, gastrointestinal bleeding or menorrhagia may be present. The BT is prolonged, usually over 20 minutes. The platelet count may be decreased markedly, and the platelets appear large on the blood smear. The platelets are unable to adhere to the subendothelial matrix mediated by von Willebrand factor because the platelet membrane lacks the glycoprotein Ib/IX, which is a von Willebrand factor receptor. The platelets aggregate poorly with ristocetin compared with normal platelets but respond normally to other agonists including ADP, epinephrine, and thrombin. If the patient is hemorrhaging, platelet transfusions are the best treatment. Desmopressin acetate (DDAVP) may shorten the BT and should be tried.

Glanzmann's thrombasthenia is inherited as an autosomal recessive trait and seen in populations in which consanguinity is frequent. It presents with mucocutaneous bleeding. BTs are markedly prolonged, although the platelet counts and morphology are normal. These platelets do not aggregate with ADP or epinephrine, although they may aggregate normally with thrombin. They are structurally abnormal, having a deficiency of glycoprotein IIb/IIIa complexes, which serve as receptors for both fibrinogen and von Willebrand factor, proteins necessary to support platelet aggregation. Treatment is instituted only for hemorrhages and is limited to transfusion of normal platelets. In contrast to Bernard-Soulier syndrome, DDAVP has no role in treatment.

Additional deficiencies of the platelet membrane are still being discovered but continue to be rare. If a patient presents with mucocutaneous bleeding and a prolonged BT, sophisticated analysis of the glycoprotein receptors on the platelet may be performed by specific laboratories.

Storage pool deficiencies encompass a variety of inherited defects of either the platelet granules or the secretory mechanism. Patients can present with mucocutaneous bleeding or increased postoperative blood loss. The platelet count is normal, but the BT is prolonged. On platelet aggregation tests, the second-wave aggregation caused by epinephrine and ADP may be absent and response to collagen decreased. Because aspirin and nonsteroidal anti-inflammatory drugs can cause very similar defects, patients should discontinue all such drugs before testing.

Alpha granule deficiency (gray platelet syndrome) presents with a mild bleeding diathesis, moderate thrombocytopenia, and a prolonged BT. Dense granule deficiency also occurs in *Hermansky-Pudlak syndrome* (oculocutaneous albinism) and *Chédiak-Higashi syndrome.* Platelet counts and morphology are usually normal, and the BT is usually prolonged.

In all the platelet release defects, if bleeding is severe, DDAVP at doses of 0.3 μg per kg intravenously is the treatment of choice. If DDAVP is not efficacious, a transfusion of normal platelets can be tried. It should be noted that in approximately 25% of patients who are found to have a prolonged BT, no defect is identified. If it is necessary to shorten the BT, as for surgery, a therapeutic attempt using DDAVP should be made.

Acquired Disorders of Platelet Function

Drug-Induced Platelet Dysfunction

Drug-induced platelet dysfunction is probably the most common type of acquired platelet disorder. Cyclooxygenase is an enzyme involved in converting arachidonic acid, found in abundance in the platelet membrane, to thromboxanes. Thromboxanes enhance platelet aggregation by causing granule release. Even at lower doses, aspirin irreversibly inactivates cyclooxygenase for the life of the platelet, thus inhibiting platelet aggregation, especially the second wave. Patients taking aspirin may have prolonged bleeding times and a slight increase in the risk of bleeding during surgery. Platelet aggregation studies may show a decreased secondary wave of aggregation. In general, patients should stop aspirin intake 4 to 6 days prior to undergoing major surgery. Nonsteroidal anti-inflammatory drugs also inhibit cyclooxygenase but not irreversibly. Thus, BTs may be prolonged and platelet aggregation affected, but if the drug is stopped for 2 to 3 days, platelet function should normalize. Ticlopidine (Ticlid), a new drug that is effective in the prevention of stroke in patients with previous transient ischemic attacks, is a more potent inhibitor of platelet aggregation than aspirin, interfering in vitro with ADP-induced aggregation.

Chronic Renal Failure

BTs may be prolonged in uremic patients; however, this may be associated with the anemia of renal failure. As the anemia is corrected with blood transfusions, or more recently erythropoietin, the BT normalizes secondary to the rheology of red cell and platelet interaction. In addition, the prolonged BT in uremia is thought to be secondary to abnormal platelet–vessel wall interactions, although the exact mechanisms have not been elucidated. Empirically, both conjugated estrogens and DDAVP at a dose of 0.3 μg per kg intravenously shorten the BT in uremic patients.

Liver Cirrhosis

Patients with liver disease also have prolonged BTs. As in renal disease, it is not clear whether the prolonged BT is due to platelet abnormalities or to the underlying disease. Patients with liver disease may be thrombocytopenic secondary to hypersplenism. Abnormalities in the multimeric structure of von Willebrand factor may also occur. DDAVP has been shown to shorten BTs in patients with cirrhosis and should be tried if normalization of the BT is a prerequisite for surgery.

Cardiopulmonary Bypass

Surgical patients on cardiopulmonary bypass may have abnormal platelet function, perhaps caused by the membrane oxygenator in the extracorporeal circulation. Thrombocytopenia can also occur secondary to hemodilution and sequestration. In some series, platelet dysfunction was thought to cause excessive bleeding, which seemed to diminish with the use of perioperative or postoperative DDAVP.

Quantitative Disorders of Platelets

The platelet count is considered decreased when it falls below 150,000 cells per mm^3, but the smear should be examined whenever there is an unexpected drop in the platelet count, because the platelets may clump with the anticoagulant. Thrombocytopenia can be secondary to increased destruction, which may be immune mediated or due to decreased production or sequestration.

Increased Platelet Destruction

DRUG-INDUCED THROMBOCYTOPENIA

Most cases of drug-induced thrombocytopenia are immune mediated. Quinidine or quinine can cause thrombocytopenia, which may be severe, with counts less than 10,000 per mm^3. Occurring approximately 2 weeks after ingestion, it is mediated by a drug-dependent IgG that binds to the platelet in the presence of the drug. The drug should be stopped as soon as thrombocytopenia is discovered. The platelet count will rebound within 7 to 10 days. Steroids have not been shown to be helpful in these cases, but intravenous gamma globulin (IVIG), 400 mg per kg per day for 4 days, can be used if there is an acute need to obtain an increased platelet count.

Gold-induced thrombocytopenia has been seen in patients with rheumatoid arthritis. It occurs in 1% to 5% of patients receiving gold therapy, appears to be HLADR3 associated, and is found mainly during the first 20 weeks of treatment. It is immune related, resolving when the drug is stopped.

Heparin-induced thrombocytopenia is a widespread problem because heparin is a commonly used drug. It occurs in patients who are receiving therapeutic or prophylactic heparin and even in those having heparin flushes for indwelling intravenous lines. Approximately 5% to 10% of patients receiving heparin develop thrombocytopenia, usually 5 to 15 days after administration begins. This side effect is more prevalent with bovine heparin than with porcine heparin. It is caused by an IgG antiheparin antibody. In about 20% of patients who develop thrombocytopenia while on heparin, arterial or venous thrombosis or both occur, paralleling the fall in the platelet count. Thrombosis is thought to be secondary to platelet activation and release caused by the binding of the antibody-heparin immune complex to the platelets. Patients receiving heparin should have daily platelet counts, and the drug should be discontinued if thrombocytopenia is noted. If the underlying thrombosis needs treatment, alternatives such as warfarin, a vena cava filter, or dextran should be considered. Ancrod, a derivative of snake venom that causes hypofibrinogenemia, has also been used at doses of 2 units per kg intravenously over 6 to 12 hours until warfarin becomes effective. Patients with heparin-induced thrombocytopenia should not be rechallenged with heparin unless absolutely necessary. Whether thrombocytopenia can be induced by the new low-molecular-weight heparins is now under study.

An abbreviated list of drugs causing thrombocytopenia is given in Table 1. If a patient develops thrombocytopenia while on multiple drugs, all drugs should be discontinued if possible, because it may be difficult to determine which particular drug is the causative one.

IDIOPATHIC THROMBOCYTOPENIC PURPURA

Idiopathic thrombocytopenic purpura (ITP) occurs most often in people between the ages of 20 and 50 years and is three times more common in females than in males. Although in children it may be associated with an acute viral infection, such a history is rarely obtained in adults. The patient may be asymptomatic or signs of mucocutaneous bleeding may be present. Platelet counts are usually below 100,000 and may be as low as 1000 to 2000 per mm^3. On peripheral smear, the platelets may be large. The hemoglobin and white blood cell counts are usually normal. Other disorders such as disseminated intravascular coagulopathy, sepsis, thrombotic thrombocytopenic purpura, systemic lupus erythematosus, drug-induced thrombocytopenia, and more recently, human immunodeficiency virus type 1 (HIV-1)–induced thrombocytopenia must be ruled out. Bone marrow examination shows normal to increased megakaryocytes, and if obtained, an antiplatelet antibody test may be positive. However, because the sensitivity of this test is poor, a negative result does not rule out the diagnosis. The disease is caused by an IgG autoantibody directed against Gp IIb/IIIa or other membrane glycoproteins. Treatment should be instituted if the platelet count falls below 30,000 to 50,000 per mm^3.

High-dose corticosteroids (prednisone 1 to 2 mg per kg per day orally) are usually the treatment of choice and should not be considered a failure until they have been given for 4 to 6 weeks. Both decrease autoantibody production and interfere with binding of the antibody to macrophage receptors. The platelet count will increase in most patients over 7 to 10 days, but only a small proportion of patients will achieve remission. Splenectomy should be considered in patients who are steroid dependent; the response rate is 60% to 80%. Danazol (Danocrine), a synthetic androgen/progesterone, at doses of 200 mg three to four times a day orally, will also increase the platelet count. Side effects include masculinization and hepatic toxicity. IVIG, 400 mg per kg per day intravenously for 4 days or 2 gm per kg per day for 2 days, has also been successful in the treatment of this disease. However, the rise in platelet count is usually transitory, making IVIG most useful when a rapid increase in the platelet count is necessary. Platelet transfusions are ineffective in elevating platelet counts and in general should not be used. If a patient with ITP who has had a splenectomy becomes thrombocytopenic again, both steroids and danazol can induce long-term remissions.

HIV-1 can induce thrombocytopenia that mimics ITP, and patients presenting with ITP should be questioned about risk factors for HIV-1 and tested if appropriate. Studies have shown that HIV-1 can induce autoantibodies against platelets as well as directly affect megakaryocyte production of platelets. Steroids and splenectomy have been successful in this setting, but fears of causing more immunosuppression have limited their use. IVIG has been used with good results, although elevation of platelet counts may be temporary. Anti-Rh factor (RhoGAM), given either intramuscularly or intravenously, also increases platelet counts in thrombocytopenic HIV-1 seropositive individuals and is much cheaper than IVIG. More recently, zidovudine has been shown to elevate platelet counts in this group, and it should be considered when CD4 lymphocyte counts fall below 500 cells per mm^3.

POST-TRANSFUSION PURPURA

Whereas the previously discussed diseases are caused by an autoantibody, post-transfusion purpura is caused by an IgG alloantibody that is seen 1 week after transfusion of red cells or other blood products. The antibody is directed against the PlA1 antigen on platelets in most cases and occurs in the small percentage of PlA1-negative patients who are receiving PlA1-positive platelets. The syndrome is thought to occur in previously sensitized individuals such as those with prior pregnancies or those who have received blood transfusions. Thrombocytopenia may last as long as 1 month. Treatment is problematic. Plasmapheresis to remove the IgG antibody has been successful in some cases, and IVIG has had some efficacy, especially in combination with corticosteroids.

Decreased Platelet Production

These disorders are covered in greater detail in other articles in this volume. The acute leukemias, infiltrative diseases of the bone marrow, and nutritional disorders such as vitamin B_{12} and folate deficiency can all cause thrombocytopenia and must be ruled out with appropriate blood tests and physical and bone marrow examination. Excessive alcohol intake can also cause thrombocytopenia by suppressing platelet production in the bone marrow.

Massive hemorrhage can cause thrombocytopenia secondary to the dilutional effects of replacement with banked blood that has few viable platelets and

TABLE 1. **Commonly Used Drugs That Can Cause Thrombocytopenia**

Heparin
Gold
Quinine/quinidine
Antibiotics
Sulfa drugs
High-dose penicillin/cephalosporins
Procainamide
Valproic acid

TABLE 2. **Treatment of Thrombocytopenia**

Treatment		Disease
Platelet transfusions	*Effective:*	TP due to decreased production, qualitative platelet disorders
	Ineffective:	TP due to immune-mediated destruction (e.g., ITP)
High-dose steroids	*Effective:*	ITP, HIV-1–induced TP
	Ineffective:	Drug-induced TP
Intravenous gamma globulin	*Effective:*	ITP, HIV-1–induced TP, drug-induced TP
	Ineffective:	Production defects or sequestration
Danazol	*Effective:*	ITP
Desmopressin (DDAVP)	*Effective:*	In some qualitative platelet disorders
	Ineffective:	In TP due to increased destruction or decreased production

Abbreviations: TP = thrombocytopenia; ITP = idiopathic thrombocytopenic purpura; HIV-1 = human immunodeficiency virus type 1.

the inability of the body to rapidly produce more platelets. Platelet concentrates should be administered after each 10 to 12 units of blood transfused to avoid this problem.

Increased Platelet Sequestration

The spleen normally acts as a reservoir for platelets and contains a large exchangeable pool (about 30% of the total platelet mass in a normal-sized spleen and up to 90% in an enlarged spleen). Thrombocytopenia can occur in splenomegaly of any origin, but usually in conjunction with leukopenia, anemia, or both. The thrombocytopenia is rarely severe and symptoms of mucocutaneous bleeding are not present. If the spleen is not palpable, diagnosis may require imaging studies. Splenomegaly can occur secondary to numerous disorders, such as congestion from liver disease, lymphoma, storage diseases, and infections. Splenectomy is rarely the treatment of choice unless it is performed for diagnosis or for relief of pain or early satiety. Because patients are rarely symptomatic, the underlying cause of splenomegaly should be found and treated.

Treatments for the various types of thrombocytopenia are summarized in Table 2.

DISSEMINATED INTRAVASCULAR COAGULATION

method of
ERIK Y. YEO, M.D., and
EDWARD M. CONWAY, M.D.
The Toronto Hospital, University of Toronto
Toronto, Ontario, Canada

Disseminated intravascular coagulation (DIC) is a potentially life-threatening coagulation syndrome characterized by an intravascular consumptive coagulopathy and thrombocytopenia that complicates an underlying disease process. Its clinical presentation is highly variable, ranging from asymptomatic laboratory abnormalities to minor or major bleeding, thrombosis, and/or hemorrhagic tissue necrosis.

The key to recognizing DIC lies in an awareness of its clinical presentation, associated diseases, and initiating mechanisms. DIC is an unregulated disruption of finely balanced procoagulant, anticoagulant, and fibrinolytic forces that otherwise maintain hemostasis in the vascular tree. The uncontrolled intravascular coagulation is usually triggered by sustained exposure of blood to a wide variety of cellular proteolytic enzymes, toxins, and cofactors, but most significantly to tissue factor (TF). Tissue injury or ischemia may lead to enhanced TF expression on and/or release from endothelial cells, leukocytes, subendothelial tissue, or malignant cells, or alternatively may result in the release of thromboplastic substances and/or various proteases such as occurs in acute promyelocytic leukemia (APL). Exogenous proteases, such as those from snake venom, or endotoxins released in bacterial sepsis cause activation of leukocytes, damage to endothelial cells, and activation of complement, all of which may also potentiate and initiate DIC.

Infection from a variety of viral, bacterial, or fungal organisms is probably the most common cause of DIC and appears to be characterized predominantly by thrombosis (purpura fulminans) rather than bleeding. The syndrome is more often associated with gram-negative infections accompanied by endotoxemia, particularly in patients who are either cirrhotic or asplenic, conditions in which clearance of invading organisms is impaired. Tissue injury/ischemia, such as occurs following trauma (especially cerebral), obstetric complications (retained dead fetus, abruptio placentae, amniotic fluid embolism, or eclampsia), and diffuse or organ-specific vascular injury (e.g., acute respiratory distress syndrome), also results in the release of tissue factors that may trigger DIC. Finally, clinical and biochemical coagulation abnormalities consistent with DIC may occur in the setting of malignant disease, including acute leukemia and many solid tumors.

As stated previously, the clinical manifestations of DIC are highly variable and largely depend on the underlying illness, the rapidity and extent of its onset, and the patient's ability to compensate for the consequent hemostatic defects. Thus, when the physiologic response of an affected individual is further compromised by, for example, hepatic disease (the site of synthesis of most clotting factors and the site of clearance of degradation products), that patient's susceptibility to DIC and its manifestations will be enhanced.

Depending on the balance between the forces of fibrinolysis and coagulation, bleeding or thrombosis may predominate, respectively. However, in severe DIC, the former process often appears to dominate. The bleeding diathesis may be caused by depletion of coagulation factors, thrombocytopenia, or hyperfibrino(geno)lysis (consumption of fibrin and fibrinogen) and is further exacerbated by the generation of fibrin(ogen) degradation products (FDPs), which inhibit fibrin polymerization and interfere with platelet function. The resultant systemic coagulopathy is most commonly manifested by bleeding at the sites of venipunctures and from the gastrointestinal tract, genitourinary tract, and pulmonary system, although devastating intracerebral bleeds can also occur. Petechiae and purpura are due to thrombocytopenia, possibly contributed to by vascular endothelial cell disruption, microvascular thrombosis, or both. Concomitant microvascular, or less commonly large-vessel, thromboses in DIC can lead to further tissue injury/ischemia with end-organ damage, including focal skin necrosis, acute renal failure, or central nervous system involvement with seizures, altered consciousness, and stroke.

DIAGNOSIS

DIC must be considered in the differential diagnosis of any acquired coagulopathy characterized by either systemic bleeding or multiorgan ischemia in a clinical situation known to trigger the syndrome. In a patient with an underlying illness such as an infection or malignancy, depleted clotting factors, thrombocytopenia, and evidence of fibrinolysis, the laboratory diagnosis can usually be made with a considerable degree of certainty and with a minimum of laboratory tests. Owing to consumption of coagulation factors, the prothrombin time (PT) and activated partial thromboplastin time (APTT) are typically prolonged. A prolonged thrombin time (TT) is evident in the presence of hypofibrinogenemia, the latter generally being clinically significant at levels below 100 grams per dL. Augmentation in circulating levels of products of fibrino(geno)lysis (FDPs, D-dimers) also contributes to prolongation of the PT, APTT, and TT. Consumptive thrombocytopenia results from thrombin activation of platelets and thrombi formation. In mild "compensated" DIC, fibrinogen and platelet levels may be normal or only mildly depressed. In these patients, circulating FDPs are a more sensitive indicator of fibrino(geno)lysis. Unfortunately, however, elevated FDPs are not specific for DIC. They can also be increased following surgery or trauma and can rise owing to diminished clearance by the liver, kidney, or both. D-Dimers are derived from the degradation of cross-linked fibrin by plasmin and are therefore a more specific marker for intravascular coagulation.

Newer assays that may be helpful in the diagnosis of DIC include decreased measurements of the physiologic anticoagulant antithrombin III (ATIII) complexed with thrombin (TAT). ATIII levels have been variably reported as an indicator of severity of disease, and rising levels may predict successful therapy. Other tests that may ultimately be diagnostically or therapeutically useful in managing these patients include the plasma levels of fibrinopeptide A, prothrombin activation peptide (F_{1+2}) and plasmin-antiplasmin complex.

Examination of the peripheral blood smear in patients with DIC may reveal evidence of red blood cell fragmentation (i.e., microangiopathy), presumably caused by shearing of the circulating erythrocytes on microvascular fibrin strands. This finding, however, is neither specific nor sensitive, but in concert with other clinical and biochemical findings may provide supportive evidence for DIC. Pathologic examination of tissue sections from patients with DIC may reveal deposition of a fibrin clot within the microvasculature with perivascular inflammation and hemorrhage.

DIFFERENTIAL DIAGNOSIS

The laboratory differential diagnosis of DIC includes clotting factor deficiencies, thrombocytopenia, or red cell fragmentation states. Liver disease causes the most difficulty in diagnosis because moderate thrombocytopenia, coagulation factor deficiencies, and raised FDPs can occur secondary to decreased hepatic clearance. Practically, hepatic disease often can be identified by evaluating the clinical setting and determining the Factor VIII level (Factor VIII is not synthesized by the liver) and the presence of D-dimers. DIC obviously can also occur in the presence of significant liver disease. Management, however, remains largely supportive (see further on) and is directed at reversing the initiating event(s). Finally, thrombotic thrombocytopenic purpura (TTP) and hemolytic uremic syndrome (HUS) may be confused with DIC. These may best be differentiated by their clinical presentation and the lack of abnormalities in PT, APTT, TT, and markers of hyperfibrino(geno)lysis.

TREATMENT

Successful management of DIC lies in the recognition and treatment of the underlying disease. A septic patient must be treated with appropriate antibiotics, infected abscesses should be promptly drained, and retained fetal products must be evacuated. Persistence of clinically significant DIC after appropriate treatment of the underlying process is an ominous prognostic sign. Therapy in all circumstances must be individualized and includes supportive measures to maintain circulation and oxygenation as priorities. While the underlying cause is being ameliorated, replacement blood products may be administered to temporarily treat the complications of bleeding and thrombosis. Blood products are *not* indicated for patients who exhibit laboratory evidence of DIC without clinical manifestations.

In the face of life-threatening bleeding and hyperfibrinogenemia (fibrinogen <100 mg per dL), fibrinogen replacement in the form of cryoprecipitate (1 unit per 3 to 5 kg of body weight) may provide temporary hemostasis, depending on the rate of clearance of the administered blood product. Coagulation factors and inhibitors may be replaced by giving fresh-frozen plasma while using the correction of the PT as a guide. Platelet transfusions (6 to 10 units) may benefit individuals with severe thrombocytopenia (<10,000 to 20,000 per μL) and should be given if there is major bleeding and the platelet count is less than 50,000 per μL. Empirical administration of vitamin K and folate is recommended because patients with DIC are often at risk of developing deficiencies.

Although heparin is generally not recommended in DIC and is of questionable benefit because of the theoretical concern over bleeding, there are selected situations in which it may be indicated. These include acute promyelocytic leukemia (APL), septic purpura fulminans, and malignancy. Low-dose continuous infusion of heparin (2 to 5 units per kg per hour) may be beneficial with increasing dose titration while monitoring the response with fibrinogen levels or FDPs. In APL, DIC will usually be exacerbated as chemotherapy is administered. Prophylactic continuous heparin is still controversial in this setting. Owing to a frequent concomitant augmentation in fibrinolysis, the addition of an antifibrinolytic agent such as ε-aminocaproic acid (Amicar), 4 to 6 grams orally every 6 hours, to the heparin may be considered. Antifibrinolytics are contraindicated for most other causes of DIC because of the risk of converting a bleeding disorder into a thrombotic disorder. DIC associated with sepsis that manifests as purpura fulminans or infarction and gangrene of the digits, extremities, and areas of fat distribution may also respond dramatically, both biochemically and clinically, to low-dose continuous intravenous heparin. Standard full-dose heparin is indicated only in cases of chronic DIC (Trousseau's syndrome) in which large-vessel thromboses occur. Other therapeutic options, such as the administration of ATIII concentrates, have recently become available and may be beneficial, but clinical experience is limited.

THROMBOTIC THROMBOCYTOPENIC PURPURA

method of
EDWARD M. CONWAY, M.D., and
ERIK Y. YEO, M.D.
The Toronto Hospital, University of Toronto
Toronto, Ontario, Canada

Thrombotic thrombocytopenic purpura (TTP) is a clinical syndrome predominantly characterized by thrombocytopenia and microangiopathic hemolytic anemia, but which also can include fever, neurologic symptoms, and renal abnormalities. Pathologically, TTP is manifested by the presence of intravascular hyaline thrombi that are primarily composed of platelets and fibrin. Since its original description in 1924, considerable progress has been made in the therapy of this disorder, although the precise etiology remains somewhat of a mystery.

The clinical course of TTP is extremely heterogeneous, and therefore a high degree of suspicion must be present in order to make the diagnosis. It may occur in both sexes at any age, although it is somewhat more frequent in females during the third and fourth decades. TTP not uncommonly follows a viral-like illness, but has also been reported with pregnancy, oral contraceptives, human immunodeficiency virus infection, a variety of drugs and chemotherapeutic agents (particularly mitomycin), neoplasia, vasculitides, including systemic lupus erythematosus (SLE), as well as bee stings, dog bites, and carbon monoxide poisoning. Thrombocytopenia, although often severe, usually results only in mild bleeding, most frequently manifested as petechiae and hematuria. The importance of examining the peripheral blood smear in patients with thrombocytopenia cannot be overemphasized. TTP is characterized by red blood cell fragmentation, a finding that may be subtle but is more often striking and diagnostic in the context of the other critical features of the syndrome. Polychromasia and an elevation in serum lactate dehydrogenase (LDH) are naturally found in this red blood cell destructive process. Neurologic abnormalities may fluctuate and vary from mild headache or confusion to major events, including focal or generalized seizures, stroke, and coma. Renal dysfunction is also extremely variable, ranging from microscopic hematuria to acute renal failure.

DIFFERENTIAL DIAGNOSIS

The differential diagnosis, although limited, is critically important in view of the urgency and complexity of therapy. Immune thrombocytopenia purpura (ITP) occasionally occurs in young women following a viral-like illness, and the symptoms may be confused with TTP. For example, a patient with ITP may present with fever, headache, and signs of thrombocytopenia and hematuria due to the low platelet count. However, the peripheral blood smear associated with ITP shows no evidence of fragmentation. Owing to the rarity of the syndrome, however, TTP is more often mistakenly misdiagnosed as ITP when the physician fails to examine the peripheral blood smear, and precious therapeutic time is lost when the patient is started on corticosteroids, rather than plasma exchange/infusion.

Disseminated intravascular coagulation (DIC) is a clinical and laboratory diagnosis that may also manifest itself with all the features of TTP. In TTP, however, coagulation parameters, including the prothrombin time (PT), activated partial thromboplastin time (APTT), and thrombin time (TT) are normal, whereas in DIC they are often prolonged due to consumption of coagulation factors and generation of soluble fibrin(ogen) degradation products. In individuals with underlying collagen vascular diseases, such as SLE, the diagnosis of TTP may be particularly difficult. Similarly, pre-eclampsia or the HELLP syndrome of pregnancy (the latter characterized by fragmentation (*H*emolysis, *El*evated *L*iver enzymes, and *L*ow *P*latelets) may resemble TTP.

Hemolytic uremic syndrome (HUS), predominantly a childhood illness, is often associated with verocytotoxin-producing strains of *Escherichia coli* in the gastrointestinal tract and is characterized by marked renal insufficiency, microangiopathic hemolysis, and thrombocytopenia, the latter two being generally less profound than in TTP. Although HUS usually follows a more benign course with considerably less mortality, the similarities between HUS and TTP suggest that they may actually be due to the same process, and they are usually treated identically.

PATHOGENESIS

TTP is characterized by intravascular aggregation of platelets that leads to microvascular thrombosis, fibrin deposition, and end-organ damage. Several theories have been proposed to explain the pathogenesis of this process. Plasma from some patients, particularly those with chronic relapsing TTP, have abnormal patterns of von Willebrand factor (vWF) whereby unusually large multimers (ULvWF) are synthesized and released by vascular endothelial cells and megakaryocytes. Evidence suggests that the circulating ULvWF multimers, which in normal individuals are reduced in size within the plasma, efficiently promote platelet aggregation and consequently lead to vascular thrombosis. Other investigators have extended this theory with the discovery that TTP plasma occasionally contains elevated levels of calpain, a cysteine protease that is postulated to enhance the formation of platelet aggregates via increased expression of platelet glycoprotein GpIIb/IIIa and proteolyzed ULvWF multimers. These and other proposed mechanisms (e.g., alterations in prostacyclin processing) are promising with respect to elucidating the pathogenesis of TTP and hopefully will lead to more specific and effective therapies.

TREATMENT

Until the last 15 to 20 years, the mortality in TTP was in excess of 75 to 80%. Currently, however, long-term survival exceeds 70%, and this reversal largely reflects dramatic improvements in therapy. In spite of progress in our understanding of the pathogenesis of TTP, treatment strategies remain largely empiric, based on the premise that there is either an excess or a lack of a factor in the plasma that results in the syndrome.

Since the early 1980s, anecdotal reports of the utility of whole blood exchange in altering the course of TTP have led to the routine use of plasma infusion and plasma exchange. Due to the rarity of TTP and the heterogeneity of the syndrome, clinical trials to determine the most efficacious treatment(s) have been difficult to design. Data from a large randomized multi-institutional study by the Canadian Apheresis Group (CAG) indicate that plasma exchange using fresh-frozen plasma (FFP) as the replacement fluid was superior to plasma infusion, although the latter clearly still has utility in many patients.

We currently recommend that all individuals suspected of having TTP be immediately started on daily plasmapheresis, exchanging 1.5 plasma volumes with FFP per day for 3 to 4 days, and then single-volume exchanges daily. If clinical and/or hematologic improvement is not apparent within 10 days, the replacement fluid is changed to cryosupernatant. This therapy is based on the following suppositions: (1) high-molecular-weight forms of vWF are absent from this blood product, and (2) a factor in cryosupernatant is important in controlling the metabolism of ULvWF multimers. Plasmapheresis is not available in some institutions, and sometimes there are delays in obtaining the necessary intravenous access. Nevertheless therapy should not be delayed, and plasma infusions of 8 to 10 units of FFP per day should be initiated promptly with careful monitoring of renal function. Fluid overload may be a complication, and occasionally individuals will require hemodialysis and/or ultrafiltration to manage the fluid load. There is little in the way of definitive data on the efficacy of antiplatelet agents. The CAG study used aspirin, 325 mg per day, and dipyridamole (Persantine), 400 mg per day, in both treatment arms, and we generally maintain patients on these drugs for 3 to 6 months from the time of diagnosis. Responses can be monitored both clinically and by laboratory measures, including serum LDH, platelet count, and renal function. Red blood cell fragments may be found in the peripheral blood smear for several weeks following remission.

In 60 to 80% of cases, the syndrome is reversible with FFP exchange or infusion. Preliminary studies suggest that cryosupernatant is the superior replacement fluid, and its increased use might further improve the therapeutic results. Varying degrees of renal or neurologic sequelae may persist. Approximately 15 to 20% of patients will develop a chronic relapsing form of the disease and will require further treatments within several months to years. Further failure to respond is an indication to resort to one of several unproven, but occasionally successful, maneuvers, including pulse corticosteroids, splenectomy, and vincristine. For particularly recalcitrant cases, intravenous gamma globulin, cyclosporine (Sandimmune), dextran, urokinase, and prostacyclin have been used by other groups, but we recommend these only as a last resort. We consider platelet transfusions to be potentially harmful for patients with TTP.

The management of TTP in pregnancy is fraught with controversy. Much of the largely anecdotal literature suggests that evacuation of the uterus is most reliably beneficial. However, successful therapy with plasma exchange/infusion has been reported, and we therefore recommend an aggressive trial of plasma exchange as detailed previously, with consideration of immediate delivery of the fetus if the therapy fails.

In summary, TTP is a rare but serious life-threatening syndrome that requires prompt diagnosis and rapid therapeutic intervention. Appropriate management can yield dramatic responses, even in those with severe hematologic, renal, or central nervous system abnormalities.

HEMOCHROMATOSIS

method of
BENJAMIN N. SMITH, M.D., and
NORMAN D. GRACE, M.D.
Tufts University School of Medicine and Faulkner Hospital
Boston, Massachusetts

In the normal adult, total body iron content is approximately 4 grams, with more than half in the form of hemoglobin. Most of the remaining iron is stored as ferritin or hemosiderin in the liver (approximately 500 mg), spleen, bone marrow, and skeletal muscle.

The human body possesses no effective means of excreting iron. Iron homeostasis is therefore dependent on close regulation of iron absorption from food. In men, approximately 1 mg of iron is absorbed from the usual daily dietary content of 10 to 20 mg, replacing iron lost through sloughing of mucosal epithelium. In women of child-bearing age, approximately 1.8 mg is absorbed per day to replace additional losses from menstruation and gestation. Iron overload develops when absorption is inappropriately high for the level of iron stores or the usual regulatory mechanisms are overwhelmed or bypassed.

Therapy for iron storage disorders is based on clinical and histologic evidence that depletion of iron stores can arrest, and sometimes reverse, the toxic sequelae of iron accumulation in the liver and other end organs.

DEFINITION AND CLASSIFICATION

Iron overload syndromes are typically classified as primary or secondary. Primary iron overload refers specifically to hereditary hemochromatosis, an autosomal recessive disorder. Secondary iron overload includes other diseases that can result in abnormal iron loading (Table 1).

TABLE 1. **Iron Overload Syndromes**

Primary Iron Overload
Hereditary hemochromatosis
Secondary Iron Overload
Anemia with ineffective erythropoiesis
Thalassemia major
Sideroblastic anemia
Anemia with chronic hemolysis
Glucose-6-phosphate dehydrogenase deficiency
Hereditary spherocytosis
Anemia associated with folic acid or vitamin B_{12} deficiency
Liver disease
Alcoholic cirrhosis
Post-portosystemic shunt
Excess iron ingestion
Dietary: e.g., Bantu siderosis
Prolonged medicinal iron ingestion
Other conditions
Multiple transfusions
Chronic hemodialysis
Porphyria cutanea tarda
Other inherited conditions
Atransferrinemia
Zellweger's cerebrohepatorenal syndrome
Neonatal iron storage disease
Childhood familial hemochromatosis

HEREDITARY HEMOCHROMATOSIS

Hereditary hemochromatosis (HHC) is inherited as an autosomal recessive disorder. It is the most common inherited disease in adults, more common than cystic fibrosis. The gene frequency is approximately 5%. In the United States, more than 10% of the white population are heterozygotes and an estimated 0.2 to 0.7% are homozygotes. Thus, there are potentially 600,000 individuals in the United States with homozygous HHC, most of whom remain undiagnosed.

Clinical Features

In homozygotes, iron accumulation begins at birth, but clinical symptoms usually do not appear until 40 to 60 years of age. Presentation is delayed in women secondary to iron losses from menstruation and gestation. The classic triad of cirrhosis, bronzed skin, and diabetes mellitus reflects severe end-organ damage and fortunately has become an unusual presentation due to increased awareness of the disease and improved diagnostic tests. Today, nonspecific symptoms of lethargy and malaise, often in association with weight loss, loss of libido, and arthritic complaints, are more common presenting complaints. Physical findings include hepatosplenomegaly, testicular atrophy, loss of body hair, and bronze or slate gray skin pigmentation.

Because the liver is the primary storage organ for iron, hepatomegaly is detected in 90% of homozygotes at initial presentation. Liver function test abnormalities include mild to moderate transaminase increase and elevation of alkaline phosphatase. Manifestations of portal hypertension occur late in the disease. Hepatic disease is reversible and life expectancy is normal if phlebotomy is instituted prior to the development of hepatic fibrosis. Untreated complications of liver disease are the most common cause of morbidity and mortality, and 15 to 20% of patients with cirrhosis at the time of diagnosis will succumb to hepatocellular carcinoma.

Iron accumulation in the pancreas leads to insulin-dependent diabetes mellitus in 60 to 70% of patients. All the complications of familial diabetes mellitus may develop, including nephropathy, neuropathy, retinopathy, and vascular disease. Thirty to fifty percent of individuals show improvement in glucose metabolism with depletion of iron stores by phlebotomy.

Two forms of cardiac disease are described: biventricular failure from iron deposition in the myocardium and cardiac arrhythmias as a result of iron deposition in the conduction system, especially the atrioventricular node. The latter usually occurs in younger patients. One-third of patients with electrocardiographic changes at diagnosis improve with therapy. Impaired left ventricular function often improves with venesection.

The pituitary is the primary endocrine organ affected by iron deposition. Clinical and laboratory manifestations are generally confined to sexual dysfunction with loss of libido in both genders and impotence and low testosterone levels in men. Only 20% of individuals with this complication improve with treatment of the iron overload, and many men require exogenous testosterone replacement.

Abnormal skin pigmentation is a frequent occurrence. Bronze coloration reflects melanin deposition in the epidermis; a slate gray color reflects iron deposition in the dermis. Scars, gums, and the cornea may also be darkly pigmented. Skin pigmentation improves with treatment in 80% of patients.

The arthropathy of genetic hemochromatosis can affect any joint, but classically involves the second and third metacarpophalangeal joints. X-rays may demonstrate chondrocalcinosis. Aspiration of joint fluid yields calcium pyrophosphate crystals characteristic of pseudogout. Unfortunately, the arthropathy usually persists despite therapy.

Iron overload is associated with an increased incidence of infection by certain organisms, including *Yersinia, Vibrio,* and *Listeria* species.

Diagnosis

Laboratory Studies. In the patient with suspected hemochromatosis, serum iron, total iron-binding capacity (TIBC) and serum ferritin should be obtained. Bassett and colleagues* determined that the combination of a transferrin saturation greater than 50% (normal 15 to 45%) and an elevated ferritin level (>150 μg per liter, female; >200 μg per liter, male) has 94% sensitivity and 86% specificity for the detection of HHC in young homozygotes. There may be a falsely elevated transferrin saturation if the patient does not fast prior to testing. The serum ferritin level is an accurate reflection of total body iron stores. However, it can be elevated in a number of chronic inflammatory conditions, acute liver disease, and certain malignancies. Symptomatic individuals usually have ferritin levels greater than 1000 mg per liter. Bassett and colleagues† found that no subject with a serum ferritin level below 700 mg per liter had hepatic fibrosis or cirrhosis on liver biopsy.

Liver Biopsy. The gold standard for diagnosing HHC is liver biopsy with quantitative determination of hepatic iron. Iron deposition is seen primarily within hepatocytes. Hepatic fibrosis and cirrhosis are associated with a decreased life expectancy and an increased risk of hepatoma. Fibrosis generally does not occur unless hepatic iron concentrations exceed 22,000 μg per gram dry weight, although cofactors such as excessive alcohol consumption and chronic hepatitis C can lower the threshold. Symptomatic patients with hereditary hemochromatosis generally have

*See Bassett ML, et al: Ann NY Acad Sci *526*:274–289, 1988.
†See Bassett ML, et al: Hepatology *6*:24–29, 1986.

hepatic iron concentrations greater than 10,000 μg per gram. In heterozygotes and individuals with alcoholic liver disease and secondary iron overload, hepatic iron concentration is usually less than 10,000 μg per gram.

Some forms of secondary iron overload may lead to serum iron levels and histologic findings that overlap with those seen in genetic hemochromatosis. The hepatic iron index, which reliably distinguishes HHC from alcoholic liver disease and other forms of secondary iron overload, is calculated by dividing the hepatic iron concentration in micrograms per gram (dry weight) by the patient's age in years. A hepatic iron index greater than two is diagnostic for HHC.

SECONDARY IRON OVERLOAD

Most forms of secondary iron overload can be distinguished from HHC by the history and liver biopsy. The etiology of iron overload is critical when deciding whether or not to treat. Patients with alcoholic liver disease and iron overload do not benefit from depletion of iron stores. Oral iron rarely raises body iron stores above 3 grams, and manifestations of tissue injury other than hepatomegaly and fibrosis are unusual. In contrast, patients with chronic anemia and secondary iron overload due to ineffective erythropoiesis can develop the full spectrum of iron-related injury seen with HHC. The major lesions associated with iron overload in thalassemia are hepatic fibrosis and occasionally cirrhosis, pituitary insufficiency, pancreatic fibrosis, and as a late manifestation, cardiac arrhythmias and cardiomyopathy. Both the liver disease and the skin lesions of porphyria cutanea tarda may improve with phlebotomy.

TREATMENT

The goal of therapy is to remove excessive amounts of tissue iron deposits as rapidly and safely as possible to avoid further organ damage.

Hereditary Hemochromatosis

Phlebotomy is the mainstay of treatment in HHC. Patients often have body iron stores of 25 to 50 grams. A 1-unit phlebotomy (500 ml whole blood) will remove approximately 250 mg of iron. The phlebotomy protocol is as follows:

1. Obtain baseline transferrin saturation, ferritin, and hematocrit counts and then begin weekly phlebotomy of 500 ml of whole blood.
2. At each subsequent visit, if the hematocrit is above 34% and at least 80% of the baseline hematocrit, proceed with weekly phlebotomy.
3. If the hematocrit falls below 80% of baseline, delay phlebotomy 1 week and repeat.
4. Obtain serum ferritin and reticulocyte counts every 3 months. The ferritin tends to fall before the transferrin saturation.
5. If the patient's hematocrit remains below 80% of initial hematocrit for 3 consecutive weeks, assess for an iron-deficient state (the goal of therapy) by obtaining
   (a) Serum ferritin (<50 mg/L);
   (b) Transferrin saturation (<15%);
   (c) Reticulocyte count (<1.5%) and red cell indices and smears consistent with iron deficiency.
6. Occasional patients with mild anemia or advanced liver disease with ascites can tolerate phlebotomy only every 2 to 3 weeks or removal of only 250 ml of blood during each session. Patients with severe anemia and/or cardiovascular disease may not tolerate phlebotomy, and a chelating agent such as deferoxamine mesylate (Desferal) will be necessary.
7. Individuals with HHC continue to absorb excess iron throughout their lifetime. Therefore, after initial depletion of iron stores, venesection every 3 to 4 months is indicated to maintain an iron-deficient state. Serum ferritin can be checked annually to estimate iron stores and to adjust the interval of maintenance phlebotomy.

HLA Typing and Family Screening

The gene determining the phenotypic expression of hereditary hemochromatosis has yet to be discovered. However, it is known that the gene lies in close proximity to the HLA locus on the short arm of chromosome 6. HLA A3, B7, and B14 are more common in patients with HHC than in the general population. Once an individual with homozygous HHC has been diagnosed, HLA A and B haplotypes of the proband can be determined from serum and compared to that of blood relatives. Those first-degree relatives, particularly siblings, who are HLA identical to the proband are at high risk of developing the disease and should be carefully followed. Siblings who are heterozygous may develop slightly increased iron stores but will not have tissue damage. Nonidentical siblings have virtually no chance of contracting this illness. We advocate performance of iron studies in all blood relatives of the proband and HLA typing of the proband and his or her siblings.

Secondary Iron Overload

Phlebotomy is clearly impractical in iron overload syndromes associated with anemia. Chelation therapy with deferoxamine must be given parenterally. The method most commonly used is continuous infusion by way of a small portable pump. Administration of 2 to 4 grams of deferoxamine over 12 hours in adults results in urinary excretion of 50 to 100 mg of iron per 24 hours. Bolus infusion is much less effective.

Ascorbic acid has been used as an adjunct to deferoxamine to increase iron mobilization. However, because deterioration of cardiac function has been reported with ascorbic acid, it should be given with caution in doses of not more than 200 mg per day orally.

Side effects of subcutaneous infusions of deferoxamine include local irritation with erythema, urticaria, and pruritus. This may be alleviated with antihistamines and/or by adding small doses of steroids to the infusion solution. Systemic effects, which are rare, include bradycardia, hypertension, photopho-

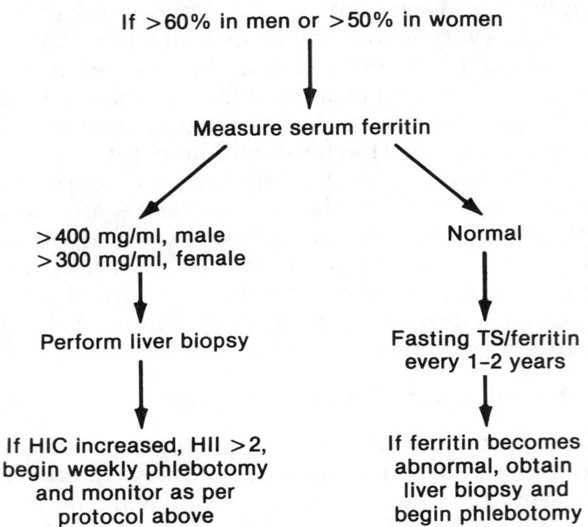

Figure 1. Screening for hereditary hemochromatosis: hypothetical algorithm. (Adapted from L. Powell and colleagues [personal communication].)

bia, headaches, auditory impairment, growth failure, and bone abnormalities.

In patients with thalassemia, treatment with deferoxamine has led to a marked prolongation of life expectancy by prevention of iron-induced cardiac disease. Studies of oral iron-chelating agents such as "L1" are ongoing.

Screening for Hemochromatosis

Many investigators have advocated inclusion of iron studies as part of routine health screening measures. A screening protocol is depicted in Figure 1. The optimum age at which to begin screening and the cost effectiveness of such an endeavor are subjects of active investigation.

HODGKIN'S DISEASE: CHEMOTHERAPY

method of
SIMON SUTCLIFFE, B.Sc., M.D.
Ontario Cancer Institute / Princess Margaret Hospital
Toronto, Ontario, Canada

Hodgkin's disease is a malignant lymphoma with a stable incidence of approximately 3.5 per 100,000 person years. It has a bimodal incidence with peaks in the early adult years and late middle life. It affects males and females equally. Despite uncertainty regarding the nature and lineage of the malignant cell and the etiology, current therapeutic approaches offer the potential for cure for 80% of patients with Hodgkin's disease. The principal goals in the management of Hodgkin's disease are (1) optimization of initial therapy regimens (radiation, chemotherapy, or combined-modality therapy) to maintain or improve on current cure rates with minimization of treatment-related side effects, (2) establishment of patient or disease attributes characterizing failure of standard therapy, and (3) determination of an optimal salvage therapy for those with disease progression despite the use of current, standard treatment.

DIAGNOSIS AND STAGING

Hodgkin's disease commonly presents as asymptomatic lymph node enlargement, most frequently in the cervical nodes and less commonly in the axillary or inguinal regions. Mediastinal adenopathy is common and frequently bulky, but it is usually asymptomatic and rarely causes vena caval or tracheal symptomatology. Presentation in extranodal sites can occur in patients with advanced disease but is unusual in the absence of clinical adenopathy. Similarly, presentation in the peripheral nodal regions (e.g., epitrochlear, occipital, submental, or preauricular) or involvement of extranodal tissues (e.g., nasopharynx, thyroid, or gastrointestinal tract) is unusual and should stimulate careful consideration of the diagnosis, because such presentations are much more common in non-Hodgkin's lymphoma.

The diagnosis of Hodgkin's disease is made by examination of appropriately prepared biopsy material, usually lymph node tissue (Table 1). Histologic subtyping is valuable insofar as it is prognostically relevant and also defines certain areas of controversy relating to the heterogeneity of Hodgkin's disease (Table 2). Biopsy of an extranodal site for diagnosis is less satisfactory and is reliable only if all histologic criteria are met or if an unequivocal diagnosis can be made from a lymph node biopsy.

PROGNOSTIC FACTORS

Traditionally, the principal determinants of therapy have been extent of disease and the presence or absence of systemic symptoms, both of which are considered in the staging of Hodgkin's disease. Based upon longer term analysis of outcome following radiation alone, chemotherapy alone, or combined-modality therapy, various other factors have been determined to influence response to therapy and survival (Table 3). In general, these prognostic factors either reflect, or are surrogates for, the tumor burden or probability of occult disseminated disease or the biologic potential of the disease and its response to therapy. The selection of optimal therapy should take into account determinants of prognosis, because the majority of factors predict primary treatment failure and thus direct the use of chemotherapy or combined-modality therapy in patients with localized presentations (clinical Stages I and II) or more intensive therapies in those with advanced disease.

The staging system for Hodgkin's disease is the Ann Ar-

TABLE 1. **Histologic Features of Hodgkin's Disease**

Effacement of normal lymph node architecture
Pleomorphic cellular infiltrate (lymphocytes, eosinophils, plasma cells)
Coarse bonds of fibrous tissue in the presence of the above cytologic features (nodular sclerosing subtyping)
Reed-Sternberg cells (multinucleated giant cells with prominent nucleoli) or variants (e.g., lacunar cells)
Reed-Sternberg cells, commonly $CD30^+$, $CD15^+$, $CD45^-$
No evidence of clonal cell population on phenotypic or genotypic analysis of whole tissue cell suspension

TABLE 2. **Histologic Subtypes of Hodgkin's Disease**

Subtype	Incidence (%)	Associated Features
Lymphocyte predominant (LP)	<10	Early disease; localized stage; adolescent and young adult incidence peak. Nodular LP subtype now considered to be a low-grade B cell non-Hodgkin's lymphoma
Nodular sclerosis (NS)	65	Mediastinal adenopathy common. Evidence for heterogeneity in NS type 1 (cellular phase, prognostically more favorable) and NS type 2 (cellular depletion, prognostically less favorable)
Mixed cellularity (MC)	25	More common in older age peak, greater tendency for disseminated nodal disease, advanced disease
Lymphocyte depletion (LD)	<10	Rare presentation previously characterized by more advanced, symptomatic disease in older age groups. In previously untreated patients, differential diagnosis includes T cell lymphoma variants. LD Hodgkin's disease should be diagnosed with caution and with phenotypic or genotypic assistance

bor Classification (Table 4), an anatomically based classification requiring clinical, radiologic, radionuclide, or tissue biopsy information (Table 5) for designation of a clinical stage (defined without tissue biopsy information other than the diagnostic node biopsy) or a pathologic stage (defined by evaluation of tissue samples taken at laparotomy and splenectomy or from biopsy of selected extranodal sites, e.g., liver, lung, bone marrow). Although the majority of patients are asymptomatic, mass lesion, specific disease-related symptomatology comprising fever, night sweats, and unexplained weight loss (i.e., B symptoms; see Table 6) should be actively elicited as it constitutes an important prognostic determinant influencing therapy.

Laparotomy series have indicated that optimal clinical staging will not detect occult abdominal disease (most often in the spleen or upper abdominal lymph nodes). In an unselected population of patients with Stages I and II supradiaphragmatic Hodgkin's disease, approximately 30% will have occult abdominal disease. Detailed analysis of prognostic factors indicates that many attributes reflect occult disease and therefore correlate with the demonstration of splenic or intra-abdominal nodal disease at laparotomy. Consequently, as treatment regimens have become established according to multiple prognostic determinants, including Ann Arbor stage and symptoms, the routine use of staging laparotomy and splenectomy in patients with early-stage disease has greatly diminished. Laparotomy remains a valid diagnostic and staging procedure for patients presenting with intra-abdominal disease and in those centers where therapy is critically dependent upon accurate intra-abdominal disease definition. Laparotomy and splenectomy no longer have any role in patients with clinical Stage IIIB or IV disease.

TREATMENT

Chemotherapy for Primary Management

Early-Stage Disease. Historically, the standard therapy for Stages I and II Hodgkin's disease has involved external-beam radiation therapy (RT) alone. Such an approach has resulted in excellent disease control with relapse-free rates of 60 to 85% and long-term overall survival rates of 70 to 85%. However, depending on selection factors, 15 to 40% of patients treated with RT alone developed recurrence of disease. Although chemotherapy has been recognized for the past two decades as the primary therapy for advanced Hodgkin's disease, a more detailed understanding of the attributes characterizing disease progression after RT has led to an increased use of combined-modality therapy (chemotherapy and RT) in selected patients with early or localized Hodgkin's disease. In practice, if patients with Stages I and II Hodgkin's disease are estimated to have a relapse risk in excess of 30% based upon analysis of pretreatment prognostic attributes, a strong case exists for combined-modality therapy. Indicators for chemotherapy as a component of primary therapy for clini-

TABLE 3. **Prognostic Factors in Hodgkin's Disease**

Prognostic Factor	Early Stage*	Advanced Stage†	Comments
Stage	I vs. II	III vs. IV	See Table 4
Symptoms	A vs. B	A vs. B	See Table 5
Histology	LP/NS vs. MC/LD	–	Impact of histology seen principally in patients treated with RT
Disease sites	≤3 nodal sites vs. >3	1 vs. multiple extranodal sites	
Tumor burden	Bulk and number of sites	Bulk and number of sites	
Large mediastinal mass	Non/small vs. large	–	Impact on intrathoracic disease control in patients treated with RT
Age	<50 yr vs. >50 yr	<50 yr vs. >50 yr	
Sex	Male < female	Male < female	
ESR	<50 mm/hr vs. >50	—	
Anemia	—	Hb <10 gm/L	
Lymphocytopenia	—	<500–1000/mm^3	

*Clinical Stages I and II.
†Clinical Stages III and IV and recurrent disease.
LP = lymphocyte predominant; NS = nodular sclerosis; MC = mixed cellularity; LD = lymphocyte depletion; ESR = erythrocyte sedimentation rate; Hb = hemoglobin; RT = radiation therapy.

TABLE 4. **Ann Arbor Staging of Hodgkin's Disease**

Stage	Involvement
I	Single lymph node region
II	Two or more lymph node regions on the same side of the diaphragm
III	Lymph nodes on both sides of diaphragm (the spleen is considered a lymph node in this classification)
IV	Disseminated involvement of one or more extralymphatic organs or tissue, with or without associated lymph node involvement

*All stages can be A (asymptomatic) or B (symptomatic). Stage III can be subdivided into III_1 (involvement of upper abdomen, i.e, spleen, splenic hilar, celiac, or porta hepatis nodes) or III_2 (involvement of lower abdomen, i.e., para-aortic, mesenteric, pelvic, or inguinofemoral nodes). Stage IV, disseminated involvement, is distinguished from E disease (applicable to Stages I to III), in which extension into an extranodal site occurs contiguous with adjacent nodal disease. The distinction of E disease from Stage IV disease is therapeutically valid only if the extranodal extension can be encompassed with the nodal disease and relevant lymphatic pathways in an appropriate irradiation field to the full therapeutic radiation dose.

TABLE 6. **Prognostically Relevant Symptomatology of Hodgkin's Disease**

Symptoms	Characteristics
Fever	>38.4° C; repeat episodes; no documented infectious cause
Night sweats	Repeated episodes, sufficient to moisten night attire or bed linens
Weight loss	>10% body weight in 6 months prior to diagnosis, in absence of other identifiable cause

*If any or all symptoms are present, disease is classified as B; if all symptoms are absent, disease is classified as A. Other relevant symptoms/history include lassitude, anorexia, generalized pruritus, alcohol-induced pain, and immunodeficiency state (congenital or acquired, e.g., HIV infection or predisposition; therapeutic immunosuppression).

cal Stages I and II Hodgkin's disease are shown in Table 7. They are predictive for an increased risk of failure following RT either locoregionally (massive mediastinal disease, extranodal intrathoracic extension) or distantly, i.e., outside the irradiated area (B symptoms,* age, histology, erythrocyte sedimentation rate, number of nodal sites). Combined-modality therapy increases remission rate and freedom from relapse, but to date has not been shown to improve overall survival over that with chemotherapy given as salvage treatment.

The rationale for combined-modality therapy is based upon (1) the ability of chemotherapy to control occult disseminated disease and to reduce the tumor bulk to optimize radiation field disposition, and (2) the effectiveness of radiation in achieving very high disease control rates within the radiation field. There is no evidence for synergy between the two therapies, but the benefits are additive. Such an approach, however, necessitates exposure to the acute and late complications of both therapies. Given increasing realization that the late complications of therapy contribute as much to mortality in early-stage Hodgkin's disease as the disease itself, the use of each component of combined-modality therapy requires critical evaluation. A recent National Cancer Institute study established equal efficacy of MOPP chemotherapy (Table 8) and radiation therapy in a randomized comparison in unselected cohorts of patients with early-stage Hodgkin's disease. If efficacy of disease control is equivalent, the principal problem becomes determining what constitutes optimal therapy when all causes of late morbidity and mortality are considered, with overall survival as the primary end point. Such a study would compare an optimized program incorporating RT alone or in combined-modality therapy with a chemotherapy regimen of established effectiveness and low late morbidity, such as ABVD (Table 9), and would require long-term follow-up to identify all principal causes of late morbidity and mortality. The results of such a study to determine optimal therapy for early-stage Hodgkin's disease are awaited.

*Fever, night sweats, weight loss (Table 6).

Advanced Disease. Chemotherapy is the primary curative treatment for patients with Stages III and IV Hodgkin's disease and for those with recurrent disease after RT. There has been controversy regarding the benefits of chemotherapy versus RT for patients with pathologic stage (PS) IIIA disease (occult abdominal disease defined at staging laparotomy and splenectomy in a patient with an asymptomatic, supradiaphragmatic presentation). The distinction of PS $IIIA_1$ disease (occult disease in spleen or nodes above the superior mesenteric artery) from PS $IIIA_2$

TABLE 5. **Staging Procedures in Hodgkin's Disease**

History—special attention to fever, night sweats, weight loss
Complete physical examination—distribution and size of peripheral nodal disease, presence of hepatosplenomegaly, evidence of extranodal disease
Laboratory examination—complete blood count, sedimentation rate, liver and renal function studies
Chest x-ray—PA and lateral
CT of thorax
Lymphangiogram—only in CT abdomen-negative cases
CT of abdomen
Bone marrow biopsy—in advanced, symptomatic, or recurrent cases or with abnormal hematology
Staging laparotomy and splenectomy, if indicated

PA = posteroanterior; CT = computed tomography.

TABLE 7. **Indications for Chemotherapy/Combined-Modality Therapy in Early Hodgkin's Disease**

Attribute	Prediction
Massive mediastinal adenopathy	Locoregional, intrathoracic failure
Extranodal extension to chest wall, lung, or pericardium	Locoregional, intrathoracic failure
B symptoms (see Table 6)*	Distant disease progression
Age >60 yr; MC and LD histology; ESR >50 mm/hr; >3 nodal sites	Distant disease progression

*B symptoms include fever, night sweats, weight loss (Table 6).
MC = mixed cellularity; LD = lymphocyte depletion; ESR = erythrocyte sedimentation rate.

TABLE 8. **MOPP Regimen***

Agent	Route	Dose (mg/m²)	Days
Mechlorethamine (Mustargen)	IV	6	1 and 8
Vincristine (Oncovin)	IV	1.4	1 and 8
Procarbazine (Matulane)	PO	100	1–14
Prednisone (Deltasone)	PO	40	1–14

*Cycle is repeated every 4 weeks; prednisone is used in cycles 1 and 4 only.

(occult disease in nodes below the superior mesenteric artery) has demonstrated the superiority of chemotherapy for patients with PS $IIIA_2$ disease. Similarly, the distinction of extent of splenic involvement (number and size of disease deposits) has underscored the importance of chemotherapy for those with extensive splenic involvement. Controversy exists regarding optimal therapy for patients with PS $IIIA_1$ disease with minimal splenic involvement or disease confined only to nodes above the superior mesenteric artery. Some investigators believe RT alone is sufficient. It is unlikely that this issue will be resolved, and in an era of declining use of laparotomy and splenectomy, this presentation will become increasingly rare.

Chemotherapy Regimens for Induction of Remission

The era of effective chemotherapy for Hodgkin's disease began in the mid 1940s with the use of nitrogen mustard as a single agent. In the 1960s, the first effective form of combination chemotherapy, the MOPP regimen, was developed at the National Cancer Institute (NCI).

MOPP and Derivative Regimens. In the first NCI study of patients with advanced Hodgkin's disease treated with MOPP regimen (Table 8), a complete remission rate was achieved in 81%, and 54% of patients remained disease free for more than 10 years. A recurrence rate of 35% was noted, with the majority occurring within the first 5 years after therapy. This experience was confirmed subsequently with a general recognition of a complete remission rate of 65 to 80%, relapse rate of 30 to 40%, and a "cure" rate of approximately 50 to 60% with MOPP. Factors influencing the success of chemotherapy for advanced disease are shown in Table 3. Recognition of these factors, which principally affect the complete remission (CR) rate (primary disease control), has stimulated continued attempts to modify the regimen to enhance effectiveness and to minimize acute and long-term side effects.

Variants of the MOPP regimen include MVPP, with substitution of vinblastine (Velban) for vincristine (Oncovin); ChlVPP; LOPP; and CVPP, with substitution of chlorambucil (Leukeran) and vinblastine (Velban) or cyclophosphamide (Cytoxan) to reduce gastrointestinal toxicity and neuropathy. Other active agents added include the nitrosoureas carmustine (BiCNU) and lomustine (CeeNU) in a five-drug regimen (BCVPP); bleomycin (Blenoxane) in a five-drug regimen (MOPP-Bleo); doxorubicin (Adriamycin) substituted for mechlorethamine (MOP BAP); and doxorubicin and bleomycin substituted for procarbazine in the MABOP regimen. These modifications have provided no consistent benefit over MOPP in terms of remission induction, although they have reduced acute morbidity. In achieving optimal results with MOPP, the NCI group stressed the necessity of adhering to the recommended dosages, particularly for vincristine, and the administration schedule.

ABVD Regimen and Alternating Sequence Regimens. The ABVD regimen (Tables 9 and 10) was introduced in the mid 1970s by Bonnadonna as an alternative regimen for salvage of MOPP failure utilizing a combination of active single agents including doxorubicin, bleomycin, vinblastine, and DTIC (dacarbazine). Because of the excellent response to ABVD in MOPP-resistant patients, this regimen has also been used in untreated patients. Studies indicate

TABLE 9. **ABVD Regimen**

Agent	Route	Dose (mg/m²)	Days
Doxorubicin (Adriamycin)	IV	25	1 and 15
Bleomycin (Blenoxane)	IV	10	1 and 15
Vinblastine (Velban)	IV	6	1 and 15
DTIC (Dacarbazine)	IV	375	1 and 15

TABLE 10. **Alternating Sequence Regimens**

Agent	Route	Dose (mg/m²)	Day(s)
*MOPP/ABVD Alternating Sequence Regimen**			
MOPP Regimen			
Mechlorethamine (Mustargen)	IV	6	1 and 8
Vincristine (Oncovin)	IV	1.4	1 and 8
Procarbazine (Matulane)	PO	100	1–14
Prednisone (Deltasone)	PO	40	1–14
After 14-day treatment-free period, then:			
ABVD Regimen			
Doxorubicin (Adriamycin)	IV	25	1 and 15
Bleomycin (Blenoxane)	IV	10	1 and 15
Vinblastine (Velban)	IV	6	1 and 15
DTIC (Dacarbazine)	IV	375	1 and 15
After 14-day treatment-free period, then repeat MOPP			
MOPP/ABV Hybrid Regimen†			
Mechlorethamine (Mustargen)	IV	6	1
Vincristine (Oncovin)	IV	1.4	1
Procarbazine (Matulane)	PO	100	1–7‡
Prednisone (Deltasone)	PO	40	1–14
Doxorubicin (Adriamycin)	IV	35§	8
Bleomycin (Blenoxane)	IV	10	8
Vinblastine (Velban)	IV	6	8

*For MOPP cycle, prednisone is given in cycles 1, 4, 7, and 10. Cycle repeats every 28 days; 12 cycles (months) of therapy complete program.

†Cycles repeat every 28 days for minimum of six cycles and two cycles beyond complete remission.

‡Note reduced duration of therapy compared with MOPP.

§Note increased dose of doxorubicin compared with ABVD.

comparable efficacy of ABVD and MOPP in controlling advanced Hodgkin's disease.

Building on the success of the MOPP and ABVD regimens, the Milan group introduced the concept of alternating sequence therapy as a means of intensifying therapy and exploiting the non–cross-resistance of the regimens. In the initial MOPP/ABVD trial, each regimen was administered in alternate months for a total of 12 months. In a randomized comparison with MOPP in patients with Stage IV Hodgkin's disease, MOPP/ABVD was superior in terms of CR rate, relapse-free rate, and overall 5-year survival. Modifications of the MOPP/ABVD regimens include the MOPP/ABV hybrid and the MM/AA (conventional alternation) and MA/MA (alternate MOPP and ABVD in each cycle) hybrids. No improvement in efficacy has been demonstrated with these changes in the MOPP/ABVD program, but reducing the duration of treatment from twelve cycles to six induction cycles to CR plus two consolidation cycles did not compromise results.

In an attempt to determine optimal therapy for advanced Hodgkin's disease, Cancer and Leukemia Group B (CALGB) recently reported the results of a randomized comparison of MOPP, ABVD, and MOPP/ABVD (Table 11). The study concluded that six to eight cycles of ABVD were as effective as 12 cycles of MOPP/ABVD and that both were superior to MOPP alone. Factors predicting a higher risk of disease progression were older age, Stage III versus IV, treatment regimen, and two or more extranodal sites of disease. Following failure of the first regimen, the crossover from ABVD to MOPP resulted in a higher CR rate than did a change from an MOPP regimen to ABVD (61% versus 35%, respectively). ABVD was less myelotoxic than MOPP or MOPP/ABVD. The incidence of second solid tumors was similar in the ABVD alone and MOPP/ABVD groups, but two cases of acute leukemia were observed in the MOPP and MOPP/ABVD groups. Overall survival of patients receiving second-line therapy was 61% at 3 years and 40% at 5 years with no differences attributable to the second-line therapy. This study has established the superiority of ABVD as the principal chemotherapy regimen for advanced Hodgkin's disease as a result of its increased efficacy, decreased myelotoxicity, and reduced incidence of gonadal dysfunction and leukemia. An intergroup study comparing ABVD with MOPP/ABV is currently ongoing.

TABLE 11. **Results of Randomized Comparison of MOPP, ABVD, and MOPP/ABVD**

	MOPP	ABVD	MOPP/ABVD
Number of patients	123	115	123
Duration of therapy (cycles)	6–8	6–8	12
Complete response rate (%)	67*	82	83
Failure-free survival at 5 yr (%)	50	61	65
Overall survival at 5 yr (%)	66†	73	75

*p = 0.006 for comparison of MOPP with other two regimens.
†p = 0.28 for comparison of MOPP with doxorubicin-containing regimens.

Assessment of Remission Status

The decision to discontinue therapy is almost as important as the decision to initiate therapy. Only those patients whose disease is eradicated have the opportunity to be cured. The assessment of disease eradication (CR) is based on the absence of symptoms, a normal physical examination, and the return of all previously abnormal parameters to normal. Tests that were abnormal initially should be monitored throughout therapy and determined to be normal at the end of the program. Initially involved extranodal tissue should, within the limits of practicality, be determined to be free of disease after therapy. Great caution should be exercised in the attribution of abnormalities to post-treatment "scarring" or "inactive disease," and every attempt should be made to establish total disease eradication before treatment is considered to be complete. Failure to secure CR may result in a reduction in treatment options and may have a prejudicial effect on long-term disease control.

Adjuvant Radiation Therapy and Maintenance Chemotherapy in Advanced Disease

Given that approximately 30% of patients who achieve CR with first-line chemotherapy will experience disease recurrence, attempts have been made to increase the overall rate of disease control, either through maintenance chemotherapy during remission or by adjuvant therapy to the previous sites of disease. No study of maintenance chemotherapy has demonstrated a survival advantage, although time to relapse may be increased, and most studies demonstrated increased toxicity. There has been no consistent, reproducible evidence that adjuvant RT affects survival rates, although the patterns of relapse in the irradiated and nonirradiated groups may differ. Although no benefit has been defined for adjuvant RT in all patients with advanced Hodgkin's disease, the therapeutic role of RT in controlling localized areas of disease after chemotherapy should not be forgotten. This is especially important in patients with a large mediastinal mass at presentation, in whom the risk of local failure is high and for whom post-chemotherapy mediastinal RT is part of standard management.

Treatment for Recurrent or Progressive Advanced Disease

Despite optimal first-line chemotherapy with ABVD or MOPP/ABVD combinations, 20% of patients with advanced or recurrent Hodgkin's disease will fail to achieve complete remission and another 20% will relapse from a state of complete remission. Thus, 30 to 40% of all patients with advanced Hodgkin's disease may require therapy beyond the initial induction regimen. The prognosis for patients who fail to achieve disease control with initial therapy (primary

TABLE 12. **Major Acute Side Effects of Chemotherapy for Advanced Hodgkin's Disease and Their Management**

Side Effect	Drug	Precautionary Measures	Treatment
Cytopenia	Doxorubicin, mechlorethamine, procarbazine, DTIC, vinblastine	Blood count supervision Prophylactic antibiotics	Blood component support G-CSF (Neupogen)
Alopecia	Doxorubicin	Ice pack on scalp	Wig, turban
Nausea and emesis	Mechlorethamine, doxorubicin, DTIC, carmustine, lomustine	Antiemetics—ondansetron (Zofran) Sedative—lorazepam (Ativan)	
Constipation	Vinca alkaloids	Diet	Laxatives
Neuropathy	Vinca alkaloids	–	Omit agent
Gastric irritation	Prednisone	Diet, antacids	Ranitidine (Zantac) Cimetidine (Tagamet)
Hyperglycemia	Prednisone	Urinalysis (Keto-Diastix)	Oral hypoglycemics Insulin
Hyperuricemia	All cytotoxics	Uric acid measurement	Allopurinol (Zyloprim)
Monoamine oxidase inhibitor effects	Procarbazine	Diet, alcohol avoidance	
Skin rash	Procarbazine Allopurinol (Zyloprim)	Omit drug if implicated Omit drug if implicated	Diphenhydramine (Benadryl) Hydroxyzine (Atarax)
Pulmonary fibrosis	Bleomycin (principally dose related)	Lung function surveillance	Omit bleomycin
Cardiotoxicity	Doxorubicin (dose related)	Cardiac function surveillance	Omit doxorubicin
Febrile reaction	Bleomycin	Bleomycin test done (1 mg IV) with monitoring	Hydrocortisone (SoluCortef)
Phlebitis	Mechlorethamine Doxorubicin Vinca alkaloids DTIC, carmustine	Good IV access IV access device	

induction failure) is considerably less satisfactory than for those who experience relapse after initial CR. Primary induction failure has a very low salvage rate with alternative therapy; the median survival is approximately 18 months. Relapse after initial CR has been classified as early (within 12 months of achieving initial CR) or late (after 12 months of CR). The second rate of CR with alternative chemotherapy is substantially lower for early relapse and the prognosis is less favorable. In the CALGB study, crossover between the MOPP and ABVD arms for all patients yielded an overall second CR rate of 46% (35% if the first regimen was MOPP, 61% if it was ABVD). Five-year failure-free survival from the time of crossover to ABVD was 15%, and 31% for crossover to MOPP. The overall 5-year survival was 40%.

Given a median failure-free period of approximately 12 to 20 months after initiation of alternative chemotherapy, and an approximate 5-year failure-free probability of 30% and survival of 40%, a number of alternative regimens employing combinations of active agents other than MOPP and ABVD have been developed.

Because no effective third-line chemotherapy (other than ABVD and MOPP) has been found, there has been a trend to consider more intensive chemotherapy requiring autologous bone marrow transplantation (ABMT) or stem cell support for patients with advanced Hodgkin's disease who fail to enter remission or who relapse following remission achieved with MOPP, ABVD, or MOPP/ABVD combinations. Because of the inherent toxicity of such regimens, eligibility for intensive chemotherapy and ABMT requires an acceptable level of performance status, age less than 60, acceptable major organ functions, patient consent, and availability of harvestable "tumor-free" bone marrow or peripheral stem cells. Many centers require evidence of chemosensitivity of the recurrent tumor, established through the use of an alternative chemotherapy regimen in vitro.

The ability to control disease substantially with alternative chemotherapy, RT, or both has been defined by some as the most important prognostic factor. High-dose chemotherapy regimens are characterized by the use of phenylalanine mustard (melphalan [Alkeran]), VP-16 (etoposide [VePesid]), cytosine arabinoside (Cytosar), carmustine (BiCNU) or lomustine (CeeNU), cyclophosphamide, and cisplatinum (cisplatin [Platinol]), either alone or in combination in doses lethal to the bone marrow. Total body irradiation is not a part of high-dose therapy, although involved field or regional radiation may be used. With current practice, procedure-related mortality approximates 5%. Morbidity is significant and requires highly specialized management in centers experienced in the support of the severely hematologically compromised patient. Although follow-up of patients treated with such protocols is still short, many centers are reporting disease-free survival rates of 30 to 40% at a median follow-up of 4 to 5 years for otherwise unselected patients undergoing intensive therapy. However, the probability of remission in patients with poor prognostic factors such as older age, poor performance status, bulky disease, and chemoresistance is low, with a failure-free probability of only 0 to 15%. However, for patients with favorable prognostic factors, the probability of durable disease control may be as high as 60 to 70%. Despite the ability of some third-line chemotherapy regimens to achieve response in patients with progressive disease, intensive therapy with ABMT or peripheral blood stem cell support is considered the only salvage approach with curative potential.

Side Effects of Chemotherapy

Chemotherapy has both acute and delayed side effects. The acute side effects reflect individual toxicities specific to the agent(s) in question and the combined toxicity on organ systems with rapid self-renewal (e.g., bone marrow, gastrointestinal tract). In general, toxicity is dose related, and although toxicity may be diminished by dose reduction or prolongation of cycle frequency, these may have adverse implications on disease control. The principal acute side effects and the strategies for their minimization are shown in Table 12. Currently, the use of hematopoietic growth factors (e.g., G-CSF [Neupogen]) permits the delivery of full-dose chemotherapy according to schedule in the majority of patients and reduces the incidence of associated infections.

Cytotoxic therapy has a profound impact on gonadal function. Patients should be advised of the effects of chemotherapy on gonadal function so that the symptoms, probabilities, and options for infertility, the role of hormonal replacement therapy, and the psychosocial and psychosexual effects of therapy are understood and managed appropriately. Azoospermia is expected with the MOPP, ABVD, and MOPP/ABVD/hybrid regimens. Recovery of spermatogenesis is remote with the MOPP regimen but may be expected 2 to 3 years after ABVD therapy. Factors influencing recovery include the state of the germinal epithelium pre-therapy, avoidance of alkylating agents, avoidance of chronic oral alkylator therapy, minimized cumulative chemotherapy exposure, and no prior radiation therapy encompassing the pelvic or inguinal nodes.

Germinal epithelial function may be inferred by measurements of follicle-stimulating hormone or semen analysis. Hypogonadism is unusual, as is a hormonal basis for impotence. Chemotherapy with alkylating agents causes a reduction of functioning ovarian life span, characterized by age-dependent premature ovarian dysfunction with consequent menstrual irregularity, amenorrhea, loss of libido, and menopausal symptomatology. Premature menopause should be treated by hormonal replacement therapy, unless medically contraindicated, to offset symptomatology and prevent excess risk of osteoporosis and atherogenesis. Although there is no indication that hormonal suppression of ovulation protects ovarian function during therapy, contraception by such means is appropriate because conception during chemotherapy would constitute strong medical grounds for termination of pregnancy.

The other major delayed complication is the induction of second malignancies in survivors of therapy for Hodgkin's disease. Acute myeloid leukemia has occurred in patients treated with MOPP therapy; there is no recognized increased risk with ABVD. The risk of acute leukemia is 5 to 15% expressed over 10 to 12 years post-chemotherapy. Cumulative chemotherapy exposure, use of alkylating agents, older age at therapy (>40 years), and prior splenectomy are associated with a higher risk of acute leukemia. Second solid tumors, including non-Hodgkin's lymphomas, also constitute a significant long-term risk, with an estimated cumulative lifetime probability approaching 10 to 20%. Unlike acute leukemia, which has a risk period of 10 to 12 years post-chemotherapy, the risk of a second solid tumor appears to be cumulative over the remaining life span. Solid tumors comprise common malignancies (e.g., lung cancer, breast cancer, skin cancer, including melanomas) as well as rare tumors (e.g., bone sarcomas, mesotheliomas, non–HIV-related Kaposi's sarcoma). Solid tumors are clearly related to exposure to both radiation and chemotherapeutic agents, and malignancies commonly occur within previously applied radiation fields. An underlying cell-mediated immunologic deficit characterizing Hodgkin's disease and its subsequent therapy may also play a role in susceptibility to second tumor development.

Thyroid function may also be influenced by prior chemotherapy, RT, or both and should be monitored through periodic surveillance of thyroid-stimulating hormone levels.

HODGKIN'S DISEASE: RADIATION THERAPY

method of
PELAYO C. BESA, M.D.
The University of Texas M. D. Anderson Cancer Center
Houston, Texas

Advances in treatment have made Hodgkin's disease a highly curable malignancy with a long-term survival rate of more than 90%. Radiation therapy is a major component of the therapy of Hodgkin's disease. Treatment planning and patient selection are based on thorough clinical staging and review of the pathology.

Adequate therapy with radiation requires pretreatment simulation and therapy with megavoltage photon beams through parallel opposed fields that deliver a tumoricidal dose in a fractionated fashion. Dosimetric calculations are made at multiple points, and doses are adjusted accordingly. Treatment reproducibility is verified periodically. After the completion of therapy, the patient is followed regularly to detect relapse and treatment-related toxic effects.

STAGING

To determine the best treatment approach, the patient needs to undergo disease staging, including a complete medical history with special attention to the tumor history and the presence of B symptoms (fever, night sweats, and weight loss). The physical examination should be thorough, with special attention to all nodal areas, Waldeyer's ring, the liver, and the spleen. The hematologic assessment should include a complete blood cell count, a platelet count, and screen chemistries, including lactate dehydrogenase. Imaging studies include x-ray films and computed tomography (CT) scans of the chest, especially in the presence of mediastinal involvement, to help design the treatment fields. The abdomen is evaluated with CT images that show the celiac complex, the liver, and the spleen, although Hodgkin's disease in the spleen is poorly demonstrated. The pelvis and the lower abdomen are evaluated with a bipedal lymphangiogram. Bone marrow biopsies are usually performed in all patients but those with early-stage (Stage I or II) disease and no B symptoms. Hodgkin's disease is staged according to the Ann Arbor staging classification system (Table 1).

RADIATION TREATMENT TECHNIQUE

Treatment planning starts by reviewing the staging evaluation and pathology report. Clinical and imaging studies are used to determine the extent of the disease. The treatment fields include the known disease area and any adjacent areas at risk. Three main areas are treated in Hodgkin's disease: the mantle or supradiaphragmatic region; the abdomen; and the pelvis, including the inguinal and femoral nodal regions (Fig. 1). The treatment plan identifies the areas to be irradiated and the order in which they will be treated. The junction between the fields must avoid splitting the tumor to prevent underdosing and must consider normal tissue tolerance to avoid organ toxicity.

After the treatment plan has been determined, the radiation therapy field is simulated and marked on the patient. The simulator is a diagnostic x-ray unit that reproduces the geometry of the therapy machine and has the ability to take verification radiographs. To optimize reproducibility of the daily set-up, patient immobilization devices are used. These are different for each treatment field; for example, a face mask of low-temperature thermal plastic (polycarbolactone) is used for the mantle. Treatment fields are determined by the anatomic landmarks on the patient and the fluoroscopic examination during simulation. Radiographs of the planned treatment fields are taken. The treatment fields include both the involved and the contiguous uninvolved lymphoid regions, and to encompass all these areas, large fields are necessary.

The simulation x-ray films are used to outline the field to be treated and to design the blocks for the areas to be protected from irradiation. Divergent blocks are constructed from the drawings on the films using a low–melting point alloy such as Lipowitz metal (Cerrobend). Also during simulation, the therapist measures the different thicknesses of the treatment field and uses the calculation method for asymmetric fields to determine the dose at all diameters. Typically, the dose is prescribed to be delivered along the central axis at the mid-plane. The dose is higher for thin areas where diameters are small. Partial transmission blocks are used to compensate for the difference in the diameters and to make the dose homogeneous throughout the treatment field.

Patients are treated on a linear accelerator at a 100-cm source-to-surface distance, usually utilizing 6-MV photons for the upper torso and 18-MV photons for the abdomen and the pelvis. The patient is seen on the treatment table by the radiotherapist to verify the proper location of the fields. Machine films for verification are taken at the beginning of treatment and weekly thereafter. The dose delivered to the visible tumor areas is 39.6 Gy in 22 fractions over 4½ weeks. The nodal areas treated prophylactically receive 30.6 Gy in 17 fractions over 3½ weeks. In general, the treatment field is arranged with parallel opposed fields, using even-weighted beams, and all fields are treated daily. When two fields are matched (e.g., mantle and abdomen), special gap calculations are used to avoid overlap. If the adjacent fields overlie the spinal cord, lateral x-ray films are taken and computer-generated isodose calculations are made to determine the dose at the cord.

TABLE 1. **Ann Arbor Staging Classification System**

Stage I	Involvement of a single lymph node region (I) or localized involvement of an extralymphatic organ or site (IE)
Stage II	Involvement of two or more lymph node regions on the same side of the diaphragm (II) or localized involvement of an extralymphatic organ or site and one or more nodal regions on the same side of the diaphragm (IIE)
Stage III	Involvement of lymph node regions on both sides of the diaphragm (III), which may be accompanied by localized involvement of an extralymphatic organ or site (IIIE)
Stage IV	Diffuse involvement of one or more extralymphatic organs with or without associated lymph node involvement

Systemic symptoms (fever, night sweats, and unexplained weight loss greater than 10% body weight): A = no; B = yes.

Mantle Field Irradiation

Radiation to the mantle field treats the supradiaphragmatic nodal regions. The mantle field extends from the mastoid and base of the mandible to the diaphragm and encompasses the submental, occipital, cervical, supraclavicular, infraclavicular, axillary, mediastinal, and hilar nodes. The patient is treated using parallel opposed anteroposterior fields, with individually contoured lung and heart blocks. Usually the cervical spine is blocked posteriorly, the larynx anteriorly, and both humeral heads anteriorly and posteriorly. The mantle is treated with equally loaded beams to a dose of 30.6 Gy in 17 fractions. At this point, treatment is stopped for the areas of prophylactic irradiation and continues only for the areas of gross involvement to a dose of 39.6 Gy. Low-dose lung irradiation is given when mediastinal masses are larger than 7.5 cm in maximum diameter or hilar nodes are involved. The lungs receive 15 Gy in 15 fractions to decrease the risk of disease relapse in the lungs.

Subdiaphragmatic Irradiation

Subdiaphragmatic nodal areas are usually divided into two treatment fields: the abdomen, which in-

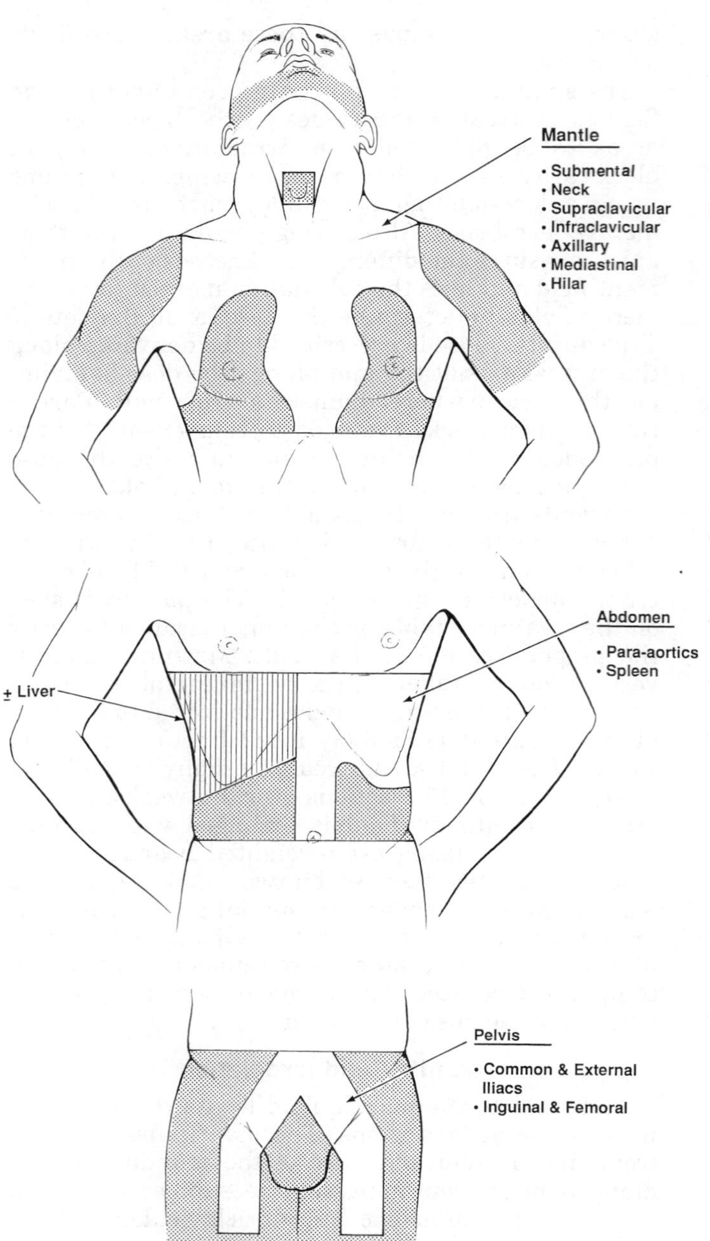

Figure 1. Radiotherapy fields.

cludes the para-aortic nodes and spleen, with or without the liver, and the pelvis, which includes the common and external iliac nodes and the inguinal/femoral regions. The field encompassing the para-aortic and spleen areas extends from the diaphragm to the bottom of the fourth lumbar vertebra; field edges are matched with those of the mantle field. Radiation is delivered using parallel opposed antero-posterior fields with equally loaded beams that deliver a dose of 30.6 Gy in 17 fractions. An additional 9-Gy boost in five fractions is given to areas with tumor involvement. When the liver is treated, a 50% transmission block is placed over it to deliver a dose of 15 Gy. Individually contoured blocks are made to protect the kidneys and bowel.

Often it is not necessary to treat the pelvic lymph nodes, and the radiation treatment stops at the level of the fourth lumbar vertebra. If needed, pelvic treatment is given through parallel opposed anteroposterior/posteroanterior fields utilizing 6-MV photons from the front (because the inguinal and femoral nodes are superficial) and 18-MV photons from the back. The pelvic field matches the para-aortic and splenic fields at the level of the fourth lumbar vertebra and extends to encompass the femoral lymph nodes. The nodal areas are well outlined by a lymphangiogram, which aids in the design of the radiation treatment.

Careful blocking is used to spare the bone marrow as much as possible and, in young females, the ovaries. The ovaries are transposed medially and placed as low as possible behind the uterus to avoid radiation-induced amenorrhea and sterility. The ovaries are marked with radiopaque clips to aid in the placement of a double-thickness block. At a distance of 2 cm from the edge of the block, the ovaries receive approximately 8% of the pelvic dose.

Combined-Modality Therapy

Many patients with Hodgkin's disease benefit from combined chemotherapy and radiation therapy. To reduce the toxicity from the combined-modality approach, special attention must be paid to chemotherapy agents and number of cycles and to radiation therapy fields and doses. Both the medical oncologist and the radiotherapist must work together from the beginning of treatment planning.

At the University of Texas M. D. Anderson Cancer Center, most patients with Hodgkin's disease are treated initially with two cycles of a combination of mechlorethamine, vincristine, procarbazine, and prednisone (MOPP), followed by radiation therapy to the tumor and areas at risk. For supradiaphragmatic presentations, the mantle and para-aortic and spleen areas are treated. This combined approach decreases the toxicity to the lungs from irradiation, especially in patients with large mediastinal masses. Six cycles of chemotherapy only are given to patients with advanced-stage disease (Stage IIIB or IV) and mediastinal masses larger than 15 cm. After the completion of the six cycles of chemotherapy, radiation is delivered to the areas of initial tumor involvement.

Gallium scanning is used to evaluate treatment response in patients receiving combined-modality therapy. The test is done before chemotherapy begins and, if positive, is repeated before radiation is delivered. Patients who have negative findings on gallium scanning have a lower relapse rate.

TREATMENT RECOMMENDATIONS AND RESULTS

Supradiaphragmatic Favorable Stages I and IIA

Upper torso presentation in patients younger than 40 years of age with four or fewer sites and no B symptoms should be treated with radiation therapy alone. Radiation is delivered to the mantle field and the para-aortic and spleen areas. Patients with mediastinal disease are excluded because they benefit from induction chemotherapy, which reduces the mediastinal mass and decreases radiation-induced pulmonary injury. Freedom from relapse for this group of patients is 80 to 90% (Table 2).

Patients with Stage IA nodular sclerosis lymphocyte-predominant Hodgkin's disease are a special subgroup in whom disease tends to be localized and has a late relapse pattern similar to that of low-grade follicular lymphomas. These patients receive radiation to the involved field (i.e., the hemineck or the axilla) only.

TABLE 2. **Treatment Results at M. D. Anderson Cancer Center**

Stage	Treatment	Survival (%)	Freedom from Relapse (%)
I–IIA favorable	XRT	92 (4 years)	78 (4 years)
I–IIA unfavorable, I–IIB	2 cycles MOPP-XRT	100 (4 years)	79 (4 years)
I–II large mediastinal mass	2 cycles MOPP-XRT	84 (4 years)	66 (4 years)
IIIA–IIIB (except III_3)	2 cycles MOPP-XRT	87 (10 years)	83 (10 years)
IV	CVPP/ABDIC	77 (4 years)	64 (4 years)

XRT = chemotherapy; MOPP = mechlorethamine/vincristine/procarbazine/prednisone combination; CVPP/ABDIC = cyclophosphamide/vinblastine/procarbazine/prednisone combination alternating with doxorubicin/bleomycin/dacarbazine/lomustine/prednisone combination.

Supradiaphragmatic Unfavorable Stages I–IIA and I–IIB

This group includes all patients with Stages I and II disease who do not meet the "favorable" criteria or who have B symptoms. These patients have an increased risk of abdominal involvement approaching 30% according to laparotomy data. At the M. D. Anderson Cancer Center, these patients are given combined-modality therapy. Chemotherapy (two cycles of MOPP) is given first, followed by radiation therapy to the mantle and the para-aortic nodes and spleen; the liver receives low-dose radiation. Patients in this group have a disease-free survival rate of 79%, and a 100% survival rate at 4 years.

Stages I and II with Mediastinal Involvement

Mediastinal involvement, which is very common in Hodgkin's disease, presents a special challenge to the radiotherapist because toxicity to lungs and heart must be avoided. The extent of mediastinal tumor involvement is determined by measuring the maximum single horizontal width of the mediastinum on a standing posteroanterior chest radiograph. Three categories are defined: tumors less than 7.5 cm are considered small, those 7.5 cm to less than 15 cm are large or bulky, and those 15 cm or more are massive.

Most of these patients receive combined-modality therapy. Chemotherapy (two cycles of MOPP) is administered first to decrease the size of the mediastinal tumor. Patients with small mediastinal masses receive radiation to the mantle field followed by treatment to the para-aortic and spleen areas. Patients with bulky tumors or hilar involvement also receive low-dose lung irradiation, using an on/off lung-block technique that delivers 15 Gy in 15 fractions. These patients have a relapse-free survival rate of 84% at 4 years. Patients with massive tumors are treated with six cycles of combination chemotherapy followed by radiation therapy to the areas of initial involvement.

Stages I and II with Subdiaphragmatic Involvement Only

Fewer than 10% of patients with Stage I or II Hodgkin's disease present with disease limited to the subdiaphragmatic areas. Lymphangiography is extremely important to determine the extent of involvement in the pelvic and para-aortic regions. CT is used to evaluate the upper abdomen, including the mesenteric nodes and spleen, and treatment is adjusted according to the extent of tumor involvement.

For a Stage IA inguinal presentation, radiation is delivered to the inguinal region and hemipelvis. More advanced cases receive combined-modality therapy. Two cycles of MOPP are given initially, followed by radiation therapy. Fields to be irradiated include the abdomen; the para-aortic and spleen areas, with or without low-dose liver irradiation; the pelvis; and the common and external iliac, inguinal, and femoral nodes. Treatment results for these patients are similar to those for patients with supradiaphragmatic presentations.

Stage III

Nodal involvement in patients with Stage III disease varies greatly. This heterogeneous group of patients is divided into subgroups according to the extent of abdominal tumor (Fig. 2). Patients with disease limited to the upper abdomen (involving the celiac region, splenic hilum, and spleen) are classified as having Stage III_1 disease. When the disease extends to the para-aortic region, it is classified as Stage III_2, and if the pelvis or inguinal region is involved, the classification is Stage III_3. At the M. D. Anderson Cancer Center, all patients with Stage III disease receive combined-modality therapy. With the exception of the few patients presenting with Stage III_3B disease, all patients with Stage III disease receive two cycles of MOPP followed by radiation therapy with the fields adjusted according to the extent of tumor involvement. Patients with Stage III_1 disease receive radiation first to the mantle and then to the para-aortic region and spleen with low-dose liver irradiation. Patients with Stages III_2 and III_3 disease receive radiation to the same fields used for patients with Stage III_1 disease and also receive radiation to the pelvis and inguinal and femoral nodal regions. At M. D. Anderson, the relapse-free rate for this group is 83% at 10 years. The few patients who present with Stage III_3B disease are treated with the Stage IV regimen described in the next section.

Stages III_3B and IV

The majority of patients with Stage III_3B disease and many with Stage IV disease receive combined-modality therapy. Treatment begins with six cycles of combination chemotherapy (cyclophosphamide, vinblastine, procarbazine, and prednisone alternating with doxorubicin, bleomycin, dacarbazine, lomustine,

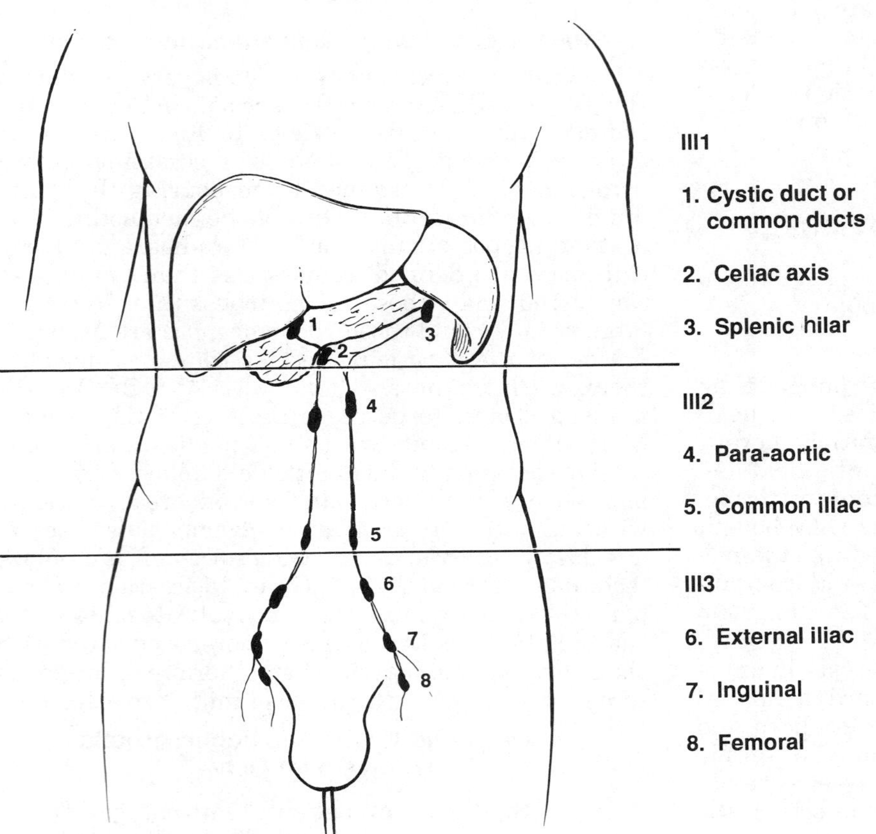

Figure 2. Abdominal substage.

and prednisone), followed by irradiation of the known sites of disease. At 4 years, the relapse-free survival rate at M. D. Anderson is 64% and the survival rate is 77%.

Complications

Complications are classified as acute or late. Acute complications occur during or shortly after the course of radiation therapy; they are treated symptomatically and resolve quickly after the completion of treatment. Late complications occur after treatment has been completed (months or years later) and tend to be permanent. Acute complications include mild skin reactions and hair loss in the irradiated areas, dysphasia, dry cough, nausea, and diarrhea. Xerostomia (mouth dryness) develops during irradiation of the mantle fields and only partially resolves in many patients. These complications are treated symptomatically with analgesics, cough suppressants, and antidiarrheal agents.

Late complications include pneumonitis, carditis, hypothyroidism, dental caries, Lhermitte's sign, and herpes zoster infection. Improvements in radiation equipment and technique have decreased cardiotoxicity; radiation carditis occurs in fewer than 2% of these patients. Pericarditis presents as an acute episode of chest pain, with fever and friction rub or sometimes a decrease in heart sounds because of pericardial effusion. The electrocardiogram is used to measure any decrease in the overall electrical potential of the patient's heart, and the echocardiogram is used to diagnose pericardial thickening and effusion. Pericarditis is managed with nonsteroidal anti-inflammatory agents and usually clears up after a few weeks. For severe cases, corticosteroids are used. Occasionally, patients present with asymptomatic pericardial effusion that usually resolves spontaneously after several months. Constrictive pericarditis and pericardial tamponade are rare complications that require surgical correction. In the long term, because there is a small increase in the incidence of coronary artery disease, patients must be encouraged not to smoke.

Radiation pneumonitis occurs infrequently, and its risk is proportional to the volume of lung irradiated, the total dose, and the fraction size. The patient typically presents 6 to 12 weeks after the completion of the radiation therapy with dry cough, pleuritic chest pain, and fever. The chest x-ray reveals interstitial infiltrates. Severe cases of pneumonitis require treatment with corticosteroids for 4 to 6 weeks, with gradual tapering to avoid recurrence of symptoms.

Subclinical hypothyroidism develops in one-third of patients who have undergone mantle irradiation. Patients are asymptomatic, and the physician is alerted by the elevation in thyroid-stimulating hormone seen on the routine yearly blood measurement. Thyroid replacement is necessary to avoid development of goiter.

Xerostomia caused by irradiation of the salivary glands produces a favorable environment for dental caries. This complication can be prevented with a pre-treatment dental evaluation, careful dental care, and the daily use of fluoride.

Herpes zoster involving the skin develops in approximately 20% of patients and is limited to one or two contiguous dermatomes. As soon as the diagnosis is made, the patient must start treatment with acyclovir (Zovirax) to decrease the duration and intensity of the infection.

Lhermitte's sign is common in patients who receive treatment to the mantle field. It manifests as an electric sensation or paresthesia along the extremities, usually the legs, when the neck is flexed anteriorly. Generally, it presents 1 to 3 months after completion of treatment and resolves spontaneously within a few months, leaving no sequelae. The cause of Lhermitte's sign is a transient demyelinization of the spinal cord. It is not related to the transverse myelitis that can occur when an overdose of radiation is given to the spinal cord.

Irradiation of the gonads can produce sterility in both men and women, but the scattered dose to the gonads from irradiated mantle and abdominal fields is very low and does not affect the patient's fertility. In men, pelvic irradiation with adequate testicular shielding produces only a transient azoospermia. In women, ovariopexy is needed before irradiation to preserve fertility. The ovaries are blocked with 10 half-value layers but even this may not preserve ovarian function, especially in women older than 30 years. Combined-modality therapy with two cycles of MOPP does not affect fertility in males or females beyond that with radiation alone.

The improved survival of patients with Hodgkin's disease has been accompanied by an increase in the frequency of second malignancies. Leukemia is very rare after radiation therapy alone or in combination with two cycles of MOPP. Solid tumors develop late (10 years or more after treatment) and occur more frequently in older patients and those with more advanced disease. Patients must avoid smoking. Workup for early detection of cancer must be included in the yearly follow-up.

Radiation therapy plays a primary role in the treatment of Hodgkin's disease. The tremendous technologic advances in radiation therapy have contributed to the improvement in patient outcome. The use of combined-modality therapy with a limited number of chemotherapy cycles has further improved the results in patients with more extensive disease and has limited treatment morbidity.

ACUTE LEUKEMIA IN ADULTS

method of
STEPHANIE J. LEE, M.D., and
LAWRENCE N. SHULMAN, M.D.
Brigham and Women's Hospital, Harvard Medical School
Boston, Massachusetts

The clinical manifestations of leukemia follow from the malignant clonal expansion of hematopoietic cells. Chronic leukemias, which usually have more indolent biology and clinical features, are addressed in another chapter. Acute leukemias are aggressive and rapidly fatal if untreated. In these disorders, normal hematopoietic differentiation appears to be interrupted, and a malignant proliferation and accumulation of immature cells occurs.

Acute leukemia is an uncommon disease in adults. The estimated incidence is 3.5 cases per 100,000 population, and it is the twentieth most common cause of cancer deaths. The two major types of acute leukemia, acute lymphoblastic leukemia (ALL) and acute myelogenous leukemia (AML), are important to distinguish because their treatment and prognosis differ.

CLINICAL PRESENTATION

Clinical signs and symptoms are often due either to the replacement or to the suppression of normal hematopoiesis by immature leukemic cells called "blasts." The decreased production of red cells, platelets, and normal leukocytes results in anemia, fatigue, bleeding, and infection. Leukemic cells can accumulate in the mediastinum, spleen, skin, or other tissues. Central nervous system (CNS) involvement may present as headache, cranial nerve palsies, stroke symptoms, or changes in mental status.

DIFFERENTIAL DIAGNOSIS

Patients often present with some combination of anemia, thrombocytopenia, and neutropenia. The differential diagnosis in such circumstances is broad and includes all forms of bone marrow failure or invasion. Aplastic anemia; myelodysplastic syndromes; invasion of the marrow cavity by carcinoma, lymphoma, or leukemia; and marrow fibrosis can all cause abnormal blood counts. Although most think of elevated white blood cell counts in leukemia, half of all patients have low or normal white cell counts on presentation, necessitating a thorough examination of the peripheral blood smear for abnormal cells. Circulating blasts may be rare and are often confused with atypical lymphocytes or monocytes. However, once leukemic blasts are identified, the differential diagnosis narrows to the acute leukemias: AML, ALL, chronic myelogenous leukemia (CML) in blast crisis, undifferentiated or biphenotypic leukemia, or the leukemic phase of lymphoma.

EVALUATION AND GENERAL TREATMENT

Once the diagnosis of acute leukemia is established, special attention should be paid to signs of infection, bleeding, CNS involvement, or tissue invasion. The history should include onset of symptoms, date of the last prior normal examination and blood counts, family history, and possible chemical or radiation exposures. Baseline laboratory studies are performed to evaluate the need for transfusion, to look for evidence of tumor lysis syndrome or disseminated intravascular coagulation (DIC), and to assess renal, cardiac, and hepatic function in preparation for chemotherapy.

Treatment of leukemia involves administration of intensive chemotherapy to destroy the malignant clone and induce marrow aplasia. If this is successful, normal hematopoiesis may take place from surviving stem cells, repopulating the bone marrow and eliminating clinical evidence of the disease. "Remission," or inability to detect the disease, must be distinguished from "cure," or eradication of disease. Advances in supportive care such as the use of indwelling central venous catheters, broad-spectrum antibiotics, antifungal agents, specialized nursing units, and improvements in blood product support have decreased the number of treatment-related deaths. However, despite initial successful remission induction in 65 to 70% of patients with AML and 70 to 90% of patients with ALL, many of these patients ultimately suffer a relapse of their disease and die. Bone marrow transplantation and other intensive therapies have been pursued in an attempt to improve the survival rate.

ACUTE MYELOGENOUS LEUKEMIA

Acute myelogenous leukemia accounts for 80% of adult acute leukemias and is a malignancy of myeloid precursors. The clonal abnormality may involve red cell, white cell, or platelet precursors. The incidence of AML rises with age without predilection for race or gender. Most cases of AML are idiopathic, although a few predisposing factors have been identified, including exposure to radiation or chemicals (e.g., benzene), genetic diseases (e.g., Down's syndrome, Bloom's syndrome, and Fanconi's anemia), and underlying abnormalities of hematopoietic cells (e.g., paroxysmal nocturnal hemoglobinuria, myelodysplastic syndrome, myeloproliferative syndromes). Prior therapy with alkylating agents or high-dose podophyllotoxins can lead to "secondary," or treatment-related, AML.

Generally, AML is not believed to be a heritable disease, although very rare families appear to have a genetic predisposition. In these families, siblings of an affected patient have a fivefold greater risk of developing leukemia than the general population, although that risk remains exceedingly low.

Diagnosis and Classification

AML blasts appear on the peripheral blood smear or bone marrow preparation as large cells with a moderately high nuclear-to-cytoplasmic ratio. The cytoplasm is often pale blue and may contain granules suggesting myeloid lineage. Auer rods are purple, cigar-shaped, cytoplasmic inclusions composed of abnormal azurophilic primary granules and are pathognomonic for AML. The nuclear chromatin often has a fine granular appearance, and numerous prominent "punched out" nucleoli may be present.

A bone marrow biopsy and aspirate are obtained

from the posterior iliac crest under local anesthesia. Failure to obtain a marrow aspirate is not uncommon and can result from a hypoplastic variant of AML, myelofibrosis as in M7 AML, or an extremely hypercellular marrow. Aspirate specimens yield the best cellular morphology for Wright-Giemsa and histochemical stains. Core biopsy is required to document aplasia and remission, because it allows determination of overall cellularity and percentage of blasts.

AML subtypes are classified according to the FAB (French-American-British) M0–M7 classification (Table 1). These subdivisions delineate different degrees of myeloid differentiation and the specific lineage involved. M2 AML displays more differentiation than M1 AML, with increased primary granule formation, and M4 AML blasts have both myeloid and monocytic differentiation. Erythroid blasts are found in M6 AML, and megakaryocytic blasts in M7 AML. With the exception of promyelocytic leukemia (M3), the FAB subtype does not determine treatment.

Histochemical stains help to identify myeloid cells by staining specific cellular contents. Myeloperoxidase and chloroacetate esterase are produced early in myeloid development, and staining for these helps in distinguishing myeloid from lymphoid cells. Nonspecific esterase stains monocytic cells including monoblasts.

Immunophenotyping utilizes fluorescence-labeled antibodies to identify cell surface markers. Specific patterns of cluster designation (CD) antigens displayed on the cell surface during different stages of development identify the lineage and degree of maturation. For example, CD11, CD13, and CD33 are present on myeloid cells and may be present on myeloid blasts. Spectrin and glycophorin A are found on the erythroleukemic blasts of M6 AML. Platelet antigens are present on megakaryocytic blasts seen in M7 leukemia.

Cytogenetic analysis can be performed using specialized tissue culture techniques to isolate metaphases for chromosomal analysis. Banding patterns identify chromosomes 1 to 22 (numbered in order of size) and allow recognition of translocations, deletions, additions, or aneuploidy. With advanced techniques, clonal karyotypic abnormalities can be identified in the majority of AML patients. Some of these chromosomal abnormalities have prognostic significance. A better prognosis is associated with leukemias bearing the t(8;21) of M2 AML and the inv 16 of the M4 subtype of AML with eosinophilia. Patients whose leukemic blasts demonstrate monosomy 5 or 7 or trisomy 8 chromosomal abnormalities have a less favorable prognosis. Specialized molecular techniques allow identification of specific products of

TABLE 1. **FAB Subtypes of AML with Clinical Correlations**

FAB Subtype	Morphology	Histochemistry Immunophenotyping	Cytogenetics	Clinical Correlation
M0 (1%)	Myeloblast—undifferentiated	MPO (−), NSE (−), PAS (−) immunophenotyping shows myeloid markers		
M1 (10%)	Myeloblast—undifferentiated, granules and Auer rods rare	MPO (+), NSE (−), PAS (−)	Trisomy 8, monosomy 5, 7	
M2 (40%)	Myeloblast—differentiation present	MPO (+), NSE (−), PAS (−)	Trisomy 8, monosomy 5, 7 t(8;21)	
M3 (10%)	Promyelocyte—abundant Auer rods, atypical primary granules	MPO (++), C (+), NSE (−), PAS (−)	t(15;17)	DIC common; may treat with ATRA; microgranular variant (20%)—same treatment and prognosis
M4 (15%)	Myelo-monocytic	MPO (+), C (+), NSE (+)	Trisomy 8, monosomy 5,7, eosinophilic variant inv (16)	Extramedullary sites common—gingiva, skin, CNS, DIC; eosinophilic variant has better prognosis
M5 (10%)	Monocytic clefted nucleus	MPO (−), C (−), NSE (+), PAS (+)	t(4;11), t(9;11)	Extramedullary sites common—gingiva, skin, CNS, HSM, DIC
M6 (5%)	Erythroleukemia	PAS (+), glycophorin A (+), spectrin (+), ABH blood type (+)	Trisomy 8, monosomy 5,7	Long prodromal phase; rheumatic signs—serositis, autoimmune phenomena
M7 (5%)	Megakaryocytic, high N/C ratio, pale cytoplasm	MPO (−), PAS (+/−), VWF, GpIb, IIb/IIIa, IIIa (+)		Elevated LDH, myelofibrosis, more common in Down's syndrome

Abbreviations: MPO = myeloperoxidase; NSE = nonspecific esterase; PAS = periodic acid–Schiff; ATRA = all-trans-retinoic acid; HSM = hepatosplenomegaly; CNS = central nervous system; C = chloroacetate; VWF = von Willebrand factor; GpIb, IIb/IIIa = platelet surface markers; DIC = disseminated intravascular coagulation; LDH = lactate dehydrogenase; N/C ratio = nuclear-to-cytoplasmic ratio.

chromosomal translocations and suggest certain subclassifications of AML. For example, the t(15;17) translocation involves the alpha chain of the retinoic acid receptor and is pathognomonic for M3 AML.

Therapy

Without treatment, AML is fatal in weeks or months from complications such as anemia, bleeding, leukostasis, and infection. Treatment is rigorous, and success declines with increasing patient age as the complication rate rises. AML therapy is divided into two phases, induction and consolidation. *Induction therapy* refers to the initial intensive chemotherapy treatment that ablates the bone marrow with the hope of allowing return of normal hematopoiesis. Successful induction therapy places the patient in a clinical remission, but only the rare patient will truly be cured after induction therapy only.

After remission induction, *consolidation therapy* is administered, consisting of multiple cycles of high-dose chemotherapy designed to eliminate subclinical residual disease. Studies have shown improved survival for patients given consolidation therapy following induction. Most regimens include two to three consolidation cycles.

Many studies have sought to determine the ideal chemotherapy drugs, dosages, and administration schedules for patients with AML. In the 1960s, a combination of cytarabine (Cytosar-U) and 6-thioguanine resulted in remission rates of 50%. In the mid-1970s, the addition of daunorubicin (Cerubidine) to cytarabine raised the remission rate to 60 to 70% and revolutionized AML treatment. These two agents remain the mainstay of AML induction therapy. Studies have shown that daunorubicin is superior to doxorubicin (Adriamycin), primarily because of a reduction in mucositis and infectious complications, and that cytarabine is most effective if given by continuous infusion or in high doses. Often cytarabine is administered by continuous infusion (100 to 200 mg per M^2 per day) over 5 to 7 days, and daunorubicin is given by bolus during the first 3 days (45 mg per M^2 per day); this is the so-called 7 + 3 regimen. Consolidation therapy usually consists of several intensive courses of multiple agents, including cytarabine, daunorubicin, and other drugs effective in AML, such as mitoxantrone (Novantrone), idarubicin (Idamycin), and etoposide (VePesid). Total treatment time is approximately 8 months, and patients may feel reasonably well between cycles. In an effort to improve cure rates, our institution and others are conducting trials with more intensive chemotherapy regimens.

At the time of initial diagnosis, patients are usually hospitalized for administration of chemotherapy and careful monitoring. Metabolic parameters are closely followed. Tumor lysis syndrome may occur with resultant hyperkalemia, hyperuricemia, hypocalcemia, and hypomagnesemia generated by lysis of blasts and is most common in rapidly progressive leukemias with large tumor burdens. Allopurinol (Zyloprim), urine alkalinization, and aggressive hydration decrease the risk of uric acid nephropathy and kidney stone formation. Care must be taken in interpreting blood potassium, glucose, and oxygen levels, because metabolically activated tumor cells can spuriously alter these laboratory values. Antileukemic therapy causes lysis of blasts, and primary lysosomal granules may release their contents, inducing a coagulopathy. Coagulation studies should be followed because several subtypes, particularly M3, M4, and M5, are prone to DIC and may require treatment with fresh-frozen plasma.

Febrile neutropenic episodes must be aggressively treated with double gram-negative antibiotic coverage including a beta-lactam antipseudomonal antibiotic and an aminoglycoside. With persistent fevers, vancomycin (Vancocin) is often added, since most patients have indwelling central venous catheters that place them at risk for coagulase-negative staphylococcal infections. Patients are at increasing risk for fungal infection as duration of neutropenia increases, and amphotericin is often added next if fever persists. Unless patients have particular risk factors for anaerobic infections, specific anaerobic coverage is added last. Antibiotics are usually continued until patients are afebrile and their absolute neutrophil count (ANC) is greater than 500 per microliter.

Transfusions are often given through leukopoor filters to decrease alloimmunization, risk of leukocyte transfusion reaction, and exposure to cytomegalovirus (CMV). Platelet products from single donors are used to minimize antigenic exposure. Blood products are usually irradiated to kill donor leukocytes; rarely, transfusion-associated graft-versus-host disease can occur in these immunocompromised hosts. Screening for CMV-negative products whenever the patient does not show signs of previous exposure helps to prevent primary infection.

Hyperleukocytosis may be a medical emergency and is associated with leukocyte blast counts in excess of 100,000 per microliter. Symptoms are attributable to stasis and sludging of large blasts as they pass through capillaries and can include dizziness, headache, stupor, stroke symptoms, dyspnea, and priapism. Treatment with cranial irradiation, leukapheresis, or immediate institution of antileukemic therapy results in dramatic lowering of the white blood cell count and resolution of symptoms.

Prognosis

Prognosis is based on a number of factors, the most important being the age and underlying physical condition of the patient. Cytogenetic abnormalities, leukemic subtype, and pre-existing bone marrow abnormalities may also have prognostic significance. Remission rates range from 45 to 75%, depending on age. Although some patients will die of treatment-related causes and some will be cured, most will eventually succumb to relapsed leukemia. Median survival is 1 year, and 10 to 20% of patients are alive at 5 years. Leukemias that arise after alkylating agent therapy or from myelodysplastic disorders are termed secondary leukemias. They appear to be more refractory to treatment and outcome is worse than in "de novo" leukemia.

Complications of treatment are numerous and increase with age. Infection, bleeding, and drug toxicity result in a treatment-related mortality rate of 5 to 25%. Alopecia, nausea, vomiting, fatigue, fevers, and rashes are expected during therapy. Anthracyclines can induce cardiomyopathy, and cardiac function should be tested by echocardiography or nuclear medicine study if doubt exists about cardiac reserve.

Therapy of Relapsed AML

Relapsed AML poses a particularly difficult clinical problem. Once relapse occurs, long-term disease-free survival is extremely unlikely. Although 25 to 50% of patients will successfully achieve a second remission, reinduction is more difficult than at diagnosis, and remission duration tends to become progressively shorter; most patients eventually develop resistant disease. Various protocols using mid- or high-dose cytarabine in combination with mitoxantrone or etoposide are undergoing study. Bone marrow transplantation may be offered to suitable candidates.

Bone Marrow Transplantation

Despite its higher initial mortality, bone marrow transplantation offers appropriate candidates their best chance of long-term disease-free survival. Patients undergoing allogeneic transplant in first remission have a 50 to 60% survival rate at 3 years, while autologous transplant yields a 40 to 50% survival at 2 years, surpassing results with conventional chemotherapy. Success of transplantation is largely due to the cytoreductive effects of intensive chemotherapy and radiotherapy. Allogeneic transplants may offer the additional benefit of a graft-versus-leukemia (GVL) effect. The GVL effect refers to the "rejection" or elimination of leukemic myeloblasts by alloreactive donor lymphocytes. Relapse of leukemia following allogeneic transplant is rare, but overall success is limited by the availability of histocompatible donors and toxicities innate to the transplant procedure. Approximately 30% of patients will have a histocompatible sibling match. Matched unrelated donor transplants result in significantly more toxicity and a lower survival rate but may be appropriate in certain circumstances.

ACUTE LYMPHOBLASTIC LEUKEMIA

Acute lymphoblastic leukemia is generally thought of as a childhood malignancy, but incidence is actually bimodal with a peak in adulthood as well. A tumor of lymphoid cells, its etiology is unknown. In 1948, Farber demonstrated that childhood ALL could be placed in remission by aminopterin,* a folic acid antagonist and forerunner of methotrexate (Folex). Current chemotherapy regimens have improved the success rate. In general, pediatric ALL is a highly curable disease, with 80 to 90% disease-free survival in good-risk patients. Adult ALL is less common and less curable than childhood ALL. However, the prognosis is slightly better than that of adult AML.

*Not available in the United States.

Diagnosis and Classification

Lymphoblasts can be identified by their extremely high nuclear-to-cytoplasmic ratio. They are usually smaller and may be more pleomorphic than myeloblasts. Cytoplasmic granules are not observed, and the cytoplasm is basophilic and scant. Nuclear chromatin is largely open with some irregularly clumped areas and may contain a few "rimmed" nucleoli. Special studies have shown 67% to be of early B cell and 33% of T cell origin.

Histochemical stains show the blasts to be myeloperoxidase-, chloroacetate esterase–, and nonspecific esterase–negative. Periodic acid–Schiff (PAS) stains polysaccharide and may be positive in a clumped, cytoplasmic pattern (myeloblasts may show diffuse positivity). Immunophenotyping may show CD3, CD5, and CD7 staining of T cells or CD10 (common ALL antigen or cALLa) and CD19 staining of pre-B cells.

Molecular genetic studies often demonstrate rearrangement of immunoglobulin genes in B cells or T cell receptor gene rearrangement in T cells. Although these rearrangements occur in normal developmental stages in lymphocytes, *clonal* rearrangements are seen in ALL.

Certain cytogenetic abnormalities are thought to portend an extremely poor prognosis, such as t(4;11), t(8;14) translocations or the Philadelphia chromosome t(9;22), which is present in about 30% of adults with ALL. Since the prognosis with standard therapy is so poor for these patients, they should be considered for bone marrow transplant in first complete remission. Standard metaphase cytogenetics are not always successful in patients with ALL because lymphoblasts sometimes do not undergo mitosis in tissue culture. Molecular diagnostic probes can identify the Philadelphia chromosome and some other translocations with more reliability. The Philadelphia chromosome usually seen in ALL yields a 190-kilodalton (p190) product, whereas in CML a different 210-kilodalton (p210) product is usually made.

Clinically, patients with ALL are less prone to DIC and may have extremely elevated leukocyte counts without symptoms of leukostasis. The lymphoblasts appear to be less "sticky" than the myeloblasts. Often, lactate dehydrogenase is elevated and patients may have adenopathy or splenomegaly. In T cell ALL, cells may have a cleaved nucleus and be associated with a mediastinal mass.

ALL is classified according to either the FAB LI-3 schema or immunophenotyping (Tables 2 and 3).

Therapy

Childhood ALL is a more easily cured disease than the adult form, and treatment utilizes primarily

TABLE 2. **FAB Classification of ALL**

FAB Subtype	Morphology	Clinical Correlations
L1 (30%)	Small uniform nucleus, scant cytoplasm, regular nucleus with inconspicuous nucleoli	Best prognosis
L2 (60%)	Larger, less uniform, prominent nucleoli	
L3 (10%)	Uniform cell, more cytoplasm, prominent vacuoles and nucleoli	Non-Hodgkin's lymphoma, small, noncleaved cell (Burkitt's or non-Burkitt's), surface immunoglobulin, t(8;14), worst prognosis

doxorubicin, vincristine (Oncovin), prednisone, and methotrexate. In adults, treatment consists of multidrug therapy often including cyclophosphamide (Cytoxan), anthracyclines, methotrexate, vincristine, L-asparaginase (Elspar), prednisone, cytarabine, 6-mercaptopurine (Purinethol), and 6-thioguanine. Multiple cycles of treatment are administered and include an intensive induction phase, CNS prophylaxis with cranial irradiation and intrathecal chemotherapy, and prolonged systemic maintenance. Without CNS prophylaxis, 50% of patients will relapse at that site in 2 years, and without systemic maintenance chemotherapy, most patients will experience bone marrow relapse.

Completion of all phases of therapy usually requires 2 to 3 years. Although the initial induction period requires 3 to 6 weeks of hospitalization, the remainder of the therapy is designed to be given on an outpatient basis.

Patients require careful follow-up after completion of therapy. Relapse may be noted first in the blood, bone marrow, CNS, or testicles. The latter two are felt to be sanctuary sites, i.e., areas where systemic therapy may not be potent enough to eradicate disease. Testicular relapse presents as painless swelling and requires radiation and systemic treatment. Bone marrow relapse may be first manifested by thrombocytopenia.

Patients with the L3 subtype represent a distinct category. Although a classification for them exists in the ALL schema, they should be neither considered nor treated as having standard ALL. This subtype is now classified as non-Hodgkin's lymphoma of the small non–cleaved-cell type and is divided into either Burkitt's or non-Burkitt's type based on morphologic characteristics. These tumors are made up of more mature B cells, and patients often have extensive bone marrow, extralymphatic, and CNS involvement. Cytogenetic analysis usually demonstrates the t(8;14) translocation. These patients have a particularly poor prognosis if treated with standard ALL regimens and should be given specially designed, high-dose regimens. As the doubling time of these tumors may approach 24 hours, prophylaxis and immediate treatment for tumor lysis syndrome are mandatory.

Prognosis and Bone Marrow Transplantation

ALL has proved to be more curable than AML, with a 30 to 40% long-term disease-free survival rate in adults. Poor prognostic factors include older age, higher initial white blood cell count, cytogenetic abnormalities such as t(4;11), t(8;14), t(9;22) translocations, shorter duration of remission, and difficulty in inducing remission. These criteria may select a subpopulation of patients who would benefit from allogeneic bone marrow transplantation in first remission, which offers a 40 to 50% chance of long-term disease-free survival. Many hematologists recommend conventional chemotherapy for standard-risk adults and reserve transplantation for patients who relapse. Second or subsequent remissions have a 20 to 30% chance of cure with transplantation, and matched unrelated donors may be pursued if a histocompatible sibling is not available. Autologous transplant has not proved to be effective despite attempts to purge the bone marrow of leukemic cells.

Long-term complications are similar to those of AML. However, cranial irradiation and intrathecal therapy may increase the incidence of late cognitive dysfunction.

TABLE 3. **Classification of ALL by Immunophenotyping**

Cell Type	Immunophenotyping	Clinical Correlations
Pre-B cell (62%)	CD19(+), CD20 (−), CALLA (+), HLA-DR (+), cytoplasmic u chain (+)	
T cell (33%)	CD2 (+), CD7 (+)	Mediastinal mass, CNS involvement, high white cell count, better prognosis
Mature B cell (5%)	CD19 (+), CD20 (+), HLA-DR (+), surface immunoglobulin (+)	Short doubling time, CNS involvement, small non–cleaved-cell lymphoma (Burkitt's and non-Burkitt's), t(8;14), poor prognosis

ACUTE LEUKEMIA IN CHILDREN

method of
MARTIN L. BRECHER, M.D.
Roswell Park Cancer Institute
Buffalo, New York

Acute leukemia can be broadly divided into two groups of diseases, both of which are characterized by the abnormal proliferation of immature hematopoietic cells. Acute lymphocytic leukemia (ALL) accounts for about 80% of cases in the pediatric age group. Acute nonlymphocytic leukemia (ANLL), also known as acute myelocytic leukemia (AML), constitutes the remaining 20%. The etiology of these diseases is unknown, although certain groups of children, such as those with Down's syndrome, are known to be at increased risk.

DIAGNOSIS

The signs and symptoms of acute leukemia most frequently result from the failure of normal hematopoiesis. Common presentations include fever, pallor, fatigue, easy bruising, and epistaxis. Infiltration of leukemic cells into extramedullary sites can produce lymphadenopathy, hepatosplenomegaly, and bone pain. The complete blood count frequently reveals anemia and thrombocytopenia. The white blood cell count can range from low to greatly increased. Leukemic cells are often present in the peripheral blood smear. Definitive diagnosis is made by examination of a bone marrow aspirate, which will demonstrate increased numbers of immature, or blast, cells, and generally a paucity of normal erythroid, myeloid, and megakaryocytic precursors.

ACUTE LYMPHOCYTIC LEUKEMIA

This most common form of childhood leukemia has its peak incidence between 2 and 5 years of age, although it can occur at any age.

Subclassification

Recent progress made in the therapy of ALL has, in part, been due to recognition of the heterogeneity of the disease, making it possible to tailor therapy based on subclassification. Morphologically, the French-American-British (FAB) classification divides ALL into three subtypes (Table 1), with the L1 variant the most common in the pediatric age group.

The ability to immunophenotype cells using monoclonal antibodies has greatly increased knowledge of leukemic cell derivation. Approximately 80 to 85% of childhood ALL is of B cell lineage: 60% can be classified as early pre-B cell leukemia, in which there is generally expression of the common ALL antigen (CALLA); 15 to 20% contains cytoplasmic immunoglobulin and is classified as pre-B cell ALL. B cell ALL, in which there is expression of surface immunoglobulin, makes up 1 to 2% of all cases and usually demonstrates the L3 morphology; it often represents bone marrow dissemination of B cell lymphoma (Table 2). T cell lineage leukemias, which occur most frequently in adolescent males, make up 15 to 20% of cases.

Cytogenetic abnormalities can be detected in the leukemic cell population in more than half of the cases, with specific chromosomal alterations characteristic of certain subsets of patients.

Prognostic Factors

The overall prognosis for childhood ALL continues to improve, with 60 to 70% of patients now achieving long-term disease-free survival. Several factors have been demonstrated to have prognostic significance.

1. The white blood cell count (WBC) at diagnosis is probably the single most important predictor of outcome; the higher the WBC, the poorer the prognosis.
2. Age remains an independent prognostic factor in most studies. Children between the ages of 2 and 10 years fare best; adolescents do less well; and infants under 1 year of age have cure rates of only 25 to 30%.
3. Patients whose leukemic cells contain specific translocations, such as t(9;22) (Philadelphia chromosome), t(1;19) (more frequent in pre-B ALL), and t(4;11) (seen frequently in infantile ALL), carry a poor

TABLE 1. **"Lymphoblastic" Leukemias**

Cytologic Features	L1	L2	L3
Cell size	Small cells predominate	Large, heterogeneous in size	Large and homogeneous
Nuclear chromatin	Homogeneous in any one case	Variable—heterogeneous in any one case	Finely stippled and homogeneous
Nuclear shape	Regular, occasional clefting or indentation	Irregular; clefting and indentation common	Regular—oval to round
Nucleoli	Not visible, or small and inconspicuous	One or more present, often large	Prominent; one or more vesicular
Amount of cytoplasm	Scanty	Variable; often moderately abundant	Moderately abundant
Basophilia of cytoplasm	Slight or moderate, rarely intense	Variable; deep in some	Very deep
Cytoplasmic vacuolation	Variable	Variable	Often prominent

Reprinted with permission from Bennett JM, Catovsky D, Daniel MT, et al: Proposals for the classification of the acute leukemias. Br J Haematol *33*:451–458, 1976.

TABLE 2. **Multivariate Analysis of the Relationship of Pretreatment Characteristics to Duration of Continuous Complete Remission in Children (1 Year or Older) with ALL, by Immunophenotype**

Factor	"Worse" Category	*P* Value*	95% Confidence Interval for Relative Risk†
Early pre-B cell disease			
Age	≥11 yr	.0001	(1.8, 4.8)
Ploidy	Pseudodiploidy	.0001	(1.7, 5.2)
White cell count	>50 × 10⁹/L	.005	(1.2, 3.6)
Sex	Male	.004	(1.2, 2.8)
	>10× 10⁹/L	.04	(1.0, 2.4)
Pre-B cell disease			
Race	Black	.003	(1.3, 4.6)
Age	≥11 yr	.0001	(1.8, 6.0)
White cell count	>10 × 10⁹/L	.005	(1.3, 3.9)

*The significance of the likelihood ratio test for the Cox life-table regression analysis, with the fit of the model evaluated in the presence and absence of a particular category.

†Confidence interval estimating the proportional increase in risk of failure at any time for a patient in the worse category of a factor relative to a patient in the better category.

From Crist W, Boyett J, Jackson J, et al: Prognostic importance of the pre-B-cell immunophenotype and other presenting features in B-lineage childhood acute lymphoblastic leukemia: A pediatric oncology group study. Blood *74*(4):1252–1259, 1989.

prognosis. Hyperdiploidy, defined as the presence of more than 50 chromosomes per cell (DNA index >1.16 by flow cytometry) appears to confer a more favorable prognosis.

4. Children with B cell leukemia associated with lymphomatous masses do poorly with conventional ALL therapy. Some, although not all, studies suggest that T cell ALL carries a less favorable prognosis.

5. The presence of central nervous system (CNS) disease at diagnosis increases the risk of subsequent relapse.

The prognostic significance of other variables, including gender, race, and extent of organomegaly, has been inconsistent across studies. Improved treatment may override prognostic features.

Treatment

Treatment of childhood ALL is undertaken with curative intent. Rapid advances in chemotherapy regimens and supportive care mandate that treatment be carried out through a pediatric cancer center. Most centers treat patients on national cooperative group protocols, both to ensure state-of-the-art therapy and to answer biologic and therapeutic questions that will permit future therapeutic advances. The treatment described by the author is that currently used by the Pediatric Oncology Group (POG) for non–T lineage ALL (B cell ALL with L3 morphology excluded).

Induction Therapy

The goal of the initial phase of therapy is to induce complete remission, defined as the absence of any detectable leukemic cells. Induction therapy is designed to rapidly reduce the leukemic cell burden.

The use of three chemotherapeutic agents, vincristine, prednisone, and L-asparaginase, will produce remission in approximately 95% of children. Vincristine is given once per week, in a dose of 1.5 mg per M^2 (maximum dose, 2 mg) intravenously for 4 weeks. Prednisone is given daily during that 4-week period, at a dose of 40 mg per M^2 per day (maximum daily dose, 60 mg) in three divided doses. L-Asparaginase is given three times weekly at a dose of 6000 units per M^2 intramuscularly for six doses. The addition of an anthracycline to the induction regimen in childhood ALL has not been proved to increase remission duration or survival. Children who fail to enter a complete remission are given an additional 2 weeks of vincristine and prednisone. The few patients who are induction failures after 6 weeks of therapy carry a very poor prognosis and require aggressive salvage therapy.

Intensification Therapy

The goal of the intensification phase is to achieve maximum cell kill of residual subclinical leukemia to prevent the emergence of drug-resistant cell clones. For patients at lower risk of relapse, consolidation involves the administration of methotrexate at a dose of 1 gram per M^2 as an intravenous infusion over 24 hours with vigorous intravenous hydration, followed immediately by 6-mercaptopurine (6-MP) given as a 6-hour intravenous infusion at a dose of 1 gram per M^2. Forty-eight hours after the start of the methotrexate infusion, leucovorin rescue is administered at a dose of 5 mg per M^2 every 6 hours times five doses. Methotrexate levels are monitored to detect patients who excrete the drug slowly and who are, therefore, at increased risk of toxicity. The following week, patients receive methotrexate, at a dose of 20 mg per M^2 intramuscularly on day 1 and take 6-MP, 50 mg per M^2 orally for 7 days. These 2-week cycles are repeated for a total of 12 courses. The goal of intravenous infusion is to achieve prolonged cytocidal levels of each drug in the blood and in sanctuary sites, including the cerebrospinal fluid. A second arm of the protocol uses an oral regimen of methotrexate, given at a dose of 30 mg per M^2 every 6 hours for six doses in place of the methotrexate infusion to determine if comparable antileukemic effect can be achieved with outpatient chemotherapy. A third arm gives intravenous methotrexate, but no intravenous 6-MP, to allow the contribution of intravenous 6-MP during consolidation therapy to be assessed.

Patients at increased risk of relapse may be randomized to an intensification arm that alternates the intravenous 6-MP and methotrexate infusions with two other drug combinations, including VM-26 (teniposide [Vumon]) plus cytosine arabinoside (Ara-C), and daunomycin, Ara-C, vincristine, prednisone, and L-asparaginase. Each of these combinations has demonstrated efficacy in relapsed ALL. The conceptual basis for this arm is the Goldie-Coldman hypothesis that rotating effective, non–cross-resistant drug combinations can prevent the emergence of drug-resistant cell clones.

Continuation Therapy

6-Mercaptopurine and methotrexate are the most effective agents for continuation (maintenance) treatment of childhood ALL. These drugs are administered as follows: 6-MP, 50 mg per M^2 per day by mouth, and methotrexate, 20 mg per M^2 per week intramuscularly. Methotrexate is given parenterally, rather than by mouth, due to the variability in absorption from the gastrointestinal tract. Although the inclusion of vincristine and prednisone reinforcement pulses during maintenance therapy has improved disease-free survival in some studies, their benefit has not been demonstrated in treatment programs that include an intensification phase.

Sanctuary Therapy

The central nervous system (CNS) is the primary sanctuary site in childhood leukemia. Intrathecal chemotherapy is the mainstay of CNS prophylaxis. Triple intrathecal therapy (methotrexate, Ara-C, and hydrocortisone) is given on day 1 of treatment, on seven occasions during the intensification phase, and every 12 weeks during continuation therapy (Table 3).

Additional CNS protection is afforded by cerebrospinal fluid (CSF) penetration of methotrexate and 6-MP during the intensification phase. Intermediate-dose methotrexate infusions appear to provide protection against leukemic relapse in the testes, which is the second most frequent sanctuary site. Cranial irradiation should be employed only in patients at very high risk of CNS relapse, such as those with T cell ALL and very high initial WBC, and those with CNS disease at diagnosis, owing to its potential serious CNS toxicities, including intellectual impairment and the induction of secondary brain tumors.

TABLE 3. **Age-Adjusted Dosage of Intrathecal Chemotherapy**

	1 Year	2 Years	>3 Years	>9 Years
Methotrexate	8 mg	10 mg	12 mg	15 mg
Hydrocortisone	8 mg	10 mg	12 mg	15 mg
Cytosine arabinoside	16 mg	20 mg	24 mg	30 mg

Treatment of Specific ALL Subgroups

Children and adolescents with T cell ALL are treated on an aggressive, multiagent chemotherapy protocol, which is also used for patients with advanced-stage T cell lymphoma. Pulses of cyclophosphamide and Ara-C, which are particularly effective against T lineage lymphoblasts, are administered throughout the 2-year treatment program. Doxorubicin (Adriamycin) and VM-26 (teniposide [Vumon]) are incorporated in the regimen, as is vigorous CNS prophylaxis.

Children with B cell ALL with FAB L3 morphology do poorly on conventional ALL regimens but may achieve long-term disease-free survival on intensive regimens employed for disseminated undifferentiated (B cell) lymphoma.

ALL in infants less than 1 year of age is often common ALL antigen (CALLA) negative, frequently contains the t(4;11) translocation, and is usually associated with other high-risk features. Improved remission durations have been achieved using regimens that include cyclophosphamide, VP-16 and Ara-C, and anthracycline.

Treatment of Relapse

Bone Marrow Relapse. Children who experience bone marrow relapse while on therapy or shortly after its completion are unlikely to be cured by conventional chemotherapy. Second remission can be achieved in 80% of patients using a 4-week schedule of vincristine, 1.5 mg per M^2 weekly (maximum dose, 2 mg) intravenously; prednisone, 40 mg per M^2 daily by mouth; daunorubicin, 25 mg per M^2 weekly intravenously; and L-asparaginase, 10,000 units per M^2 intramuscularly three times per week.

Unfortunately, these remissions are rarely durable, and the best chance for cure is with ablative therapy and allogeneic bone marrow transplantation, using an HLA-identical sibling, if available, as the donor. Such an approach cures approximately one-third of patients. In the absence of an HLA-compatible family member, an unrelated donor may be located through the National Bone Marrow Registry, or a single-locus mismatched donor may be used. The results of autologous bone marrow transplantation in this setting have been disappointing, although recent reports suggest possible benefit for patients who have had long first remissions. Children for whom a bone marrow donor is not available should be treated with an intensive chemotherapy regimen that contains effective agents not used during the first remission. Approximately 25% of children who suffer a bone marrow relapse more than 1 year after initial elective cessation of therapy can be salvaged with aggressive chemotherapy regimens, although bone marrow transplantation may offer the best chance for cure in this group of patients as well.

Central Nervous System Relapse. Isolated CNS relapse should be treated with weekly triple intrathecal therapy until the CSF has been cleared of leukemic cells. Intrathecal therapy is then continued on a monthly schedule. Systemic reinduction and intensification therapy, using drugs that penetrate the CSF, such as high-dose methotrexate and high-dose Ara-C infusions, both consolidates the CNS remission and prevents subsequent bone marrow relapse. Craniospinal irradiation is administered following the completion of the intensive phase of the therapy. Approximately one-third of these patients can be salvaged by this approach.

Testicular Relapse. Isolated testicular relapse occurring during therapy or shortly after its discontinuation indicates the presence of drug-resistant cells and is often a harbinger of subsequent bone marrow relapse. These patients require aggressive reinduction and intensification therapy and additional CNS prophylaxis, as well as testicular irradiation. Testicular relapse occurring more than 6 months after the completion of therapy carries a less ominous prognosis. Many of these children can be salvaged utilizing regimens similar to the initial treatment protocol combined with radiation to the testes.

ACUTE NONLYMPHOCYTIC LEUKEMIA

Acute nonlymphocytic leukemia (ANLL) is relatively rare in children, accounting for 15 to 20% of childhood leukemia cases. Therapy is similar to that for adults with ANLL and requires intensive cycles of chemotherapy producing profound bone marrow aplasia. The most active chemotherapeutic agents are cytosine arabinoside (Ara-C) and the anthracyclines. Standard therapy includes daunorubicin, 45 mg per M^2 intravenously daily for 3 days, and Ara-C, given as a continuous intravenous infusion at a dose of 100 mg per M^2 per day for 7 days. 6-Thioguanine has been included in some induction regimens, but its efficacy remains unproved. Approximately 80% of children achieve complete remission.

Consolidation therapy includes one or more courses of high-dose Ara-C, given at a dose of 3 grams per M^2 every 12 hours for six or more doses. Additional cycles of the initial induction therapy are often incorporated into the consolidation regimens. Other agents, including VP-16, 5-azacitidine,* mitoxantrone (Novantrone), and amsacrine,* are included in some regimens.

CNS relapse is less frequent in ANLL than in ALL, and only a few doses of intrathecal therapy are administered during the course of treatment. The FAB M5 (monoblastic) subtype has a higher incidence of CNS involvement and requires more aggressive CNS prophylaxis. Intrathecal Ara-C should not be given simultaneously with high-dose Ara-C due to the risk of encephalomyelitis.

Long-term disease-free survival rates of approximately 40% are achieved with current chemotherapy regimens. Some studies have suggested that allogeneic bone marrow transplantation during first remissions can cure 60% of pediatric patients with ANLL. Because of the acute and long-term toxicities associated with bone marrow transplantation, the best initial therapy for patients with an available sibling donor remains controversial. The role of autologous bone marrow transplantation following remission induction as front-line therapy is currently being investigated.

Approximately 50% of children with ANLL who relapse can achieve a second remission with anthracyclines and Ara-C. However, subsequent bone marrow transplantation offers the only realistic chance for cure in this setting.

*Investigational drug in the United States.

Supportive Care

The provision of vigorous supportive care is essential for the successful management of children with leukemia being treated with intensive chemotherapy regimens.

Fluid and Electrolyte Management

During the first few days of induction therapy, large numbers of leukemic cells are destroyed, resulting in the release of a large purine load. Children with large tumor burdens, such as those with very high WBC or massive organomegaly, are at particularly high risk of tumor lysis syndrome during this period of massive tumor breakdown. High serum levels of uric acid may lead to uric acid nephropathy and renal shutdown. Vigorous hydration should be administered during this period, consisting of twice-maintenance intravenous hydration, unless there is evidence of congestive heart failure. Allopurinol (Zyloprim) is given at a dose of 300 mg per M^2 per day by mouth or intravenously, in three divided doses, to block uric acid formation. Sodium bicarbonate is added to the intravenous solution to maintain urine pH above 6.5 to prevent crystallization of uric acid in the kidneys. Intravenous solutions *without* potassium should be used until the risk of hyperkalemia secondary to tumor cell lysis and renal dysfunction has subsided. Serum electrolytes, including calcium and phosphorus, as well as potassium, should be monitored closely, as should the patient's fluid status. Urine output should be measured frequently in patients at high risk of massive tumor lysis. Renal dialysis should be available for those patients who develop oliguria unresponsive to diuretic therapy.

Management of Infectious Complications

Infection is the leading cause of death in children with leukemia. Neutropenia, either from replacement of bone marrow by leukemic cells or from myelosuppressive chemotherapy, greatly increases the risk of severe bacterial or fungal infection. Children with absolute neutrophil counts of less than 1000 per mm^3 and fever of greater than 38.3° C (101° F) should have appropriate cultures, including blood cultures, performed and should be started on broad-spectrum antibiotic therapy. Our initial regimen includes an aminoglycoside and an antipseudomonal penicillin. Third-generation cephalosporins, such as ceftazadime (Fortaz), and thienamycin antibiotics, such as imipenem-cilastatin (Primaxin), may be used as monotherapy, especially in the presence of renal dysfunction. Alteration of the antibiotic regimen may be necessary based on culture results. Indwelling central venous catheters are often used during the intensive phases of therapy, and coagulase-negative staphylococci and alpha-hemolytic streptococci are seen with increased frequency in this setting, requiring the addition of vancomycin to the antibiotic regimen. Children who remain febrile and neutropenic should have amphotericin-B added empirically to provide antifungal coverage.

Even in the absence of neutropenia, children on intensive immunosuppressive therapy are at increased risk of opportunistic infections, including *Pneumocystis carinii* pneumonia. Trimethoprim-sulfamethoxazole (Bactrim, Septra) is given in a dose of 5 mg per kg per day of trimethoprim in two divided doses on three successive days each week for prophylaxis against *Pneumocystis* infections. Varicella-zoster infections may be extremely severe in the immunosuppressed host. Susceptible children with a known exposure should receive a dose of varicella-zoster immune globulin (VZIG) intramuscularly within 48 hours of the contact. Established cases of varicella should be treated with acyclovir (Zovirax), every 8 hours intravenously for 5 to 7 days. These children should be monitored closely for the development of varicella pneumonia, a potentially life-threatening complication.

Blood Component Therapy

Children with acute leukemia may require the administration of blood products during induction therapy, following intensive myelosuppressive chemotherapy, or in the setting of leukemic relapse. We have become more conservative in our criteria for transfusion in an effort to reduce the risk of transmitting infectious agents. Packed red blood cells are given if the hemoglobin level is less than 8 grams per dL and is not expected to recover quickly on its own. Platelet transfusions are given to thrombocytopenic patients who have evidence of clinical bleeding. Platelets are administered prophylactically to patients with platelet counts of less than 20,000 per cubic milliliter, unless they are refractory to such transfusions due to prior alloimmunization. Granulocyte transfusions have not been documented to be of benefit in infected neutropenic patients and are rarely used. All blood products should be irradiated to avoid development of graft-versus-host disease from the infusion of foreign lymphocytes into an immunosuppressed host. Patients who are cytomegalovirus (CMV) negative and who may be candidates for bone marrow transplantation should receive only CMV-negative blood products.

Nutritional Support

Children with standard-risk ALL rarely require medical intervention to maintain adequate caloric intake. However, the same is not true for patients on intensive chemotherapy regimens for ANLL or those undergoing bone marrow transplantation. In these settings, oral mucositis and prolonged periods of general debilitation may necessitate the administration of parenteral hyperalimentation to maintain adequate nutrition. Patients must be monitored for excessive weight loss and biochemical evidence of malnutrition.

Psychosocial Support

There is a great need for psychologic support for children with leukemia and for their families. The entire family dynamic is upset. The emotional reaction of the child is, in part, age dependent. Economic difficulties frequently add to the turmoil. A team approach, using physicians, nurses, clinical nurse specialists, psychologists, social workers, and when available, child life specialists, is generally required to provide comprehensive care to the child and family.

CHRONIC LEUKEMIAS

method of
TED P. SZATROWSKI, M.D.
Cornell University Medical College and New York Hospital
New York, New York

CHRONIC MYELOGENOUS LEUKEMIA

Chronic myelogenous leukemia (CML), one of the myeloproliferative diseases, is a clonal malignancy involving the hematopoietic stem cell of the bone marrow. CML is characterized by increased numbers of maturing myeloid cells and their progenitors in the peripheral blood, bone marrow, spleen, and liver. The disease has a biphasic pattern; an initial, or chronic, phase lasting a median of about 3 years is followed by a terminal, or blast, phase whose median duration is about 3 months. The blast phase may be heralded by a period of quickening disease tempo, sometimes referred to as the accelerated phase.

CML accounts for about one-fifth of all leukemias, having an annual incidence of about 1.4 per 100,000. No etiology is known, but there is an increased incidence 7 to 10 years following heavy radiation exposure. There is no concordance in monozygotic twins.

In over 90% of cases, the Philadelphia (Ph^1) chromosome can be demonstrated in cells of hematopoietic origin, including lymphocytes. The Ph^1 chromosome arises from a translocation of genetic material from the long arm of chromosome 9 to the long arm of chromosome 22, designated t(9;22)(q34;q11); the resulting 22q− is the Ph^1 chromosome. At the level of the gene, the Abelson oncogene (ABL) from chromosome 9 is juxtaposed onto a restricted area (*bcr,* for breakpoint cluster region) of the BCR gene on chromosome 22, producing a chimeric mRNA and a novel fusion protein of 210 kilodaltons (p210). The latter has increased tyrosine kinase activity relative to the 145-kilodalton protein encoded by the normal

ABL gene. Whether the BCR/ABL gene rearrangement is the initiating event in CML is not entirely clear. Mice injected with bone marrow transfected with the BCR/ABL gene rearrangement develop a CML-like syndrome. The role of the SIS oncogene reciprocally translocated from chromosome 22 to chromosome 9 is unknown. Many patients who appear to have CML but lack the Ph^1 chromosome will demonstrate the BCR/ABL gene rearrangement by Southern blotting or polymerase chain reaction (PCR) methods. In addition, either simple or complex variant forms of the Ph^1 translocation (including some that may mask the Ph^1 chromosome) are present in about 5% of CML cases.

Closely related disorders include BCR/ABL-negative CML, chronic neutrophilic leukemia, chronic monocytic leukemia, chronic myelomonocytic leukemia (a myelodysplastic disease), and juvenile CML.

Clinical Manifestations and Diagnosis

Patients with CML often present with hypermetabolic symptoms, such as weight loss, night sweats, or, rarely, fever; lethargy or fatigue associated with anemia; abdominal fullness or early satiety due to splenomegaly; or bleeding or thrombosis due to platelet dysfunction, often with thrombocytosis. Symptoms of hyperleukocytosis and leukostasis are much rarer and may correlate better with the absolute peripheral blood blast count. In some 20 to 30% of patients with CML, the diagnosis is made in the absence of symptoms when a routine blood test done for unrelated reasons shows an elevated white blood cell (WBC) count, anemia, or thrombocytosis.

Over 80% of patients will have a palpable spleen, and splenomegaly may be pronounced even at presentation. Hepatomegaly occurs in about half of all patients. Lymphadenopathy is rare in the absence of accelerated or blast phase disease.

The median age at presentation is 45 to 50 years, with a peak incidence in the sixth decade; there is a slight male predominance. CML is rare before the age of 5, but juvenile CML, which is Ph^1-negative and carries a poor prognosis, can occur in infants.

In the presence of (1) leukocytosis with a marked shift to the left (but less than 5% blasts) and increased numbers of nucleated red blood cells, basophils, or eosinophils and (2) the Ph^1 chromosome, the diagnosis is not difficult to make. In addition to the symptoms, signs, and laboratory features described, the serum B_{12} and B_{12} binding capacity are usually elevated, while the leukocyte alkaline phosphatase (LAP) level is markedly depressed. Although other myeloproliferative diseases and a leukemoid reaction may mimic the clinical picture of CML, the presence of the Ph^1 chromosome or other evidence of the BCR/ABL gene rearrangement and a low LAP score will usually differentiate CML from other myeloproliferative diseases.

Based on certain clinical features present at diagnosis, it is possible to determine the relative prognosis of a given patient, and a staging system for CML has recently been proposed. Major factors associated with a worse prognosis include older age, larger numbers of blasts in the peripheral blood, either a very high or a very low (relative to the normal range) platelet count, and splenomegaly. Whether the precise location of the breakpoint within the *bcr* is predictive of the time to blast phase is controversial.

Findings that may signal accelerated disease are numerous and include difficulty controlling the WBC or platelet count with conventional doses of cytoreductive agents, new anemia or thrombocytopenia, more than 10% blasts (more than 20% blasts plus promyelocytes) in the blood or marrow, a WBC doubling time of less than 5 days, bone marrow fibrosis or dysplasia, worsening splenomegaly, new constitutional symptoms, the development of extramedullary leukemia such as chloroma, and the development of new chromosomal abnormalities (evolving new clone). Typically, an accelerated phase can be controlled with appropriate treatment for several months, but inevitably there is a progression to frank blast phase, defined as more than 30% blasts plus promyelocytes in the blood or marrow. The phenotype of blast phase may be either lymphoid (20 to 30%) or myeloid (70 to 80%); occasionally an undifferentiated or biphenotypic pattern is seen. Rarely, patients may present in frank blast crisis. Acute lymphoblastic leukemia may be Ph^1-positive in up to 30% of cases, but the breakpoint within the *bcr* and the resulting fusion protein (p190) are different than in CML. The median duration of survival from the onset of blast phase is about 6 months.

Treatment

Chronic Phase

The initial management of newly diagnosed CML in the chronic phase centers on the alleviation of symptoms and rarely involves emergency measures. Reducing the WBC count to below 100,000 per microliter and the platelet count to below 600,000 per microliter is a reasonable initial goal. This may also lead to correction of anemia and thrombohemorrhagic complications.

The traditional treatment goal in the chronic phase has been to control CML with oral cytoreductive agents, particularly hydroxyurea, a cycle-specific inhibitor of DNA synthesis, and busulfan, an alkylating agent. Hydroxyurea (Hydrea) is given orally at doses in the range of 20 to 50 mg per kg per day; a maintenance dose to keep the WBC count below 20,000 per microliter, for example, is then selected. Busulfan (Myleran) is given orally at doses in the range of 2 to 8 mg per day until the WBC count falls below 20,000 per microliter and restarted when it rises above 50,000 per microliter again. Although control of WBC count is less complete than with busulfan and it must be given continuously, hydroxyurea has been associated with longer overall patient survival than busulfan in recent randomized trials in patients with previously untreated CML. Busulfan also has major toxicities including pulmonary fibrosis, prolonged aplasia despite cessation of therapy, skin hyperpigmentation, a syndrome resembling Addison's disease, and permanent infertility.

Recently the use of recombinant interferon-α (IFN-α) in the treatment of chronic phase CML has generated considerable interest. Given at a dose of 5×10^6 IU per M^2 subcutaneously per day, it produces normalization of peripheral blood counts, as well as improvement in splenomegaly and bone marrow cellularity, in about 70% of patients. IFN-α therapy also produces relatively long suppression of the Ph^1-positive clone to less than 50% of metaphases in 20 to 30% of patients; while the ultimate importance of the latter effect with respect to overall survival is not entirely clear, results from a few randomized trials suggest that IFN-α in previously untreated patients results in longer overall survival compared to hydroxyurea or busulfan. Control of disease may take several months, and the putative survival benefit may be at least partly dependent on aggressive reduction of blood counts to near-cytopenic levels and concomitant bone marrow hypoplasia. Some patients will develop resistance to IFN-α therapy, which may be related to anti–IFN-α neutralizing antibodies. More importantly, IFN-α is not inexpensive and its side effects are not trivial. Most patients develop flulike symptoms, including fever, chills, myalgias, arthralgias, fatigue, and anorexia; neurologic, neuropsychiatric, gastrointestinal, and liver function abnormalities are less common. Side effects tend to diminish with time if the patient continues therapy.

A number of other agents such as thiotepa, 6-thioguanine, melphalan, daunorubicin, and cyclophosphamide are effective in CML but have no demonstrated advantage over hydroxyurea or busulfan. The role of cytoreductive agents in combination with IFN-α is under investigation.

While dose-intensive and combination chemotherapy can bring about more rapid hematologic control of disease and even produce transient suppression of the Ph^1-positive clone, no overall survival advantage has been realized with such protocols.

The subset of patients who are under the age of 50 and have an HLA-identical sibling donor should be considered for bone marrow transplantation (BMT). It is believed that the shorter the interval between diagnosis and time of transplant in chronic phase, the better the long-term survival. Indications and timing of transplant in older patients or those without a match remain controversial. The overall survival at 3 years after allogeneic BMT is approximately 60%, when the several large transplant series are considered in the aggregate. It is important to recall when advising patients about transplant options that there is considerable early mortality (approximately 25% at 2 years) after BMT and that graft-versus-host disease, which may be a source of considerable morbidity, occurs in more than half. The use of various immunosuppressive therapies post-transplant to reduce the incidence and severity of graft-versus-host disease, without destroying the beneficial graft-versus-leukemia effect that has been observed to occur in transplanted patients, is under active investigation. Patients who experience hematologic relapse of chronic-phase CML (not merely the presence of the BCR/ABL gene rearrangement) may benefit from the use of IFN-α. Second BMT carries a high mortality.

Thrombohemorrhagic complications can occur in any phase of CML, usually in the presence of platelet dysfunction and refractory thrombocytosis, which may manifest as a persistently elevated platelet count with a very low WBC count. Agents hindering platelet function have not been particularly effective. A change in cytoreductive agents is usually required. Specific thromboreductive drugs remain investigational.

Accelerated Phase

Management of the accelerated phase should be individualized. In general, however, it necessitates more aggressive measures to control blood counts and disease activity. Disease control may require larger doses of a given agent, a switch to a different agent, or the addition of an agent to the chronic phase regimen. Patients whose splenomegaly becomes difficult to control with chemotherapy may benefit from splenic irradiation or splenectomy. Similarly, patients who develop isolated bulky extramedullary disease may benefit from radiotherapy for local control. In the absence of options for definitive treatment of accelerated-phase disease, such as allogeneic BMT, patients should be monitored closely for signs of frank blast-phase disease.

Blast Phase

The standard approach to treatment of blast phase is to use chemotherapy in a manner analogous to that in acute leukemia, though responses in blast-phase CML are quite brief, and the goals of therapy must be limited. Nonetheless treatment of blast-phase CML requires hospitalization, blood product support, and experienced oncology support staff. The initial choice of chemotherapy is then dictated by the type of transformation.

Patients with lymphoid blast phase respond (by a return to chronic phase) in about 60% of cases to vincristine (Oncovin)– and prednisone-containing regimens, but overall duration of survival remains very short. Maintenance chemotherapy in responsive patients should probably resemble maintenance regimens in acute lymphoblastic leukemia; such regimens usually contain methotrexate, 6-mercaptopurine, and L-asparaginase. Central nervous system (CNS) prophylaxis with intrathecal methotrexate and possibly cranial irradiation may also be reasonable in this setting.

Patients with myeloid blast phase usually have a weaker response, even when regimens resembling those used in induction therapy for acute myeloid leukemia are used.

Because allogeneic BMT in blast phase results in perhaps 15% long-term survival, it is certainly an option worth pursuing when it is available, given the poor prognosis associated with all other currently available therapies for blast crisis.

Complications occurring frequently in patients with acute leukemia should be prevented wherever possible in blast-phase CML. These include complications of leukocytosis, which may affect the lungs and CNS when the peripheral blood blast count exceeds 100,000 per microliter. Chemotherapy or large doses of hydroxyurea should be administered immediately to reduce the blast count. Leukapheresis has been employed to this end, but it must be performed frequently while waiting for the effect of more definitive chemotherapy. Low doses of cranial irradiation have also been tried as CNS prophylaxis against leukostasis. Tumor lysis syndrome can also occur in blast-phase CML, usually during chemotherapy for very large tumor burdens, with hyperuricemia, hyperkalemia, hyperphosphatemia, acidosis, and renal failure. Prophylaxis with allopurinol (Zyloprim) prior to chemotherapy is indicated.

HAIRY CELL LEUKEMIA

Hairy cell leukemia (HCL) is a chronic lymphoproliferative disorder characterized by peripheral blood pancytopenia, splenomegaly, and morphologically typical lymphocytes with cytoplasmic projections. HCL is of B cell origin; the surface antigen profile typically includes mature B cell markers, such as CD19 and CD20, as well as CD11c and CD25, the β-chain of the IL-2 receptor. Rare T cell variants have been reported.

Infection remains the leading cause of death in patients with HCL, and the profile of infections to which they are susceptible is noteworthy. In particular, HCL patients frequently develop tuberculosis, atypical mycobacterial disease, *Legionella* pneumonitis, nocardiosis, toxoplasmosis, histoplasmosis, and pyogenic infections.

Clinical Manifestations and Diagnosis

More than 80% of patients are male, and most are over 40 years old (median age 55). Formerly often elusive, the diagnosis should be considered in the patient in this demographic group with cytopenias and splenomegaly, which is often massive, without lymphadenopathy. The differential diagnosis includes acute lymphoblastic leukemia, chronic lymphocytic leukemia, lymphomas primarily involving the spleen, aplastic anemia, agnogenic myeloid metaplasia, and Waldenström's macroglobulinemia. Characteristic hairy cells are seen in the blood (frequently at the feather edge of a peripheral smear) and bone marrow, although the marrow is often difficult to aspirate because of fibrosis. The hairy cells stain positive for tartrate-resistant acid phosphatase (TRAP). Associated manifestations include erythema nodosum, cutaneous nodules from perivasculitis, and polyarteritis nodosa. Constitutional symptoms and bruising from thrombocytopenia are also common. A few patients are diagnosed without symptoms on the basis of an abnormal routine blood count.

Treatment

The advent of recombinant cytokines and the purine nucleoside analogues has broadened enormously the treatment options for hairy cell leukemia. Formerly the median overall survival time from diagnosis was 53 months; presently it is estimated to be at least 8 years, but the precise impact of recently developed treatments on the long-term survival of these patients is still to be determined.

Since it remains to be shown that HCL can be cured, it is reasonable to follow without specific treatment those patients who are asymptomatic without serious cytopenia (absolute granulocyte count below 1500 per microliter, platelet count below 100,000 per microliter, or hemoglobin below 10 grams per dL) in order to ascertain the pace of their disease.

The adenosine analogue 2-chlorodeoxyadenosine (cladribine [Leustatin]) given at a dose of 0.1 mg per kg per day as a continuous 24-hour intravenous infusion appears to result in a durable complete clinical response in about 80% of patients. While experience with this new agent is relatively limited, toxicity is minimal except for leukopenia and culture-negative fever. 2-CdA is immunosuppressive, and its mechanism of action is unknown. An oral preparation and alternative dosing schedules are under investigation.

Deoxycoformycin (DCF, pentostatin [Nipent]), an adenosine analogue with adenosine deaminase inhibitory activity, produces durable complete responses in about 75% of patients when given at a dose of 4 mg per M^2 intravenously every other week for 3 to 6 months. Toxicity associated with DCF is significant, and includes renal impairment, nausea, vomiting, immunosuppression and myelosuppression with secondary infection, skin rash, and conjunctivitis. Overall poor performance status, recent infection, or renal insufficiency may preclude immediate use of DCF in favor of an alternative therapeutic agent.

IFN-α is highly active in the treatment of HCL. The usual dose is 2×10^6 IU per M^2 subcutaneously three times per week of interferon alpha-2b or 3×10^6 IU subcutaneously daily of interferon alpha-2a for up to 1 year. Overall response rates approach 90%, but it has lower complete response rates (about 10%) than the adenosine analogues, suggesting that its curative potential may be limited. Toxicity, as described for CML, is frequent, although at this dose it is often mild and subject to tachyphylaxis.

Although less frequently a first-line treatment for HCL, splenectomy nonetheless is an effective treatment for this disease and produces partial responses, particularly in terms of blood count improvement, in over 90% of patients. Because such surgery is not without risk, and because splenectomized patients often require further therapy within 1 year, the role of splenectomy in HCL is diminishing.

It should be noted that there is relatively little cross-resistance among the various therapeutic options described, such that prior treatment with one is not likely to decrease a patient's chances of benefiting from another. The roles of combination and alternating therapies are under investigation.

While the cytopenias and the predisposition to infection in this B cell disorder would suggest that colony-stimulating factors, such as granulocyte colony-stimulating factor, might be ideal adjuncts to treatment, their role is still undefined.

CHRONIC LYMPHOCYTIC LEUKEMIA

Chronic lymphocytic leukemia (CLL) is characterized by the proliferation of mature-appearing lymphocytes in the bone marrow, peripheral blood, lymph nodes, and spleen. It is the most common type of leukemia in the Western Hemisphere.

Clinical Manifestations and Diagnosis

Recently convened working groups have attempted to standardize the criteria for the diagnosis of CLL, which in nearly all cases is easily recognized. These criteria require (1) lymphocytosis of more than 10,000 per microliter or lymphocytosis of more than 5000 per microliter of cells with low-density cell-surface light-chain immunoglobulin or CD5 antigen for at least 4 weeks; (2) bone marrow involvement of more than 30% lymphocytes; and (3) mature lymphocytes with no more than 55% atypical or immature-appearing lymphocytes. Painless rubbery lymphadenopathy is also frequently present at diagnosis.

The differential diagnosis of CLL includes prolymphocytic leukemia, hairy cell leukemia, splenic lymphoma, leukemic phase of non-Hodgkin's lymphoma, and Waldenström's macroglobulinemia. Because the overwhelming majority (over 95%) of CLL cases are B cell, a T cell phenotype should prompt an effort to rule out another T cell disease, such as adult T cell leukemia/lymphoma, Sézary syndrome, T prolymphocytic leukemia, large granular lymphocyte leukemia, or leukemic phase of T cell non-Hodgkin's lymphoma. Similarly, if the patient's lymphocytes do not express CD5, the diagnosis of CLL should be questioned.

The median age at presentation is 55 years, but CLL is being diagnosed in younger individuals more and more frequently. Two-thirds of patients are male. No clear etiology has been identified, but a few occupational associations and familial aggregations have been described.

Some 50% of cases will be found to have an abnormal karyotype; the most common abnormality is trisomy 12, followed by abnormalities of 14q+.

Autoimmune phenomena occur frequently in association with CLL, including autoimmune hemolytic anemia, Coombs' positivity, pure red cell aplasia, and immune thrombocytopenia; cytopenias may be caused by marrow infiltration as well. Susceptibility to infection is multifactorial and relates to hypogammaglobulinemia and abnormal T cell and natural killer cell activity. Leukostatic complications of hyperleukocytosis, though described, are very rare.

The value of clinically available prognostic factors in CLL has been recognized for some time, and well-established staging systems provide the clinician with useful treatment guidelines. Table 1 shows that the three-stage modified Rai system is roughly comparable to the Binet staging system in terms of the separation of prognostic groups. In addition to the parameters comprising these staging systems, other clinical manifestations have independent prognostic value: a worse prognosis is associated with (1) a lymphocyte doubling time of less than 12 months, (2) increasing peripheral blood lymphocyte count, (3) a diffuse pattern of infiltration, (4) an abnormal karyotype, (5) increasing age, and (6) male gender.

Only a small number of patients with CLL will demonstrate evolution of their disease to a more aggressive form (carrying a very poor prognosis), namely, a diffuse large cell lymphoma (Richter's syndrome) or prolymphocytic leukemia. Prolymphocytes are larger than CLL cells and have a convoluted nucleus, immature-appearing nuclear chromatin, and large nucleoli. Prolymphocytic leukemia may arise de novo as well, and clinically is characterized by a median age of 60 years, prominent splenomegaly, minimal lymphadenopathy, extreme leukocytosis, and karyotypic abnormalities involving chromosome 14.

Treatment

It has become clear that a subset of Binet stage A patients with a lymphocyte count of less than 30,000 per microliter, a lymphocyte doubling time of more

TABLE 1. **Staging Systems in CLL**

Stage		Clinical Features	Median Survival (years)
Modified Rai	*Rai*		
Low risk	0	Lymphocytosis in blood (>5000/μL) and marrow (>30%) only	>10
Intermediate risk	I	Lymphocytosis and enlarged lymph nodes	8
	II	Lymphocytosis and enlarged liver and/or spleen	
High risk	III	Lymphocytosis and hemoglobin <11 gm/dL	1.2
	IV	Lymphocytosis and platelet count <100,000/μL	
Binet			
A		Less than three lymphoid sites involved	>10
B		Three or more lymphoid sites involved	6.3
C		Hemoglobin <10 gm/dL or platelet count <100,000/μL	1.3

than 12 months, a hemoglobin concentration of greater than 13 grams per dL, and a nondiffuse marrow histology have a life expectancy approaching that of an age- and gender-matched control population and probably do not require any form of treatment.

Among patients with more advanced disease, findings that suggest the need for treatment include (1) disease-related systemic symptoms, such as significant weight loss, extreme fatigue, fever without evidence of infection, or night sweats; (2) massive or progressive organomegaly or lymphadenopathy; and (3) rapidly progressive lymphocytosis with an increase in blood lymphocyte count of more than 50% over a 2-month period or an anticipated doubling time of less than 12 months.

Traditionally the first-line treatment of CLL has consisted of chlorambucil (Leukeran), an alkylating agent, 30 mg per M^2 (or 0.7 mg per kg) orally on day 1, with or without prednisone, 40 mg per M^2 per day on days 1 through 5, repeated every 4 weeks; alternatively, chlorambucil may be administered at a continuous daily dose of 0.1 mg per kg. Allopurinol may prevent the consequences of hyperuricemia. The principal potential toxicity of chlorambucil is myelosuppression, which may be easier to avoid on the intermittent schedule. Steroid-related side effects are well described. The goal of treatment is control of symptoms and blood counts, as complete remission is rare in CLL.

Fludarabine monophosphate (Fludara) is an adenosine analogue that has recently become available for the treatment of refractory CLL. It is given at a dose of 25 mg per M^2 per day intravenously over 10 minutes on days 1 through 5, with concomitant allopurinol, repeated every 4 weeks. Up to one-third of patients so treated may experience a complete remission (keeping in mind that the quantitation of response in CLL is not defined since complete responses have historically been very rare). Fludarabine-related toxicity is not uncommon and includes myelosuppression, infection, and low-grade neuropathies. The role of fludarabine as first-line therapy in CLL, as well as in combination with chlorambucil, is under investigation. The role of other adenosine analogues, namely, 2-chlorodeoxyadenosine and deoxycoformycin, which appear to have therapeutic activity in CLL, is likewise being defined.

Alternative treatment for patients with CLL who have failed chlorambucil includes cyclophosphamide, 300 mg per M^2 per day orally on days 1 through 5, or 750 mg per M^2 intravenously on day 1, repeated every 4 weeks. Cyclophosphamide has been used in combination with prednisone, with vincristine and prednisone (CVP and COP), and with vincristine, prednisone, and doxorubicin (CHOP), but the therapeutic benefit to be derived from the addition of such agents is controversial, while toxicity may be greater.

Standard therapy for autoimmune hemolytic anemia or immune thrombocytopenia is oral prednisone, 60 mg per day (or its equivalent in intravenous corticosteroids) adjusted according to the response in blood counts; 2 to 3 weeks of such treatment may be required. Intravenous gamma globulin (IVGG), 400 mg per kg per day intravenously over 3 hours for 5 days, may be added in patients whose response to steroids is poor. Autoimmune cytopenias should prompt systemic therapy as well in those patients not so treated previously.

Infections occurring in patients with CLL should be treated aggressively; the use of IVGG as prophylaxis in patients with a major or recurrent infection has been proposed, but the cost-effectiveness of such an approach has been questioned.

Additional therapeutic modalities in CLL have included splenic irradiation and splenectomy, usually employed in the setting of massive splenomegaly and autoimmune cytopenias. Effective therapy for transformation to prolymphocytic leukemia has not been described, but intensive CHOP-based chemotherapy is probably reasonable.

NON-HODGKIN'S LYMPHOMA

method of
JULIE M. VOSE, M.D.
University of Nebraska Medical Center
Omaha, Nebraska

The non-Hodgkin's lymphomas (NHL) are a heterogeneous group of lymphoid malignancies that can present clinically as an asymptomatic slow-growing neoplasm, a symptomatic moderately aggressive neoplasm, or a rapidly progressive malignancy. The incidence of NHL has been consistently rising over the past two decades in the United States. In 1993, 43,000 new cases of NHL were diagnosed in the United States. Although the incidence is rising in all age categories, the increase is most pronounced in patients over 60 years of age. In addition, as patients infected with the human immunodeficiency virus (HIV) are living longer due to improvements in supportive care, the incidence of HIV-associated lymphomas is rising steadily. Furthermore, the incidence of newly diagnosed NHL is increasing in patients outside of these two categories.

No etiologic agent is identified in most cases of NHL. Some congenital immunologic disorders, such as ataxia telangiectasia, severe combined immunodeficiency disorder, and Sjögren's syndrome, are associated with an increased incidence of NHL. In addition, acquired immunodeficiency due to HIV infection or the use of chronic immunosuppressive agents following transplantation carries an increased incidence of NHL. African Burkitt's lymphoma is associated with the Epstein-Barr virus, and the human T cell leukemia virus I is the causative agent of T cell leukemia-lymphoma endemic in southern Japan and some islands in the Caribbean. No viral etiologic agent has been identified in the majority of cases of NHL diagnosed in the United States. Some studies have found an increased incidence of NHL in humans exposed to certain chemical agents used in the agricultural industry.

Depending on the type of NHL, patients may present with asymptomatic painless lymphadenopathy, constitutional "B" symptoms such as fever, weight loss, or night sweats, or various regional symptoms depending on the location of the NHL. An accurate and timely diagnosis of NHL is important for proper medical management.

PATIENT EVALUATION

When patients present with symptoms that suggest the diagnosis of NHL, an adequate biopsy from an affected area is necessary. Fine-needle aspirates are often difficult to assess for the initial diagnosis of NHL. An experienced hematopathologist should review the incisional biopsy and staging material for accuracy. Specialized immunohistochemical assessment of surface markers, cytogenetics, and molecular biology evaluation of biopsy material are often necessary to establish the diagnosis of NHL or its subclassification.

Many histologic systems have been used for the classification of various subtypes of NHL. The system most frequently used in the United States over the last decade has been the International Working Formulation (Table 1), which classifies NHL into low, intermediate, and high-grade categories based on clinical outcomes.

After the histologic diagnosis of NHL has been confirmed, appropriate staging evaluation including computerized tomography of the chest, abdomen, and pelvis, complete blood count, chemistry profile, and a bone marrow biopsy must be done to complete the clinical evaluation. Other clinical tests may be appropriate in certain patients, such as spinal fluid analysis, magnetic resonance imaging, and gallium scanning. Following the completion of the staging evaluation, appropriate planning of therapy should ensue promptly.

The staging system currently used for NHL is the Ann Arbor system originally developed for the staging of Hodgkin's disease. Stage I represents involvement of a single lymph node region; Stage II, involvement of two or more lymph node regions on the same side of the diaphragm; Stage III, involvement of lymph node regions on both sides of the diaphragm; and Stage IV, widespread involvement of extralymphatic sites. An isolated extralymphatic lesion is designated as an "E" lesion.

A number of different prognostic factors have been found to be predictive of overall outcome. These include stage of disease, age, constitutional symptoms, tumor bulk, number of extranodal sites, serum lactate dehydrogenase (LDH) level, and performance status at the time of diagnosis.

TREATMENT

Treatment must be specifically tailored to the individual patient, depending on histologic subtype, stage, and other prognostic factors mentioned previously.

TABLE 1. **International Working Formulation**

Low-Grade Non-Hodgkin's Lymphomas
Small lymphocytic
Follicular small cleaved cell
Follicular mixed small and large cleaved cell
Intermediate-Grade Non-Hodgkin's Lymphomas
Follicular large cleaved cell
Diffuse small cleaved cell
Diffuse mixed small and large cleaved cell
Diffuse large cleaved cell
High-Grade Non-Hodgkin's Lymphomas
Immunoblastic
Lymphoblastic
Small non–cleaved cell

Low-Grade NHL

Patients diagnosed with low-grade NHL typically present with painless lymphadenopathy and are often found to have bone marrow involvement at the time of staging. The natural history of low-grade NHL includes an average survival of 5 to 8 years with or without standard therapeutic intervention. Low-grade lymphoma frequently converts to a more aggressive diffuse NHL over an extended time period. Autopsy series have reported up to an 80% conversion of low-grade lymphomas to aggressive NHL.

Localized or symptomatic low-grade NHL can often be successfully treated with radiotherapy. Single-agent or combination chemotherapy has not been found to be curative for extensive low-grade NHL; therefore, many physicians advocate a "watch and wait" strategy until the patient becomes symptomatic. When treatment is initiated, single-agent therapy with oral alkylating agents, such as chlorambucil (Leukeran) or cyclophosphamide (Cytoxan), is often used. Another initial therapy frequently employed in this clinical situation is the CVP (Cytoxan, vincristine, prednisone) regimen.

The use of aggressive combination chemotherapy regimens usually used for the intermediate and high-grade NHL can lead to a more rapid therapeutic response in low-grade lymphoma. Despite the high rate of response to combination chemotherapy, no changes in long-term survival have been documented to date in patients treated with this modality compared with patients treated with less aggressive therapy. Some institutions are now utilizing high-dose myeloablative chemoradiotherapy and autologous bone marrow transplantation (ABMT) or peripheral stem cell transplantation (PSCT) for the treatment of low-grade NHL. Extended follow-up of these patients will be necessary for evaluation of the curative potential of this approach.

Monoclonal antibodies directed against lymphocyte-specific antigens have been evaluated for the treatment of NHL. These agents have been assessed as isolated agents, tagged with toxins, chemotherapeutic agents, radioisotopes, or immunotherapeutic molecules. Preliminary trials with radiolabeled antibodies for the treatment of low-grade NHL have had some promising results.

Intermediate-Grade NHL

Diffuse mixed (DM) cell and diffuse large cell (DLC) lymphoma constitute the two most commonly diagnosed intermediate-grade lymphomas. In addition, immunoblastic NHL, which technically falls in the high-grade NHL category in the Working Formulation, is often considered with DM and DLC lymphomas due to their similar clinical behavior. Other histologies included in the intermediate-grade category are follicular large cell NHL and diffuse small cleaved cell NHL. These two histologic types often behave clinically in a more indolent manner than diffuse mixed cell, diffuse large cell, and immunoblastic lymphoma.

Patients who present with diffuse large cell, diffuse mixed cell, or immunoblastic NHL should be treated with curative intent. For the past two decades, combination chemotherapy has been the basis for curative therapy for intermediate-grade NHL. The first-generation chemotherapy regimens, formulated in the early 1970s, include CHOP, COMLA, and CHOP-Bleo (Table 2). These regimens were the first to produce long-term disease-free survival in NHL. Second- and third-generation regimens were developed by adding new agents to the original CHOP regimen to take advantage of alternative modes of administration or by alternating non–cross-resistant chemotherapeutic agents. These regimens include COP-BLAM, CAP-BOP, ProMACE-MOPP, m-BACOD, MACOP-B, and ProMACE-CytaBOM (Table 2).

With multiagent chemotherapy, 5-year survival rates are approximately 75 to 85% in patients with localized Stage I or Stage II intermediate-grade NHL. Involved-field irradiation can also be used for localized disease either alone or in combination with short-course multiagent chemotherapy. Survival for patients with localized disease is similar with these therapies. Patients with bulky Stage II, Stage III, or Stage IV disease have 5-year survival rates of 30 to 50% in most series. A large multicenter trial has recently been completed that compared the four most popular combination chemotherapy regimens—CHOP, m-BACOD, MACOP-B, and ProMACE-CytaBOM. The preliminary analysis of this prospectively randomized trial did not demonstrate any difference in duration of remission or survival among the different cohorts.

Prognostic factors found to predict for a poorer outcome include older age, the presence of systemic symptoms, elevated LDH, bulky disease, and extranodal sites of disease. Lymphoma in certain locations necessitates adjuvant therapy. For example, NHL in the paranasal sinuses and epidural spaces is often associated with CNS lymphoma, and CNS prophylaxis should be used. In addition, radiation of the contralateral testicle is necessary in primary testicular NHL.

Recurrent intermediate-grade NHL has a poor prognosis with routine salvage chemotherapy. Multiagent chemotherapy regimens such as DHAP, MINE, IMVP-16, and ESAP have been evaluated in this setting. However, despite a 20 to 30% complete response rate with most of these regimens, fewer than 5% of the patients are long-term disease-free survivors (Table 3). In recent years, the use of high-dose chemotherapy and ABMT or PSCT for patients with relapsed NHL has led to an increase in long-term disease-free survival in this patient population. In patients with chemotherapy-sensitive relapsed NHL, high-dose chemotherapy and ABMT or PSCT has produced 5-year disease-free survival rates of 35 to 45% in several series. Many transplant centers are now using high-dose chemotherapy and ABMT or PSCT as first-line therapy for high-risk patients rather than waiting for a relapse.

Alternative therapies that are currently being evaluated for patients who are not transplant candidates include infusional chemotherapy, modulation of the multidrug resistance (MDR) gene, and monoclonal antibody therapy, either alone or with conjugated toxins, chemotherapy, or radiolabeled isotopes. Figure 1 outlines a possible treatment strategy for patients with intermediate-grade NHL.

TABLE 2. **Combination Chemotherapy Regimens Commonly Used in Non-Hodgkin's Lymphoma**

CHOP: Cyclophosphamide, doxorubicin, vincristine, prednisone
COMLA: Cyclophosphamide, vincristine, methotrexate, leucovorin, cytarabine
CHOP-Bleo: Cyclophosphamide, doxorubicin, vincristine, prednisone, bleomycin
COP-BLAM: Cyclophosphamide, vincristine, procarbazine, bleomycin, doxorubicin, prednisone
CAP-BOP: Cyclophosphamide, vincristine, procarbazine, bleomycin, doxorubicin, prednisone
ProMACE-MOPP: Prednisone, methotrexate, doxorubicin, cyclophosphamide, etoposide, nitrogen mustard, vincristine, procarbazine
M/m-BACOD: Methotrexate, bleomycin, doxorubicin, cyclophosphamide, vincristine, dexamethasone
MACOP-B: Methotrexate, doxorubicin, cyclophosphamide, vincristine, prednisone, bleomycin
ProMACE-CytaBOM: Prednisone, methotrexate, doxorubicin, cyclophosphamide, etoposide, cytosine arabinoside, bleomycin, vincristine
VACOP-B: Etoposide, doxorubicin, cyclophosphamide, vincristine, prednisone, bleomycin
CNOP: Cyclophosphamide, mitoxantrone, vincristine, prednisone

High-Grade Lymphoma

Lymphoblastic lymphoma and small non–cleaved cell lymphoma constitute the high-grade lymphomas in the Working Formulation. These lymphomas are seen most frequently in the pediatric population; however, adolescents and adults are also occasionally affected. Both of these lymphomas have a rapid doubling time, and patients often present with rapidly progressive symptoms. Tumor lysis syndrome can occur with the initiation of therapy, particularly with small non–cleaved cell NHL. Because the high-grade lymphomas are biologically different, the chemotherapeutic regimens used for their treatment are also quite specific.

Lymphoblastic NHL is most frequently diagnosed in adolescent males who present with a large mediastinal mass. CNS and bone marrow involvement are frequent and are associated with a poor prognosis. Intensive chemotherapeutic regimens similar to those used in acute lymphocytic leukemia produced the best long-term disease-free survival in patients with lymphoblastic NHL. CNS prophylaxis is a part

TABLE 3. **Salvage Chemotherapy Regimens**

DHAP: Cisplatin, cytarabine, dexamethasone
MINE: Ifosfamide, mitoxantrone, etoposide
IMVP-16: Ifosfamide, methotrexate, etoposide
ESAP: Etoposide, cisplatin, cytarabine, dexamethasone
CEPP: Cyclophosphamide, etoposide, procarbazine, prednisone

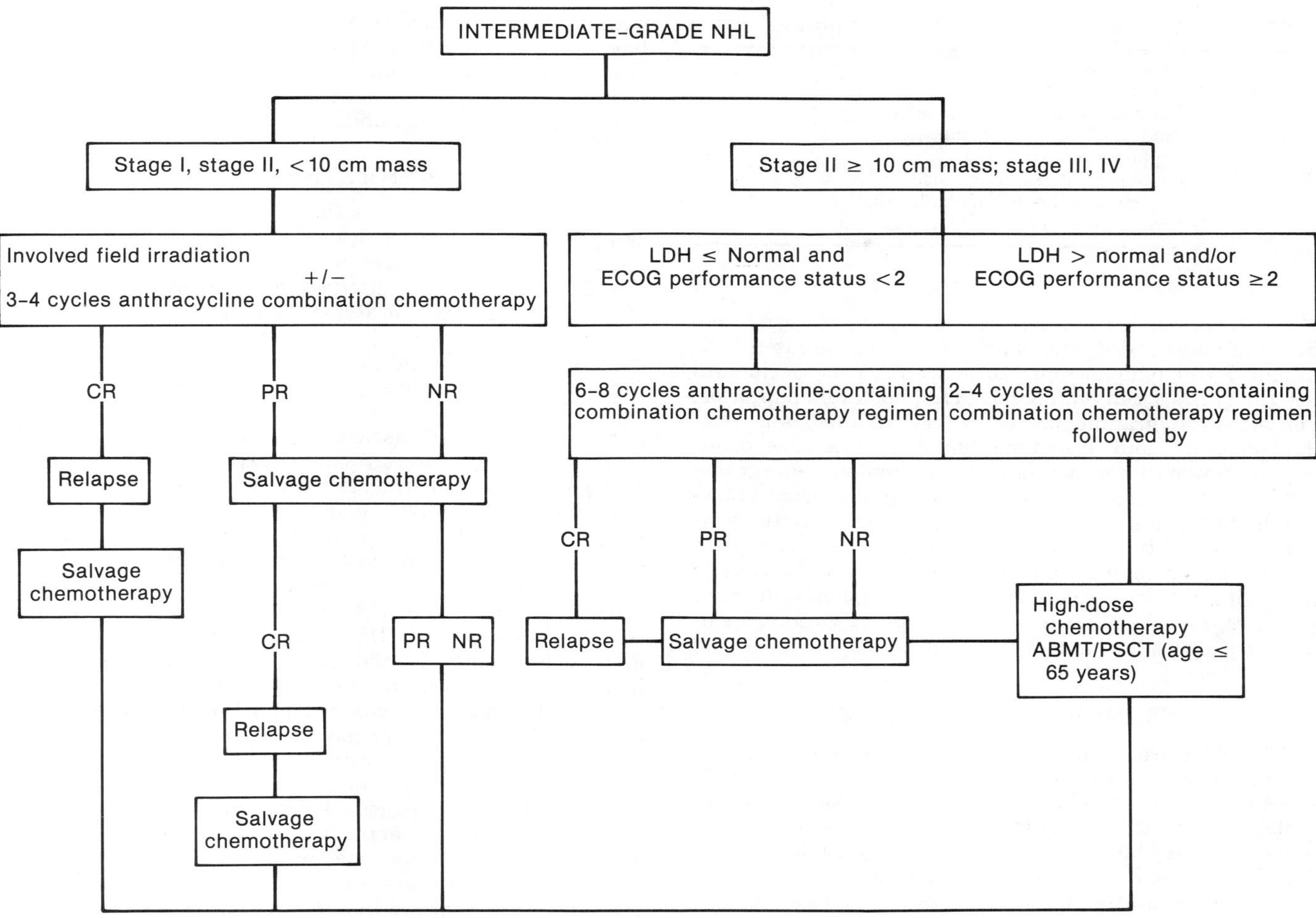

Figure 1. Treatment strategy for patients with intermediate-grade NHL.

of most of the regimens for lymphoblastic NHL due to the high propensity for CNS relapse if not properly treated. Particularly in adult patients, bone marrow involvement, CNS involvement, and elevated LDH at the time of diagnosis are poor prognostic signs. In many protocols, if these characteristics are present, high-dose chemotherapy and marrow or peripheral stem cell transplantation is done after the initial induction chemotherapy. Some series have shown that the use of an HLA-identical sibling donor results in an increased chance of long-term disease-free survival in young patients.

Small non–cleaved cell lymphomas must be treated with aggressive combination chemotherapy regimens, including CNS prophylaxis, owing to a high propensity for CNS disease in this histologic type. As with patients diagnosed with lymphoblastic NHL, patients with small non–cleaved cell NHL who present with CNS or bone marrow involvement or elevated LDH have a poor prognosis with conventional chemotherapy. High-dose chemotherapy and bone marrow transplantation are often used as part of the planned initial therapy in this patient subset. Most protocols use an initial induction program followed by high-dose chemotherapy and transplantation if these high-risk characteristics were present at the time of diagnosis. The use of high-dose chemotherapy and transplantation for relapsed high-grade lymphomas produces few long-term disease-free survivors.

T CELL LYMPHOMA
(Mycosis Fungoides and Sézary's Syndrome)

method of
TIMOTHY M. KUZEL, M.D., and
STEVEN T. ROSEN, M.D.
Robert H. Lurie Cancer Center, Northwestern University Medical School
Chicago, Illinois

Nowhere in hematology or oncology is the careful clinical evaluation of a patient's history, examination of the presenting lesion or lesions, and review of the histology as important as in determining the approach to the adult patient with a T cell lymphoma or leukemia involving the skin. A number of different disorders have been included within the spectrum of cutaneous T cell lymphomas

TABLE 1. **Cutaneous T Cell Lymphomas**

Mycosis fungoides
Sézary's syndrome
Adult T cell leukemia/lymphoma
Peripheral T cell lymphoma
Lymphomatoid papulosis
Lymphomatoid granulomatosis
Angioimmunoblastic lymphadenopathy
T gamma lymphoproliferative disorders

(Table 1): mycosis fungoides (MF) and Sézary's syndrome (SS), the adult T cell leukemia/lymphoma associated with human T cell lymphotropic virus I (HTLV I), peripheral non-Hodgkin's T cell lymphomas, lymphomatoid papulosis, lymphomatoid granulomatosis, angioimmunoblastic lymphadenopathy, and T gamma lymphoproliferative disorders. Although these diseases share a common presentation with skin involvement, they have widely disparate etiologies, histologic appearances, prognoses, and indications for and results of treatment. In this article, we attempt to describe salient clinical and histologic features we use in diagnosing the most common of these lymphoproliferative disorders, namely MF and SS, and suggest various treatment modalities that may be of benefit.

EPIDEMIOLOGY AND ETIOLOGY

MF and SS are the most common primary lymphomas of the skin. The average age at presentation is approximately 50 years. One thousand new cases are diagnosed each year in the United States. The incidence of MF increases with advancing age, but presentation in individuals younger than 30 is becoming more common as well.

The etiology of MF remains unknown. Investigators have suggested that genetics, infectious agents, or environmental exposures may play a role. Clusters of cases within families have been reported, as has an association with certain histocompatibility antigens (B8 and BW35). Cytogenetic analyses have demonstrated no consistent abnormality, but numeric and structural abnormalities of chromosomes 1 and 6 are most common. A variety of putative oncogenes such as *Erb-A, K-ras,* and *v-fps* may be activated by deletions, translocations, or amplifications of these chromosomes. The *lck* proto-oncogene, a member of the *src* gene family, is located on chromosome 1 at the site of frequent deletions or translocations.

The linkage of MF with exposures to industrial or environmental toxins has recently been refuted. Despite anecdotal cases that certainly seem to be work related, several well-designed case-control studies failed to support the concept. Other investigators have postulated that prolonged exposure to contact allergens may lead to enhanced immune responses leading directly or indirectly to the development of the lymphoproliferative state. Again, a case-control study demonstrated no significant differences in skin allergy to plants, metals, cosmetics, topical or nontopical medications, food, or insect bites between cases and controls.

Finally, a retroviral etiology for MF has been postulated. The similarity between the cutaneous lesions in MF and adult T cell lymphoma/leukemia has been noted, although the clinical courses are dramatically different. Several case reports have identified antibodies to HTLV I in patients with MF, and investigators have recently identified a significantly increased percentage of MF patients with retroviral gene elements in circulating lymphocytes compared with controls. It remains unclear whether these patients have true MF or rather atypical indolent examples of adult T cell lymphoma/leukemia. Given the heterogeneity in appearance and behavior of these diseases, more than one etiology is a distinct possibility.

HISTOPATHOLOGY

At present, it is thought that MF initially involves the skin; with time, however, wide dissemination to the lymph nodes, the spleen, the liver, or other visceral organs occurs. The diagnosis of MF is based on light microscopic evidence of a dermal infiltrate of atypical lymphocytes with hyperconvoluted cerebriform nuclei, epidermal exocytosis of these cells, and the presence of Pautrier microabscesses. This classic histopathologic presentation may vary, however. SS is an erythrodermic variant associated with a leukemic phase of the disease. Review of peripheral blood smears or biopsy material with an experienced dermatopathologist or hematopathologist is essential.

The development of monoclonal antibodies directed against specific cluster of differentiation (CD) antigens has allowed for much more exact identification of surface markers on the neoplastic cell. In most cases, the cells express the pan T cell antigens CD2, CD3, CD5, and CD6. Early T cells may also express CD7 on the cell surface. This marker may be frequently deleted in MF, a finding that may be helpful in differentiating neoplastic conditions from reactive lymphocytic involvement. The majority of cases are of the T helper/inducer phenotype ($CD4^+$, $CD45RA^-$, and $CDw29^+$), but occasional cases expressing a suppressor ($CD8^+$) phenotype have been described. Recent immunoconjugate trials have suggested that interleukin-2 receptor (CD25) expression is common in MF also. Because typical MF cases have been described with aberrant immunophenotypes, cell surface marker analysis may be of limited value for diagnostic purposes but may provide some prognostic information with regard to treatment outcomes.

Techniques have also been developed to detect the presence of T cell receptor (TCR)–associated antigens on the surface of the neoplastic cells. The mature TCR has at least two subunits, alpha and beta, connected by a disulfide bond. This protein dimer is in association with the CD3 molecule, a collection of small protein subunits. With the advent of molecular genetic techniques, such as Southern blotting, it is possible to detect the clonal somatic gene rearrangement associated with the TCR-beta subunit in cases of malignancy. This sensitive technique has improved the ability of pathologists to identify cells with the identical rearrangement in peripheral blood or lymph nodes. More sophisticated methods using the polymerase chain reaction should allow for the detection of residual or recurrent malignant disease in treated patients' skin, lymph nodes, or even peripheral blood, and may result in earlier diagnoses in atypical cases. However, the recent discovery of similar T cell gene rearrangements in patients with lymphomatoid papulosis, an indolent disease associated with cutaneous T cell proliferations, suggests that equating these rearrangements with neoplasia may be erroneous.

A number of other techniques remain investigational, including flow cytometry, cytogenetic analysis, calculation of epidermal Langerhans' cell densities in biopsy specimens, and determination of nuclear contour indices using electron microscopy.

STAGING

In 1979, the staging committee at an international workshop on MF proposed a staging system based on the international tumor-node-metastasis (TNM) system (Table 2). This classification was based on the evaluation of 347 patients and a multivariate analysis of potential prognostic factors. This group identified several independent prognostic factors: extent of skin disease at diagnosis (T), type of lymph node involvement (N), presence or absence of peripheral blood involvement (PB), and presence or absence of visceral (M) involvement. They also translated these categories into a recommended clinical staging system (Table 2).

PROGNOSIS

The initial course of patients with MF is usually indolent. Many patients give a history of antecedent skin lesions, usually nonspecific erythematous dermatoses. In many cases, there is an orderly progression from limited patches to more generalized patches, plaques, tumors, and finally, nodal or visceral involvement. The characteristic patch lesion is typically macular, lightly erythematous, and usually on the trunk or the extremities. Plaque lesions are more erythematous and have well-demarcated margins with some scaling. They frequently resemble psoriasis. Plaques can arise from patch lesions or previously uninvolved areas of skin. Tumor lesions tend to develop later, frequently associated with previous patches or plaques. They can be located on any part of the body. Ulceration of these lesions is common, and secondary infection is a major cause of morbidity.

At initial diagnosis, approximately 42% of patients have plaque skin disease covering less than 10% of the body surface, 30% have more extensive plaques, 16% have cutaneous tumors, and 12% have generalized erythroderma. In some reports, palpable lymphadenopathy has been noted in as many as 60% of patients at diagnosis. Light microscopic study of these nodes frequently shows dermatopathic lymphadenopathy, which is thought to be a reactive lymphoid hyperplasia associated with intranodal deposition of melanin released from areas of severe cutaneous damage. More sophisticated immunophenotypic, chromosomal, and molecular studies have detected involvement by neoplastic cells in up to 85% of these nodes. Sausville and colleagues* have described a system of grading of lymph node involvement in patients with MF based on the number and distribution of atypical lymphoid cells in paracortical zones and evaluation of lymph node architecture. LN-1, LN-2, and LN-3 nodes have preserved architecture, but the number of cells ranges from single infrequent atypical lymphocytes to small clusters of these cells to large clusters of atypical cells, respectively. LN-4 nodes demonstrate partial or total effacement of the normal architecture by the abnormal cells.

Peripheral blood involvement can be demonstrated in all stages of skin disease: 12% of patients with plaque disease, 16% of patients with tumor lesions, and nearly 100% of those with generalized erythroderma. Approximately 50% of patients with blood involvement have palpable lymphadenopathy, whereas most patients with visceral involvement have circulating malignant cells and palpable lymphadenopathy. Lymphopenia has been noted in patients with MF, although there is no definite prognostic significance. However, patients with eosinophilia have a shortened survival time compared with patients without eosinophilia.

Visceral involvement is generally associated with short survival times (median 25 months). The liver, spleen, and lung are most commonly involved at autopsy. There appears to be a predilection for other epithelial surfaces as well, such as those of the oral cavity, airway, gastrointestinal tract, or genitourinary tract. At presentation, few patients have evidence of bone marrow involvement by light microscopy.

Occasional patients may develop a more clinically aggressive lymphoma concurrent with a change in the histologic appearance of the neoplastic cells. This progression from typical small, convoluted lymphocytes to larger lymphocytes such as those associated with large cell lymphoma has been described. Whether this conversion is secondary to prior therapeutic modalities or reflects progressive genetic alterations in the neoplastic cell population remains unknown.

Infection remains the major cause of death (approximately 50% mortality rate) in patients with MF, regardless of the presence of systemic disease. Bacteremia due to *Staphylococcus aureus, Staphylococcus epidermidis,* and *Pseudomonas aeruginosa* is most common; infected skin lesions or intravenous catheter sites are usually the initial site of infection.

TABLE 2. **TNM Staging of Mycosis Fungoides and Sézary's Syndrome**

T (Skin)	
T0	Clinically or histopathologically suspicious lesion
T1	Limited plaques, papules, or eczematous patches covering 10% or less of the skin surface
T2	Generalized plaques, papules, or eczematous patches covering greater than 10% of the skin surface
T3	Tumors (one or more)
T4	Generalized erythroderma
Note:	Pathology of only T1–4 is diagnostic of MF. When more than one T stage exists, both are recorded, but the higher one is used for staging. Record other features, if appropriate
N (Lymph Nodes)	
N0	No clinically abnormal peripheral lymph nodes
N1	Clinically abnormal peripheral lymph nodes (record #)
NP1	Biopsy performed, not MF
NP2	Biopsy performed, MF
PB (Peripheral Blood)	
PB0	Atypical circulating cells not present (Sézary cells <5%)
PB1	Atypical circulating cells present (Sézary cells >5%)
M (Visceral Organs)	
M0	No visceral organ involvement
M1	Visceral involvement; must record organ involved

Staging Classification: Stage IA = T1N0PB0M0, IB = T2N0PB0M0, IIA = T1–2N1PB0M0, IIB = T3N0NP1PB0M0, III = T4N0NP1PB0–1Mo, IVA = T1–4N0–1NP2M0, IVB = T1–4N0–1NP1–2M1.

MANAGEMENT

The focus of the treatment of MF and SS is on control of the skin disease and, thus, palliation of symptoms. Multiple modalities have now been described that are effective (Table 3). These modalities include nonspecific moisturizers, antipruritics, and topical steroids. Specific antineoplastic therapy traditionally has involved ultraviolet light (UVA or UVB), with or without photoactivated psoralen compounds, topical chemotherapeutic agents, radiation therapy (either total-skin electron beam or photon), and systemic chemotherapy. Complete responses, especially in the early stages of the disease, are observed with all of the above-mentioned therapies, but long-term remissions are rare and it is debatable whether or not a cure can be achieved.

---

*Sausville EA, Worsham GF, Matthews MJ, et al: Histologic assessment of lymph nodes in mycosis fungoides/Sézary syndrome (cutaneous T-cell lymphoma): Clinical correlations and prognostic import of a new classification system. Hum Pathol *16*:1098–1109, 1985.

TABLE 3. **Therapeutic Alternatives for Mycosis Fungoides and Sézary's Syndrome**

Photochemotherapy (PUVA)
Topical chemotherapy (HN2; BCNU)
Electron-beam or photon radiation therapy
Systemic chemotherapy
Corticosteroids
Interferon
Purine analogs
Photopheresis
Retinoids
Monoclonal antibodies
Recombinant toxins
Cyclosporine

Photochemotherapy (PUVA)

8-Methoxypsoralen (OxSoralen-Ultra) is a member of a family of photoactivated compounds (furocoumarin derivatives), which may inhibit both DNA and RNA synthesis through formation of monofunctional or bifunctional thymine adducts, gene mutations, or sister chromatid exchanges. These drugs are active only if the tissue containing the psoralen compound is exposed to UVA light. Early preliminary trials suggested benefit; thus, at Northwestern University, patients with early-stage patch and plaque disease are often treated with PUVA alone. Long-term follow-up of 82 patients demonstrated complete clearing in 59% overall. No patients with tumors or nodal involvement attained a complete response.

Phototherapy units with UVA lamps emit a continuous spectrum of long UVA in the range of 320 to 400 nanometers, with peak emission between 350 and 380 nanometers. Initial exposure times of patients to high-output UVA are based on the degree of pigmentation before therapy, the history of the patient's ability to tan, and the output of the phototherapy units. Exposure times are increased with each treatment depending on the patient's response and evidence of erythema. The initial UVA dose is between 1.5 to 3.0 joules per cm^2, and it can be increased by approximately 0.5 joule per cm^2 per treatment, as tolerated. UV light–blocking eyeglasses should be worn for 24 hours after administration of 8-methoxypsoralen (8-MOP). Therapy is typically given three times weekly until complete clearing occurs. The frequency of treatments can then be reduced, but some maintenance therapy (ranging from 1 to 4 times per month) appears to prolong the duration of remission. Relapse can often be initially treated by increasing the frequency of treatment to two to three times per week.

Relatively few side effects have been witnessed. They include occasional nausea due to the psoralen ingestion, erythema, pruritus, and chronic dry skin. A more significant concern is the possibility that long-term PUVA exposure may be associated with abnormal amyloid deposition in the skin, an increased incidence of cutaneous carcinomas (especially squamous cell cancers of the skin and male genitalia), or cataract formation. Despite these problems, the long remissions induced, the ease of administration, and the lack of interactions with other therapeutic modalities make PUVA an attractive early intervention.

Topical Chemotherapy

Mechlorethamine hydrochloride (Mustargen)*† was the first topical agent evaluated to demonstrate efficacy in advanced MF. The solution used for topical application contains 10 to 20 mg of mechlorethamine dissolved in 50 to 100 mL of tap water (no vesicant activity at this low concentration). Recently, an ointment-based (Aquaphor or polyethylene glycol) preparation has been described that provided results similar to those obtained with the water-based solutions but may be easier to apply and have a lower incidence of cutaneous sensitivity.

Complete remissions are seen in 80%, 68%, and 61% of patients with limited plaque, extensive plaque, and tumor lesions, respectively. The corresponding median durations of remissions are in excess of 15, 5, and 12 months. It is difficult to make definite conclusions from these data because many patients included in the analysis also received intravenous mechlorethamine or methotrexate, and some may have received radiation therapy. Several patients have experienced a relapse as long as 8 years after treatment, suggesting that long follow-up times are essential before claims of cure should be made. For early-stage disease, however, topical mechlorethamine offers an efficient, convenient, and relatively inexpensive treatment option. A number of investigators have compared the results of topical mechlorethamine with total skin electron beam radiation therapy (nonrandomized comparisons), and there does not seem to be significant differences in terms of long-term outcomes.

Side effects consist of delayed hypersensitivity in approximately 35% of patients, although ointment-based solutions appeared to offer a reduced risk of contact dermatitis. Once hypersensitivity develops, patients can be desensitized by injecting minute daily doses of mechlorethamine over a period of several weeks or by starting at a low concentration applied topically with gradual weekly increments in dose. This procedure should be performed only in an appropriate medical setting because of the risk of anaphylaxis. There has been an increased incidence of skin cancers in patients receiving long-term administration of mechlorethamine. Of recent concern is the safety of family members of health care workers exposed to the topical solutions, although we are unaware of any documented adverse outcomes.

Several other topical agents have been tested and shown to be of benefit in MF, including corticosteroids, cytarabine, dianhydrogalactitol,‡ dacarbazine, guanazole,‡ teniposide, hydroxyurea, thiotepa, methotrexate, and carmustine.

*Not available in the United States.
†Not FDA approved for this indication.
‡Investigational drug in the United States.

Radiation Therapy

There has been extensive testing of total skin electron beam radiation therapy as the primary treatment modality for MF. Linear accelerator-generated electron beams are scattered by a penetrable plate placed at the collimator site. This reduces the energy of the electrons to approximately 4 to 7 MeV and allows adequate field distribution. The beam penetrates the surface only several millimeters to 1 centimeter (into the dermis). Patients may receive radiotherapy using six-field or rotational treatments. Thus, the total skin surface can be treated without significant internal organ toxicity. Total radiation doses of approximately 3000 to 3600 cGy over an 8- to 10-week period are tolerable.

Most patients who receive radiotherapy (80 to 90%) achieve a clinical remission. Approximately 50% of patients with limited-stage disease and 25% of those with generalized plaques had long-term remissions (3-year disease-free survival). Patients with tumor lesions, generalized erythroderma, peripheral blood or nodal involvement, or visceral spread can be successfully palliated with electron beam radiation, as well. Alternatively, external beam radiation can adequately control areas of otherwise resistant MF and provide palliation in cases of bulky tumor lesions. Unfortunately, the cumulative dosage that can be given to patients over time is limited owing to organ toxicity.

Side effects associated with electron beam therapy may be extreme, including scaling, dryness of skin, erythema, extremity edema, telangiectasia formation, skin ulceration, and hair loss or sweat gland atrophy (which is frequently permanent). Careful radiation dosimetric techniques are required to ensure adequate skin treatment without excessive normal tissue toxicity. Thus, this therapy should be given only at centers with extensive experience. Electron beam radiotherapy should not be used early in the disease course now that other topical therapies have been developed that yield similar response rates with less potential toxicity. Side effects associated with external beam photon radiation include leukopenias, thrombocytopenias, and radiation dermatitis, all of which may prevent long-term therapy with other modalities.

Systemic Chemotherapy

Systemic chemotherapy should be reserved for those patients who have relapsed or who have disease refractory to topical interventions, or for those with nodal or visceral disease at the time of diagnosis. Single-agent chemotherapy with alkylating agents, methotrexate, cisplatin (Platinol), VP-16 (etoposide [VePesid]), bleomycin (Blenoxane), doxorubicin (Adriamycin), vincristine (Oncovin), vinblastine (Velban), or oral corticosteroids has been used for the treatment of MF and SS. Complete response rates have ranged from 20 to 50% in most trials, but the duration of response is short, averaging several months.

Combination chemotherapy has also been used. Combinations of chlorambucil (Leukeran) and prednisone (CP); cyclophosphamide (Cytoxan), doxorubicin, vincristine, and prednisone (CHOP); cyclophosphamide, vincristine, prednisone, and bleomycin (COP-bleo); and doxorubicin, vincristine, and prednisone (HOP) have all been tested. Higher response rates of 80 to 100% have been achieved and have been associated with longer durations of remission. However, no trial has demonstrated survival benefit in patients treated early with aggressive interventions. Thus, we reserve combination chemotherapy agents for patients whose disease has demonstrated more aggressive behavior.

Combined Approaches

A number of combinations of topical and systemic approaches for the treatment of early-stage MF have been tested. Most trials have demonstrated significant improvement in the overall response rate achieved, especially in the subgroups of patients with advanced disease. However, there does not appear to be a prolongation of survival, nor has conclusive evidence of cure been demonstrated. The most definitive trial was performed at the National Cancer Institute. Patients with all stages of disease and levels of performance status were randomized to either aggressive combination chemotherapy and total-skin electron-beam or sequential palliative topical and systemic interventions. After a median follow-up of 75 months, the National Cancer Institute was able to demonstrate significant differences between the treatment groups in rates of complete remission induction (combined treatment was more effective than conservative treatment) but not in disease-free or overall survival. In addition, combined therapy was associated with considerable toxicity. Therefore, such approaches should remain investigational.

Biologics and Other Investigational Approaches

Interferon-alpha* remains one of the most active modalities in MF and SS. Multiple trials with high or low doses have been performed, with complete response rates ranging from 10 to 27% in heavily pretreated individuals. In trials of less heavily pretreated patients, response rates of 76 to 92% have been reported. Toxicity is most pronounced at the high doses, including fever, chills, myalgias, malaise, anorexia, and cytopenias. In light of this, we rarely give more than 12 million units per M^2 daily, and this dose frequently needs to be reduced over time.

Interferons have also been combined with other agents. Combining interferon-alpha 3 times weekly with PUVA therapy has been associated with response rates of approximately 90%; the majority are complete remissions. If the disease clears completely, the PUVA frequency should be reduced to the maintenance dose every 2 to 4 weeks. Other investigators

*Not FDA approved for this indication.

have combined the purine analog 2′-deoxycoformycin* (an adenosine deaminase inhibitor) with interferon-alpha in a small phase II trial. The overall response rate was 44% (one complete remission and 10 partial remissions), with a median duration of response of 11 months. Toxicity consisted of fever, malaise, myalgias, and reversible mental status changes.

Additional purine analogs including fludarabine* and 2-chlorodeoxyadenosine (cladribine)* have demonstrated significant clinical activity in patients with MF. Several trials have demonstrated response rates of 30 to 40%. Toxicity is primarily related to myelosuppression, with thrombocytopenia being most problematic for the patient. Trials with 2-chlorodeoxyadenosine combined with interferons are anticipated.

Photopheresis is a new adaptation of the use of psoralens with UVA light. In standard fashion, patients ingest the 8-methoxypsoralen prior to treatment. They then undergo leukapheresis with isolation of the mononuclear cell fraction. The cells are then exposed to UVA light ex vivo within a special chamber within the pheresis device and the damaged cells are subsequently re-infused. These treatments can be given every 2 to 4 weeks as needed for control of the disease. The mechanisms by which extracorporeal treatment of malignant and normal lymphocytes with psoralens and UVA light results in skin clearing in patients with MF and SS remain speculative.

Retinoids also have been used to treat MF with limited success. Trials reporting response rates of approximately 40% and minimal toxicity with a variety of compounds suggest a use for these agents in combination with other drugs or as maintenance therapy. Newer retinoids with enhanced activity are being developed. Insight into retinoid biology may lead to more rational uses for these drugs in MF.

A variety of other approaches remain investigational. These approaches include autologous bone marrow rescue following high-dose chemotherapy, monoclonal antibody therapy, targeted fusion toxin therapy, anti-thymocyte globulin, interleukin-2,† cyclosporine, and acyclovir.

In conclusion, several effective therapies have now been developed. However, no one treatment can be described as most beneficial or curative. Therefore, for most patients, treatment should be directed at palliation of cutaneous disease with topical therapies or PUVA. Further definite treatment recommendations must await the results of prospective randomized trials.

*Not FDA approved for this indication.
†Investigational drug in the United States.

MULTIPLE MYELOMA

method of
BART BARLOGIE, M.D., Ph.D.,
DAVID VESOLE, M.D., Ph.D., and
SUNDAR JAGANNATH, M.D.
University of Arkansas for Medical Sciences
Little Rock, Arkansas

Multiple myeloma is a clonal B cell malignancy in which terminal B cells (plasma cells) are the dominant phenotype, although more immature B cells are also involved and may contribute to the dissemination of the disease via the peripheral blood. Multiple genetic abnormalities have been observed including *N-ras, c-myc, bcl-1,* and the suppressor genes *Rb* and *p53.* An intricate cytokine network seems to be operating, with interleukin-6, interleukin-1, and tumor necrosis factor featured prominently, which explains some of the clinical manifestations, such as lytic bone disease, anemia, and hypoalbuminemia. The disease etiology is unknown, but an increased frequency among farmers suggests chemical carcinogenesis in some patients. The delayed occurrence of myeloma after more than 20 years in Japanese atomic bomb survivors is consistent with a long subclinical course, which may also explain the low rate of progression (1 to 2% per year) from benign monoclonal gammopathy to overt myeloma.

Approximately 12,000 new cases of myeloma are reported annually in the United States. The median age is 65 years, blacks are afflicted more often than whites, and males more frequently than females. Myeloma is one of the few malignancies for which an increase in both incidence and mortality has been reported.

Presenting features include weakness, bone pain, recurrent infections, and symptoms resulting from hypercalcemia or renal failure. With increased use of routine laboratory testing, more asymptomatic patients are being diagnosed because of elevated serum protein levels, proteinuria, anemia, or mild renal failure. Some patients suffer from tissue deposition of light chain (AL) amyloid or light chains in visceral organs, which can cause death in the absence of major tumor mass–related symptoms.

DIAGNOSIS

The standard work-up for a patient suspected of having multiple myeloma should include a peripheral hemogram, blood chemistry, complete bone survey, bone marrow aspirate, and biopsy as well as serum and urine electrophoresis, and quantitative serum immunoglobulin analysis. Immunoelectrophoresis or immunofixation of serum and urine is needed to confirm the presence of monoclonal immunoglobulin secretion. A 24-hour urine collection should be performed to quantitate the excretion of total protein and monoclonal light chains.

The diagnosis of multiple myeloma is obvious in the presence of marked bone marrow plasmacytosis (>20%), lytic bone lesions, and a monoclonal protein. However, difficulties may arise in the absence of lytic bone disease or monoclonal protein production or when bone marrow involvement is focal. Magnetic resonance imaging (MRI) has been helpful in detecting patchy bone marrow involvement, and computed tomography (CT) is helpful in the detection of early lytic lesions. Isotope bone scanning is usually not

Supported in part by CA 55819 from the National Institutes of Health, Bethesda, Maryland.

useful and is positive mainly in the case of healing fractures as a result of increased osteoblastic activity. The diagnosis of a solitary plasmacytoma of bone or soft tissue requires the absence of bone marrow plasmacytosis and, more recently, of abnormal MRI signals suggesting bone marrow involvement. Benign monoclonal gammopathy, or MGUS (*M*onoclonal *G*ammopathy of *U*ndetermined *S*ignificance), should not be confused with multiple myeloma, as the former condition is merely a laboratory syndrome of monoclonal plasma cell proliferation with monoclonal protein production usually of limited extent (<10% plasma cells in the bone marrow). Some cases fulfilling the criteria of multiple myeloma are considered to be indolent disease that can follow a smoldering course not requiring therapy for months to years.

TUMOR STAGING

Staging has been performed according to the criteria of Durie and Salmon, but the serum beta$_2$-microglobulin level represents the single most important prognostic variable that is readily obtainable in a quantitative and reproducible fashion. In addition, the plasma cell labeling index and the serum C-reactive protein level (reflecting in vivo interleukin-6 activity) have been recognized as independently helpful parameters. Plasmablastic morphology portends a rapidly fatal course, associated with high tumor cell labeling index and elevation of serum lactic dehydrogenase (LDH).

TREATMENT

Therapy of Newly Diagnosed Myeloma

In the absence of curative therapy due to marked resistance of tumor cells to standard doses of drugs, it is important that both physicians and patients be aware of new therapeutic developments. Inquiry at specialized treatment centers about promising new therapies under investigation is recommended, especially for treatment of patients under age 60.

The mainstays of treatment are glucocorticoids, especially in high doses; alkylating agents; radiation; and interferon-alpha. Among the alkylating agents, differences exist in efficacy and toxicity. Melphalan is the most active alkylator. However, as is the case with nitrosoureas, prolonged use of melphalan (≥1 year) can induce bone marrow damage and, potentially, myelodysplasia or acute myeloid leukemia. Cyclophosphamide, on the other hand, targets more differentiated hematopoietic cells (i.e., spares normal stem cells) and hence is less leukemogenic. When given in high doses, cyclophosphamide is effective for peripheral blood stem cell mobilization and collection.

Much debate has centered on the optimal *standard alkylating agent regimen,* especially melphalan plus prednisone (MP) versus combination chemotherapy with additional alkylating agents and/or anthracyclines. This topic has been addressed in large randomized trials, and even when statistical differences were noted, the clinical benefit from combination chemotherapy was measured in only a few months. Thus, provided adequate doses of melphalan are used (e.g., 8 mg per M^2 daily for 4 days), with dose escalation according to hematologic toxicity in succeeding cycles, response rates and survival match those of any combination regimen.

Patients up to age 65 lacking other significant health problems should remain candidates for autotransplant trials currently under investigation. The preservation of adequate hematopoietic stem cell function is assured with regimens such as dexamethasone (DEX) alone or in combination with vincristine and doxorubicin (VAD) (Table 1). VAD affects tumor cytoreduction more rapidly than any other treatment currently available. This approach is especially useful when hypercalcemia or renal failure with light-chain cast nephropathy requires prompt intervention. Depending on the response definitions used (≥50% or ≥75%), 50 to 70% of patients achieve remission, and maximum antitumor effect is usually obtained within four cycles of such therapy. Remissions can be maintained with DEX pulsing, interferon, or both. When considering autologous bone marrow transplantation (ABMT), peripheral blood stem cells (PBSC) or autologous bone marrow should be collected prior to initiation of chronic alkylating agent or interferon therapy because of stem cell impairment.

Patients over age 65 can also be treated with DEX or VAD, although side effects such as irritability, depression, hyperglycemia, and immunosuppression with infectious complications are more common and pronounced. Standard MP is certainly appropriate until a stable plateau phase has been attained. There is no value to maintenance therapy, since responses can be reinduced upon disease relapse.

Transplants

The duration of bone marrow aplasia associated with marrow-ablative therapy such as melphalan, 200 mg per M^2 or 140 mg per M^2 with added total body irradiation (TBI) (850–1200 cGy), can be shortened markedly when PBSC are used that have been collected after high-dose cyclophosphamide (HDCTX) priming with granulocyte-monocyte colony-stimulating factor (GM-CSF [Leukine]) or granulocyte colony-stimulating factor (G-CSF [Neupogen]). Thus, severe neutropenia (≤500/μL) and thrombopenia (≤50,000/μL) usually do not last longer than 1 week. Mortality is less than 5%. The most crucial determinant for adequate stem cell function is the duration of prior alkylating agent therapy, especially with melphalan or nitrosoureas. Significant compromise of hematopoietic stem cell function is seen in more than 50% of patients who have had more than 1 year of prior therapy with such drugs. When applied within 1 year of diagnosis, autotransplant regimens achieve complete remission (CR) rates (immunofixation negative, normal bone marrow aspirate and biopsy) in up to 50% of patients. Depending on prognostic factors, event-free and overall survival durations are on the order of 3 and 5 years, respectively, from transplant. Post-transplant interferon maintenance is still under investigation.

TABLE 1. **Treatment Regimens in Use for Myeloma**

	Regimen	Doses	Schedule
Standard Dose Therapy	IFN DEX	3–5 mu/M^2 qd or TIW 40 mg days 1–4, 9–12, 17–20	q 35 days
	V A D	VCR 0.5 mg days 1–4 CI ADR 10 mg/M^2 days 1–4 CI DEX 40 mg days 1–4, 9–12, 17–20	q 35 days
	E D A P	VP16 100–200 mg/M^2 days 1–4 CI DEX 40 mg days 1–5 ARA-C 1 gm/M^2 × 1 on day 5 DDP 25 mg/M^2 days 1–4 CI	q 21–28 days
		± G-CSF or GM-CSF 0.25 mg/M^2 day 6 → hematopoietic recovery	
	M P	MEL 8 mg/M^2 days 1–4 PO PRED 40 mg/M^2 days 1–7 PO	q 28–42 days
	V M C P	VCR 1.0 mg day 1 IV MEL 6 mg/M^2 days 1–4 PO CTX 125 mg/M^2 days 1–4 IV PRED 60 mg/M^2 days 1–4 PO	q 28–42 days
	V B A P	VCR 1.0 mg day 1 IV BCNU 20 mg/M^2 day 1 IV ADR 30 mg/M^2 day 1 IV PRED 60 mg/M^2 days 1–4 PO	q 28–42 days
	V B M C P	VCR 1.2 mg/M^2 day 1 IV BCNU 20 mg/M^2 day 1 IV MEL 8 mg/M^2 days 1–4 PO CTX 400 mg/M^2 day 1 IV PRED 40 mg/M^2 days 1–7 PO	q 35–42 days
Myeloablative Therapy	Autologous	Single MEL 200 mg/M^2 MEL 140 mg/M^2 + TBI 850–1200 cGy Double (within 3–6 months) MEL 200 mg/M^2 q 3–6 months × 2 MEL 200 mg/M^2 followed in 3–6 months by MEL 140 mg/M^2 + TBI 850–1200 cGy	+ PBSC/ABMT + G/GM-CSF
	Allogeneic	MEL 140 mg/M^2 + TBI 850–1200 cGy BU 1 mg/kg/dose q 6 h × 4 days PO (16 mg/kg) + CTX 60 mg/kg × 2 days (120 mg/kg)	+ Allogeneic BMT

Abbreviations: IFN = interferon; DEX = dexamethasone; VCR = vincristine; ADR = Adriamycin (doxorubicin); ARA-C = cytosine arabinoside; DDP = cisplatin; MEL = melphalan; CTX = cyclophosphamide; PRED = prednisone; TBI = total body irradiation; BU = busulfan; TIW = three times a week; CI = continuous infusion; PBSC = peripheral blood stem cells; ABMT = autologous bone marrow transplant; VP16 = etoposide; BCNU = carmustine.

Salvage Therapy

DEX or VAD

Salvage treatment is needed for patients who have developed resistance to first-line treatment, either due to primary refractoriness or as a result of resistant relapse after remission. The scope of available salvage regimens narrows with the number of regimens to which resistance has been established. In the presence of resistance restricted to alkylating agents, DEX alone induces responses in about 30% of patients regardless of whether a response had been obtained previously. VAD benefits about 50% of relapsing patients and about 30% of those with primary unresponsive disease.

Transplants

With additional resistance to DEX or VAD (beyond alkylating agents), tumor control can be established with dose-intensive therapy using autotransplants. With melphalan-TBI (or similar combinations) and especially with two successive autotransplants 3 to 6 months apart, almost 80% of patients achieve greater than 75% tumor cytoreduction including true CR rates of 15 to 20% with a median survival on the order of 2 to 3 years post-transplant. Because of the usually palliative use of myeloablative therapy in this setting, subsequent DEX pulsing and/or interferon-alpha may be useful in further extending the duration of disease control.

Refractory myeloma with plasmablastic features, increased tumor cell labeling index (>2%), or elevated serum LDH usually relapses soon, even after intensive myeloablative therapy. A lymphoma-oriented regimen such as EDAP (etoposide, dexamethasone, cytarabine, and cisplatin; see Table 1) induces objective responses (≥75% tumor cytoreduction) in approximately 40% of patients, even during relapse after recent myeloablative therapy. Two to three cycles of EDAP are recommended prior to autologous transplant in order not to further compromise hematopoietic stem cell function.

Overcoming Drug Resistance

The multidrug resistance (MDR) phenotype is present in varying tumor cell proportions even at diagnosis in both marrow and peripheral blood. Trials with calcium channel blockers, quinine, or cyclosporin A have been performed mainly in refractory disease with no clinical benefit.

Prognostic Factors in Refractory Myeloma

The frequency of antitumor effect, especially with DEX and VAD salvage regimens, declines with the duration of resistance to prior therapy. Event-free and overall survival are shortened in the presence of increased beta$_2$-microglobulin or LDH levels prior to salvage therapy. Patients with resistant relapse have a significantly worse prognosis than those who fail to respond initially; this may be attributable to differences in tumor cell kinetics (i.e., greater proliferative activity with resistant relapse).

Interferon-alpha

Interferon-alpha is the only interferon (IFN) with documented clinical activity in multiple myeloma. There is no role for IFN-alpha as salvage therapy for chemotherapy-refractory disease except as maintenance treatment once salvage cytotoxic therapy has achieved remission.

The role of IFN-alpha for the management of newly diagnosed myeloma is still evolving. Trials with thrice-weekly or daily administration of 2 to 5 megaunits subcutaneously have been explored during remission induction with standard MP or combination regimens such as M2 (VBMCP) or VMCP/VBAP (see Table 1). Other trials have evaluated, in a randomized fashion, IFN-alpha maintenance versus no treatment. Collectively, these data show longer durations of disease control in patients receiving IFN-alpha, but overall survival is usually not extended. The emphasis has shifted toward exploration of IFN-alpha after autologous transplants when tumor bulk is markedly reduced so as to make IFN-alpha more effective in a minimal residual disease setting.

Transplants

Allogeneic Transplants

The treatment-related mortality for bone marrow transplants in myeloma is on the order of 25 to 30%, with about 50% of patients surviving for 1 year. Compared to autotransplants, additional antitumor effect may result from a graft-versus-myeloma effect. Late relapses, unfortunately, have been observed, especially when allotransplants were used in the salvage setting and when true complete remissions were not attained. Overall, some 30% of patients survive beyond 5 years, often with residual disease.

Transplant Preparatory Regimens

For both autologous and allogeneic transplants, the optimal conditioning regimen has yet to be established. Even in the setting of consolidation therapy for first remission, the frequency of true CR usually does not exceed 50%. Further improvements can be anticipated from multidrug combinations, escalation of TBI, or repeated applications of myeloablative regimens, all of which are under investigation.

Autologous Bone Marrow Transplantation versus PBSC

Tumor cells are present in both bone marrow and peripheral blood, even in newly diagnosed patients, so that PBSC does not necessarily constitute a preferred source of normal hematopoietic stem cells containing fewer tumor cells. Tumor cell removal strategies include the use of monoclonal antibodies, immunotoxins, and chemotherapy. As long as CR rates do not exceed 50%, it is doubtful that such purging approaches will significantly alter the clinical course. Positive selection of normal hematopoietic cells using CD34 antigen expression is being evaluated on the assumption that myeloma cells do not express this marker.

Hematopoietic Growth Factors

Although potentially stimulating myeloma cell replication and extending tumor cell survival in vitro, GM-CSF and G-CSF have not been shown to induce tumor cell proliferation in vivo. These factors are useful alone or in combination with high-dose cytoxan (HDCTX) for collecting PBSC and can further shorten the period of bone marrow aplasia when applied after transplant as well.

Supportive Care Strategies

Hypercalcemia

Hypercalcemia in myeloma is mediated by a variety of cytokines, most notably IL-6, IL-1-beta, and TNF-beta, all of which are effectively down-regulated by glucocorticoids. Thus, there is a good biologic explanation for the observed clinical efficacy, especially of high-dose DEX. Such therapy can be combined with calcitonin, which usually obviates the need for excessive hydration. With this regimen, hypercalcemia is controlled rapidly in over 95% of individuals. Hypercalcemia should not recur once effective tumor control is established with front-line or salvage therapies. Biphosphonates have a later onset of activity but are useful when symptomatic control of hypercalcemia remains the only therapeutic goal in patients no longer responsive to available salvage treatments.

Renal Failure

The renal failure of myeloma is multifactorial but results most frequently from light-chain cast nephropathy, hypercalcemia, or both. As with hypercalcemia, effective tumor control is crucial and can be achieved readily in recently diagnosed patients with DEX or VAD. Over 50% of recently diagnosed patients presenting with renal failure will regain normal renal function. Clinical intervention associated with dehydration, such as intravenous pyelography or preparation for barium enema, may precipitate renal failure. This can be further accentuated by interstitial nephritis with the use of nonsteroidal anti-inflammatory drugs.

Hemodialysis may be required as an acute measure or as chronic therapy if medical management is ineffective. Patients with a good long-term prognosis, especially after bone marrow transplant, may be considered for renal transplantation as well.

Anemia

The pathogenesis of anemia in multiple myeloma is multifactorial. In addition to physical replacement of normal hematopoiesis by tumor cells in the bone marrow, cytokines (e.g., IL-6) and renal failure are contributing factors. Cytokines can interfere with erythropoietin production, which is also impaired in renal failure and possibly also in the presence of hyperviscosity. More than two-thirds of patients respond briskly to exogenous erythropoietin (EPO) administration at a usual dose of 10,000 units thrice weekly subcutaneously, with maximum responses typically observed within 4 to 6 weeks. EPO seems to be more effective when endogenous EPO levels are low and duration of potentially stem cell–damaging alkylating agent therapy is limited to less than 1 year. When anemia develops as a result of myelodysplastic disease due to prolonged alkylating agent therapy, EPO is usually ineffective.

Anemia typically improves once tumor control is established. Patients with refractory myeloma seem to derive marked clinical benefit when their anemia is improved with EPO. Maintenance schedules of weekly or biweekly administration are sufficient to maintain adequate hemoglobin concentrations.

Infections

Infections result from profound suppression of both B and T cell functions. Such immunoparalysis is further aggravated by the use of high doses of DEX. Recurrent bacterial infections require broad-spectrum antibiotic prophylaxis with ciprofloxacin or trimethoprim-sulfamethoxazole. With high doses of glucocorticoids and prolonged neutropenia, the possibility of fungal or viral infections has to be considered, which may present as esophagogastroduodenitis. Acyclovir (Zovirax) should be instituted promptly when herpes simplex or herpes zoster infection is suspected. In the latter case, high daily doses exceeding 2 grams intravenously may be required for the initial 7 days. Fluconazole (Diflucan) is useful for the control of *Candida* infections at a dose of 100 mg orally. When aspergillosis occurs in invasive disease, amphotericin B (Fungizone) should be instituted promptly. Concurrent intravenous administration of high-dose immunoglobulins may also be helpful.

Pain Control

Pain associated with lytic bone disease improves rapidly once effective chemotherapy has been instituted. Rather dramatic responses within hours are sometimes observed with high doses of DEX alone or with VAD. Such therapy is also useful to control symptoms of spinal cord compression due to extradural disease, so that laminectomy or local radiotherapy can be deferred. Responses typically occur within 24 to 48 hours. In case of persistent pain and especially when neurologic deficits develop, local radiation therapy at a total dose of approximately 3000 cGy should be instituted. Failure of the patient to improve within a few days should alert the physician to the possibility of radiation resistance, requiring surgical decompression. Intramedullary rod fixation of impending long bone fractures has produced good results.

All patients with multiple myeloma, especially those with extensive bone disease, should be encouraged to be as active as possible, and analgesics should be administered generously for effective pain control.

Hyperviscosity Syndrome

Serum viscosity is occasionally increased as a result of high levels of monoclonal protein, more often with IgA than with IgG myeloma. Symptoms result from impaired circulation, leading to blurred vision, mental status changes, and cardiac or pulmonary compromise, as well as renal insufficiency. Although, generally, there is a correlation between myeloma protein concentration and serum viscosity, the physicochemical characteristics of the individual immunoglobulin molecules may favor aggregation and polymerization, further increasing serum viscosity. Prompt symptomatic relief can be obtained with plasmapheresis using cell separator devices, although durable symptom control requires effective cytotoxic therapy that reduces tumor burden and hence immunoglobulin production.

Special Clinical Presentations

Solitary Plasmacytoma of Bone or Soft Tissue (Extramedullary Plasmacytoma)

Local radiotherapy at a dose of 4000 to 5000 cGy can eradicate local disease effectively. Cure rates on the order of 50% have been reported with soft tissue plasmacytoma. In contrast, systemic disease develops more commonly in presumed solitary plasmacytoma of bone, reflecting either undetected systemic disease from the outset or metastatic spread due to inadequate local tumor control. Diagnostic precision has been improved with the use of MRI for the detection of occult bone marrow tumor deposits. Persistence of a monoclonal protein peak despite adequate local radiotherapy signifies persistence of viable tumor cells at the irradiated site because of tumor cell resistance or systemic disease.

Plasma Cell Leukemia

The presence of circulating plasma cells at a frequency of 2000 or more per microliter is diagnostic for plasma cell leukemia, which can occur de novo or develop during the course of multiple myeloma (seccondary plasma cell leukemia). Most patients, even those with low tumor mass, do have circulating tumor cells, although they are present at a low frequency and apparently do not adversely affect prognosis. Primary plasma cell leukemia requires intensive systemic therapy, and myeloablative treatment requiring transplants should be considered early on, especially for younger patients. Secondary plasma cell leukemia is usually highly refractory to salvage attempts, including transplant.

Meningeal Plasma Cell Disease

Meningeal involvement by myeloma is exceedingly rare and usually occurs in patients with advanced disease that has become refractory to multiple treatment regimens. The EDAP regimen (see Table 1) should be considered because plasmablastic morphology is most common and this regimen exhibits activity in patients with central nervous system manifestations of lymphoma. Intrathecal administration of glucocorticoids, cytarabine, and methotrexate is appropriate.

Perspective

The treatment of currently incurable malignancies such as multiple myeloma requires a research-oriented approach, so that progress and therapy can be evaluated properly. Reproducible staging is required for comparisons of different treatments. More stringent and quantitative response definitions are needed in order to recognize potentially more effective therapies. An early treatment goal should be the induction of true complete remission, which is feasible in about one-half of newly diagnosed patients using myeloablative regimens. The need for exercise cannot be overemphasized, especially in patients with painful lytic lesions who, for fear of aggravating their disease, tend to limit their activity. Swimming or aqua-exercise, in conjunction with effective medical therapy, is exceedingly helpful. An attitude of resignation and an emphasis on palliation on the part of physicians assures lack of therapeutic advances and can cause a feeling of abandonment in an already distressed patient.

POLYCYTHEMIA VERA

method of
RICHARD T. SILVER, M.D.
Cornell University Medical College
New York, New York

Polycythemia vera (PV) is a clonal myeloproliferative disease that develops from a pluripotent stem cell. It is characterized not only by proliferation within the marrow of erythroid progenitors, which causes an absolute increase in red cell mass (i.e., an absolute increase in red blood cells), but also by proliferation of myeloid and megakaryocytic elements, which results in elevation of the peripheral white blood cell and platelet counts. Initially thought to be a disease restricted to the elderly, routine automated blood cell counts have disclosed individuals with this disease in their third and fourth decades. Thus, an increasing percentage of cases are being detected prior to the development of symptoms. Close questioning may indicate, however, that these individuals have had mild headaches and plethora for years prior to the diagnosis. As the disease progresses, symptoms develop that are related to hypervolemia and hyperviscosity, often accentuated by the increase in platelet count. Headache, tinnitus, lightheadedness, vertigo, blurred vision, and both arterial and venous thromboses are frequent. Epistaxis, spontaneous bruising, peptic ulcer, and gastrointestinal hemorrhage may be seen as the disease progresses. A troublesome symptom is pruritus, which is often worse after a hot bath or shower. As an expression of increased nucleoprotein breakdown, uric acid levels are increased in the blood and urine, and secondary gout and uric acid stones are relatively frequent.

This study was supported in part by grants from the United Leukemia Fund, Inc., and the Cancer Research and Treatment Fund, Inc.

PHYSICAL FINDINGS

Virtually all patients show some evidence of the increase in red cell mass. Plethora and slight red-purplish discoloration of the tips of the fingers are frequent. Mild hypertension is noted in about a third of the patients. Depending upon the degree and duration of disease, about three-quarters of the patients have an enlarged spleen.

LABORATORY FINDINGS

In addition to the elevated red blood cell count, examination of the peripheral blood smear and determination of red blood cell indices reveal hypochromic microcytic cells with a reduced mean corpuscular volume indicating iron deficiency. This is further supported by a low serum iron level and absence of iron stores in the bone marrow, abnormalities that may be accentuated by prior gastrointestinal bleeding. As the disease progresses and as an expression of extramedullary hematopoiesis, abnormally sized and shaped red blood cells, nucleated erythroid cells, and immature granulocytes are noted in the peripheral blood. Approximately 60% of patients with PV have an increased white blood cell count at the time of diagnosis. Usually this is of modest degree, involving increased numbers of neutrophils and bands. Basophils and eosinophils are likewise often more numerous. A simple diagnostic test to distinguish PV from chronic myeloid leukemia is the leukocyte alkaline phosphatase (LAP) stain. In PV, there is usually an increased LAP score, reflecting increased activity of this enzyme within circulating granulocytes. (The leukocyte alkaline phosphatase is *not* the same as the serum alkaline phosphatase manufactured by the liver.) As an expression of the increased white blood cell mass in PV, serum vitamin B_{12} and serum unbound vitamin B_{12} binding capacity are increased. In the majority of cases, the platelet count is elevated. Coagulation studies indicate that abnormalities of platelet function are virtually always present. The bone marrow is typically hypercellular and shows hyperplasia of all three marrow elements (i.e., megakaryocytes, erythroid cells, and granulocytes). The marrow findings are not specific and are also seen in patients with chronic myeloid leukemia, essential thrombocythemia, and the cellular phase of agnogenic myeloid metaplasia. The reticulin stain, reflecting early marrow fibrosis, is increased in intensity. Consistent cytogenetic abnormalities are not found in PV. Trisomy of chromosomes 8 and 9 and loss of chromosome 7 are the most frequently observed abnormalities; in contrast to chronic myeloid leukemia, however, no unique cytogenetic abnormality is diagnostic of PV.

DIAGNOSIS

"Polycythemia" means an increase in red cell mass; this must be demonstrated unequivocally by a chromium-51 red cell mass determination. The use of the hematocrit alone to diagnose an increased red cell mass will yield false-positive results in those cases characterized by restricted plasma volume.

The diagnostic criteria for PV are classified into two general categories (Table 1). Using the criteria of the Polycythemia Vera Study Group, the diagnosis can be made with reasonable certainty if A-1, A-2, or A-3 are present or if A-1 and A-2 are present with any two items from category B. The serum erythropoietin level is almost always below normal, and this can help to distinguish true PV from secondary polycythemia, which may have strikingly similar clinical and laboratory findings. Thus, the diagnosis of PV is made after elimination of all the diseases that cause or are associated with secondary polycythemia.

TREATMENT

The initial step in treating any newly diagnosed patient with PV is phlebotomy. Since blood viscosity correlates with the elevation of the hematocrit, every effort should be made to reduce the hematocrit to below 45%, at which point the problems associated with hypervolemia and hyperviscosity lessen. Usually, the amount of whole blood removed is approximately 400 to 500 mL, although smaller amounts should be removed in elderly patients, especially those with coexistent cardiovascular and/or respiratory disease. Phlebotomy can be performed once or twice weekly. Since most patients have associated iron deficiency, red blood cell production gradually is reduced; eventually, patients may require two to five phlebotomies a year, although many will require more. Phlebotomy is not a completely benign procedure as it often increases the degree of thrombocytosis and consequently the risk of thrombotic complications.

Table 1. **Diagnostic Guidelines of the Polycythemia Vera Study Group**

A-1	Increased red cell mass Male: ≥36 mL per kg Female: ≥32 mL per kg
A-2	Normal O_2 saturation (≥92%)
A-3	Splenomegaly
B-1	Thrombocytosis Platelet count >400,000/μL
B-2	Leukocytosis >12,000/μL Absence of fever or infection
B-3	Leukocyte alkaline phosphatase score (LAP >100)
B-4	Increased serum B_{12} vitamin (>900 pg per mL) Increased unbound B_{12} binding capacity (>2200 pg per mL)
Criteria No. 1	A-1 + A-2 + A-3
Criteria No. 2	A-1 + A-2 + any two from Category B

Although some form of myelosuppression traditionally has been used in PV, radioactive phosphorus (^{32}P) and alkylating agents, such as chlorambucil* or busulfan,* all have significant side effects. In a randomized controlled study of 431 patients by the Polycythemia Vera Study Group, median survival was 13.9 years for patients receiving phlebotomy, 11.8 years for ^{32}P, and 8.9 years for chlorambucil; however, the difference became statistically significant only after 10 years of treatment. Nevertheless, there was a significant difference in the causes of death in each treatment arm. Patients managed with phlebotomy only had a significant excess incidence of severe and often fatal thrombotic complications, particularly during the first 2 to 4 years of treatment, especially those older than 70 years and those with a phlebotomy requirement of more than four to six treatments per year. The use of ^{32}P or alkylating agents significantly decreased the risk of thrombotic complications early in the disease; however, both chlorambucil and ^{32}P were associated with a statistically significant increased risk of acute leukemia, particularly after 5 to 7 years of treatment. Further, increased frequency of carcinoma of the skin and gastrointestinal tract and intra-abdominal lymphomas were also seen in patients treated with chlorambucil.

Because of the significant secondary effects of chlorambucil and similar agents, alternative drugs for myelosuppression have been employed. The antimetabolite hydroxyurea* currently is the cytoreductive agent most commonly used, although it still has the potential to cause leukemia. The incidence of leukemia in 51 patients with PV treated with hydroxyurea for a median duration of 5 years was 5.8%, compared with 1.5% for patients treated with phlebotomy only. Other side effects of hydroxyurea include hepatic and renal toxicity, fever, skin rash, and gastrointestinal intolerance. Further, the dose must be carefully administered, because excess myelosuppression may occur. The main indication for hydroxyurea therapy is an elevated platelet count of more than 800,000 per microliter, which, particularly in the elderly patient, places the individual at risk. Hydroxyurea may reduce the size of the spleen, although not dramatically in my experience. Splenomegaly often persists even when the red blood cell count reverts to normal. The usual dose of hydroxyurea is 500 to 1500 mg daily, but it can be modified upward and downward. Prompt relapse occurs upon discontinuation, and therefore maintenance therapy must be continued indefinitely.

It is noted that phlebotomy alone does not stop the natural course of PV, which includes progressive myelofibrosis and splenomegaly. Recombinant interferon has myelosuppressive activity. Platelet-derived growth factor (PDGF), a product of megakaryocytes, initiates proliferation of fibroblasts, which may be involved in the development of secondary myelofi-

*Not FDA approved for this indication.

brosis in PV. Interferon-alpha* antagonizes the action of PDGF by inhibiting the activation of G_0 cells for G_1 traverse and S-phase entry. Additionally, PDGF stimulates the proliferation of early and late erythroid progenitor cells, which interferon-alpha inhibits in vitro. Thus, interferon provides a physiologic basis for treating PV without the risk of leukemia. In patients with active disease, interferon-alpha controlled and then normalized red blood cell values within 6 to 12 months, eliminating the need for phlebotomy. No thrombohemorrhagic event occurred, and in fact thrombocytosis and splenomegaly were reversed in the majority of patients. Pruritus and other constitutional symptoms also abated. Recombinant interferon has side effects that can be troublesome, particularly during the first 6 months of treatment; these include muscle aches and pains, fever, diarrhea, depression, and somnolence. Acetaminophen or aspirin usually brings relief. Long-term effects of interferon that have been reported in the literature include nephrotic syndrome, a lupus-like syndrome, and peripheral neuropathy, but I have not encountered these.

For patients who do not or cannot undertake interferon therapy, the addition of anagrelide to phlebotomy can be considered. Anagrelide, an aminoquinolone derivative, is a potent platelet inhibitor that consistently lowers platelet counts in patients with PV and other myeloproliferative diseases. It does have side effects, such as headache, gastrointestinal toxicity, and palpitations, but patients usually find these tolerable. Anagrelide is contraindicated in elderly patients with clinical arteriosclerotic heart disease.

I have no objection to the use of radioactive phosphorus (^{32}P) in patients who are elderly or who have coexistent cardiac, respiratory, hepatic, or renal disease. Its activity is smooth and relatively predictable. The initial dose is 2.5 mCi per M^2 intravenously with maximum effect seen in 8 to 10 weeks. Supplemental doses may be required.

Because of the relative risk of secondary gout, allopurinol (Zyloprim) should be used in all patients at a dose of at least 100 mg per day. Low-dose aspirin (80 mg), but not high-dose aspirin (325 mg), should be employed as a platelet antiaggregating agent.

Pruritus can be treated with cyproheptadine (Periactin) in doses of 8 to 10 mg per day orally as needed. (Note that interferon* relieves pruritus.)

Treatment of Spent-Phase PV

As myelofibrosis develops and intensifies, the spleen becomes larger, and eventually, the patient with PV becomes anemic. Coexistent iron or folic deficiency should be corrected. Although androgens may stimulate erythropoiesis, increasing splenomegaly sometimes occurs as a result of their use. Massive splenomegaly rarely responds to hydroxyurea* or radiation therapy, and in some patients it produces significant thrombocytopenia. Splenectomy is hazardous and in a recent review of our cases has not led to an increased life span. The treatment of secondary acute leukemia developing in patients with PV is extraordinarily unsuccessful and is usually not worth an intensive chemotherapeutic trial. Supportive therapy is recommended for these patients.

*Not FDA approved for this indication.

THE PORPHYRIAS

method of
PETER V. TISHLER, M.D.
Veterans Affairs Medical Center
Brockton, Massachusetts

The eight porphyrias result from seven distinct inborn errors of heme biosynthesis. Two clinical types of porphyria are recognized: those with acute neuropathic manifestations (acute attacks), and those with a cutaneous syndrome. In intermittent acute porphyria (IAP) and ALA dehydratase deficiency porphyria (ALAD-P), the two porphyrias whose enzyme defects result almost exclusively in the accumulation and excretion of the porphyrin precursors delta-aminolevulinic acid (ALA) and porphobilinogen (PBG), the manifestations are neuropathic only. The porphyrias in which only porphyrins accumulate have cutaneous manifestations: congenital erythropoietic porphyria (CEP), porphyria cutanea tarda (PCT), hepatoerythropoietic porphyria (HEP), and erythropoietic protoporphyria (EPP). Coproporphyria (CP) and variegate porphyria (VP), in which both porphyrins and porphyrin precursors are excreted in excess, can have both acute and cutaneous manifestations. All diseases are inherited. The genes responsible for the porphyrias (Table 1) have been mapped and, in most instances, isolated. Diagnosis by characterization of the gene is a research procedure for now but will probably become the diagnostic method of choice in the next few years.

THE ACUTE PORPHYRIAS

Patients may present with symptoms suggestive of an acute attack: pain, usually in the abdomen or back; sensory or motor peripheral neuropathy, with paresthesias and progressive motor changes (similar to the Guillain-Barré syndrome) that may lead to paralysis and bulbar palsy; autonomic manifestations—constipation, tachycardia, hypertension; an organic brain syndrome with psychosis; and hyponatremia due to inappropriate secretion of antidiuretic hormone (SIADH). Patients may also present with or without these symptoms and with a history of a previous diagnosis of porphyria or of a relative with a porphyria. Patients themselves are often well informed about their illness, and information they provide should not be ignored (although, regrettably, it often is). Precipitation of an acute attack by the cavalier use of drugs must be avoided. A full-blown acute

TABLE 1. **Schema of Porphyrin Biosynthesis, Including Porphyrias Resulting from Genetically Determined Deficiencies of Specific Enzymes***

Heme Metabolism		Porphyria	
Substrate/Product	*Enzyme*	*Full Name*	*Abbreviation*
Succinyl coenzyme A + glycine			
↓	ALA synthase		
δ-Aminolevulinic acid (ALA)			
↓	ALA dehydratase	ALA dehydratase deficiency	ALAD-P
Porphobilinogen (PBG)			
↓	PBG deaminase	Intermittent acute porphyria	IAP
Hydroxymethylbilane			
↓	Uro'gen III synthase	Congenital erythropoietic porphyria	CEP
Uroporphyrinogen (8)			
↓	Uro'gen decarboxylase	Porphyria cutanea tarda Hepatoerythropoietic porphyria	PCT HEP
Coproporphyrinogen (4)			
↓	Copro'gen oxidase	Coproporphyria	CP
Protoporphyrinogen (2)			
↓	Proto'gen oxidase	Variegate porphyria	VP
Protoporphyrin IX + Fe^{++}	Ferrochelatase	Erythropoietic protoporphyria	EPP
↓			
Heme			

*The small molecule substrates condense to form porphyrinogens, nonaromatic cyclic tetrapyrroles that undergo enzymatic decarboxylation (numbers in parentheses = numbers of carboxyl groups). The resultant porphyrin, the aromatic cyclic tetrapyrrole protoporphyrin IX, incorporates iron to form heme. Uroporphyrinogen (= uro'gen) and coproporphyrinogen (= copro'gen) are also oxidized to the corresponding porphyrins, which are the substances that are measured. The natural products of this pathway are all members of the III isomer series.

attack with progressive neuropathy is a potentially fatal event and *must be considered a medical emergency.* Unfortunately, general physicians so rarely encounter a porphyria that they may not entertain the diagnosis. This can lead to irreversible neurologic sequelae or death.

The diagnosis of an acute porphyria should be entertained on the basis of historical information mentioned previously; an unexplained, possibly neurologic-type illness after taking certain medications (e.g., sulfonamides, barbiturates, estrogens, anticonvulsants); unexplained episodes of burgundy-colored urine; or hyponatremia and SIADH. The absence of any or most of these indicators does not rule out an acute porphyria. In patients who are having an acute attack, the single most important diagnostic exercise is testing the urine for ALA and PBG. Both porphyrin precursors are excreted in greatly increased amounts (usually more than 20 mg per day, or 20 to 40 mg per day greater than the baseline excretion) during an acute attack in all acute porphyrias except ALAD-P, in which only ALA excretion is augmented. These elevations are *not* subtle. Conversely, the absence of a marked increase in urinary porphyrin precursor excretion rules out the presence of an acute porphyric attack. The range of excretion of PBG can be estimated quickly in urine samples with the Watson-Schwartz test or a more recently developed derivative-column qualitative method. These tests require only a spot urine sample. A negative test in all but the most dilute urine makes an acute porphyric attack very unlikely. The results should be confirmed by quantitation of the amounts in a 24-hour urine sample. For patients who are not having an acute attack, the excretion of ALA or PBG may be elevated or may approximate normal levels, particularly in VP and CP.

If a diagnosis of an acute porphyria is likely, because of a positive test for porphyrin precursors or other factors (e.g., family history), further studies are required to determine the exact porphyria. These include measurement of the activity of the erythrocyte enzymes ALA dehydratase and PBG deaminase and of the excretion of fecal porphyrins. ALA dehydratase activity is reduced by more than 90% in patients with ALAD-P, which has thus far been described in only a few individuals (often children). PBG deaminase activity is usually (but not always) about 50% of normal in IAP. The finding of reduced activity of PBG deaminase and increased urinary excretion of porphyrin precursors is diagnostic of IAP. Stool is analyzed by high-performance liquid chromatography (the only acceptable method) for porphyrin fractions, identified by the number of carboxyl groups. In VP and CP, respectively, the fecal excretion of 2-carboxyl porphyrin (protoporphyrin) and 4-carboxyl porphyrin (coproporphyrin) is markedly increased. These porphyrin excretion patterns persist at all times and are rarely seen in the other porphyrias. Thus, one ultimately makes the diagnosis of a specific acute porphyria. This is important prognostically, in evaluating other family members, and in genetic counseling.

Treatment of the acute attack requires meticulous attention to detail. Success is measured by both normalization of clinical manifestations (reduced pain, pulse rate, blood pressure, psychiatric manifestations; increased bowel peristalsis, measures of pulmonary function, and deep tendon reflexes) and reduction in the urinary excretion of PBG or ALA. ALA and/or PBG must be measured daily until the attack is in remission. These values must be available with little delay. Treatment must include the following components:

1. Removal of the precipitating agent, by changing

the patient's environment (i.e., via hospitalization) and strictly regulating all input.

2. Careful monitoring and, if necessary, treatment of the patient's vital functions, in an intensive care unit. This may include use of beta blockers in moderate doses for hypertension (propranolol [Inderal], 120–160 mg per day), endotracheal intubation and artificial ventilation, and other supportive measures. Severe pain can be treated with narcotic analgesics (which can aggravate constipation) and/or phenothiazines (prochlorperazine [Compazine] or chlorpromazine [Thorazine]) in standard doses.

3. Treatment of any acid-base, electrolyte, or volume disturbances (e.g., SIADH, the hyponatremia of which may be severe) by standard means.

4. Treatment of any intercurrent illness, using medications that are safe for patients with an acute porphyria. *All medications, however innocuous they may seem, must be scrutinized before use for their safety in patients with an acute porphyria.* A very incomplete list of safe and unsafe medications is presented in Table 2. The author can provide more information upon request.

5. Treatment of seizures if they occur. The best treatment is purely symptomatic, with proper attention to issues of airway patency and safety. This is practical if the seizures are the result of hyponatremia. If they persist, magnesium sulfate can be given intravenously. The initial dose of 3 to 6 grams infused over 30 minutes is followed by a maintenance dose of 1 to 2 grams per hour. The aim is to maintain a serum magnesium level of 4 to 8 mEq per liter. This treatment should be maintained for about 24 hours after the seizures stop and then tapered. Since these doses of magnesium have curare-like paralytic effects, patients must be monitored and given appropriate ventilatory and other support. Bromides are safe and effective, but current experience with the use of this toxic anticonvulsant is very limited. Clonazepam (Klonopin) may also be used, with initial doses of 0.5 mg three times daily and increasing to a 3 to 4 mg total daily dose. Urine porphyrin precursors should be monitored and clonazepam discontinued if their excretion increases.

TABLE 2. **Drug Experience in the Acute Porphyrias***

Safe / Probably Safe Drugs
Vaccines, vitamins, minerals, cholestyramine, niacin
Penicillins, cephalosporins, gentamicin, tetracycline
Aspirin, acetaminophen, ibuprofen, naproxen
Insulin, glipizide, corticosteroids, thyroxine
Warfarin, heparin
Narcotic analgesics, chloral hydrate, phenothiazines, lithium
Adrenalin, beta blockers, glyceryl trinitrate, digoxin, thiazide diuretics, furosemide
Suxamethonium, fentanyl, nitrous oxide, propofol, procaine
Bromides, clonazepam
Possibly / Definitely Unsafe Drugs
Sulfonamides, erythromycin
Barbiturates
Hydantoins, carbamazepine, valproate
Estrogens, oral contraceptives
Tricyclic antidepressants
Benzodiazepines
Calcium channel blockers

*Compiled from printed lists and the author's experience, which may differ from published information. *All* drugs must be used with caution in patients with acute porphyrias, since responses are not necessarily predictable.

6. Treatment of the attack with carbohydrate. The *prompt* addition of high carbohydrate intake will abort a large percentage of attacks. Patients should receive 300 to 500 grams of carbohydrate daily, by intravenous and oral routes (10% dextrose, high-carbohydrate meals and between-meal high-carbohydrate drink [Polycose]). Glycosuria should be minimized.

7. Treatment with hemin (Panhematin). Indications for hemin include any of the following: (a) intractable signs and symptoms that are unresponsive over days to the aforementioned forms of therapy; (b) progression of manifestations to include involvement of the peripheral nervous system (sensory or motor neuropathy, or loss of deep tendon reflexes); or (c) any acute or progressive, potentially life-threatening event (e.g., progressive reduction in pulmonary function or respiratory paralysis). Early treatment for any of these indications maximizes the chances of favorable therapeutic response. Hemin can be obtained by telephoning Abbott Laboratories (800-255-5162, or 708-937-7970 after hours). It is reconstituted in saline *immediately* before use and given intravenously at a dosage of 2 to 4 mg per kg one or two times daily in a large vein over 10 to 15 minutes. Treatments should be continued until urinary porphyrin precursor excretion returns toward pre-attack levels and the patient has experienced clear clinical improvement (especially of any life-threatening manifestations), or there is no response to an adequate trial. Courses of hemin usually range from 3 to 13 days. Rare side effects include local phlebitis, thrombocytopenia, prolongation of bleeding parameters, and renal dysfunction. Because any general physician's experience with this treatment is limited, *hemin should be used only with the active collaboration (if only by telephone) of a clinician familiar with its use.* A list of such physicians is available from the author.

8. A long-term commitment to rehabilitation. Although some individuals may be left with major neurologic residua after an acute attack, they should be offered skilled rehabilitation. Recovery from the neuropathy of an acute porphyric attack may be a long, slow process, taxing the dedication of both the patient and the health care team. Nonetheless, recovery of most if not all function is the rule, and thus rehabilitation should be pursued with vigor.

Simple but important measures should be adopted in the care of porphyric patients during asymptomatic or chronic phases of their illness. Of utmost importance is education: the patient must assume the role of his or her own best advocate, by learning all there is to know about the porphyria, exercising extreme caution in taking medications or being exposed to environmental chemicals (including alcohol and cigarette smoke), challenging physicians to make sure that they provide informed and responsible care, and carrying appropriate identification (Medic-Alert). Membership in the American Porphyria Foundation (P.O. Box 22712, Houston, TX 77227) provides both information and group support. Women may develop disabling, cyclic symptoms in relation to menstrual periods. These manifestations can often be eliminated with agonists of luteinizing hormone–releasing hormone (LRH). Because experience with this therapy is limited, treatment should be carried out according to a protocol, which the author can make available. Patients must also avoid strict weight-reducing diets, maintain immunizations, and contact an informed physician early in the course of an intercurrent illness. When offered medications, every patient must *insist that the safety of the drugs be corroborated by an expert.* An incomplete list of safe and unsafe medications, compiled largely on an anecdotal basis and including few new entities, is included in Table 2. If a patient must be given a medication of uncertain safety, urinary excretion of ALA or PBG must be monitored during its administration.

Surgery poses special problems. Certain anesthetic agents, muscle relaxants, hypnotics, and analgesics can be used safely. Nonetheless, the patient must be observed closely during the postoperative period for any manifestations of an acute attack. This author is especially attentive to the deep tendon reflexes (especially ankle jerks) and also monitors the urinary excretion of PBG by means of a bedside-modified Watson-Schwartz test. The details of this are available upon request.

IAP, VP, and CP are all inherited as autosomal dominant diseases. Thus, the probability is 0.5 that each first-degree relative (child or sibling) of an affected individual has inherited the gene. Only a minority of individuals who inherit the gene will actually develop the clinical syndrome, however. ALAD-P is inherited in an autosomal recessive fashion, with a probability of 0.25 that each sibling of an affected individual will have this genotype. Because the pharmacologic implications of having any of these genes are potentially extreme, appropriate relatives should be screened for chemical evidence of the porphyria. Affected but asymptomatic individuals should receive the same preventive counseling as their symptomatic relatives.

PORPHYRIAS WITH CUTANEOUS MANIFESTATIONS

The six photosensitivity porphyrias fall into three clinically distinct groups. In EPP, the rather immediate symptoms include burning, swelling, itching, and redness of the sun-exposed skin; scarring follows repeated exposure. CEP and the very rare HEP are characterized by severe blistering, leading ultimately to disfiguring scarring and resorption of the nose, auricles, and fingers. The photosensitivity of PCT and the two acute porphyrias VP and CP involves much milder blistering and fissuring in exposed areas, leading to scarring, hyperpigmentation, increased skin fragility, and facial hypertrichosis.

In patients (often children) in whom EPP is suspected on clinical grounds, the diagnosis is substantiated by finding increased quantities of free protoporphyrin in erythrocytes and plasma. This syndrome is inherited as an autosomal dominant trait; relatives can be screened by the same biochemical means even if they are asymptomatic. Treatment is with oral beta carotene (Solatene), initially at dosages of 30 to 60 mg per day. The dosage is increased progressively over 1 to 2 months (to 180 to 240 mg per day, in single or divided doses) until the photosensitivity is ameliorated. Both a carotenemic hue to the skin and a serum carotene concentration of at least 600 μg/dL are usually necessary for therapeutic effect. Although the photosensitivity may not be totally relieved, the positive effect of beta carotene treatment may be dramatic: a normal lifestyle for a patient who might otherwise have been required to stay indoors. A second and dire problem, severe hepatic dysfunction that can progress rapidly to liver failure, affects a minority of patients. Liver function tests must be monitored periodically, and liver biopsy in individuals with persistent abnormalities is useful for prognosis. Medical treatment with cholestyramine (Questran,* 12 to 15 grams per day in divided doses) to reduce the body burden of protoporphyrin is reasonable but of unproved benefit. Hepatic failure is an indication for liver transplantation.

CEP and HEP are associated with virtually identical photomutilating syndromes that can also include hemolysis and hypersplenism. The diagnoses may be made with high confidence on the basis of the clinical findings. Both are also characterized chemically by markedly increased quantities of 8-carboxyl porphyrin (uroporphyrin) in urine and erythrocytes. They can be differentiated from each other only by assay of the two specific enzymes (see Table 1), the activities of which are usually less than 10% of normal. Both syndromes are inherited in an autosomal recessive manner. Parents who carry a single copy of the gene for the porphyria may be normal or, in the case of HEP, may have PCT. They may benefit from genetic counseling and prenatal diagnosis (if a research laboratory agrees to assay the gene or enzyme). Treatments are not satisfactory but are evolving. Avoidance of excessive sun exposure by the use of protective clothing, sunscreens with an SPF of greater than 30, and tinted glass (Scotchtint in automobiles) is essential. Some reduction in photosensitivity may be afforded with beta carotene, used as outlined previously. Experimental therapies include oral charcoal* (to increase porphyrin removal) and erythropoietin* (to decrease porphyrin production). Patients should be referred for study of these therapies.

---

*Not FDA approved for this indication.

The cutaneous syndromes of PCT, VP, and CP are indistinguishable. As mentioned previously, VP and CP are also acute porphyrias. Their cutaneous manifestations bear no temporal relation to any acute manifestations. The manifestations of PCT often develop secondary to excessive alcohol intake, estrogen therapy, iron overload (e.g., chronic hemodialysis), and environmental exposure to halogenated hydrocarbons. The diagnosis of PCT is substantiated by the finding of a markedly increased urinary excretion of uroporphyrin but essentially normal fecal porphyrin content (when assayed by clinical laboratories). Reduced activity (about half of normal) of the erythrocyte enzyme uroporphyrinogen decarboxylase will confirm the diagnosis in patients with one form of PCT that is inherited in an autosomal dominant manner; but in the more common sporadic form, activity of the erythrocyte enzyme is normal. Patients with symptomatic PCT invariably have tissue iron overload, indicated by increased serum ferritin, iron, or percent transferrin saturation. An unfixed liver biopsy illuminated by a Wood's lamp exhibits an intense red autofluorescence. The histology is characterized by needle-like inclusions of crystallized porphyrin.

The usual treatment of symptomatic PCT is to reduce the body burden of iron. One unit of blood is removed by phlebotomy every 2 weeks, with monitoring of the hemoglobin (biweekly), serum ferritin, and 24-hour urinary uroporphyrin (monthly). With time, the serum ferritin level, urinary uroporphyrin excretion, and cutaneous manifestations diminish. When the serum ferritin concentration and urine uroporphyrin excretion reach normal levels, phlebotomy is discontinued. If the patient becomes anemic before these parameters normalize, the frequency of phlebotomy is decreased (e.g., to monthly or every 6 weeks). In most circumstances, however, hematopoiesis can keep pace with phlebotomy. If the patient becomes persistently or severely anemic before the other parameters normalize, one should suspect that the diagnosis is incorrect. When the biochemical parameters are normal and clinical manifestations are minimal, the patient is followed with 24-hour urine uroporphyrin determinations at 3- to 6-month intervals. If and when the urinary porphyrin progressively increases, the iron studies should be repeated and treatment reinstituted.

Patients with untreated PCT may be at risk for the development of hepatoma. Contributory intrinsic factors include the increased hepatic iron and porphyrin content. In addition, patients with PCT are often infected with the hepatitis C or B virus. The presence of so many oncogenic stimuli dictates that these individuals be treated promptly as outlined previously and monitored carefully for signs of hepatic cancer. In addition, patients with hepatitis C or B and persistently abnormal liver chemistries despite normalization of porphyrin and iron economy should be considered for treatment with interferon-alpha-2b* (Intron-A).

*Not FDA approved for this indication.

THERAPEUTIC USE OF BLOOD COMPONENTS

method of
CAROLYN F. WHITSETT, M.D.
Emory University School of Medicine
Atlanta, Georgia

Blood products available for clinical use have been traditionally classified as components and derivatives. Blood components are made using centrifugation techniques, and blood derivatives are made from large pools of human plasma using chemical fractionation, often followed by other purification procedures. Recently, recombinant DNA techniques have been used in the production of blood proteins, and a recombinant form of one coagulation factor, Factor VIII, is now available for clinical use.

Although donated blood is thoroughly screened to reduce the possibility of transmitting infectious diseases by transfusion, there is still a very small risk of disease transmission with blood components. Whenever possible, the risks associated with transfusion should be discussed with the patient and/or family members and written consent obtained for transfusion therapy. Blood derivatives are either heated or chemically treated to inactivate contaminating infectious agents and are generally transfused without obtaining specific consent. However, some religious groups prohibit the use of these products as well as blood transfusion, and consent may be needed for some patients. A thorough transfusion history should be obtained prior to the administration of blood and blood components because information provided in the history could influence product selection (e.g., the use of leukocyte-depleted products in a patient with recurrent febrile reactions). The indications for transfusion and the patient's response to transfusion should be clearly documented in the medical record.

The component therapy guidelines presented in the following sections were developed from information provided in *Standards for Blood Banks and Transfusion Services* (15th ed), and the *Technical Manual* (11th ed) published by the American Association of Blood Banks, as well as the recent scientific literature.

BLOOD COMPONENTS

Whole Blood

Indication: • Simultaneous replacement of plasma volume and red cell mass

Whole blood is usually collected in CPDA-1 (citrate-phosphate-dextrose-adenine) anticoagulant and stored between 1° and 6° C. It has an expiration date of 35 days. Most units of whole blood collected are used for component preparation, and whole blood is not always available.

Reconstituted whole blood, a product that is made

by resuspending red cells in fresh-frozen plasma, is sometimes prepared by hospital transfusion services for use in neonatal exchange transfusion.

Whole blood represents 450 ± 45 mL of blood collected in 63 mL of anticoagulant. At least 24 hours are required for completion of routine laboratory testing. Even though the blood is refrigerated during this time, the granulocytes, platelets, and labile coagulation factors (Factors V and VIII) deteriorate. Thus, whole blood is not a reliable source of these components and may need to be supplemented with platelets, fresh-frozen plasma, and other coagulation products if there are abnormalities in hemostasis.

Red Cells

Indication:
- Replacement of red cell mass

Red cells, prepared from whole blood by centrifugation, have a shelf life of 35 days when maintained in CPDA-1 anticoagulated plasma or 42 days when suspended in additive solutions that enhance red cell survival.

A unit of CPDA-1 red cells has a volume of approximately 220 mL and a hematocrit of 70 to 80%; red cells in additive solutions have a volume of approximately 320 mL and a hematocrit of 55 to 60%. Red cells in additive solutions can be infused more rapidly than CPDA-1 red cells; however, the volume infused is greater and may create a risk of volume overload. Although the indications for the two types of red cell products are the same, it is generally believed that newborn infants receiving large-volume transfusions or exchange transfusions may not tolerate the additional volume or some of the components of the additive solutions. The red cells may be washed and the hematocrit of the washed red cell product adjusted to the desired level.

The hemoglobin level at which tissue oxygenation is impaired by a reduced red cell mass has been the subject of debate since the publication of the NIH Consensus Conferences guidelines, which suggested that, in many patients, the hematocrit can be allowed to fall to 21% before transfusion is required. Symptoms of anemia or the presence of cardiovascular or pulmonary disease must be taken into consideration when making the decision to initiate transfusion therapy. The indications for transfusion and the patient's response to the transfusion should be documented in progress notes. If the hemoglobin level is above the guidelines recommended by the institutional transfusion committee or markedly different from national standards of transfusion practice, a more detailed entry may be desirable. In general, transfusion of a unit of red cells will increase the hemoglobin by 1 gram per dL, or the hematocrit by 3%, in a 70-kg adult male.

Modified Red Cell Products

Washed Red Cells

Indications:
- Prevention of allergic reactions by removal of plasma proteins
- Prevention of febrile reactions by reducing leukocyte content
- Red cell transfusions in IgA-deficient patients when blood from IgA-deficient donors is not available

Red cells are washed with 0.9% (normal) saline, which removes plasma proteins, microaggregates, and white cells. Automated washing is more efficient than manual washing, but it is not as effective in removing leukocytes as the new generation of high-efficiency leukocyte depletion filters. Red cells that have been washed five times are reported to be suitable for use in IgA-deficient patients. The shelf life for washed cells is 24 hours.

Frozen-Deglycerolized Red Cells

Indications:
- Replacement of red cell mass in patients with rare blood types and IgA deficiency
- Used as an alternative form of leukocyte-depleted red cells
- When long-term storage of autologous blood is desired

Using glycerol as a cryopreservative, red cells can be stored frozen for 10 years. After thawing, the glycerol is removed by washing, and the red cells are resuspended in an isotonic electrolyte solution containing glucose. The shelf life of this product is 24 hours. Most hospitals do not have facilities for preparing or storing frozen red cells, and these procedures are usually performed at blood centers. Deglycerolization takes 30 to 40 minutes, and additional time is required to transport the product to the hospital. Freezing of red cells is usually reserved for rare blood types, but it may also be used to store blood for patients desiring autologous blood for elective surgery.

Platelets

Indication:
- To prevent or control bleeding caused by a reduced platelet count or abnormal platelet function

Platelets are provided as random-donor platelet concentrates obtained from whole blood donations by centrifugation or as single-donor platelets obtained with apheresis techniques. The pheresis donor may be selected to have an HLA type similar to that of the patient to provide an HLA-matched platelet product.

Each unit of random donor platelets contains approximately 5.5×10^{10} platelets. For the average adult patient, each unit of concentrate transfused will increase the platelet count 5 to 10×10^{9} per liter. A plateletpheresis product contains a minimum of 3×10^{11} platelets, which is equivalent to about six platelet concentrates. Platelets are stored at 20° to 24° C with continuous agitation and are usually usable for 5 days. To facilitate transfusion, random-donor concentrates can be pooled just prior to transfusion. Pooled platelets have an expiration time of 4 hours.

Platelet products contain lymphocytes and may also contain some red cells. When frequent platelet transfusions are given, the contaminating lymphocytes may immunize patients to HLA antigens, making them refractory to subsequent platelet transfusions. When platelets from Rh-positive individuals must be transfused to Rh-negative individuals, immunization to Rh may result because of contamination of platelet products with small numbers of red cells. Rh immunization in these circumstances can be prevented by the use of Rh immune globulin.

Platelets contain ABO blood group antigens, HLA antigens, and platelet-specific antigens. Routine platelet transfusions are usually ABO compatible, but satisfactory increases in platelet count can be obtained with ABO-incompatible platelets. Over time, patients who receive multiple platelet transfusions frequently fail to obtain adequate increases in their platelet counts with products from random donors, a development that is usually associated with the appearance of anti-HLA antibodies, although antibodies to platelet-specific antigens are also observed. Selecting platelet donors who have HLA types similar to that of the patient or using a platelet crossmatch to select products for transfusion is frequently helpful.

Granulocytes

Indication: • Severe neutropenia or neutrophil dysfunction with sepsis

Granulocyte concentrates are prepared with apheresis techniques except when transfused to neonates. For neonates, adequate numbers of cells may be collected from freshly donated units of whole blood. Products prepared with apheresis contain a minimum of 1.0×10^{10} granulocytes. Granulocytes should be transfused as soon as possible after collection, but storage at 20° to 24° C is permitted for up to 24 hours. Granulocytes are usually contaminated with significant numbers of red cells, so donors should be ABO and Rh compatible and negative for any clinically significant antibodies found in the patient's serum. If Rh-negative donors are unavailable and Rh-positive granulocytes must be used in an Rh-negative patient, Rh immune globulin administration should be considered.

Patients with granulocyte counts below 0.5×10^9 per liter and sepsis or severe bacterial infections unresponsive to therapy are candidates for granulocyte transfusions. Patients with hereditary disorders of neutrophil function may be candidates for granulocyte transfusion at higher counts. Prophylactic granulocyte transfusions are no longer given because they were ineffective at the doses given and were associated with adverse reactions. In many patients who are at risk for chemotherapy-induced neutropenia, severe neutropenia can be avoided by the administration of granulocyte colony-stimulating factor (G-CSF) or granulocyte-macrophage colony-stimulating factor (GM-CSF).

Fresh-Frozen Plasma

Indications:
- Deficiencies of multiple clotting factors
- Deficiencies of any congenital coagulation factor for which concentrate is unavailable
- Replacement therapy in plasma exchange, especially in the treatment of thrombotic thrombocytopenic purpura and hemolytic-uremic syndrome.

Plasma separated from blood within 8 hours and stored at −18° C or less is called fresh-frozen plasma. The product retains full activity of labile and stable clotting factors for 1 year. Most units of fresh-frozen plasma are prepared from whole blood donations, but the product can also be prepared by apheresis. Units prepared by apheresis have a volume of 400 mL, whereas the standard product has a volume of approximately 200 mL.

Fresh-frozen plasma is thawed to between 30° and 37° C and must be transfused within 24 hours when used as a source of labile coagulation factors. Fresh-frozen plasma can be thawed rapidly with microwave technology, but most hospitals still use water baths. The thawing time with the latter method is approximately 30 minutes, and this lag time must be taken into account when ordering the product.

Coagulation tests should always be performed to document the extent of the clotting deficiency and the adequacy of correction following treatment.

Cryoprecipitate

(Cryoprecipitated Antihemophilic Factor)

Indication: • Correction of coagulation abnormalities caused by deficiency of Factor VIIIc, Factor VIIIvWF, or fibrinogen

A unit of cryoprecipitate is the cold-insoluble portion processed from the unit of fresh-frozen plasma obtained from a whole blood donation. Cryoprecipitate is frozen immediately after production and placed at −18° C or below. Each unit contains 80 to 100 units of Factor VIII/von Willebrand factor and 100 to 250 mg of fibrinogen in a volume of 10 to 15 mL.

Units of cryoprecipitate are usually selected to match the patient's ABO type because small amounts of ABO isoagglutinins are present. The dose transfused is a function of the severity of the coagulation deficiency. Cryoprecipitates are usually thawed and pooled to facilitate transfusion. The product must be given within 6 hours of thawing and 4 hours of pooling if it is to be used as a source of Factor VIII.

Cryoprecipitate can be used to correct the coagulation abnormality in hemophilia A and all forms of von Willebrand's disease except type III, in which platelets or DDAVP may also be required. Cryoprecipitate is also used to correct congenital or acquired afibrinogenemia or hypofibrinogenemia. It contains fibronectin and is used to prepare fibrin glue, a biologic adhesive.

Leukocyte-Depleted Blood Products

Indications:
- Prevention of febrile transfusion reactions
- Prevention of immunization to HLA antigens

Leukocyte-reduced red blood cells are prepared by washing or filtration using special leukocyte depletion filters. Frozen deglycerolized red cells are also considered leukocyte-reduced products. Leukocyte-reduced platelet products are also prepared using special leukocyte depletion filters. Single-donor platelet products prepared with some apheresis equipment also have a lower leukocyte count than a comparable number of platelet concentrates.

When leukocyte-reduced products are used to prevent febrile transfusion reactions, the degree of leukocyte reduction required is not as great as that needed to prevent immunization to HLA antigens. The leukocyte number in the final component must be less than 5×10^8. However, only products prepared with special leukocyte depletion filters and some methods for producing frozen deglycerolized red cells consistently reduce the component leukocyte content to less than 5×10^6, the level considered useful for preventing immunization to HLA antigens.

CMV Seronegative Blood Products

Indication:
- Prevention of transfusion-transmitted cytomegalovirus (CMV) infections in CMV-seronegative patients in the following categories: infants weighing less than 1200 grams; pregnant patients; patients who are candidates for, or who are currently undergoing, bone marrow transplantation; patients who have had splenectomy

Blood centers routinely provide red cells, platelets, and granulocytes from CMV-seronegative donors for transfusion to patients in the categories listed above. The list of patients who should be considered for CMV-seronegative blood products may include any CMV-seronegative recipient who will be rendered immunologically deficient by disease or treatment. Although morbidity from CMV is less in solid organ transplant recipients than in bone marrow transplant recipients, there is reason to believe that morbidity caused by CMV in such individuals is sufficient to warrant the use of seronegative blood when the organ is from a CMV-seronegative donor. In some regions, the demand for seronegative blood products exceeds the supply. CMV is transmitted in the mononuclear cells of donor blood. The current generation of highly efficient leukocyte depletion filters removes more than 99% of such contaminating cells. CMV-safe red cells and platelets (i.e., blood with a lower risk of transmitting CMV) can be prepared by filtration leukodepletion.

Irradiated Blood Products

Indication:
- Prevention of transfusion-induced graft-versus-host disease

T lymphocytes found in cellular blood components and in plasma that has not been frozen can cause graft-versus-host disease (GVHD) when transfused to individuals who are immunologically deficient or to immunologically competent individuals who share HLA antigens with the blood donor. Currently, the minimum recommended dose of irradiation is 2500 cGy (1 cGy = 1 rad). This dose inactivates the lymphocytes, but does not affect the function or survival of platelets or granulocytes. Irradiated red cells release potassium during storage and may require washing when used for pediatric patients. The expiration period of irradiated red cells is ≤ 28 days from the date of irradiation.

Irradiated blood components are absolutely indicated for the following categories of patients: fetuses receiving intrauterine transfusion; patients with congenital immunodeficiency syndromes (severe combined immune deficiency, DiGeorge's syndrome, Wiskott-Aldrich syndrome); recipients who have undergone allogeneic or autologous bone marrow transplantation; recipients of blood products known to be from a blood relative; and recipients with Hodgkin's disease. There are several other patient groups in whom there is an increased risk of transfusion-induced GVHD (Table 1), but the scientific data do not fully support irradiation of blood products for all patients.

Facilities for blood irradiation are available in most large blood centers and hospitals that perform allogeneic bone marrow transplantation.

TABLE 1. **Indications for Irradiated Blood Components**

Indicated (irradiation mandatory)	Intrauterine transfusion
	Bone marrow transplantation
	Congenital immunodeficiency syndromes
	Directed donations from blood relatives
	Hodgkin's disease
Possibly indicated (irradiation indicated for some patients)	Infants receiving exchange transfusion
	Premature newborns
	Other hematologic malignancies
	Solid tumors with intensive chemotherapy
	Solid organ transplant recipients
	Recipients of HLA-matched platelets
Not indicated (no evidence of risk at this time)	Term newborns
	Acquired immune deficiency syndrome (AIDS)

BLOOD DERIVATIVES

Plasma Volume Expanders (Albumin and Plasma Protein Fraction)

Indication:
- Plasma volume expansion

Albumin is provided as 5% and 25% solutions. Plasma protein fraction (PPF) is primarily albumin but contains trace amounts of alpha- and beta-globulins. These natural plasma volume expanders prepared from pooled plasma using cold ethanol fractionation are heat treated and have been safely used for many years. Although synthetic volume expanders such as hydroxyethyl starch (hetastarch [Hespan]) are suitable for use when short-term support of blood volume is anticipated, albumin and PPF are preferable when chronic use of a volume expander is required. Although colloid and crystalloid volume expanders can cause a dilutional coagulopathy, hydroxyethyl starch and Dextran can cause other coagulation problems not observed with albumin and PPF.

Clotting Factor Concentrates

Indication: • Replacement of specific factor deficiencies.

Pooled plasma is the source material for clotting Factor concentrates with the exception of recombinant Factor VIII, which is produced by cloning of the human factor VIII gene into either Chinese hamster ovary cells or baby hamster kidney cells. Clotting concentrates are provided as a lyophilized powder that is reconstituted with sterile water immediately before use. They are either heated or chemically treated to reduce the risk of transmission of viral diseases. The human immunodeficiency virus is inactivated with current treatment. However, hepatitis A and B-19 parvovirus may be transmitted. Table 2 summarizes the clotting factor concentrates that are widely available.

Factor VIII Products. The Factor VIII concentrates manufactured today are highly purified products with vastly reduced amounts of contaminating serum proteins. The products are primarily a source of Factor VIIIc and are designed for use in patients with hemophilia A, unlike cryoprecipitate, which can be used to treat hemophilia A and von Willebrand's disease. Each vial of concentrate comes with information about Factor VIII content. The dose of Factor VIII to be given is a function of the patient's baseline level and the clinical circumstances requiring treatment. Therapy should be monitored with either Factor VIII levels or a partial thromboplastin time (PTT). Recombinant Factor VIII is free from the risk of disease transmission associated with Factor VIII concentrate but is much more expensive. It is the product of choice for previously untreated patients with hemophilia A. Following treatment with plasma, cryoprecipitate, or Factor VIII concentrate, some patients develop Factor VIII inhibitors. Patients with low-titer inhibitors (<10 Bethesda units) respond to increased doses of Factor VIII concentrate. When high-titer inhibitors are present, treatment with activated prothrombin complex concentrate (APCC) or porcine Factor VIII may be necessary. Prothrombin complex concentrate and APCC carry a risk of thrombosis and disseminated intravascular coagulation (DIC), and allergy to the porcine product may limit its usefulness.

Factor IX Products. Prothrombin complex concentrate (PCC) contains Factor IX and other vitamin K–dependent coagulation clotting factors, some of which may be present in activated form. Factor IX concentrate and PCC may be used for the treatment of hemophilia B. The more purified concentrates appear to have less activated clotting factors, and the risk of thrombosis and DIC should be less when they are used. As in hemophilia A, patients with hemophilia B may develop inhibitors, and APCC concentrate is also useful in these patients.

Antithrombin III Concentrates. Antithrombin III (AT-III) inhibits thrombin and other activated coagulation factors. Congenital deficiency of AT-III is associated with venous thrombosis and thromboembolic phenomena. Acquired deficiencies of AT-III may also occur in liver disease, severe nutritional deficiency, and DIC along with other factor deficiencies. The primary indication for treatment with AT-III concentrate is congenital deficiency of AT-III, but its use in acquired forms of the deficiency is under clinical investigation.

Immune Serum Globulin

Indications: • Diseases in which congenital or acquired deficiencies in B lymphocyte function result in deficiency in humoral immunity (e.g., congenital or acquired agammaglobulinemia or hypogammaglobulinemia)

TABLE 2. **Clotting Factor Concentrates**

Product Name	Description	Indication
Antihemophilic factor (Factor VIII)*	Purified Factor VIII made from pooled cryoprecipitate using affinity chromatography; monoclonal antibodies used in purification process	Hemophilia A
Recombinant Factor VIII	Produced by DNA recombinant techniques	Hemophilia A
Prothrombin complex concentrate	Contains Factors II, VII, IX, and X and some activated forms of these factors	Hemophilia B
Factor IX concentrate	More purified form of Factor IX; contains fewer activated factors	Hemophilia B
Anti-inhibitor complex (activated prothrombin complex)	Specially activated prothrombin complex to bypass need for Factor VIII or Factor IX	Hemophilia A and B patients with inhibitors
Antithrombin III concentrates	Purified, heat-treated antithrombin III	Congenital AT-III deficiency

*Some intermediate-purity Factor VIII products may contain sufficient Factor VIII VWF for use in patients with von Willebrand's disease.

- Passive prophylaxis against infections
- Immune modulation in autoimmune cytopenias, autoimmune neurologic diseases, and Kawasaki syndrome

Products Available: 5% and 10% solutions of immune globulin for intravenous use, immune serum globulin for intramuscular use, and specific immune globulins (usually for intramuscular use) designed to provide high titers of antibody to specific antigens or pathogens (e.g., Rh immune globulin, tetanus immune globulin, varicella-zoster immune globulin [VZIG]).

Immune serum globulin is made by ethanol fractionation of pooled plasma. The plasma pools generally contain a minimum of 6,000 to 10,000 donors, and the antibodies in the product reflect immunity in the donor population. The product is primarily IgG with small amounts of IgM and IgA. Many products contain enough IgA to trigger anaphylaxis in patients with IgA deficiency. Thus, only some manufacturers' products will be suitable for use in these patients. The product designed for intravenous use is treated to disrupt aggregates of IgG formed during the preparative process. The product designed for intramuscular use contains IgG aggregates and should not be used intravenously. The preparative procedures for immune globulin include steps that inactivate many viruses, and some manufacturers have added additional chemical treatments for that purpose.

Immune serum globulin for intravenous use is the product of choice for replacement therapy in humoral immunodeficiencies and as an immunomodulatory agent. The dose and frequency of administration for immunodeficiency is usually 200 mg per kg per month. When used for immune modulation, as in idiopathic thrombocytopenic purpura, the dose is much higher and is individualized. A standard induction dose might be 400 mg per kg for several days with a maintenance dose based on the disease and the patient's response to induction.

The use of specific immune globulins such as tetanus immune globulin is covered in chapters dealing with the treatment of the various infections. However, a word about Rh immune globulin is indicated because it is sometimes given when Rh-positive blood products are inadvertently or unavoidably given to Rh-negative patients. Rh immune globulin was originally developed to prevent hemolytic disease of the newborn. A 1-ml full-dose vial of Rh immune globulin (300 μg anti-D) will eliminate the immunizing effect of 15 mL of red cells. Platelet products and granulocytes may contain considerable numbers of red cells. Unsensitized Rh-negative patients who have received Rh-positive cellular products should be considered for treatment with Rh immune globulin.

ADVERSE REACTIONS TO BLOOD TRANSFUSIONS

method of
LAURIE J. SUTOR, M.D., and
HAROLD S. KAPLAN, M.D.
University of Texas Southwestern Medical Center
Dallas, Texas

Reactions to infusion of blood components are relatively common, occurring in 1 to 2% of transfusion episodes, the vast majority of which are benign and self-limited. Adverse outcomes include those of immune etiology (antibody-antigen interactions), infections, and those caused by other means (Table 1). Reactions may also be characterized as acute (occurring in the first 24 hours) or chronic (Table 1).

Transfusion-related adverse effects must be recognized by the transfusionist so that the following four goals can be attained:

1. Interruption of transfusion and investigation of suspected reaction
2. Administration of appropriate treatment
3. Prevention of future reactions in the same patient
4. Identification of blood donors carrying infectious diseases to avoid further spread.

The transfusion service must be promptly notified of all adverse transfusion outcomes other than localized urticaria and volume overload. Chronic adverse effects, including suspected infectious disease transmission, must be reported along with the more acute reactions.

COMPLICATIONS OF IMMUNE ETIOLOGY

Immune-Mediated Hemolysis

Acute. Immune hemolysis in the acute setting generally results from the administration of ABO blood group–incompatible blood. Transfusion of ABO-incompatible red blood cells (RBCs) is potentially life-threatening for several reasons: (1) Virtually all individuals have preformed circulating antibodies to

TABLE 1. **Adverse Effects of Blood Transfusion**

	Acute	Chronic
Immune	Acute hemolysis Febrile, nonhemolytic reaction Allergy/anaphylaxis Noncardiogenic pulmonary edema (TRALI)	Delayed hemolysis Graft-vs.-host disease (GVHD) Alloimmunization Post-transfusion purpura Immune suppression
Nonimmune	Volume overload Bacterial contamination Citrate toxicity Hyperkalemia Coagulopathy Mechanical hemolysis	Iron overload Viral transmission Parasitic transmission

the antigens they lack in the ABO system (for example, group O individuals have pre-existing anti-A and anti-B antibodies). (2) Anti-A and/or anti-B antibodies are potent complement-fixing antibodies that cause immediate damage to the RBC membrane with intravascular cell lysis. (3) A cascade-type reaction is set off with the activation of complement, involving the kinin system and coagulation cascade, leading to widespread vascular dilation, hypotension, and disseminated intravascular coagulation (DIC) triggered by only a small initial amount of incompatible blood.

Signs and symptoms include hypotension/shock, red urine, fever, chills, vague malaise or discomfort, frank chest or back pain, or pain at the infusion site. Not all patients receiving an ABO-incompatible transfusion will manifest profound signs and symptoms, so any individual finding should be viewed with caution. A work-up should be initiated in all cases involving significant hypotension, red urine, or fever to evaluate whether incompatible blood may have been transfused.

Treatment is immediate. The transfusion must be stopped and generous crystalloid fluid replacement begun. Diuretics may be administered to maintain good renal function. In general, supportive care should be maintained as appropriate. Do not administer more blood until the proper ABO type has been ascertained, or, if necessary for emergencies, use group O RBCs until the investigation has been completed.

Nearly all ABO-incompatible transfusions occur because of misidentification of the original blood sample or of the recipient at the time of infusion. Therefore, if an ABO-mismatched transfusion is discovered, it is important to identify, if possible, any other patient who was misidentified so that he or she does not receive an ABO-mismatched transfusion also.

Blood group antibodies other than anti-A and anti-B can occasionally cause acute intravascular hemolysis, although not usually with the severity of ABO incompatibility. Of the other blood groups, an antibody to a Kidd RBC antigen (Jk), which can also activate the complement cascade, is the most frequent cause of acute hemolysis.

Delayed. When blood is inadvertently transfused that is incompatible for other RBC antigens, delayed immune hemolysis may occur. Diagnosis of a delayed hemolytic transfusion reaction is often made by the transfusion service. The clinical team may note the dropping hematocrit and send a new specimen to the transfusion service for crossmatching of additional units. At that time, several days after the original transfusion, the transfusion service personnel will detect one or more RBC antibodies whose titers have risen anamnestically after the immune stimulation of transfused blood expressing the antigens targeted by the antibodies. These antibodies were present but undetectable prior to the original transfusion and generally were formed following transfusion or pregnancy in the distant past.

Antibodies to RBC antigens of the Rh (C, c, D, E, e), Ss, Duffy, and Kell systems typically do not fix complement, but rather sensitize the cell to clearance by the macrophage/monocyte system. Breakdown of the antibody-coated cells then occurs extravascularly, such as in the spleen. Such hemolysis occurs slowly, often only becoming recognizable 7 to 10 days after transfusion. Symptoms are mild or nonexistent and accompany a slowly dropping hematocrit and mild elevation in bilirubin and lactate dehydrogenase.

Treatment of a delayed hemolytic transfusion reaction is often unnecessary or consists of additional transfusions with blood negative for the offending antigen(s). When clinical circumstances allow, it is prudent to delay further transfusion until subsequent blood samples show no other evidence of emerging previously unrecognized antibodies. Rarely, particularly with anti-Kidd antibodies, a delayed severe hemolytic reaction may occur that must be treated as an acute hemolytic transfusion reaction.

Fever Not Associated with Hemolysis

Fever of at least 1° C above normal is a common complication of transfusion, occurring in approximately 1 to 2% of all transfusion recipients. The fever may be accompanied by other symptoms such as chills, flushing, or malaise. If other causes of fever can be excluded, such as underlying disease, infection, or a bacterially contaminated unit of blood, a febrile nonhemolytic transfusion reaction is presumed to have occurred.

Fever accompanying transfusion is generally seen in patients with a history of prior transfusion. Antibodies to leukocyte antigens present in transfused blood are formed in the recipient. Symptoms occur during infusion of the blood or within 1 to 2 hours after completion of the transfusion.

Administration of antipyretics prior to transfusion helps prevent febrile symptoms. Patients in whom repeated febrile reactions occur despite antipyretics may benefit from blood components with a reduced number of leukocytes. Such components are generally prepared by filtration. Current filtration methods reduce the number of leukocytes in units of RBCs or platelets by 3 to 4 logs. Rarely, a patient with high titers of leukocyte antibodies will manifest fever despite receiving leukocyte-reduced blood components.

Allergic Reactions

Allergic signs and symptoms range from the common rash or urticaria with itching to anaphylactoid reactions. Allergic reactions generally occur shortly after the start of the transfusion and are caused by preformed recipient antibodies to a plasma protein in the donor plasma. Fever is unusual.

Mild symptoms involving only the skin can be treated by temporarily halting the transfusion and administering antihistaminic agents. Once the rash or urticaria subsides, the transfusion can be resumed. Reactions with additional symptoms such as facial swelling, laryngeal edema, or dyspnea should be treated more cautiously and transfusion of the donor unit immediately discontinued. Full-fledged anaphylaxis is an emergency and requires epinephrine injection and appropriate support. Subsequent transfusions should be approached with great care and autologous blood used whenever possible. Washed RBCs are a possible alternative when patients cannot donate blood for their own use.

The classic cause of anaphylaxis is the reaction of antibodies in an IgA-deficient recipient with IgA molecules in transfused plasma. Patients with severe allergic reactions should be tested for IgA deficiency, but antibodies to other proteins can also cause severe symptoms. Blood from IgA-deficient donors can be used for transfusion in IgA-deficient patients, but such units often take significant time to procure.

Pulmonary Symptoms

Dyspnea can occur in several clinical settings involving transfusion. Most commonly it may accompany circulatory overload when the volume of transfused blood and other fluids cannot be tolerated by the patient. Dyspnea can also be caused by antibodies to transfused leukocytes and can accompany febrile transfusion reactions. A severe form of transfusion-induced dyspnea called transfusion-related acute lung injury (TRALI), or noncardiogenic pulmonary edema, occurs when high-titer leukocyte antibodies from a blood donor (usually a multiparous female) are transfused in a plasma-containing component. Such antibodies attack recipient leukocytes, cause them to agglutinate, and the agglutinates become lodged in the pulmonary capillaries. Breakdown of leukocytes occurs with release of enzymes and damage to the pulmonary capillary bed, and a clinical syndrome resembling adult respiratory distress syndrome is seen. Treatment is supportive.

Graft-Versus-Host Disease

Certain immunosuppressed patients receiving transfusion are at risk for injury from viable T lymphocytes in transfused blood. Such donor T cells are not destroyed by the host and can proliferate, attacking tissues throughout the body. Such a reaction is seen in the first month following transfusion and consists of rash, gastrointestinal symptoms, and hepatosplenomegaly. In addition, transfusion-related graft-versus-host disease (GVHD) is a more serious illness than the GVHD that follows bone marrow transplantation: there is severe pancytopenia of the bone marrow, treatment is difficult, and mortality exceeds 90%. GVHD can be prevented by gamma irradiation of RBCs and platelet concentrates prior to infusion in susceptible patients.

Recently, rare immunocompetent recipients have been described with transfusion-associated GVHD. Such individuals generally received blood donated by relatives. Shared HLA haplotypes are thought to be the reason why the recipient's system does not recognize the donor's lymphocytes as foreign. Irradiation of blood components donated by relatives is now recommended as a preventive measure.

Post-Transfusion Purpura

This rare complication of transfusion is seen predominantly in women and is manifested by severe thrombocytopenia 7 to 10 days after transfusion. It most frequently occurs following transfusion of red cell components. The etiology is not clear but is presumed to involve antibodies to platelet-specific antigens. Treatment consists of administration of intravenous immunoglobulin concentrate or plasmapheresis. Platelet transfusion should be avoided whenever possible.

Alloimmunization

Primary antibody formation to RBC antigens occurs in approximately 1% of transfusion recipients overall and in up to 20% of selected groups, such as sickle cell anemia patients. The formation of the antibody itself causes no problem as the RBCs of the inciting transfusion are generally out of circulation, but units of blood for future transfusions must be carefully selected to avoid the targeted antigens.

Antibody formation to platelet antigens also occurs frequently and can cause destruction of subsequent platelet transfusions and refractoriness to such therapy. Treatment includes use of HLA-matched platelets or donated blood from relatives. Platelet cross-matching may improve the success of transfusion. Prevention of platelet alloimmunization is thought to be accomplished by leukoreduction of RBC and platelet components with filters.

Immune Suppression

Recent reports suggest that blood transfusion can cause general immunosuppression. The strongest evidence demonstrates improved survival of renal allografts in transfused patients. Other reports indicate that transfused patients are more likely to have postoperative infections. Most controversial is the theory that transfused patients undergoing cancer resection have more frequent or earlier tumor recurrence. Use of leukoreduced blood may prevent immunosuppressive effects.

NONIMMUNE, NONINFECTIOUS COMPLICATIONS

Volume Overload

One of the most common complications, this is easily treated in most patients with administration of diuretics.

Complications of Massive Transfusion

Patients receiving a transfusion volume in excess of their baseline blood volume in an emergency situation can experience several complications. Citrate toxicity (hypocalcemia) can result from the accumulation of anticoagulant from numerous transfused units. Hypothermia can occur if refrigerated RBCs are infused rapidly without rewarming, especially when infused into a central line. Potassium excess in the plasma of stored RBCs can cause hyperkalemia. Finally, coagulopathies can develop because of dilutional loss of clotting factors in the setting of serious underlying illness.

Iron Overload

Patients receiving more than 100 units of RBCs over their lifetime are at risk for deposition of excess iron in organs such as the heart, liver, and pancreas. Such deposition can ultimately cause organ failure and the death of the patient. Treatment with iron chelating agents (deferoxamine mesylate [Desferal]) can help but is often not completely successful in eliminating the excess iron.

INFECTIOUS COMPLICATIONS

Bacterial Contamination

Bacteria can proliferate in stored blood components and cause sepsis in the recipient upon infusion. The most serious complications occur when psychrophilic, gram-negative, endotoxin-producing bacteria proliferate in stored RBCs. Infusion of the unit after 20 days or more of storage results in an immediate septic shock, with high mortality. The most frequent pathogens are *Yersinia enterocolitica* and some *Pseudomonas* species. Prevention is difficult and treatment is supportive.

Because platelets are stored at room temperature, they not uncommonly harbor detectable bacteria. However, such contamination rarely causes clinical symptoms: the organisms do not make endotoxin, and the recipients are often receiving antibiotics already.

Parasites

Transmission of malaria via blood transfusion is well documented worldwide. Recent reports of transmission of both *Babesia microti* (babesiosis) and *Trypanosoma cruzi* (Chagas' disease) via transfusion in the United States have generated concern.

Viral Infections

Hepatitis C. Non-A, non-B hepatitis continues to be the most common clinically significant infection transmitted by blood transfusion in the general hospital population. The incidence of infection has been estimated recently to be 1 in 3000 transfusion episodes. Most of the transfusion-transmitted viral hepatitis is probably type C, but some experts suspect that another yet unnamed (hepatitis F?) parenteral form of viral hepatitis may be responsible for some cases seronegative for hepatitis C.

Post-transfusion hepatitis C leads to chronic infection in approximately 60% of cases. Sequelae can include chronic active hepatitis, cirrhosis, and hepatocellular carcinoma.

Hepatitis B. The risk of acquiring hepatitis B from transfusion has been greatly reduced in the last decade with the addition of donor testing for antibodies to hepatitis B core and alanine aminotransferase levels in 1986. Hepatitis B surface antigen testing has been in place for over 20 years. Although hepatitis B infection from transfusion can still occur, an individual with acute hepatitis B should be carefully evaluated for risk factors other than transfusion.

Cytomegalovirus. Cytomegalovirus (CMV) is said to be the most common infection transmitted by transfusion, with 45 to 80% of U.S. blood donors having evidence of prior CMV infection. Fortunately, CMV transmission seldom has clinical significance. Recipients with intact immune systems generally have few if any symptoms. Only immunosuppressed patients are at risk for serious, even life-threatening, complications of CMV infection. Such patients (e.g., transplant recipients and fetuses), if CMV seronegative, should receive blood that is either obtained from CMV-seronegative donors or is leukocyte reduced.

Human Immunodeficiency Virus Type 1 (HIV-1). With current donor screening practices and donor testing, the risk of HIV-1 transmission through transfusion is very small. Theoretically, it still can occur if a donor gives blood early in the course of the infection and prior to seroconversion. The risk is estimated to be between 1 in 100,000 and 1 in 250,000 per unit administered.

Parvovirus B-19. This virus, the etiologic agent of fifth disease, is known to be transmitted by blood components, including current manufactured plasma derivatives (e.g., clotting factor concentrates). The chief risk is in patients with chronic compensated anemic states, such as sickle cell anemia or hereditary spherocytosis. The virus causes a period of bone marrow aplasia for which individuals with chronically stressed marrows cannot compensate, leading to marked anemia and the need for more transfusions.

Section 6

The Digestive System

CHOLELITHIASIS AND CHOLECYSTITIS

method of
DAN I. N. GIURGIU, M.D., and
JOEL J. ROSLYN, M.D.
Medical College of Pennsylvania
Philadelphia, Pennsylvania

Calculus disease of the biliary tract continues to be a major health problem in the United States and throughout the world. Current estimates suggest that over 20 million Americans, in excess of 10% of the population, have gallstones. Each year, an estimated one million patients will be diagnosed with cholelithiasis. Approximately 700,000 patients in the United States will undergo cholecystectomy in this coming year, and the overall treatment cost will surpass the $5 billion mark in 1994.

Gallstones can be classified based on composition, location, and site of origin. It is generally accepted that there are three types of gallstones: pure cholesterol, pigment, and mixed stones. Although pigment stones are the most common type of stone worldwide, cholesterol and mixed stones account for the majority of gallstones found in the United States. The hepatic secretion of cholesterol-saturated bile is a prerequisite for cholesterol gallstone formation. This type of bile induces a series of changes in gallbladder function that ultimately results in nucleation of crystals and gallstone formation. Predisposing factors in cholesterol gallstone disease include female gender, increasing age, diabetes, obesity, rapid weight loss, and other less well-defined genetic factors.

Throughout the world, pigment stones are the most prevalent type of calculi found in the gallbladder. These stones form when calcium bilirubinate and insoluble salts precipitate as a result of altered solubilization of unconjugated bilirubin. Pigment gallstones are further classified as either black or brown stones. Black pigment stones are generally found in patients with hemolytic disorders, such as sickle cell disease or hereditary spherocytosis, as well as in patients with cirrhosis, whereas brown stones are associated with infection.

NATURAL HISTORY OF GALLSTONE DISEASE

Over the years, considerable controversy has surrounded the issue of how best to manage patients with asymptomatic gallstones. This is particularly important, given the fact that between 40 and 60% of patients with cholelithiasis are asymptomatic. Three separate studies have attempted to identify the incidence of subsequent development of symptoms in patients with asymptomatic gallstones. The results indicate that between 10 and 30% of patients with asymptomatic gallstones will develop some symptoms from their biliary tract disease over the ensuing decade, the majority of which are secondary to biliary colic. Approximately 20% of patients developing symptoms will present with acute cholecystitis as their initial symptom, and a smaller percentage will present with jaundice, cholangitis, or pancreatitis. Hospitalization culminating in death as the initial manifestation is a rare occurrence. Based on our current understanding of the natural history of asymptomatic gallstone disease, prophylactic cholecystectomy is rarely indicated in these patients.

A related, and perhaps more difficult, question is how to manage those patients with documented cholelithiasis who complain of nonspecific dyspeptic symptoms without specific evidence of biliary colic. Recent studies indicate that up to 70% of such patients derive significant benefit from cholecystectomy, suggesting that these nonspecific symptoms may in fact be due to biliary calculi. Early or prophylactic cholecystectomy should be considered, or at least discussed with the patient, in certain specific clinical settings. One must be cognizant of the potential for symptom development, life expectancy, and associated operative morbidity and mortality in order to determine whether cholecystectomy is appropriate for a given patient. There are no data to suggest that medical dissolution with oral agents, contact dissolution, or biliary lithotripsy should be employed in patients with truly asymptomatic stones.

DIAGNOSTIC EVALUATION

Although supine and upper right abdominal radiographs are essential in the early evaluation of patients with an acute abdomen, their usefulness is limited in patients with cholelithiasis. Gallstones are detected on plain abdominal radiographs in only 20% of patients whose gallstones are grossly calcified. For many years, the gold standard for the diagnosis of gallstone disease has been the oral cholecystogram (OCG). While this is a very accurate test in patients with chronic cholelithiasis and cholecystitis, its utility is particularly limited in patients with acute inflammation of the gallbladder. Factors that can result in a false-negative study include acute illness, poor patient compliance, and inability to absorb tablets as a result of emesis, nonabsorption, diarrhea, jaundice, and hepatic dysfunction.

Over the last 15 years, abdominal ultrasonography has emerged as the preferred test for the evaluation of patients with suspected cholelithiasis or acute cholecystitis. Abdominal ultrasonography is highly accurate, with a sensitivity and specificity approaching 98%. In addition, ultrasound can yield important information regarding the size of the common bile duct, the presence of pericholecystic fluid collections, gallbladder wall thickness, and other upper abdominal masses. Hepatobiliary scintigraphy, which involves intravenous administration of specific radionuclide agents that are cleared from the blood by hepatocytes and excreted in an unconjugated form directly into the biliary ductular system, can provide very specific information about cystic duct patency. While this finding may definitively diagnose acute cholecystitis (which is characterized by cystic duct obstruction), it nonetheless does not specifically identify the presence or absence of gallstones. This test has little utility in the patient with uncomplicated biliary colic and its usefulness in acute cholecystitis has been the subject of some debate. The diagnosis of acute cholecystitis is typically a clinical one, and in most instances, the presence of cholelithiasis in the patient who has right upper quadrant tenderness, mild leukocytosis, and fever is sufficient to confirm the diagnosis without a hepatobiliary scan. Biliary drainage with cholecystokinin (CCK) cholecystography is helpful in the occasional patient who presents with what appear to be classic symptoms of biliary colic but with no evidence of cholelithiasis on either OCG or abdominal ultrasonography. The vast majority of patients who have an abnormal biliary drainage and CCK cholecystographic examination will in fact benefit from cholecystectomy.

CHRONIC CHOLECYSTITIS

Clinical Presentation

Intermittent, postprandial, right upper quadrant pain is the classic complaint of patients with chronic cholelithiasis and cholecystitis. Biliary colic results from the presence of an impacted stone in the cystic duct or passage of a stone through this ductular structure. Characteristically, the pain of biliary colic is of sudden onset, builds in intensity, plateaus for several hours, and then resolves within 3 to 6 hours. Although the pain is typically located in the right upper quadrant, many patients with biliary colic localize their pain to the midepigastrium, back, or other sites within the abdomen. These episodes are often associated with nausea and emesis. Although biliary colic has classically been associated with fatty meals, it is quite apparent that virtually any food can precipitate such an attack.

Treatment

Since 1882, open cholecystectomy has been the gold standard for the treatment of patients with symptomatic gallstone disease. This operation continues to be a safe and effective means of treating gallstones and is performed in most hospitals throughout the world. The operative mortality associated with this procedure in patients, is significantly less than 1% regardless of patient age.

The surgical approach to patients with chronic gallstone disease has been revolutionized by the introduction and development of laparoscopic cholecystectomy. This surgical procedure has become the preferred treatment modality for patients with gallstone disease. Laparoscopic cholecystectomy has numerous potential advantages over the open procedure, including reduction of postoperative pain and intestinal ileus, rapid return to full activity and employment, improved patient satisfaction secondary to cosmesis, rapid discharge from the hospital, and reduced cost. Over the last several years, considerable experience has been gained with this procedure, and morbidity and mortality rates have been found to differ little from those for traditional, open cholecystectomy. There continues to be some lingering concern about a learning curve and a slight increase in risk of bile duct injury during this period. A recent consensus conference sponsored by the National Institute of Diabetes and Digestive and Kidney Diseases focusing on laparoscopic cholecystectomy and traditional surgical and nonsurgical approaches to the management of gallstones concluded that while most patients with asymptomatic gallstones should not be treated, those individuals developing symptoms require prompt treatment. Moreover, laparoscopic cholecystectomy has become the treatment of choice for many patients for the reasons outlined previously. The outcome of laparoscopic cholecystectomy is dependent on the training and skill, as well as the judgment, of the surgeon performing the procedure. Laparoscopic cholecystectomy, as with any other innovation, should be compared to the standard therapy, which continues to be open cholecystectomy.

During the last 20 years, a number of nonsurgical modalities for the treatment of gallstone disease have been introduced. These include dissolution of gallstones by both oral agents (chenodeoxycholic acid [Chenix] and ursodeoxycholic acid [Actigall]), as well as by agents instilled directly into the gallbladder (methyl *tert*-butyl ether [MTBE]). Oral dissolution therapy is effective only for cholesterol gallstones and even in carefully selected patients results in complete dissolution in only 40%. These oral agents can be expensive and a prolonged course of therapy is typically required. An additional concern with this treatment modality includes the need for lifelong maintenance therapy to avoid recurrence of stones. Gallstone recurrence occurs at a rate of approximately 10% per year after discontinuation of therapy and then plateaus at approximately 50 to 60% after 5 years. Contact dissolution with MTBE is appropriate only for patients with cholesterol gallstones, and its usefulness is limited by the invasive nature of the procedure, as well as the documented recurrence, which is similar to that for oral dissolution therapy.

Although there was initial enthusiasm for biliary lithotripsy (ESWL), a number of factors, including technical limitations, rigid criteria for patient selection, and stone recurrence, have provided clinicians with considerable cause for reflection.

ACUTE CHOLECYSTITIS

Presentation

Cystic duct obstruction and acute inflammation of the gallbladder continue to be the most common complications of gallstone disease, affecting 20 to 30% of patients with symptomatic disease. In most cases, acute cholecystitis results from impaction of a stone in the cystic duct, although stones that lodge in Hartman's pouch can cause a similar clinical picture. The pain associated with acute cholecystitis is similar to that of biliary colic in terms of onset and character; however, unlike biliary colic, in which the pain lasts for a limited period of time, the pain of acute cholecystitis persists and may be unremitting for several days. These patients typically complain of persistent right upper quadrant pain, nausea, vomiting, anorexia, and fever. The classic physical finding of acute cholecystitis is a positive Murphy's sign—inspiratory arrest during deep palpation of the right upper quadrant. Clinical experience suggests that there is a wide variation in the spectrum of complaints and physical findings in acute cholecystitis. While many patients have right upper quadrant pain, leukocytosis, and fever, others may have only persistent, unremitting right upper quadrant pain. Mild jaundice, even in the absence of choledocholithiasis, may be present in up to 10 to 20% of patients and is secondary to contiguous inflammation.

The primary event in the development of acute cholecystitis is biochemical in nature; bacterial infection plays only a minor role in the genesis of this disease. Nonetheless, between 30 and 70% of patients with the clinical diagnosis of acute cholecystitis will have positive bile cultures. Most of the bacteria cultured from these patients are of enteric origin, with *Escherichia coli* the most common organism. The presence of bacteria in the bile of patients with acute cholecystitis is a source of potential morbidity insofar as most of the organisms cultured from wound infections are identical to those found in the patient's bile.

Treatment

Cholecystectomy remains the preferred treatment for patients with acute cholecystitis. For many years, these patients were managed expectantly during their initial hospitalization, discharged, and then brought back after 6 weeks for elective cholecystectomy. Subsequently completed prospective randomized studies demonstrated that delayed surgery was associated with a 20% chance of recurrent symptoms requiring hospitalization during this period, increased length of hospitalization and associated cost, and greater technical difficulty. Current dogma suggests that early cholecystectomy, performed within 24 to 72 hours after onset of symptoms, is the most efficacious way of treating patients with acute cholecystitis. Upon admission to the hospital, these patients should be managed with appropriate antibiotics and bowel rest, with surgery undertaken at the optimum time based on the surgeon's best judgment.

The role of laparoscopic cholecystectomy in the management of patients with acute cholecystitis is evolving. Early experience with laparoscopic cholecystectomy suggested that the presence of acute cholecystitis was a contraindication for this procedure. This was based primarily on technical considerations and concerns over bleeding and injury to the bile duct. More recent anecdotal experience indicates that laparoscopic cholecystectomy can be performed safely in selected patients with acute cholecystitis. Although cholecystectomy remains the standard treatment for patients with acute cholecystitis, cholecystostomy has been advocated for certain high-risk groups and can generally be performed under local anesthesia. Recent interest has focused on ultrasound-guided percutaneous transhepatic cholecystostomy and endoscopic transpapillary drainage of the gallbladder as alternatives to surgical cholecystostomy.

CHOLECYSTITIS IN SPECIFIC CLINICAL SETTINGS

Acalculous cholecystitis is an infrequent but often fatal complication of gallbladder disease, with an estimated incidence of 6% of all patients who present with acute inflammation of the gallbladder. Most patients with this entity are, in fact, critically ill, having sustained trauma or significant burn or undergone major surgery. The diagnosis in these patients is often quite challenging but can be confirmed ultrasonographically. The finding of a thickened gallbladder wall with pericholecystic fluid in the appropriate clinical setting is highly suggestive of acalculous disease. Treatment requires prompt surgical intervention.

It has long been thought that acute cholecystitis in diabetics is associated with increased morbidity and mortality. More recently completed studies, however, suggest that this may not be the case. Although many diabetics are at increased risk of morbidity and mortality secondary to underlying cardiovascular disease, there is little evidence that diabetics are in fact more likely to develop acute cholecystitis or have a greater incidence of postoperative infectious complications.

The incidence of gallstones increases with age, and elderly patients tend to have a more virulent course than younger patients when they develop acute cholecystitis. The overall mortality for cholecystectomy in elderly patients is probably five to ten times greater than in younger populations. However, most of these patients succumb to unremitting sepsis or cardiovascular disease. The incidence of choledocholithiasis, emphysematous cholecystitis, and gallbladder perforation is significantly increased in the older age group. A number of authors have suggested that a general reluctance on the part of physicians to care for elderly patients because of their underlying disease may be responsible for the increased rate of complications of biliary tract disease, as well as for the overall increase in morbidity and mortality. It has therefore been recommended that strong consideration be given to early cholecystectomy in elderly patients with symptomatic gallstone disease.

A number of studies have clearly demonstrated increased risk of gallstone formation in patients with cirrhosis. Moreover, cholecystectomy in this patient population has been associated with increased morbidity and mortality. In most patients, this is secondary to underlying portal hypertension, and complications are typically due to bleeding as a consequence of thrombocytopenia, portal hypertension, and impaired hepatic function. The indications for cholecystectomy in a cirrhotic patient should be carefully considered.

COMPLICATIONS OF ACUTE CHOLECYSTITIS

A number of specific clinical entities have been identified as complications of cholecystitis, including emphysematous cholecystitis, empyema of the gallbladder, and gallbladder perforation. Emphysematous cholecystitis is an unusual but potentially lethal complication of cholecystitis that is characterized by the radiographic demonstration of gas within the gallbladder lumen or wall. This disease is more common in elderly men, especially those with diabetes. The demonstration of gas within the lumen of the gallbladder wall is indicative of infection with a gas-producing bacterium, typically *Clostridia perfringens*. These patients can be gravely ill with sepsis, and the potential for serious morbidity and mortality is such that emergent cholecystectomy is warranted. The pathogenesis of empyema of the gallbladder is similar to that of acute, uncomplicated cholecystitis, the major difference being the presence of actual pus and purulent material within the gallbladder lumen. As in emphysematous cholecystitis, the patient is often quite toxic, and emergent cholecystectomy is required. Gallbladder perforation, which occurs in approximately 3 to 10% of all patients with acute cholecystitis, has been classified as either type 1 (acute free perforation with bile-stained peritoneal fluid, type 2 (subacute perforation with pericholecystic or right upper quadrant abscess formation), or type 3 (chronic perforation with formation of either cholecystenteric or cholecystocutaneous fistulas). The clinical suspicion of acute perforation of the gallbladder warrants prompt and aggressive treatment with fluid resuscitation, nasogastric decompression, intravenous administration of broad-spectrum antibiotics, and expeditious laparotomy. Patients with a cholecystenteric fistula may present with small bowel obstruction, an entity called gallstone ileus. This relatively rare condition accounts for fewer than 5% of all cases of intestinal obstruction. Patients with gallstone ileus are best managed as if they had a mechanical small bowel obstruction, with aggressive fluid resuscitation, broad-spectrum antibiotics, and early laparotomy. Since many of these patients are elderly and quite ill at the time of presentation, the primary goals of surgical intervention are correction of the obstruction and removal of the offending stone.

CIRRHOSIS

method of
VICTOR IDROVO, M.D., and
K. RAJENDER REDDY, M.D.
Center for Liver Diseases, University of Miami School of Medicine
Miami, Florida

Cirrhosis and fibrosis are not synonymous. Cirrhosis is a chronic pathologic state of the liver in which parenchymal necrosis has occurred, followed by regeneration and scarring. As a result, regenerating nodules surrounded by fibrous tissue with or without ongoing necrosis occur, with the development of distortion of the normal liver architecture. Once cirrhosis is established, it is irreversible, and progression is dependent on the underlying etiology and whether there is continuing necrosis.

The etiology of cirrhosis is variable, with alcohol being responsible for most cases in the Western world, while chronic viral hepatitis B and C are the leading causes worldwide. Hepatitis C has emerged as a major cause of cirrhosis and is responsible for many of the cases previously diagnosed as cryptogenic. Other etiologies for cirrhosis are shown in Table 1. On a morphologic basis, cirrhosis has

TABLE 1. **Etiology of Cirrhosis**

Alcohol	
Viral hepatitis B, C, and D	
Biliary cirrhosis:	Primary
	Secondary
Venous outflow obstruction:	Budd-Chiari syndrome
	Veno-occlusive disease
	Cardiac cirrhosis
Metabolic:	Hemochromatosis
	Wilson's disease
	$Alpha_1$-antitrypsin deficiency
	Nonalcoholic steatonecrosis
	Other metabolic disorders
Autoimmune chronic active hepatitis	
Drugs and toxins:	Alpha-methyldopa (Aldomet)
	Methotrexate (Rheumatrex)
	Isoniazid (INH)
	Nitrofurantoin (Macrodantin)
	Amiodarone (Cordarone)
	Trichloroethylene
	Hypervitaminosis A
Miscellaneous:	Syphilis
	Hereditary hemorrhagic telangiectasia
	Sarcoidosis
	Bowel bypass
	Indian childhood cirrhosis
Cryptogenic	

been traditionally classified into three groups: (1) micronodular—nodules having a uniform size, usually less than 3 mm in diameter; (2) macronodular—variation in the size of the regenerating nodules, usually greater than 3 mm in diameter and up to several centimeters; and (3) mixed—micronodules and macronodules are present with equal frequency. Although it is possible to suspect the etiology of cirrhosis on a morphologic basis (e.g., alcohol in micronodular cirrhosis, post-necrotic in macronodular cirrhosis), there may be a lack of good correlation.

The clinical manifestations of cirrhosis are primarily the result of the associated complications. These include portal hypertension with bleeding esophagogastric varices or portal hypertensive gastropathy, or both; hepatic encephalopathy; ascites; spontaneous bacterial peritonitis; functional renal failure (hepatorenal syndrome); hypersplenism; coagulopathy; hepatocellular carcinoma; pruritus; and bone disease.

TREATMENT

Cirrhosis may have a specific therapy depending on the etiology. Alcoholics who abstain from further alcohol consumption often have better survival. Nutritional supplementation is an important aspect of treatment in patients with superimposed alcoholic hepatitis, with a select role for corticosteroids in severely ill patients. Corticosteroids can be considered for patients with alcoholic hepatitis who have a discriminant factor index of greater than 32 (calculated as [patient prothrombin time minus control prothrombin time × 4.6] plus total bilirubin) in the absence of infection, pancreatitis, gastrointestinal bleeding, and renal failure, and such treatment has been associated with improved short-term survival. Vitamin and mineral deficiencies are common in these patients, and supplementation with a high-potency multivitamin that includes vitamin B_{12}, folic acid, thiamine, pyridoxine, vitamin A, vitamin D, and minerals such as zinc, magnesium, calcium and phosphorous should be provided. Oral colchicine 0.6 mg two times a day may be of benefit in a patient with cirrhosis who has undergone long-term treatment. Given that it is relatively safe and inexpensive, it would be a good choice in patients with cirrhosis but is of no benefit in patients with alcoholic hepatitis.

Individuals with hemochromatosis often benefit from phlebotomies and iron depletion. While undergoing phlebotomies, pharmacologic doses of ascorbic acid should be avoided because they may cause deterioration in cardiac function, although small doses may actually facilitate urinary excretion of iron. Patients may require several phlebotomies depending on the degree of iron accumulation, and maintenance phlebotomies are required.

Wilson's disease can be managed with chelating agents such as penicillamine. Up to 20% of patients may develop a hypersensitive reaction characterized by fever, rash, pruritus, malaise, lymphadenopathy, leukopenia, and thrombocytopenia, which necessitates withdrawing the drug. Desensitization with incremental doses of D-penicillamine under corticosteroid coverage is well tolerated. An alternative chelating agent, trientine hydrochloride (Syprinel) appears to be effective, and the use of zinc has been advocated because of its ability to decrease copper absorption. D-penicillamine, however, is the mainstay treatment.

Interferon-alpha-2b is the only approved drug for treatment of chronic viral B and C hepatitis. Patients with replicative stage hepatitis B virus (DNA positive and HBeAg positive) and well-compensated liver disease can be treated either with 5 million units subcutaneously daily or 10 million units three times a week for 4 months. Close monitoring of hemotologic parameters (white cell count and platelet count) is essential while the patient is undergoing treatment, and the patient's ultimate response is based on loss of viral replication, as indicated by loss of HBeAg and HBV-DNA, which can be expected in approximately 35% of patients. Most often, the response is sustained. Patients with decompensated chronic hepatitis B infection should not be treated with interferon-alpha because the disease could potentially get worse due to the immunostimulatory effect of the drug. Favorable features for response are female gender, short duration of infection, negative anti-HIV, white race, and an abnormal alanine aminotransferase (ALT) with low HBV-DNA. Asians who most likely have acquired this infection perinatally do not respond well, particularly if they have immune tolerance to the virus as noted by a normal ALT. The recommended dose for chronic hepatitis C is 3 million units subcutaneously three times a week for 6 months. Unfortunately, sustained response has been found in only 15% of patients. High rates of relapses and associated side effects of interferon have made this less than an ideal form of treatment for chronic C hepatitis.

Autoimmune chronic active hepatitis can go into remission with corticosteroid therapy. Maintenance therapy is often a small dose of corticosteroids, along with azathioprine. While the patient is on corticosteroids, attention should be given to bone disease in women, particularly those who have passed the stage of menopause, and it would be prudent to supplement the therapy with vitamin D and oral calcium.

Cardiac cirrhosis may improve if the underlying heart disorder is controlled.

The two cholestatic chronic liver conditions, primary sclerosing cholangitis and primary biliary cirrhosis, may benefit from ursodiol (Actigall), which is a relatively safe drug. The management of the complications of cirrhosis and liver transplantation is discussed in the following section.

MANAGEMENT OF THE COMPLICATIONS OF CIRRHOSIS

Treatment of cirrhotic patients has been focused primarily on the management of complications of this disorder. Advances in the understanding of the pathophysiology of these complications have expanded the number of therapeutic alternatives currently available.

Portal Hypertension

Cirrhosis of the liver is the most common cause of portal hypertension in the United States. It is defined as a sustained elevation of the portal venous pressure, leading to the development of portal-systemic collaterals diverting the blood from the splanchnic bed to the systemic circulation, bypassing the liver. Portal hypertension in cirrhotics is a result of two pathologic features: (1) high resistance to hepatic outflow and (2) elevated splanchnic flow related to a hyperdynamic circulation secondary to endogenous vasodilators (glucagon, nitric oxide) and to an avid retention of sodium and water. An elevation of the portal pressure above 12 mmHg may produce serious consequences including gastrointestinal bleeding, hepatic encephalopathy, ascites, and splenomegaly with hypersplenism.

Gastrointestinal Bleeding

The subject of esophageal variceal bleeding is discussed elsewhere.

Portal Hypertensive Intestinal Vasculopathy

Over the past decade, awareness of the association between portal hypertension and changes in the gastrointestinal mucosa has increased. Portal hypertensive intestinal vasculopathy (PHIV) is the result of changes in the intestinal microcirculation, mainly the development of numerous vascular ectasias and arteriovenous communications in the absence of inflammatory infiltration. PHIV most frequently involves the stomach (portal hypertensive gastropathy [PHG]) and occasionally the small bowel and colon (portal hypertensive enteropathy and colopathy respectively). PHG accounts for over 5% of all bleeding episodes in cirrhotics. This hemorrhage from the gastric mucosa can range from insidious to massive. Endoscopically, the features may show mild (mosaic, reticular pattern) to severe changes in the gastric wall (cherry red spots or diffuse hemorrhagic pattern).

Treatment

These patients do not respond to medication used to neutralize or reduce gastric acid secretion (sucralfate [Carafate], H_2-blockers, proton-pump inhibitors, antacids). The reduction of splanchnic flow associated with beta blockers has been shown to be effective in the prevention of bleeding in patients with PHG. Propranolol (Inderal) should be given in a dose that is high enough to reduce the resting heart rate by 25%, monitoring blood pressure and the occurrence of any side effects. Portal-systemic shunting has also been used to control bleeding in PHG patients. A radiologically placed portosystemic shunt called TIPS is gaining in popularity for the management of portal hypertension–related bleeding, and this approach may offer benefit in recalcitrant PHG bleeding.

Portosystemic Encephalopathy

Cirrhotics are prone to develop this potentially reversible neuropsychiatric disorder as a consequence of both hepatic insufficiency and portal hypertension. The presence of portal-systemic shunting permits the passage of blood with protein products normally metabolized by the liver, into the systemic circulation. The final result may be a depression of the central nervous system, secondary to the toxic effect of these substances. The pathogenesis of portosystemic encephalopathy (PSE) is not clearly understood. Several theories imply that ammonia produced by the colonic flora is the main source. Other possible mechanisms include an increased ratio of aromatic amino acids to branched chain amino acids, leading to the development of false neurotransmitters, and an increased sensitivity of gamma-aminobutyric acid benzodiazepine receptors in the central nervous system. There is a wide spectrum of signs and symptoms in the clinical presentation of PSE, which varies from subtle personality changes to deep coma. The diagnosis is easily made if the physician maintains a high index of suspicion.

Treatment

In the initial approach to a patient with PSE, it is important to exclude other causes for this neurologic disorder such as drug overdose, acute alcoholism, delirium tremens, subdural hematoma, or a cerebrovascular accident. Once the diagnosis has been made, all efforts are directed toward identifying and avoiding any precipitating factors (Table 2). Sedatives, tranquilizers, and narcotics must be discontinued. Any evidence of gastrointestinal bleeding and electrolyte abnormalities should be recognized and treated appropriately. Patients that are comatose must be started on parenteral nutrition, and an establishment of an airway is essential. Protein intake must be restricted depending on the degree of encephalopathy. A restriction of 40 to 60 grams per day may be sufficient in a patient with a mild case of PSE. More severe cases need a further reduction, as much as 20 grams per day. Patients in coma should receive no protein at all. According to the patient's response, protein intake may be increased in amounts of 10 to 20 grams per day every 3 to 5 days to a maximum of 60 grams. Vegetable protein sources are preferred over animal protein sources. Dietary counseling is necessary, and at least 1500 calories should be given daily to prevent tissue catabolism, which will increase the production of ammonia. Patients who are prone to encephalopathy or who are in coma and require nutritional support would be better served with

TABLE 2. **Precipitating Factors in Portosystemic Encephalopathy**

Sedative or hypnotic drugs
Gastrointestinal bleeding
Hypokalemia/alkalosis
Hyponatremia
Dietary protein excess
Azotemia (diuretic-induced)
Infections (including spontaneous bacterial peritonitis)
Constipation
Exacerbation of underlying liver disease

either enteral or a parenteral form that is high in branched chain amino acids.

Administration of a gut-cleansing enema is a useful maneuver in patients with PSE, particularly those with GI bleeding and constipation. Enemas should be administered until the return is clean. Water and sodium status should be monitored carefully. Lactulose (Cephulac) is a disaccharide compound that has a cathartic action and is neither absorbed nor metabolized in the upper gastrointestinal tract. In addition to its laxative effects, it has been shown that lactulose prevents the absorption of ammonia from the gastrointestinal tract, thereby reducing the levels of ammonia in the blood. This effect is a consequence of the degradation of lactulose by the intestinal flora, leading to a low colonic pH. It may be given orally or via nasogastric tube in a dose of 30 mL, two to three times a day, adjusting the dosage to produce two to three semiformed stools per day. For patients not able to receive lactulose orally, it may be given as an enema (300 mL of lactulose in 700 mL of tap water as a retention enema, two to three times a day). Because of cathartic action, care must be taken to avoid volume contraction, metabolic acidosis, and hypokalemia, which may further exacerbate the PSE.

Neomycin is a poorly absorbed aminoglycoside that can be given alone or in conjunction with lower doses of lactulose. Its mechanism of action in PSE may be reducing the gut content of ammonia-producing bacteria. The dosage ranges from 2 to 4 grams orally per day in divided doses. Because 3% of neomycin is absorbed systemically, there are potential risks for nephrotoxicity and ototoxicity, and intestinal malabsorption with the development of steatorrhea. A good alternative to neomycin is metronidazole (Flagyl) in a dosage of 250 mg orally three times per day, especially in patients with renal impairment. The mechanism of action appears to be the same as that for neomycin.

Other therapies used in PSE have not consistently been proved to be beneficial. L-Dopa and bromocriptine have been used on the basis of their presumed ability to displace false neurotransmitters responsible for the PSE. These therapies are not currently recommended, and more controlled trials should be conducted to prove their efficacy. Studies using benzodiazepine receptor antagonists (flumazenil) are opening a new field in the management of PSE.

Assessment of a therapeutic response is performed mainly by a careful clinical examination, with additional aids such as the number-connection test, which is an important tool in the detection of very mild neuropsychiatric alterations. The level of blood ammonia does not correlate with the severity of PSE.

Pruritus

Pruritus is a frequent complication of chronic liver disease, particularly cholestatic liver diseases. The etiology is unknown but may be related to the accumulation in plasma of substances (pruritogens) that are normally secreted in bile. Pruritus can be mild and tolerated without interference of normal activities, or it may be severe and incapacitating. It can be localized, especially to the palms and soles, or it may be generalized and may not be relieved by scratching.

Treatment

The pruritogens responsible for pruritus have not been identified yet, and current therapeutic modalities are used empirically. The most widely used treatment for pruritus is the anion exchange resin cholestyramine. Cholestyramine binds to bile acids and other compounds (probably pruritogenic) and facilitates their fecal excretion. Most patients experience an initial response. However, in some, this response may be transient. Side effects such as bloating, constipation, and diarrhea are frequent. The maximum dose is 16 grams orally per day in divided doses. Concomitant medications must be taken at least 2 hours apart to ensure their absorption. Another anion exchange resin, colestipol, appears to be better tolerated than cholestyramine.

Other medications used in the management of pruritus are antihistamines and phenobarbital. Apparently, they do not have direct antipruritic effects but have sedative properties. Other therapeutic modalities and medications that have been studied in the management of pruritus are listed in Table 3. All of these modalities have shown results of varying degrees, and the response is usually transient. Plasmapheresis can be tried in extreme cases, and benefit has been reported. Patients not relieved by any of the available measures can be considered for liver transplantation, particularly if they have evidence of decompensated liver disease.

Recent studies have demonstrated that cholestasis is associated with increased opiotergic neurotransmission and that pruritus may be related to increased activity of endogenous opioids. The mecha-

TABLE 3. **Therapeutic Modalities for Pruritus in Liver Disease**

Anion Exchange Resins:
Cholestyramine
Colestipol
Medications with Sedative Effects:
Antihistamines
Phenobarbital
Hepatic Enzyme Inducers:
Rifampicin
Opiate Antagonists:
Naloxone
Nalmefene*
Plasmapheresis
Miscellaneous:
Phototherapy
Lignocaine
Androgens
Carbamazepine
Propofol
Charcoal hemoperfusion
Liver Transplantation

*Not available in the United States.

nism by which the opiate system is activated in cholestasis is unknown. Naloxone (Narcan), an opiate antagonist, has proved effective in controlling severe, intractable cholestatic pruritus. The route of administration is parenteral, and it is recommended for the management of intractable pruritus in emergency situations. Naloxone is given as an intravenous infusion in doses of 0.2 μg per kg per minute over 24 hours. Subcutaneous injections may be an alternative to the intravenous route. Preliminary results with an orally administered opiate antagonist, nalmefene,* are encouraging, but the long-term effect of this medication on cholestatic pruritus is uncertain and still under evaluation.

Bone Disease

Osteopenia is a well-known complication of chronic liver disease and is usually caused by either osteomalacia or osteoporosis. Osteomalacia is characterized by defective bone mineralization secondary to vitamin D or calcium deficiency, or both. Osteoporosis is characterized by bone mass loss without alterations in the mineral components. The cause of osteopenia in cirrhosis, particularly in primary biliary cirrhosis, has not been well defined. Vitamin D deficiency and inadequate calcium absorption may occur with cholestasis because of malabsorption of vitamin D. Impaired hydroxylation of vitamin D by the diseased liver may be a contributing factor. Unidentified factors normally metabolized and excreted by the liver but retained in cholestasis may be responsible for a defective osteoblast function, leading to decreased bone formation.

Patients with osteopenia may present with muscular weakness, bone fractures, and subsequent pain. Radiographic studies of the bone may show a decrease in bone density, loss of trabeculae, thinning of the bone cortex, and fractures, if present. Evaluation of bone mass may be performed by measuring bone densitometry through computed tomography (CT) scanning or photon absorptiometry, or both. Definite diagnosis can be established by bone biopsy.

Treatment

No specific treatments have been proved to be of benefit for osteopenia in chronic liver disease. General recommendations include exercise and calcium and vitamin D supplementation when deficiencies are present. Alcoholics are encouraged to abstain because alcohol might be responsible for osteoblastic dysfunction and reduced bone formation. Medications under investigation for the management of osteopenia in liver disease, particularly in primary biliary cirrhosis (PBC), include estrogens, sodium fluoride, calcitonin, biphosphonates, and ursodeoxycholic acid (UDCA). Bone density may improve in PBC patients and after liver transplantation. UDCA has very few side effects, is well tolerated, and may be effective in the long-term management of PBC. Liver transplantation may decrease bone mass and increase the incidence of bone fractures in the first 6 months, probably secondary to the high doses of corticosteroids used and to the lack of exercise. However, 1 year after transplantation the bone density may return to normal, most likely due to the effects of the new healthy liver.

*Not available in the United States.

Ascites

The presence of ascites in patients with cirrhosis is usually an indication of significant hepatic insufficiency. During the last decade, new concepts about the pathogenesis and treatment of ascites have evolved. Initially, ascites was thought to be only a consequence of portal hypertension due to altered mechanisms of the Starling's Law (high hydrostatic pressure and low albumin). New theories that might explain more clearly the pathogenesis of ascites in cirrhotics have emerged from recent studies. The so-called underfill theory states that the first event for the formation of ascites is a depletion of the effective intravascular volume secondary to the passage of fluid to the peritoneal cavity, leading to stimulation of kidney baroreceptors and activation of the renin-angiotensin-aldosterone (RAA) system. This produces retention of sodium and water that will further augment the ascites. The so-called overflow theory is probably the more accepted one at present. The first event in this setting is the stimulation of kidney baroreceptors with activation of the RAA system due to a low hepatic outflow found in cirrhotics plus a diminished peripheral vascular resistance in the presence of endogenous vasodilators. This leads to fluid retention which, in the presence of portal hypertension, leads to the formation of ascites. Another feature of cirrhotics with ascites is the presence of high levels of atrial natriuretic factor (ANF). Normally, ANF produces a high urine volume and sodium excretion, and increases the glomerular filtration rate. However, cirrhotic patients are resistant to ANF, and no response to this hormone is observed. As ascites progresses and vasodilatation with low peripheral vascular resistance persists, the effective arterial blood flow will decrease further, producing impairment of renal function with the development of hepatorenal syndrome. This is a terminal event in the cirrhotic patient with ascites, and it is discussed later.

Clinical examination is the key for the diagnosis of ascites. When there is uncertainty about the presence of ascites, ultrasonography and CT are very sensitive and specific for detecting small amounts of fluid. A diagnostic paracentesis should always be performed. Evaluation of the total protein and the albumin gradient (serum albumin–ascitic albumin) of the ascitic fluid is helpful in the initial differential diagnosis (Table 4). Usually, the cirrhotic ascitic fluid has a low protein content (< 1.5 grams per dL) with an albumin gradient (serum albumin–ascitic albumin) greater than or equal to 1.1. Approximately 10% of cirrhotics with ascites may develop a pleural effusion referred

TABLE 4. **Differential Diagnosis of Ascites**

Etiology	Total Ascitic Protein (grams per dL)		Albumin Gradient	
	≤1.5	*≥1.5*	*≥1.1*	*<1.1*
PORTAL HYPERTENSIVE			+	
Sinusoidal:	+		+	
Cirrhosis				
Post-sinusoidal:		+	+	
Cardiac ascites				
Veno-occlusive disease				
Budd-Chiari syndrome				
Inferior vena cava block				
NON-PORTAL HYPERTENSIVE				+
Peritoneal carcinomatosis		+		+
Peritoneal inflammation		+		+
Infection: Tuberculosis (TB)				
Fungal				
Viral				
Bacterial				
Serositis: Connective tissue disease		+		+
Oncotic: Nephrotic syndrome		+		+
Protein-losing enteropathy				
Kwashiorkor				
MIXED		+	+	
Cirrhosis and peritoneal TB				
Cirrhosis and liver metastases				
Cirrhosis and peritoneal carcinomatosis				

to as hepatic hydrothorax. It usually occurs in the right side, but may occur on both sides or only on the left side. Evidence favors a defect in the diaphragm as the etiology, permitting the passage of ascitic fluid from the abdomen into the pleural space. The negative intrathoracic pressure is a contributing factor. Occasionally, the transport of the ascitic fluid into the pleural space overcomes its production in the abdomen, leading to pleural effusion without ascites. Hepatic hydrothorax is usually asymptomatic but may produce respiratory compromise requiring prompt treatment, which is often difficult.

Treatment

The initial treatment for cirrhotic ascites is based on dietary sodium restriction (no more than 0.5 grams per day) and the use of diuretics that inhibit sodium reabsorption at different tubular levels. Patients with ascites without peripheral edema should be given the aldosterone antagonist spironolactone (Aldactone) at a starting dose of 50 mg twice daily, and increasing the dose according to response to a maximum of 400 mg daily. In the presence of ascites plus peripheral edema, a loop diuretic such as furosemide (Lasix) should be given concomitantly with spironolactone. The dose should be started at 40 mg daily and may be increased to a maximum of 120 mg daily. Once the peripheral edema is resolved, furosemide is discontinued. The goal of diuretic treatment is to produce reduction of fluid of no more than 500 mL (1 pound of weight) daily (assessed by measuring weight daily). If there is concomitant pedal edema, weight loss of more than 1 pound a day can be achieved without compromising renal function. Electrolyte status should be monitored frequently. Alcoholic cirrhotics should be encouraged to stop drinking. Nonsteroidal anti-inflammatory agents should be avoided while diuresis is being achieved, because they significantly impair the ability to diurese.

The majority of patients with cirrhotic ascites respond to the low-sodium and diuretic regimen. However, 20% of patients are refractory to management, and usually this group has a urinary sodium level of less than 10 mEq per liter. Therefore, other therapeutic measures must be taken. Large-volume paracentesis with plasma expander replacement has proved effective in the treatment of refractory ascites. With this approach, adverse effects, mainly hypovolemia, hyponatremia, azotemia, and hypotension, are prevented, and patients may be discharged from hospital earlier. Up to 6 liters daily or even total paracentesis may be performed in a single session, with concomitant infusion of 6 to 8 grams of albumin per liter of ascites removed. Many European countries are using Dextran 70 as a plasma expander, obtaining a response similar to that obtained with albumin but being more cost effective. Diuretics must be continued between each session of paracentesis. Use of a peritoneovenous shunt is an alternative for refractory ascites, and this method should be reserved when all other modalities of treatment have failed due to a high incidence of complications, most of them life-threatening (disseminated intravascular coagulation and sepsis). It is recommended to perform a total paracentesis prior to the shunting to prevent disseminated intravascular coagulation. Contraindications for a peritoneovenous shunt are infected ascites, recent variceal bleeding, severe coagulopathy (prothrombin time greater than 4 sec over control), hyperbilirubinemia (total bilirubin greater than 5 mg per dL), intrinsic renal disease, and cardiac failure. Shunt patency must be frequently monitored because the rate of obstruction is very high (greater than 40% in the first year).

Other alternatives have been shown to be effective in the management of refractory ascites. The transjugular intrahepatic portosystemic stent shunting has proved effective for the treatment of refractory ascites in some patients, but long-term follow-up needs to be taken before it is accepted as a definite measure. Recirculation consists of infusing ascites itself or protein concentrates from the ascitic fluid. Results are encouraging, but comparative studies with other treatment modalities must be performed.

Elimination of ascites is sufficient to control most cases of hepatic hydrothorax. Therapeutic thoracentesis, together with paracentesis, may be necessary if respiratory distress occurs. Tube thoracostomy is contraindicated in refractory cases. Obliteration of the pleural space by instillation of sclerotic agents is usually unsuccessful. Peritoneovenous shunting may control a refractory hydrothorax accompanied by ascites. Recent evidence has demonstrated that transjugular intrahepatic portosystemic stent shunting may also control intractable pleural effusion in cirrhotics. Successful hepatic transplantation is associated with total resolution of hepatic hydrothorax that is unresponsive to all the above-mentioned measures.

Spontaneous Bacterial Peritonitis

Spontaneous bacterial peritonitis (SBP) is a frequent complication found in cirrhotic patients with ascites. It occurs in 10 to 25% of hospitalized individuals, and carries a mortality rate of almost 50%. SBP is defined as a bacterial infection of the ascitic fluid without a known intra-abdominal source. The main route of colonization of ascites is hematogenous owing to the passage of bacteria from the intestinal lumen or other extraintestinal infectious focus to the bloodstream. Once bacteremia is present, the organisms cannot be cleared from the circulation because of the impaired phagocytic activity of the reticuloendothelial system found in cirrhotics, and finally the ascitic fluid is colonized. Transmural migration of organisms through the intestinal mucosa is another possible source.

Most patients with SBP present with fever and abdominal pain. However, these symptoms may be absent, and the physician must be aware of the clinical diagnosis of this entity in the presence of cirrhotic ascites, which is complicated by deterioration of the patient's clinical status with onset of encephalopathy or worsening of hepatic and renal function. Up to one-third of patients may be asymptomatic.

Early diagnosis and the prompt institution of appropriate antibiotics has decreased the mortality rate due to SBP. Paracentesis should be performed, and 10 mL of fluid must be cultured at bedside into blood culture bottles. The presence of more than 250 polymorphonuclear (PMN) leukocytes per μL of ascitic fluid, together with a positive culture (usually monobacterial), confirms the diagnosis of SBP. When the PMN count is less 250 per μL of ascitic fluid with a positive culture (bacterascites), the prognosis is much better, with two-thirds of patients experiencing spontaneous recovery and only one-third developing classic SBP. If the PMN count is greater than 250 per μL of ascitic fluid, even in the presence of a negative culture (culture-negative neutrocytic ascites), the mortality rate is as high as SBP and must be treated as such.

Treatment

Treatment should be started with an antibiotic effective against gram-negative aerobic bacteria and gram-positive cocci, until culture results are obtained. A third-generation cephalosporin (cefotaxime [Claforan]) is the antibiotic of choice. With a dose of 2 grams intravenously two to three times daily for 5 days, most cases of SBP are resolved. Once treatment is instituted, the fluid should be re-examined after 48 hours. If the PMN count decreases by 50%, together with clinical improvement of the patient, recovery can be expected. On the other hand, a worsening of symptoms, with an increasing PMN count in ascitic fluid, must raise the suspicion of a secondary cause for peritonitis. Aminoglycosides must be avoided to prevent worsening of the renal function.

Whether or not a patient with cirrhotic ascites requires prophylactic intestinal decontamination to prevent SBP remains controversial. However, consideration for this approach could be given in the following groups: (1) those with gastrointestinal bleeding, (2) those with a history of more than one episode of SBP, (3) low-protein (less than 1 gm per dL) in ascitic fluid, (4) low complement (C_3) in ascitic fluid (less than 16 mg per dL), and (5) patients with ascites awaiting liver transplantation. The antibiotic of choice in this setting is norfloxacin (Noroxin), 400 mg/day orally. Of course, treatment of ascites per se must be continued because SBP only develops in the presence of fluid in the peritoneal cavity.

Functional Renal Failure and Hepatorenal Syndrome

Functional renal failure (FRF) is defined as a renal failure in patients with hepatocellular failure. However, some patients have associated primary kidney disease or have developed acute tubular necrosis due to hemorrhage or infection. FRF is the most severe alteration of renal function that occurs in patients with cirrhosis and ascites. It is present in 15% of these patients admitted to the hospital and has a very poor prognosis.

Although it is incompletely understood, FRF involves severe renal vasoconstriction resulting in reduced glomerular filtration rate and ultimately in renal failure. There are mechanisms involved, all leading to a reduction of effective renal circulation. The most important are the presence of a hyperdynamic circulation, increased preglomerular vascular resistance, and the presence of endotoxins and possibly of other mediators. The hyperdynamic circulation found in cirrhosis produces a redistribution of blood to the skin, splanchnic area, spleen, and brain, whereas the renal plasma flow is reduced. This event leads to a low glomerular filtration rate, and plasma renin rises producing diversion of blood flow away from the renal cortex.

The finding of a preglomerular vascular resistance may be due to an imbalance between systemic vasodilators and renal vasoconstrictors. Alterations in metabolites of arachidonic acid have been described. Thromboxane A_2, a potent vasoconstrictor, is raised in FRF, whereas the vasodilator prostaglandin (PGE_2) is reduced.

Endotoxins produced by gram-negative aerobic bacilli are increased in cirrhotics. In these patients, the reticuloendothelial system fails to remove toxins absorbed from the gut, and the toxins are shunted to the systemic circulation through portal-systemic collaterals. They have potent vasoconstrictive effects that are probably responsible for the stimulation of thromboxane A_2 and leukotrienes (LTC_4 and LTD_4).

Other mediators have been implicated in the development of FRF. The most important is probably adenosine, which produces a potent systemic vasodilatation together with renal vasoconstriction. Bradykinin, with its vasodilatating effects, may also play a role. Whatever the mechanism is playing the most important role, the final result is reduced renal blood flow with the onset of oliguria and azotemia.

The presence of FRF must be suspected in all patients with cirrhosis and ascites that develop oliguria and slow onset of azotemia with a plasma creatinine level greater than 1.5 mg per dL. Renal studies show evidence of a good tubular function, with a urine-to-plasma osmolarity ratio greater than 1, a urine-to-plasma creatinine ratio greater than 30, and a urinary sodium concentration less than 10 mEq per dL.

Treatment

To date, all attempts to improve renal function in patients with FRF have been unsuccessful. Therefore, preventive measures must be taken. Diuretic overdose should be avoided, and ascites must be treated slowly. Also, the patient must be monitored for the development of electrolyte imbalance or development of infection. Care must be taken with the administration of lactulose in order to prevent excessive diarrhea. Medications such as nonsteroidal anti-inflammatory drugs and aminoglycosides should be avoided.

Once FRF develops, there is little that can be done. Expansion of the intravascular space has shown no sustained benefit. Dialysis does not improve survival and may precipitate gastrointestinal bleeding resulting in shock. The infusion of renal vasodilators, such as dopamine, although producing a moderate increase in plasma flow, does not modify the glomerular filtration rate. Misoprostol with albumin infusion may improve kidney function temporarily but does not improve survival. Linoleic acid, an essential fatty acid able to increase renal prostaglandin synthesis in healthy individuals, has not been shown to modify renal function in patients with FRF. Peritoneovenous shunting may improve renal function, but it has no effect on survival. Finally, patients with FRF should be considered candidates for liver transplantation, although the mortality rate in this setting is very high. This group of patients is usually unresponsive to all forms of therapy.

Coagulopathy

All coagulation proteins and protease inhibitors of coagulation are synthesized by the liver, with the exception of von Willebrand factor. Therefore, it is expected that patients with severe liver impairment exhibit hemostatic problems. Also, patients with cirrhosis have quantitative or qualitative defects, or both, in platelets. Thrombocytopenia is often observed and is the result of platelet sequestration in a congested spleen. Bone marrow suppression and folic acid deficiency in an alcoholic cirrhotic may contribute.

Patients with alterations in hemostasis are frequently asymptomatic but can present with evidence of spontaneous bleeding in the form of ecchymoses and petechiae, or they may experience major blood loss resulting from hemorrhage (e.g., gastrointestinal) or an invasive procedure such as liver biopsy. Evidence of coagulopathy in cirrhotics includes a prolonged prothrombin time, low platelet count, prolonged bleeding time, and in the presence of disseminated intravascular coagulation, a low plasma fibrinogen with increased fibrin degradation products.

Treatment

All patients with a prolonged prothrombin time should receive vitamin K (AquaMEPHYTON), in a dose of 10 mg daily subcutaneously for three consecutive days. If prolongation of the prothrombin time is the result of reduced concentrations of vitamin K–dependent factors (II, V, VII, IX, and X), secondary to vitamin K deficiency as in intestinal bile salt deficiency, malnutrition, or antibiotic therapy, the prothrombin time should be corrected.

In the presence of severe liver insufficiency, the prolonged prothrombin time cannot be corrected with vitamin K. Fresh frozen plasma can be administered, if necessary, especially in the presence of active gastrointestinal bleeding or prior to an invasive procedure such as a liver biopsy. It is indicated if the prothrombin time is prolonged more than 4 seconds. Platelet transfusions are rarely necessary. They are indicated in severe bleeding with a platelet count of less than 50,000 per mm^3. Splenectomy for hypersplenism is usually not indicated. Desmopressin, a vasopressin analogue, can be used when control of bleeding is necessary in patients with cirrhosis. It causes transient shortening of bleeding time and PTT, and increases factor VIII and von Willebrand factor. The dose is 0.3 μg per kg diluted in 50 mL of saline, and it is infused intravenously over 30 minutes. Plasmapheresis has been effective prior to invasive procedures. Disseminated intravascular coagulation is usually mild and rarely requires the transfusion of fresh blood, or fresh frozen plasma and packed red blood cells. The underlying precipitating cause should be corrected. Heparin therapy is usually not necessary.

Hepatocellular Carcinoma

Cirrhosis is the most frequent underlying liver disorder associated with hepatocellular carcinoma (HCC), being present in more than 80 to 90% of patients. The sequence of liver necrosis, followed by repair and nodular regeneration in cirrhosis, may induce mutations and expansion of abnormal cells into frank neoplasms.

Nonalcoholic post-hepatic cirrhosis of the macronodular type is more frequently associated with HCC than alcoholic cirrhosis of the micronodular variety. Hepatitis B virus infection has been strongly associated with the development of HCC, but recently this trend has shifted toward hepatitis C virus–associated cirrhosis. There is no evidence that hepatocarcinogens such as aflatoxins induce cirrhosis before HCC develops. Metabolic disorders (e.g., hemochromatosis) usually develop HCC when cirrhosis is present.

Every cirrhotic should be routinely screened for HCC in the hope of detecting lesions amenable for surgical excision before they are already far advanced. Of the carcinofetal proteins, alpha-fetoprotein has proved to be the most useful. Any level above 400 nanograms per mL, or a rising level even below 400 nanograms per mL is highly suspicious for HCC. Diagnostic imaging studies can detect lesions as small as 1 cm. Ultrasonography is the most widely available, the most cost effective, and has the advantage of being radiation free. When ultrasound is nondiagnostic, CT without and with contrast, and CT with Lipiodol angiography may be helpful in defining the malignant nature of a lesion. It is recommended that every cirrhotic patient should be followed-up at least with measurement of the alpha-fetoprotein level every 6 months and performance of an ultrasound once a year. Once a suspicious lesion is detected, the diagnosis can be confirmed by liver biopsy, performed under direct visualization by laparoscopy or guided by ultrasound or CT.

Treatment

Despite recent advances in treatment for HCC, the outlook is usually hopeless. The 3-year survival rate, even in patients with small tumors (less than 3 cm), is less than 15%. Resection of the tumor remains the best therapeutic option for cure in HCC. However, surgical excision is frequently limited by the size and multinodular character of the tumor, by extrahepatic spread at the time of diagnosis, and by the presence of severe hepatocellular insufficiency. Therefore, surgical resection is attempted only if a solitary tumor is found in a liver with good hepatic synthetic function. Liver transplantation is pursued in selected patients. Other therapeutic alternatives such as chemoembolization, alcohol injection, immunotherapy, and hormone manipulation have shown results of varying degree and have not improved survival.

Liver Transplantation

All cirrhotics should be considered for liver transplantation, although the timing of the procedure may be difficult. Transplant centers would like to evaluate patients earlier than later, because that would give them an idea of what the case entails and they can design an appropriate follow-up plan. The more severe the hepatic insufficiency, the poorer the outcome after liver transplantation. On the other hand, in cirrhotic patients capable of having a relatively normal life for a prolonged period, transplantation is not necessary on an urgent basis. Alcoholic cirrhotics have also been transplanted successfully as have patients with other etiologies for cirrhosis. The decision of whether or not to perform liver transplant surgery on an alcoholic patient is a matter of debate, but it is generally agreed that at least 6 months of alcohol abstention on the part of the patient is required in order to consider it. Furthermore, strong family support, factors such as previous attempts at rehabilitation, and the presence or absence of alcohol-related cardiomyopathy, pancreatitis, peripheral neuropathy, and cerebral atrophy are features that are evaluated thoroughly and incorporated in the decision process. Transplantation for chronic B hepatitis is associated with high incidence of graft re-infection and graft failure. Of special concern are patients with chronic hepatitis B in whom re-infection of the transplanted liver is followed by a severe cholestatic fibrosing hepatitis with a poor outcome and a high mortality rate. Long-term immunization with hepatitis B immune globulin may reduce the recurrence of infection. Hepatitis C–related chronic liver disease is a leading indication for liver transplantation. However, recurrence of infection is invariable, although the long-term consequences in the post-transplant period are unclear. Patients transplanted for end-stage Wilson's disease generally do well, as do patients with primary biliary cirrhosis and primary sclerosing cholangitis.

BLEEDING ESOPHAGEAL VARICES

method of
KENRIC M. MURAYAMA, M.D., and
LAYTON F. RIKKERS, M.D.
University of Nebraska Medical Center
Omaha, Nebraska

Variceal hemorrhage is the most serious complication of portal hypertension. Only one-third to one-half of patients with portal hypertension and varices ever bleed from the varices. However, the risk of a second bleeding episode is greater than 70%, usually occurring within 6 weeks of the first episode. Mortality associated with the first episode of variceal hemorrhage ranges from 15% to greater than 50%, depending on the status of the underlying liver disease.

Portal hypertension can be caused by a variety of problems. In the United States, the most common cause of portal hypertension is alcoholic cirrhosis, while the most common cause worldwide is schistosomiasis.

The majority of patients with esophageal varices have cirrhosis and virtually all have portal hypertension (varices develop when the portal pressure is 12 mmHg or greater). Elevated portal pressure induces portosystemic collateralization wherever splanchnic and systemic venous systems are in close apposition. Esophageal varices, gastric varices, and portal hypertensive gastropathy account for 80 to 90% of upper gastrointestinal bleeding episodes in patients with portal hypertension. Because treatment varies depending on the source of bleeding, early endoscopy is essential in the management of these patients. In addition, treatment in the form of sclerotherapy or banding of varices can be initiated at the time of initial endoscopy. The degree of portal pressure elevation and esophagitis does not correlate with the risk of variceal rupture. While varix appearance (red wale markings, cherry-red spots, diffuse redness) and size may correlate with the likelihood of bleeding, there is no reliable predictive factor.

Visceral angiography and duplex ultrasound examination are the best methods for evaluation of the portal venous system and for qualitative assessment of hepatic portal perfusion. If shunt surgery is considered, visceral angiography is necessary to define the vascular anatomy.

TREATMENT

Management of variceal hemorrhage due to portal hypertension can be divided into three phases: (1) treatment of acute hemorrhage, (2) prevention of recurrent hemorrhage, and (3) prophylaxis against an initial hemorrhage.

Management of Acute Hemorrhage

An organized approach to the patient with acute upper gastrointestinal bleeding and portal hypertension is essential. The management scheme for acute portal hypertensive bleeding used at the University of Nebraska is outlined in Figure 1.

Acute variceal hemorrhage is associated with a high mortality. Due to the presence of chronic liver disease and other complications of portal hypertension, these patients are generally considered at high risk for surgical intervention. Therefore, in most centers nonoperative treatment is undertaken first, often at the time of initial endoscopy. Endoscopic sclerotherapy results in nonoperative control of hemorrhage in more than 80% of patients. Recently, rubber-band ligation has been found in some studies to be more effective and associated with fewer complications than sclerotherapy.

Early endoscopy is essential since a significant number of patients with portal hypertension and esophageal varices bleed from another source (e.g., gastric varices, portal hypertensive gastropathy, or peptic ulcer). Prior to endoscopy, restoration of circulating blood volume should be accomplished. Endoscopic sclerotherapy has decreased the role of pharmacotherapy, balloon tamponade, and emergency surgery in the management of esophageal variceal hemorrhage. However, when bleeding results from gastric varices or portal hypertensive gastropathy, sclerotherapy is not effective and pharmacotherapy and emergency surgery play more predominant roles.

Currently, the mainstay of pharmacotherapy is simultaneous administration of vasopressin* (Pitressin), bolus 20 units over 20 minutes followed by continuous infusion of 0.4 unit per minute; can be increased to a maximal dose of 0.6 unit per minute), and nitroglycerin* (start at 40 μg per minute; can be increased 40 μg per minute every 15 minutes to a maximum of 400 μg per minute). Although nitroglycerin was initially thought to simply protect against the adverse effects of vasopressin, it appears to lower portal pressure independently of vasopressin. The combination of vasopressin and nitroglycerin controls bleeding in approximately 50% of cases of portal hypertensive bleeding.

Balloon tamponade, usually with a Sengstaken-Blakemore tube, results in immediate control of variceal hemorrhage in 80 to 90% of patients. However, it is uncomfortable for the awake patient and can

*Not FDA approved for this indication.

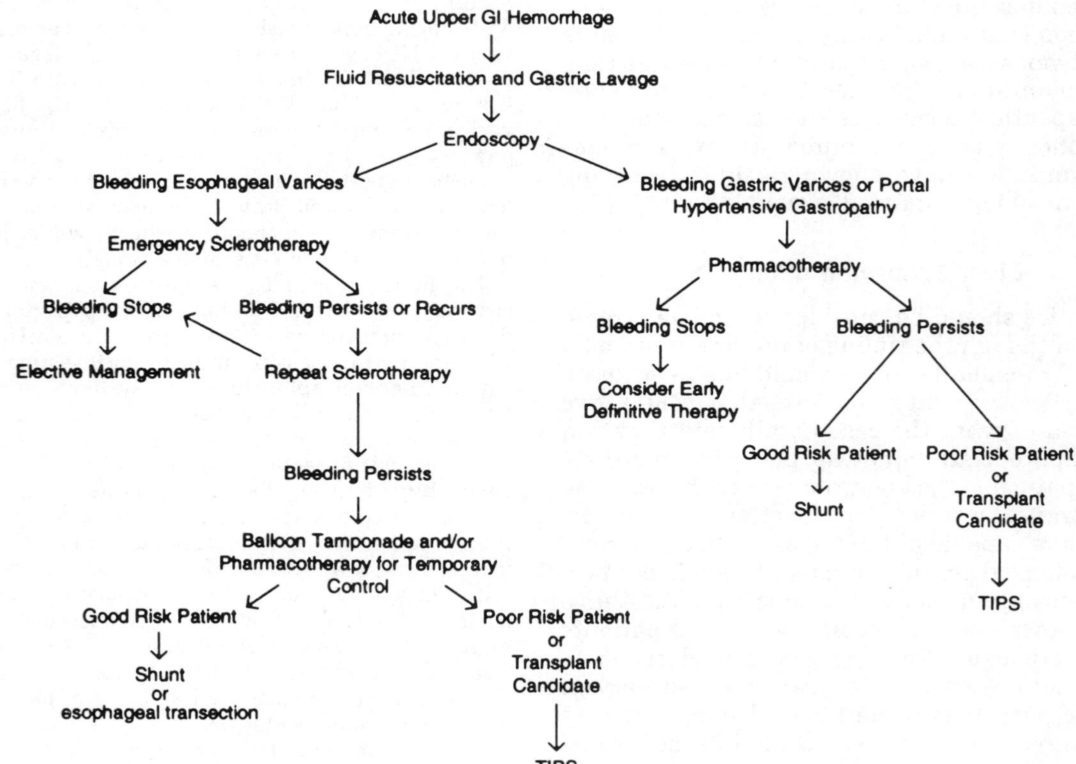

Figure 1. Algorithm for management of acute portal hypertensive bleeding that is used at the University of Nebraska Medical Center.

result in major complications when used by inexperienced personnel. In addition, bleeding recurs in 20 to 60% of patients soon after the balloons are deflated. Balloon tamponade is still indicated in a few circumstances: massive variceal hemorrhage uncontrolled by sclerotherapy, acute hemorrhage in patients who have failed sclerotherapy, and during transport of patients with active hemorrhage to a center where sclerotherapy and surgery are available.

Recently, a fluoroscopically placed transjugular intrahepatic portosystemic shunt (TIPS) has become available in many institutions. Initial reports indicate that this approach is safe and effective in the management of portal hypertensive bleeding. In addition, TIPS provides an effective method of managing refractory acute variceal hemorrhage in patients awaiting liver transplantation and in patients who either refuse surgery or are prohibitive surgical risks. The major disadvantage of TIPS is development of shunt occlusion or stenosis in a high proportion of patients within 1 year.

Emergency operations should be reserved for the 10 to 15% of patients in whom nonoperative therapy fails to stop hemorrhage. Failure of nonoperative methods must be clearly defined so that when necessary, an emergency operation can be promptly performed. A reasonable definition of sclerotherapy failure is lack of bleeding control after two attempts. When faced with this situation, either TIPS or an emergency operation should be considered. The most commonly performed operations in the emergency setting are the portacaval shunt, the interposition mesocaval shunt, and esophageal transection with a stapling device. A selective shunt such as the distal splenorenal shunt, which has the advantage of a lower likelihood of postoperative encephalopathy, can be considered if the patient has medically controllable ascites and there is temporary control of bleeding. Although not as effective as portal decompression, esophageal transection can be performed more rapidly and is more familiar to a greater number of surgeons.

Prevention of Recurrent Hemorrhage

The likelihood of recurrent bleeding after the initial variceal hemorrhage is controlled is greater than 70% if no additional therapy is instituted. The advantages and disadvantages of current options for prevention of recurrent hemorrhage are listed in Table 1.

Available Therapies

Pharmacotherapy. Administration of nonselective beta blockers (e.g., propranolol) has been advocated for the prevention of recurrent portal hypertensive hemorrhage; however, success requires patient compliance and rebleeding is frequent (greater than 50%). Information is accumulating regarding other pharmacologic agents (e.g., serotonin antagonists, calcium channel blockers). Pharmacotherapy has the advantage of being noninvasive and readily accessible, but the strict compliance required would be formidable for alcoholic patients.

Chronic Endoscopic Sclerotherapy. Chronic sclerotherapy (or banding) is the most commonly used definitive treatment to prevent recurrent variceal hemorrhage. Although controlled clinical trials have demonstrated that sclerotherapy results in significantly fewer bleeding episodes than medical management, 40 to 60% of sclerotherapy patients experience rebleeding. Rebleeding is most frequent during the first year, with rates decreasing to 15% per year thereafter. Surgical shunts more reliably control bleeding (rebleeding in fewer than 10%); however, sclerotherapy is less invasive than surgery and better preserves hepatic portal perfusion. Patients who fail chronic sclerotherapy are candidates for shunt surgery or liver transplantation.

Portosystemic Shunts. Decompression of the por-

TABLE 1. **Prevention of Recurrent Variceal Hemorrhage**

Therapy	Advantages	Disadvantages
Propranolol*	Noninvasive; widely available; few side effects	Frequent rebleeding (50%); compliance required
Sclerotherapy	Nonoperative; widely available; maintains portal perfusion (95%)	Frequent rebleeding (50%); compliance required; not for gastric varices
Nonselective shunts	Reliable bleeding control (95%); good ascites control	Loss of portal perfusion; encephalopathy (20–50%)
Selective shunts	Reliable bleeding control (90%); maintain portal perfuson (50%)	May aggravate ascites; technically difficult
Nonshunting procedures	Maintain portal perfusion (95%); relieve hypersplenism; technically easy	Frequent rebleeding (20–40%); prevent future selective shunt
TIPS	Nonoperative; good option for sclerotherapy failures who are unacceptable operative risks; good bridge to transplantation	High shunt stenosis and occlusion rate; can predispose to encephalopathy
Hepatic transplantation	Reliable bleeding control (95%); restores hepatic function	Limited donor supply; not applicable to many patients; expensive; requires compliance

*Not FDA approved for this indication.

tal circulation is the most effective means of preventing recurrent hemorrhage. Nonselective shunts, such as the portacaval and mesocaval shunt, divert all portal blood away from the liver. Although rebleeding is reliably prevented, elimination of hepatic portal perfusion may have adverse consequences including hepatic failure and encephalopathy.

The distal splenorenal shunt, the most commonly performed selective shunt operation, provides selective decompression of esophagogastric varices and preserves hepatic portal perfusion in some patients. The major advantage of the distal splenorenal shunt over nonselective shunts is a lower incidence of postshunt encephalopathy. Some studies have demonstrated a survival advantage to selective variceal decompression in patients with nonalcoholic cirrhosis. Recurrent bleeding occurs in fewer than 10% of patients after both nonselective and selective shunts. Another advantage of the distal splenorenal shunt is that dissection of the porta hepatis is avoided, making subsequent liver transplantation less formidable than after a portocaval shunt.

Nonshunt Procedures. The most commonly performed nonshunt operation for prevention of recurrent variceal bleeding is esophageal transection and re-anastomosis. The advantage of this procedure is that it maintains portal perfusion, is technically easy, and is familiar to most surgeons. However, esophageal transection is associated with frequent rebleeding (20 to 40%). A nonshunt operation may be the only option for sclerotherapy failures with diffuse splanchnic venous thrombosis as the cause of their portal hypertension.

TIPS. The role of TIPS in the long-term treatment of portal hypertension has yet to be defined. Whether TIPS is preferable to either endoscopic sclerotherapy or operative shunts for prevention of recurrent bleeding needs to be determined in controlled randomized trials. What has been shown is that TIPS effectively decreases portal pressure and that it is an effective bridge to transplantation in patients with portal hypertension and variceal bleeding. TIPS is also preferable for patients with advanced hepatic functional decompensation, because the operative mortality rate in this group is as high as 50%. Because a functioning TIPS is a nonselective shunt, it may predispose to encephalopathy.

Liver Transplantation. Liver transplantation is not a therapy for variceal hemorrhage per se, but rather the ultimate treatment for selected patients with end-stage chronic liver disease. It not only returns portal pressure to normal but also restores hepatic functional reserve. In most centers, liver transplantation is reserved for nonalcoholic cirrhotics and abstinent patients with alcoholic cirrhosis. Unfortunately, the majority of variceal bleeders in this country are active alcoholics; sclerotherapy and shunt operations remain the best management alternatives for them.

Selection of Therapy

After the episode of acute variceal bleeding has been controlled, the appropriate therapy should be chosen for each individual patient. The first step is to determine whether the patient is a transplant candidate (nonalcoholic cirrhotics and abstinent alcoholic cirrhotics). Transplantation should be accomplished as soon as possible in patients with advanced hepatic functional decompensation and in those with a poor quality of life secondary to their liver disease (e.g., fatigue, encephalopathy, ascites). Individuals with good hepatic functional reserve and with bleeding as the only symptom of their liver disease should undergo either initial sclerotherapy or a shunt operation. Chronic sclerotherapy is a good choice for patients who live in close proximity to their sclerotherapist and surgeon. Individuals living in remote areas and those who will not be compliant with a sclerotherapy schedule are probably better served by an initial shunt operation. Likewise, patients who bleed from gastric varices and portal hypertensive gastropathy are not good sclerotherapy candidates and should undergo a shunt procedure. Patients undergoing chronic sclerotherapy should be closely followed and receive either a shunt or transplantation if sclerotherapy should fail, as it does in approximately 20 to 33% of the patients.

Shunt candidates with appropriate anatomy (splenic vein >7 mm in diameter) and absent or minimal ascites should receive a distal splenorenal shunt because the frequency of postshunt encephalopathy is less than after a nonselective shunt. Individuals with medically intractable ascites in addition to variceal bleeding should undergo a nonselective shunt, because these operations are effective in relieving ascites as well as preventing recurrent bleeding.

TIPS is an excellent short-term bridge to transplantation. Another good candidate for TIPS is the patient with severe liver disease who would be unlikely to survive a shunt operation and who is not a transplant candidate.

Nonshunt operations are seldomly done in the elective setting in the Western world. However, esophagogastric devascularization combined with splenectomy may be the only option for patients with diffuse splanchnic venous thrombosis, which makes both nonoperative (TIPS) and operative shunts impossible.

Finally, pharmacotherapy thus far has not played a major role in the definitive treatment of portal hypertensive bleeding. Strict compliance is necessary and most trials have shown only a marginal decrease in the likelihood of recurrent bleeding with nonselective beta blockade. Clinical research with drugs other than beta blockers as well as with combinations of agents is actively being pursued.

Prophylactic Treatment

The aim of prophylactic therapy is to prolong survival by preventing the first bleeding episode. The natural history of varices that have never bled is unpredictable, and it has been shown that only one-third to one-half of patients with varices will ever bleed. Therefore, because of the potential adverse effects of surgical procedures and endoscopic sclerotherapy, prophylactic treatment of varices that have never bled cannot currently be recommended. The prophylactic use of beta blockers to prevent first bleeding episodes has been effective in some trials and can be recommended for selected patients.

DYSPHAGIA AND ESOPHAGEAL OBSTRUCTION

method of
REZA SHAKER, M.D.
Medical College of Wisconsin and Froedtert Memorial Lutheran Hospital
Milwaukee, Wisconsin

Swallowing is a highly coordinated physiologic event that involves sequential and overlapping contractions of the facial, cervical, oral, pharyngeal, laryngeal, and esophageal muscular apparatus and results in transit of ingested material and saliva from the mouth into the stomach. For descriptive purposes, swallowing can be divided into four consecutive phases: (1) preparatory, (2) oral, (3) pharyngeal, and (4) esophageal. Dysphagia, or difficulty in swallowing, may involve one or more of these phases.

ORAL/PHARYNGEAL DYSPHAGIA

From a functional point of view, events that take place during the oral/pharyngeal phase of swallowing contribute to the following: (1) transit of the bolus into the esophagus, and (2) protection of the airway. The transit and protective aspects of oral/pharyngeal swallowing are highly coordinated. Recent studies have shown that oral/pharyngeal transit occurs during the full activation of the protective aspect of swallowing. A successful oropharyngeal swallow requires the effective and coordinated actions of the anatomic elements involved in these two functions. Oral/pharyngeal dysphagia can develop when the efficacy and/or coordination of either the transport or the protective aspect of oral/pharyngeal swallowing is compromised. The true prevalence of oral/pharyngeal dysphagia is not known, but studies have shown a prevalence of 59 to 66% in nursing homes and 10 to 30% in general medical wards.

Symptoms

Except for patients with silent aspirations who present with frequent pneumonia, most oral/pharyngeal dysphagia patients seek help because of symptoms. These symptoms reflect the abnormalities in the transport or protective function during oral/pharyngeal swallowing (Table 1). Dysphagia symptoms are highly specific and should not be labeled as functional or psychogenic. Subtle abnormalities may escape detection, but every effort needs to be made to arrive at a diagnosis.

TABLE 1. **Symptoms of Oral/Pharyngeal Dysphagia**

Inability to keep the bolus in the oral cavity
Difficulty gathering the bolus on the back of the tongue
Hesitation or inability to initiate the swallow
Food sticking in the throat
Nasal regurgitation
Inability to propel the food bolus caudad into the pharynx
Difficulty swallowing solids
Frequent repetitive swallowing
Frequent throat clearing
"Gargley" voice after meal
Hoarse voice
Nasal speech and dysarthria
Swallow-related cough: before, during, or after swallowing
Avoidance of social dining
Weight loss
Recurrent pneumonia

A frequently reported symptom is a sensation of inadequate clearance of the bolus from the pharynx, described as "food sticks in the throat." This sensation may be caused by the presence of large residue in the pyriform sinus or valleculae; it may also be a referred sensation from obstruction of the distal esophagus. Patients with strictures of the proximal esophagus may also present with cervical symptoms. For this reason, in patients with complaints of cervical symptoms, evaluation of the esophagus must be a part of the dysphagia work-up. Because inflammation, abrasion, or tumors of the hypopharyngeal area and the larynx can produce the same sensation, a careful examination by direct visualization of this area is also necessary.

Etiology

Because of the number of organs involved in oral/pharyngeal swallowing, dysphagia can result from many defects of the muscular apparatus of the oropharynx and its related neuromuscular plate, the peripheral nervous system, and the central nervous system. These diseases may affect the oral/pharyngeal transport, deglutitive airway closure, or both (Table 2). Neuromuscular diseases are responsible for approximately 80% of the cases, with local structural lesions of the oropharynx accounting for the rest. Oral/pharyngeal dysphagia has been reported in approximately 25% of adults following head injury, of whom 94% have been reported to recover in about 3 months.

Cricopharyngeal muscle dysfunction is becoming an increasingly recognized cause of dysphagia. Primary neurogenic cricopharyngeal muscle dysfunction includes cricopharyngeal achalasia and discoordination of upper esophageal sphincter relaxation and opening with pharyngeal peristalsis due to a variety of neurogenic causes, such as cerebrovascular hemorrhage and Parkinson's disease. Primary myogenic cricopharyngeal dysfunction includes loss of elasticity and fibrotic changes that prevent adequate opening during swallowing. A variety of causes, including gastroesophageal reflux and aging, have been suggested.

In secondary cricopharyngeal dysfunction, the pa-

TABLE 2. **Causes of Oral/Pharyngeal Dysphagia**

Peripheral and Central Nervous System	*Local Structural Lesions*
Cerebrovascular accident	Surgical resection of oropharynx/larynx
Head injury	Oropharyngeal carcinoma
Parkinson's disease	Laryngeal carcinoma
Huntington's chorea	Zenker's diverticulum
Multiple sclerosis	Extrinsic compression
Amyotrophic lateral sclerosis	Enlarged thyroid gland
Central nervous system tumor	Senile ankylosing hyperostosis of cervical spine
Tabes dorsalis	Rheumatoid cricoarytenoid arthritis
Central nervous system disorders (e.g., Alzheimer's disease)	Radiation injury
Bulbar poliomyelitis	Neuromuscular damage
Peripheral neuropathies	Salivary gland damage
Post-traumatic abnormalities	Cricopharyngeal abnormalities
Friedreich's spastic ataxia	Achalasia
Familial dysautonomia	Fibrosis
Muscular / Neuromuscular	Esophageal webs
Inflammatory muscle diseases	*Pharmacologic Agents*
Polymyositis	Antihistamines
Dermatomyositis	Anticholinergics
Inclusion body myositis	Phenothiazines
Muscular dystrophies (myotonic oculopharyngeal)	
Kearns-Sayre syndrome	
Metabolic myopathy (thyroid-associated myopathy)	
Alcoholic myopathy	
Myasthenia gravis	

thology lies within the suprahyoid muscles. This includes inflammatory changes such as those seen in inclusion body myositis. In these patients, the suprahyoid muscles are incapable of exerting traction force during swallowing that is adequate to pull the upper esophageal sphincter open. These patients typically lack normal laryngeal elevation. Excitatory impulses to the cricopharyngeal muscle are inhibited normally during swallowing, resulting in manometric relaxation of the upper esophageal sphincter. However, the upper esophageal sphincter does not open adequately due to insufficient traction. Depending on the severity of the condition, patients who have upper esophageal sphincter dysfunction may present with aspiration pneumonia, swallow-related coughing, choking, repeated swallowing, food sticking in the throat, and weight loss.

Increasing evidence indicates that inadequate opening of the upper esophageal sphincter or its incoordination with pharyngeal peristalsis plays a pathogenic role in the development of Zenker's diverticulum. Depending on its size, Zenker's diverticulum causes symptoms that range from sensation of a foreign body in the throat and/or difficulty swallowing to regurgitation and aspiration.

Video fluoroscopic recording of a modified barium swallow is the diagnostic modality of choice for patients with oral/pharyngeal dysphagia. Because of the radiation exposure and the difficulty in moving some patients to the radiology suite, a video endoscopic approach has recently been developed.

Only a minority of the patients with oral/pharyngeal dysphagia are amenable to medical/surgical therapy. Cricopharyngeal dilatation and myotomy has been performed for a variety of neurogenic and myogenic causes of oral/pharyngeal dysphagia with variable results. Cricopharyngeal myotomy with diverticulectomy or diverticulum suspension is the treatment of choice for symptomatic Zenker's diverticulum.

However, the majority of patients who have oral/pharyngeal dysphagia require specialized rehabilitation of their swallowing function. Maintaining adequate nutrition during this period is essential, otherwise the vicious cycle of malnutrition and oral/pharyngeal dysphagia complications will continue.

Several therapeutic maneuvers are used to improve oral/pharyngeal bolus transport and airway safety. A change in bolus size and/or consistency is helpful in some patients, whereas in others swallowing with the head in a specific position may help provide safe passage of the bolus through the hypopharynx. Flexion of the head reduces the chance of aspiration by displacing the larynx under the epiglottis, whereas rotating the head toward the weaker side will improve pharyngeal transit and prevent aspiration.

Patients with predeglutitive and deglutitive aspiration may benefit from specific therapeutic maneuvers, such as supraglottic swallow. In this maneuver, patients take a deep breath and hold it, then swallow. Swallowing is followed by a voluntary cough before resumption of respiration that clears the larynx of aspirated material.

In patients with impaired pharyngeal transit and post-deglutitive aspiration, Mendelsohn's maneuver may improve pharyngeal emptying and prevent aspiration. Patients are taught to generate a sustained laryngeal and hyoid bone elevation during swallowing in order to increase upper esophageal sphincter traction and prolong its opening. This results in improved pharyngeal emptying. Observing the fluoroscopy monitor during this maneuver greatly enhances the patient's learning and compliance.

When abnormal closure of the vocal cords causes deglutitive aspiration, injection of the defective cord with Teflon or gel foam is done. Medialization of the cord is also used to prevent aspiration. In severe unrelenting cases, laryngeal closure and tracheostomy or laryngectomy may be necessary to prevent devastating pulmonary complications of aspiration.

ESOPHAGEAL DYSPHAGIA

Transport of ingested material from the proximal esophagus to the stomach may be impaired by two mechanisms: (1) motor abnormalities of the esophagus and its lower sphincter, and (2) structural abnormalities of the esophagus. Disorders of the former type commonly produce difficulty in swallowing liquids as well as solids, progress slowly, and can occur intermittently (Table 3). On the other hand, structural lesions of the esophagus, unless they induce near complete or complete obliteration of the lumen, usually cause solid food dysphagia only. Rapid progression of dysphagia is suggestive of malignancy, whereas slow progression is more common in a benign condition such as peptic strictures. A thorough history and physical examination are extremely helpful, but diagnostic tests are required to establish the specific diagnosis. A history of chronic heartburn with dysphagia suggests peptic stricture. However, the possibility of Barrett's esophagitis with malignant transformation resulting in dysphagia needs to be ruled out. In addition, queries need to be made about odynophagia (painful swallowing), which suggests infectious esophagitis. Ingestion of quinidine, tetracycline, doxycycline, or potassium chloride pills can induce mucosal lesions and odynophagia. Evidence of significant weight loss favors malignancy. Raynaud's phenomenon or sclerodactyly may indicate esophageal involvement in systemic sclerosis.

Evaluation of the dysphagic patient needs to be systematic. The history and physical examination dictate the diagnostic test, which is tailored to the patient's needs. Single- and double-contrast x-ray studies of the esophagus are done to look for structural lesions, such as webs, rings, strictures, masses, external compression, and diverticuli.

TABLE 3. **Causes of Esophageal Dysphagia**

Structural Abnormalities (Mostly Solid Food Dysphagia)	Motor Abnormalities (Solid and Liquid Food Dysphagia)
Strictures	Achalasia
Reflux-related (most common)	Diffuse esophageal spasm
Radiation-induced	Nonspecific motility disorders
Pill-induced	Scleroderma esophagus
Caustics-induced	
Malignancy	
Rings and webs	
Peptic rings	
Schatzki's ring	
Plummer-Vinson syndrome	
Esophageal carcinoma	
Extrinsic compression	

Upper gastrointestinal endoscopy directly visualizes the mucosa for evaluation of reflux-induced or infectious injuries and is used to obtain tissue samples from masses or suspicious strictures for pathological testing. It is also used for transendoscopic balloon dilation of strictures under direct vision and concurrently with fluoroscopy for placing guidewires across the stricture for subsequent wire-guided bougienage.

If radiography and endoscopy are nonrevealing, esophageal motor disorders should be suspected and manometry performed. More sophisticated tests, such as computerized tomography, are done to evaluate an extrinsic cause of esophageal dysphagia, such as malignant lymph nodes, thymoma, or thyroid gland or vascular compression.

ACHALASIA

Achalasia, the best characterized esophageal motility disorder, presents with liquid as well as solid food dysphagia. It may be accompanied by a retrosternal burning sensation or pain. Dysphagia in achalasia patients is chronic and worsens gradually. The pathophysiology of achalasia includes loss of ganglionic cells in the myenteric plexus. Manometrically typical achalasia is characterized by a lack of esophageal peristalsis and lower esophageal sphincter relaxation. During swallowing, resting lower esophageal sphincter pressure is commonly abnormally high, but it can be within the normal range. These changes induce a functional obstruction that on barium esophagraphy appears as an esophageal dilation that tapers into a bird beak at the gastroesophageal junction. Carcinoma of the gastric cardia may present with similar manometric features and should be ruled out by upper GI endoscopy.

Therapy in achalasia is directed toward elimination of esophageal outflow obstruction by reduction or abolition of lower esophageal sphincter pressure. In some cases, this can be achieved medically by agents that reduce the lower esophageal sphincter pressure; these include calcium channel blockers such as nifedipine* (Procardia), 10 mg by mouth 30 minutes before each meal. Depending on the presence or absence of side effects, such as headache and flushing, the dose may be increased to 20 mg before each meal.

Alternatively, isosorbide dinitrate* (Isordil), 5 to 10 mg sublingually 10 to 20 minutes before each meal, can be used. However, headache may be a limiting factor to its use. Unfortunately, although close to 70% of patients initially respond to these measures, their effect is short lived and generally partial. However, pharmacologic therapy can be used as a temporary measure in patients who are unable to undergo more definitive treatments.

The next step in treatment of dysphagia is balloon dilatation of the lower esophageal sphincter with the goal of disrupting its circular muscle. This is achieved in over 75% of cases by distending a balloon dilator

*Not FDC approved for this indication.

positioned within the gastroesophageal junction. A diameter of 3.0, 3.5, or 4.0 cm may be used with increasing efficiency as well as complications. Perforation requiring surgery occurs in about 2 to 5% of cases and commonly is heralded by pain and fever.

The day before balloon dilatation, the esophagus is lavaged and cleared of residual food and secretions. Patients are placed on antifungal agents such as nystatin (Mycostatin) (swish and swallow), as well as prophylactic intravenous antibiotics. The procedure is done in the fluoroscopy suite. A complete endoscopic examination of the esophagus and gastroesophageal junction is done first to rule out malignancy. A guidewire is then placed into the stomach through the biopsy channel and the endoscope is removed. Subsequently, the balloon dilator is inserted over the guidewire and placed within the lower esophageal sphincter under fluoroscopic control. Dilatation is done while the balloon is observed continuously by fluoroscopy. The balloon is kept distended for 1 minute. Initially, the lower esophageal sphincter area is seen as a "waist" on the dilating balloon. This will disappear gradually. If the "waist" does not disappear, the procedure is repeated after several minutes. Pneumatic dilatation produces a successful outcome in approximately 75% of cases. However, up to a third of these patients may require a second dilatation.

If balloon dilatation is unsuccessful or unacceptable to the patient, Heller myotomy can be offered, a procedure that is effective in over 90% of patients. An antireflux procedure is also done during the same operation to prevent gastroesophageal reflux.

ESOPHAGEAL SPASM

Esophageal spasm includes several constellations of abnormalities, ranging from derangement of esophageal peristalsis, in the form of simultaneous intermittent contractions, to diffuse esophageal spasm, to abnormally high amplitudes of peristaltic waves or hypertensive lower esophageal sphincter with normal relaxation response to swallowing. Diffuse esophageal spasm may present with significant dysphagia, because simultaneous intermittent contractions result in ineffective propulsion. Other common symptoms include chest pain and odynophagia. The pathophysiology of this group of esophageal motor disorders is not well understood; however, an abnormality in visceral pain sensitivity and response to esophageal distention has been suggested. Since gastroesophageal reflux can play an etiologic role, 24-hour pH monitoring can be done to establish the correlation of symptoms with the reflux episodes. Alternatively, a Bernstein test may reproduce the patient's symptoms. Therapy should include reassurance of the patient about the benign nature of the disorder. A variety of medications have been used with varying degrees of success in treatment of diffuse esophageal spasm, including hyoscyamine sulfate (Levsin), belladonna alkaloids, dicyclomine hydrochloride (Bentyl), calcium channel blockers, and nitrates. Antidepressants, antianxiety agents such as trazodone (Desyrel), and amitriptyline (Elavil), have been used with varying results. Long esophageal myotomy has been reported to be successful in alleviating refractory symptoms in a selected group of patients.

THE ESOPHAGUS IN COLLAGEN VASCULAR DISEASES

The esophagus is involved to varying degrees in a variety of collagen vascular diseases. In progressive systemic sclerosis, a mixed connective tissue disease, fibrotic and degenerative changes result in absent or diminished peristalsis in the distal two-thirds of the esophagus and an incompetent patulous lower esophageal sphincter. These abnormalities commonly lead to gastroesophageal reflux disease with symptoms of heartburn and regurgitation. The reflux insult can cause stricture and mechanical dysphagia. Distinctive radiographic and manometric features can be documented in two-thirds of cases. Before attributing the dysphagia to motor abnormalities of the lower esophagus, structural lesions, such as stricture, need to be ruled out by endoscopy or esophagraphy and treated accordingly. Patients are advised to chew their food completely and take extra fluids with meals. Prokinetic agents are generally not helpful regardless of the presence or absence of reflux symptoms or injuries. Antireflux measures such as elevation of the head of the bed, avoidance of eating within 3 to 4 hours of bedtime, and acid suppressive agents such as H_2 antagonists or proton pump inhibitors need to be instituted to prevent reflux injuries.

Dermatomyositis/polymyositis, on the other hand, primarily involves the proximal striated muscle of the esophagus and upper esophageal sphincter and pharynx. In some cases, impairment of suprahyoid muscle contractility reduces upper esophageal sphincter opening, further increasing cervical dysphagia. If this pathology is suspected, a modified barium swallow study should be obtained, which may show pharyngeal/vallecular residue, nasopharyngeal reflux, and tracheal aspiration. Involvement of the swallowing apparatus is part of the general spectrum of the disease. Swallow rehabilitation techniques may be helpful in preventing aspiration while patients are being treated for their systemic disease.

STRUCTURAL ABNORMALITIES

Peptic Stricture

Reflux-induced esophageal stricture is the most common benign stricture of the esophagus, occurring in about 10% of patients with severe reflux disease. The incidence of esophageal stricture is increased in patients with Barrett's esophagitis and scleroderma esophagus. Peptic strictures commonly involve the distal esophagus and induce esophageal dysphagia. However, they can also occur in the proximal esophagus, causing symptoms of cervical dysphagia such as aspiration and choking. A variant of reflux-induced esophageal dysphagia is the loss of esophageal wall compliance due to inflammation. These patients may present with solid food dysphagia without evidence of stricture, narrowing, or mucosal injury. However, a marshmallow swallow will document impaction of the bolus in the distal esophagus and will reproduce the patient's symptoms. Interestingly, heartburn may diminish as the stricture increases. However, esophageal peptic stricture may be present in the absence of a clinical history of heartburn.

Diagnosis of peptic stricture is usually established by a barium esophagram; however, endoscopic examination is needed to rule out malignancy. Mechanical dilation of the esophagus remains the mainstay of treatment for peptic strictures. A variety of mercury-filled, rounded- or tapered-tip dilators are used for bougienage. However, if the stricture is eccentric or severe, bougienage must be done over a guidewire placed through the stricture under fluoroscopic control. Several gradual dilatations are performed to avoid perforation. Dysphagia is usually relieved when the stricture is dilated to 14 mm (42 French). Patients with peptic strictures need to be vigorously treated for reflux disease during and after dilatation to avoid stricture recurrence. Antireflux therapy includes elevating the head of the bed 4 to 6 inches, avoiding food 3 to 4 hours before retiring, and avoiding substances that reduce lower esophageal sphincter pressure such as alcohol, chocolate, caffeine, and smoking. Acid-reducing medications such as H_2 receptor antagonists and proton pump inhibitors are the mainstay of management. Patients with stricture and Barrett's esophagus pose exceptional clinical problems. A 6- to 12-month interval surveillance approach is advocated by some for patients with Barrett's esophagus to look for high-grade mucosal dysplasia, a premalignant lesion.

ESOPHAGEAL CARCINOMA

Malignant dysphagia is due to esophageal squamous cell carcinoma in 80 to 90% of instances. The most common site is the midthoracic segment of the esophagus. Esophageal carcinoma generally is well extended submucosally before it extends into the lumen; thus, by the time dysphagia develops, the cancer is well spread. Adenocarcinoma of the esophagus seems to be on the rise, and often originates in Barrett's esophagus. Benign tumors of the esophagus are rare and include leiomyomas, lipomas, and papillomas. The esophagus may receive metastatic spread from breast cancer, melanoma, oat cell carcinoma of the lung, and Hodgkin's lymphoma. Diagnosis is suggested by radiography and confirmed with endoscopy and biopsy of the lesion. Brushing for cytology along with biopsy increases the diagnostic yield to almost 100%. In recent years, endoscopic ultrasound has increased the yield for evaluation of local spread. Since more than 95% of esophageal carcinomas are not amenable to curative surgery at the time of diagnosis, management generally consists of palliation and supportive care. Chemotherapy generally has not been helpful. Surgical palliation and radiation therapy have similar 5-year survival rates of about 10%.

The primary purpose of therapy for malignant esophageal dysphagia is to alleviate the esophageal stricture and restore luminal diameter sufficient enough to allow the patient to resume oral feeding. Esophageal dilatation has a success rate of about 90% in restoring adequate lumen to maintain nutrition. Newer modalities for alleviating malignant strictures include endoprosthesis placement (plastic or expandable wire mesh stents) and endoscopic tumor ablation using laser or tumor probes.

ESOPHAGEAL RINGS AND WEBS

Esophageal webs and rings can be classified according to the site of origin. Proximal esophageal webs, as seen in Plummer-Vinson or Paterson-Brown-Kelly syndrome, occur in the upper 2 to 4 cm of the esophagus and are associated with iron deficiency anemia. Dysphagia is often associated with aspiration symptoms. There have been reports of an association between these webs and postcricoid carcinoma.

Diagnosis is usually made by barium swallow study in the lateral projection. Treatment is by dilatation, either by bougienage or endoscopic balloon dilatation. Iron stores need to be replenished to prevent recurrence. Proximal esophageal webs may be associated with Zenker's diverticulum and graft-versus-host disease following bone marrow transplantation.

Distal esophageal ring, as described by Schatzki and Gary in 1953, is a thin ring located at the junction of the squamous and columnar mucosa. It is usually accompanied by a hiatal hernia. Dysphagia is intermittent and occurs with ingestion of solid foods. Schatzki's ring is seen in 9% of autopsy studies and produces dysphagia when the lumen becomes narrower than 13 mm. Treatment consists of single bougienage with a 50 French dilator. A few patients require a second dilatation. Bougienage should be done under fluoroscopy to assure the safe passage of the dilator into the stomach. Alternately, transendoscopic balloon dilatation can be used to break the ring.

PILL-, CHEMICAL-, AND RADIATION-INDUCED STRICTURES

A variety of medications in tablet form have been reported to induce esophageal mucosal injury and potential stricture. Pill-induced esophageal injury is usually associated with retrosternal pain on swallowing. Some patients will slowly develop dysphagia if the offending agent is continued. These agents include tetracycline, doxycycline, potassium chloride, iron preparations, quinidine, and analgesics such as aspirin and nonsteroidal anti-inflammatory drugs. Diagnosis is suggested by the history. A barium esophagram may show ulcer, stricture, or mass. Endoscopy and biopsy will confirm the diagnosis. Therapy includes cessation of the offending agent. Stricture is generally resolved by dilatation; the technique is similar to that described earlier for peptic strictures.

Esophageal stricture can follow ingestion of caustic chemicals. Endoscopy yields accurate assessment of the damage. In the acute phase, patients with esophageal injury are managed with antibiotics, intravenous fluids, and acid-suppressing medications and are advised to avoid oral intake. Stricture formation occurs in about half of the victims and can be followed by barium esophagraphy. These strictures are dilated in a manner similar to that for peptic strictures. However, in severe cases, esophageal resection and gastric pull-up or colonic interposition may be necessary.

Radiation therapy can induce esophageal symptoms in a dose-dependent fashion. Stricture formation usually occurs after 6000 cGy delivered to the mediastinum. Concurrent chemotherapy potentiates radiation-induced esophageal complications. These strictures are treated with esophageal dilatation.

FOREIGN BODIES

Acute obstruction of the esophagus is usually caused by food impaction. A bolus of food, usually meat, becomes lodged at the level of a stricture, a ring, or a mass. Accidental swallowing of pieces of bone, toothpicks, pins, or dentures is more serious and can result in esophageal perforation, hemorrhage, and sepsis with a fatal outcome. The cervical esophagus, a point level with the aortic arch, and the gastroesophageal junction are common lodging sites. Ingestion of disk batteries poses a special danger because of their alkaline content; they should be removed from the esophagus immediately. Plain x-ray films with soft tissue techniques are indicated to localize the foreign body. However, failure to visualize a foreign body by x-ray does not rule out its presence, and if symptoms persist, endoscopic examination is indicated.

Intravenous glucagon, 0.5 to 1.0 mg, may help an impacted food bolus to pass into the stomach. Use of enzymatic dissolution should be avoided owing to the risk of esophageal perforation and aspiration of the enzyme. If a conservative approach is unsuccessful, endoscopic removal is indicated. Similarly, impacted foreign bodies are best removed endoscopically. This may be done by flexible upper endoscopy under conscious sedation with use of a variety of retrieving forceps and snares. An over tube facilitates multiple passes and prevents accidental aspiration of the foreign body during its removal. However, in cases of razor blade ingestion or very proximal impaction, rigid esophagoscopy and general anesthetic may be required.

DIVERTICULA OF THE ALIMENTARY TRACT

method of
GEORGE AHTARIDIS, M.D.
The Graduate Hospital
Philadelphia, Pennsylvania

Diverticula are mucosal pouches in the gastrointestinal tract. They can involve any area of the gastrointestinal tract and can be classified as true or false. True diverticula include all layers of the intestinal wall; false diverticula are formed by herniation of mucosa and submucosa through a defect in the muscular wall of the gut. Some authors classify the diverticula according to etiology as congenital, pulsion, or traction or as arising from motility disorders.

Diverticula are usually asymptomatic. Patients can present with dysphagia, bleeding, perforation, or intestinal stasis and malabsorption depending on the anatomic location in the gastrointestional tract.

HYPOPHARYNGEAL DIVERTICULA

The hypopharyngeal diverticulum (Zenker's, or pharyngoesophageal) is the most common diverticulum of the esophagus. It is defined as a protrusion of hypopharyngeal mucosa between the oblique fibers of the inferior pharyngeal constrictor and the transverse fibers of the cricopharyngeus muscles caused by incoordination of the upper esophageal sphincter, achalasia (spasm) of the upper esophageal sphincter, or weakness of the esophageal wall. It occurs in 2% of patients with dysphagia and reaches its peak incidence after the sixth decade.

The main symptom of Zenker's diverticulum is transient dysphagia when the sac is relatively small. When the sac becomes relatively large and retains contents, the patient may experience regurgitation of food into the mouth, pharyngeal dysphagia, pulmonary aspiration, gurgling in the throat, or even appearance of a mass in the neck. Esophageal obstruction from retained food into a very large sac has been described. In addition to the previously mentioned symptoms, a Zenker's diverticulum may produce other rare complications such as fistula between the diverticulum and the trachea, bleeding, and squamous cell carcinoma.

Treatment

Patients with asymptomatic diverticula, usually discovered incidentally during x-ray examination, do not require treatment. However, when persistent symptoms are present, surgery is recommended. Procedures include (1) excision of the diverticulum (diverticulectomy); (2) cricopharyngeal myotomy; (3) suspension of the diverticulum (diverticulopexy); and (4) endoscopic resection of the esophagodiverticular wall. Results are very good with any one of these procedures, but wound infection and fistulization can occur as complications of diverticulectomy.

MIDESOPHAGEAL DIVERTICULA

The pathogenesis of midesophageal diverticula remains uncertain, but the increasing use of motility techniques has demonstrated that motility disorders play a causal role. The theory that fibrous adhesions from granulomatous diseases of the mediastinum cause traction diverticula has not been confirmed by autopsy studies. The diverticula are usually small and do not retain food. They do not require any form of treatment. If the patient has symptoms of dysphagia or chest pain, attention should be directed toward possible motility disturbances.

INTRAMURAL DIVERTICULOSIS

Intramural diverticula are very rare. Dysphagia is caused by numerous 1- to 3-mm outpouchings of the esophagus that are usually associated with hiatal hernia, upper esophageal stricture or webs, and in some cases with *Candida* infection. The diverticula represent dilated submucosal glands that can be present in the proximal or distal esophagus and are lined with squamous epithelium. The diagnosis is established by barium esophagram, but endoscopy is useful in the evaluation of strictures, possible candidiasis, and esophagitis.

EPIPHRENIC DIVERTICULA

Epiphrenic diverticula are located in the distal esophagus and can be single or multiple. About two-thirds of patients with these diverticula have esophageal motility disorders. Symptoms, which include dysphagia, chest pain, and regurgitation, are usually secondary to underlying motor disorders, but a small number of patients experience characteristically large-volume food regurgitation at night while in the recumbent position. Complications of epiphrenic diverticula include phlegmonous esophagitis, bezoar, squamous cell carcinoma, perforation, aspiration, and bleeding. The diagnosis is established by barium esophagram. Esophageal manometry is necessary to rule out motility disorder.

Asymptomatic diverticula do not require treatment. In patients who present with dysphagia, regurgitation of food, or complications such as tumor, surgical treatment should be considered. Several surgical procedures may be used, including diverticulopexy, diverticulectomy, short and long myotomy, and antireflux procedures. Simple excision of diverticula is associated with high morbidity and mortality and should be avoided.

GASTRIC DIVERTICULA

The etiology of these rare diverticula is unknown. Located on the posterior wall of the cardia, they are single lesions, about 3 cm in diameter. Occasionally they are found in the prepyloric antrum. They are usually asymptomatic, but fullness or epigastric pain has been attributed to them. Complications are uncommon, but bleeding, perforation, and torsion have been described. Treatment is rarely indicated.

SMALL INTESTINAL DIVERTICULA

Duodenal Diverticula

Duodenal diverticula are extraluminal (most common) or intraluminal (rare). Extraluminal duodenal diverticula are quite common, especially in the older population, with an overall incidence of 6% on barium x-rays and about 20% on endoscopic retrograde cholangiopancreatography. About 75% occur within 2 cm of the ampulla of Vater.

In general, duodenal diverticula are asymptomatic, and no treatment is indicated unless they cause bleeding, perforation, or obstruction. Bleeding from the diverticulum can be massive and difficult to diagnose.

Duodenal diverticulitis presents as upper abdominal pain radiating to the right upper quadrant or back with nausea, abdominal tenderness, fever, and leukocytosis. A computed tomographic (CT) scan may be helpful in establishing the diagnosis. Duodenocolic fistula, bacterial overgrowth, and enterolith formation have been reported.

Periampullary diverticula are associated with increased incidence of gallstones and common bile duct stones. Stasis within the diverticula and sphincter of Oddi dysfunction can lead to contamination of the duodenum and biliary tree.

Duodenal diverticula can create diagnostic difficulties and have been mistaken for pancreatic pseudocysts or abscess or even carcinoma on CT, since they are sometimes located in the same area of the pancreas and contain air, fluid, and debris.

Treatment

Duodenal diverticula rarely require therapy except when there is bleeding or perforation. Surgery is indicated after supportive measures fail. In cases of perforated diverticula, several techniques have been advocated, including excision and serosal patch or diversion of enteric flow with gastrojejunostomy or duodenojejunostomy with extra care to avoid injury of the ampulla of Vater.

Jejunal and Ileal Diverticula

Diverticula of jejunum and ileum are much less common than duodenal diverticula, with an incidence of about 0.5 to 1% on small bowel examinations. Jejunal diverticula are usually multiple and are larger than ileal diverticula, varying in size from a few millimeters to 10 cm. Located within the leaves of the mesentery, they are easily overlooked at operation. Jejunal diverticula are acquired and are frequently associated with motility disorders of the small intestine, such as scleroderma and visceral myopathies and neuropathies.

Patients commonly present with chronic abdominal pain, early satiety, and bloating, and bleeding, intestinal perforation, and obstruction can also occur. Intestinal stasis, bacterial overgrowth, and malabsorption frequently lead to steatorrhea, weight loss, and associated fat-soluble vitamin deficiencies.

The diagnosis is made on the basis of the clinical presentation and can be confirmed by a D-xylose test, mucosal biopsy, growth tests, small bowel x-rays, and sometimes a Schilling test.

Treatment

Asymptomatic diverticula require no treatment. If the patient presents with malabsorption secondary to bacterial overgrowth, treatment with broad-spectrum antibiotics for both aerobic and anaerobic infections should be instituted.

Meckel's Diverticulum

Meckel's diverticulum is the most common congenital anomaly of the intestinal tract with an incidence of 0.3 to 3.0% on autopsy. The cause is the incomplete obliteration of the vitelline duct, and the diverticulum can be found in the antimesenteric border of the ileum, usually within 100 cm of the ileocecal valve. This true diverticulum is approximately 5 cm in length and has a wide mouth. About 45% contain ileal mucosa, but the great majority contain gastric mucosa.

Complications include bleeding, obstruction, and perforation. Bleeding, the most common complication, is caused by ulceration of ileal mucosa adjacent to ectopic gastric mucosa. It occurs most often in children less than 2 years of age and presents as melanotic or dark red stools. Intestinal obstruction can be secondary to either intussusception or volvulus around the vitelline duct or fibrous cord remnant of the duct. Diverticulitis may be indistinguishable from acute appendicitis.

Treatment

A technetium-99m scan will implicate ectopic gastric mucosa as the source of bleeding. Diverticulectomy is the indicated procedure. A Meckel's diverticulum discovered incidentally during surgery should not be removed because the morbidity from such incidental removal of asymptomatic diverticula may well exceed the risk of possible complications later in life.

DIVERTICULAR DISEASE OF THE COLON

Diverticular disease of the colon is the most common colonic disease in the Western world with an incidence of 50% in individuals over 70 years of age. Colonic diverticula are false diverticula that represent herniations of the mucosa and submucosa through the muscular layer of the bowel wall at the point where the nutrient arteries penetrate the wall of the colon. The diverticula vary in number from one to several hundred. It is estimated that 90% of patients with diverticulosis have involvement of the sigmoid colon. Solitary diverticula are usually found in the ascending colon and cecum and are true diverticula with a different etiology.

Definitions

The term *diverticulosis* suggests a multiplicity of diverticula and a segment of affected bowel with or without symptoms. *Diverticulitis* is a descriptive term applied when the bowel shows pathologically or surgically verified inflammation. *Diverticular disease* refers to the symptom complex produced by diverticula.

Diverticulosis

Uncomplicated diverticulosis is asymptomatic and requires no treatment. A small percentage of patients with diverticulosis present with symptoms of low abdominal pain or colic, usually in the left lower quadrant. The pain is often worse after eating, and relief is often obtained by passage of a bowel movement or flatus. The differential diagnosis of this pain includes a long list of conditions producing similar symptoms, such as irritable bowel syndrome, lactose intolerance, gynecologic and urologic disorders, and carcinoma of the colon and rectum.

Diets high in vegetable fiber have been shown to have a beneficial effect on painful diverticulosis. The same effect can be achieved by use of hydrophilic colloid laxatives and, to a lesser extent, by antispasmodics (anticholinergics).

Diverticular Bleeding

Diverticular disease is the most common cause of massive lower gastrointestinal bleeding. It is estimated that 30 to 50% of massive colonic bleeding is due to diverticulosis, while angiodysplasia is responsible for another 20 to 30%. Diverticular bleeding arises from the right colon in 70 to 90% of patients. The bleeding stops spontaneously in 75 to 80% of patients with diverticular hemorrhage. The risk of rebleeding is 25% but increases to 50% in patients who have suffered a second episode of hemorrhage. The herniation of the diverticulum carries one of the penetrating vessels with it. Eventually the vessel becomes draped over the dome of the diverticulum, separated from the colonic lumen by only the thin mucosal layer. This predisposes to injury with subsequent rupture.

Treatment

If the patient is actively bleeding and is hemodynamically stable, attempts at localization of the bleeding site should be made by selective mesenteric angiography, radioisotope scanning, or colonoscopy.

Selective mesenteric angiography successfully identifies the site of bleeding in 40 to 60% of patients. The low positive rate is due to the high incidence of spontaneous cessation of bleeding. Also, bleeding must be active at a rate of 0.5 mL per minute in order for arteriography to be diagnostic. Radioisotope scans, preferably with labeled erythrocytes (tagged red blood cell scan), can be useful in detecting chronic or intermittent bleeding with bleeding rates as low as 0.1 mL per minute. If a bleeding site is located with arteriography, selective intra-arterial vasopressin* (Pitressin), 0.1 to 0.4 units per minute, usually stops the bleeding.

During the last few years, colonoscopy has proved to be extremely effective in localizing the site of bleeding after adequate cleansing of the bowel.

Partial colectomy (i.e., excision of the segment that contains the bleeding diverticula) is indicated when medical treatment fails to arrest the bleeding. Emergent surgical intervention is necessary in patients who are hemodynamically unstable. Blind subtotal colectomy should be reserved for patients with recurrent bleeding, because this procedure has an operative mortality of 30 to 50%. Elective colon resection is recommended in any patient with a history of previous diverticular bleeding who presents with a second episode of bleeding.

Diverticulitis

Diverticulitis is the most common complication of diverticulosis; between 10 and 25% of patients with diverticulosis will develop symptoms and signs of diverticulitis. The term *diverticulitis* implies inflammation of one or more diverticula. The disease spectrum ranges from mild, well-localized inflammation to a fulminant process causing free perforation and generalized peritonitis. In more than 90% of patients, the inflammation is limited to the sigmoid colon; the right colon is involved in only 5% of patients.

Diverticulitis is believed to occur secondary to inflammation of the wall of a diverticulum, with subsequent microperforation or macroperforation. With microperforation, a small paracolonic abscess or area of fibrosis can be found. In most settings, even with macroperforation, the inflammatory process is mild and the perforation is walled off by the pericolic fat and surrounding mesentery. Involvement of other organs occasionally leads to intestinal obstruction or fistulization.

Clinical Features

The presenting clinical features vary according to the location of perforation and the severity of the process, ranging from mild low abdominal pain to severe pain in the left lower quadrant or right lower quadrant, to generalized abdominal pain. Nausea, vomiting, and urinary tract symptoms are present in a smaller number of patients. Fever and leukocytosis with marked predominance of polymorphonuclear leukocytes are invariably present. Physical examination reveals abdominal tenderness, usually in the left lower quadrant. A tender abdominal mass may be palpable and the abdomen is often distended and tympanitic.

Routine chest and abdominal radiographs are usually unremarkable. Free air under the diaphragm is unusual in diverticulitis. Contrast radiography or colonoscopy should be undertaken with caution in patients with suspected diverticulitis because of the risk of worsening the perforation with introduction of air or contrast material. CT scanning is probably the most useful and versatile diagnostic procedure for diverticulitis and can be used in the early stages of the disease.

The differential diagnosis includes painful diverticulosis, carcinoma of the colon, Crohn's disease, ulcerative colitis, and ischemic colitis.

Treatment

A small number of patients with minor episodes of diverticulitis can be treated as outpatients with oral antibiotics and a clear liquid diet, but the great majority require hospitalization for medical or surgical treatment. It has been estimated that 70 to 85% of patients will recover with medical treatment; the remainder require surgical intervention.

Medical therapy consists of bowel rest, NPO status, nasogastric suction especially if nausea, vomiting, or abdominal distention is present, and intravenous antibiotics and fluids. Since the bacterial spectrum includes gram-negative aerobic and anaerobic organisms, the antibiotic regimen should provide coverage for these flora.

The patient should be followed carefully with frequent abdominal examinations and laboratory studies to determine the response to the treatment. The antibiotic regimen may be changed depending on the blood culture results.

In most cases, the symptoms and signs of diverticulitis abate in 3 to 4 days, but sometimes it may be 7 to 10 days before the acute process resolves. Oral intake can be instituted gradually and barium enema or colonoscopy should be postponed until several weeks after the acute episode.

Urgent surgical treatment may be required for patients who fail to respond or who deteriorate within 24 or 48 hours after hospitalization. Indications for surgery include generalized peritonitis, persistence or progression of an abscess despite antibiotic therapy, intestinal obstruction, persistent urosepsis secondary to colovesical fistula, and disease in patients under the age of 40 and those who are immunocompromised.

Resection of the involved segment and primary anastomosis is the procedure of choice (one stage procedure) for patients with a history of recurrent attacks and those undergoing elective surgery, due to the low mortality and morbidity.

In patients presenting with fulminant disease, two- and three-stage procedures are usually used. The two-stage procedure consists of resection of the involved bowel segment and creation of an end-colostomy (using the proximal end of the bowel) with the distal end brought up as a mucus fistula or closed and left in the pelvis (Hartman's procedure). The colostomy is closed in a subsequent procedure after 8 to 12 weeks.

*Not FDA approved for this indication.

The three-stage procedure consists of drainage of the diseased region with formation of a diverting colostomy followed by resection of diseased colon with primary anastomosis and finally closure of colostomy several weeks later. This procedure is rarely justified and is now of largely historical interest.

ULCERATIVE COLITIS

method of
SUMNER C. KRAFT, M.D.
University of Chicago Medical Center
Chicago, Illinois

Nonspecific ulcerative colitis is a chronic inflammatory disease of the colon of unknown etiology; it must be diagnosed by excluding Crohn's disease, specific microbial infections, ischemia, the effects of antibiotics and other drugs, and various systemic disorders. In acute ulcerative colitis, the colonic mucosa and perhaps the submucosa show diffuse vascular congestion, capillary dilatation, edema, hemorrhage, superficial ulceration, and cellular infiltration with neutrophils, lymphocytes, plasma cells, and eosinophils. Crypt abscesses are common and consist of accumulations of neutrophils, eosinophils, and cellular debris. In chronic ulcerative colitis, inflammation, edema, muscular hypertrophy, and the deposition of fibrous tissue and fat can lead to thickening, contraction, narrowing, and shortening—a "lead-pipe" appearance. Inflammatory polyps are often noted as mucosal remnants or accumulations of granulation tissue with or without overlying colonic epithelial cells.

The patient with acute ulcerative colitis may be seriously ill with 20 or more watery, bloody stools per day, dehydration, anemia, hypoproteinemia, and fever. In many patients the disease follows a chronic course with frequent exacerbations, but this may vary considerably and prolonged remissions are not unusual. The onset may be mild and insidious, with no more than four bowel movements per day, minimal gross bleeding, and perhaps only vague abdominal discomfort. The general physical examination may be normal but fever, tachycardia, pallor, and wasting are not uncommon. The abdomen may be tender and distended, perhaps with signs of peritoneal irritation, although the absence of abdominal findings is not unusual even in the presence of total colonic involvement. The anorectal examination may disclose perianal erythema, hemorrhoids, and simple fissures without the perirectal abscesses, fistulas, extensive fissure formation, and profuse scarring that are common in patients with Crohn's disease. Colonic complications include massive hemorrhage, toxic dilatation, "pericolitis," perforation, stricture, and neoplasia; extracolonic complications involve the liver, skin, eyes, joints, kidneys, cardiovascular system and, occasionally, the lungs. In approximately 20% of cases, the process is limited to the rectum at diagnosis; these individuals tend to remain in good general health without overt manifestations of systemic disease.

Anemia frequently results from combinations of blood loss, iron or folic acid deficiency, hemolysis, and chronic inflammation. The leukocyte count and erythrocyte sedimentation rate may be elevated, especially in the presence of complications, while prolonged diarrhea may lead to depressed serum levels of albumin, potassium, chloride, sodium, and magnesium. The feces usually contain no identifiable pathogenic bacteria, and occult blood persists for long periods after clinical symptoms subside. Proctosigmoidoscopy (without preparation) is a most valuable diagnostic procedure; the mucosal appearance may range from mild hyperemia, fine granularity, petechiae, and minimal pinpoint bleeding after cotton wiping to more severe abnormalities such as increased friability, edema, mucopurulent exudate, and frank ulceration with spontaneous bleeding. Colonic x-rays reveal abnormalities in the vast majority of patients but should not be performed in the presence of very active or fulminant colitis. Mucosal detail is especially well seen in air-contrast barium enemas, and frequent findings are ulceration, diminished or absent haustrations, straightening, narrowing, shortening, diminished distensibility, spasm, an irregular mosaic pattern due to mucosal edema, and an increase in the retrorectal soft-tissue space. Although total fiberoptic colonoscopy should not be a routine diagnostic procedure, it has proven useful in selected cases for demonstrating the extent of mucosal involvement, excluding dysplasia and overt carcinoma in high-risk categories of patients, and more precisely differentiating ulcerative colitis from Crohn's disease that is limited to the colon.

TREATMENT

An adequate diagnostic assessment is critical in patients with ulcerative colitis since treatment varies with the proximal extent of the involvement, the acuteness or chronicity of the process, the initial response to therapy, and the presence of extracolonic manifestations. The approach must be individualized for each patient, often proving to be both comprehensive and prolonged; the ultimate goal is a return to an active, normal life. In pursuit of this objective, the broad categories of medical management are rest, diet, and medication.

Rest

Both physical and mental rest are important features of the overall therapeutic plan; a careful psychosocial history should serve as a guide to a common-sense approach, e.g., limiting daily activities when indicated, getting more sleep, and indulging in pleasant recreation. Bed rest is an important measure in the early treatment of active disease; with chronicity, fatigue, malnutrition, and a poor state of general health, some patients may require hospitalization. A gradual increase in physical activity is permitted as recovery proceeds. At the other extreme, patients with mild disease and those in remission require little or no restriction.

Emotional support should be provided, aided by psychological and social evaluations, as anxiety and depression may be prominent. However, intensive psychotherapy may be hazardous during acute exacerbations of the bowel disease. Awareness of the psychological impact of frequent symptoms, potent medications, deleterious environmental factors, and the patient's relationship with family and peer groups is of great importance in the successful care of the patient. In short, the patient-doctor relationship becomes an important part of any successful therapeutic program in ulcerative colitis; an informed, sympathetic physician should furnish continuous support and reassurance both to patients and their families.

Diet/Nutrition

Specific dietary recommendations, if indeed indicated, will vary with the extent of disease activity and tissue involvement, the presence of diarrhea and/or abdominal pain, the results of a detailed nutritional assessment, and a history of intolerance to certain foods. The primary purpose of dietary recommendations is to alleviate or prevent symptoms while providing adequate nutrition. In addition to causing significant weight loss, malnutrition can hinder responses to medications and increase both the risk of infection and the morbidity of possibly indicated surgery. In the adolescent, growth is inhibited when caloric intake has been reduced and the inflammatory process has increased metabolic needs and caused enteric losses of important nutrients. The patient should be counseled to choose foods that are palatable; protein, caloric, and micronutrient supplements should be used as needed.

In mild or quiescent disease, the diet may be unrestricted or merely bland and nonlaxative. The patient often is in the best position to decide which foods, if any, need be eliminated. Those that commonly are avoided include prunes, figs, cabbage, highly spiced foods, excessively fatty products, raw fruits and vegetables, fruit juices, and foodstuffs that contain nuts, hulls, kernels or seeds. Caffeinated and carbonated beverages and alcoholic drinks can be permitted in moderation in some patients, especially if their total elimination would create undue emotional stress. Cooked, canned, or peeled fruits and vegetables may be added as diarrhea subsides. Constipation can actually occur in patients with limited distal proctitis and can be helped by increasing dietary bulk, even including a preparation containing psyllium or methylcellulose. Patients known to be intolerant of milk or other dairy products should avoid them. Of course, milk intolerance may be merely the result of chronic diarrhea and a secondary disaccharidase deficiency. Therefore, this excellent source of calcium and protein may be continued in many of these patients with the prior addition of yeast-derived lactase (Lactaid). If appetite is poor, peroral or enteral-tube alimentation with chemically defined mixtures may result in improved nutritional status and decreased residue in the inflamed colon.

Vitamins and Minerals

In patients eating a reasonably balanced diet, specific vitamin deficiency is unusual and vitamin supplementation rarely is needed. Folic acid in a dose of 1 mg daily generally is prescribed for individuals taking sulfasalazine because this anti-inflammatory agent competitively inhibits the enzyme system required for dietary folate absorption. In the presence of anorexia and diminished food intake, a once-daily multivitamin supplement does not seem unreasonable. In the presence of extensive diarrhea, impaired electrolyte and mineral absorption may require careful monitoring in order to initiate appropriate replacement of potassium, sodium, chloride, and magnesium. Of course, electrolyte imbalances are more common in patients receiving corticosteroids. Although iron deficiency is prevalent in ulcerative colitis, oral iron products often are poorly tolerated, even when taken with meals, and parenteral iron therapy may be needed. While fluid replacement in general is indicated during acute exacerbations of disease, oral alimentation should be encouraged as soon as possible as a means of keeping up with vitamin, electrolyte, and mineral requirements.

Parenteral Alimentation

When oral alimentation is not feasible and there is an obvious need for increased caloric and protein intake, a parenteral approach may be very useful in conjunction with bowel rest. This is especially important in patients with severe, acute ulcerative colitis and those with "pericolitis" or toxic dilatation of the colon. Strict attention must be directed to proper fluid and electrolyte balance. Although an immediate operation may be avoided by this technique, and perhaps even a period of remission induced in those with less extensive colitis, progressive megacolon, massive hemorrhage, or perforation may still develop and can be masked by corticosteroid therapy and the reduced oral intake. A several-week period of parenteral alimentation may be useful in youngsters with growth retardation who want to avoid surgery, as well as in others in whom surgery is not yet an acceptable option. However, it should not be inferred that improved nutrition will necessarily result in a better clinical outcome. Hyperalimentation may prove quite useful in nutritionally-depleted ulcerative colitis patients during the perioperative period.

Medications

Supportive Agents: Antidiarrheal Preparations

The general supportive approach is to treat the symptoms and findings with as-needed medications such as sedatives, tranquilizers, antispasmodic agents, antidiarrheal preparations, vitamins, hematinics, albumin and other blood products, and electrolyte, mineral, and trace-metal supplements. The most frequently used antidiarrheal preparations are diphenoxylate hydrochloride with atropine sulfate (Lomotil) and loperamide hydrochloride (Imodium). Especially helpful for patients with mild disease that results in cramping and refractory diarrhea, these compounds generally are given as one or two tablets or capsules every 4 to 6 hours as needed. Since there are differences in the activities of these two drugs, patients who do not respond well to one might try the other. Diphenoxylate is chemically related to meperidine and is obviously better for long-term use than morphine, codeine, and opium. Side effects may include increased cramping, even with decreasing diarrhea, and anticholinergic effects are possible when larger doses are used. Loperamide specifically inhibits peristalsis by a direct effect on the gastrointestinal wall, interacting locally with cholinergic as well as noncholinergic mechanisms; it is poorly absorbed and excreted mainly in the feces. However, both agents should be used cautiously in patients with acute and severe disease to avoid colonic dilatation. The more potent antidiarrheal agents of the opiate class (e.g., codeine, tincture of opium, and paregoric) should be reserved for highly selected situations; in most cases, narcotic analgesics should be considered only for preoperative management.

Anticholinergic Agents

In patients with limited disease manifestations, including those with mild abdominal cramping, diarrhea, and nocturnal defecation, there may be enhanced control and regularity of bowel habits with the use of low-dose belladonna-containing preparations. However, a risk of toxic dilatation exists and thus anticholinergic agents should be used judiciously in patients with unstable or increasing symptoms, especially in the presence of nutritional depletion. Such preparations clearly are contraindicated in patients with severe ulcerative colitis.

Sedatives/Tranquilizers

Adjunctive therapy with low doses of a sedative such as phenobarbital or a mild tranquilizer may be useful in highly anxious patients, but the indication for their continued use should be closely monitored, especially since these patients often require multiple drugs. The use of phenobarbital in combination with anticholinergic agents such as belladonna alkaloids and dicyclomine hydrochloride (Bentyl) is contraindicated in patients with moderate to severe disease because of the risk of colonic dilatation.

Analgesics

Pain medications and narcotics rarely are required for the treatment of ulcerative colitis, and the onset of significant and persistent pain may be a harbinger of toxic dilatation and perforation. Nonsteroidal anti-inflammatory drugs and aspirin and its derivatives should be used with caution, since antiplatelet and other untoward effects can exacerbate mucosal hemorrhage, and the patient's already precarious situation may be aggravated by the development of gastric irritation, peptic ulceration, and upper gastrointestinal hemorrhage. Nonsteroidal anti-inflammatory drug–induced disease in the distal ileum and large bowel is another problem that is under active investigation.

Sulfasalazine and Newer Aminosalicylates

Sulfasalazine (Azulfidine) has been used for about 50 years for the treatment of ulcerative colitis, including long-term maintenance therapy. As indicated by its earlier generic name, salicylazosulfapyridine, the drug is a combination of 5-aminosalicylic acid and sulfapyridine. Bacteria in the distal bowel split the diazo bond and liberate the 5-aminosalicylic acid (5-ASA), which exerts a local mucosal anti-inflammatory effect, i.e., it reduces the amount of leukotriene B_4 and inhibits local interleukin-1 production and platelet activating factor—important constituents of the inflammatory reaction. Most of the sulfapyridine component is absorbed and acetylated/hydroxylated in the liver prior to conjugation with glucuronic acid. While the sulfapyridine appears to protect the combined molecule from degradation until it reaches the colon, it is also this moiety that is responsible for most of the side effects and untoward reactions to sulfasalazine, e.g., headache, fever, gastric irritation, nausea, and anorexia as well as oligospermia with temporary male infertility. A positive test for the slow-acetylator phenotype often correlates with higher blood sulfapyridine levels and a greater likelihood of adverse reactions to the drug. Although the conventional route of administration is oral, topical forms of sulfasalazine or its newer analogues have resulted in beneficial effects in acute distal forms of ulcerative colitis (Table 1).

Sulfasalazine is used to induce remission in patients with mild to moderate ulcerative colitis and as indefinite maintenance therapy for preventing relapses; patients often are maintained for two or more years on dosages between 2 and 4 grams daily in divided amounts. Some have suggested that intermittent sulfasalazine is an effective alternative to continuous therapy for the maintenance of remission in this condition. The drug usually is withheld in severe disease in favor of systemic steroids and parenteral antibiotics. It is common practice to start with 500 mg twice daily with meals and temporarily add 500 mg daily until the anticipated dose has been achieved. Mild side effects may be minimized by temporarily reducing the dosage with more gradual increases every few days.

Discontinuation of sulfasalazine for relatively short periods with reinstitution using a dilute suspension and a slowly increasing dosage regimen (so-called desensitization) has been advocated in patients who have only mild side effects; this approach clearly should not be used in patients who have experienced agranulocytosis, hemolytic anemia, anaphylactoid reactions, Stevens-Johnson syndrome, and other more serious sequelae. The liquid preparation of sulfasalazine is a convenient form with which to attempt desensitization. Starting with as little as 1 to 10 mg given once daily, the dosage can be doubled every three days if there are no adverse reactions, until the desired maintenance dose is achieved. If a mild skin rash occurs, an antihistaminic may be prescribed and the sulfasalazine withheld until this resolves. Then, the drug may be administered again, resuming the process from the initial dose but allowing longer intervals between increments.

Both topical and oral preparations of 5-ASA (mesalamine) are presently available for patients with ul-

TABLE 1. **Guidelines for the Use of Anti-Inflammatory Medications in Ulcerative Colitis**

Drug	Proctitis/Distal Colitis	Extensive Colitis	Severe Colitis
Active Disease			
Oral anti-inflammatory			
Sulfasalazine	2–6 gm/day	2–6 gm/day	2–6 gm/day
Mesalamine	1.6–4.8 gm/day	1.6–4.8 gm/day	1.6–4.8 gm/day
Topical anti-inflammatory			
Mesalamine	1–4 gm/day	1–4 gm/day	
Hydrocortisone	100–200 mg/day	100–200 mg/day	100–200 mg/day
Systemic anti-inflammatory			
Prednisone	20–60 mg/day*	40–60 mg/day	40–60 mg/day
ACTH			80–120 U/day†
Maintenance			
Oral anti-inflammatory			
Sulfasalazine	2–4 gm/day	2–4 gm/day	
Mesalamine	0.8–4 gm/day	0.8–4 gm/day	
Olsalazine	0.75–1.5 gm/day	0.75–1.5 gm/day	
Topical anti-inflammatory			
Mesalamine	500 mg suppository at bedtime 4 gm enema at bedtime		

*Avoid steroids for proctitis.
†Used only for patients not receiving steroids.

cerative colitis in whom adverse side effects have occurred with sulfasalazine as a result of sulfapyridine toxicity. These non–sulfa-containing aminosalicylates are worthy of consideration as alternatives in any patient who has demonstrated some degree of sulfasalazine intolerance. More than half of the patients with distal ulcerative colitis who are refractory to conventional therapy (sulfasalazine and topical or oral corticosteroids) respond to 4-gram 5-ASA enemas (Rowasa) once or twice daily, and they may be more effective than hydrocortisone retention enemas in the treatment of mild to moderate distal ulcerative colitis. Suppositories containing 500 mg of 5-ASA (Rowasa) are effective in active ulcerative proctitis when given two or three times daily. Since the disease can flare relatively quickly when the 5-ASA is withdrawn, the use of reduced-frequency topical mesalamine in maintaining remission also has been advocated.

Since enemas and suppositories are unlikely to benefit most patients with more extensive proximal ulcerative colitis and may not be preferred for chronic use as a maintenance regimen, oral forms of 5-ASA are now available to deliver an intact form of the anti-inflammatory agent to the lower intestine (see Table 1). The advantage of the oral 5-ASA preparations lies primarily in the reduction of adverse effects rather than in enhanced therapeutic benefit. Although there is the potential for salicylate-induced renal side effects, nephrotoxicity thus far has been limited to rare allergic-type reactions. All formulations that deliver 5-ASA can infrequently cause an acute exacerbation of diarrhea and other colitis symptoms.

Asacol consists of 400 mg of mesalamine coated with an acrylic-based resin that prevents release of the active ingredient until the intestinal pH rises above 7 (roughly correlating with the terminal ileum or right colon). The preparation was designed to release mesalamine in a similar manner to sulfasalazine, although absorption is somewhat higher because of some small bowel availability. Asacol is effective in divided doses of 1.6 to 4.8 grams daily* for active disease and in doses of between 800 mg and 2.4 grams daily for maintenance of remission in ulcerative colitis.

Pentasa is a preparation of mesalamine incorporated into semipermeable ethylcellulose microspheres that gradually release 5-ASA along the length of the small and large intestine in a time- and pH-dependent manner. Based on urinary excretion data, 20 to 30% of the 5-ASA in Pentasa is absorbed. The drug has been effective in active ulcerative colitis in doses of 2 to 4 grams daily and for the maintenance of remission in doses of 1.5 to 4 grams daily. Other preparations of mesalamine (Claversal, Salofalk) are currently in use to treat ulcerative colitis in various parts of the world but are not commercially available in the United States at this time.

Olsalazine (Dipentum) consists of two 5-ASA molecules linked by the same azo bond present in sulfasalazine. This compound affords the delivery of two 5-ASA molecules directly into the colon without significant systemic absorption. Olsalazine has successfully maintained remissions in adult patients with ulcerative colitis who have been intolerant of sulfasalazine. The usual dosage is 500 mg twice daily to four times daily. About 15% of patients with quiescent disease have reported loosening of the stools or diarrhea. A gradual upward titration of olsalazine administered with food, beginning with 250 mg daily with a gradual increase to the desired dose, may minimize this secretory diarrhea that the dimer generates in the small bowel. Future therapeutic ap-

*Exceeds dosage recommended by the manufacturer.

proaches may include the use of Zileuton,* eicosapentaenoic acid,* or different still-to-be-tested selective inhibitors of leukotriene B_4 and other 5-lipoxygenase-related products of arachidonic acid—considered part of the cascade of inflammatory mediators in ulcerative colitis.

Antibiotics

For patients with ulcerative colitis who fail to achieve remission with sulfasalazine or its analogues, antibiotics sometimes are used, primarily on an empiric basis. Antimicrobial agents that have been tried in this clinical setting include ampicillin, tetracycline, trimethoprim-sulfamethoxazole, ciprofloxacin, and metronidazole. While certain patients seem to have done well on maintenance therapy with some of these agents, it must be emphasized that conclusive, controlled evidence of efficacy has not been established. Furthermore, these drugs may have significant side effects, and many antibiotics actually promote the overgrowth of *Clostridium difficile,* which can increase diarrhea and cause a superimposed specific colitis. The development of bacterial resistance, the undetermined long-term effects on the gut microflora, and the variable clinical responses are other important limitations to antibacterial therapy for ulcerative colitis. Of course, appropriate antibiotics are used when there is impending or definite colonic perforation or clear evidence of suppuration.

Corticosteroids

The decision to use topical, oral, or parenteral corticosteroids is based upon disease location and activity; it is the principal type of medication used to achieve remission in patients with severe ulcerative colitis (see Table 1). Topical preparations are quite beneficial in the treatment of distal disease or proctosigmoiditis, with diminished bleeding, urgency, diarrhea, and inflammation occurring after 1 to 3 weeks of such therapy. The enema form is best administered at bedtime and should be retained for at least 2 hours, and preferably overnight. The most commonly used preparation is the hydrocortisone retention enema (Cortenema), which is usually begun as a once-a-night treatment and continued for 2 to 3 weeks provided progress is made; in patients with tenesmus and other more severe distal symptoms, a twice daily regimen may be useful initially. With the induction of satisfactory remissions, topical steroid therapy can be decreased to an alternate night basis for 3 to 4 weeks and then to twice weekly for another 4 to 6 weeks. At this point, long-term topical therapy is generally not required in the vast majority of patients.

Topical therapy is used most frequently in conjunction with sulfasalazine for mild to moderate cases of ulcerative colitis, especially when limited to the left colon. While the effect would seem to be "local," some of the retained enema may reach at least the splenic flexure and a substantial amount may be absorbed

*Not available in the United States.

systemically. As a result, new types of topical corticosteroids are being investigated, including beclomethasone diproprionate, budesonide* and tixocortol pivalate.* Beclomethasone does not appear to suppress the pituitary-adrenal axis, while the reported absence of systemic effects with tixocortol relates more to its rapid metabolism in the blood and liver than to its poor absorption. Hydrocortisone acetate foam (Cortifoam; Epifoam; Proctofoam-HC) may be useful in the context of limited distal proctitis, because these aerosol preparations can be instilled and retained without the patient's needing to go to bed. Some have used high-potency steroid suppositories (Cort-Dome) containing 25 mg of hydrocortisone acetate as a daytime supplement to the nocturnal steroid retention enema or for convenience once symptoms are controlled.

The most frequently used oral corticosteroid is prednisone in divided doses totaling from 40 to 60 mg per day during the treatment of acute active disease. When a response occurs, it is usually evident within 10 days to 2 weeks, and the dosage can be decreased by 10 mg per week until the patient is taking 30 mg per day. The drug is then reduced by 5 mg per week until 20 mg per day is being given, provided the patient continues to do well. A return of symptoms may be related to too-rapid tapering and may require an upward adjustment of the dosage. The specific regimen for subsequent steroid tapering has to be carefully individualized, e.g., decrease the dosage by 2.5 mg approximately every 2 weeks to 10 mg per day; then decrease by 2.5 mg every month to 5 mg per day; then switch to a regimen such as 7.5 mg every other day. Although the drug ordinarily may be reduced further and discontinued over the next few months, some people seem to require a more prolonged alternate-day regimen. Repeated efforts may be made to decrease and, if possible, eliminate oral corticosteroids completely. Sulfasalazine (or a 5-ASA analogue) is often used concomitantly. By contrast with sulfasalazine, long-term prophylactic therapy with prednisone does not appear to prevent relapses in patients with ulcerative colitis in remission.

When patients do not respond to an outpatient program at the higher dosage levels of prednisone, consideration should be given to hospitalization for more intensive therapy and a re-evaluation of the entire treatment program. For example, a failure to respond may indicate poor nutritional status, limited compliance, or inadequate bioavailability of a particular steroid product. In the latter instance, a trial of a different preparation, such as methylprednisolone or hydrocortisone, may be useful. Likewise, consideration of the long-term metabolic and immunologic side effects must be weighed against the potential for a surgical cure.

Intravenous corticosteroids are used in the presence of severe disease manifestations, such as fever, marked abdominal pain, frequent bloody diarrhea, dehydration, abdominal rebound tenderness, anemia,

*Not available in the United States.

hypoalbuminemia, and other evidence of malnutrition. In these situations, intravenous hydrocortisone, 200 to 400 mg daily in divided doses, or methylprednisolone, 30 to 50 mg daily, may be required. Many of these patients are also receiving parenteral nutrition either peripherally or centrally. Careful observation of the patient, including plain films of the abdomen, is essential because this potent therapy can mask the presence of an abscess, progressive dilatation of the colon, or spontaneous perforation. The optimal duration of parenteral corticosteroid therapy is considered to be between 5 and 10 days.

Corticotropin hormone (ACTH) is still used in some centers, but hydrocortisone appears to be superior for patients who received prior steroid therapy. ACTH can be given intravenously in a dose of 40 units in 1000 mL of 5% dextrose in water slowly over 8 hours. This is done for 16 hours a day, resulting in a total dose of 80 units intravenously slowly over each 24-hour period. After 3 to 4 days, the dosage is decreased to 40 units over 8 hours and then changed to 40 units administered intramuscularly every 12 hours. At this point, the maintenance dose of 40 units daily of intramuscular ACTH generally is replaced by a regimen of oral corticosteroids.

Immunosuppressive Agents

Evidence of the effectiveness of immunosuppressive agents such as 6-mercaptopurine (Purinethol) and azathioprine (Imuran) in the treatment of ulcerative colitis is incomplete. Even in a clinical research setting, caution is necessary in the use of these agents for this condition because they can suppress host defenses, and these individuals already are vulnerable to many local and systemic problems, including infections. There may be added risks of neoplasms in those patients with ulcerative colitis who already are more vulnerable to colonic carcinoma. Certainly, such therapy must be supervised carefully to insure that the prospective benefits to the patient exceed the potential short- and long-term risks. The use of these medications in ulcerative colitis perhaps should be limited to individuals whose disease has been refractory to the previously mentioned drugs and who refuse surgery or are poor surgical risks. Yet randomized controlled trials continue to be reported, and some now believe that purine analogues should be accepted as part of the armamentarium for corticosteroid-dependent, active ulcerative colitis and in the maintenance of remission.

6-Mercaptopurine and azathioprine in doses of 50 to 150 mg daily are generally well tolerated, but the blood count should be closely monitored to see if dose reduction is necessary. Pancreatitis can be anticipated in up to 15% of patients, usually within the first month of therapy, and virtually always resolves with discontinuation of the drug. Patients should be warned about the possibility of new abdominal pain and instructed to discontinue the medication if any new symptoms arise. The time course to response may be 3 to 6 months, and a flare-up can be expected in responding patients when the immunosuppressives are discontinued. Immunosuppressive therapy should not be prescribed for patients with possible dysplasia or neoplasia, nor continued if patients are unable to discontinue steroids gradually. The potential long-term effects must be balanced against the potential for cure by colectomy.

Surgery

The usual indications for surgery in ulcerative colitis are intractability, massive hemorrhage, perforation, persistent toxic dilatation despite maximum medical therapy, obstruction, carcinoma, or a high risk of cancer, often preceded by a finding of severe dysplasia. Relative indications for surgery include certain extraintestinal manifestations that threaten to become disabling and are uncontrollable, or unacceptable side effects of maintenance medications.

The standard operation is a total proctocolectomy with conventional ileostomy, although other surgical options include proctocolectomy with a continent ileostomy (Kock pouch) and sphincter-saving abdominal colectomies with rectal mucosectomy, ileoanal anastomosis, and various ileal reservoirs or pouches. One must be careful not to perform these newer procedures in any patient in whom the colitis is of an indeterminate nature and when the possibility remains that the diagnosis is in fact Crohn's disease of the colon. These more demanding techniques usually lengthen the perioperative period and may be associated with local complications, including adhesive obstructions, pouch leaks or fistulas, or strictures at the anastomosis. Another complication seen with increasing frequency is "pouchitis," an inflammation of the reservoir that is correlated with bacterial proliferation within the pouch and often responds to metronidazole. In some cases, "pouchitis" may be resistant, requiring continued therapy with metronidazole, other antibiotics, aminosalicylates, or corticosteroids. As alluded to above, this complication can also be a manifestation of previously unsuspected Crohn's disease.

In patients with a percutaneous ileostomy, the assistance of an attentive enterostomal therapist, a well-educated and prepared patient, and perhaps guidance from other patients who have undergone the same type of operation are of great benefit. Self-help organizations, such as the Crohn's and Colitis Foundation of America, the United Ostomy Association, and other local associations can provide support and education.

Special Considerations

Toxic Dilatation of the Colon

So-called toxic megacolon is one of the most dreaded complications of ulcerative colitis and represents transmural inflammation that may follow overexuberant use of anticholinergic/narcotic/antidiarrheal agents, a barium or colonoscopic examination in a patient with a severely inflamed colon, or hypokalemia. This local complication should be presumed in any patient with persistent abdominal pain, direct and especially rebound abdominal tenderness, diminished bowel sounds, fever, tachycardia, greatly reduced stool output, and progressive dilatation of the colon on plain radiographs of the abdomen. Attempts to stabilize the patient should include nothing by mouth, nasogastric suction, intravenous fluids and electrolytes, broad-spectrum antibiotics, and high-dose corticosteroids. If there is no improvement within perhaps 24 hours, and especially if there is a suggestion of intramural or free intra-abdominal air, surgery should be urgently considered; indeed, these patients should be followed from the outset by an experienced surgeon. Improvement is manifested by diminution in the diameter of the colon by x-ray examination and signs of decreasing toxicity, including decreasing fever, white blood cell count, and abdominal tenderness. In our experience, approximately one-third of patients with toxic dilatation of the colon will have concomitant severe colonic hemorrhage.

At surgery, the transmurally necrotic colon is often paper thin and very friable, often with microperforations. Once colonic perforation occurs, mortality can be as high as 80%. Although a small proportion of patients with colonic dilatation who experience remission with medical therapy have relatively mild, easily controllable disease over the long term, the majority of ulcerative colitis patients who develop this complication ultimately require total proctocolectomy. If the toxic dilatation improves with medical management, surgery should be postponed because elective proctocolectomy done later has a much lower surgical morbidity.

Cancer Surveillance

Ulcerative colitis is a premalignant condition, and the incidence of adenocarcinoma of the colon occurs at a rate approaching 20% per decade after the first 10 years of the condition. Risk factors include childhood onset and involvement of the entire colon. Cancer can also develop in patients with relatively quiescent disease who have been off treatment for many years. Nevertheless, 10 to 15% of such cancers are found after only 5 to 10 years of known disease.

Carcinoma as a complication of ulcerative colitis is often flat, with plaquelike lesions that may be difficult to recognize on barium enema or even colonoscopic examinations. Furthermore, these cancers are often multicentric, occur more commonly beyond the reach of the sigmoidoscope, and may not produce clear-cut symptoms before the neoplasm is advanced. These factors make cancer surveillance a difficult but important task. Detailed characterization of epithelial dysplasia, the precancerous lesion, is a valuable diagnostic tool. This involves the detection of well-defined cytologic and other histologic abnormalities in random colorectal biopsies; these changes frequently are present when a colonic carcinoma exists nearby or elsewhere in the bowel. Up to 50% of patients in whom severe dysplasia is seen in several biopsies may harbor colorectal cancers. When high-grade dysplasia or a dysplastic mass is identified, the recommendation for colectomy rests on a solid foundation. Indefinite changes require follow-up and repeat colonoscopic examinations at short intervals (6 to 12 months) and treatment of the inflammation to reduce confusion between inflammatory and neoplastic changes.

Colonic strictures can occur in the presence of active or inactive disease. Strictures in the setting of active colitis are reversible and usually are due to muscular hypertrophy rather than fibrosis. Strictures that persist as the inflammation is treated are usually dysplastic or neoplastic, and colonoscopy with biopsies and cytologic brushings should be performed at short intervals (6 months) to screen for neoplasia. The presence of dysplasia in a stricture is a definite indication for colectomy.

Growth Retardation

This is a special complication of ulcerative colitis occurring in childhood. It can be the first manifestation of the disease, presenting as a decline or falling off in the expected growth curve. Reversal of the growth retardation requires greater therapeutic control over the underlying disease, special attention to adequate nutritional support, including periods of parenteral nutrition, and the use of alternate-day corticosteroid therapy and alternative medications when appropriate. If the disease cannot be brought into remission and normal growth does not resume, surgery may be indicated. Colectomy should not be withheld for so long that the optimum time for growth has passed with permanent diminution of stature. Aseptic necrosis can occur in any age group after high-dose steroid therapy but may be of special concern in children.

Extra-intestinal Manifestations

Extra-intestinal features are common in ulcerative colitis and may even be the dominant or presenting manifestation. A useful classification relates these systemic problems to the major site of bowel involvement:

1. A "colitis-related" group, in which the severity of the extra-intestinal disorder is more likely to vary directly with the activity of the bowel disease (e.g., peripheral arthritis, pyoderma gangrenosum, erythema nodosum, oral lesions, iritis, uveitis, and episcleritis).
2. A group of disorders related to impaired nutrition (and thus seen more commonly in Crohn's disease than in ulcerative colitis).
3. Miscellaneous nonspecific complications (e.g., a variety of hepatic problems such as primary sclerosing cholangitis, nonspecific triaditis, and an increase in parenchymal fat deposition). The liver pathology may run a course independent of the ulcerative colitis, including progression after colectomy.

Generally, resolution of extra-intestinal complications is achieved by treatment of the bowel disease itself, although ankylosing spondylitis and sacroiliitis follow a course independent of the colitis and require long-term therapy even after proctocolectomy. Pyoderma gangrenosum requires topical steroids and antibiotics, while topical steroids may be of use in certain patients with the more severe eye manifestations in addition to treatment of the underlying colitis. Ulcerative colitis may be considered a systemic disorder predominantly affecting the gastrointestinal tract but manifesting a wide variety of extra-intestinal associations. Early recognition of these extraintestinal manifestations should help guide therapy so that overall morbidity is reduced.

Prognosis

The short-term prognosis for an initial attack of ulcerative colitis is determined by the severity and extent of the disease, the age and physical condition of the patient, the response to medical therapy, and the results of various laboratory and x-ray parameters. For example, the onset of ulcerative colitis in elderly or postpartum patients often is associated with a more stormy course. Factors associated with poorer long-term prognosis are extensive involvement of the colon, a severe initial attack, and onset either in childhood or after the age of 60 years. However, initial observations may not always be predictive of the subsequent course, and the most severely ill patient may undergo remarkable improvement. Medical advances, such as the availability of corticosteroids, control of infection, and better surgical techniques, have led to an improved prognosis in recent years. Exacerbations can be precipitated by upper respiratory infections, infectious gastroenteritis, and other intercurrent illnesses, emotional stress, oral antibiotics, oral contraceptives, physical fatigue, dietary indiscretions, and local anorectal surgery.

Most pregnant patients with pre-existing ulcerative colitis have normal deliveries and healthy infants. Although the pregnancy per se may not affect the course of the bowel disease, relapses occur in 25 to 50% of pregnant patients, especially during the first trimester and puerperium. Every attempt should be made to control the woman's symptoms and nutritional status during gestation to provide the best setting for a successful outcome of the pregnancy. While ulcerative colitis is not a contraindication to pregnancy, it is advisable to delay pregnancy until the disease is in remission.

Clearly, ulcerative colitis requires careful teamwork among experienced medical and surgical colleagues working in concert with the patient and family. At each point, medical therapy and its consequences must be weighed against the potential operative cure. More than 80% of individuals are able to tolerate prolonged medical therapy while maintaining a normal lifestyle, family status, and occupation. Although total proctocolectomy is a curative option for selected patients with ulcerative colitis, current and emerging medical regimens afford a favorable prognosis for most patients. Despite concerns regarding cancer and the other local complications of ulcerative colitis, the primary reason for recommending colectomy continues to be failure to respond to a comprehensive, sustained medical program. It is vital that the affected patient be able to maintain the quality of life to which he or she aspires.

CROHN'S DISEASE

method of
ASHER KORNBLUTH, M.D., and
DAVID B. SACHAR, M.D.
The Mount Sinai School of Medicine
New York, New York

The approach to therapy for the patient with Crohn's disease is determined by the dominant presentation of the disease: inflammatory, fistulizing, or fibrostenotic.

INFLAMMATORY PRESENTATIONS

Inflammatory disease, whether in the small bowel or colon, is best treated with anti-inflammatory drugs, antibiotics, or both. The presenting symptoms are usually lower abdominal pain, diarrhea, and weight loss. When the inflammatory process in the colon is mild to moderate, appropriate drugs include sulfasalazine (Azulfidine) or another aminosalicylate; for ileitis, preparations that deliver mesalamine to the small bowel (e.g., Pentasa or Asacol) may be the best choice. The efficacy of all these drugs is dose related, so that they must be given a trial with sufficient dosage before they are deemed ineffective. For sulfasalazine, the maximum tolerated daily dose is usually 4 to 6 grams; for olsalazine (Dipentum), 2 to 4 grams*; for Pentasa, 4 grams; and for Asacol, 4.8 grams.*

Metronidazole (Flagyl) has also been found to have therapeutic benefit roughly equivalent to that of sulfasalazine and presumably of the other aminosalicylates as well. The usual starting dose is 250 mg three to four times daily. Although few other broad-spectrum antibiotics have been subjected to controlled trials in Crohn's disease, ciprofloxacin (Cipro) and others, such as ampicillin and cephalexin, are widely used and recommended.

If these medications prove inadequate, or if the inflammatory process is severe or associated with constitutional symptoms, a short course of steroids is often warranted. The initial dose must be high enough to induce a rapid remission; a typical starting dose of prednisone is 40 to 60 mg per day. In this respect, the approach to severe Crohn's disease is virtually the same as for ulcerative colitis, with the exception of a possibly greater role for antibiotics and for bowel rest in Crohn's disease. As an alternative to steroids in small bowel Crohn's disease, bowel rest by

*Exceeds dosage recommended by the manufacturer.

means of total parenteral or defined enteral nutrition seems to reduce the intestinal inflammation, but long-term remission is rare once a regular diet is resumed.

If a remission in Crohn's disease cannot be maintained without dependence on unacceptably high doses of steroids, antimetabolites are indicated for their steroid-sparing effect. Although not approved in the United States for this indication, 6-mercaptopurine (6-MP) (Purinethol) or azathioprine (Imuran) allow steroid withdrawal in about two-thirds of cases. The starting dose should be 1.5 mg per kg per day, which can be increased by 25 mg per day every 1 to 2 months until a dose of 2.5 mg per kg per day is reached or mild leukopenia is seen (white cell count 3500 to 4500 per mm^3), whichever occurs first. The white blood cell count should be monitored monthly or bimonthly when stable dose levels are achieved but more frequently at times of dosage increase. Other adverse drug effects include a 5% incidence of allergic reactions, which generally occur within the first few weeks of therapy. Allergies appear in the conventional form of fever, rash, or joint pain in about 2% of patients, but in another 3% manifest as an acute self-limited pancreatitis. Late development of drug-induced hepatitis (as long as several years after the start of therapy) occurs in about 1% of patients. Unusual infections have been reported in approximately 7%, but their relationship to treatment has not always been clear and none has proved fatal.

In some patients with Crohn's disease, the predominant symptoms are those of neuromotor disturbances (i.e., intestinal irritability and spasm, urgency, diarrhea) rather than of mucosal inflammation per se. In such circumstances, it is a common mistake to pursue treatment with high-potency anti-inflammatory drugs when simple symptomatic measures (e.g., antidiarrheals, tranquilizers, antispasmodics, psychoactive agents) are effective.

Two particular types of inflammatory presentation, toxic megacolon and massive hemorrhage, may require early surgery, because prolongation of ineffective medical therapy may lead to disaster. Likewise, when chronic inflammatory manifestations of pain, fever, and weight loss persist despite optimal medical therapy, surgery may be necessary. Despite the high rate of postoperative recurrence, operation in such cases is preferable to continuing an ineffective regimen of high-dose steroids or immunosuppressive drugs. Early introduction of 5-aminosalicylates or low-dose antimetabolites may reduce the incidence of recurrence.

Symptomatic inflammatory Crohn's disease of the stomach or duodenum is fortunately uncommon and may respond to antacids, H_2 blockers, or omeprazole (Prilosec). In more resistant cases, anti-inflammatory treatment with steroids or antimetabolites may be indicated.

FISTULIZING PRESENTATIONS

Fistulizing presentations encompass a wide spectrum, but for practical purposes can be classified into three principal categories.

The *innocent fistula* does not produce any major signs or complications and its mere presence therefore does not mandate any particular therapy. This category includes simple ileoileal, ileocecal, and ileosigmoid fistulas, which might not produce much diarrhea and may remain asymptomatic without any specific treatment for many years.

The *nuisance fistula* needs to be closed due to annoying symptoms or troublesome pathophysiologic consequences, but neither the complication nor the underlying bowel disease is so advanced as to compel surgery. The category includes enterovesicular, enterocutaneous, and cologastric or coloduodenal fistulas. In an effort to close a fistula or to at least reduce the associated infection, antibiotics should be the first step; metronidazole in a dose of 1 to 2 grams per day has sometimes been effective when tolerated. When single or multiple antibiotics are insufficient, immunosuppressive therapy with 6-MP or azathioprine should be used. The action of these antimetabolites is very slow, and they may need to be administered in doses up to 2.5 mg per kg per day for up to 6 months (inducing mild leukopenia) before they are declared unsuccessful. Bowel rest by means of total parenteral nutrition (TPN) may accelerate the healing process while one waits for an antimetabolite to "kick in," but TPN alone is generally a waste of time and money as reinstitution of oral intake generally leads to prompt reopening of the fistula.

More severe is the *complicated fistula*, which is associated with severe underlying bowel disease (either ulcerating inflammation or distal obstruction) or abscess. In these advanced cases, the role of medical therapy is simply to control the obstructing, inflammatory, or suppurative process before definitive surgery. The goal of surgery in these instances is evacuation of the abscess and, if not contraindicated by associated sepsis, resection of the diseased bowel.

Another form of fistulizing Crohn's disease that needs to be considered distinct from intra-abdominal disease is perianal fistulization. In the absence of an abscess, a simple or complex fistula, including rectal or vaginal fistulas, can be treated initially with metronidazole. In more refractory cases, 6-mercaptopurine may be better tolerated for longer periods than metronidazole. Early experience with cyclosporine (Sandimmune) suggests that it may be useful in treating fistulas that are refractory to all other medical therapy.

If an abscess is present, surgery is required for immediate palliation of symptoms. A localized perianal or perirectal abscess may be treated by simple incision and drainage. An intermuscular abscess is best managed by a partial interanal sphincterotomy that unroofs the intersphincteric component, which is presumed to be the focus of origin of the abscess.

In patients with perineal manifestations in association with severe proctitis, intensive medical therapy with antibiotics, topical therapy, and 6-MP, if necessary, should be given to control the proctitis. If medical therapy fails, a proctectomy may be required.

Local conservative therapy is appropriate for anal

fissures, skin tags, and hemorrhoids. Similarly, large external skin tags ("elephant ears") are usually not a cause of significant symptoms and so should be left alone to avoid the possibility of a poorly healing perineal wound. Hemorrhoidal surgery is contraindicated due to the likelihood of complications. Most anal strictures can be managed by periodic dilatation under anesthesia with a finger, endoscope, balloon, or small bougie.

FIBROSTENOTIC PRESENTATIONS

The fibrostenotic form of Crohn's disease produces bowel obstruction. Since mechanical problems demand mechanical solutions, fibrostenotic obstruction is manageable only by surgery. However, before surgery is considered inevitable, obstruction secondary to fibrostenosis must be distinguished from obstruction secondary to the inflammatory or fistulous forms of disease described previously. With fibrostenotic obstruction, signs and symptoms of inflammatory disease are usually absent. Indeed, the patient with fibrostenotic obstruction may enjoy a long period of remission before presenting with the signs of progressive intestinal obstruction.

Although the onset of partial obstructive symptoms may be abrupt, fibrostenotic Crohn's disease virtually never presents catastrophically as sudden and total bowel obstruction. Appearance of complete obstruction implies another etiology, such as adhesion or volvulus and accordingly requires emergency surgery. By contrast, obstruction due to fibrostenotic Crohn's disease almost invariably resolves spontaneously in a day or two without any specific treatment except for strictly conservative and supportive management (intravenous fluids, nothing by mouth, and intestinal tube decompression for the most advanced cases). It is almost unheard of for surgery to be required for relief of the obstructive episode itself. However, a continuing pattern of recurrent fibrostenotic obstruction indicates the need for elective surgery.

The goal of surgery in fibrostenotic Crohn's disease should be resection of the frankly obstructed segment or segments of bowel. Widespread areas or distant "skip lesions" of nonobstructing inflammatory disease should be left alone. In order to limit the extent of resection when multiple strictures are scattered extensively throughout the bowel, strictureplasty has become the preferred procedure.

MAINTENANCE OF REMISSION

Treating an acute attack of Crohn's disease is a relatively simple matter compared to the challenge of preventing relapses over the long term. Aminosalicylates seem to be of benefit in maintaining both medically and surgically induced remissions of Crohn's disease if introduced in relatively high doses (5-ASA, 2 to 4 grams per day) early in the course of the remission. Corticosteroids and cyclosporine, for all their potency in inducing acute remission in many cases, appear to be both ineffective and toxic when used for long-term maintenance therapy.

Antimetabolites, on the other hand, seem to be quite effective for long-term steroid-sparing maintenance of remissions. Specifically, continuing therapy with 6-MP or azathioprine in doses of 1.5 to 2.0 mg per kg per day help to prevent relapses in those patients whose initial remissions have already been induced with these agents. Their role in maintaining remissions when newly introduced, especially after surgery for Crohn's disease, appears promising but has yet to be established.

THE IRRITABLE BOWEL

method of
W. GRANT THOMPSON, M.D.
University of Ottawa
Ottawa, Ontario, Canada

Epidemiologic surveys in many countries suggest that 10 to 20% of adults have the symptoms of irritable bowel syndrome (IBS). The variation in prevalence is due to the use of different definitions. In the general population, females with IBS symptoms outnumber males by two to one. However, only a minority of IBS subjects consult physicians, and even fewer are referred to specialists. Females are more likely than males to seek medical attention in Western countries, yet the opposite is true in India and other underdeveloped countries. These facts suggest that issues other than the severity of the symptoms may be important in the decision to consult a doctor, thereby converting a person with IBS symptoms into a patient. It is the common experience, supported by the few available longitudinal studies, that IBS usually commences in youth and continues or recurs over many years. Some patients date the onset of their symptoms from an attack of gastroenteritis or traveler's diarrhea.

PATHOGENESIS

The variable symptoms of IBS are explained, at least in part, by disordered motility, but the exact nature of the dysfunction remains to be elucidated. Few now believe that dysmotility is the only, or even the primary, event. The most consistent physiologic observation in IBS patients is that the rectum, colon, and small bowel are hypersensitive to a variety of stimuli, such as balloon distension, emotional or physical stress, eating, hormones, and drugs. This phenomenon, however, has only been recorded in patients referred to tertiary care centers. We know less about those who are seen only in primary care or those who seek no help at all. Recent work on the enteric nervous system (ENS) and its many vagal and sympathetic connections with the central nervous system (CNS) has disclosed a myriad of ganglia, neurons, neurotransmitters, and hormones that govern the motor, secretory, and probably the immune functions of the gut. The ENS shares many characteristics with the CNS and is sometimes known as the "gut brain." Currently, many believe that IBS is due to a disturbance in the ENS, probably involving the afferent as well as the efferent connections with the brain and spinal cord. Thus signals from the gut may be misinterpreted or overinterpreted by both the ENS and the CNS, resulting in an efferent reaction and disturbed motility.

PSYCHOLOGICAL FACTORS

It was once believed that IBS was a psychosomatic disease, and certainly, a high prevalence of psychopathology has been found in patients studied by gastroenterologists and psychiatrists. However, among those nonpatients in the community fulfilling the symptom criteria for IBS, no associated psychological or personality disorder is recognized. Presumably, the situation in primary care is intermediate. The lesson is clear: life events, psychosocial stresses, or personality disorders may in many cases underlie the patient's decision to consult with or be referred to a specialist. Thus a graded response to IBS is necessary if we are to address each patient's needs. Whereas most primary care patients may respond satisfactorily to a firm diagnosis, reassurance, and dietary advice, more severely affected patients may need drugs for pain or diarrhea, while those most disabled may require more concentrated attention to psychosocial issues.

DIAGNOSIS

Symptom Criteria

With experience, a physician can diagnose IBS with a high degree of accuracy. It is not just a diagnosis of exclusion; there are identifiable symptom characteristics. The Manning criteria (Table 1) have been widely used, but recently a series of international working teams have developed the Rome criteria (Table 2). These are recommended for selection of subjects for physiologic studies or clinical trials but can also serve as a useful guide for clinical diagnosis. IBS should be distinguished from other functional bowel diseases (Table 3), or even non–bowel disorders, such as functional dyspepsia, which have other diagnostic and therapeutic imperatives. Through meticulous history taking and physical examination, the careful physician will be alert for symptoms such as bleeding, weight loss, fever, anemia and even recent onset that are not explained by IBS. Remember, in a condition that affects 15% of the population, by chance a few will have another disorder.

Relevant Investigations

Tests must be prompt, direct, and kept to a minimum. The patient should understand that the results will likely be negative so that expectations that a curable disease will be found are minimized. A complete blood count is advisable, and should be normal if only IBS is present. Sigmoidoscopy is also important, not only to exclude proctitis, perianal disease, and melanosis coli (a darkly pigmented colon due to anthraquinone laxatives), but also for its reassurance value. At sigmoidoscopy, one might observe scybala, or "sheep stools," frequently found in IBS and reproduce the patient's pain by insufflation of air, thereby adding credibility to the notion that gut symptoms can occur without structural disease.

Over the course of a career, one may see many patients with IBS symptoms. Although the symptoms are *not* those of colon cancer, a polyp or small malignancy may be coincidently present. Older patients or those with a family history of colon cancer should therefore be reassured that their colon is free of disease at the outset. This is best accomplished by an air-contrast barium enema.

For most patients the investigation should stop there. However, special circumstances may dictate special testing. In endemic areas, stools may be tested for *Giardia lamblia*. Lactose intolerance is common in non-Caucasians; a trial period on a milk-free diet is usually adequate, but some may require a lactose tolerance test or breath test. Those with a family history of inflammatory bowel disease may need a small bowel enema. Many IBS patients with pelvic pain first consult gynecologists. Symptom criteria should help identify IBS, but in doubtful cases, a pelvic examination or ultrasound may be required. Further tests are usually unnecessary. Intravenous pyelography, computed tomography, laparoscopy, and other tests are expensive, sometimes hazardous, and serve only to undermine the patient's confidence in the diagnosis. The diagnosis of IBS is a safe one, rarely requiring modification over time. Therefore repeat tests are necessary only if new clinical evidence comes to light.

TABLE 1. **The Manning Criteria**

Abdominal pain relieved by defecation
More frequent bowel movements with pain onset
Looser stools with pain onset
Abdominal distension
Mucus in the stool
Feeling of incomplete emptying after defecation

In persons with abdominal pain and altered bowel habits, two or more of these criteria support the diagnosis of the irritable bowel syndrome. The more of these criteria that are present, the more likely the IBS. However, other symptoms such as bleeding, fever, weight loss, or anemia suggest a coexistent structural disease.

From Manning AP, Thompson WG, Heaton HW, Morris AF: Towards positive diagnosis of the irritable bowel. Brit Med J 2:653–654, 1978.

TABLE 2. **Rome Diagnostic Criteria for the Irritable Bowel**

At least 3 months' continuous or recurrent symptoms of:

1. Abdominal pain or discomfort which is:
   (a) relieved with defecation,
   (b) and/or associated with a change in frequency of stool,
   (c) and/or associated with a change in consistency of stool, and
2. Two or more of the following, at least a quarter of occasions or days:
   (a) altered stool frequency,*
   (b) altered stool form (lumpy/hard or loose/watery stool),
   (c) altered stool passage (straining, urgency, or feeling of incomplete evacuation),
   (d) passage of mucus,
   (e) bloating, or feeling of abdominal distension.

*For research purposes "altered" may be defined as >3 bowel movements/day or <3 bowel movements/week.

From Thompson WG, Creed F, Drossman DA, et al: Working team report: Functional bowel disease and functional abdominal pain. Gastroenterol Int 5:75–91, 1992.

TABLE 3. **Functional Bowel Disorders**

Irritable bowel syndrome
Functional abdominal bloating
Functional constipation
Functional diarrhea
Unspecified functional bowel disorder

Adapted from Thompson WG, Creed F, Drossman DA, et al: Working team report: Functional bowel disease and functional abdominal pain. Gastroenterol 5:75–91, 1992.

MANAGEMENT STRATEGY

A Graduated Response

Most IBS clinical trials are done on patients attending tertiary care centers. However, the above discussion suggests that in primary care, or, at least on the first presentation, a firm diagnosis, reassurance, and diet and lifestyle advice are adequate treatment in most cases. Those patients with a dominant symptom, such as diarrhea or pain, may require a drug specific for that symptom. Those disabled with severe symptoms are often psychologically ill and require special measures and continuing care. The following strategy addresses these gradations in severity.

The First Clinical Encounter

It is important to arrive at a confident, positive diagnosis of IBS as soon as possible. Many patients may be frightened by the possible significance of their symptoms, and suitable reassurance can be given only if the physician is diagnostically secure. Tests should be completed promptly and not redone or added to with each visit. Assurance that no significant disease exists may be the physician's most powerful therapeutic weapon. It is also important to explain how an apparently normal bowel can generate such symptoms: an analogy to headaches may be helpful. Research indicates that time spent early on explaining the role of diet, stress, drugs, early life experience: reassuring the patient; and exploring psychosocial interactions with the somatic symptoms produces a better long-term outcome.

Point out that caffeine, alcohol, or sorbitol-containing gum and soft drinks may compound IBS symptoms. Although dietary fiber has not been consistently effective in IBS trials, it does improve constipation and even diarrhea and gives the patient a sense of control over some of the symptoms. It is also a cheap, safe means of eliciting the placebo response. A truly high-fiber diet is difficult to achieve. To convince the patient of the efficacy of fiber, I advise 1 teaspoonful of raw bran three times a day with meals. From there the dose may be titrated to achieve the desired effect. Once the stools are bulkier, softer, and more easily passed, the fiber may then be worked into the normal diet. Some patients simply continue the raw bran. For those who cannot tolerate bran, one of the plain psyllium products (Metamucil, Perdiem, Fiberall* is a more expensive substitute. Beware that some other psyllium compounds include laxatives.

Follow-Up Visit

At least one follow-up appointment should be arranged in about 6 to 8 weeks. Patients whose symtoms have improved may be instructed to work the fiber into their diet but warned that the symptoms may recur periodically. If there is no improvement, the symptoms should be reviewed, but further tests resisted unless there are new developments. Comprehension of the symptoms and compliance with treatment suggestions should be explored. Often, lack of improvement is due to insufficient fiber. No medication has proved to be universally effective in IBS, but sometimes a symptom such as diarrhea (plus incontinence) or abdominal pain may respond to a drug (Table 4). In all cases, continuing care should be assured. IBS symptoms recur, and some patients will try alternative treatments such as restrictive diets, some of which can be harmful.

*Not available in the United States.

The Difficult or Unresponsive Patient

A small number of patients will have no improvement despite the family doctor's best efforts. At this point, several referral options can be considered. If insecurity with the diagnosis is a problem for the patient or the doctor, consultation with a gastroenterologist is appropriate. Rather than perform exhaustive investigations, this specialist should carefully review the history, physical examinations, and available test results and do only what is required to exclude a complicating organic disease and gain the confidence of the patient. In most cases, the consulting physician will confirm the diagnosis and reinforce the management plan. A new, exhaustive round of tests, on the other hand, implies uncertainty (a diagnosis of exclusion) and undermines confidence in the diagnosis. It may also temporarily raise false hopes that a curable lesion will be found. The consultant must also confront the psychosocial difficulties that referred patients also suffer and support the primary care physician's efforts to deal with these.

A physician can achieve much by genuine interest and concern, discussion of the symptoms, and reassurance of their benign nature. Regular, well-

TABLE 4. **Drugs for Specific Complaints**

Indication	Drug
Diarrhea predominant/ incontinence	Loperamide (Imodium), 1–2 tabs tid, antidiarrheal, tightens anal sphincter Cholestyramine (Questran),* binds bile salts
Constipation predominant	Bran, 1 tbsp tid and adjust Psyllium, 1 tbsp tid and adjust
Gas/bloat/flatus	Simethicone Beano (α-galactosidase) with meals
Pain predominant	
Post-meal pain	Dicyclomine (Bentyl), 10–20 mg before meals
Chronic pain syndrome	Amitriptyline (Elavil),* individualized dose

*Not FDA approved for this indication.

From Drossman DA, and Thompson WG: Irritable bowel syndrome: A graduated multicomponent treatment approach. Ann Intern Med 116:1009–1016, 1992.

spaced visits facilitate this. There are a number of psychological and behavioral treatment approaches, each of which has its enthusiastic proponents, but few data support efficacy beyond the placebo response. In very disabled patients, one may consider referral for biofeedback, hypnosis, stress management, relaxation therapy, or psychotherapy, if the appropriate facilities are available in the patient's community. In all cases, however, long-term management is the responsibility of the family doctor, and the emphasis should be on improved social and employment functioning rather than cure.

Epidemiology teaches us that IBS is a common disorder, that most people with IBS symptoms do not consult doctors, and that many of those who do may have reasons other than the symptoms themselves. These reasons may include worry about serious disease, threatening life events, depression or other psychosocial difficulties. Because the cause of IBS is unknown, treatment must be empirical. The diagnosis must be confidently based upon the history, physical examination, and minimal diagnostic testing. Therapy should be graded to the patient's needs. In primary care, most patients will be satisfied and even improved with sympathetic reassurance and dietary advice stressing bulk for the constipation. At a follow-up visit, non-responders should have a case review, but no further testing without a clear indication. The symptoms, course, and treatment of IBS should be again painstakingly explained. Those with a dominant symptom may respond to a specific drug. Those who continue to complain of symptoms, are disabled, or demand treatment need continuing care by the doctor, whose aim is to restore social function rather than cure IBS. Consultation can be sought for confirmation of the diagnosis or for psychological or behavioral treatment.

HEMORRHOIDS, ANAL FISSURE, AND ANORECTAL ABSCESS AND FISTULA

method of
PETER A. CATALDO, M.D.
Wright-Patterson Air Force Base
Dayton, Ohio

An understanding of perineal anatomy is essential to properly diagnose and treat anorectal problems. The area of discussion encompasses the distal rectum, the anal canal, and the perianal spaces. The dentate line divides the rectal mucosa above (generally insensate and lined with columnar mucosa) and the anoderm below (highly sensitive due to somatic innervation provided by the inferior hemorrhoidal nerve and lined with modified squamous mucosa). The anal canal is surrounded by two muscles. The internal sphincter, innervated by the autonomic nervous system, maintains the resting anal tone and is under involuntary control. The external sphincter, innervated by somatic nerve fibers, generates the voluntary anal squeeze and is most important in maintaining anal continence.

The area surrounding the anorectum is divided into four spaces. Knowledge of these spaces is particularly important when evaluating perirectal abscesses and fistulas. The *perianal* space is a subcutaneous space between the dentate line and the superficial-most fibers of the external sphincter. The *ischiorectal* space surrounds the perianal space and extends into the fat of the buttock. The *supralevator* space is adjacent to the rectum and proximal to the levator ani, the muscle that serves as the pelvic floor. Finally, the *intersphincteric* space is the area between the internal and external sphincters within the anal canal. All these spaces may be sites for perirectal abscesses.

HISTORY AND PHYSICAL EXAMINATION

In diagnosing and treating anorectal disorders, a dedicated history and physical is essential. In most instances, the diagnosis can be predicted by the nature of the patient's reports and only needs to be confirmed at physical examination. Four areas must be investigated:

1. Pain—the character of the pain (e.g., knifelike or achy) and its relationship to bowel movements, its duration, and causative factors.
2. Bleeding—the quantity and timing of bleeding (e.g., mixed with stool, dripping into the toilet with bowel movements, or occurring between bowel movements).
3. Bowel habits—Constipation, diarrhea, incontinence, straining at stool, or change in bowel habits.
4. Masses—prolapsing masses with bowel movements, tender perianal masses, and nontender perianal masses.

Nearly all patients with anal problems dread visiting their physicians, not only because of the embarrassing nature of the problem but mostly because of the fear of physical examination. Reassurance and gentle handling are required. Explaining the details of the examination in advance alleviates the patient's anxiety. Examination in a left lateral decubitus, or Sims', position is preferred because it is more comfortable and less humiliating to the patient than lithotomy, prone, or the jackknife position.

The examination starts with visual inspection. Spreading the buttocks alone may reveal anal pathology (e.g., perianal abscess, thrombosed external hemorrhoid, prolapsing hemorrhoids). Gently everting the anoderm at the anal verge in the posterior midline often allows an anal fissure to be identified. This procedure should be followed by careful palpation of the perianal area, looking especially for abscesses. Following all of this, the digital examination can then be performed. Asking the patient to bear down in a manner similar to pushing out a bowel movement relaxes the sphincters and makes the digital examination more comfortable. Following this procedure, anoscopy can be performed (a side-viewing anoscope is best) to evaluate internal hemorrhoids. A rigid sigmoidoscopy can also be performed to examine the mucosa of the distal rectum to rule out inflammatory bowel disease.

It is important to remember that every patient does not require every aspect of the anorectal examination just described. For example, a patient with an acute anal fissure may only require visual inspection with gentle eversion of the anoderm; in this case, digital examination and anoscopy do not add information and only causes the patient discomfort.

ANAL FISSURE

An anal fissure is a tear or split in the anoderm just distal to the dentate line. The exact cause is unknown. Fissures are characterized as either acute or chronic. Not surprisingly, all chronic fissures begin as acute fissures but for various reasons remain unhealed. An acute fissure is generally caused by the mechanical force of a large, hard bowel movement being passed through an anal canal too small to accommodate safe, easy passage (although diarrhea can also cause anal fissures). These forces usually cause a split to occur in the posterior midline (90% of fissures in females and 99% of fissures in males are located posteriorly). Decreased local blood flow or increased mechanical stress may account for the propensity for these fissures to occur posteriorly.

Patients suffering from anal fissures present with characteristic reports of pain and bright red rectal bleeding associated with bowel movements. The pain may persist for several hours following each bowel movement, and it is described as a knifelike pain or tearing sensation. The bleeding is usually minor and seen mainly on the toilet tissue. Physical examination is difficult because patients experience tenderness and are fearful. It is important to provide reassurance. Often, visual inspection with gentle eversion of the anoderm in the posterior midline is all that is required. Physical findings include an approximately 1-cm split in the anoderm in the posterior midline just distal to the dentate line. In chronic fissures, the classic triad may be present: (1) hypertrophy of the anal papilla; (2) anal fissure; and (3) sentinel skin tag. Once an anal fissure has been diagnosed, further examination is very painful, unrewarding, and unnecessary. More extensive investigation can be performed after the fissure has healed.

Multiple fissures, or fissures occurring away from the anterior or posterior midline, are unusual and should raise suspicion for other problems such as inflammatory bowel disease, acquired immune deficiency syndrome (AIDS), or tuberculosis.

Acute fissures are arbitrarily defined as those present for less than 6 weeks and are treated nonoperatively. Fiber supplements, stool softeners, and generous intake of water, along with sitz baths and local anesthetic ointments, improve symptoms rapidly and usually result in complete healing. Anal suppositories are to be avoided because they are painful, and once inserted, they rest in the rectum rather than the anal canal.

Chronic fissures are fissures have been present for more than 6 weeks and are more likely to have an associated hypertrophied papilla and skin tag. They respond poorly to nonoperative treatment, although in some cases a short course of therapy similar to that for an acute fissure may be indicated. The most common surgical treatment for fissures is *lateral internal sphincterotomy.* In this procedure, the internal sphincter distal to the dentate line is cut in a lateral aspect of the anal canal. This allows for relaxation of the forces keeping the fissure from healing and results in cure in 90 to 95% of the patients.

ABSCESS

Anorectal abscesses, like abscesses elsewhere in the body, are the result of local, walled-off infections. The majority of perirectal abscesses have a cryptogenic origin. That is, they begin as infections in the anal glands that surround the anal canal and empty into the anal crypts at the dentate line. The ducts leading to and from these glands become obstructed with feces and infection secondarily develops and follows a path of least resistance, resulting in an anorectal abscess.

Abscesses are characterized as either perianal, ischiorectal, intersphincteric, or supralevator. Perianal abscesses are the most common and, together with the ischiorectal abscesses, make up greater than 90% of all perianal infections. Perianal abscesses occur in the perianal space immediately adjacent to the anal verge. Ischiorectal abscesses are larger and often more complex than their perianal counterparts, and they present as a tender buttock mass. Supralevator abscesses occur above the levator ani muscles and are exceedingly rare. Intersphincteric, or intermuscular, abscesses occur in the plane between internal and external sphincters, high within the anal canal. The location of these abscesses is important because it dictates subsequent therapy.

Regardless of their location, anorectal abscesses are associated with a constant dull perirectal ache. Accompanying symptoms may include fever, chills, and malaise. In rare cases, systemic toxicity may be evident. History reveals a gradual onset of rectal pain that has progressively increased until time of presentation. Occasionally, spontaneous drainage may have developed in which case the abscess has become decompressed and the patient will report the presence of a purulent discharge.

Again, visual inspection of the perineum often clinches the diagnosis. A fluctuant, erythematous, tender area identifies the abscess. In the rare case of supralevator or intersphincteric abscesses, there may be no external manifestations, and a tender mass on digital examination either above the anal canal, adjacent to the rectal ampulla (supralevator abscess), or within the anal canal (intersphincteric abscess) provides the only clue to diagnosis.

Treatment for anorectal abscesses, similar to abscesses elsewhere, is adequate drainage. These abscesses may be drained in either the office (or emergency room) or in the operating room. In general, simple perianal and small ischiorectal abscesses can safely be drained in the office setting. However, recurrent or complex abscesses, abscesses in immunocompromised hosts (including diabetics), and intersphincteric and supralevator abscesses should all be drained in the operating room.

When draining an abscess in the office or emergency room setting, there are several important points to remember. (1) Local anesthetic works poorly in the presence of infection (owing to acidity within the tissues) and the addition of one part sodium bicarbonate to 10 parts local anesthetic may improve effectiveness. (2) Wide drainage is far superior to minimal drainage. Making a small incision with the patient's best interest at heart does him or her a disservice and often results in the need for repeat drainage procedures. (3) Packing of anal abscess cavities is always painful and almost always unnecessary, and usually indicates that the drainage incision is too small. Following drainage, antibiotics are rarely needed and repeat packing of the wound is meddlesome. Patients should be discharged with fiber supplements and stool softeners, pain medications, and instructions for sitz baths two to three times daily.

FISTULA-IN-ANO

An anal *fistula* is a communication from the anal canal to the perianal skin found in association with 40% to 80% of anorectal abscesses. The fistula most commonly begins in a crypt at the dentate line and follows a course between the internal and external sphincters (most common location) resulting in a perianal abscess, or across the external sphincter resulting in a ischiorectal abscess, or above the sphincters leading to a supralevator abscess.

Following acute drainage of an abscess, if a fistula is present, one of three things may occur. (1) The fistula may heal spontaneously and the patient experience no further symptoms. (2) The abscess may completely heal only to recur in the future. (3) The abscess may heal leaving a chronic draining anal fistula or fistula-in-ano. Only the third scenario is discussed here. Usually following the drainage of one or more abscesses, a fistula is associated with chronic serosanquinous to seroperulent drainage. As long as the fistula remains open and draining, the patients report very little pain. But should the fistula close externally, an anorectal abscess may develop. Physical examination reveals a small BB shot–sized opening in the perianal skin with surrounding induration. Often, a fistula tract can be palpated as a firm cord running between the external opening and the anal canal.

Essentially, all chronic fistulae require surgical treatment, which consists of unroofing the entire fistula track and leaving the wound open to heal secondarily. Rarely, fistulae that course through significant amounts of sphincter muscles cannot be opened entirely or incontinence will result. These fistulae are partially opened, and the anal musculature is left intact and is encircled with a seton.

HEMORRHOIDS

Hemorrhoids are fibrovascular cushions that line the anal canal and are classically found in three locations—right anterior, right posterior, and left lateral. Contrary to popular belief, hemorrhoidal location in the anal canal has no relationship with the terminal branches of the superior hemorrhoidal artery, and pathologic hemorrhoids are not engorged perianal varices. Hemorrhoids are part of normal anal anatomy and become engorged during straining or the performance of the Valsalva maneuver as a component of the normal mechanism of fecal continence. Hemorrhoidal engorgement most likely completes the occlusion of the anal canal and prevents stool loss associated with nondefecatory straining. However, when the term hemorrhoid is used in medical literature, it almost exclusively refers to pathologic hemorrhoids and it will be used as such in the following paragraphs.

Hemorrhoids are divided between internal and external components. Internal hemorrhoids are found proximal to the dentate line, whereas external hemorrhoids occur distally. External hemorrhoids are redundant folds of perianal skin generally related to prior perianal swelling, remain asymptomatic unless they are thrombosed, and are treated entirely differently from internal hemorrhoids. Internal hemorrhoidal disease is demonstrated by two main symptoms—painless bleeding and protrusion. Pain is rarely associated with internal hemorrhoids because they originate above the dentate line in insensate rectal mucosa. The most popular etiologic theory states that hemorrhoids result from chronic straining at defecation (upright posture and heavy lifting may also contribute). This straining not only causes hemorrhoidal engorgement but also creates forces that decrease the fixation between the hemorrhoids and the rectal muscular wall. Continued straining causes further engorgement and bleeding as well as hemorrhoidal prolapse. Internal hemorrhoids are categorized into four grades based on symptoms: (I) bleeding without prolapse, (II) prolapse that spontaneously reduces, (III) prolapse requiring manual reduction, and (IV) irreducible prolapse.

Questioning often reveals a long history of constipation and straining at defecation. These patients commonly are extensive bathroom readers, spending many hours in the bathroom each week. Symptoms start with painless bleeding and may progress to anal protusion. Hemorrhoidal prolapse must be distinguished from true full-thickness rectal prolapse. The physical examination again begins with visual inspection and may reveal prolapsing hemorrhoidal tissue as a rosette of three distinct pink-purple hemorrhoidal groups. If prolapse is not present, anoscopy reveals redundant anorectal mucosa just proximal to the dentate line in the classic locations.

The majority of patients with internal hemorrhoids can be treated without surgical intervention. All patients with grade I or II hemorrhoids and most patients with grade III hemorrhoids should be treated initially with efforts to correct their constipation. Recommendations should include a high-fiber diet, liberal water intake (six to eight 8-ounce glasses of water daily), and fiber supplements such as Metamucil or Citrucel. Sitz baths are recommended for their soothing effect. Hemorrhoidal creams may be added but have never been proved effective. Suppositories should be avoided because they deliver medication to the rectum and not the anus. Patients should be instructed to avoid prolonged trips to the bathroom and all reading materials should be removed.

If these measures are not effective there are a number of nonoperative therapies available such as rubber band ligation, infrared coagulation, sclerotherapy, and others. These methods are equally effective and most successful when applied to grade I and grade II hemorrhoids, but they also cure some patients with grade III hemorrhoids. All may be performed in the office setting. Patients with grade II and grade III internal hemorrhoids that are refractory to nonoperative measures, patients with grade IV hemorrhoids, and patients with combined internal and external hemorrhoids are candidates for operative hemorrhoidectomy. Hemorrhoidectomy can be performed under local, regional, or general anesthesia, and it can be either an inpatient or an outpatient procedure. Recurrence following hemorrhoidectomy varies from 2 to 5%.

Hemorrhoids commonly flare during pregnancy, related to constipation and local effects of the gravid uterus. The majority of these patients improve dramatically following delivery. Therefore, efforts to control constipation are usually all that is required.

THROMBOSED EXTERNAL HEMORRHOIDS

External hemorrhoids are asymptomatic except when secondary thrombosis occurs. Thrombosis may be the result of defecatory straining, or it may be a random event. Patients present with acute onset of constant anal pain, and often report a sensation of sitting on a tender marble. The physical examination identifies the external thrombosis as a purple mass at the anal verge. The treatment is dependent on the patient's symptoms. In the first 48 hours following the onset of thrombosis, the pain generally increases and excision is warranted. After 48 hours, the pain is generally diminishing and expectant treatment is all that is necessary. If operative treatment is chosen, the entire thrombosed hemorrhoid should be excised under local anesthesia. Incision and evacuation of the clot are never indicated because this results in rethrombosis and worsening symptoms.

GASTRITIS

method of
ROBERT A. KOZOL, M.D.
*Veterans Affairs Medical Center
Allen Park, Michigan and
Wayne State University
Detroit, Michigan*

Gastritis refers to inflammation of the gastric mucosa. Unfortunately, there is no pathognomonic symptom complex and no gold standard imaging test for the disease. The definitive diagnosis can only be made endoscopically or by biopsy. Fortunately, gastritis is usually a mild self-limited disorder; therefore, it is not necessary to perform endoscopy on every patient suspected of having gastritis.

Patients with gastritis can be symptomatic or asymptomatic. Symptomatic patients usually present with epigastric pain (dyspepsia), while others will have anemia due to slow but steady occult blood loss in stool. Severe cases may present with hematemesis. Patients with mild disease (often due to aspirin or alcohol) will respond to over-the-counter medications such as antacids. Patients with persistent epigastric pain or dyspepsia (longer than a week) should be suspected of having an etiology other than gastritis. Additional causes of epigastric pain include pancreatitis, reflux esophagitis, and atypical angina pectoris. Patients with persistent or recurrent bouts of dyspepsia should be evaluated for gallstones (ultrasound) or peptic ulcer (endoscopy). Dyspepsia accompanied by early satiety or significant weight loss suggests gastrointestinal malignancy; the diagnosis should be ruled out by barium upper gastrointestinal series or by endoscopy (esophagogastroduodenoscopy). The latter has the potential advantage of obtaining biopsy tissue. Patients with mild to moderate dyspepsia should be evaluated endoscopically only after failure of empiric treatment (avoidance of alcohol and aspirin plus treatment with antacid or H_2 blocker). Symptoms persisting after several weeks of therapy should trigger a work-up as described. Treatment for gastritis causing dyspepsia depends on the cause of the gastritis (see further on).

Gastritis presenting with hematemesis is diagnosed by endoscopy. Patients should be hospitalized, and those with continued hematemesis or signficant hypovolemia require close observation, fluid resuscitation, and possibly blood transfusion. Regardless of the etiology, this disorder almost always responds to antacid therapy (H_2 blockers or antacids) or the mucosal protective agent sucralfate* (Table 1). It is rare that upper gastrointestinal hemorrhage from gastritis resists medical management and requires surgical intervention.

ACUTE GASTRITIS/GASTROENTERITIS

Acute gastritis due to ingestion of bacteria, virus, or toxins or to "food poisoning" may present with

*Not FDA approved for this indication.

TABLE 1. **Common Drugs Used in the Treatment of Gastritis***

Drug	Oral Dose	IV dose
Antacids	2 tablespoons qid	
Cimetidine (Tagamet)	300 mg qid or 400 mg tid	300 mg q 8 h
Famotidine (Pepcid)	40 mg hs	30 mg q 12 h
Ranitidine (Zantac)	150 mg qid	50 mg q 8 h
Sucralfate (Carafate)	1 gm qid	

*These recommendations are for active acid-peptic disease; duration of therapy varies according to clinical circumstances. Long-term maintenance dosages (for patients with proven peptic ulcer) will differ. Please consult the *Physicians' Desk Reference* for further information.

severe, often crampy, upper abdominal pain accompanied by vomiting. These patients may have fever, which is unusual with other types of gastritis. With gastroenteritis, the syndrome eventually includes significant diarrhea. These illnesses are usually self-limited, lasting from 24 hours to 3 or 4 days. In severe cases, dehydration may require hospitalization for parenteral rehydration.

ALCOHOLIC GASTRITIS

Alcoholic gastritis is commonly associated with binge drinking. If a patient presents with epigastric pain after an alcohol binge, serum amylase and lipase levels should be determined to assess for pancreatitis. If the patient is not vomiting, there is no advantage to nasogastric suction. Empirical therapy for gastritis with an H_2 blocker is appropriate, and endoscopy is unnecessary in these cases. With appropriate therapy and avoidance of alcohol, alcoholic gastritis resolves rapidly, as the gastric mucosa reconstitutes itself within 72 hours.

If the patient has hematemesis, endoscopic examination will determine whether gastritis, peptic ulcer, esophageal varices, or a Mallory-Weiss tear is the source of bleeding. If gastritis is the cause, it can be treated with H_2 blockers, antacids, or sucralfate.*

ASPIRIN AND NONSTEROIDAL ANTI-INFLAMMATORY DRUG GASTRITIS

Aspirin and nonsteroidal anti-inflammatory drugs (NSAIDs), such as ibuprofen, cause erosive gastritis via the inhibition of protective prostaglandin production and by direct toxic action on gastric mucosal cells. Risk factors for the development of gastric mucosal injury in patients taking NSAIDs or aspirin include age over 60, regular tobacco or alcohol usage, and a past history of peptic ulcer disease. As in alcoholic gastritis, patients may present with epigastric pain or hematemesis. Once the diagnosis is made, aspirin or NSAIDs should be stopped and the patient treated with an H_2 blocker,* antacids, or sucralfate.* Patients who must continue taking aspirin or NSAIDs (e.g., in severe rheumatoid arthritis) may be placed on the prostaglandin analogue misoprostol (Cytotec), 100 to 200 μg four times daily. To avoid diarrhea begin with the lower dose. Misoprostol should not be given to women in the childbearing years. Patients with gastritis who must continue NSAIDs may be given high-dose H_2 blockers plus antacids* as an alternative to misoprostol. Patients on NSAIDs are also at increased risk for the development of peptic ulcer disease.

*Not FDA approved for this indication.

HELICOBACTER PYLORI–ASSOCIATED GASTRITIS

Helicobacter pylori infection is the most common cause of gastritis. Acute infection can cause nausea, vomiting, and epigastric pain. This phase is self-limited and indistinguishable from other forms of acute gastritis, including "food poisoning." After the acute phase (2 to 5 days), symptoms often subside. Long-term infection can ensue, with infiltration of acute and chronic inflammatory cells into the gastric mucosa in response to the presence of the organism. *H. pylori* is detected by a commercially available rapid urease test of gastric mucosal biopsy tissue, or it can be diagnosed noninvasively with a urea breath test. The organism is also readily detectable histologically. Giemsa staining is best, but *H. pylori* is readily seen on hematoxylin-eosin stained tissue by pathologists familiar with the organism. *H. pylori* is detectable by culture with very good specificity but poor sensitivity; therefore, this technique is not recommended.

After the discovery of *H. pylori,* it was hoped that infection from this organism would prove to be the most common cause of nonulcer dyspepsia, and in fact 35 to 85% of patients with nonulcer dyspepsia have *H. pylori*–associated gastritis. Unfortunately, there is very poor correlation between eradication of *H. pylori* and relief of symptoms. At this time, it is not appropriate to treat every case of *H. pylori*–associated gastritis (this disorder is often present in asymptomatic persons). However, there are two situations in which treatment for *H. pylori* is indicated: (1) patients with peptic ulcer who are *H. pylori* positive, in whom treatment lowers the ulcer recurrence rate; and (2) symptomatic patients with *H. pylori*–associated gastritis in whom all other potential causes of dyspepsia have been ruled out.

H. pylori is sensitive to antibiotics and to bismuth, and combined therapy is much more successful than single-drug therapy for eradication of the organism. Acceptable therapy for eradication of *H. pylori* is bismuth subsalicylate* (Pepto-Bismol), 2 tablespoons or 2 tablets four times daily, plus amoxicillin,* 500 mg by mouth four times daily, or bismuth subsalicylate plus tetracycline,* 500 mg by mouth four times daily. Treatment should continue for 14 days. In refractory cases, metronidazole* (Flagyl), 250 mg by mouth three times a day, may be added to these regimens.

*Not FDA approved for this indication.

BILE REFLUX GASTRITIS

This disorder is most commonly seen after surgery for peptic ulcer disease. Destruction or bypass of the pyloric sphincter by pyloroplasty or gastroenterostomy results in bile reflux into the stomach in some patients. Symptomatic patients have bilious vomiting, dyspepsia, or both. The diagnosis is confirmed by endoscopy with biopsy. Endoscopically, the mucosa is often bile coated, hyperemic, and edematous. Biopsy in bile reflux gastritis reveals foveolar hyperplasia with minimal inflammatory cell infiltration.

Treatment with bile salt–binding agents such as cholestyramine (Questran) has been ineffective. The mucosal protectant sucralfate (Carafate), 1 gram four times daily, relieves symptoms in some patients. Sucralfate can be combined with a prokinetic agent such as metoclopramide (Reglan), 10 to 15 mg by mouth 30 minutes prior to each meal. If medical therapy fails, bile diversion via a Roux-en-Y bypass procedure can be performed. This can result in dramatic relief in severe cases.

STRESS GASTRITIS

Significant erosive gastritis is not a true inflammatory disorder but instead represents loss of the gastric mucosal surface epithelium accompanied by petechial hemorrhage, shallow ulcers, or both. These lesions are seen in patients suffering severe physiologic insults. Populations at risk include patients in intensive care units, those with severe burns, postoperative patients, or patients under severe stress. Endoscopically, there are scattered mucosal erosions often confined to the proximal stomach. This disorder can result in massive upper gastrointestinal hemorrhage. Prophylaxis with H_2 blockers, antacids,* or sucralfate* is now standard practice in intensive care units. Maintenance of intragastric pH above 4 prevents gastric mucosal bleeding in the majority of stressed patients. Treatment consists of control of the insult (e.g., antibiotics for infection), appropriate nutritional support, and intravenous H_2 blockers. Rarely, surgery is needed for hemorrhagic gastritis that is unresponsive to medical therapy.

PORTAL HYPERTENSIVE GASTROPATHY

Many patients with cirrhosis and portal hypertension have gastric mucosal pathology. Of patients with esophageal varices presenting with upper gastrointestinal hemorrhage, 10 to 20% will be bleeding from a gastric or duodenal mucosal source. Endoscopically, portal hypertensive gastropathy may appear as rugal edema and erythema (mosaic or snakeskin appearance) or as patchy erythema with or without cherry red spots. These endoscopic appearances are not specific for this type of gastropathy, however.

Intravenous vasopressin*† (Pitressin), 0.4 to 1.0 units per minute, may arrest hemorrhage in this condition. Patients on vasopressin must be monitored for acute cardiac arrhythmias. Rebleeding from portal hypertensive gastropathy may be prevented by treatment with propranolol* (Inderal), 20 to 160 mg by mouth twice daily. Octreotide* (Sandostatin), a somatostatin analogue, may be of benefit because it can lower azygous blood flow. Patients with recurrent hemorrhage or hemorrhage unresponsive to medical therapy may require portosystemic shunting or the relatively new TIPS (transjugular intrahepatic portal shunt) procedure.

*Not FDA approved for this indication.
†Exceeds dosage recommended by the manufacturer.

ATROPHIC GASTRITIS

Patients with this autoimmune disease have one or more of the following findings: pernicious anemia, hypergastrinemia, achlorhydria or hypochlorhydria (gastric pH consistently above 3.5), or antibodies to intrinsic factor, parietal cells, or both. Endoscopically, the gastric mucosa is flattened and pale. The diagnosis is confirmed with gastric biopsy. Histologic examination shows mucosal thinning, lymphocytic or eosinophilic infiltration, dysplasia, and/or intestinal metaplasia. The mucosal changes are most pronounced in the proximal stomach. Patients with atrophic gastritis are at increased risk for development of gastric cancer. There is no specific treatment for atrophic gastritis but patients may need parenteral vitamin B_{12} and/or iron depending on their pattern of anemia.

*Not FDA approved for this indication.

ACUTE AND CHRONIC VIRAL HEPATITIS

method of
STEVEN A. ROGERS, M.D., and
LAWRENCE S. FRIEDMAN, M.D.
Massachusetts General Hospital and Harvard Medical School
Boston, Massachusetts

The clinical spectrum of viral hepatitis is quite diverse, accounting for both acute and chronic liver disease. Of the five currently identified hepatitis viruses (A through E), all can cause acute hepatitis, whereas only hepatitis B virus (HBV), hepatitis C virus (HCV), and hepatitis D virus (HDV, delta agent) can cause chronic hepatitis. Mortality from all types of viral hepatitis is well below 1%, except for delta hepatitis, in which the mortality rate may be as high as 5%, and pregnant women with hepatitis E, in whom the mortality rate is 10 to 20%. In the majority of cases, acute viral hepatitis is a self-limited illness; approximately 85% of hospitalized patients and over 95% of outpatients recover completely and uneventfully within 3 months. Additionally, a majority of patients never develop jaundice; the illness is often interpreted as a nonspecific viral syndrome unless liver function tests and serologic tests for viral hepatitis are obtained. In a large proportion of patients, particularly children, the episode of acute hepatitis remains clinically silent. In the elderly and in those with immunologic disorders, however, acute illness can be severe or protracted.

In typical acute viral hepatitis, prodromal symptoms occur after an incubation period that varies with the viral agent (Table 1). Characteristic symptoms include malaise, anorexia, nausea, vomiting, low-grade fever, alteration in taste and smell, and right upper quadrant or epigastric discomfort. These symptoms typically last for 1 to 2 weeks and are coincident with peak elevations in the serum aminotransferase levels. When jaundice occurs, it does so as the prodromal symptoms abate. After approximately 6 to 8 weeks of symptomatic illness, the majority of patients recover fully without any residual hepatic impairment.

There are several variations to this characteristic clinical course of acute viral hepatitis. Rarely, acute hepatitis can lead to rapid hepatic deterioration associated with coagulopathy and encephalopathy, a condition known as fulminant hepatic failure. Fulminant hepatic failure can be a consequence of acute infection caused by any of the viral agents and is associated with a mortality rate of up to 80%, depending on the severity.

Another possible consequence of acute viral hepatitis B, C, or D is chronic hepatitis, which is characterized by abnormal liver function tests with or without clinical evidence of liver disease persisting for at least 6 months and associated with histologic evidence of ongoing hepatic inflammation. The probability of developing chronic hepatitis varies with the viral agent (see Table 1). Chronic viral hepatitis may be associated with a clinical course marked by relapsing episodes of acute hepatitis, persistent or progressive liver dysfunction, or an asymptomatic carrier state. Histologically, chronic hepatitis is often divided into two general types: chronic persistent hepatitis and chronic active hepatitis. *Chronic persistent hepatitis* denotes mononuclear cell inflammation limited to portal tracts without erosion of the periportal limiting plate of hepatocytes. *Chronic active hepatitis* is characterized by the presence of a mononuclear cell portal infiltrate that extends beyond the portal tracts into the adjacent periportal space and results in erosion of the limiting plate of periportal hepatocytes, so-called piecemeal necrosis.

Distinguishing chronic active from chronic persistent hepatitis has some prognostic implications. In general, chronic persistent hepatitis is usually nonprogressive; the prognosis is excellent and cirrhosis is rare. In contrast, chronic active hepatitis often progresses to cirrhosis and, in some cases, to hepatocellular carcinoma. The distinction between chronic persistent and chronic active hepatitis is not absolute, in part because percutaneous needle biopsy of the liver is associated with some degree of sampling error and in part because the course of chronic hepatitis, whether chronic persistent or chronic active, is unpredictable and variable.

ETIOLOGIC AGENTS AND DIAGNOSIS

Hepatitis A Virus

The five identified hepatitis viruses differ widely in their respective molecular structures and modes of transmission, as does the clinical course of the respective form of hepatitis (see Table 1). Hepatitis A virus (HAV) is an RNA virus that can cause acute but not chronic hepatitis. It is transmitted almost exclusively by the fecal-oral route and may be associated with outbreaks as well as sporadic cases of acute hepatitis traced to contaminated food, water, milk, and shellfish. Epidemiologic surveys suggest that acute hepatitis A is most likely to occur in the late fall and early winter. Symptoms usually appear after an incubation period of approximately 1 month. Because fecal shedding of virus has been found to be maximal during the late incubation period, patients are most infectious just before or shortly after the onset of symptoms of liver disease. The age of the infected individual influences the clinical presentation and severity of illness. In young children, especially those under the age of 2 years, acute hepatitis A is frequently asymptomatic and often passes unnoticed. On the other hand, in the majority of adults infected with HAV, the illness is symptomatic and may be associated with jaundice.

Diagnosis of acute hepatitis A is supported by serologic detection of specific viral antibodies (Table 2). Antibody to HAV (anti-HAV) of the IgM class is often detectable in serum at the time symptoms appear and is a reliable marker of acute or recent infection. The IgM anti-HAV response is typically short-lived, persisting for approximately 3 to 6 months after the onset of acute illness, rarely longer. During convalescence, anti-HAV of the IgG class becomes the predominant anti-HAV antibody. Following recovery, IgG anti-HAV persists indefinitely and signifies immunity to reinfection.

The prognosis of acute hepatitis A is excellent. With resolution of the acute infection, liver function returns to normal. In a small proportion of cases, biochemical and serologic relapse can occur weeks or occasionally months after apparent recovery. A few patients experience several such flares, but ultimate recovery is the rule. Occasional cases of acute hepatitis A are associated with profound cholestasis, mimicking biliary obstruction. Management involves supportive care during acute infection and protection of contacts who are not immune to the virus (see further on).

Hepatitis B Virus

The hepatitis B virus (HBV) is a DNA virus associated with a wide spectrum of clinical outcomes. It has long been recognized that a major route of hepatitis B viral transmission is percutaneous. Additional nonpercutaneous (or covertly percutaneous) routes that contribute to the spread of

TABLE 1. **The Hepatitis Viruses**

	Hepatitis A	Hepatitis B	Hepatitis C	Hepatitis D	Hepatitis E
Nucleic acid	RNA	DNA	RNA	RNA	RNA
Incubation period	15–45 days	30–180 days	15–160 days	21–140 days	14–63 days
Fecal-oral transmission	+ + +	–	–	?	+ + +
Percutaneous transmission	+ (rarely)	+ + +	+ + +	+ + +	?
Chronic hepatitis (frequency)	No	Yes (1–90%)*	Yes (>50–60%)	Yes	No
Fulminant hepatitis	~0.1%	<1%	<1%	Up to 17%	10–20% in pregnant women
Risk of hepatocellular carcinoma	No	Yes	Yes	?No	No

*Depends on age and immunocompetence of patient.

TABLE 2. **Common Serologic Patterns**

	Anti-HAV	HBsAg	Anti-HBs	Anti-HBc	HBeAg	Anti-HBe	Anti-HCV	Anti-HDV
Acute hepatitis A	IgM	–	–	–	–	–	–	–
Acute hepatitis B	–	+	–	IgM	+	–	–	–
Resolved hepatitis B	–	–	+	IgG	–	±	–	–
HBV vaccine response	–	–	+	–	–	–	–	–
Chronic HBV infection, high infectivity	–	+	–	IgG	+	–	–	–
Chronic HBV infection, low infectivity	–	+	–	IgG	–	+	–	–
Acute or chronic hepatitis C	–	–	–	–	–	–	+	–
Acute hepatitis D and B	–	+	–	IgM	+	–	–	+
Chronic hepatitis D and B	–	+	–	IgG	–	±	–	+

HBV are intimate (especially sexual) contact and perinatal transmission from an infected mother to her neonate at the time of or just after delivery.

Acute infection with HBV is clinically silent in up to 90% of cases, particularly when acquired early in life. In patients with acute hepatitis and jaundice, the risk of fulminant liver failure is less than 1% but significantly higher than the risk associated with HAV or HCV. Hepatitis B may also be associated with a variety of immune-complex phenomena, including arthritis, a serum sickness–like illness, polyarteritis nodosa, and glomerulonephritis.

The major risk of acute hepatitis B is progression to chronic hepatitis B, which occurs in up to 90% of acutely infected neonates or immunocompromised persons, irrespective of the presence of symptoms during acute infection, but in less than 1 to 2% of acutely infected immunocompetent adults. In patients with chronic active hepatitis B, the risk of developing cirrhosis may be as high as 25 to 40%; the delay between infection with HBV and the development of cirrhosis may be as long as 10 to 30 years or more. In addition, patients with cirrhosis caused by HBV have a substantially increased risk of developing hepatocellular carcinoma. The risk of tumor development is higher in men than in women and is largely a consequence of cirrhosis but is also related to integration of the viral genome into the host genome of infected hepatocytes.

Serologic markers of HBV infection have been well characterized (Table 2). Hepatitis B surface antigen (HBsAg) becomes detectable in the serum before the onset of acute illness and persists through early convalescence. In typical cases, as acute hepatitis resolves, HBsAg becomes undetectable and antibody to HBsAg (anti-HBs) appears in the serum. Antibody to HBsAg is a neutralizing antibody that confers lifelong immunity; it is the sole antibody produced in response to hepatitis B vaccination. Persistence of circulating HBsAg is suggestive of progression to chronic hepatitis B.

Hepatitis B core antigen (HBcAg) is a nonsecreted nucleocapsid protein contained in the inner core of the virion and usually not found freely circulating in serum. However, antibody to HBcAg (anti-HBc) usually appears in serum early in the course of infection, just after HBsAg, and persists indefinitely. During acute hepatitis B, anti-HBc of the IgM class predominates; as the infection resolves, levels gradually decline and are often undetectable within 6 months. Thereafter, anti-HBc of the IgG class predominates and remains detectable indefinitely. In a patient with acute hepatitis and HBsAg in serum, the detection of IgM anti-HBc in serum suggests acute hepatitis B, whereas the detection of IgG anti-HBc suggests chronic hepatitis B and superimposed acute hepatitis due to another agent. Rare cases of acute hepatitis B in which either HBsAg levels fall below the detection threshold of the diagnostic assay or the loss of HBsAg is not followed promptly by the appearance of anti-HBs can be diagnosed as hepatitis B by the detection of IgM anti-HBc in serum.

Another readily detectable hepatitis B serologic marker, hepatitis B e antigen (HBeAg), usually appears in the serum of patients at the same time as HBsAg. The presence of HBeAg in serum correlates with viral replication in the liver. Typically, HBeAg is detectable early in acute infection and disappears within several weeks, as acute hepatitis resolves. When HBeAg persists for more than 3 to 4 months, progression to chronic hepatitis B is likely. In chronic hepatitis B, HBeAg may remain detectable for months or even years, signifying continued active replication of the virus. In most cases, testing for HBeAg is of little value during acute infection but is useful in patients with chronic hepatitis B, in whom HBeAg is an important marker of viral replication, infectivity, and ongoing liver injury.

Antibody to HBeAg (anti-HBe) appears as HBeAg becomes undetectable in serum. The detection of anti-HBe is associated with a high likelihood of spontaneous resolution of acute infection.

In recent years, a variant of HBV has been identified, especially in Mediterranean regions, that produces a different serologic profile than that described previously. This variant form of HBV arises from a single nucleotide mutation in the pre-core region of the viral genome, which results in a premature termination signal. The consequence of this mutation is the absence of synthesis of HBeAg. Patients infected with this pre-core mutant have high serum levels of HBV DNA, despite the absence of HBeAg and presence of anti-HBe in serum. The clinical course of infection with the pre-core mutant is characterized by severe chronic hepatitis B with a rapid progression to cirrhosis and with a limited response to antiviral therapy. The mutant form of HBV may arise during the course of chronic infection by wild-type HBV. In addition, sporadic cases and outbreaks of fulminant acute hepatitis B in Israel and Japan have been attributed to the pre-core mutant.

The conventional serologic markers of hepatitis B infection described previously can be complemented by newer commercially available molecular methods to detect HBV DNA in serum. Testing for HBV DNA provides a quantitative estimate of the level of HBV replication and is more sensitive than HBeAg in detecting HBV infection. Determination of serum HBV DNA levels can also be used to identify patients likely to respond to antiviral treatment and to monitor HBV replication in response to therapy (see later discussion). Additionally, in certain situations in which the diagnosis of HBV infection may be difficult, the highly sensitive technique of polymerase chain reaction

(PCR) can be used to amplify trace quantities of HBV DNA, which would otherwise be undetectable by standard hybridization techniques.

Hepatitis C Virus

Hepatitis C virus is an RNA virus that accounts for a substantial proportion of cases previously designated non-A, non-B hepatitis. To date, HCV has been divided into at least four classes based upon nucleotide and amino acid sequencing; the various genotypes appear to differ with respect to geographic prevalence and response to antiviral therapy. Hepatitis C is often characterized by a waxing and waning pattern of serum aminotransferase elevations, high rate of chronicity following acute infection, and a propensity for progression to cirrhosis. Transmission of HCV is primarily by the percutaneous route. Hepatitis C accounts for most cases of transfusion-associated hepatitis; however, transfusion-associated cases account for only about 4% of all cases of hepatitis C. Up to 50% of cases of hepatitis C are the result of intravenous drug use, sometimes in the remote past. Perinatal and sexual transmission of HCV is thought to be uncommon but may occur when circulating levels of HCV RNA are high. The risk of sexual transmission also correlates with the duration of marriage.

Acute hepatitis C is clinically silent in approximately 95% of individuals but is associated with a high rate (at least 50 to 60%) of progression to chronic hepatitis. Moreover, patients with chronic HCV infection are at significant risk of developing cirrhosis, with a frequency of over 20% by 10 to 15 years, and such patients are at increased risk of hepatocellular carcinoma. Recently, extrahepatic complications of HCV infection have been reported to include cryoglobulinemia, Sjögren's syndrome, and autoimmune thyroiditis. The risk of fulminant liver failure in patients with HCV infection appears to be low, although the precise role of HCV in this clinical entity requires further study.

Diagnosis of HCV infection has been made possible by the development of assays that identify antibodies to specific hepatitis C viral antigens (see Table 2). The first-generation radioimmunoassay was designed to detect an antibody directed against a recombinant polypeptide called C100-3. Detection of the C100-3 antibody proved to be insensitive in diagnosing early acute infection; it appeared in serum no earlier than several weeks and often months after the onset of acute hepatitis and did not become detectable in 30 to 40% of patients with acute, self-limited hepatitis C.

A number of more sensitive, second-generation enzyme immunoassays (EIAs) for HCV have been developed. A commercially available assay incorporates a polypeptide (C200) that is a composite of C100-3 and an adjacent nonstructural protein, C33c, and another polypeptide, C22-3, a nucleocapsid core protein. Typically, antibodies against the C22-3 and C33c viral antigens are detected 30 to 90 days before anibody to C100-3 during the course of acute hepatitis C. The overall sensitivity of the second-generation assay is 10 to 20% higher than that of the first-generation assay.

The first-generation anti-HCV assay also suffered from a lack of specificity, with false-positive results occurring in some patients with elevated serum globulin levels or after prolonged storage of serum specimens. Nonspecificity is also a problem, although to a lesser extent, with second-generation EIAs. For example, among healthy blood donors with a positive second-generation anti-HCV result but normal serum aminotransferase levels, the anti-HCV result proves to be falsely positive in up to 50% of cases. Confidence in the specificity of the second-generation anti-HCV EIA can be improved with the use of a supplemental recombinant immunoblot assay (RIBA). The second-generation (RIBA-II) assay consists of a nitrocellulose strip impregnated with separate bands of recombinant viral polypeptides incorporating both first- and second-generation assay proteins (C100-3, C33c, and C22-3). The primary use of RIBA-II testing is to "confirm" positive anti-HCV results on first- and second-generation EIA testing when there is a high likelihood of a false-positive result. In particular, RIBA-II testing is useful in "confirming" positive anti-HCV results in low-risk populations, such as asymptomatic blood donors with normal serum aminotransferase levels. Additionally, in persons at high risk of having HCV infection, RIBA-II testing, like second-generation anti-HCV EIA testing, improves the sensitivity of detecting HCV infection.

The most sensitive method of diagnosing HCV infection is by polymerase chain reaction (PCR) to detect HCV RNA in serum. Use of PCR for HCV RNA is generally not necessary in routine practice but may be of particular value in immunocompromised patients with falsely negative anti-HCV EIA and RIBA-II results.

Hepatitis D Virus

Hepatitis D virus (HDV), or the delta agent, is an RNA virus that requires the helper function of HBV to cause infection; therefore, HDV infection is not encountered in the absence of HBV infection. Infection caused by HDV can occur concurrently with acute HBV infection (co-infection) or, more commonly, superimposed on chronic HBV infection (superinfection). Cases of superinfection with HDV tend to be more severe, with more rapid progression to cirrhosis than occurs in cases of chronic hepatitis B alone. In addition, HDV superinfection is associated with an increased risk of fulminant hepatic failure.

There are two distinct epidemiologic patterns of HDV transmission. In certain areas of the world, such as the Mediterranean region, where HDV is endemic, transmission usually occurs by nonpercutaneous routes, presumably by intimate contact. In nonendemic areas, such as North America and western Europe, HDV transmission is primarily through percutaneous routes and is generally confined to specific high-risk groups, namely intravenous drug users and multiply transfused hemophiliacs.

Diagnosis of hepatitis D is based on the detection of antibody to HDV (anti-HDV) in serum (see Table 2). In acute HDV/HBV coinfection, anti-HDV may be present in serum only transiently or in low titers. In HDV superinfection of a patient with chronic hepatitis B, however, anti-HDV titers are high and sustained. Prevention of HDV infection is advanced through efforts at preventing HBV infection (see further on).

Hepatitis E Virus

Hepatitis E virus (HEV) is an RNA virus that can cause acute but not chronic hepatitis. Like HAV, HEV is spread primarily by the fecal-oral route. Hepatitis E virus is an important cause of epidemic and sporadic hepatitis in parts of India, Asia, Africa, and Central America. Hepatitis caused by HEV is self-limited; there is no chronic carrier state. For unknown reasons, the mortality rate is particularly high (10 to 20%) in pregnant women. Whether this form of hepatitis occurs outside of recognized endemic areas, such as North America, and whether in North America HEV accounts for any of the sporadic cases of hepatitis not caused by HAV, HBV, or HCV remain to be determined. Specific serologic tests to diagnose HEV infection are not generally available.

PRINCIPLES OF MANAGEMENT

Acute viral hepatitis is typically a benign and self-limited illness, which in most cases can be managed on an outpatient basis. Hospitalization generally should be reserved for certain high-risk patients or for patients with severe illness. High-risk patients include the elderly, persons with immunocompromised states, and patients with underlying illnesses that may be difficult to manage in the setting of acute hepatitis. A severe course is suggested by marked prolongation of the prothrombin time (>5 seconds prolonged), encephalopathy, ascites, edema, inability to maintain adequate hydration or oral intake, hypoglycemia, or hypoalbuminemia. No specific therapy for acute viral hepatitis exists that will shorten the symptomatic phase or prevent complications from occurring. Therefore, management centers on maintenance of adequate nutrition, amelioration of symptoms, avoidance of further hepatic injury, if possible, and prevention of the spread of infection to others.

The course of acute viral hepatitis, whether uncomplicated or severe, is not altered by dietary manipulations or strict bed rest. A high-caloric diet is recommended, and because many patients experience nausea late in the day, larger meals are usually tolerated best in the morning. Exercise does not interfere with convalescence, although many patients feel better with restricted physical activity. Corticosteroid therapy has no value in acute viral hepatitis and in some cases may be hazardous. The value of corticosteroids in treating cholestatic hepatitis A, as suggested by some authorities, is unproved. Alcohol intake should be avoided, and the use of drugs associated with liver injury should be avoided or closely monitored; in general, however, oral contraceptives need not be discontinued.

The symptoms associated with acute viral hepatitis can be quite debilitating and may require pharmacologic intervention. Nausea and vomiting can be controlled by judicious use of antiemetics. Because phenothiazines can cause cholestatic hepatitis in up to 1% of patients, other agents such as trimethobenzamide (Tigan) or metoclopramide (Reglan) should be used. In patients with cholestasis and pruritus, cholestyramine (Questran), up to 1 packet in a glass of water four times a day, may give relief.

It is usually not necessary to isolate patients with acute viral hepatitis, except perhaps in the case of a patient with hepatitis A and fecal incontinence or a patient with hepatitis B or C and excessive bleeding. Although fecal shedding of virus is minimal or absent during the symptomatic phase of HAV infection, it is still prudent to recommend simple hygienic precautions to the patient, including thorough handwashing, particularly after a bowel movement. For patients with acute hepatitis B or C, caregivers should avoid direct contact with blood or other body fluids. Sexual activity should be avoided until the illness resolves; chronic HBV carriers, even those who are negative for HBeAg, should practice "safe sex."

Patients with acute viral hepatitis should be assessed for the severity of symptoms and the presence of other chronic illnesses. Generally, an office visit 2 to 3 weeks after the initial presentation is advisable in ambulatory patients. Thereafter, the frequency of follow-up visits depends on how well the patient is managing. Serum aminotransferase and bilirubin levels and the prothrombin time may need to be assessed several times a week in severely ill patients or every few weeks in stable patients. Serum aminotransferase levels are particularly helpful in detecting ongoing inflammation, but the absolute values do not correlate with the severity of disease in the acute phase of illness. The prothrombin time and serum albumin levels are good determinants of hepatocellular synthetic function. If symptoms or laboratory values of disease activity persist beyond 3 months after presentation, repeated assessments at monthly intervals are warranted. In cases of hepatitis B, HBsAg should be repeated after resolution of acute illness and then monthly, until seroconversion. Liver biopsy may be considered in patients with evidence of disease activity persisting for longer than 6 months if antiviral therapy is contemplated (see further on).

Immunoprophylaxis

To prevent spread of infection, immunoprophylaxis should be considered for contacts of patients with viral hepatitis. In the case of hepatitis A, passive immunization of all intimate (household, institutional) contacts with immune globulin in a dose of 0.02 mL per kg intramuscularly is indicated. Because immune globulin is safe and inexpensive, potential recipients need not be tested for anti-HAV before immunoprophylaxis. Passive immunization may be effective even when administered as late as 2 weeks after exposure. Generally, prophylaxis with immune globulin is not necessary for casual contacts, such as co-workers. In some areas of the world, elderly individuals are likely to be immune to HAV and may not need immune globulin.

Several vaccines derived from inactivated HAV have been shown to be highly effective in providing protection from clinically apparent disease in both adults and children and are likely to become commercially available in the near future. Guidelines for administration of HAV vaccine have not yet been established, although particular groups likely to benefit from vaccination include travelers to endemic regions, military recruits, and individuals residing in institutional settings.

Available modalities to prevent HBV infection include passive immunoprophylaxis with high-titered anti-HBs immune globulin and active immunization with the HBV vaccine (Recombivax HB, Engerix-B) (Table 3). Pre-exposure prophylaxis to prevent infection in individuals at high risk due to frequent or occupational exposure consists of three intramuscular injections (deltoid, not gluteal) of hepatitis B vaccine at 0, 1, and 6 months. High-risk individuals include health care workers exposed to blood products, dialysis patients, intravenous drug users, hemophil-

TABLE 3. **Guidelines for Immunoprophylaxis Following Percutaneous Exposure**

Status of Exposed Individual	Source of Exposure*			
	HSsAg+	*HBsAg−*	*Unknown Serologic Status*	*Anti-HCV+*
Unvaccinated	Hepatitis B immune globulin + HBV vaccine	HBV vaccine	HBV vaccine	Immune globulin
Previously vaccinated	Test for anti-HBs—if titer less than 10 ml U/mL, treat as unvaccinated	No treatment	No treatment	

**Abbreviations:* HBsAg = hepatitis B surface antigen; HBV = hepatitis B virus.

iacs, persons with a history of sexual promiscuity, and household and sexual contacts of chronic HBV carriers. Because many persons who contract HBV infection do not fall into a defined high-risk group, it is now recommended in the United States that hepatitis B vaccination be incorporated into the standard immunization program for all children, preferably before adolescence.

The currently available HBV vaccine is a genetically engineered recombinant vaccine, and the recommended dose for each injection is 10 to 20 μg for adults, 40 μg for immunosuppressed persons (the precise dose depending on the formulation). Because there is a small but significant failure rate (5 to 10%) in achieving protective antibody titers after a three-dose course of the vaccine, particularly in older recipients, anti-HBs titers should be determined in serum at approximately 1 month after the third injection if confirmation of seroconversion is considered desirable. Adverse effects from the vaccine are uncommon and are usually limited to soreness at the injection site, malaise, and occasionally low-grade fever.

For those unvaccinated individuals who are exposed to HBV, postexposure prophylaxis with hepatitis B immune globulin and the hepatitis B vaccine is recommended (see Table 3). The dose of hepatitis B immune globulin in adults is 0.06 mL per kg intramuscularly. For persons experiencing a direct inoculation, such as from a needlestick with HBsAg-positive blood or body fluids, a single dose of hepatitis B immune globulin administered as soon after exposure as possible followed by a complete course of hepatitis B vaccine beginning in the first week is recommended. The first dose of vaccine can be administered at the same time as (but at a different site from) the hepatitis B immune globulin. Similar guidelines are recommended for persons exposed by sexual contact to a patient who is a chronic HBV carrier or to an infant born to an HBsAg-positive mother. In the event that an unvaccinated individual has a percutaneous exposure to a source for which the HBV status is unknown, administration of the complete course of hepatitis B vaccine is indicated. If the exposed individual has been previously vaccinated against HBV, serum anti-HBs levels should be obtained prior to vaccination to determine if protective antibody levels are still present. An individual with an inadequate antibody level of less than 10 mIU per mL should be treated as an unvaccinated person.

Currently, there is little to offer an individual exposed to HCV that is proven to reduce the risk of transmission. Administration of immune globulin probably has no role in preventing HCV after a blood transfusion but is often advised (without proof of efficacy) in individuals who sustain percutaneous, sexual, or perinatal exposure to the virus. Generally, two intramuscular injections of 0.06 mL per kg each within the first 2 weeks is recommended.

Medical Therapy of Chronic Viral Hepatitis

The only drug approved for the treatment of chronic viral hepatitis in the United States is interferon-alpha. Interferons are a chemically heterogeneous family of proteins that have been grouped together because of similarities in structure, antiviral effects, and mechanisms of modulating the immune system. There are three different classes of interferon, referred to as alpha, beta, and gamma. Interferon-alpha is produced primarily by B lymphocytes, interferon-beta by fibroblasts, and interferon-gamma by T lymphocytes. Interferons bind to specific receptors found on a wide variety of cells and have a multitude of effects: they increase the activity of macrophages, natural killer cells, and cytotoxic T cells, which mediate the direct destruction of virus-infected cells; in addition, the interferons have specific antiviral effects, which include inhibition of viral entry into cells and reduction of viral RNA and protein synthesis.

Because of their immunomodulatory and antiviral properties, interferons have been administered in pharmacologic doses for the treatment of chronic hepatitis B and C. Most published studies have reported on trials of interferon-alpha (Table 4). Interferon-alpha in a dose of 5 million units daily given subcutaneously for 4 to 6 months induces remission in 25 to 40% of patients with chronic hepatitis B infection as compared to a spontaneous remission rate of 5 to 15% in untreated controls. Remission is defined as the loss of HBV DNA and HBeAg from serum, events that are almost invariably associated with resolution of symptoms, normalization of serum aminotransferase levels, and improvement in liver inflammation. Typically, response to interferon is heralded by an elevation, or "flare," in serum aminotransferase levels, most commonly after approximately 8 to 10 weeks of treatment. This characteristic response is thought to represent immune clearance of HBV-infected hepatocytes and generally predicts a long-term remission.

Responders to interferon-alpha may ultimately clear HBsAg from serum and develop anti-HBs, indicating resolution of infection; in one study, the apparent "cure" rate in responders was 65% at 5 years.

Several variables have been recognized that identify those patients with the greatest likelihood of responding to interferon. These include female sex, a serum alanine aminotransferase level greater than 100 units per liter, serum HBV DNA level less than 200 picograms per mL, liver histology consistent with chronic active hepatitis, onset of disease in adulthood, and absence of antibody to human immunodeficiency virus and anti-HDV. Nevertheless, in an individual case, predicting response to interferon or the occurrence of adverse effects is impossible.

Because response to interferon occurs in only a minority of patients with chronic hepatitis B, other approaches aimed at increasing the remission rate have been explored. In patients with serum aminotransferase levels of less than 100 units per liter, a tapering course of prednisone for 6 weeks prior to treatment with interferon-alpha may improve the response rate to interferon by enhancing viral replication and immune responsiveness to interferon therapy. However, use of prednisone in patients with chronic hepatitis B is fraught with hazards and may precipitate deterioration in liver function, which is occasionally fatal. Higher doses of interferon have been tried in nonresponders to standard doses but are associated with increased toxicity without a substantive increase in response rate.

Most patients experience side effects during treatment with interferon (Table 5). Common initial side effects are dose dependent and include chills, malaise, myalgia, headache, and fever. These flulike symptoms can be ameliorated by administration of acetaminophen before each dose of interferon. In most cases, symptoms do not persist beyond the first few weeks of treatment. Additional side effects of interferon include diarrhea, alopecia, lethargy, anorexia, nausea and vomiting. Adverse neuropsychiatric effects include irritability, insomnia, difficulty in concentrating, and depression; rarely, frank delirium and suicidal ideation occur. Interferon can induce autoimmune disease, including autoimmune thyroiditis, although this is less common in patients with chronic hepatitis B than in those with chronic hepatitis C.

TABLE 4. **Suggested Regimens of Interferon-alpha for Chronic Hepatitis B and C**

Hepatitis B
- 5 million units daily or 10 million units three times a week
- Treat for 4 months (? 6 months)
- Monitor serum aminotransferase, HBeAg, HBV DNA levels

Hepatitis C
- 3 million units three times a week
- Treat for 6–12 months if serum aminotransferase levels improve by 3 months and if HCV RNA is decreasing or absent
- If serum aminotransferase levels do not improve by 3 months and HCV RNA is not decreasing, consider increasing interferon dose to 5 million units three times a week for another 3 months

TABLE 5. **Side Effects of Interferon-alpha**

Constitutional	*Immunologic*
Flulike symptoms	Autoantibodies
Fever	Thyroid disease
Myalgias	*Neuropsychiatric*
Arthralgias	Decreased concentration
Headache	Depression
Fatigue	Irritability
Hematologic	
Granulocytopenia	
Leukopenia	
Thrombocytopenia	

Blood counts need to be monitored during interferon treatment, weekly for 2 to 4 weeks, then monthly. It is typical to observe a 25 to 40% reduction in peripheral granulocyte and platelet counts during interferon therapy, and occasionally profound granulocytopenia or thrombocytopenia occurs. The interferon dose should be decreased by 50% when the granulocyte count drops below 750 per mm^3 or the platelet count drops below 50,000 per mm^3. The drug should be discontinued when these counts fall below 500 per mm^3 and 30,000 per mm^3, respectively.

The decision to treat a patient with chronic hepatitis B with interferon must be individualized. The patient should be fully informed about the potential merits and shortcomings of therapy. On the one hand, interferon is a carefully tested therapy that can eradicate the virus in a minority of individuals, thereby presumably preventing the potential for progression to cirrhosis or primary liver cancer. Remission can also result in recovery from the often incapacitating symptoms of chronic viral hepatitis. On the other hand, interferon fails to produce a sustained response in most patients and can have potentially serious side effects in patients who were previously asymptomatic. Additionally, interferon-alpha is expensive, with a 6-month course of therapy costing over $1500.

Interferon therapy has also been applied to the treatment of chronic hepatitis C (see Table 4). At a dose of 3 million units three times a week for 6 months, therapy with interferon-alpha results in normalization of serum aminotransferase levels and improvement in liver histology in approximately 50% of patients with chronic hepatitis C. However, at least 50% of responders experience a relapse, often within 1 year of stopping the drug. Consequently, the long-term, sustained response rate in all individuals treated with interferon is only 15 to 25%. Few variables have been identified that predict which patients will respond to therapy. These include the absence of cirrhosis, shorter duration of infection, low pretreatment serum HCV RNA levels, and HCV genotype. Whether higher doses or more prolonged therapy will result in higher long-term remission rates is still unclear.

Because of the limitations of therapy with interferon, several other antiviral agents are actively being investigated. These include interferon-beta, the antiviral cytokine thymosin,* and nucleoside analogues such as ribavirin and lamivudine.* However, none of these is yet approved for routine use.

MALABSORPTION

method of
RONALD E. MASON, M.D., and
RALPH A. GIANNELLA, M.D.
University of Cincinnati Medical Center and Veterans Affairs Medical Center
Cincinnati, Ohio

In clinical practice, malabsorption is used as a global term to encompass all aspects of impaired digestion and absorption. More strictly speaking, *malabsorption* refers to defective mucosal absorption of nutrients, whereas *maldigestion* denotes impaired nutrient hydrolysis. These terms reflect two distinct pathophysiologic entities.

Numerous pathologic processes, congenital or acquired, can lead to malabsorption of fat, protein, carbohydrate, and specific vitamins and minerals. This chapter focuses on the diagnostic work-up, and briefly reviews the mechanisms, salient clinical and laboratory features, and general principles of management of malabsorptive disorders. It concludes with a brief description of various malabsorptive-maldigestive disorders.

CLINICAL FEATURES

The signs and symptoms of malabsorption are varied. Mild malabsorption may be asymptomatic, and the classic manifestations of flatulence, bulky, greasy, foul-smelling stools, and weight loss may not be apparent. Malabsorption should be suspected in any patient with weight loss, diarrhea, or signs and symptoms of specific vitamin or nutrient deficiency, including visual disturbances, neuropathies, anemias, osteopenic bone diseases, tetany, hemorrhagic diathesis, or infertility (i.e., manifestations of malabsorption of folate, and vitamins A, B_{12}, D, E, and K). The pathophysiologic basis for the various signs and symptoms manifest in malabsorptive disorders, and the resultant laboratory abnormalities, are listed in Table 1.

DIAGNOSTIC EVALUATION

Malabsorption can be divided into three broad categories: (1) mucosal malabsorption, (2) intraluminal maldigestion, and (3) postmucosal lymphatic obstruction. After a detailed history and physical examination, specific screening and diagnostic studies should be done to document malabsorption and to define the pathologic process responsible for the clinical syndrome.

Several important differences distinguish maldigestion produced by diseases of the pancreas or biliary tract from malabsorption caused by small intestinal disorders (Table 2). Anemia, moderate steatorrhea, hypocalcemia, and an abnormal D-xylose test are suggestive of small intestinal disease, whereas marked steatorrhea, normal serum calcium, and an abnormal bentiromide test are typical of advanced pancreatic or biliary disease. The small intestinal biopsy is usually abnormal in small intestinal disease and normal in pancreatic disease.

Clinical Tests for Malabsorption

Screening Serologic Tests

Several simple blood tests can provide clues to the presence of malabsorption (see Table 1). A complete blood count may identify anemia. A low mean cell volume (MCV) is seen in iron deficiency; whereas a high MCV can result from malabsorption of folate or vitamin B_{12}. Low serum folate concentrations are common in alcoholism, malnutrition, and intestinal malabsorptive syndromes. However, normal or high folate levels are seen in the small intestinal bacterial overgrowth syndromes. Low vitamin B_{12} levels may indicate malabsorption of vitamin B_{12} secondary to pernicious anemia, pancreatic disease, bacterial overgrowth, or small intestinal diseases involving the terminal ileum. Low levels of serum carotene suggest malabsorption of vitamin A and fat and should precipitate more definitive testing.

Fecal Fat Determination

Because the absorption of fat is a complex process requiring hepatic synthesis of bile salts, a patent bile duct, normal pancreatic digestive function, normal small intestinal enterocytes, and an unobstructed intestinal lymphatic system, malabsorption of fat is usually the most sensitive and common indicator of malabsorption. Thus, when malabsorption is suspected, the absorption of fat should be assessed.

The Sudan stain for fecal fat is a useful qualitative screening test. It is reasonably reliable when positive, but a negative stain does not rule out malabsorption. A quantitative determination of fecal fat is more accurate and reliable. Specimens are collected over a 72-hour period while the patient ingests approximately 100 grams of fat per day. Stool fat in excess of 6 grams in 24 hours indicates malabsorption.

Plain and Barium Abdominal X-Rays

Plain abdominal films may show pancreatic calcification indicating chronic pancreatitis. Barium examination of the upper gastrointestinal tract may reveal thickened intestinal folds caused by an infiltrative process (Whipple's disease, lymphoma, or amyloidosis). A narrowed terminal ileum is suggestive of Crohn's disease. Diverticula, fistulae, and surgical alterations may also be evident on these studies.

*Investigational drug in the United States.

TABLE 1. **Correlation of Clinical Manifestations, Pathophysiology, and Laboratory Findings in Malabsorptive Processes**

Signs and Symptoms	Pathophysiologic Mechanism	Laboratory Abnormalities
Gastrointestinal		
Diarrhea	Malabsorption of fat, carbohydrate, and protein; increased secretion due to crypt hyperplasia, inflammatory mediators, bile and fatty acids	Stool weight >200 g Stool weight ↓ to normal with fast Stool osmotic gap >100 mOsm/kg H_2O [Na] <60 mmol/L
Weight loss	Nutrient malabsorption, anorexia in mucosal diseases	Increased stool fat, decreased serum proteins
Flatulence, borborygmi, abdominal distention, foul-smelling stools	Bacterial fermentation of malabsorbed carbohydrates and proteins Increased flatus production	
Bulky, greasy stools	Fat malabsorption	Increased stool fat, low serum carotene
Abdominal pain	If severe, due to chronic pancreatitis; if mild, distention of bowel and inflammation	
Hematopoietic		
Anemia	Iron, pyridoxine, folate, and vitamin B_{12} deficiency	Microcytic, macrocytic, or dimorphic anemia
Hemorrhagic diathesis	Vitamin K deficiency	Prolonged prothrombin time
Musculoskeletal		
Bone pain (osteopenic bone disease)	Calcium, vitamin D, and protein malabsorption	Hypocalcemia, hypophosphatemia, increased serum alkaline phosphatase
Tetany	Calcium, magnesium, vitamin D malabsorption	Above plus hypomagnesemia
Endocrine		
Amenorrhea, infertility, impotence	Malabsorption with protein-calorie malnutrition	Low serum proteins; may have abnormalities in gonadotropin secretion
Secondary hyperparathyroidism	Probably vitamin D and calcium deficiency	Increased alkaline phosphatase, increased serum parathyroid hormone
Skin and Mucous Membranes		
Cheilosis, glossitis, stomatitis	Iron, riboflavin, niacin, folate, and vitamin B_{12} deficiency	Low serum iron, folate, and vitamin B_{12}
Purpura	Vitamin K deficiency	Prolonged prothrombin time
Follicular hyperkeratosis	Vitamin A deficiency	Low serum carotene
Scaly dermatitis or acrodermatitis	Zinc and essential fatty acid deficiency	Low serum or urinary zinc
Hyperpigmented dermatitis	Niacin deficiency	
Edema and/or ascites	Protein malabsorption or protein-losing enteropathy	Hypoalbuminemia
Nervous System		
Xerophthalmia and night blindness	Vitamin A deficiency	Decreased serum carotene
Peripheral neuropathy	Vitamin B_{12}, thiamine deficiency	Decreased serum vitamin B_{12}

Modified from Powell D: Approach to the patient with diarrhea. *In* Yamada T, Alpers DH, Owyang C, et al (eds): Textbook of Gastroenterology, vol 1. Philadelphia, JB Lippincott Co, 1991.

D-*Xylose Absorption Test*

D-Xylose is a five-carbon sugar absorbed in the jejunum. Detection of diffuse small intestinal disease can be achieved by observing decreased serum and urine levels of this sugar after ingestion of a standard 25-gram dose. However, falsely low urinary excretion can be seen in patients with small intestinal bacterial overgrowth, delayed gastric emptying, renal failure, ascites, or pleural effusions.

Pancreatic Function Tests

The "gold standard" for evaluating pancreatic function remains the secretin-CCK test, which requires duodenal intubation and pharmacologic stimulation of pancreatic and enzyme secretion with intravenously administered secretin and cholecystokinin (CCK). Bicarbonate concentrations of less than 70 mEq per liter and secretion volume below 2 mL per kg body weight are abnormal. While this remains the most sensitive test of pancreatic exocrine function, it is invasive, expensive, and not generally available. Other, simpler tests are readily available but are insensitive; abnormalities are evident only when pancreatic disease is advanced.

Bentiromide is a synthetic peptide that is cleaved by pancreatic chymotrypsin into benzoyl-L-tyrosine and para-amino benzoic acid (PABA). Free PABA is then absorbed by the intestine and the serum level and urinary excretion are measured. Less than 60% urinary excretion of PABA suggests pancreatic insufficiency. In the face of steatorrhea, a normal bentiromide test effectively excludes pancreatic insufficiency.

Breath Tests

Although bile acid breath tests (^{14}C-glycocholate) can be useful in determining bacterial overgrowth

TABLE 2. **Differential Features of Malabsorption and Maldigestion**

	Site of Involvement	
	Small Intestine	*Pancreas or Biliary Tract*
Weight loss	Marked because of associated anorexia	Mild: most patients maintain a low normal weight unless carcinoma has developed
Signs of vitamin deficiency	Smooth tongue margins and cheilitis are common	Rare unless malnutrition is present
Anemia	Frequent, often megaloblastic	Not common unless there is associated alcoholism
Steatorrhea	Moderate (20 to 35 g)	Marked (40 to 80 g)
Hypocalcemia and hypomagnesemia	Common in severe disease	Rare in chronic disease; may be seen in acute pancreatitis
Vitamin B_{12} deficiency	Present if ileal disease is severe	Rare and usually not associated with anemia
Xylose absorption	Reduced	Normal unless there is marked bacterial overgrowth
Bentiromide test	Normal	Reduced PABA release, absorption, and urinary excretion
Jejunal mucosa	Abnormal with flattening of villi and increased subepithelial inflammatory cells	Normal

From Gray G: Malabsorption and maldigestion. Scientific American 2:2, 1988.

(the radiolabeled ^{14}C-glycocholate is deconjugated by bacteria in the small bowel, leading to early detection of $^{14}CO_2$ in expired air), this test is generally not available. Hydrogen breath testing after the ingestion of 10 to 12 grams of lactulose is more readily available and is useful in the diagnosis of small intestinal bacterial overgrowth. An excessive early (1 to 2 hours) breath hydrogen peak (greater than 10 ppm above baseline values) is due to bacterial fermentation of this nonabsorbable sugar. This test does have a significant false-negative rate.

Schilling Test

The Schilling test (absorption of orally administered radioactive vitamin B_{12}) is useful in the differential diagnosis of pernicious anemia, small intestinal bacterial overgrowth, pancreatic insufficiency, and ileal disease (Table 3).

Luminal Aspiration and Mucosal Biopsy

Aspiration of jejunal contents during endoscopy can aid in diagnosing giardiasis (duodenal aspiration for trophozoites), strongyloidiasis (duodenal aspiration for larval forms), and small bowel bacterial overgrowth (see Bacterial Overgrowth Syndrome). Endoscopically guided or blind suction biopsy taken at sites distal to the duodenal ampulla may reveal characteristic morphologic lesions of specific diseases (Table 4). In some disorders, the histologic features are pathognomonic and in others are suggestive of a particular disease process. Several biopsy specimens should be taken.

In view of the large number of tests that are available to study patients suspected of having malabsorption, we suggest an algorithm (Fig. 1) to arrive at a diagnosis expeditiously. While a 72-hour fecal fat analysis is usually the most sensitive test for malabsorption, similar information can be obtained with simpler, more convenient tests, such as a Sudan stain of a stool specimen or a ^{14}C-triolein breath test. If these are abnormal, a D-xylose and small bowel barium series should be done. These often delineate small intestinal mucosal disease and also define structural lesions (strictures, diverticula, fistulas) that may be present. An abnormal D-xylose test and a normal barium study suggests either bacterial overgrowth or a specific mucosal disease and should prompt a small bowel biopsy. A normal small bowel biopsy suggests bacterial overgrowth, which can be confirmed by jejunal culture or specific breath tests. If both the D-xylose and the small bowel series are normal, pancreatic insufficiency should be considered and specific tests carried out. Finally, an abnormal small bowel series suggests a specific diagnosis, such

TABLE 3. **Schilling Test Interpretation**

Stage	Pernicious Anemia	Bacterial Overgrowth	Ileal Dysfunction	Chronic Pancreatitis
I B_{12} alone	Low	Low	Low	Low
II B_{12} + intrinsic factor	Normal	Low	Low	Low
III B_{12} + antibiotics	Low	Normal	Low	Low
IV B_{12} + pancreatic enzymes	Low	Low	Low	Normal

From Giannella RA: The small intestine. *In* Rogers AI (Ed): Medical Knowledge Self-Assessment Program in the Specialty of Gastroenterology and Hepatology. American College of Physicians. Philadelphia, 1993, p 79.

TABLE 4. **Diagnostic Reliability of Peroral Small Intestinal Biopsy**

Diagnostic histology; diffuse lesions; should be present on endoscopic biopsy	
Whipple's disease	PAS-positive lamina propria macrophages
Mycobacterium avium–intracellular	Acid-fast lamina propria macrophages
Abetalipoproteinemia	Vacuolated, lipid-laden enterocytes with normal architecture
Agammaglobulinemia	Sprue-like histology with *Giardia* or absence of plasma cells
Abnormal, but not diagnostic, histology; diffuse lesions; should be present on endoscopic biopsy	
Celiac, refractory, and tropical sprue	Varying degrees of villus atrophy and crypt hyperplasia with lamina propria inflammation
Viral enteritis	Same as mild–moderate sprue
Bacterial overgrowth	Same as mild–moderate sprue
Severe, prolonged folate and B_{12} deficiency	Same as sprue, reduced mitoses in crypts
Pericryptic eosinophilic enterocolitis	Infiltration of eosinophils and mast cells; normal villi and superficial mucosa
Diagnostic histology; patchy distribution; therefore may be missed on endoscopic biopsy	
Lymphoma	Villi widened and lamina propria filled with malignant lymphoma cells
Lymphangiectasia	Dilated lymphatics in lamina propria and submucosa
Eosinophilic enteritis	Lamina propria infiltrated with eosinophils and neutrophils; mucosa normal to flat
Mastocytosis	Lamina propria infiltrated with mast cells, eosinophils, and neutrophils; mucosa normal to flat
Amyloidosis	Amyloid in lamina propria and submucosa with Congo red stain; normal mucosa and architecture
Crohn's disease	Varying inflammation and ulceration with subepithelial granulomas
Giardiasis, coccidia, *Strongyloides*	Mucosa normal to flat; *Giardia, Cryptosporidium,* or *Strongyloides* on surfaces of villi or crypts; *Eimeria, Isospora,* or Microsporidia within enterocytes
Abnormal but not diagnostic; patchy distribution; may be missed on endoscopic biopsy	
Acute radiation enteritis, enteropathy of dermatitis herpetiformis	Sprue-like lesion of varying severity
AIDS enteropathy	Nonspecific changes, apoptosis

Abbreviations: AIDS = acquired immune deficiency syndrome; PAS = periodic acid–Schiff stain.
Modified from Powell DW: Approach to the patient with diarrhea. *In* Yamada T, Alpers DH, Owyang C, et al (eds): Textbook of Gastroenterology, vol 1. Philadelphia, JB Lippincott Co, 1991.

as Crohn's disease or surgical alterations leading to malabsorption. This sequence of tests is usually sufficient to establish the cause of malabsorption, although other tests may be indicated.

MUCOSAL MALABSORPTION

Celiac Sprue

Celiac sprue, also referred to as nontropical sprue or gluten-sensitive enteropathy, is a prototypical immunologic disease of the small intestinal mucosa. It is characterized by malabsorption of nutrients, distinctive lesions of the affected small bowel, and prompt clinical improvement following withdrawal of the antigenic stimulant found in certain grains and cereals (gluten). Histologic examination typically reveals villus atrophy, crypt hyperplasia, mononuclear infiltrates involving the lamina propria, cuboidal transformation of the normal columnar epithelial cells, and intraepithelial lymphocytes. The ileum is frequently normal, and thus vitamin B_{12} absorption is usually normal.

Clinical symptoms are determined by the severity and the proximal-distal extent of the lesions. Symptoms often manifest in childhood but may disappear and recur in adulthood. In some patients, the disease presents initially in the fifth or sixth decade of life. Gastrointestinal symptoms include diarrhea, flatulence, weight loss, and fatigue. Extra-intestinal manifestations include anemia, osteopenic bone disease, neurologic dysfunction, secondary hyperparathyroidism, and amenorrhea. The diagnosis is made by demonstrating the characteristic pathologic changes on small bowel biopsy and the response to gluten withdrawal. Various antibodies (anti-gliadin, anti-reticulin, anti-endomysium) are present in patients with celiac sprue. The diagnostic sensitivity and specificity of these antibody tests vary considerably from laboratory to laboratory. They may prompt further testing for sprue but should not replace biopsy as the essential procedure in establishing the diagnosis. These antibodies can be used to follow therapeutic responses as they decrease in titer when patients adhere to a gluten-free diet.

Therapy consists of gluten withdrawal, i.e., avoiding products containing wheat, barley, rye, or oats. A small percentage of patients relapse, most often because of dietary noncompliance. In a small group, the clinical and morphologic abnormalities do not improve despite a strict gluten-free diet. These patients may benefit from a short course of prednisone, starting with 40 mg per day with gradual reduction to 10 to 15 mg per day maintenance. Rarely azathioprine may be added to steroids with some benefit. Collagenous sprue or small bowel lymphoma should be suspected in continued nonresponders.

Dermatitis Herpetiformis

Patients with this subepidermal blistering skin disease have a celiac-like intestinal morphology and as-

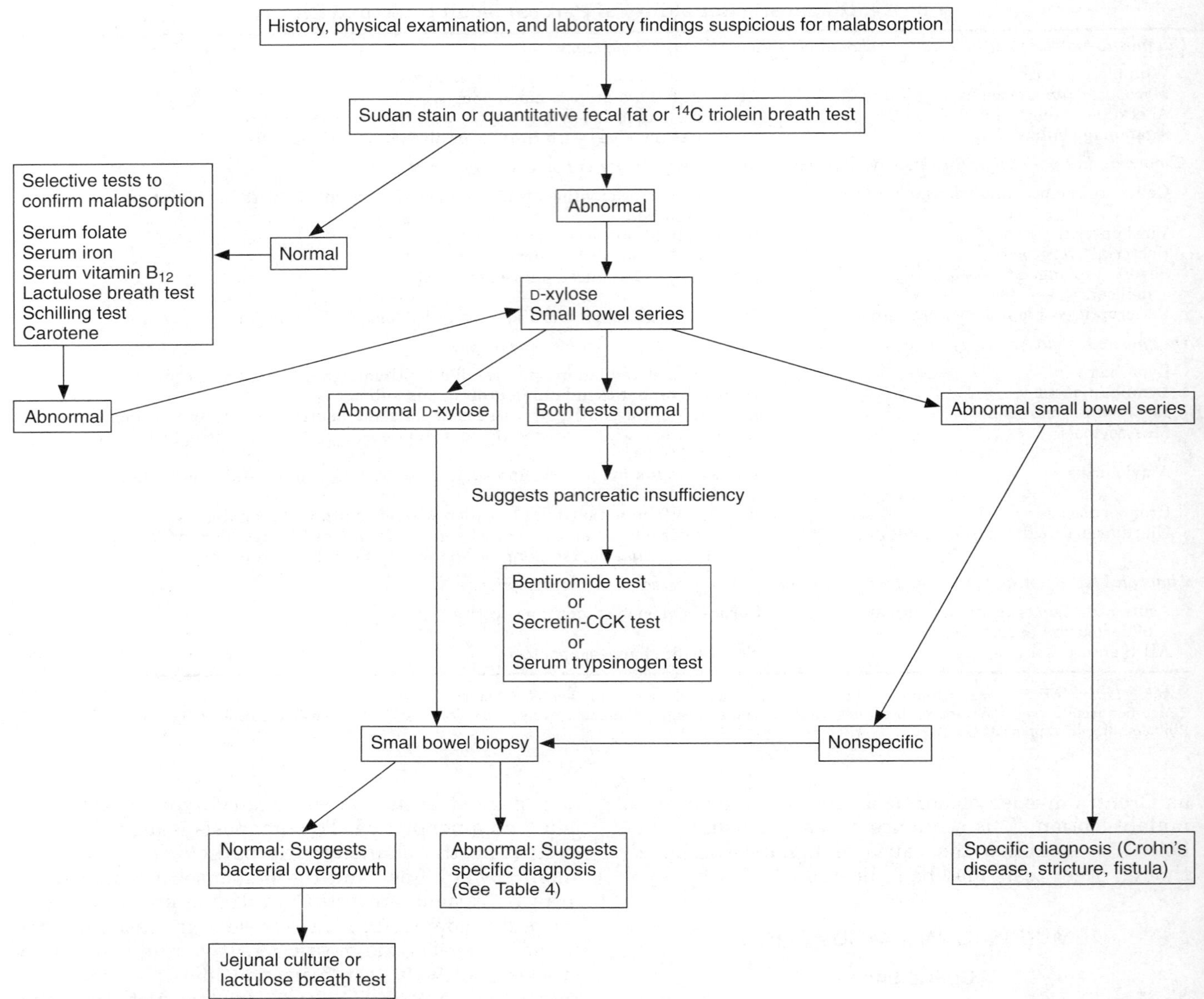

Figure 1. Algorithm for investigation of suspected malabsorption. (Modified from Levine, J.: Decision Making in Gastroenterology, 2nd ed. St. Louis, Mosby–Year Book Inc., 1992.)

sociated malabsorption. The skin lesions usually respond to dapsone, while the mucosal lesions respond to a gluten-free diet. The diet has a beneficial effect on the skin lesion, and 50% of patients will be able to stop taking dapsone.

Tropical Sprue

This disease of unknown etiology is endemic in certain tropical regions, including Puerto Rico, Cuba, Central and South America, the Far East, and Central and South Africa. It can occur in visitors residing in these areas for as little as 1 to 3 months. Its acute onset suggests an infectious agent. Most cases occur after an acute diarrheal illness and are followed by mild chronic diarrhea. The natural history of tropical sprue is variable. After 1 month, jejunal villus blunting and malabsorption occur. At 3 months, folate deficiency develops, and after 6 months anemia and clinical signs of malabsorption are apparent. Laboratory abnormalities such as folate and vitamin B_{12} deficiency, hypocholesterolemia, hypocalcemia, D-xylose malabsorption, and steatorrhea are common. A small bowel biopsy that reveals short blunted villi and a chronic inflammatory infiltrate in the lamina propria confirms the diagnosis. It is imperative to rule out other causes of chronic diarrhea, specifically giardiasis, strongyloidiasis, and coccidiosis. The illness may resolve spontaneously if the villus atrophy is mild and the patient is removed from the area of exposure.

The optimal therapy is a combination of folic acid, 5 mg by mouth per day, and tetracycline, 250 mg by mouth 4 times a day, or sulfonamides. If vitamin B_{12} deficiency is detected, treatment should include 1000 μg of this vitamin parenterally for several days, then 1000 μg intramuscularly monthly until stores are repleted. A clinical response is usually seen within 2 to 4 weeks. Native inhabitants of tropical areas may require up to 6 months of therapy, and the relapse rates are high in this population.

Whipple's Disease

This systemic infectious disease primarily involves the small intestine but can affect virtually any organ of the body. Clinical manifestations include diarrhea, malabsorption, weight loss, arthralgias, cardiac symptoms (congestive heart failure, pericarditis), lymphadenopathy, edema, and central nervous system (CNS) involvement (headache, convulsions, sensory deficits, dysarthria, deafness). Involved tissues are infiltrated with PAS-positive glycoprotein containing macrophages and small rod-shaped bacilli, *Tropheryma whippleii*. The diagnosis is established by the characteristic clubbed villi with PAS-positive macrophages in the lamina propria on small bowel biopsy. Treatment is by the administration of effective antibiotic therapy. The optimal therapeutic regimen has not been established. Initial treatment is with 1.2 million units of intramuscular procaine penicillin G plus 1 gram of intramuscular streptomycin for 2 weeks followed by trimethoprim-sulfamethoxazole (TMP-SMX [Bactrim, Septra]) double strength by mouth twice a day for 1 year. If allergy to sulfonamides is present, oral penicillin-VK, 250 mg by mouth four times a day for 1 year, can be substituted, as can chloramphenicol. Relapses can occur, and follow-up small bowel biopsy yearly for 5 years has been suggested as histologic relapse generally precedes clinical relapse. CNS relapses have a poor prognosis; hence, initial therapy should be aggressive.

Crohn's Disease

Crohn's disease is characterized by a chronic transmural inflammatory process that can involve any part of the alimentary tract from mouth to anus. It is most frequently associated with abdominal pain, diarrhea, and occasionally malabsorption. Pathogenetic mechanisms include diffuse inflammation of the small bowel, high enteric fistulas leading to intestinal blind loops, and strictures with partial or complete obstruction, all of which lead to stasis and bacterial overgrowth. Crohn's disease with extensive surgical resection, specifically of the terminal ileum, can lead to bile salt depletion and steatorrhea. Treatment should be directed at reducing inflammation with steroids (prednisone), immunosuppressive drugs (6-mercaptopurine), or both. Surgical repair of mechanical defects (stricture, fistula) may be necessary. Nutritional supplements should include vitamins (vitamins A, B_{12}, D, E, K, and folate) and minerals (calcium, magnesium, zinc). When bacterial overgrowth is suspected, metronidazole, 250 mg by mouth four times a day for 7 days, should be given.

Radiation Enteritis

Radiation in doses of 4500 to 5000 cgy can cause damage to the small intestine. Acute changes occurring immediately after irradiation include villus shortening, decreased mucosal thickness, hyperemia, edema, and extensive inflammation. Subacute changes that can occur 2 to 12 months after radiation therapy include obliterative arteriolar changes and progressive ischemia. Late changes are the direct result of ischemia, which can lead to ulceration, fibrosis, and fistula and stricture formation. Malabsorption in the first or second week of radiation therapy may be due to direct damage to ileal mucosa with reduced bile salt reabsorption. In general, these symptoms resolve shortly after completion of radiation therapy. Cholestyramine (Questran), a low-fiber diet, and antidiarrheal agents (loperamide [Imodium], atropine-diphenoxylate [Lomotil]) are generally all that is required. Malabsorption during late stages may be due to extensive ileal damage and resultant bile salt malabsorption or fistula or stricture formation with bacterial overgrowth. Management of late complications should begin with delineation of anatomic abnormalities by barium studies. Suspected bacterial overgrowth should be treated with antibiotics. Surgical correction of fistulas or strictures may be necessary. Bile salt malabsorption from ileal damage can be treated with cholestyramine. Elemental formulas and medium chain triglycerides may be beneficial. If extensive small bowel disease or damage is present, total parenteral nutrition may be required.

Infectious Diseases

Parasitic infection can cause malabsorption, particularly the protozoal *Isospora* and *Giardia* and the helminth *Strongyloides stercoralis*. These organisms are ingested and eventually adhere to the small intestinal brush border, leading to malabsorption. The mechanisms for malabsorption and diarrhea are unknown. Giardiasis can be diagnosed by microscopic examination of the stool or duodenal contents and per oral biopsy. Many patients who harbor *Giardia* are asymptomatic. Either quinacrine (Atabrine),* 100 mg by mouth three times a day for 7 days, or metronidazole (Flagyl), 250 mg by mouth three times a day for 7 days, is effective. In immunodeficient patients, longer treatment periods may be necessary. *Isospora* may also be detected with per oral intestinal biopsy and stool examination. Treatment is of questionable benefit. Trimethoprim, 160 mg, and sulfamethoxazole, 800 mg by mouth four times a day for 10 days then twice a day for 3 weeks, are recommended. For patients allergic to trimethoprim-sulfamethoxazole, furazolidone (Furoxone), 100 mg by mouth four times a day, can be used. Strongyloidiasis is best diagnosed by microscopic examination of duodenal secretions. The helminth can also be found in stool specimens

*Not available in the United States.

and duodenal biopsy. Thiabendazole (Mintezol), 25 mg per kg orally twice a day for 2 days, is effective. Therapy should be continued for 5 days or longer if disseminated disease (hyperinfection syndrome) is suspected.

Immune System Diseases

Inflammatory diseases, including systemic mastocytosis and eosinophilic gastroenteritis, are rare disorders that can lead to gross distortion of intestinal mucosa and malabsorption. Eosinophilic gastroenteritis may present with a protein-losing enteropathy. The diagnosis is best made by peroral small bowel biopsy, which reveals eosinophilic mucosal infiltration. Treatment with dietary manipulation may be beneficial in patients who report a history consistent with food intolerance. Steroids are the mainstay of therapy. Prednisone, 20 to 40 mg a day for 7 days with slow tapering toward a maintenance dose of 5 to 10 mg per day, will keep symptoms under control. There have been scattered reports of benefit with sodium cromoglycate in eosinophilic gastroenteritis and systemic mastocytosis.

Drugs

A careful drug history should be taken as a wide range of drugs can lead to malabsorption. Colchicine inhibits crypt cell division and disaccharidase activity, which can lead to malabsorption. Other drugs, such as neomycin, methotrexate, laxatives, cholestyramine, and alcohol, can cause malabsorption by a variety of mechanisms, including enterocyte damage and binding of bile salts. Malabsorption disappears with discontinuation of the drug.

Abetalipoproteinemia

Abetalipoproteinemia is a rare congenital autosomal recessive disorder that manifests in childhood as anorexia, malabsorption, and failure to thrive. The absence of apoprotein B, which is essential for chylomicron formation and transport, leads to engorgement of epithelial cells with lipid droplets. Spinocerebellar degeneration, retinitis pigmentosa, and red cell acanthosis are secondary to cell membrane abnormalities seen in apoprotein-B deficiency. The diagnosis rests on small bowel biopsy revealing lipid-laden epithelial cells and very low triglyceride and cholesterol levels in serum. Treatment includes low-fat diet, fat-soluble vitamin supplementation, and medium-chain triglycerides, which are absorbed into plasma without lipoprotein formation.

Alpha Heavy Chain Disease

Alpha heavy chain disease is characterized by plasma cell infiltration of the lamina propria of the small intestine and malabsorption. It is an immunoproliferative B cell disorder seen in patients from the Mediterranean region and the Middle East. In some instances, malabsorption and weight loss have remitted with antibiotic therapy, particularly tetracycline. Whether this is due to treatment of coexistent bacterial overgrowth or parasitic infection with *Giardia* is unknown.

Idiopathic Diffuse Ulcerative Nongranulomatous Enteritis

Idiopathic chronic ulcerative jejunoileitis, or unclassified sprue, is a disease whose pathogenesis is unknown. Gluten sensitivity does not seem to play a role in causing the flattened jejunal mucosa. Gluten withdrawal and steroids have not altered the course of the disease. The clinical picture is one of severe malabsorption and protein-losing enteropathy. Most of the patients have died within 1 or 2 years after recognition of intestinal ulceration. Some patients may develop lymphoma. Chemotherapy and radiation may be of benefit in some.

INTRALUMINAL MALDIGESTION

Chronic Liver Disease and Bile Duct Obstruction

Biliary duct obstruction from cholangiocarcinoma and cancer in the head of the pancreas can cause steatorrhea, presumably through bile salt insufficiency and pancreatic lipase deficiency, respectively. Mild steatorrhea and malabsorption can develop in cirrhosis and other parenchymal liver diseases owing to inadequate micelle formation secondary to bile salt deficiency. In most forms of chronic liver disease and malignancies, weight loss is usually multifactorial. Treatment is directed at relieving the bile duct obstruction and improving the liver disease.

Bacterial Overgrowth Syndrome

Bacterial overgrowth is characterized by diarrhea, steatorrhea, and frequently macrocytic anemia. This syndrome results from proliferation of aerobic and anaerobic bacteria along the length of the small intestine. Lesions predisposing to bacterial overgrowth include motor or structural abnormalities of the small intestine that result in intestinal stasis. Ingested bacteria colonize and proliferate to reach populations of 10^6 to 10^9 organisms per mL. Structural disorders that predispose to bacterial overgrowth include Billroth II anastomosis (stasis in afferent limb), multiple jejunal diverticula, enteroenteric fistula, intestinal stricture, and anastomosis with bypassed segments of intestine (jejunoileal bypass). Predisposing motility disorders include intestinal scleroderma, idiopathic pseudo-obstruction, and diabetic enteropathy.

The two primary manifestations of this disorder, macrocytic anemia and steatorrhea, are a direct consequence of bacterial metabolic activity. Consumption of vitamin B_{12} by the bacteria leads to depletion and deficiency. Steatorrhea occurs because anaerobic bacteria deconjugate bile salts, rendering them inefficient detergents for emulsification and absorption of fat. The diagnosis should be suspected in patients with diarrhea, malnutrition, malabsorption, macrocytic anemia, vitamin B_{12} deficiency, or increased serum folate concentrations.

The gold standard for diagnosis is the demonstration of increased levels of bacteria in the lumen of the proximal small intestine. Quantitation of total aerobic and anaerobic flora (greater than 10^6 colony counts per mL) by small bowel aspirate confirms bacterial overgrowth. Various hydrogen breath tests (lactulose, glucose) are also available for diagnostic purposes. An early peak (1 to 2 hours) in breath hydrogen excretion following ingestion of the sugar is highly suggestive.

Treatment should be supportive, and specific drug therapy employs broad-spectrum antibiotics (tetracycline, 250 mg orally four times a day for 7 days, or metronidazole, 250 mg a day for 7 days). Repeated courses of antibiotics may be required if relapses occur. If a correctable anatomic lesion is found (Billroth II anastomosis with an afferent blind limb, intestinal stricture, or enteroenteric anastomosis with bypassed small intestine), surgical resection and reconstruction should be considered.

Pancreatic Exocrine Insufficiency

Chronic alcoholism is by far the most common cause of chronic pancreatitis in the Western world. Other etiologies include tropical-nutritional pancreatitis, inherited pancreatitis, hypertriglyceridemia, hypercalcemia, idiopathic pancreatitis, and benign or neoplastic pancreatic obstruction. When at least 90% of the secretory capacity is lost, chronic pancreatic exocrine insufficiency supervenes and diarrhea, malabsorption, and weight loss develop. Treatment consists of oral pancreatic enzyme therapy (Viokase, Ilozyme, Cotazym). To eliminate malabsorption, the concentration of enzymes delivered to the duodenum need only be 5 to 10% of the concentration secreted by a maximally stimulated pancreas. This means that 30,000 units of lipase must be present in the duodenum with each meal. The best commercial preparations contain only 3000 to 4000 units of lipase per tablet, therefore 6 to 10 tablets per meal are needed to eliminate steatorrhea. If the patient fails to improve, gastric acidity may be destroying the enzymes; this can be avoided by co-administration of H_2 antagonists. Alternatively, enteric coated enzyme preparations (Pancrease, Creon, Entolase) can be utilized.

Zollinger-Ellison Syndrome

Zollinger-Ellison Syndrome (ZES) results from a gastrin-secreting tumor causing increased output of highly acidic gastric juice. The increased acid neutralizes the bicarbonate and inactivates the pancreatic enzymes secreted into the duodenum and damages the small intestinal mucosa. The resulting diarrhea is complicated by malabsorption and bile salt–fatty acid stimulated colonic secretion. A fasting gastrin level of greater than 1000 picograms per mL in the presence of gastric acidity is virtually diagnostic of ZES. Lower levels of hypergastrinemia may require provocative testing with intravenous secretin. The two goals of management are control of acid hypersecretion and removal of tumors. If patients cannot be cured surgically, medical therapy with omeprazole (Prilosec), a proton-pump inhibitor, is the treatment of choice. Twenty to 120 mg daily may be necessary for adequate acid reduction and amelioration of diarrhea and acid-induced diarrhea/malabsorption.

POSTMUCOSAL OBSTRUCTION

Intestinal Lymphangiectasia

Intestinal lymphangiectasia is either a congenital or an acquired (cardiac disease, Whipple's disease, Crohn's disease, mesenteric tuberculosis and sarcoid, lymphoma and retroperitoneal fibrosis) disease that causes protein-losing enteropathy and steatorrhea. Obstructed lymphatic channels are unable to absorb fat. Carbohydrate absorption is usually unaffected. Clinical manifestations include peripheral edema, chylous ascites, protein loss, and steatorrhea. Diagnosis should be suspected in patients with classic physical findings, lymphocytopenia, and peritoneal or pleural fluid with triglyceride elevations. Lymphangiography may show hypoplastic lymph vessels with gut extravasation in secondary disease. Treatment aims at correcting the underlying disease responsible for the protein-losing enteropathy. Medium chain triglycerides, which do not require intestinal lymphatic transport, can reduce enteric protein and fat loss. A low-fat diet should also be instituted.

Lymphoma

Lymphomas are most common in the ileum and can be either a primary small intestinal process or part of a disseminated lymphomatous process. Intestinal lymphomas can complicate celiac disease or chronic immunosuppression in organ transplant patients. Clinical manifestations include severe abdominal pain, weight loss, fever, diarrhea, and malabsorption. The diagnosis is very difficult to make. It should be suspected in patients with nonresponsive celiac disease, intestinal perforation complicating celiac disease, or in a setting of a malabsorptive disorder with a diffuse abnormality seen on small bowel barium study. The diagnosis can sometimes be made by small bowel biopsy but frequently requires an exploratory laparotomy with a full-thickness intestinal biopsy. Radiation and chemotherapy may be of some benefit.

MIXED CAUSES OF MALABSORPTION

Short Bowel Syndrome

The short bowel syndrome is a malabsorption syndrome that results from extensive intestinal resec-

TABLE 5. **Systemic Diseases Associated with Malabsorption**

Diseases	Mechanisms
Thyrotoxicosis	Hyperphagia and rapid transit; minor mucosal changes
Hypothyroidism	Variable villus atrophy; pancreatic insufficiency
Addison's disease	Unclear
Hypoparathyroidism	Minor mucosal changes; occasional monilial infection
Diabetes mellitus	Pancreatic insufficiency; autonomic neuropathy and bacterial overgrowth
SLE, PAN, vasculitis	Variable villus atrophy
Rheumatoid arthritis	Amyloidosis
Systemic sclerosis	Bacterial overgrowth and lymphatic obstruction
Extraintestinal malignant disease	Unknown

Abbreviations: SLE = systemic lupus erythematosus: PAN = polyarteritis nodosa.

Modified from Riley SA, Turnberg LA: Maldigestion and malabsorption. *In* Sleisenger MH, Fordtran JS (eds): Gastrointestinal Disease. 5th ed. Philadelphia, WB Saunders Co, 1992.

tion, usually as a consequence of intestinal gangrene due to vascular accidents (e.g., superior mesenteric artery thrombosis or embolism, superior mesenteric venous thrombosis, or profound low flow states such as chronic congestive heart failure), strangulated hernias, prolonged intestinal obstruction, repeated intestinal resection in Crohn's disease, and jejunoileal bypass for obesity. The severity of malabsorption depends on five factors: (1) extent of resection, (2) site of resection (ileum, jejunum, colon), (3) presence or absence of the ileocecal valve, (4) adaptation of the remaining intestine, and (5) extent of residual disease in retained bowel. Patients who have lost more than 70% of their small bowel generally require total parenteral nutrition for survival. Removal of 50 to 100 cm of terminal ileum may lead to mild bile salt malabsorption and diarrhea (bile salt diarrhea), whereas removal of more than 100 cm of ileum leads to severe bile salt malabsorption, bile salt depletion, and steatorrhea (fatty acid diarrhea). If the ileocecal valve is sacrificed, bacterial overgrowth can occur and contribute to malabsorption. With limited ileal resection, malabsorption is minimal and inconsequential, and cholestyramine, 2 to 4 grams orally three times a day, is effective in controlling diarrhea. If the terminal ileum has been resected, vitamin B_{12}, 1000 μg intramuscularly, should be given monthly. Extensive ileal resection is more difficult to manage. If fat malabsorption has been documented, dietary fat reduction to 30 to 40 grams per day is necessary: medium chain triglycerides can also be utilized. Fat-soluble vitamin, calcium (1500 mg per day), and magnesium supplements should be given. A low-oxalate diet may help to prevent kidney stone formation. Some patients may only benefit from home total parenteral nutrition with adequate vitamin and mineral supplementation.

Systemic Diseases

Diseases such as thyrotoxicosis, adrenal insufficiency, and protein-calorie malnutrition can result in malabsorption. Thyrotoxicosis causes a decrease in intestinal transit time; adrenal insufficiency disturbs intraluminal and mucosal absorption as does protein-calorie malnutrition. Other systemic illnesses have also been associated with malabsorption (Table 5).

Malabsorption and the Acquired Immune Deficiency Syndrome (AIDS)

AIDS is a major cause of gastrointestinal symptoms, particularly diarrhea. Almost 50% of AIDS patients develop diarrhea, weight loss, and malabsorption when the CD4 count is less than 50 cells per mm^3. An infectious agent (*Giardia*, mycobacteria, cytomegalovirus, cryptosporidia, microsporidia, and *Isospora*) can be identified in 60 to 70% of these patients. Malabsorption is mild but can contribute to the morbidity of AIDS patients when it occurs in combination with anorexia, fever, and systemic infections.

Treatment is usually unsatisfactory because an infectious agent often can neither be identified nor eradicated by antibiotic therapy. Symptomatic therapy includes antidiarrheals (diphenoxylate-atropine and loperamide) and octreotide (Sandostatin) at doses of 50 to 500 μg subcutaneously every 8 hours. AIDS enteropathy may improve with zidovudine (Retrovir).

ACUTE PANCREATITIS

method of
SCOTT M. BERRY, M.D.
University of Cincinnati Medical Center
Cincinnati, Ohio

and

AARON S. FINK, M.D.
Emory University Medical Center and Atlanta Veterans Affairs Medical Center
Atlanta, Georgia

Pancreatitis results from a diffuse array of insults: metabolic disorders, structural abnormalities, exogenous chemicals, and trauma have all been implicated in this disease process. Symptomatology ranges from imperceptible to severe and is often defined not by the underlying disease process but rather by the severity of the pancreatic inflammation. Certain causes may predispose to more severe forms of the disease. However, once incited, pancreatic inflammation can rapidly lead to fulminant multiple organ system failure and death, regardless of the etiology.

Many papers have discussed the management of acute pancreatitis. Given the previous lack of a clinically based classification system, however, comparison of results is difficult, if not impossible. Another confusing factor is the paucity of research models that accurately reflect the pathophysiology operative during pancreatitis: While multiple acute pancreatitis models exist, their clinical course may vary widely. Therefore, study results must always be interpreted with respect to the particular model used, as findings may or may not be applicable to the human situation. Although pain is usually the most prominent presenting symptom, its origin remains obscure. Thus, even the most basic questions about pancreatitis persist.

With such a broad range of etiologies, presentations, and clinical courses, formulating a treatment plan can be difficult. Fortunately, certain principles apply to the management of all cases. Described herein is the format we have found useful for planning management: recognition, resuscitation, evaluation, classification and treatment, and complications.

RECOGNITION

Recognizing pancreatitis solely on clinical grounds may be exceedingly difficult. Sudden, constant aching abdominal pain in the left upper quadrant, midepigastrium, left flank, or back is the most common presentation. However, the pain can be perceived as pleural, cardiac, scapular, or periumbilical. The patient will occasionally report pain radiating straight through to the back, and this subjective symptom is very suggestive of acute pancreatic inflammation, but it is not invariably present and certainly is not necessary to entertain the diagnosis. Patients may experience pain relief by assuming a forward sitting position or the fetal position, although many are unable to obtain relief in any position. Nausea is also common and may or may not be accompanied by emesis. The emesis is thought to be in response to the pain, rather than mechanical duodenal obstruction; like most reflexive retching, it usually produces little volume. Anorexia is invariably present in the early phases of pancreatitis and may contribute to the severe dehydration often present in these patients. Objective signs include tachypnea, tachycardia, and often hypotension. Mild to moderate (100°–101.5° F) fever is usually present. When temperatures exceed this range, either a complication of pancreatitis has occurred (e.g., necrosis) or comorbid conditions exist (e.g., pneumonia, urinary tract infection).

Although the physical findings of acute pancreatitis seldom suggest the etiology, some useful clues may be obtained from the physical examination. Icterus or excoriations from scratching suggest common duct obstruction; xanthomas around the eyes or a corneal arcus suggests hyperlipidemia; band keratopathy suggests hypercalcemia. Testicular atrophy, hypothenar wasting, gynecomastia, spider angiomata, and hepatomegaly may all be present with alcoholism. Finally, when Grey Turner's or Cullen's sign is present, a particularly severe hemorrhagic pancreatitis is evolving.

Abdominal findings range from a silent, tender abdomen, to board-like rigidity. Epigastric fullness is seldom discovered on physical examination unless the patient has a preexisting pseudocyst. However, it is unusual for a patient to permit such deep palpation early during the acute attack. Decreased breath sounds with dullness on percussion may occur over the left lower chest if sympathetic effusion is present. Alternatively, if pancreatitis is severe and if there is a pancreatic ductal disruption, these findings may indicate a pancreatopleural fistula.

Pancreatitis should be considered in any patient with complaints that involve the area between the nipples and the knees. The diagnosis usually rests on the demonstration of serum hyperamylasemia. Serum amylase is very sensitive (85%), but not specific, for pancreatitis. Other causes of hyperamylasemia (Table 1) should be excluded. Often, the patient's history coupled with a thorough physical examination will distinguish causes of hyperamylasemia.

TABLE 1. **Common Nonpancreatic Causes of Hyperamylasemia**

Macroamylasemia	Ischemic bowel
Renal failure	Small bowel obstruction
Diabetic ketoacidosis	Ectopic pregnancy
Perforated duodenal ulcer	Mumps

After the history and physical examination, a complete blood count (CBC); coagulation profile (prothrombin time, partial thromboplastin time); renal profile; measurements of liver enzymes, lactate dehydrogenase (LDH), serum amylase, calcium, phosphorus, magnesium, and beta-human chorionic gonadotropin (beta-hCG) (in all women with abdominal pain); urinalysis; arterial blood gas analysis; and 12-lead electrocardiogram are obtained. All women with a negative beta-hCG and all men should have chest and abdominal radiographs. This battery of tests not only helps to document pancreatitis and determine its severity (see further on) but also helps to rule out other causes of abdominal pain and hyperamylasemia (Table 1). It must be remembered that amylase can be normal in as many as 20% of cases. When doubt still exists, a serum lipase assay can be obtained, which increases diagnostic sensitivity to 95% when combined with serum amylase measurement. Lipase is not useful as the sole initial screening test because its sensitivity is less than that of serum amylase. However, when clinical suspicion is high and amylase is normal, lipase's specificity will allow definitive diagnosis in two-thirds of equivocal, normoamylasemic cases.

Other diagnostic tests that may be helpful include ultrasound, computed tomography, and abdominal exploration. Although an inflamed, edematous, or hemorrhagic pancreas can be accurately diagnosed by any of these means, none is appropriate as an initial screening test. However, they may all prove necessary when the diagnosis is in question and misdiagnosis will likely result in mortality (e.g., ischemic bowel).

RESUSCITATION

Volume deficits become more profound as the pancreatitis worsens. In general, resuscitation should proceed with balanced salt solutions such as normal saline. Potassium-containing fluids should be avoided until adequate urine output is established and renal filtering capabilities are documented by a renal chemistry profile. In the acute setting, glucose-containing fluids should also be avoided as electrolyte abnormalities may be worsened without appreciable metabolic benefit. Similarly, so long as the acidosis does not impair cardiac function, we withhold bicarbonate-containing fluids since the acidosis is usually due to hypoperfusion. Correction of the acidosis by hydration can be used as a clinical marker of adequate resuscitation.

Colloid resuscitation with albumin, hetastarch, or fresh-frozen plasma provides no benefit over adequate balanced salt solution resuscitation. While resuscitation with salt solutions requires approximately three times the volume required with colloid, the latter's theoretical benefit of retaining volume in the intravascular space by improving plasma oncotic pressure has never been proved. Furthermore, in the absence of adequate nutritional repletion, exogenously administered albumin is rapidly metabolized, making its serum half-life too short to realize oncotic benefit. In addition to increased expense, albumin may be detrimental to the pulmonary parenchyma should pulmonary capillary leak occur.

Upon presentation, all patients with pancreatitis should be placed on nothing-by-mouth (NPO) status. Because these patients are anorectic and nauseated, this is usually not a problem. Proscribing oral intake not only provides a margin of safety should emergency procedures be necessary, but also expedites the work-up, as many tests require NPO status. Hyperdynamic starvation leads to severe, additive nutritional deficits each day the patient is without adequate nutrition. Thus, some form of nutritional therapy should be initiated as soon as feasible and safe (see later). It is seldom necessary, and may be unwise, to do this within the first 48 hours after presentation, however. Permitting time to pass allows preliminary determination of disease severity, which, in turn, may then dictate the most appropriate form of nutritional support.

Nasogastric suction is not required for every patient with pancreatitis. No study has shown that gastric decompression lessens the severity or shortens the clinical course of pancreatitis. In general, a nasogastric decompression tube should be used symptomatically. If the patient is vomiting or has persistent nausea, nasogastric intubation may provide considerable relief. This measure is particularly helpful in "severe" attacks.

The decision to place a urinary catheter to monitor volume resuscitation depends upon disease severity and the initial response to volume challenge. In the absence of co-morbid conditions, urinary output is the most reliable means of evaluating resuscitative efforts. If the pancreatitis appears mild and the patient responds rapidly to a small resuscitative volume (500 mL), urinary catheterization may be unnecessary. However, this is often the exception. Because volume deficits can develop rapidly and be severe, urinary output should initially be monitored every 1 to 2 hours.

When pancreatitis is severe and/or co-morbid conditions exist (e.g., renal failure, congestive heart failure), Swan-Ganz hemodynamic monitoring may become necessary. The high volumes required for resuscitation coupled with pancreatitis-induced pulmonary changes make physical and radiographic evaluation of interstitial pulmonary edema unreliable. Pulmonary capillary wedge pressures will differentiate pulmonary edema from pulmonary changes secondary to pancreatitis and allow optimal hemodynamic resuscitation.

Antibiotics are indicated only for severe necrotizing pancreatitis and as an adjunct during surgical intervention for established infectious complications (e.g., infected pseudocyst, pancreatic abscess). Other patients should be treated with antibiotics as co-morbid conditions dictate (e.g., urinary tract infection, pneumonia).

All metabolically stressed, fasting patients should be placed on an ulcer prophylaxis regimen. This practice not only helps to decrease stress gastritis/ulceration, but may also decrease pancreatic stimulation evoked by acid-induced secretin release. Maintaining the gastric pH above 4 should decrease pancreatic stimulation from this mechanism. However, what effect the elevated gastrin levels, which occur with H_2 receptor antagonist or H^+-K^+ pump inhibitor therapies, have on pancreatic stimulation is unknown.

The pain associated with acute pancreatitis is rarely relieved by mild analgesics. Pain is often particularly difficult to manage in alcoholic pancreatitis due to the combination of severe visceral pain and high narcotic tolerance. Because morphine has been shown to increase common bile duct pressure and biliary sphincter pressure, use of parenteral nonsteroidals, such as ketorolac (Toradol), or opioid-like analgesics that do not affect sphincter pressure (e.g., meperidine, [Demerol], buprenorphine [Buprenex], tramadol* [Crispin]) should be considered. Frequently, however, these measures prove inadequate, and ancillary measures may be necessary.

When the serum amylase level is normal and their pain has abated, patients can be started on clear liquids. After this, the patient is put on a low-fat diet without the intermediate step of full liquids. Although nutritive, full-liquid diets consist of heavy creams and soups that are maximally stimulatory to pancreatic and biliary secretions. There will be patients, especially those with alcohol-induced pancreatitis or small stable pseudocysts, whose amylase levels will never completely normalize and whose pain may not subside. They can be judiciously fed throughout their pain or hyperamylasemia, provided their clinical status does not worsen. As the diet is advanced, the patient's clinical status and serum amylase should be followed daily. If either worsens significantly, the patient's diet is downgraded stepwise until relief is obtained.

EVALUATION

Clinical parameters that assist the clinician in determining the severity of disease are necessary for planning diagnostic evaluation and treatment course. The most popular set of criteria is that established by Ranson (Table 2). After evaluating over 400 factors, he discovered 11 criteria, five determined on admission and six determined up to 48 hours after admission, that correlate with mortality in pancreatitis patients. When less than three criteria are present, mortality is around 1%; when three to seven are present, mortality is 15%, with 50% of patients requiring admission to the intensive care unit (ICU); when more than seven criteria are present, mortality is 50% and virtually all patients require ICU admission. The initial criteria sensitize the physician to the severity of disease, while the 48-hour criteria define remote organ system involvement. If 48 hours have elapsed before the diagnosis of pancreatitis is made or if pancreatitis persists for longer than 48 hours, Ranson's criteria may no longer be useful for prognostication and for guiding therapy. In these cases, APACHE II scores or CT evaluation may have greater diagnostic and therapeutic utility.

*Investigational drug in the United States.

TABLE 2. **Ranson's Criteria**

On Admission	Within 48 Hours of Admission
Age >55	≥6 L volume requirement
Blood sugar >200 mg/dL	BUN increase >5 mg/dL
LDH >350 IU/L	PaO_2 <60 mmHg
SGOT (AST) >250 U/L	HCT decrease by ≥10%
WBC >16,000/mm^3	Base deficit >4 mEq/L
	Serum calcium <8 mg/dL

<3 criteria: 1% mortality
3–7 criteria: 15% mortality and 50% require ICU admission
>7 criteria: 50% mortality and virtually all require ICU admission

Abbreviations: LDH = lactate dehydrogenase; SGOT = serum glutamic-oxaloacetic transaminase; AST = aspartate aminotransferase; WBC = white blood cells; BUN = blood urea nitrogen; HCT = hematocrit.

CLASSIFICATION AND TREATMENT

As stated, one of the problems surrounding the diagnosis and treatment of acute pancreatitis has been the lack of standardized terminology. To remedy this, a symposium of internationally recognized experts from six different disciplines published its consensus on a clinically based classification system for acute pancreatitis.* Clinical classification systems are useful as initial screening tools; they allow management planning and may predict mortality based on physiologic severity, irrespective of etiology. Etiologic classification systems are more useful for planning long-term, definitive therapy. Although knowledge of etiology may be useful, this information is neither available nor required for the early phases of acute pancreatitis management.

Clinical Classification

Acute pancreatitis is defined as an acute inflammatory process of the pancreas with variable regional and remote organ system involvement. *Mild acute pancreatitis* is associated with minimal organ dysfunction and an uneventful recovery; it correlates with fewer than three Ranson criteria or eight APACHE II points. *Severe acute pancreatitis* is associated with organ failure and/or local complications (e.g., necrosis, abscess, or pseudocyst formation) and correlates with three or more Ranson criteria or eight or more APACHE II points.

Local complications resulting from pancreatitis, such as acute fluid collections, pseudocysts, pancreatic necrosis, and pancreatic abscess are also defined. *Acute fluid collections* are any fluid collections in proximity to the pancreas that lack a wall of granulation or fibrous tissue. A *pseudocyst* is a collection of pancreatic juice enclosed by a granulation or fibrous tissue wall. A *pancreatic abscess* is a collection of purulence in proximity to the pancreas that contains little or no necrotic pancreatic tissue. A diffuse or focal area of nonviable pancreatic parenchyma defines *pancreatic necrosis,* which may or may not be infected. Computed tomography (CT) criteria for the latter include nonenhanced zones of pancreatic tissue greater than 3 cm or involving more than 30% of the pancreas. Terms such as phlegmon, infected pseudocyst, and hemorrhagic pancreatitis do not exist in this clinical classification system.

For all cases of pancreatitis, initial treatment is supportive. Definitive therapy should be directed at the etiologic agent responsible for the pancreatitis, as discussed in the next section. Many management issues have been previously addressed in the section on resuscitation. One of the most often debated questions is the role of nutritional support. The premise that parenteral nutrition therapy is indicated for all patients with pancreatitis is clearly erroneous. When fewer than three Ranson criteria or eight APACHE II points are assessed, enteral therapy by mouth or feeding tube should be considered. If support is required because of prolonged nausea, a postpyloric tube may prove adequate. A formula that requires minimal hepatobiliary or gastrointestinal tract function for assimilation is preferred. This usually mandates a lipid-based formula with medium-chain triglycerides as the major calorie source and protein provided as dipeptides and tripeptides.

When parenteral nutrition is required in more severe attacks, specialized formulas should be chosen based on co-morbidities or remote organ system involvement. Pancreatitis does not mandate specific nutritional therapy with two exceptions: pancreatitis known to be due to hyperlipidemia or pancreatitis of unknown etiology. In these cases, only 100 mL of 10% lipid should initially be provided weekly to prevent essential fatty acid deficiency. Once hyperlipidemia has been excluded as a cause of idiopathic pancreatitis, lipids can be given in a standard fashion.

Etiologic Classification

Gallstones account for approximately two-thirds of pancreatitis cases in private institutions and one-third of those in county and Veterans Affairs medical centers. The pancreatitis tends to be self-limited and is seldom complicated by necrosis, hemorrhage, pseudocyst, or abscess formation. Amylase levels often exceed 1000 units per mL. When renal function is adequate, the serum amylase level will usually decline by 50% each day. Gallbladder ultrasound generally shows stones with echogenic shadowing if intestinal gas allows visualization of the gallbladder. CT is usually unnecessary in this setting, but may be useful for ruling out distal common duct or pancreatic head pathology. Although less sensitive than ultrasound, CT may prove complementary when clinical suspicion is high and other studies are equivocal. After resolution, double-dose oral cholecystography may document stones when clinical suspicion remains high and ultrasound or CT scan is equivocal.

Patients with gallstone pancreatitis should undergo cholecystectomy with intraoperative cholangiography performed after resolution of their pancreatitis but before discharge from the hospital. If allowed to go home before definitive therapy, up to 35% of patients will have a second attack of pancreatitis (with all its attendant morbidity) while awaiting operation.

Ethyl alcohol is the other major cause of pancreatitis in the United States. The mechanism(s) mediating alcohol-induced pancreatitis remains unclear. Alcoholic pancreatitis can be quite severe, although the amylase level seldom reaches 1000 units per mL. Many patients become so sensitized to ethyl alcohol that a single drink can cause recrudescence of their pancreatitis. This is the only common form of pancreatitis that leads to pancreatic calcifications; hyperparathyroidism, parasitic infestation, and familial pancreatitis are much rarer causes of calcifying pancreatitis. Complications, such as pseudocysts and ductal strictures, are common and usually require

*See Arch Surg 128:586–590, 1993.

surgical intervention. Definitive treatment requires abstinence from ethyl alcohol.

Pancreatitis associated with hyperlipidemia types I, IV, and V can be quite severe, although the exact pathogenetic mechanism remains unclear. Like other forms of pancreatitis associated with metabolic disorders, hyperlipidemia-associated pancreatitis tends to run a prolonged course, seldom exhibits a serum amylase level greater than 1000 units per mL, and is frequently followed by significant complications. Definitive treatment is directed at the hyperlipidemia and is dependent upon the particular type of hyperlipidemia present. Dietary restriction and drug therapy to lower serum triglycerides may prevent recurrence.

The mechanism mediating the pancreatitis associated with hyperparathyroidism is obscure. Because hypercalcemia from other causes does not lead to pancreatitis, a direct effect of parathyroid hormone has been speculated. Initial screening should include serum calcium, phosphorus, and chloride measurements. Because parathyroid hormone has a direct effect on the renal tubules, causing phosphorus excretion and chloride reabsorption, the chloride-phosphorus ratio is usually greater than 33 when hyperparathyroidism is present. An inappropriately elevated serum parathyroid hormone level is necessary for diagnosis of hyperparathyroidism; elevated calcium is usual but not universal. Parathyroidectomy is curative.

Medications known to cause pancreatitis are legion (Table 3). Drug-induced pancreatitis should be a diagnosis of exclusion. When patients on multiple medications are admitted to the hospital with pancreatitis, all nonessential drugs should be discontinued. If the metabolic and structural work-up is inconclusive, medications should be reviewed and those known to cause pancreatitis discontinued. The pancreatitis is treated symptomatically after the offending agent has been discontinued.

Although hyperamylasemia occurs in up to 20% of patients undergoing endoscopic retrograde cholangiopancreatography (ERCP), clinical pancreatitis occurs in only 1 to 3% of cases. Those most predisposed to ERCP-induced pancreatitis include patients with pancreatic pathology, patients with prior pancreatitis, and those undergoing endoscopy by inexperienced endoscopists. Maneuvers that may decrease the likelihood of pancreatitis include slow, low-pressure contrast injections and limiting the volume and number of injections. This type of pancreatitis is usually mild and self-limited, although pancreatic hemorrhage and necrosis can occur. Treatment is supportive, with surgery for complications.

TABLE 3. **Medications Known to Cause Pancreatitis**

Hydrochlorothiazide	Nitrofurantoin
Furosemide	Pentamidine
Estrogens	Sulfonamides
L-Asparaginase	Procainamide
Azathioprine	Tetracycline
6-Mercaptopurine	Valproic acid
Methyldopa	

Various structural abnormalities have been associated with pancreatitis. Most cases present as recurrent acute pancreatitis and often are labeled idiopathic because the metabolic work-up for pancreatitis is repeatedly negative. Ampullary stenosis, dominant dorsal duct syndrome (pancreas divisum), choledochal cyst, duodenal diverticulum, annular pancreas, and malignant ductal obstruction are all associated with pancreatitis. Upper gastrointestinal endoscopy with retrograde pancreatography of both major and minor pancreatic ducts coupled with CT scan will diagnose most of these disorders. Endoscopic sphincterotomy is the treatment of choice for pancreatitis caused by ampullary stenosis, while surgical sphincteroplasty is currently the preferred management technique for pancreas divisum. The remaining anatomic defects require surgical correction: choledochal cyst requires choledochoduodenostomy, duodenal diverticula should be resected, annular pancreas should be bypassed with a gastrojejunostomy, and malignant ductal obstructions should be resected when possible or bypassed when unresectable.

Infections with varicella-zoster, coxsackievirus, echovirus, Epstein-Barr virus (EBV), and cytomegalovirus (CMV) have all been associated with pancreatitis. However, other than CMV, these viruses have never been cultured from human pancreatic tissue, leaving questions about the mechanisms involved. The pancreatitis tends to be self-limited and complications are uncommon. Viral cultures or serum immunoglobulin titers will document viral presence or exposure.

Parasitic infestation with *Clonorchis sinensis* or *Schistosoma mansoni* has been reported to cause pancreatitis. The organisms inhabit the pancreatic ducts, causing ductal dilatation, squamous metaplasia, and ductal fibrosis. In addition, *Ascaris* spp and *Echinococcus* spp can obstruct the ampulla of Vater, causing subsequent pancreatitis. Treatment is directed at the offending organism.

Envenomation from a scorpion sting is a common cause of pancreatitis in Trinidad. Organophosphates are also known to cause pancreatitis. Massive cholinergic neurotransmitter stimulation of the pancreas may represent a common mechanism mediating pancreatitis from these two causes. Such toxin-related pancreatitis may be particularly severe with a high degree of complications. Treatment is supportive with removal of the offending agent.

While pregnancy was at one time considered to be an etiologic agent for pancreatitis, review suggests that most cases were probably attributable to other causes. Thus, when a pregnant woman develops pancreatitis, common etiologic agents should be sought. Gallstones are often the cause of pancreatitis in this setting. If the risk of prolonged observation is deemed inordinate, cholecystectomy can be safely performed during the second or late third trimester.

Vasculitides such as systemic lupus erythematosus,

thrombotic thrombocytopenic purpura, Henoch-Schönlein purpura, and polyarteritis nodosa have all been associated with acute pancreatitis. In these cases, medication-induced pancreatitis may also be implicated since many agents used to treat vasculitides can cause pancreatitis.

In about 5% of pancreatitis cases, no etiologic agent can be identified, culminating in the diagnosis of idiopathic pancreatitis. If aggressive evaluation does not reveal an etiologic agent, supportive care is all that can be offered.

Complications

Complications of acute pancreatitis can occur after the initial episode or any subsequent episodes. Some complications make their presence obvious, while others will not be diagnosed unless specifically sought. Although alcoholic hepatitis and alcoholic pancreatitis can occur in the same individual, this is rather unusual. Thus, we feel that an alcoholic patient with pancreatitis and an enlarged spleen or ascites should be evaluated for splenic vein thrombosis and pancreatic ascites, respectively. Splenic vein thrombosis can be diagnosed by CT scan and treated by splenectomy. Pancreatic ascites occurs after ductal disruption with leak of pancreatic fluid into the abdominal cavity. Because CT scan will not demonstrate the ductal disruption, ERCP is necessary. When ductal disruption is in the tail of the pancreas, distal pancreatectomy is curative; when disruption occurs in the pancreatic head, Roux-en-Y pancreaticojejunostomy is the treatment of choice. Preliminary reports have described endoscopic insertion of pancreatic endoprostheses as definitive therapy for pancreatic ascites. At this time, such treatment should be considered experimental and reserved for expert endoscopists.

Most (85%) acute pancreatic fluid collections noted immediately after an episode of acute pancreatitis will resolve. However, if a fluid collection persists for more than 6 weeks, it most likely represents a pseudocyst. Symptomatic or enlarging pseudocysts usually require internal drainage. At the time of surgery, multiple biopsies of the cyst wall should be taken to ensure that the collection is not a true pancreatic cystic lesion, since the malignant potential of mucinous cystic pancreatic neoplasms necessitates pancreatic resection. When pseudocysts form around the head of the pancreas, the stomach often forms the anterior wall of the pseudocyst. This anatomic proximity can often be exploited by performing a cystogastrostomy or cystoduodenostomy with pyloroplasty. When pseudocysts occur in the body or tail of the pancreas, pancreaticojejunostomy or resection should be performed.

Pancreatic abscess discussed previously usually represents a secondarily infected bland fluid collection that, by definition, does not contain necrotic pancreatic debris. These collections are not adequately treated by broad-spectrum antibiotics alone; drug therapy must be combined with surgical or CT-guided drainage, both of which have been used successfully to treat these collections.

Pancreatic necrosis is diagnosed by contrast-enhanced CT. When an area of 3 cm or 30% of the pancreas fails to become enhanced with injection of intravenous contrast media, pancreatic necrosis has occurred. While there is debate on the most appropriate management of these patients, CT-guided fine-needle aspiration is being utilized more frequently. When the necrotic area is sterile, treatment is symptomatic with the addition of broad-spectrum antibiotics. When it is infected, urgent pancreatic débridement is indicated, because the patient will not likely survive without surgery. If multiple organ system failure occurs, pancreatic débridement may also be performed in hopes of reversing this complication, even without evidence of infected pancreatic necrosis. We perform serial pancreatic débridements with peripancreatic packing, leaving the abdomen open until the area will allow closure with insertion of closed suction drains; silastic window abdominal closure may be required early in the intervention of these patients.

CONCLUSIONS

Although pancreatitis can arise from a diffuse array of insults, the initial therapy is dictated more by severity than by etiology. Most (85%) cases of pancreatitis are mild, with more severe forms carrying significant morbidity and mortality. Clinical classification systems are helpful in management planning and may portend mortality. Once the etiology is determined, definitive therapy can be initiated when appropriate. Complications, which rarely occur with mild attacks, carry their own significant morbidity and mortality and often require surgical intervention.

CHRONIC PANCREATITIS

method of
HOWARD A. REBER, M.D., and
DAVID W. McFADDEN, M.D.
UCLA Center for the Health Sciences and Sepulveda Department of Veterans Affairs Medical Center
Los Angeles, California

Chronic pancreatitis is an inflammatory disease of the pancreas that is marked by gradual destruction of pancreatic exocrine and endocrine tissues and replacement of the pancreatic parenchyma by fibrous scar tissue. In the United States, most cases are found in chronic alcoholics, who are 20 to 50 times more likely to suffer from the disease. Chronic unrelenting abdominal pain and back pain are the primary reasons for surgical therapy. Other specific complications of chronic pancreatitis that may require surgery include pseudocysts, biliary and intestinal obstruction, and mesenteric venous thrombosis.

Gallstone pancreatitis, the most common cause of acute

pancreatitis, rarely leads to chronic pancreatitis. Indeed, the pancreas is believed to return to normal between attacks. It is this difference in the capacity of the pancreas to recover that forms the basis for the classification of pancreatitis into acute and chronic forms (Table 1). Nevertheless, patients with chronic pancreatitis may suffer episodes of acute pancreatitis clinically identical to an attack of gallstone pancreatitis.

Surveillance studies of patients with chronic pancreatitis suggest that few die as a direct result of the disease. Prognosis is determined by the adequacy and availability of medical care, socioeconomic conditions, intellectual capacity, and continued alcoholism and narcotic addiction. Several large cohort studies have revealed that chronic pancreatitis is the direct cause of death in only 20% of patients, with most succumbing from alcoholic liver disease, cancer, or postoperative mortality. Between 25 and 35% of patients operated upon for chronic pancreatitis have died within 4 to 6 years of surgery. The mortality rate is higher in patients who continue to drink alcohol (63% versus 25% at 6 years).

ETIOLOGY

Alcoholism is the cause of 75% of the cases of chronic pancreatitis in the United States and other developed countries. Pancreatic calcifications are seen in one-third of patients with alcoholic chronic pancreatitis. Significant degrees of weight loss are common, as eating tends to worsen the pain. Narcotic addiction is common. The usual age of onset is in the mid-thirties, and men are affected more commonly than women. Cessation of alcohol use may slow the continued deterioration in pancreatic function, but abstinence does not stop disease progression. Abstinence may increase the chance of pain relief after surgical intervention, however.

Symptomatic chronic pancreatitis can be diagnosed as early as 2 years after substantial alcohol consumption begins, but a decade or more of significant ethanol ingestion is more commonly seen. Daily consumption averages 100 to 150 grams. A high-protein and high-fat diet may increase the risk of chronic pancreatitis. An estimated 10 to 15% of chronic alcoholics develop chronic pancreatitis; a similar percentage develop cirrhosis of the liver. The factors that control individual susceptibility are unknown.

Mechanical obstruction of pancreatic secretion is a less common primary cause of chronic pancreatitis. It is important to quickly establish obstruction as the cause, however, since reversal of some of the damage to the pancreas is possible if the obstruction is removed early enough. Obstruction as a cause of chronic pancreatitis occurs in a variety of clinical settings. For example, fusion of the ventral and dorsal pancreatic ducts occurs during fetal development, and narrowing of the duct at the point of fusion occurs in 3% of patients. If seen on endoscopic retrograde cholangiopancreatography (ERCP), it should be considered significant only if proximal ductal dilation exists. Chronic pancreatitis has been reported in patients with severe strictures. These are typically young adults who present with significant weight loss and abdominal pain. Other areas of the pancreatic duct may develop strictures, usually from trauma or secondary to scarring from acute pancreatitis.

Cystic fibrosis, an autosomal recessive trait, is the most common lethal genetic disease in the United States. Pancreatic insufficiency is present in up to 95% of patients, usually manifesting as steatorrhea and azotorrhea. Recurrent episodes of acute or chronic pancreatitis occasionally develop in older children or adults with this disorder. The surgical management of these patients is the same as in those with chronic pancreatitis from other causes, but their chronic pulmonary disease puts them at higher risk for perioperative complications.

Pancreas divisum is an anatomic variant of the pancreatic ductal system in which most of the pancreatic juice enters the duodenum through the minor papilla and only the secretions from the uncinate process of the gland (the ventral pancreas) empty through the major papilla. This variant occurs in about 7% of the population and in most is not associated with disease. In some patients, the opening at the minor papilla may be too small for the large amount of pancreatic juice secreted, and the relative obstruction results in repeated episodes of acute pancreatitis or chronic

TABLE 1. **Classification of Pancreatitis**

Classification	Clinical Characteristics	Morphologic Characteristics
Acute Pancreatitis		
Exocrine and endocrine functions are temporarily and variably impaired. Functional restitution to normal usually occurs. Rarely leads to chronic pancreatitis.	Acute abdominal and/or back pain. Increased pancreatic enzymes in blood and/or urine. Usually benign course, but can be severe and fatal. May be a single episode or recurrent.	Gradation of lesions from mild (interstitial edema, periglandular fat necrosis) to severe (peripancreatic and pancreatic necrosis and hemorrhage). Clinical features and morphologic findings may not correlate.
Chronic Pancreatitis		
Irreversible morphologic changes lead to progressive and permanent deficits in endocrine and exocrine function. In obstructive chronic pancreatitis, improvements are noted after the obstruction is removed.	Persistent and recurrent abdominal pain in most patients. Evidence of pancreatic insufficiency, e.g., steatorrhea or diabetes.	Irregular sclerosis, with destruction and permanent loss of exocrine parenchyma in focal, segmental, or diffuse patterns. Varying degrees of ductular and ductal dilatation. Cysts, pseudocysts, and intraductal calculi are common, as is edema and focal necrosis. Islets of Langerhans appear relatively well preserved. In obstructive chronic pancreatitis, the ductal system is dilated proximal to the point of occlusion (by tumor or scarring), with diffuse atrophy and fibrosis. Calculi are uncommon.

obstructive pancreatitis. In patients with chronic pancreatitis and pancreas divisum, efforts to relieve the obstruction at the minor papilla are ineffective.

Cancer of the head of the pancreas is almost always circumscribed by areas of chronic pancreatitis. At surgery, it is common to find a firm pancreas with a dilated pancreatic duct proximal to the malignant obstruction. Clinically significant chronic pancreatitis is unusual in this setting. Episodes of acute pancreatitis may also occur. These patients are usually older than those with alcoholic chronic pancreatitis and often have no apparent cause for the pancreatitis. A high index of clinical suspicion is necessary to make a correct diagnosis.

A specific type of chronic pancreatitis is seen in children with severe protein-calorie malnutrition and kwashiorkor. Adequate dietary replenishment is curative, provided parenchymal fibrosis is minimal. Another kind of chronic pancreatitis, possibly related to malnutrition, occurs only in certain tropical areas. The pancreatic ducts are usually dilated and obstructed. Nutritional repletion does not reverse this process.

Hypercalcemic states, most commonly hyperparathyroidism, can cause acute pancreatitis and chronic pancreatitis via unclear mechanisms. Hypercalcemia may encourage the intraductal precipitation of calcium stones, seen in nearly 50% of these patients. Calcium also influences the activation of certain pancreatic enzymes and acinar cell synthetic and secretory events. Acute hypercalcemia increases pancreatic ductal permeability, which may allow enzyme leakage into the parenchyma.

Hereditary, or familial, pancreatitis is a rare form of chronic pancreatitis associated with a variable clinical course. It is inherited as an autosomal dominant trait with incomplete penetration. Symptoms begin in early adolescence and are typical of acute pancreatitis. Relentless progression is the rule, and calcifications, diabetes, and steatorrhea are seen in up to 75% of patients. Most patients have dilated pancreatic ducts, and lateral pancreaticojejunostomy has provided effective pain relief. An increased incidence (9 to 20%) of pancreatic carcinoma has been noted in these patients, requiring close follow-up.

No definitive cause of chronic pancreatitis is found in 10% of patients in the United States and up to 30 to 50% in countries with low alcohol intake. Idiopathic chronic pancreatitis usually occurs in an older age group than does alcoholic pancreatitis. ERCP generally documents dilated pancreatic ducts, and pancreatic calcifications are less common. Patients with idiopathic chronic pancreatitis usually have less pain; disease progression and complications also occur less frequently.

PATHOLOGY

Early in the disease, the pancreas is grossly normal in appearance and endoscopic evaluation may reveal normal ducts. As the disease progresses, the pancreas may become enlarged, indurated, and edematous. The ducts may be normal, or slight dilation may be seen. Later, the pancreas is usually small, with rounded edges, and rubbery or firm in consistency. By this time, endoscopy usually reveals dilated ducts. Occasionally, narrowing with distortion or even normal ducts may be seen. Ductal calculi are common, and their size varies from 1 mm to over 1 cm in diameter. All pancreatic calcifications are intraductal in location. At surgery, large dilated ducts are often palpable as a longitudinal soft depression on the anterior surface of the gland, whereas in the healthy pancreas the main duct is posterior and not palpable.

Microscopically, the disease initially is scattered irregularly throughout the gland and is characterized by sclerosis of the exocrine parenchyma. Protein deposits, which may later calcify to form stones, are seen to obstruct the ducts. As the disease advances, fibrosis extends through the gland, although normal lobules may still be found. In the most advanced stages, the pancreas is almost completely replaced with fibrous tissue. Islets of Langerhans appear well preserved and hyperplastic, despite functional deficiencies. Intrapancreatic nerves are preserved but are more densely distributed secondary to parenchymal contraction and fibrosis. Perineural sheaths appear destroyed, possibly allowing noxious substances to contact and irritate them.

DIAGNOSIS

The presenting symptom in up to 95% of patients with chronic pancreatitis is abdominal pain (Table 2). The intensity of the pain can be severe, and it is often described as boring, dull, cramping, or aching in quality. Although usually located in the epigastrium, it is also felt in the back in about 50% of patients. The pain may be partially relieved by sitting with the trunk bent forward or lying prone. The pain may be episodic or constant. In most cases, the pain-free intervals shorten and the painful attacks become longer. When the disease is so far advanced that the majority of exocrine function is lost, about one-third of patients will experience spontaneous pain relief; another 10 to 20% have temporary remissions that last from 1 to 3 years. The "burnout" theory of pain has led many clinicians to postpone surgical consultation for these patients in the hope that the pain will eventually subside spontaneously. Unfortunately, there is no way to predict those patients in whom this will occur.

The aggravation of pain by eating is characteristic of both chronic pancreatitis and carcinoma of the pancreas and is probably related to food-stimulated pancreatic secretion. Drinking ethanol may worsen the pain, although many patients claim that pain develops after 12 to 24 hours of abstinence; thus they continue to drink. Patients often fear eating, and about 75% lose weight because of decreased intake. Significant weight loss from malabsorption or diabetes is less common, since most of these patients are able to maintain their weight by eating more frequently and in greater quantities. Narcotic addiction is common and correlates with a worsened surgical prognosis. Painless chronic pancreatitis accounts for 5 to 10% of cases and is more likely to be of the idiopathic variety.

Diarrhea, steatorrhea, and azotorrhea are hallmarks of significant pancreatic exocrine insufficiency, but usually do not occur until 90% of the secretory capacity of the pancreas is lost. These symptoms can be the result of either progressive parenchymal destruction or major ductal obstruction. Steatorrhea is an earlier and more troublesome problem than azotorrhea, as diarrhea usually accompanies significant fat malabsorption. Carbohydrate digestion is unaffected because salivary amylase production continues normally. Patients complain of bulky, offensive, fatty, or oily stools. Fat-soluble vitamins are rarely deficient, however.

Almost 70% of patients with chronic pancreatitis have abnormal glucose tolerance, and half of these have diabetes mellitus. Some degree of malabsorption is also present. The diabetes is usually easily controlled with insulin, but hypoglycemia may be a problem in alcoholics with irregular eating habits. Generally, most patients with chronic pancreatitis have failed to adapt to societal stresses and have inadequate personalities. The stresses of the disease often

TABLE 2. **Clinical Features of Chronic Pancreatitis**

Feature	Incidence	Etiology	Remarks
Pain	85%	Unknown. Fibrosis, low blood flow, neural encasement are suggested reasons	Back/abdominal pain; postprandial in nature, relieved by postural changes
Weight loss	Common	Fear of eating because of pain (sitophobia); malabsorption	Typically gradual; if rapid, consider pancreatic cancer
Malabsorption	Subclinical in almost all patients	Exocrine insufficiency	Diarrhea, steatorrhea, azotorrhea
Diabetes	Glucose intolerance common, frank diabetes rare	Endocrine insufficiency	Ketoacidosis, nephropathy rare; retinopathy and neuropathy have similar incidences

result in depression and anxiety. These psychosocial factors must be recognized and addressed by the treating physician.

Unusual physical findings are rare in patients with chronic pancreatitis. There may be some epigastric tenderness and evidence of weight loss. Occasionally jaundice is present. A palpable mass is usually a pancreatic pseudocyst. Painful nodules over the lower extremities, from subcutaneous fat necrosis, and polyarthritis of the small hand joints are occasionally seen.

Laboratory Findings

Standard blood studies are rarely of benefit in chronic pancreatitis. Leukocytosis, hyperamylasemia, and hyperlipasemia can be seen during acute exacerbations but may not be present later in the course of the disease. The reasons for normal serum pancreatic enzymes include acinar cell destruction that limits the amount of enzyme available for release and the chronic fibrosis that restricts leakage of enzymes during inflammation. Nearly 70% of patients with alcoholic chronic pancreatitis have abnormal liver function studies, usually manifested as mild elevations of serum levels of bilirubin, alkaline phosphatase, and aspartate aminotransferase.

A number of pancreatic function tests have been used to establish the diagnosis and/or prognosis in chronic pancreatitis. These include measurements of serum concentrations of trypsin, elastase, pancreatic isoamylase, and pancreatic polypeptide, as well as tests of pancreatic function, including CCK/secretin stimulation tests and test meals (Lund test). These tests are rarely indicated in patients with overt chronic pancreatitis, as they seldom influence therapy, but they may be of some value in the evaluation of patients in whom the presence of pancreatic disease is suspected but for which no direct evidence exists.

Imaging Studies

The finding of calcifications within the pancreas on plain abdominal radiographs is diagnostic of chronic pancreatitis and is seen in 30 to 50% of patients. Accordingly, plain films of the abdomen are often the first imaging procedure performed. Ultrasound is the next simplest and cheapest radiographic modality. Dilated pancreatic ducts greater than 4 to 5 mm in diameter, cavities greater than 1 cm in diameter, pseudocysts, and calcification can all be detected with overall sensitivities of 70% and specificities of 90%.

Computed tomographic (CT) scanning is 10 to 20% more sensitive than ultrasound for diagnosing chronic pancreatitis, but has similar specificity. Although more expensive and requiring radiation, it provides the most reliable overall assessment of the pancreas and peripancreatic area, and should be performed in all patients in whom surgery is contemplated. The most common CT findings in chronic pancreatitis include duct dilatation, calcifications, and cystic lesions. Less commonly, enlargement or atrophy of the gland, heterogenous parenchymal density, and splenic venous thrombosis are seen. When the duct is dilated, it usually can be seen traversing the gland. Biliary dilation is also seen clearly.

The accuracy of endoscopic retrograde cholangiopancreatography diagnosing chronic pancreatitis increases with the duration of disease, reaching 92% in patients who have had the disease over 5 years. ERCP should also be done in most patients with chronic pancreatitis who are being evaluated for operation. The radiologic appearance of the ductal system may show caliber variations, strictures, obstructions, ductal filling defects consistent with stones, and areas of dilatation. If preoperative ERCP cannot be obtained, intraoperative pancreatography may be performed. This is usually done by needle puncture of the main pancreatic duct through the anterior surface of the gland. Occasionally, duodenotomy and cannulation of the duct through the ampulla is required. Intraoperative ultrasound should also be considered in cases where the main pancreatic duct is difficult to localize.

In the majority of patients with advanced chronic pancreatitis, the main pancreatic duct is dilated up to 1 cm in diameter, often with intermittent points of obstruction (chain of lakes appearance). The common bile duct is usually opacified during ERCP. This may reveal common duct obstruction and influence the choice of therapy.

DIFFERENTIAL DIAGNOSIS

The diagnosis of chronic pancreatitis is usually straightforward, but occasionally it is difficult to differentiate pancreatitis from cancer of the head of the pancreas. Although CT and ERCP help to distinguish the two, laparotomy and biopsy may ultimately be required. Even then it may not be possible to diagnose a small cancer situated deeply within an indurated, enlarged, and chronically inflamed head of the pancreas. The decision to resect must then be based on the surgeon's judgment and the ability to perform the Whipple operation with an acceptably low mortality rate. Since chronic pancreatitis primarily affecting the head of the pancreas is also effectively treated by the same operation, resection may be an acceptable approach even when cancer has not been proved to be present.

TREATMENT

Pancreatic Insufficiency

Fat malabsorption, causing steatorrhea and diarrhea, is the principal problem requiring treatment in these patients. Protein digestion is aided by gastric pepsin and small intestinal brush border enzymes, and salivary amylase facilitates carbohydrate digestion. Diarrhea can be eliminated and steatorrhea minimized if approximately 30,000 IU of lipase are supplied with each meal. The least expensive of the available preparations should be chosen. If diarrhea continues, a histamine receptor antagonist should be added to decrease gastric acidity, which may be so high that it inactivates the lipase. Another approach is to change the enzyme preparation to one that is enteric coated. This prevents the release of enzymes until they are in the small bowel where the pH is more alkaline.

Diets for patients with chronic pancreatitis should supply 3000 to 6000 calories per day, emphasizing carbohydrate (40 grams or more) and protein (100 to 150 grams). In general, fat intake should not exceed 100 grams per day, divided among four meals. Fat malabsorption can never be eliminated, but diarrhea should cease and weight gain should occur in most patients.

Diabetes Mellitus

Patients with diabetes from chronic pancreatitis are quite sensitive to exogenous insulin, and hypoglycemia can result from even small doses. The absence of endogenous glucagon is probably a factor. Conversely, ketoacidosis is rare, even if blood glucose levels are high. Fasting blood glucose levels of less than 250 mg per dL should not be treated, and maintenance of fasting levels around 200 mg per dL is acceptable. Usually less than 20 to 30 units of insulin per day are required. Oral agents are rarely effective.

The chances of developing diabetes after pancreatic resection are directly related to the preoperative glucose tolerance and the amount of pancreas resected. Most patients with abnormal glucose tolerance before operation will require insulin after a resection of 50% or more of the pancreas.

Pain

Up to 75% of patients experience pain relief by simply stopping the intake of alcoholic beverages, but more than 50% continue to drink despite chronic pain. Oral enzyme replacement can reduce pain by suppressing endogenous pancreatic enzyme synthesis and secretion. Although several studies have shown improvement in up to 75% of patients, most responders were middle-aged women with idiopathic chronic pancreatitis. Celiac plexus block by percutaneous alcohol injection, using either ultrasound or CT guidance, has produced inconsistent results in chronic pancreatitis. Benefits may last only a few months, and repeated injections tend to be less effective.

Analgesics remain the mainstay of pain control in these patients. Initially, non-narcotic agents should be used, and taking them before meals to decrease postprandial pain is suggested. Later, mild narcotics such as codeine or hydrocodone are used in combination with acetaminophen. In severe cases, potent opiates are required, and addiction is common. All too often, patients are denied surgical treatment until they have become addicted and are severely depressed from the constant pain. Operation earlier in the course of the disease should be considered for most patients.

Surgical Treatment

The aims of surgery in chronic pancreatitis are to relieve intractable pain, to treat complications, and to preserve as much functioning pancreatic tissue as possible. Several points must be clarified to the patient and family. First, surgery will probably not affect the relentless deterioration of pancreatic function in most patients. Second, no single operation is appropriate for all patients. Third, unreformed drug addicts or alcoholics have the worst results from surgery.

The majority of operations for chronic pancreatitis are performed for the associated intractable pain, which interferes substantially with a patient's quality of life. Factors that are considered include employability, frequency of hospitalizations, weight loss, psychiatric disturbances (usually depression), deterioration of family life, and narcotic addiction.

Historically, there have been three surgical approaches to the management of pain in chronic pancreatitis: ductal drainage, pancreatic resection, and denervation procedures. The choice of operation is dictated by ductal anatomy and co-morbid conditions.

Drainage Operations

The normal diameter of the main pancreatic duct is 4 to 5 mm in the head, 3 to 4 mm in the body, and 2 to 3 mm in the tail of the gland. When the diameter in the head and body enlarges to 7 to 8 mm or more, an anastomosis between the pancreatic duct and the jejunum, also known as a pancreaticojejunostomy or Puestow procedure, is technically feasible and has a good chance of producing lasting pain relief. Results are poor in glands with smaller ducts, possibly because of anastomotic stricturing.

The anastomosis should extend to within 1 cm of the duodenum and well out into the tail of the gland. All identifiable ductal stones should be removed. It is important to demonstrate patency of the pancreatic ducts into the duodenum to assure that the dissection has progressed far enough. The incision in the head of the gland may need to be rather deep, since the duct to the uncinate process may be quite posterior, especially when the head of the gland is enlarged. Excision of some of the pancreatic tissue may be useful in that circumstance to improve anastomotic patency and pancreatic drainage. Pseudocysts occur in nearly 40% of patients, and they should be drained into the same jejunal limb used for the pancreaticojejunostomy.

Most series have reported operative mortality rates from Puestow procedures to be 0 to 5%, with morbidities ranging from 7 to 30%. Diabetes does not result directly from the operation, as little or no pancreatic tissue is removed. Several studies have suggested that the operation slows the deterioration of pancreatic function. A small randomized trial of drained versus undrained patients suggested an advantage for pancreatic duct drainage in terms of maintenance of existent exocrine function. Clinical improvement in malabsorption is rare, but most patients with pain relief gain weight because they eat more. Pain is relieved completely or substantially in 75 to 80% of patients for the first few years after surgery. Unfortunately, pain recurs in up to 50% of patients after 5 years. Recurrence of pain is an indication for ERCP and CT scan. If stenosis of the pancreaticojejunal anastomosis is present, revision is reported to be successful in 71% of patients. If the anastomosis is widely patent, and no other cause for the pain is apparent, then pancreatic resection should be considered.

Pancreatic Resection

Resection is the treatment of choice when operation is indicated in patients whose ducts are normal or narrow in diameter. As a rule, the portion of the gland where the disease is most severe should be resected. Often, the head of the pancreas is significantly involved, making a pancreaticoduodenectomy a reasonable option. The traditional Whipple pancreaticoduodenectomy offers an 85% chance of long-term pain relief. The operative mortality rate is now less than 5% in major centers. Alternatives to the standard Whipple operation include the pylorus-preserving Whipple operation and the duodenum-preserving resection of the head of the pancreas.

Distal resections (50 to 60% of the gland) are indicated less often, when the disease is concentrated in the body or tail. This may be the case in patients who develop chronic pancreatitis after traumatic stricturing of the main pancreatic duct in the body of the gland. Subtotal (80 to 95%) or total pancreatectomy may be considered in those with diffuse disease, or if pain persists after more limited resection or drainage. Extensive resections may be complicated by brittle diabetes, and they should be done infrequently for that reason.

Many patients have extensive disease that predominantly involves the head of the pancreas, which may be swollen to 5 to 6 cm in diameter or more and contain multiple cysts and calcifications. The bile duct and/or duodenum also may be obstructed by chronic fibrosis associated with the inflammatory process, and in these circumstances, a Whipple resection may be appropriate. Pancreaticoduodenectomy also is indicated if there is clinical suspicion that pancreatic cancer is present.

Duodenum-Sparing Resections of the Head of the Pancreas. Beger and colleagues from Ulm, Germany, have described a duodenum-preserving resection of the head of the pancreas for patients with chronic pancreatitis and inflammatory masses in the head of the gland. Normally, these patients would be candidates for a Whipple resection. The body and tail of the pancreas, along with a thin rim of the head of the gland along the duodenum, are preserved. In 141 patients, the hospital mortality was only 0.7%, and 77% of patients were pain free (average follow-up of 3.6 years). Glucose metabolism was unchanged or improved in 90% of patients. The results appear promising, but longer follow-up and confirmation of these results in other centers are needed.

Another resection procedure for patients with chronic pancreatitis associated with an enlarged pancreatic head and a dilated pancreatic duct was recently described by Frey. In this procedure, the head of the pancreas is cored out rather than resected. The operation is easier than the one described by Beger because the neck of the pancreas is not divided, and dissection near the mesenteric vessels is avoided. As with the Beger procedure, a 0.5 to 1.0 cm rim of pancreatic tissue is left in situ next to the duodenum to maintain duodenal viability. The pancreatic duct is opened along its length and drained along with the cored-out head as in the usual side-to-side pancreaticojejunostomy. In both operations, the intrapancreatic segment of the common bile duct can be freed from the surrounding fibrosis, thus frequently avoiding the need for biliary bypass.

A 95% distal pancreatectomy entails removal of all but a thin rim of pancreatic tissue that lies within the C-loop of the duodenum. Usually the spleen is also removed, although it may be preserved by either maintaining the integrity of the short gastric vessels or meticulous ligation of the pancreatic vessels communicating with the splenic artery and vein, preserving them as well. This operation is rarely indicated today because of the endocrine and exocrine insufficiency that results. Pain relief is afforded to 60 to 80% of patients with 4 to 8 years of follow-up.

Total pancreatectomy is rarely performed because it uniformly results in diabetes and exocrine insufficiency, and pain relief can usually be accomplished by a less radical operation. It is most often employed when a previous Whipple procedure or distal pancreatectomy has failed to provide pain relief. If possible, the pylorus should be preserved. The results appear to be satisfactory, although only a few series are available to evaluate. Pain relief occurs in 56 to 86% of this select group of patients in whom previous operations have failed.

Denervation Procedures

Surgical sympathectomy and celiac ganglionectomy have relieved pain effectively in several series, but not in others. Recently, Stone reported encouraging results in a small group of patients treated by left transthoracic splanchniectomy and bilateral truncal vagotomy. One-third of patients subsequently required right transthoracic splanchnicectomy. Over 90% of patients had excellent results, albeit with a mean follow-up of only 16 months. The intriguing aspect of this procedure is its potential to be performed thoracoscopically.

A denervated splenopancreatic flap procedure for chronic pancreatitis has also been described. The operation consists of a subtotal resection of the head of the pancreas, division of the gland at the junction of the neck and body, and complete mobilization of the distal pancreas and spleen from the retroperitoneum with division of the splenic artery and vein. The blood supply to the spleen and distal pancreas is maintained retrograde via the short gastric vessels, and the pancreatic remnant is drained into a Roux-en-Y limb of jejunum. This operation theoretically severs all neural pathways to the pancreas, excises the scarred pancreatic head, and drains the duct. Longer follow-up is needed, and the success of the original small series needs to be confirmed by others.

Pancreatic Autotransplantation

To avoid the complication of diabetes, autotransplantation of the distal pancreas has also been performed. After a 95% pancreatectomy, the duct of the distal 50 to 60% of the pancreas is injected with neoprene and ligated. The pancreatic remnant is placed in a subcutaneous pocket overlying the vastus lateralis muscle in the thigh. Vascular anastomoses are performed to the distal common femoral vessels. The number of patients is small and the length of follow-up is limited, so this procedure must still be regarded as experimental.

Islet Cell Autotransplantation

The University of Minnesota group has reported their series of patients who underwent total or near-total pancreatectomy with autotransplantation of dispersed islet tissue. Prepared islet cells are injected slowly into a mesenteric vein. There was one perioperative death in 26 patients and a 44% operative morbidity rate. Ninety percent of patients experienced partial or complete pain relief, and 20% are insulin independent at a mean follow-up of 5.7 years. Insulin independence correlated with the number of islets recovered, which was less when pancreatic fibrosis was more severe. Although still experimental, islet autotransplantation may prove to be a useful adjunct to extensive pancreatic resection.

Nonsurgical Approaches

Percutaneous neurolysis of the celiac ganglia by injection of ethanol or phenol may be valuable in patients with small pancreatic ducts who are not candidates for drainage or resective procedures. The procedure is effective in about two-thirds of patients, but pain recurs within 1 year in most. Although the procedure may be repeated, it is less likely to be effective.

PEPTIC ULCER DISEASE

method of
ARTHUR J. DECROSS, M.D., and
DAVID A. PEURA, M.D.
University of Virginia
Charlottesville, Virginia

There are approximately 4 million individuals with peptic ulcer disease (PUD) in the United States, with an annual incidence of about 350,000 new cases. Approximately 1.2 million individuals were hospitalized for PUD in 1990. Total yearly health care and indirect costs (e.g., time lost from work) associated with ulcer disease are estimated to be more than 3.2 billion dollars.

PATHOPHYSIOLOGY

The pathophysiology of PUD, which includes duodenal ulcers (DUs) and gastric ulcers (GUs), can be viewed as an imbalance between mucosal aggressive and defensive factors. Historically, gastric acid and peptic enzyme secretion were felt to be the major aggressive factors leading to ulceration. It was assumed that hypersecretion of acid simply overwhelmed mucosal defense mechanisms, resulting in an ulcer. However, only about one-third of patients with DU, and far fewer with GU, secrete excess gastric acid. Although extraordinary acid hypersecretion can occur in patients with gastrinoma (Zollinger-Ellison syndrome), these account for fewer than 0.1% of ulcers. Therefore, weakened mucosal defense has emerged as the major factor in the pathophysiology of PUD. Mucosal defense mechanisms are thought to include bicarbonate secretion, mucosal blood flow, prostaglandin synthesis, special properties of gastric mucus, and epithelial cell regeneration. Physiologic stress, as well as exogenous factors such as cigarette smoking, alcohol, and nonsteroidal anti-inflammatory drugs (NSAIDs), can impair these defensive mechanisms, thereby increasing mucosal susceptibility to the damaging effects of gastric acid and peptic activity.

Until recently, the treatment of PUD focused on re-establishing mucosal balance through the inhibition of acid (antacids, type 2 histamine receptor antagonists [H_2-RAs], or acid pump inhibitors) or the enhancement of mucosal protection (prostaglandin analogues or site protectants that coat ulcers). Smoking cessation and NSAIDs have also been shown to improve initial healing and maintenance management of PUD. Although these measures provide symptomatic relief and promote ulcer healing, they do little to alter the chronic relapsing natural history of the condition.

The discovery of *Helicobacter pylori* (HP) in 1982, a bacterium that leads to chronic infection and inflammation of the gastric mucosa, shed new light on the pathophysiology of peptic disease and revolutionized its therapeutic management. The role of HP in PUD is no longer speculative, but now well substantiated. A review of this relationship is beyond the scope and intent of this article, but may be found elsewhere.*

Although acid and pepsin still retain an important role as cofactors in the pathophysiology of PUD, the two most important etiologic factors are now considered to be HP and NSAIDs. Therefore, we will be referring to DUs and GUs as secondary to either HP or NSAIDs (e.g., HP-DU, NSAID-GU). The impact of this etiologic classification on the management of PUD is profound. While there is still a place for the traditional acid-suppressive or mucosal site–protective medications, the focus of management has shifted from the palliation of a chronic relapsing condition to (1) the cure of an infectious disease (for HP) or (2) the prevention and treatment of a drug-induced injury (for NSAIDs).

In addition to diagnostic and pharmacologic considerations, management strategies relevant to the initial therapy, follow-up, and maintenance therapy of PUD, as well as therapy for refractory ulcers, is discussed. However, the special situation of ulceration in critically ill patients, referred to as stress ulcer or stress-related mucosal damage,

*DeCross AJ, Marshall BJ: The role of *Helicobacter pylori* in acid-peptic disease. Am J Med Sci 306:381, 1993.

and very rare causes of ulcers, including extreme acid hypersecretion (e.g., gastrinoma, mastocytosis), anatomic abnormalities (e.g., duodenal webs), Crohn's disease, and non-*Helicobacter* infections in the immunocompromised and children (e.g., herpes simplex virus infection, cytomegalovirus infection) are beyond the scope of this article.

DIAGNOSIS

It is worth emphasizing the simple principle that an inaccurate diagnosis will probably result in ineffective treatment. This is particularly true in PUD, where the erroneous impression persists that DU and GU can be accurately diagnosed based on "classic" symptom presentation. The traditional symptom complex of DU is burning epigastric pain relieved by meals or antacids, often occurring 1 to 3 hours after a meal or awakening the patient at night. Epigastric pain in older patients that is not relieved by meals and is sometimes accompanied by weight loss is often attributed to GU. However, these clinical symptoms have repeatedly been shown to lack sensitivity and specificity for PUD. The rational treatment of PUD requires confirmation of an ulcer by either barium contrast radiography or, preferably, endoscopy. Although barium contrast radiography is almost as sensitive as endoscopy in identifying active ulceration, endoscopy has several important advantages. It permits biopsy of GUs to exclude malignancy, biopsy of the gastric antrum to assess for HP infection, differentiation of a re-epithelialized (inactive) ulcer scar from an acute ulcer, and diagnosis of nonulcer etiologies of dyspeptic symptoms (e.g., esophagitis).

Dyspepsia is a symptom complex of persistent or recurrent abdominal discomfort (commonly described as gnawing, burning, aching, or stabbing pain, tightening, or soreness), centered in the upper abdomen, often accompanied by some combination of belching, bloating, flatulence, distention, heartburn, nausea, or satiety. So defined, dyspepsia affects 20 to 40% of the population at some time and accounts for 2 to 3% of all visits to the primary care physician. The crucial decision is when to investigate dyspeptic complaints. In an otherwise healthy, reliable patient for whom follow-up is assured, dyspepsia can be managed initially with a short-term trial of empiric therapy. As will be discussed later, this usually consists of either antacids, H_2-RAs, or sucralfate (Carafate). Investigation of dyspeptic symptoms is recommended when (1) empiric therapy fails to relieve symptoms after 2 weeks, (2) symptoms recur after completion of a 6-week trial of empiric therapy, (3) patients are older than 45 to 50 years, (4) patients have risk factors for gastric cancer, or (5) dyspepsia is accompanied by symptoms and signs such as anorexia, early satiety, weight loss, anemia, or gastrointestinal bleeding.

MANAGEMENT

General Nonpharmacologic Considerations

Patients with PUD invariably ask for dietary recommendations. Diet is no longer considered to play a major role in the etiology or management of peptic ulcer disease, so patients should feel free to enjoy any foods they wish without fear of promoting new ulcers or delaying ulcer healing. Spicy foods, in particular, do not need to be deliberately excluded from the diet. Patients should be counseled, however, that certain foods can aggravate their symptoms, but this is highly individual and unpredictable. The best advice is to avoid particular foods that are troublesome. Although alcohol can cause mucosal injury, and alcohol abuse can interfere with compliance, there is no need to prohibit alcoholic beverages in moderation, especially if buffered with a meal. While caffeinated beverages are acid secretagogues, there is also no need to prohibit modest consumption of coffee, tea, or caffeinated sodas with meals. Despite its reputation, milk has been shown to be neither helpful nor harmful in the management of PUD.

Smoking is a risk factor for the development, recurrence, and impaired healing of HP-PUD; no data specifically link smoking with NSAID-PUD. Interestingly, following eradication of HP, smoking ceases to be a risk factor for ulcer recurrence. Cessation of smoking during acute and maintenance ulcer treatment has as great an impact on healing and recurrence as the use of routine pharmacologic measures. The poor compliance with smoking cessation, however, limits its therapeutic usefulness.

Pharmacologic Considerations

Antacids are more effective than placebo, and comparable to H_2-RAs, in providing symptom relief from PUD and in healing DUs. There are no good data to support antacid use to heal GUs. Unfortunately, most available data suggest that antacids are most effective when given in doses of 30 mL 1 and 3 hours after meals and at bedtime. The cost of such therapy approaches that of H_2-RAs, and in addition to their inconvenient dosing schedule, antacids can interfere with the absorption of other medications. Aluminum-based antacids can cause constipation, and magnesium-based preparations, diarrhea. Some antacids are particularly high in sodium and should be used cautiously by individuals with sodium and fluid restrictions. Renal insufficiency represents a relative contraindication to the use of magnesium-containing compounds.

There are four H_2-RAs in use: cimetidine (Tagamet), ranitidine (Zantac), famotidine (Pepcid), and nizatidine (Axid). All are equally effective in the treatment of PUD and are considered safe medications. Therapeutic doses (oral) for the healing of acute peptic ulceration are cimetidine, 400 mg twice daily; ranitidine, 150 mg twice daily; famotidine, 20 mg twice daily; or nizatidine, 150 mg twice daily. For DU, but not for GU, the total daily dose (oral) can be taken after the evening meal or at bedtime as follows: cimetidine, 800 mg; ranitidine, 300 mg; famotidine, 40 mg; or nizatidine, 300 mg. The H_2-RAs are also used for the prevention of recurrence in the following maintenance doses (oral): cimetidine, 400 mg at bedtime; ranitidine, 150 mg at bedtime; famotidine, 20 mg at bedtime; or nizatidine, 150 mg at bedtime. The most frequent side effect of the H_2-RAs is headache, which occurs in fewer than 10% of patients. Uncommonly, these drugs can cause idiosyncratic hepatotoxicity, cardiac conduction abnormalities, mental confusion, and thrombocytopenia. Cimetidine has antiandrogenic effects and has been reported to rarely cause gynecomastia and testicular atrophy. Additionally, cimetidine and to a lesser extent, ranitidine interfere with cytochrome P-450 metabolism of several classes of drugs, most significantly warfarin (Coumadin), anticonvulsants, and theophyllines.

Omeprazole (Prilosec) is currently the most potent acid-suppressing medication available in the United States. A therapeutic dose (oral) of 20 mg once daily heals PUD faster than the H_2-RAs, although this is of questionable clinical significance. For a patient with a bleeding complication, it seems rational to heal the ulcer as quickly as possible to reduce the chance of rebleeding. However, omeprazole has no proven superiority in this setting. Omeprazole can heal ulcers refractory to treatment with H_2-RAs, but a 40 mg once-daily dose (oral) is required. Since omeprazole works best on actively secreting parietal cells, it should be taken at mealtime. Omeprazole capsules contain enteric coated beads; the medication is broken down by acid, and absorption takes place in the small intestine. For these reasons, although the capsule can be opened and the beads administered via nasogastric tube, they should not be crushed. The enteric coating will dissolve in a suspension of neutral or basic pH, and it is, therefore, recommended that the beads be suspended in citrus juice for nasogastric administration. Omeprazole has few side effects. There is concern, based only on animal studies, that prolonged hypergastrinemia secondary to hypochlorhydria can cause gastric carcinoid tumors. This complication has never been seen in humans and almost a decade of experience in Europe confirms the safety of long-term administration. Nevertheless, omeprazole is currently approved for only 8 weeks of treatment in the United States, and more prolonged use should be limited to special clinical situations such as gastrinoma or severe gastroesophageal reflux disease in which alternative therapies are associated with significant morbidity or mortality.

Sucralfate (Carafate) is a sulfated polysaccharide complexed with aluminum hydroxide; its mechanism of action in promoting symptom relief and mucosal healing is not well understood. However, it is as effective as the H_2-RAs in healing and maintenance therapy of DU. There are insufficient data to support its use in healing or maintenance of GU. Early claims that sucralfate offered an advantage over H_2-RAs in patients who smoked have not been substantiated. For DU, the therapeutic dose (oral) is either 1 gram four times daily or 2 grams twice daily; the maintenance dose (oral) is 1 gram twice daily. Since sucralfate is poorly absorbed, it is theoretically safer to use in pregnant or lactating women. Side effects include constipation and interference with the absorption of other medications, although the clinical consequences appear to be minor.

Misoprostol (Cytotec) is a prostaglandin E_1 analogue that can heal ulcers but is primarily indicated for the prophylaxis of NSAID-PUD. The usual dose (oral) is 200 μg four times daily. Side effects of abdominal cramping and diarrhea are so frequent that patients are often started on 100 μg four times daily and slowly advanced to the 200 μg dose, which diminishes these symptoms. The drug is also an abortifacient and should never be prescribed to women who might be, or might become, pregnant.

There are no circumstances in which the combination of any of these medications has been shown to be superior to single-drug treatment. The particular practice of combining sucralfate and H_2-RAs or omeprazole and H_2-RAs needlessly increases the cost of therapy and should be discouraged.

When it is appropriate to treat an HP infection, as will be discussed later, standard therapy ("triple therapy") consists of the simultaneous 2-week administration (oral) of bismuth subsalicylate (Pepto-Bismol) two tablets four times daily, tetracycline, 500 mg four times daily, and metronidazole (Flagyl), 250 mg four times daily. Doxycycline (Vibramycin) cannot be substituted for tetracycline. For patients intolerant of tetracycline, amoxicillin, 500 mg four times daily, may be substituted. In patients with previous exposure to metronidazole, and thus in whom metronidazole-resistant organisms are likely, one of the following alternative therapeutic regimens may be used: a 2-week course (oral) of either omeprazole, 20 mg twice daily with amoxicillin, 500 mg four times daily; or omeprazole, 20 mg twice daily with clarithromycin (Biaxin), 500 mg three times daily. Omeprazole and the antibiotic should be started at the same time since pretreatment with an acid pump inhibitor reduces the likelihood of eradication. While the side effects of each antibiotic will not be reviewed here, it should be noted that up to half of the patients treated with "triple therapy" experience minor malaise, nausea, and loose stools, whereas the combination of omeprazole and an antibiotic is usually better tolerated. When clinically necessary, documentation that the infection has been eradicated should be pursued no earlier than 1 month after the completion of therapy (i.e., 6 weeks after the start of treatment).

Specific Recommendations

HP-DU

More than 90% of duodenal ulcers are due to *Helicobacter pylori* infection (HP-DU). The goals of initial therapy of HP-DU are to relieve symptoms and heal the ulcer, and these can be accomplished with therapeutic doses of antacids, sucralfate, H_2-RAs, or omeprazole given for 4 to 8 weeks. Selection of a particular therapy should be based on comparative costs and expected compliance. Eradication of HP is also an appropriate adjunctive treatment option, especially if the HP-DU is complicated or recurrent. If a patient is still symptomatic after 8 weeks, documentation (preferably by endoscopy) that the DU persists (and is therefore refractory to therapy) should be obtained; this will avoid continued PUD management for symptoms that may be due to a different etiology. Eradication of HP is appropriate for refractory HP-DUs. Alternatively, omeprazole, 40 mg daily for 8 weeks, will heal almost all HP-DUs failing treatment with therapeutic doses of H_2-RAs or sucralfate.

Once an HP-DU is healed, the goal is to prevent symptomatic recurrences and complications. If HP is not eradicated, the annual recurrence rate for HP-DU is about 70%, compared to about 10% following bacterial eradication. For recurrent or complicated HP-DU, anti-*Helicobacter* treatment is strongly recommended. An alternative approach to prevent recurrence and complications is continuous maintenance dose antiulcer treatment. For complicated HP-DU, such maintenance therapy should probably be continued indefinitely, even after eradication of HP has been confirmed.

NSAID-DU

The most important principle in treating peptic ulcers caused by nonsteroidal anti-inflammatory drugs (NSAID-PUD) is to discontinue the NSAID whenever possible. Often, these medications are prescribed for pain relief rather than for their anti-inflammatory effects. If analgesia is all that is required, then the PUD patient should be given a non-NSAID analgesic such as acetaminophen.

Whether or not the NSAID is discontinued, therapeutic doses of H_2-RAs, omeprazole or sucralfate for 6 to 8 weeks, will heal most NSAID-DUs. However, omeprazole, 40 mg once daily, may be appropriate for complicated, large, or slow healing NSAID-DUs, especially if the NSAID cannot be stopped.

If NSAIDs are restarted or continued, then the maintenance strategy for NSAID-DUs that healed with H_2-RAs involves continued therapeutic doses of the H_2-RAs (not maintenance doses). Misoprostol, 200 μg four times daily may also be used for this purpose. If a patient with a NSAID-DU also has HP infection, the bacteria should be eradicated.

HP-GU

About 70% of gastric ulcers are due to *Helicobacter pylori* infection (HP-GUs). Therapeutic doses of H_2-RAs or omeprazole for 12 weeks will heal most HP-GUs. The role of eradication of HP during initial therapy of GU is still controversial. Two key principles underlie the management of any GU: endoscopic biopsies should be obtained to exclude malignancy, and complete healing should be documented. A GU that does not heal after 12 weeks should be rebiopsied and NSAID use excluded. Refractory HP-GU is treated with omeprazole, 40 mg once daily for 8 weeks, and HP eradication. As with HP-DU, recurrence can be reduced by HP eradication or continuous maintenance treatment with full-dose (not maintenance dose) H_2-RAs.

NSAID-GU

The management of NSAID-GU is virtually identical to that of NSAID-DU with several exceptions. First, a NSAID-GU needs to be biopsied to exclude malignancy and its healing documented. Next, omeprazole, 20 mg or 40 mg once daily, is the preferred therapy if the NSAID cannot be stopped. Finally, the only effective prophylaxis against recurrence of NSAID-GU is misoprostol, 200 μg four times daily.

Surgical Considerations

Surgical intervention for DU is primarily indicated for complications such as perforation, uncontrollable hemorrhage, or unremitting obstruction. The need for elective surgery to control symptoms and recurrence is now rare. Consideration of elective surgery should prompt consultation with a gastroenterologist.

In addition to intervention for acute complications, elective surgery for GU is indicated for lesions completely refractory to medical treatment, even when multiple biopsies are benign. However, as outlined previously, a GU should not be considered completely refractory until medical therapy has included (1) 12 weeks of treatment with therapeutic doses of H_2-RAs or omeprazole; (2) 8 additional weeks of treatment with high-dose omeprazole (40 mg once daily); (3) eradication of HP; and (4) discontinuation or exclusion of NSAID use.

GASTRIC TUMORS

method of
BARBARA A. POCKAJ, M.D., and
BRUCE AVERBOOK, M.D.
Case Western Reserve University
Cleveland, Ohio

Benign tumors of the stomach represent only 2% of all gastric neoplasms. Benign lesions include mucosal epithelial polyps (40%), leiomyomas (40%), and other rare tumors. These benign tumors may appear in a variety of ways clinically. The patient may develop iron deficiency anemia secondary to tumor ulceration, epigastric pain, or intermittent obstruction. The diagnosis is usually made by endoscopy or radiographic evaluation. Indications for excision include tumor-related symptoms and exclusion of malignancy.

Gastric polyps are uncommon. Seventy-five percent of gastric polyps are hyperplastic. These polyps result from glandular proliferation and are not neoplastic. In contrast, adenomatous polyps may become malignant. Adenomatous polyps are either sessile or pedunculated and are usually located in the antrum. Like intestinal polyps, they can be tubular adenomas, tubulovillous adenomas, or villous adenomas. The association between these polyps and gastric cancer is related to their size. There is only a 4% incidence of malignancy in polyps less than 2 cm and a 20% incidence of malignancy in polyps greater than 2 cm. Endoscopic removal of all gastric polyps is indicated for pathologic evaluation. Open surgical excision is indicated when (1) a pedunculated polyp greater than 2 cm cannot be completely excised endoscopically, (2) a sessile polyp greater than 2 cm exists, and (3) in patients with multiple polyps that are either sporadic in nature or secondary to a polyposis syndrome. No additional treatment is required if there is no malignancy or if carcinoma-in-situ or cancer limited to the surface of the polyp is present. Formal gastrectomy is required, however, if invasion is found in the stalk, mucosa, or submucosa of the underlying stomach. Patients with a history of gastric polyps may have an increased risk for cancer. These patients need planned lifetime endoscopic surveillance to screen for early disease.

GASTRIC CANCER

In the United States, the incidence of gastric cancer has dramatically decreased over the last 50 years from 30 per 100,000 to seven per 100,000. Although the incidence has declined, survival after surgical resection remains unchanged. Gastric cancer is the sixth leading cause of cancer deaths in the United States. The overall 5-year survival is only about 10%. The disease is usually diagnosed at a late stage, which contributes to the lack of improved survival. Only 6 to 15% of cases are diagnosed as early gastric cancer, and 17 to 42% are regarded as unresectable at presentation. This is in contrast to the incidence in Japan, where gastric cancer is endemic, representing an incidence of 55 per 100,000 and the most common cause of cancer deaths. Massive screening programs have been carried out in Japan (accounting for the diagnosis of early cancer in 30 to 60% of patients), which contribute to an overall 5-year survival of 50%.

Epidemiology

Gastric cancer is more common in men than in women (2:1). In the United States, it is more common in blacks than in whites. Worldwide, there is a high incidence of gastric cancer in Japan, Iceland, Chile, and Costa Rica. The incidence increases with age and peaks in the seventh decade.

The varying incidence of gastric carcinoma from country to country supports an environmental etiology. Studies of migrant populations who are at high risk and then move to a low-risk area reveal that the first generation is still at twofold risk for gastric cancer but the second generation carries the same risk as the indigenous population. Diets high in salted or smoked meats or fish that are high in nitrates combined with diets low in animal protein and fat have been associated with an increased incidence of gastric cancer. A higher incidence of gastric cancer is found in certain miners and in workers exposed to some chemicals (nitrates), asbestos, and heavy metals. *Helicobacter pylori* has been reported in 90% of noncancerous tissue from patients who underwent resection for gastric cancer. Studies with matched controls have shown a 61 to 70% infection rate with *H. pylori,* suggesting that other factors contribute to the pathogenesis of gastric cancer.

There is some evidence for a genetic component to gastric cancer. People with blood group A have a higher incidence of gastric cancer. A first-degree relative of an individual with gastric cancer has a twofold to threefold increased risk of developing gastric cancer.

Other clinical conditions predispose individuals to the development of gastric cancer. Six to ten percent of patients with pernicious anemia develop gastric cancer. Chronic atrophic gastritis is a disease of decreased or absent normal gastric glands with hypochlorhydria or achlorhydria. Patients with chronic atrophic gastritis are at increased risk when intestinal metaplasia is present, especially the large intestinal variant. After 20 years, approximately 10% of patients will develop gastric carcinoma. Gastric cancer may complicate 10% of the cases of hypertrophic gastropathy (Ménétrier's disease). Gastric polyps represent a premalignant lesion, with the incidence of gastric cancer increasing with increasing tumor size. There is a 2 to 6% increased risk for gastric stump cancer in patients who undergo partial gastrectomy for benign disease. This is observed only after a latency period of 15 years. Most observed cases occur in patients operated on for gastric ulcers. There is also a higher incidence in women and those undergoing a Billroth II anastomosis. Patients with the above-mentioned risk factors should be followed carefully and screened to detect gastric cancer at an early stage.

Pathophysiology

The initial staging system for gastric cancer was introduced by Lauren in 1965. He divided the cases of gastric cancer into two distinctive subtypes: intestinal and diffuse. This system provides correlation between pathologic features, metastatic spread, and prognosis. The intestinal type has the tendency to form glands and resembles colon cancer with profuse inflammatory cell infiltration. It arises in a background of chronic gastritis, gastric atrophy, metaplasia, and dysplasia and is seen in the countries with a high incidence of gastric cancer. Most metastases are blood borne (most commonly liver and lungs). This form suggests an environmental etiology and is believed to be the epidemic form of the disease. The diffuse type forms tiny clusters of small uniform cells that spread more widely through the mucosa. This type is more commonly seen in women, younger patients, and in association with blood type A. The incidence is relatively constant and represents the endemic disease type. Spread is by transmural extension into the peritoneal cavity or adjacent organs and lymphatic invasion.

Most cancers are staged by the American Joint Commission TNM system. This system is largely based on pathological evaluation. The TNM system can accurately predict 5-year survival but the cancer cannot be accurately assessed before surgical resection.

The five-year survival rate of gastric cancer is poor (10%). Survival depends on many factors. The most important factor is depth of tumor penetration into the stomach wall. Early gastric cancers are those that penetrate only the mucosa or submucosa. These cancers have approximately a 10 to 15% incidence of lymph node metastases and a 5-year survival rate of 70 to 90%. Those patients with serosal penetration (late cancers) have only a 20% 5-year survival rate. Patients with positive lymph nodes demonstrate a 17% 5-year survival rate. Survival is further influenced by the number of lymph nodes involved with metastatic disease. Those patients with three or fewer metastatic lymph nodes or with tumors that measure 5 cm or less have an improved 5-year survival. A positive margin after surgical resection is a poor prognostic indicator, with no survivors usually found 2 years after surgery. The age and sex of the patients have no significant impact on survival.

Previously, most gastric cancers were located in the antrum of the stomach. These cancers have the best survival rates. Recently, the incidence of proximal carcinomas has increased from approximately 30% to 60%. Proximal carcinomas have a much worse prognosis than their more distal counterparts.

Diagnosis

Most patients with early gastric cancer are asymptomatic. Patients usually develop symptoms when the cancer becomes advanced. The most common presenting symptom is weight loss, occurring in 60% to 80% of patients. Thirty to sixty percent of patients develop abdominal pain that is usually epigastric in origin, unremitting, and aggravated by food. Presenting symptoms include nausea (30 to 40%); anorexia (30%); dysphagia, especially when lesions are located in the cardia (20 to 25%); and early satiety, especially with lesions of diffuse mucosal infiltration such as linitis plastica (17%). In addition, melena (12 to 20%), hematemesis (10 to 15%), gastric outlet obstruction in the presence of an enlarged antral tumor, and gastric perforation may be presenting signs. Therefore, symptoms of fatigue and dyspepsia with weight loss or anemia in patients older than 40 years of age should raise an index of suspicion that requires diligent examination to exclude gastric cancer.

Physical findings usually denote incurable disease. These include an abdominal mass (23%), cachexia (20%), hepatomegaly (17%), a Virchow's (supraclavicular) node (4%), ascites (3%), a Krukenberg (ovarian) tumor (5%), and a Blumer's (rectal) shelf (1%).

Radiographic evaluation by upper gastrointestinal series can detect 95% of advanced gastric cancers, but it may miss 20 to 40% of early gastric cancers. At present, upper gastrointestinal endoscopy is the mainstay of diagnosis and should be performed in all patients with suspected gastric cancer. A biopsy should be performed at the time of endoscopic evaluation for pathologic confirmation of the diagnosis. Six to ten biopsies should be performed to increase the yield of diagnosis to greater than 95%. Approximately 10% of all gastric ulcers are malignant, and the diagnosis cannot be made on gross appearance. All patients undergoing endoscopic evaluation for gastric ulcer should also have multiple biopsies to ensure a diagnosis of cancer is not missed.

After the diagnosis of gastric cancer is made, further metastatic work-up should include a chest x-ray study and abdominal (computed tomography) CT scan. The CT scan can overestimate or underestimate extragastric involvement in 50% of the cases; therefore, resectability of the tumor is only assessed by an exploratory laparotomy. A new method of preoperative evaluation is endoscopic ultrasound, which uses a high-frequency transducer at the end of an endoscope. It can accurately determine depth of invasion of the primary tumor and lymph node status. Endoscopic ultrasound has proved to be more accurate than CT scans in determining the local T and N status. This method can also accurately evaluate metastases to the left lobe of the liver and direct extension of the tumor into contiguous organs. It can be used to study patients with advanced cancer who are potential candidates for preoperative chemotherapy. The limitation of endoscopic ultrasound has been the size of the instrument. The endoscope cannot be passed through the tumor in 25 to 40% of patients because of stricture. Endoscopic ultrasound cannot be used to assess distant metastases and thus does not replace the CT scan in the preoperative evaluation. Others have advocated laparoscopic cytologic evaluation to determine those patients at high risk of recurrence and those that may benefit from adjuvant therapy. There are no biochemical markers that are useful for gastric cancer.

Therapy

The only potentially curative modality for localized gastric cancer is surgery. Overall, the biggest advance in gastric cancer therapy is decreased operative mortality over the last 20 years from 10 to 20% to 5 to 7%. Randomized trials have not documented differences in operative mortality or overall survival between subtotal versus total gastrectomy for distal carcinomas. The rationale for a total gastrectomy is that there may be extensive submucosal extension of tumor, and in 6% of patients, there are multiple carcinomas. For proximal lesions, total gastrectomy with a roux-en-Y anastomosis is superior to proximal subtotal gastrectomy because roux-en-Y anastomosis alleviates postoperative alkaline reflux gastritis. Another group of patients who will benefit from a total gastrectomy includes those with diffuse lesions (linitis plastica), large tumors, mucosal lesions with malignant potential (e.g., chronic atrophic gastritis), a strong family history, and diffuse gastric polyposis syndromes.

Controversy exists among surgeons whether extended (radical) lymphadenectomy improves survival in patients with gastric cancer. The Japanese routinely perform extended lymphadenectomy at the time of resection for gastric cancer and believe this has led to their improved long-term survival. Studies conducted in Western nations have not conclusively linked improved survival with radical lymphadenectomy. The greatest difficulty is in determining who may benefit from the radical surgery preoperatively. The extended lymphadenectomy employed by the Japanese includes not only resection of N1 nodes (perigastric) but also resection of the greater and lesser omentum; the superior leaf of the transverse mesocolon; the pancreatic capsule; and the hepatic, common hepatic, celiac, and splenic lymph nodes. In addition, the left gastric artery is ligated en bloc with the gastrectomy specimen.

Other therapies currently under investigation include laser fulguration and photodynamic laser ablation for early gastric cancers limited to the mucosa. These modalities are also being used for palliation in advanced gastric cancers with bleeding or obstruction. Early reports from Japan suggest that these forms of ablation are reasonable alternatives, especially in patients who are poor surgical candidates.

Some patients with advanced gastric cancer at the time of laparotomy benefit from palliative gastrectomy. In several studies, most patients report improvement of their symptoms, and the investigators document improved rates of survival. Selected patients, with a good premorbid status, can tolerate the gastrectomies with acceptable morbidity and mortality.

There have been several trials of adjuvant chemotherapy for gastric cancer. Thus far, most trials have not shown a survival advantage in the treatment group. Currently trials are ongoing for patients at high risk for recurrence. Neoadjuvant studies are now being investigated for patients with locally advanced gastric cancers, and early reports have shown promise. A neoadjuvant trial at the Surgery Branch of the National Cancer Institute (NCI) has shown a partial response rate of 38% and comparable resectability rates of 65 to 70% after a regimen of 5-fluorouracil (5-FU), leucovorin, and interferon-alpha. Recurrences that developed after treatment were primarily confined to the peritoneal cavity and accounted for most deaths. Overall, previous data have shown local relapse occurs in 40 to 80% of patients after undergoing potentially curable gastrectomy.

In efforts to address the problem of peritoneal recurrences and after review of Japanese data with intraperitoneal mitomycin-C, preclinical studies were conducted at the Surgery Branch, NCI, using continuous hyperthermic peritoneal perfusion (CHPP) with tumor necrosis factor-alpha (TNF-α) in pigs. These studies demonstrated that high levels of TNF-α were maintained in the peritoneal cavity and detected serum levels were not toxic to the animals. A new Phase I study for peritoneal carcinomatosis from gastrointestinal malignancy (especially from gastric cancer) is under way using CHPP, a fixed dose of cisplatin, and escalating doses of TNF-α. The peritoneal perfusion is performed at a temperature of 42° to 43°C (107.6° to 109.4°F) using a roller pump circuit with a heat exchanger.

Because of the high local failure rate of gastric cancer chemotherapy, radiation therapy is also an attractive adjuvant therapy to consider. At present, there have been few reported studies using external beam or intraoperative radiation therapy. The use of radiation therapy is constrained secondary to the proximity of normal tissues near the tumor mass, thus limiting the dose that can be delivered.

Systemic chemotherapy is used to treat metastatic gastric cancer. 5-Fluorouracil (5-FU) is the most extensively studied single agent, with a response rate of 21%. The most common multidrug regimen includes 5-FU, doxorubicin, and mitomycin-C (FAM) with a response rate of 30%. Although various multidrug chemotherapeutic regimens have been studied, none has had decisively superior survival to 5-FU alone.

GASTRIC LYMPHOMA

Gastric lymphomas represent the most common site for lymphoma of the gastrointestinal tract. Gastric lymphomas account for less than 5% of all gastric cancers. The presentation of gastric lymphoma is similar to gastric adenocarcinoma. Most patients are older than 50 years of age. Men are affected twice as often. Most patients present with abdominal pain, weight loss, nausea, vomiting, and anorexia. The diagnosis is made by endoscopic evaluation with biopsy. Accuracy of this technique has been reported at 50 to 90%. Because of the difficulty in diagnosis, a combination of biopsy and brush cytology has been used to increase the yield of diagnosis. Systemic lymphoma needs to be ruled out in the work-up, which includes a chest x-ray study, abdominal CT scan, and bone marrow biopsy. In contrast to other lymphomas, gastric lymphoma has a pattern of spread similar to gastric adenocarcinoma. Local spread to contiguous organs and lymph nodes is followed by distant metastases. The most common types of lymphoma encountered are diffuse histiocytic of mixed lymphocytic and histiocytic type. Prognosis is improved in those patients with a nodular pattern and low nuclear grade, whereas a poorer prognosis is found in patients with diffuse pattern, tumor size greater than 5 cm, serosal involvement, regional lymph node metastases, and distant metastases.

The treatment of gastric lymphoma is controversial. There are few prospective studies that evaluate the primary role of surgery, chemotherapy, or radiation therapy. In studies using Cox regression analyses to remove selection bias and variables that alter prognosis, surgical resection appears to be the primary treatment modality with a significant impact on survival. Most medical centers resect gastric lymphomas and use radiation therapy and chemotherapy (usually Cytoxan, Adriamycin, vincristine, and prednisone [CHOP]) for patients at a high risk for recurrence or with incomplete resection. Chemotherapy is indicated in the presence of diffuse metastatic disease. Because new therapeutic modalities are emerging, it is advisable for a primary care physician to elicit opinions from the surgical, radiation, and medical oncologists so that the optimal treatment plan can be offered to a patient.

MALIGNANT DISEASES OF THE COLON AND RECTUM

method of
STEVEN D. WEXNER, M.D., and
JUAN J. NOGUERAS, M.D.
Cleveland Clinic Florida
Ft. Lauderdale, Florida

In the United States, an estimated 149,000 new cases of carcinoma of the colon and rectum will be diagnosed this year, and an estimated 56,000 persons will die of the disease. Colorectal cancer is surpassed only by lung cancer as a cause of cancer mortality. The age-adjusted incidence rates of colon cancer and rectal cancer are 40.6 and 18.1 per 100,000 males and 29.6 and 10.6 per 100,000 females, respectively. Although the sigmoid colon remains the most common site, an increased incidence of right-sided lesions has recently been described. Moreover, the National Cancer Institute has reported a decline in both incidence and mortality rates for colorectal cancer in the United States during recent years. Many factors may be responsible for this decline, including increased public and professional awareness, endoscopic removal of precursor colonic adenomas, and improved dietary habits (i.e., either a reduction in ingestion of carcinogenic agents, an increase in intake of "protective" agents, or both).

Among 46 industrialized nations reporting cancer data to the World Health Organization, the United States ranked twentieth and nineteenth for males and females, respectively, in age-adjusted death rates per 100,000 population for carcinoma of the colon and the rectum. Czechoslovakia and New Zealand ranked first among males and females, respectively, whereas Mexico and Ecuador ranked lowest among these 46 nations.

PATHOGENESIS

Population studies of Japanese and Chinese immigrant families reveal an increase in incidence of colorectal carcinoma after migration to the United States. Among the many environmental factors that may be responsible for this phenomenon is the adoption of a westernized diet. Numerous studies confirm that increased consumption of dietary fat, especially animal fat, is associated with the development of colorectal cancer. Other factors, such as obesity and a sedentary lifestyle, are also associated with colorectal cancer. Recently, cigarette smoking has been implicated in the development of colorectal adenomatous polyps.

Diet may also play a role in the prevention of colorectal neoplasia. Increased consumption of dietary fiber, especially insoluble or grain fiber, has been associated with a lower risk of colorectal cancer. The Melbourne Colorectal Cancer Study concluded that all types of fiber are probably protective against colorectal neoplasia, and this has been corroborated by other studies. In addition to fiber, other dietary factors, such as calcium, selenium, and vitamins A, D, C, and E, may also play a protective role. Large-scale clinical trials are under way to examine the effects of nutritional factors on the development of colorectal neoplasia. The National Cancer Institute–sponsored Large Bowel Adenomatous Polyp Dietary Intervention Study will evaluate the recurrence rate of colorectal adenomas. The rate in subjects with a history of adenomatous polyp who receive a low-fat, high-fiber diet will be compared with that of a control group. Another large study sponsored by the American Cancer Society will examine the effects of a fat-reduced and fiber-enriched diet on polyp recurrence.

Based on current information, certain dietary recommendations can be made. Dietary fat should comprise less than 30% of total caloric intake, and the intake of animal (saturated) fat should be reduced. Dietary fiber intake should be no less than 20 grams per day, including ample raw vegetables and fruits. Patients should be advised to exercise, control obesity, avoid smoking, and limit alcohol consumption.

Adenomatous polyps are regarded as the precursor lesion of colorectal cancer. There is abundant circumstantial evidence to support the adenoma-to-carcinoma sequence. For example, most adenocarcinomas arise from adenomatous tissue, and the occurrence of de novo cancers is exceedingly rare. Adenomas are common in populations with a high incidence of colorectal cancer but are unusual in those with a low cancer incidence. Moreover, adenomas and carcinomas share some genetic characteristics, such as *ras* gene mutations and allelic loss of chromosomes 5 and 18.

The risk of malignancy in an adenomatous polyp increases with the size, degree of dysplasia, and extent of villous component of the adenoma. The vast majority of polyps can be colonoscopically removed. Histopathologic evaluation of these lesions generally reveals them to be entirely benign. Those few lesions in which a carcinoma is noted must be assessed as to the level of invasion of the neoplasm as well as the adequacy of the electrocautery margin. For these reasons, endoscopic polypectomy with adequate surveillance may reduce the long-term risk of developing colorectal cancer.

Most cases of colorectal cancer are sporadic, but certain inherited conditions predisposing to cancer exist. Familial adenomatous polyposis (FAP) represents approximately 1% of all cases of colorectal cancer. In this autosomal dominant inherited condition, there is a generalized growth disorder heralded by multiple adenomatous polyps in the large intestine. The majority of untreated patients develop colorectal carcinoma by the fourth decade of life. Occasionally, the condition is diagnosed in the older patient. FAP patients are also prone to develop tumors at other locations, including periampullary duodenal neoplasms and desmoid tumors. The value of an organized registry in monitoring affected families is well documented.

Hereditary nonpolyposis colorectal cancer (HNPCC) syndromes are manifested by a family history of colorectal cancer at an early age. These cancers are frequently located on the right side of the colon, and are often mucinous. In addition to colorectal cancer (Lynch I syndrome), HNPCC patients are at increased risk of developing cancers of the ovary, breast, and endometrium (Lynch II syndrome).

During the past decade, exciting molecular discoveries at the genetic level have increased our understanding of the events leading to colorectal tumorigenesis. It is apparent that the genetic alterations function as a multistep process, with both suppressing and proliferating events. In patients with FAP, there is an inherited deletion of the long arm of chromosome 5 (5q). The gene responsible for FAP, which has been isolated on 5q is termed the APC gene. Moreover, another gene sequence on 5q, termed MCC, has been identified and may be responsible for sporadic colorectal cancers. In addition to alterations in chromosome 5, other genetic events may be responsible for the development of colorectal cancer. These include *ras* gene mutation, and allelic deletions of chromosomes 17 and 18. Further research at the genetic level will hopefully guide development of newer targeted therapies.

SCREENING

The rationale for screening an asymptomatic population is to improve survival by detecting the neoplastic process at a point in its natural history when it will be most responsive to therapeutic intervention. An effective screening program will employ tests with a low rate of false-positive and false-negative results and therefore high sensitivity and specificity and positive predictive value. The end result of such a program should be a decrease in cancer-related mortality. Data from large colorectal cancer screening trials document that the diagnostic yield is 70% higher in a screened group than in a control group. Moreover, 60% of the cancers found in the screened group are node negative (Stage I or II), compared with only 45% of lesions in the control group. In addition, more premalignant adenomas are found in the screened group.

The current recommendations of the American Cancer Society for asymptomatic individuals include an annual digital rectal examination beginning at age 40 and a sigmoidoscopic examination every 3 to 5 years in conjunction with an annual fecal occult blood test after age 50. Those patients with a first-degree relative with colorectal cancer diagnosed at age younger than 55 years are recommended to have colonoscopy every 5 years starting at age 35 to 40 years. The exact age of the first recommended colonoscopy is partially determined by the age at which the relatives had their carcinoma. In general, if a single first-degree relative had a tumor discovered at an advanced age, screening can begin later in life than if two first-degree relatives developed colorectal neoplasia in their fourth decade.

The peroxidase test (Hemoccult) is the most widely used test to detect fecal occult blood. The test has a false-positive rate of approximately 3% and a false-negative rate approaching 31% with an overall predictive value of 22% and 58% for adenoma and carcinoma, respectively. Recent data support the utility of the peroxidase fecal occult blood test for colorectal cancer screening. The University of Minnesota study demonstrated a 33% reduction in mortality from colorectal cancer by annual fecal occult blood testing with rehydrated slides combined with colonoscopy in patients with positive results. Other studies have also shown similar rates of reduction in colorectal cancer mortality with fecal occult blood screening. It is crucial not to assume that random fecal occult blood testing has the same value as routine population screening. Numerous studies have documented that up to 60% of patients in whom fecal occult blood is noted have no colorectal pathology. Perhaps more significant is the fact that 50% of patients with known colorectal carcinoma have false-negative fecal occult blood tests.

Digital rectal examination alone will detect only those tumors within reach of the examining finger and will therefore miss 85 to 90% of all colorectal cancers. The rigid proctosigmoidoscope will reach approximately 28% of all colorectal cancers, and although this examination can be uncomfortable for the patient, it is relatively quick and easy and is less expensive than other endoscopic examinations. However, up to 64% of tumors can be detected with a flexible sigmoidoscope inserted to the splenic flexure. Flexible sigmoidoscopy has a much higher yield, is probably more comfortable for the patient, and requires little extra time. However, it does require additional training and the purchase of expensive equipment. Complete visualization of the colon is achieved in the majority of patients with a colonoscopy to the cecum. This procedure is expensive, reliant on specially trained personnel, and associated with a 0.1 to 0.3% complication rate.

SYMPTOMS

The majority of patients with symptomatic colorectal tumors have advanced disease. The most common symptoms are rectal bleeding and changes in bowel habits. Left-sided colonic tumors are more prone to present with obstructive symptoms for a variety of reasons. The lumen of the left colon is narrower than the lumen on the right side, and because it carries a more solid stool load is more prone to obstruction from an intraluminal tumor. Tumors of the right side, especially in the cecum, can grow to a large size before affecting bowel habits. More often, these tumors will present with hematochezia, melena, or occult fecal bleeding. A history of rectal bleeding in patients within the population at risk for developing colorectal cancer mandates complete colonic evaluation.

TREATMENT

Preoperative Evaluation

Once a diagnosis of colorectal carcinoma is established, the goals of preoperative evaluation include exclusion of synchronous colonic lesions, assessment of perioperative risk factors, and staging of the tumor. A thorough cardiopulmonary and medical evaluation will assess the condition of the patient and help to minimize perioperative risk. In addition to routine preoperative blood studies, a serum carcinoembryonic antigen (CEA) level is obtained. Elevated preoperative CEA may have adverse prognostic significance, and postoperative monitoring of the CEA level may help to detect otherwise clinically undetectable recurrent disease. The incidence of synchronous carcinoma is between 2% and 6%. Thus, total colonic evaluation is necessary with either colonoscopy or double-contrast barium enema in order to exclude synchronous lesions.

Accurate preoperative staging of a colorectal tumor helps to guide surgical therapy. Surgical resections for colonic malignancies are standard for tumor location and independent of the depth of tumor penetration or the presence of enlarged pericolic lymph nodes. If there are distant metastases, palliative colonic resection is performed in order to prevent obstruction or bleeding. Therefore, preoperative staging of a colonic tumor is not as important as it is with rectal tumors. Preoperative computerized axial tomography may be helpful in documenting liver metastases or adjacent organ invasion and therefore useful for specific protocols, such as placement of a hepatic artery infusion pump or insertion of ureteral catheters.

As mentioned, preoperative staging of rectal cancers helps in selecting among the various surgical options available for the management of rectal tumors. This is especially true for distal rectal cancers, for which the options range from local excision to abdominoperineal resection. Although the procedure can be selected at the time of surgery, failure to take advantage of advanced planning is unfair to the patient. Thus maximum information about tumor height, size, mobility, and depth of invasion should should be gleaned prior to surgery. Rigid proctoscopy is performed in order to accurately measure the level of the tumor with respect to the dentate line; tumor appearance can be assessed and biopsies obtained. Endorectal ultrasonography can help to determine the depth of tumor penetration through the rectal wall, and the presence of any enlarged pararectal lymph nodes. In experienced hands, endorectal ultrasonography has an accuracy rate of nearly 90% in determining depth of penetration of the tumor and an accuracy rate of 70% in predicting nodal metastases. Such information is helpful in selecting appropriate patients for local therapy, major resective surgery, and preoperative adjuvant therapy. Computerized axial tomography or magnetic resonance imaging are more expensive tests that are helpful in delineating pelvic anatomy and the relation of the tumor to the surrounding viscera. However, both of these tests are inadequate in assessing depth of invasion.

Surgical Therapy

Surgical resection is the primary modality for the management of colonic carcinoma. The goal of surgery is to maximize the chance for cure through en bloc removal of the tumor and the lymphatic nodal basin with margins that are adequate to ensure removal of the entire locoregional tumor burden. Resection of a tumor located in the right colon should include the ileocolic, right colic, and right branch of the middle colic artery. Resection of a tumor at the hepatic or splenic flexure or in the transverse colon should include the entire distribution of the middle colic artery. For tumors in the descending colon, a left hemicolectomy is performed that includes the left branch of the middle colic and the left colic artery. Sigmoid carcinomas can be resected with a sigmoid colectomy. None of these operations are controversial as all have withstood the test of time.

Colotomy and disc excision or wedge resection have no role in the curative treatment of colonic adenocarcinoma. The advent of the laparoscope has led many to champion its use for colonic cancer, despite irrefutable proof of the inadequacy of such limited resections. Until the conclusion of prospective, randomized trials and the subsequent assessment of 5-year recurrence and survival data, it is premature to recommend "routine" laparoscopic resections for cure of colon cancer.

A variety of options are available for the management of rectal carcinoma. Surgical procedures include transanal resection, anterior resection, sphincter-preserving coloanal resection, and abdominoperineal resection. Among the nonoperative options are electrocoagulation, endocavitary irradiation, and laser photoablation. The choice of surgical procedure is dependent upon a variety of factors, including the level of the tumor from the dentate line. The rectum is 15 cm in length and is traditionally divided into 3- to 5-cm long surgical segments: upper, middle, and lower. In general upper third lesions are managed by an anterior resection with colorectal anastomosis. Middle third lesions fall in the "zone of controversy": a variety of procedures are recommended. Sphincter-preserving procedures are technically feasible for many tumors at this level. The creation of colonic reservoirs with coloanal anastomosis may improve early functional results. Lower third rectal tumors are best assessed with endorectal ultrasonography in order to determine the depth of penetration through the rectal wall and the presence of any perirectal nodal metastases. The surgeon must choose among transanal techniques, coloanal anastomosis, or abdominoperineal resection.

Controversial issues in the operative management of rectal carcinoma include level of vessel ligation, distal margin of resection, and extent of lateral margins. High ligation of the inferior mesenteric artery (IMA) at its takeoff from the aorta was initially advocated by Moynihan in 1908. To date, there are no controlled studies that document a survival advantage to high ligation of the IMA compared to other resective techniques. With the widespread use of sphincter-saving anterior resections, the length of the distal rectal margin of clearance from the tumor has been the focus of renewed interest. The traditional 5-cm margin has been challenged by recent data that fail to show a survival advantage over a 2-cm margin. The curative intent of an operation for rectal carcinoma will not be compromised if a 2-cm margin of distal clearance is obtained.

There is mounting evidence that an adequate curative resection for rectal carcinoma must envelop clear lateral margins of resection in addition to a minimum distal margin. Heald and co-workers advocate total mesorectal excision (TME) for low-lying rectal carcinomas, believing that this extended technique will decrease the incidence of local pelvic recurrence. Heald's published series of 218 patients who underwent curative resection of rectal carcinoma with TME and no adjuvant radiation therapy with a mean follow-up period of 10 years documented a local recurrence rate of 5%. These results were achieved at some cost, however, because all patients had temporary diversion. The postoperative complication rate was 19% with an anastomotic leak rate of 13%. The principles of total mesorectal excision imply that in order to achieve a curative resection and diminish the chance for local recurrence, the lateral lymphatic margins must be cleared. Quirke and Williams have confirmed that adequate lateral resection margins are very important as independent variables in predicting local recurrence. These data support the notion that the technique and conduct of the operation is an important prognostic variable that needs to be considered when results of adjuvant therapy trials are evaluated.

Transanal local excision of rectal carcinomas is an acceptable option for selected tumors. Criteria include tumors that are exophytic, less than 3 cm in size, well- to moderately well-differentiated, and involving less than one-half of the rectal circumference. Endorectal ultrasound is useful for determining the depth of tumor penetration through the rectal wall.

Local excision should be reserved for tumors that are confined to the rectal wall, in the absence of enlarged pararectal lymphadenopathy.

Adjuvant Therapy

The purpose of adjuvant therapy in colonic neoplasia after curative resection is to eradicate occult and viable tumor cells that have the potential for implantation at local and distant sites. The recent study by the North Central Cancer Treatment Group, with a median follow-up of 5 years, documents significantly decreased recurrence rates, cancer deaths, and overall death rate with a combination of 5-fluorouracil (5-FU) (Adrucil) and levamisole (Ergamisol) for Stage III colon carcinoma when compared to those patients receiving levamisole only or surgery only. Debate persists regarding the need for levamisole or other 5-FU modulators, the role of adjuvant therapy in Stage II disease, and the efficacy of portal vein infusion.

Controversial issues in the adjuvant therapy of rectal carcinoma include timing of radiation therapy (preoperative, intraoperative, or postoperative), dosages of radiation therapy, and benefit from combining radiation therapy with chemotherapy. The rationale for radiation therapy in rectal carcinoma is to effect a reduction in locoregional recurrence that will result in improved survival rates. A number of clinical trials involving adjuvant radiation therapy for rectal carcinoma have been completed. Some studies have demonstrated a reduced incidence of local recurrence with either preoperative or postoperative radiation therapy when compared to surgery alone. In studies comparing preoperative versus postoperative radiation therapy, preoperative irradiation was better tolerated and associated with fewer complications. Despite reduced rates of local recurrence, there are no data documenting improved survival with adjuvant radiation therapy alone for rectal carcinoma. However, combinations of chemotherapy and radiation therapy have realized advantages in survival and reductions in cancer recurrence rates when compared to surgery alone or postoperative radiation alone. Some of the studies involved the use of 5-FU and semustine (methyl-CCNU)* with postoperative radiation. The complications of this combined modality regimen are significant, and there is a reluctance to use semustine because of its toxicity, particularly blood dyscrasias. Newer combinations will be the focus of future trials.

*Investigational drug in the United States.

INTESTINAL PARASITES

method of
RICHARD D. PEARSON, M.D.
University of Virginia School of Medicine
Charlottesville, Virginia

Enteric parasites are prevalent among persons who live in developing areas of the world where sanitation is poor, and these parasites pose a risk to international travelers. A number of enteric parasites are endemic in North America. Several have emerged as important causes of disease in persons with the acquired immune deficiency syndrome (AIDS). Enteric parasites can be classified as either protozoa or helminths. Protozoa are single-celled organisms with the capacity to divide and multiply within humans. Theoretically, infection with even one protozoan can lead to life-threatening disease. Helminths, on the other hand, are multicellular organisms with internal organs and complex life cycles. With two important exceptions, *Strongyloides stercoralis* and *Hymenolepis nana,* which are capable of autoinfection, helminths do not multiply in humans. The severity of helminthic disease is usually correlated with the magnitude of the worm burden, although a single adult worm or larva can on occasion cause life-threatening disease, as in the case of an adult *Ascaris lumbricoides* that migrates into and obstructs the pancreatic duct.

In most instances the diagnosis of an intestinal parasitic infection is made by identifying ova, larvae, or adult worms in stool. Eosinophilia is common when helminths migrate through tissues, but it is frequently absent when adult worms are confined to the gastrointestinal tract. In contrast, eosinophilia is not typically a feature of protozoal infections. In a few parasitic infections, the finding of antibodies in serum allows for a presumptive diagnosis. New techniques to detect coproantigens are being developed for several of the enteric parasites.

Effective drugs are available for the treatment of all but a few of the enteric parasites. Specific recommendations for the treatment of protozoal infections are listed alphabetically in Table 1 and for helminthic diseases in Table 2 and are discussed in detail in the text.* They are based on the consensus recommendations of *The Medical Letter on Drugs and Therapeutics* (35:111–122, 1993). In some instances the drug of choice for a given parasitic disease has been licensed by the United States Food and Drug Administration (FDA) but for different indications. In others the drug of choice is not licensed in the United States. Many such drugs are available from the CDC Drug Service at the Centers for Disease Control and Prevention (see Tables 1 and 2). A full description of the life cycles, clinical manifestations and diagnostic approaches is available elsewhere.† Therapeutic issues are discussed in the following sections.

INTESTINAL PROTOZOA

Giardia lamblia is an important cause of acute and chronic diarrhea in North Americans. Large waterborne outbreaks have been reported from communities in the Rocky Mountains and the Appalachian Mountains. Infection is occasionally acquired by hikers who drink unboiled ground water, and *G. lamblia* is a relatively common pathogen among children in day care centers. Giardiasis can be acquired during international travel. It has historically been a problem for Americans who visit Moscow and other cities

*In this article, adult dosages are given in the text; pediatric dosages can be found in Tables 1 and 2.

†Jernigan J, Guerrant RL, Pearson RD: Parasitic infections of the small intestine. *Gut,* 35:289–293, 1994; Pearson RD: Parasitic diseases: helminths. *In* Yamada T, et al (eds): Textbook of Gastroenterology. Philadelphia, JB Lippincott Co, 1994, in press; Guerrant RL: Schwartzman JD, Pearson RD: Intestinal nematode infections. *In* Strickland GT (ed): Hunter's Tropical Medicine, 7th ed. Philadelphia, WB Saunders Co, 1991, pp 684–711.

TABLE 1. **Drugs for the Treatment of Protozoal Infections**

Infection	Drug	Adult Dosage	Pediatric Dosage
Amebiasis *(Entamoeba histolytica)*			
Asymptomatic			
Drug of choice	Iodoquinol	650 mg tid × 20 d	30–40 mg/kg/d in 3 doses × 20 d
	or		
	Paromomycin	25–30 mg/kg/d in 3 doses × 7 d	25–30 mg/kg/d in 3 doses × 7 d
Alternative	Diloxanide furoate†	500 mg tid × 10 d	20 mg/kg/d in 3 doses × 10 d
Mild to moderate intestinal disease			
Drug of choice	Metronidazole	750 mg tid × 10 d	35–50 mg/kg/d in 3 doses × 10 d
	or		
	Tinidazole*	2 grams/d × 3 d	50 mg/kg (max 2 g) qd × 3 d
Followed by iodoquinol, paromomycin, or diloxanide furoate as above			
Severe intestinal disease			
Drugs of choice	Metronidazole	750 mg tid × 10 d	35–50 mg/kg/d in 3 doses × 10 d
	or		
	Tinidazole*	600 mg bid × 5 d	50 mg/kg (max 2 g) qd × 3 d
Alternative	Dehydroemetine†	1 to 1.5 mg/kg/d (max 90 mg/d) IM for up to 5 d	1 to 1.5 mg/kg/d (max 90 mg/d) IM in 2 doses for up to 5 d
Followed by iodoquinol, paramomycin, or diloxanide furoate as above			
Blastocystis hominis Infection			
Drug of choice	See text		
Cryptosporidiosis *(Cryptosporidium parvum)*			
Drug of choice	See text		
Cyclospora species			
Drug of choice	Trimethoprim-sulfamethoxazole	TMP 160 mg, SMX 800 mg bid × 3 d	TMP 5 mg/kg, SMX 25 mg/kg bid × 3 d
Dientamoeba fragilis			
Drug of choice	Iodoquinol	650 mg tid × 20 d	40 mg/kg/d in 3 doses × 20 d
	or		
	Paromomycin	25–30 mg/kg/d in 3 doses × 7 d	25–30 mg/kg/d in 3 doses × 7 d
	or		
	Tetracycline	500 mg qid × 10 d	40 mg/kg/d (max 2 gm/d) in 4 doses × 10 d (not recommended for children less than 8 yr)
Entamoeba polecki Infection			
Drug of choice	Metronidazole	750 mg tid × 10 d	35–50 mg/kg/d in 3 doses × 10 d
Giardiasis *(Giardia lamblia)*			
Drug of choice	Metronidazole	250 mg tid × 5 d	15 mg/kg/d in 3 doses × 5 d
Alternatives	Quinacrine HCI*	100 mg tid after meals × 5 d	6 mg/kg/d in 3 doses after meals × 5 d (max 300 mg/d)
	or		
	Tinidazole*	2 gm once	50 mg/kg once (max 2 gm)
	or		
	Furazolidone	100 mg qid × 7–10 d	6 mg/kg/d in 4 doses × 7–10 d
	or		
	Paromomycin	25–30 mg/kg/d in 3 doses × 7 d	
Isosporiasis *(Isospora belli)* Drug of choice	Trimethoprim-sulfamethoxazole	160 mg TMP, 800 mg SMX qid × 10 d, then bid × 3 wk	
Microsporidiosis			
Intestinal *(Enterocytozoon bieneusi, Septata intestinalis)*			
Drug of choice	See text		

*Not available in the United States.
†Available from the CDC Drug Service, Centers for Disease Control and Prevention, Atlanta, GA 30333; 404-639-3670 (evenings, weekends, or holidays, 404-639-2888).
Modified from Drugs for parasitic infections. Med Lett Drugs Ther 35:111–122, 1993.

in the former Soviet Union. Although *G. lamblia* is prevalent among children living in developing tropical areas, it does not appear to be a major cause of disease among them.

Metronidazole (Flagyl), administered at the relatively low dose of 250 mg three times a day for 5 days, is the drug of choice for the treatment of adults with giardiasis, although it has not been approved for this specific indication by the FDA. Patients must be warned against the use of alcohol while taking metronidazole because of its disulfiram-like effect. Gastrointestinal disturbances, headache, dry mouth, and a metallic taste are relatively frequent side effects. On rare occasions, metronidazole has been associated with seizures, encephalopathy, peripheral neuropathy, ataxia, and pancreatitis.

Quinacrine* (Atabrine), 100 mg three times a day after meals for 5 days, has similar efficacy in giardiasis, but it is frequently associated with gastrointes-

*Not available in the United States.

TABLE 2. **Drugs for the Treatment of Helminth Infections**

Infection	Drug	Adult Dosage	Pediatric Dosage
Angiostrongyliasis *(Angiostrongylus costaricensis)*			
Drug of choice	Thiabendazole	75 mg/kg/d in 3 doses × 3 d (max 3 gm/d); toxicity may require dosage reduction	75 mg/kg/d in 3 doses × 3 d (max 3 gm/d); toxicity may require dosage reduction
Anisakiasis *(Anisakis* and other genera)			
Treatment of choice	Surgical or endoscopic removal		
Ascariasis *(Ascaris lumbricoides)*			
Drug of choice	Mebendazole	100 mg bid × 3 d	100 mg bid × 3 d
	or		
	Pyrantel pamoate	11 mg/kg once (max 1 gm)	11 mg/kg once (max 1 gm)
	or		
	Albendazole*	400 mg once	400 mg once
Capillariasis *(Capillaria philippinensis)*			
Drug of choice	Mebendazole	200 mg bid × 20 d	200 mg bid × 20 d
Alternative	Albendazole*	200 mg bid × 10 d	200 mg bid × 10 d
	or		
	Thiabendazole	25 mg/kg/d in 2 doses × 30 d	25 mg/kg/d in 2 doses × 30 d
Cysticercosis, see Tapeworm Infection			
Enterobius vermicularis (Pinworm) Infection			
Drug of choice	Pyrantel pamoate	11 mg/kg once (max 1 gm); repeat after 2 wk	11 mg/kg once (max 1 gm); repeat after 2 wk
	or		
	Mebendazole	A single dose of 100 mg; repeat after 2 wk	A single dose of 100 mg; repeat after 2 wk
	or		
	Albendazole*	400 mg once; repeat in 2 wk	400 mg once, repeat in 2 wk
Flukes (Intestinal Infection)			
Fasciolopsis buski			
Drug of choice	Praziquantel	75 mg/kg/d in 3 doses × 1 d	75 mg/kg/d in 3 doses × 1 d
	or		
	Niclosamide	A single dose of 4 tablets (2 gm) chewed thoroughly	11–34 kg: 2 tablets (1 gm); >34 kg: 3 tablets (1.5 gm)
Heterophyes heterophyes			
Drug of choice	Praziquantel	75 mg/kg/d in 3 doses × 1 d	75 mg/kg/d in 3 doses × 1 d
Metagonimus yokogawai			
Drug of choice	Praziquantel	75 mg/kg/d in 3 doses × 1 d	75 mg/kg/d in 3 doses × 1 d
Nanophyetus salmincola			
Drug of choice	Praziquantel	60 mg/kg/d in 3 doses × 1 d	60 mg/kg/d in 3 doses × 1 d
Hookworm Infection *(Ancylostoma duodenale, Necator americanus)*			
Drug of choice	Mebendazole	100 mg bid × 3 d	100 mg bid × 3 d
	or		
	Pyrantel pamoate	11 mg/kg (max 1 gm) × 3 d	11 mg/kg (max 1 gm) × 3 d
	or		
	Albendazole*	400 mg once	400 mg once
Oesophagostomum bifurcum			
Drug of choice	See text		
Pinworm, see *Enterobius vermicularis*			
Schistosomiasis (Bilharziasis)			
Schistosoma haematobium			
Drug of choice	Praziquantel	40 mg/kg/d in 2 doses × 1 d	40 mg/kg/d in 2 doses × 1 d
S. japonicum			
Drug of choice	Praziquantel	60 mg/kg/d in 3 doses × 1 d	60 mg/kg/d in 3 doses × 1 d
S. mansoni			
Drug of choice	Praziquantel	40 mg/kg/d in 2 doses × 1 d	40 mg/kg/d in 2 doses × 1 d
Alternative	Oxamniquine	15 mg/kg once	20 mg/kg/d in 2 doses × 1 d
S. makongi			
Drug of shoice	Praziquantel	60 mg/kg/d in 3 doses × 1 d	60 mg/kg/d in 3 doses × 1 d
Strongyloidiasis *(Strongyloides stercoralis)*			
Drug of choice	Thiabendazole	50 mg/kg/d in 2 doses (max 3 gm/d) × 2 d; ≥5 d for hyperinfection	50 mg/kg/d in 2 doses (max 3 gm/d) × 2 d; ≥5 d for hyperinfection
	or		
	Ivermectin†	200 μg/kg/d × 1–2 d	
Tapeworm Infection—Adult (Intestinal Stage)			
Diphyllobothrium latum (fish), *Taenia saginata* (beef), *Taenia solium* (pork), *Dipylidium caninum* (dog)			
Drug of choice	Praziquantel	5–10 mg/kg once	5–10 mg/kg once
	or		
	Niclosamide	A single dose of 4 tablets (2 gm), chewed thoroughly	11–34 kg: a single dose of 2 tablets (1 gm); >34 kg: a single dose of 3 tablets (1.5 gm)

Table continued on following page

TABLE 2. **Drugs for the Treatment of Helminth Infections** *Continued*

Infection	Drug	Adult Dosage	Pediatric Dosage
Hymenolepis nana (Dwarf Tapeworm)			
Drug of choice	Praziquantel	25 mg/kg once	25 mg/kg once
Alternative	Niclosamide	A single daily dose of 4 tablets (2 gm), chewed thoroughly, then 2 tablets daily × 6 d	11–34 kg: a single dose of 2 tablets (1 gm) × 1 d, then 1 tablet (0.5 gm)/d × 6 d; >34 kg: a single dose of 3 tablets (1.5 gm) × 1 d, then 2 tablets (1 gm) × 6 d
Cysticercus cellulosae (Cysticercosis)			
Treatment of choice	Albendazole*	15 mg/kg/d in 3 doses × 28 d, repeated as necessary	15 mg/kg/d in 3 doses × 28 d, repeated as necessary
	or		
	Praziquantel	50 mg/kg/d in 3 doses × 15 d	50 mg/kg/d in 3 doses × 15 d
Alternative	Surgery		
Trichinosis *(Trichinella spiralis)*			
Drug of choice	Steroids for severe symptoms plus mebendazole	200–400 mg tid × 3 d, then 400–500 mg tid × 10 d	
Trichostrongylus Infection			
Drug of choice	Pyrantel pamoate	11 mg/kg once (max 1 gm)	11 mg/kg once (max 1 gm)
Alternative	Mebendazole	100 mg bid × 3 d	100 mg bid × 3 d
	or		
	Albendazole*	400 mg once	400 mg once
Trichuriasis *(Trichuris trichiura,* Whipworm)			
Drug of choice	Mebendazole	100 mg bid × 3 d	100 mg bid × 3 d
	or		
	Albendazole*	400 mg once; may require 3 d for heavy infection	400 mg once; may require 3 d for heavy infection.

*Available in the U.S. only from the manufacturer.
†Available from the CDC Drug Service, Centers for Disease Control and Prevention, Atlanta, GA 30333; 404-639-3670 (evenings, weekends and holidays, 404-639-2888).
Modified from Drugs for parasitic infections. Med Lett Drugs Ther 35:111–122, 1993.

tinal side effects such as nausea, vomiting, and diarrhea, as well as dizziness and headache. On occasion, quinacrine is responsible for toxic psychoses and other neuropsychiatric effects including insomnia and bizarre dreams, yellow skin, blood dyscrasias, urticaria, or a psoriasis-like rash. Rarely, quinacrine causes acute hepatic encephalopathy, convulsions, exfoliative dermatitis, or ocular toxicity. For these reasons many physicians prefer to use metronidazole for giardiasis in adults. Furazolidone (Furoxone) is available in liquid form and is often used to treat children. Furazolidone is frequently associated with nausea and vomiting. Allergic reactions occur occasionally as do hypoglycemia and headache. On rare occasions, furazolidone has been associated with hemolytic anemias in patients with glucose-6-phosphate dehydrogenase deficiency and in neonates, disulfiram-like reactions, polyneuritis, and adverse interactions with monoamine oxidase inhibitors. Tinidazole* (Fasigyn), a nitroimidazole like metronidazole, is effective when given as a single dose of 2 grams. Tinidazole is generally well tolerated, but on occasion it causes nausea, vomiting, rash, or a metallic taste. Paromomycin (Humatin), 25 to 30 mg per kg per day in three divided doses for 7 days, is not well absorbed and not highly effective against *G. lamblia,* but it has been used by some to treat giardiasis during pregnancy.

Entamoeba histolytica is an important cause of colitis and liver abscesses in areas where sanitation is poor. Stools are almost always positive for gross or occult blood in persons with amoebic colitis, but fecal leukocytes are frequently absent because they are lysed by trophozoites. In North America, amebiasis is most likely to be diagnosed in immigrants, returning American travelers, and institutionalized psychiatric patients with no history of travel. Asymptomatic *E. histolytica* infection is treated with a luminally active agent. Iodoquinol (Yodoxin) or paromomycin is the drug of choice. On occasion, iodoquinol causes rash, slight thyroid enlargement, or gastrointestinal side effects. It is contraindicated in persons with known iodine sensitivity. Rarely, iodoquinol has been associated with optic neuritis, optic atrophy, and loss of vision after prolonged use at high doses. In order to avoid these side effects, the dose and duration of iodoquinol should never exceed 650 mg three times a day for 20 days (adult recommendation). Paromomycin is a poorly absorbed aminoglycoside that is associated with gastrointestinal disturbances. In patients with renal insufficiency, paromomycin can cause eight-nerve and renal damage. Diloxanide furoate* (Furamide), which is not licensed for use in the United States, is a well-tolerated alternative. Flatulence is relatively frequent, and on rare occasions, diloxanide furoate is associated with diplopia, dizziness, urticaria, or pruritus.

Intestinal disease due to *E. histolytica,* or on rare

*Not available in the United States.

*Investigational drug in the United States.

occasion *Entamoeba polecki,* should be treated with high-dose metronidazole, 750 mg three times a day for 10 days. Although metronidazole frequently eradicates the cysts as well as the trophozoites in patients with amebic colitis, most physicians follow treatment with metronidazole with a course of one of the luminally active agents discussed previously. Outside of the United States, tinidazole is often used to treat *E. histolytica;* the dose and duration depend on the severity of infection as shown in Table 2. Tinidazole appears to be at least as effective as metronidazole and better tolerated.

Other intestinal protozoa are occasionally identified in the stools of persons with diarrhea. The significance of *Blastocystis hominis* is controversial, but clinical responses have been anecdotally reported with metronidazole, 750 mg three times a day for 10 days, or iodoquinol, 650 mg three times a day for 20 days. The finding of *B. hominis* in the stool is suggestive of fecal-oral contamination. Since *G. lamblia* is easily missed on microscopic examination of stools and may accompany *B. hominis,* metronidazole is a good therapeutic choice for persons with diarrhea and *Blastocystis* identified in the stool. *Dientamoeba fragilis* infections respond to iodoquinol, paromomycin, or tetracycline. Tetracycline is usually well tolerated but can cause gastrointestinal disturbances, photosensitivity dermatitis, vaginal candidiasis, and on rare occasions, pseudomembranous colitis. In addition, it cannot be used in children under 8 years of age.

Over the past decade, *Cryptosporidium parvum* has been increasingly recognized as a cause of enteric disease. It is endemic throughout the world and was recently responsible for a large waterborne epidemic in Wisconsin. *Cryptosporidium* has emerged as a major pathogen in patients with human immunodeficiency virus (HIV) infection. The organism typically causes self-limited diarrhea in immunocompetent persons, but it can cause severe, large-volume, chronic diarrhea in persons with concurrent HIV infection. Despite extensive studies of a large number of drugs, none has emerged as the treatment of choice for cryptosporidiosis. Octreotide* (Sandostatin) has been used to control diarrhea, but it does not eradicate infection, and its efficacy has recently been questioned. Paromomycin has been used successfully to treat a small number of HIV-infected persons with cryptosporidiosis. Preliminary data suggest that azithromycin (1250 mg daily for 2 weeks followed by 500 mg daily)† may be effective in some patients. The treatment of cryptosporidiosis remains an area of intense research interest.

The HIV epidemic has brought attention to several other enteric protozoa. *Isospora belli,* which is common in some tropical areas but encountered infrequently in the United States, can produce self-limited disease in immunocompetent patients and severe, chronic diarrhea in patients with concurrent HIV infection. *I. belli* is susceptible to trimethoprim-sulfamethoxazole. Relapses are common in patients with HIV infection, and long-term suppressive therapy may be necessary. In sulfonamide-sensitive individuals, pyrimethamine, 50 to 75 mg daily, has been effective.

Microsporidiosis due to *Enterocytozoon bieneusi* or *Septata intestinalis* has been identified in HIV-infected persons with diarrhea. Although the precise pathogenic role of microsporidia in persons with HIV and diarrhea has been questioned, albendazole (400 mg twice a day), which is not licensed for use in the United States, has brought symptomatic relief to some persons with *E. bieneusi* and cured others with *S. intestinalis.* The side effects of albendazole and its other indications are discussed in the next section.

Cyclospora species, recently described coccidian parasites that were previously known as cyanobacterium-like bodies, have caused severe diarrhea in normal as well as immunocompromised persons in the United States and abroad. Recent reports suggest that *Cylospora* species are susceptible to trimethoprim (160 mg)/sulfamethoxazole (800 mg) (Bactrim, Septra), given twice a day for 3 days.

INTESTINAL NEMATODES

The intestinal helminths can be classified as nematodes (roundworms) or platyhelminths (flat worms), which are further subdivided into trematodes (flukes) and cestodes (tapeworms). This classification is helpful not only in organizing the parasites, but also in planning chemotherapy since members of these groups are frequently susceptible to the same drugs or family of drugs.

Ascaris lumbricoides, hookworms, *Trichuris trichiura,* and *Strongyloides stercoralis* are prevalent throughout the world in areas where sanitation is poor. In North America, they are most frequently encountered among immigrants and returning travelers, but on occasion they are found in North Americans who have not traveled abroad. Ova of *A. lumbricoides,* hookworms, and/or *T. trichiura* are often found in the stool of the same person. The benzimidazoles, which are generally well tolerated but are contraindicated in pregnancy, are widely used for the treatment of these nematodes. Mebendazole (Vermox), 100 mg twice a day for 3 days, is effective against all three. It is usually well tolerated, but on occasion mebendazole is associated with diarrhea, abdominal pain, or migration of *Ascaris* through the mouth or nose. Rarely, it has been associated with leukopenia, agranulocytosis, or hypospermia.

Albendazole, which is not licensed in the United States, is also active against these nematodes and has the advantage that it can be given as a single dose (400 mg). Albendazole has been used successfully as a single dose in mass treatment programs resulting in an increased rate of weight gain and in improved performance by children with *A. lumbricoides, T. trichiura,* and/or hookworms. However, in the case of heavy *T. trichiura* infestation, it may be

*Not FDA approved for this indication.
†Exceeds dosage recommended by the manufacturer.

necessary to give albendazole, 400 mg daily for 3 days. Albendazole is usually well tolerated but sometimes causes diarrhea, abdominal pain, or migration of *Ascaris* through the mouth or nose. Rarely leukopenia, alopecia, or elevated serum transaminase levels have been reported. Pyrantel pamoate (11 mg per kg body weight to a maximum dose of 1.0 gram), a depolarizing neuromuscular blocker, is effective against *A. lumbricoides* and hookworms, but it is not active against *T. trichiura*. It, too, is generally well tolerated, although gastrointestinal disturbances, headache, dizziness, rash, or fever occur on occasion.

Enterobius vermicularis, the pinworm, is common in North America and other industrialized countries among children of all socioeconomic classes. The diagnosis is usually made by finding ova or adult worms in the perianal region. The ova are occasionally identified in stool or in ectopic sites in the urogenital tract of females. Pinworms can be treated with a dose of either pyrantel pamoate (11 mg per kg body weight to a maximum of 1.0 gram), mebendazole (100 mg), or albendazole (400 mg) followed by a second dose 2 weeks later. If pinworm infections recur and there is more than one young child in the household, empiric therapy for all children should be considered. Clothing and bedding must be washed and the house thoroughly cleaned to prevent reinfection.

Strongyloides stercoralis is found in the southern part of the United States and in many developing areas of the world. It is periodically diagnosed in immigrants, returning travelers, military personnel including former prisoners of war, and residents of endemic areas in North America. *S. stercoralis* is important because it produces autoinfection, can persist for decades after a person leaves an endemic area, and in immunocompromised patients can produce life-threatening disseminated hyperinfection. The hyperinfection syndrome has been associated with steroid use, immunosuppression following organ transplantation, and malnutrition. Hyperinfection with *S. stercoralis* has not been as prevalent in HIV-infected persons as might have been predicted on the basis of their T cell defects.

Thiabendazole (Mintezol), has been the treatment of choice for strongyloidiasis. The dose is 50 mg per kg body weight (maximum 3 grams per day) administered in two divided doses for 2 days for intestinal disease and for at least 5 days for the hyperinfection syndrome. Thiabendazole is well absorbed. Nausea, vomiting, and vertigo are frequent, and rash, erythema multiforme, leukopenia, hallucinations, and olfactory disturbances are occasionally seen. Rare side effects include shock, tinnitus, intrahepatic cholestasis, convulsions, angioneurotic edema, and the Stevens-Johnson syndrome. Recent studies suggest that ivermectin, which has been widely used abroad for the treatment of onchocerciasis and other filarial diseases, is equally effective against *S. stercoralis* but much better tolerated. Ivermectin has not been licensed in the United States.

Trichinella spiralis is acquired through ingestion of inadequately cooked or raw pork, bear, walrus, or other contaminated meat. Abdominal pain and diarrhea can occur during the early phases of infection. Invading larvae are responsible for the classic picture of myalgia, periorbital edema, and eosinophilia. Chronic diarrhea due to *Trichinella nativa* has been reported among Inuit populations in Canada who have evidence of prior *Trichinella* infection. Mebendazole,* 200 to 400 mg three times a day for 3 days, then 400 to 500 mg three times a day for 10 days, is recommended. It eradicates adult *Trichinella* in the intestinal tract, and animal studies suggest that mebendazole has activity against invading larvae in muscle. Albendazole may also be effective. Steroids are frequently used to reduce the inflammatory symptoms that accompany larval invasion.

A number of less common intestinal nematodes may be encountered among returning travelers, immigrants, or residents of endemic areas. *Capillaria philippinensis* is acquired by ingesting improperly cooked, contaminated fish in the Philippines or other endemic areas. Infection is associated with malabsorption, diarrhea, and severe wasting. High-dose, prolonged treatment with mebendazole,* 200 mg twice a day for 20 days, is the treatment of choice based on studies in animals; albendazole, 200 mg twice a day for 10 days, or thiabendazole,* (25 mg per kg body weight daily in two divided doses for 30 days, is an alternative.

Trichostrongylus species are important pathogens of cattle, and they are periodically acquired through fecal-oral contamination by people living in cattle raising areas. Human infection is usually mild or asymptomatic. The drug of choice is pyrantel pamoate, 11 mg per kg body weight to a maximum of 1 gram. Mebendazole, 100 mg twice a day for 3 days, or albendazole, 400 mg, are alternatives. *Oesophagostomum* species, common parasites of monkeys and gorillas, have been reported to cause intestinal disease in humans in Africa and Indonesia. They may be susceptible to albendazole or pyrantel pamoate.

Angiostrongylus costaricensis, which is endemic in scattered areas of Latin America, is acquired through ingestion of raw snails or snail-contaminated food. *Angiostrongylus* invades mesenteric arterioles and results in the formation of granulomatous, eosinophilic, inflammatory masses. Patients are often initially thought to have appendicitis or a neoplasm, and the diagnosis is frequently made at the time of surgical exploration when involved tissue is resected. Thiabendazole, 75 mg per kg body weight per day to a maximum dose of 3 grams given in 3 divided doses for 3 days, is the treatment of choice, although its effectiveness has been documented only in animals. This dose of thiabendazole is likely to be toxic and the dosage may have to be decreased.

Anisakiasis follows ingestion of raw or inadequately treated fish that are infected with *Anisakis* species or related genera. The larvae elicit painful, inflammatory responses when they attempt to invade the wall of the stomach, small intestine, or colon. On

---

*Exceeds dosage recommended by the manufacturer.

many occasions the larvae can be visualized and removed endoscopically, but some cases require surgery.

CESTODES (TAPEWORMS)

Humans are the definitive host for a number of tapeworms; that is, the adult tapeworm resides in the human gastrointestinal tract. *Diphyllobothrium latum,* the fish tapeworm, is acquired by eating raw or inadequately cooked fresh water fish and competes with humans for vitamin B_{12}. *Taenia saginata,* which is acquired from contaminated beef, grows to incredible lengths in the human intestine but usually does so without producing significant symptoms. On occasion the dog tapeworm, *Dipylidium caninum,* is acquired by children. Praziquantel (Biltricide), 5 to 10 mg per kg body weight as a single dose, or niclosamide (Nicloside), 2 grams chewed thoroughly, are effective for the treatment of these cestodes. Praziquantel is reasonably well tolerated and without serious long-term sequelae. Short-term side effects, including malaise, headache, and dizziness, are common; sedation, abdominal pain, sweating, fever, nausea, and fatigue occur occasionally. On rare occasions, rash or pruritus accompany praziquantel use. Very little niclosamide is absorbed, and it is usually well tolerated. Patients occasionally experience nausea and abdominal pain.

Hymenolepis nana, the dwarf tapeworm, is among the most prevalent of the human cestodes, and it is capable of autoinfection. A single dose of praziquantel, 25 mg per kg body weight, is effective for treating *Hymenolepis nana.* Niclosamide can also be used, but a 7-day course is required (2 grams chewed thoroughly the first day followed by 1 gram daily for 6 days).

Humans can be both the definitive and the intermediate host for *Taenia solium.* When adult worms are present in the human intestine, a single dose of praziquantel, 10 to 15 mg per kg body weight, or niclosamide, 2 grams, is effective. When humans ingest *T. solium* ova in fecally contaminated food or water, the ova excyst in the intestine. The larvae can invade the brain, resulting in neurocysticercosis, or other organs. Albendazole (15 mg per kg body weight per day in three doses for 28 days) or long-term treatment with praziquantel,* (50 mg per kg body weight per day for 15 days) is recommended for neurocysticercosis. Albendazole (three or more cycles of 400 mg twice a day for 28 days followed by a 2-week rest period) has emerged as the treatment of choice for inoperable echinococcal liver cysts, a condition in which humans serve as the intermediate host for *Echinococcus granulosus* or *Echinococcus multilocularis.* Albendazole should be taken with a fatty meal to enhance absorption.

INTESTINAL TREMATODES AND SCHISTOSOMIASIS

Trematodes have complex life cycles involving snails as intermediate hosts. Several trematode species reside in the lumen of the human gastrointestinal tract. They include *Fasciolopsis buski,* which is acquired by eating contaminated water plants such as the water chestnut; *Heterophyes heterophyes* and *Metagonimus yokogawai,* which are acquired through ingestion of contaminated freshwater fish; and *Nanophyetus salmincola,* which is acquired by eating raw or uncooked salmon or other fish. All of these trematodes are thought to be susceptible to praziquantel, although the treatment data are anecdotal in some instances. The recommended dosage and duration of therapy are summarized in Table 2. As noted, praziquantel is associated with a number of transient side effects but has no known major long-term toxicity. The abdominal discomfort, fever, eosinophilia, and rash that are occasionally associated with praziquantel are probably due at least in part to the release of worm antigens.

Adult *Schistosoma* species live in the mesenteric venules of humans. Ova are produced there and pass through the mucosa into the lumen of the bowel, resulting in mucosal inflammation, hypertrophy, and ulceration. The major intestinal pathogens are *Schistosoma mansoni,* which is endemic in many areas of Africa, Latin America, and the Middle East, and *Schistosoma japonicum* and *Schistosoma mekongi,* which are endemic in Southeast Asia. *Schistosoma hematobium* typically resides in the vesical plexus, producing urinary tract pathology, but on occasion it involves the appendix or other areas of the intestine. All of the *Schistosoma* species are susceptible to praziquantel. *S. japonicum* and *S. mekongi* require a higher dosage (60 mg per kg body weight divided into 3 doses and given in 1 day) than *S. mansoni* and *S. haematobium* (40 mg per kg body weight divided into two doses and given in 1 day). Oxamniquine (Vansil), is an alternative drug for the treatment of *S. mansoni:* a single dose of 15 mg per kg body weight has generally been recommended, but higher doses are necessary to treat *S. mansoni* acquired in East Africa, South Africa, and Egypt. Oxamniquine is occasionally associated with headache, fever, dizziness, somnolence, nausea, diarrhea, rash, insomnia, hepatic enzyme elevations, electrocardiographic changes, or orange-red discoloration of the urine. Seizures and neuropsychiatric disturbances are rare side effects.

SUMMARY

A diverse array of parasites can produce intestinal disease in humans. *Entamoeba histolytica* and *Giardia lamblia* have long been recognized as pathogens, and over the past decade, increasing attention has been paid to the importance of *Cryptosporidium,* which is endemic worldwide. *Cryptosporidium* has caused large, waterborne outbreaks of diarrheal illness among immunocompetent persons and has emerged as an important cause of severe, chronic diarrhea in patients with HIV infection. Recent studies have pointed to the importance of *Cyclospora* species and microsporidia such as *Enterocytozoon bi-*

*Exceeds dosage recommended by the manufacturer.

eneusi as causes of diarrhea in immunocompetent persons as well as those with concurrent HIV infection. With the important exception of *Cryptosporidium,* effective chemotherapy is available for *E. histolytica, G. lamblia* and most of the other enteric protozoal pathogens.

Pyrantel pamoate and the benzimidazoles, mebendazole and albendazole, are active against a number of intestinal nematodes (roundworms). These drugs, all relatively well tolerated, are effective for the treatment of *Enterobius vermicularis* (pinworm), *Ascaris lumbricoides,* and hookworms. Only mebendazole and albendazole, which is not licensed in the United States, are effective against *Trichuris trichiura.* Albendazole can be administered in a single dose and has been used effectively in mass treatment programs in developing areas for persons infected with *A. lumbricoides,* hookworms, and/or *T. trichiura.* Thiabendazole is well absorbed and effective for the treatment of *Strongyloides stercoralis* infections, but side effects are frequent. Although not licensed in the United States, ivermectin also appears to be effective. It is much better tolerated than thiabendazole, and it is likely to become the treatment of choice for strongyloidiasis.

Praziquantel and niclosamide are highly effective against adult cestodes (tapeworms) in the human gastrointestinal tract. Praziquantel has a number of short-term side effects, but they are transient and tolerable. Niclosamide, which is poorly absorbed, is well tolerated. Albendazole and praziquantel are effective against the tissue stage of *Taenia solium* (pork tapeworm) and are used for the treatment of neurocysticercosis. Praziquantel is also very effective for the eradication of *Schistosoma* species or intestinal trematodes (flukes). In summary, safe, effective drugs are available for the treatment of most of the intestinal helminths.

Section 7

Metabolic Disorders

DIABETES MELLITUS IN ADULTS

method of
WILLIAM C. DUCKWORTH, M.D.
University of Nebraska Medical Center
Omaha, Nebraska

THE DIABETES CONTROL AND COMPLICATIONS TRIAL

With the publication of the results of the Diabetes Control and Complications Trial (DCCT), the care of the patient with diabetes has reached a new standard. No longer should there be questions about the importance of glucose control; instead, efforts to achieve the best possible control should predominate. This 10-year study (terminated after 9 years because of definitive results) of 1441 patients with Type I diabetes (IDDM) randomized to conventional or intensive glucose control demonstrated a remarkably beneficial effect of "tight" glucose control. A summary of the results of this study is shown in Table 1. All of the specific complications of diabetes (retinopathy, nephropathy, and neuropathy) were improved by intensive therapy.

Although all of the subjects in the DCCT had Type I diabetes, there are no reasons to question the extrapolation of these results to patients with Type II diabetes (NIDDM), at least with regard to the specific complications. Cardiovascular complications are more complex with multifactorial causes, especially in patients with NIDDM, and glucose control alone may not produce as marked a benefit as with the specific complications. Nevertheless, glucose control is the major priority in all patients with diabetes.

CLASSIFICATION AND PATHOGENESIS

Diabetes mellitus is a syndrome. This syndrome is characterized by sustained inappropriate hyperglycemia and is associated chronically with microvascular and macrovascular complications. This definition allows for several causes of the clinical state and emphasizes the association of glucose and complications. The current classification of diabetes (Table 2) also recognizes the heterogeneity of the disease.

Although originally described by its clinical presentation, IDDM is now generally recognized as an autoimmune process with a genetic predisposition and precipitated by only partially characterized environmental factors. The genetic predisposition involves variations in the HLA-DQ region and differs in different racial types. IDDM susceptibility, for example, is associated with the absence of aspartic acid at residue 57 in the HLA-DQB chain in Caucasians but not in Japanese. The autoimmune process results in destruction of the pancreatic beta cells and total or near total insulin deficiency.

NIDDM is a group of diseases with different causes but generally similar clinical presentations. The primary pathogenetic features include insulin resistance and abnormalities in insulin secretion of varying degrees. In most studies of populations that are at risk for developing NIDDM but lack the presence of clinical glucose intolerance, the initial lesion is insulin resistance, typically characterized by decreased glucose uptake by muscle.

The development of glucose intolerance or overt diabetes mellitus is accompanied by worsening of the defect in muscle glucose uptake, increased hepatic glucose output, and qualitative defects in insulin secretion. The early changes in insulin action typically are accompanied by increased serum insulin levels with later decreases in the hormone.

Epidemiologic, family, and twin studies have led most investigators to conclude that NIDDM is a heterogeneous group of genetic abnormalities resulting in a similar clinical profile. The search for the NIDDM gene or genes has led to convincing evidence of the involvement of the glucokinase gene in a subgroup of NIDDM patients, the syndrome of maturity-onset diabetes of youth (MODY). This syndrome is characterized by early onset of relatively mild diabetes mellitus with an autosomal dominant inheritance and lesser degrees of insulin resistance than are seen in the typical NIDDM patient. Because glucokinase is a pancreatic and hepatic enzyme, abnormalities in these organs predominate over muscle abnormalities.

Evidence of the involvement of glucokinase in the more common type of NIDDM is limited, and attention has focused on other candidate genes. The list of candidate genes is extensive, and it is highly likely that many different genetic abnormalities will ultimately be shown to be able to produce the clinical syndrome.

The genetic nature of NIDDM and the progressive changes that occur have led to the suggestion that staging of the disease could facilitate both research efforts and clinical management. The advantages of such an approach appear to be clear for research studies but are outside the purpose of this presentation. The clinical usefulness of staging is currently limited by the small number of therapeutic approaches available in this country. The introduction of additional pharmacologic agents (e.g., metformin,* insulin sensitizers, and so on) could enhance the clinical usefulness of staging approaches, but even today some theoretical advantages are present. A simplified staging protocol will be used (Table 3) for discussion purposes in the therapy portion of this presentation.

DIAGNOSIS

Although diabetes is a complex disease that includes abnormalities in lipid and protein as well as carbohydrate metabolism, the clinical diagnosis is based on blood glucose elevation. Some suggestions have been made about the potential usefulness of glycosylated proteins such as hemoglobin A_{1C} in diagnosis, but the only currently accepted criteria are shown in Table 4. The fasting glucose is the most useful measurement and is the most frequent means of diagnosis.

---

*Not available in the United States.

TABLE 1. **Summary of Results from the Diabetes Control and Complications Trial (DCCT)**

	Primary Prevention Risk Reduction*	Secondary Intervention Risk Reduction*	Combined Risk Reduction*
Retinopathy	76%	54%	63%
Nephropathy	44%	56%	54%
Neuropathy	69%	57%	60%

*The decrease in risk for development or progression of the specified complication in patients with intensive glucose control (mean blood glucose 155 mg/dL) versus conventional glucose control (mean blood glucose 231 mg/dL).

Oral glucose tolerance tests can be used for early cases and for diagnosis of glucose intolerance. The prevalence of specific complications of diabetes (nephropathy, retinopathy, and neuropathy) is very low at glucose levels below the diagnostic cutoff for diabetes, but patients with glucose intolerance are at greater risk for cardiovascular complications than subjects with normal glucose tolerance.

Much interest has been generated about the possibility that individuals with genetic insulin resistance but without clinical abnormalities of glucose metabolism (Stage 0 in Table 3) may be at increased risk for cardiovascular disease or hypertension. If so, then approaches to the diagnosis and management of this group would be of considerable clinical importance.

MANAGEMENT OF DIABETES

General Principles

Although specific approaches to therapy vary with the type of diabetes and, in the case of NIDDM, with the stage of the disease, certain general principles are valid for all types of diabetes. Diabetes is a chronic disease and requires extensive patient participation in the proper management of the disease. Education of the patient and the patient's family is thus a cornerstone of successful long-term management of this disease. The list of topics necessary to be covered in an educational program is extremely broad, ranging from diet and physical activity to foot care and self-medication. Education is a continuing need in patients with diabetes and should be given by a certified diabetes educator (CDE).

The long-term care of the patient with diabetes also requires extensive input from a wide variety of professional health care deliverers. The importance of patient and family participation, the need for many types of professional input, and the chronic nature of the disease are best handled by a team approach in which the patient and the patient's family join with a variety of health care givers who interact continuously to establish a treatment program and long-term maintenance of the patient with diabetes.

TABLE 2. **Classification of Diabetes Mellitus**

Type I	Insulin-dependent diabetes mellitus (IDDM)
Type II	Non–insulin-dependent diabetes mellitus (NIDDM)
Glucose Intolerance	
Gestational Diabetes	

TABLE 3. **Simplified Clinical Staging of NIDDM**

Stage 0:	Genetic defect present but no clinical abnormalities in glucose metabolism
Stage 1:	Glucose intolerance or early NIDDM (fasting glucose less than 140 mg/dL). Characterized by insulin resistance and peripheral hyperinsulinemia
Stage 2:	Overt diabetes mellitus (fasting glucose 150–200 mg/dL). Insulin resistance. Insulin levels slightly increased or decreased compared with normal but relatively inadequate
Stage 3:	Insulin-deficient NIDDM. Endogenous insulin levels clearly insufficient for degree of insulin resistance

The ability to achieve glucose control in patients with diabetes has been revolutionized by techniques developed to monitor glucose control. Glycosylated hemoglobin and other glycosylated proteins provide information about the intermediate- to long-term glucose levels, but self–blood glucose monitoring is essential to determine daily patterns of glucose fluctuation. This information is necessary to tailor therapy to maintain a near-normal glycemia with reduced risks of hypoglycemia. Daily adjustments in insulin doses are required in most patients with IDDM and in many insulin-requiring patients with NIDDM. Without information about the daily fluctuations in glucose, these adjustments are impossible. The general consensus is that all insulin-requiring diabetic patients; most, perhaps all, sulfonylurea-treated patients; and many patients treated by diet and exercise require self–blood glucose monitoring. In general, all patients with diabetes should have the capability to measure their blood glucose levels, but the frequency of measurement may vary greatly, depending on the clinical status, from weekly to four to eight times daily. Many different systems are now available for self–blood glucose monitoring, and the technology is changing so rapidly that specific recommendations are not possible. Patient education and maintenance of quality control of the measurements are essential and again depend on a team approach involving the patient, certified diabetes educators, and others to maintain the quality of the measurements and thus their clinical usefulness.

TABLE 4. **Diagnostic Criteria for Diabetes Mellitus**

1. Random blood glucose greater than 200 mg/dL accompanied by symptoms (e.g., polyuria, polydipsia, polyphagia)
2. Fasting blood glucose greater than 140 mg/dL on at least two separate occasions
3. Elevated blood glucose levels after a 75-gm glucose load at least twice. The 2-hour level is greater than 200 mg/dL, and at least one other value between 0 and 2 hours exceeds 200 mg/dL.

Glucose Intolerance

During an oral glucose tolerance test the 2-hour value is between 140 and 199 mg/dL, and one value between 0 and 2 hours exceeds 200 mg/dL.

Goals of Therapy

The goal of therapy of diabetes mellitus is to prevent acute and chronic complications while maintaining the patient's quality of life. The cornerstone of prevention of complications is the achievement of as near normal a glucose level as possible. True euglycemia, however, is a virtual impossibility in most patients with our current approaches, and thus individual goals must be set for each patient depending on a realistic appraisal of the specific situation. Defined, specific goals should be established for every patient.

The establishment of goals for glucose levels requires consideration of many factors. As with almost all aspects of diabetic management, the team approach is essential. Educational, social, psychological, and medical aspects are important factors. The patient and the patient's family must be actively involved in these decisions. The diabetes professionals may set a goal of euglycemia, but if the patient is not motivated or if there are barriers to achieving this goal, frustration and disillusionment may prevent any progress. Medical problems must be considered. A patient with hypoglycemic unawareness or a history of repeated severe hypoglycemic episodes is not a candidate for intensive glucose control. The goal of therapy in an elderly patient with severe cardiovascular disease is very different from that in a young, motivated patient with no or minimal complications.

Goals should also be set for aspects other than glucose levels, such as diet and exercise. Control of associated abnormalities such as hypertension and hyperlipidemia is also essential.

Therapy of IDDM

The conceptual basis for therapy of IDDM is simple. The abnormality that produces the disease is beta cell destruction and insulin deficiency. Thus, the therapeutic approach is to provide insulin replacement in as near a physiologic fashion as possible. Because insulin requirements are altered by dietary intake, exercise, stress, and so on, consideration of these factors is essential and, as discussed earlier, requires the assistance of a team of professionals. Specific aspects of diet are discussed subsequently. Despite these considerations, an insulin program that provides for a basal insulin level and mealtime increments is required. Much has been published on intensive insulin regimens, and an extensive discussion of these is beyond the scope of this presentation. Rather, a brief description of the different insulin programs and their advantages and disadvantages is given followed by my own choices. Table 5 shows selected insulin preparations and their characteristics.

Mixed or Split Program

A mixed or split program consists of a morning (breakfast) and evening (supper) injection of a mixture of intermediate (NPH or lente) and short-acting (regular) insulin. This is the absolute minimum requirement for even adequate glucose control in IDDM. The rationale is that the morning regular dose will provide for breakfast coverage and the intermediate dose will provide daytime basal and lunchtime coverage. Similarly, the evening regular dose will cover food intake at supper, and the intermediate will provide overnight basal requirements. Thus, if glucose monitoring data show unacceptable glucose levels prior to the evening meal, the morning intermediate insulin dose is increased. Pre-bedtime elevations would be managed by increasing the evening regular dose. Morning fasting hyperglycemia indicates a need for additional evening intermediate.

TABLE 5. **Insulin Preparations**

Type	Characteristic	Onset of Action (h)	Maximal Effect (h)
Regular	Short-acting	0.5–1	2–4
Semi-lente	Short-acting	1–2	3–5
NPH	Intermediate-acting	3–4	8–14
Lente	Intermediate-acting	3–4	8–14
Ultralente	Long-acting	6–8	12–18

Although each patient's insulin requirement must be established individually in terms of both amount and distribution, an initial dose of 0.3 to 0.5 unit per kg is a reasonable starting point in IDDM patients. The traditional distribution in a mixed or split program is two-thirds in the morning and one-third in the evening, with two-thirds of each dose being intermediate insulin and one-third being regular insulin. Adjustments are then made based on the glucose monitoring data as described previously.

The major disadvantage of this program is that with the currently available purified intermediate insulins the effective duration of action is shorter than the usual 12- to 14-hour period between supper and breakfast, resulting in fasting hyperglycemia in most patients. Increasing the evening intermediate insulin results in a significant risk of nocturnal (2 to 4 A.M.) hypoglycemia.

Three-Injection Intermediate-Regular Program

This regimen consists of a pre-breakfast intermediate-regular injection, a pre-supper regular injection, and a bedtime intermediate injection. This provides better overnight coverage with less risk of nocturnal hypoglycemia, although occasional 3 A.M. glucose measurements are still recommended. This program is also effective in patients with the dawn phenomenon, an early morning increase in insulin requirements due to growth hormone pulses. This program is superior to the two-injection mixed-split approach. The primary drawback of this approach is the lack of a true insulin bolus at lunch and thus the potential for hyperglycemia after this meal.

Four-Injection Intermediate-Regular Program

This is an intensive insulin program. It adds a prelunch, regular injection to the three-injection regimen that provides coverage for this meal. If this regimen is used, the morning intermediate dose should be reduced.

Ultralente-Regular Program

Basal insulin requirements are provided by two injections of long-acting ultralente insulin daily with regular insulin injections before each meal to provide for mealtime glucose excursions. This program provides the greatest flexibility of all multiple injection schemes. If the ultralente doses are appropriate, meals can be altered in time or amount with little risk of loss of control. This is the preferred program for patients with varying work schedules. It also eliminates the need for a rigid, inflexible meal plan.

This approach is my preferred method for most patients. Again, insulin doses and distribution must be individualized, but, in general, half of the total dose is long-acting insulin given in two equal parts, one before breakfast and one before supper, and half of the total dose is given as regular insulin. The distribution of the regular insulin depends on the eating preferences of the patient. Adjustments in the long-acting insulin are made on the basis of fasting glucose levels but should not be made more often than every 4 to 6 days. Adjustments in regular insulin can be made at each dose if necessary. Patients should have an individualized algorithm for alterations in the regular dose.

Subcutaneous Insulin Infusion Pumps

Subcutaneous insulin infusion pumps provide a constant infusion of regular insulin for basal requirements and can be programmed to provide different rates at different times throughout the day and night (e.g., to cover a dawn phenomenon). Boluses are given prior to meals and, if necessary, snacks. This approach is the most effective way to obtain intensive glucose control. Fifty-nine percent of intensively treated patients in the DCCT required the use of a pump for at least a portion of their therapy, and approximately one-third used a pump for the entire study. Pump therapy provides the greatest flexibility of all the approaches generally used and may reduce the frequency of hypoglycemia.

Pump therapy is not without problems. It requires a motivated and well-educated patient and an experienced team. Infections and abscesses at the infusion site are the most common problems. Mechanical difficulties can occur, and mild diabetic ketoacidosis episodes can occur when interruptions of the basal insulin infusion occur, as, for example, with displacement of the needle during the night. Cost is also a factor because the initial investment for the pump is significant. Nevertheless, for appropriately selected patients in the proper setting this is the best intensive program currently available.

Pancreas Transplantation

Pancreas transplantation has now become an accepted mode of therapy in selected patients with IDDM. Although relatively little long-term experience with the current transplant methods is available, short-term success rates (1 to 3 years) are now well over 90% (graft and patient survival) with combined kidney-pancreas transplants. Thus, all IDDM patients needing a kidney transplant should be evaluated for a combined kidney-pancreas procedure. Solitary pancreas transplants are less successful (70% in experienced centers) but are appropriate in certain selected cases. The criteria for pancreas transplants alone vary considerably in different centers.

Management of NIDDM

Diet

Diet remains the cornerstone of management of established NIDDM and plays an important role in preventing or delaying the onset of the disease. Unlike IDDM, in which dietary management is necessary to coordinate with insulin peaks, prevent excessive glucose excursions, and maintain overall health status, such as the prevention of vascular disease, dietary therapy in NIDDM is a direct therapeutic modality. Insulin resistance is a primary pathologic feature of NIDDM, and obesity increases insulin resistance. Because more than 80% of NIDDM patients are obese, correction of obesity may improve insulin action sufficiently to allow the remaining endogenous insulin secretion to maintain normal or near-normal glucose levels. Thus, diet alone may be sufficient for the management of many patients with NIDDM during the early stages of the disease (Stage 1, see Table 3). Hypocaloric diets, even before significant weight loss occurs, may improve glucose levels significantly. Relatively minor changes in weight, such as a 5 to 10% loss, will produce major changes in glucose levels in many patients. Thus, dietary therapy is important even in patients with moderate to extreme obesity, in whom the chances of obtaining normal body weight are remote.

Dietary therapy must be individualized and requires the participation of a registered dietitian. Simply giving a patient a standard diet sheet is inadequate and ineffective. The established American Diabetes Association (ADA) dietary recommendations include 50 to 60% carbohydrates, 12 to 20% protein, and less than 30% fat, with restrictions on cholesterol and saturated fat intake. Increased fiber intake is encouraged, although the exact role of fiber remains controversial. This overall dietary plan will need to be adjusted for many patients, for example, those who have carbohydrate-sensitive hypertriglyceridemia or those with hypercholesterolemia. Most NIDDM patients require a hypocaloric diet. There is no perfect approach to weight loss, and success depends on persistence and support. There is no substitute for an experienced dietitian in the management of patients with NIDDM.

Exercise

Exercise has long been considered an adjunctive therapy to diet in managing patients with NIDDM.

Exercise has a number of beneficial effects in these patients. Exercise can improve cardiovascular fitness and reduce the risk of cardiovascular events, and an exercise program can be very useful in combination with a diet and weight reduction program. Exercise can also be beneficial in helping to control hypertension, a common problem in patients with NIDDM. In addition, however, exercise has a significant effect on insulin resistance. A regular exercise program can increase insulin sensitivity even between sessions. Thus, regular exercise can produce overall persistent improvements in insulin action. Particularly in the early stages of NIDDM (Stage 1) or, in fact, prior to the development of hyperglycemia in patients with the genetic abnormality (Stage 0), exercise may be the most effective approach to delaying the onset of hyperglycemia or the progression from mild to moderate hyperglycemia. Thus, an aerobic exercise program carried out at least every other day for 20 to 40 minutes, is an important component of the therapy of NIDDM. Resistance training, that is, increasing muscle mass, is somewhat less well established, but several studies suggest that a benefit accrues from such a program. Ideally, then, a combination of aerobic/resistance exercise may produce extra benefits in patients who are willing to make this commitment.

Oral Agents

At the time of this writing, the only pharmacologic agents available in this country for controlling glucose, outside of insulin, are sulfonylureas (Table 6). The actual role of these agents remains somewhat ill defined. Given the pathologic features of NIDDM, namely, insulin resistance and abnormalities in endogenous insulin secretion, their pharmacologic properties are extremely attractive. Sulfonylureas increase endogenous insulin secretion and have an effect on peripheral insulin action. In practice, these theoretical advantages of sulfonylureas are not always realized. Although the sulfonylureas may be extremely helpful in many patients with NIDDM, they are also among the most misused drugs available. Many patients who fail to respond to a diet and exercise program may respond to sulfonylureas with adequate control of blood glucose levels, although both primary and secondary failures of the agents are not infrequent. Far too often patients with NIDDM are placed on oral agents and considered "treated" without consideration of the fact that there may be no response or an inadequate response, or that the initial response may be lost. Patients on sulfonylureas should be monitored in the same way as patients on insulin, and treatment should be adjusted or altered if the desired effect is not seen or is lost.

TABLE 6. **Sulfonylureas Available in the United States**

	Initial Dose (mg)	Maximal Dose (mg)	Duration of Action (h)
First-Generation			
Tolbutamide (Orinase)	500	2500	6–12
Chlorpropamide (Diabinese)	100	750	60
Tolazamide (Tolinase)	100	1000	12–24
Acetohexamide (Dymelor)	250	1500	12–24
Second-Generation			
Glyburide (Micronase, Diabeta)	2.5	20	12–24
(Glynase)	1.25	12	12–24
Glipizide (Glucotrol)	5.0	40	12–24

Table 6 lists the sulfonylureas currently available in this country and some of their properties. In my opinion, the role of the so-called first-generation agents is limited. My approach is to use the second-generation agents with the rare exception of the elderly patient who may respond to tolbutamide. The two second-generation agents, glyburide and glipizide, are not identical, although both increase endogenous insulin secretion and have effects on peripheral insulin action. Much overlap exists, but glyburide has greater effects on fasting insulin levels and basal glucose output than glipizide, which has greater effects on stimulated insulin secretion and post-prandial glucose levels. Although each patient should be considered individually, glyburide tends to be the agent of choice for patients with fasting hyperglycemia, and glipizide is the first choice for patients whose fasting glucose level is acceptable but who have unacceptable post-prandial glucose excursions.

In either case, therapy is initiated with the minimally effective dose and increased in steps at 1- to 2-week intervals. It requires this period of time to achieve the maximum effect of each dose of oral agent, and exceeding this rate can result in hypoglycemia or, in some cases, in reduced effectiveness. During sulfonylurea therapy it is essential to continue to stress the importance of diet and exercise, which greatly enhance the effectiveness of these agents.

Insulin

The established importance of glucose control requires that insulin therapy be used in patients who do not achieve targeted glucose levels with diet, exercise, and sulfonylurea therapy. Given the importance of hepatic glucose output in the progressive hyperglycemia of NIDDM, a rational and experimentally proved approach for the initiation of insulin therapy is to administer an intermediate-acting insulin at bedtime to control overnight glucose output. An initial dose of 10 to 15 units is a reasonable start for most patients, with adjustments of 2 to 3 units being made every 2 to 3 days based on the morning fasting glucose. In many patients, this therapy alone will reduce fasting glucose levels to normal and, combined with endogenous insulin secretion, will maintain acceptable glucose levels throughout the day. For patients who do not respond to this simple approach, combination therapy, discussed later, or additional insulin doses are required. Information obtained from self–blood glucose monitoring is invaluable for making therapeutic adjustments. For patients who require additional insulin, a reasonable approach is to add a regular-intermediate insulin injection in the morning. The great majority of insulin-requiring patients with NIDDM can be maintained with this approach—that is, either a single intermediate insulin injection at bedtime, or a combination of intermediate at bedtime and intermediate-regular in the morning. A small percentage of NIDDM patients with severe insulin deficiency may require intensive insulin programs similar to those used for patients with IDDM. Alternative insulin programs for NIDDM patients include the use of long-acting, ultralente insulin injections in place of bedtime intermediate injections, and "mixed-split" injections before breakfast and before supper in place of morning mixed-split and bedtime NPH. If twice-a-day mixed-split programs are used, monitoring for nocturnal hypoglycemia (i.e., 3 A.M. blood glucose levels) should be performed initially and intermittently with therapy.

It is important to recognize that NIDDM patients who require insulin may need very large amounts to control glucose to near-normal levels. Several large studies have shown that the average dose needed to achieve near-euglycemia is approximately 100 units per day.

Combination Therapy

Combination therapy composed of insulin plus sulfonylureas remains controversial. Recent studies, however, have reinforced both the theoretical and the practical desirability of using this combination in selected patients. First, with the importance of glucose control now established, a casual approach to glucose levels, that is, accepting fasting levels of about 200 mg/dL, is no longer acceptable. Sulfonylureas by themselves frequently fail to achieve glucose levels in or near the normal range. Insulin therapy alone in patients with Type II diabetes may require very large doses to achieve blood glucose levels in the normal range. In addition to the theoretical disadvantage of hyperinsulinemia (see later discussion), this dose of insulin almost inevitably results in weight gain and frequently in increases in blood pressure as well. Thus, the use of a sulfonylurea to reduce the total amount of insulin required for reaching the ideal glucose level is attractive. A combination of bedtime intermediate insulin and daytime sulfonylurea therapy has been shown to result in lower peripheral insulin levels and less weight gain than various combinations of insulin therapy alone or than evening sulfonylurea and daytime insulin. Given the importance of controlling hepatic glucose output overnight and maintaining glucose levels during the day, bedtime intermediate insulin with daytime sulfonylurea appears to be a reasonable approach for many patients.

A different type of combination therapy is being used by some diabetologists. This approach takes advantage of the differences between glyburide and glipizide, namely, that glyburide has a better effect on fasting levels, and glipizide tends to achieve better normalization of post-prandial glucose levels. In some patients who either have failed to improve with a maximum dose of sulfonylurea alone or will not or cannot start on insulin, bedtime glyburide with morning glipizide has been successful in achieving glucose goals. This combination is not recommended for general use; however, in the patient who absolutely refuses to take or cannot take insulin for whatever reason, and who maintains unacceptable glucose levels on maximum doses of individual sulfonylureas, this approach may be worth a try. As with any therapeutic approach, the patient should be monitored for the effectiveness of the therapy, and if it is ineffective it should not be continued. If both drugs are used, the dose of each agent should not exceed half the usual dose of that agent.

STANDARDS OF CARE

The care of the patient with diabetes is a major commitment. Because appropriate care can greatly reduce the morbidity and mortality of this disease, standards of medical care for patients with diabetes have been developed by the ADA. Tables 7 and 8 summarize some of these recommendations, and the reader is referred to the full statement referenced in Tables 7 and 8. These are minimum requirements, and many patients require far more intensive therapy. Insulin-treated patients undergoing therapeutic adjustments may require daily contact, for example.

COMPLICATIONS OF DIABETES

The complications of diabetes can be divided into two types—specific, that is, those that for practical purposes do not occur except in diabetes (e.g., hyper-

TABLE 7. **Standards of Care for Patients with Diabetes Mellitus**

Initial Visit
Complete history and physical examination
Laboratory determinations:
- Fasting plasma glucose
- Glycosylated hemoglobin
- Fasting lipid profile
- Serum creatinine
- Urinalysis
- Quantitative urine protein (microalbuminuria)
- Thyroid function tests
- ECG

Management plan (by diabetes team)

Continuing Care
Visit frequency—as needed for stabilization, then:
- For insulin-treated patients, at least quarterly
- For other patients, at least semiannually

Education and support at each visit
Complete history and physical examination annually
Eye examination by ophthalmologist annually
Glycosylated hemoglobin at least semiannually; quarterly in insulin-treated patients
Lipid profile annually
Urinalysis annually
Urine protein (microalbuminuria) annually
Creatinine clearance (or other assay) annually

Extracted from Standards of medical care for patients with diabetes mellitus. Diabetes Care 12:365–368, 1989.

glycemia), and nonspecific, that is, those that occur with increased frequency in patients with diabetes. Table 9 lists the specific and a few of the nonspecific complications.

It seems beyond question now that the specific complications of retinopathy, nephropathy, and neuropathy are due to hyperglycemia. Furthermore, the higher the glucose level, the greater the risk of development or progression of the complications, which is analogous in many ways to blood pressure or serum cholesterol. From this it follows that the primary approach to the early management of these complications is improvement in glucose control. Achievement of true euglycemia is exceedingly difficult, and thus complications of diabetes will continue to occur. It is essential to detect and treat these complications to reduce further morbidity and mortality. Monitoring requirements for these complications are included in Table 7. Effective treatment approaches require assistance from a variety of professionals, e.g., ophthalmologists for retinopathy, nephrologists and transplant surgeons for nephropathy, and urologists, podiatrists, orthopedic surgeons, and others for neuropathy. With an integrated approach, the morbidity and mortality resulting from these complications can be reduced. Patient education (e.g., on foot care) is an important part of this approach, as is attention to factors that may accelerate progression (e.g., hypertension, smoking). Of the nonspecific complications cardiovascular disease is by far the most important. This is the cause of death in 70% of patients with diabetes. The development of cardiovascular disease is clearly multifactorial. Hyperglycemia is an important factor, as shown by the DCCT in patients with IDDM. Hyperglycemia undoubtedly is a significant contributor to atherosclerotic heart disease in NIDDM, but other factors must also be considered. Hyperglycemia in NIDDM is frequently only a component of a syndrome that includes hypertension, hypertriglyceridemia, reduced high-density lipoproteins, central obesity, hyperinsulinemia, and various other components. This syndrome was named syndrome X and was attributed by Reaven and collaborators to a genetic abnormality that produced insulin resistance. This syndrome is characterized by a high prevalence of cardiovascular disease. Although controversial, several components of this syndrome, including hypertension, hypertriglyceridemia, and accelerated atherosclerotic heart disease, have been considered secondary to the hyperinsulinemia. Although it is possible that the primary lesion, insulin resistance, may also be the direct cause of these components, strong evidence exists that insulin itself can produce increases in blood pressure, triglycerides, and atherosclerotic changes in blood vessels.

TABLE 8. **Components of Management Plan**

- Statement of goals
- Medications
- Individualized nutrition recommendations and instructions
- Recommendations for lifestyle changes (e.g., exercise)
- Patient and family education
- Monitoring instructions
- Consultation for specialized services as needed
- Agreement on support and follow-up
- Discussion of contraception and pregnancy for women of childbearing age.

Extracted from Standards of medical care for patients with diabetes mellitus. Diabetes Care *12*:365–368, 1989.

TABLE 9. **Complications of Diabetes**

Specific	Nonspecific (partial list)
Retinopathy	Cardiovascular
Nephropathy	Hypertension
Neuropathy	Infections
	Growth defects
	Glaucoma
	Periodontitis

The considerations discussed earlier have led many diabetologists, including myself, to conclude that although lowering glucose is essential in patients with NIDDM, attention must also be paid to insulin levels. Diet and exercise programs therefore achieve an even greater importance. Antihypertensive agents (e.g., diuretics) that increase insulin levels or requirements should be avoided, as should agents that may increase lipids (beta blockers). Short-acting insulin (i.e., regular with meals) is preferred over long-acting insulins, which produce prolonged basal hyperinsulinemia. Combination therapy (sulfonylureas plus insulin) may be preferable to simply increasing exogenous insulin doses to very high levels. Much of the discussion of therapeutic approaches is predicated on the concept of the potentially deleterious effects of hyperinsulinemia.

The importance of controlling factors that accelerate diabetic complications cannot be overstressed. Cessation of smoking, therapy for hypertension, and treatment of hyperlipidemia are essential components of the management of diabetes.

TYPE I DIABETES MELLITUS IN CHILDREN AND ADOLESCENTS

method of
STEPHEN C. DUCK, M.D.
Northwestern University Medical School
Chicago, Illinois

Type I diabetes mellitus is a multifactorial disease that occurs throughout life but is especially prevalent during the first 2 decades. The incidence is increasing worldwide. In the United States the yearly incidence is 14 to 18 cases in 10^5 persons under age 21 years. The prevalence is 1 of 600 high school children. The cause varies with the age at diagnosis: pancreatic (islet cell) agenesis in the neonatal period; aggressive autoimmune destruction of the beta cells in children under the age of 5 years; and an indolent (slow) autoimmune destruction of the beta cells among a genetically defined risk group throughout life. Currently, over 90% of newly diagnosed children have beta cell–specific autoantibodies. Genetic markers of interest are the DR, DQ-beta, and DQ-alpha alleles of the HLA system located on chromosome 6. Environmental factors are very strongly suggested and include geography, lifestyle, viruses, and early introduction of cow milk protein feedings.

Detection of an at-risk population includes the measurement of islet-specific autoantibodies and of the first-phase release of insulin (1- and 3-minute values) to an intravenous glucose challenge. Intervention studies to prevent diabetes in those with "pre-diabetes" are under way, and interventions include the use of the antioxidant nicotinamide (vitamin B_3) and subclinical doses of insulin (pancreatic "rest").

DIAGNOSIS

The clinical signs of polyuria, polydipsia, polyphagia, and weight loss are cardinal. Fatigue, enuresis, or vaginal candidiasis may be noted. Abdominal pain, vomiting, rapid deep breathing with a fruited scent, and depressed consciousness are indicative of ketoacidosis.

A child with symptoms and a random blood glucose level of more than 200 mg/dL has diabetes. Postprandial glucose values are sufficient to resolve most confusing signs in diagnosis. Oral glucose tolerance tests are rarely indicated, last only 120 minutes, and include blood glucose and insulin values determined from blood drawn every 30 minutes.

Presentation of type II diabetes in childhood should be suspected in a child with a strong family (three-generation) history of diabetes or in the presence of acanthosis nigricans and obesity.

MANAGEMENT PHILOSOPHY

Publication of the results from the Diabetes Control and Complications Trial (DCCT) forever changed the definition of care of patients with Type I diabetes. Intensive therapy effectively delayed the onset and slowed the progression of diabetic microangiopathic complications in patients with Type I diabetes. Blood glucose control with protection from severe hypoglycemia is normative. The goals of management should reflect that norm.

INITIAL EDUCATION

Most parents and patients can be educated in 3 to 5 days following recovery of the patient from an episode of ketoacidosis. Managed competition will create the environment for this to be done exclusively in the outpatient setting—an appropriate location provided that personnel and facilities are available. The best outcome involves referral to the Diabetes Team at diagnosis, reinforcing the importance of continuity and building a bridge of trust.

The educational program usually involves a multidisciplinary team of physicians, nurse educators, dietitians, social workers, and clinical psychologists. The initial program focuses on insulin therapy, glucose monitoring and control, the use and impact of diet and exercise, hyperglycemic and hypoglycemic reactions, and management of intercurrent illness.

Catalyzing the grief process for the parents and patient is essential to the long-term success of an educational program. Successfully coping with the psychological impact of diabetes is a primary goal of both the initial and the comprehensive educational programs. This goal dictates the active intervention practiced by the Diabetes Team, whose task it is to foster the normal growth and development as well as the independence and self-confidence of the patient.

DIET

The "prudent diet" is the preferred meal plan for the child with diabetes. Supported by the American Heart, Pediatric, and Diabetic Associations, this diet provides the total distribution of calories as 55 to 60% carbohydrate, 30% or less fat, and 15 to 20% protein. Total cholesterol is limited to 300 mg per day and saturated fats to 10% of the total calories. Excessive intake of protein is avoided because of the detrimental impact on the kidney; restrictive intake is avoided because of the adverse effect on growth. Moderation in salt intake is encouraged (3 grams or less daily).

Balanced with these goals is the requirement to build the diet around the ethnic, social, and financial constraints of the family. Food choices (what and how much) are too often the battlefield that dooms adherence and control. The Diabetes Team is committed to supporting the child's lifestyle, including food choices, but in a way that maximizes glycemic control.

Introduction of intensive insulin treatment allows greater flexibility in the composition of the diet and the timing of meals. This is especially true for patients under age 5 and for patients in late adolescence. When predictability of food intake is unlikely to be experienced, the use of frequent doses of regular insulin provides a creative alternative to the "split and mix" regimen of insulin administration.

Snacks are rarely required to maintain glucose control. Their presence is initially dictated by the prevailing family lifestyle, not by the Team. An after-school snack is a nearly universal time for eating. Mid-morning and bedtime snacks are prudent if all the other children or family members are snacking also. Snacks with a significant amount of fat or fiber content generally allow slower absorption of the carbohydrate content than those without.

INSULIN THERAPY

The preferred therapy for children with diabetes mellitus is human (recombinant) insulin. The rare patient with maturity-onset diabetes of youth (MODY) may be the exception and is managed preferably by oral hypoglycemic agents and weight reduction. Published concerns about the benefit of pork insulin to prevent hypoglycemic unawareness are not substantial enough to justify its use.

Glycemic control is achieved with greater success when regular insulin is used to control the glycemic excursion of meals and larger snacks and when intermediate insulin (Lente or NPH) is used to provide basal insulin through the night. Lente insulin is slower in onset and longer acting but quickly adsorbs and alters the release characteristics of regular insulin. NPH is widely used because of its stability when mixed with regular insulin; however, its onset of action is often too rapid and its duration too short to be used successfully. Ultralente is not widely used among pediatric patients because of its time action profile and the need for an injection separate from that of regular insulin.

The concentration of insulin is 100 units. However, if less than 2 units are prescribed, the use of dilute (e.g., 10-unit) insulin is required for accuracy and precision. This is true when using syringes that have only 25- or 30-unit capacities.

Insulin penlike injectors are useful for independent adolescents who want to take regular insulin inconspicuously. Insulin pumps are superb for those mature young people who truly wish to maximize their blood glucose control but are usually not required during the first year of the disease.

Synthetic (monomer) regular insulin preparations allow more rapid absorption and a shorter duration of action following the injection. The immediate convenience is to allow the patient to shorten the time between the injection and the initiation of eating.

The patient and family tend to accept the frequency of injections used at diagnosis. Therefore, a considered choice is made to select the dosing regimen that will provide the best control once the partial remission is past. For the elementary school-aged child, twice daily combinations of regular and intermediate (NPH) are prudent; for the teenager and the pre-school-aged child, the combination of regular insulin before breakfast and dinner with intermediate insulin before breakfast and at bedtime is a better regimen.

At diagnosis, owing to peripheral insulin resistance, glycemic control generally requires 0.7 to 1.3 units of insulin per kg per day. Within a few days, insulin sensitivity returns, and the total daily dose drops toward 0.3 to 0.6 unit per kg per day. Following the complete loss of endogenous insulin, prepubertal diabetic patients often require 0.7 to 1.0 unit per kg per day and post-pubertal patients 1.0 to 1.3 units per kg per day.

Not infrequently, 67% of the total daily dose is given in the morning and the rest during the evening. A common split of intermediate and regular is a combination of 2/1 in the morning and 1/1 during the evening. The availability of premixed insulin preparations (NPH and regular) in 70/30 and 50/50 concentrations supports this general trend; however, the freedom to adjust the two insulins independently provides better control in patients.

Algorithms for alternative doses of insulin based on activities, phases of the menstrual cycle, illness, or degree of control are invariably needed but should be created by the patient or parent rather than handed down "from on high" by the Diabetes Team! Maintaining the family unit as the center of the Team is necessary. Initial use of a fixed dosing regimen facilitates the family's ability to create the algorithm: When and why did that dose succeed or not succeed?

TARGET GLYCEMIC CONTROL

The DCCT suggested a level of 70 to 130 mg/dL (3.9 to 7.2 millimoles per liter) before meals and at bedtime, more than 65 mg/dL (>3.6 millimoles per liter) during sleep, and less than 180 mg/dL (<10 millimoles per liter) 1 or 2 hours after eating. These are worthy targets for children of all ages unless they are proved in a given patient to be too stringent, as defined by the presence of severe hypoglycemia. The pre-school-aged child may be noncommunicative and noncooperative enough to require higher averages (≤180 mg/dL; ≤10 millimoles per liter).

Assessment of control requires analysis of the individual data and also of the trend over time (the "modal" day data). The period of glycemic control produced by each component (regular or intermediate) of an insulin dose is unique and limited. That reality dictates that multiple and sequential (consecutive) glucose monitoring be performed daily. Because of the risk of nocturnal hypoglycemia and of an exaggerated dawn phenomenon, monitoring periodically at 3 A.M. is prudent or even required.

Insulin and the "period" that is controlled:

A.M. regular	Pre-breakfast *to* pre-lunch
A.M. intermediate	Pre-lunch *through* P.M. snack *to* pre-dinner
P.M. regular	Pre-dinner *to* pre-bedtime
P.M. intermediate	Pre-bedtime *through* 3 A.M. *to* pre-breakfast
Pre-snack regular	Pre-snack *to* +2 to 3 hours afterward

Adjustment of an insulin dose (by 10% of the dose) is undertaken following detection of a single unexplained hypoglycemic value or after a consistent (3 to 5 days) pattern of hyperglycemia. If no pattern is evident, the physician should wait and gather more information, especially about what and how much is being eaten.

Development of infrared technologies that allow assessment of the glucose level without direct sampling of blood will enhance compliance with monitoring and minimize the risk of undetected nocturnal hypoglycemia.

Glycohemoglobin analyses reflect in a single value the ambient glucose values during the past 4 to 8 weeks. They measure the nonenzymatic linkage of glucose to a free amino group on the alpha and beta chains of hemoglobin (Maillard reaction). Many different methodologies are currently used for this analysis; they are not alike, although they are similar and should give concordant results. Specific measures of hemoglobin HbA_{1c} and for total glycosylated hemoglobin are preferred.

The glycohemoglobin value confirms the validity of glucose self-monitoring and has no "best" value for a given patient. A practical assessment of glycemic control as defined by a glycohemoglobin value is the following: (20 to 30) × (Ghb%) = average glucose values in mg/dL, with a value of 20× to be used at the lower end of abnormal glycohemoglobin and 30× at the higher end. Families and patients are instructed that glucose and glycohemoglobin monitoring is performed to allow them to solve problems. Shaming and blaming are defective applications of this process and indicate an urgent need for psychosocial intervention. Here is the dilemma: to be "within the normal range" is the goal, and the "best" value of glycohemoglobin for any patient is the "best" that he or she can obtain at this time.

The availability of assays of advanced Maillard products (fluorescent collagen and the advanced glycosylated end-products, pentosidine and pyrraline) in tissues and body fluids will likely provide information about organ damage and individual susceptibility to cardiovascular and renal complications.

TIME AND LOCUS OF INJECTION

Insulin is injected before food is eaten. The lead time between injection and eating allows standard, hexameric regular insulin to dissolve to monomers and to be absorbed into the circulation and allows the insulin to transform the liver into an organ used for "storage" rather than one of "production." The particular lead time must be empirically determined but may exceed 60 minutes in patients with moderately elevated glucose values.

The abdomen is the preferred locus of injection for constancy and rapidity of absorption. Site rotation is prudent but not necessary if the whole area is used rather than just the silver dollar–sized region. Abuse of the injection site is easily detected by palpation of an indurated and raised area. Months of site avoidance are required to restore the lipodystrophic tissue to normal. The more deeply the insulin is injected, the more rapidly it is absorbed. The same is true of injection over a muscle mass that will be exercised significantly.

MORNING HYPERGLYCEMIA

Four causes of pre-breakfast hyperglycemia are frequently encountered:

1. Too small an insulin dose to last through the night. This is often the case with intermediate insulin given at dinner or NPH given at bedtime.
2. Too much food given as a bedtime snack (or as "rescue" during the night). Children often prefer to eat a "meal" before going to bed; initiation of a dose of regular insulin to cover the snack is prudent. Parents tend to refeed their child until the symptoms of hypoglycemia clear. Educational reinforcement is required.
3. Worsening insulin resistance from 3 A.M. until 8 A.M.: the "dawn phenomenon." This situation is exaggerated in patients with poor glucose control and is the reason why bedtime intermediate insulin is required for many individuals to achieve control in the morning.
4. Mild blood sugar rise in response to a low blood sugar reaction during the night: "Somogyi (rebound) reaction." The mean glucose value before breakfast is 150 to 160 mg/dL. Values above this range should be considered the result of one of the three reasons noted previously.

MANAGEMENT OF INTERCURRENT ILLNESS

In the event of significant illness (infectious, posttraumatic, or surgical), two concerns are paramount for the patient with diabetes: hydration and glucose control.

The sick patient who is vomiting is better served by intravenous hydration in an outpatient setting (2 to 4 hours of lactated Ringer's solution at a rate of twice the maintenance dose). The sick patient who is able to drink should be instructed about a "liquid diet" that is free of protein and fat yet delivers the full daily allotment of carbohydrate calories and 100 mL of fluid per kg (about 2.5 liters per m^2 per day). The usual choices are clear sugar-containing sodas or drinks (Seven-Up, Sprite, Kool Aid, and so on), apple or cranberry juice, and sweetened Jello.

The stress of intercurrent illness augments the release of counterregulatory hormones and causes a decrease in peripheral insulin sensitivity. Hepatic glycogenolysis, gluconeogenesis, and ketogenesis increase. Peripheral glucose uptake declines. As a result, the need for additional insulin may be marked.

Frequent monitoring of blood glucose values and of urinary ketone body concentrations during such an illness is mandatory. The availability of reagent-strip analysis of beta-hydroxybutyrate allows for easy, accurate assessment of ketoacidosis in the outpatient clinic setting.

Blood glucose values of over 150 mg/dL aggravate the risk of dehydration through glucosuria. Values of over 200 mg/dL require intervention. Illness with glucose values of over 200 mg/dL invariably requires supplemental insulin administration in addition to the usual maintenance insulin requirements. The amount of the supplement can be estimated by using either a dose equal to 15 to 20% of the normal total daily insulin dose or the dose of regular insulin usually taken at breakfast or dinner. This supplemental insulin is injected as deeply as possible (intramuscular injection is allowed) and as often as needed (every hour if indicated) to keep the glucose value below 150 mg/dL. Deeply injected regular insulin usually acts for just 4 hours.

Failure to monitor for the consequences of treatment places the patient at unnecessary risk of both ketoacidosis and hypoglycemia. Monitoring is performed hourly to ensure appropriate intervention with fluids and insulin but may be delayed once control has been sustained for several hours. Families that have been instructed to monitor and treat patients aggressively in this way will obviate most admissions for ketoacidosis.

The exception to the reaction to illness just described is the child, usually young, who still has significant endogenous insulin reserves. Such a child when sick eats less and risks hypoglycemia from exogenous insulin administration. Treatment with glucose-containing fluids or intravenous hydration is warranted in such cases.

HYPOGLYCEMIA

The apparent price of improved control is an increased frequency of hypoglycemia. Nevertheless, this is to be avoided whenever possible. Fortunately, the long-term consequences of hypoglycemia are minimal to nonexistent, although cognitive ability is severely affected when glucose falls below 65 mg/dL (3.6 millimoles per liter). Seizures usually cause no permanent harm; however, the fear and consternation generated by a single hypoglycemic coma or seizure are not overcome for years.

Warning signs and symptoms of hypoglycemia are of two types: adrenergic and neuroglycopenic. The former include trembling, a pounding heart, sweatiness, and cold hands and feet. The latter include difficulty in concentrating, confusion, slurred speech, blurred vision, numb lips, uncoordinated movements, hunger and weakness, and nervous or tense feelings. The more reliable symptoms, in ranked order, are difficulty in concentrating, trembling, uncoordinated movements, pounding heart, slowed thinking, nervousness and tenseness, and sweatiness.

Hypoglycemia during sleep may be but is not usually detected by the patient and so requires periodic monitoring during the night. Further, any episode increases the risk for the next. This occurs because any hypoglycemic episode is associated with depressed adrenomedullary (epinephrine) and sympathetic hormone release, leading to the need to achieve a lower glucose level to trigger the counterregulatory hormone release; thus, reduced release of counterregulatory hormones and fewer neuroglycopenic symptoms occur. It appears, therefore, that hypoglycemia may induce the state of hypoglycemic unawareness.

Treatment depends on the ability of the patient to cooperate. If he or she can drink (help hold the cup) or chew (and swallow), ingestion of 10 to 20 grams of glucose is the most effective measure. Flavored tablets (5 grams) and gels are available that are easily carried on the person and are not likely to invite unnecessary ingestion. Fruit juices or sugar-containing soft drinks are less effective. The time needed for recovery is 15 to 20 minutes; peak glycemic response may not occur for 30 to 45 minutes. If the next scheduled meal is not for 45 minutes, ingestion of an additional 10 to 20 grams of carbohydrate is prudent; the choices are milk, cookies, or bread and butter.

If the patient is unable to help himself, is comatose, or is seizing, the use of intramuscular glucagon is indicated. Children under 5 years are given 0.5 mg, and others are given 1.0 mg. Even glucagon takes about 15 minutes to elevate blood glucose values; the duration of action is 45 to 60 minutes. Because of the risk of glucagon-induced vomiting, immediate follow-up in a physician's office or emergency room is prudent. The one circumstance of hypoglycemia that glucagon will not correct is ethanol-induced hypoglycemia. Adolescents must be educated about this risk.

In the absence of glucagon, the child must be treated with intravenous glucose. Infusion of 250 mg per kg (0.5 ml of 50% dextrose solution per kg) is adequate under most circumstances.

The cause of the hypoglycemic episode must be determined. The usual events include decreased food intake and increased exercise. The former is self-evident and requires intervention only if the circumstance is repeated regularly. Aerobic exercise can affect insulin sensitivity and glucose control for up to 8 hours afterward. Additional testing and the use of snacks during strenuous exercise are required to ensure glycemic control. Documentation of glucose values of less than 65 mg/dL before breakfast should lead to an immediate adjustment in the evening insulin regimen. Most nighttime hypoglycemic seizures are heralded by measured low glucose values before breakfast.

PSYCHOSOCIAL ISSUES

Growing up successfully in our culture is difficult; growing up successfully while saddled with a chronic disease is almost impossible. To support the child and his or her family, both clinical psychologists and social workers are on the Diabetes Team. The stress of diabetes on the integrity of the family and on the coping skills of the child is immense. There is no shame in reaching out for help. Eating disorders are frequent among adolescent patients. Appreciation of this fact can explain the erratic glycemic control sometimes seen in these patients. Discontinuation of insulin therapy is used to promote weight loss and is the main cause of recurrent ketoacidosis among diabetic patients.

Rest from the tasks of diabetic care is needed periodically by both the patient and the family. Camping and vacation experiences are to be encouraged. Having the parents contract to perform the requisite tasks of testing and recording for the young person is helpful to prevent the child's sense of abandonment by the parents once the child can perform those tasks for himself.

CHRONIC COMPLICATIONS

Microangiopathic and macroangiopathic complications appear to share common pathways, and their progression can be prevented or slowed. Although the clinical presentation may be delayed for 10 to 30 years, evidence of these complications can now be detected in time for medical intervention to make a significant difference.

Renal disease must be anticipated by assessment for microalbuminuria and documentation of a trend toward rising blood pressure. Distal symmetrical, primarily sensory neuropathy is well marked by abnormalities in assessment of light touch, pinprick, and ankle jerk reflexes and also by decreases in sural sensory-evoked amplitude and slowed peroneal motor conduction velocity. Detection of retinal pathology requires the performance of a dilated ophthalmologic examination.

Three hypotheses are emerging that integrate what is known about the evolution of nerve, renal, retinal, and large vessel disease: (1) accelerated oxidation by glucose, glycoxidation (Maillard) end-products, or free radicals; (2) the presence of intracellular pseudohypoxia as defined by the imbalance of the cytosolic ($NADH^+$/NAD) ratio; and (3) the presence of sorbitol accumulation and toxicity.

Therapy is first directed toward achieving glycemic control. Intervention trials with anti-oxidants (probucol*, nicotinamide*, and aminoguanidine*†), antihypertensive medications (captopril*, enalapril*), and aldose reductase inhibitors (tolrestat*‡) have continually established that the early biochemical consequences of diabetes can be prevented with interventions that are independent of glycemic control.

ROUTINE CARE AND MONITORING

Following the initial education and therapy of the patient, careful follow-up is needed to build confidence and trust with the Team. Immediate return to school or to the child's normal routine is important. Phone contact with the nurse educator should be maintained at least weekly. Medical clinic visits commence within 6 weeks of the diagnosis and recur quarterly. Review of the educational goals for the family may require additional nurse education visits on an "as needed" basis. The experience of recurrent, protracted phone contact is an indicator that an additional clinic visit is needed.

A period of partial remission of endogenous insulin production is expected for most patients and lasts about a year. In children under age 5 years the remission may be brief; in patients in whom onset of diabetes occurred at 20 years of age or older, the remission may be longer. An intervention that has been proved to extend the remission is early, aggressive, and tight glucose control. Although 10% of all patients have measurable C-peptide after 5 years of disease, glucose control in them is no better than in those without C-peptide.

For most pediatric patients, the quarterly visits are indicated primarily to build and reinforce the educational goals and objectives. After the first decade of disease, clinic visits are more important to monitor for diabetic complications. Contract making and goal setting at each visit promote accountability within the family and identify which family units will need psychosocial intervention early in the follow-up process.

At each visit, an interval history and a focused examination are performed. Height, weight, blood pressure, and mean arterial pressure are noted. Evidence of interphalangeal joint contractures, thyroid enlargement, retinopathy, and pubertal staging are recorded. A comprehensive examination of the patient with emphasis on the peripheral nervous and vascular systems is performed annually.

Diabetic patients are at increased risk for the consequences of hypertension. The functional definition of hypertension among pediatric diabetic patients is in question but may be practically defined as either a mean arterial pressure of over 90% for age and gender or as a steadily increasing pressure over time. If documented, treatment with angiotensin-converting enzyme inhibitors is indicated.

The glycohemoglobin value is measured at each visit, and measurement can now be performed within 9 minutes by capillary blood sampling. This procedure allows confirmation of the authenticity of the self-monitoring results while the family and patient are present and receptive.

Semiannual measurement of fractionated cholesterol (total, high-density lipoprotein [HDL], and low-density lipoprotein [LDL]) and total triglyceride values is recommended. If these are normal at diagnosis, this degree of attention probably is unnecessary unless control deteriorates or the child's condition progresses through puberty. Values of total cholesterol of over 200 mg/dL and of LDL cholesterol of over 130 mg/dL invite intensive dietary intervention. Intervention with medication is indicated if the cholesterol values are over 240 mg/dL (total) or over 150 mg/dL (LDL).

Although 20 to 25% of newly diagnosed patients have thyroid antibodies, only 3 to 4% develop clinical thyroid disease. Antibodies against thyroglobulin and thyroid (microsomal) peroxidase are better measured by radioimmunoassay than by hemagglutination titers. At diagnosis, if antibody levels are negative and a goiter is absent, the likelihood of disease is remote. If antibodies are noted at diagnosis, annual assessment of thyroxine and thyroid-stimulating hormone is indicated. Detection of a goiter should initiate a full assessment of the thyroid.

Renal disease that occurs before 5 years' duration of diabetes is rarely due to diabetes and is screened by routine urinalysis annually. After 5 years, an overnight timed (12-hour) urine collection for microalbuminuria is indicated annually. If microalbuminuria is present, treatment with an angiotensin-converting enzyme inhibitor is indicated to preserve function.

Formal eye examination with dilation is indicated annually after the fifth year of disease. Background

*This drug has not been approved by the Food and Drug Administration (FDA) for this indication (diabetes).

†Not available in the United States.

‡Investigational drug in the United States.

retinopathy is unusual before puberty but can occur in 10% of patients at 5 years if careful documentation (fundus photography) is performed. Medical intervention currently includes only improved glycemic control, a maneuver that may be associated with short-term worsening of the stage of retinopathy. Anti-oxidants may prove safe enough to use in children to minimize this problem.

Nerve conduction velocity studies document the presence of peripheral neuropathy at a time when improved glycemic control can make a beneficial difference. Deterioration within the normal range of velocity or deterioration of amplitude indicates the need for intervention. Aldose reductase inhibitors and aminoguanidine are effective if they are started early in the clinical course of this complication.

DIABETIC KETOACIDOSIS

method of
WILLIAM T. CEFALU, M.D.
Bowman Gray School of Medicine of Wake Forest University
Winston-Salem, North Carolina

Diabetic ketoacidosis (DKA) represents a life-threatening acute decompensation of diabetes and is reported to be extremely common in young patients, with a reported annual incidence of 14 per 100,000 general population, of which 20% may represent newly diagnosed cases. The events that lead to the development of DKA are multifactorial, and as such, DKA can be described as a condition in which catabolism is accelerated in three tissues (liver, fat, and muscle). In general, these tissues are associated with breakdown of glycogen stores, hydrolysis of triglycerides (in the adipose tissue), and mobilization of the amino acids (from muscle). The fuels released by these tissues are used by the liver for accelerated gluconeogenesis and ketogenesis, two important processes that define the disorder of DKA. Therefore, the diagnosis of DKA is generally made by demonstrating the presence of hyperglycemia and metabolic acidosis in a previously treated or newly diagnosed Type I diabetic.

PATHOPHYSIOLOGY

Hyperglycemia

Absolute insulin deficiency or relative insulin deficiency resulting from excess counterregulatory hormone secretion (e.g., cortisol, glucagon, epinephrine) can initiate the metabolic decompensation. In the past it was thought that only insulin deficiency was necessary to initiate hyperglycemia and metabolic acidosis. However, recent data suggest that it is insulin deficiency coupled with glucagon excess that is the operative mechanism. When Type I diabetic patients are withdrawn from insulin, rapid elevations in plasma glucagon, glucose, and ketone levels occur. These changes in glucose and ketones have been shown to be blunted when glucagon release is blocked by somatostatin. Furthermore, it has been shown that a strong correlation exists between blood glucose and glucagon levels during clinical studies. Therefore, there appears to be substantial evidence that elevated glucagon levels in association with low circulating insulin levels are responsible for the hyperglycemia seen in DKA.

Ketogenesis

The characteristic and defining metabolic abnormality of DKA is a marked overproduction of acids (e.g., acetoacetate, beta-hydroxybutyrate), which results in a metabolic acidosis. As has been demonstrated for hyperglycemia, absolute or relative insulin deficiency associated with excess counterregulatory hormones is the major factor responsible for the increased acid production in DKA. Insulin deficiency has been demonstrated to result in a marked release of free fatty acids from adipose tissue. However, the increased ketogenesis observed in the liver is caused not only by increased substrate for this process (i.e., increased free fatty acids) but also by other hepatic processes that promote acid formation. Insulin is important in this process because elevated insulin levels prevent release of free fatty acids from adipose tissue and suppress hepatic ketogenesis. In contrast, a deficiency of insulin increases adipose tissue breakdown, resulting in an increase in free fatty acid levels and hepatic metabolic processes that promote acid formation. Regardless of cause, when there is an increase in free fatty acid release from adipose tissue, as in DKA, and when hepatic processes that normally metabolize these substrates are exceeded, excess metabolic acids (e.g., acetoacetate, beta-hydroxybutyrate) are formed, producing the characteristic metabolic acidosis. These ketoacids generally circulate in a ratio of 3:1, favoring beta-hydroxybutyrate. Acetone, however, is formed by the spontaneous decarboxylation of acetoacetate and does not contribute to the metabolic acidosis. Acetone is excreted by the lungs and, because of its fruity odor, may be detected on the breath of a patient who is experiencing DKA.

PRECIPITATING FACTORS

In the initiation and progression of the DKA state, the lack of insulin action in peripheral tissues to suppress the responsible metabolic abnormalities is of utmost importance. Therefore, a deficiency of insulin action (secondary to a relative or absolute lack of circulating insulin) is a key and primary feature of DKA (Table 1).

An absolute deficiency of insulin is considered the major precipitating factor in newly diagnosed Type I diabetic patients presenting with DKA, and it has been estimated that approximately 20% of newly diagnosed patients present with DKA. In previously treated patients, an absolute deficiency of insulin would be considered the major precipitating cause in patients who inadvertently (due to equipment failure when using an insulin pump) or deliberately omit their insulin. This deficiency of insulin action in peripheral tissues leads to an increase in glucagon and other counterregulatory hormones that are responsible for the biochemical mechanisms that initiate and maintain ketoacidosis. Relative insulin deficiency should also be considered in situations in which insulin is being administered but because increased amounts of insulin are required (secondary to the stress associated with an active infection, inflammatory process, trauma, or other endocrinologic disorder), the amount of insulin being delivered is inadequate to suppress peripheral catabolism.

Table I lists the precipitating factors that may initiate DKA. Among these, infection has been reported to be the most common, accounting for 27 to 56% of cases. Active infection, therefore, should be ruled out in every patient with DKA who comes to the hospital.

SYMPTOMS AND SIGNS

Thirst, polyuria, fatigue, and weakness are common complaints given during the initial evaluation by patients with DKA. Hyperglycemia induces an osmotic diuresis and results in thirst and polyuria. Vomiting may occur secondary to gastric stasis and may result from a direct central effect of ketones. As would be expected, recurrent vomiting contributes to a negative fluid balance and hypovolemia, and the hypovolemic state may then be exacerbated by peripheral vasodilation secondary to both sepsis and acidosis. In addition, systemic acidosis may have a negative inotropic effect that contributes further to hypotension.

Variable physical signs are usually present in patients with DKA. Tachycardia is generally present in most patients, but it is not unusual for mean blood pressure to be normal. However, a low blood pressure secondary to the mechanisms outlined earlier has been demonstrated to be a poor prognostic sign because approximately 20% of patients who succumb to DKA can be expected to present initially with hypotension or shock. In contrast, hypotension has also been shown to be present in 10% of patients who survive DKA. If an elevated temperature is present initially in patients with DKA, the likelihood of infection is extremely high. Conversely, the patient may present with hypothermia, presumably secondary to peripheral vasodilation.

Abdominal pain with tenderness is a recognized symptom of DKA, particularly when acidosis is severe. Therefore, the clinician must be able to differentiate the abdominal pain of DKA from medical conditions such as pyelonephritis, pancreatitis, or acute appendicitis that may have precipitated the ketoacidotic state. The clinician should recognize that the abdominal pain should resolve rapidly with successful treatment of the ketoacidosis if the pain is secondary to DKA. A confounding factor in the management of abdominal pain is that a diagnosis of pancreatitis may be difficult given the fact that the serum amylase may be nonspecifically elevated. However, persistent pain in the abdomen during the course of treatment of ketoacidosis mandates medical attention. Finally, mental status may be a variable finding in DKA. True coma may be present in an estimated 10% of cases, whereas the majority show signs of clouding of consciousness. The decreased mental status may correlate with the degree of hyperosmolality.

TABLE 1. Precipitating Factors in Diabetic Ketoacidosis

- Absolute insulin deficiency
  - Newly diagnosed insulin-dependent diabetes mellitus
  - Omission of insulin therapy
    - Inadvertent (i.e., insulin pump failure)
    - Deliberate
- Relative insulin deficiency
  - Active infection
  - Acute abdominal disease
    - Pancreatitis
    - Pyelonephritis
    - Appendicitis
  - Acute myocardial or cerebral infarct
  - Trauma
  - Endocrine disorders
    - Hyperthyroidism
    - Pheochromocytoma
    - Somatostatinoma
  - Drugs
    - Steroids
    - Adrenergic agonists (e.g., epinephrine)
    - Pentamidine
    - Phenytoin (Dilantin)

Adapted from Walker M, Marshall SM, Alberti KG: Clinical Aspects of Diabetic Ketoacidosis. Diabetes Metab Rev 5:651–663, 1989. Reprinted by permission of John Wiley & Sons, Ltd.

LABORATORY ABNORMALITIES

Hyperglycemia and glucosuria are generally present in DKA, but extreme variability is noted. A review of laboratory values in DKA reported that blood glucose levels were in the 28- to 33-millimolar range (500 to 600 mg/dL), but the values can be extremely variable among individual cases. If severe hyperglycemia is observed (i.e., glucose levels of over 1000 mg/dL), marked dehydration should be considered as a major factor responsible for this extreme level. Furthermore, continual fluid losses (osmotic diuresis secondary to the hyperglycemia) lead to intravascular volume depletion and a decreased urine output. As a result, increased blood urea nitrogen and creatinine levels are common. Furthermore, if the creatinine is measured with an autoanalyzer in which acetoacetate interferes, the creatinine level reported may be spuriously elevated.

The serum sodium level has been reported to be low, normal, or high in DKA initially despite volume depletion, and the causes of this observation are multifactorial. First, the degree of hyperglycemia influences the measured sodium concentration (e.g., causing water movement from the intracellular to the extracellular space), resulting in a lower sodium concentration. A 1-millimolar drop in plasma sodium for every 3-millimolar increase in glucose has been proposed as a correction for this observation. A second reason for an extremely low sodium concentration may be hypertriglyceridemia. Insulin deficiency results in reduced clearance of triglycerides, and the elevated triglycerides displace plasma water, causing a low sodium concentration.

Usually there is a universal depletion of total body potassium stores in patients with DKA; however, the initial potassium concentration in DKA is also highly variable. Many reasons have been proposed for this variable finding, such as a shift of potassium from the intracellular to the extracellular compartment in response to acidosis and a decrease in sodium and potassium exchange across the cell membrane secondary to insulin deficiency. In addition, intracellular potassium depletion is promoted by both hyperglycemia and elevated glucagon levels. In all cases, potassium entering the intravascular space is lost because of the osmotic diuresis, and this effect is compounded by losses secondary to recurrent vomiting.

Overproduction of acetoacetate and beta-hydroxybutyric ketoacids by the liver with accumulation in the plasma is the hallmark of DKA, and these acids are generally present in plasma in a 3:1 ratio of beta-hydroxybutyric acid to acetoacetate. Unmeasured anions ("anion gap") are therefore noted in the plasma, and these can be quantitated by employing the formula, Anion gap $= Na^+ - (HCO_3 + Cl^-)$ (normal range 8 to 16 mEq per liter). Serum lactate secondary to poor tissue perfusion and increased anaerobic metabolism may contribute to the anion gap and metabolic acidosis. A semiquantitative estimate of the ketones in plasma can be made by employing reagent tablets using nitroprusside. In this reaction, nitroprusside reacts with acetoacetate but not with beta-hydroxybutyrate to produce a purple color.

Like potassium, the initial phosphate level in DKA may be low, normal, or high despite total body depletion. As a result of hypophosphatemia, a marked deficiency of erythrocyte 2,3-diphosphoglycerate may occur and may hinder oxygen delivery to tissues. Finally, an elevated white blood cell count may be present but does not always indicate active infection in patients with DKA.

INITIAL EVALUATION

During the initial evaluation the physician's history should focus on the duration and type of symptoms that the patient has been experiencing. If the patient has a history of Type I diabetes, questions regarding the events leading up to the presentation should be sought. These may include questions about the previous level of diabetic control, the quantity and frequency of insulin injections, and whether any concurrent illness had been present during the last several days. As stated earlier, a patient with pre-existing diabetes may be taking insulin regularly, but because of the increased stress of an infection or other process, the insulin levels achieved may be inadequate to prevent metabolic processes in peripheral tissues that promote diabetic ketoacidosis. If the patient is not a known diabetic, the combination of hyperglycemia and acidosis, particularly in a young patient, makes the diagnosis of Type I diabetes. At this stage, the patient's treatment will certainly consist of lifelong insulin administration after successful treatment of the acute event.

On physical examination, emphasis should be placed on noting the respiratory rate and depth, determining mental status level, and searching for signs of active infection. Laboratory tests should consist of routine serum chemistries to assess the degree of hyperglycemia, blood urea nitrogen (BUN), creatinine, electrolytes, complete blood count, and urinalysis. Assessment of blood gases is generally helpful to estimate the degree of metabolic acidosis, and a semiquantitative analysis of blood ketones can be made initially. Other considerations, as suggested by the physical examination and history, would be an electrocardiogram, chest radiograph, and blood culture if the suspicion of infection is high. Baseline liver function tests and amylase levels, should be done, particularly if abdominal pain is present. As stated previously, amylase may be nonspecifically elevated in this state.

TREATMENT

The goals of treatment of DKA should be twofold: (1) identify and eliminate the precipitating factor, and (2) reverse the metabolic abnormalities. Generally, this is accomplished by administering vigorous hydration, providing adequate insulin, replacing electrolytes, and when warranted, administering bicarbonate therapy. Identification and early treatment of an underlying infection should be considered in every case of DKA.

Fluid Replacement

Restoration of intravascular volume is a primary goal for the clinician because as much as 4 to 10 liters may be estimated to be the initial fluid deficit. Restored vascular volume will lower hyperglycemia through a process of hemodilution and will increase renal perfusion, thereby increasing the glucose that is excreted into the urine. Second, restored intravascular volume will allow optimal tissue perfusion to ensure delivery of administered insulin to tissues. The initial choice of fluid should be dictated by several factors, such as (1) the age of the patient, (2) the clinical hemodynamic status of the patient on admission, (3) the underlying medical conditions, and (4) consideration of the precipitating event (i.e., myocardial infarction or sepsis). Generally, rapid fluid replacement (i.e., 1 to 2 liters during the first hour followed by 1 liter per hour for the first several hours) is indicated. However, clinical factors may dictate modification of this approach, especially in older patients with underlying cardiac dysfunction in an intensive care unit; specific monitoring of intravascular volume may be necessary in these cases. The use of isotonic saline or Ringer's lactate has been recommended for initial therapy because these fluids are better for restoring intravascular volume than hypotonic fluids. The clinician should recognize, however, that patients with DKA ultimately require free water for normalization because they are in a state of hypotonic dehydration. As such, once the patient's vascular status has been stabilized, intravenous fluids should be changed to half normal saline.

With successful therapy, the serum glucose level will fall to a relatively normal or high normal range before the ketones are completely cleared from the circulation. At this stage, insulin therapy is still needed and should continue to be delivered to suppress the ketogenic mechanisms, yet hypoglycemia should be avoided by providing intravenous glucose-containing solutions. Therefore, when it is observed that the blood glucose level has fallen to approximately 250 mg/dL (13.9 millimoles), intravenous fluids should be switched to a 5% dextrose solution. The end-point of fluid management is stabilization of the intravascular volume such that blood pressure, urine output, and tissue perfusion (brain, heart) are maintained. Fluid overload should be avoided.

Insulin

At the same time that aggressive fluid management is being planned and implemented, the administration of insulin should be considered as well. Insulin is of paramount importance in reversing the metabolic and hormonal abnormalities of DKA. As such, insulin decreases glucagon release from the alpha cells of the pancreas and counteracts the hepatic effects of glucagon, resulting in a suppression of gluconeogenesis and ketogenesis in the liver. Enhancement of glucose uptake and utilization in muscle and fat and peripheral inhibition of adipose tissue breakdown are other important actions of insulin. Because of the increased levels of counterregulatory hormones in DKA, significantly more insulin is needed to treat DKA than would be needed for maintenance doses after the acute event. As a result, clinical insulin resistance is universally present in all patients with ketoacidosis.

Intravenous insulin should be used in the initial treatment of DKA because it allows a steady-state level of insulin to be reached in approximately 25 to 30 minutes, especially when the intravenous infusion is preceded with a bolus injection of insulin. Using this approach, effective insulin concentrations can be achieved immediately, and the intravenous route also allows rapid dosing changes, given that the half-life of intravenous insulin is only approximately 5 minutes. Therefore, an initial intravenous insulin bolus of 0.1 to 0.4 unit per kg body weight is suggested, followed by a continuous infusion delivering 0.1 unit per kg per hour. In the average adult, this amounts to approximately 5 to 10 units of insulin per hour.

Regardless of the initial insulin dose, careful clinical and biochemical observation of the patient is required during the course of treatment. One of the goals of treatment is to lower the patient's glucose level by approximately 75 to 100 mg/dL per hour (4.1 to 5.6 millimoles per hour) and to adjust insulin therapy if this goal is not achieved. An increased insulin requirement, greater than that existing before the event, is to be expected. However, an increased insulin requirement may also indicate a severe underlying infection or inadequate expansion of the intravascular volume such that peripheral tissue hypoperfusion may be present.

It is essential that insulin therapy be continued even when normal blood sugar levels are approached because the acidosis in DKA may take longer to correct than the hyperglycemia. The management of fluid and insulin therapy at this point may be combined so that intravenous insulin is given with glucose-containing solutions. One suggested approach is to add 10 to 16 units of insulin to a liter of 10% dextrose solution and deliver it at 100 mL per hour once the blood glucose level has reached approximately 270 mg/dL (15 millimoles per liter). However, a different approach would be to continue the peripheral insulin infusion and change the fluids to a 5% dextrose solution. The goal of both approaches is to deliver adequate insulin to inhibit the ketogenic pathway while maintaining an adequate glucose level. The patient may be started on subcutaneous insulin only after the ketones have cleared and near-normal or slightly elevated glucose levels are maintained.

Potassium

As explained earlier, although total body potassium stores are generally depleted, plasma values may be normal or even high on the initial evaluation because of the metabolic acidosis that shifts potassium from the intracellular to the extracellular spaces. This may occur in the presence of potassium deficits ranging from 300 to 1000 millimoles. Therefore, immediate institution of intravenous potassium is required if the initial serum concentration is low in the presence of systemic acidosis. Potassium chloride solution may be given at an initial rate of 20 to 30 mEq per hour, and the rate of administration should be dictated by the level of potassium at hourly checks. Rates as high as 60 mEq per hour may be required, but careful monitoring in intensive care unit settings may be required. A slower rate of 10 to 30 mEq per hour may be suggested if the patient is found to have normal potassium levels on admission. Intravenous potassium may be withheld initially if the value is elevated, but replacement should be initiated during the next several hours because the potassium level will drop as fluids and insulin are administered. The clinician must be aware that there will be a steep decline in potassium concentration immediately after the institution of therapy, the lowest levels being reported within the first few hours of therapy. Hypokalemia carries the risk of cardiac arrhythmias and respiratory failure, whereas hyperkalemia may predispose the patient to life-threatening arrhythmias. Therefore, close monitoring of the patient and the potassium levels is required.

Phosphates

It has been suggested that phosphate therapy be initiated when the serum level falls toward the lower limit of normal and that phosphate be replaced at a rate not exceeding 10 millimoles per hour (provided as a sodium or potassium salt). Although it is well established that total body phosphate stores may be markedly depleted in DKA, there has been no evidence that phosphate therapy contributes significantly to the patient's clinical outcome.

Bicarbonate

Severe acidosis is a major manifestation of DKA, and its presence may cause confusion, stupor, coma, and arrhythmias, which may lead to heart failure or hypotension. In addition, acidosis may result in a negative inotropic effect on the heart and may produce direct peripheral vasodilation contributing to hypotension. Yet bicarbonate therapy remains controversial in the management of DKA. Although it is understood that treatment of severe acidosis is necessary, the efficacy of the routine use of intravenous bicarbonate for this purpose has not been clearly established. Furthermore, successful treatment of patients with DKA with fluids and insulin will correct the acidosis. At present, there seems to be little evidence to support the routine use of bicarbonate in patients with DKA unless they are severely acidotic. Therefore, it has been suggested that bicarbonate therapy be reserved for patients with severe acidosis (pH less than 7) or severe acidosis associated with mental status changes, coma, respiratory failure, or cardiac arrhythmia.

HYPERURICEMIA AND GOUT

method of
SHANNON HOWE, M.D., and
N. LAWRENCE EDWARDS, M.D.
University of Florida
Gainesville, Florida

Gout is one of the most frequently encountered forms of arthritis and has a prevalence in the United States of 1%

for all ages. The disease is much more common in men than in women, but the prevalence in both sexes increases with age. In men over the age of 65 years the prevalence exceeds 5%. Effective drug therapy for treating acute gout and preventing chronic tophaceous gout has been available for almost 30 years, but widespread misconceptions about when and how to start therapy persist.

Acute gout commonly becomes manifest as a monarticular or pauciarticular arthritis, classically involving the first metatarsophalangeal joint, mid-foot, ankle, or knee, with fever, leukocytosis, and exquisite tenderness. The diagnosis is based on a suggestive clinical history, an elevated serum urate level, and an analysis of the synovial fluid from the involved joint that shows strongly negative birefringent crystals within polymorphonuclear leukocytes. This last finding is a sine qua non for the definitive diagnosis of acute gout, and we rely heavily on this finding because the most common error in the management of gout is an initial misdiagnosis. Occasionally, the serum uric acid (urate) level is found to be in the normal range during an acute attack. This is most likely due to the temporary uricosuric effect of stress associated with the acutely painful process. In time, untreated acute intermittent gout can progress to a chronic polyarticular arthropathy involving any number of joints including "unusual" joints such as the small joints of the hand, elbows, and sternoclavicular joints. Urate crystals are often identified in the synovial fluid during asymptomatic periods between acute gouty attacks or by needle biopsy of suspected tophaceous deposits.

Hyperuricemia is a biochemical condition associated with increased body mass, hypertension, and hypertriglyceridemia. Weight loss counseling is generally a good idea in obese hyperuricemic individuals. Such patients should be discouraged from excessive alcohol intake, especially beer, and the consumption of organ meats such as sweetbreads, tongue, liver, and kidney. Other than these recommendations, there is no reason for more severe restrictions on purine intake in the diet. Hyperuricemia is also associated with lead toxicity (saturnine gout) and certain drugs—diuretics, ethambutol, pyrazinamide, moderate to low-dose aspirin, and nicotinic acid. Substitution or elimination of the offending drugs, when practical, is preferable to adding a drug to treat the hyperuricemia. It is important to remember that hyperuricemia is a common biochemical abnormality that will result in clinical gout in only a small percentage of cases. Therefore, treating asymptomatic hyperuricemia is rarely justified.

The presence of hyperuricemia in unusual clinical settings, such as teenage males or premenopausal females, or in association with renal stones requires an aggressive diagnostic work-up. In these patients one should consider inborn metabolic disorders, renal disturbances, and "high-turnover" states such as lympho- and myeloproliferative disorders and psoriasis. A 24-hour urinary uric acid measurement is helpful in these circumstances to distinguish "overproducers" from "underexcretors" of uric acid. In the typical middle-aged man with hyperuricemia and gout the urinary uric acid quantitation rarely adds any useful information.

THERAPY FOR ACUTE GOUT

Therapy for acute gout is based on decreasing the inflammatory response to the urate crystals as rapidly as possible while minimizing drug toxicity. There are few patients as miserable as those stricken with acute gout. This is especially true of elderly or postsurgical patients who find their activities of daily living or rehabilitation hampered. Untreated acute gout typically takes 5 to 7 days to resolve completely, and in patients with chronic tophaceous gout the acute flares can last up to several weeks. All forms of therapy for acute gout described in this section are effective in shortening the duration of symptoms. The success of treatment has much more to do with how soon after the onset of symptoms the therapy is begun than on which drug is chosen.

Nonsteroidal anti-inflammatory drugs (NSAIDs) are among the easiest and most accessible drugs for treating the inflammation of acute gout. Contraindications may exist for NSAIDs in individual patients, such as NPO status, gastrointestinal bleeding, renal insufficiency, congestive heart failure, anticoagulation therapy, or an allergic reaction to aspirin. Although any NSAID can be effective, NSAIDs with a short half-life (ibuprofen*, tolmetin sodium*, diclofenac*) may be associated with more rapid onset of action and fewer risks. Indomethacin (Indocin), 50 to 75 mg every 6 to 8 hours, remains our first choice among NSAIDs, although in elderly patients it may be associated with vestibular symptoms, drowsiness, and headache. High initial doses of these NSAIDs are used to treat acute gout for the first several days until the symptoms have declined dramatically; reduced (maintenance) doses of NSAIDs are then continued for a 2-week course (Table 1).

Oral colchicine therapy for acute gout has traditionally been given in doses of one tablet (0.6 mg) hourly or every 2 hours until one of the following occurs: gastrointestinal toxicity (nausea, vomiting, diarrhea, or cramps, which occur in 80% of patients); the maximum allowable dose has been taken (usually 8 to 10 mg orally over 24 hours, then no more for 7 days); or relief occurs. Significant gastrointestinal side effects place an undue burden on a patient who may have ambulation difficulties from the gout itself or from medical illness that has contributed to the acute attack. There are sufficient therapeutic alternatives so that such potentially toxic therapy is unnecessary. Although intravenous colchicine avoids

*This drug has not been approved by the FDA for this indication.

TABLE 1. **Dosages of NSAIDs in the Management of Gout**

Drug	Dosage (mg)	
	Acute	*Prophylaxis*
1. Indomethacin (Indocin)	100 then 50 qid	50 tid
2. Ibuprofen (Motrin, Rufen)	800 qid	600 tid
3. Diclofenac (Voltaren)	100 then 50 qid	75 bid
4. Meclofenate (Meclomen)	100 qid	50 tid
5. Ketoprofen (Orudis)	75 qid	50 tid
6. Flurbiprofen (Ansaid)	100 tid	100 bid
7. Tolmetin (Tolectin)	800 then 600 tid	400 tid
8. Naproxen (Naprosyn)	750 then 500 bid	375 bid

Abbreviations: bid = twice daily; tid = three times daily; qid = four times daily.

the gastrointestinal toxicity, bone marrow toxicity remains a serious possibility. This is especially true in elderly, infected, debilitated, postoperative, and marrow-suppressed individuals in whom bone marrow suppression with colchicine can have fatal consequences. Precautions especially are in order for those patients with renal and hepatic insufficiency. We no longer recommend using colchicine by either route for the treatment of acute gout because other less toxic and more effective medications are available.

Perhaps an underutilized therapeutic option for acute gout is adrenocorticotrophic hormone (ACTH).* We have found it to be useful for patients who are elderly or seriously ill or have severe gastrointestinal or renal disease or polyarticular gout. We often use it when NSAIDs cannot be administered, such as for patients with NPO status. Because it can be given intravenously, intramuscularly, or subcutaneously, there is an appropriate route of administration for all patients. The onset of relief is achieved more quickly than with NSAIDs (approximately 3 ± 1 hours compared with 24 ± 10 hours for indomethacin), and there are fewer side effects. A typical starting dose is 40 to 80 units given parenterally every 6 to 12 hours for 1 to 2 days. Because "rebound" effect can occur, prophylactic NSAIDs or low-dose oral colchicine (0.6 mg twice a day) should be added after relief is obtained. ACTH is contraindicated in patients who are pregnant or have congestive heart failure.

Intra-articular steroids can also be effective in blunting an acute gouty attack and may afford the most rapid relief when they are combined with a local anesthetic (lidocaine or bupivacaine). Soluble, noncrystalline forms of steroids (for example, Depo-Medrol) are preferred. In acutely inflamed gouty joints it is important to keep the volume of steroid and anesthetic injected into the joint to a minimum because large volumes will worsen the symptoms. In a knee joint we use 40 mg of prednisolone or the equivalent in 1.5 to 2 mL total volume; for an ankle, 20 mg in 1 mL; and for a first metatarsophalangeal joint, 5 mg in 0.3 mL.

PROPHYLAXIS FOR ACUTE GOUT

By using the approaches described in the previous section we can generally achieve good symptomatic control of acute gout during the first 24 to 36 hours of therapy. If antiarthritic prophylaxis is not maintained for at least 10 to 14 days during this critical period, gouty symptoms may promptly return. If we have used NSAIDs to achieve initial control, we simply reduce the high doses used in the first 2 days and continue with a lower "maintenance" dose of the NSAID for a total of 2 weeks. If initial control has been achieved with either ACTH injections* or intra-articular steroids, we then place the patient on either maintenance doses of NSAIDs or low-dose oral colchicine. The typical dose of colchicine in this situation is 0.6 mg given twice daily. About 20% of patients experience gastrointestinal hypermobility on this dose that requires dose reduction.

*This drug has not been approved by the FDA for this indication.

Long-term daily use of NSAIDs or colchicine is helpful in decreasing the frequency and severity of acute attacks in patients with intermittent gout and in diminishing chronic pain in patients with tophaceous gout. The decision about when to initiate this type of maintenance anti-inflammatory therapy is quite variable, with some patients requesting it after their first acute episode, whereas others totally eschew chronic therapies of any type. We like to delay chronic prophylaxis until the patient has had at least several acute gouty attacks, and in general we do not encourage this therapy until the attacks are occurring every 6 to 8 months. The mean interval between the first and second gouty attack is approximately 11 months, but this period varies greatly. Many patients go 2 to 3 years between episodes, but it is rare for a patient to have early attacks more frequently than every 6 months. This latter pattern of recurrence is, however, typical of patients with myelo- or lymphoproliferative disorders or those taking cyclosporine (Sandimmune) following organ transplantation. During this early period of acute intermittent gout, while we are determining the frequency of acute episodes, the patient is encouraged to keep a supply of a NSAID (such as indomethacin) close by so that at the first symptom of a gouty flare he or she can begin therapy and ideally minimize the attack.

NORMALIZATION OF URIC ACID LEVELS

The medications we have discussed so far, including NSAIDs, colchicine, corticosteroids, and ACTH,* are all effective in treating the symptoms of gout but have no beneficial effect on the immediate cause of gout—i.e., hyperuricemia. The drugs discussed in this section are effective in reducing serum urate levels but have no short-term benefit in reducing the pain and swelling that bring the patient into the physician's office. The decision to begin drugs like allopurinol (Zyloprim) or the uricosuric agents (probenecid [Benemid] or sulfinpyrazone [Anturane]) is therefore not made in the presence of active gouty symptoms but rather after the gout has become quiescent and the entire clinical course of the patient's disease can be examined. Not all patients with acute intermittent gout ultimately require uric acid–lowering drugs, but we feel that they are indicated in subjects with (1) more than two attacks per year despite prophylactic therapy, (2) the presence of joint deformities or radiographic evidence of joint damage, (3) the presence of subcutaneous tophi, or (4) a history of recurrent kidney stones or renal insufficiency.

We mentioned earlier that treating asymptomatic hyperuricemia with uric acid–lowering drugs is rarely indicated. This is because only a small percentage of asymptomatic subjects eventually go on to develop urate-related symptoms. An exception to this rule occurs in patients with serum urate levels in

*This drug has not been approved by the FDA for this indication.

excess of 12 mg/dL. Urate levels in this range are usually secondary to drugs or other known or occult diseases, and these precipitating causes should be investigated and rectified if possible. An untreated serum urate level of greater than 12 mg/dL will probably result in clinical symptoms of gout or renal stones during the next 12 months and should therefore be treated empirically.

A special group of hyperuricemic patients are those taking cyclosporine, which is known to affect renal handling of uric acid. The transplant population on cyclosporine who have elevated uric acid levels generally should be taking uric acid–lowering drugs to avoid further renal function decline attributable to uric acid nephropathy. Allopurinol is the preferred drug in this instance. In transplant patients taking azathioprine, however, allopurinol can lead to toxic elevations of purine analogues, and this possibility should be carefully monitored.

The drugs used to lower uric acid levels can be divided into two categories: the uricosuric agents, which enhance renal clearance of uric acid, and the xanthine oxidase inhibitors, which block uric acid formation. Because the majority of patients with primary gout are hyperuricemic on the basis of renal underexcretion, one might assume that the uricosurics are an ideal remedy to the problem. However, because of multiple drug-drug interactions, difficult long-term dosing schedules, and the potential for precipitating nephrolithiasis, the uricosurics, probenecid and sulfinpyrazone, are used relatively sparingly. Allopurinol is the only xanthine oxidase inhibitor currently available and is very effective in rapidly reducing serum urate levels with only one dose per day. Its good safety record when used carefully (see following section) and the better compliance achieved with a once daily dose make allopurinol the most popular method for lowering uric acid levels. It should be remembered that any acute alterations in uric acid concentration within the joint (either increasing it or decreasing it) can precipitate a gouty flare. For this reason, a patient should be at least 2 to 3 months past the most recent attack before starting any form of uric acid–lowering drug. We typically maintain our patients on a prophylactic regimen of colchicine or a NSAID for 6 months after initiating either allopurinol or one of the uricosurics.

Allopurinol

Allopurinol is a convenient and extremely effective drug for inhibiting the production of uric acid. It is the preferred agent (1) in patients with renal insufficiency (although the dose must be adjusted for creatinine clearance); (2) if the urinary uric acid on a normal diet is more than 800 mg per day; (3) when previous uricosuric therapy has failed; (4) when there is a history of renal stones; and (5) if there is a need to prevent acute uric acid nephropathy secondary to "tumor lysis" in the course of chemotherapy. We start with 100 mg per day orally (or 50 mg if the creatinine clearance is less than 30 mL per minute) and accelerate the therapy based on the clinical assessment and serum urate response. The goal of all forms of uric acid–lowering drugs is to reduce the serum urate level to a range of 5 to 6 mg/dL. It is during initiation of therapy that severe toxic side effects are most common. These include severe hypersensitivity reactions manifested by rash, eosinophilia, interstitial nephritis, hepatic injury, fever, leukocytosis, and bone marrow suppression. Such reactions have been associated with death and are most commonly seen in patients with mild renal failure and concomitant thiazide diuretic therapy treated initially with full doses (300 mg per day) of allopurinol. Other mild dermatologic reactions include an erythematous rash on the shin or dorsal foot that generally requires only a reduction in the allopurinol dose. The ultimate therapeutic maintenance dose can range widely, depending on the clinical response, which must be monitored closely once allopurinol therapy is begun. Important drug interactions include those with 6-mercaptopurine, azathioprine, theophylline, and possibly oral anticoagulants.

Uricosuric Agents

Uricosuric agents are also effective in treating tophaceous gout but are not recommended when renal insufficiency is present. They are generally a second-line choice for us because of long-term problems with patient compliance. Probenecid (Benemid) is initiated as a dose of 250 mg twice a day and gradually increased up to 2 gm per day in two or three divided doses. Sulfinpyrazone (Anturane) is given as a dose of 100 mg twice a day to start and increased to 800 mg per day in three to four divided doses. Probenecid can interfere with renal handling of weak anionic drugs such as penicillin, digoxin, and other drugs, leading to toxicity. Sulfinpyrazone has some antiplatelet effects and therefore has been proposed as a preferred drug for patients with secondary hyperuricemia and gout resulting from diuretic therapy for hypertension because these patients have additional risks for coronary artery disease. Adding uricosuric agents to allopurinol tends to decrease the serum concentration of oxypurinol, the long-acting active metabolite of allopurinol, thereby reducing the therapeutic effectiveness of allopurinol. Oral fluids should be encouraged with the initiation of any uricosuric agent to avoid the development of renal stones.

HYPERLIPOPROTEINEMIAS

method of
CONRAD B. BLUM, M.D.
Columbia University College of Physicians and Surgeons
New York, New York

Elevations of plasma cholesterol and triglyceride levels are caused by elevated levels of the plasma lipoproteins, the transport vehicles for the otherwise insoluble plasma lipids. The disorders of lipoprotein metabolism achieve their importance because of their clinical sequelae. Elevated levels of low-density lipoprotein (LDL) and low levels of high-density lipoprotein (HDL) increase the risk of development of atherosclerotic vascular disease, and high levels of very-low-density lipoproteins (VLDL) may also indicate increased risk. Extremely high levels of the triglyceride-rich lipoproteins VLDL and chylomicrons can cause pancreatitis and xanthomatosis.

METABOLISM OF THE PLASMA LIPOPROTEINS

There are four major classes of lipoproteins in plasma (Table 1). The lipoproteins are spherical particles with a core composed primarily of triglyceride or cholesteryl ester and a surface coat of unesterified cholesterol, phospholipid, and specific apolipoproteins. The various apoproteins function as detergents, solubilizing the lipids in plasma; additionally, some act as recognition sites for cell-surface receptors, and some are cofactors for enzymes involved in lipid metabolism.

The plasma lipoproteins contain varying amounts of all of the lipids of plasma. LDL and HDL are rich in cholesterol and contain very little triglyceride. Normally, LDL is the major carrier of cholesterol in human plasma, accounting for approximately 70% of total plasma cholesterol. Chylomicrons and VLDL are triglyceride rich. Chylomicrons are the transport vehicle for dietary triglyceride. VLDLs, secreted by the liver, are the transport vehicle for endogenous triglyceride. In the circulation, lipoprotein lipase hydrolyzes triglyceride in the core of VLDL and chylomicrons, yielding a smaller, shrunken remnant particle. The remnant lipoproteins are thought to be atherogenic. Chylomicron remnants are rapidly taken up by the liver. Most VLDL remnants undergo further conversion to form LDL particles.

The clearance of LDL from plasma occurs largely through a specific receptor-mediated process involving the recognition of apoB-100, the sole apoprotein of LDL. Normally, this process accounts for two-thirds of the clearance of LDL from plasma. Clearance of LDL through this mechanism is antiatherogenic. Another receptor, the scavenger receptor of macrophages, recognizes oxidized and other chemically altered forms of LDL. Clearance of LDL through the scavenger receptor may contribute to the development of atherosclerotic plaque.

HDL particles originate in both the liver and the intestine. Processes associated with the metabolic degradation of VLDL and chylomicrons further contribute to the formation of HDL. The mechanisms responsible for the inverse relationship between HDL concentration and coronary heart disease (CHD) risk are not fully understood. They may involve (1) facilitation by HDL of transport of cholesterol from the periphery to the liver ("reverse cholesterol transport"), (2) stimulation of prostacyclin synthesis by vascular endothelium, (3) HDL's capacity to act as a scavenger for polar surface active components released during lipolysis of triglyceride-rich lipoproteins, and (4) associations between low HDL levels and elevated concentrations of particularly atherogenic lipoproteins (e.g., VLDL remnants, chylomicron remnants, or small dense LDL particles).

DIAGNOSIS OF THE HYPERLIPOPROTEINEMIAS

Although total plasma cholesterol and HDL cholesterol levels are not substantially altered by fasting or eating, assessment of the plasma LDL and triglyceride levels requires a fasting blood sample. Acute injury or illness such as myocardial infarction or major surgery can lead to substantial reductions in LDL and HDL levels lasting as long as 2 to 3 months. Thus, blood samples for assessment of lipoprotein levels should be taken when the patient is in a metabolic steady state and taking his or her usual diet.

All of the cholesterol in fasting plasma is normally found in VLDL, LDL, and HDL. Because the known composition of VLDL allows us to approximate its cholesterol content as one-fifth of the triglyceride level, LDL cholesterol is generally calculated as [C − Tg/5 − HDL], where C is the total plasma cholesterol, Tg is the fasting plasma triglyceride level, and HDL is the measured HDL cholesterol level. The approximation of VLDL cholesterol as one-fifth the plasma triglyceride level loses its validity when chylomicrons are present (e.g., in a nonfasting sample), when the plasma triglyceride level exceeds 400 mg/dL, and in the rare patient with Type III hyperlipoproteinemia (dysbetalipoproteinemia). Thus, these are circumstances when LDL cannot be approximated by this formula.

Because all of the plasma lipoproteins contain cholesterol, hypercholesterolemia can be associated with elevation of any of the lipoprotein classes. However, marked elevation of cholesterol with a normal triglyceride level generally indicates elevation of LDL and increased risk of CHD. Lesser elevations of cholesterol with normal triglyceride levels can also be due to elevations of HDL, a circumstance associated with reduced CHD risk. Genetically determined elevations of LDL may be due to familial hypercholesterolemia (caused by defective or deficient LDL receptors), familial defective apoprotein B (caused by mutant apoB, which is poorly recognized by LDL receptors),

TABLE 1. **Major Classes of Plasma Lipoproteins**

Lipoprotein Class	Origin	Catabolism	Clinical Correlates of Elevation
Chylomicrons (>95% triglyceride)	Intestine	Lipoprotein lipase, remnants cleared by liver	Pancreatitis Eruptive xanthomas Hepatosplenomegaly
VLDL (60% triglyceride)	Liver	Lipoprotein lipase, conversion to LDL	Glucose intolerance Hyperuricemia
LDL (50% cholesterol)	VLDL	LDL receptor	Atherosclerosis Corneal arcus Xanthelasma Tendinous xanthoma
HDL (50% protein, 25% cholesterol)	Liver and intestine	??Liver	Decreased CHD risk (increased risk with low HDL)

familial combined hyperlipidemia (caused by increased secretion of apoB-100 in VLDL, the precursor of LDL), or polygenic hypercholesterolemia (a heterogeneous group of imperfectly understood disorders). Additionally, LDL levels may be elevated by diets high in cholesterol and saturated fats, obesity, hypothyroidism, diabetes mellitus, and nephrotic syndrome. Treatment with thiazide diuretics, glucocorticoids, or cyclosporine A (Sandimmune) can also elevate LDL levels.

Elevations of VLDL and chylomicrons appear in laboratory tests as hypertriglyceridemia. Triglyceride levels can be categorized as borderline high (200 to 400 mg/dL), high (400 to 1000 mg/dL), and very high (over 1000 mg/dL). Very high plasma triglyceride levels are generally due to elevations of VLDL and chylomicrons (Type V hyperlipoproteinemia); such very high triglyceride levels can cause pancreatitis. Very high triglyceride levels warrant drug therapy when nonpharmacologic measures are not sufficiently effective. One should attempt to reduce the fasting plasma triglyceride level to below 500 mg/dL, although this is not always possible. Borderline high and high triglyceride levels are most commonly associated with obesity and alcohol consumption. Triglyceride elevations in the range of 200 to 1000 mg/dL can also result from treatment with estrogens, *cis*-retinoic acid, diuretics, beta-blocking medications, and glucocorticoids. Additionally, borderline high or high triglyceride levels can result from diabetes, uremia, nephrotic syndrome, or hypothyroidism. There is an increased risk of CHD when hypertriglyceridemia is associated with diabetes or is due to either familial combined hyperlipidemia or Type III hyperlipoproteinemia. In familial combined hyperlipidemia elevated levels of cholesterol and triglycerides or both are found in various members of the family. Rarely, hypertriglyceridemia is a consequence of familial Type III hyperlipoproteinemia (dysbetalipoproteinemia). The pathogenesis of this very uncommon disease involves homozygosity for a mutation in apolipoprotein E, rendering it poorly recognizable to cell surface receptors. As a consequence, highly atherogenic remnants of VLDL and chylomicrons accumulate in plasma.

TREATMENT OF ELEVATIONS OF LDL IN ADULTS

A large number of clinical trials have shown that reduction of LDL levels by dietary and pharmacologic measures reduces CHD risk in hypercholesterolemic patients. Furthermore, these trials show that cholesterol reduction reduces the frequency of fatal and nonfatal CHD events in patients who have already suffered an acute myocardial infarction. In these large studies, the risk of CHD fell by 2% for every 1% reduction in serum cholesterol levels. Additionally, angiographic studies have demonstrated that aggressive cholesterol reduction retards the growth of established atherosclerotic lesions and enhances the regression of these lesions. These studies provide the experimental underpinning for the current approach to treatment of elevated LDL levels.

The Adult Treatment Panel of the National Cholesterol Education Program issued reports in 1988 and 1993 focusing on reduction of plasma levels of LDL, the major atherogenic lipoprotein. Plasma LDL cholesterol levels are categorized as desirable (under 130 mg/dL), borderline high risk (130 to 159 mg/dL), and high risk (160 mg/dL or more). The approach taken involves more aggressive therapy for those at higher risk. Individuals are considered to be in one of three categories of CHD risk. More than 80% of deaths in persons who have survived a myocardial infarction are due to CHD. Therefore, the category of highest risk includes those who have already developed CHD or symptomatic peripheral vascular or cerebrovascular disease. An intermediate category of risk includes those with at least two risk factors for CHD (other than elevated LDL cholesterol) (Table 2). A high HDL cholesterol level (at least 60 mg/dL) is considered to be a negative risk factor for CHD, reducing by one the total number of risk factors present. Obesity is associated with increased risk of CHD, but much of the increased risk of obesity is due to other conditions that are secondary to obesity; these include hypertension and low HDL cholesterol. Thus, although obesity should be earmarked for intervention, its presence is not a factor in determining the aggressiveness of LDL reduction. Similarly, physical inactivity is a target of intervention but is not used in determining the aggressiveness of LDL reduction.

Before initiating intensive treatment of hyperlipoproteinemia with diet or medication, it is important to determine whether the lipoprotein disorder is secondary to another disease (e.g., hypothyroidism, nephrotic syndrome, diabetes mellitus) or to treatment with a medication. If it is, attention to the primary cause may be the most appropriate treatment for the hyperlipoproteinemia.

Dietary Therapy for Elevated LDL Levels

Most patients with mild or moderate degrees of primary hypercholesterolemia due to elevated LDL levels can be treated satisfactorily with diet alone; cholesterol-lowering medications are not needed for these individuals. The threshold for initiation of intensive therapy to reduce LDL cholesterol by diet or drugs depends on an individual's overall risk of CHD (Table 3). Saturated fats and cholesterol in the diet suppress LDL receptor activity, thereby retarding the clearance of LDL from plasma and elevating LDL levels in plasma. Obesity is associated with increased hepatic secretion of VLDL, the metabolic precursor of LDL. Thus, the principles of dietary treatment are (1) restriction of dietary saturated fats, (2) restriction of

TABLE 2. **CHD Risk Factors**

Positive Risk Factors
1. Low HDL cholesterol (<35 mg/dL)
2. Current cigarette smoking
3. Hypertension (BP ≥140/90 mmHg or drug treatment for hypertension)
4. Family history of premature CHD (myocardial infarction or sudden death in male first-degree relative <55 years of age or female <65 years of age)
5. Diabetes mellitus
6. Age (male ≥45 years of age, female ≥55 years of age or menopausal without estrogen replacement)

Negative Risk Factor
High HDL cholesterol (≥60 mg/dL)

TABLE 3. **Treatment of High LDL Cholesterol in Adults**

CHD Risk Status	LDL Level to Initiate: Diet Therapy	LDL Level to Initiate: Drug Therapy	LDL Goal
No CHD and fewer than two other risk factors	≥160 mg/dL	≥190 mg/dL	<160 mg/dL
No CHD and at least two other risk factors	≥130 mg/dL	≥160 mg/dL	<130 mg/dL
CHD present	>100 mg/dL	>130 mg/dL	≤100 mg/dL

dietary cholesterol, and (3) achievement and maintenance of ideal body weight. The approach to diet involves two steps. In the Step I diet fat is limited to a maximum of 30% of calories, saturated fat to 8 to 10% of calories, and cholesterol to 300 mg daily. If the Step I diet proves to be inadequate, the Step II diet is instituted, with saturated fat limited to 7% of calories and cholesterol limited to 200 mg daily. Individuals with established CHD or other atherosclerotic disease should begin immediately with the Step II diet. A registered dietitian is usually needed to initiate the Step II diet.

Drug Therapy for Elevated LDL Levels

When LDL cholesterol cannot be controlled satisfactorily with dietary measures, the use of cholesterol-lowering medications should be considered. In patients without CHD, intensive dietary measures should usually be pursued for at least 6 months before cholesterol-lowering medications are considered. However, it is appropriate to use medication sooner in those with CHD or marked elevation of LDL cholesterol (over 220 mg/dL). The use of cholesterol-lowering medication should usually be deferred in young men (under 35 years of age) and premenopausal women with LDL cholesterol levels of less than 220 mg/dL who do not have evidence of atherosclerotic disease and do not have multiple CHD risk factors. It is important to assess the changes in plasma lipoproteins and to monitor for potential adverse effects 4 to 6 weeks after initiating treatment with a lipid-altering medication.

The major drugs used for reduction of LDL cholesterol levels are the bile acid sequestrants, the inhibitors of 3-hydroxy-3-methylglutaryl coenzyme A reductase (HMGRIs), and nicotinic acid. Estrogens play an important role in reducing LDL levels in postmenopausal women. Other drugs that are less effective for reducing LDL cholesterol are the fibric acid derivatives (gemfibrozil and clofibrate) and probucol.

Bile Acid Sequestrants. The bile acid sequestrants, cholestyramine (Questran) and colestipol (Colestid), are anion exchange resins. They speed the clearance of LDL from plasma by increasing LDL receptor activity. As a consequence, plasma LDL levels can be reduced by 15 to 30%. The usual dose is 1 to 2 packets (or scoops) twice daily. The bile acid sequestrants are particularly useful in combination regimens along with an HMGRI or nicotinic acid. Because the bile acid sequestrants act within the intestine and are not systemically absorbed, they are thought to be quite safe. The most common side effects are constipation, bloating, and abdominal pain. These drugs interfere with the intestinal absorption of a variety of other medications; thus, other medications should not be given simultaneously with bile acid sequestrants. The bile acid sequestrants stimulate VLDL secretion and may thereby cause or exacerbate hypertriglyceridemia. Thus, baseline hypertriglyceridemia is a relative contraindication to the use of a bile acid sequestrant.

3-Hydroxy-3-Methylglutaryl Coenzyme A Reductase Inhibitors. The HMGRIs are the most effective agents for reducing plasma LDL levels. Four of these drugs are now available: lovastatin (Mevacor), simvastatin (Zocor), pravastatin (Pravachol), and fluvastatin (Lescol). Their mechanism of action depends primarily on stimulation of LDL receptor activity in hepatocytes. All of these drugs are targeted to the liver by extensive first-pass hepatic extraction. In the maximum recommended dose, LDL reductions of 40% occur with lovastatin and simvastatin, 27% with pravastatin, and 25% with fluvastatin. Small reductions in triglyceride levels and small increases in HDL cholesterol also occur. The HMGRIs are very well tolerated. The most important side effects are transaminase elevation (about 1% of patients) and acute myositis (about 0.1% of patients). These adverse effects are dose related. Theoretical considerations and animal experiments suggest that these drugs may be teratogenic; thus, they should not be used during pregnancy.

Nicotinic Acid. Nicotinic acid (niacin) is a B vitamin; in doses greatly exceeding those needed to prevent deficiency syndromes it has a beneficial effect on the plasma levels of VLDL, LDL, and HDL. Its primary action as a lipid-modifying medication involves a reduction in the secretion of VLDL, the metabolic precursor of LDL. In doses of 3 to 4.5 grams daily, nicotinic acid typically reduces LDL cholesterol by 25% and triglycerides by 50% and increases HDL cholesterol by 25 to 50%. Adverse effects prevent about one-third of patients from taking nicotinic acid over the long term. These include cutaneous flushing, ichthyosis and itching, gastritis and peptic ulcer disease, hepatitis, hyperglycemia, and hyperuricemia. Flushing, which is prostaglandin mediated, can be mitigated or abolished by aspirin taken 30 minutes before the nicotinic acid. Sustained-release forms of nicotinic acid cause less flushing but are more likely to cause hepatitis.

Estrogens. In postmenopausal women with elevated LDL cholesterol levels, estrogen treatment should often be considered before other lipid-altering agents are used. Estrogens reduce LDL levels by increasing LDL receptor activity; they also increase HDL cholesterol levels. Epidemiologic studies suggest that estrogen replacement therapy reduces the risk of CHD. Clinical trials designed to prove that estrogen replacement therapy can reduce CHD risk have not been completed. Because estrogens increase triglyceride levels, they are relatively contraindicated in women with baseline hypertriglyceridemia. Estrogens should be avoided in those with severe hypertriglyceridemia.

Fibric Acid Derivatives. The fibric acid derivatives (gemfibrozil [Lopid] and clofibrate [Atromid-S]) act primarily to reduce VLDL levels by increasing lipoprotein lipase activity. They also enhance the clearance of remnant lipoproteins. They generally cause a modest reduction in LDL (about 10%) and a modest increase in HDL (also about 10%). In hypertriglyceridemic persons, these drugs often lead to an *increase* in LDL cholesterol levels. In the Helsinki Heart Study, gemfibrozil caused a 34% reduction in the incidence of acute myocardial infarction and death due to CHD.

The fibric acid derivatives increase cholesterol secretion in bile, thereby increasing the risk of cholelithiasis and cholecystitis. The most common side effects of these drugs are gastrointestinal distress and decreased libido. When used in combination with an HMGRI, there is a substantial increase in the risk of myositis.

Probucol. Probucol (Lorelco) reduces LDL cholesterol levels by about 10% by stimulating the clearance of LDL through nonreceptor mechanisms. It has antioxidant activity that may be beneficial. Unfortunately, it also causes marked reductions in HDL levels. This drug did not reduce CHD in the one large clinical trial in which it was used. It can increase the electrocardiographic QT interval, and rarely it can cause sudden death. Although it tends to be well tolerated, probucol's role is limited by its weakness as an LDL reducer, its marked reduction of HDL, and the absence of any clinical trials demonstrating that it can prevent CHD.

Combination Drug Therapy. Certain combinations of these medications can be useful in treating markedly elevated LDL cholesterol levels. Combination therapy can maximize the reduction in LDL levels. It can also allow us to limit the dosage of individual LDL-reducing drugs, thus limiting side effects. For patients with elevation of both triglycerides and LDL, the addition of nicotinic acid or a fibric acid derivative to control triglyceride levels can allow the use of a bile acid sequestrant (otherwise precluded by hypertriglyceridemia) to help reduce LDL levels. The most effective combinations for lowering LDL are (1) bile acid sequestrant plus nicotinic acid, (2) bile acid sequestrant plus HMGRI, and (3) nicotinic acid plus HMGRI (although this last combination may increase the risk of myopathy). The combination of a fibric acid derivative with an HMGRI should usually be avoided because this increases the risk of myopathy.

TREATMENT OF ELEVATIONS OF LDL IN CHILDREN

Children generally have lower levels of total and LDL cholesterol than adults. Thus, the pediatric criteria for categorizing LDL cholesterol levels differ from the adult criteria. For children, acceptable LDL cholesterol levels are considered below 110 mg/dL, borderline LDL cholesterol 110 to 129 mg/dL, and high LDL cholesterol at least 130 mg/dL. For children 1 to 19 years of age, an LDL level of 130 mg/dL approximates the 95th percentile of the population distribution.

In pediatric populations much recent debate has focused on the issue of when to screen for lipid disorders. Children should be tested if premature CHD has occurred in a parent or grandparent, if a parent has an elevated cholesterol level (240 mg/dL or higher), if the family history is not available, or if the child has at least two other risk factors for CHD.

Because of concern about the possible adverse effects of therapy given during periods of growth and development, the approach to treatment in children is much more conservative than that in adults. No therapy whatsoever (not even diet) should be applied to children below the age of 2 years. For children at least 2 years of age, dietary therapy is warranted for borderline or high LDL cholesterol levels. In children who are at least 10 years old, drug therapy is recommended if the LDL cholesterol remains above 190 mg/dL despite dietary measures; in those with two or more other risk factors for CHD, drug therapy is recommended when LDL cholesterol remains above 160 mg/dL despite dietary modification. Because of their safety, the bile acid sequestrants are the only cholesterol-lowering medications recommended for routine use in children. Other cholesterol-lowering drugs should be prescribed to children only after referral to a lipid specialist.

TREATMENT OF ELEVATIONS OF TRIGLYCERIDES

Nonpharmacologic therapy is advisable for nearly all patients with hypertriglyceridemia. This involves weight reduction for those who are overweight, exercise, and restriction of alcohol. Additionally, hypertriglyceridemic patients should follow the Step I diet. When elevations of triglycerides are due to a medication (e.g., estrogen) or to a specific disease, correction of the primary cause of hypertriglyceridemia may be all that is necessary. When very high triglyceride levels (over 1000 mg/dL) persist despite these measures, drug therapy is warranted to prevent pancreatitis. Borderline high (200 to 400 mg/dL) and high (400 to

1000 mg/dL) triglyceride levels that persist despite treatment with nonpharmacologic measures warrant consideration of triglyceride-lowering drugs in patients with established CHD, diabetes mellitus, Type III hyperlipoproteinemia, and familial combined hyperlipidemia. However, the benefits of such treatment remain unproved.

The most effective drugs for reducing triglyceride levels are nicotinic acid, the fibric acid derivatives, and somatic fish oils. Because nicotinic acid has beneficial effects on VLDL, LDL, and HDL, it is the preferred agent when side effects do not preclude its use. The fibric acid derivatives often have the undesirable effect of raising LDL levels in hypertriglyceridemic patients. However, they do reduce triglyceride levels, and they raise HDL levels effectively.

The somatic fish oils contain large amounts of highly polyunsaturated omega-3 fatty acids. When given in large doses (9 to 16 grams daily), they reduce hepatic secretion of VLDL. Fasting triglyceride levels may fall by over 50% in response to the fish oils. Unfortunately, therapeutic doses of fish oils also provide a significant burden of dietary calories (80 to 150 kcal daily). Additionally, treatment with fish oils can raise LDL levels.

TREATMENT OF CONCURRENT ELEVATION OF VLDL AND LDL

Considerations for treatment of concurrent elevation of VLDL and LDL are similar to those for isolated elevations of LDL and isolated elevations of triglyceride. These patients generally have moderate elevations of both cholesterol and triglyceride. When associated with a low HDL level, this pattern appears to confer a particularly high risk of CHD. Dietary management involves restricting saturated fats, cholesterol, and alcohol; calories are limited to achieve and maintain ideal weight. When drug therapy is needed, certain special considerations apply. Nicotinic acid is the most effective drug for these patients because it is potent in reducing both VLDL and LDL levels while raising HDL levels. HMGRIs are also good choices, although they are much less effective in reducing triglyceride levels. A bile acid sequestrant often cannot be used as the sole agent because it has the potential to elevate triglyceride levels. Conversely, fibric acid derivatives are often not ideal as the sole drug because they frequently raise LDL levels in hypertriglyceridemic patients. A bile acid sequestrant can often be used to reduce LDL levels in combination with another agent (e.g., nicotinic acid, gemfibrozil, or fish oil) that controls triglyceride levels.

TREATMENT OF LOW HDL LEVELS

In many epidemiologic studies, low HDL levels have been associated with increased CHD risk. Furthermore, in several clinical trials designed to test the benefits of reduced LDL levels, small increases in HDL cholesterol were independently associated with improved CHD risk. However, no clinical trials have been designed specifically to test the effects of modifying HDL levels, and no clinical trials have been conducted in which the principal lipoprotein change was in HDL. Thus, the base of knowledge supporting treatment to raise HDL levels is not as firm as that supporting treatment to reduce LDL levels. Nonetheless, we can advise nearly everyone to pursue nonpharmacologic measures for raising HDL levels. These include cessation of cigarette smoking, weight loss in the obese, and increased exercise. Furthermore, it is reasonable to attempt to avoid HDL-lowering medications in patients who already have low HDL levels. These medications include androgenic and most progestational steroids, thiazide diuretics, beta blockers, retinoids, and probucol.

HDL levels can often be increased substantially by treatment with nicotinic acid and, in patients with hypertriglyceridemia, with fibric acid derivatives. Lesser increases in HDL levels (about 10%) occur when fibric acid drugs are taken by normotriglyceridemic persons and when HMGRIs are taken in high doses. For patients who warrant treatment to reduce LDL levels, a low HDL level (under 35 mg/dL) may influence the choice of an LDL-reducing drug. In these high-risk patients with high LDL and low HDL, nicotinic acid may be the drug of first choice. Drug therapy designed specifically to raise low HDL levels (under 35 mg/dL) may be considered for patients with established CHD and for those with strong risk factor profiles. Isolated low HDL levels, in the absence of CHD or risk factors for CHD, often occur in vegetarian populations in whom CHD rates are low. Thus, patients with isolated low HDL levels but no other CHD risk factors should not be given medication specifically to raise HDL levels.

OBESITY

method of
STEVEN B. HEYMSFIELD, M.D., and
KATHY HOY, ME.D., R.D.
St. Luke's-Roosevelt Hospital
New York, New York

According to National Health and Nutrition Examination Survey II, conducted from 1976 to 1980, approximately 28% of adults between the ages of 20 and 74 were found to be overweight, and more than 37% were severely obese. Preliminary statistics from NHANES III suggest that the prevalence of obesity has increased in the past 15 years and can now be diagnosed in over one-third of Americans. There is a higher prevalence of overweight and obesity in females than in males, especially among African Americans and Hispanics.

CO-MORBID CONDITIONS

Obesity alone carries a substantial social and psychological burden. Additionally, obesity increases the risk of high blood pressure, cardiovascular disease, non–insulin dependent diabetes mellitus, hepatobiliary diseases, and possibly some forms of cancer. Obesity may also exacerbate other medical conditions such as arthritis, back pain, sleep apnea, and gout.

Obesity can exist without medical complications, although the prevalence of related conditions increases with increasing levels of obesity. Morbidly obese individuals are at higher risk for complications. Generally, the risk of obesity-related complications increases when the body mass index (BMI, in kg/M^2) exceeds about 30. At BMIs above 40, the health risks are high.

Additionally, in a culture where extraordinary emphasis is placed on thinness, the stigma of obesity is great. These social and physical consequences of obesity impinge on the patient's physical health and on the overall quality of life.

UNDERLYING MECHANISMS

Obesity is recognized as a problem of long-term positive energy balance, in which energy intake exceeds expenditure. A variety of factors influence intake and expenditure, and an imbalance can have different origins. Certain medical conditions can cause obesity of varying severity, including hypothyroidism, Cushing's syndrome, hypothalamic injury, and gonadal failure. Medications can cause an energy imbalance by increasing appetite or lowering metabolic rate. Medications that can induce weight gain include corticosteroids, some hormonal preparations, and psychotropic medications. Certain genetic conditions, although rare, are associated with obesity and include Prader-Willi, Bardet-Biedl, Cohen's, and Carpenter's syndromes.

The most common cause of obesity is excess intake of calories in relation to expenditure that is not attributable to known organic causes or to medications. This has previously been referred to as endogenous obesity, but it is now more appropriately called dietary obesity.

The etiology of obesity is multifactorial. Genetically mediated factors are important in the development of obesity, possibly through an effect on adipose cell number and size, on metabolic rate, or on satiety and hunger-regulating mechanisms. However, it is also clear that environmental factors contribute significantly to the development of obesity; these include family and cultural food habits, lifestyle factors, availability of foods (particularly snack foods), diet composition, and food attitudes. There may also be genetic-environmental interactions such that environmental factors potentiate a genetic predisposition to obesity.

DIAGNOSIS

The current clinical definitions of obesity using anthropometric data are presented in Table 1. It is important to distinguish among patients who are overweight, overfat, and obese. An individual is classified as overweight when body weight is above a defined standard. The most commonly used weight standard is the Metropolitan Life Insurance Height-Weight Tables, first published in 1959 and updated in 1983. Other tables have been developed that consider age-related increases in body weight observed in population studies. However, weight tables do not provide the only indication of health risk. A person may be overweight according to these charts, but may not be overfat, as might be the case with a highly muscular trained athlete. An individual can also be within the normal weight range, but the percentage of body fat may be high. Obesity is technically defined as an excess of adipose tissue; however, in most cases, at body weights defined as obese, the percentage of body weight that is fat will also be high. Specific standards for ideal percentage of fat are not yet available; the normal percentage of body weight as fat for men is between 15 and 25% and for women, between 20 and 30%. Generally, obesity is present when the percent of body weight as fat is above 25% for men and 35% for women.

Population studies of United States citizens demonstrate that body weight tends to increase with age. Recent cross-sectional studies suggest that a modest increase in body weight with age is not detrimental to health and that the body weights associated with lowest mortality increase with age. Some controversy surrounds this concept, and more research is needed before final recommendations can be made. The height-weight tables shown in Table 2 consider the increases in body weight observed with age and compare them to the weight ranges from the 1983 Metropolitan Life Insurance Company tables.

Body weight alone is not the only factor that can be used to judge an obese patient's risk of morbidity and mortality. Other salient factors include the distribution of adipose tissue and the percent of body weight as fat. The distribution of adipose tissue is indirectly inferred from the waist/hip circumference ratio. A distribution in which adipose tissue is primarily abdominal versus truncal is associated with most of the obesity-related co-morbid conditions, including hyperinsulinemia and Type II diabetes mellitus, elevated serum levels of low-density and very-low-density lipoproteins, and low levels of high-density lipoprotein cholesterol. Abdominal obesity is a stronger predictor of mortality than either body weight or BMI.

A high percentage of body weight as fat has not been directly associated with health risks but may be indicative of habits that have been linked to some diseases, including a diet that is high in fat and sugar and low in fiber and a sedentary lifestyle.

CLINICAL ASSESSMENT

Assessment of the obese patient and recommendation of appropriate treatment require a global assessment of risk,

TABLE 1. **Definitions of Overweight and Obesity Using Different Anthropometric Methods***

	% Ideal Body Weight†	Body Mass Index	% Body Fat	
			Male	*Female*
Overweight	>110–120	25–28	>25	>35
Moderate obesity	>120–150	28–35	>30	>40
Severe obesity	>150–200	35–40	>35	>45
Morbid obesity	>200	40	>40	>50

*The relationships among ideal body weight, body mass index, and percent of body weight as fat are estimates. Fat as a percent of body weight also varies with gender and age.

†Ideal body weight is based on the 1983 Metropolitan Life Insurance Tables.

TABLE 2. **Comparison of the Weight-for-Height Tables from Actuarial Data (Build Study): Non–Age-Corrected Metropolitan Life Insurance Company and Age-Specific Gerontology Research Center Recommendations***

	Metropolitan 1983 Weights for Ages 25–59†		Gerontology Research Center Weight Range for Men and Women by Age (Years)				
HEIGHT	MEN	WOMEN	25	35	45	55	65
FT-IN	LB						
4-10	—	100–131	84–111	92–119	99–127	107–135	115–142
4-11	—	101–134	87–115	95–123	103–131	111–139	119–147
5-0	—	103–137	90–119	98–127	106–135	114–143	123–152
5-1	123–145	105–140	93–123	101–131	110–140	118–148	127–157
5-2	125–148	108–144	96–127	105–136	113–144	122–153	131–163
5-3	127–151	111–148	99–131	108–140	117–149	126–158	135–168
5-4	129–155	114–152	102–135	112–145	121–154	130–163	140–173
5-5	131–159	117–156	106–140	115–149	125–159	134–168	144–179
5-6	133–163	120–160	109–144	119–154	129–164	138–174	148–184
5-7	135–167	123–164	112–148	122–159	133–169	143–179	153–190
5-8	137–171	126–167	116–153	126–163	137–174	147–184	158–196
5-9	139–175	129–170	119–157	130–168	141–179	151–190	162–201
5-10	141–179	132–173	122–162	134–173	145–184	156–195	167–207
5-11	144–183	135–176	126–167	137–178	149–190	160–201	172–213
6-0	147–187	—	129–171	141–183	153–195	165–207	177–219
6-1	150–192	—	133–176	145–188	157–200	169–213	182–225
6-2	153–197	—	137–181	149–194	162–206	174–219	187–232
6-3	157–202	—	141–186	153–199	166–212	179–225	192–238
6-4	—	—	144–191	157–205	171–218	184–231	197–244

*Values in this table are for height without shoes and weight without clothes. To convert inches to centimeters, multiply by 2.54; to convert pounds to kilograms, multiply by 0.455.

†The weight range is the lower weight for small frame and the upper weight for large frame.

Gerontology Research Center information from Andres R: Mortality and obesity: the rationale for age-specific height-weight tables. *In* Andres R, Bierman E, Hazzard WR (eds): Principles of Geriatric Medicine. New York, McGraw-Hill, 1985, pp 311–318.

with consideration of health, emotional factors, and general impact of obesity and of dieting on the individual's quality of life.

The first step in assessment is to determine the patient's relative weight and the degree of risk associated with that weight. Adipose tissue distribution, based on the waist/hip circumference ratio, also helps to classify the patient's risk of adverse health outcomes. Risk and suitability for treatment are then further elaborated upon by examining the various social and co-morbid conditions that may be present. A format for a comprehensive medical examination is provided in Table 3.

TREATMENT

The goal of obesity treatment is to safely produce long-term medically significant weight loss. Generally, long-term results of obesity treatment do not appear favorable, although treatment programs may not be long enough or sufficiently comprehensive to produce substantial weight losses that can be maintained.

To improve outcome, treatment recommendations should be made based on consideration of the patient's general medical condition, immediate medical need, and prior history of weight loss. It is also essential to consider lifestyle and personality factors, including occupation, family and financial factors, and ability to prioritize weight reduction efforts. An individualized treatment plan should include referral to appropriate programs or professionals: more than a simple recommendation to lose weight is needed.

Currently, there are several options available for obesity treatment. The more conservative and traditional approach is a low-calorie diet combined with behavior modification instruction. However dietary recommendations and behavioral approaches have broadened to include lifestyle management strategies and an increased emphasis on exercise.

Alternatively, more aggressive treatments are available that include very-low-calorie diets (VLCD), usually as liquid formulas, pharmacologic therapy, and surgery. These vary in the degree of associated risk, and the selection of a particular treatment option requires careful evaluation. The patient will ultimately need to implement dietary strategies and behavior management techniques to maintain weight loss achieved by any of these methods.

Diet

Conventional Approach. A calorie deficit provided by a diet will result in weight loss. A good diet plan provides structure and guidance and educates the patient to select a healthful diet of appropriate composition and adequate caloric and nutrient content. However, the effectiveness of diets is limited by their perceived restrictiveness, which can predispose to "all or nothing" thinking, leading to abnormal eating patterns, bingeing, and subsequent abandonment of weight loss efforts. Ideally, the patient will use the diet plan as a guide for making food selections and will learn how to include favorite foods in a balanced diet. Diet plans are usually based on the exchange lists developed by the American Diabetes Associa-

TABLE 3. **Recommended Comprehensive Physical Assessment**

Physical/Anthropometric
Body weight
Height
Relative weight (actual weight/ideal weight)
BMI (kg/M²)
Adipose tissue distribution (waist/hip circumference ratio)
Percent body fat (optional)
Medical
Medical history
Weight loss history
Previous weight loss programs
Amount of weight lost
Time weight loss maintained
Family history of obesity and related conditions
Medications that can influence weight loss
Medical Examination
ECG, blood pressure
Blood work
Thyroid panel
Fasting glucose
Lipid profile
Liver enzymes
Electrolytes
Uric acid
CBC
Urinalysis
Diet History
Dietary intake
Lifestyle factors (occupation, cultural food habits and beliefs, eating patterns)
Compulsive overeating and/or bulimia
Physical Activity
Current level of physical activity
Capabilities for exercise/physical limitations
Barriers to exercise
Psychological
Depression/anxiety
Stress
Other

Abbreviations: BMI = body mass index; ECG = electrocardiogram; CBC = complete blood count.

tion. It is best if the diet is individualized for the patient based on food preferences and meal patterns.

The best recommendation is a balanced low-calorie diet in which 25 to 30% (or less), 55 to 60%, and 20 to 25% of total calories come from fat, carbohydrate, and protein, respectively. For many people, this represents a modification of their usual diet. Americans typically derive 35 to 45% of their calories from fat. A recommendation that 25 to 30% of calories be provided from fat is reasonable in terms of providing a diet that is palatable and that is beneficial for weight loss. A low-fat, high-fiber diet is less calorically dense and tends to produce a greater degree of satiety compared to isocaloric amounts of a high-fat diet.

The food guide pyramid was developed by the United States Department of Agriculture as a tool for consumers to select a healthful diet. The pyramid is also useful for planning a well-balanced diet for weight loss. It emphasizes the importance of complex carbohydrates, including whole grains and whole grain products, legumes, fruits, and vegetables. Foods that derive most of their calories from fat, such as meats and poultry, dairy products, and oils, should be used sparingly. Diet plans for weight loss based on the food pyramid are shown in Table 4.

The ideal low-calorie diet causes a negative caloric balance that leads to a weight loss of 1 to 3 pounds per week or 1% of body weight. A daily caloric deficit of 500 kcal will result in approximately a 1 pound per week weight loss. Generally, weight loss in sedentary to moderately active men and women will occur with intakes of 1500 to 1800 kcal per day and 1200 to 1500 kcal per day, respectively.

Another method of determining the calorie level for weight loss is to estimate energy expenditure using equations to predict resting or basal metabolic rate (BMR). A commonly used set of equations based on age and gender developed by the World Health Organization is shown in Table 5. A calorie intake equivalent to the BMR will usually produce an average weight loss of at least 1 pound per week over time. This is because total energy expenditure and thus energy requirements are about 33% above those of the basal rate for a sedentary person. Extra calories can be included if an individual is very active. For weight maintenance, the estimated calories expended in physical activity are added to the estimated BMR.

TABLE 4. **Diet Plans Based on the Food Guide Pyramid**

	Calorie Level (kcal/d)		
	About 1600	*About 2200*	*About 2800*
Bread group servings	6	9	11
Vegetable group servings	3	4	5
Fruit group servings	2	3	4
Milk group servings	2–3	2—3	2–3
Meat group servings	2, for a total of 5 oz	2, for a total of 6 oz	3, for a total of 7 oz
Total fat (gm)	53	73	93

Examples of Food Choices

Bread, Cereal, Rice, and Pasta Group

1 slice bread	1 oz ready-to-eat cereal	½ cup cooked cereal, rice, or pasta
3–4 small crackers		

Vegetable Group

1 cup raw leafy vegetables	½ cup other vegetables, cooked or chopped raw
¾ cup vegetable juice	

Fruit Group

1 medium apple, banana, orange	1½ cup chopped, cooked, or canned fruit
¾ cup fruit juice	

Milk, Yogurt, and Cheese Group

1½ oz natural cheese	1 cup lowfat milk or yogurt
2 oz processed cheese	

Meat, Poultry, Fish, Dry Beans, Eggs, and Nuts Group

2–3 oz cooked lean meat, poultry, or fish

½ cup cooked dry beans, 1 egg, ⅓ cup nuts, or 2 Tbsp peanut butter (count as 1 oz lean meat)

TABLE 5. **Prediction Equations for Basal Metabolic Rate Suggested by the World Health Organization**

Men	
18–30 years	= 0.063 × wt (kg) + 2.8957
31–60 years	= 0.0484 × wt (kg) + 3.6534
>60 years	= 0.0491 × wt (kg) + 2.4587
Women	
18–30 years	= 0.0621 × wt (kg) + 2.0357
31–60 years	= 0.0342 × wt (kg) + 3.5377
>60 years	= 0.0377 × wt (kg) + 2.7545
Caloric requirement	
BMR × 1.3	= kcal for sedentary patients
BMR × 1.5	= kcal for active patients

Abbreviations: wt = weight; BMR = basal metabolic rate.

It is difficult to select a diet that meets the recommended dietary allowances (RDAs) if the calorie level is less than 1000 to 1200 calories per day, and foods must be chosen carefully. Most moderately active people will find these diets too restrictive and inflexible. At these low energy intake levels, hunger and preoccupation with food may increase, diminishing the likelihood of long-term adherence. Sedentary individuals may not find these energy intake guidelines as difficult to follow but should be encouraged to increase physical activity as part of their weight loss efforts.

Fads. As with other patients who have a disabling chronic illness that is refractory to treatment, obese patients are susceptible to quackery and fads. The uninformed consumer who is looking for novel and painless ways to lose weight is highly vulnerable to fad diets. Examples are the Beverly Hills Diet, the Fit for Life Diet, and the Atkins Diet, to name a few. While some of these diets may not be harmful, they do not teach long-term food and weight management, are generally restrictive and inflexible, and are founded on specious scientific claims. They also create the illusion that something magical is needed to lose weight, and fad diets distort the fact that food and food-related behaviors need only to be modified and managed. Patients should be taught to be skeptical of any diet that purports to have a special effect or magical quality.

Meal Replacement Products. Meal replacement products, usually beverages, provide low-calorie, well-balanced nutrition in place of self-selected regular foods. They are usually used in place of one or two meals a day, and a calorie-controlled meal consisting of regular foods is consumed as the third meal. These products are not formulated to be the sole source of nutrition and should not be used exclusively. Meal replacement products are convenient because they incorporate portion control and calorie control and require minimal involvement with regular foods. Since they are fortified with vitamins and minerals, the daily intake can be set around 1000 to 1200 calories, and the RDAs for vitamins and minerals can be met. Meal replacement products are usually used by patients outside conventional treatment programs, but they may under some circumstances be incorporated into a medically supervised weight loss program.

Prepackaged Foods. These convenient portion-controlled products are generally low in fat and sodium. As with meal replacement products, they typically fit well with prescribed diet plans and are convenient for the patient.

Exclusive long-term use of meal replacement products and prepackaged foods leads to monotony and limits the individual's ability to learn how to manage a normal diet and its attendant temptations. These products should therefore never constitute the entire diet. They are best used in the short term while other longer term treatments are being introduced or during periods of relapse to get the patient "back on track."

Very-Low-Calorie Diets. Very-low-calorie diets (VLCDs) provide 400 to 800 kcal per day and are intended to produce a large weight loss while minimizing depletion of lean body tissue. They usually come in powder form and are reconstituted with water. VLCDs are usually consumed in three to six servings per day. At least 64 ounces of fluids should be consumed with the formula, and some noncaloric beverages (e.g., carbonated water) and food items may be allowed.

The currently available VLCD products are safer than the earlier formulations as they provide all essential nutrients and contain appropriate amounts of high-quality protein. A formula should provide at least 75 grams or more of high-quality protein per day to minimize protein catabolism and nitrogen losses. Additionally, the formula should provide at least 50 grams of carbohydrate per day to prevent ketosis and 10 grams of fat per meal to stimulate gallbladder contraction and thereby reduce the risk of cholesterol gallstone formation.

VLCDs are indicated in patients who are severely obese or who are moderately obese with serious comorbid conditions requiring rapid and significant weight loss. Despite the appeal to those who wish to lose weight rapidly, VLCDs should not be recommended to patients who are less than 130% over ideal body weight or who have a BMI of approximately 30 or less. Mildly obese individuals may lose more lean body mass during VLCD treatment than the severely obese, which can lead to cardiac disturbances and other adverse side effects.

Before implementing a VLCD, the patient should have a thorough medical examination that includes laboratory work and an electrocardiogram (see Table 3). Contraindications for VLCD treatment are myocardial infarction within the previous 6 months, prolonged electrocardiographic QT interval adjusted for heart rate, serious arrhythmias, a history of cerebrovascular, renal, or hepatic disease, cancer, Type I diabetes mellitus, or significant psychiatric disturbance.

Patients on VLCDs should be examined by the physician weekly and weight and vital signs should be monitored. Electrolyte levels should also be evaluated weekly or biweekly. In addition, changes in cardiac electrical activity should be monitored with an electrocardiogram at regular intervals and re-evaluation should be done in patients with a prolonged or lengthening heart-rate–corrected QT interval. The patient should be asked about side effects, which can include fatigue, dizziness, muscle cramping, headache, gastrointestinal distress, and cold intolerance. Other risks associated with VLCD, particularly with unsupervised use, are dehydration, electrolyte imbalances, orthostatic hypotension, elevated uric acid levels, and cholesterol gallstones.

With VLCDs, women will lose up to 1.5 kg per week and men, 2.0 kg per week. Weight loss in the first 2 weeks may be more rapid owing to initial loss of water with high protein and low calorie intake. Heavier people have a higher lean body mass, retain nitrogen better, and can diet safely on VLCDs for longer periods. If patients lose weight too rapidly, caloric intake should be increased. The length of treatment is usually 12 to 16 weeks, followed by 3 to 6 weeks of gradual refeeding. During this time, the patient should receive nutrition education and counseling on lifestyle management in order to maintain the weight loss. This should continue with experienced providers for at least 3 to 4 months after food is introduced, and ideally the patient should have some contact with health care professionals for up to a year or longer.

Behavior Management

The primary purpose of behavior management is to eliminate or modify habits that lead to excess caloric intake and weight gain. Principles that are incorporated into a behavior management program for weight loss and maintenance are derived from several disciplines in the field of psychology.

Classical behavior modification strategies are based on the principles of operant conditioning and include stimulus control, cue elimination, and reinforcement. Examples of these strategies as they relate to weight control are putting the fork down between bites and modifying the environment to reduce food cues that can lead to overeating (e.g., storing food out of sight). Self-awareness and self-monitoring are also an integral part of behavior modification and are accomplished by keeping daily records of food intake and physical activity. Additionally behavior is "shaped" using goal setting to focus on problematic eating behaviors. The new behaviors are reinforced with a reward system that is usually developed and implemented by the patient.

Cognitive behavioral approaches acknowledge the influence of thoughts on behavior and help the individual to develop coping skills and problem-solving strategies for selected situations. These strategies focus on individuals' attitudes, beliefs, and perceptions about their ability to manage food and to incorporate exercise into their lifestyle. Identifying negative thoughts and changing them into positive thoughts through affirmations and visual imagery are examples of these techniques.

External situations can also influence eating through the emotional responses invoked, which differ for each person. Patients learn to identify the emotional situations that trigger eating so that they can then develop alternative ways of handling feelings rather than suppressing them by eating. Treatment strategies include meditation, stress management, and assertiveness training.

The importance of social support and management of relapse has been recognized, and they have been incorporated into behavior management programs. With relapse management, the patient learns that inappropriate or unplanned eating does not signify failure or inability to lose weight. The person is taught how to refocus on weight loss efforts rather than giving up because of perceived failure. Social support is important because the individual can learn from the experiences of others and actions can be affirmed and reinforced. Individuals who have a good support system as part of their treatment and in their own environment are more likely to successfully lose weight and maintain their weight loss.

Physical Activity

The beneficial effects of added physical activity and a specific exercise program include increased exercise-related energy expenditure, increased lean body mass and associated metabolic rate, cardiovascular conditioning, enhanced strength, greater flexibility, increased self-esteem, decreased stress, and in some cases reduced appetite. A combination of diet and exercise appears to be most effective for weight loss.

It is useful to distinguish between physical activity and exercise. Physical activity refers to the overall level of activity that an individual engages in on a daily basis, including the activities of daily living, occupational activity, and recreational activity. Exercise usually refers to activities that include aerobic and anaerobic exercises and that are carried out for the specific purpose of improving some aspect of fitness.

It is beneficial for patients to begin exercise programs by making incremental changes in routine physical activities, which then become incorporated into their lifestyles. Examples are walking and stair climbing, avoiding labor-saving devices, and reducing sedentary activities such as watching television. These efforts will help patients become more comfortable with moving their bodies and will also add to the calorie deficit produced by dieting. Additionally, some studies have shown a health benefit of exercise in patients who are more physically active in their daily routines and in recreational activities. These benefits include improved cardiovascular fitness, increased high-density lipoprotein cholesterol levels, and improved glucose tolerance.

Energy is best dissipated during aerobic activity performed 3 to 5 times a week at a low to moderate intensity for at least 20 to 30 minutes. The sedentary patient should build up to this level gradually. Patients should find an activity that they are comfortable performing and that they will enjoy for a long period of time. Consistent exercise appears to be an important factor in weight maintenance.

Psychological Counseling

The notion that obesity is a direct result of specific psychopathologies was dispelled many years ago. However, psychological factors may contribute to a patient's inability to lose weight or to maintain weight loss. For selected patients, referral for psychological counseling may be indicated to treat problems that arise during weight loss therapy. Psychological therapy may help the individual to better understand the associations among psychological status, food intake, and body weight. Serious problems, such as compulsive or binge eating, can be examined. Lastly, many obese patients, up to 50% in some referral clinic series, are clinically depressed. This is often a source of great distress, and appropriate evaluation and treatment may be indicated.

Obesity is not classified in the Diagnostic and Statistics Manual of Mental Disorders IV (DSM-IV) as a psychological disorder nor as an eating disorder. However, a distinct subgroup of obese persons have been identified as having binge eating disorder. Provisional criteria are delineated in the DSM-IV, and evaluation by a licensed psychologist is necessary to establish the diagnosis.

Pharmacologic Therapy

Over one dozen prescription and over-the-counter medications are now used in obesity treatment. Drug treatment was generally not well regarded until recently for at least four reasons: tolerance sometimes develops, side effects are recognized, relapse often occurs with medication discontinuation, and addiction and abuse potential exist. Another practical concern is that treatment duration is often limited by federal and state regulations.

This view of pharmacologic treatment of obesity is now changing with the publication of long-term studies showing good weight maintenance and with accumulating evidence that combining medications with differing modes of action can bring improved efficacy and reduced side effects. It is being increasingly recognized that, like many other chronic illnesses, obesity requires lifelong treatment, and drug therapy may be required indefinitely. This view is not held by all experts, and as already mentioned, some medications cannot be legally prescribed beyond several months.

Medications can be classified according to mode of action (e.g., anorectics or satiety enhancers) or biochemical sites of action (e.g., serotonergic or adrenergic). The usual practice is to prescribe a medication to patients with medically significant obesity only after other forms of treatment have failed to produce weight loss or weight maintenance. If there are no contraindications, a medication is prescribed from one of the various classes. As of yet, no algorithm is available for medication selection, and patients who are most likely to benefit from a specific drug cannot be easily identified beforehand. Monitoring for side effects is continued throughout the active treatment period.

As mentioned, certain drug combinations have proved effective, particularly fenfluramine (Pondimin) and phentermine (Ionamin) resin. Fenfluramine is a serotonergic agonist, and phentermine acts on the adrenergic nervous system. The treatment protocol used in our clinic is shown in Table 6. A number of promising medications are currently under development.

Surgery

As with medications, surgical treatment is reserved only for obese patients who fail on conventional therapy. The primary surgical procedures currently used for weight loss are vertical banded gastroplasty and the Roux-en-Y gastric bypass. In the vertical banded gastroplasty, a small pouch is constructed with a restricted outlet along the lesser curvature of the stomach. The Roux-en-Y gastric bypass involves construction of a proximal gastric pouch whose outlet is a Y-shaped limb of small bowel of varying lengths. These procedures are irreversible, although the capacity of the stomach may expand over time. Rates of weight loss have been reported to be slightly higher with the Roux-en-Y procedure. There is usually a substantial weight loss, which peaks at 18 to 24 months; most patients will regain some weight within 2 to 5 years after surgery. Since high-caloric-density foods can still be consumed, there is no absolute guarantee of weight loss if the patient is noncompliant with dietary recommendations.

Potential candidates for surgery are those whose BMI is greater than 40 and whose quality of life is severely impaired by obesity. In some cases, certain

TABLE 6. **Combination Treatment Protocol with Phentermine and Fenfluramine**

Day	Medication	Timing
1 and 2	Phentermine (Ionamin) 15 mg	One before breakfast
3 and 4	Phentermine 15 mg	One before breakfast One at 4 P.M.
5–8	Phentermine 15 mg	One before breakfast One at 4 P.M.
	Fenfluramine (Pondimin) 20 mg	½ before dinner
9	Phentermine 15 mg	One before breakfast One at 4 P.M.
	Fenfluramine 20 mg	½ before lunch ½ before dinner
10–12	Phentermine 15 mg	One before breakfast One at 4 P.M.
	Fenfluramine 20 mg	½ before breakfast ½ before lunch ½ before dinner

high-risk persons whose BMI is 35 to 40 may be considered for surgery; this may include patients with life-threatening cardiopulmonary problems (e.g., sleep apnea, Pickwickian syndrome, or cardiomyopathy), severe diabetes mellitus, joint diseases treatable but for obesity, or other disorders that impair quality of life.

These procedures are severe interventions that should be done only when other approaches have failed. The patient should be carefully evaluated by an experienced team of medical, surgical, psychiatric, and nutritional professionals, and the risk versus benefits of surgical intervention should be discussed with the patient. Patients who undergo surgery for obesity should have tried other methods of weight loss and should have a good knowledge of nutrition, food composition, and behavioral techniques.

Behavioral management techniques are critical after surgery, and patients should have insight into their eating behavior problems. Those patients who have a history of binge eating and craving sweets may have problems with implementing behavior modification strategies. Additionally, prospective patients should be psychologically competent, should understand the ramifications of the procedure and how their lives may or may not change after the operation, and should be able to take responsibility for integrating the necessary changes into their lives.

After the surgery, the patient will initally be able to ingest only approximately 1 tablespoon of food over a 15-minute interval. He or she should be instructed to eat slowly and to consume liquid and solid foods separately, usually with a 15 to 30 minute interval between. The amount of food ingested will gradually be increased to 8 ounces per meal over 4 to 6 months. The foods tolerated by individuals will vary, and the patient must learn what foods work well.

Surgical procedures are now relatively safe when performed by experienced teams at centers equipped to manage morbidly obese patients. Vomiting, electrolyte abnormalities, vitamin deficiencies, and gallstones are all associated with obesity surgery, again emphasizing the importance of selecting only those patients in whom the benefits of weight loss substantially outweigh the surgical risks.

WATER-SOLUBLE VITAMIN DEFICIENCY STATES

method of
STEPHEN R. NEWMARK, M.D.
University of Nevada School of Medicine
Las Vegas, Nevada

Vitamins generally included in the "water-soluble" group include vitamins C, B_1 (thiamine), B_2 (riboflavin), B_6 (pyridoxine), niacin, biotin, and pantothenic acid. Folic acid and vitamin B_{12} are not included in this review because they are considered elsewhere. This group of nutrients is classified as water-soluble because they do not require fat absorption to be transferred across the gut mucosa; they pass directly to the blood, where they are transported to the appropriate target tissues. Nevertheless, factors that impair absorption of the "fat-soluble" or lipid-soluble group, such as malabsorption states, can also impair absorption of the water-soluble vitamin group in severe cases. Excretion of water-soluble vitamins takes place mainly in the kidney. Water-soluble vitamins, with the exception of vitamin B_{12}, are not appreciably stored in body tissues.

Most causes of vitamin deficiency of the water-soluble group can be ascribed to either dietary deficiency with or without alcoholism, dietary faddism, severe malabsorption, or special increases in vitamin metabolism due to metabolic states, malignancies, or interference by certain pharmacologic preparations. It should be emphasized that isolated vitamin deficiencies are unusual and that multiple deficiency states may be found in the same individual. Thus, even when a specific vitamin deficiency syndrome is diagnosed, treatments incorporating most if not all of the other vitamins and nutrients should be considered.

Table 1 summarizes the dietary sources and recommended daily allowances (RDA) of the water-soluble vitamins, whereas Table 2 provides a summarized version of deficiency states and suggested treatments.

VITAMIN C

Vitamin C (ascorbic acid) is important as a cofactor for the transfer of hydroxyl groups to amino acids, particularly proline and lysine, which are essential for maintaining collagen structure. In addition, vitamin C may aid in the absorption of iron and in the metabolism of certain steroid hormones. Vitamin C deficiency or scurvy is usually encountered as a result of a dietary deficiency in which citrus fruits or vegetables are not ingested. Long-term parenteral nutrition without associated parenteral vitamin infusion was previously observed but now is fortunately rare. Alcoholism and chronic illnesses are also associated with vitamin C deficiency. Infantile scurvy presents with severe pain, hemorrhage in the periosteum, bleeding, and associated infections. Adults with scurvy have symptoms of fatigue, hyperkeratotic hair follicles, and gastrointestinal or genitourinary bleeding. Bleeding gums are common. The diagnosis of scurvy can be made on the basis of the clinical signs and symptoms as well as decreased plasma ascorbic acid levels (less than 0.1 mg per liter).

Treatment is simple and consists of oral vitamin C at doses of 100 mg three to five times per day until the signs and symptoms of scurvy are relieved. Although large doses of vitamin C have been proposed to prevent respiratory infections or to treat certain other conditions, at the time of this writing the data on such treatments are still inconclusive.

VITAMIN B_1 (THIAMINE)

Vitamin B_1 (thiamine) deficiency states are usually observed in individuals with chronic alcoholism.

TABLE 1. **Description of Water-Soluble Vitamins**

Vitamin	Common Name	Source	Recommended Daily Allowance*
C	Ascorbic acid	Citrus fruits, vegetables	Adult: 60 mg Child: 45 mg Lactation: 90 mg Pregnancy: 70 mg
B_1	Thiamine	Meats, cereals, legumes	Male: 1.2–1.5 mg Female: 1.0–1.1 mg Increase by 0.2–0.3 mg for pregnancy or lactation Child: 0.7–1.0 mg
B_2	Riboflavin	Meat products, dairy products	Male: 1.3–1.5 mg Female: 1.2–1.3 mg Pregnancy: 1.5 mg Lactation: 1.6 mg Child: 0.8–1.2 mg
B_6	Pyridoxine	Chicken, fish, liver, pork, eggs, oats, wheat, walnuts	Male: 1.7–2.0 mg Female: 1.4–1.6 mg Pregnancy: 2.2 mg Lactation: 2.1 mg Child: 1.1–1.7 mg
Niacin		Cereals, legumes, meats; tryptophan is converted to niacin at a ratio of 60:1 Milk and eggs contain tryptophan	1 mg per 1000 kcal (6.6 niacin equivalents per 1000 kcal); add 2–5 niacin equivalents for pregnancy or lactation
Biotin		Liver, egg yolks, soy flour, cereals	30–100 μg (estimated)
Pantothenic acid		Widely distributed in foods	4–7 mg (estimated)

*RDA is based on the recommendations of the National Academy of Science Food and Nutrition Board (1989).

TABLE 2. **Clinical Aspects of Water-Soluble Vitamin Deficiency Conditions**

Vitamin	Etiology of Deficiency State	Clinical Description of Deficiency	Treatment
C (ascorbic acid)	Dietary deficiency	Fatigue, hyperkeratotic hair follicles, petechial bleeding, subperiosteal hemorrhaging in young children, bleeding from gastrointestinal and genitourinary systems	Ascorbic acid 100 mg three to five times daily for 1 week; then maintenance doses
B_1 (thiamine)	Alcoholism; increased metabolic states such as hyperthyroidism or malignancies Severe malabsorption	Peripheral neuropathy, edema, high-output cardiac failure, Wernicke's encephalopathy (nystagmus, confusion, ataxia, ophthalmoplegia)	Parenteral thiamine (100 mg) in cases of cardiac disorder; otherwise, thiamine is given orally 25 mg per day with follow-up maintenance dose
B_2 (riboflavin)	Dietary deficiency, alcoholism, severe malabsorption	Dermatitis, alopecia, cheilosis, glossitis, neuropathy, anemia	Oral replacement at three to four times replacement dose until symptoms abate
B_6 (pyridoxine)	Alcoholism, malabsorption	Neuropathy, possible seizures	Oral replacement with 10–20 mg per day until stable; avoid large doses of pyridoxine, which may cause irreversible neuropathic changes
Niacin	Dietary deficiency, malabsorption, carcinoid syndrome, alcoholism	Diarrhea, dermatitis, psychosis	20–125 mg per day until symptoms abate; then maintenance doses. In patients with carcinoid, large doses may be needed to prevent reccurrence of pellagra
Biotin	Malabsorption, long-term total parenteral nutrition without vitamins, ingestion of large amount of egg whites	Dermatitis	In suspected cases, oral replacement at 50 to 100 μg per day; then maintenance doses
Pantothenic acid	Malabsorption, long-term total parenteral nutrition without vitamins	Possible neuritis, fatigue, nausea and vomiting	In suspected cases 10–20 mg per day are given, followed by maintenance doses

Thiamine is a major catalytic cofactor in carbohydrate metabolism for the formation of thiamine pyrophosphate, which is important in the oxidative decarboxylation of alpha-keto acids, and for the activity of transketolase in the pentose phosphate pathways. A deficiency state of thiamine can impair intermediary metabolism and energy metabolism, producing subsequent organ failure. Hyperthyroidism may accelerate the metabolism of thiamine and rapidly precipitate cardiac failure. The clinical state of beriberi can present with high-output cardiac failure with vasodilatation along with dermatitis and neuropathy. Central nervous system dysfunction occurs in thiamine deficiency and may be manifested as Wernicke's encephalopathy, consisting of nystagmus, ophthalmoplegia, truncal ataxia, and confusion.

The diagnosis of thiamine deficiency can be made by finding a decrease in urinary thiamine excretion. Reduced thiamine pyrophosphate saturation of erythrocyte transketolase has also been observed in deficiency states.

In suspected cases of thiamine deficiency, parenteral thiamine (100 mg per day) for several days can prevent or rapidly treat incipient cases. In cases of high-output cardiac failure or severe hyperthyroidism, prophylactic administration of thiamine can be given even when no symptoms of deficiency states are present. All patients with a history of chronic alcohol abuse should be treated with a multivitamin containing thiamine.

VITAMIN B_2 (RIBOFLAVIN)

Vitamin B_2 (riboflavin) deficiency can be observed in cases of inadequate diets or with severe malabsorption. Riboflavin forms coenzymes such as flavin mononucleotide and flavin adenine dinucleotide, which are important cofactors in many enzymatic reactions. Severe dermatitis, which can appear as a scrotal rash in males, may be observed. Angular stomatitis and glossitis are encountered along with anemia and neuropathy. Although the data are inconclusive, it has been suggested that tricyclic antidepressants and oral contraceptives may impair riboflavin metabolism.

Diagnosis of riboflavin deficiency is made by assessing the increase in erythrocyte glutathione reductase (EGR) when flavin adenine dinucleotide is added in vitro. A ratio of 1:2 of EGR activity in erythrocytes both with and without added flavin adenine dinucleotide may suggest riboflavin deficiency. Other tests include the direct measurement of urinary riboflavin.

Treatment consists of oral replacement of riboflavin at doses of 5 to 20 mg per day until symptoms resolve.

VITAMIN B_6 (PYRIDOXINE)

Pyridoxine forms an important coenzyme of which glycogen phosphorylase–bound pyridoxal phosphate is the most important. Vitamin B_6 (pyridoxine) deficiency is usually observed in individuals with chronic alcoholism or in severe protein-calorie malnutrition. In addition, it has been suggested that oral contraceptives, primidone, cycloserine, isoniazid, hydralazine, and some diuretics may cause pyridoxine deficiency. Symptoms of deficiency states include neuritis and possible induction of seizures.

The diagnosis of pyridoxine deficiency can be made by direct measurement of pyridoxine in blood or urine or by assessment of the response of tryptophan metabolites after oral tryptophan ingestion.

Although oral pyridoxine, 10 to 20 mg per day, is indicated in the therapy of these disorders, one must be careful to avoid high daily doses of pyridoxine (over 200 to 500 mg) because irreversible neurologic changes including ataxia have been observed with such high doses. Once the individual has been successfully treated, daily replacement doses are indicated.

NIACIN

Niacin is cycled through the nicotinamide adenine dinucleotide pathway to nicotinamide. The nicotinamide coenzymes are important in the dehydrogenase reactions that play a role in the metabolism of carbohydrates, fats, and amino acids. Niacin deficiency is encountered in chronic malabsorption and in individuals who are ingesting a diet composed primarily of corn, which is low in tryptophan, a niacin precursor. Symptoms of niacin deficiency or pellagra include diarrhea, a scaly dermatitis, and dementia. Rarely, the carcinoid syndrome has been reported to cause pellagra because the tryptophan is diverted away from niacin synthesis into other metabolic pathways.

Diagnosis of niacin deficiency can be made by measuring the urine levels of N^1-methylnicotinamide and 2-pyridone. Treatment includes oral replacement of niacin in doses of 20 to 125 mg per day.

BIOTIN AND PANTOTHENIC ACID

Clinical deficiency states of biotin and pantothenic acid are extremely unusual. Biotin is a cofactor for carboxylases, whereas pantothenic acid is the important intermediary component in the formation of coenzyme A, which, in turn, is necessary for many important biochemical reactions involving enzymes such as pyruvic dehydrogenase, alpha-ketoglutarate dehydrogenase, fatty acid oxidase, and fatty acid synthetase. Rarely, biotin deficiency can be caused by ingestion of large amounts of egg whites, which contain the protein avidin, which binds dietary biotin. Specific biochemical tests for biotin and pantothenic acid deficiency states are not generally available. When biotin and pantothenic acid deficiency states are suspected, the individuals involved usually have been previously supported on total parenteral nutrition for several weeks to months. With modern intravenous vitamin supplementation, this deficiency state has all but disappeared. Patients in whom this deficiency is suspected can be treated with a multivitamin containing biotin and pantothenic acid.

VITAMIN K DEFICIENCY

method of
ROBERT E. OLSON M.D., PH.D.
State University of New York at Stony Brook
Stony Brook, New York

Vitamin K is the generic name for a family of fat-soluble vitamins required for normal hemostasis. Compounds with vitamin K activity all contain the 2-methyl-1,4-naphthoquinone nucleus with a lipophilic side chain at position three. Vitamin K_1, named phylloquinone, has a phytyl side chain at position 3 and is the only homologue of vitamin K found in plants. The first member of the vitamin K_2 family was isolated from bacterially fermented fish meal and identified as 2-methyl-3-heptaprenyl-1,4-naphthoquinone in 1939. This family, principally of bacterial origin, contains a large number of vitamin K homologues that have side chains composed of multiple isoprenyl groups at position 3 numbering from 4 to 13. They are now designated as menaquinones-n (MK-n), in which n represents the number of isoprenyl units in the side chain. Menaquinone-4 is synthesized in animals and birds from the vitamin K precursor 2-methyl-1,4-naphthoquinone, previously designated vitamin K_3 and now called menadione.

Vitamin K is widely distributed in both animal and vegetable foods and varies from less than 1 μg per 100 grams in milk, potatoes, and oranges to over 400 μg per 100 grams in spinach, kale, and turnip greens. The concentration of vitamin K in plasma (which is 90% phylloquinone) in healthy persons is less than 1 ng per mL, and the body pool of phylloquinone in humans is about 1 μg per kg of body weight. Menaquinones synthesized in the gut may make up 50% of the vitamin K found in the liver but are mobilized more slowly than phylloquinone.

Vitamin K is essential for the synthesis of six liver proteins involved in the coagulation cascade, namely factors II (prothrombin), VII, IX, and X and proteins C and S plus at least two other proteins present in bone and at least one other present in kidney. The total number of vitamin K–dependent proteins is no doubt larger than this because evidence of new ones is appearing periodically. The function of vitamin K is to act as a cofactor for the gamma carboxylation of glutamate residues in vitamin K–dependent proteins. This reaction occurs cotranslationally in the rough reticulum of liver and other cells that contain the vitamin K–dependent gamma glutamyl carboxylase. The active form of vitamin K in the carboxylation reaction is its hydroquinone (KH_2). The addition of carbon dioxide to glutamate residues to form gamma carboxyglutamate (Gla) facilitates the binding of Ca^{2+} ions, which is essential for the action of these vitamin K–dependent proteins in metabolism. Factors II (prothrombin) VII, IX, and X are procoagulants and are proenzymes that are converted to serine hydrolases during activation. Protein C is an anticoagulant that serves as a break on the speed of the intrinsic cascade through a feedback loop involving thrombin. While thrombin is producing fibrin it is also activating protein C, which in turn inactivates factors V and VIII, thus slowing its own production. Protein S enhances the activity of protein C in the presence of phospholipid.

Vitamin K is conserved in the liver and other tissues by recycling the product of the carboxylation reaction vitamin K-2,3-epoxide to vitamin KH_2. This vitamin K cycle contains three enzymes, the gamma glutamyl carboxylase, a vitamin K epoxide reductase, and a vitamin K reductase. The coumarin anticoagulant drugs block both reductases in this cycle, thus preventing the formation of KH_2, which is essential for the carboxylation reaction. Large doses of vitamin K are required to overcome the blockade of this cycle by coumarin drugs.

The two vitamin K–dependent proteins in bone, osteocalcin or bone-Gla protein (BGP) and matrix Gla-protein (MGP), are induced by vitamin D hormone and mediate, through their calcium-binding properties, some actions of vitamin D in bone metabolism. Reduced plasma levels of both phylloquinone and MK-7 and MK-8 are found in patients with advanced osteoporosis.

CLINICAL MANIFESTATIONS

Bleeding is the major manifestation of vitamin K deficiency whether the cause is inadequate dietary intake or the antagonism of vitamin K by drugs. Easy bruisability and mucosal bleeding (especially epistaxis, gastrointestinal hemorrhage, menorrhagia, and hematuria) occur in vitamin K deficiency. Oozing of blood from puncture sites or incisions may occur following trauma, and life-threatening intracranial hemorrhage can occur in infants.

LABORATORY FEATURES

Reduction in the activity of prothrombin and other vitamin K–dependent factors is an accepted indicator of vitamin K deficiency or antagonism. The prothrombin time (PT) and the activated partial thromboplastin time (PTT) are usually prolonged if factor levels drop below 50%. The fibrinogen level, thrombin time, platelet count, and bleeding time are in the normal range. The measurement of plasma phylloquinone and menaquinones, which requires reverse phase high-pressure chromatography, does not correlate well with vitamin K status in an individual. The normal range of plasma phylloquinone is 0.2 to 1.0 ng per mL.

The most sensitive indicator of vitamin K deficiency is the presence of des-gamma-carboxyprothrombin (DCP), also known as PIVKA (protein induced in vitamin K absence or antagonism), in plasma, which can be measured by appropriate antibodies. Undercarboxylated prothrombin (DCP) is absent from the plasma of healthy persons. The amount of urinary excretion of gamma carboxyglutamic acid (Gla) is not a reliable indicator of vitamin K lack.

CAUSES OF VITAMIN K DEFICIENCY

Primary vitamin K deficiency is uncommon in healthy adults. Several factors protect adults from a lack of vitamin K. These include (1) widespread distribution of vitamin K in plant and animal tissue, (2) the vitamin K cycle, which conserves the vitamin, and (3) the microbiologic flora of the normal gut, which synthesizes menaquinones. On the other hand, vitamin K deficiency in breast-fed infants remains a major worldwide cause of infant mortality and morbidity.

Newborn infants represent a special case of vitamin K nutrition because (1) the placenta is a relatively poor organ for transmission of lipids, (2) the neonatal liver is immature with respect to prothrombin synthesis, (3) breast milk is low in vitamin K, containing only 1 to 3 μg per liter (although cow milk contains 5 to 10 μg per liter), and (4) the infant gut is sterile during the first few days of life. Hemorrhagic disease of the newborn (HDN) generally occurs 1 to 7 days postpartum and may be manifested by cutaneous, gastrointestinal, intrathoracic, or, in the worst cases, intracranial bleeding. Late hemorrhagic disease (LHD) occurs 1 to 3 months postpartum and has the same clinical manifestations as HDN. It is usually associated with malabsorption or liver disease. If the mother has ingested hydantoin anticonvulsants, cephalosporin antibiotics, or coumarin anticoagulants, the incidence of all types of HDN is increased.

In otherwise normal adults, vitamin K deficiency can occur in persons with marginal dietary intake who undergo trauma, extensive surgery, or long-term parenteral nutrition with or without treatment with broad-spectrum antibiotics. Patients with biliary obstruction, malabsorption, and parenchymal liver disease also have a higher risk of vitamin K deficiency. As already mentioned, persons who ingest certain drugs including anticonvulsants, anticoagulants, certain antibiotics (particularly those of the cephalosporin type), salicylates, and megadoses of vitamin A and E are vulnerable to vitamin K–related hemorrhagic disease.

PREVENTION AND TREATMENT

Prevention of vitamin K deficiency in healthy persons is easily accomplished by consumption of a reasonably well balanced diet containing green leafy vegetables. The requirement for vitamin K_1 in humans ranges from 0.2 to 0.6 μg per kg per day. The recommended dietary allowance (RDA) for vitamin K, set for the first time in 1989 by the National Academy of Sciences, averaged 1.0 μg per kg per day for persons from infancy to adulthood. According to the American Academy of Pediatrics, neonates should receive 1 mg of vitamin K intramuscularly within 1 hour of birth to prevent HDN. Oral vitamin K is not recommended because it is variably absorbed and unpredictably retained. A recent epidemiologic study that claimed that intravenous (but not oral) vitamin K at birth was associated with a later twofold increase in childhood leukemia has not been confirmed and is not grounds for altering the practice of protecting newborns with intramuscular vitamin K.

For patients with life-threatening hemorrhage due to vitamin K lack or antagonism, blood transfusion or administration of 10 to 15 mL per kg body weight of fresh frozen plasma or factor concentrates may be necessary. Plasma fractions may rarely be contaminated with pathogenic viruses, so their benefit must outweigh the risk in each case. Less severe cases, requiring correction within 6 to 24 hours, should be treated by 10 mg of phylloquinone (Aqua-MEPHYTON, Konakian) given intramuscularly. In patients with coumarin overdosage, 15 to 25 mg of phylloquinone given intramuscularly may be indicated.

Patients receiving total parenteral nutrition should also receive 1 mg of phylloquinone intramuscularly per week. Patients with malabsorption may require oral doses of 1 to 2 mg of phylloqinone per day. Patients with severe liver disease that is refractory to oral vitamin K should be given 10 mg intravenously at weekly intervals. It is not necessary to repeat high doses daily. Intravenous vitamin K should be given cautiously (not over 1 mg per minute) to prevent any allergic reactions, which are encountered infrequently.

Phylloquinone is not toxic at 500 times the RDA (0.5 mg per kg per day). Menadione, the vitamin K precursor, however, has a finite toxicity owing to its reaction with sulfhydryl groups and has been reported to cause hemolytic anemia, hyperbilirubinemia, and kernicterus in infants. Menadione (Synkayvite) should not be employed in the therapy of vitamin K deficiency states.

OSTEOPOROSIS

method of
ERNEST SCHWARTZ, M.D.
Bronx Veterans Administration Medical Center
Bronx, New York

A simplistic concept of uncomplicated osteoporosis postulates a continuous senescent involution of bone in both sexes with the superimposition in the female of a time-limited post-menopausal acceleration of bone loss. Typically, the diagnosis is applied to a 60-year-old, otherwise healthy woman with osteopenia and vertebral compression fractures. The common denominator may be described as sufficient loss of bone mass to increase vulnerability to fractures of the axial and appendicular skeleton. Such loss of bone mass may be due either to disease and various extrinsic factors or to a normal physiologic process. Most healthy 90-year-old humans have lost enough bone mass to be susceptible to fractures. Because trabecular bone constitutes only about 20% of the skeletal mass and is more labile than cortical bone, post-menopausal acceleration weakens the distal radius and vertebrae long before aging bone loss seriously compromises the cortical bone of the femur. A state of mild secondary hyperparathyroidism due to declining 1,25-dihydroxyvitamin D production may contribute to senescent bone loss, but it seems doubtful that this mechanism is more than a minor factor. Before assuming that osteopenia and its consequences are due to senescence and menopause, one must carefully consider the multitude of diseases and environmental factors that weaken bone and that may be correctable. A short list is presented in Table 1. Among endocrine causes, corticosteroid excess is responsible for a common and particularly fulminant variety of osteoporosis, which is attributed to a dual pathogenic mechanism of impaired bone formation and increased resorption. Whether there is major permanent bone loss in hyperthyroidism has been debated. Likewise, although hyperparathyroid patients have a somewhat lower bone mass than normals, their bone mass apparently does not rapidly diminish with time, and osteopenia is generally not severe. In men with osteoporosis, alcoholism should be the first differential diagnosis. However, in alcoholics in general, severe pre-senile osteoporosis is infrequent and is probably dose related because moderate alcohol consumption in a few clinical studies did not seem to produce significant bone loss. In some patients, alcoholism is associated with adrenocortical hyperfunction (alcoholic pseudo-Cushing's syndrome), which may contribute to major bone loss. Direct toxic effects of excessive alcohol consumption on bone cells may also be involved.

Finally, it is important to realize the significance of "idiopathic" pre-senile and pre-menopausal osteoporosis. These disorders probably reflect a heterogeneous mixture of inborn errors of metabolism, which resemble the numerous defects described in osteogenesis imperfecta and result in low bone mass and abnormal structure. The concept of peak bone mass is also highly significant because a very low peak bone mass is a major risk factor for osteoporosis in later life. The fact that females have a lower peak bone mass than males is probably the major determinant of greater female susceptibility to osteoporosis. The determinants of peak bone mass appear to be intrinsic as well as extrinsic and have yet to be fully defined. A major role for genetic factors in the pathogenesis of uncomplicated osteoporosis is suggested by the recent demonstration of strong correlations of bone turnover and density with allelic variants of the vitamin D receptor gene.

CLINICAL FEATURES AND DIAGNOSIS

Classically, the presence of osteoporosis is announced by the sudden occurrence of a painful vertebral compression fracture or of a wrist or hip fracture. Radiography then reveals the characteristic osteopenia, which is quantitated by bone densitometry studies. It is important to recognize that the majority of vertebral fractures are asymptomatic and are incidental findings in radiographs obtained for other reasons. Some spine radiographs are obtained because of obvious developing kyphosis or height loss. In the Mayo survey of 762 women in Rochester, Minnesota, the prevalence of vertebral fractures in women older than 50 years of age was 25.3 in 100 patients. The annual incidence of new vertebral deformities in this group was 17.8 per 1000 patient-years. In contrast, hip fracture incidence in the 50- to 59-year age group was only about 0.3 in 1000 patient-years, rising only to 5 in 1000 patient-years at age 70 to 74, and then to 33 in 1000 patient-years at age 85 or greater. Despite the overwhelming domination of mortality and medical costs incurred by hip fracture, the great majority of patients with osteoporosis are 1 to 3 decades younger than hip fracture patients and are being followed for vertebral osteoporosis. At this time, it is still not possible to determine the effect of most therapies on the "bottom line"—the prevention of hip fractures.

The classic presentation of a new vertebral fracture is acute back pain, often radicular in nature, which immobilizes the patient because of its severity. Characteristically, the most frequently involved vertebrae are those at the thoracolumbar junction. The syndrome is usually self-limited, lasting a few months and rarely up to 6 months. Neurologic sequelae or residuals are rare. However, most vertebral fractures are found incidentally by radiographs. Radiologic diagnosis at this time depends on measurements of vertebral deformity or bone density. There has been considerable debate about the criteria used to define significant vertebral deformity owing to the considerable variation that exists in normal anatomic structure. Many reported therapeutic trials, otherwise impeccable in experimental design, can be contested because of arguable major deficiencies in the particular definitions of new fractures.

Bone densitometry methodology has become progressively more refined during the past decade. Radiograph-generated dual-photon densitometry (DEXA or DPX) is capable of 1% precision. Considerable data have now been accumulated from normal and osteoporotic populations, and correlations have been attempted with fracture incidence. In one study of 380 post-menopausal patients, the vertebral fracture incidence increased sixfold between the highest 20th percentile and the lowest 20th percentile in bone density. In this study, the prevalence in patients of one or two vertebral fractures increased the incidence of new fractures sevenfold. Densitometry data have been used to define, or rather, propose, a "fracture threshold" of approximately 1 gram per square centimeter. Because of the difficulties and controversies involved in defining fracture incidence by vertebral anatomical measurements, there has been increasing dependence on serial bone densitometry studies to judge the effect of therapies for osteoporosis. Densitometry data have clearly defined the post-menopausal acceleration of bone loss and are helpful in deciding on the need for estrogen replacement. Although densitometry is a useful surrogate in clinical trials, one must always remember that the major objective of therapy is to reduce fractures and, in particular, to reduce hip fractures occurring in the distant future.

TABLE 1. **Major Causes of Bone Loss**

Endocrine causes
Cushing's disease; steroid excess
Hyperthyroidism; thyroxine excess
Primary hypogonadism
Secondary amenorrhea (hypoestrogenism): lack of exercise, anorexia nervosa, oophorectomy, prolactinoma
Bone toxins
Alcohol excess
Chemotherapy
Anticonvulsants
Heparin
Bone marrow and lymphatic disease
Multiple myeloma, lymphoproliferative disease, chronic anemias
Miscellaneous causes
Rheumatoid arthritis
Subtotal gastrectomy
Smoking

PATHOPHYSIOLOGY AND LABORATORY EVALUATION

Uncomplicated osteoporosis may be viewed as a progressive decompensation of the complex system involved in maintaining bone mass and architecture. Bone and bone marrow contain a variety of cells that communicate by humoral messengers and that also respond to hormones secreted by endocrine tissues elsewhere. Furthermore, because bone serves as a protective supporting scaffold, its response to stressing forces implies the existence of an internal transducing mechanism, like the piezoelectric effect, which influences bone cell function. The purposeful interaction of all these elements has been simply described as the coupling of formation and resorption, which is carefully regulated. In early life, during which active bone growth occurs, the coupling axis is tilted toward a net formation excess, although resorption is also quite active. The result of the bone formation tilt of the coupling axis during growth is reflected in the peak bone mass. Once peak bone mass is attained at maturity, a state of equilibrium ensues in which the continuing remodeling process results in no loss or gain of bone. This implies a relatively steady state of tonic stress and a net equality of bone cell formative and resorptive functions. The steady state persists in the human for only a few years and is followed by a slow tilt of the coupled formation-resorption axis toward resorptive excess, resulting in net bone loss. This tilt toward resorption is temporarily increased at the menopause. The overall activity of the formation-resorption axis has been designated "turnover." Only one third of osteoporotic patients manifest high turnover as shown by bone histomorphometry and chemical indices of bone cell activity. In these patients both bone resorption and bone formation are increased, but the axis is tilted toward net resorption. The osteoblast apparently responds to what seems to be a primary increase in resorptive activity, but the response is not sufficient to maintain bone mass. One mechanism that potentiates the increased resorption of aging may be mild secondary hyperparathyroidism due to inadequate calcium intake. In addition, possible mechanisms of menopause-accelerated resorption may be the withdrawal of a tonic positive estrogenic effect on bone cell performance, possibly by antagonism of parathormone action or by modulation of marrow cell cytokines. Most therapeutic agents under investigation have primarily antiresorptive activity and can be expected to be most effective in patients with high turnover. Because bone histomorphometry is available at only a few specialized laboratories, increasing attention has been paid to noninvasive biochemical markers of bone.

The most readily available marker of resorption is the 24-hour urine calcium determination. High or high-normal urine calcium levels (over 200 mg per day) may reflect bone lysis due to high turnover. Idiopathic hypercalciuria must be excluded. Patients with low turnover usually have urine calcium levels well below 100 mg per day. The 24-hour urinary hydroxyproline concentration largely reflects dissolution of bone collagen and has been widely used as an index of resorption, chiefly in Paget's disease. At present the quantitation of urinary pyridinoline and deoxypyridinoline cross-links is considered to be a more sensitive index of bone collagen breakdown in metabolic bone disease and is commercially available. Immunoassays for serum free pyridinoline and tartrate-resistant acid phosphatase (TRAP), which is a bone-specific osteoclastic enzyme, are under development. If these methods prove useful, it may soon be possible to measure most biochemical markers of bone formation and resorption in a single serum specimen. For appraisal of bone formation, the time-honored test has been the serum alkaline phosphatase level in patients without liver disease. About 30% of osteoporotic patients have mildly elevated alkaline phosphatase values, apparently reflecting high turnover. The values are also frequently elevated for several weeks following fractures. A monoclonal assay for bone-specific alkaline phosphatase has recently become available. Serum osteocalcin has come into use as an index of bone formation. This is a noncollagen matrix protein, also termed bone Gla-protein, which is a product of the osteoblast. Its level in serum probably reflects mostly osteoblastic activity, although some of it may be derived from dissolution of bone matrix. Like alkaline phosphatase, osteocalcin is elevated in high-turnover osteoporosis. Another marker of bone formation, serum carboxy terminal propeptide of type I procollagen (PICP), seems to be highly sensitive and is undergoing clinical evaluation. At present, the screening tetrad used to ascertain the state of bone turnover includes 24-hour urine calcium and pyridinium cross-links, serum alkaline phosphatase (or bone-specific alkaline phosphatase), and serum osteocalcin.

THERAPY OF ACUTE COMPRESSION FRACTURES

Osteoporotic patients may be classified by a triad of clinical presentations: the painful vertebral fracture syndrome, the hip fracture, and the asymptomatic radiologic vertebral deformity or osteopenia. Acute onset and disabling back pain are the classic manifestations of sudden vertebral damage and usually require temporary bed rest. The syndrome is generally self-limited in that full symptomatic recovery is expected within weeks or months. Early progressive ambulation is advisable and generally practicable. Except for unusually severe episodes, particularly those with painful radiculopathy, bracing is not considered desirable. After recovery from the most painful phase, assuming that the final diagnosis is uncomplicated osteoporosis, the patient should undergo further testing for qualitative and quantitative classification.

Calcitonin Therapy, Early and Late

Because of its central psychotropic action on pain, calcitonin is often employed in the initial therapy of the acute compression fracture syndrome. Salmon calcitonin (Calcimar, Miacalcin) is preferred to human calcitonin* because of its greater potency and longer half-life. The effective dose is 50 to 100 units given subcutaneously daily, preferably at bedtime. One hundred units daily provide little additional benefit, increase the side effects (nausea and flushing), and double the expense. The use of calcitonin for acute pain should be regarded as a temporary expedient pending a final decision on the mode of long-term therapy, which may or may not include calcitonin. Calcitonin received early approval from the Food and Drug Administration (FDA) as an effective agent in osteoporosis based on clinical studies that demonstrated modest increases in spinal bone density, reaching a plateau after 2 to 3 years of therapy. As a potent antiresorptive agent, calcitonin appears to blunt post-menopausal bone loss and corticosteroid-induced bone loss. Calcitonin has been thought

*This drug has not been approved by the FDA for this indication.

to be most effective in patients with high-turnover osteoporosis as defined by elevated bone marker measurements and histomorphometry. Its usefulness in low-turnover disease is doubtful, and, as with all agents, there is a heterogeneous response among individual patients. The longevity of antiresorptive calcitonin effects and its effect on fracture incidence are uncertain. In long-term therapy, calcitonin is generally used in a daily or alternate-day regimen at a dosage of 50 to 100 units. Nasal calcitonin* and an oral absorbable calcitonin analogue* are being investigated. The chief advantage of calcitonin therapy is the absence of serious toxicity. The chief disadvantages are parenteral administration and the lack of convincing evidence for fracture prevention, particularly in the hip.

ASYMPTOMATIC OSTEOPOROSIS

The majority of osteoporotic patients with or without spinal compression fractures are asymptomatic. Regardless of the absence of symptoms, the patient with radiographic evidence of a spinal fracture is considered a candidate for prompt therapeutic intervention. Whether any intervention can affect the natural course of disease in such a patient has been disputed. At the point of spontaneous vertebral fracture, perhaps 30 to 50% of bone mass has been lost throughout the spine with loss of connectivity and perforation of the trabecular plates. All other vertebrae are implicitly at risk for fracture because of architectural defects, and it is doubtful whether a simple cessation of further bone loss or even augmentation of defective structure will prevent new fractures. Nonetheless, the usual choice is to pursue, at the least, antiresorptive therapy for whatever benefit the stabilization of bone mass may produce.

The other class of patients with osteoporosis is the osteopenic group without compression fractures, probably the "silent majority" of osteoporotic patients, whose disease usually remains undetected until fractures appear. It is assumed that patients with relative osteopenia in the immediate perimenopausal period are prone to major complications consequent to accelerated bone loss in the post-menopausal years. Abnormalities in this group are now being detected by bone densitometry screening. Age-related normal values have been established for male and female populations, and values have been suggested as "fracture thresholds" for the lumbar spine and hip. Perimenopausal patients who have densitometry readings greater than two standard deviations below the mean normal, or whose values are below the fracture threshold, are considered at major risk in the post-menopausal years. The finding of low bone mass at this time is considered an indication for estrogen replacement therapy or other antiresorptive therapy if estrogen is contraindicated or rejected by the patient. Some investigators have suggested the need for bone augmentation therapy at this time as a prophylactic measure.

ESTROGEN

Estrogen has long been considered the gold standard of antiresorptive therapy for osteoporosis in the female. There is general agreement that post-menopausal bone loss is arrested and that vertebral and hip fracture incidence are reduced by as much as 50%. The minimum effective dose of conjugated equine estrogens (Premarin) is believed to be 0.625 mg daily. Because the risk of uterine carcinoma is increased severalfold with unopposed estrogen therapy, cyclic therapy with medroxyprogesterone (Provera), 5 to 10 mg daily for the last 12 to 14 days of the cycle, is commonly employed. With respect to breast cancer, the consensus at present is that the risk is modestly increased with a risk ratio of perhaps 1.2 to 1.3. However, it is also believed that the risk increases progressively with prolongation of estrogen therapy. Prolonged estrogen therapy appears to be necessary to gain the bone-protective effect of estrogen. It now seems clear that discontinuance of estrogen after any time period of therapy results in a menopause-like acceleration of resorption with a rapid decline in bone density. In the Framingham study, by the age of 75, bone density fell to that characteristic of the untreated group. Because the risk of hip fracture rises rapidly after the age of 70, it has been predicted that time-limited estrogen therapy at menopause will have only a modest effect on the overall incidence of hip fracture in the general population. The implication of such data is that lifetime estrogen therapy would be necessary to reduce hip fracture risk significantly. Such lifetime therapy would be expected to increase the risk of breast cancer significantly, posing a therapeutic dilemma. A possible solution may be the use of antiestrogens such as tamoxifen, which appears to have an estrogen-agonist action on bone resorption. With respect to other actions of estrogen, the reduction in cardiovascular risk has been estimated to be about 50%, which is attributed in part to the favorable effects on the blood lipid profile. The consequent benefits to mortality and morbidity have been considered by some to far outweigh any negative influence of estrogen on breast cancer and uterine risk. Perhaps the most significant deterrent to estrogen therapy is patient noncompliance. It appears that many women do not wish to start estrogen therapy. Of those who do start, the majority discontinue therapy. Possibly a clinically inoffensive antiestrogen will solve the compliance problem.

CALCIUM THERAPY

A time-honored health proverb states that "milk (calcium) is good for the bones" on the simple assumption that more calcium enters the bone and makes more bone. On the other hand, it has also been assumed that calcium deficiency results in less bone

*These drugs are not available in the United States.

and may eventually produce osteoporosis. There may be a germ of truth in these hypotheses, in that high calcium intake during growth has been thought by some to increase peak bone mass. However, Stanley Garn, using precise anatomic methods, showed years ago that the mean values of bone morphometric measurements were the same in matched population groups who habitually had high and low calcium intakes despite the wide spread of bone mass in any single group. Of course, other nutritional factors may influence peak bone mass as well. Careful prospective studies are needed to settle this controversy.

The effects of calcium supplementation and deficiency have been attributed to modulation of parathyroid hormone secretion. The reduction in bone turnover by high calcium intake was convincingly demonstrated by radiocalcium kinetic studies conducted 30 years ago. Although some of the studies reported in recent years speak to the contrary, the prevailing weight of evidence demonstrates a significant reduction in the rate of bone loss with calcium supplementation. There are grounds for believing that an intake of at least 1.5 to 2 grams of calcium daily is necessary. In a recent double-blind study of sodium fluoride* therapy lasting 4 years, vertebral bone loss was essentially totally arrested in the control group, who took a 1.5-gram calcium supplement daily. The subjects of this study were older women 50 to 75 years of age with vertebral fractures, most of them presumably beyond the phase of accelerated bone loss. The effect of very high calcium intake on perimenopausal acceleration of bone loss has been debated. The apparent lysis of bone following estrogen withdrawal seems to be accompanied by parathyroid suppression, which would temper any benefit from further parathyroid suppression by high calcium intake. It seems clear that estrogen is much more potent in arresting perimenopausal acceleration of bone loss. However, there is some evidence of an estrogen-calcium synergism in that a calcium supplement of 1.5 grams daily added to a half dose of estrogen (Premarin, 0.3 gram daily) seems to be as effective as the usual minimum Premarin dose of 0.625 gram daily. During the later decades of life when hip fractures begin to appear, such high calcium intakes may be of considerable value in slowing the component of aging bone loss attributed to calcium deficiency and mild secondary hyperparathyroidism. Poor bioavailability has been a problem with many calcium tablets. Chewable calcium carbonate preparations (Tums) are preferred for more reliable absorption.

BISPHOSPHONATE THERAPY

Sodium etidronate (Didronel)† has been a highly effective therapy for Paget's disease, which is considered a multicentric disease of excessive resorption produced by increased numbers of abnormal osteoclasts. The mechanisms of resorption inhibition by the bisphosphonates have still not been fully defined, but they are thought to involve direct effects on the osteoclast. Because prolonged therapy with sodium etidronate can produce osteomalacia, intermittent therapy regimens were tried, usually involving daily doses of 400 mg for about 14 days of every 90 days. Numerous studies have now documented resorption-suppression by this regimen, leading to cessation of bone loss and a modest increase in bone mass over at least a 2-year period. In most studies, the bone mass then stabilizes owing to eventual down-regulation of bone formation by the coupling mechanism. Although some investigators have claimed that this regimen reduces the fracture rate, the evidence is weak for any significant effect on fractures. The bone mass in most patients at the therapeutic plateau is usually still well below the fracture threshold. A heterogeneous response has been described with etidronate,* and perhaps as many as 20% of patients are nonresponders. As with calcitonin therapy, high-turnover disease is believed to respond best to bisphosphonates. The long-term usefulness of these agents in preventing hip fractures is somewhat doubtful and is impossible to predict at this time. Several new bisphosphonates are now under investigation, and it will require many years to define the comparative usefulness of these drugs in the treatment of osteoporosis. The bisphosphonates appear to share with estrogen and calcitonin the rebound acceleration of bone loss that occurs after discontinuation of therapy. The new bisphosphonates have much lower inhibitory effects on bone formation and less propensity to produce osteomalacia. Consequently, the experimental regimens have usually involved continuous daily doses, which may afford some advantage over the intermittent regimens necessary with sodium etidronate.

SODIUM FLUORIDE THERAPY

Fuller Albright realized the possible significance of sodium fluoride* as a therapy for osteoporosis when he came upon the syndrome of fluorosis. The preponderance of experience with fluoride favors its usefulness as the only agent capable of producing a continuous progressive increase in bone mass. The effect is most striking on the vertebral bone mass, which is largely trabecular, and somewhat less on the femur, which has varying proportions of trabecular bone. The fluoride controversy intensified with the completion of two prospective double-blind studies, which claimed to show no significant diminution in vertebral fracture rate despite a progressive increase in vertebral density. Unfortunately, both treated and control groups received what we now realize to be a significant therapy—a 1.5-gram calcium supplement daily. Furthermore, no attempt was made in either study to separate bone mass responders from nonresponders despite the evidence that 25 to 30% of

*This drug has not been approved by the FDA for this indication.
†Didronel is an investigational drug in the United States.

*This drug has not been approved by the FDA for this indication.

fluoride-treated patients are nonresponders. When responders were segregated, the data from a large retrospective study showed a striking reduction in vertebral fracture rate. Most of the other published studies have also shown reduced fracture rates. The issue of hip fracture remains undecided. There appears to be no change or even a slight increase in hip fracture incidence during the early years of fluoride therapy. However, very few hip fractures occurred in these study populations, which have mostly not yet reached the eighth decade when hip fracture incidence begins to rise sharply. The toxic effects of fluoride therapy include gastrointestinal upset and a lower extremity pain syndrome that occurs in 10 to 30% of patients and requires temporary cessation of therapy. This is apparently due to increased bone turnover at weight-bearing sites and perhaps to some stress fractures. A narrow "therapeutic window" has been postulated for fluoride, and most investigators now favor a daily dose of not more than 45 mg of sodium fluoride* daily, compared with the 75-mg dose used in the two double-blind studies. The desirable pre-dose level of serum fluoride is considered to be about 10 μM after 2 to 3 months of therapy. Because of the high frequency of nonresponse with sodium fluoride, bone formation markers are needed to determine response. Serum alkaline phosphatase and osteocalcin rise with successful fluoride therapy. Serial bone densitometry at 6-month intervals is important to establish response. Fluoride is still considered an investigational drug and should be used only with a meticulous experimental protocol. If the evidence at 1 year of therapy indicates nonresponse, the drug should be discontinued.

THE HIP FRACTURE PATIENT

When a hip fracture occurs, osteoporosis is usually at end-stage. Hip fracture is predominantly an event of the eighth and ninth decades. Vertebral fractures are usually pre-existent, and all bone densities are below the fracture threshold. There has been extensive cortical bone loss, which is especially nonsusceptible to antiresorptive or augmentation therapy. Hip fracture is an absolute contraindication to fluoride therapy. Conservative therapy with calcium supplementation is usually employed to reduce bone turnover.

The main issue with respect to hip fracture is prevention. The paramount problem is falling owing to the assortment of neurologic and muscular impairments associated with aging. The measures employed for prevention are largely environmental and extrinsic, including the recent development of "hip protectors" to cushion the hip of an aged patient against impact. The major pharmacotherapeutic options for stabilizing or increasing bone mass must be used much earlier in life. At present, there is considerable doubt that any of the therapies now in use will be able to prevent hip fracture in the last decades of life.

*Exceeds dosage recommended by the manufacturer.

OTHER THERAPIES

Calcitriol, 1α-hydroxyvitamin D_3, hydrochlorothiazide, and daily human parathormone injections have been reported to produce favorable effects. A combined parathormone-estrogen regimen has also recently been studied. All of these regimens are investigational at present.

MALE OSTEOPOROSIS

Although primary or secondary hypogonadism is associated with male osteoporosis, the normal male does not suffer a "male menopause." Other pathogenic factors accelerating bone loss in the male include endogenous or exogenous Cushing's syndrome, alcoholism, and subtotal gastrectomy. In the absence of pathogenic factors, mean male bone density does not reach the nominal vertebral fracture threshold until the ninth decade. At age 85+, the cumulative incidence of hip fracture in the male is 15% as opposed to 35% in the female. Osteoporotic vertebral fractures in the male are generally asymptomatic. Few data are available on treatment of male osteoporosis. The role of antiresorptive therapy in male osteoporosis has not been defined. Calcium supplementation of 1.5 grams of calcium daily is usually employed. Because alcoholic osteoporosis and steroid-induced osteoporosis are characterized by impaired bone formation, sodium fluoride therapy has been used in males with these syndromes to stimulate osteoblastic activity.

RECOMMENDATIONS

The major lesson to be learned from the osteoporosis experience to date is that the patient population is heterogeneous and the response to any therapy is heterogeneous as well. Practically all of the reported studies have used cross-sectional data, which obscure the heterogeneity of individual longitudinal responses. There are low and high peak bone masses, strong and weak bone microstructures, high and low bone turnover rates, slow and fast bone losers, and, most significantly, responders and nonresponders to every therapy. Densitometry at the menopause is particularly important and may serve to stratify very-low-risk and very-high-risk patients early on. Whatever therapeutic course is selected, it is extremely important to make serial measurements of biochemical bone markers and use serial bone densitometry to separate responders from nonresponders. Osteoporosis therapy is prolonged and expensive, and the effectiveness of any therapy should generally be determinable within 1 year of commencement. If the patient is a nonresponder, the therapeutic approach should be promptly changed. Finally, the rebound acceleration of bone loss following discontinuance of antiresorptive agents may require a strategy of lifetime therapy to maintain improved bone mass.

PAGET'S DISEASE OF BONE

method of
ALISON A. MOY, M.D., and
WILLIAM J. BURTIS, M.D., PH.D.
Yale University School of Medicine
New Haven, Connecticut

Paget's disease affects approximately 3% of the United States population over the age of 55 and is the second most frequent disease of bone after osteoporosis in this age group. Paget's disease is most common in persons from England, France, North America, New Zealand, and Australia; it is rare in Africa and Asia. In the United States it is slightly more common in the northeastern states than in the midwest or southern states. There is also a slight male predominance with the usual onset of disease in the fifth to sixth decade. Some studies show an increased frequency of HLA-DQW1 antigen, and Paget's disease is seven times more likely to develop in a patient whose first-degree relative has the disease, but only about 30% of cases are familial.

Paget's disease is characterized by rapid bone turnover, that is, increased bone resorption followed by increased but abnormal bone formation. The abnormal bone formed is larger and less compact than normal bone and has disorganized lamellar units, a chaotic woven structure, and increased vascularity. The pathognomonic microscopic feature of pagetic bone is the distorted architecture, in which lytic and blastic lesions often occur at adjacent sites. Overall, pagetic bone does not have the same tensile strength as normal bone and is more prone to deformity and fracture. Paget's disease may occur in a localized area of one bone (monostic disease) or in several sites in one bone or asymmetrically in several bones (polyostic disease). The bones most commonly involved include the skull, pelvis, tibia, femur, spine, humerus, and clavicles. Most patients at presentation have a "stable" number of bones involved; that is, once the disease is established it rarely spreads to a distant site. However, it commonly spreads within an involved bone. There may be concern about possible osteosarcomatous change if a patient with established Paget's disease develops increased symptoms in a known previous site.

The etiology of Paget's disease is probably multifactorial and involves both a genetic predisposition and slow viral infection of the osteoclast. The viral inclusions found in the osteoclasts of pagetic bone share similarities with the paramyxovirus family. Specifically, researchers have found viral particle inclusions that share sequence homology with respiratory syncytial virus, measles virus, and canine distemper virus. It appears that virally infected osteoclasts fuse into multinucleated giant cells more quickly than noninfected osteoclasts, and this results in the accelerated bone resorption that then leads to increased bone formation. The presence of viral particles is also believed to cause an increase in the differentiation of pre-osteoclasts into mature osteoclasts. Viral infection may also stimulate bone macrophages to produce more interleukins such as interleukin-6. Production of interleukins along the ruffled border of the osteoclast enhances bone resorption, and interleukins may serve a paracrine function in signaling the osteoblast to enter the resorbed lacune.

DIAGNOSIS

The diagnosis of Paget's disease is made from the history (which may indicate a familial predisposition), physical examination, and supporting laboratory and radiologic abnormalities. The majority of patients with Paget's disease are asymptomatic; however, many patients have symptoms of bone pain. The bone pain may originate at the site of pagetic involvement or from the abnormal mechanics that occur as a result of bowing and enlargement of the bone. Pain may also result from the development of osteoarthritis at joints adjacent to the involved bone. The pain may occur at rest or may become worse with ambulation. Many patients describe an uncomfortable sensation and local increased warmth at the involved sites. This correlates with increased blood flow. If microfractures occur at advancing osteolytic borders or on convex surfaces of deformed bones, these may produce pain. Patients occasionally present with fracture.

The lumbar spine is another common area of pain, with increased blood flow and bony overgrowth causing altered vertebral alignment or nerve compression. A rare presentation of Paget's disease is paraplegia, which results from the vascular steal syndrome. The vascular steal syndrome occurs when vertebral blood flow supersedes that delivered to the spinal cord. The result is diminished spinal cord blood flow and subsequent paraplegia. This is a neurosurgical emergency. Increased blood flow to pagetic bone may rarely result in high-output congestive heart failure.

If the skull is involved, a patient may develop deafness or complain of headache, vertigo, or enlarging hat size. Deafness is most likely multifactorial as the result of eighth nerve entrapment in the skull (rare) and possibly changes in the auditory ossicles and cochlea as well. Severe skull thickening may lead to obstructive hydrocephalus due to thickened basilar skull bone, basilar invagination, and blocked outflow of cerebrospinal fluid. From the hydrocephalus, dorsal column disease may ensue, and the patient may have altered gait and proprioception. A patient with Paget's disease can develop hypercalcemia when immobilized. Patients with Paget's disease also have an increased risk of kidney stones (calcium and urate stones) and gout.

Although it occurs in less than 1% of pagetic bone, osteosarcoma is a dreaded complication of the disease. In a Mayo Clinic review, the bone most likely to undergo malignant transformation is the pelvis, followed by the femur and humerus respectively. A patient with established disease who develops a new symptom of disease may have osteosarcoma at that site. Giant cell tumors also occur with increased frequency in pagetic bone, and, although less common than osteosarcomas, they are much more responsive to treatment.

Pagetic bone may be localizable by physical examination. An enlarged cranium, with so-called frontal bossing, indicates skull involvement. Other affected bones may be deformed, such as the anterolateral bowing of long bones. Patients often have increased local warmth or, less commonly, pain on palpation of the involved bones. Those with lower extremity involvement or with hydrocephalus may have a broad-based gait. A combination of conductive and sensorineural deafness is commonly seen with skull involvement.

When Paget's disease is suspected from the history and physical examination, measurement of appropriate biochemical markers and radiologic plain films will substantiate the diagnosis. Biochemical markers include elevated serum alkaline phosphatase and urinary hydroxyproline levels. For the clinician, the most reliable biochemical marker is an elevated serum alkaline phosphatase concentration. The clinician should confirm that the elevated alkaline phosphatase is of bony origin by evaluating the liver enzymes, namely, aspartate aminotransferase and alanine aminotransferase and 5′ nucleosidase. The degree of elevation of alkaline phosphatase usually corresponds to disease severity and may be used to follow a patient's response to treatment. Other biochemical markers of bone formation, such as osteocalcin and bone-specific alkaline phosphatase, are also elevated but are not necessary to make the diagnosis or to follow the response to treatment. Newer markers of bone resorption include serum and urinary pyridinoline crosslinks. These are also elevated in patients with Paget's disease, but they are not routinely available in most laboratories and again are not necessary for clinical management.

There are also pathognomonic radiologic changes in pagetic bone. These include (1) bowing deformities, (2) cotton-wool appearance of skull, (3) osteolytic wedge along the shaft of the long bones, or osteoporosis circumscripta in the skull, (4) thickened bony cortex with blurring of the corticomedullary junction, (5) osteolytic and osteoblastic changes adjacent in a bony area, and (6) overall enlargement of affected bones. The constellation of clinical, biochemical, and radiologic findings is almost always sufficient to diagnose Paget's disease. Bone biopsy, which is difficult in thickened, vascular pagetic bone, is rarely necessary.

Another helpful radiologic tool for detecting involved bones is the bone scan. Because of the increased osteoblastic activity, a bone scan will reveal the areas of disease. This is often a more efficient way of documenting the extent of disease than plain films because the bone scan evaluates the whole skeleton with one image. A plain film may be of more diagnostic significance in evaluating new bone pain in a patient with established disease. In this situation, the plain film may reveal a new lesion or a partial fracture or may show extracortical calcification in an established site that raises concern about osteosarcomatous transformation.

TREATMENT

The reasons for medical treatment of Paget's disease are (1) to control pain, (2) to prevent progressive deformity, (3) to treat hypercalcemia that can result when patients are immobilized, (4) to treat vascular steal syndrome, and (5) to decrease blood flow to bone prior to orthopedic surgery. Treatment may also minimize the risk of developing complications of disease such as deafness and bone deformities. Pharmacologic therapy aimed at the osteoclast usually relieves pain that is the direct result of pagetic involvement, headache from skull involvement, low back pain from vertebral involvement, and increased bone warmth. The pain that results from arthritic changes, the deafness, and the bowing do not improve with pharmacologic treatment, but their rate of progression may be slowed. Many clinicians treat even asymptomatic patients who have alkaline phosphatase concentrations that are elevated three or four times higher than normal, skull involvement (to prevent or retard deafness), or disease of the tibia or femur. In this last situation, treatment is aimed at preventing progressive bowing deformities and osteoarthritis.

Calcitonins

Calcitonin is available in the United States as a subcutaneous injection, and both human and salmon preparations are Food and Drug Administration (FDA) approved for treatment of Paget's disease. Salmon calcitonin is more potent and less expensive than human calcitonin; however, in patients who are allergic to salmon preparations, human calcitonin should be used preferentially. Salmon calcitonin is manufactured by Rhone-Poulenc-Rorer as Calcimar and by Sandoz as Miacalcin. Each vial of Calcimar contains 400 units or 2 mL, and each 1-mL vial of Miacalcin contains 100 units. Human calcitonin is manufactured by Ciba-Geigy as Cibacalcin. Human calcitonin is distributed in pre-filled syringes of 0.5 mg, which is equivalent to 150 to 200 units of salmon calcitonin. Calcitonin acts on distinct calcitonin receptors on osteoclasts and thus inhibits osteoclastic bone resorption. Salmon calcitonin is more potent than human calcitonin in inhibiting osteoclastic bone resorption. Both salmon and human calcitonin provide analgesic relief to some patients as well.

Prior to initiating full-dose therapy with salmon calcitonin, a 1-unit test dose is given subcutaneously. In the rare hypersensitive patient, a wheal and flare reaction develops at the local site of injection. If there is no allergic reaction, one may proceed with a dose of 100 units a day. The equivalent dose of human calcitonin is injection of one half of the pre-filled syringe. During the first few months of therapy, daily calcitonin administration usually decreases the alkaline phosphatase level to approximately 50% of its pre-treatment level and also alleviates pain. Maintenance therapy can then be continued at a dose of 50 units given subcutaneously every other day or three times a week. However, if a patient has severe disease or continued pain, daily therapy may be used indefinitely. The use of salmon calcitonin is complicated by the possible development of anticalcitonin-neutralizing antibodies. These antibodies will result in a decrease in the effectiveness of calcitonin. Neutralizing antibodies are not seen with human calcitonin.

Another reason for loss of effectiveness of calcitonin is down-regulation of calcitonin receptors on osteoclasts as a result of the prolonged exposure to calcitonin. Administration on alternate days may allow escape from this down-regulation. Calcitonin therapy has other side effects, including nausea, vomiting, facial flushing, and paresthesias, which may occur in about 20% of patients. These effects are not considered true allergic effects because they are mediated by the biochemical effects of calcitonin on the autonomic nervous system. Patients often become tolerant to these effects with repeated use. The need for subcutaneous injection and the cost of treatment make the use of calcitonin less than ideal for treating patients with Paget's disease. Calcitonin given as an intranasal solution is currently being studied in clinical trials and should be available soon, but it may not be as efficacious when administered by this route.

Bisphosphonates

Bisphosphonates are derivatives of naturally occurring bone pyrophosphate. A carbon substitution for oxygen in the phosphate backbone prevents degradation of the bisphosphonate by bone phosphatases. The bisphosphonates, which have a high affinity for calcium phosphate, are tropic to bone and are rapidly cleared from the circulation. They act as antiresorptive agents by "poisoning" the osteoclast. This results from the degradation of the bony matrix and endocytosis of the bisphosphonate by the osteoclast. The bisphosphonate, once intracellular, appears to inhibit the osteoclast from resorbing bone further.

The first bisphosphonate to be widely used to treat Paget's disease was etidronate. This drug is FDA approved and is still commonly used for this indication. Unfortunately, however, in addition to acting as an antiresorptive agent by inhibiting the osteoclast, etidronate also inhibits mineralization of newly formed bone. For this reason, etidronate must be given in limited doses on a cyclic basis. Etidronate is manufactured by Procter and Gamble as Didronel. It is available in 200- and 400-mg tablets. The dose is 5 to 10 mg/kg body weight daily for a 6-month period. Higher doses are associated with an increase in bone pain from osteomalacia and increased risk of fractures. After each 6-month course of therapy, the patient must not take etidronate for at least 6 months to prevent the development of osteomalacia.

Etidronate should be taken either 1 hour before meals or 2 hours after meals to improve gastrointestinal absorption. Gastrointestinal absorption is low and ranges between 2 and 10%. At least 60% of patients respond to etidronate with reduced levels of alkaline phosphatase and urine hydoxyproline. The decreases in symptoms and biochemical markers are equivalent to those seen with calcitonin. Dyspepsia, diarrhea, bloating, and abdominal discomfort are other known side effects of etidronate. Etidronate may be more convenient for many patients because of its oral administration. It is also less expensive than calcitonin. However, calcitonin may be preferable in certain clinical situations. These include (1) patients with severe pain, (2) patients with advancing lytic lesions, (3) patients about to undergo orthopedic surgery, and (4) patients with healing fractures. In these patients, calcitonin works more quickly to alleviate pain and decrease vascular blood flow and does not impair mineralization of new bone.

Although not FDA approved at this time, other bisphosphonates have been used to treat Paget's disease. These include pamidronate, alendronate, and others under development. Although it has been approved by the FDA only for hypercalcemia of malignancy, intravenous pamidronate (Aredia) (developed by Ciba-Geigy) seems to be effective in the treatment of Paget's disease. It does not have the side effect of impaired bone mineralization characteristic of etidronate. Given intravenously, its bioavailability is better than that of etidronate. The best dose and treatment schedule are not clearly defined at this time. Pamidronate has a prolonged effect in halting osteoclastic bone resorption, and some patients have achieved disease remission for up to one year with treatment.

Other Modalities

A multidisciplinary approach to the treatment plan often provides the most benefit to the patient. This includes appropriate physical therapy, orthopedic consultation, and medical intervention. Simple preventive measures include the use of nonsteroidal anti-inflammatory agents or salicylates to control pain and the use of canes and walkers to steady gait. Shoe lifts may also be used to equalize leg length and prevent mechanical loading abnormalities. It is important for patients to remain mobilized because immobilization may lead to hypercalcemia. Although it is uncommon for a patient to have concomitant primary hyperparathyroidism and Paget's disease, surgical intervention to remove either the parathyroid adenoma or hyperplastic parathyroid glands is necessary to prevent further rapid bone turnover and to control hypercalcemia in this setting.

For patients whose disease is refractory to calcitonin and bisphosphonates, plicamycin* (Mithracin) is occasionally used. Plicamycin acts on osteoclasts to inhibit bone resorption. The dose is 15 μg per kg given as an intravenous infusion over 6 to 8 hours. If needed in a situation of acute spinal cord compression, additional infusions can be given on the second and third days. Some patients require up to five infusions in these settings. As stated earlier, in nonresistant patients calcitonin may be equally effective in this clinical situation and may be preferred, especially if a neurosurgical or orthopedic procedure is planned. Especially with repeated use, plicamycin can be hepatotoxic and may cause renal insufficiency. It also affects platelets and thus prolongs the bleeding time. Nausea and vomiting are often associated with infusions of plicamycin. Because of its rapid onset of action in arresting bone resorption, plicamycin may cause falls in serum calcium and phosphorus with each infusion. To obviate this effect, concomitant supplementation with calcium and vitamin D may be necessary.

Analgesics such as nonsteroidal anti-inflammatory agents and salicylates may be used at any point during the course of illness. They may be particularly helpful if the patient has arthritic pain in addition to pagetic bone pain. Orthopedic surgery is also used if pagetic involvement is severe and gait is impaired. Specifically, patients may require shoe lifts, osteotomy, total hip replacement, or total knee replacement. If osteosarcomatous change occurs, therapy is aimed at tumor ablation through resection followed by chemotherapy and possibly radiation therapy, but mortality remains high. There is, however, some preliminary evidence that bisphosphonate therapy may reduce the risk of osteosarcomatous transformation.

Overall, the treatment aims are directed at controlling progression of disease and symptoms. The best approach to providing thorough care involves the use of a multidisciplinary team of physical therapists, orthopedic surgeons and neurosurgeons, and internists

*This drug has not been FDA approved for this indication.

and family practioners. An important resource for physicians and patients alike is the Paget Foundation (200 Varick Street, Suite 1004, New York, NY 10014), an active nonprofit organization that supports research and publishes a newsletter and other patient-oriented literature on Paget's disease. Of the available pharmacalogic agents, etidronate is typically administered first. If the patient does not respond with reduced symptoms and a decreased alkaline phosphatase level within 3 or 4 months, calcitonin may be given. Also, calcitonin is more helpful when acute intervention is necessary as in vascular steal syndrome or prior to orthopedic surgery. Patients who do not respond to one agent or become resistant to one agent may respond to another. Plicamycin may also be used in emergency situations, but it has more side effects than calcitonin. Pamidronate is another agent that will most likely be used once more data are available about the dosing regimens. Newer bisphosphonates may also play a role in treating Paget's disease, as may intranasal calcitonin. Therapy usually improves the quality of life in symptomatic patients with Paget's disease, and it is hoped that early pharmacologic intervention will prevent many of the long-term complications of this disease.

PARENTERAL NUTRITION IN ADULTS

method of
ROLANDO H. ROLANDELLI, M.D., and
JOAN R. ULLRICH, R.D.
University of California at Los Angeles School of Medicine
Los Angeles, California

Over the past 25 years, parenteral nutrition has evolved from a new, sophisticated form of therapy, only available in major university medical centers, to a routine practice in most hospitals and even at home. During this time, every aspect of parenteral nutrition has been improved and simplified with a concomitant reduction in morbidity. The dismal prognosis of short bowel syndrome has been dramatically improved with the use of home parenteral nutrition. It is estimated that nearly 275,000 patients are leading relatively normal and productive lives while receiving parenteral nutrition at home. The use of the parenteral route as the sole means of nutrition over prolonged periods of time has also led to the identification of previously unknown essential nutrients, such as trace elements.

Recent investigations have demonstrated an association between parenteral nutrition and increased permeability of the intestinal barrier. These observations have led to the belief that bowel rest (as the result of parenteral nutrition) may be the origin of sepsis and multiple organ system failure in critically ill patients. The current emphasis on cost containment, the renewed interest in enteral nutrition, and the belief that bowel rest can lead to severe complications have limited the indications for the use of parenteral nutrition. However, it remains a life-saving therapy for many patients.

INDICATIONS AND CONTRAINDICATIONS FOR PARENTERAL NUTRITION

Nutritional support can reduce the mortality of multiple illnesses in patients who present with chronic malnutrition or develop malnutrition in the course of an acute illness. Patients at risk for chronic malnutrition are those with reduced dietary intake due to cancer, mental illness, advanced age, or poverty; gastrointestinal obstruction of benign or malignant cause; and malabsorption due to impaired digestion or absorption. Chronic organ insufficiencies also predispose patients to malnutrition.

In catabolic situations, such as multiple trauma, burn wounds, sepsis, and major surgery, a sudden increase in energy expenditure with protein loss can result in acute malnutrition. Acute malnutrition can be predicted in patients who have had inadequate nutrient intake for 5 days and who are likely to suffer an additional 5 days of inadequate intake. The severity of acute illness correlates with the degree of hypermetabolism and, consequently, with depletion of cellular mass and nutrients. Patients who develop organ insufficiencies during the course of acute illnesses require nutrient formulas specifically designed to maintain metabolic balance and preserve organ function.

Malnutrition impairs the body's resistance to infection, delays healing and rehabilitation, and increases morbidity and mortality after surgery. It also increases the risk of complications such as wound dehiscence, anastomotic leakage, and infection and the need for prolonged ventilatory support. Therefore, nutritional support should be instituted when nutritional risk is suspected or anticipated. However, the likelihood of a short life expectancy and poor quality of life, the clinical judgment of the attending physician, and the wishes of the patient or legal guardian should all be considered before instituting nutritional support. Contraindications for nutritional support include hemodynamic instability, hypoxemia, and metabolic imbalance.

CONTRAINDICATIONS TO ENTERAL NUTRITION

In general, enteral nutrition is preferred over parenteral nutrition when feasible and safe. The most common obstacle to enteral nutrition is lack of gastrointestinal access. Enteral nutrition is contraindicated in patients with gastroparesis, a common phenomenon in acute illness, unless combined access to the stomach for decompression and to the jejunum for feeding can be established. Other contraindications include acute inflammation of the pancreas or intestine, malabsorption due to massive small bowel resection, enterocolitis due to radiation or chemotherapy, and gastrointestinal bleeding or obstruction (Tables 1 to 3). Finally, in many patients the volume of enteral nutrients needed to provide sufficient calories and protein is not well tolerated and results in diarrhea.

NUTRITIONAL ASSESSMENT

Chronic malnutrition is assessed by considering the history of dietary intake and weight change, the presence of gastrointestinal symptoms, and results of the physical examination (which includes anthropometric measurements) and laboratory testing. Analysis of diet reveals adequacy of caloric and protein intake, as well as any prescribed or self-imposed restrictions. A history provides information regarding usual body weight and recent weight changes. A loss of 10% of body weight over 6 months or 5% over 1 month is indicative of malnutrition. The basal energy expenditure (BEE) is estimated using the Harris-Benedict equations, which take into consideration gender, weight, height, and age.

BEE equations—kilocalories per day:

$$\text{Men} = 66.47 + 13.75 \times (\text{wgt–kg}) + 5 \times (\text{hgt–cm}) - 6.76 \times (\text{age–years})$$

$$\text{Women} = 655.6 + 9.56 \times (\text{wgt–kg}) + 1.85 \times (\text{hgt–cm}) - 4.68 \times (\text{age–years})$$

Gastrointestinal symptoms associated with malnutrition include dysphagia, recurrent vomiting, chronic diarrhea, and unusual gastrointestinal losses (such as those produced by enterocutaneous and enterovaginal fistulas). Muscle wasting and edema are indicative of hypoproteinemia. Ascites and hepatomegaly are seen in advanced kwashiorkor and protein malnutrition. Essential nutrient deficiencies produce typical lesions in the skin and oral mucosa.

Laboratory blood parameters used to assess nutritional status include serum albumin, cholesterol, iron, total iron-binding capacity, zinc, and vitamin levels. Numerous studies confirm the predictive value of low serum albumin for malnutrition-related complications, and various prognostic nutritional indexes have been developed combining albumin levels with other factors, such as triceps skinfold thickness, skin testing for delayed immunity, and weight change. When statistical analysis is applied to these indexes, serum albumin level is found to carry the greatest weight of any factor.

TABLE 1. **Nutritional Risk Factors and Indications for Nutritional Support**

- Chronic malnutrition
  - Reduced dietary intake
  - GI obstruction
  - Malabsorption
  - Organ insufficiency
- Acute malnutrition
  - Prior reduced intake (5 days)
  - Future reduced intake (5 days)
  - Hypermetabolism
  - Organ insufficiency

TABLE 2. **Contraindications for Nutritional Support**

- Grim prognosis
- Against patient/family wishes
- Hemodynamic instability
- Hypoxemia
- Metabolic imbalance
  - Uncontrolled hyperglycemia
  - Hypokalemia, hypophosphatemia
  - Fluid overload, dehydration

Most of the nutritional assessment parameters used in chronic malnutrition lose sensitivity in the context of acute malnutrition. Weight change during acute illnesses is more commonly due to fluid shifts than to changes in body protein and fat. Albumin levels also vary with fluid status. The use of serum proteins to assess nutritional status depends upon the constant protein renewal, which, in turn, depends on nutrient availability. The half-life of albumin ranges from 14 to 21 days, creating a delay between an acute insult in nutritional status and the descent of albumin levels in serum. Therefore, serum proteins with a shorter half-life are more representative of acute changes in nutritional status. These proteins include prealbumin, transferrin, retinol-binding protein, and thyroxine-binding protein.

In acute illnesses, clinical judgment plays an important role in nutritional assessment. Malnutrition is more likely to result in complications following gastrointestinal surgery than after cardiac or vascular surgery. Furthermore, gastrointestinal procedures requiring anastomoses increase the risk of nutrition-related complications, more so than a resection procedure with end ileostomy or colostomy. Preoperatively, a surgeon can surmise what effect malnutrition might have on the outcome of an operation and prescribe preoperative parenteral nutrition. During an operation a surgeon can predict, for example, whether a patient will have a prolonged ileus and can prescribe parenteral nutrition early in the postoperative period before the nutritional status is further compromised.

ASSESSING NUTRIENT NEEDS

Information gained through nutritional assessment is used to estimate nutrient needs. A correction factor is added to the BEE depending on the degree

TABLE 3. **Indications for Parenteral Nutrition and Contraindications for Enteral Nutrition**

- Lack of access to the GI tract
- GI bleeding or obstruction
- Acute pancreatitis
- Acute enterocolitis
  - Crohn's disease
  - Ulcerative colitis
  - Radiation
  - Chemotherapy
- Massive small bowel resection
- Inability to tolerate sufficient enteral nutrition

TABLE 4. **Stress Factors in Acute Illnesses**

Illness	Stress Factor
Uncomplicated surgery	1.00–1.05
Long bone fracture	1.25–1.30
Complicated surgery	1.25–1.30
Sepsis or multiple trauma	1.30–1.50
Burn wounds	1.50–2.00

of metabolic stress on the patient (Table 4). These factors provide only a rough estimate of the additional energy expenditure induced by stress. In clinical practice, there is significant overlap of various conditions that increase energy expenditure, such as organ failure, hemorrhage, and the effects of inotropic drugs. These adjustments are made based upon clinical judgment. In patients who are not severely ill, an additional 25% of calories are added to the energy expenditure to provide for physical activity and to promote weight gain. In critically ill patients, however, especially those developing multiple organ failure, the hormonal milieu creates unfavorable conditions for anabolism, and an excess of calories can create further metabolic derangements. Therefore, the amount of calories supplied to these patients is limited to no more than 1.20 to 1.30 times the BEE. In patients with severe chronic malnutrition, especially elderly patients, calories should be introduced very gradually to avoid the refeeding syndrome, which consists of fluid overload and electrolyte imbalance on initiation of nutritional support.

In some patients, precise determination of caloric requirements is crucial, and they should not simply be estimated. For instance, in patients with short bowel syndrome who depend entirely on parenteral nutrition to maintain nutritional status, indirect calorimetry should be done before hospital discharge. A portable machine samples inhaled and exhaled air and measures oxygen consumption and carbon dioxide production. The machine calculates both resting energy expenditure (REE) and the respiratory quotient (RQ). REE is computed according to the Weir formula:

$$\text{REE (kcal/day)} = [3.9(VO_2) + 1.1(VCO_2)] \times 1.44$$

The RQ is simply the VCO_2/VO_2 ratio and represents the type of fuel being oxidized or synthesized by the body. A low RQ, approximately 0.7, is indicative of fat oxidation; an RQ closer to 1 is indicative of carbohydrate oxidation, while a high RQ (RQ >1) indicates lipogenesis. Determination of both the REE and the RQ assists in monitoring the metabolic effects of parenteral nutrition. For instance, an RQ of more than 1 reveals an excessive caloric intake and can be demonstrated by comparing the amount of calories supplied with the measured REE.

The "gold standard" in assessing protein needs is nitrogen balance, which is calculated by subtracting nitrogen loss from nitrogen intake. Nitrogen intake is obtained by dividing protein and amino acid intake by 6.25. Nitrogen is lost primarily in the urine, and in much smaller proportions, in feces and through the skin. Urea accounts for 85% of urinary nitrogen; the remaining 15% consists of ammonia, creatinine, and some amino acids. Although the Kjeldahl method can be used to measure the total nitrogen in any sample, it is cumbersome, time consuming, and unsuitable to hospital laboratories. In clinical practice, nitrogen losses can be calculated based on the urinary urea nitrogen (UUN) measured in a 24-hour urine collection. Non–urea nitrogen compounds and nonurinary nitrogen losses are accounted for by the addition of a correction factor of 4:

$$\begin{gathered}\text{Nitrogen balance (day)} = \\ \text{protein intake (grams per 24 hours)/6.25} \\ - \text{UUN (grams per 24 hour)} + 4\end{gathered}$$

This estimated nitrogen balance assumes normal fecal and cutaneous losses and no abnormal losses of nitrogenous compounds from fistula output, exudate through open wounds, proteinuria, amino aciduria, or similar sources. Regardless of the relative value of this estimation of nitrogen balance, UUN has its own value as an index of catabolism. Protein turnover normally generates approximately 5 grams of UUN in 24 hours. A UUN of 5 to 10 grams per 24 hours indicates mild catabolism, 10 to 15 grams per 24 hours, moderate catabolism, and more than 15 grams per 24 hours, severe catabolism.

Normal protein turnover is approximately 100 grams per 24 hours in a 70-kg adult. Most of the nitrogen derived from proteolysis is recycled into new protein. In order to replace the obligatory loss of nitrogen, a healthy adult requires 0.6 to 0.8 grams of protein per kg of body weight per 24 hours. In nonstressed patients a ratio of 0.8 to 1.0 grams of nitrogen per kg of body weight per day is used to calculate the total amount of amino acids to be included in the parenteral formula. Calculation of caloric and protein requirements is illustrated in Table 5.

TABLE 5. **Calculation of Caloric and Protein Requirements**

40-year-old man (wgt 154 lbs, hgt 5′8″) with intra-abdominal abscess following a laparotomy for blunt abdominal trauma
BEE = 66.47 + 13.7 (70) + 5 (170) − 6.76 (40) = 1600 kcal/d
Adjusted BEE = 1600 + 400 = 2000
Activity/wgt gain = 2000 + 500 = 2500 kcal/d (35.7 kcal/kg)
Protein requirements = 70 × 1 = 70 gm/d (11.2 gm nitrogen)
Calorie:nitrogen = 223:1
75-year-old woman (wgt 143 lbs, hgt 5′) with Ogilvie's syndrome (colonic pseudo-obstruction) following hip replacement
BEE = 655.6 + 9.56 (65) + 1.85 (150) − 4.68 (75) = 613.4 kcal/d
Adjusted BEE = 1200 + 150 = 1350
Activity/wgt gain = 1350 + 135 = 1485 kcal/d (14.4 kcal/kg)
Protein requirements = 65 × 1 = 65 gm/d (10.4 gm nitrogen)
Calorie:nitrogen = 140:1

Abbreviation: BEE = basal energy expenditure.

MACRONUTRIENTS IN PARENTERAL SOLUTIONS

Carbohydrates

The main caloric source used in parenteral solutions is dextrose. Some tissues in the body (e.g., nervous system, renal medulla, white blood cells) selectively use dextrose as a fuel. The body has only a small reserve of carbohydrates in the form of glycogen (approximately 400 grams in an adult). After this reserve is exhausted, usually after 24 to 36 hours of starvation, the body synthesizes glucose de novo via gluconeogenesis. The carbon skeleton precursors for gluconeogenesis are amino acids obtained from muscle proteolysis, and since the early studies of Gamble in starving men, it has been well known that the exogenous administration of dextrose can spare protein from destruction. Other fuels presently available for parenteral use, such as long chain triglycerides in fat emulsions, have a higher caloric density; however, at equimolar concentrations, dextrose has a greater protein-sparing capacity than fat emulsions. The need for carbohydrates is even greater after trauma or surgery, since wounds also selectively utilize glucose in the healing process.

The use of glucose as a calorie source is associated with some practical problems. The addition of dextrose to parenteral solutions raises the osmolality, precluding the use of peripheral veins at concentrations greater than 10 to 15%. During stress and infection, increased insulin resistance causes hyperglycemia and glucosuria when large amounts of dextrose are administered. This can be corrected with the concomitant administration of insulin, but careful monitoring is required since glucose tolerance can change as the underlying disease improves or worsens. An excess of intravenous dextrose can also result in hypercarbia and liver dysfunction. At equimolar amounts, there is greater production of carbon dioxide with administration of dextrose than fat emulsions. In patients with normal pulmonary function, this is compensated for by increased minute ventilation and carbon dioxide excretion in exhaled air. However, in patients with borderline pulmonary function, a high carbohydrate load can precipitate respiratory failure. Similarly, in patients receiving mechanical ventilation, a high production of carbon dioxide may interfere with weaning from the respirator.

Carbohydrate calories that exceed the energy needs of the body are used for lipogenesis. In parenteral nutrition, lipid mobilization is inhibited by hyperinsulinemia. Synthesized fat is retained in the liver, infiltrating the parenchyma and producing intrahepatic cholestasis. To avoid this complication, the amount of parenteral glucose administered should not exceed the hepatic oxidation capacity, which is estimated at 5 mg of glucose per kilogram of body weight per minute.

Lipids

Fat emulsions consist of long chain triglycerides containing linoleic acid, an essential fatty acid. Administration of fat-free parenteral nutrition results in the syndrome of essential fatty acid deficiency. This can be prevented with the administration of two bottles of 500 cc of 10% lipid emulsion per week. Indications for increasing the proportion of lipids in the formula are glucose intolerance, respiratory failure, and sepsis. The isotonicity of fat emulsions makes them the ideal fuel source for parenteral nutrition via peripheral veins.

Extensive research is presently being conducted on various aspects of lipid metabolism. One area of great interest is the role of fat emulsions on the synthesis of prostaglandins and leukotrienes and their consequent effect on the immune response. Some investigators advocate the use of fat emulsions in patients with acquired immune deficiency syndrome. Another area of research involves the combination of medium chain triglycerides with long chain triglycerides for intravenous administration. While long chain triglycerides require carnitine-mediated transport into mitochondria for oxidation, transport of medium chain triglyceride into mitochondria is independent of carnitine. Also, medium chain triglycerides seem to have a greater protein-sparing capacity than long chain triglycerides. Another new frontier in lipid research is the selection and combination of various fatty acids in the creation of a triglyceride. Probably the most exciting area in lipid research involves the discovery of the different effects of 3-omega versus 6-omega fatty acids. Three-omega fatty acids are obtained from fish oils and seem to prevent inflammation and atherosclerosis.

Protein

Commercially available parenteral solutions use crystalline amino acids as the nitrogen source. Standard solutions contain all essential amino acids and most nonessential amino acids. The ratio of essential to nonessential amino acids is 1.0:1.3, which matches the ratio of amino acids in proteins of high biologic value. Early solutions of crystalline amino acids had a high chloride content to solubilize acidic amino acids, but this caused metabolic acidosis in some patients. Present standard solutions of crystalline amino acids consist of equivalent amounts of chloride and acetate, resulting in a neutral pH. In addition to the standard crystalline amino acid formula, there are three other commercially available formulas: a hepatic formula (HepatAmine), a renal formula (RenAmin), and a formula enriched in branched chain amino acids (BranchAmin) (Table 6).

Joseph Fischer developed a formula to reduce the risk of hepatic encephalopathy when providing parenteral nutrition to patients in liver failure. Aromatic amino acids induce encephalopathy when a diseased liver is not able to remove them from the bloodstream and they compete with branched chain amino acids to pass through the blood-brain barrier; consequently, the formula, called FO-80, is enriched with branched amino acids and omits the aromatic amino acids and methionine. The formula supplies a heavier load of

TABLE 6. **Composition of Amino Acid Solutions**

	Total AA (gm/100 mL)	Essential AA (%)	BCAA (%)
Standard	3, 3.5, 7, 8.5, 10, 15	42–47	18–24.9
Renal	5.2, 5.4, 6	66.5, 88.5, 100	29.5, 33, 39
Hepatic	8	52.2	35.6
High BCAA	6.9, 7	63.8, 60.2	44.9, 45.1
BCAA only	6	100	100

Abbreviations: AA = amino acids; BCAA = branched chain amino acids.

amino acids to patients in liver failure without precipitating encephalopathy and can reverse encephalopathy that has already developed; however it was never demonstrated to improve outcome in patients with liver failure and it fell into disuse. With the success of liver transplantation, the formula may well enjoy a resuscitation, acting as a bridge to transplantation by providing adequate amounts of amino acids to the end-stage liver failure patient awaiting transplant.

The renal formula was developed based upon the Giordano-Giovanetti theory of urea nitrogen recycling. Although urea is the end product of protein metabolism for human enzymes, a proportion of urea circulating through the colon hydrolyzes into ammonia via bacterial ureases. Ammonia returned to the liver via the portal circulation enters a nitrogen pool used for synthesis of nonessential amino acids. The renal formula supplies essential amino acids and histidine, which, when combined with adequate calories, can promote protein synthesis using recycled urea nitrogen as a precursor of nonessential amino acids. Protein anabolism is induced, while the need for dialysis is reduced. However, routine use of hemodialysis for treatment of patients in acute renal failure has almost eliminated the need for this solution. As with the hepatic formula, there is now renewed interest in renal amino acids formulas. Hemofiltration is a new method, much simpler than hemodialysis, that removes water and electrolytes but not nitrogen compounds. Since the protein intake of patients in acute renal failure undergoing hemofiltration is still restricted, a renal formula can supply enough nitrogen to achieve equilibrium.

The branched chain amino acids, valine, leucine, and isoleucine, are the only amino acids not metabolized by the liver. They reach muscle tissue directly and become precursors for protein synthesis. Standard amino acid solutions contain approximately 24% branched chain amino acids. Enrichment to 45% branched chain amino acid content has been shown to improve nitrogen retention in severely stressed patients. The solutions have not changed the clinical outcome of stressed patients but have allowed better preservation of protein stores. Criteria for use of branched chain amino acid solutions are not well defined, but such solutions can be beneficial for severely hypercatabolic patients when standard solutions do not reverse negative nitrogen balance.

Glutamine, a nonessential amino acid, is excluded from standard amino acid formulas because it spontaneously converts to toxic compounds when stored in aqueous solutions. Yet, recent research has demonstrated glutamine to be the preferred fuel for enterocytes and cellular concentration fall during critical illness. Experimental studies have shown that glutamine is stable when added to a solution of amino acids as long as the solution is used within a few days. Prospective randomized trials have proved that glutamine supplementation in patients undergoing bone marrow transplantation results in fewer infections and shorter hospital stays. Nevertheless, glutamine is still commercially unavailable, and its use is restricted to a few research centers. The instability of glutamine as a free amino acid has led to investigations on the effects of dipeptides for intravenous use. These studies have been conducted in Europe and have shown that dipeptides are hydrolyzed by endothelial enzymes, rendering glutamine available to the body.

Other amino acids currently being investigated include arginine and taurine. Taurine is essential in premature infants and appears to reduce liver dysfunction associated with parenteral nutrition. Arginine has long been known to be an intermediary in the urea cycle, but only recently has it become apparent that it acts as an immune stimulant, inducing secretion of growth hormone from the hypophysis and acting as the precursor of nitric oxide, a regulator of vascular tone.

Micronutrients

Over the past 25 years there has been an evolution in the understanding of the role of various micronutrients in metabolism and their deficiency syndromes. At first only sodium, potassium, and vitamins were added to the intravenous dextrose-protein hydrolysate solution. This practice led to acute hypophosphatemia, so phosphates were incorporated. Magnesium and calcium were recognized as essential soon thereafter. As parenteral nutrition was used to treat more patients over longer periods of time, new deficiencies were demonstrated, including zinc, copper, manganese, and chromium. Presently, these elements are all included in parenteral nutrition solutions (Table 7). Other micronutrients are administered as needed in each patient. Vitamin K is given to some patients receiving parenteral nutrition in the form of a subcutaneous injection of 10 mg monthly. Iron dextran (InFeD), is administered to parenteral nutrition patients who develop iron deficiency ane-

TABLE 7. **Vitamins and Minerals in Parenteral Nutrition Solutions**

Vitamins	Dose
A (IU)	3300
D (IU)	200
E (IU)	10
Ascorbic acid (mg)	100
Folic acid (μg)	400
Niacin (mg)	40
Riboflavin (mg)	3.6
Thiamine (mg)	3
B_6 (pyridoxine) (mg)	4
B_{12} (cyanocobalamin) (μg)	5
Pantothenic acid (mg)	15
Biotin (μg)	60
Minerals (mg)	
Zinc	2.5–5.0
Copper	0.5–1.5
Manganese	0.15–0.8
Chromium	0.01–0.015

mia. An iron deficit can be calculated according to the following formula:

Iron dextran needed (mL) = (normal hemoglobin − patient's hemoglobin) × (0.0476 × kg body weight) + (1 mL for every 5 kg body weight)

Each mL of iron dextran supplies 50 mg of iron. This amount is administered in fractionated doses after a test dose (10 mg) is administered to rule out allergy. Several other micronutrients are currently under investigation with regard to intravenous requirements.

FORMS OF PARENTERAL NUTRITION

Peripheral Parenteral Nutrition (PPN)

The only advantage to PPN is that placement of a central line is not necessary. A mildly hypertonic solution can be infused via an arm vein; however, regardless of tonicity, peripheral veins only tolerate catheterization for short periods of time, usually from 3 to 5 days. The availability of peripheral veins is further restricted, since most hospitalized patients already have had multiple venipunctures. Usually after 7 to 10 days of PPN, peripheral vein access is impossible. Therefore, PPN is indicated in only a few rare clinical situations. PPN may be appropriate when there is a short-term need for parenteral nutrition (e.g., postoperative ileus) along with a contraindication for central line placement (e.g., incorrigible coagulopathy) or high risk for pneumothorax (e.g., severe emphysema). Fortunately, these clinical situations are rare.

Total (Central) Parenteral Nutrition (TPN)

In TPN, the high flow of central veins allows rapid dilution of hyperosmolar solutions. The preferred site for infusion of TPN is the superior vena cava, which is accessed by direct puncture of the subclavian or internal jugular vein and the advancement of a catheter into the superior vena cava by the Seldinger technique. Silastic catheters for long-term TPN can be placed by direct puncture of the same veins, subclavian and internal jugular, or by cutdown of the cephalic or external jugular vein. Central access can also be achieved by placing a long catheter in an antecubital (basilic) vein and advancing it into the superior vena cava; this is known as a peripherally inserted central catheter (PICC) line.

TPN solutions are prepared in the hospital pharmacy under sterile conditions (laminar flow hood) by mixing dextrose and amino acid solutions. The solution can be made in large batches and fractionated for individual patients. Electrolytes, minerals, vitamins, and trace elements are added to the TPN solution daily. Fat emulsions are administered through a separate intravenous line or are "piggybacked" with the TPN line. At some centers, TPN and all additives are delivered in a single plastic bag. These three-in-one solutions are prepared with an automated mixing device.

Home TPN

Patients requiring long-term parenteral nutrition include those with intestinal failure due to short bowel syndrome, radiation enteritis, chronic bowel obstruction or pseudo-obstruction, active inflammatory bowel disease, or enterocutaneous fistulas. In evaluating a patient for home parenteral nutrition, the following issues should be assessed: dexterity, physical and mental impairment, home environment, family support, health insurance, and other concomitant home therapies. Most patients are able to learn home TPN administration in a 5- to 7-day training period in the hospital.

Vascular Devices

The intravenous devices used for delivery of TPN are classified as temporary catheters or long-term vascular access devices. Temporary catheters can have a single, double, or triple lumen and are composed of polyurethane. Long-term vascular access devices can consist of a Silastic catheter that exits through the skin or is connected to a subcutaneous reservoir. Long-term vascular access devices can also have a single or a double lumen. As a rule, in both temporary and long-term access, the fewer number of lumens the lower the risk of infection; however, multilumen catheters are unavoidable in patients who require additional intravenous therapies, such as chemotherapy, antibiotic therapy, or blood transfusion.

Placement of Temporary Catheters

Temporary catheters can be placed at the bedside. However, TPN catheters should be placed under strict sterile conditions. The preferred technique is percutaneous catheterization of the subclavian vein via the infraclavicular approach. The approach via the right subclavian vein sidesteps the thoracic duct, which enters the venous system at the junction of the left subclavian and internal jugular veins; however, a guidewire through the right subclavian vein is more likely to enter the right jugular vein than the superior vena cava, whereas this is not true with left subclavian vein catheterization. This is probably due to the steeper arch of the right subclavian with the ostium of the internal jugular into the subclavian vein at the apex of this arch. The arch in the left side, however, is smoother, which allows the guidewire to circumvent the ostium of the internal jugular vein. The major advantage of the subclavian over the internal jugular approach is that the catheter in the subclavian vein exits on the chest, a much more stable surface than the neck.

Before infusion of a hypertonic solution, the position of the catheter should be confirmed roentgenographically. Multiple studies have shown the importance of catheter care in preventing catheter infection. Types of dressings and frequency of dressing changes vary among institutions, but in all cases, good technique in catheter care is more important than the dressing material or the frequency of dressing changes.

Placement of Long-Term Access Devices

Placement of long-term vascular access devices should be undertaken in the operating room. Patients who require long-term vascular access are likely to require several catheters in their lifetime. Reasons for catheter exchange include infection, rupture, and thrombosis. In patients with previous catheterizations of subclavian veins it is advisable to obtain a Doppler study of these veins prior to device placement. Thrombosis may be asymptomatic and can result in unsuccessful attempts at cannulation of the subclavian veins, increasing the possibility of complications. Subcutaneous devices have the advantage of freeing the patient from the external apparatus while TPN is not being administered, although in practice an angled needle is left in place. A major disadvantage to these devices is that removal requires a substantial surgical intervention. Silastic catheters, however, can be removed in the office or at the bedside in an emergency. In addition, Silastic catheters are much more easily accessed by the patient and can be repaired in case of dysfunction since they are external devices.

Placement of long-term vascular access devices can be made via a percutaneous approach through the subclavian or internal jugular vein or by cutdown of the cephalic or external jugular veins. The percutaneous approach may be easier to accomplish and carries a lower risk for thrombosis. Since for many patients these catheters are their lifeline for many years, preservation of vascular access is crucial.

Administration of Parenteral Nutrition

Prior to initiating TPN, baseline blood parameters, including electrolytes, glucose, blood urea nitrogen (BUN), and creatinine; liver function tests; and albumin and prealbumin levels are obtained. After correction of any electrolyte imbalance, TPN is started at a rate of 40 mL per hour, which in most adults is about half of the nutritional requirement. In severely malnourished patients and in diabetic patients, the starting rate should be lower. During the first 2 or 3 days glucose tolerance is assessed by measurement of blood glucose levels every 6 hours and by examination of the urine for glucose. Hyperglycemia is corrected with subcutaneous administration of regular insulin on a sliding scale. When the patient is stable and the glycemia is under control, the rate of TPN administration is increased to meet the patient's nutritional requirement. In patients requiring insulin, the average daily amount of insulin given subcutaneously during the second and third days is administered via the TPN solution.

Training is begun immediately for those patients who will be discharged on home TPN. Most patients prefer to receive TPN in cycles during the night. The transition from continuous infusion to 12-hour cycles is carried out gradually by increasing the rate of infusion. In one suggested compression sequence, TPN infusion is first reduced to 18 hours, then to 15 hours and then to 12 hours or less. After each cycle of TPN administration, before discontinuing infusion, the rate should be tapered by half over the last 30 minutes. Blood glucose levels should be checked 30 minutes later: if a patient develops hypoglycemia, a 15-minute taper to one-fourth of the full rate of infusion is added to the regimen. Electrolytes, glucose, BUN, and creatinine should be checked biweekly after the initiation of TPN and liver function tests performed weekly.

TPN infusion should be tapered and discontinued in patients undergoing major surgery. Experimental studies have shown that brain damage during hypotension occurred more frequently in animals who received concentrated dextrose as compared to a solution of electrolytes.

Complications

Patients receiving TPN are at risk for complications related to the central venous catheter, macronutrient imbalance, micronutrient imbalance, and liver dysfunction.

Central Venous Catheter Complications

The most feared complication at the time of insertion of a central venous catheter (CVC) is pneumothorax. This is more common with the subclavian approach than the internal jugular approach. Unless asymptomatic and very small in magnitude ($<10\%$), most pneumothoraces require a tube thoracostomy for pleural drainage. Usually the air leak will subside immediately after drainage and the tube can be removed within 24 to 48 hours. When the CVC is maintained after production of pneumothorax, the air leak may persist, indicating that the catheter is piercing the pulmonary parenchyma and perpetuating the pleuropulmonary fistula. In such case, the catheter should be immediately removed and replaced on the same side using a different approach. Bilateral attempts are dangerous when attempted without a chest x-ray prior to use of the contralateral subclavian vein approach. Other serious complications associated with CVC placement include arterial puncture, air embolism, and thoracic and brachial plexus injury.

All indwelling CVCs carry the risk of catheter-related infection. The effective monitoring of inpatients and outpatients by multidisciplinary teams has contributed to the reduction of catheter infection. Infection most often occurs after exchange of intravenous tubing, when the nidus is at the catheter hub. Other sites and sources of infection include the exit site through the skin, contaminated parenteral solutions, and bacteremia from other sources. The microorganisms circulating in the bloodstream settle on the fibrin coating in the intravascular portion of the catheter.

Whenever a TPN patient develops a fever, catheter infection should be suspected, but other sources should be investigated before the catheter is removed. Blood cultures should be obtained through the catheter and through a peripheral vein. The type of microorganisms detected in cultures may provide a clue to the source of infection. The most common organisms involved in catheter infections are *Staphylococcus aureus, S. epidermidis,* and *Candida albicans.* In patients with inflammatory signs at the exit site, in those with no other potential sources of infection, and in those who remain febrile despite a full course of antibiotics, the catheter should be removed and replaced. In patients with no inflammatory signs at the catheter site, the treatment varies depending on the type of catheter and the patient's clinical condition. Patients with long-term vascular access devices can be treated with long courses of antibiotics as long as there are no signs of severe infection present (e.g., persistent high fever and hemodynamic compromise).

With a temporary CVC, the catheter can be exchanged over a guidewire without incurring the risks of de novo CVC placement. In most patients, infection will promptly subside after catheter exchange and administration of antibiotics, but if it persists, the catheter should be removed and a new one placed at a different site.

Another common complication of CVC is venous thrombosis. Subclinical thrombosis is usually detected by the failure of infusion of lipid emulsion by gravity, indicating the presence of a blood clot. Manifestations of thrombosis vary from unilateral arm edema to superior vena cava syndrome. Unless contraindicated, thrombosis is first treated by urokinase (Abbokinase) infusion followed by heparin and warfarin (Coumadin). Catheter removal is not absolutely essential, especially in patients who have had thrombosis of other veins.

Thrombosis can lead to a lack of vascular access in patients receiving prolonged parenteral nutrition, such as those with short bowel syndrome. In exceptional cases, the only recourse is direct catheterization of the right atrium via a thoracotomy. Fortunately, because of aggressive treatment with thrombolytic agents and placement of endovascular stents, this is very seldom required.

Macronutrient Imbalance

The most common macronutrient imbalance is hyperglycemia. Patients at risk include not only diabetics but also patients under stress, especially those with serious infection. Persistent hyperglycemia can lead to the development of nonketotic coma and ketoacidosis. These conditions can be prevented by close monitoring of glucose levels and correction of hyperglycemia with insulin. The appropriate amount of insulin to add to the TPN solution is determined by using a sliding scale for subcutaneous insulin replacement. Patients with nondiabetic glucose intolerance must continue to be closely monitored clinically and with serial blood glucose assays even while in recovery from infection or stress, since insulin resistance can subside and an excess of exogenous insulin can cause hypoglycemia.

Hypoglycemic complications are also seen in patients receiving cyclic TPN after the infusion is stopped, but this can easily be prevented by gradual tapering of the glucose infusion. For example, in a TPN patient receiving 25% dextrose at 100 mL per hour, the rate should be reduced by half for the last 30 minutes of infusion. If hypoglycemia continues, the rate should be decreased again by half.

Uremia and hyperammonemia are potential side effects of amino acid infusions. Amino acid–induced uremia can occur in patients with renal insufficiency or in those under severe catabolic stress. The amount and type of amino acids to be administered to patients with renal failure depend on the concomitant use of hemodialysis or hemofiltration. If a patient is undergoing periodic hemodialysis, the suggested amount and type of amino acids to be administered are similar to those for patients with normal renal function (i.e., standard amino acids at approximately 1 gram per kg body weight per day). Hemodialysis is usually indicated for acidosis, fluid overload, or dangerous electrolyte elevation in plasma. When a patient does not require hemodialysis, the amount of amino acids should be decreased to 0.6 gram per kg body weight per day. If BUN levels continue to rise when a standard amino acid formula is used, a renal formula (containing only essential amino acids) can be used in combination with large amounts of carbohydrate calories.

In highly catabolic conditions such as multiple trauma, burns, sepsis, and complicated surgery, uremia can develop despite normal renal function. This may indicate insufficient caloric intake leading to the oxidation of amino acids as a calorie source. One way to investigate this situation is to measure the resting energy expenditure (REE) by indirect calorimetry and to obtain a 24-hour urinary urea nitrogen level (UUN). By comparing the amount of calories administered with the value of REE obtained, one can determine whether the patient is receiving adequate amounts of calories. This will also be reflected in the respiratory quotient (RQ), with high values seen in patients receiving excessive calories and low values in patients receiving insufficient calories. The UUN indicates the severity of metabolic stress and the adequacy of amino acid intake. When severely stressed patients continue in negative nitrogen balance despite adequate amounts of calories and total nitrogen, the use of a branched chain amino acid–enriched solution should be considered.

Fat emulsion consists of long chain triglycerides, which are hydrolyzed by endothelial lipases. If fat emulsion is infused at a rapid rate, a high concentration of triglycerides and fatty acids can accumulate in plasma. Side effects of fat emulsions include pulmonary infiltration and hypoxemia, hemolytic anemia, thrombocytopenia with associated coagulopathy, and hepatic and renal dysfunction, all of which can be exacerbated by hyperlipidemia. In order to avoid these complications, the infusion rate of triglycerides should not exceed 0.1 gram per kg body weight per hour in hospitalized patients and 0.15 gram per kg body weight per hour in patients receiving cyclic TPN at home.

Fat emulsion contains phospholipids as emulsifiers. A 10% and a 20% emulsion solution contain the same amount of phospholipids, 1.2 grams per 100 mL. In a 10% solution, there are more liposomal particles containing phospholipids at equal amounts of triglycerides than in a 20% solution. Liposomal particles can interfere with the metabolism of fatty acids and can modify cell membrane lipid composition. Therefore, of the two concentrations, the 20% fat emulsion is preferred.

Micronutrient Imbalance

Acute hypokalemia and hypophosphatemia can be precipitated by TPN infusion, especially in patients with chronic malnutrition. As malnutrition develops, the cellular stores of potassium and phosphorus are depleted to maintain serum levels. When anabolism is induced with TPN, these cations acutely migrate from the serum inside the cells. Hypomagnesemia is due to high gastrointestinal loss, diabetic ketoacidosis, or in those receiving aminoglycosides, diuretics and cisplatin.

Disorders of calcium metabolism are more common during long-term parenteral nutrition. Hypocalcemia can develop due to hypercalciuria and lead to osteopenia and bone pain. Hypercalcemia results from excessive vitamin D administration.

Zinc deficiency is also common, especially in patients with high gastrointestinal losses. Zinc deficiency syndrome is quite characteristic, consisting of vesiculopustular dermatitis around body orifices, particularly the mouth and nares, hair loss, anosmia and dysgeusia, cerebellar dysfunction, and depression. Copper deficiency can lead to anemia, leukopenia, neutropenia, and impaired wound healing. Chromium deficiency is associated with glucose intolerance, peripheral sensory neuropathy with ataxia, and mental confusion. Selenium deficiency results in muscle cramps, muscle weakness, and cardiomyopathy.

Deficiencies of fat-soluble vitamins (A, D, E, and K) are rare because body stores are large. Hypervitaminoses A and D are more common and more serious. Signs of vitamin A toxicity include dry skin; pseudotumor cerebri with headaches, vomiting, diplopia, and papilledema; hypertriglyceridemia; and hypercalcemia. Signs of vitamin D toxicity include anorexia, nausea, vomiting, and fatigue. At high doses (>75,000 IU), vitamin D can cause precipitation of calcium in soft tissues, joints, and renal tubules.

Abnormalities in serum sodium levels are secondary to fluid imbalance. Hyponatremia is associated with fluid overload, while hypernatremia is caused by dehydration.

Liver Dysfunction

Fatty infiltration of the liver with cholestasis develops in 25 to 30% of patients receiving long-term TPN, and especially in those with inflammatory bowel disease and short bowel syndrome. The causes of liver dysfunction associated with TPN are multiple and include excess calories, excess carbohydrates, inadequate protein, relative deficiencies in amino acids, essential fatty acid deficiency, and bacterial overgrowth of the small bowel. The administration of adequate amounts of protein and calories, inclusion of fat calories, carbohydrates under 5 mg per kg body weight per minute, and administration of metronidazole to treat small bowel bacterial overgrowth can help to reduce the incidence of TPN-associated liver dysfunction.

In a few patients, liver dysfunction evolves to liver failure with jaundice, coagulopathy, and portal hypertension. Approximately 20 patients have received a combined liver–small bowel transplant for short bowel syndrome and TPN-induced liver failure. With new immunosuppressive drugs, patient survival is over 80% with graft survival of 70%.

PARENTERAL FLUID THERAPY FOR INFANTS AND CHILDREN

method of
CHARLES L. STEWART, M.D., and
FREDERICK J. KASKEL, M.D., PH.D.
SUNY Stony Brook School of Medicine
Stony Brook, New York

Parenteral fluid and electrolyte therapy in infants and children is used for a wide variety of reasons but usually has two major goals. The first is to provide fluid and electrolytes to replace the amount usually lost by the normal functioning of the respiratory and gastrointestinal systems, the skin, and the urinary tract ("maintenance" fluid and electrolytes). The second is to repair a deficit or an excess of fluid or electrolytes that has resulted from a disease process or behavior (by the patient or caretaker) and is usually called "replacement" fluid and electrolytes. Physicians caring for children should recognize that, whenever feasible, the enteral route should be used for maintenance and replacement fluid therapies in children; parenteral therapies should be reserved for children in whom medical or surgical reasons argue against use of the enteral route. If the parenteral route of fluid and electrolyte administration is chosen, several important concepts should be remembered:

1. The results of all parenteral fluid therapies should be monitored often. This includes frequent assessment of vital signs, especially body weight measured on the same zeroed scale in the same state of undress. Blood pressure and heart rate should be carefully measured, and notations are made about the patient's state of alertness and mental status (e.g., crying, irritable behavior, sleeping).
2. Frequent physical examination should be carried out, and close attention is paid to signs of peripheral and central perfusion (capillary refill, heart rate, skin color, blood pressure) as well as to auscultation of the lungs and assessment of peripheral edema.
3. If abnormalities in serum electrolytes exist prior to starting parenteral therapy, these should be reassessed at reasonable intervals depending on their severity.
4. Enteral nutrition should be resumed as soon as feasible.

MAINTENANCE REQUIREMENTS

Most children admitted to a hospital will be receiving maintenance fluids, usually administered by the enteral route. Prior to undergoing major surgical procedures, some children may need parenteral administration of fluids and electrolytes, as do many children who are recovering from major surgery, especially abdominal and thoracic procedures. Depending on the surgical procedure, some patients may require more fluids than just the "normal" maintenance amount. In addition, many acute and chronic diseases impair a child's ability to ingest food and water or may make oral consumption of fluids dangerous. Maintenance fluids are designed to keep total body water and electrolytes at zero balance—i.e., the amount of fluid and electrolytes expended by the body (skin losses, respiratory losses, stool losses, and urine output) should equal the amount given to the child intravenously.

Numerous methods have been used to estimate maintenance fluid and electrolyte requirements in children. In the two most commonly used methods the fluid and electrolyte computations are based on metabolic rate ("caloric" method of Holliday) and body surface area ("per meter squared" method). Both methods yield similar results, and it must be remembered that both methods are only estimates of actual requirements, thus necessitating frequent reassessment of each patient after instituting this type of therapy. This chapter will outline the caloric method of fluid therapy.

Insensible water losses are related to energy expended, with 1 mL of water used ("lost") by the child for each kilocalorie metabolized. In basal conditions two-thirds of insensible water losses occur through the skin (note: not as sweat, which is an additional fluid loss), and one-third is lost through the respiratory tract. Together, these account for about 45 mL of fluid lost per 100 kcal metabolized per day. Note that no electrolytes are lost through these insensible routes.

The remainder of normal maintenance fluid requirements is composed of urine output, which normally varies depending on the daily solute load and oral fluid intake. The solute load is determined by the rate of metabolism and by solute intake. The value used to calculate parenteral fluid requirements is a value that does not allow the kidney to maximally dilute or maximally concentrate the urine (thus permitting the excretion of urine that is more or less isoosmolar with extracellular fluid). This value ranges between 55 and 75 mL of urine per 100 kcal metabolized.

TABLE 1. **Caloric Requirements Based on Body Weight**

Body Weight (kg)	Calories Expended (kcal/kg Body Weight/Day)
3–10	100
10–20	1000 calories + 50 per kg for each kg >10
>20	1500 calories + 20 per kg for each kg >20

When the estimated insensible water loss (45 mL per 100 kcal metabolized) is added to the estimated urine loss (55 mL per 100 kcal metabolized), a one-to-one relationship (100 mL of fluid per 100 kcal metabolized) emerges that simplifies the calculation of maintenance fluid requirements based on caloric expenditure. The estimation of caloric requirements is based on body weight in kilograms (Table 1). These are reasonable estimates for infants older than several weeks of age and do not apply to small premature infants. For the first 10 kg of body weight the child requires 100 kcal per kg (and thus 100 mL of fluid per kg). The next 10 kg of body weight (10 to 20 kg) require an additional 50 kcal per kg (and thus an additional 50 mL of fluid per kg body weight). These children require 1000 kcal (or 1000 mL) for the first 10 kg of body weight and 50 kcal (or 50 mL for each kg of body weight between 10 and 20 kg. In children weighing over 20 kg, an additional 20 kcal (or 20 mL) per kg of body weight is added to the 1500 kcal (or 1500 mL) required for the first 20 kg of body weight.

It must be emphasized that although parenteral fluid requirements are easily determined using this formula, supplying the actual caloric requirements is quite difficult. The usual intravenous fluids, composed of 5% dextrose per 100 mL of fluid, supply only 20% of the calculated caloric needs. However, for short-term use, this is adequate to prevent severe ketosis and tissue catabolism. If the patient is not expected to be able to receive enteral nutrition for several days, total parenteral nutrition should be considered.

In addition to maintenance water needs, parenterally administered fluids must also supply electrolytes (Table 2). No electrolyte losses occur during ventilation, and insensible skin losses of electrolytes are negligible (unlike sweat, see Table 4). Urinary losses of electrolytes do occur and are estimated to be between 2 and 3 mEq per 100 kcal metabolized (alternatively, they are often estimated at 2 to 3 mEq of sodium per kg body weight per day, and between 1 and

TABLE 2. **Electrolyte Requirements Based on Caloric Expenditure**

Electrolyte Requirements (mEq/100 Calories Metabolized/Day)
Sodium = 2.5–3.0
Potassium = 2.0–2.5
Chloride = 4.5–5.5

2 mEq of potassium per kg body weight per day). Electrolytes may continue to be lost ("ongoing losses") through diarrhea, vomiting, nasogastric tubes, surgical drains, and medications, and these need to be replaced (see the next section Ongoing Losses). The usual maintenance fluid and electrolyte therapy is hypotonic relative to electrolyte composition. Table 3 summarizes the components of normal maintenance fluid requirements, and Table 4 outlines the various conditions that affect maintenance fluids and ongoing losses.

Example 1. A 17-kg toddler is expected to require intravenous fluids and electrolytes while recovering from an illness. There have been no unusual fluid or electrolyte losses, and the patient's serum electrolytes and kidney function are normal. Calculate the child's maintenance parenteral fluid and electrolyte needs for 24 hours assuming that no unusual ongoing losses occur.

1. Maintenance fluids are calculated as 1000 mL (100 kcal or mL per kg body weight for the first 10 kg body weight) plus 350 mL (50 mL or kcal for each kg body weight over 10) = 1350 mL of maintenance fluid is needed each day.
2. Maintenance electrolytes. With 1350 kcal metabolized, 2.5 mEq of sodium (and potassium) per 100 kcal = $2.5 \times 13.5 = 33.75$ mEq of sodium (and potassium). This amount of electrolytes is given in the total daily infusion of fluids as calculated in step 1.
3. Ongoing losses: none.
4. Deficits: none.
5. The final 1-liter fluid infusion "bag" should therefore contain 5% dextrose with 25 mEq of sodium and 25 mEq of potassium and should be infused at 56.25 mL per hour. (Note: It is unreasonable to prescribe this type of fluid infusion rate; "rounding off" to 55, 56, or 57 mL per hour is more reasonable.) If this solution is given for 24 hours it will provide 1350 mL of fluid containing the maintenance electrolytes as calculated in step 2.

ONGOING LOSSES

Many children who appear at a physician's office or hospital who have already experienced significant loss of bodily fluids continue to experience these losses as maintenance and replacement fluids are given. These ongoing losses of fluids and electrolytes must be measured or estimated and replaced to achieve normal body fluid homeostasis in the infant or child. Some of these additional ongoing losses (including losses due to sweat, fever, and polyuric conditions) are outlined in Table 4; estimates of gastrointestinal electrolyte losses are given in Table 5. Persons caring for the child should be instructed to measure all ongoing losses so that accurate fluid replacement can be given. Measurements of the electrolyte and bicarbonate concentrations of vomitus and liquid stool can be obtained from many clinical laboratories, allowing more accurate replacement of these fluids in children with more prolonged or difficult illnesses.

TABLE 3. **Components of Maintenance Fluid Requirements**

Water Requirements (mL/100 Calories/Day)
Insensible
Skin = 30
Lungs = 15
Stool = 5
Urine = 50

TABLE 4. **Conditions Altering Maintenance Requirements and Ongoing Losses**

Condition or Factor	Type of Adjustment to Be Made
Increased metabolic rate	
Fever	Increase caloric estimate by 12% per degree centigrade rise in body temperature
Hypermetabolic states (hyperthyroidism, salicylism)	Increase caloric estimate by 25 to 50%
Decreased metabolic rate	
Hypothermia	Reduce caloric estimate by 12% per degree centigrade fall in fever
Hypometabolic states	Reduce caloric estimate by 5 to 15%
Sweat requirements	
Mild to moderate sweating	Increase water allowance by 5–25 mL per 100 kcal; increase sodium by 0.5–1.0 mEq per 100 kcal
Mild to moderate sweating in cystic fibrosis	Increase water as above; increase sodium by 1–2 mEq per 100 kcal
Urinary requirements	
Obligatory oliguria	Adjust water allowance to replace output
Obligatory polyuria	Increase water allowance to replace output (watch for hyperglycemia)
Sodium- or potassium-wasting states	Increase sodium or potassium to equal losses
Sodium- or potassium-retaining states	Reduce or eliminate potassium or sodium intake

Modified from Winters RW: Principles of Pediatric Fluid Therapy, 2nd ed. Boston, Little Brown, 1982, pp 75, 78.

If ongoing losses are significant, fluids should be replaced frequently (every 1 to 4 hours), especially if previous fluid losses have been incurred.

DEHYDRATION

The most common reason for the use of replacement fluid and electrolyte therapy in children is the loss of these substances through the gastrointestinal tract as with diarrheal stools, which are often accompanied by vomiting. This type of disorder is usually due to bacterial (e.g., *Salmonella, Shigella, Vibrio cholerae*), or viral (e.g., rotavirus, Norwalk virus) infection of the gastrointestinal tract. However, the physician should be alert for indications of other systemic conditions that may cause fluid losses through the gastrointestinal tract, such as diabetes mellitus, increased intracranial pressure, or gastrointestinal obstruction. Other causes of dehydration are presented in Table 6.

TABLE 5. **Gastrointestinal Losses of Water and Electrolytes**

Fluid	Na (mEq/L)	K (mEq/L)	Cl (mEq/L)	HCO_3 (mEq/L)
Gastric juice	50	5–15	110	0
Pancreatic juice	140	5	75	110
Small bowel	140	5	110	30
Ileostomy	130	10	110	30
Diarrhea	50–140	5–15	55–110	15–50

Modified from Feld FG, Kaskel RJ, and Schoeneman MJ: The approach to fluid and electrolyte therapy in pediatrics. Adv Pediatr 35:497–536, 1988.

TABLE 6. **Causes of Dehydration in Children**

Inadequate intake
- Altered mental status (comatose, lethargic)
- Physical impairment (debilitated, restrained)
- Altered thirst (central nervous system lesion)
- Dysphagia

Excessive insensible water loss
- Fever
- Burns
- Cystic fibrosis
- Sweating
- Increased ambient temperature
- Hyperventilation

Increased gastrointestinal loss
- Vomiting
- Diarrhea
- Ileostomy

Increased renal water loss
- Osmotic diuresis (diabetes mellitus, mannitol, glycerol)
- Diabetes insipidus (central or renal)
- Renal tubular concentrating defect (sickle cell disease, hypokalemia, hypercalcemia, congenital nephropathy)

Modified from Feld LG: Parenteral fluid therapy for infants and children. *In* Rakel RE (ed): Conn's Current Therapy, Philadelphia, WB Saunders, 1993, pp 589–595.

When evaluating a child with fluid losses, attention to several important questions and concepts are helpful in guiding the formulation of an appropriate therapeutic response.

1. Is the child dehydrated, and if so, how much fluid has he or she lost?
2. Is there an osmolar (usually sodium) disturbance accompanying the fluid loss?
3. Is there an acid-base disturbance accompanying the fluid loss?
4. Is there a potassium abnormality accompanying the fluid loss?
5. Is the renal response to the fluid deficit appropriate?

All dehydrated infants should be evaluated with consideration of these points.

Volume Deficits

Unfortunately, there is usually no precise mechanism that can be used to assess fluid volume deficits accurately in dehydrated children. The most accurate method requires a knowledge of the child's body weight immediately prior to the onset of the disease process causing the volume deficit; however, this information is frequently not available. If it is, the amount of water lost in an acute illness (or, more accurately, the percentage of dehydration) can then be estimated in percentages as:

$$\text{Degree of dehydration (\%)} = \frac{\text{Pre-illness weight} - \text{Admission weight}}{\text{Pre-illness weight}} \times 100$$

Because pre-illness body weight is not always available, estimations of the percentage of body weight lost (as fluid) are based on a careful bedside examination of the child as well as on historical information provided by the child's parent or caretaker. Items included in this evaluation are listed in Table 7. The most reliable signs used in estimating severity of dehydration are peripheral perfusion and skin turgor; lack of tears and dry mucous membranes are less reliable signs and may cause less experienced physicians to overestimate the degree of dehydration significantly.

With a real body volume deficit of 5%, 50 mL per kg body weight have been lost and need to be replaced. It must be re-emphasized that the great majority of these children do not need parenteral therapy and usually do very well with oral rehydration. Children with a 10% volume deficit have lost 100 mL per kg body weight, and children with a 15% volume deficit, who usually appear very ill, have lost 150 mL per kg body weight. Estimates of percentage of dehydration, although subjective in nature, provide a starting point for estimating the infant's or child's fluid needs. In addition, these percentages can be used to estimate the pre-illness weight. The difference between the pre-illness weight and the current weight in children with acute gastrointestinal illnesses generally reflects the amount of body fluid lost.

Example 2. A child is brought to the emergency room with a 2- to 3-day history of decreased appetite, poor fluid intake, and watery diarrhea. The last known weight was 37.5 pounds 1 week ago on a bathroom scale. No fever has been noted. The child has decreased urine output, a rapid pulse, dry mucous membranes, slightly decreased skin elasticity, and slight coolness of the skin; capillary refill time is about 2 seconds, and there is no skin mottling or cyanosis. Blood pressure is normal, and the child is responsive but is crying and slightly irritable. Based on the history and physical examination, you quickly estimate the amount of dehydration as about 10%. The current weight is 15.3 kg.

QUESTION 1. How would you calculate the fluid losses sustained by this patient?

ANSWER 1. If the bathroom scale was reasonably accurate (often they are not), the weight in pounds measured 1 week before the illness would correspond to about 17 kg. Seventeen kilograms minus the current weight indicates a weight loss (and therefore a fluid loss) of 1.7 kg. By this method, an exact loss of 10% of original pre-illness weight is esti-

TABLE 7. **Evidence of Dehydration on Physical Examination**

Signs and Symptoms	Mild	Moderate	Severe
Body weight loss			
Infant <20 kg	5%	10%	15%
Older child	3%	6%	9%
Mucous membranes	Normal	Dry	Very dry
Tears	Normal	Absent	Absent
Eyes	Normal	Sunken	Very sunken
Urine output	Normal	Decreased	Scant or none
Blood pressure	Normal	Normal or increased	Low
Heart rate	Normal or slightly increased	Increased or orthostatic changes	Increased; often thready pulses
Capillary refill time	Normal (<2 sec)	Normal or increased	Increased (>2 sec)
Skin elasticity	Normal retraction	Slow retraction	Delayed retraction, tenting

mated, and 1.7 liters of fluid should be replaced (along with maintenance fluids and ongoing losses).

If the prior weight is unknown, it can be estimated based on the physical examination findings indicating 10% dehydration using the formula:

$$\frac{\text{X (Rehydrated weight)}}{\text{Current weight}} = \frac{100}{100 - \text{Estimated percent dehydration}}$$

In this patient, this would be:

$$\frac{\text{X}}{15.3 \text{ kg}} = \frac{100}{90}$$

Therefore, X = 17 kg. Again, 17 kg minus 15.3 kg would give a weight (fluid) loss of 1.7 kg. Thus, deficit fluid replacement should include 1.7 liters, added to ongoing losses and maintenance fluids. Fluid loss due to diarrhea or vomiting also contains electrolytes, which should be estimated or measured and replaced.

Osmolar Disturbances

An infant's or child's dehydrated state is often divided into three different categories depending on the serum sodium concentration (or, more importantly, the osmolality, which is usually estimated by the serum sodium). In the most common form, isonatremic dehydration, the serum sodium concentration is normal or near normal (between 130 and 150 mEq per liter). In this situation, the amounts of water and electrolytes lost from the body are proportional in concentration to the concentrations present normally in the extracellular fluid, or in other words, hypotonic fluid is lost and replaced orally with hypotonic fluid, so that the serum sodium concentration remains "physiologic." Proportional sodium losses are estimated in Table 8.

Infants with hyponatremic dehydration are usually thought to have a greater loss of solute (sodium) relative to water loss. However, it seems likely that in many of these infants replacement of iso-osmolar losses is begun orally (or intravenously) with hypotonic solutions. Hypotonic dehydration tends to have a greater impact on the child because additional fluid is lost from the intravascular compartment into the now more hypertonic intracellular compartment to maintain osmolar equilibrium. These infants appear sicker and may have clinical evidence of shock out of proportion to the degree of fluid loss. The additional losses of sodium can be estimated by the formula:

$$(135 - \text{Serum sodium}) \times \text{Body weight in kg} \times 0.6$$

The formula 0.6 × body weight is used to estimate the body water distribution of sodium.

TABLE 8. **Estimated (Proportional) Deficits in Children with Dehydration**

Degree of Dehydration	Water (mL/kg)	Na (mEq/kg)	K (mEq/kg)	Cl (mEq/kg)
5%	50	4	3	3
10%	100	8	6	6
15%	150	12	9	9

In children with hypernatremic dehydration, who have had a proportionately greater loss of water than sodium, the osmolality of the intravascular and extracellular fluid spaces will rise. This causes a shift of fluid from the intracellular compartment to the extracellular compartment, thus helping to maintain intravascular volume and organ perfusion. These children appear ill but have fewer overt signs of dehydration and are much less likely to be in a shocklike state. With the shift of intracellular water to the extracellular space, the brain cells begin to produce new osmoles ("idiogenic" osmoles such as taurine), which serve to reduce additional water loss. These new osmoles are important in formulating therapy for hypernatremic dehydration. Osmolar differences can sometimes be determined based on physical examination findings as outlined in Table 9.

Acid-Base Abnormalities

Infants and children who have had a diarrheal illness for several days are very likely to have a simple normal anion gap metabolic acidosis due to stool losses of bicarbonate ions and renal "retention" of chloride anion to maintain electrochemical neutrality. This acidosis, even if severe (with serum bicarbonate levels of less than 15 mEq per liter), rarely requires the addition of alkali to the parenteral replacement fluid. If alkali administration is considered necessary, inclusion in the parenteral fluid rather than "bolus" administration of hypertonic sodium bicarbonate seems more reasonable. In addition, children with prolonged lack of enteral feeding and fluids may develop ketosis, which will create a high anion gap acidosis, or, in extreme cases, patients may have such poor perfusion that a lactic acidosis develops. These children are best treated by replacing intravascular volume without the addition of intravenous alkali therapy. Infants with chronic lung disease or sepsis-induced respiratory depression may have a mixed respiratory acidosis along with a metabolic acidosis, and ventilatory assistance may be needed. Other, more complex acid-base abnormalities may be present, and these often require the simultaneous assessment of serum chemistries (with the anion gap), blood gases, and urinalysis (occasionally with urine chemistries and urinary anion gap).

TABLE 9. **Osmolar Disturbances—Physical Examination Findings**

Signs and Symptoms	Hyponatremic	Isonatremic	Hypernatremic
Mental status	Very lethargic	Lethargic	Very irritable
Capillary refill time	>3 sec	1.5–3.0 sec	Normal–3.0 sec
Skin texture	Moist, clammy	Dry	Doughy
Blood pressure	Low (for age)	Normal or orthostatic	Normal or orthostatic
Heart rate	Markedly increased	Increased	Orthostatic or somewhat increased

Potassium Abnormalities

Most infants with diarrheal dehydration or dehydration secondary to vomiting and poor oral fluid intake have total body potassium deficiencies. Estimates of typical sodium and potassium deficiencies in various types of dehydration are given in Table 8. It should be noted that the serum potassium level is a relatively poor indicator of total body potassium and may appear normal or even slightly high owing to the presence of acidosis. If the serum potassium level is high and the patient is oliguric or anuric, the possibility of acute renal failure should be considered. Potassium is usually added to intravenous fluids after urinary voiding is established on admission to the hospital. If the child is oliguric secondary to dehydration or shock and is also hypokalemic, a small dose of potassium may be given (for example, 0.3 to 0.5 mEq per kg) over 1 to 3 hours. Cardiac conduction abnormalities are unusual in children with hypokalemia and may involve conduction delays and heart block. These children should be treated with parenteral potassium, and continuous monitoring of the electrocardiogram and frequent serum or plasma potassium levels should be performed. As a general guideline, potassium should not be added to parenteral fluids until the presence of urinary voiding has been established.

Renal Function in Children with Dehydration

The major differential diagnosis in infants with oliguria remains "pre-renal" azotemia, usually due to dehydration, or intrinsic renal insufficiency (as in acute tubular necrosis). Several "indices" have been proposed, and these are indeed useful in distinguishing between pre-renal oliguria and oliguria due to acute renal failure (Table 10). The most used indicator is the fractional excretion of sodium (FE_{Na}), which conceptually is the clearance of sodium divided by the glomerular filtration rate estimated by creatinine clearance, multiplied by 100:

$$FE_{Na} = \frac{U(Na)/P(Na)}{U(Cr)/P(Cr)} \times 100$$

U(Na) and P(Na) are urine and plasma concentrations of sodium, and U(Cr) and P(Cr) are urine and plasma concentrations of creatinine, respectively. A FE_{Na} of less than 1 to 2% suggests pre-renal azotemia; numbers greater than 2 to 3% suggest acute renal insufficiency. Patients with acute renal insufficiency resulting from primary glomerular disease who have intact renal tubular function may initially have a low urinary sodium and a low FE_{Na}.

THERAPY

Intravenous maintenance fluid therapy has been described previously. Several phases of fluid therapy are usually considered when treating children with dehydration. These phases include:

1. Emergency Fluids. If an infant or child is severely dehydrated and has impaired peripheral perfusion or other evidence of shock, emergency management is needed, including the rapid administration of isotonic fluid (regardless of subsequent serum sodium determinations). Usually between 10 and 20 mL per kg body weight of isotonic saline or lactated Ringer's solution is given as rapidly as possible (usually over 10 to 20 minutes) as the patient is being monitored, perfusion and vital signs are assessed, and other diagnostic and therapeutic interventions are considered. The great majority of children with dehydration do not require this phase of therapy.

2. Maintenance Fluids and Electrolytes. All children on intravenous fluid therapies require maintenance fluids. For most children, these may be calculated as described previously. In children with hypernatremic dehydration, maintenance fluids are modified as described later.

3. Ongoing Losses. In many children with diseases causing diarrhea and vomiting a significant reduction, and often complete cessation, of these fluid losses occurs after intravenous therapy is started and oral intake is reduced or eliminated. However, in some disease states ongoing losses of fluids from liquid stools, vomitus, nasogastric drainage, and other sources may occur and must be replaced. The electrolyte content of these losses should be measured and replaced appropriately; estimates of these losses are given in Table 5.

4. Deficit Fluids and Electrolytes. The amount of fluid lost by the child is sometimes difficult to estimate. The best data are obtained from body weight measurements taken on the same scale; however, many previously healthy children who develop an intestinal infection with resultant diarrhea and dehydration have not had an accurate or recent body weight assessment. Therefore, the degree of deficit should be estimated by the physical examination criteria outlined in Table 7, and fluid should be given accordingly. The electrolyte losses depend on the osmolar state of the child, and these can be estimated by the values given in Table 8.

TABLE 10. **Renal Failure Indices**

Laboratory Parameter	Pre-Renal Oliguria	Acute Renal Failure/Tubular Necrosis
Urine Na (mEq/L)	<15	>40
Urine osmolality (mOsm/L)	>500	<350
U/P osmolality	>2	<1.2
U/P creatinine	>20	<10
FE_{Na} (%)	<2	>3

Abbreviation: U/P = Urine values divided by plasma values (must be the same units (e.g., mg/dL for creatinine).

ISONATREMIC (ISOTONIC) DEHYDRATION

Most infants with dehydration are found to be isonatremic; the fluid lost from the extracellular space contains sodium and potassium in proportional amounts, or, more likely, hypotonic fluids lost through the gastrointestinal tract are replaced with similarly hypotonic oral fluids. Table 8 describes the usual sodium and potassium deficits in children with isonatremic dehydration.

Example 3. A previously well toddler developed diarrhea and occasional vomiting and had decreased oral intake of food and fluids. This persisted for several days, and the parents took the child to an emergency room. The child is noted to have dry mucous membranes, slight tenting of the skin, slightly sunken eyes, and no tears; capillary refill time is about 2 seconds. The child is still voiding but in small amounts and less frequently than usual, and the urine has a specific gravity of 1.032. Serum chemistries show a sodium concentration of 134 mEq per liter, potassium 3.8 mEq per liter, chloride 114 mEq per liter, bicarbonate 14 mEq per liter, serum urea nitrogen 32 mg/dL, and creatinine 1.0 mg/dL. You estimate that the child has about a 10% dehydration; no recent body weights are available for comparison. The child's current weight is 15.3 kg, his blood pressure is 100/62 mmHg, and his heart rate is 130 beats per minute.

QUESTION 1. Does this child need emergency fluids?

ANSWER 1. Probably not. Although the child is clearly dehydrated, capillary refill and blood pressure are normal, heart rate is slightly high, and the child is voiding a concentrated urine.

QUESTION 2. Calculate the fluid deficit, the maintenance fluid requirements, electrolyte deficits, and maintenance electrolyte requirements and decide on the appropriate intravenous fluid to be administered.

ANSWER 2. The fluid deficit (see Example 2) is 1700 mL, and the sodium deficit is about 136 mEq (see Table 8; with 10% dehydration the sodium deficit is 8 mEq per kg). Maintenance fluid requirements (based on rehydrated weight; see Example 1) are 1350 mL per day, with a maintenance sodium requirement of 33.75 mEq. The total fluid volume is 3050 mL per day, and the total sodium requirement (deficit plus maintenance) is 169.75 mEq per day. The fluid to be administered will be 5% dextrose with 53 mEq of sodium per liter, which is very close to the commercially available solution known as D5 one-third normal saline. In most dehydrated children a potassium deficit exists, and after urinary voiding has been established, potassium can be added to the parenteral fluids. Maintenance potassium has been described (see Example 1) and is 33.75 mEq. Potassium loss in the diarrheal stools can be estimated (see Table 8) as 102 mEq. Total potassium to be added is 135.75 mEq; this would be just over 40 mEq of potassium added to a liter of parenteral fluids (40 mEq of potassium chloride is usually the largest amount of potassium added to intravenous fluids on a "routine" basis; with more severe acidosis, potassium acetate may be considered). A combination of replacement fluid plus maintenance fluids results in an intravenous infusion rate of 127 mL per hour (which can be rounded off to 130 mL per hour), given for 24 hours.

QUESTION 3. What should be monitored in this child after parenteral fluid therapy is begun?

ANSWER 3. The personnel providing this child's care should continue to monitor vital signs, body weight, blood pressure, peripheral perfusion, and mental status and should examine the child frequently, paying special attention to auscultation of the lungs and heart. Urine and stool output should be measured and recorded on a bedside chart; the assessment of urine specific gravity may also be helpful. When the child is ready (often after less than 24 hours), oral fluids should be introduced and parenteral fluids reduced accordingly. If the child is not able to resume oral fluids within 24 hours, reassessment of serum electrolytes, urea nitrogen, and creatinine is reasonable.

HYPONATREMIC DEHYDRATION

A large number of disorders can result in hyponatremia; if the clinical history is not available or is unclear, it may be useful to assess serum osmolality to differentiate between the usual hypotonic hyponatremia seen with gastrointestinal fluid losses and the isotonic "pseudo-hyponatremia" that occurs in individuals with severe hyperlipidemia or hyperproteinemias. This will also exclude the unusual child who has hypertonic hyponatremia due to hyperglycemia or ingestion of mannitol or glycerol. Volume status should be assessed in all children, and dividing the hypotonic hyponatremias into hypovolemic, euvolemic, and hypervolemic states will help in determining the underlying reason for the hyponatremia as well as the appropriate therapy (Fig. 1). It is also helpful to measure urinary sodium in these patients. Because hypovolemic hyponatremia secondary to gastrointestinal losses of fluids (often with hypotonic fluids given orally contributing to the hyponatremia) is by far the most common pediatric scenario for hyponatremia, discussion will be limited to that example.

Example 4. A previously well 10-kg infant with diarrhea and vomiting is found on examination in the emergency room to weigh 9 kg and to have sunken eyes, poor capillary refill (3 to 4 seconds), dry mucous membranes, and significant lethargy and irritability. Blood pressure is 55/38 mm Hg, and heart rate is 140 beats per minute. Laboratory evaluation includes a serum sodium concentration of 125 mEq per liter, potassium 4.1 mEq per liter, chloride 115 mEq per liter, and bicarbonate 9 mEq per liter.

QUESTION 1. Does this child need emergency fluids?

ANSWER 1. Yes. This child has evidence of poor perfusion with altered mental status, poor capillary refill, and decreased blood pressure. The usual emergency fluids are 20 mL per kg of isotonic saline or lactated Ringer's solution given rapidly (over 10 to 15 minutes) and repeated if the response is not sufficient.

QUESTION 2. Calculate the fluid and electrolyte replacement requirements appropriate for this child, after seeing that the child responds to the first infusion of 20 mL per kg of isotonic saline with a decrease in heart rate to 110 beats per minute, an increase in blood pressure to 88/50 mm Hg, and a decrease in capillary refill to about 2 seconds.

ANSWER 2. The maintenance fluid requirement for a child whose rehydrated weight is 10 kg is 1000 mL (see Table 3); this child is 10% dehydrated. The maintenance sodium requirement is 25 mEq (2.5 mEq of sodium per 100 kcal). Because the child lost one kg of body weight (or 10%), the fluid deficit is 1000 mL. Proportional sodium losses (as in isonatremic dehydration) are given in Table 8 and in this example are

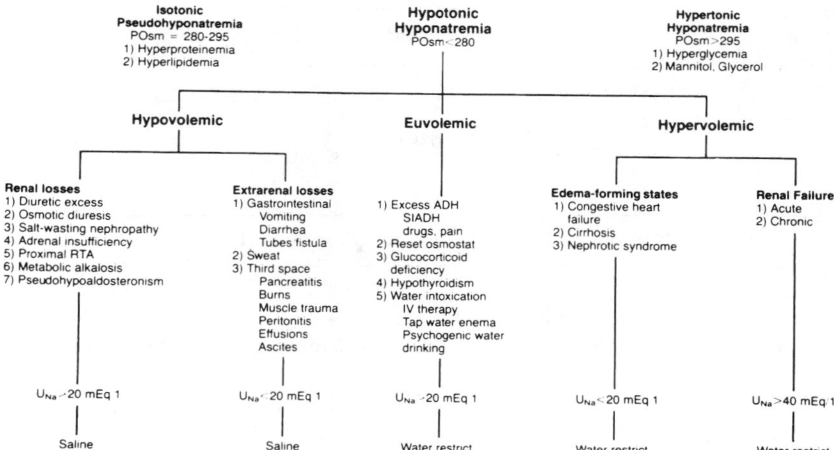

Figure 1. Diagnosis and treatment of hyponatremia. (From Berry PL, Belsha CW: Hyponatremia. Pediatr Clin North Am *37*[2]:354, 1990.)

80 mEq. Additional sodium losses are calculated using the sodium deficit formula:

$$(135 - 125) \times 10 \times 0.6 = 60 \text{ mEq sodium}$$

The 24-hour fluid and sodium requirements are then 2000 mL of fluid and 25 + 80 + 60 = 165 mEq of sodium. The final solution would then be 5% dextrose with 82.5 mEq sodium per liter; most children with hyponatremic dehydration have significant potassium deficits, and 40 mEq of potassium (as the chloride salt) can be added to the parenteral fluids after urinary voiding occurs. This parenteral solution is very close to the commercially available 5% dextrose with one-half normal saline. The infusion rate in this child would be 84 mL per hour (2000 mL given over 24 hours).

HYPERNATREMIC DEHYDRATION

Causes of hypernatremia are listed in Table 11; central and nephrogenic diabetes insipidus as well as diabetes mellitus are usually easily recognized based on clinical and laboratory findings. The loss of hypotonic fluid without adequate water intake is the most common cause of hypernatremic dehydration. In these children, both sodium and water are lost from the body, but water content is decreased proportionately more than sodium content. In several reports a higher than normal content of breast milk sodium may have contributed to hypernatremia. In most children, loss of sodium in diarrheal stool ranges between 30 and 65 mEq per liter; if oral intake is limited, these losses will result in both sodium and water losses from the body, with water in excess of sodium, and hypernatremia may occur. The importance of replacing fluid deficits slowly and adjusting maintenance fluids appropriately cannot be overemphasized; giving fluids too rapidly frequently results in a sudden decline in serum sodium and then in seizure activity. In some cases, permanent neurologic sequelae may result from hypernatremic dehydration and its therapy.

Example 5. A child previously weighing 10 kg develops diarrhea and occasional vomiting. He becomes very irritable and begins a high-pitched crying. The skin has a "doughy" texture; mucous membranes are dry, and muscle tone seems somewhat increased. The child now weighs 9 kg, and serum electrolyte measurements include a sodium level of 165 mEq per liter. The child's blood pressure is 82 mm Hg systolic and 54 mm Hg diastolic, and heart rate is 125 beats per minute. Urine output has been described as very little for the past 36 hours.

QUESTION 1. Does this child require emergency fluids?

ANSWER 1. Probably. Although blood pressure is normal, the decrease in urine output and other physical signs suggest significant losses that may benefit from volume replacement. Children with hypernatremic dehydration may have a relative preservation of intravascular (extracellular) water because osmotic shifts result in fluid removal from the intracellular compartment to the extracellular space. Thus, typical signs of shock may be delayed or lessened for a given percentage of volume loss. In addition, individuals with hypernatremia have maximal secretion of antidiuretic hormone (arginine vasopressin). Although significant volume loss stimulates the secre-

TABLE 11. **Causes of Hypernatremia**

Water deficit in excess of sodium deficit
Diarrhea
Osmotic diuresis
Diabetes mellitus
Obstructive uropathy
Renal dysplasia
Water deficit
Diabetes insipidus
Central
Nephrogenic
Sweating
Increased insensible losses
Lack of access to water
Lack of thirst
Diabetes mellitus
Sodium excess
Improperly mixed infant formula
Ingestion of sea water
Excessive parenteral sodium administration

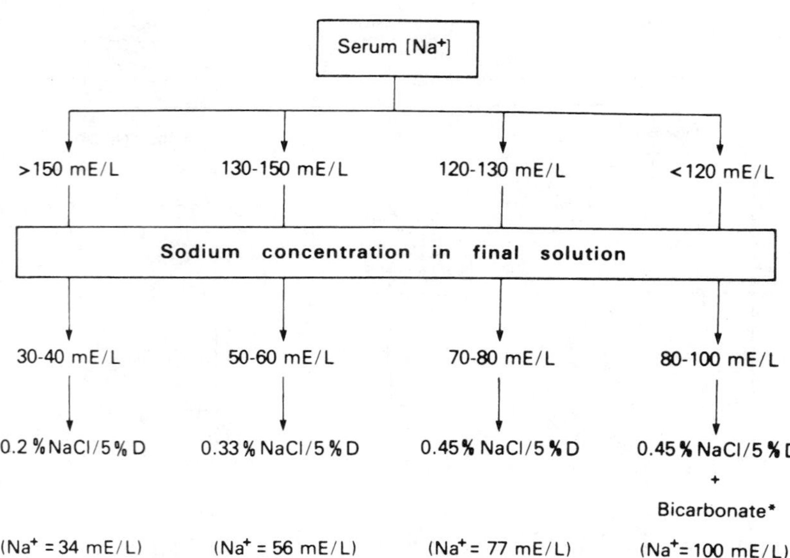

Figure 2. Decision tree for fluid therapy in children with diarrheal dehydration. (From Kallen RJ: The management of diarrheal dehydration in infants using parenteral fluids. Pediatr Clin North Am *37*[2]:274, 1990.)

tion of antidiuretic hormone, hyperosmolality stimulates it much sooner; thus, urine output will be low and cannot be considered an accurate assessment of intravascular volume status. It is probably reasonable to give 10 to 20 mL per kg of normal saline as a fluid bolus; however, many infants with hypernatremic dehydration may not require early vigorous fluid resuscitation.

QUESTION 2. How would you formulate maintenance and replacement fluid and electrolyte requirements for this infant?

ANSWER 2. Maintenance fluids in children with hypertonic dehydration should be modified. Remember that in the calculation of maintenance fluids, 55 mL per 100 calories metabolized are estimated to allow the excretion of urine that is neither maximally dilute nor maximally concentrated. With the strong antidiuretic hormone secretion from hyperosmolality, urine output is obligatorily small. It is therefore reasonable to allow 65 or 70 mL per 100 calories metabolized for maintenance water requirements. Studies have shown that 100 mL per 100 calories metabolized (which sounds like "normal" maintenance requirements) provides both maintenance and a small replacement requirement. The sodium content should be small (0.2 to 0.3% isotonic saline). When this fluid administration protocol was compared with those using more fluid and more sodium, or the same amount of fluid but more sodium, it was found that infants given the very hypotonic fluid recovered better very slowly and had a lower frequency of seizures and edema. Therefore, children with hypernatremic dehydration who are given calculated maintenance fluid volumes of low sodium (0.2% isotonic saline) usually do reasonably well and have less morbidity. Children with hypernatremia often develop hypocalcemia, and therapy with calcium chloride or calcium gluconate is then indicated. Some infants with hypernatremia also develop hyperglycemia; decreasing the dextrose concentration in the parenteral fluid to 2.5 grams per 100 mL (2.5% rather than 5% dextrose) is all that is usually necessary.

QUESTION 3. How often is follow-up evaluation needed for a child being treated for hypernatremic dehydration?

ANSWER 3. In general, these children should be monitored more frequently than children with isonatremic or hyponatremic dehydration. Because the rate of decline of serum sodium seems to be an important factor, one should aim for a reduction in serum

TABLE 12. **Guidelines for Oral Rehydration Therapy**

Patient Eligibility
All ages
Any cause of dehydration
Avoid if patient has:
  Shock or near shock
  Intractable vomiting ("ordinary" vomiting is not a contraindication)
  Altered mental status
Method
Estimate fluid deficit based on:
  Previous weight (if known)
  Percentage of dehydration (see Table 7)
Use rehydration solution
  Glucose content 2.0–2.5 gm/dL
  Sodium content 60–75 mEq/L
Give 6 to 8 hours of maintenance therapy plus deficit fluid volume over 6 to 8 hours
If stool losses continue, replace with rehydration formula
After rehydration, reassess. If still dehydrated, estimate deficit fluid, add maintenance fluids, and give over 6 to 8 hours
May breast feed
If rehydration is successful, change to maintenance formula
Do not use rehydration solution for more than 4–12 hours
If hypernatremic, give replacement fluids over 24 hours
Maintenance Phase
Use solution with 2.0–2.5 gm/dL glucose and 40 to 60 mEq/L sodium
Give as tolerated, making sure enough is taken to supply maintenance needs and ongoing losses
Offer half-strength formula within 24 hours after starting rehydration therapy; advance to full strength within 24 hours

sodium of 10 to 12 mEq per liter per day. It therefore seems reasonable to obtain serum electrolyte measurements every 2 to 8 hours, depending on the original serum sodium level and the clinical response to intravenous fluid therapy. It should also be remembered that urine output may be low until the serum sodium level is near the normal range despite fluid administration (due to antidiuretic hormone stimulation and activity); in this case, urine output is not an adequate assessment of the results of therapy. As mentioned earlier, calcium and glucose should be assessed at the beginning of therapy and once or twice a day during therapy; some patients need supplemental calcium. The dextrose concentration in the parenteral fluid may have to be reduced if the child becomes hyperglycemic. Finally, for most of these children potassium should be added to the parenteral fluid at 20 to 40 mEq per liter.

SUMMARY OF FLUID NEEDS IN DEHYDRATION

A simplified approach to fluid therapy for children with diarrheal dehydration is presented in the decision tree shown in Figure 2. With this approach the physician needs to calculate the fluid volume required for maintenance needs and calculated deficits; the type of fluid to be given then depends on the measured serum sodium level as shown in Figure 2. The type of parenteral fluids needed in children with various types of dehydration are fairly standard, and this decision-tree approach is quite useful. Again, it should be emphasized that oral fluids should be given whenever possible. The advantages of oral rehydration therapy seem obvious, i.e., lower cost, less need for hospitalization, and reduced need for intravenous access. General guidelines for oral fluid rehydration are presented in Table 12.

Section 8

The Endocrine System

ACROMEGALY

method of
MARK E. MOLITCH, M.D.
Northwestern University Medical School
Chicago, Illinois

PRETREATMENT EVALUATION

Acromegaly is an insidious disorder that is usually present for years before the diagnosis is made. It is important to establish the activity of the disease prior to instituting therapy for two reasons: (1) A small percentage of growth hormone (GH)–secreting tumors undergo spontaneous infarction. This causes the condition known as "burned out" or "fugitive" acromegaly, in which GH levels are normal by the time the diagnosis is made and no therapy is indicated. (2) Tumor activity post-therapy can then be compared with that documented pre-therapy to determine whether additional treatment is needed.

The definition of an abnormal basal serum GH level has been difficult to ascertain because of the low sensitivity of the GH radioimmunoassay and the episodic secretion of GH. Some patients with active acromegaly may have basal GH levels of less than 5 nanograms per milliliter. Except for the episodic secretory surges, a level of 2 nanograms per milliliter may well be the upper limit of normal for basal GH levels. For establishing the diagnosis and clinical activity of acromegaly it is necessary to document both an elevated basal level of GH and a failure to suppress GH levels to less than 2 nanograms per milliliter with an oral glucose load. Elevation of levels of insulin-like growth factor I (IGF-I, also known as somatomedin C) has also become accepted as a criterion for the diagnosis of active acromegaly. IGF-I levels correlate with indices of disease activity better than GH levels in most but not all studies.

About 35 to 40% of patients with acromegaly have elevated prolactin (PRL) levels. Uncommonly, patients present with symptoms caused by hyperprolactinemia, such as decreased libido, impotence, galactorrhea, or amenorrhea, rather than the normal symptoms of acromegaly.

Almost all patients with acromegaly have GH-secreting pituitary adenomas. The size and degree of any extrasellar extension of the adenoma are assessed by magnetic resonance imaging (MRI) or, when that is unavailable, high-resolution computed tomography (CT) scanning. Compression of the optic chiasm by the adenoma can be determined with Goldmann visual field testing. About 80% of patients have macroadenomas (more than 10 mm in diameter) and 15 to 20% have suprasellar extension of the adenoma. Large adenomas may cause hypopituitarism by directly compressing the normal pituitary or interfering with stalk function. Less commonly, such large adenomas may cause diabetes insipidus (DI). A detailed evaluation of anterior and posterior pituitary function will determine whether hormone replacement is necessary.

Acromegaly may cause hypertension, diabetes mellitus, and a hypertrophic cardiomyopathy. Colonic adenomatous polyps and colon cancer occur more frequently than expected, especially in males, those over the age of 50 years, and those with more than six skin tags. Should surgery be chosen as therapy, these complications may need assessment and treatment preoperatively.

Rarely, no evidence of pituitary adenoma is found, and, if surgery is performed, hyperplasia of the somatotropes may be found. Such patients may have a syndrome in which GH-releasing hormone (GHRH) is being secreted by a pancreatic, carcinoid, hypothalamic, or other tumor. If one of these GHRH-secreting tumors is suspected, GHRH blood levels can be measured.

Virtually all GH-secreting adenomas arise de novo in the pituitary and are not due to underlying hypothalamic dysfunction. In about 40% of cases mutations have been found in the guanine nucleotide regulatory protein that couples the GHRH receptor to adenylyl cyclase, resulting in a constitutive unregulated stimulation of the somatotropes to secrete GH. In other cases, the specific mutations causing the tumors have not been identified. The clinical importance of these findings with respect to therapeutic goals lies in the fact that once a tumor is ablated in its entirety, it is not expected to recur because of some underlying hypothalamic dysfunction.

Goals of therapy include (1) elimination of effects due to the mass of the tumor (hypopituitarism, visual field defects, and so on), (2) reduction of elevated GH levels to normal; (3) amelioration of the end-organ effects of the elevated GH levels; (4) avoidance of damage to remaining normal hypothalamic or pituitary function; and (5) reduction of other potential adverse effects of therapy.

TREATMENT

Transsphenoidal Adenomectomy

Transsphenoidal surgery offers the patient a chance for cure. Even when "cure" is not achieved, surgery may effect a significant reduction in GH levels and considerable amelioration of clinical symptoms. As expected, the smaller the tumor and the lower the basal GH levels, the better the surgical result. The actual cure rates depend on the criteria used. Using the criterion of postoperative GH levels of less than 5 nanograms per milliliter, "cure" rates of 60 to 80% can be expected for intrasellar lesions and 40 to 50% for larger tumors when the operation is performed by experienced neurosurgeons. Adding criteria such as suppressibility by glucose, nonresponsiveness to thyrotropin-releasing hormone (TRH), basal GH levels of less than 2 nanograms per milliliter, and normal IGF-I levels substantially reduces these numbers. Relapses occur in 5 to 10% of patients who initially achieve GH levels of less than 5 nanograms per milliliter.

With microadenomas, the risks of surgery are very small. The mortality from surgery approaches that of anesthesia alone. Transient DI may occur in 10 to 20% of patients, but it is rare for the patient to need treatment following discharge from the hospital. Hypopituitarism occurs in less than 1% of patients, and other complications such as meningitis and cerebrospinal fluid leak also occur in less than 1%. The total complication rate for this surgery by an experienced pituitary neurosurgeon, except for transient DI, is less than 3%.

The complication rate is higher for larger tumors. Because acromegaly carries a twofold excess mortality, primarily cardiovascular, one should consider whether in some patients with big tumors the normal pituitary should be sacrificed in an effort to remove the adenoma in toto. This decision must be made on an individual basis, and the risk of hypopituitarism should be weighed against the potential benefit of a better chance at total tumor removal.

Rarely, patients with very large tumors may need craniotomy and a subfrontal lobe approach. This may be necessary if the tumor has a large suprasellar extension with a dumbbell configuration. Risks are much higher with craniotomy, and mortality reaches 5% in some series.

Pituitary function tested 6 to 8 weeks postoperatively determines whether the patient is cured or whether there is persistent GH hypersecretion. Testing involves obtaining basal GH and IGF-I levels and showing suppression of GH with glucose. Patients who appear to be cured need to be followed to detect potential relapse. Testing of other pituitary functions will detect other hormonal deficiencies that may need treatment. We routinely place patients with macroadenomas on maintenance glucocorticoids (5 to 7.5 mg daily of prednisone) until this time of postoperative testing in case loss of adrenocorticotropic hormone (ACTH) function has occurred. Because loss of ACTH is very unlikely following surgery for microadenomas, we usually do not prescribe maintenance glucocorticoids for these patients unless the patient is symptomatic or is found to be deficient on the formal testing carried out at 6 to 8 weeks.

Irradiation

Conventional irradiation, given at a dose of 4500 to 5000 cGy through two or three fields over 5 weeks will lower GH levels substantially in over 80% of patients. The destructive effects of the irradiation are cumulative over time, levels of GH continuing to decrease for up to 20 years of follow-up. GH levels decrease to less than 5 nanograms per milliliter in 15 to 20% of treated cases by 2 years, in about 40% by 5 years, and in about 70% of patients by 10 years. Because the progressive reduction in GH levels appears to be a percentage function regardless of the initial GH levels or tumor size, it is obvious that the lower the initial GH levels the faster GH levels will return to normal.

At the same time that irradiation affects tumor function it also affects the normal pituitary. By 10 years after irradiation, about 20% of patients are hypothyroid, 35 to 40% are hypoadrenal, and about 50% are hypogonadal.

During irradiation therapy some patients complain of fatigue. If a patient is deficient in ACTH and is taking glucocorticoid replacement therapy, a doubling of the glucocorticoid dose is sometimes needed during radiation therapy. In some patients, irradiation may cause subtle but permanent cognitive and short-term memory deficits. Patients may complain of difficulty in concentrating, poor memory, and lack of initiative.

Tumor infarction is more common following irradiation. Tumor infarction usually causes a sudden onset of severe headache and often coma and vascular collapse, a syndrome referred to as "pituitary apoplexy." CT or MRI usually shows evidence of hemorrhage. Such patients must be supported with glucocorticoids in stress doses, and consideration should be given to emergency transsphenoidal decompression. Lesser degrees of tumor infarction may also occur, and the patient may have either no symptoms or a mild headache, evidence of infarction being found only later on scan or at surgery.

Proton beam therapy may offer some advantage over conventional irradiation in that it requires only a single large dose of irradiation and may have a somewhat better therapeutic benefit-risk ratio. With this treatment GH levels of less than 5 nanograms per milliliter are achieved in 28% by 2 years, 56% by 5 years, 76% by 10 years, and 93% by 20 years. Complications of proton beam therapy include diplopia resulting from oculomotor nerve dysfunction in 1.6%, visual field defects in 1.6%, and blindness in 0.2%. By 5 years after proton beam therapy, 10% of patients have developed hypothyroidism, 9% have adrenal insufficiency, and 7% have hypogonadism. As of 1994, such treatment is available only in Boston. Recently, patients have been treated with a new technique known as stereotactic radiosurgery ("gamma-knife"), in which radiation is also given as a single dose through hundreds of ports adjusted to the size and configuration of the tumor by computer analysis. Although this technique seems promising, at present there are few data available to show that it is better than conventional irradiation.

Medical Therapy

Dopamine Agonists. About 70 to 75% of patients respond to dopamine agonists such as bromocriptine (Parlodel) or pergolide (Permax) with some decrease of GH levels, although in only 10 to 20% do GH levels actually reach levels of less than 5 nanograms per milliliter. Despite only modest reductions in GH levels, substantial clinical improvement is sometimes seen, such as a reduction in ring size and improvement in glucose tolerance. In contrast to their documented high efficacy in shrinking the tumor size of PRL-secreting macroadenomas, dopamine agonists are much less effective in shrinking GH-secreting tumors. The dose needed to lower GH levels is much higher than that used to lower PRL levels. The effective daily dose of bromocriptine is usually in the 10- to 40-mg range given in divided doses, although doses greater than 30 mg are rarely necessary. The starting dose is 1.25 to 2.5 mg daily, given with a snack at bedtime to avoid nausea and orthostatic hypotension. The dose is raised by 2.5-mg increments every 2 to 4 days as tolerated. With each dose increase, nausea and lightheadedness may recur, but these symptoms usually resolve within 1 to 2 days. Constipation, digital vasospasm, nasal congestion, and alcohol intolerance may become problems at higher doses.

Patients who do not tolerate or respond to bromocriptine may rarely respond to pergolide, another dopamine agonist that has not been approved at the time of this writing for the treatment of acromegaly by the Food and Drug Administration (FDA). When patients do not respond to dopamine agonists, they are then given octreotide.

Octreotide. A somatostatin analogue, octreotide (Sandostatin),* has a 40-fold greater activity in suppressing GH compared to insulin. After subcutaneous injection, octreotide causes an acute decrease in GH levels, the nadir occurring within 2 to 3 hours and the suppressive effects lasting for 6 to 12 hours. Long-term studies suggest that substantial reductions of GH and IGF-I occur in 80 to 90% of patients, and IGF-I levels can be brought into the normal range in about 60%. In most cases a dosing frequency of every 6 to 8 hours is usually necessary, beginning at 100 μg at each dose and increasing as necessary up to 1500 μg per day. In some patients, more frequent administration, such as every 2 hours using a pump, will provide more sustained lowering of GH levels at lower octreotide doses. Some patients respond better to the combination of octreotide plus bromocriptine than to either drug alone. CT and MRI scans have demonstrated tumor size reduction as a result of therapy in about 20% of patients.

Side effects include mild abdominal bloating, nausea, moderate diarrhea, steatorrhea, and gastritis related to *Helicobacter pylori.* Cholelithiasis due to poor gallbladder contractility occurs in 5 to 20% of patients.

CONCLUSIONS

In patients with microadenomas and intrasellar macroadenomas, transsphenoidal surgery offers a 60 to 80% chance of cure, depending on the experience of the neurosurgeon. The recurrence rate after apparent cure is less than 10%. Thus, this appears to be the best choice of primary therapy for such patients. In patients with larger tumors with lower chances of cure, surgery may still result in a considerable debulking of the tumor with a concomitant reduction in GH levels. Preliminary studies suggest that a 3- to 6-month course of octreotide to reduce tumor size may be beneficial in some patients. Because radiotherapy appears to cause a fractional rate of decrease in GH levels, the lower the initial GH level, the more rapidly this mode of treatment results in decreasing GH levels to normal. This appears to hold true regardless of whether GH levels were low to begin with or were low as a result of prior surgery. Thus, an operation performed before radiotherapy also appears to be beneficial for larger tumors. Because radiotherapy may take 5 to 10 years to bring GH levels to normal, I believe it should be regarded as a second-line therapy to be used if an operation does not result in cure or is contraindicated. Bromocriptine, other dopamine agonists, and octreotide are best reserved for patients not cured by surgery or radiotherapy or in whom ablative therapy is contraindicated. Additionally, these drugs may be useful while the patient awaits the eventual destructive effects of irradiation.

*Octreotide has not been approved by the FDA for this indication.

ADRENOCORTICAL INSUFFICIENCY

method of
WILLIAM F. YOUNG, JR., M.D.
Mayo Medical School
Rochester, Minnesota

Clinical recognition and appropriate management of adrenocortical insufficiency are lifesaving, but misdiagnosis or inappropriate management can be fatal. The disease is referred to as "primary" adrenal insufficiency (or Addison's disease) when it is caused by a disease or disorder of the adrenal glands. "Secondary" adrenal insufficiency is caused by adrenocorticotropin (ACTH) deficiency due to hypothalamic-pituitary insufficiency. The causes of primary and secondary adrenal insufficiency are listed in Table 1. The most common forms of primary and secondary adrenal insufficiency are autoimmune adrenal disease and recent exogenous glucocorticoid therapy, respectively.

TABLE 1. **Causes of Adrenocortical Insufficiency**

Causes
Primary adrenal insufficiency (Addison's disease)
Autoimmune
Hemorrhagic
Infectious
Fungal
Human immunodeficiency virus
Bacterial
Enzymatic deficiencies
Congenital: 21-, 11-, or 17-hydroxylase
Iatrogenic: ketoconazole, metyrapone, aminogluthethimide
Surgical: bilateral adrenalectomy
Metastatic disease
Secondary adrenal insufficiency (ACTH deficiency)
Exogenous glucocorticoid withdrawal
Pituitary or hypothalamic tumors
Iatrogenic
Hypophysectomy
Sellar radiation
Lymphocytic hypophysitis
Granulomatous disease
Sarcoidosis
Histoplasmosis
Tuberculosis
Hemochromatosis
Hemorrhage

PRESENTATION

The recognition of adrenal insufficiency may be difficult because of the nonspecific nature of its symptoms. Adrenal insufficiency should be considered in patients with unexplained weakness, weight loss, and hypotension, especially in the following clinical situations: (1) glucocorticoid therapy that has been administered within the last year, (2) acquired immune deficiency syndrome [AIDS], (3) metastatic malignancy, (4) failure of one or more endocrine glands, and (5) coagulopathy or administration of anticoagulant therapy.

The presentation of adrenal insufficiency is determined by the clinical setting, rate of onset, and whether it is primary or secondary. The presentation of acute adrenal insufficiency, or adrenal crisis, is dominated by dehydration and cardiovascular collapse. In most patients, adrenal insufficiency develops gradually, with symptoms of muscle weakness, myalgias, fatigue, weight loss, anorexia, emesis, diarrhea, abdominal pain, postural hypotension, hyponatremia, and fasting hypoglycemia. The hyponatremia is dilutional in nature and is caused by inappropriate secretion of antidiuretic hormone and decreased renal free-water clearance. ACTH has a melanocyte-stimulating effect, and patients with primary adrenal insufficiency (high ACTH levels) have a "muddy" type of hyperpigmentation (especially in the palmar creases and over the extensor surfaces) and tan easily in the sun. In contrast, secondary adrenal insufficiency (low ACTH levels) is associated with relative pallor and sun sensitivity. In addition to the cortisol deficiency associated with primary adrenal insufficiency, there is a loss of aldosterone and adrenal androgens. Therefore, primary adrenal insufficiency is also associated with hyponatremia and hyperkalemia. The loss of axillary and pubic hair in women is due to a deficiency of ACTH-dependent adrenal androgen secretion. Aldosterone secretion and normokalemia are maintained in secondary adrenal insufficiency because the renin-angiotensin-aldosterone axis is intact.

DIAGNOSIS

An accurate diagnosis is critical for both the immediate and lifelong treatment programs. In the emergent or acute clinical setting, patients with possible acute adrenal insufficiency, or adrenal crisis (dehydration and cardiovascular collapse), should be treated immediately (see later discussion), and the diagnostic evaluation should be postponed until after recovery. In the urgent or subacute clinical setting, blood may be drawn for measurement of cortisol and ACTH, and dexamethasone, 4 mg, may be given intravenously. Also, the short ACTH stimulation test may be performed (see later).

The condition of most patients is clinically stable, and treatment can be deferred until the results of diagnostic studies are available. If, in clinically stable patients, the 0800-hour plasma cortisol level is less than 10 μg/dL or the 24-hour urinary free cortisol is less than 50 μg, further studies are needed to establish the diagnosis of adrenal insufficiency. However, even these levels of plasma and urinary cortisol *do not exclude* the diagnosis of adrenal insufficiency (Fig. 1). The three most frequently used tests are the ACTH stimulation test, the metyrapone test, and the insulin-induced hypoglycemia test. First, the baseline level of plasma ACTH is determined and the short cosyntropin test is performed. Insulin-induced hypoglycemia testing is performed if the baseline level of plasma ACTH is low and the peak response to cosyntropin administration is subnormal or delayed. A subnormal glucocorticoid response to insulin-induced hypoglycemia confirms the diagnosis of hypothalamic-pituitary insufficiency. No further testing is necessary in patients with classic primary adrenal failure (e.g., hyperpigmentation, high baseline level of plasma ACTH, and lack of cortisol response to short cosyntropin stimulation). However, if the clinical presentation is atypical or the patient has received long-term glucocorticoid replacement therapy, then the 3- to 5-day ACTH stimulation test may be necessary to make a conclusive diagnosis of primary adrenal failure.

Testing Protocols

ACTH Stimulation Test. This test may be performed over 1 hour or 3 days. The short or rapid ACTH-stimulation test is carried out by administering synthetic α1,24-ACTH (cosyntropin) at a dosage of 250 μg (25 units) either intravenously or intramuscularly. Plasma cortisol levels are determined just before and at 30 and 60 minutes after cosyntropin administration. The normal response is defined by (1) baseline levels of plasma cortisol greater than 5 μg/dL, (2) an increment of at least 7 μg/dL over the baseline value, and (3) an increase in plasma cortisol to at least 18 μg/dL. Failure to meet these criteria suggests a deficiency at either the adrenal or hypothalamic-pituitary level. A baseline plasma ACTH determination is required to distinguish between these two possibilities. *Some patients with mild secondary adrenal insufficiency may respond normally to the rapid ACTH test.*

The 3- to 5-day ACTH stimulation test is required in equivocal cases and in patients who have received glucocorticoid replacement therapy for presumed primary adrenal failure that was never documented. 1,39-ACTH is administered in the form of Acthar gel, 40 units given intramuscularly twice daily for 3 to 5 days. Before the test, blood specimens are obtained to determine the baseline level of ACTH and cortisol and 24-hour urine specimens are obtained to determine the baseline level of free cortisol and creatinine. Blood specimens are collected daily during the test for measuring cortisol levels, and 24-hour urine collections are needed for measuring free cortisol and creatinine levels. If the patient has received long-term treatment with glucocorticoids, treatment should be discontinued at the start of the test. The patient instead receives dexamethasone (0.5 mg once or twice daily). If a subnormal glucocorticoid response is evident on the third day, the test should be continued for the full 5 days. A normal adrenocortical response is an increase in the serum cortisol level to more than 50 μg/dL and an increase in the urinary free cortisol level to two to four times the baseline value. Patients with primary adrenocortical insufficiency fail to demonstrate a normal response. Patients with secondary adrenocortical insufficiency have a delayed response but one that eventually reaches the criteria just outlined by day 5.

Insulin-Induced Hypoglycemia and Metyrapone Tests. Readers are referred to textbooks on endocrinology for the protocols of these two tests.

Imaging Studies. Imaging studies may reveal the cause of adrenal insufficiency. Computed tomographic adrenal or pituitary imaging is indicated in patients with confirmed primary or secondary adrenal insufficiency, respectively.

PRINCIPLES OF TREATMENT

Maintenance Therapy

ACTH is not used for replacement therapy because it requires parenteral administration, has a potential

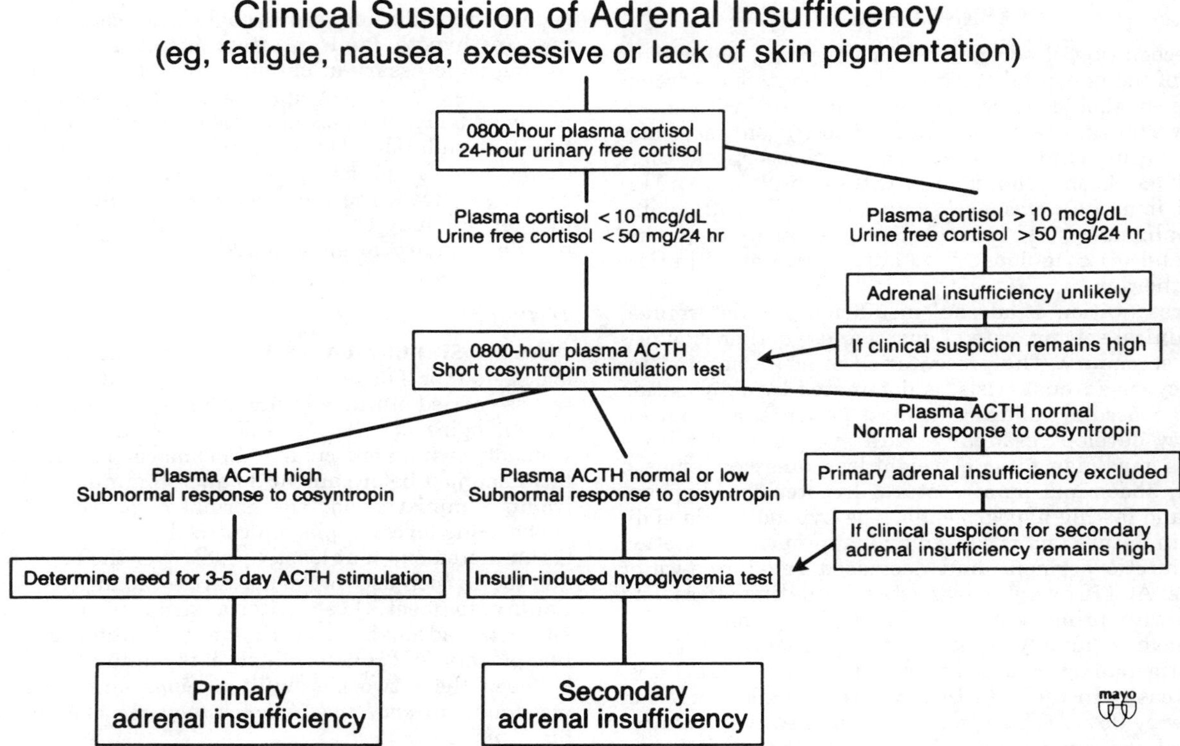

Figure 1. Algorithm for the diagnostic approach to patients with suspected adrenal insufficiency.

for allergic reactions, and is costly. Hydrocortisone (Hydrocortone), cortisone acetate (Cortone), and prednisone (Deltasone) are the most frequently used preparations in standard replacement therapy. The catabolism of synthetic steroids is affected by interindividual variability and the effects of concomitantly administered drugs. I prefer the major glucocorticoid secreted by the adrenal cortex, hydrocortisone. In an attempt to replicate the normal glucocorticoid circadian rhythm, two-thirds of the glucocorticoid dose (hydrocortisone, 20 mg, or cortisone acetate, 25 mg) is administered in the morning and one-third (hydrocortisone, 10 mg, or cortisone acetate, 12.5 mg) before the evening meal. Giving the afternoon dose later in the evening may cause insomnia. Lower doses (e.g., hydrocortisone, 10 mg twice daily) may be given to the majority of patients. Clinical judgment and lack of symptoms of glucocorticoid deficiency or excess are the primary means of determining dose adequacy. Hepatic enzyme inducers such as rifampin and phenobarbital may accelerate hepatic glucocorticoid catabolism and necessitate an increased maintenance dose. Because of the short half-life of hydrocortisone, serum cortisol concentration is not a useful index for dose adequacy. A 24-hour urinary cortisol measurement may be helpful in some cases.

In secondary adrenal failure (ACTH deficiency), the renin-angiotensin-aldosterone axis is intact, and mineralocorticoid replacement is not needed. However, in primary adrenal insufficiency, mineralocorticoid replacement is important. Aldosterone is not available for therapeutic use. Fludrocortisone (Florinef), a very potent steroid, is the only medication commonly used for this purpose. Typically, 0.05 to 0.2 mg (0.1 mg daily is the usual dose) is administered orally in a single dose daily. The dosage is titrated to a normal serum level of potassium. Inadequate dosage causes dehydration, hyponatremia, and hyperkalemia. Excessive dosage results in hypertension, weight gain, and hypokalemia. Most patients are advised to maintain a sodium intake of approximately 150 mEq per day.

Patients with Newly Diagnosed Adrenocortical Insufficiency. Initial treatment with standard replacement or higher doses of glucocorticoid for patients with chronic ACTH-glucocorticoid deficiency who are not in adrenal crisis may precipitate euphoric or even psychotic behavior. This side effect is assumed to be due to glucocorticoid receptor "up-regulation." Therefore, the initial glucocorticoid doses should be lower (e.g., hydrocortisone, 5 to 10 mg twice daily) than the eventual maintenance dose.

Instructions for Patients. Patients should be told to (1) increase the replacement dose of glucocorticoids twofold to threefold during major physical stress (e.g., fever over 101° F, acute illness, tooth extraction), (2) seek medical care if more than 3 days of stress glucocorticoid coverage is required, (3) avoid long-term supraphysiologic doses because of the potential for iatrogenic Cushing's syndrome, (4) be aware that increased glucocorticoid dosage *is not* required for mental stress, headaches, or minor illness, (5) administer the increased oral glucocorticoid dose intramuscularly if it cannot be taken orally because of nausea or emesis, and (6) carry and wear medical identification (wallet card and bracelet or necklace) that includes the diagnosis (adrenal insufficiency) and the words "give cortisone" so that appropriate glucocorticoid treatment can be given if he or she is found unconscious (Medic Alert Foundation International, P.O. Box 1009, Turlock, CA 95381-1009; telephone 1-800-344-3226). Complete patient understanding of these instructions is the key to successful treatment.

Three syringes, each filled with 4 mg (4 mg/mL) of dexamethasone, should be prescribed for patients to keep at home, at work, and with them if possible (avoiding exposure to extreme heat). A single dose may be repeated in 8 hours if symptoms of the underlying illness persist and a physician is not available. Instructions on self-injection technique should be given and periodically reviewed. Expired medication should be replaced promptly.

Perioperative Glucocorticoid Therapy

Surgical procedures with general anesthesia require coverage with high doses of glucocorticoid. Our standard glucocorticoid preparation preoperatively is 40 mg of methylprednisolone sodium succinate (Solu-Medrol) administered intramuscularly the morning of the operation and again on the evening of the operation; the dose is tapered to 20 mg and 10 mg intramuscularly every 12 hours on the first and second postoperative days, respectively. The patient's clinical condition is the guide to how much further the dose should be tapered to parallel clinical improvement and when to reinstate maintenance glucocorticoid therapy. Patients who take fludrocortisone daily do not usually require supplemental mineralocorticoid until oral intake is resumed postoperatively.

Adrenal Crisis

Adrenal crisis is found in patients with undiagnosed adrenal insufficiency or in those with known disease who have become acutely stressed. Treatment should be considered in all severely ill patients with shock that is refractory to volume expansion and pressor agents. If adrenal insufficiency has not been diagnosed, the following guidelines for treatment *should not be postponed* pending the results of tests for diagnosing adrenal insufficiency. The therapeutic approach to acute adrenal insufficiency should include (1) hydrocortisone sodium succinate (Solu-Cortef) at a dose of 100 mg administered intravenously as a bolus; (2) rapid intravascular volume repletion with dextrose in isotonic saline (approximately 2 to 4 liters given over the first 4 hours) depending on the degree of dehydration, the presence of other cardiovascular or renal disorders, and the clinical response; (3) diagnostic assessment of the precipitating cause (e.g., infection); and (4) frequent monitoring of serum electrolyte, acid-base balance, blood glucose level, and renal function. Hydrocortisone sodium succinate is continued at a dose of 100 mg intravenously every 6 hours until remission of the underlying illness; the dosage may then be decreased by 50% per day until maintenance doses are achieved.

Glucocorticoid Withdrawal

The most common form of adrenal insufficiency is withdrawal from glucocorticoid therapy. Exogenous glucocorticoids suppress the secretion of hypothalamic corticotropin-releasing hormone (CRH) and pituitary ACTH; this is termed hypothalamic-pituitary-adrenal (HPA) axis suppression. HPA axis suppression can occur with high doses (over 100 mg of hydrocortisone or equivalent per day) of glucocorticoid therapy for more than 1 week or lower doses (over 50 mg of hydrocortisone or equivalent per day) for more than 4 weeks (Table 2). Full HPA axis recovery may require hours to months. The recovery of hypothalamic CRH secretion is the primary and limiting determinant for recovery. Some degree of adrenal insufficiency must occur during recovery from HPA axis suppression.

If the goal is to discontinue glucocorticoid therapy, then the patient may be given a "replacement" dose of hydrocortisone (e.g., 20 mg in the morning and 10 mg in the evening). If this modification is well tolerated, it is important to change the dose to a single morning dose (e.g., 20 mg of hydrocortisone every morning). This lower dose of hydrocortisone facilitates HPA recovery by causing relative cortisol deficiency in the afternoon and evening. If the symptoms of adrenal insufficiency cannot be tolerated, the dosage of hydrocortisone should be increased to the previous level and then tapered by smaller decrements over a longer period. Morning plasma cortisol concentrations are measured every 1 to 2 months to assess HPA axis recovery. When the daily dosage of hydrocortisone is 20 mg, it is rarely necessary to taper this

TABLE 2. **Steroid Hormone Preparations***

Preparation	Glucocorticoid Activity	Mineralocorticoid Activity	Duration of Action (hr)	Cost per Day ($)
Hydrocortisone	1.0	1.0	4 to 8	0.15
Cortisone	0.8	0.8	4 to 8	0.13
Prednisone	4.0	0.25	6 to 12	0.05
Dexamethasone	30	0	12 to 20	0.47
Fludrocortisone	10	250	12 to 20	0.38

*The glucocorticoid and mineralocorticoid activities are expressed relative to hydrocortisone, which is assigned an activity value of 1.0.

dose further. When the basal level of plasma cortisol is 10 μg/dL or greater, therapy may be discontinued. Depending on the degree of HPA suppression, it may take up to 1 year before the plasma cortisol concentration becomes normal. Cosyntropin stimulation testing is not helpful in monitoring recovery because this test determines only the status of the adrenal gland. Also, alternate-day glucocorticoid administration is usually not necessary or helpful in the withdrawal process. Patients should receive stress glucocorticoid coverage and wear Medic Alert identification for 1 year after the use of exogenous glucocorticoids have been discontinued.

Treatment of Underlying Disease and Associated Conditions

For each patient, all the causes of adrenal insufficiency listed in Table 1 should be considered. In patients with adrenal insufficiency the possibility of autoimmune adrenal disease should be considered, and patients should be assessed for other glandular dysfunction (primary thyroid failure, diabetes mellitus, hypoparathyroidism, and gonadal failure). Vitiligo may also be present in these patients. Adrenal crisis may be precipitated by other acute illnesses, such as infectious diseases. Each patient should be evaluated for an underlying triggering disease.

CUSHING'S SYNDROME

method of
PAUL C. CARPENTER, M.D.
Mayo Clinic
Rochester, Minnesota

The Cushing syndromes are caused by prolonged exposure to excessive exogenous or endogenous glucocorticoid hormones. This can result from exogenous administration of adrenocorticotropic hormone (ACTH) or glucocorticoids, or endogenous increased secretion of cortisol, ACTH, or corticotropin-releasing hormone (CRH). The manifestations of exogenous Cushing's syndrome are controlled by regulation or discontinuation of drug administration. Definitive therapy of endogenous Cushing's syndrome is surgical except in patients in whom definitive surgery is not feasible.

Endogenous Cushing's syndrome is conventionally divided into ACTH-dependent (80 to 85%) and ACTH-independent (15%) forms. The former is caused by excess pituitary ACTH secretion (Cushing's disease, 80%) and ectopic ACTH or CRH secretion (20%) from nonpituitary neoplasms, the great majority of which are due to ACTH excess. Cushing's disease comprises 65% of all Cushing's syndrome patients and is more common in women (at a ratio of 2.5:1). Ninety-five percent of patients with Cushing's disease have corticotroph-secreting pituitary adenomas, the remainder have corticotroph hyperplasia. ACTH-independent Cushing's syndrome is caused by benign or malignant adrenocortical neoplasms in most instances. A minority of cases are attributed to ACTH-independent micronodular or macronodular adrenocortical disease in which the adrenals contain multiple autonomous cortisol-secreting adenomas. This form can be a familial disease. Ectopic production of ACTH is most commonly caused by malignancies such as bronchial or thymic carcinoid tumors and small cell lung cancer, these two accounting for 85% of cases. The remainder may be due to pancreatic neoplasms, medullary thyroid carcinoma, and a variety of other tumors. Ectopic CRH has been found in several small and often atypical neoplasms. Co-secretion of CRH and ACTH from malignancies is also seen.

DIAGNOSTIC STRATEGY

The importance of precision in diagnosis and differential diagnosis of Cushing's syndrome cannot be overemphasized. Appropriate treatment relies on accurate diagnoses. Many cases of Cushing's syndrome can be diagnosed precisely by combining the clinical and laboratory assessment. However, in some cases of ACTH-dependent Cushing's syndrome the differential diagnosis is challenging because many ectopic CRH- or ACTH-secreting tumors (particularly bronchial and thymic carcinoid tumors) suppress cortisol with high-dose dexamethasone testing and have other biochemical parameters that mimic pituitary-dependent disease. Also, it has become more obvious that periodic hormonogenesis is more common than was once thought.

All forms of endogenous Cushing's syndrome involve an increased secretion of cortisol. Virtually all patients with Cushing's syndrome have increased urinary cortisol levels at some point in their clinical course. The first step in diagnosis is the establishment of hypercortisolism. The single best laboratory test for this purpose is the measurement of urinary free cortisol, preferably with a chomatograph-purified assay (high-pressure liquid chromatography [HPLC]) because the binding assay for urine cortisol is subject to interference by other steroids. The precision is demonstrated simply in the upper normal ranges of the two assays, the HPLC assay at less than 55 μg per day and the binding assay commonly up to 100 μg per day; the difference in the binding assay exists because it detects a variety of noncortisol products in the urine. Measurement of urinary 17-ketogenic or 17-hydroxysteroid levels, corrected for daily creatinine excretion, is useful but produces more false-negative results than the urinary free cortisol and is also subject to interference from a number of drugs. The precision of plasma cortisol determinations is limited because of the wide normal range and the pulsatile nature of cortisol production. The highest precision is found in late afternoon measurements.

Baseline cortisol measurements may be elevated by alcoholism, depression, severe illness, and a variety of stressful states. This must be kept in mind because the demonstration of true cortisol excess is the hallmark of the disease. Equivocal results should be reconfirmed by remeasurement and demonstration of autonomy with low-dose dexamethasone testing (1 mg overnight with early morning plasma cortisol measurement, or 0.5 mg every 6 hours for 2 days with collection of urinary cortisol during 24 hours). In my experience the failure to confirm cortisol excess is the most common error in diagnosis.

A variety of symptoms and physical or laboratory findings may aid in the differential diagnosis independent of the information found in dynamic testing. Rapid onset of severe symptoms and signs of cortisol excess suggests an adrenal neoplasm or aggressive ectopic ACTH secretion. Virilization in women with Cushing's syndrome is the hallmark of adrenal malignancy. Similarly, disproportionate elevations of plasma dehydroepiandrosterone (DHEA/DHEA-S) or urine 17-ketosteroids relative to cortisol and its metabolites are often found with adrenal carcinoma. Severe hypokalemia is very rare in pituitary-dependent Cushing's syndrome and suggests ectopic hormonogenesis, as does marked elevation of the basal ACTH level.

When hypercortisolism has been demonstrated, tests are then performed to establish the differential diagnosis of Cushing's syndrome. These tests include (1) static and dynamic tests to determine the condition of the pituitary-adrenal axis and (2) imaging techniques to detect pituitary or adrenal neoplasms and search for ectopic ACTH- or CRH-secreting neoplasms.

The major components of the diagnostic testing algorithm have been in place for more than 25 years and include low- and high-dose dexamethasone suppression testing. In the presence of typical clinical symptoms and signs of cortisol excess accompanied by evidence of excessive cortisol secretion, low-dose dexamethasone testing is superfluous. The presence of suppressed or undetectable basal ACTH levels identifies ACTH-independent Cushing's syndrome (adrenal neoplasm). More recently, CRH stimulation testing and petrosal sinus venous sampling (PSS) to determine ACTH levels have been added to improve diagnostic precision in ACTH-dependent disease.

The general features of differential diagnostic testing focus on the fact that, in the majority of patients with Cushing's disease, plasma and urine cortisol levels are suppressed with high-dose dexamethasone testing. If the urinary cortisol level is suppressed more than 90% with high-dose dexamethasone testing, a diagnosis of Cushing's disease can be made with high sensitivity and precision. Lesser degrees of suppression (e.g., 50%) lower the precision of the test substantially and need confirmation with CRH testing or PSS to differentiate Cushing's disease from ectopic ACTH syndromes.

Advances in computed tomographic (CT) scanning and magnetic resonance imaging (MRI) have improved the capability of detecting neoplasms in adrenal and pituitary glands. Adrenal neoplasms causing Cushing's syndrome are now found easily with high-quality imaging.

TREATMENT

The discussion of therapy is organized under specific differential causes of Cushing's syndrome. Some therapeutic techniques are more relevant to particular types of Cushing's syndrome, and some can be used regardless of cause. Medical therapy is discussed separately because the specific medications overlap the various forms of Cushing's syndrome. Therapy should also address management of the effects of excess cortisol and mineralocorticoid hormones.

Surgical Therapy

Cushing's Disease

More than half of patients with Cushing's disease with pituitary microadenomas have negative CT scans and nearly one-third have negative MRI studies. When the diagnosis is firm this lack of demonstration of a definitive mass should not argue against surgical intervention because long-term surgical cure rates are actually higher in patients with negative imaging. Transsphenoidal surgical (TSS) removal of pituitary microadenomas by accomplished pituitary surgeons generally yields a remission in Cushing's disease (in 80 to 95% of patients) and minimal chance of recurrent disease (5 to 8%) in centers with a large surgical experience. It is my opinion that TSS for Cushing's disease should be performed only by neurosurgeons who have a large experience in this disease. Significantly lower short- and long-term remission rates are reported from centers that have a limited number of cases.

Very selective adenomectomy seems to carry a higher recurrence rate than removal of visible adenoma along with adjacent pituitary tissue. Failure to obtain remission is generally due to the presence of an invasive pituitary tumor or the infrequent anterior pituitary corticotropin hyperplasia. Marked suppression of plasma cortisol levels postoperatively and for many weeks afterward correlates with long-term remission.

The addition of PSS to the diagnostic tools contribute to pituitary tumor localization. The primary information obtained from PSS is confirmation of the source of ACTH (central vs. peripheral), but it can also give some information on lateralization to guide the neurosurgeon (70% accuracy). When no tumor is found on exploration of the sella, hemihypophysectomy of the side indicated on PSS has been curative.

In patients with recurrence of Cushing's disease surgical re-exploration of the sella is often warranted and leads to subsequent remission in 70% of patients. This magnitude of benefit also depends on the breadth of the surgeon's experience. Imaging is often less helpful in these cases because of prior surgical intervention and the resulting alteration in sellar anatomy.

Reconfirmation of the diagnosis is the first step in planning longitudinal treatment in patients in whom complete clinical remission does not occur following transsphenoidal pituitary surgery for Cushing's disease. If the diagnosis is confirmed, several choices of therapy are available.

Bilateral adrenalectomy, preferably using a posterior or flank approach, produces clinical remission in Cushing's disease and can be used as primary therapy as it was before 1973 and the advent of selective pituitary microsurgery. However, these patients face a long-term risk of development of an aggressive ACTH-secreting pituitary adenoma (Nelson-Salassa syndrome), which often is difficult to manage with both surgical and nonsurgical means. Therefore, most centers try to avoid bilateral adrenalectomy and favor other treatments.

Following adrenalectomy the patient is clearly obligated to take replacement glucocorticoid medication. Surprisingly, surveillance and periodic reassessment of adrenal function must be continued after bilateral adrenalectomy because as many as 25% may eventually be shown to have functioning adrenocortical tissue.

For many years adrenal allografts have been attempted by means of reimplantation of small adrenocortical tissue remnants at the time of adrenalectomy to obtain relief from chronic replacement steroid. This practice has miserable success rates and, when executed, may lead to recurrent disease because the primary defect in ACTH secretion has not been addressed. This procedure should probably be limited to the rare patient who undergoes surgery for bilateral adrenal medullary neoplasm.

Radiotherapy of the pituitary (conventional radiotherapy, 40 to 50 Gy) can be used as primary therapy for Cushing's disease, but the cure rates are dismal (less than 40%). Over time there is a 40% risk of pituitary hormone deficiency, and some patients develop subtle changes in cognitive function. Remission rates are significantly higher if radiation is used adjunctively following failed transsphenoidal pituitary surgery. Rates of disease remission using conventional radiotherapy are also higher in children. Success in radiation therapy for Cushing's disease seems to parallel the hospital's or physician's case load volume, as is true of the surgical outcomes cited earlier.

Remission is achieved gradually and may take over 1 year to reach maximal extent, leaving the patient with the risk of continued exposure to excess cortisol during that time. Better results are achieved with stereotactic charged-particle radiation using a proton beam or, more recently, a helium ion beam. One-third of these patients develop anterior pituitary hormone losses, and the technique carries a 1% risk of injury to the temporal lobe or optic nerves. The technique is available at only a few centers around the world.

Adrenal Neoplasm

Complete extirpation of adrenocortical neoplasms is the preferred therapy for ACTH-independent forms of Cushing's syndrome. Unilateral adrenalectomy is curative for benign adrenocortical adenomas causing Cushing's syndrome. A posterior approach is preferred because of the lessened perioperative morbidity and shortened hospital stays associated with it. Overall morbidity and mortality for unilateral adrenalectomy should be less than 2%. Bilateral adrenalectomy through the flank or posterior approach is used to manage ACTH-independent bilateral nodular adrenocortical hyperplasia.

An anterior abdominal surgical approach should be used when an adrenocortical carcinoma is suspected. This suspicion arises from the magnitude and patterns of steroid excretion plus the size of the lesion. The majority of adrenal masses over 6 cm in diameter are cancers. Unfortunately, many individuals with adrenocortical carcinoma producing Cushing's syndrome are found to have distant metastatic spread of disease at the time of the original diagnosis. Repeated surgery for removal of recurrent adrenocortical carcinoma still leads to the highest survival rates despite the use of medical or radiation therapy.

Ectopic ACTH Syndrome

Removal of the neoplastic tissue secreting CRH or ACTH eliminates the ectopic forms of Cushing's syndrome. However, as with adrenocortical malignancy, metastatic spread of the sources of ectopic peptides can make surgical cure untenable. Embolization of residual tumor, particularly hepatic metastases, has been used to diminish ectopic peptide production. Intraoperative focal radiation therapy and direct organ infusion chemotherapy are other options for some neoplasms. When laboratory evaluation indicates a diagnosis of ectopic ACTH syndrome and no tumor is found with imaging or localization techniques, the patient should be periodically re-evaluated with attempts to find the occult tumor source. If cortisol overproduction causes significant Cushing's syndrome, bilateral adrenalectomy can be considered. Adrenalectomy is also warranted when long-term survival with a tumor burden is anticipated in patients with unresectable malignancies causing ectopic ACTH syndrome. Individuals with small cell lung cancer accompanied by ectopic ACTH syndrome have a lower survival rate than those without the hormone secretory component. Disease-specific chemotherapy may yield remission in a minority of cases.

Medical Therapy

Pharmacologic therapy of Cushing's syndrome has had limited use but in some instances can become an important component in the management of hypercortisolism. The agents used are of three types: (1) drugs that modify pituitary ACTH release, (2) agents that interfere with the production of adrenocortical hormones, and (3) drugs that modify the cellular effects of glucocorticoids (cortisol) or mineralocorticoids (aldosterone, deoxycorticosterone).

It should be noted that the use of the various drugs cited subsequently should always be done under the supervision of a physician experienced in their use because significant toxicity can occur with each. Several of these agents are considered investigational drugs and therefore are used only under established research therapeutic protocols. Many clinicians routinely put patients on small doses of dexamethasone (0.25 to 0.50 mg per day) when these drugs are used to avoid clinical adrenocortical insufficiency if the drug therapy is highly effective. Table 1 lists some common doses and features of the drugs available or under investigation that have been used in the adjunctive management of Cushing's syndrome.

The antiserotoninergic properties of cyproheptadine (Periactin) and the investigative drug metergoline* appear to be the origin of the effect of these agents. Both have been used for short- and long-term management of selected cases of Cushing's disease but have had minimal success, and, even when successful, remissions have been incomplete in most instances. They have generally not been effective in altering the secretion of ACTH from ectopic sources.

Bromocriptine (Parlodel) may lower ACTH production from the pituitary in a few patients with Cushing's disease. Some long-term control of cortisol excess has been reported, but even larger numbers of cases seem to become refractory to the drug over

*This is an investigational drug in the United States.

TABLE 1. **Drugs Potentially Used in Treatment of Cushing's Syndrome***

Drug	Common Doses	Side Effects (Major)
Bromocriptine (Parlodel)	10–20 mg/day	Sedation, nausea, sleep disorders
Octreotide acetate (Sandostatin)	600–3000 μg/day	Diarrhea, gallstones
Cyproheptadine (Periactin)	4–16 mg/day†	Sedation, weight gain
Reserpine	0.25–2 mg/day	Sedation, depression, nasal stuffiness
Valproic acid (Depakene)	250–2000 mg/day†	Hepatic toxicity, nausea, thrombocytopenia, teratogenic tendency, sedation
Ketoconazole (Nizoral)	600–1600 mg/day†	Liver toxicity, gynecomastia, gastrointestinal upsets
Mitotane (Lysodren)	0.5–4 gm/day	Liver toxicity, gastrointestinal rashes
Aminoglutethimide (Cytadren)	0.75–2 gm/day	Sedation, nausea, rash
Metyrapone (Metopirone)	1–4 gm/day	Acne, hirsutism, dizziness, edema, hypertension
Spironolactone (Aldactone)	0.5–2 gm/day	Gynecomastia
Mifepristone (RU-486)†‡	5–20 mg/kg/day	

*All drugs must be used with caution.
†Doses above usual recommendations.
‡Not available in the United States.

time. Prediction of who might respond by giving a single large dose appears to be imprecise. It has been suggested that the pituitary neoplasm in these patients originates in the neural elements of the pars intermedia of the pituitary, unlike the much more common eosinophilic corticotroph adenomas, which originate in the anterior pituitary. This type of tumor occurs in less than 5% of all patients with Cushing's disease, thereby explaining the limited utility of bromocriptine.

On an investigational basis, octreotide acetate (Sandostatin) and some of the longer-acting somatostatin analogues also diminish ACTH production in Cushing's disease patients following repeated subcutaneous administration. These agents are also under current investigation for the adjunctive management of ectopic ACTH production.

Rare patients with Cushing's disease have been treated with valproic acid (Depakene), which appears to inhibit CRH production.

Singular cases of Cushing's disease may respond to reserpine treatment. This drug may increase the response rate to pituitary irradiation in patients with Cushing's disease. The same has been suggested for bromocriptine.

A substantial experience has accumulated in the use of drugs that interfere with adrenocortical steroid production and release. Metyrapone, aminoglutethimide, trilostane, and ketoconazole can all diminish adrenocortical steroid production by interfering with one or more of the enzymatic steps involved in adrenocortical steroid biosynthesis. Mitotane (Lysodren) is an adrenal cytolytic agent that can inhibit adrenal steroid synthesis and destroy normal and neoplastic adrenocortical cells.

The best tolerated of these drugs is ketoconazole, which is currently the most popular drug for the management of hypercortisolism, particularly because it is relatively free of side effects. Individual sensitivity to ketoconazole varies widely among patients, necessitating close monitoring of steroid production and dose adjustment. Substantial hepatic toxicity may be noted, particularly with high doses. This effect is generally reversible when the dosage is lowered or the drug is discontinued.

The highest yield for cortisol reduction with ketoconazole and the best clinical benefits are seen in patients with Cushing's disease and adrenal adenomas. Ectopic ACTH production occasionally is reduced, but the drug is no help in patients with adrenal carcinoma. Some patients with Cushing's disease eventually override the enzymatic blockade of ketoconazole, and the drug becomes ineffective. Most commonly the drug is used as an adjunctive therapy during and after pituitary radiation therapy. Ketoconazole paired with octreotide acetate appears to produce greater reductions in cortisol production than either agent used alone.

The primary effect of ketoconazole is derived from the inhibition of the 17,20-desmolase enzyme in the adrenal cortex (P450C17). It also has some 11β-hydroxylase inhibiting activity. Steroid secretion patterns produced by this drug include decreased cortisol but increased deoxycorticosterone, 11-deoxycortisol, and aldosterone, which explains the increased hypertension seen in patients taking the drug.

Metyrapone's major effect is inhibition of 11β-hydroxylation in the adrenal cortex. Diminished cortisol production is achieved at the expense of an accumulation of androgenic cortical products, resulting in virilization in women and excess deoxycorticosterone with resultant hypertension and hypokalemia. Many patients with Cushing's disease respond to the diminished cortisol levels created by metyrapone with an increase in ACTH, resulting in an effective override of the competitive enzymatic blockade. This phenomenon is less often seen with aminoglutethimide, mitotane, or ketoconazole.

The primary problem with the use of mitotane is the presence of gastrointestinal symptoms including anorexia, nausea, and vomiting. Skin rashes are common. Symptoms of depression, excess somnolence, and lightheadedness occur in one-third of patients.

The drug may affect the zona glomerulosa in the adrenal cortex, leading to mineralocorticoid deficiency that may require replacement with oral fludrocortisone in doses of 50 to 250 μg daily. Mitotane can also be used as an adjunctive therapy with pituitary radiotherapy while the patient is awaiting clinical and biochemical improvement, which can be delayed several months following radiation therapy. The drug can be used in divided doses ranging from 1 to 4 grams daily to gain more rapid control of the patient's hypercortisolism. The dose can be diminished as the effects of pituitary irradiation become more prominent with the passage of time. The practice of tracking plasma drug levels seems to have merit. Blood levels of 5 to 10 μg per mL are therapeutic, whereas concentrations below that range are ineffective in reducing cortisol production. Higher levels are very toxic.

Aminoglutethimide (Cytadren) combined with ketoconazole has been used to prepare patients for surgical resection of functioning adrenal adenomas. The drug also has significant gastrointestinal side effects. To many patients the most bothersome side effects, however, are the significant lethargy and sedation that occurs. One peculiar side effect of aminoglutethimide is hypothyroidism, which occurs in a small number of patients. A maculopapular skin rash is often seen during the first 2 weeks of therapy but generally resolves despite continuation of treatment. Similar problems were observed with the use of trilostane, an inhibitor of 3β-hydroxysteroid dehydrogenase, when it was under investigation.

There has been a long search for agents that specifically interfere with the glucocorticoid effect on target cells. The search has focused predominantly on drugs that block the cortisol receptor. Most drugs developed in the past have had very limited success and have been abandoned. Currently, mifepristone (RU-486)* has been used in some clinical trials of hypercortisolism in children and adults with limited success. There have been no long-term trials. Modification of the steroid-receptor complex interaction with nuclear protein is another area of research.

Many individuals with severe hypercortisolemia, particularly those with adrenocortical malignancy or ectopic ACTH production, may have substantial hypertension and severe hypokalemia as a result of the overproduction of mineralocorticoid in the form of deoxycorticosterone, aldosterone, or even cortisol. Spironolactone (Aldactone) specifically interferes with the renal mineralocorticoid effect, and its use is often necessary and very efficacious. Additionally, spironolactone is known to block androgen receptors partially in various tissues, and it can diminish the skin oiliness, acne, and hirsutism that occurs in patients with Cushing's syndrome accompanied by androgen excess. Most individuals require 100 to 200 mg per day to obtain significant benefit, and amounts as high as 400 mg per day in divided doses may be necessary. In severe instances, potassium supplementation may be necessary, but its need is markedly diminished when spironolactone is used.

*Not available in the United States.

All of the preceding agents are used in patients with the various forms of Cushing's syndrome predominantly as adjunctive or temporizing therapy. In some instances drugs that diminish steroid production either by interference with ACTH or by a direct adrenocortical effect are used to try to improve the patient's condition prior to surgical intervention. To date there is no definitive study that shows that this delay produces specific benefits in surgical outcomes. These drugs are also used on a short-term basis while awaiting the effects of pituitary irradiation. In patients with inoperable adrenocortical carcinoma with Cushing's syndrome, mitotane has been the only drug shown to have relatively consistent antitumor effects, but even then it has not significantly altered the long-term prognosis for this malignancy. Mitotane used for 6 to 12 months in patients following resection of adrenocortical malignancy has not proved to be of any benefit in extending life, even in those patients with no apparent residual disease. Patients with no apparent residual disease following resection of adrenal cancer still have less than a 50% 3-year survival.

In some cases of Cushing's syndrome, combined therapy using adrenolytic agents and steroidogenic enzyme inhibitors might be of benefit, but to date long-term clinical trials have been reported rarely. Because metyrapone, mitotane, and aminoglutethimide inhibit different steroidogenic enzymes and have different side effects, combinations using low doses of these drugs may lead to effective therapy with diminished side effects due to the lower doses.

THERAPEUTIC GOALS

The goal of therapy in patients with Cushing's syndrome, like the goals in other therapeutic endeavors, is to use therapeutic modalities involving minimal risk, obtain complete remission from the hypercortisolism or other steroid excesses, and, ideally, allow the patient to lead a medication-free life. Selective transsphenoidal adenomectomy for Cushing's syndrome generally produces these results. Following pituitary surgery, patients are ACTH deficient presumably because hypercortisolism suppresses normal CRH production and perhaps directly inhibits normal anterior pituitary corticotroph function. These patients require glucocorticoid but not mineralocorticoid replacement. Intraoperatively and during the first 2 or 3 postoperative days, parenteral glucocorticoid (hydrocortisone or equivalent water-soluble steroid) is given at a rate of approximately 100 mg per square meter per day. This can be given by continuous intravenous infusion or by intramuscular injection every 12 hours. We routinely use methylprednisolone (Solu-Medrol) perioperatively giving 40 mg parenterally every 12 hours on the day of surgery. The dose is tapered rapidly over 2 or 3 days by halving the dose daily and then starting oral replacement with hydrocortisone or cortisone (12 to 15 mg per square meter per day) or prednisone (5 mg per square meter per day in divided doses). This regimen is maintained for 1 month and then tapering begins. Diminishing the dose can be accomplished by either discontinuing the lower afternoon doses of glucocorticoid replacement for 1 or 2 months and then tapering the morning doses, or the daily doses can be doubled but given on an every-other-day basis for 1 or 2 months.

Recovery of the pituitary-adrenal axis can be monitored by measuring the morning plasma cortisol levels before administering the morning steroid doses or monitoring the response to a short ACTH stimulation test (cosyntropin, 250 μg intramuscularly, with cortisol measurements taken at 0 and 60 minutes). If the response to stimulation is normal (doubling of plasma cortisol levels or absolute values above 20 μg/dL), replacement steroid can be discontinued in most instances. If suboptimal plasma levels are noted or if ACTH stimulation is insufficient, steroid therapy can be continued for another 1 or 2 months and then the test should be repeated. In our experience, most patients are able to stop glucocorticoid replacement in 3 or 4 months, but some require therapy for as long as 1 year. During the recovery time, stress illnesses should be treated by doubling the daily dose of glucocorticoid, and major stresses such as major trauma, substantial body burns, or surgery with general anesthesia should be covered with parenteral steroid injections at four to ten times the daily replacement dose. Following extirpation of unilateral benign cortisol-secreting adenomas, a similar tapering of the glucocorticoid schedule and testing can be used.

Last, there is a growing concern that the doses of glucocorticoid used for long-term management of adrenal insufficiency may be excessive. This concern has arisen from observations of reduced bone mineral density, difficult weight control, and other problems in patients on "conventional" replacement doses. Although 25 to 35 mg of cortisol or cortisone per day is commonly cited as a replacement steroid dose, it has been shown that most patients do very well on approximately 18 mg per day in divided doses. Proportional success has been noted with prednisone in doses of around 5 mg per day.

DIABETES INSIPIDUS

method of
IRWIN SINGER, M.D., and
JAMES R. OSTER, M.D.
Department of Veterans Affairs Medical Center
Miami, Florida

Diabetes insipidus (DI) is characterized by excessive urinary losses of solute-free water (water diuresis), usually resulting in polyuria and polydipsia. Polyuria can be defined operationally as a 24-hour urine volume greater than that appropriate for a patient's effective circulating volume and plasma sodium concentration (usually a urine volume of more than 3 liters). If water intake fails to keep up with water loss in patients with DI, hypertonicity (due to hypernatremia) and volume depletion can result. Primary polydipsia can also produce a large volume of dilute urine but not the hypernatremia or volume depletion seen in patients with DI. In central diabetes insipidus (CDI), the plasma level of arginine vasopressin (AVP) does not increase sufficiently in response to a rise in plasma tonicity. CDI may be "partial" (plasma AVP subnormal) or "complete" (AVP absent). In nephrogenic diabetes insipidus (NDI), AVP levels are sufficient, but renal sensitivity to the hydro-osmotic effect of AVP is impaired (partial NDI) or lacking (complete NDI). Disorders characterized by excessive destruction of AVP ("vasopressinase syndromes") are sometimes considered a separate category. In these syndromes, the production of AVP may be normal or elevated, but increased destruction may lead to subnormal levels and thereby to partial or complete DI.

CDI is caused by congenital or acquired lesions that disrupt the hypothalamic–posterior pituitary axis. Severe NDI is most often hereditary and congenital, but relief of chronic urinary obstruction or therapy with lithium (or other drugs) may cause an acquired form severe enough to warrant treatment. NDI due to hypokalemia or hypercalcemia is usually mild and responds to correction of the electrolyte abnormality.

In addition to primary polydipsia, polyuria can be caused by solute diuresis (electrolytes, e.g., NaCl, or nonelectrolytes, e.g., glucose, mannitol, or urea); diuretic use and resolving acute renal failure are specific examples. Solute diuresis can be excluded by demonstrating that the urine osmolality is below 150 mOsm per kg of water or that the urine specific gravity is below 1.005.

For patients with suspected DI, a formal water deprivation test is sometimes dangerous and unnecessary if significant hypertonicity is already present, but such testing may be required to diagnose partial diabetes insipidus or patients already under treatment. Assessment of the response to hypertonic saline is indicated only infrequently. The urinary response to exogenous AVP should not be used for the diagnosis of DI, but it differentiates CDI from NDI in most cases. Plasma AVP levels are confirmatory and important in equivocal cases.

Several different types of DI (central, vasopressinase-induced, and nephrogenic) may be seen during and following pregnancy. Pre-existing CDI (or NDI) may appear to become worse during pregnancy, and the dosage requirements for AVP or desmopressin (DDAVP) may increase. One type of transient DI of pregnancy is secondary to markedly enhanced activity of plasma vasopressinase, and thus plasma AVP levels may be unmeasurable during dehydration. Polyuria, which may be massive, usually begins during gestation and remits after delivery. Although little or no response to large intravenous doses of AVP occurs, a satisfactory antidiuretic response to DDAVP is observed because DDAVP is vasopressinase resistant.

TREATMENT

The general goals of treatment are to correct any pre-existing water deficits and to reduce any ongoing excessive urinary water losses. The specific therapy required varies with the clinical situation. Awake, ambulatory patients with normal thirst and free access to water have little body water deficit but benefit greatly from relief of the polyuria and polydipsia that disrupt normal activity. Handicapped, demented, and physically restricted patients and comatose patients with acute DI after head trauma are often unable to drink in response to thirst; in such individuals, progressive hypertonicity may become life threatening. Patients who are significantly volume depleted may initially require saline infusions to maintain blood pressure.

Correction of Water Deficit

The established water deficit (in liters) may be estimated from the following formula:

$$\text{Water deficit} = 0.6 \times \text{premorbid weight} \times (1 - 140/[\text{Na}])$$

in which [Na] is the serum Na concentration in millimoles per liter. This formula depends on three assumptions: Premorbid total body water is approximately 60% of body weight (kilograms); no net body solute was lost as hypertonicity developed; and the premorbid serum [Na] was 140 millimoles per liter. Adjustments for the premorbid sodium concentration and percentage of body weight are readily made, but estimating net body solute loss is very difficult.

To reduce the risk of central nervous system damage from protracted exposure to severe hypertonicity in symptomatic patients, the serum osmolality should be lowered aggressively by 1 to 2 millimoles per liter per hour to the range of 330 mOsm per kg H_2O (serum [Na] equals approximately 160 millimoles per liter). In such patients, an initial rapid decrement of serum [Na] of only 3 to 4 millimoles per liter over 1 to 2 hours will often terminate seizures if they are present.

Tonicity may be estimated as twice the serum Na concentration if there is no hyperglycemia (or any abnormal solute such as mannitol), and measured osmolality may be substituted for tonicity if azotemia is not present. (Note: Urea contributes to osmolality but not to tonicity.) In response to continuing hypertonicity, brain cells increase their content of a variety of organic osmolytes; because these osmolytes cannot be immediately dissipated as hypertonicity resolves, correction of serum Na into the normal range (after initial therapy to reverse symptomatic hypernatremia) should be conducted gradually over the next 48 hours to avoid producing cerebral edema. The water deficit formula given earlier does not take into account ongoing water losses and is only a rough estimate. Frequent serum and urine electrolyte determinations should be made, and all water losses should be measured; the administration rate of oral water or 5% dextrose in water (D_5W) should be adjusted accordingly.

If administered fluid is to result in a reduction of serum [Na], it must have an [Na] less than that of any ongoing [Na] losses (usually urinary). Thus, in many patients, replacement fluid containing 0.45% NaCl may have an [Na] that is too high (75 millimoles per liter) to reduce serum [Na]. Urine K losses (in addition to Na losses) should be taken into account in correcting the serum [Na] only if the excretion of K represents a net loss from the body. Similarly, if K is added to intravenous fluids (and is retained within the body), it will tend to increase tonicity unless the amount of Na given is reduced proportionately.

Because of the risk of hyperglycemia when very large amounts of D_5W are given intravenously, water should, as much as possible, be administered by the enteral route; a nasogastric tube may be used, if needed. Alternatively, if a central vein is cannulated, 0.25% NaCl, $D_{2.5}W$, or, in a true emergency, sterile distilled water can be infused (the last-mentioned should be given at a rate not to exceed 10 mL per minute).

Meticulous attention to initial and subsequent clinical (e.g., blood pressure, body weight, edema, mental status, and so on) and laboratory data, and careful individualization of treatment are critical to therapeutic success.

Pharmacologic Agents

The agents and usual dosages currently recommended for treatment of DI are listed in Table 1. Only AVP and DDAVP are specifically recommended by their manufacturers for use in DI.

Arginine Vasopressin (AVP, Pitressin Synthetic). Aqueous AVP has a relatively short half-life and often increases blood pressure when given intravenously. Frequent or continuous administration is required, and the dose must be continually titrated to achieve the desired reduction in urine output. AVP is used mainly in acute situations, such as postoperative CDI. AVP is not useful in patients with vasopressinase syndromes.

DDAVP. Desmopressin (1-deamino-8-D-arginine vasopressin) was developed for therapeutic use because it has a longer half-life than the native hormone and is largely devoid of the latter's pressor activity. In normal persons DDAVP may produce certain extrarenal effects: an increase or decrease in blood pressure, an increase in plasma renin activity, and a stimulation of the release of coagulation factor VIIIc and von Willebrand factor. DDAVP is the drug of choice for chronic administration in patients with CDI or vasopressinase syndromes, but it is expensive. The intranasal aqueous solution is provided in two different formulations:

1. In a bottle with a calibrated rhinal tube. The tube is filled to the appropriate graduation line and bent in a U shape. Taking care to retain the fluid within the tube, one end is placed in the mouth and the other is inserted approximately 1 cm into the anterior nares. The drug is then puffed into the midportion of the nose, deep enough to avoid runoff out of the nose but not so far back as to propel the solution into the throat. Patients require training in how to use the catheter reliably; not all patients have the required dexterity.

2. As a nasal spray delivering a single metered

TABLE 1. **Pharmacologic Treatment of Diabetes Insipidus**

Drug	Usual Total Daily Dose*	Usual Frequency of Administration (times per day)	Usual Onset of Action (h)	Usual Duration of Action (h)	Comments (see text for important details)
Arginine vasopressin (Pitressin) 20 units per mL	5–10 units subcutaneously	q 2 h to q 4 h	1–2	2–6	Avoid intravenous use because of risk of acute hypertension
Desmopressin (DDAVP) 10 μg per 0.1 mL for intranasal use	10–40 μg (0.1–0.4 mL) intranasally	qd or bid	1–2	8–12	Drug of choice for chronic treatment of CDI; higher doses may be helpful in some patients with NDI
4 μg per mL for injection	2–4 μg intravenously or subcutaneously	qd or bid	1–2	8–12	
100- or 200-μg tablets†	100–300 μg orally	bid or tid	1–2	8–10	
Chlorpropamide (Diabinese) 100- or 250-mg tablets	100–500 mg	qd or bid	Delayed (days)	24–48	Potentiates renal effect of AVP; particularly useful in partial CDI
Hydrochlorothiazide (HydroDIURIL) 50-mg or 100-mg tablets	50–100 mg	qd or bid	2–4	24–48	Reduces renal water clearance; useful in NDI: equivalent doses of other thiazides are equally effective
Amiloride (Midamor) 5-mg tablets	5–20 mg	qd or bid	2	24	Particularly helpful in lithium-induced DI but may be useful in other types of NDI
Indomethacin (Indocin) 50- or 75-mg capsules	100–150 mg	bid or tid	2–4	6–8	Decreases renal water clearance; useful adjunctive therapy in NDI

*Wide variations, outside the usual values shown above, occur; dose size and frequency must be matched to action, onset, and duration for each individual.
†Oral form not yet approved for use in United States.

dose of 0.1 mL (10 μg) or multiples thereof. This simplified dosing has the disadvantage of requiring fixed doses, which may be more than needed by some patients.

The absorption of nasally administered DDAVP may be erratic, and its usefulness is diminished in the presence of nasal mucosal atrophy, scarring, congestion, blockage, or discharge. Its duration of action is decreased by swimming without nose plugs. At high doses, DDAVP may cause angina or increase blood pressure; thus it should be used with caution in patients with coronary artery disease or hypertensive cardiovascular disease or in association with vasopressor agents. The side effects of DDAVP are uncommon and are generally dose related.

Dosages of DDAVP must be individualized according to the response and daily activities of the patient so that the duration of sleep is adequate and the turnover of water is adequate without being excessive. If two doses are needed, the morning and evening doses should be titrated separately. The usual practice is to begin with and titrate the evening dose; a second (morning or other time) dose should be added only if it is needed for the patient's comfort. Disease in adults is commonly controlled with an intranasal dose of 10 μg twice a day; the duration of action varies from 6 to 24 hours. Some patients (perhaps one-fourth to one-third) may need only a single daily dose (typically given at night). The parenteral form of DDAVP may be given by the intravenous, intramuscular, or subcutaneous routes; it is approximately five to ten times more potent than the intranasal preparation. For both the intranasal and parenteral preparations, an increase in the administered dose generally increases the duration rather than the magnitude of the antidiuresis; consequently, altering the dose can be a useful maneuver in reducing the required frequency of administration.

It appears likely that an oral formulation of DDAVP will soon be marketed in the United States.

Chlorpropamide (Diabinese). This oral hypoglycemic agent also potentiates the renal hydro-osmotic effect of AVP and stimulates the hypothalamic release of AVP. It is of no value in NDI (or in most patients with complete CDI) but can be useful in patients with partial CDI. Hypoglycemia is a concern, particularly in patients with anterior pituitary insufficiency. Four or more days of treatment are often required before the maximal effect is seen.

Other sulfonylureas share the effects of chlorpropamide but are less potent. The newer generation of oral hypoglycemic agents, e.g., glipizide (Glucotrol) and glyburide (Micronase), are largely devoid of any AVP-potentiating effects.

Thiazide Diuretics. The natriuretic effect of the thiazide class of diuretics is conferred by their ability to block sodium absorption in the cortical diluting site; when combined with dietary sodium restriction, the drugs cause modest hypovolemia and diminish distal solute delivery. Because these effects markedly diminish the kidney's diluting ability and free water clearance independent of any action of AVP, agents of this class are the mainstay of therapy for NDI. Any drug of the thiazide class may be used with equal potential for benefit; the physician is advised to use the one with which he or she is most familiar. The main limitations of using diuretics to treat DI are symptomatic volume depletion and relatively KCl-resistant potassium depletion. Special care must be exercised in treating patients who are taking lithium as well as diuretics because the induced plasma volume contraction may decrease lithium excretion, possibly producing lithium toxicity.

Amiloride. The potassium-sparing diuretic amiloride (Midamor) is now considered to be the pharmacologic agent of choice for the specific management of lithium-induced NDI. Amiloride ameliorates lithium-induced NDI, probably by blocking lithium uptake in the distal tubules and collecting ducts.

Nonsteroidal Anti-inflammatory Drugs (NSAIDs). Prostaglandins increase renal medullary blood flow and diminish medullary solute reabsorption, effects that modestly decrease the tubular-interstitial gradient for water reabsorption. Prostaglandins also antagonize the antidiuretic actions of AVP at the cellular level. By blocking renal prostaglandin synthesis, NSAIDs can increase non–AVP-mediated water reabsorption and minimal urine osmolality, thus reducing electrolyte-free water clearance and urine output. Although these agents can be effective in patients with partial CDI, their main usefulness is as an adjunctive therapy in those with NDI, for which more direct antidiuretic therapies are limited. Indomethacin (Indocin), tolmetin (Tolectin), and ibuprofen (Motrin) have been used beneficially. Unfortunately, the side effects of these agents (e.g., gastrointestinal ulceration, decreased glomerular filtration rate, and hyperkalemia) limit their chronic use.

Other Agents. Clofibrate (Atromid-S), 500 mg four times a day, and carbamazepine (Tegretol), 200 to 600 mg per day, augment the release of vasopressin in partial CDI, but significant side effects preclude recommending their routine use.

Clinical Situations

Acute Postsurgical or Post-traumatic CDI. Post-traumatic CDI is usually obvious from the clinical situation but should not be treated until the diagnosis is clear. Hypernatremia may develop rapidly, is likely to be severe, and warrants specific therapy with intravenous D_5W at a rate estimated from the deficit calculation described previously. Parenteral AVP in a dose of 5 units subcutaneously or DDAVP in a dose of 1 to 2 μg intramuscularly or subcutaneously should be given to reduce urine flow and simplify fluid management and should be repeated at intervals determined by frequent monitoring of urine output (volume and electrolytes) and serum electrolytes. Dose size and frequency are usually based on the desired hourly urine flow (e.g., 100 mL per hour); the next dose is usually given when the urine flow exceeds the desired rate by more than 25% for 1 to 2 hours.

After the acute phase, partial or complete resolution of post-traumatic DI often occurs and should be sought. In some patients there is a triphasic pattern: (1) An initial phase of DI is followed by (2) axonal necrosis of vasopressin-secreting neurons with uncontrolled AVP release, potentially leading to water retention and hyponatremia, and then by (3) axonal death with cessation of AVP production and recurrent (and usually persistent) DI. AVP requirements may vary at different times. To ensure detection of recovery from DI or a period of inappropriate antidiuresis, the dosage interval for parenteral DDAVP or AVP should be empirically tailored to allow a brief recurrence of polyuria (see next section on chronic CDI). Postsurgical patients who do not recover need chronic outpatient therapy, usually with DDAVP. Very late recovery from surgical CDI occurs, which should be ascertained by periodic DDAVP withdrawal.

Chronic CDI. Unless the hypothalamic thirst center is also affected, patients with CDI become thirsty when they are hypertonic. Severe hypertonicity is therefore not a risk in the patient who is alert, has access to water, and is able to drink. Polyuria and polydipsia are inconvenient and disruptive but not life threatening in such patients. The treatment of choice in patients with complete CDI is intranasal DDAVP. Following initiation of therapy with DDAVP, hypotonicity is uncommon (in part because the decline in serum Na leads to suppression of thirst) and usually asymptomatic, but it may be progressive if water intake continues during a relatively long period of continuous antidiuresis. Therefore, treatment must be designed to minimize polyuria and polydipsia without incurring an undue risk of hyponatremia from overtreatment. To reduce the likelihood of hyponatremia and to be able to recognize the unusual instances of disease remission, it is important to permit brief, intermittent polyuric episodes. Ideally, withdrawal should be done on a daily basis but no less often than weekly, at the patient's convenience; this is commonly accomplished by omitting or reducing the morning dose of DDAVP on a weekend day.

Treatment must be individualized, sometimes with an in-hospital trial to determine the optimal dosage and intervals between doses. This also permits careful education of the patient about how to administer the drug intranasally and how to ensure a polyuric phase. Starting with doses of 10 μg once a day or 5 μg twice a day, the doses that result in 12 to 24 hours of control should be determined; for some patients, once-daily dosing suffices. In compliant patients two or three small doses daily are sometimes more cost-effective than a single very large dose. With a great deal of caution, chlorpropamide (or NSAIDs) may be used to lower the required DDAVP dose and produce an additional economy; chlorpropamide alone may be sufficient and simpler in some patients with partial CDI. A trial-and-error approach with different regimens is often needed to establish the most satisfactory arrangement for each patient.

Nephrogenic Diabetes Insipidus. If relevant, any underlying disorder (e.g., hypercalcemia) should be treated. Some specific causes of NDI (e.g., lithium administration) can also be treated "specifically" (e.g., with amiloride). Useful general treatment measures include sodium restriction and thiazides combined with a NSAID.

Physicians caring for patients with NDI must be prepared to use several agents concurrently. For example, patients with lithium-induced DI who do not respond to amiloride alone may also be given hydrochlorothiazide and/or indomethacin. Combinations including amiloride may obviate the need for potassium supplementation. The combination of a thiazide and an NSAID may not increase urinary osmolality above that of plasma, but the lessening of polyuria is nonetheless beneficial. Finally, although DDAVP is usually not effective in patients with NDI, some patients experience appreciable increases in urine osmolality after an intranasal dose of 10 μg of this agent. Of course, in such instances it is possible that the patient may also have a component of CDI.

Vasopressinase Syndromes. Because DDAVP is resistant to vasopressinase, it is the ideal agent for treatment of these syndromes. Clinical experience suggests that somewhat larger doses than those usually needed for CDI are required, but treatment should follow the same principles as described previously.

GOITER

method of
JOHN J. ORLOFF, M.D., and
GERARD N. BURROW, M.D.
Yale University School of Medicine
New Haven, Connecticut

The term goiter is defined as an enlargement of the thyroid gland to at least twice the normal size (i.e., greater than 40 grams). Nontoxic goiter may be classified as either endemic, sporadic, or compensatory, and may be diffuse or nodular, containing one or more nodules. Endemic goiter, which by definition occurs in more than 10% of a defined geographic population, is the most common type of goiter worldwide. It usually results from iodine deficiency, but occasionally dietary goitrogens containing thiocyanate (e.g., cassava) can contribute. Iodine deficiency as a cause of goiter in the United States has been largely eliminated by the introduction of iodized salt. However, even in areas of adequate iodine intake, the prevalence of goiter remains significant (4% in the Framingham Study). The term simple or sporadic goiter is used to refer to benign thyroid enlargement occurring in a nonendemic region. A compensatory goiter may develop following subtotal thyroidectomy. Autoimmune Hashimoto's thyroiditis is a common cause of goiter in nonendemic areas, and viral subacute thyroiditis may result in transient enlargement of the thyroid. Thyroid function is usually normal in patients with simple goiter. However, hyperthyroidism may be seen with toxic nodular goiter (Plummer's disease) following exposure to contrast agents or iodine (jodbasedow phenomenon), or with subacute thyroiditis; hypothyroidism may be due to Hashimoto's thyroiditis, dyshormonogenesis, some drug-induced goiters, or the recovery phase of subacute thyroiditis. Amiodarone therapy for cardiac arrhythmias may be associated with hypothyroidism (more common in iodine-replete areas such as the United States) or hyperthyroidism. Finally, nodular and occasionally diffuse thyroid enlargement may result from thyroid cancer, which is discussed in another article.

The cause of benign nontoxic goiter in iodine-replete areas is not clear. Inherited disorders of thyroid hormone biosynthesis are probably uncommon and often present in childhood with hypothyroidism. Periodic increases in secretion of thyroid-stimulating hormone (TSH) have been postulated to play a central role in the development of nodular hyperplasia. Factors other than TSH, including epidermal growth factor, insulin-like growth factors, and fibroblast growth factors, may also stimulate thyroid growth. The role of activated oncogenes and other growth factors in the development of multinodular goiter remains unclear. Other factors include genetic predisposition, exposure to certain medications such as lithium, and exposure to ionizing radiation to the head and neck.

CLINICAL EVALUATION

Clinical evaluation of goiter requires assessment of thyroid size and function and of whether the enlargement may represent a malignancy. The clinical presentation of patients with goiter is usually that of thyroid enlargement without a change in thyroid function. However, some patients do present with hypothyroidism (e.g., Hashimoto's thyroiditis), and others have hyperthyroidism due to Graves' disease or autonomous function of thyroid nodules. A careful history and physical examination may reveal signs and symptoms of thyroid dysfunction. The goiter may be diffuse or nodular and may be a solitary prominent nodule or multinodular. Local complications of thyroid enlargement include dysphagia, a sense of obstruction on raising the arms over the head (in patients with a substernal goiter [Pemberton's sign]), dyspnea resulting from tracheal narrowing, and hoarseness due to compression of the recurrent laryngeal nerves. The presence of hoarseness or cervical adenopathy, a history of childhood neck irradiation, or recent growth of a solitary or dominant nodule raises the clinical suspicion of malignancy. Very rapid painful growth (days) suggests hemorrhage into a benign or neoplastic lesion.

Laboratory tests should include an evaluation of thyroid function. The screening test of choice is an ultrasensitive assay for thyroid-stimulating hormone (TSH), which can distinguish hyperthyroidism (TSH less than 0.05 milliunit per liter) from normal function. Abnormal screening TSH values should be confirmed with thyroid indices. Some multinodular goiters may produce triiodothyronine (T_3) rather than thyroxine (T_4), resulting in a normal free T_4 index and a suppressed TSH level associated with an elevated total T_3. The presence of autoimmune thyroiditis may be indicated by elevated titers of antimicrosomal (peroxidase) and antithyroglobulin antibodies. Serum calcitonin and carcinoembryonic antigen (CEA) should not be obtained at the initial evaluation unless there is a family history of medullary carcinoma of the thyroid or multiple endocrine neoplasia type 2A or 2B. Serum thyroglobulin is not helpful in the diagnosis of thyroid cancer.

The challenge to the clinician in evaluation of a nodular goiter is to determine which patients from the great majority with benign thyroid lesions require surgical management. Thyroid nodules are extremely common, but only a very small percentage (~5%) represent malignancies. It is not cost effective to operate on all such lesions, so several tests have been developed to help determine which lesions represent the greatest risk of thyroid cancer. The desired outcomes for the ideal test include the fewest number of missed malignancies, the fewest operations for benign disease, and the lowest cost. The test that most closely approaches this ideal is the fine-needle aspiration (FNA) biopsy. Decision analysis studies have determined that it is more cost effective and efficient to begin with an FNA rather than the traditional radionuclide scan. Radionuclide scans demonstrate that a majority of nodules (benign or malignant) are "cold." Surgical referrals based on scan results and clinical suspicion have resulted in an incidence of thyroid carcinoma in thyroid nodules of approximately 10 to 20% in most surgical series. Use of the FNA has been shown to decrease the amount of thyroid nodule surgery by one-half and to double the proportion of nodules found to be malignant at surgery. Recent studies indicate that FNA is also accurate in rural practices provided that biopsies are concentrated with as few operators as practical and that slides are read by an experienced cytopathologist. Approximately two-thirds of patients have a benign cytologic analysis, with false-negative results ranging from less than 1% to 3%. FNA can reliably diagnose papillary, medullary, and anaplastic carcinomas with very few false-positive readings. The cytologic features of follicular carcinoma are similar to those of benign follicular neoplasms and therefore cannot be distinguished by FNA. Such biopsies account for about 20% of all FNAs and are categorized as suspicious or indeterminate. Approximately 20 to 25% of these are found to be malignant at surgery. Patients who have indeterminate findings on FNA should have a radionuclide scan to determine the functional status of the nodule, because the presence of a "hot" nodule on a radioiodine scan essentially rules out follicular carcinoma. Nodules that are shown to be functional by technetium scanning should probably be reevaluated with an iodine-123 scan, because rare nodules may trap technetium but fail to organify iodine, thus appearing "cold" only on iodine scanning. The fourth type of interpretation of a biopsy is inadequate, and it is commonly observed with aspiration of cyst contents that do not contain any cellular elements for analysis. Such biopsies should be repeated, under ultrasound guidance if necessary.

The role of thyroid ultrasound in the initial evaluation of a solitary or dominant thyroid nodule is limited. High-resolution studies demonstrate that the overwhelming majority of nodules are solid or partially solid (complex cysts) and require a biopsy. Pure, simple cysts are truly rare and should be diagnosed equally well with a biopsy, which also provides definitive therapy in approximately half the cases. Ultrasound may be used as a guide in performing the FNA, especially for nodules in difficult locations or complex nodules with a small solid component, but it is expensive. Ultrasound may have a role in objective assessment of the size of a nodule in response to therapy, although the cost effectiveness of this approach compared with simple palpation is questionable. Finally, ultrasound may provide evidence of a multinodular goiter, which may slightly lessen the likelihood of cancer. However, a dominant nodule within a multinodular gland carries a risk of malignancy that is similar to that for a solitary nodule, and therefore it should be approached in the same way.

Visualization of thyroid size and relationship to vital structures in the neck may be pursued if there are significant local compressive symptoms. This is best accomplished with a computed tomography (CT) or magnetic resonance imaging (MRI) scan. These studies allow assessment of a substernal component of the goiter and can show whether there is critical narrowing of the airway, especially in the noncartilaginous portion of the trachea below the thoracic inlet. A flow-volume loop can demonstrate functional upper airway obstruction, and esophagrams may help to establish that a goiter is causing dysphagia. Vocal cord paralysis due to compression or invasion can be demonstrated by laryngoscopy.

TREATMENT

Thyroxine Suppression Therapy

Thyroxine suppression therapy should be considered in all patients with diffuse or nodular nontoxic goiter. Because TSH provides a potent stimulus for thyroid cell growth, suppression of endogenous TSH secretion may arrest goiter growth. Although thyroxine therapy has been widely utilized for this purpose, recent prospective data suggest that the majority of benign solitary thyroid nodules do not respond to suppressive therapy during the short term. Others have reported more favorable responses to suppressive therapy. Likewise, experience with the treatment of multinodular goiter has varied widely, with some concluding that many multinodular goiters do not respond to such therapy. Treatment failures may be due to fibrosis within long-standing goiters or to the presence of growth stimulators other than TSH. The response to thyroxine suppression has also been widely employed in the past to distinguish benign from malignant nodules; however, occasional thyroid cancers have been documented to shrink with suppressive therapy, and autonomous benign nodules may continue to grow. Nevertheless, documented growth of a lesion while the patient is on suppressive therapy warrants surgical intervention. Selection of patients for suppressive therapy rests on several factors. In patients with long-standing stable multinodular goiter, elderly patients with cardiovascular disease or tachyarrhythmias and those with thyroid gland autonomy and a suppressed baseline TSH, the physician may consider observation without treatment. Chronic suppression of TSH to less than 0.1 milliunit per liter is associated with decreased cortical bone mass, so treatment of patients at risk for osteoporosis should avoid complete suppression of TSH unless there are compelling reasons to do so (e.g., thyroid cancer). Nonpalpable nodules that are identified incidentally by ultrasound, MRI, or CT scan performed for other reasons should also probably be observed. In patients with benign cytopathologic findings on FNA, a trial of thyroxine suppression therapy may be reassuring if the nodule decreases in size. Similarly, a time-limited trial of suppression could be considered in a patient with a long-standing multinodular goiter and an indeterminate biopsy, although such an FNA reading in most other clinical settings should prompt referral for surgical resection.

Levothyroxine (T_4) (Synthroid, Levothroid) is the drug of choice for goiter therapy. Desiccated thyroid hormone preparations and synthetic combinations of T_4 and T_3 cause excessive elevations of serum T_3 concentration and are not physiologic. Once a decision has been made to proceed with suppressive therapy, the physician must establish treatment goals. In patients with diffuse goiters or with benign cytopathologic findings, complete suppression of TSH is not necessary; the TSH level should be suppressed to the low but detectable range (0.1 to 0.5 milliunit per liter). An initial T_4 dose of 100 to 150 μg daily, depending on patient age and weight, is usually sufficient. The TSH should be monitored with a sensitive second- or third-generation TSH assay. This approach should avoid the long-term complication of osteoporosis. We recommend a minimum of 6 to 12 months of T_4 therapy before declaring that a goiter has failed to respond because regression is more likely to occur with a longer period of treatment. If therapy is successful in decreasing or arresting growth of the nodule or goiter, the physician is left with the option of continuing therapy indefinitely or discontinuing treatment after several years. The rationale for continued therapy is that it may prevent emergence of new nodules or prevent further growth of the existing goiter if it has not disappeared completely with therapy. Discontinuation of therapy should be followed by close observation, and if regrowth is noted, lifelong suppressive therapy should be instituted.

Postsurgical treatment of patients with thyroid cancer, on the other hand, should aim for complete suppression of TSH into the undetectable range using a sensitive TSH assay. Further documentation that the T_4 dose is adequate may be provided by a blunted TSH response to administered thyrotropin-releasing hormone (TRH), although a suppressed ultrasensitive TSH value should suffice. Suppression therapy, however, should avoid inducing thyrotoxic symptoms. Lifelong therapy is indicated.

Surgery

Surgical treatment of nontoxic goiter that fails to respond to adequate T_4 suppression may be required if continued growth is noted, particularly if there is a concern about malignancy or if upper airway obstruction or other local compressive symptoms supervene. Although the practice should not be encouraged, some patients may request surgery as the initial approach for asymptomatic goiters for cosmetic reasons. Postoperatively, thyroid hormone is prescribed to prevent goiter recurrence.

Surgical excision may also be appropriate for some thyroid nodules. Patients whose FNA biopsies reveal malignant cells or reveal indeterminate findings along with suspicious clinical features should be referred for surgery. Nodules that grow with thyroxine suppression therapy should also be managed surgically. Recurrent thyroid cysts that do not respond to reaspiration can be excised, or they can be observed if they are small, simple cysts. The surgical management of thyroid cancer, as well as the management of toxic adenoma and toxic nodular goiter with surgery or radioactive iodine, is discussed in other articles.

HYPERPARATHYROIDISM AND HYPOPARATHYROIDISM

method of
JOHN P. BILEZIKIAN, M.D.
College of Physicians and Surgeons
Columbia University
New York, New York

DIAGNOSIS

The Hyperparathyroid States

Primary Hyperparathyroidism. Primary hyperparathyroidism is one of the more common endocrine disorders and has an incidence that approaches 1 in 1000. It occurs at all ages but peaks in the decade between 50 and 60 years. Women are affected more frequently than men by a ratio of 3:2. Primary hyperparathyroidism seems to surface most regularly among women within the first decade after the menopause. The disorder is due to excessive secretion of parathyroid hormone from one or more parathyroid glands. A single adenomatous gland is responsible for the disease in about 80% of cases, whereas hyperplasia affecting all four parathyroid glands is seen in about 15 to 20% of patients. Parathyroid carcinoma is exceedingly rare and is seen in only about 0.5% of patients with hyperparathyroidism. The sine qua non for diagnosis of primary hyperparathyroidism is hypercalcemia and elevated levels of parathyroid hormone. Most patients come to medical attention because of the discovery of hypercalcemia in the course of a routine multichannel screening test. Thus, primary hyperparathyroidism has an important role in the differential diagnosis of hypercalcemia. In this regard, the elevated serum parathyroid hormone concentration not only helps to confirm primary hyperparathyroidism but also rules out virtually all other causes of hypercalcemia. Experience with the two-site immunoradiometric and immunochemiluminometric assays (IRMA and ICMA, respectively) for intact parathyroid hormone and with the radioimmunoassay for midregion fragments of parathyroid hormone has shown that levels of PTH are elevated in about 90% of patients with primary hyperparathyroidism. In the remaining 10%, the PTH concentration is at the upper limits of normal, which can be regarded as abnormally elevated when hypercalcemia is present.

Hypercalcemia of malignancy is the other most common cause of hypercalcemia. Parathyroid hormone levels are suppressed in this setting because the parathyroid glands are inhibited when hypercalcemia is not caused by the parathyroid glands. This is also true when hypercalcemia of malignancy is caused by parathyroid hormone–related protein (PTHrP). PTHrP circulates in abnormally high levels in the syndrome of humoral hypercalcemia of malignancy, but it is not detected in any of the available assays for parathyroid hormone.

The more uncommon causes of hypercalcemia, such as those due to granulomatous disease, vitamin D or A toxicity, thyrotoxicosis, immobilization, and so on, are also associated with reduced levels of PTH. The only settings, besides primary hyperparathyroidism, in which PTH may be elevated in association with hypercalcemia are those related to thiazide or lithium use and familial hypocalciuric hypercalcemia. Appropriate historical information or family screening, if indicated, helps to rule out these causes. The unusual situation of hypercalcemia, markedly elevated levels of PTH, and renal failure (tertiary hyperparathyroidism) is discussed subsequently.

Secondary Hyperparathyroidism. The parathyroid glands are stimulated by hypocalcemia from any cause. This is a normal response of the parathyroids. By increasing parathyroid hormone production in response to a hypocalcemic stimulus, the serum calcium is returned toward normal by virtue of the physiologic actions of parathyroid hormone to conserve calcium in the renal tubules and to stimulate calcium release from bone. There are many causes of secondary hyperparathyroidism: any gastrointestinal disorder associated with deficient calcium absorption; any vitamin D deficiency state; some vitamin D–resistant states; any disorder leading to significant renal dysfunction; and states of parathyroid hormone resistance (pseudohypoparathyroidism—see later discussion). The essential difference between primary hyperparathyroidism and secondary hyperparathyroidism is the serum calcium level.

The serum calcium is elevated in primary hyperparathyroidism and is normal or reduced in secondary hyperparathyroidism.

Tertiary Hyperparathyroidism. This term refers to a situation of prolonged stimulation of the parathyroids due to a secondary cause that eventually leads to autonomous production of parathyroid hormone and hypercalcemia. It is a term that fell into disfavor but now has returned because it does accurately describe a pathophysiologic process and a clinical reality. The most common cause of tertiary hyperparathyroidism is long-standing, poorly controlled renal insufficiency. It is also seen, but more rarely, in situations of uncontrolled or unrecognized gastrointestinal tract malabsorption syndromes. Tertiary hyperparathyroid states are usually fairly obvious and are readily differentiated from primary hyperparathyroidism. PTH levels in tertiary hyperparathyroidism are on average much higher (more than fivefold above normal) than PTH levels in primary hyperparathyroidism (two- to threefold above normal). There is also usually an obvious cause.

The Hypoparathyroid States

Hypoparathyroidism. The sine qua non for diagnosis of hypoparathyroidism is hypocalcemia. By definition, also, PTH levels are inadequate to normalize the serum calcium concentration. In most situations, the PTH concentration is below normal or frankly undetectable. With the highly sensitive IRMA and ICMA assays for PTH, a diagnosis of hypoparathyroidism can be readily established. Most patients with hypoparathyroidism also have a high normal or frankly elevated phosphorus level. The causes of hypoparathyroidism are conveniently divided into those due to surgical removal of parathyroid tissue (postsurgical hypoparathyroidism) and those due to autoimmune destruction of parathyroid tissue (idiopathic hypoparathyroidism). Hypoparathyroidism can also occur in severe magnesium deficiency. Rarely, hypoparathyroidism may be caused by infiltration of the parathyroids by malignant tissue, iron (hemochromatosis), copper (Wilson's disease), or amyloid.

Postsurgical hypoparathyroidism is usually obvious by virtue of the history or evidence of prior neck surgery. The neck surgery need not have been prior parathyroid surgery. It could have been prior thyroid surgery or other neck surgery. Postsurgical hypoparathyroidism may develop soon after surgery or may not develop until many years have passed. In situations of delayed-onset postoperative hypoparathyroidism, it is believed that vascular compromise at the time of the surgery may place such a patient at risk and that, with the passage of years and the aging process, further reductions in vascular competence render the remaining parathyroid tissue insufficient.

Idiopathic hypoparathyroidism, which occurs at all ages, may be seen as an isolated endocrine deficiency state or in conjunction with the autoimmune end-organ endocrine deficiency syndrome. When seen as a component of the multiglandular insufficiency syndrome, the hypoparathyroidism may be the harbinger of subequent endocrine deficiencies such as hypothyroidism, hypoadrenalism, hypogonadism, diabetes mellitus, and hypopituitarism. Sometimes mucocutaneous candidiasis is associated with the hypoparathyroid state. The sequence, time course, and extent of endocrine gland involvement are all unpredictable.

The hypoparathyroidism of magnesium deficiency is virtually always associated with markedly reduced circulating levels of magnesium and an obvious cause such as severe malabsorption syndrome or alcoholism. The magnesium deficiency must be marked because mild reductions in magnesium levels actually stimulate the production of parathyroid hormone. In severe magnesium deficiency the cellular machinery that facilitates the secretion of parathyroid hormone into the extracellular space is impaired; thus, this is a true but reversible hypoparathyroid state.

The Pseudohypoparathyroid States

Pseudohypoparathyroidism is actually a form of secondary hyperparathyroidism (see earlier discussion). It is a state of resistance to the actions of parathyroid hormone. In most situations, pseudohypoparathyroidism is associated with hypocalcemia, hyperphosphatemia, and elevated levels of parathyroid hormone. Pseudohypoparathyroidism describes a number of different clinical and genetic abnormalities that are distinguished by their presentation and associated biochemical defects. The classic form of pseudohypoparathyroidism (Type IA) is associated with a phenotype known as Albright's hereditary osteodystrophy (AHO). Patients afflicted with AHO are short and have rounded facies with short necks and foreshortened metacarpal and metatarsal bones. They are hypocalcemic and hyperphosphatemic and show modestly elevated levels of PTH. These patients have a deficiency in the guanine nucleotide–binding protein Gs that is important in the biochemical coupling between the PTH receptor and the adenyl cyclase effector. The variant known as pseudohypoparathyroidism Type IB is not associated with the AHO phenotype, but the biochemical hypoparathyroidism is indistinguishable from that in Type IA. There is no defect in Gs in these patients. In both Type IA and IB pseudohypoparathyroidism, an infusion of PTH does not lead to the expected phosphaturia and an increase in urinary cyclic AMP excretion. Other variants of pseudohypoparathyroidism include Type II, in which cyclic AMP responsiveness is normal but there is no phosphaturia following PTH infusion. Pseudopseudohypoparathyroidism describes the unusual situation of the classic phenotype, namely AHO, without any biochemical abnormality.

TREATMENT

The Hyperparathyroid States

Primary Hyperparathyroidism

Most patients with primary hyperparathyroidism do not have signs or symptoms that can be clearly or commonly attributed to hypercalcemia or to excessive secretion of parathyroid hormone. They do not present with the classic manifestations of the disease such as kidney stones or overt skeletal demineralization. The condition is most often discovered in the course of a routine medical evaluation. Thus, the disease presents most often as asymptomatic primary hyperparathyroidism. Recognition that these patients constitute the majority of patients with primary hyperparathyroidism today presents a dilemma in management. When primary hyperparathyroidism used to be invariably associated with some complication that could be attributed to the hyperparathyroid state, the obvious therapeutic approach was to remove the offending parathyroid adenoma. Now, however, the clinician is faced with the nagging problem of a disease that is completely curable by surgery on the one hand, and a disorder that may well not eventually lead to any complications on the other hand.

Appreciating the dictum that surgery is usually reserved for those situations in which it is lifesaving or is necessary to improve the quality of life, patients with asymptomatic primary hyperparathyroidism often do not appear to be surgical candidates. No longitudinal studies of asymptomatic primary hyperparathyroidism have yet been carried out for a long enough period of time to know whether patients who do not undergo surgery are at significant risk for complications. Nevertheless, it appears that if patients have no accepted indications for surgery at the time they are first evaluated, their course is stable without progression or development of complications. Accepted surgical guidelines are shown in Table 1. If one follows these guidelines, approximately 50% of patients will be surgical candidates. It should be duly noted that the majority of patients who are candidates for surgery are asymptomatic in that they have hypercalciuria and reduced bone density (i.e., signs but no symptoms).

Surgery for primary hyperparathyroidism is relatively straightforward in the hands of an expert parathyroid surgeon. It has been written elsewhere that the most predictive element of successful localization and removal of abnormal parathyroid tissue is the expertise of the parathyroid surgeon. Parathyroid surgeons are successful in over 95% of cases. Parathyroid glands, however, are elusive, and there is an incidence of unsuccessful surgery. Among surgeons who are not intimately familiar with the nuances of parathyroid surgery and the favorite "hiding places" of ectopically located parathyroid tissue, the success rate is lower. It is the judgment of most experts in the field that noninvasive preoperative localization tests should be reserved for situations in which previous parathyroid surgery has been unsuccessful or in which the patient has had previous neck surgery for other reasons. In these situations, even the expert parathyroid surgeon is helped by preoperative localization. There are five noninvasive localization approaches in use: ultrasound, CT scanning, MRI, dual isotopic imaging with technetium and thallium, and a new isotopic imaging test involving technetium-labeled sestamibi. The approach is to gain localization by at least two of these noninvasive tests before embarking on repeat neck surgery for primary hyperparathyroidism. If localization is not achieved by these maneuvers, one might resort to invasive studies such as arteriography or selective venous catheterization of the neck. For invasive localization, it is recommended that patients be referred to centers that have experience in performing these tests.

For patients who are not operative candidates, a conservative approach is taken. They are seen twice yearly, at which time the serum calcium level is obtained. At yearly intervals a 24-hour urine collection (for calcium excretion) and bone mineral densitometry are performed. Any trend toward worsening hypercalcemia or hypercalciuria or a reduction in bone mass is an indication to proceed with surgery. Patients are recommended to keep ambulatory and well hydrated. They should avoid diuretics, especially thiazides. Their diet should be moderate in calcium-containing foods.

TABLE 1. **Guidelines for Surgical Treatment of Primary Hyperparathyroidism**

Serum calcium >1 mg/dL above the upper limits of normal
Presence of signs or symptoms (at any hypercalcemic level)
Hypercalciuria
Reduced cortical bone mineral density (>2 SD below controls)
Age (<50 years)
Difficulty in ensuring adequate medical follow-up

There are no specific medical approaches for inhibiting parathyroid hormone secretion and thus controlling the hyperparathyroid state. However, oral phosphate (1 to 1.5 grams daily) reduces the serum calcium concentration in patients with primary hyperparathyroidism. With phosphate therapy, one is concerned about ectopic soft tissue calcifications, especially if long-term therapy is contemplated. If there seems to be a real need to consider long-term phosphate therapy, it might be wise to consider parathyroid surgery. In postmenopausal women with primary hyperparathyroidism, estrogens have been advocated. The serum calcium level will decline when estrogens are administered, but the serum phosphorus concentration will not increase nor will the serum parathyroid hormone concentration be reduced. Nevertheless, estrogen therapy (0.625 mg daily of conjugated estrogens [Premarin] or the equivalent) may well be indicated in postmenopausal women for other reasons and will ameliorate the hypercalcemia. As is true for virtually all uses of estrogens in postmenopausal women who still have a uterus, a cyclic regimen with a progestational agent like medroxyprogesterone (Provera) (2.5 to 5.0 mg daily) is recommended.

When primary hyperparathyroidism is complicated by an episode of acute life-threatening hypercalcemia, patients are treated initially as they would be for any cause of hypercalcemia. They should then be promptly referred for definitive operative intervention.

Secondary Hyperparathyroidism

It is self-evident that the most effective way to treat secondary hyperparathyroidism is to treat the underlying cause of the hypocalcemic stimulus. However, the most common cause of secondary hyperparathyroidism, namely, renal insufficiency, is not usually reversible. Judicious medical management of the renal insufficiency in these patients includes a low phosphate diet (less than 1 gram daily), which helps to reduce the tendency to hyperphosphatemia and ectopic calcium-phosphate deposition in soft tissues. Additionally, phosphate binders can be useful to reduce gastrointestinal phosphate absorption. The most commonly used phosphate binders are calcium carbonate and calcium acetate instead of aluminum-containing compounds like aluminum hydroxide. The calcium salts, which are given with meals, bind phosphate without subjecting the patient to an excessive burden of aluminum that can be absorbed and can lead to a picture of aluminum osteodystrophy. Total daily calcium (dietary plus supplemental) is recommended to be 1 to 1.5 grams. It is particularly important to avoid citrated forms of calcium because aluminum absorption is heightened and can be a major problem if aluminum-containing phosphate binders are also being used. Depending on the serum calcium, phosphorus, and PTH levels, 1,25-dihydroxyvitamin D therapy can be very helpful. This active form of vitamin D is usually low in these patients because the renal 1α-hydroxylase activity that converts 25-hydroxyvitamin D to 1,25-dihydroxyvitamin D is either diminished in amount or inhibited. 1,25-Dihydroxyvitamin D (0.25 to 1.5 μg daily) facilitates calcium absorption and thereby reduces the stimulus to PTH production. If intact PTH levels are markedly elevated (more than three- to sixfold above normal), vitamin D therapy should be considered seriously. 1,25-Hydroxyvitamin D (calcitriol [Rocaltrol]) also inhibits gene transcription of PTH, but this gene effect is usually not demonstrable when modest daily doses (less than 1 μg) of the oral form of 1,25-dihydroxyvitamin D are used. However, pulse therapy with larger intermittent oral doses of 1,25-dihydroxyvitamin D (1 to 3 μg twice or thrice weekly) has been associated with significant reductions in circulating levels of PTH. In patients who are undergoing chronic dialysis, intravenous 1,25-dihydroxyvitamin D after each dialysis session (1 μg) is another effective approach to help control the secondary hyperparathyroidism associated with renal failure. If pulse oral therapy or postdialysis intravenous 1,25-dihydroxyvitamin D is to be used, the serum calcium and phosphorus concentrations must be monitored carefully. The implicit danger of this therapy is to increase both calcium and phosphorus levels, which could lead to ectopic calcium-phosphate deposition in soft tissues. Careful attention to dialysate calcium concentration, oral phosphate binders, and dietary restrictions can help to ensure the safety and efficacy of this therapy.

Tertiary Hyperparathyroidism

When the stimulus to produce PTH is long-standing and the underlying cause (i.e., renal insufficiency) is not successfully managed, hyperparathyroidism may become a major problem. Patients may manifest the classic bone changes of primary hyperparathyroidism, namely, osteitis fibrosa cystica with subperiosteal bone resorption, bone cysts, brown tumors, and generalized osteopenia. Bone pain is often a prominent disconcerting symptom. Parathyroid hormone levels by IRMA or ICMA, which reflect intact hormone and are not affected appreciably by the accumulation of inactive PTH fragments in renal insufficiency, may be extraordinarily high. In this situation, it is exceedingly difficult to apply the guidelines for management noted earlier for secondary hyperparathyroid states. Even if one were to control the excessive parathyroid glandular activity, it could well take years, during which time the patient might sustain marked further reductions in bone mass. These patients are best advised to undergo subtotal parathyroidectomy. At the time of parathyroidectomy, all four parathyroid glands are typically enlarged. Not uncommonly, however, a single gland may have become adenomatous and may in fact resemble the adenomatous gland of a patient with primary hyperparathyroidism. It may well be the case that prolonged stimulation of parathyroid tissue does lead, in some cases, to an autonomous hyperparathyroidism. Parathyroidectomy consists of removing most of the functional parathyroid tissue (3.5 glands) or performing a total parathyroidectomy and transplanting a small portion of tissue into the forearm. It is important not to render the patient truly hypoparathyroid because there is a greater risk to patients in this situation of developing other manifestations of renal osteodystrophy such as aluminum intoxication. One immediate benefit of parathyroidectomy in patients who are so afflicted is a rather immediate reduction in bone pain.

The Hypoparathyroid States

Chronic Hypoparathyroidism

The treatment of chronic hypoparathyroidism consists of adequate dietary and supplemental calcium along with vitamin D. This approach is applicable to patients with postsurgical, idiopathic, and pseudohypoparathyroidism. Calcium intake should be at least 1 to 1.5 grams daily. This is hard to achieve by dietary calcium alone, so supplemental calcium is usually prescribed. The most efficient preparation is calcium carbonate because calcium comprises a greater percentage of the compound (40%) than in any other formulation of calcium. In older patients, who may have a reduction in gastric hydrochloric acid, or in those who have known hypo- or achlorhydria, calcium citrate is preferred because it does not require hydrochloric acid for absorption.

It is very unusual for a patient with hypoparathyroidism to maintain normal calcium levels with calcium alone. The defect in production of 1,25-dihydroxyvitamin D (due to the inhibiting effects of high phosphorus and low PTH levels) usually means that patients need supplemental vitamin D as well. A popular preparation is 1,25-dihydroxyvitamin D, the active metabolite of vitamin D. The use of 1,25-dihydroxyvitamin D in amounts of 0.5 to 1.0 μg will facilitate calcium absorption from the gastrointestinal tract. This form of vitamin D is preferred because it is relatively fast-acting and is not stored appreciably in fat. Use of the other compounds that are available and could be used, 25-hydroxyvitamin D and cholecalciferol itself (vitamin D), may present problems because they must first be activated in the kidney and thus must be administered in pharmacologic amounts. The large quantities given may then lead to substantial storage in fat, especially of vitamin D, and at some point to a period of vitamin D toxicity.

Therapy of Acute Hypocalcemia

When hypocalcemia is accompanied by signs and symptoms of tetany, emergency therapy with parenteral calcium is usually indicated. The amount of calcium and the dispatch with which it is administered depend on the nature of the symptomatology and the actual level of the serum calcium. As is true for any electrolyte abnormality, the presence of clinical features is due not only to the actual level of the serum calcium but also to the rate of change. A patient who has experienced a sudden reduction in the serum calcium may be more symptomatic than one whose serum calcium reaches the same level more slowly. The use of calcium gluconate in a dose of 15 mg per kg given over 4 to 10 hours usually leads to a 2- to 3-mg/dL increase in the serum calcium concentration and provides satisfactory relief. In the presence of a life-threatening emergency with laryngospasm or seizure, administration of a 10-mL ampule of 10% calcium gluconate given intravenously over 5 to 10 minutes is indicated.

Hypoparathyroidism Due to Magnesium Deficiency

Patients with magnesium deficiency may present with marked hypocalcemia. If they have symptoms of tetany, the same approach with parenteral calcium gluconate is used as with any patient who has acute hypocalcemia. Obviously, magnesium therapy is important, but it should not be used alone in the presence of symptomatic hypocalcemia. This is because the hypoparathyroidism of hypomagnesemia is due not only to an inhibition of PTH secretion, a block that is overcome literally within seconds, but also to a peripheral resistance to the actions of PTH. This latter problem takes several days to overcome despite the fact that PTH levels rise rapidly after magnesium administration. The goal of magnesium therapy in this setting is to raise the serum magnesium but not to raise the serum calcium acutely or to replace total body magnesium stores. Effective therapeutic regimens include 2 grams of magnesium sulfate (200 mg of elemental magnesium) given as a 50% solution every 8 hours intramuscularly over several days. To avoid the pain associated with this route, magnesium sulfate can be given by intravenous infusion, 600 mg of elemental magnesium over 24 hours. The challenge of replacing total body magnesium stores is best met by ensuring an adequate diet and addressing the underlying cause of the magnesium deficiency. In situations of chronic gastrointestinal or renal losses, oral magnesium can be given as one of several different salts (oxide, chloride, lactate, and so on) to achieve a dose of 300 mg of elemental magnesium. Divided doses avoid the cathartic effect of magnesium.

Hypoparathyroidism in Pregnancy

Management of hypoparathyroidism in pregnancy is a special situation that requires careful monitoring. One wants to avoid any substantial period of hypocalcemia or hypercalcemia. Hypocalcemia in the early phases of pregnancy can conceivably lead to a heightened irritability of the uterus, thus placing the patient at risk for a spontaneous abortion. Hypercalcemia poses a risk of certain congenital abnormalities such as supravalvular aortic stenosis. These patients, however, can usually be managed by continuing their usual regimen of supplemental calcium and 1,25-dihydroxyvitamin D. It is important to recognize, however, that the placenta has the capability to synthesize 1,25-dihydroxyvitamin D and will do so toward the end of the second trimester and the beginning of the third. As the placenta begins to produce 1,25-dihydroxyvitamin D, the need for supplemental vitamin D therapy may be reduced. In some patients, the need for 1,25-dihydroxyvitamin D may actually be eliminated entirely during the third trimester. If management of the hypoparathyroidism has been successful, the offspring usually shows no untoward evidence of maternal hypoparathyroidism. Theoretically, however, chronic hypocalcemia in the mother could lead to a temporary hyperparathyroid state in the infant, a point that should obviously be checked if there has been any difficulty in this regard during the pregnancy.

PRIMARY ALDOSTERONISM

method of
DIANA L. MAAS, M.D., and
MAHENDR S. KOCHAR, M.D.
Medical College of Wisconsin and
Clement J. Zablocki Veterans Affairs Medical Center
Milwaukee, Wisconsin

Primary aldosteronism occurs in less than 1% of unselected hypertensive patients and is most common in the third through the fifth decades. Aldosterone is a mineralocorticoid hormone produced and secreted by the outer layer, the zona glomerulosa, of the adrenal gland's cortex. Its major site of action is at the distal tubule and collecting duct of the nephron, where it causes sodium reabsorption and potassium and hydrogen ion excretion. Key clinical and biochemical features of this syndrome include hypertension, hypokalemia, alkalosis, low plasma renin activity, and high aldosterone levels. The associated hypertension tends to be moderate, only rarely progressing to the accelerated or malignant phases, and is secondary to the sodium-retaining effects of this mineralocorticoid. From a practical perspective, the best screening test for primary aldosteronism is a serum potassium level obtained from blood drawn while the patient is ingesting an adequate salt intake and is not taking a potassium-sparing diuretic. Eighty to 90% of patients with primary hyperaldosteronism have a serum potassium level of less than 3.5 mEq per liter. Forty percent of hypertensive patients with spontaneous hypokalemia have a variant of primary hyperaldosteronism. Although rarely prominent, symptoms associated with hyperaldosteronism include polyuria, easy fatigability, anorexia, muscle weakness, and cramps. These features are secondary to the hypokalemia.

CAUSES OF PRIMARY ALDOSTERONISM

Causes of mineralocorticoid hypertension include primary hyperaldosteronism, real or apparent mineralocorti-

TABLE 1. **Causes of Mineralocorticoid Hypertension**

Primary hyperaldosteronism
1. Aldosterone-producing adenoma
2. Idiopathic hyperaldosteronism
3. Glucocorticoid-suppressible hyperaldosteronism
4. Adrenocortical carcinoma

Real or apparent mineralocorticoid excess not due to aldosterone
1. 11β-Hydroxysteroid dehydrogenase deficiency
   a. Ulick syndrome (genetic generalized)
   b. Induced-licorice (glycyrrhizic acid) carbenoxolone ingestion
2. Cushing's syndrome
   a. Deoxycorticosterone (DOC) excess
   b. 19-Nor-DOC excess
   c. Ectopic ACTH and adrenocortical tumors
3. 11β-Hydroxylase deficiency (DOC excess)
4. 17-Hydroxylase deficiency (DOC and 19-nor-DOC excess)
5. Liddle's syndrome

coid excess not due to aldosterone (Table 1), and secondary hyperaldosteronism. Unlike patients with primary hyperaldosteronism, patients with secondary hyperaldosteronism have hyperreninemic hyperaldosteronism and are not always hypertensive. Disorders leading to secondary hyperaldosteronism with hypertension include renal artery stenosis, renin-secreting tumors, malignant hypertension, and, in some instances, chronic renal disease. In hypertensive secondary hyperaldosteronism the elevated blood pressure is more likely to be related to increased angiotensin II rather than to aldosterone. Hyperreninemic hyperaldosteronism in patients with normotensive secondary hyperaldosteronism is due to decreased cardiovascular function with subsequent ineffective circulating blood volume. Patients with primary hyperaldosteronism typically have an increase in intravascular volume. Causes of normotensive secondary hyperaldosteronism include renal tubular acidosis, renal tubulopathies (Bartter's syndrome), hepatic cirrhosis, cardiac failure, gastrointestinal disorders, and diuretic abuse.

There are four major pathologic causes of primary hyperaldosteronism. They are aldosterone-producing adrenocortical adenomas (APA), idiopathic hyperaldosteronism (IHA), glucocorticoid-suppressible hyperaldosteronism, and aldosterone-producing adrenocortical carcinoma. The first two subtypes are the most common, APA accounting for 60 to 80% of cases of primary hyperaldosteronism. These adenomas are usually solitary, unilateral, small (0.5 to 2.5 cm), and benign. IHA is characterized by bilateral adrenocortical hyperplasia of the zona glomerulosa and accounts for 20 to 40% of cases of primary hyperaldosteronism. Although the pathogenesis of IHA is unknown, it is thought to result from hypersecretion of an unidentified aldosterone-stimulating factor, possibly of anterior pituitary origin.

Recently, the biochemical and genetic defects of glucocorticoid-suppressible hyperaldosteronism have been elucidated. Biochemical abnormalities include accumulation in the adrenal cortex's zona fasciculata of two unusual metabolites of cortisol, namely, 18-hydroxycortisol and 18-oxocortisol. Aldosterone synthase activity, an enzyme ordinarily restricted to the adrenal zona glomerulosa, has been isolated in the zona fasciculata of these patients. The genetic mutation causing this biochemical phenotype has recently been identified. Specifically, a hybrid gene containing the promoter region of the 11β-hydroxylase gene and the biochemically active portion of the aldosterone synthase gene has been isolated. Because this hybrid gene has the promoter region of the 11β-hydroxylase gene, it is under the control of adrenocorticotropin hormone (ACTH), but the enzymatic activity is that of aldosterone synthase. This enzyme allows synthesis of aldosterone and the hybrid steroids 18-hydroxycortisol and 18-oxocortisol. This excess mineralocorticoid activity suppresses plasma renin activity and with it, normal zona glomerulosa activity. Because this hybrid enzyme is under ACTH control, its activity can be suppressed with glucocorticoids.

Aldosterone-secreting adrenocortical carcinomas are a very rare cause of primary hyperaldosteronism. Typically, these tumors are plurihormonal-secreting mineralocorticoids, glucocorticoids, or sex steroids. In addition, unlike benign adenomas, the malignant tumors are usually large at the time of diagnosis (more than 3 cm).

DIAGNOSIS

There are two steps in the diagnosis of primary hyperaldosteronism. The first step is to confirm the presence of primary hyperaldosteronism, and the second step is to differentiate among the four causes of primary hyperaldosteronism. The tests for diagnosing primary hyperaldosteronism are improved by ensuring adequate salt intake and by treating the hypokalemia. Additionally, diuretics should be discontinued for at least 4 weeks, and spironolactone and estrogens should be stopped for at least 6 weeks. Other drugs that could affect the test results should be withheld for at least 1 to 2 weeks (Table 2). A hypertensive patient with either spontaneous hypokalemia (serum potassium of less than 3.5 mEq per liter) or marked provoked (diuretic-induced) hypokalemia (serum potassium of less than 3.0 mEq per liter) should be screened with the following tests: (1) 24-hour urine collection for potassium while the patient is hypokalemic, and (2) a simultaneous plasma renin activity (PRA) determination and plasma aldosterone concentration (PAC) (Table 3).

At this point, in a hypertensive patient taking no medication who has spontaneous hypokalemia, inappropriate kaliuresis, a suppressed upright PRA, and an elevated plasma aldosterone concentration, the diagnosis of primary hyperaldosteronism can be confirmed with one or more of the following tests after correcting the hypokalemia.

1. Upright PAC/PRA ratio. A 4-hour upright PAC/PRA ratio of greater than 20 is consistent with primary hyperaldosteronism. During the week prior to this test, the pa-

TABLE 2. **Drugs Potentially Interfering with the Renin-Angiotensin-Aldosterone Axis**

	PRA	**PAC**
Spironolactone	↑	↑
Estrogens	↑	↑
Diuretics	↑	↑
Prostaglandin synthase inhibitors	↓	↓
Angiotensin-converting enzyme inhibitors	↑	↓
Vasodilators	↑	↑
Sympathomimetics	↑	↑
Adrenergic inhibitors	↓	↓
Calcium channel blockers	↑	↓

Antihypertensive Drugs That Can Be Used During Testing for Primary Hyperaldosteronism

Central α_2-agonists such as methyldopa (Aldomet) and clonidine (Catapres)

Peripheral α_1-antagonists such as prazosin (Minipress)

Abbreviations: PAC = plasma aldosterone concentration; PRA = plasma renin activity.

TABLE 3. **Diagnostic Tests for Primary Hyperaldosteronism Due to Aldosterone-Producing Adenoma and Idiopathic Hyperaldosteronism**

Screening	
24-hour urinary potassium	>30 mEq/day
Plasma renin activity	<2 ng/mL/h
Plasma aldosterone concentration	>14 ng/dL
Confirmatory	
4-hour upright PAC/PRA	>20
Captopril suppression test	
PAC/PRA	>50
Plasma aldosterone	>15 ng/dL
4-hour saline infusion test	
Plasma aldosterone	>10 ng/dL
Localizing	
CT scan of the adrenals	
Adrenal vein catheterization	

Abbreviations: PAC = plasma aldosterone concentration; PRA = plasma renin activity.

tient is directed to maintain an intake of at least 100 mEq of sodium daily (5 to 6 grams of salt per day). The posture study is started at 8:00 A.M. after the patient has been kept recumbent overnight. A supine blood sample at 8:00 A.M. and 4-hour upright samples for PAC and PRA determinations are drawn. Because up to 30% of patients with essential hypertension may have a subnormal upright PRA (less than 3.0 ng per mL per hour), the concomitant measurement of an elevated PAC increases the diagnostic significance of the low PRA.

2. Captopril (Capoten) suppression test. The specificity of the PAC/PRA ratio is increased further with the addition of a PAC/PRA ratio taken 90 minutes after 25 to 50 mg of captopril is ingested. After captopril ingestion, a ratio of greater than 50 suggests primary hyperaldosteronism. In normal subjects receiving captopril, an angiotensin-converting enzyme (ACE) inhibitor, plasma aldosterone levels fall below 15 ng/dL.

3. Saline infusion test. A volume of 1250 to 2000 mL of normal saline is infused over 4 hours. In a normal patient this infusion suppresses PRA and, secondarily, PAC to less than 10 ng/dL. This test is contraindicated in patients who have had a recent myocardial infarction or stroke or who have congestive heart failure.

After a diagnosis of primary hyperaldosteronism has been established, one must determine the cause of this biochemical defect. Generally, this involves distinguishing between APA and IHA. This differentiation is made both biochemically and radiologically.

1. An initial assessment should be made using an adrenal computed tomography (CT) scan. CT scanning localizes the aldosterone-producing adenoma in 70 to 80% of cases. If an adenoma is not found with a CT scan, there is no advantage in performing an MRI scan.

2. The aforementioned 4-hour upright posture study can also be of benefit in differentiating APA from IHA in 90% of cases. Generally, individuals with APA have an ACTH-dependent circadian fall in plasma aldosterone concentration with upright posture. In contrast, patients with IHA respond with an increase in plasma aldosterone at the end of 4 hours owing to a posture-generated rise in angiotensin II. The adenomas are generally not responsive to angiotensin II stimulation. Measuring a plasma 18-hydroxycorticosterone (18-OHβ) level during the posture study may further aid in distinguishing between APA and IHA. Unlike patients with IHA, plasma 18-OHβ levels are generally greater than 100 ng/dL in APA patients.

3. The most definitive method of distinguishing between APA and IHA is bilateral adrenal vein catheterization for measurement of cortisol and aldosterone levels. This test is reserved for those relatively few patients in which CT scanning and posture studies are equivocal. Prior to proceeding with this invasive study, one should consider the patient's surgical risk. Cortisol levels are determined to confirm catheter placement and to correct aldosterone values for dilution by blood of extra-adrenal origin. Basal and ACTH-stimulated aldosterone-cortisol ratios are calculated from blood samples obtained from both adrenal veins and a peripheral site. An aldosterone ratio greater than 10 in the presence of a symmetrical ACTH-induced cortisol response is diagnostic of APA.

Because glucocorticoid-suppressible hyperaldosteronism is inherited in an autosomal dominant pattern, if several family members have a history of childhood-onset hypertension and spontaneous hypokalemia, this disorder should be suspected. The diagnosis is made by determining the response of urinary aldosterone to dexamethasone. Dexamethasone is given every 6 hours for 3 days at a dose of 0.5 mg and will decrease urinary aldosterone to 1 to 2 μg per day by the second or third day of treatment. These patients will also have an elevated serum 18-oxocortisol and 18-hydroxycortisol.

The diagnosis of adrenal aldosterone-producing carcinomas depends on the histologic demonstration of capsule and blood vessel invasion of tumor cells.

TREATMENT

The treatment of choice for patients with APA is surgical resection of the involved adrenal gland. One year after surgery, 70 to 80% of patients are cured of their hypertension and hypokalemia. Interestingly, although the patients remain normokalemic after the fifth postoperative year, only approximately 50% remain normotensive. In patients with a high surgical risk, medical management should be undertaken. In these cases medical management is initiated with spironolactone (Aldactone), a competitive inhibitor of the aldosterone cytosolic receptor. The dosage of spironolactone ranges from 50 to 400 mg daily. Generally, it is better to start at a higher dose, such as 200 mg daily, and titrate the dose downward. Although serum potassium levels are quickly restored to normal, blood pressure may remain elevated for 4 to 8 weeks. Side effects of spironolactone include impotence, decreased libido, gynecomastia, breast tenderness, and menometrorrhagia owing to its antiandrogen and progestational effects. Because of these antiandrogen effects, amiloride (Midamor) is often used as the initial treatment in men. In doses of 10 to 30 mg per day (initial dosage 5 mg twice daily), amiloride corrects hypokalemia in the majority of patients with APA and IHA but has little antihypertensive effect. Side effects of amiloride include fatigue, headache, impotence, increased serum uric acid concentration, and gastrointestinal disturbances. A third choice for hypokalemic correction is triamterene (Dyrenium). The initial dose is 100 mg twice daily, and the maximum dosage should not exceed 300 mg daily. Again, this drug also has little effect on blood pressure control.

The principal therapy for IHA is medical because bilateral adrenalectomy is usually ineffective in controlling hypertension. Medical therapy is aimed at correcting the hypokalemia and treating the hypertension. As with all hypertensive patients, therapy with a low-sodium diet (less than 80 mEq per day), regular exercise, and maintenance of ideal body weight significantly enhance the effects of pharmacologic therapy. Hypokalemia can be normalized with spironolactone as mentioned earlier. Not infrequently, another antihypertensive drug must be added to spironolactone to achieve optimal blood pressure control.

Agents with the best antihypertensive effects in patients with both APA and IHA are the calcium channel blockers. Specifically, nifedipine (Procardia, Adalat) seems to offer the best control of hypertension in APA. Because calcium is involved in the final steps of aldosterone production, these agents represent an alternative pharmacologic treatment strategy. Side effects include dizziness, flushing, headaches, peripheral edema, weakness, and constipation. If the elevated blood pressure persists after treatment with calcium channel blockers, other classes of antihypertensive agents can be tried empirically and are generally equally effective.

Although one would not expect ACE inhibitors, which block the formation of angiotensin II, to be effective in controlling blood pressure in patients with primary hyperaldosteronism, in fact they are effective in treating hypertension and hypokalemia in patients with IHA. Because the zona glomerulosa is very sensitive to angiotensin II stimulation, this antihypertensive effect of ACE inhibitors suggests that IHA may be dependent on angiotensin II. Side effects include cough, headache, dizziness, fatigue, gastrointestinal disturbance, impaired renal function, and hyperkalemia.

Long-term treatment with physiologic doses of glucocorticoid is used to manage hypertension and hypokalemia in patients with glucocorticoid-suppressible hyperaldosteronism. Alternatively, these patients may be treated effectively with one of the potassium-sparing diuretics or spironolactone, which does not disrupt the hypothalamic-pituitary-adrenal axis.

Surgical resection is the treatment of choice for aldosterone-secreting adrenal carcinoma. Mitotane (Lysodren) and cisplatin (Platinol) have very limited effects in stopping progression of disease in advanced cases.

HYPOPITUITARISM

method of
MARY LEE VANCE, M.D.
University of Virginia
Charlottesville, Virginia

Pituitary insufficiency, or hypopituitarism, may have disastrous consequences for the patient unless it is recognized and treated promptly. Without hypothalamic releasing hormones, stimulation of the anterior pituitary and subsequent release of trophic anterior pituitary hormones (adrenocorticotropic hormone [ACTH], thyroid-stimulating hormone [TSH], luteinizing hormone [LH], and follicle-stimulating hormone [FSH]), adrenal, thyroid, and reproductive functions cease. If growth hormone secretion is compromised during childhood, growth failure occurs. In contrast to the other anterior pituitary hormones, prolactin secretion may increase if there is interference with hypothalamic dopamine secretion or transport to the pituitary; prolactin is normally tonically inhibited by dopamine. When the supraoptic or paraventricular hypothalamic nuclei or posterior pituitary function is compromised, diabetes insipidus results. The most common causes of hypopituitarism are a large pituitary tumor, hemorrhage into a pituitary tumor (pituitary apoplexy), pituitary surgery, and pituitary radiation. Less common causes include metastatic disease, infections, granulomatous disease, trauma, intrasellar aneurysm, and cranial radiation during childhood.

Symptoms and signs of hypopituitarism usually develop insidiously and often sequentially. Exceptions include spontaneous hemorrhage into a tumor or hemorrhage resulting from pituitary surgery. The most common deficiencies in patients presenting with a large pituitary mass are of the gonadotropins (LH, FSH) and growth hormone. Gonadotropin deficiency in adults is characterized by menstrual abnormalities or infertility in women of reproductive age and by diminished libido or impotence in men. Symptoms of ACTH deficiency, resulting from secondary adrenal insufficiency (cortisol), include nonspecific complaints of fatigue, anorexia, and, in some patients, weight loss. Serum electrolyte abnormalities often include mild hyponatremia. Because mineralocorticoid (aldosterone) secretion is not regulated primarily by ACTH, the classic electrolyte abnormalities of hyperkalemia and hyponatremia of primary adrenal failure are usually absent. Physical examination may reveal only orthostatic hypotension; hyperpigmentation does not occur with ACTH deficiency. In women with long-standing ACTH deficiency, axillary and pubic hair may be absent. Symptoms of secondary hypothyroidism are the same as those of primary thyroid gland failure. More common symptoms include fatigue, weight gain or difficulty in losing weight, cold intolerance, and constipation. Physical examination may demonstrate periorbital puffiness, yellowish, doughy skin, and a delayed relaxation phase of deep tendon reflexes. Diabetes insipidus is characterized by polyuria and polydipsia; several liters of fluid per day may be ingested if the thirst center is intact. A striking feature is frequent, often hourly, nocturia. Physical examination is unremarkable if the patient has maintained adequate fluid intake and avoided dehydration and hypernatremia.

The biochemical diagnosis of hypopituitarism is straightforward if the target gland hormone concentrations are undetectable or inappropriately low. However, diagnosis of partial pituitary hormone deficiencies requires a stimulation test. The most important deficiencies are secondary adrenal insufficiency and secondary hypothyroidism because cortisol and thyroxine are necessary for life. Screening tests for pituitary insufficiency should include a *morning* serum cortisol, serum L-thyroxine (T_4), serum insulin-like growth factor 1 (IGF-1), somatomedin C (a measure of integrated growth hormone [GH] secretion), and serum testosterone (men). Some investigators recommend measurement of serum estradiol in women of reproductive age; a low serum concentration of estradiol is expected in a woman with amenorrhea and also occurs during the follicular phase of the menstrual cycle. The menstrual history is probably more useful to ascertain the onset of reproductive system problems. Levels of the pituitary hormones (ACTH, TSH, LH, and FSH) and growth hormone may be in the "normal" range but inappropriately low for the target gland hormone concentration; thus pituitary hormone concentrations should not be used to exclude pituitary failure. The serum prolactin concentration is often a useful indicator of pituitary dysfunction; an elevated serum prolactin suggests either a prolactin-secreting tumor or interference with normal dopaminergic inhibition of prolactin by a pituitary lesion.

HORMONE REPLACEMENT

The goals of replacement therapy are to relieve clinical symptoms, emulate normal physiology as much as possible, and avoid the side effects of over-replacement. Patients with adrenal or thyroid failure should always wear a medical identification bracelet or necklace in case of emergency (Medic Alert Foundation, Turlock, CA 95381; telephone 800-ID-ALERT).

ACTH Deficiency

Drugs include hydrocortisone, 20 mg on awakening, 10 mg in the evening; cortisone acetate, 25 mg on awakening, 12.5 mg in the evening; prednisone, 5 mg on awakening, 2.5 mg in the evening; dexamethasone, 0.5 to 0.75 mg once daily. The most physiologic drug is hydrocortisone. Some patients develop mild cushingoid features while taking a longer acting glucocorticoid (prednisone, dexamethasone). Conversely, because of the short half-life of hydrocortisone (4 to 8 hours), patients may develop fatigue, usually in the afternoon, which is relieved by a small third dose (usually 5 to 10 mg). During times of intercurrent illness or severe stress, the patient should be instructed to double the replacement dose for the duration of the illness. During hospitalization for severe illness or surgery, an appropriate stress regimen is hydrocortisone, 100 mg intravenously every 6 hours. Unfortunately, there is no blood or urine test to assess the appropriateness of glucocorticoid replacement; clinical features are used to determine the adequacy of the regimen.

TSH Deficiency

Drugs include L-thyroxine (T_4), which is the preferred and most physiologic preparation because it is deiodinated in the peripheral tissues to the active hormone, triiodothyronine (T_3), the rate of which is probably highly individual. The usual L-thyroxine (Synthroid) replacement dose in women ranges from 0.1 to 0.125 mg per day, and in men from 0.125 to 0.15 mg per day. Older adults (over 60 years), particularly those with a history of angina or coronary artery disease, should be started with a very small dose (0.0125 mg per day or every other day), which is increased gradually (0.0125 mg per week) over 4 to 6 weeks until the patient is clinically euthyroid. Biochemical monitoring of the thyroxine dose is best done by assessing clinical symptoms and measuring T_4 or T_3; serum TSH measurements are of no value in secondary hypothyroidism. One caveat: Thyroid hormone increases the metabolism of endogenous cortisol; thus, it is necessary to exclude partial ACTH deficiency before beginning thyroxine replacement.

Gonadotropin Deficiency

In *females* gonadal steroid replacement consists of estrogen and progesterone preparations when fertility is not desired. Estrogen and progesterone are contraindicated if there is a history of breast or endometrial cancer, recurrent thromboembolism, recent myocardial infarction or stroke, or liver disease. The goals of gonadal steroid replacement are to reduce the risk of osteoporosis and coronary artery disease and to prevent hot flashes, diminished libido, and vaginal and urethral atrophy. Various regimens are available; the minimum estrogen dose to prevent bone loss is 0.625 mg of conjugated estrogens (Premarin) or the equivalent (ethinyl estradiol [Estinyl], 20 or 50μg). Estrogen is given daily from days 1 to 25 of the month, and medroxyprogesterone acetate, 5 to 10 mg, is added on days 15 to 25, which allows endometrial sloughing and withdrawal bleeding. Another option is to give 0.625 mg of conjugated estrogen plus 2.5 mg of medroxyprogesterone acetate continuously; intermittent spotting may occur for a few months with amenorrhea later developing; this regimen is thought to prevent endometrial hyperplasia. Transdermal estrogen (4-mg patch applied twice weekly) is suitable for preventing accelerated bone loss, but it is not yet known whether the cardiovascular protective effect occurs with this preparation. If the woman has undergone a hysterectomy, progesterone is not required. In addition to estrogen and progesterone replacement, women should also ingest an adequate amount of elemental calcium (1000 to 1500 mg daily) to minimize the risk of bone loss. Side effects of oral estrogen include weight gain, headache, hypertension, breast tenderness, spotting, glucose intolerance, and increase in serum lipids (triglycerides, cholesterol); these effects are usually dose dependent and may diminish with a smaller estrogen dose.

If fertility is desired, a more complicated and expensive regimen is necessary to stimulate ovarian function. A combination of exogenous human chorionic gonadotropin (hCG) and FSH is necessary to stimulate gonadal steroid production and ovulation. Alternatively, pulsatile administration of gonadotropin-releasing hormone may be used if the pituitary gland is intact. Administration of these drugs is complex and produces a risk of ovarian hyperstimulation (ovarian enlargement, multiple pregnancy) and thus should be supervised only by physicians experienced in their use.

In *males,* if fertility is not desired, gonadal steroid replacement consists of a long-acting testosterone ester, testosterone cipionate or testosterone enanthate. Testosterone enanthate is administered by intramuscular injection, usually 200 to 300 mg every 3 weeks. Oral and buccal androgens are not as effective in restoring libido, sexual function, maintenance of secondary sexual characteristics, prevention of bone loss, or ejaculate volume (without spermatogenesis); additionally, they can produce cholestatic jaundice and possibly hepatic neoplasms. It is anticipated that a transdermal testosterone preparation will soon be available. Side effects of testosterone include mood changes, gynecomastia, breast tenderness, acne, and lowering of high-density lipoprotein (HDL) cholesterol concentrations. It is prudent to begin therapy with a small dose (testosterone enanthate, 50 or 100 mg) and increase it over 1 to 2 months. Hot flashes may develop if the interval between injections is too long. Because of the potential deleterious effect of testosterone on serum HDL cholesterol, the minimum dose that provides normal sexual function should be used. Testosterone has become a controlled drug, and prescriptions can be given for only 6 months.

If fertility is desired, testosterone is discontinued, and the man is treated with exogenous gonadotropins. If gonadotropin deficiency occurs after puberty, there may be some residual LH and FSH secretion; in this situation, the LH-like preparation, human chorionic gonadotropin (hCG), may be sufficient to promote testosterone production and spermatogenesis. hCG is administered as 500 international units three times per week intramuscularly for a month and may be increased to 5000 international units three times per week as necessary. Spermatogenesis requires approximately 76 days. Thus, after 3 months of treatment, sperm should be present in the ejaculate; a sperm count of 5 to 10 million per milliliter is usually adequate for fertility. If the patient has not completed puberty before hypopituitarism develops, a combination of LH (hCG) and FSH (e.g., Metrodin) is required to promote testosterone production and spermatogenesis. FSH is given as 75 international units intramuscularly three times a week. The appropriateness of the regimen is monitored by measuring monthly testosterone and estradiol concentrations; an increase in the hCG dose is indicated after 3 months if the testosterone level remains below 200 ng per dL, and a decrease is indicated if the estradiol level is over 50 pg per mL or if gynecomastia develops. Gonadotropin-releasing hormone (GnRH) is a suitable therapy for the patient with hypogonadism secondary to a hypothalamic GnRH deficiency. GnRH stimulates pituitary LH and FSH production with resulting testicular growth, testosterone production, and spermatogenesis. This hormone is administered in a pulsatile fashion every 2 hours subcutaneously, using a portable programmable pump and an indwelling subcutaneous catheter. The usual GnRH dose needed to produce normal serum testosterone levels ranges from 26 to 600 ng per kg for each bolus. GnRH therapy for fertility must be considered long-term treatment and may require 1 to 2 years to achieve an adequate sperm count. As in females, this treatment is complex and expensive and should be supervised only by a physician experienced in its use.

Growth Hormone Deficiency

Growth hormone replacement is currently approved only for children with short stature secondary to GH deficiency. In pre-pubertal children, recombinant human GH therapy (once nightly subcutaneous injection) accelerates linear growth. The greatest degree of linear growth acceleration occurs in children diagnosed at an early age; thus, early diagnosis is an important determinant of the ultimate treatment outcome. If a child is diagnosed as GH deficient relatively late (i.e., just before expected puberty), it is possible to delay the onset of puberty and epiphyseal closure with a long-acting GnRH agonist (e.g., Lupron) to enable GH therapy to produce a more beneficial effect on linear growth. Growth hormone replacement in adults is currently experimental and under investigation; it is not yet approved by the Food and Drug Administration (FDA) for adults. Short-term studies (up to 18 months) of GH replacement indicate that GH decreases adipose mass, increases muscle mass, and increases muscle strength in GH-deficient adults. Long-term effects and side effects are not yet known. Side effects such as edema, increased blood pressure and blood glucose, and arthralgias appear to be dose-dependent.

Antidiuretic Hormone Deficiency

If hypopituitarism involves the posterior pituitary (more common in patients with craniopharyngioma or after pituitary surgery), antidiuretic hormone (ADH or vasopressin) replacement is required to relieve the symptoms of diabetes insipidus (DI). Although a patient with DI may be able to maintain a euvolemic and normonatremic state, this occurs only with excessive urination and excessive ingestion of fluids with considerable disruption of the patient's activities. The diagnosis of DI is made on the basis of clinical features, especially a history of frequent urination, particularly at night, accompanied by thirst and frequent fluid (usually water) ingestion. The random serum sodium and serum osmolality are normal if fluid intake is adequate; morning urine osmolality is usually very low, which, along with a history of pituitary disease or surgery, suggests DI. Definitive diagnosis may require a water deprivation test (during hospitalization under close physician supervision). If DI is present, the most simple replacement therapy is the nasally administered vasopressin analogue, DDAVP. The dose of DDAVP must be titrated to relieve symptoms of polyuria and polydipsia; some patients require twice-daily doses (one spray in each nostril), whereas others achieve control with a once-daily spray in each nostril. The patient can usually estimate the need for a DDAVP dose based on the onset of polyuria. The side effect of over-replacement is hyponatremia; altered mental status occurs if the serum sodium is sufficiently low. The consequence of under-replacement is uncontrolled polyuria and hypernatremia and hypovolemia if inadequate fluid ingestion occurs.

HYPERPROLACTINEMIA

method of
EUGENE KATZ, M.D.
Greater Baltimore Medical Center
Baltimore, Maryland

Prolactin, a polypeptide hormone secreted by the anterior pituitary, is under tonic inhibition by hypothalamic dopamine, which reaches the anterior pituitary by way of the pituitary-portal system. Until recently prolactin was thought to be essentially a mammotropic hormone but is now believed to play a role in the modulation of the immune system as well.

Hyperprolactinemia can result from physiologic, pharmacologic, and functional (idiopathic) causes (Table 1). Commonly, hyperprolactinemia is suspected in the presence of an abnormal menstrual cycle (oligomenorrhea, amenorrhea) or galactorrhea. The severity of these signs varies because of two factors. One is the presence of dimers (big-prolactin) and tetramers (big-big prolactin) of the hormone, which are immunoreactive (recognized as prolactin when the hormone is measured in radioimmunoassay) but possess little biologic activity. The second factor is the existence of variable proportions of glycosylated and nonglycosylated circulating prolactin of different biologic activities. In addition to the specific signs associated with hyperprolactinemia of any origin, patients may present with endocrine manifestations specific to the pathologic condition underlying the disorder (hypothyroidism, hypothalamic failure, pituitary failure, acromegaly, and so on) as well as with signs associated with compression by a prolactinoma on adjacent structures. In turn, these signs may be nonspecific (e.g., headaches) or specific (e.g., temporal hemianopsia, oculomotor dysfunction, facial pain, seizures).

Both CT scans and magnetic resonance imaging (MRI) are highly effective in delineating pituitary tumors and, in the case of MRI, in defining the structural relationships of the pituitary gland with the adjacent structures.

Prolactinomas are classified radiologically into microadenomas (less than 10 mm in diameter) and macroadenomas. In general, larger tumors are associated with circulating prolactin levels in excess of 100 ng per mL. In addition, in the absence of pregnancy, most patients with prolactin levels of over 200 mg per mL harbor a pituitary tumor.

TREATMENT OF HYPERPROLACTINEMIC DISORDERS

Treatment of hyperprolactinemia of pharmacologic origin consists in eliminating, if possible, the drug implicated in lactotroph hyperactivity. When alternative medications are not available, the effects of hyperprolactinemia must be weighed against the consequences of discontinuing the drug altogether. The treatment of pathologic conditions other than prolactin-producing pituitary adenomas and idiopathic hyperprolactinemia should be directed toward correction of the underlying pathology (e.g., hypothyroidism, hypernephroma).

TREATMENT OF PROLACTIN-PRODUCING PITUITARY ADENOMAS

Theoretically, prolactinomas can be managed with radiotherapy, surgery, dopaminergic agents, or combinations thereof. Furthermore, if small, prolactinomas can be managed with observation alone.

Radiotherapy is effective in shrinking most tumors. However, given the slow rate of response and, more important, the potential development of secondary panhypopituitarism, radiotherapy is reserved only for large tumors that fail to respond to medical treatment and for which surgery has failed or is not possible.

Surgical treatment consists of excision of the tumor through a transsphenoidal approach. Although safe in experienced hands, it carries the risk of infection, postoperative cerebrospinal fluid leak, and transient diabetes insipidus.

Bromocriptine, a dopamine agonist, was first introduced as a therapeutic agent in 1969 and remains the only agent available for treatment of hyperprolactinemic disorders in the United States since it was approved for clinical use in this country in 1979. Bromocriptine (Parlodel) is a semisynthetic product derived from a family of ergot alkaloids. Bromocriptine exerts a direct effect at the pituitary level, competing with dopamine for binding to the anterior pituitary. In addition, bromocriptine inhibits the secretion of prolactin by isolated and heterotopic pituitary glands and lactotroph proliferation.

After an oral dose of bromocriptine mesylate, 28% of the drug is absorbed. Of that fraction, 94% is metabolized after the first passage through the liver and excreted in the bile and feces. Following a single oral dose of 2.5 mg, drug levels tend to peak at 3 hours and then fall; the half-life is 3.3 hours. The effect of the drug is almost immediate, and prolactin levels remain low for at least 8 hours. Attempts to administer vaginally the same tablet of bromocriptine mesylate designed for the oral route have also proved successful. Given in this fashion, the drug bypasses the liver, and serum levels of bromocriptine display a continuous rise over a period of 8 hours accompanied

TABLE 1. **Causes of Hyperprolactinemia**

I. Physiologic	Pregnancy, excessive breast stimulation, stress, surgery, venipuncture, etc.
II. Pharmacologic*	
Depletion of dopamine stores	Reserpine
Blockade of dopamine binding	Phenothiazines: chlorpromazine (Thorazine), thioridazine, (Mellaril), prochlorperazine (Compazine), perphenazine (Trilafon), trifluoperazine (Stelazine), pimozide (Orap)
	Thioxanthenes: chlorprothixene (Taractan)
	Butyrophenones: haloperidol (Haldol)
	Benzamines: metoclopramide (Reglan),
	Alpha-methyldopa (Aldomet)
	Dibenzazepine antidepressants: amoxapine (Asendin)
Inhibition of dopamine release	Opiates: methadone, morphine, meperidine (Demerol), etc.
Blockade of H_2 receptor binding	Cimetidine (Tagamet), ranitidine (Zantac), famotidine (Pepcid)
Estrogen-containing preparations	Oral contraceptives, estrogens
Others	Tricyclic antidepressants: imipramine (Tofranil), amitriptiline (Elavil, Etrafon)
	Papaverine (Pavabid)
	Verapamil (Calan, Isoptin, Verelan)
III. Pathologic	
Primary hypothyroidism	Neoplastic, infectious, vascular, degenerative or granulomatous lesions
Hypothalamic disorders	Prolactin-secreting adenoma, acromegaly, Cushing's disease, Nelson's syndrome
Pituitary stalk section	
Pituitary disorders	
Ectopic production	Bronchogenic cancer, hypernephroma, cervical cancer
Chronic renal failure	
Chest wall lesions	Surgical scars, herpes zoster
IV. Functional	
Idiopathic (no demonstrable tumor)	

*Partial list. In general, suspect any drug that affects the central nervous system.

by a concomitant decrease in serum prolactin levels. Oral doses as low as 1.25 mg per day are often sufficient to normalize serum prolactin levels in patients with mild idiopathic hyperprolactinemia, whereas most patients with tumors respond to less than 10 mg per day. Bromocriptine is not without adverse effects. Some unwanted reactions to bromocriptine appear to be associated with the initiation of therapy, whereas others appear to be the result of long-term administration. Initially, bromocriptine may induce nausea, vomiting, postural hypotension, headaches, and nasal stuffiness. These side effects are transient and can be minimized by administering the drug at bedtime, by avoiding large increments in dosage, and by providing the drug in conjunction with meals. For instance, 1.25 mg can be initiated at bedtime and the dose then increased to 2.5 mg after 5 to 7 days. Vaginal administration of bromocriptine is effective and may be better tolerated than oral bromocriptine. Bromocriptine mesylate may produce alcohol intolerance and gastrointestinal bleeding, and very high doses (as prescribed for Parkinson's disease) may result in cold-induced digital vasospasm (not "ergotism"), erythromelalgia, hallucinations, delusions, dementia, and depression. To date, there is no evidence of long-term harmful effects of bromocriptine mesylate on hepatic, renal, or hematologic functions. Parlodel crosses the placenta but does not appear to have a significant teratogenic potential. However, for patients attempting to become pregnant, some practitioners advocate discontinuation of therapy after ovulation to avoid exposure of the embryo to bromocriptine. The only other dopamine agonist available in the United States is pergolide mesylate, which is approved for use in Parkinson's disease. Although it is less well tolerated than bromocriptine, some patients who are intolerant to bromocriptine prefer it.

A long-acting form of bromocriptine has been developed for intramuscular injection (Parlodel-LAR) but is not available in the United States. A single 50-mg intramuscular injection of Parlodel-LAR suppresses prolactin for 28 days, with a gradual return to pre-injection levels thereafter. Also not available in the United States is another long-acting bromocriptine preparation (Parlodel-SRO), which requires a single daily dose.

Newer nonergot dopamine agonists (also not available in the United States) include pramipexole, cabergoline, and quinagolide (CV 205-502). Cabergoline can be administered orally once weekly, and CV 205-502 requires a single daily dose that produces less severe side effects than bromocriptine. However, as is often seen in clinical practice, tolerability to one medication or another is an individual matter, and some patients who are unable to tolerate a newer preparation tolerate bromocriptine better.

TREATMENT OF MACROADENOMAS

Macroadenomas, defined as tumors that exceed 10 mm in diameter, can be managed surgically or medically. Although capable of effecting immediate (albeit transient) resolution in up to 60% of cases with relatively low morbidity and mortality rates, the surgical approach is associated with an unacceptable recurrence rate that can reach 91%. Consequently, this mode of therapy is not curative, strongly suggesting that the more conservative (albeit equally noncurative) medical approach may be superior. Bromocriptine effectively reduces the size of macroadenomas in 33 to 100% of patients, including those with suprasellar extension. Rapid tumor shrinkage occurs during the first 3 months with continued slower shrinkage for 12 months or more. Although serum prolactin values appear to reach normal levels in 50 to 100% of cases, a significant but not necessarily complete reduction in the circulating levels of the hormone is observed in practically all cases. Although the effect of bromocriptine is dramatic, regrowth can occur when the drug is discontinued. Patients resistant to one dopaminergic agonist may respond to treatment with another.

In summary, bromocriptine constitutes the initial treatment of choice for all macroprolactinomas, particularly in view of the limitations and potential complications of alternative forms of therapy. During pregnancy, symptomatic macroadenomas respond dramatically to bromocriptine as well.

TREATMENT OF MICROADENOMAS

Transsphenoidal resection of microprolactinomas results in correction of hyperprolactinemia in 54 to 93% of cases. Although the morbidity associated with surgery is low, it is certainly higher than the morbidity associated with bromocriptine. Even in experienced hands, recurrence rates after surgery can reach 50%. On the other hand, bromocriptine represents a highly effective noninvasive alternative to surgery. Bromocriptine reduces prolactin levels in 94 to 100% of patients with microprolactinomas, although not always to within the normal range. Nevertheless, even such an apparently incomplete response is, in most cases, adequate to bring about the return of ovulation and fertility. Although in some cases the remission of hyperprolactinemia is permanent, in most patients discontinuation of treatment results in elevated prolactin levels.

In selecting the appropriate treatment, particularly when fertility is not a consideration, it is important to remember that the natural history of the disease is not completely understood. Microadenomas, left untreated, display a slow rate of progression. It is not known what proportion of smaller tumors progress to macroadenomas. However, the fact that microadenomas are so prevalent whereas invasive macroadenomas are seldom seen suggests that prolactinomas are in most cases nonprogressive. Therefore, in patients with a microprolactinoma, simple observation without treatment appears to be an acceptable management option when symptoms are not unacceptable and fertility is not being sought. One possible exception to this rule, however, is the hyperprolactinemic hypoestrogenic patient or the one in whom bone loss is observed.

During pregnancy, less than 2% of microprolactinomas and less than 10% of macroadenomas show significant re-expansion. Their behavior can be monitored with serial visual field examinations or MRI. If re-expansion threatens adjacent structures, bromocriptine therapy can be safely reinstituted.

BROMOCRIPTINE IN IDIOPATHIC HYPERPROLACTINEMIA

The term idiopathic hyperprolactinemia is used to refer to those hyperprolactinemic patients in whom there is no radiologically proven pituitary tumor. In these cases, bromocriptine is highly effective in correcting the hyperprolactinemia. However, as with microprolactinomas, if symptoms are not unacceptable to the patient and fertility is not being sought, expectant management constitutes an acceptable option. However, decreased bone density has been reported to occur in hyperprolactinemic women. Although the lack of estrogen probably contributes to the bone loss, hypoestrogenism in itself may not fully account for the development of osteoporosis. Rather, prolactin may also affect bone economy either directly or indirectly. Because the correction of hyperprolactinemia restores bone density, patients who choose not to be treated must be counseled about the effects of high levels of prolactin on bone density.

Recently, prolactin has been shown in animals to exert a profound effect on the immune system. Indirect evidence in the human suggests that prolactin has a stimulatory effect on the immune system. In fact, hyperprolactinemia is more commonly found in patients with rheumatoid arthritis and systemic lupus erythematosus. Therefore, when considering the option of observation alone, hyperprolactinemic patients should be advised that prolactin may play a role in the pathogenesis of autoimmune disorders.

HYPOTHYROIDISM

method of
BEN PATAROQUE, M.D., and
DAVID S. COOPER, M.D.
Sinai Hospital of Baltimore
Baltimore, Maryland

Hypothyroidism is a clinical and biochemical state in which the supply of thyroid hormones to the tissues is inadequate for cellular needs. Because the metabolic effects of thyroid hormone are ubiquitous, its absence may adversely affect almost all body functions. Clinically, hypothyroidism is a spectrum of disease, ranging in severity from unrecognized subclinical hypothyroidism to life-threatening myxedema coma. Hypothyroidism is usually caused by primary failure of the thyroid gland itself; the absence of pituitary thyroid-stimulating hormone (TSH), or, more rarely, hypothalamic thyrotropin-releasing hormone (TRH) deficiency, is far less common. A rare defect is tissue resistance to thyroid hormone. In the United States the most common cause of hypothyroidism is chronic lymphocytic thyroiditis, or Hashimoto's thyroiditis, which is most prevalent in women over 50 years of age; the patient presents with a diffuse goiter and positive antithyroid antibodies. Primary hypothyroidism also occurs commonly after radioactive iodine treatment or thyroidectomy. Other causes include ingestion of goitrogenic drugs, especially lithium carbonate and amiodarone, and congenital absence of the thyroid. Whatever its cause, the treatment remains the same: replacement therapy with exogenous thyroid hormone.

DIAGNOSIS

The classic signs and symptoms of hypothyroidism include fatigue, dry hair and skin, weight gain, constipation, cold intolerance, and delayed relaxation of the deep tendon reflexes. Some patients with mild or subclinical hypothyroidism may be asymptomatic. The diagnosis of primary hypothyroidism is confirmed by a low free thyroxine (T_4) or free T_4 index and an elevated serum TSH concentration. In subclinical hypothyroidism, serum thyroxine levels are normal, but the TSH concentration is elevated, with levels usually less than 20 milliunits per liter. In this situation, the pituitary gland perceives the levels of thyroxine to be inadequate, even though they may be within the broad range of normal. The great sensitivity of the pituitary enables the physician to detect a seemingly minor impairment in thyroid function. Secondary hypothyroidism should be suspected if the free T_4 or free T_4 index and the TSH level are low or low-normal. Patients with diffuse goiter secondary to Hashimoto's thyroiditis usually have elevated antithyroid antibody titers (antimicrosomal antibody, also called antithyroid peroxidase or antiTPO, and antithyroglobulin antibody).

TREATMENT

Preparations

Synthetic L-thyroxine (levothyroxine sodium [Synthroid]) is the only drug currently recommended for the chronic treatment of hypothyroidism. Once a day therapy provides stable levels of both T_4 and the more active triiodothyronine (T_3) because of peripheral T_4 to T_3 conversion. A wide range of tablet strengths permits precise titration of the dose. The goal of L-thyroxine therapy is to normalize TSH levels and correct clinical symptoms. Desiccated thyroid preparations may yield variable serum thyroid hormone concentrations, which could result in undesirable symptoms and problems in biochemical monitoring. We do not recommend their use. Patients taking these medications should be switched to L-thyroxine. The metabolic equivalent of 1 grain of desiccated thyroid hormone is 0.1 mg of synthetic L-thyroxine. However, a better way of switching to L-thyroxine is to base the dose on the patient's body weight (see subsequent section). Liothyronine (synthetic L-T_3 [Cytome]) has no role in chronic therapy. However, it is often used for short-term therapy of patients with thyroid cancer after thyroidectomy in preparation for ^{131}I scanning, and it may be useful in the management of myxedema coma.

Dosage

Before initiating L-thyroxine treatment, one should consider the patient's age and underlying medical problems as well as the severity and cause of the hypothyroidism. L-Thyroxine is generally started at a dose of 50 to 75 μg per day, with 25-μg increments until a euthyroid state is achieved. A full replacement dose is approximately 1.6 μg per kg per day, which is usually 75 to 100 μg per day for women and 100 to 150 μg per day for men. Patients who develop hypothyroidism after radioiodine therapy or thyroidectomy for Graves' disease may require a lower dose than this because of persistent autonomous thyroid function. In otherwise healthy individuals, the full L-thyroxine dose may be given at the outset; a lower starting dose of 25 μg per day is recommended for patients with severe hypothyroidism and the elderly, in whom cardiac disease is often present. Because the half-life of L-thyroxine is 6 to 7 days, steady-state levels are not achieved until 6 weeks after therapy is initiated. On average, TSH levels should normalize within this time. Patients should be told that complete resolution of symptoms may take months, even when biochemical parameters have become normal.

Side Effects and Adverse Reactions

True allergic reactions have not been documented except in the rare patient who might conceivably have a reaction to the excipients in the thyroxine tablets. Vague complaints that may be psychosomatic in origin can sometimes be alleviated by administering the drug with meals or in divided doses.

Hypothyroid women who are infertile should be cautioned that therapy may restore fertility. An increase in insulin requirement may also occur in diabetics, and anticoagulant dosage may need to be reduced. Because L-thyroxine can increase the metabolism of cortisol, any patient with suspected adrenal insufficiency should be evaluated before L-thyroxine therapy is initiated. If adrenal insufficiency is documented, the patient should be receiving full steroid replacement treatment before thyroid hormone is begun.

Most problems related to thyroid hormone replacement are due to overtreatment. Anxiety, headache, tremors, and palpitations are the usual complaints in this situation. L-Thyroxine-induced hyperthyroidism can be confirmed by a suppressed serum TSH level; it can be managed by temporary cessation of therapy with resumption at a lower dose 1 week later.

Chronic Therapy

The adequacy of thyroxine therapy should be confirmed by annual measurement of the serum TSH. Routine free T_4 or free T_4 index measurements are usually not necessary to monitor the treatment of stable primary hypothyroidism, but they are needed in patients with central hypothyroidism. Because TSH cannot be used as a guide in these patients, the free T_4 or free T_4 index should be adjusted so that it is in the middle of the normal range. An increase in L-thyroxine replacement dose may be necessary in hypothyroid patients with malabsorption or in patients treated with drugs that accelerate L-thyroxine metabolism such as phenytoin (Dilantin), carbamazepine (Tegretol), and rifampicin (Rifampin). Certain drugs such as cholestyramine (Questran), colestipol (Colestid), ferrous sulfate, and sucralfate (Carafate) may interfere with L-thyroxine absorption. In patients taking these agents, L-thyroxine administration should be temporally spaced far apart from the other drugs. Patients in whom hypothyroidism persists despite adequate L-thyroxine dosage and in whom malabsorption or drug interactions can be ruled out are usually noncompliant with their medication. Occasionally, patients taking generic L-thyroxine preparations have an inadequate response owing to lower bioavailability or potency than in the proprietary products, and it is for this reason that we prefer to prescribe nongeneric L-thyroxine. Overzealous L-thyroxine therapy may also adversely affect bone metabolism (i.e., osteoporosis), especially in postmenopausal women. Overtreatment can also exacerbate cardiac symptoms. Therefore, patients taking L-thyroxine replacement therapy should be monitored with TSH measurements to prevent the adverse consequences of iatrogenic hyperthyroidism. With the use of sensitive TSH assays that can determine TSH concentration to as low as 0.05 milliunit per liter, overtreatment with L-thyroxine can be easily detected and should be avoided. TSH levels should be maintained within the normal range, which is between 0.5 and 5 milliunits per liter in most laboratories.

It should be recalled that thyroid hormone production normally declines with age. Therefore, the requirement for L-thyroxine also decreases as patients get older. In general, a 10 to 15% decrease in the replacement dose is anticipated in patients over the age of 65 or 70 years.

SPECIAL TREATMENT SITUATIONS

Myxedema Coma

Myxedema coma is a medical emergency. It typically occurs in hypothyroid patients with longstanding disease that may have been unrecognized or inadequately treated. It is often precipitated by concomitant systemic disease, surgery, or drugs such as narcotics and hypnotics. Treatment is directed not only toward reestablishing normal thyroid hormone levels but also toward ventilatory support, correction of fluid and electrolyte balance, treatment of infection, and reversal of hypothermia by passive (not active) warming. The proper method of treatment in this condition remains controversial. Treatment with large doses of L-T_3 (Cytomel) to restore metabolic function rapidly may be appropriate but may also lead to higher cardiovascular mortality. However, severely ill patients may have impaired T_4 to T_3 conversion, so that L-thyroxine therapy may be relatively ineffective. There is currently no consensus of opinion about the most appropriate therapy for myxedema coma. Administration of L-thyroxine in loading doses of 300 to 500 μg given intravenously, followed by daily intravenous doses of 100 to 150 μg, is standard therapy. Intravenous L-T_3 (Triostat) in doses of 10 to 12.5 μg every 4 to 6 hours may prove to be equally or even more effective than L-thyroxine, but further studies are necessary before L-T_3 administration can be recommended as routine therapy.

Pregnancy

Hypothyroidism may develop during pregnancy, but more often it exists in pregnant women with previously treated hypothyroidism. During pregnancy the L-thyroxine dose should be periodically assessed because a higher dosage may be necessary beginning in the first trimester. It is recommended that serum TSH be assessed at 8 weeks' and again at 6 months' gestation. After delivery, the replacement dose will need to be reduced to prepregnancy levels to avoid iatrogenic hyperthyroidism. L-Thyroxine can be safely taken during nursing because little is transferred to breast milk.

Coronary Artery Disease

Treatment of elderly hypothyroid patients with coronary artery disease requires caution. However, in most patients, angina remains stable, and it may even improve. For any cardiac patient, L-thyroxine treatment should be initiated with 12.5 to 25 μg per day, with increasing increments of 12.5 to 25 μg at 6-week intervals. If anginal symptoms become worse, the medications should be discontinued or the dosage lowered. Treatment of coronary artery disease with agents such as aspirin, nitrates, beta blockers, and calcium channel blockers should be used to maximize medical therapy. Some patients may require angiography and subsequent bypass surgery or angioplasty if maximal cardiac therapy does not allow restoration of a euthyroid state. If invasive cardiac testing or therapy is not warranted, "compromise therapy" with L-thyroxine will at least partially alleviate symptoms of hypothyroidism.

Surgery or Emergency Surgery in Hypothyroid Patients

Surgery is generally well tolerated by hypothyroid patients, but they may be at increased risk for perioperative complications, including fluid and electrolyte abnormalities, increased sensitivity to anesthetics, and prolonged ileus. Fever is less likely to occur with infection in hypothyroid patients. Thus, they may require lower anesthetic doses, fluid balance and electrolytes must be monitored vigilantly, and infection must be considered even in the absence of fever. Emergency surgery should not be postponed in hypothyroid patients, but it is reasonable to defer elective surgery until a euthyroid state is achieved.

Transient Hypothyroidism

Transient hypothyroidism occurs as part of the evolution of subacute thyroiditis and painless thyroiditis. The latter is also called postpartum thyroiditis because of its propensity to develop in the postpartum period. Because the hypothyroidism in these conditions is usually self-limited and mild, therapy is often not needed. Some patients may require L-thyroxine therapy for 6 to 12 months to alleviate hypothyroid symptoms. Approximately 25% of patients with painless or postpartum thyroiditis develop permanent hypothyroidism and may require lifelong replacement therapy.

Subclinical Hypothyroidism

Subclinical hypothyroidism is at the far end of the spectrum of hypothyroidism. In these patients thyroxine levels are normal, but TSH levels are slightly to modestly elevated. It may be the most common thyroid disease in the United States, with a prevalence rate of 10 to 15% in women over age 60. Treatment of this entity is controversial because patients typically have few or no symptoms. However, two randomized placebo-controlled trials have shown modest improvements in hypothyroid symptoms in mildly symptomatic patients who receive thyroxine. Also, patients with subclinical hypothyroidism may have subtle reversible abnormalities of low-density lipoprotein (LDL) and high-density lipoprotein (HDL) cholesterol. Serum TSH can usually be normalized with relatively small doses of thyroxine (i.e., 50 to 100 μg daily). Another reason to consider treatment even when patients are asymptomatic is the high rate of progression to overt thyroid failure (5 to 20% of patients per year) in patients with subclinical hypothyroidism and positive antithyroid antibodies. If therapy is not begun, annual thyroid function testing is recommended, particularly in elderly patients with circulating antithyroid antibodies, who have a particularly high rate of thyroid failure on follow-up.

REASSESSMENT OF HYPOTHYROIDISM

The clinician may occasionally encounter a patient taking thyroid hormone without prior documentation of hypothyroidism. In selected situations, it may be reasonable to discontinue L-thyroxine in such patients, particularly if the reasons for its use appear to have been inappropriate (e.g., for treatment of obesity, infertility, or fatigue). If the initial serum TSH concentration is normal, the dose can be decreased by 50% and levels measured 6 weeks later. An elevated TSH level confirms the presence of hypothyroidism, and therapy should be reinstituted. If the TSH level remains normal, the dose can be reduced or discontinued and the patient reevaluated in 6 more weeks. In this manner, patients who are truly hypothyroid can be distinguished from euthyroid patients who have been inappropriately treated.

HYPERTHYROIDISM

method of
GILBERT H. DANIELS, M.D.
Massachusetts General Hospital
Boston, Massachusetts

Hyperthyroidism is a clinical *syndrome* characterized by excess amounts of thyroid hormone and its clinical consequences. Symptoms include weight loss with preserved appetite, heat intolerance, fatigue, palpitations, shortness of breath, increased frequency of bowel movements, decreased menstrual flow or irregular menses, weak muscles, tremor, emotional lability, anxiety, and difficulty in sleeping. Shortness of breath is common in the absense of congestive heart failure, presumably due to weakness of the respiratory muscles. Some hyperthyroid patients gain rather than lose weight. In the elderly, weight loss and constipation without tachycardia may occur. Some patients are surprisingly asymptomatic despite severe chemical hyperthyroidism ("apathetic hyperthyroidism"). Signs include widened pulse pressure, tachycardia, hyperreflexia, tremor, warm moist skin, onycholysis, and weak muscles. Goiter need not be present. Proptosis, inflammatory eye findings, and pretibial myxedema are specific for Graves' disease. Signs and symptoms of underlying heart disease including angina, tachyarrhythmias, and congestive heart failure are often exacerbated by hyperthyroidism.

THYROID FUNCTION TESTING

Ultrasensitive thyroid-stimulating hormone (TSH) measurements have revolutionized thyroid function testing. A low TSH is the hallmark of hyperthyroidism, with the rare exception of TSH-induced hyperthyroidism. Early TSH radioimmunassays (RIAs) could not distinguish normal (0.5 to 5.0 microunits per milliliter) from low TSH concentrations. Currently available TSH assays measure TSH concentrations as low as 0.1 microunit per milliliter (second-generation assays), 0.01 microunit per milliliter (third-generation assays), or even 0.001 microunit per milliliter (fourth-generation assays). Any useful assay must be able to distinguish hyperthyroid patients from normal, and this must be verified by the physician's own laboratory.

A low TSH cannot distinguish degrees of hyperthyroidism! The serum free thyroxine (T_4, or free thyroxine index) and total serum triiodothyronine (T_3) (by RIA) are measured when a low TSH is noted. These studies determine the degree of hyperthyroidism and are necessary to monitor therapy. The presence of a normal free T_4 and total T_3 with a consistently low serum TSH is called *subclinical hyperthyroidism.*

In inpatients TSH alone is less useful as a screening study because ill patients are often found to have low serum TSH concentrations without hyperthyroidism. In addition, cortisol excess and pituitary disease may cause lower than normal TSH concentrations.

Before appropriate therapy can be considered, the cause of the hyperthyroidism must be determined. The mechanisms and types of hyperthyroidism are summarized in Table 1. The diagnosis is obvious in some patients (e.g., the presence of a diffuse goiter with a bruit and exophthalmos equals Graves' disease); however, in most cases the situation is less clear. A 24-hour radioiodine uptake and radionuclide (^{123}I or ^{99}m-technetium) scan are very helpful. It is most useful to divide patients into those with a low versus

TABLE 1. **Mechanisms of Hyperthyroidism**

Exogenous Hormone	Thyroid Stimulators	Autonomous Production	Excess Release of Hormone
L-Thyroxine L-Triiodothyronine	Antibodies (Graves' disease) Thyroid-stimulating hormone* Human chorionic gonadotropin*	Hot nodule Toxic multinodular goiter Struma ovarii*	Painful subacute thyroiditis Silent thyroiditis

*Rare.

those with a normal or high radioactive iodine uptake (Table 2). For example, hyperthyroidism due to excess thyroid hormone is treated by decreasing or stopping the hormone. Hyperthyroidism due to silent or painful subacute thyroiditis resolves spontaneously and generally does not require therapy.

THERAPY

Despite the usefulness of TSH measurements in the diagnosis of hyperthyroidism, TSH measurements may be misleading during therapy of hyperthyroidism. A suppressed TSH may remain low for weeks to months, even though the patient is euthyroid. Serum free T_4 (or free thyroxine index) and total T_3 must be monitored during therapy of hyperthyroidism. In some treated patients the free T_4 (or free T_4 index) returns to normal while the T_3 remains elevated ("T_3 toxicosis"). In others, the free T_4 and T_3 return to normal, indicating effective therapy, even though the TSH remains suppressed.

The choice of therapy for Graves' disease is most problematic and is the major focus of this discussion. Graves' hyperthyroidism is due to antibody stimulation of TSH receptors (thyroid-stimulating immunoglobulins). In some patients (around 5%) both the antibodies and the hyperthyroidism spontaneously disappear; in others, antithyroid drug therapy is associated with loss of these antibodies and disease remission. Therapeutic choices include inhibition of hormone production (antithyroid drugs), thyroid gland destruction (radioiodine, ^{131}I), or thyroid gland removal (surgery).

The underlying rationale for selecting antithyroid drug therapy in most patients is the hope that a sustained remission will occur when therapy is stopped. After 1 year of therapy approximately 50% of patients enter a remission of 4 months or longer. Unfortunately, approximately 50% of those in remission subsequently undergo a relapse with recurrence of hyperthyroidism. Ultimately, 15% of those previously treated with antithyroid drugs develop *hypothyroidism.*

Radioiodine is the ultimate therapy of choice for most hyperthyroid adults, based on a 50-year record of safety and efficacy. Radioiodine does not cause cancer or infertility. Subsequent pregnancies in women treated with radioactive iodine are normal by all criteria. Radiation exposure to the ovaries is comparable to that of many common radiologic procedures (e.g., several barium enemas) and less than that of other procedures used to evaluate infertile women (e.g., hysterosalpingogram). Although many endocrinologists favor antithyroid drugs as the initial therapy for children, radioactive iodine is a safe and effective alternative for those with allergies or poor compliance.

Surgery is an uncommon choice for treatment of patients with Graves' hyperthyroidism. It remains an important alternative therapy if a skilled thyroid surgeon is available.

All the therapeutic options are effective, but none are perfect. Therefore, patient education and dialogue are extremely important. Patients must understand all the options and be comfortable with their choice of therapy. Patients must not be forced into a choice of therapy that frightens them.

Patients with subclinical hyperthyroidism are at increased risk for atrial fibrillation and bone loss. Although short-term observation (months) may be appropriate for young asymptomatic patients, persistent hyperthyroidism should be treated.

Adjunctive Therapy

Therapy for hyperthyroidism works slowly. When tachycardia, palpitations, or tremor is disturbing to the patient, long-acting beta blockers provide symptomatic relief. Atenolol (Tenormin), metoprolol (Lopressor),* nadolol (Corgard),* and long-acting propranolol (Inderal-LA)* are all effective and probably superior to the shorter-acting agents (e.g., propranolol (Inderal).*

Antithyroid Drugs

The antithyroid drugs methimazole (Tapazole) and propylthiouracil (PTU) rapidly block the synthesis of

*This drug has not been approved by the FDA for this indication.

TABLE 2. **Causes of Radioactive Iodine Uptake**

Low or Zero Radioactive Iodine Uptake	Normal or High Radioactive Iodine Uptake
Painful subacute thyroiditis Silent thyroiditis Factitious (exogenous) hyperthyroidism Iodide excess* Struma ovarii†	Graves' disease Toxic nodular goiter Hot nodule Human chorionic gonadotropin– or TSH-induced

*Recent exposure to excess iodide can cause a low or normal radioactive iodine uptake in all disorders characterized by normal or high radioactive iodine uptake.

†Uptake will be low over the neck but not the pelvis.

thyroid hormone. However, because these drugs do not inhibit the release of thyroid hormone, the time needed to achieve euthyroidism will vary greatly, depending in part on thyroid hormone stores (average time to euthyroidism is 4 to 12 weeks). Compliance is very important; if the drug is missed for 1 to several days, thyroid hormone stores are replenished, delaying the therapeutic effect.

I prefer methimazole because of its longer half-life. Single daily dose therapy with methimazole is effective in almost all compliant patients. I generally begin therapy with 30 mg, although lower initial doses may suffice in some patients. Initially, patients are followed at 6-week intervals. If the 30-mg daily dose is continued, hypothyroidism usually results. Therefore, as the patients become euthyroid (generally after about 6 to 12 weeks), two choices are available. I generally prefer to taper the dosage of methimazole, initially to 15 mg and subsequently to 10 or even 5 mg. Alternatively, a block-replace regimen can be used, continuing the methimazole at a dose of 30 mg and adding full therapeutic doses of L-thyroxine (e.g., 1.7 μg per kg, usually 0.1 to 0.125 mg per day). This latter approach is particularly useful with patients who are away at school or who cannot return for frequent blood studies.

Many endocrinologists prefer PTU because it blocks the conversion of T_4 to T_3. Unfortunately, the bulk of the circulating T_3 in hyperthyroid patients comes from the thyroid gland rather than from peripheral conversion. Because of its shorter half-life, propylthiouracil often fails to control the thyroidal production of T_3 unless multiple daily doses are used. PTU is one-tenth as potent as methimazole; the usual starting dose is 100 mg three or four times daily.

The monthly cost of methimazole at a dosage of 30 mg per day is about $29; PTU at 300 mg per day costs about $14.00. Once maintenance dosages have been established, the cost of the two drugs is comparable.

Side effects of antithyroid drugs are uncommon. Fever, rash, or joint pains occur in 5% of patients. Patients with these minor allergies may switch from methimazole to PTU (or vice versa) with small risk of cross-reactivity. Agranulocytosis occurs in 0.2 to 0.4% of patients, generally within the first 3 months of starting or restarting therapy. A low white cell count (3000 to 4000) is common in untreated patients with Graves' disease and is not a contraindication to therapy. I usually check the white count and differential at each follow-up visit or if symptoms suggestive of agranulocytosis develop (fever, sore throat, mouth ulcerations). Some endocrinologists check the white cell count and differential every 2 weeks while the patient is on therapy. If agranulocytosis develops, hospitalization is necessary. Granulocyte colony-stimulating factor (Filgrastim)* may facilitate the return of granulocytes and shorten the usual 7- to 14-day recovery period. Agranulocytosis precludes further antithyroid drug therapy! Less common side effects include toxic hepatitis (methimazole), hepatic necrosis (PTU), and lupus-like reactions (PTU).

Antithyroid drugs are generally administered for a period of 1 to 2 years, but there is no absolute time limit. Some patients prefer to remain on these drugs for much longer periods of time rather than experience frequent relapses. A recent Japanese study reported a very high remission rate when levothyroxine (0.1 mg) was added to methimazole at the 6-month point; the two drugs were continued together for 1 year, and the levothyroxine was continued for 18 months after methimazole was stopped. Although further study is necessary, this is a reasonable alternative to just stopping antithyroid drugs. Relapse after antithyroid medication has been stopped may be treated by restarting the drug or choosing an alternative therapy such as radioiodine or surgery.

Patients in remission after antithyroid drug therapy need careful, lifelong follow-up. Thyroid function is tested annually or whenever symptoms develop. Relapse of Graves' disease is very common during the postpartum period. Preliminary studies suggest that levothyroxine in patients with Graves' disease during pregnancy may prevent such relapses.

Patients with hot nodules or toxic nodular goiters do not enter remission after treatment with antithyroid drugs. Methimazole or PTU may be used to treat hyperthyroidism prior to initiating definitive therapy with radioiodine or surgery.

Radioiodine Therapy

Radioiodine (^{131}I) is administered by mouth as a liquid or a capsule. Pregnancy is a strict contraindication to its use. There are no immediate aftereffects of its administration. Patients do not become sick. Allergy to iodinated contrast materials is not a contraindication to radioiodine use. Radioiodine has a half-life of 8 days; after 40 days virtually no radioactivity remains in the body.

Radioiodine works slowly. Patients become euthyroid over 12 to 26 weeks. Approximately 20% of patients require a second dose of radioiodine. The dose is selected to deliver 5000 to 15,000 rads to the thyroid. Pain or tenderness over the thyroid gland is uncommon. During the days or weeks after radioiodine administration, increased release of thyroid hormone may result in worsening of the hyperthyroidism. Beta blockers are often employed during this time. Some endocrinologists pretreat all patients with antithyroid drugs (weeks to months) to deplete the stores of thyroid hormone and prevent post-radioiodine exacerbation of hyperthyroidism. I generally reserve this pretreatment for the elderly or those with serious heart disease.

Return to the euthyroid state may be accelerated after radioiodine administration when persistent hyperthyroidism is symptomatic or is considered dangerous. After radioiodine therapy, patients with Graves' disease are particularly sensitive to the effects of iodine on inhibition of hormone release. The addition of supersaturated solution of potassium io-

*This drug has not been approved by the FDA for this indication.

dide (SSKI), 3 drops twice daily beginning 1 week after radioiodine administration, shortens the average time to euthyroidism from 12 to 6 weeks. Alternatively, methimazole or PTU can be added 4 to 7 days after radioiodine.

Hypothyroidism is the expected outcome for most patients with Graves' disease treated with radioiodine, although 20% remain euthyroid. Approximately 50% become hypothyroid at 1 year with 2 to 3% becoming hypothyroid each additional year. Long-term follow-up of all radioiodine-treated patients is therefore mandatory. Some clinicians begin levothyroxine therapy as soon as patients become euthyroid, and others wait until hypothyroidism develops. Hypothyroidism after radioiodine administration in patients with Graves' disease is usually transient if a goiter persists.

Surgery

Surgery is rarely performed in patients with Graves' hyperthyroidism. Less than 1% of our patients opt for this therapy. Who are these patients? Pregnant women who are allergic to antithyroid drugs, patients who are allergic to antithyroid drugs and afraid of radioiodine, patients with concomitant Graves' disease and suspicious thyroid nodules, and young patients with very large goiters who may require multiple treatments with radioiodine after drug failure or allergy comprise most of these patients.

A surgeon skilled at performing a bilateral thyroidectomy is absolutely necessary. A small amount of thyroid remnant can remain, but too much residual thyroid tissue results in persistent or recurrent hyperthyroidism (in 5% of patients or more). Mortality is rare in properly prepared patients. Complications include temporary and permanent hypoparathyroidism, temporary or permanent hoarseness (recurrent laryngeal nerve involvement), bleeding, wound infection, and keloid or unsightly scar formation. Hypothyroidism occurs in 10 to 60% of patients initially, and in 1 to 3% more per year thereafter.

It is best to operate when the patient is euthyroid, but this is not always possible. In compliant nonallergic patients, methimazole or PTU is prescribed until the patient is euthyroid. SSKI (10 drops twice daily) is added for 10 days prior to surgery to decrease the vascularity of the thyroid gland. If pretreatment is not possible, surgery can be performed under beta-adrenergic blockade. I generally prescribe propranolol* (Inderal) in high doses for 3 to 4 days before surgery to decrease the resting and post-walking pulse to 70 beats per minute or less. Oral dosages of 60 to 240 mg four times daily (total 240 to 960 mg) are employed. Because of the long half-life of thyroxine (7 days), beta blockade must be continued after surgery. In emergency situations, beta blockers can be administered intravenously.

Iodine is not used for preoperative preparation of patients with toxic multinodular goiters or hot nodules. I prefer to prepare these patients for surgery with antithyroid drugs, although some major centers operate without preparation.

*This drug has not been approved by the FDA for this indication.

EFFECT OF THERAPY ON GRAVES' EYE DISEASE

It is uncertain whether the course of Graves' eye disease is influenced by any of the conventional modalities of therapy. Some centers report worsening of eye problems after radioiodine therapy, particularly in patients with severe initial eye disease. Other groups report eye improvement when the thyroid is ablated with radioiodine. For most patients, therapy can be chosen independent of the eye findings. For patients with *severe* inflammatory eye changes, I generally prefer to start with antithyroid drugs and defer radioiodine therapy until the eye problems are quiescent.

HYPERTHYROID PREGNANCY

When therapy is necessary, antithyroid drugs are the first choice during a hyperthyroid pregnancy; radioiodine is contraindicated, and surgery is best avoided. Antithyroid drugs cross the placenta and affect both the maternal and fetal thyroid, although placental passage is less complete with PTU. PTU is preferred during pregnancy, although methimazole is a reasonable alternative. Maternal thyroid function should be maintained in the high normal to slightly high range because low normal maternal free T_4 concentrations cause fetal hypothyroidism. The minimal dose of PTU should be used; doses less than 150 mg per day rarely cause fetal thyroid dysfunction. The immunosuppressive effects of pregnancy often cause Graves' disease to improve, and progressive tapering or even discontinuation of PTU is often possible in the third trimester. Mild hyperthyroidism may be observed without therapy. If antithyroid drugs can be discontinued during pregnancy, the addition of levothyroxine may prevent postpartum recurrent hyperthyroidism. If necessary, beta-adrenergic blocking agents can be employed early in pregnancy for symptomatic relief.

SEVERE HYPERTHYROIDISM OR THYROID STORM

Thyroid storm, characterized by severe hyperthyroidism, fever, and altered mental status, is rare. However, severe hyperthyroidism requiring emergency therapy due to concomitant illness (e.g., myocardial infarction) is more common and is treated in a similar fashion.

Large doses of antithyroid drugs are used to block the synthesis of thyroid hormone. PTU (200 mg by mouth every 4 hours) is preferred because of its effect on T_4 to T_3 conversion. If necessary, PTU can be administered by nasogastric tube or rectally. Release of thyroid hormone from the thyroid is inhibited by iodine. Antithyroid drugs should be administered first to prevent an increase in the stores of thyroid hormone. Iodine can be given intravenously (sodium iodide 1 to 2 grams per 24 hours) or by mouth (SSKI [5 drops four times a day] or iopanoic acid [Telepaque,* 1 to 3 grams per day in divided doses, or ipodate sodium (Oragrafin), 1 to 3 grams in divided doses. Iopanoic acid and ipodate sodium are particularly useful because they serve as sources of iodine and are potent inhibitors of T_4 to T_3 conversion.

Beta-adrenergic blocking agents provide the most immediate relief. Oral propranolol (Inderal)* in doses of 40 to 160 mg every 6 hours or intravenous propranolol (2 to 5 mg every 4 hours or as an infusion at a rate of 5 to 10 mg per hour) controls the heart rate in most patients. When the blood pressure is low or when the patient has underlying pulmonary disease, the shorter-acting esmolol (Brevibloc)* is the initial therapy of choice. Reserpine,* guanethidine,* and calcium channel blockers have all been employed in patients who are intolerant of beta blockers. Stress dosages of glucocorticoids are usually administered, largely based on historical precedant rather than on a clear rationale. In high doses, glucocorticoids do inhibit the conversion of T_4 to T_3. Plasmapheresis, peritoneal dialysis, or charcoal resin hemoperfusion is rarely necessary. In children with accidental overdoses of thyroid hormone, the addition of cholestyramine* to prevent enterohepatic circulation is effective. Cholestyramine may be effective in endogenous thyroid storm as well.

*This drug has not been approved by the FDA for this indication.

THYROID CANCER

method of
GARY B. TALPOS, M.D.
Henry Ford Hospital
Detroit, Michigan

There are approximately 12,000 new cases of thyroid cancer in the United States each year, accounting for about 3% of all new cancers. Although the mortality rate averages 10 to 20% for all thyroid malignancies, there is a clear difference in death rate between the different types of thyroid cancer and, with differentiated thyroid cancer, between patients with different ages of onset. The prolonged natural history of early-onset differentiated thyroid cancer is such that the patient sometimes has outlived the treating physician by the time a recurrence becomes apparent.

Finally, there are more board-certified surgeons trained to treat thyroid cancer than new cases of the disease each year. Because resection is the mainstay of treatment and most treating surgeons operate on relatively few new cases each year, there are marked differences in basic approach, terminology, extent of resection, morbidity, and mortality independent of the highly variable biologic behavior of the disease. Other than tumor resection and thyroid hormone replacement, few strategies are commonly agreed on by treating physicians.

CLASSIFICATION OF THYROID CANCER

Thyroid cancer develops in different forms. Table 1 lists the most common types. Two important criteria used in separating the types are the degree of differentiation and the cell of origin. Well-differentiated tumors developing from the thyroid hormone-producing cells are the most common. They also share the same favorable prognosis owing to their iodine uptake (initially for thyroid hormone production) and their usual lack of biologic aggressiveness.

These differentiated thyroid cancers account for approximately 90% of all thyroid carcinomas. The most common variant is papillary thyroid carcinoma, which is usually found in 70% of patients, whereas follicular cancer is seen in the remaining 20%. Papillary cancer has various morphologies, although they are not always considered mutually exclusive. (There are approximately the same number of board-certified pathologists as new cases of thyroid cancer each year.) The lack of consensus on terminology limits attempts to correlate prognosis with morphologic subtype. Papillary cancer has a bimodal age distribution with one peak in the second and third decades and the other peak in the sixth and seventh decades of life. It is bilobar or multifocal in up to 25% of cases. Metastasis usually occurs first through the lymphatics, with distant metastasis found infrequently. When found, however, distant metastasis invariably occurs late, in the elderly, or in a dedifferentiated form of the disease.

Morphologic subtypes include the follicular variant, tall cell, sclerosing, and the recently described microfollicular type. Incidental or occult papillary cancers are those measuring less than 1 centimeter in diameter. The term incidental is something of a misnomer, however; no patient with such a cancer considers it incidental. Although autopsy series have demonstrated that up to 13% of individuals harbor a thyroid malignancy at death, only very limited evidence exists to suggest that these tumors would not have progressed had the patient lived longer. In younger patients these sometimes nonpalpable primary tumors are identified only when a metastasis is diagnosed correctly. Although mistakenly considered clinically insignificant, these incidental cancers have caused death in some individuals. In general, the prognosis of papillary thyroid cancer is considered

TABLE 1. **Classification of Thyroid Cancer**

Differentiated	**Medullary**
Papillary	Sporadic
"Incidental cancer"	Hereditary
Follicular variant	**Lymphoma**
Sclerosing	**Anaplastic**
Tall cell	
Insular	
Follicular	
Hürthle cell	

very good, especially in patients under the age of 40, because the majority of papillary malignancies concentrate radioactive iodine after appropriate surgery and are therefore subject to ablation. Five-year survival exceeds 95%. However, after the age of 40, individuals begin to lose their capacity to concentrate iodine, rendering ^{131}I therapy less reliable. Postoperative thyroglobulin production by metastatic deposits has provided a good estimate of iodine uptake specifically and the degree of differentiation in general, as well as of the increasing tumor burden. Some tumors, usually in older patients, change their morphology and function and become less differentiated. Some that have islands of follicles within the malignancy are termed insular cancers. Others completely dedifferentiate and become very poorly differentiated in morphology and function. Neither these anaplastic cancers nor the insular tumors concentrate iodine, and this fact is reflected in the reduced survival rates of patients with these tumors.

Follicular thyroid carcinoma occurs mainly in the fifth and sixth decades of life and is uncommon prior to age 30. It frequently presents as a solitary tumor similar to the benign follicular adenoma except that capsular or angioinvasion has occurred. Metastasis or marked cellular atypia is less commonly seen. Hematogenous dissemination, though uncommon, occurs at an earlier stage than with papillary cancer and consequently distant metastasis, usually to the lung or bone, is seen earlier. As with papillary cancer, age of onset greater than 45 and tumor diameter greater than 5 cm are regarded as independent risk factors owing to their adverse effects on iodine concentration, dedifferentiation, and survival. Despite this, 5-year survival is at least 90%. Hürthle cell carcinoma is regarded as a subset of follicular cancer. Although the morphology follows that of follicular neoplasms, the dense oxyphilic staining and dense uniform appearance immediately characterize these tumors as distinct. In our experience, 60% of Hürthle cell tumors are benign. However, 40% show either localized invasion or more aggressive behavior. An additional 16% of patients with benign Hürthle cell tumors also have associated differentiated thyroid malignancies. Survival correlates with completeness of excision. Patients with unresectable tumors have a limited survival because iodine uptake and concentration are poor, as is the response to conventional adjuvant chemotherapy or external beam irradiation.

The other types of thyroid malignancies are not considered differentiated because they do not arise from the follicular epithelium, the cells that produce thyroid hormone, and they concentrate neither iodine nor radioiodine. Medullary thyroid cancer arises from the parafollicular cells, which elaborate calcitonin. They are usually highly differentiated tumors, although typically they become less differentiated in their preterminal phase. Medullary thyroid cancer occurs in sporadic and hereditary forms and accounts for approximately 5% of thyroid cancers in general hospitals. The sporadic form usually appears in the fifth or sixth decade of life as a hard solitary nodule. Metastasis to regional lymph nodes is found at the time of diagnosis in 50% of individuals. Medullary cancer also occurs in hereditary forms that have autosomal dominant transmission and apparent complete penetrance. Three separate forms have been recognized: multiple endocrine neoplasia Type 2A (MEN-2A) syndrome, MEN-2B syndrome, and familial medullary thyroid cancer (FMTC). MEN-2A syndrome includes bilobar medullary cancers, bilateral pheochromocytoma, and possibly parathyroid disease. (It is not clear whether the primary hyperparathyroidism that occurs with this entity is a primary or secondary manifestation of the syndrome because it rarely if ever develops following curative thyroidectomy.) The gene mutations for MEN-2A have recently been located on chromosome 10 by both Wells and Ponder, and clinical testing for the presence of the abnormal gene in an infant of an affected family should become clinically available in the near future. Interestingly, different gene mutations are seen in the same RET proto-oncogene region of chromosome 10 in both the MEN-2B syndrome and FMTC.

The thyroid malignancy associated with the MEN-2A variant is almost always evident biochemically by the age of 30 through pentagastrin and calcium stimulation of serum CT levels. It is essential to remove the thyroid preemptively in affected individuals because no patient has been cured once the malignancy is palpable.

The MEN-2B syndrome is characterized by bilobar medullary thyroid cancer, bilateral adrenal pheochromocytomas, mucosal neuromas, and an earlier age of onset than the MEN-2A variant. Doubling time estimates of the thyroid malignancy also show a more aggressive growth rate in this group. Mucosal neuromas and abnormal stimulated calcitonin values are invariably present by age 4. In this group also preemptive thyroidectomy is essential for cure. Genetic identification of patients with this condition is still not widely available. Thyroidectomy is usually performed when either the mucosal neuromas or elevated stimulated calcitonin levels first appear.

FMTC is a related condition, although it is genetically distinct. It is characterized by bilobar thyroid cancer transmitted in an autosomal dominant pattern. The peak age of biochemical identification is usually the sixth decade, and the tumor appears to have a more indolent course. Other endocrine disorders have not been consistently associated with this entity.

Survival of patients with medullary thyroid cancer frequently extends for decades even in individuals first identified with metastasis. Some patients with the familial variant seem to live out normal lifespans. In individuals with the MEN-2A and MEN-2B syndromes survival is directly correlated with the method of diagnosis; patients identified through regular screening programs of families at risk prior to the onset of palpable cancer are probably cured if they have a complete and total thyroidectomy. Patients who have lesser operations or are first identified with metastatic disease have a more variable course, although MEN-2B patients possess a faster growing tumor. It is not evident whether this is due to inherent increased biologic aggressiveness of the cancer or the presence of growth factors in these younger patients. Finally, patients with sporadic tumors also have a less predictable course because half of them have metastasis at the time of diagnosis. Calcitonin and carcinoembryonic antigen (CEA) determinations provide significant insight into the amount and aggressiveness of residual disease. Shorter doubling times of these products or a fall in calcitonin while the CEA level continues to rise is an ominous sign and usually heralds rapidly progressive disease and a preterminal state. Chemotherapy is not highly effective and is reserved for symptomatic patients. Radiation therapy likewise is frequently ineffective. Re-operation, whether guided by scintigraphy and tomography or by selective venous sampling, appears to offer the only significant palliation and possible cure at this time.

Thyroid lymphoma accounts for 3 to 4% of thyroid malignancies. Typically, this is a non-Hodgkin's diffuse large cell tumor and accounts for 40% of all thyroid lymphomas. Diffuse mixed and diffuse small cell variants each account for another 20%. Patients usually present with these tumors in the seventh decade of life; approximately 70% of them are females. The major discriminating factor in survival has been found to be tumor extent. Tumors confined to the thyroid gland are associated with an 85% 5-year survival with surgery and irradiation, whereas patients with extrathyroidal tumors have only a 40% 5-year survival despite irradiation and some form of surgery ranging from biopsy to extirpation. Combination chemotherapy appears to confer some additional advantage, as does bone marrow transplant. However, long-term follow-up of large series of patients treated with chemotherapy and bone marrow transplantation is not yet available.

Anaplastic thyroid cancer can arise de novo or as a dedifferentiated papillary or follicular malignancy and accounts for about 2% of all thyroid cancers. Previously, anaplastic cancer represented a larger proportion of thyroid cancers, the majority of which occurred in neglected well-differentiated malignancies. More recently, this rapidly growing cancer has had a peak incidence in the seventh decade. Males and females are affected approximately equally. Median survival formerly was 6 months, with only a few patients living 5 years or more after diagnosis. New programs combining radiotherapy and chemotherapy with surgery, sometimes preoperatively as well as postoperatively, appear to have improved at least short-term survival, although further evaluation of these protocols is necessary.

DIAGNOSIS AND TREATMENT OF THYROID CANCER

Fine-needle aspiration biopsy (FNA) allows definitive diagnosis of the majority of thyroid nodules. With other nodules (such as follicular neoplasms), FNA can only narrow the range of diagnostic possibilities, but it still provides important information that helps to determine whether surgery is indicated. For thyroid cancer, surgery is the primary treatment. The most feared surgical complications are permanent hypoparathyroidism and recurrent or superior laryngeal nerve injury. Some endocrinologists believe that either of these complications is worse than the typical well-differentiated tumor. To reduce the risks of these complications and to plan surgery better, we support liberal use of FNA with any thyroid nodule. Experienced cytologists can usually alert the surgeon to thyroid nodules that are worrisome for malignancy and even specify the type of cancer. The extent of surgery can be planned accordingly.

Currently, most surgeons perform a thyroid lobectomy (for biopsy or treatment), a subtotal thyroidectomy, or a near-total thyroidectomy. There are no operational definitions to specify the extent of resection more accurately in the latter cases. A total thyroidectomy performed by some surgeons leaves behind more thyroid tissue than a subtotal thyroidectomy performed by others when seen at reoperation or on postoperative scan. Comparing results of treatment of specific types of thyroid cancer is complicated when this factor is taken into account. In particular, the term subtotal thyroidectomy lacks precision. For this reason, we define that operation as a removal of the entire ipsilateral lobe, isthmus, and some of the contralateral lobe, leaving behind at least 1 gram of thyroid tissue, which is sufficient to provide a postoperative uptake of 10%. Smaller remnants with lower uptakes are reserved for near total or total thyroidectomy. Most surgeons are able to perform near-total thyroidectomy consistently with minimal risk to two parathyroid glands and one recurrent laryngeal nerve and achieve postoperative uptakes of 5%. This is adequate surgical treatment for the majority of *well-differentiated papillary or follicular malignancies* because it should result in tumor extirpation with minimal risk of permanent hypoparathyroidism or bilateral laryngeal nerve injury. Near-total thyroidectomy also has the advantage of leaving a remnant small enough to allow easy performance of radioiodine ablation, if desired, prior to assessing the patient for well-differentiated metastatic disease by radioisotope scanning.

Because most U.S. surgeons who operate on the thyroid gland do so fewer than 10 times per year, some surgeons may feel compelled to perform only a hemithyroidectomy for papillary or follicular cancer to minimize the risk of surgical complications. We agree that this approach is satisfactory (and preferable to subtotal thyroidectomy) for treatment of a unilobar tumor because it should leave untouched the anatomic planes around the contralateral lobe. More experienced surgeons should continue to perform near-total or total thyroidectomy for differentiated tumors if their rates of major complications are less than 2 to 3%. This approach not only effectively removes any likelihood of incomplete excision of a multifocal papillary cancer but also allows rapid postoperative scanning and ablation for both papillary and follicular tumors alike. We also support a more extensive approach to Hürthle cell carcinomas because surgery is the only effective therapy for this tumor, and 20% of patients with Hürthle cell tumors are found to have malignancy in the contralateral lobe as well.

FNA also allows preoperative identification of index patients with *medullary thyroid cancer* and those with the sporadic form of the disease. Ideally, nonindex individuals with the hereditary form have been identified through screening with stimulated calcitonin determinations or genetic testing. In addition, preoperative calcitonin and CEA determinations allow some generalizations about tumor size and possible extent of metastasis when compared with postoperative levels. More important, preoperative identification of patients with medullary thyroid cancer should be sought to evaluate patients for the pheochromocytomas associated with the MEN-2A and MEN-2B variants of the disease. Induction of general anesthesia in a patient with a pheochromocytoma who is unprepared with alpha-adrenergic blocking drugs may prove lethal. In the operating room, excision of all tumor as well as total thyroidectomy has been the procedure of choice because all C cells are considered pre-malignant in the hereditary variant of medullary thyroid cancer. The C cells are clustered in the upper and middle thirds of the thyroid along Berry's ligament, and meticulous and precise technique is required to remove all thyroid tissue while leaving the laryngeal nerves and parathyroid glands intact. Lymphatic drainage of this area includes the lymph nodes of the central and lateral neck. Both sets of nodes should be surgically evaluated for metastasis. The optimum extent of lymphadenectomy has yet to be determined in this disease because very few patients, if any, are cured once the disease has progressed to this point. Radical neck dissection or a less disfiguring modified neck dissection is sometimes indicated. Postoperatively, serial calcitonin and CEA measurements and scans are obtained on follow-up. Reoperation is warranted to prevent worsening symptoms and airway or vascular invasion. The role of reoperation for treatment of bulky metastasis or microdissection remains to be better defined.

Lymphoma confined to the thyroid is best treated with thyroidectomy. The addition of irradiation or chemotherapy to the treatment of small tumors without extrathyroidal extension has been controversial. Many individuals have fared well on long-term follow-up without adjuvant treatment. More extensive lymphomas involving the thyroid gland are usually treated with open biopsy and then aggressive chemotherapy. Tracheostomy has not been uniformly necessary with the newer protocols even in patients presenting with vocal cord palsy because airway compression has rarely been observed.

Surgical management of *anaplastic cancer* remains challenging. Although improvements in survival have been reported with the addition of irradiation and chemotherapy, surgical therapy usually includes a classic en bloc dissection including at least a hemithyroidectomy and radical neck dissection on the affected side. Removal of the uninvolved contralateral lobe has not been helpful because radioiodine administration postoperatively has not been beneficial. Because the laryngeal nerves and parathyroid glands on the ipsilateral side are frequently encompassed by tumor, leaving the uninvolved contralateral lobe preserves the functioning laryngeal nerves and parathyroid glands on that side, thereby diminishing morbidity. Tracheostomy has been performed judiciously.

Routine postoperative imaging of patients with differentiated thyroid cancer has largely been supplanted by a selective treatment policy. Risk factors favoring scanning of differentiated tumors include large, multifocal, or metastatic malignancy. Thyroxine replacement is stopped until thyroid-stimulating hormone (TSH) is greater than 50 micro international units per milliliter. A low iodine diet is also used prior to radioiodine scintigraphy and ablation. Afterward, adequate thyroxine is given to suppress TSH to subnormal levels, if tolerated, although some physicians believe that a normal TSH is adequate. Others attempt to reduce TSH to undetectable levels to eliminate any hormonal stimulus for tumor recurrence. Increased experience is also being gained with serial thyroglobulin determinations. These measures are primarily beneficial in patients with differentiated thyroid cancer. They occasionally confer some cytoreductive benefit in individuals with Hürthle cell, medullary, or anaplastic carcinoma, although complete ablation has not been observed in those with metastasis. Nor has any benefit been observed in patients with these tumors or thyroid lymphomas with thyroxine replacement designed to lower TSH to subnormal or undetectable levels.

Finally, patients with medullary thyroid cancer and Hürthle cell cancer are periodically assessed with computed tomography and, in those with medullary thyroid cancer, with thallium-technetium scintigraphy to identify recurrences. Judicious reoperation has been used for local tumor control in selected individuals.

FUTURE DIRECTIONS

Studies in progress will provide knowledge that may allow consensus on some aspects of current thyroid cancer management including the extent of resection, indications for radioiodine scanning and ablation, and the degree of TSH suppression to be used postoperatively. In the future, more complete understanding of thyroid tumor biology may allow recognition of some cancers that truly are clinically insignificant. Better understanding may also lead to control of the tumor's genetic code, allowing a tumor to be inactivated genetically or converted to a tumor that can be more successfully treated by conventional means.

PHEOCHROMOCYTOMA

method of
WILLIAM F. YOUNG, Jr., M.D.
Mayo Clinic and Mayo Foundation
Rochester, Minnesota

Pheochromocytoma is a tumor frequently sought and rarely found. It is associated with spectacular cardiovascular disturbances and, when correctly diagnosed and properly treated, it is curable; however, when it is undiagnosed or improperly treated, it can be fatal. Catecholamine-producing tumors that arise from chromaffin cells of the adrenal medulla and sympathetic ganglia are termed pheochromocytomas and paragangliomas, respectively. However, the term pheochromocytoma has become the generic name for all catecholamine-producing tumors and will be used in this chapter to refer to both adrenal pheochromocytomas and paragangliomas.

PRESENTATION

Prevalence estimates for pheochromocytoma range from 0.01% to 0.1% of the hypertensive population. These tumors occur equally in men and women, primarily in the third through fifth decades. Patients harboring these tumors may be asymptomatic. However, symptoms usually are present and are due to the pharmacologic effects of excess circulating catecholamines. Episodic symptoms include abrupt onset of throbbing headaches, generalized diaphoresis, palpitations, anxiety, chest pain, and abdominal pain. These episodes can be extremely variable in their presentation and may be spontaneous or precipitated by postural changes, anxiety, exercise, or maneuvers that increase intra-abdominal pressure. The episode may last 10 to 60 minutes and may occur daily to monthly. The clinical signs include hypertension (paroxysmal in half of the patients and sustained hypertension in the other half), orthostatic hypotension, pallor, grade I to IV retinopathy, tremor, and fever. Pheochromocytoma of the urinary bladder is associated with painless hematuria and paroxysmal attacks induced by micturition or bladder distention.

A rule of 10 has been quoted for pheochromocytomas: 10% are extra-adrenal, 10% occur in children, 10% are multiple or bilateral, 10% recur after surgical removal, 10% are malignant, and 10% are familial. The familial syndromes include familial pheochromocytoma, multiple endocrine neoplasia (MEN) type IIA (with pheochromocytoma, medullary carcinoma of the thyroid, and primary hyperparathyroidism), and MEN type IIB (with pheochromocytoma, medullary carcinoma of the thyroid, mucosal neuromas, thickened corneal nerves, intestinal ganglioneuromatosis, and marfanoid body habitus). Neurofibromatosis (von Recklinghausen's disease) and von Hippel–Lindau syndrome (retinal angiomatosis and cerebellar hemangioblastoma) also are associated with increased incidence of pheochromocytoma. Familial types of pheochromocytoma frequently involve both adrenal glands.

DIAGNOSIS

The diagnostic approach to catecholamine-producing tumors is divided into two series of studies (Fig. 1). First, the diagnosis of a catecholamine-producing tumor must be suspected and then confirmed biochemically by the presence of increased urine or plasma concentrations of catecholamines or their metabolites. Suppression testing with clonidine or provocative testing with glucagon, histamine, or metoclopramide rarely are needed. The differential diagnosis for pheochromocytoma is summarized in Table 1.

The next step is to localize the catecholamine-producing tumor to guide the surgical approach. Computer-assisted adrenal and abdominal imaging (magnetic resonance imaging or computed tomography) is the first localization test. Approximately 90% of these tumors are found in the adrenal glands and 98% are in the abdomen. If the results are negative on abdominal imaging, then scintigraphic localization with iodine 123–meta-iodobenzylguanidine (^{123}I-MIBG) is indicated. This radiopharmaceutical accumulates preferentially in catecholamine-producing tumors; however, this procedure is not as sensitive as was initially hoped (sensitivity 88% and specificity 99%). Computer-assisted chest, neck, and head imaging and central venous sampling are additional localizing procedures that can be used, although they are rarely required. Thorough discussions of the diagnostic investigation of catecholamine-producing tumors are found elsewhere.

The emphasis of this chapter is on the therapeutic approach to pheochromocytomas. Hypertension usually is cured by excision of the tumor, and careful preoperative pharmacologic preparation is crucial to successful treatment.

PRINCIPLES OF TREATMENT

The treatment of choice for pheochromocytoma is surgical resection. Most of these tumors are benign and can be totally excised. However, prior to the operation, the chronic and acute effects of excess circulating catecholamines must be reversed.

Preoperative Management

Combined alpha- and beta-adrenergic blockade is required preoperatively to control the blood pressure and to prevent intraoperative hypertensive crises (Table 2). Alpha-adrenergic blockade should be started 7 to 10 days preoperatively to allow for expansion of the contracted blood volume. A liberal salt diet is advised during the preoperative period. Once adequate alpha-adrenergic blockade is achieved, beta-adrenergic blockade is initiated (e.g., 3 days preoperatively).

Alpha-Adrenergic Blockade

Phenoxybenzamine (Dibenzyline) is an irreversible long-acting alpha-adrenergic blocking agent. Approximately 25% of an oral dose of phenoxybenzamine is absorbed. Phenoxybenzamine is available as 10 mg capsules. The initial dosage is 10 mg orally two times daily; the dosage is increased by 10 to 20 mg every 2 to 3 days as needed to control the blood pressure and spells. The effects of daily administration are cumulative for nearly a week. The average dosage is 20 to 100 mg per day. Side effects include postural hypotension, tachycardia, miosis, nasal congestion, inhibition of ejaculation, diarrhea, and fatigue.

Prazosin (Minipress), terazosin (Hytrin), and doxazosin (Cardura) are selective alpha$_1$-adrenergic blocking agents. After oral administration, they are highly bound to plasma proteins. Metabolism occurs primar-

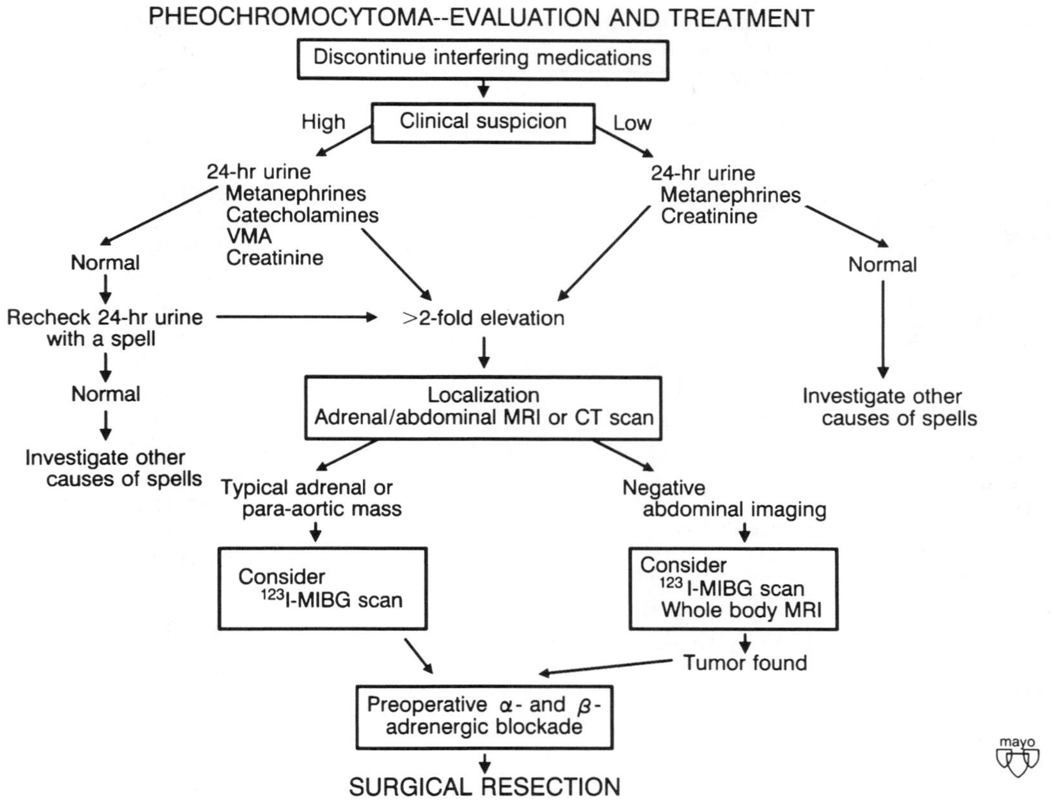

Figure 1. Evaluation and treatment of catecholamine-producing tumors. The details are discussed in the text. *Abbreviations:* VMA = vanillylmandelic acid; CT = computed tomography; MRI = magnetic resonance imaging; ^{123}I-MIBG = ^{123}I-metaiodobenzylguanidine.

ily in the liver, and the majority of the drug is excreted in the bile and feces. The plasma half-lives of prazosin, terazosin, and doxazosin are approximately 3, 12, and 22 hours, respectively. These agents are available as 1-, 2-, 4-, 5-, 8- and 10-mg tablets or capsules. The initial dose is 1 mg orally at bedtime to avoid the occasional syncope that follows the first dose. The dosage, up to 20 mg orally (in divided doses for prazosin), is then increased every 2 days as needed to control the blood pressure. The side effects with these selective alpha$_1$-adrenergic blocking agents include dizziness, drowsiness, headache, fatigue, palpitation, nausea, blurred vision, nasal congestion, peripheral edema, and somnolence. Because of the more favorable side effect profiles of prazosin, terazosin, and doxazosin, these agents may be preferable to phenoxybenzamine when long-term pharmacologic treatment is indicated (e.g., for metastatic pheochromocytoma).

Phenoxybenzamine is the preferred drug for preoperative preparation because it provides alpha-adrenergic blockade of long duration. Effective alpha-adrenergic blockade permits expansion of blood volume, which usually is severely decreased as a result of excessive adrenergic vasoconstriction.

Beta-Adrenergic Blockade

The beta-adrenergic antagonist should be administered only after alpha-adrenergic blockade is effective because beta-adrenergic blockade alone may result in more severe hypertension owing to the unopposed alpha-adrenergic stimulation. Preoperative beta-adrenergic blockade is indicated to control the tachycardia associated with both the high circulating catecholamine concentrations and the alpha-adrenergic blockade. Caution is indicated if the patient is asthmatic or has congestive heart failure. Chronic catecholamine excess can produce a myocardiopathy, and beta-adrenergic blockade can result in acute pulmonary edema. Noncardioselective beta-adrenergic blockers such as propranolol (Inderal and Inderal LA) and nadolol (Corgard) or cardioselective beta-adrenergic blockers such as atenolol (Tenormin) and metoprolol (Lopressor) may be used. (Mechanisms of action, routes of metabolism, dosages, and side effects are discussed elsewhere in this text.) When administration of the beta-adrenergic blocker is begun, the drug should be used cautiously and at a low dose. For example, propranolol is usually started at 10 mg orally twice daily at least 5 days after the initiation of alpha-adrenergic blockade. The dose is then increased as necessary to control the tachycardia.

Labetalol (Normodyne, Trandate) exhibits both selective alpha$_1$-adrenergic and nonselective beta-adrenergic blocking activities in a ratio of approximately 1:3. It is well absorbed after oral administration and is metabolized primarily in the liver; its metabolites are excreted in the urine. Labetalol is available as

TABLE 1. **Differential Diagnosis for Pheochromocytoma Episodes**

Endocrine
- Thyrotoxicosis
- Menopausal syndrome
- Hypoglycemia
- Hyperadrenergic episodes

Cardiovascular
- Essential hypertension—labile
- Cardiovascular deconditioning
- Pulmonary edema
- Syncope
- Orthostatic hypotension
- Paroxysmal cardiac arrhythmia
- Angina and myocardial infarction
- Aortic dissection
- Renovascular hypertension

Psychologic
- Anxiety and panic attacks
- Hyperventilation

Pharmacologic
- Withdrawal of adrenergic-inhibiting medications (e.g., clonidine)
- Monoamine oxidase inhibitor treatment and concomitant ingestion of tyramine or a decongestant
- Sympathomimetic ingestion
- Illegal drug ingestion (e.g., cocaine, phencyclidine, lysergic acid)
- Gold myokymia syndrome
- Acrodynia (mercury poisoning)

Neurologic
- Migraine headache
- Diencephalic epilepsy
- Fatal familial insomnia
- Stroke
- Cerebrovascular insufficiency
- Autonomic neuropathy

Other
- Mastocytosis (systemic or activation disorder)
- Carcinoid syndrome
- Idiopathic flushing spells
- Acute intermittent porphyria

100-, 200-, and 300-mg tablets. The dose is 100 mg orally twice a day initially and is increased in increments of 100 mg twice daily every 2 days up to 1200 mg per day if necessary for control of hypertension and spells. Labetalol is contraindicated in patients with nonallergic bronchospasm or congestive heart failure. It has been shown to be an effective agent for the treatment of hypertension associated with catecholamine-producing tumors. However, some instances of paradoxical hypertensive responses have been reported, presumably due to incomplete alpha-adrenergic blockade. Therefore, its safety as primary therapy is controversial. Hepatic and cholestatic jaundice have been associated with labetalol therapy on rare occasions. Side effects include dizziness, fatigue, nausea, nasal congestion, and impotence. Its role in the therapy of pheochromocytoma may be in the chronic pharmacologic management of patients with metastatic disease.

Catecholamine Synthesis Inhibitor

Alpha-methyl-L-tyrosine (metyrosine; Demser) inhibits the synthesis of catecholamines by blocking the enzyme tyrosine hydroxylase. It is rapidly absorbed from the gastrointestinal tract, and most of it is excreted in the urine unchanged. Metyrosine is available as 250-mg capsules. The initial dosage is 250 mg orally four times daily. The dosage may be increased by 500 mg per day every 2 days to a maximum of 4 grams per day (1 gram four times per day) as needed for blood pressure control. Side effects include sedation, diarrhea, anxiety, nightmares, crystalluria and urolithiasis, galactorrhea, and extrapyramidal manifestations. Therefore, this agent should be used with caution and only when other agents have been ineffective. The extrapyramidal effects of phenothiazines and haloperidol may be potentiated, and their use concomitantly with metyrosine should be avoided. High fluid intake to avoid crystalluria is suggested for any patient taking more than 2 grams daily. Although some centers have used this agent preoperatively, we have reserved it primarily for those patients who have persistent catecholamine-producing tumors that (for cardiopulmonary reasons) cannot be treated with combined alpha- and beta-adrenergic blockade.

Potential Alternative Agents

Calcium channel antagonists and angiotensin-converting enzyme inhibitors have been reported to control the hypertension associated with pheochromocytoma. Further experience will be needed with these agents before any therapeutic recommendations can be made.

Acute Hypertensive Crises

Acute hypertensive crises may occur before or during operation and should be treated with nitroprusside (Nipride) or phentolamine (Regitine) administered intravenously. Phentolamine is a short-acting nonselective alpha-adrenergic blocker. It is available in lyophilized form in vials containing 5 mg. An initial test dose of 1 mg is administered and, if necessary, this is followed by repeat 5-mg boluses or a continuous infusion. The response to phentolamine is maximal in 2 to 3 minutes after a bolus injection and lasts 10 to 15 minutes. A solution of 100 mg of phentolamine in 500 mL of 5% dextrose and water can be infused at a rate titrated for blood pressure control. The use of nitroprusside is discussed subsequently.

Anesthesia and Surgery

This is a high-risk surgical procedure requiring an experienced surgeon and anesthesiologist. The last oral doses of alpha- and beta-adrenergic blockers can be administered early in the morning on the day of operation. Cardiovascular and hemodynamic variables must be monitored closely. Continuous measurement of intra-arterial pressure and heart rhythm is required. In the setting of congestive heart failure or decreased cardiac reserve, monitoring of pulmonary capillary wedge pressure is indicated. Premedication includes minor tranquilizers and barbiturates. Fentanyl and morphine should not be used because of the potential for stimulating catecholamine release

TABLE 2. **Orally Administered Drugs Used to Treat Patients with Pheochromocytoma**

Drug (Trade Name)	Dosage (mg/day)*	Side Effects
Alpha-Adrenergic Blocking Agents		
Phenoxybenzamine (Dibenzyline)	20–100†	Postural hypotension, tachycardia, miosis, nasal congestion, diarrhea, inhibition of ejaculation, fatigue
Prazosin (Minipress)	1–20‡	First-dose effect, dizziness, drowsiness, headache, fatigue, palpitations, nausea
Terazosin (Hytrin)	1–20†	First-dose effect, asthenia, blurred vision, dizziness, nasal congestion, nausea, peripheral edema, palpitations, somnolence
Doxazosin (Cardura)	1–20	First-dose effect, orthostasis, peripheral edema, fatigue, somnolence
Combined Alpha- and Beta-Adrenergic Blocking Agent		
Labetalol (Normodyne, Trandate)	200–1,200†	Dizziness, fatigue, nausea, nasal congestion, impotence
Catecholamine Synthesis Inhibitor		
Alpha-methyl-p-L-tyrosine (Demser)	1,000–4,000‡	Sedation, diarrhea, anxiety, nightmares, crystalluria, galactorrhea, extrapyramidal symptoms

*Given once daily unless otherwise indicated.
†Given as two doses daily.
‡Given in three or four doses daily.

from the pheochromocytoma. In addition, parasympathetic nervous system blockade with atropine should be avoided because of the associated tachycardia. Induction usually is accomplished with thiopental (Pentothal), and general anesthesia is maintained with a halogenated ether such as enflurane (Ethrane) or isofluorane (Forane). Hypertensive episodes should be treated with phentolamine (2 to 5 mg intravenously) or nitroprusside intravenous infusion (0.5 to 1.5 μg per kg per minute). Lidocaine (50 to 100 mg intravenously) or esmolol (Brevibloc) (50 to 200 μg per kg per minute intravenously) is used for cardiac arrhythmia.

Because intra-abdominal pheochromocytoma may be multiple and extra-adrenal, an anterior midline abdominal surgical approach is used. If the pheochromocytoma is in the adrenal gland, the entire gland should be removed. If the tumor is malignant, as much tumor as possible should be removed. Because of the bilateral nature of pheochromocytomas (10% in sporadic cases and more than 50% in familial syndromes), the contralateral adrenal should be palpated and removed if it is believed to be abnormal. If a bilateral adrenalectomy is planned preoperatively, the patient should receive glucocorticoid stress coverage while awaiting transfer to the operating room. Glucocorticoid coverage should be initiated in the operating room if unexpected bilateral adrenalectomy is necessary. The entire abdomen should be inspected carefully. Ligation of the tumor vasculature and then extirpation is indicated. Paragangliomas of the neck, chest, and urinary bladder require specialized approaches.

Hypotension may occur after surgical resection of the pheochromocytoma and should be treated with fluids and colloids. Postoperative hypotension is less frequent in patients who have had adequate alpha-adrenergic blockade preoperatively. If both adrenal glands had been manipulated, adrenocortical insufficiency should be considered as a potential cause of postoperative hypotension. Hypoglycemia can occur in the immediate postoperative period and, therefore, blood glucose levels should be monitored and the fluid given intravenously should contain 5% dextrose.

Blood pressure usually is normal by the time of dismissal from the hospital. Some patients remain hypertensive for up to 8 weeks postoperatively. Long-standing persistent hypertension does occur and may be related to accidental ligation of a polar renal artery, resetting of baroreceptors, established hemodynamic changes, structural changes of the blood vessels, altered sensitivity of the vessels to pressor substances, renal functional or structural changes, or coincident primary hypertension.

Approximately 2 weeks postoperatively, a 24-hour urine sample should be obtained for measurement of catecholamines and metanephrines. If the levels are normal, the resection of the pheochromocytoma can be considered to have been complete. In major centers, the surgical mortality rate is less than 2%. At Mayo Clinic, the 30-day perioperative mortality rate in 110 patients operated on from 1980 to 1989 was 0.9%. The survival rate after removal of a benign pheochromocytoma is nearly that of age- and sex-matched controls. The 24-hour urinary excretion of catecholamines should be checked annually for at least 5 years as surveillance for recurrence in the adrenal bed, metastatic pheochromocytoma, or delayed appearance of multiple primary tumors.

Malignant Pheochromocytoma (Pheochromoblastoma)

The distinction between benign and malignant catecholamine-producing tumors cannot be made on clinical, biochemical, or histopathologic characteristics. Malignancy is based on finding direct local invasion or disease metastatic to sites that do not have chromaffin tissue, such as lymph nodes, bone, lung, and liver. Metastatic lesions should be resected, if possible. Painful skeletal metastatic lesions can be treated with external radiation therapy. In initial studies, local tumor irradiation with ^{131}I-MIBG has proved to be of limited therapeutic value. Further studies with ^{131}I-MIBG may help define a subset of patients with malignant pheochromocytoma that may benefit from this treatment. Although the 5-year survival rate is less than 50%, many of these patients have prolonged survival and minimal morbidity. If the tumor is considered to be aggressive and the quality of life is affected, then combination chemotherapy may be considered. A chemotherapy program consisting of cyclophosphamide (Cytoxan, Neosar), vincristine (Oncovin, Vincasar), and dacarbazine (DTIC-Dome) given cyclically every 21 days has proved to be beneficial but not curative in these patients. Hypertension and spells can be controlled with combined alpha- and beta-adrenergic blockade or inhibition of catecholamine synthesis with metyrosine.

Pheochromocytoma in Pregnancy

Pheochromocytoma in pregnancy can cause the death of both the fetus and the mother. The treatment of hypertensive crises is the same as for nonpregnant patients. Although there is some controversy regarding the most appropriate management, pheochromocytomas should be removed immediately if they are diagnosed during the first two trimesters of pregnancy. Preoperative preparation is the same as for the nonpregnant patient. If medical therapy is chosen or if the patient is in the third trimester, cesarean section and removal of the pheochromocytoma in the same operation is indicated. Spontaneous labor and delivery should be avoided.

THYROIDITIS

method of
TERRY F. DAVIES, M.D.
Mount Sinai Medical Center
New York, New York

AUTOIMMUNE THYROIDITIS

Background

Autoimmune thyroiditis (Hashimoto's disease) results in thyroid decompensation in 1 to 3% of the population. The disease satisfies the classic criteria for an autoimmune disease, including its association with autoreactive T cells and autoantibodies to thyroglobulin, thyroid peroxidase (the microsomal antigen), and, less commonly, the TSH receptor. Because many people with apparently normal thyroid function may have detectable thyroid autoantibodies and autoreactive T cells, we have recently reclassified autoimmune thyroiditis into Type 1 (euthyroid), Type 2 (hypothyroid), and Type 3 (hyperthyroid) (Table 1). Type 2 thyroiditis includes the different grades of hypothyroidism—subclinical, mild, and overt. The term subclinical hypothyroidism refers to a condition marked by an increased serum thyroid-stimulating hormone (TSH) level but a serum free thyroxine (T_4) level that is within the normal range and few or no clinical symptoms. Such patients with thyroid autoantibodies progress to overt thyroid failure at a rate of 3 to 5% per year. Mild thyroid failure refers to increased TSH levels with below-normal free T_4 in the presence of a variety of nonspecific symptoms that remit with T_4 replacement therapy. Overt hypothyroidism presents with obvious clinical features, a major elevation of serum TSH level, and a low free T_4 concentration. Patients with autoimmune thyroiditis may present with an obvious firm rubbery thyroid enlargement (goitrous thyroiditis as in classic Hashimoto's disease) or without a palpable thyroid at all (atrophic thyroiditis or primary myxedema). The atrophic variety may be associated with TSH receptor–blocking antibodies.

TABLE 1. **Classification of Human Thyroiditis**

Type 1 Autoimmune Thyroiditis (Hashimoto's disease Type 1)
1A Euthyroid—goitrous
1B Euthyroid—nongoitrous
Type 2 Autoimmune Thyroiditis—(Hashimoto's disease Type 2)
2A Hypothyroid—goitrous (classic Hashimoto's disease)
2B Hypothyroid—nongoitrous (primary myxedema, atrophic thyroiditis)
2C Transient aggravation (post partum)
Type 3 Autoimmune Thyroiditis (Graves' disease)
3A Hyperthyroid Graves' disease
3B Euthyroid Graves' disease
3C Hypothyroid Graves' disease
Type 4 Thyroiditis (nonautoimmune)
4A Acute thyroiditis
4B Subacute thyroiditis

Treatment of Autoimmune Thyroiditis

In my opinion, all forms of thyroid failure should be treated, including the "subclinical" variety. Various data have suggested that patients with the mildest degree of thyroid failure show subtle cardiac abnormalities that are corrected with therapy. Treatment consists of L-thyroxine (T_4, most commonly Synthroid) as replacement therapy (to be distinguished from T_4 suppression therapy). This should increase the serum T_4 value and suppress the increased TSH level into the lower half of the normal range (which is 0.2 to 5 microunits per milliliter). Such treatment effectively removes all symptoms related to thyroid disease and may additionally prevent the development of more severe thyroid failure in the future even if residual tissue remains. Treatment should continue to be guided by the normalization of serum TSH levels on a supersensitive third-generation immunoassay that is capable of distinguishing normal from suppressed TSH levels (below 0.2 microunits per milliliter). Most patients require less than 150 μg of T_4 per day as a once-daily medication for the rest of their lives (1.7 μg per kg body weight), and the correct replacement dose may require repeatedly titrating the patient's T_4 dose against the serum TSH level. Any need for higher doses should be well documented by consistent T_4 intake in the presence of a persistently raised TSH. It is wise to allow 4 to 6 weeks for TSH normalization after a change in the dose of T_4. There is little to distinguish between the different commercial preparations available except that it is important for the patient to remain on the *same* reliable preparation because the patient's TSH level should be titrated carefully to avoid the long-term side effects of excess T_4 including potential bone demineralization. Changing the T_4 preparation requires a reevaluation of the patient's thyroid status. Hence, generic preparations can be a problem unless the patient can ensure a consistent supply from the same source. Caution should also be exercised when initiating T_4 therapy in the elderly and those with coronary artery disease. The initial dosage should be 25 μg daily for 7 days with a subsequent very gradual increase to avoid the development of arrhythmias. Thyroid extract preparations should no longer be used. The commonly raised serum triiodothyronine (T_3) levels found in patients on thyroid extract preparations appear to me to be an unnecessary risk when T_4 therapy is available to everyone. Combination preparations of T_4 and T_3 (Thyrolar) are also still available, but indications for them are beyond my understanding. Similarly, T_3 (Cytomel) is still used as thyroid replacement therapy, but it has a three times daily dosage regimen that makes it unpopular (T_3 has a shorter half-life than T_4), and it tends to cause tachycardia in an unacceptably high proportion of patients.

Surgery is rarely indicated in patients with autoimmune thyroiditis, although particularly firm areas of a goiter may appear as hard nodules and are a common reason in some hospitals for mistaken and unnecessary surgery, which could be avoided by prior aspiration biopsy. However, occasionally a large goiter due to Hashimoto's thyroiditis causes pressure effects on the trachea that are best relieved by a careful surgeon.

POSTPARTUM THYROIDITIS

Background

Pregnancy is associated with a period of generalized immunosuppression. Thyroid antibody titers consistently fall as parturition approaches and then rebound after delivery, sometimes to concentrations greater than those seen before pregnancy. Titers peak at about 3 to 6 months after delivery, and at this period a variety of postpartum thyroid syndromes may be observed in up to 8% of women. The most common presentation is lethargy in the postpartum period associated with an increased TSH and high titers of antibodies to thyroid peroxidase (the microsomal antigen). Diagnosis can be confirmed in the nonbreast-feeding mother by a low or absent 24-hour radioiodine uptake, indicating thyroiditis. Treatment depends on severity. Most episodes are transient, and rapid recovery can be expected over a 2- to 4-month period.

Treatment

Symptoms of thyroid failure, combined with reduced serum T_4 levels and raised TSH, can be relieved by administration of 100 to 150 μg of T_4 once daily. Thyroid antibody titers should be monitored as well as the TSH level. As antibody titers begin to fall, it should be possible to withdraw T_4 completely. However, in some patients such a presentation may indicate the onset of chronic autoimmune thyroiditis. Even the long-term outlook for patients with the transient syndrome is at present uncertain. We do know that it may recur after a subsequent pregnancy, and data suggest that 20 to 30% of such patients eventually develop permanent thyroid failure. The early phase of the disease may be associated with hyperthyroidism because of widespread thyroid cell destruction. This appears to be more common in the postpartum period than in patients with traditional autoimmune thyroiditis and may be related to the marked immunologic rebound that occurs in such patients. Usually the mild hyperthyroidism associated with suppressed serum TSH (less than 0.2 microunits per milliliter) settles into thyroid gland failure before treatment is necessary, although propranolol (20 to 40 mg four times per day) may be helpful for tachycardia. Finally, Graves' disease may occasionally present in the postpartum period and requires appropriate treatment.

SUBACUTE THYROIDITIS

Background

Subacute (DeQuervain's) thyroiditis has a varied prevalence in different countries. It appears to be common in North America, although there are no epidemiologic data. Often, a viral type of pharyngitis is associated with general malaise, headache, fever, and a unique localized tenderness of the thyroid gland, usually affecting both lobes but unilateral tenderness may occur. It is likely that many individuals experience a mild form of the disease but only with more severe neck discomfort do they present for treatment. Indeed, a painless variety is sometimes observed. The disorder is considered viral in etiology, and probably many viruses have such a propensity, although there are few data to confirm this.

Treatment

Most patients do not require treatment apart from aspirin to relieve the neck pain. Severe thyroidal tenderness is sometimes devastating, and in this situation prednisone, 30 to 40 mg daily for a 5-day period with gradual reduction during the subsequent 2 to 4 weeks, is very effective. During the period of acute tenderness, massive destruction of thyroid tissue occurs, and biochemical hyperthyroidism may be present, requiring beta blockade with propranolol,* 20 to 40 mg four times daily. This is followed by a period of hypothyroidism while the gland is undergoing regeneration and may itself require T_4 supplementation depending on the serum TSH values obtained. A dose of 100 μg of T_4 daily for a period of 8 weeks should be sufficient to allow subsequent withdrawal and monitoring of the return to normal function. We find that serum thyroglobulin levels are effective for monitoring the activity of the thyroiditis.

Some patients have a transient thyroid abnormality associated with no thyroid tenderness, the so-called painless thyroiditis. Such a diagnosis can be made during the hyperthyroid phase of the thyroiditis by the absence of radioiodine uptake into the thyroid. Treatment of the hyperthyroid phase is best accomplished with beta blockade using propranolol and then, as the hypothyroid phase ensues, with T_4 if it is necessary to replace thyroid function until recovery occurs.

SUPPURATIVE THYROIDITIS

Background

Now rare, this once more common disease is usually associated with *Staphylococcus aureus, Streptococcus,* or *Escherichia coli* infection in parallel with obvious infective loci elsewhere, often nearby. The gland is generally enlarged and acutely tender, and the patient is sick with fever, tachycardia, and often a septicemia. There may be thrombophlebitis of the external jugular veins.

Treatment

Treatment involves high-dose antibiotics and incision and drainage when appropriate. Thyroid function should be monitored throughout the illness and appropriate replacement therapy provided if necessary.

*Not approved by the FDA for this indication.

RIEDEL'S THYROIDITIS

I have never seen a case that was convincing enough to be called just Riedel's thyroiditis. This suggests to me that this presentation is most likely the end point of a chronic disease that is now arrested by modern treatment. It is associated with marked destruction of the thyroid gland and fibrous replacement. There may be fibrosis of adjacent tissues in the neck and fibrous mediastinitis or retroperitoneal fibrosis. Treatment with thyroxine and corticosteroids does not apparently arrest the development of fibrosis, and any obstruction must be relieved surgically. The disease may be a variant of autoimmune thyroiditis, but few cases have been reported with immunologic data.

PERINEOPLASTIC THYROIDITIS

Pathology reports often contain mention of an associated thyroiditis around a benign or malignant thyroid neoplasm. The significance of this is uncertain, although thyroid antibodies have an increased prevalence in patients with thyroid cancer. Such tumors are not tender but rather are firm on examination. Similarly, Hashimoto's gland may have areas of more severe fibrosis and feel clinically like a suspicious nodule. Removal of suspicious areas such as this is a not uncommon mistake, which can be avoided by performing thyroid antibody assessment and aspiration biopsy prior to surgery. Sometimes thyroid cell aspiration biopsy reveals the diagnosis, but such cells may also be reported as atypical, thus confirming the investigator's mistaken first impression.

Section 9

The Urogenital Tract

BACTERIAL INFECTIONS OF THE URINARY TRACT IN MALES

method of
FREDRIC J. SILVERBLATT, M.D.
Providence Veterans Administration Medical Center
Providence, Rhode Island

In children under the age of 1, urinary tract infections (UTIs) occur four times more often in males than in females. However, beyond the first year, symptomatic infections are 13-fold higher in girls. Although UTIs are rare among young and middle aged men, they can occur spontaneously in normal healthy individuals. Lack of circumcision, interceptive rectal sexual activity, and vaginal intercourse with a woman who is colonized by uropathogens have been shown to predispose young men to UTI. In older men, prostatic obstruction contributes to an increasing risk of colonization. Elderly men are four times more likely than women to have asymptomatic bacteriuria.

MICROBIOLOGIC EVALUATION

Escherichia coli is the predominant uropathogen in men, but it occurs less frequently than in women. Other gram-negative organisms, such as *Proteus* species, and gram-positive organisms, such as enterococci and coagulase-negative staphylococci, account for up to 50% of episodes. *Staphylococcus saprophyticus,* the second most common pathogen in women, is rarely responsible for UTIs in men. Because uropathogens other than *E. coli* are less likely to be susceptible to commonly used oral antibiotics, it is especially important in men to obtain a urine specimen for culture and sensitivity before starting therapy. Urine is rarely contaminated by periurethral flora in men, so a random voided specimen is adequate for culture. The presence of at least 10^3 colonies per mL of a single or predominant pathogen is indicative of infection.

TREATMENT

Cystitis and Pyelonephritis

Cystitis can be treated with a number of oral agents such as trimethoprim-sulfamethoxazole (Bactrim, Septra), amoxicillin, an oral first-generation cephalosporin, or a fluoroquinolone (Table 1). Males with infection of the lower urinary tract should be treated for 7 to 10 days. Patients with pyelonephritis should be admitted to the hospital for treatment with parenteral antibiotics if septicemia is suspected or if the patient cannot tolerate oral antibiotics. I use gentamicin in addition to ampicillin as empiric therapy and treat for 2 weeks until the sensitivity results are known.

Because of the high likelihood of structural or physiologic abnormalities of the urinary tract, males under 1 year and those over age 50 should be referred to a urologist for evaluation of their first UTI. Children under 1 year are at especially high risk for renal scarring after UTIs. Appropriate treatment of symptomatic episodes and investigation for surgically re-

TABLE 1. **Antibiotic Therapy for Male Urinary Tract Infections**

Antibiotic	Recommended Dose	
	Adult	*Child*
Oral Therapy		
Amoxicillin	250 mg PO q 8 h	30 mg/kg/d PO in 3 divided doses
Trimethoprim-sulfamethoxazole (Bactrim, Septra)	1 double-strength tablet PO q 12 h	8 mg/kg/d of trimethoprim and 40 mg/kg/d of sulfamethoxazole in 2 divided doses
First-generation cephalosporin (e.g., cephradine [Velosef])	500 mg PO q 6 h	25–50 mg/kg/d PO in 4 divided doses
Fluoroquinolone (e.g., ciprofloxacin [Cipro])	250–500 mg PO q 12 h	Not recommended for use in children
Parenteral Therapy		
Gentamicin sulfate*	3–4 mg/kg IV in 2 divided doses	6 mg/kg IV in 3 divided doses
Ampicillin	1–2 gm IV q 4 h	50–100 mg/kg/d IV q 6 h
Candida Infections		
Amphotericin B bladder irrigation	50 mg/L intermittent irrigation for 3 days	Not recommended for use in children
Fluconazole (Diflucan)	200 mg PO on first day followed by 100 mg q d for 3 d	Not recommended for use in children

*Dose must be adjusted with renal failure.

mediable abnormalities are essential to prevent progressive loss of renal function. It is usually not necessary to investigate the urinary tract of a young man presenting with a single episode of UTI; however, recurrent infections or clinical suspicion of a structural abnormality should prompt a urologic evaluation. Asymptomatic bacteriuria (ABU) should be treated if the individual has an abnormal urinary tract. There is little evidence, however, to support routine treatment of elderly men with ABU, because these episodes are usually self limited.

UTIs in Patients with Indwelling Urinary Catheters

The risk of UTI is increased in patients with indwelling urinary catheters. While prophylactic antibiotics can prevent acquisition of bacteriuria in patients with short-term catheterization, it is my practice to try to prevent acquisition of bacteriuria by minimizing the number of days of catheterization. Newer and more costly methods to prevent nosocomial UTIs, such as use of silver-impregnated catheters, have not been proved effective in men. Patients who require prolonged catheterization, such as those with spinal cord injury or obstructive uropathy, almost invariably develop colonization of their bladder and experience intermittent or recurrent symptomatic infections. Prophylactic antibiotics and treatment of asymptomatic colonization do not reduce the number of symptomatic episodes but do increase the likelihood that a more antibiotic-resistant population will become established. Efforts should be directed at preventing obstruction of the lumen of the catheter. The catheter should be replaced at regular intervals and anatomic obstruction surgically corrected.

For incontinent patients, permanent indwelling catheterization should be instituted only after the cause of the incontinence is identified and appropriate medical or behavioral methods of management tried (see the article on urinary incontinence). Intermittent self- or assisted catheterization will greatly diminish the incidence of UTI. Patients with indwelling urethral catheters, especially those who have received multiple courses of antibiotics, may develop *Candida* cystitis. Whenever possible, I remove the catheter and stop antibiotic therapy. For those patients who fail conservative measures, amphotericin B bladder washouts or oral fluconazole (Diflucan) is effective.

BACTERIAL INFECTIONS OF THE URINARY TRACT IN WOMEN

method of
A. R. RONALD, O.C., M.D.
St. Boniface General Hospital
University of Manitoba
Winnipeg, Manitoba, Canada

Bacteriuria refers to the presence of bacteria in the urinary tract regardless of bacterial numbers or of any host response such as symptoms or pyuria. Urinary tract infections (UTIs) are further classified by the presence of underlying disease. An uncomplicated infection is infection of the bladder or kidney occurring in an ambulatory, otherwise healthy host without structural or functional urinary tract abnormalities. Table 1 classifies complicated urinary tract infections in women.

Women present with either (1) lower tract symptoms (i.e., *cystitis*) or (2) upper tract symptoms (i.e., *pyelonephritis*) or (3) are found by screening programs or follow-up urine cultures to have "incidental" infection (i.e., *asymptomatic bacteriuria*). The management of each of these categories of infections will be outlined.

TREATMENT

Urinary infections do not always require treatment, but treatment is indicated:

To reduce duration and severity of symptoms
To prevent sepsis and death in patients with invasive pyelonephritis
To prevent complications during pregnancy
To prevent bacterial dissemination during manipulation of the urinary tract
To prevent stone formation or retard stone growth
To prevent renal impairment
To treat illness made more serious by concomitant UTI (e.g., diabetes mellitus)

If indications are not present, treatment should not be given. However, few studies exist for many categories of infection, and the decision to prescribe antimicrobial treatment must be based on individual circumstances until adequate prospective treatment studies can determine if any advantage is to be gained by treatment.

Acute Cystitis

About one-third of women have a history of an episode characteristic of acute cystitis during their years of sexual activity. About 10% of these, or 3% of women overall, have recurring episodes (two or more each year). UTI pathogens generally originate from the fecal flora. Bacterial adherence to uroepithelium is a prerequisite for most UTIs, and women with a history of recurrent UTIs are more likely to be nonsecretors of ABO and Lewis blood group antigens. Nonsecretors synthesize unique glycolipid receptors on epithelial cells that bind *Escherichia coli.* Most *E. coli* urinary tract pathogens possess adhesions that are virulence factors and facilitate both infection and invasion of the urinary tract.

Behavioral risk factors are also important in UTI. Coitus frequently precedes acute infection, and

TABLE 1. **Complicated Urinary Tract Infections**

Catheterization—indwelling or intermittent	Diabetes mellitus
Nonambulatory and elderly women	Renal transplantation
Urinary calculi	Immunosuppression
Renal impairment (unilateral or bilateral)	Neutropenia
Neurogenic bladder	Cystic renal disease

women who are sexually inactive have a three-fold reduced risk of infection compared to women experiencing regular penile vaginal intercourse. In addition, both diaphragm and spermicide use significantly increase the risk of UTI. Other behavioral factors, including daily fluid intake, frequency of micturition, interval between intercourse and urination, tampon use, douching practices, perianal hygiene, direction of wiping after defecation, or type of undergarments have not been shown to alter the risk of urinary infections.

Historically, cranberry juice has been used to prevent UTIs. Cranberry juice contains a chemical that inhibits *E. coli* fimbrial adhesion and may prevent colonization of the perineum with virulent strains. Among seven different fruit juices tested, only blueberry and cranberry juice contained this substance.

The diagnosis of acute cystitis is made primarily by the patient and confirmed by the presence of pyuria and bacteriuria and an appropriate response to treatment. About 15% of women diagnosed clinically with acute cystitis actually have another disorder, such as chlamydial or gonococcal urethritis, interstitial cystitis, vaginitis, or other inflammatory disorders of the lower genital tract. Women with recurring cystitis are able to self-diagnose recurrences quite specifically. As a result, the necessity of laboratory investigation, including urine culture, to confirm bacteriuria in women with recurrent acute cystitis is under review. However, most clinicians still routinely obtain a urine culture and a urinalysis.

Pyuria is demonstrated by microscopic demonstration of pus cells or by the leukocyte esterase test and is present in over 95% of women with acute bacterial cystitis. However, about one-third of women who present with acute cystitis have fewer than 10^5 colony-forming units (cfu) of a urinary pathogen. As a result, laboratories may screen these cultures as "negative" and fail to detect bacteriuria. Culture technology must identify at least 10^3 cfu to prevent false-negative urine cultures in patients with bacterial cystitis. *E. coli* is responsible for 90% of acute bacterial cystitis episodes, with *Staphylococcus saprophyticus* accounting for most of the remainder. Approximately 10% of patients have pyuria and no demonstrated pathogen; most will respond to antibacterial treatment, providing presumptive evidence of an unidentified bacterial pathogen. However, searches for fastidious organisms, such as *Lactobacillus* spp, *Gardnerella vaginalis,* or *Mycoplasma hominis,* are not indicated in women with acute cystitis.

Acute cystitis is readily cured with a variety of regimens. As treatment shortens the natural course of the illness, it should be routinely prescribed. Over 100 studies have shown that single-dose therapy cures 80 to 95% of women with acute cystitis. However, many women find single-dose regimens unsatisfactory as symptoms often persist for 2 or 3 days; as a result, most physicians and their patients now prefer a 3-day regimen. These regimens tend to be associated with a very low incidence of side effects (<2% requiring a medical visit) and a cure rate of more than 95%. In nonpregnant women, the agent of choice is either trimethoprim-sulfamethoxazole (Bactrim, Septra), one double-strength tablet daily for 3 days, or a fluoroquinolone (norfloxacin [Noroxin], 400 mg; ciprofloxacin [Cipro], 250 mg; ofloxacin [Floxin], 200 mg, each twice daily for 3 days; or lomefloxacin [Maxaquin], 400 mg, or fleroxacin,* 400 mg, each once daily). The urinary excretion kinetics of all these agents ensure antibacterial levels far in excess of the minimal inhibitory concentration of UTI pathogens throughout each 24-hour period. Over 95% of patients will be free of symptoms by the third day.

Conventional wisdom dictates that all women with acute cystitis have a repeat urine culture 1 to 2 weeks after completion of a treatment regimen to prove cure, but the cost-effectiveness has not been proved. Over 75% of recurrences in this population will be symptomatic, and unless patients have underlying pathology that makes it necessary to find and treat asymptomatic infection, strategies to treat only symptomatic recurrences are probably appropriate and follow-up urine cultures are unnecessary. However, if the patient has any risk factors for occult renal infection (hospital-acquired infection, recent urinary tract instrumentation, acute presentation to an urban emergency department, functional or anatomic abnormality of the urinary tract, symptoms for more than 7 days at presentation, diabetes, or immunosuppression) a follow-up urine culture should be obtained. The quinolones can persist for 4 to 7 days in the urine following cessation of treatment, so a urine culture for "proof of cure" should be obtained at least 1 week after a 3-day regimen.

Routine investigation with imaging or urologic studies in women with acute cystitis is not warranted. Women with risk factors for occult renal infections should be followed and given a longer course of therapy if symptoms recur. Continued, closely spaced recurrences should be investigated with renal ultrasound and the determination of residual urine volumes. Cystoscopy and excretory pyelography are rarely necessary.

Women with three or more episodes of cystitis within a year require further evaluation. If the episodes are related to any known risk factor (e.g., spermicide use) or are temporally associated with coitus, prophylaxis with intercourse may prevent most recurrences. Trimethoprim-sulfamethoxazole (80 mg/400 mg) is an effective regimen. The fluoroquinolones are also useful (norfloxacin, 400 mg; ciprofloxacin, 250 mg; ofloxacin, 200 mg). Other women will choose to take continuous prophylaxis with one of these drugs. Studies have shown that trimethoprim-sulfamethoxazole (40 mg/200 mg) or the fluoroquinolones taken thrice weekly will prevent over 95% of recurrences. Continuous prophylaxis for as long as 5 years has not been associated with emergence of resistance or cumulative adverse effects in women with recurrent acute cystitis.

Investigators have recently shown that local topi-

*Not available in the United States.

cal estradiol cream (Estrace) (0.1%) reduces by 10-fold the cystitis recurrence rate in postmenopausal women with frequent urinary infections. This regimen also permits reappearance of lactobacilli and a "normalization" of vaginal pH. Further studies are needed on hormonal strategies for preventing UTIs.

Acute Pyelonephritis

Women with invasive infection of the upper urinary tract can present with overwhelming sepsis and shock, may only complain of mild flank pain and/or low grade fever, or may seek help for a variety of symptoms. Older women can present with increasing confusion, functional deterioration, or hypothermia. About one-quarter of women who are diagnosed with acute pyelonephritis in the emergency room or a physician's office are subsequently found to have some other illness. As a result, this clinical diagnosis, which has substantial significance to the patient and to subsequent management decisions, must be confirmed with laboratory support.

All women with presumed acute pyelonephritis require urinalysis, an assessment of renal function, and urine and blood cultures. In many instances, a chest x-ray and a flat plate of the abdomen should also be obtained. The latter will identify renal stones and other intra-abdominal illnesses that can mimic acute pyelonephritis and allow assessment of renal size. Urinalysis will almost invariably show pyuria, and bacteria may also be seen. One patient in five will have a urine culture with fewer than 100,000 organisms per mL; blood cultures will be positive in as many as one-third of women.

Treatment should commence as soon as possible once cultures have been obtained. For mild to moderately ill women, trimethoprim-sulfamethoxazole (one double-strength tablet STAT, followed by one every 8 hours until the patient is afebrile and then one twice daily to complete a 14-day course) or ciprofloxacin (500 mg every 8 hours until the patient is afebrile, followed by 500 mg twice daily to complete a 14-day course) are appropriate choices. Other effective drugs include oral ofloxacin, fleroxacin,* lomefloxacin, and cefixime (Suprax).

For moderately ill patients, initial therapy should be provided parenterally. Ceftriaxone (Rocephin) (1 gram intravenously or intramuscularly every 24 hours) is an excellent initial choice and can be administered out of hospital. Parenteral therapy can be modified to an oral regimen as soon as the diagnosis is confirmed and the patient has responded to treatment.

Severely ill patients require hospitalization; a large number of treatment regimens have been found to be effective. Gentamicin with or without ampicillin, ciprofloxacin, trimethoprim-sulfamethoxazole, imipenem (Primaxin), and ceftriaxone are all suitable parenteral choices.

Many patients with acute pyelonephritis will have responded within 24 hours with markedly reduced toxicity and symptomatic improvement. Any patient who is deteriorating after 24 hours or has not begun to respond by 48 hours needs careful review. Although occasionally failure may be due to an inappropriate choice or route of antimicrobial treatment, more often it is due to an incorrect initial diagnosis, urinary obstruction, suppuration with the development of a renal or perinephric abscess, or renal impairment often localized to the infected kidney. Careful assessment of these causes of failure are essential before treatment is modified. In a large series of patients with acute pyelonephritis, over 95% of patients responded to treatment within 48 hours when the organism was susceptible.

Imaging studies, including computed tomography, urologic consultation, and modification of antimicrobial therapy, should all be considered if women with acute pyelonephritis fail to respond within 72 hours.

Although many women with acute renal infection are treated for 4 to 12 weeks, this has not been shown to be necessary in most instances. A 14-day course is probably optimal therapy, and at least 80% of women with uncomplicated pyelonephritis will be cured with a 7-day course. Patients with recurrence within 2 weeks need to be evaluated for renal calculi and other underlying conditions that might portend a complicated urinary infection.

Acute pyelonephritis of pregnancy is usually preventable if bacteriuria screening and treatment programs are carried out. However, 0.5 to 1.0% of screened pregnant women will develop renal infection during pregnancy. Trimethoprim-sulfamethoxazole (do not use at term or during lactation) or cephalexin (Keflex) is appropriate oral treatment for mild to moderately ill women and gentamicin can be used for more severely ill patients. Women may take 2 to 3 days to respond to treatment, and ultrasound evaluation is often necessary to exclude underlying pathology.

Asymptomatic Bacteriuria

Asymptomatic bacteriuria is common in adult women, increasing from a rate of about 2% at age 20 to as high as 40% in nonambulatory elderly women in nursing home settings. The diagnosis of asymptomatic bacteriuria should be made only if two urine cultures yield more than 10^5 cfu per mL of the same organism. About 80% of asymptomatic infections are due to *E. coli,* which often lacks virulence traits associated with acute pyelonephritis.

Asymptomatic bacteriuria and symptomatic UTI are not totally distinct entities. About 30% of women with asymptomatic infection develop symptoms within 1 year. Further questioning of patients with "asymptomatic" bacteriuria often elicits symptoms, and these should be treated. However, truly asymptomatic bacteriuria has not been shown to cause renal damage or hypertension in individuals with otherwise normal urinary tracts. Overall, evidence is lacking that asymptomatic infection must be rou-

*Not available in the United States.

tinely treated in healthy women. In most women, bacteriuria will recur within a year, and some studies have suggested that recurrences can occur with more invasive organisms. Permanent eradication is difficult and, as far as is known, is nonrewarding in nonpregnant women with no functional or structural abnormalities of the urinary tract.

"Search and treat" activities are worthwhile in all pregnant patients. The changes in the urinary tract during pregnancy appear to facilitate upper tract invasion and third-trimester pyelonephritis. About 75% of these cases can be prevented by detecting bacteremia during the first trimester, treating adequately, and following the patient with monthly urine cultures throughout the pregnancy. A 3-day course of cephalexin, trimethoprim-sulfamethoxazole, or amoxicillin (Amoxil) is effective in over 90% of women if the organism is susceptible. If infection with the same organism occurs within 2 weeks, a 2-week course should be prescribed. Women who frequently become reinfected during pregnancy can be given continuous nitrofurantoin prophylaxis (50 mg at bedtime) through until term.

Asymptomatic bacteriuria has a three-fold higher prevalence in women with diabetes. The consequences are unknown, but pyelonephritis is also far more common in women with diabetes. Most physicians treat bacteriuria in women with diabetes, assuming that control of diabetes may be more readily achieved and that symptomatic urinary infection will be prevented. However, no substantive published studies have shown that treating asymptomatic bacteriuria in this population favorably alters any measurable outcomes.

Complicated Urinary Tract Infection

The natural history of infection in anatomically or functionally abnormal urinary tracts is poorly defined, and the evidence that treatment alters the natural history or prevents complications is sparse.

Women with indwelling catheters have a mean of one febrile episode per 100 days of catheterization, and one-half or more of these episodes appear to arise from the urinary tract. A 5- to 7-day course of therapy, either oral or parenteral depending upon illness severity, is usually adequate to treat the infection. Longer courses have no proven value and encourage superinfection with highly resistant pathogens. Prophylaxis has not been shown to be useful in women with indwelling catheters; however, once a catheter has been removed, treatment to cure the infection should be prescribed.

Patients with neurogenic bladders being managed by intermittent catheterization should be treated whenever infection is diagnosed either by routine culture or by symptoms. Prophylaxis in these patients has not been proved to be useful.

Urinary tract infection complicating renal or bladder calculi should be managed with long-term continuous suppressive regimens. Stone removal, in most instances, is a prerequisite for cure.

All infections, regardless of symptoms, should be treated in patients who are immunosuppressed or have had a transplant. Optimal treatment regimens have not been established, but a 2-week course of either trimethoprim-sulfamethoxazole or a fluoroquinolone is appropriate. Urinary infections occur in about two-thirds of women with polycystic renal disease. Prolonged courses of treatment with lipophilic agents that gain access to cyst fluids, such as trimethoprim-sulfamethoxazole or the fluoroquinolones, can achieve symptomatic improvement, and often these infections can be cured if treatment is continued for 6 to 12 weeks.

Complicated infections are far more frequently associated with antibacterial-resistant pathogens and encompass a wide spectrum of underlying illness. As a result, empirical treatment must be chosen with care. Third-generation cephalosporins, imipenem, and the fluoroquinolones are all appropriate choices for invasive febrile UTIs until susceptibility results are known.

Conclusions

Sound rationale now exists for the treatment of most women with urinary infection. Effective prevention initiatives can thwart recurrences and markedly reduce the number of symptomatic episodes. However, management of complicated urinary infections has not been adequately investigated, and many treatment regimens are empirical and controversial.

The overall health costs of urinary infection in women have been substantially decreased over the past 20 years owing to less frequent hospitalization, the use of prophylactic regimens, and markedly reduced imaging and urologic investigation. The strategies are cost effective and should be routinely used by all physicians who care for women with urinary infection.

BACTERIAL INFECTIONS OF THE URINARY TRACT IN GIRLS

method of
ANTHONY J. CASALE, M.D.
University of Louisville School of Medicine
Louisville, Kentucky

It has been estimated that 3% of girls will have a symptomatic urinary tract infection in the first 11 years of life and that 5% will suffer one prior to graduation from high school. The yearly incidence demonstrates two peaks: one at the time of toilet training and one in late adolescence. Urinary tract infections occur in 2% of female infants and are often serious and require hospitalization. This chapter deals with urinary tract infections (UTIs) in girls and adolescents but not with the specific problems of infants with UTIs.

SYMPTOMS AND SIGNS

Symptoms of children with UTIs are varied and often unreliable. Toddlers may complain of vague abdominal or perineal discomfort. Decreased appetite and lethargy may be present. Often the first sign of infection will be a change in voiding habits or the onset of enuresis. As children grow older, their ability to describe the familiar symptoms of dysuria, frequency, and urgency improves as does their ability to localize flank and pelvic pain.

Fever generally is limited to infection of the upper urinary tract, that is, pyelonephritis, and can be extremely high, leading to febrile seizures in some cases. Back pain, chills, nausea, and vomiting are almost exclusive to pyelonephritis. Children with pyelonephritis quickly become dehydrated, and if treatment is delayed, bacterial sepsis can follow. Because of the unpredictability of symptoms in girls with UTI, the clinician must have a high index of suspicion and be quick to obtain a urine specimen for analysis and culture.

SEQUELAE

Aside from the obvious discomfort of the illness itself, the sequelae of urinary tract infection are important to consider. If treatment is delayed, the bacteria responsible for pyelonephritis can gain access to the bloodstream, leading to bacterial sepsis and potential seeding of other organs. In addition, pyelonephritis in children carries a significant risk of permanent scarring of the renal parenchyma, particularly in girls under the age of 5 years. Recurrent infection can retard renal growth and cause small kidneys. It has been estimated that scarring occurs in as many as 25% of children with pyelonephritis. Extensive scarring can lead to hypertension and renal insufficiency. In fact, renal scarring and chronic pyelonephritis account for 10% of new patients entering end-stage renal disease programs. Early diagnosis and appropriate treatment can, in some cases, prevent or decrease scarring, and this fact makes the management of UTI in children most important.

DIAGNOSIS

The diagnosis of urinary tract infection relies upon the urine culture. Urinalysis is only a guide to be used to initiate treatment, and the high rate of false positives and negatives makes a culture mandatory. The most common indicator of infection on urinalysis is the presence of leukocytes and nitrites. Unless the physician personally examines the urine, the microscopic observation of bacteria is often unreliable.

The most common cause of a false-positive urinalysis is vaginitis. Symptoms of dysuria and perineal irritation mimic UTI, and leukocytes are often washed into the urine during voiding for a clean catch specimen. False-negative urinalyses can occur very early in the course of the infection, and as many 30% of patients with bacteriuria and UTI will not demonstrate a significant number of white cells. Not only does the culture identify the bacteria, but an antibiotic sensitivity panel provides invaluable information for current and future treatment as well. *Escherichia coli* is the bacteria responsible for 80% of UTIs in children. The common bacteriologic definition of a UTI (colony count >100,000 colonies/mL) is based upon a voided clean-catch specimen and should be considered only a guide. Lower colony counts may be significant and require treatment.

The proper method of urine collection depends on the age and cooperation of the child. Cultures obtained from a specimen bag applied to a toddler's perineum are reliable if either sterile or infected with a significant growth of a single organism. Cultures with low colony counts, multiple organisms, different organisms obtained in serial samples, or organisms that are uncommon urinary pathogens are likely contaminated. The same is true with voided specimens obtained from older girls. Antiseptic cleansing prior to collection of samples is generally not necessary but it is essential to have the girl's legs spread to minimize perineal contamination. If there is any question about the validity of the specimen or if the child is particularly ill, a catheterized specimen should be obtained. Even very small girls can be safely catheterized with small pediatric feeding tubes and catheters with minor discomfort. The urine culture should be obtained prior to initiating any antibiotic therapy.

TREATMENT

Acute Cystitis

In children with signs of lower urinary tract irritability (dysuria, frequency, urgency, enuresis, and without signs of pyelonephritis) who have a positive urinalysis, it is appropriate to initiate oral outpatient antibiotics after the culture has been obtained. Pending the culture results, the patient may be started on trimethoprim-sulfamethoxazole (Bactrim, Septra), amoxicillin (Amoxil), or nitrofurantoin (Macrodantin) as first-line drugs. A 5- to 7-day course of full-strength antibiotics should be used, depending upon the severity of the symptoms. After this initial period, the dosage should be dropped to approximately 25% of the total daily dose given every evening at bedtime until complete evaluation of the infection. She should return in 10 to 14 days for a repeat urinalysis and if clear should then be scheduled for radiographic evaluation after another 2 weeks.

Acute Pyelonephritis

Pyelonephritis is usually a debilitating illness with high fever, back and abdominal pain, and nausea and vomiting in addition to the usual signs of lower tract infection. Often the girls are dehydrated and their inability to drink and tolerate oral antibiotics may require admission to the hospital. Broad-spectrum parenteral antibiotics should be started along with intravenous fluids to correct dehydration. If the child is particularly ill, blood cultures should be obtained along with the routine chemistries and blood counts. Of course, a urine culture should be obtained prior to initiating antibiotics, and in pyelonephritis a catheterized specimen is often advisable.

The optimal duration of treatment is a matter of debate. We hospitalize patients until they are afebrile for 48 hours and are tolerating oral feedings and medication. By that time the culture and sensitivities are completed and the antibiotic coverage can be adjusted and simplified. A renal ultrasound study is performed during the hospitalization to rule out hydronephrosis, abscess, and other renal anomalies. Parenteral antibiotics, if necessary because of sensitivities, can be continued on an outpatient basis under the care of a home health agency for a total of 10 to 14 days, and then the child is placed upon nightly prophylaxis with an oral antibiotic until the radiographic evaluation is completed 2 weeks later. If sensitivities reveal that an oral antibiotic will adequately treat the infection, the child may be discharged home on full-strength treatment for 7 to 10 days before starting prophylaxis.

Radiographic Evaluation

The likelihood of recurrent infection in as many as 80% of girls and the high incidence of genitourinary anomalies, particularly vesicoureteral reflux, in as many as 35% of all girls with infection make radiographic evaluation necessary in any girl with a documented urinary tract infection. Both the upper urinary tract (kidneys and ureters) and the lower tract (bladder) must be evaluated. Today renal ultrasound has all but replaced the intravenous pyelogram as the initial study of choice for the upper tracts. It can be done during the acute infection and provides a wealth of information with no significant risk or discomfort. The presence of hydronephrosis, stones, abscesses, and variations in the size and shape of the kidneys can be assessed along with the presence and extent of renal scarring.

In cases in which clinical indications for pyelonephritis are equivocal and it is important to establish the diagnosis, a nuclear imaging study of the kidneys may be helpful. DMSA renal scans outline an area of hypoperfusion within the kidney corresponding to the area of the kidney involved with pyelonephritis. Renal scarring can also be evaluated with DMSA and MAG-3 scans which, in addition, visualize the collecting system and provide differential functional data.

Evaluation of the lower urinary tract is the single most important examination because of the incidence of vesicoureteral reflux in 35% of girls with urinary infections. Reflux (passage of bladder urine in a retrograde manner back into the upper urinary tract) places the kidneys at particular risk for recurrent infection and scarring. Unfortunately, the only way to test for reflux requires catheterization for a voiding cystourethrogram (VCUG) or a nuclear cystogram. Our preference is for the VCUG because it provides information about the shape and size of the bladder, and new technology has decreased the radiation dose so that the nuclear cystogram has little of the advantage that it once had.

Natural History

Regardless of the radiographic findings, there is a high likelihood of recurrent infection after UTI. The risk of recurrence in school-age girls is 50% in the first year after the first infection, 27% in the second year, 18% during the third year, and 5% at the end of the fourth year. The fact that one-third of recurrences after a symptomatic infection will be asymptomatic makes follow-up examination of the urine necessary.

Etiology

If infection recurs in the face of a normal radiographic evaluation, it is necessary to look further for a correctable cause for the infections. The most common contributing factor in these cases is a problem with toilet habits termed dysfunctional voiding. Girls with dysfunctional voiding problems often present with UTI but usually have additional problems of daytime and nighttime wetting, constipation and encopresis, urgency, and dysuria. A detailed voiding history will reveal either a habit of very infrequent trips to the toilet (twice per day) or frequent voids (>six or eight per day). The children often display behavior of squatting or posturing to prevent unwanted voiding and denial of the need to void.

Dysfunctional voiding must be treated with a program of behavioral modification relying upon the parents to implement a system of rewards and a timed voiding schedule (four or five times per day). These children must be maintained on antibiotic prophylaxis until their toilet habits are corrected. Other medications, such as anticholinergics to help control the bladder, may be necessary. Constipation must be corrected at the same time and prevented with diet and a change in stooling habits. Once the child's dysfunctional voiding has been corrected, antibiotics can be stopped and the infections will usually not recur.

Asymptomatic Bacteriuria

Girls with asymptomatic bacteriuria must undergo complete radiographic evaluation and evaluation of their voiding habits. In cases in which these evaluations are negative, most pediatric urologists now suggest that no further treatment be rendered. It appears that colonization of the bladder in these otherwise normal children prevents symptomatic UTI and its sequelae. Infrequent periodic evaluation of the urinary tract with ultrasound, blood chemistries, and urinalysis is prudent.

CHILDHOOD ENURESIS

method of
EDMOND T. GONZALES, Jr., M.D.
Baylor College of Medicine
Houston, Texas

Delay in acquiring satisfactory urinary control is a common problem in childhood that frequently prompts parents to seek medical evaluation and attention. At age 4, nearly 25% of children have some voiding dysfunction or difficulties with urinary control, and 12% of 6-year-olds still have problems with urinary incontinence. As children get older, there is a gradual reduction in the number of children who wet at a rate of about 15% per year, with the spontaneous resolution of urinary incontinence occurring in a relatively straight-line slope throughout childhood. Enuresis can be defined as any abnormality in urinary control beyond an age in which control is expected to have been achieved.

Incontinence can occur only at night (nocturnal enuresis), can involve both day and nighttime wetting, or can occur only in the daytime (diurnal enuresis). Wetting disorders in children are also commonly classified as primary enuresis (when a child has never achieved satisfactory urinary control from the age at which parents initiated toilet training) and secondary, or onset, enuresis (the onset of urinary incontinence following a period of dryness, usually 3 to 6 months in duration). While there is a great deal of overlap among these various categories of childhood incontinence, it is convenient to discuss separately those children who have nighttime wetting only and those who wet both day and night.

NOCTURNAL ENURESIS

Incidence and Etiology

Persistent nocturnal enuresis is the most common disorder of bladder control in childhood. As noted above, it affects nearly one in four 4-year-olds and one in eight 6-year-olds. Nocturnal enuresis is known to cluster in family groups. In one study in which both the mother and father had a lengthy history of nocturnal wetting, 77% of their children wet the bed. However, the exact genetic causation remains unknown. Nighttime wetting is somewhat more common in males than in females in a ratio of 1.5 to 1.

Two and three decades ago psychological problems were thought to be the cause of enuresis, but this is no longer believed to be the case in the overwhelming majority of children. While it is possible that stressful episodes can precipitate a pattern of behavior that results in enuresis, there is no convincing evidence that lingering psychological problems perpetuate the voiding dysfunction. In many ways, nocturnal enuresis suggests a simple delay in overall maturation. The spontaneous resolution rate in these children speaks to a developmental disorder. In addition, children with nighttime wetting often exhibit other patterns of immaturity, such as sleepwalking and nightmares, at an incidence greater than a same-aged control population of children who do not wet.

Recent experimental data suggests that a significant proportion of children with nocturnal enuresis may have an abnormally high urinary output during sleep because of a lack of the normal increase in antidiuretic hormone secreted at night. It is postulated that children with this disorder rapidly overfill their bladders during sleep but presumably fail to awake because of the propensity of children to have longer and more frequent phases of deep sleep than normal adults. Nocturnal enuresis can be associated with any high-output urinary disorder, such as diabetes mellitus, diabetes insipidus, and psychogenic water drinking. However, these disorders should also manifest recognizable daytime frequency associated with high urine outputs with each void.

Evaluation

The evaluation of children with nocturnal enuresis only is office based. Assessment must include a thorough investigation into the many aspects of voiding dysfunction that can occur in children. The interviewer should seek a parental history of enuresis, should explore carefully any disorder of daytime urinary control, and should ask specifically about past urologic abnormalities, particularly problems with urinary tract infection. The examining physician should entertain the possibility of a neurologic abnormality, especially in relation to the lower extremities or bowel control. Discussion regarding family stress and isolated traumatic events should be addressed, particularly in cases of secondary enuresis, as mentioned, although it is difficult to know just what relationship these issues have to the ongoing problem of nocturnal enuresis.

A complete and thorough physical examination should then be undertaken with special attention to those areas pertinent to bladder and urinary physiology. A careful examination of the abdomen for the presence of palpable renal enlargement or a distended bladder should be performed. A complete examination of the genitalia in both boys and girls is essential. A rectal examination should be a routine part of this evaluation with particular attention being paid to anal sphincter tone as well as the presence of pelvic masses, bladder distention, or an apparent thickening of the detrusor musculature. A thorough neurologic examination of the lower extremity and the perineum, including sensory and motor aspects, should also be performed. Inspection of the lower lumbosacral region may reveal deformities in the sacrococcygeal anatomy or the presence of dimples, hairy patches, or abnormal angiomatous lesions that might suggest a defect in lumbosacral development and related maldevelopment of the distal end of the spinal cord. Finally, a complete urinalysis should be done as well as a urine culture of any suspicious microscopic sediment.

If the child presents with only nocturnal enuresis and has a completely normal history and physical examination in all other regards, further diagnostic evaluation is not indicated.

Treatment

Since the specific cause of nocturnal enuresis is unknown, treatment remains empiric. Also, since enuresis is exceedingly common until 6 years of age, it is difficult to justify active intervention in that age group. At any age, decisions regarding treatment should consider to what extent the problem affects the child and the social aspects of the child's development. Many young children and their parents are better served by reassurance that there is no physical abnormality than by long-term and expensive therapy of uncertain efficacy.

Pharmacologic Management

There are two pharmacologic approaches for managing the child with nocturnal enuresis. The first drug to be used was imipramine (Tofranil). Originally introduced as a tricyclic antidepressant, it was subsequently recognized that patients on high doses of imipramine exhibited difficulties with micturition. Subsequent studies confirmed an anticholinergic, and perhaps an alpha-adrenergic, effect on detrusor and bladder neck musculature that increased bladder volume, decreased detrusor irritability, and tightened bladder neck tone. The drug remains very useful in managing complex bladder disorders, particularly in children with significant neurologic abnormalities such as spina bifida. The effect of imipramine in treating nocturnal enuresis is presumed in most cases to result from detrusor relaxation and increased bladder capacity. However, imipramine has also been shown to alter sleeping patterns, and other more central effects may also play a role. The drug is effective in only about 50% of children. In addition, a successful result with imipramine does not appear to lessen the duration of the wetting problem. The drug benefits the child only on the night taken, but cessation of nocturnal enuresis still requires the neurophysical maturation and ultimate spontaneous resolution that would have occurred without the use of imipramine.

Imipramine has been associated with several side effects, including emotional instability, sleep disturbances, lethargy, and mild gastrointestinal disturbances. Overdoses can lead to cardiac arrhythmias, respiratory depression, and convulsions, which have resulted in fatalities. Parents need to be warned to keep the drug away from other children in the family. The usual dosage is 25 mg for children 6 to 8 years of age and 50 mg for children 9 years of age or older. It is usually given 1 hour before bedtime.

Recently, desmopressin acetate (DDAVP) nasal spray, an analogue of the naturally occurring antidiuretic hormone (ADH), has been successfully employed in the management of nocturnal enuresis. This use of DDAVP was based on the observation that a significant number of children who wet at night have blunted secretion of normal levels of ADH and subsequent high urinary output during sleep. The drug is easy to give, has few significant side effects when administered properly, and is successful in 60 to 70% of children with nocturnal enuresis. It is usually administered at a dosage of 20 to 40 μg (two to four sprays) and is given just before retiring and after the child empties the bladder completely before going to bed. However, as with imipramine, relapse is high when the drug is discontinued. It is usually recommended that it be used for 3 to 4 months if successful and then tapered gradually over several weeks to see whether there will be resumption of the enuresis. The drug is also relatively expensive. It has been my experience that many parents want to use desmopressin only when wetting would be especially inconvenient (sleepovers, vacations or summer camp, or visits with relatives). It is easy to administer, although any rhinitis (especially if chronic, as in allergic disorders) can temporarily interfere with its absorption and, hence, reduce its effectiveness. It is important that the drug be used only when the child retires to reduce the risk of fluid overload and electrolyte abnormalities.

Other anticholinergic agents, especially drugs commonly used in urology, such as oxybutynin (Ditropan), have not been shown to significantly improve nighttime wetting, despite the effectiveness of imipramine. Their use is rarely recommended in this disorder.

Behavioral Modification Therapy

Although many approaches to treating nocturnal enuresis have included behavioral modification, by far the most effective has been the use of alarm units. Introduced decades ago as large grids placed beneath the bed sheets, they have been modified and miniaturized within the last 15 years so that now the units are self-contained, are worn on the shoulder or the wrist, and are activated by a small electrode sewn directly onto the child's underclothing. When a decision is made to initiate behavioral modification therapy with one of these alarm units, it is important that the physician take the time to introduce the concept and the equipment to the parent and the child, to emphasize the principles of behavioral modification and the rationale for this therapy in uncomplicated enuresis, and to offer support during the conditioning program. The major cause of failure of behavioral modification is poor compliance on the part of the child and the parents. It must be emphasized that this is truly family therapy, and the parents must be willing to accept the responsibility of supervising the conditioning therapy. When the program is rigidly adhered to, as many as 70 to 80% of children will ultimately demonstrate improved nighttime urinary control, although the period of time required to achieve this may be as long as 3 months or more.

The principle of conditioning therapy is that repetitively arousing the child at the time of the wetting episode can ultimately condition the child to recognize that micturition is about to occur and subsequently to teach the child to inhibit the voiding reflex. As the child begins to achieve periods of whole-night dryness, the unit should continue to be worn for several more weeks. Occasional intermittent episodes of enuresis will reinforce the conditioning system. Likewise, should wetting recur some months or so later, reinitiating the conditioning program can often reinforce the previous therapy and blunt the tendency for long-term recurrence.

The major problems associated with conditioning are the length of time it takes to demonstrate an adequate response, the disruption of the entire family's sleep pattern, and the fact that many children react sluggishly to the alarm unit. It is essential during the first few weeks that the parents adequately arouse the child when the alarm signals.

Methods often tried by parents before they seek medical attention, such as withholding fluids before retiring, awakening the child at night at random, and reward-punishment strategems, are generally ineffective. Likewise, specific psychotherapy, common two to three decades ago, is not felt to be appropriate for the child with uncomplicated primary enuresis.

The effectiveness of hypnotherapy remains controversial.

My approach to treating the child with primary enuresis without any daytime symptoms whatsoever is to first initiate a trial of DDAVP. This is offered after a thorough discussion of the various options discussed previously. As noted, the advantage of a trial of DDAVP is that it provides the child with a treatment option that should assure dryness during times when nocturnal enuresis would be particularly inconvenient or traumatic, thereby allowing the child to participate in all normal activities without the fear of wetting the bed. However, after a trial of DDAVP, I generally recommend that the parents consider a subsequent trial with one of the behavioral modification units. Success with this device offers the benefits of control of enuresis without long-term drug usage.

DAY AND NIGHT URINARY INCONTINENCE

When children present with daytime symptoms, either alone or, more often, in association with nocturnal enuresis, the possibility of underlying urologic pathology must be excluded. The great majority of children with this type of urinary incontinence will not be found to have any recognizable anatomic or neurologic pathology and will fall into the large group of children said to have voiding dysfunction. However, a small percentage will have specific urologic and/or neurologic disorders responsible for their incontinence. In addition to a thorough history and physical examination, one would generally consider obtaining certain specific imaging studies in these children.

Certain aspects of the history and physical examination can suggest a certain diagnosis. Constant dampness despite a normal voiding pattern should raise suspicion of an ectopic ureter. Sudden urgency with precipitant leakage associated with squatting in an effort to hold back the urinary flow (the curtsey sign) is typical of uninhibited detrusor contractions. Primary female epispadias can be easily missed if the cardinal finding of a bifid clitoris is not recognized.

A renal ultrasound is a useful screening procedure. In girls with ectopic ureter, renal ultrasound usually shows the typical dilated ureter behind the bladder, most often associated with a duplication anomaly of the ureter. Male children with urethral obstruction, most often mildly obstructing posterior urethral valves, develop detrusor hypertrophy with subsequent detrusor instability and incontinence. A renal ultrasound in this situation can suggest urethral obstruction by demonstrating detrusor thickening, but a voiding cystourethrogram is necessary to confirm the diagnosis. A child who has urinary incontinence because of a neurogenic abnormality will commonly also have difficulties with bowel control (encopresis) and may have recognized neurologic abnormalities of the lower extremities. Nonetheless, there is the occasional child who has a subtle neurologic deficit in which the most prominent symptomatology is abnormal bladder control. In addition to careful neurologic examination and inspection of the lower lumbosacral region, imaging genitourinary studies as well as select views of the lower lumbosacral spine are appropriate. The recognition of a spina bifida occulta should prompt further consideration of other possible neurologic problems. Today, the most definitive test for evaluation of the lower lumbosacral region of the spinal cord is magnetic resonance imaging. Urodynamic testing may also be required to define the specific bladder dysfunction. However, such testing rarely provides a specific etiology for the recognized bladder abnormality.

When additional work-up fails to yield an obvious etiology for the incontinence, it is usually best to initiate treatment first for the daytime incontinence and then deal with the nighttime wetting later if it persists. Children without recognized anatomic or neurologic deficits to explain their incontinence most often demonstrate an uninhibited bladder similar in function to that of the young child before potty training. Whether these abnormal bladder patterns simply represent delayed maturation or are actually another example of a primary learned disorder in the acquisition of urinary control remains unclear and somewhat controversial. Behavioral modification therapy has been tried but with limited success. The most successful approach has been anticholinergic therapy, usually with oxybutynin or hyoscyamine sulfate (Levsin), although any number of anticholinergic drugs may be helpful. Interestingly, anticholinergic therapy is often much more helpful for the daytime wetting than in nocturnal enuresis. The length of therapy is conjectural, although it is appropriate to taper the medication every 6 months to assess how the child will do without pharmacologic support.

Children with voiding dysfunction, particularly girls, are especially susceptible to the development of urinary tract infection. When managing a child with voiding dysfunction, it is prudent to screen for urinary tract infection on a regular basis. The presence of infection makes the bladder more irritable and will certainly be associated with increasing difficulty in controlling the enuresis.

URINARY INCONTINENCE

method of
MARKO R. GUDZIAK, M.D., and
DELBERT C. RUDY, M.D.
The University of Texas Health Science Center at Houston Medical School
Houston, Texas

Urinary incontinence affects an estimated 10 to 12 million individuals in the United States. Up to 18% of children 5 to 14 years of age are incontinent. The rate of incontinence is about 4 to 5% in middle-aged men and 20 to 25% in middle-aged women, and approximately 38% of women and 19% of men over 60 years of age experience urinary incontinence. Over half of the institutionalized elderly experience urinary incontinence. The cost of treating incontinence in 1987 was $10.3 billion and exceeded the total spent on dialysis and coronary bypass surgery combined. Fewer than 1 in 10 incontinent patients seeks medical assistance for this problem and more than half of those feel they are not adequately helped.

Incontinence is obviously well-suited to self-diagnosis by the patient. However, the problem can be due to diverse etiologies, including some that are potentially or overtly life threatening. Bladder cancer can present with irritative voiding symptoms and urge incontinence. Bladder outlet obstruction from benign prostatic hyperplasia (BPH) or prostate cancer can present similarly or with overflow incontinence, an intermittent or continuous dribbling. Local inflammatory conditions such as acute cystitis or bladder calculus can also lead to irritative voiding symptoms and urge continence. Pelvic pathology, such as tumors, infections, and pelvic floor relaxation, can cause incontinence of various types. The treatment of pelvic pathology, particularly tumors, can have profound adverse effects on lower urinary tract function that can present with incontinence. Prime examples include pelvic irradiation and radical pelvic surgery (e.g., abdominoperineal resection or radical hysterectomy). Also to be considered are congenital defects (e.g., epispadias, ectopic ureter) and fistulas. Neurologic lesions of the spinal cord and brain often result in various types of incontinence. Unfortunately, previous procedures on the lower urinary tract can also result in continued, altered, or de novo incontinence. So-called transient causes of incontinence include diarrhea, altered mental state, drug therapy, and impaired mobility. Because of the multiple potential etiologies, it is easiest to conceptualize the problem as one of bladder dysfunction, urethral dysfunction, or a combination of both.

DIAGNOSTIC EVALUATION OF URINARY INCONTINENCE

There are several steps in the evaluation of the incontinent patient. A thorough history, emphasizing the nature of the incontinence, should be taken. The type (urge, associated with a precipitant desire to void; stress, associated with continuous or with intermittent increases in intra-abdominal pressure as with coughing, laughing, or straining), frequency, duration, pattern (nocturnal, diurnal, drug-related), amount, and associated symptoms (dysuria, hematuria, pain, straining to void, incomplete emptying, polydipsia, polyuria) should be ascertained. Alterations in bowel habits, sexual function, and somatic function along with other relevant history (heart disease, diabetes, cancer, neurologic disease, previous surgery or radiation) should be elicited. A list of all medications, including nonprescription drugs, should be noted. On physical examination, particular attention should be paid to the genitourinary abdominal and rectal and neurologic examinations, especially of the sacral reflexes and lumbosacral sensory dermatomes. A properly collected urine specimen should be sent for urinalysis and the postvoid residual measured. Further evaluation, depending on the clinical situation, can include an intravenous pyelogram (IVP) or renal ultrasound in patients with hematuria, suspected neoplasm, recurrent infections, or suspected neurogenic bladder. Urine cytology and cystoscopy are indicated for the evaluation of hematuria, suspected bladder calculus, fistula, or tumor. While all of the previously mentioned aspects of evaluation are necessary, frequently the information obtained is sufficient to establish the etiology and secondary complications due to the bladder and/or urethral dysfunction but inadequate to define the optimal therapy.

Bladder and urethral function can be objectively assessed only via urodynamic evaluation. This diagnostic modality includes a range of techniques from totally noninvasive procedures to urethral/bladder instrumentation with sophisticated multiport pressure transducer catheters, needle electromyographic (EMG) electrodes in various locations, and transrectal catheters/pressure transducers. The addition of fluoroscopy, with utilization of a contrast agent to fill the bladder, can provide simultaneous anatomic and functional information as well. Ideally, all aspects of evaluation are integrated appropriately in the work-up of the incontinent patient.

INCONTINENCE DUE TO BLADDER DYSFUNCTION

Areflexic or Hyporeflexic Bladder

Detrusor (bladder) areflexia refers to the absence of a reflex-induced bladder contraction. *Hyporeflexic bladder* refers to poor quality bladder contraction. Conceptually, there are three potential etiologies for this type of bladder dysfunction. First, such dysfunction can be a result of an anatomic or functional abnormality in the innervation of the bladder; examples include conus medullaris or sacral nerve outflow lesions from spinal stenosis, disc disease, tumor, autonomic neuropathies, myelodysplasia, spinal cord injury, or multiple sclerosis. In addition, radical pelvic procedures such as abdominoperineal resection or radical hysterectomy can also result in pelvic nerve injuries. Medications with anticholinergic, sedative, or alpha-agonist effects can inhibit bladder contractility or increase bladder outlet resistance, leading to an inability to void and overflow incontinence. Stool impaction can cause reflex bladder inhibition through rectal distention. Second, end-organ (i.e., bladder) pathology can also result in an areflexic or hyporeflexic bladder; examples include bladder overdistention injury, pelvic surgery, and radiation therapy to the pelvis. Finally, bladder function is under a significant degree of voluntary cortical control, and psychologic factors can play a significant role in urinary retention and detrusor areflexia/hyporeflexia in certain clinical circumstances. However, this is a difficult diagnosis to make and should be entertained with caution.

The type of incontinence associated with this type of bladder dysfunction is generically termed *overflow incontinence.* Overflow incontinence results when pressure in the overdistended bladder exceeds urethral resistance and leakage occurs. Any maneuver that increases intra-abdominal pressure, such as coughing, sneezing, or exercise, will typically exacerbate this type of incontinence, and the patient may complain of stress incontinence.

The diagnosis of an areflexic or hyporeflexic bladder is best made by urodynamic evaluation via cystometrography (CMG). Typically, no bladder contraction or only low amplitude and/or poorly sustained contractions are identified. The initial mainstay of therapy is clean intermittent catheterization (CIC) to empty the bladder, usually every 4 to 6 hours, with sufficient frequency to keep bladder volumes below 400 to 500 mL in adults. Concomitant treatment should be aimed at correctable etiologies such as discontinuing medications with anticholinergic effects or resolving fecal impaction. Chronic overdistention injuries from any etiology will require continued intermittent bladder drainage indefinitely until bladder function recovers. Although recovery of bladder function does not always occur, it does so in the vast majority of instances. In the absence of an adequate bladder contraction, definitive management of causes of bladder outlet obstruction, such as BPH, are generally inappropriate. Unfortunately, the neurologically mediated areflexic bladder (e.g., in lumbar disc disease) rarely recovers following therapy directed at the neurologic lesion. The usual reason for such intervention is to promote recovery of lost somatic function and to prevent further functional loss. It should be noted that external catheters are generally contraindicated in the management of overflow incontinence since they do not ensure adequate bladder emptying. In addition, it must be emphasized that the use of oral cholinergic agents (e.g., bethanechol (Urecholine)) is unwarranted since the clinical ineffectiveness of such agents is well documented in the literature.

The areflexic bladder, with time, is not uncommonly associated with poor bladder compliance, particularly with conus medullaris, cauda equina, and peripheral pelvic nerve lesions or injury. This is easily demonstrable on CMG. Poor bladder compliance is a particularly dangerous situation for the patient, because it can readily lead to upper tract renal compromise, including hydronephrosis, renal infection, renal stone disease, and renal failure. This combination is also optimally treated with intermittent catheterization, usually in conjunction with an anticholinergic or alpha-adrenergic blocking agent to try to improve the low bladder compliance. Failure to urodynamically demonstrate pharmacologic control of low bladder compliance usually correlates clinically with failure to control incontinence. This should lead to consideration of surgical intervention. The standard procedure is augmentation cystoplasty using a segment of bowel. We have had modest experience to date with detrusor myomectomy, in the management of low bladder compliance with encouraging results. This is a much simpler surgical procedure and has several theoretic advantages over augmentation cystoplasty.

Hyperreflexic Bladder and Detrusor Instability

An involuntary bladder contraction can cause the loss of urine and is termed *detrusor hyperreflexia* when the patient has a causative neurologic lesion. Examples of such lesions include spinal cord injury, stroke, multiple sclerosis, dementia, and closed head injury. The diagnosis of hyperreflexia requires urodynamic evaluation (at least a simple CMG) for proper management. In the absence of any functional or mechanical bladder outlet obstruction, the main problems seen clinically are the social consequences of incontinence. However, in some circumstances, such as multiple sclerosis and spinal cord injury, a functional bladder outlet obstruction can coexist (external sphincter dyssynergia), which can lead to upper urinary tract compromise and significant morbidity and even mortality. In this situation, optimum management consists of intermittent catheterization and anticholinergic medication: oxybutynin (Ditropan), 2.5 to 10 mg three to four times daily; hyoscyamine (Levsin), 0.125 to 0.375 mg three to four times daily; or propantheline (Pro-Banthine), 7.5 to 30 mg three to four times daily. Caution should be taken in using these agents in patients with glaucoma and input from an ophthalmologist is well advised. In children and elderly patients, imipramine (Tofranil) is often useful at a dose of 10 to 25 mg, usually twice a day. Other agents such as dicyclomine (Bentyl) have been clinically less useful in our experience. Failure of pharmacologic intervention to control the incontinence can lead to consideration of surgical intervention. Sacral dorsal root rhizotomy can eliminate hyperreflexia, and augmentation cystoplasty and detrusor myomectomy are also useful in increasing the reservoir capacity of the bladder at acceptable pressures. In each of these cases, CIC is usually necessary. Continent or incontinent urinary diversions, optimally maintaining the bladder as part of the drainage system, are indicated in very select instances in which problems with performance of routine CIC are encountered.

Detrusor instability (DI), involuntary bladder contractions in the absence of an identifiable neurologic lesion, is an especially common cause of incontinence in the elderly. Typically, there are associated symptoms of urgency, frequency, voiding of small amounts, and urge incontinence. The differential diagnosis includes inflammatory conditions of the bladder (e.g., acute cystitis), foreign bodies (e.g., bladder stones), bladder tumors, bladder outlet obstruction, stress urinary incontinence, and idiopathic causes. Urine culture and, often times, cystoscopy are usual components of the initial evaluation. Urodynamic evaluation, at least a simple CMG, is also frequently useful. Obviously, therapy should be directed at any specifically identifiable etiologies. Anticholinergic medications or tricyclic antidepressants can be useful in increasing the volume threshold of the bladder (i.e., the volume at which bladder contraction is reflexly induced) but only in the absence of significant bladder outlet obstruction. In conjunction with this, a timed voiding schedule should be followed by the patient. The medication will typically not give the patient any more warning time, just increased capacity. Ideally, the patient will voluntarily void on a reasonable schedule before the bladder reaches its "automatic threshold." The intervals of timed voiding may initially need to be shorter than desired but often can be progressively lengthened. Such bladder training, assisted by a voiding diary, can be very helpful but requires a dedicated therapist and patient.

Decreased Bladder Compliance

Normally, bladder filling over the physiologic range of bladder capacity is associated with a relatively small increase in bladder pressure. This is termed *normal bladder compliance.* In the case of decreased bladder compliance, bladder filling is associated with what can be very large increases in bladder pressure over actually quite small changes in bladder volume. As noted previously, this situation is frequently associated with significant morbidity and even mortality because the high intravesical pressures lead to upper urinary tract compromise. Decreased bladder compliance can be associated with bladder areflexia or with normal or abnormal reflex bladder contractions. The mainstay of therapy is anticholinergic agents in conjunction with CIC. Alpha-$_1$ adrenergic blockade (e.g., terazosin [Hytrin]) has also been used with some success. Failure of such conservative management may lead one to consider the surgical interventions noted previously.

INCONTINENCE DUE TO URETHRAL DYSFUNCTION

Urethral Hypermobility

Stress urinary incontinence (SUI) in women is most commonly associated with laxity of bladder and urethral support, which results in increased vesicourethral motion with elevations in abdominal pressure. Consequently, there is decreased ability of the urethra to withstand the expulsive force of abdominal pressure on urine in the bladder. On physical examination, one may see or feel laxity of the anterior vaginal wall. SUI can be documented on the examining table with a Valsalva maneuver. The most accurate method of assessing the cause of stress incontinence and determining optimal management is videourodynamic studies that combine fluoroscopy with bladder pressure measurement. Such evaluation is necessary to differentiate incontinence due to pelvic floor laxity and inappropriate descent of the vesicourethral junction, particularly with Valsalva maneuvers, from intrinsic urethral sphincteric insufficiency. This differentiation has crucial implications regarding optimal management. For urethral hypermobility (pelvic floor laxity), pelvic floor exercise (i.e., Kegel exercises), vaginal cones, and biofeedback have all had variable success. They are probably best suited to very mild forms of incontinence and for patients in whom other forms of therapy are unacceptable for whatever reasons. Tricyclic antidepressants (imipramine, 10 to 25 mg two times daily) or alpha-adrenergic agonists (pseudoephedrine, 30 mg three times daily) may be of some benefit. An often overlooked factor is precipitation of stress incontinence by marked weight gain. Weight loss in such circumstances may be helpful, and it provides health benefits with minimal risk. Retropubic or needle suspension procedures are highly effective and provide the most reliable definitive cure rate (short-term, 90 to 95%; long-term, 60 to 70%). Timed voiding to avoid a full bladder, which predisposes to stress urinary incontinence, can be helpful, but typically by the time patients present to the physician they have already discovered this on their own.

Intrinsic Sphincter Deficiency

When the functional ability of the smooth muscle portion of the urethra is inadequate to provide sufficient resistance to prevent incontinence, the diagnosis of intrinsic sphincter deficiency (ISD) is appropriate. Common clinical settings include post-prostatectomy incontinence, myelodysplasia, incontinence in women following multiple incontinence procedures, radical pelvic surgery, and spinal cord injury or lesions involving the T11-L2 portion of the spinal cord. In men, confirmed stress incontinence has only two causes: a neurologic lesion or injury affecting function of the smooth muscle–mediated sphincteric function of the urethra or direct injury to the urethral sphincter itself (e.g., transurethral resection of the prostate and radical prostatectomy). In women, intrinsic sphincteric insufficiency can occur de novo and may or may not be associated with hypermobility of the vesicourethral junction. Conceptually, ISD can be due to a functional deficit or to fibrosis and scarring that prevents mucosal apposition. A mild variant of ISD is associated with atrophic vaginitis, which is not uncommonly seen in post–menopausal women. In such circumstances, urethral vascularity that normally contributes about a third of the urethral closure pressure is markedly diminished. This can be treated with oral estrogens or vaginal estrogen cream. Appropriate precautions should be observed when administering unopposed estrogen in post-menopausal women.

The diagnosis of ISD is best made urodynamically, utilizing both bladder and urethral pressure recordings, sphincter EMG activity recording, and fluoroscopic monitoring. Typically, fluoroscopically documented incontinence due to ISD is associated with minimal to mild increases in abdominal pressure (e.g., Valsalva maneuvers). When ISD in women is associated with minimal to no vesicourethral hypermobility, the best initial treatment is transurethral or periurethral injection of glutaraldehyde cross-linked collagen. This major advance in the treatment of ISD was only recently approved by the FDA for this purpose. This is also appropriate therapy in many men with ISD. The major advantage of the procedure is that it can be done in the office under local anesthesia. Collagen injections are associated with minimal morbidity and are especially useful in elderly and debilitated patients who are not candidates for other surgical procedures. The majority of patients will need more than one injection. There is a possibility that with time re-injection will be necessary. When ISD in women is associated with significant urethral hypermobility, the best treatment is a pubovaginal sling procedure. The artificial urinary sphincter is another option; however the potential for infection or mechanical failure, and the high reoperation rate make this a secondary mode of therapy. In men, an artificial urinary sphincter is currently the treatment of choice for those who fail collagen injection or in whom collagen is inappropriate for anatomic or technical reasons. It should be clear from this discussion that proper urodynamic evaluation is essential in selecting the appropriate therapy in patients with ISD.

OTHER CAUSES OF INCONTINENCE

The elderly are particularly prone to incontinence because of associated illnesses and their therapies. Psychologic problems or depression can also lead to urinary incontinence. Excessive urine output and incontinence can be due to hyperglycemia, diabetes insipidus, congestive heart failure, hypercalcemia, or diuretic use. As mentioned previously, multiple medications, both prescribed and over-the-counter, can contribute to incontinence: these include diuretics, anticholinergic agents, sedative hypnotics, calcium channel blockers, sympathomimetics, and sympatholytics. Restricted mobility secondary to arthritis, orthopedic injury, fear of falling, or restraints can prevent a patient from reaching the bathroom in time. Provisions for assistance, treating the underlying condition, and improving access to a bathroom or bedside commode will usually help, but this may be difficult depending on the level of achievable nursing care or help.

EPIDIDYMITIS

method of
JOHN A. HEANEY, M.B., B.Ch.
Dartmouth Medical School and Dartmouth-Hitchcock Medical Center
Lebanon, New Hampshire

Epididymitis is a common affliction of younger men. A painful scrotal swelling is the main complaint in acute epididymitis, and the pain may spread up the spermatic cord into the lower abdomen. A sensation of scrotal heaviness is usual, and some patients develop systemic symptoms such as pyrexia, chills, and malaise. Severe inflammation can lead to an enlarged indurated epididymis that is indistinguishable from the testicle. This can present diagnostic difficulties in differentiating epididymitis from testicular torsion, testicular tumor, or both. A urethral discharge or symptoms of prostatitis or urinary tract infection may also be present. Epididymitis is usually unilateral.

Epididymitis is caused by infection from bladder urine or the prostatic fluid or from an ascending urethral infection. Infected urine or prostatic secretions can reflux into the ejaculatory duct, reach the epididymis, and result in inflammation. In men younger than 35 years of age, epididymitis is usually due to chlamydial infection, and symptoms of urethritis (e.g., urethral discharge) are frequent. Infection in men older than 35 years of age arises from bladder bacteriuria secondary to coliform organisms, and patients may have signs and symptoms of cystitis or prostatitis. "Sterile" epididymitis, associated with vigorous physical activity, is caused by vasal reflux of sterile urine, which causes a chemical inflammation of the epididymis and clinical findings indistinguishable from infectious epididymitis. Epididymitis in boys may be the presenting feature of congenital urologic anatomic abnormalities, such as ectopic ureter or posterior urethral valves.

Epididymitis is a potential complication of indwelling Foley catheters. Bacteria migrate in the pericatheter space from the external meatus to the prostatic urethra and into the vas deferens and epididymis. Bacteriuric men who undergo lower tract instrumentation, catheterization, or surgery (e.g., prostatectomy) are at increased risk for developing epididymitis.

Epididymitis due to syphilis, gonorrhea, or tuberculosis is uncommon, but the recent increased prevalence of tuberculosis may result in more cases of tuberculous epididymitis. Opportunistic bacterial and fungal (e.g., *Candida albicans*) epididymal infections are also becoming more prevalent in the patient population immunosuppressed for transplantation or by acquired immune deficiency syndrome or cancer chemotherapy.

Epididymitis has to be distinguished clinically from hydroceles, testicular tumors, and testicular torsion. The epididymis lies posterior to the testis, and this demarcation is preserved in all but the most severe cases of epididymitis. "Reactive" hydrocele formation may render the palpation of intrascrotal structures difficult. Although transillumination frequently identifies hydroceles, scrotal ultrasonography with or without Doppler imaging is much more accurate and can also diagnose testicular tumors. Acute epididymitis in young boys can be confused with testicular torsion, and careful clinical evaluation and diagnostic imaging may be needed to distinguish these disorders. Scrotal ultrasonography, and if time permits, noninvasive nuclear scanning may help in reaching a correct diagnosis. Whenever in doubt, scrotal exploration to exclude torsion should be done within 4 to 6 hours if testicular viability is to be preserved. Following treatment, boys with epididymitis deserve full urologic evaluation with intravenous urography, cystourethroscopy, and voiding cystourethrography.

TREATMENT

Epididymitis is usually treated on an outpatient basis. Symptoms are relieved by scrotal elevation, support, and bed rest. Patients with systemic symptoms of infection (e.g., leukocytosis and fever) require hospital admission for parenteral antibiotics and more vigorous supportive treatment.

Treatment with nonsteroidal anti-inflammatory drugs (e.g., ibuprofen [Motrin], 400 mg orally four times daily) provides satisfactory analgesia. Antipyretics, such as acetaminophen or aspirin, are also usually prescribed. Severe pain may necessitate a spermatic cord local anesthetic block with lidocaine (Xylocaine), bupivacaine (Marcaine), or both.

Antibiotic therapy is based on the patient's age and the presence of symptoms of urinary tract infection. In younger men, epididymitis is usually due to sexually transmitted bacteria, such as *Neisseria gonorrhoeae* or *Chlamydia trachomatis.* A Gram's stain of the urethra may reveal the gram-negative intracellular diplococci characteristic of gonococcal urethritis. Gonococcal epididymitis is far less common than chlamydial epididymitis. Preferred treatment of nongonococcal urethritis is doxycycline, 100 mg orally twice a day, or minocycline (Minocin), 100 mg twice a day for 10 to 14 days. Some of the newer fluoroquinolones, such as ofloxacin (Floxin) and ciprofloxacin (Cipro), merit consideration for the treatment of epididymitis in younger men, although they are not approved for treatment of sexually transmitted diseases.

In older men, particularly if the urinalysis shows bacteria, broad-spectrum antimicrobial therapy is indicated. Treatment with a third-generation quinolone (e.g., ciprofloxacin [Cipro], 250 mg twice a day for 10 days, or trimethoprim-sulfamethoxazole [Septra, Bactrim], one double-strength tablet twice a day for 10 days) is recommended. If there is evidence of an underlying bacterial prostatitis, antimicrobial therapy should be continued for 4 weeks. In severe cases of epididymitis associated with fever, leukocytosis, and other systemic symptoms, parenteral antibiotic therapy (e.g., an aminoglycoside or cephalosporin) is needed until the patient defervesces, at which time a longer course of oral antimicrobial therapy is instituted. The fluoroquinolones may obviate the need for parenteral antibiotics because of their broad-spectrum potency and the high tissue levels achieved after oral administration.

Most patients experience relief of their symptoms within 48 hours. However, it is not uncommon for swelling and discomfort to persist for weeks or months following eradication of the infecting organism. The epididymis may remain enlarged and/or indurated indefinitely. If fever continues in spite of suitable broad-spectrum antimicrobial therapy, an abscess should be excluded by scrotal ultrasonography. Surgical drainage, epididymo-orchiectomy, or both are indicated for patients with abscess or fistula formation.

Epididymitis can be complicated by the development of testicular necrosis, testicular atrophy, or infertility. Chronic epididymitis associated with inflammation and fibrosis can result in blockage to the ductal cord structures and impaired sperm production. This is more likely to occur with bilateral epididymitis. The swelling associated with acute epididymitis can compromise testicular blood flow and result in loss of seminiferous tubules and testicular atrophy. If there is a persistent mass, the possibility of an underlying testicular tumor must be considered.

THE PRIMARY GLOMERULOPATHIES

method of
LEE A. HEBERT, M.D.
The Ohio State University Medical Center
Columbus, Ohio

CLASSIFICATION

The Primary Glomerulopathies

In this category of glomerulopathy, the pathologic process is thought to be confined to the kidney; that is, there is no evidence of a systemic disorder that, in addition to causing glomerular injury, is injuring other organs as well. Generally, the primary glomerulopathies are idiopathic. The most common forms of primary glomerulopathy are minimal change disease, idiopathic membranous glomerulonephritis, and idiopathic focal glomerulosclerosis.

The Secondary Glomerulopathies

In this category of glomerulopathy, the glomerular injury is a manifestation of a systemic disorder that is causing, or has caused, injury to multiple organs including the kidney. The most common forms of secondary glomerulopathy are those caused by diabetes, systemic lupus erythematosus (SLE), primary or secondary amyloidosis, acute or chronic infections, or immune-mediated systemic vasculitis.

The classification of the glomerulopathies as primary and secondary glomerulopathies is, in many respects, arbitrary and unsatisfactory. Each of the histologic patterns seen in the primary glomerulopathies can also be seen in the secondary glomerulopathies. For example, membranous glomerulonephritis can be seen in SLE, focal glomerulosclerosis can be seen in human immunodeficiency virus (HIV) nephropathy, and membranoproliferative glomerulonephritis can be seen in chronic infections. Nevertheless, the classification of glomerulopathies as primary or secondary is a useful organizing principle for teaching purposes.

The remainder of this article deals with the primary glomerulopathies.

NEPHROTIC SYNDROME

This condition is present when the process affecting the glomerulus results in a marked increase in urine protein excretion, particularly albumin. Because virtually any of the glomerulopathies can cause nephrotic syndrome, a classification of glomerulopathies according to whether nephrotic syndrome is present is of limited usefulness. Nevertheless, a diagnosis of nephrotic syndrome, regardless of the nature of the glomerulopathy that is causing the nephrotic syndrome, has important implications.

There are numerous clinical definitions of the nephrotic syndrome. Some of these definitions (and their limitations) are as follows:

1. In the adult, 24-hour protein excretion of more than 3.5 grams per 24 hours in which the bulk of the urine protein is albumin.

Critique: The weakness in this widely accepted definition of nephrotic syndrome is that it does not take into account the size of the patient or the extent to which the plasma albumin concentration contributes to proteinuria. For example, a patient with a 24-hour urine protein excretion of 3.5 grams and a serum albumin level of 1.0 grams per dL has a much greater increase in glomerular capillary permeability to albumin than a patient with a 24-hour protein excretion of 3.5 grams and a serum albumin level of 3.0 grams per dL.

2. Proteinuria of greater than 3.5 grams per 24 hours, hypoalbuminemia, hyperlipidemia, and edema.

Critique: This too is a widely accepted definition. The flaw in this definition is that the presence of hyperlipidemia and edema may have little or nothing to do with the severity of the glomerular process that leads to heavy proteinuria. For example, the presence or absence of edema depends upon the patient's salt intake, extent of venous or lymphatic disease of the lower extremities, and the prevailing posture, e.g., a waitress who is on her feet all day versus a bedridden patient. Similarly, the extent to which the patient is hypoalbuminemic depends not only on the degree of glomerular capillary permeability but also on the patient's nutritional status and ability of the liver to synthesize albumin.

3. A "spot" urine protein/urine creatinine ratio exceeding 3.0.

Critique: This, too, is a reasonable definition of the nephrotic syndrome. The advantage of this definition is that it does not require a 24-hour urine collection. To translate this estimate of proteinuria to the 24-hour rate of proteinuria, the ratio is multiplied by the expected amount of creatinine in a 24-hour urine sample. For example, in a 70-kg person (who excretes 1400 mg of creatinine in the urine per 24 hours) a urine protein/urine creatinine ratio of 3.0 corresponds to 4.2 grams of protein per 24 hours. The use of "spot" urine to estimate 24-hour urine protein excretion has been shown to be accurate and is particularly useful in pediatric populations in which collection of 24-hour urine samples may be difficult. The shortcomings of this definition are the same as those of Definitions 1 and 2.

4. Twenty-four hour urine protein excretion exceeding 50 mg per kg body weight.

Critique: This is a reasonably good definition that adjusts for body size but, like Definition 1, does not take into account the patient's serum albumin level.

5. Albumin clearance of greater than 150 mL per 24 hours.

Critique: This is the most rigorous of the clinically available definitions of nephrotic syndrome, particularly if this value is adjusted for glomerular filtration rate (GFR) (creatinine clearance). Albumin clearance is the amount of *protein* excreted per 24 hours divided by the serum *albumin* level. This ratio can also be divided by the GFR (creatinine clearance) expressed per 1.73 M^2. An albumin clearance of 150 mL per 24 hours corresponds to 4.5 grams of proteinuria per 24 hours in a patient with a serum albumin level of 3.0 grams per dL.

Complications

The principal complications of nephrotic syndrome are as follows:

Protein Malnutrition. In patients with massively increased glomerular capillary permeability, urine protein excretion rates of 20 grams per 24 hours or more can be seen. The loss of protein actually exceeds that of the proteinuria, because a substantial fraction of the filtered proteins are absorbed and catabolized by the renal tubules. In patients with poor nutrition, the proteinuria of massive nephrotic syndrome can rapidly lead to severe protein malnutrition.

Predisposition to Infection. In patients with severe nephrotic syndrome, it is common to see profound hypogammaglobulinemia as a result of massive losses of IgG in the urine. Such patients may be susceptible to infections, particularly with encapsulated organisms (e.g., *Streptococcus, Haemophilus, Klebsiella*). In addition, the protein malnutrition of nephrotic syndrome may predispose to infection because of a generalized suppression of immunity.

Predisposition to Arterial and Venous Thromboses. This is a particular problem in patients with nonselective proteinuria (e.g., membranous glomerulonephritis, amyloidosis, focal glomerulosclerosis). Interestingly, diabetic glomerulosclerosis is rarely associated with renal vein thrombosis. Renal vein thrombosis should be suspected in nephrotic patients who

1. Have severe nephrotic syndrome (serum albumin <2 grams per dL and 24-hour proteinuria >10 grams) and have a glomerulopathy that is known to be nonselective (e.g., membranous nephritis). In such patients an empirical search for renal vein thrombosis is justified.
2. Develop the sudden onset of flank pain or the acute onset of a varicocele of the left testicle (the result of occlusion of the gonadal vein, which empties into the midportion of the left renal vein).
3. Develop an unexplained increase in serum creatinine, proteinuria, or both.
4. Have large and/or asymmetrical kidneys (kidney size increases with renal vein thrombosis).

A renal vein angiogram is the gold standard for diagnosis of renal vein thrombosis. More recently magnetic resonance imaging (MRI) (very expensive) and Doppler flow ultrasound have also been used with success.

Thrombi in the renal vein are thought to emanate from thrombi formed in the postglomerular circulation, which then propagate outward into the renal vein until the renal vein is completely occluded. Although renal vein thrombosis is the type most commonly associated with nephrotic syndrome, other forms of thrombosis, including deep venous thrombosis in the legs and pelvis, can occur. Thromboembolism is an uncommon but well-recognized complication of the venous thrombosis associated with the nephrotic syndrome. Arterial thromboses also appear to occur more frequently in patients with nephrotic syndrome. These arterial thromboses can take such forms as myocardial infarction, stroke, or bowel infarction.

The mechanism of the thrombotic state in nephrotic syndrome includes the loss of antithrombin III in the urine and increased aggregation of platelets (which may be the result of loss in the urine of a factor that stabilizes platelets). In the great majority of nephrotic patients with thrombosis, an identifiable mechanism for the thrombosis is *not* present. If antithrombin III levels are low, patients may respond poorly or not at all to heparin therapy.

Hyperlipidemia. Severe nephrotic syndrome is commonly complicated by an increase in total cholesterol and triglycerides. When blood lipids are fractionated, there are marked increases in very-low-density and low-density lipoproteins, but decreases in high-density lipoprotein cholesterol. It is now widely believed that hyperlipidemia of chronic nephrotic syndrome accelerates the development of atherosclerosis.

The mechanism of the hyperlipidemia of nephrotic syndrome appears to be the result of reduced plasma oncotic pressure and/or increased loss of a regulator of lipoprotein synthesis in urine. These factor(s) result in increased hepatic production of plasma lipids. There also appears to be decreased peripheral utilization of lipoproteins in patients with the nephrotic syndrome. Some of the plasma lipids may undergo filtration at the glomerulus and become oval fat bodies or fatty casts in the urine sediment.

Edema. Edema in the nephrotic syndrome is the result of the hypoalbuminemia. Edematous patients with nephrotic syndrome generally have serum albumin levels of less than 3 grams per dL, although this is quite variable depending upon the patient's salt intake, the presence or absence of lymphatic or venous disease of the lower extremities, and the patient's dominant posture (sitting versus supine).

In some nephrotic patients, sodium and water retention can be explained by the reduction in intravascular volume that occurs when plasma oncotic pressure is decreased. However, there is good evidence that in many forms of the nephrotic syndrome, sodium retention is a direct intrarenal event related to the hypoalbuminemia. For example, it has been suggested that a high filtration fraction associated with hypoalbuminemia can lead to enhanced salt and water reabsorption by the nephron. Children with minimal change nephrotic syndrome tend to have high renin levels associated with their edema, suggesting that renal sodium retention is the result of contraction in intravascular volume caused by the hypoalbuminemia. On the other hand, adults with membranous nephropathy or focal glomerulosclerosis tend to have normal to low renin levels. In these patients, it may be that intrarenal mechanisms are more important in the sodium retention.

Renal Tubular Dysfunction. Patients with severe nephrotic syndrome commonly have renal glycosuria as well as evidence of generalized proximal tubular defects, such as hyperphosphaturia, amino aciduria, and bicarbonate wasting.

Risk Factors for Progressive Loss of GFR. Recent large-scale clinical trials indicate that in a wide variety of glomerulopathies, the greater the proteinuria, the greater the likelihood that the patient will experience progressive loss of renal function. Although the mechanism is not clear, there is much evidence that certain components of the filtered proteins are nephrotoxic.

Management

Edema

Generally, moderate edema is of cosmetic significance only. The exception is the patient who has underlying heart disease, in whom the accumulation of edema during the day may lead to its resorption at night and the development of nocturnal pulmonary edema. Edema can also be harmful in patients in whom it is so severe that breakdown of the skin over the lower extremities occurs. This can rapidly lead to severe cellulitis of the lower extremities.

When it is necessary to reduce edema in patients with the nephrotic syndrome, the following steps are recommended:

1. *Reduce sodium chloride intake.* To assess the patient's dietary salt intake, it is recommended that 24-hour urine creatinine and sodium be measured periodically. In patients with problematic edema, 24-hour urine sodium excretion should be no more than 100 to 120 mEq per 24 hours, measured under conditions in which a steady state is present as documented by a stable body weight. Reduced salt intake can be most easily managed by having the patient follow a low-salt diet, e.g., 2.0 grams Na (88 mEq) per 24 hours. Patients are allowed to add surface salt to their food: salt added to the surface of food gives a much more salty taste than salt mixed with food. Sodium chloride 1 gram (about ¼ tsp) is equivalent to approximately 17 mEq of sodium. This amount of salt can be added to a salt shaker to provide the daily allotment of added salt. The commonly used salt packets also contain about 1 gram of NaCl.

2. *Administer diuretics.* Generally, furosemide (Lasix), in doses of 40 to 120 mg daily, is sufficient to control edema. If more intensive diuretic therapy is needed, metolazone (Zaroxolyn), 2.5 to 20 mg daily in association with furosemide (40 to 400 mg daily), both given twice daily, is usually effective in controlling the edema of the nephrotic syndrome. Avoid giving diuretics after 5 P.M. to avoid excessive nocturia and loss of sleep.

Development of metabolic alkalosis suggests that the patient has become volume depleted as a result of excessive diuretic therapy. In such patients, it is generally not advisable to add acetazolamide (Diamox) to induce further diuresis and to correct the metabolic alkalosis because this can result in a dangerous reduction in intravascular volume with fall in blood pressure, decline in renal function, and worsening of hypokalemia. Instead, the loop and thiazide diuretics should be decreased.

The addition of spironolactone (Aldactone), 100 to 200 mg daily in a single or divided dose, is also useful in inducing diuresis in nephrotic patients, particularly those who have become hypokalemic from loop and thiazide diuretics.

3. *Reduce protein intake.* A high protein intake can actually worsen the edema of nephrotic syndrome by causing renal vasodilatation, which results in increased proteinuria and decreased serum albumin.

Generally, a dietary protein intake of about 0.8 grams per kg per day is appropriate in patients with the nephrotic syndrome. Estimation of dietary protein intake from urinary urea nitrogen excretion can be done according to the protocol shown in Table 1.

4. *Control hypertension, particularly with antihypertensive agents that may be especially effective in reducing proteinuria.* Hypertension worsens proteinuria in patients with the nephrotic syndrome. Angiotensin-converting enzyme (ACE) inhibitors and first- and second-generation calcium channel blockers (e.g., verapamil and diltiazem) are more effective than other antihypertensive agents in reducing proteinuria. However, in patients with severe proteinuria, these agents are less effective. Perhaps the most important consideration in the management of hypertension in the nephrotic patient is not whether ACE inhibitors or first-generation calcium channel blockers are used, but rather whether blood pressure is well controlled. The National Institutes of Health Modification of Diet in Renal Disease (MDRD) Study has shown that maintaining a blood pressure of 125/75 mmHg is superior to a blood pressure of 135/85 mmHg in slowing progression of glomerulopathies.

Thrombotic Disorders

The thrombotic tendency persists as long as severe nephrotic syndrome persists. Thus, it is not uncommon for patients with renal vein thrombosis to require coumadin therapy for several years. Thrombolytic therapy with streptokinase* or urokinase* can be considered in patients with *acute* onset of serious thrombotic disease, e.g., acute onset of renal vein thrombosis. The addition of low-dose aspirin (e.g., baby aspirin or one-fourth of an adult aspirin daily) is a logical step in the management of the thrombotic tendencies of nephrotic syndrome.

Hyperlipidemia

Dietary control of the hyperlipidemia of nephrotic syndrome is usually ineffective, but it should be tried nonetheless. Usually, it is necessary to use an hMG Co A reductase inhibitor such as lovastatin (Mevacor) in patients with severe hyperlipidemia. Cholestyramine to sequester cholesterol in stool can also be an effective adjunctive therapy.

*Not FDA approved for this indication.

TABLE 1. **Calculation of Dietary Protein Intake from the Measurement of Urinary Urea Nitrogen Excretion**

Dietary protein intake (in grams) for the previous 24 h

$$= \left[(UUN)_{24UC} + [0.031 \times \text{body weight (in kg)}] \right] \times 6.25$$

where

$(UUN)_{24UC}$ = urinary urea nitrogen excretion in grams as measured in a 24-h urine

0.031 = gm of fecal nitrogen + urinary nonurea nitrogen/kg body weight/day

6.25 = gm of protein/gm of nitrogen in protein

Sample calculation:

A 70-kg person provides you with a 24-h urine containing 8 gm of urea nitrogen. That patient's dietary protein intake over the previous 24 h is calculated as follows:

$$\text{Dietary protein intake (in grams)} = \left[(8 + (0.031 \times 70) \right] \times 6.25$$

which = 63.6 gm

MINIMAL CHANGE DISEASE (LIPOID NEPHROSIS, NIL DISEASE)

Clinical Presentation

The onset of edema may be sudden and preceded by a viral upper respiratory tract infection (unusual) or some other antigenic exposure such as in allergy or immunization (rare). Renal function tends to be normal. Plasma renin levels are generally elevated because of decreased intravascular volume. Despite the decrease in intravascular volume, blood pressure may be mildly elevated. Some patients develop acute renal failure with severe exacerbation of the minimal change nephrotic syndrome. The mechanism is not clear; however, it appears *not* to be related simply to decreased intravascular volume.

The urine sediment shows the typical nephrotic changes: oval fat bodies, fatty casts, many hyaline casts. In addition, microscopic hematuria and even red cell cast formation can be seen in patients with steroid-responsive nephrotic syndrome. Gross hematuria is not a manifestation of minimal change nephrotic syndrome. In patients with severe nephrotic syndrome, IgG and IgA levels can be profoundly decreased, predisposing to infection, particularly with encapsulated organisms. Immunoglobulin infusion is of little value in preventing infection because the immunoglobulins are rapidly lost in the urine. However, in patients with active severe infections, immunoglobulin infusion* may be of value.

Diagnosis

The diagnosis of minimal change nephrotic syndrome requires renal biopsy: there is no combination of clinical findings that absolutely includes or excludes the diagnosis. Nevertheless, renal biopsy is generally not indicated in children who present with idiopathic nephrotic syndrome. The reasoning for not performing renal biopsy in pediatric patients who *present* with idiopathic nephrotic syndrome is that the prevalence of lipoid nephrosis is high (85%), and if minimal change nephrotic syndrome is present, the diagnosis can be virtually confirmed by a dramatic response to a course of prednisone therapy. Many pediatric nephrologists will consider renal biopsy in children with idiopathic nephrotic syndrome, but only if their nephrotic syndrome is resistant to the usual course of steroid therapy.

In adults with idiopathic nephrotic syndrome, some centers first provide an empirical course of prednisone therapy, and only if it is ineffective is renal biopsy performed. Other centers, such as ours, proceed

*Not FDA approved for this indication.

directly to renal biopsy in adults with idiopathic nephrotic syndrome. Our reasoning is that the renal biopsy is safe (especially with the newer approaches to imaging of the kidney for biopsy and the use of automated biopsy needles) and usually yields a definitive diagnosis. Furthermore, the informational content of the biopsy is great with respect to selecting therapy and assigning prognosis. Examples are as follows:

1. The finding of membranous nephropathy on renal biopsy mandates a search for an underlying cancer. In about half of the cancer-related membranous nephropathies (1 to 5% of all membranous nephropathy cases), the cancer is not clinically evident when the patient presents with nephrotic syndrome.
2. In our program, patients who experience relapse of the nephrotic syndrome after an initial favorable response to prednisone are more likely to receive a course of cyclophosphamide (Cytoxan) for the relapse if renal biopsy shows focal glomerulosclerosis (FGS) rather than minimal change disease. Our reasoning is that the presence of FGS is evidence that the process is capable of inducing glomerular sclerosis. For this reason we intervene sooner with cyclophosphamide (or other cytotoxic therapy) in such patients.
3. Unexpected and highly relevant findings are sometimes present on renal biopsy. Examples are amyloidosis (primary or secondary), fibrillary glomerulonephritis, light chain glomerulopathy, and allergic interstitial nephritis.
4. Type I membranoproliferative glomerulonephritis associated with hepatitis C may be present. Such patients will not benefit from an empirical course of prednisone therapy.

In light of these considerations, a strong argument can be made for renal biopsy at initial presentation in adults with idiopathic nephrotic syndrome who do not have contraindications to renal biopsy. A single caveat is that if the nephrotic syndrome occurred during regular use of nonsteroidal anti-inflammatory drugs (NSAIDs), they should be stopped for at least 2 weeks to determine if the nephrotic-range proteinuria declines. A rapid decline in proteinuria after cessation of an NSAID suggests that the drug was responsible for the proteinuria.

Management

In recent years, a reasonably coherent picture has emerged regarding appropriate use of prednisone, cyclophosphamide,* and chlorambucil* in the management of minimal change nephrotic syndrome. Based on accumulated experience, the following general principles of management apply:

1. *Treatment of the initial episode of nephrotic syndrome should last approximately 12 weeks.* Shorter periods of treatment make relapse more likely. For children, the recommended dose of prednisone is 60 mg per M^2 per day for 6 weeks (maximum dose, 80 mg daily), followed immediately by a switch to alternate-day prednisone at 40 mg per M^2 *every other day* (maximum of 60 mg per kg qod) for a total of 6 more weeks (total of 12 weeks of prednisone therapy). The prednisone is then abruptly stopped.

In adults, this amount of prednisone is probably more than is necessary. A more appropriate dose for adults with minimal change nephrotic syndrome is as follows:

Prednisone, 1 mg per kg of ideal body weight daily (maximum of 80 mg daily) for 2 weeks, then,
prednisone, 40 mg daily for 2 weeks, then,
switch to qod prednisone, 40 mg qod for 6 weeks, then,
prednisone, 20 mg qod for 2 weeks, then stop.

In patients who are obese and/or diabetic, less prednisone may be given or alternate-day prednisone therapy can be used for the entire course. A typical regimen is 80 to 120 mg of prednisone *every other day* for the first 2 to 4 weeks, then taper until 12 weeks of treatment has been given.

In patients who have neuropsychiatric disturbances with the high dose of prednisone (e.g., nervousness, sleeplessness), administration in divided doses can alleviate those symptoms. It should be recognized, however, that giving the prednisone in divided doses increases its immunosuppressive effects and other side effects (e.g., increased appetite).

2. *Relapses do not need to be treated as aggressively as the initial episode.* In children, prednisone 60 mg per M^2 per day (not to exceed 80 mg daily) can be given until the urine is protein free for a period of 3 days (as assessed by dipstick testing for proteinuria). Prednisone is then switched to 40 mg qod for 4 weeks, then stopped.

For adults, less prednisone is usually effective. For example, 40 mg daily until the urine is protein free for 3 days, followed by an abrupt switch to alternate-day prednisone, which is tapered over 4 weeks (for example, prednisone 30 mg qod for 2 weeks, then prednisone 20 mg qod for 2 weeks, then stop).

Over 90% of patients with minimal change nephrotic syndrome will become protein free within 8 weeks of therapy, and the great majority of patients will be protein free within 14 days of therapy. Adults may respond more slowly to prednisone and may require more than 12 weeks of therapy before complete remission is achieved.

About two-thirds of patients with minimal change nephrotic syndrome will relapse within 6 months of the initial treatment. Approximately 20% of such patients (15% of total) will experience infrequent relapses (<1 per yr), and approximately 40% (30% of total) will experience frequent relapses (>1 per yr).

3. In patients with frequent relapses, a course of cyclophosphamide*, 1.5 to 2.0 mg per kg per day for 8 weeks, or chlorambucil, 0.15 mg per kg per day for 8 weeks, may be advisable. Long-term remission following cytotoxic therapy is more likely to be achieved

*Not FDA approved for this indication.

*Not FDA approved for this indication.

if patients are in steroid-induced remission at the time the cytotoxic drugs are used.

4. In patients with steroid-dependent minimal change nephrotic syndrome (i.e., prednisone therapy cannot be stopped without causing relapse), a 12-week course of cyclophosphamide or chlorambucil is recommended.

In general, no more than two courses of cyclophosphamide or chlorambucil are recommended in patients with steroid-dependent minimal change nephrotic syndrome.

5. In children who develop frequent relapsing minimal change nephrotic syndrome and/or steroid-dependent nephrotic syndrome after cytotoxic therapy, some pediatricians recommend a 6- to 12-month course of cyclosporine* at 100 to 150 mg per M^2 per day. Such treatment should be regarded as experimental and not without hazard, particularly in light of the nephrotoxicity of cyclosporine.

6. In patients with steroid-resistant minimal change disease, there is increasing interest in the use of prolonged alternate-day moderate-dose prednisone or azathioprine* (Imuran) therapy (see further on).

IDIOPATHIC FOCAL GLOMERULOSCLEROSIS (FGS), [FOCAL SEGMENTAL GLOMERULOSCLEROSIS (FSG), FOCAL AND SEGMENTAL GLOMERULOSCLEROSIS (FSGS)]

In the context of a renal biopsy, a focal process is one that involves some glomeruli but not others; a segmental process is one that involves only a portion of the glomerulus. The term *focal glomerulosclerosis* (FGS), used to describe renal biopsy findings, is a nonspecific descriptor. FGS can also be seen in Alport's syndrome, reflux nephropathy, heroin abuse, HIV nephropathy, and other conditions. However, when FGS is seen in a patient with idiopathic nephrotic syndrome, it is now widely believed that this constitutes a distinct form of glomerulopathy about which a great deal is known concerning the natural history and response to treatment. Some, including myself, believe that idiopathic FGS is a more aggressive form of minimal change disease, which is thought to be a disorder of T lymphocytes.

Clinical Presentation

Nephrotic syndrome is the principal clinical manifestation. Progressive disease can be seen in adults with only moderate proteinuria (e.g., 2 grams per 24 hours). Urinary red cell cast formation and gross hematuria are well-described but unusual manifestations of idiopathic FGS. Renal biopsy is required for diagnosis. There is no combination of clinical findings that can conclusively include or exclude the diagnosis of idiopathic FGS.

*Not FDA approved for this indication.

Management

In patients with normal renal function (normal serum creatinine level) a course of prednisone similar to that used in minimal change disease should be undertaken. In adults, approximately 30% of patients with FGS can be expected to respond to prednisone therapy. If the patient becomes protein free on prednisone therapy, a good prognosis can be inferred.

In idiopathic FGS with impaired kidney function (e.g., serum creatinine >2.5 mg per dL) and renal biopsy evidence of extensive glomerulosclerosis, response to prednisone is unlikely. (Such patients should probably not undertake a course of prednisone therapy.)

Several studies have examined the effects of adding cytotoxic drugs (in particular, chlorambucil* or cyclophosphamide*) to steroid therapy in the management of idiopathic FGS, but no clear picture has emerged. It is our impression, however, that an 8- to 12-week course of cyclophosphamide (see later in this section) along with prednisone therapy may favorably influence the course of idiopathic FGS in many patients.

A controlled prospective multicenter trial is currently examining the effect of cyclosporine* in steroid-resistant idiopathic FGS. This North American Nephrotic Syndrome (NANS) Study is not slated for completion for at least 2 years.

Mendoza† has suggested the use of long-term high-dose alternate-day prednisone in children with steroid-resistant FGS. Usually, the high-dose alternate-day prednisone is preceded by pulse methylprednisolone (30 mg per kg qod for 2 weeks, maximum dose 1 gram) plus cyclophosphamide* (2 mg per kg for 8 weeks). Long-term oral prednisone therapy consists of 2.0 mg per kg qod (maximum 80 mg qod) for 18 months. In children, a 60% complete remission rate was noted by the end of the course of prednisone therapy.

As discussed previously, control of blood pressure and blood cholesterol level and avoidance of a high protein intake may be important in slowing progression of FGS. Patients with heavy proteinuria are more likely to progress than those with mild proteinuria (<1 gram per 24 hours), but spontaneous remission of FGS can occur, even in patients with heavy proteinuria.

FGS recurs in 20 to 30% of renal allografts. In at least one-third of such patients, recurrence leads to accelerated graft loss. FGS may be more likely to recur when a living related donor is used rather than a cadaveric donor. Use of cyclosporine does not prevent recurrence of idiopathic FGS in allografts. Patients with severe FGS that rapidly leads to end-stage kidney failure are more likely to have recurrence of the FGS in the renal graft than patients with more mild FGS that progresses more slowly to end-stage kidney failure.

*Not FDA approved for this indication.
†Clin Neph 35, Suppl 1, 8–15, 1991.

IDIOPATHIC MEMBRANOUS GLOMERULOPATHY (MEMBRANOUS GLOMERULONEPHRITIS, MEMBRANOUS NEPHROPATHY)

Clinical Presentation

Proteinuria usually develops insidiously; however, there are some patients in whom the onset of edema is explosive, suggesting a recent rapid worsening of proteinuria. Microscopic hematuria is seen in the majority of patients, but gross hematuria is not a part of idiopathic membranous nephropathy *unless* the patient develops renal vein thrombosis causing renal infarction (a rare phenomenon). C3 and C4 levels are normal in idiopathic membranous nephropathy; if low values for C3 and C4 are seen, SLE should be suspected. Renal biopsy is necessary for diagnosis. There is no combination of laboratory studies that can definitively include or exclude the diagnosis of idiopathic membranous nephropathy.

Management

Idiopathic membranous nephropathy is usually an indolent disorder with a high rate of spontaneous remission (20 to 40%). In as many as 10% of cases, there may be spontaneous exacerbations and remissions of the disease that resemble those seen in minimal change nephrotic syndrome. In some patients, idiopathic membranous nephropathy has an aggressive course with end-stage kidney failure occurring within 5 to 10 years of onset.

Because of the variable course, there is considerable controversy as to the appropriate therapy for membranous nephropathy. Some centers recommend no therapy. However, in patients who have an increased likelihood of progressive disease (males over age 50 with severe proteinuria [>10 grams per day], hypertension, and elevated serum creatinine), therapy is generally recommended. Several recent meta-analyses of previously reported clinical trials demonstrate that therapy, particularly with cyclophosphamide* or chlorambucil,* is effective in inducing remission of nephrotic syndrome and stabilizing or improving renal function. Our own considerable experience strongly supports the beneficial effect of immunosuppressive therapy in idiopathic membranous nephropathy.

When a decision is made to treat membranous nephropathy, it is appropriate to begin with high-dose, alternate-day prednisone, as described in the Adult Nephrotic Syndrome Study.† This form of therapy is particularly appropriate for those who have little or no elevation in serum creatinine level. Treatment consists of prednisone, 120 mg qod for 8 weeks and then tapered over 3 months. In the controlled trial, the principal outcome was that the patients who received prednisone were less likely to have diminished renal function, compared to the patients who received placebo. The prednisone therapy appeared to be benign as shown by a similar profile of side effects in the placebo group.

*Not FDA approved for this indication.
†N Engl J Med 301:1301, 1979.

If patients do not respond to prednisone and appear to be at risk for developing progressive renal failure (on the basis of heavy proteinuria, male sex, hypertension, and elevated serum creatinine level), a strong argument can be made for using cytotoxic therapy as reported by Ponticelli*: methylprednisolone, 1 gram intravenously on 3 consecutive days, then oral methylprednisolone, 0.4 mg per kg per day for 1 month. The glucocorticoid is discontinued, then chlorambucil* (Leukeran), 0.2 mg per kg per day is given for the second month. This cycle—a month of prednisone and a month of chlorambucil—is continued for a total of 6 months of therapy (3 months of prednisone and 3 months of chlorambucil). Such therapy can control the nephrotic syndrome and even partially reverse the impaired kidney function of membranous nephropathy. In our experience with the Ponticelli protocol, it was not necessary for a successful outcome to use the intravenous glucocorticoids to initiate the protocol. In addition, we have found it useful to include a moderate dose of prednisone (e.g., 10 to 20 mg daily) during the cycle of chlorambucil therapy in order to avoid leukopenia.

Low-dose aspirin therapy (e.g., ½ or a full baby aspirin or ¼ of an adult aspirin daily) seems appropriate in patients with membranous nephropathy because of their tendency to experience arterial and venous thromboses.

Cyclosporine therapy† of idiopathic membranous nephropathy is undergoing trial in the NANS Study. Uncontrolled experiences suggest that it may be effective.

Idiopathic membranous nephropathy can recur in renal transplants; however, this is unusual and generally does not result in accelerated loss of graft function.

IDIOPATHIC MEMBRANOPROLIFERATIVE GLOMERULONEPHRITIS (MPGN), (MESANGIAL CAPILLARY GLOMERULONEPHRITIS, HYPOCOMPLEMENTEMIC GLOMERULONEPHRITIS, LOBULAR GLOMERULONEPHRITIS)

There are two main forms of idiopathic MPGN, Type I and Type II. These glomerulopathies are considered together because of similarities in the renal biopsy findings by light microscopy. However, pathophysiologically, these are separate diseases as shown by the immunofluorescent and electron microscopy findings.

Clinical Presentation

Most patients present with the nephrotic syndrome. Microscopic hematuria is almost universally

*N Engl J Med 320:8, 1989.
†Not FDA approved for this indication.

present, and some patients have one or more bouts of gross hematuria. Twenty percent of patients present with an acute nephrotic syndrome; it is more common in Type II disease, and an upper respiratory tract infection may precede its onset. Partial lipodystrophy can be seen in Type II MPGN.

Low C3 is common in both Type I and Type II MPGN. The low C3 levels in Type I MPGN appear to be the result of both classical pathway activation (C4 is also low) and alternative pathway activation by C3 nephritic factor. In Type II MPGN, low C3 is primarily a result of alternative complement pathway activation by a C3 nephritic factor. C4 tends to be normal in Type II MPGN. C3 levels can fluctuate without any change in the clinical status of the patients. The lowest C3 levels are seen in Type II MPGN. C3 nephritic factor is found in over 60% of patients with Type II MPGN and in about 20% of patients with Type I MPGN. C3 nephritic factor is not diagnostic of MPGN; it can be seen in other forms of glomerulonephritis. Anemia out of proportion to the level of renal functional impairment is frequent in these disorders, and platelet turnover is also increased; the clinical significance of these findings is not clear. Although a renal biopsy is required for diagnosis, the combination of nephritic syndrome, low C3 and normal C4 levels, and C3 nephritic factor is highly suggestive of MPGN Type I or II.

Hepatitis C infection, with or without cryoglobulins, has been implicated in the pathogenesis of Type I MPGN.

Management

Patients with Type I MPGN and persistent nephrotic syndrome have a poor prognosis: 60% progress to kidney failure within 10 years. By contrast, only 15% of patients with no evidence of nephrotic syndrome at biopsy progress to kidney failure in 10 years. Spontaneous remissions occur occasionally. The prognosis in children and adults is approximately the same.

In children, long-term (1 year or more) moderate-dose alternate-day prednisone has been associated with stabilization of renal function and remission of nephrotic syndrome in many patients. However, these studies are uncontrolled. A controlled trial did not confirm a favorable effect of long-term alternate-day prednisone; however, blood pressure control was not adequate in that study.

A large controlled trial of prednisone combined with cyclophosphamide* in adults with Type I MPGN showed no benefit from the treatment. Aspirin and dipyridamole* (Persantine) therapy, although initially encouraging, has not proven to be effective in long-term follow-up. Recent evidence suggests that Type I MPGN associated with hepatitis C may benefit from recombinant interferon-alpha.

*Not FDA approved for this indication.

IDIOPATHIC RAPIDLY PROGRESSIVE GLOMERULONEPHRITIS (RPGN), (IDIOPATHIC CRESCENTIC GLOMERULONEPHRITIS TYPE I, II, OR III)

Glomerular crescents can complicate almost any form of glomerulopathy, even noninflammatory glomerulopathy such as diabetic glomerulosclerosis or membranous nephropathy. However, in these forms, the crescents tend to be fibrotic rather than cellular. Active inflammatory glomerulopathies complicated by crescent formation have *cellular* crescents, indicating an active process that has not yet gone on to scarring. The mechanism of crescent formation is thought to be a marked increase in glomerular capillary permeability leading to filtration of growth factors and inflammatory factors, including fibrinogen. This leads to fibrin deposition in Bowman's space, and proliferation of the epithelium of Bowman's capsule. In addition, Bowman's capsule may rupture, allowing ingress of interstitial macrophages, which contribute to the cellularity of crescent formation. Glassock has classified idiopathic crescentic glomerulonephritis as Type I (anti-glomerular basement membrane disease, without lung hemorrhage), Type II (immune complex–mediated disease), and Type III ("pauci-immune" glomerulonephritis in which few or no deposits are seen on immunofluorescence or electron microscopy). Type III is by far the most common form of idiopathic RPGN. Anti-neutrophil cytoplasmic antigen (typically perinuclear ANCA) is seen in many cases of Type III immune RPGN. Renal biopsy is required for diagnosis.

Clinical Presentation

These forms of idiopathic primary glomerulopathy probably represent limited forms of a systemic disease. For example, Type I RPGN probably represents a limited form of Goodpasture's syndrome; Type II, a limited form of a systemic immune complex–mediated vasculitis; and Type III RPGN, a limited form of Wegener's granulomatosis. Indeed, Type III RPGN patients frequently have p-ANCA. These patients commonly present with prodromic arthralgias, fever, malaise, hemoptysis, and abdominal pain.

Usually the urinary sediment findings are indicative of an inflammatory glomerulonephritis showing proteinuria, red cells, and red cell and leukocyte casts. However, it is well established that in some patients with severe crescentic GN, the urinary findings may be minimal, consisting of only a few red cells and minor proteinuria. Thus, absence of an "active" urine sediment does *not* exclude the diagnosis of RPGN.

Characteristically, the proteinuria is modest (2 to 3 grams per 24 hours); however, frank nephrotic syndrome can be seen. Serum C3 and C4 levels are normal in Types I and III RPGN but can be decreased in Type II.

Management

If these patients present with oliguria, the prognosis is usually poor. Nevertheless, if infection can be ruled out as the cause of the RPGN, high-dose immunosuppressive therapy (see following discussion of prednisone/cyclophosphamide therapy) is indicated.

In patients with anti-GBM disease, a course of plasmapheresis (e.g., 3- to 4-liter plasmaphereses, three or four times weekly for 2 weeks) may be of benefit. Monitoring the effect of plasmapheresis and immunosuppressive treatment by serial measurement of anti-GBM antibodies is appropriate.

Anti-GBM glomerulonephritis and the pauci-immune form of glomerulonephritis can recur post-transplant. Treatment with cyclophosphamide* and an intensified course of prednisone is probably appropriate, particularly for the Type III pauci-immune, Wegener's type RPGN.

IGA NEPHRITIS (BERGER'S DISEASE, IGA MESANGIAL NEPHROPATHY, IGA NEPHROPATHY)

Clinical Presentation

In most patients, the disease is indolent, manifesting itself as microscopic hematuria, red cell cast formation, and minor proteinuria. However, in some patients, a malignant course can be pursued with heavy proteinuria, hypertension, and progression to renal failure. In 10 to 20% of patients, gross hematuria occurs 24 to 48 hours after onset of a respiratory or gastrointestinal infection. The prognosis is generally good for these patients. Acute renal failure with exacerbations of IgA nephritis (e.g., after upper respiratory infection) can occur with recovery of renal function.

As a group, patients with IgA nephritis have a reasonably benign prognosis. One estimate is that approximately 20% will have impaired kidney function (including end-stage kidney failure) within 20 years. Familial forms of IgA nephritis have been documented; a renal biopsy is required for diagnosis. However, most patients with IgA nephritis do not undergo renal biopsy because, although the presence of glomerulonephritis will be evident from the urinary findings, the fact that they have no evidence of a systemic disorder and have normal renal function and minimal proteinuria, generally makes renal biopsy unnecessary.

Management

The treatment of IgA nephritis has been disappointing. Therapy that appears ineffective includes long-term phenytoin, short-term prednisone and cyclophosphamide,* danazol,* aspirin plus dipyridamole* (used because of the association of dermatitis herpetiformis with IgA nephropathy), and gluten-restricted diet (used because of the association of IgA nephritis with celiac disease).

Because most patients follow an indolent course, generally aggressive measures that involve immunosuppression are not recommended. However, because stimulation of the mucosal immune system appears to be important in the pathogenesis of IgA nephritis, it seems appropriate to advise patients to avoid upper respiratory tract infections as much as possible (e.g., by frequent handwashing during colds season, wearing masks when other family members have colds), avoidance of foods that produce gastrointestinal upset (this may be a sign of hypersensitivity), and avoidance of excessive alcohol intake (because of the evidence that alcohol may enhance gastrointestinal absorption of certain antigens). Nonspecific measures such as careful control of blood pressure, avoidance of a high-protein intake, and control of blood cholesterol may also be important in the management of patients with IgA nephritis.

ACUTE POSTINFECTIOUS GLOMERULONEPHRITIS

This type of primary glomerulopathy develops 1 to 3 weeks after an acute infection. Immune complex formation or deposition occurs in the kidney, leading to acute glomerulonephritis. Classically, this form of glomerulonephritis is associated with infection with certain strains of group A beta-hemolytic streptococci. However, streptococcal pneumonia and meningococcal infections have also been associated with postinfectious glomerulonephritis (GN).

Clinical Presentation

Postinfectious GN, particularly poststreptococcal glomerulonephritis, is primarily a disease of young people, although it can occur at any age. Indeed, when acute poststreptococcal glomerulonephritis occurs in the elderly, it may present as congestive heart failure due to fluid overload.

Typically there is a latent period between the recognizable streptococcal infection and the first manifestation of the glomerulonephritis. The average latent period is 10 days but intervals of up to 3 weeks have been seen.

Patients often present with gross hematuria, which in acid urine may appear brownish green. Edema and hypertension due to fluid overload are found in about 75% of cases. Congestive heart failure due to fluid overload can occur in patients with acute poststreptococcal glomerulonephritis *without* resulting in severe increases in blood pressure or renal function impairment.

The urinalysis usually shows abundant hematuria and in some instances marked pyuria in the absence of urinary tract infection. Both red cell and leukocyte casts can be seen. Low C3 levels are found in almost all cases, and in some instances, the levels are profoundly low (<30 mg per dL). The C4 level may be normal or slightly decreased. Cryoglobulins repre-

*Not FDA approved for this indication.

senting Type III cryoglobulinemia (polyclonal rheumatoid factors) may be present. The diagnosis of a group A beta-hemolytic streptococcal infection can be made by culture and should be confirmed by a rising ASO titer. Anti-DNase B titers are more sensitive for streptococcal skin infection than are ASO titers.

Generally, a renal biopsy is not necessary to make a diagnosis of acute poststreptococcal glomerulonephritis. Instead, the combination of a documented infection with a group A beta-hemolytic streptococci, a rising ASO titer, low C3 levels, normal C4 levels, and a nephritic picture on urinalysis are usually sufficient to make the diagnosis.

Management

The prognosis in acute poststreptococcal glomerulonephritis (poststrep GN) is generally very good, particularly in children, in whom complete clearing of the glomerulonephritis can be expected. Proteinuria can persist for up to 6 months, and microscopic hematuria for up to 1 year after onset of the GN. However, eventually all urinary findings should disappear, hypertension should subside, and renal function should return to normal.

Adults with post-strep GN may have a poorer prognosis, particularly older adults and those who develop severe impairment of renal function during the episode of acute glomerulonephritis. There is no good evidence that immunosuppressive or anti-inflammatory therapy is of benefit in this disease. Perhaps that is because the disease is inherently self-limited; that is, after the antigen clears from the circulation, the process is destined to wane. Nevertheless, there are reports of patients with severe manifestations of poststrep GN who appear to have benefited from high-dose steroid therapy and other measures, such as cytotoxic drugs and plasmapheresis. Perhaps the strongest argument for drug therapy in acute poststreptococcal glomerulonephritis is for the anti-inflammatory effect of short-term, high-dose prednisone.

PREDNISONE AND IMMUNOSUPPRESSION IN THE MANAGEMENT OF THE GLOMERULOPATHIES

Prednisone

Shown in Table 2 is the prednisone taper schedule that was used in the National Institutes of Health (NIH) multicenter trial of plasmapheresis in severe lupus nephritis.* This degree of prednisone therapy should be reserved for patients with the severest forms of RPGN, SLE, Wegener's granulomatosis, and Goodpasture's syndrome.

High-Dose Prednisone

Rarely should the prednisone dose exceed that shown in Table 2. However, it has become customary

TABLE 2. **High-Dose Prednisone Therapy**

Reference Point	Weeks	Patient <80 kg	Patient >80 kg
A.	1–4	60 mg/day (2 divided doses)	80 mg/day (2 divided doses)
B.	5–6	50 mg (begin single A.M. dose)	70
	7–8	50	60
	9–10	40	50 (single dose)
	11–12	40	40
C.	13–14	30	40
D.	15	30–25 (begin taper alternate day)	40–35
	16	30–20	40–30
	17	30–15	40–25
	18	30–10	40–20
	19	30–5	40–15
	20	30–0	40–10
	21	25–0	40–5
	22	20–0	40–0
	23	20–0	30–0
	23–52	20–0	25–0
	53	20–0	25–0

From Lewis EJ, Hunsicker LG, Lan S-P, et al: A controlled trial of plasmapheresis therapy in severe lupus nephritis. N Engl J Med *326*:1373, 1992.

in many centers to start high-dose prednisone therapy with intravenous glucocorticoids for the first 3 days. For example, in place of the oral prednisone, 1000 mg of prednisolone or 800 mg of methylprednisolone (Solu-Medrol) is given intravenously for each of the first 3 days of therapy.

Whether the short-term use of high-dose intravenous glucocorticoids improves the efficacy of long-term high-dose prednisone is not clear. However, 3 days of the high-dose intravenous glucocorticoid is generally well tolerated. It is likely that such massive doses of intravenous glucocorticoid do *not* increase the *immunosuppressive effect* of glucocorticoids; that is, there is evidence that the maximum immunosuppression from prednisone is achieved at a dose of about 1 mg per kg of ideal body weight.* However, the *anti-inflammatory effects* of glucocorticoids (the ability of glucocorticoids to suppress lysosomal enzyme release from phagocytes, decrease migration and activity of phagocytes, and decreased capillary permeability) may increase with increasing doses of glucocorticoids. Thus, the advantage of short-term high-dose intravenous glucocorticoids may be that their anti-inflammatory effects are maximized. This might be important in patients with acute severe manifestations of RPGN, SLE, Wegener's granulomatosis, or Goodpasture's syndrome. It should be recognized, however, that if such high doses of glucocorticoids are continued for prolonged periods, the fact that the patients are severely immunosuppressed and have severe inhibition of inflammatory mediators makes it more likely that infection will soon supervene. Thus, if high-dose intravenous glucocorticoids are used in adults, they should not be given for 3 consecutive days.

*N Engl J Med *326*:1373, 1992.

*Transplantation *33*:578–585, 1982.

When using prednisone to treat the severest forms of RPGN, SLE, Wegener's granulomatosis, or Goodpasture's syndrome, a cytotoxic drug such as cyclophosphamide* or chlorambucil* should be added, as discussed later.

High-dose prednisone therapy will result in a marked cushingoid appearance (indicating marked steroid effects) and, when combined with a cytotoxic drug, results in an approximately 40% incidence of significant infection in the first 9 weeks of therapy.† Thus, *high-dose* prednisone therapy with cytotoxic therapy should be used only in patients with the most severe manifestations of diseases and with a high degree of surveillance. For example, if patients are being managed as outpatients, they should be seen at 1- to 2-week intervals for the first 8 to 12 weeks of follow-up.

Moderately High-Dose Prednisone

For moderately severe manifestations of RPGN, SLE, Wegener's granulomatosis, or Goodpasture's syndrome, or in older or debilitated patients with severe manifestations of these diseases, it is more appropriate to use moderately high-dose prednisone therapy (with or without cytotoxic agents). Moderately high-dose prednisone therapy is achieved by using the schedule shown in Table 2 but shortening the periods from A to C from 14 weeks to 7 weeks.

General Guidelines for Prednisone Therapy

1. Do not use "stress doses" of prednisone (e.g., 20 mg three times daily) in patients who develop a severe infection and have been receiving adrenal suppressive doses of prednisone (>10 mg daily). In treating the severely infected renal patient who has been receiving prednisone therapy, the first priority is to treat the infection. Our experience is that all signs of significant glucocorticoid insufficiency (hypoglycemia and/or hypotension) can be avoided in adrenal-suppressed patients by doses of prednisone equivalent to 10 to 20 mg daily. If there are concerns about oral absorption in the severely ill patient, the drug can be given intravenously. The use of stress doses of glucocorticoid (e.g., hydrocortisone, 100 mg tid, equivalent to prednisone, 20 mg tid) may severely compromise the effectiveness of the antimicrobial therapy, worsen catabolism, and predispose to new infection and to gastroduodenal ulceration.
2. The biologic effects of prednisone are decreased by at least 50% when it is administered concomitantly with drugs that induce the hepatic p450 system (phenytoin, phenobarbital, carbamazepine, rifampin). Thus, the prednisone dose needs to be at least doubled to maintain therapeutic effectiveness in patients receiving these drugs.
3. Permanently disfiguring striae of the upper arms, abdomen, and thighs can develop within weeks of high-dose steroid therapy, particularly in young patients with severe nephrotic syndrome. Severe edema (or obesity), which stretches the skin, exacerbates striae formation. To minimize striae formation in patients on high-dose steroids, edema and obesity should be controlled as much as possible, and the steroid dose should be tapered as soon as is feasible.
4. Peptic ulcer disease develops in some patients on high-dose steroids. Consider the use of H_2 blockers or antacids, particularly in patients who are debilitated or have a prior history of peptic ulcer disease.
5. Symptomatic hyperglycemia can emerge unexpectedly in patients on high-dose steroids.

*Ann Intern Med *114*:924, 1991.
†Not FDA approved for this indication.

IMMUNOSUPPRESSIVE THERAPY

*Cyclophosphamide** is indicated in patients with the most severe manifestations of RPGN, SLE, Wegener's granulomatosis, and Goodpasture's syndrome. In recent years, there has been considerable interest in the use of intravenous (IV) cyclophosphamide.† Usual doses are 750 mg per M^2 given at 4-week intervals for 6 months. The rationale for intravenous cyclophosphamide is that it may decrease the incidence of bladder cancer and infection. However, the evidence that intravenous cyclophosphamide is safer than oral cyclophosphamide is not firm, and indeed, there are several reports of severe infection following intravenous cyclophosphamide that caused severe, persistent leukopenia. Irreversible cardiomyopathy has also been reported with the use of high-dose intravenous cyclophosphamide. This form of therapy is more expensive than oral cyclophosphamide therapy, and it is probably not as effective in treating immune disorders. Some consider the main indication for intravenous cyclophosphamide to be in patients with gastrointestinal intolerance of oral cyclophosphamide.

To treat the severe manifestations of immune-mediated renal disease, cyclophosphamide can be given orally in doses of 1.5 to 2.0 mg per kg of ideal body weight (maximum 150 mg daily) for a period of 8 to 12 weeks. Cyclophosphamide is given concomitantly with the appropriate dose of prednisone, as discussed previously.

Chlorambucil‡ is used increasingly in place of cyclophosphamide in treating severe manifestations of immune mediated disorders. At present, the published experience with chlorambucil in these disorders is relatively small and does not provide an adequate basis for comparison with cyclophosphamide. However, there are certain advantages to chlorambucil, which include apparent absence of bladder toxicity (cystitis and bladder cancer). In addition, scalp hair loss does not usually follow chlorambucil therapy whereas it usually does follow cyclophosphamide therapy, particularly when given for more than 8 weeks. Chlorambucil may be less potent than cyclophosphamide in inducing immunosuppression. When chlorambucil is used in place of cyclophosphamide,

*Not FDA approved for this indication.
†Quart J Med New Series *81*(296):975, 1991.
‡Not FDA approved for this indication.

generally 1 mg of chlorambucil substitutes for 10 mg of cyclophosphamide.

General Guidelines for Immunosuppressive Therapy

1. Cyclophosphamide is an alkylating agent and its effects are cumulative. Most men and women who are treated with cyclophosphamide in full doses for more than 6 months become sterile, although a few may recover gonadal function. Chlorambucil also causes sterility, although its effects are less well studied.
2. When full-dose cyclophosphamide is given for the equivalent of 1 year or more, there is a measurable increase in the incidence of cancers. Thus, it is important not to give more cyclophosphamide than is actually needed. Chlorambucil is a known carcinogen, but use of cyclophosphamide or chlorambucil in renal patients for 2 to 4 months has not been associated with an increased incidence of cancer.
3. Although cyclophosphamide can cause cystitis and bladder cancer, these are rare occurrences if the entire dose is given in the morning and the patient is advised to approximately double fluid intake at each meal and to take an extra glass of fluid at bedtime (personal unpublished observations).
4. Allopurinol (Zyloprim) therapy prolongs the biologic effects of cyclophosphamide, chlorambucil, and azathioprine.* The dose of these drugs must be decreased by about 50% when allopurinol is used simultaneously.
5. White blood cell counts (WBC) should be measured periodically to avoid leukopenia (neutrophil count <2000/mm^3). In patients receiving cyclophosphamide or chlorambucil, it is useful to measure the WBC at 1- or 2-week intervals during the entire period of therapy. In patients on azathioprine, WBC measurement at 1- or 2-month intervals is usually sufficient because of the lesser tendency for the usual doses of azathioprine to cause leukopenia. If leukopenia develops, reducing the dose of the immunosuppressive drug will correct the leukopenia, usually within 1 to 2 weeks.

Patients who become leukopenic while receiving cyclophosphamide or chlorambucil should discontinue the drug until the neutrophil count is greater than 2000 per mm^3. At that point the drug can be started at one-half to two-thirds of the previous dose. Such an approach usually prevents the development of severe leukopenia.

Patients who become leukopenic while receiving azathioprine can have more gradual reduction in dose because of the lesser tendency for azathioprine to cause severe leukopenia in usual therapeutic doses. For example, in a patient who becomes mildly leukopenic on azathioprine, decreasing the dose by 25% is usually sufficient to avoid progression of the leukopenia.

*Not FDA approved for this indication.

PYELONEPHRITIS

method of
MARK G. MARTENS, M.D.
Emory University School of Medicine
Atlanta, Georgia

Pyelonephritis is an inflammatory response to an infection of the renal parenchyma that is characterized clinically by flank pain, fever, and pyuria. Upon microscopic examination of the urine, an offending organism is usually seen and subsequently cultured.

Pyelonephritis is differentiated from glomerulonephritis on the basis of the former's infectious etiology. Pyelonephritis is classified as hematogenous, intrinsic, or ascending.

INTRINSIC INFECTION

Intrinsic infection is often related to transplantation or other surgical interventions. The clinical syndrome and the organisms responsible are varied owing to the manipulations of the host's immune system following transplant and the extent and route of the surgical intervention. For transplant patients, all bacterial species, even those considered mildly pathogenic, need to be taken seriously if they grow in culture owing to the immunosuppressive medications that transplant patients must take. In addition, nonbacterial species such as fungi are also important, and the presence of yeast on urinalysis should not be considered insignificant. Treatment of bacterial infection should be based on culture and sensitivity reports. The standard treatment for fungal infections remains amphotericin B; however, reports on the efficacy of ketoconazole and, more recently, fluconazole and itraconazole are promising.

Intrinsic surgical infections should have their source determined, and surgical site infections such as abscesses or infected nephrostomy sites or tubes should be débrided and treated with appropriate systemic antimicrobials.

HEMATOGENOUS INFECTION

While ascending infection is most common, pyelonephritis from hematogenous spread is often very serious as it frequently is related to, or can result in, a life-threatening situation. As the site of blood filtration, the kidneys are frequently exposed to pathogenic bacteria, especially in serious disease states such as sepsis. If the patient survives the initial septic insult, bacteria that may have infiltrated the kidney can either proliferate to form an abscess or progress to chronic infection and inflammation, termed *chronic pyelonephritis.* Chronic infection is a major cause of renal failure in the elderly that is often overlooked because of its subtle clinical presentation and the difficulty in making the diagnosis of a persistent infection with noninvasive techniques.

The bacteria involved in hematogenously acquired pyelonephritis can easily be identified by culture of the blood and urine. Treatment should be based on the results of sensitivity testing of the blood and urine isolates. It is imperative that repeat cultures be done after clinical improvement is noted, as a positive follow-up culture in an improved patient signals a persistent infection. A positive urine culture with a negative blood culture may indicate chronic pyelonephritis, and longer term antibiotic therapy may be required to eradicate this soft tissue infection. A positive urine culture with a positive blood culture in a clinically improving patient may signal the formation of a renal abscess and intermittent bacterial seeding of the blood. Confirmation of an abscess can usually be made by ultrasonography, selected x-rays, computed tomography, or, more recently, magnetic resonance imaging. Treatment usually requires long-term (2 to 6 weeks) parenteral antibiotic therapy, with the exact duration determined by the results of the often-needed surgical drainage.

ASCENDING INFECTION

Ascending infection is the most common cause of pyelonephritis. Its etiology is varied, and is more easily understood if considered in relation to age, sex, and clinical condition.

Men

Pyelonephritis in the young adult is rare, especially in males. Its presence in a previously healthy young male may signal the presence of a serious, if not fatal, underlying disease. In the absence of prior surgery, intrinsic and hematogenous sources should be investigated by culture and radiographic techniques. Sometimes renal calculi are noted, and their elimination is necessary if positive cultures persist or obstructive changes are noted.

Ascending infections in the young male are rare in the absence of an obstructive or neurologic condition. In males younger than 45 years of age, a tumor should be aggressively ruled out; the most likely malignancies are renal or bowel cancer. Prostatic cancer is rare in this age group; however, prostatic or epididymal infections are not uncommon and need to be ruled out.

In older men, pyelonephritis may likewise signal serious conditions. The most common etiology is obstruction due to prostatic enlargement. However, calculi, cancer (including prostatic cancer), and neurologic causes also need to be evaluated. The presence of diabetes mellitus should be evaluated if a neurologic cause is suspected.

In males, management consists of diagnosis and treatment of the underlying cause, with antimicrobial therapy directed against the offending organism. If obstruction is the cause, and the patient's age or medical condition do not permit surgical correction, chronic catheterization is often required and is a common cause of recurrent pyelonephritis. (Frequent, careful changes of the catheter are required, which may be accompanied by antibacterial irrigation and strict hygienic handling.) Continuous antibiotic prophylaxis is usually unsuccessful in the long term, and often leads to colonization and infection by multiple resistant organisms.

In the past, treatment of the acute episode of pyelonephritis required hospitalization and administration of systemic antibiotics. If uncomplicated pyelonephritis has been diagnosed, the organism and sensitivity have been documented, and the patient is stable, outpatient parenteral antibiotic administration can be efficacions and cost effective. In order to maximize cost savings, longer acting parenteral antimicrobial agents should be used, as noted in Table 1.

Antibiotics are chosen on the basis of culture and sensitivity results. If an aminoglycoside is to be used, it is important to routinely check the patient's renal status and aminoglycoside levels, as these patients often have underlying renal disease or damage from previous or chronic infections. Decreasing renal function may result in elevated, toxic levels of the aminoglycosides. For these reasons, alternatives to aminoglycosides have been developed, including aztreonam (Azactam) and the quinolones.

Women

Unlike men, young women frequently have urinary tract infections, and acute episodes of pyelonephritis are not uncommon. It has been demonstrated that 1 to 2% of all young women chronically harbor bacteria in their urine without symptoms, a condition termed *asymptomatic bacteriuria.* This incidence appears to double with each decade of age in women. Asymptomatic bacteriuria is thought to be due to the shorter urethra in women. Recent research has demonstrated that female hormone interaction with specific pathogenic bacterial strains may also be important.

It is this asymptomatic bacteriuria that is believed to be the source of ascending infection into the kidney in young women. Strategies to prevent colonization of the bladder and ascension of bacteria up the ureters are usually helpful in decreasing episodes of acute cystitis ("honeymoon cystitis") and pyelonephritis. These strategies include immediate urination following intercourse, antibiotic prophylaxis (single oral dose of nitrofurantoin, 100 mg, or trimethoprim-sulfamethoxasole, 80/400 mg) following intercourse, and/or increased hydration.

The primary risk factor for pyelonephritis in young

TABLE 1. **Long-Acting Parenteral Antibiotics**

Cephalosporins		
Cefotaxime (Claforan)	1–2 grams	IV every 8–12 hours
Ceftizoxime (Cefizox)	1–2 grams	IV every 8–12 hours
Cefotetan (Cefotan)	1–2 grams	IV every 12 hours
Ceftriaxone (Rocephin)	1–2 grams	IV every 12–24 hours
Quinolones		
Ofloxacin (Floxin)	300–400 mg	IV every 12 hours
Ciprofloxacin (Cipro)	500–750 mg	IV every 12 hours

women is pregnancy. Originally, this was believed to be related to the compression of the ureters and bladder by the enlarging uterus. However, the risk is increased even before the uterus grows out of the pelvis, and subsequent research has demonstrated an effect of pregnancy hormones on ureteral function and genitourinary tissue receptors for bacterial attachment.

The bacteria responsible for pyelonephritis in pregnancy are predominantly the Enterobacteriaceae, although approximately 5% of species are gram-positive bacteria, such as the enterococcus or group B streptococcus.

Because of reports of an association of pyelonephritis with preterm labor and delivery, sepsis, and a small risk of adult respiratory distress syndrome (ARDS), it is imperative that diagnosis and treatment be initiated quickly. One of the most common bacterial causes of fever in pregnancy is pyelonephritis. All pregnant patients with fever should have a urinalysis and culture. A urinalysis positive for bacteria and white blood cells in the presence of fever and flank pain is diagnostic for pyelonephritis. After determining whether the organism is gram-positive or gram-negative, treatment should be initiated with ampicillin, 2 grams intravenously every 6 hours for gram-positive bacteria, and a parenteral cephalosporin should be used for gram-negative organisms. Some practitioners use an aminoglycoside; however, the pharmacokinetics and safety of aminoglycosides in pregnancy have not been well documented, making monitoring or interpretation of levels difficult.

Cephalosporins are generally given because of their effectiveness against gram-negative organisms and their broad safety margin. Ampicillin's usefulness for treatment of gram-negative infections has declined in most areas owing to the development of resistance, and cefazolin, 1 to 2 grams intravenously every 6 to 8 hours has generally been used as the first line agent. However, there has been a similar increase in resistance to cefazolin in some areas of the United States; advance-generation cephalosporins, such as cefotaxime, 2 grams intravenously every 8 hours, have been demonstrated to be effective substitutes. The quinolones should not be given to pregnant women, nor should sulfa compounds be used in late pregnancy, because of safety considerations.

Because of a higher (>10%) incidence of urogenital anatomic abnormalities in patients with pyelonephritis in pregnancy, some researchers recommend radiographic or ultrasonographic evaluation of the urinary tract. If the patient improves on therapy, this may be omitted. However, intravenous pyelograms (IVPs) or ultrasound may be used postpartum or if the patient fails to respond to initial therapy.

Older women, especially those in nursing homes, also have an increased risk of pyelonephritis due to the frequent use of catheters. The catheterization of these women is not the result of obstructions as in older men, but rather of bladder descensus common in women after child-bearing. Patients in whom surgical correction of urinary incontinence is not advised or has failed often require long-term catheterization; The catheters become colonized, resulting in an ascending infection just as in men.

Young women who undergo radical surgery for early cervical cancer will often be unable to void spontaneously and will need intermittent catheterization. Bacteruria can result from frequent catheterization, and pyelonephritis can develop because the early signs of cystitis are often absent owing to the surgical denervation of the bladder.

Treatment for all the catheter-related infections is based on culture and sensitivity reports. Empiric treatment for patients with recurrent pyelonephritis can be initiated based on the susceptibility patterns in the previous episode. However, it must be emphasized that resistance to antibiotic therapy occurs often and rapidly, and therefore cultures must be taken for each new episode.

TREATMENT ALTERNATIVES

As noted previously, the most important aspect of treating pyelonephritis is the diagnosis of the cause, which is often treatable (e.g., calculi, bladder descensus, poor catheter hygiene). Antibiotic treatment is often initiated empirically, but Gram's stains, and resistance patterns in previous infections should all help in determining the correct antimicrobial.

Some clinicians advocate oral antimicrobial therapy for uncomplicated pyelonephritis. Short courses or single doses of antibiotics have been used to differentiate upper urinary tract disease from lower urinary tract disease in patients in whom the distinction between severe cystitis and pyelonephritis is hazy. However, true pyelonephritis is probably best managed initially with parenteral (hospitalization or home intravenous) therapy followed by oral therapy to complete a 2-week course. Up to 6 weeks of therapy can be given for chronic or recurrent pyelonephritis; however a thorough search for underlying complicating causes must be made.

In some cases of uncomplicated pyelonephritis in relatively healthy, nonpregnant patients, outpatient oral therapy can be used from the start. The quinolones appear to be quite effective orally; agents for which there is extensive clinical experience include cinoxacin (Cinobac), norfloxacin (Noroxin), ciprofloxacin (Cipro), and ofloxacin (Floxin). Penicillins, cephalosporins, and sulfa agents can also be administered, either before or after the return of the culture and susceptibility results.

Pyelonephritis is a significant bacterial infection, especially in the older patient and in pregnant women. Fortunately, with early diagnosis and appropriate antimicrobial therapy, the prognosis is excellent. However, follow-up examination and cultures are imperative if chronic pyelonephritis and its serious sequelae are to be avoided.

GENITOURINARY TRAUMA

method of
JOE Y. LEE, M.D., and
ALEXANDER S. CASS, M.D.
Hennepin County Medical Center
Minneapolis, Minnesota

Genitourinary injuries account for 10% of traumatic injuries seen in the emergency room and have a 10% mortality. Ninety-eight percent of the fatalities, however, result from associated injuries to other organ systems. Genitourinary injuries are managed within the protocols of the multiply injured patient to control associated life-threatening injuries.

A thorough history and physical examination provide insight into the patient's clinical situation as it pertains to the genitourinary system. For example, blunt trauma often causes pelvic fractures with concomitant bladder and urethral injuries, whereas rapid deceleration may be associated with renal injuries. The radiographic evaluation is tailored to the clinical findings and proceeds in a caudad to cephalad direction (e.g., urethrogram, cystogram, intravenous urogram).

The indications for radiographic evaluation of genitourinary trauma continue to evolve. Previously, patients with any degree of hematuria, gross or microscopic, required a complete radiographic evaluation. In adult patients with blunt trauma and only microscopic hematuria, the diagnostic yield of significant urologic injuries was extremely low. Presently, adult patients with blunt trauma who have either gross hematuria or microscopic hematuria that is associated with either shock or significant nongenitourinary injuries are evaluated radiographically. Adults with penetrating trauma require radiographic studies regardless of the degree of hematuria. On the other hand, pediatric patients require radiographic studies with any degree of hematuria with either blunt or penetrating trauma. With these criteria, more than 99% of patients with significant urinary injuries are staged correctly. Clinical assessment may mandate further evaluation. For example, patients with major deceleration injuries, significant fractures of the transverse spinal processes, and severe or anterior pelvic fractures should undergo radiographic evaluation.

KIDNEY INJURIES

The kidneys are protected in the retroperitoneum by the overlying ribs and are surrounded by perinephric fat, Gerota's fascia, and renal capsule. The mobility of the kidney is also a factor in resisting injury. Nevertheless, the kidney is the most commonly injured organ in the genitourinary system.

Eighty-five percent of renal injuries are blunt injuries, with the most common cause being motor vehicle accidents. Other causes of blunt renal trauma include sports injuries, falls, blunt assaults, and deceleration or crushing mechanisms. The principal causes of penetrating renal injuries are gunshot and stab wounds.

The most common sign of renal injury is hematuria, either gross or microscopic. Renal injuries in the vast majority of patients without hematuria are minor and can be managed conservatively. Significant renal injuries without hematuria, however, are usually associated with other serious injuries that prompt further evaluation. Other signs and symptoms suggestive of renal injuries include flank masses, pain, ecchymosis, hypotension, and fractures of the lower ribs and transverse processes of the lumbar vertebrae.

After initial assessment, examination, and resuscitation, stable patients suspected of having significant renal injuries are evaluated radiographically. Traditionally, intravenous urography is used to evaluate suspected renal injuries. In the hemodynamically unstable patient requiring immediate surgical intervention, the intraoperative intravenous urogram remains essential in assessing contralateral renal function. Computed tomography (CT), however, is often the primary study obtained in stable adult and pediatric patients who are multiply injured. In addition to assessing associated injuries, CT accurately stages the extent of renal injury by demonstrating depth of laceration, devascularized renal segments, and urinary extravasation.

There are four major classifications or stages of renal injuries: (1) renal contusions, which involve ecchymosis or subcapsular hematomas associated with an intact renal capsule and collecting system; (2) minor renal cortical lacerations that do not involve the medulla or collecting system; (3) major renal parenchymal lacerations that extend deep into the collecting system and frequently are associated with devitalized parenchyma; and (4) critical renal injuries, which include shattered kidneys and renal pedicle injuries involving laceration, avulsion, or thrombosis of the renal artery or vein.

In renal contusions, CT demonstrates delayed function and renal parenchymal swelling. The renal outline is smooth, intact, and without extravasation of contrast material. Subcapsular hematomas appear as flattened portions of the renal cortex compressed by the hematoma collecting under the renal capsule. Minor renal lacerations appear as a disruption of the renal cortical outline but do not extend into the collecting system. Major renal lacerations manifest as severe disruption of the renal cortical outline, extravasation of contrast material, and/or nonfunction of large segments of the renal parenchyma. Renal pedicle injuries appear as a nonenhanced kidney with minimal peripheral enhancement from the renal capsular vessels (rim sign).

Treatment

Eighty-five percent of blunt renal trauma consist of minor injuries that can be managed conservatively with bed rest and hydration. Blood counts and vital signs are monitored. Patients with gross hematuria remain on bed rest until the gross hematuria resolves. The long-term sequelae from minor renal injuries are minimal.

Patients with major renal and critical injuries may require surgical exploration. The absolute indication for operative management is persistent retroperitoneal bleeding with hemodynamic instability. Relative indications for operative management in stable patients include extensive urinary extravasation, large devitalized fragments, and renal pedicle injuries. These patients are at risk for long-term complications even if they remain hemodynamically stable with conservative therapy. Operative management consists of transperitoneal exploration, early control of the renal vessels, reflection of the colon, and repair if possible. Control of the renal vessels through an incision in the retroperitoneum over the aorta just medial to the inferior mesenteric vein decreases the nephrectomy rate in potentially salvageable kidneys. Both renal arteries are easily exposed and controlled through this incision. However, nephrectomy may be necessary in the unsalvageable kidney or unstable patient.

The management of renal artery injuries is controversial. A complete loss of renal function can result from a warm renal ischemia time of only 60 minutes. Thus, even with aggressive surgical management, renal salvage is unusual. Indications for repair of renal pedicle injuries include bilateral renal artery lesions, lesions in solitary kidneys, and isolated renal artery injuries in the stable patient. Patients with complete renal pedicle avulsion generally present with multiple life-threatening injuries and require emergent nephrectomy. Isolated segmental artery injuries can be managed conservatively and are monitored for the occasional case of renal hypertension.

In contrast to blunt renal injuries, 80% of patients with penetrating renal injuries have associated intra-abdominal injuries. Penetrating renal injuries generally are surgically explored. High-velocity, hollow-point, and tumbling bullets are associated with more significant soft tissue destruction and require more extensive intraoperative débridement. Stab wounds to the kidneys may have their entrance points in the lower thorax, flank area, or upper abdomen. With stab wounds confined to the flank, nonoperative management is reasonable if CT shows only minor renal injury. Stab wounds to the anterior abdomen carry a high incidence of associated intra-abdominal injuries and require operative exploration.

The long-term complications of renal trauma include arteriovenous fistula, hydronephrosis, hypertension, and renal atrophy. Arteriovenous fistulas are seen mainly with penetrating renal injuries. Hydronephrosis and hypertension are usually caused by fibrosis around the affected kidney. The hypertension that results from renal ischemia due to compressive fibrosis in this setting is mediated by renin. In order to detect these complications, patients with renal injuries are followed with radiographic studies and monitoring of vital signs.

URETERAL INJURIES

Injuries of the ureter are uncommon owing to its protected position. The two main types of ureteral injury are lacerations from penetrating trauma and avulsion, generally at the ureteropelvic junction. A high index of suspicion must be maintained because ureteral injuries are easily overlooked and may present without hematuria. Unrecognized injuries may be complicated by urinary extravasation, fistula formation, infection, electrolyte imbalances, and kidney loss.

Blunt trauma is a rare cause of ureteral injury, but disruption of the upper ureter, usually within 4 cm of the ureteropelvic junction, can be seen after hyperextension injuries. This is most common in children because they have more pliable spinal columns, and for unclear reasons it occurs more often on the right. With penetrating injuries, the most common site of ureteral involvement is the midureter. Penetrating ureteral injuries are usually associated with other internal injuries that require treatment. Diagnosis of a ureteral injury is made radiographically or upon surgical exploration. Radiographic evidence includes hydronephrosis, urinary extravasation, and nonvisualization of the ureter. If the initial radiographic studies are equivocal, retrograde pyelography is diagnostic.

Treatment

Treatment of ureteral injuries depends on the site, severity, and cause. Partial and complete injuries of the middle and upper ureter are best managed by surgical débridement and either suture repair of the laceration or ureteroureterostomy. With high-velocity gunshot wounds, it is critical that the ureteral edges are débrided adequately. Injuries in the distal third of the ureter are best managed with débridement and neoureterocystostomy. In critically ill patients, ureteral injuries may be treated temporarily by percutaneous drainage of the kidney until the patient is stabilized.

BLADDER INJURIES

Blunt bladder trauma, the principal cause of bladder injury, results most frequently from motor vehicle accidents; less common causes are falls, pelvic crush injuries, and blows to the lower abdomen. Injuries to other pelvic and abdominal organs may accompany penetrating bladder trauma. In the setting of blunt trauma, pelvic fractures accompany bladder rupture in 80% of cases. Conversely, about 15% of all pelvic fractures are associated with bladder or urethral injuries. Bladder injuries are generally classified as intraperitoneal or extraperitoneal. A direct blow to a full urinary bladder can result in rupture of the bladder, generally at the dome, leading to intraperitoneal extravasation of urine. Delayed diagnosis can result in peritonitis, azotemia, or metabolic acidosis. Most bladder ruptures, however, are extraperitoneal and are thought to be due to laceration from bony spicules associated with a pelvic fracture. A high index of suspicion should be maintained in patients with pelvic fractures, lower abdominal trauma, hematuria, or inability to void.

Suspected bladder injuries are evaluated radiographically. Intravenous urography is inadequate for evaluating bladder injuries because of the 20% false-negative rate. Abdominal plain films are obtained to demonstrate fractures of the pelvis. Cystography with adequate retrograde filling of the bladder with contrast media is essentially 100% accurate in the evaluation of possible bladder injuries. After a scout film, 400 mL of contrast material is instilled into the bladder under gravity from 2 feet above the table and a plain film of the abdomen is obtained. In children, the bladder is filled to capacity (age in years + 2 = capacity in ounces; maximum of 400 mL). In both adults and children, the instillation is halted if a detrusor contraction is elicited. A washout film is then obtained after the bladder is drained of contrast material and rinsed with normal saline. With an intraperitoneal rupture of the bladder, free contrast material can be seen in the abdominal cavity, initially in the cul de sac posterior to the bladder, then following the pericolic gutters, and finally outlining loops of bowel. In extraperitoneal ruptures, the contrast medium has a feathery appearance as it streaks through the perivesical tissues. Frequently extravasation is seen only on the washout films. Concomitant intraperitoneal and extraperitoneal ruptures can occur.

Treatment

With blunt trauma, intraperitoneal bladder ruptures should be meticulously repaired with two to three layers of absorbable suture. The bladder is drained via a large suprapubic tube positioned in the extraperitoneal space. Extraperitoneal bladder ruptures are managed nonoperatively with antibiotics and catheter drainage. A follow-up cystogram is obtained 10–14 days before catheter removal. Rarely, persistent extravasation or hematuria will result from a retained bone fragment in the bladder wall or from orthopedic complications from the surgical reduction of the pelvic fracture.

Incidents of complicated orthopedic fungal infections have been reported with massive urinary extravasation into complex closed pelvic fractures. To decrease the risk of complicated orthopedic infections, the bladder is meticulously repaired at the time of the orthopedic surgery. The bladder is drained with a large urethral catheter, and the closed prevesical drain (placed contralateral to the orthopedic injury) is discontinued early.

Penetrating bladder injuries and associated internal organ injuries are managed surgically.

In children, both extraperitoneal and intraperitoneal bladder ruptures are managed by surgical repair and suprapubic tube drainage to avoid urethral catheter complications and inadequate drainage of the lacerated bladder.

URETHRAL INJURIES

Urethral injuries in the male are classified as anterior and posterior. The anterior urethra consists of the bulbous and pendulous portions of the urethra; the posterior urethra consists of the prostatic and membranous portions, i.e., those portions proximal to the urogenital diaphragm.

The site of urethral injury is localized with retrograde urethrography. Urethrography before urethral catheterization prevents the conversion of a partial laceration to a complete laceration. Ten to 15 mL of isotonic contrast material is injected through a small catheter placed 1 to 2 cm into the urethra. The urethra is imaged with either fluoroscopy or plain radiographs of the pelvis.

Anterior Urethral Injuries

The anterior urethra is distal to the urogenital diaphragm. The most common site of anterior urethral injury is the bulbous urethra and the most common cause is a kick or straddle injury. These patients present with urethral bleeding, voiding difficulties, pain, swelling, and tenderness. Injuries to the pendulous urethra are rare owing to its mobility; when they do occur, they are generally the result of penetrating trauma, most commonly gunshot wounds. Urethral lacerations can also occur with instrumentation or concomitantly with penile fractures.

Anterior urethral injuries are classified as contusions, partial lacerations, or complete lacerations. In urethral contusions, the urethral mucosa is intact and there is no extravasation of urine. In partial urethral lacerations, the retrograde urethrogram demonstrates contrast material extravasating into the periurethral tissues at the site of injury and flowing into the urethra proximally. With complete injuries, the contrast media does not flow proximal to the injury.

Posterior Urethral Injuries

Injuries to the posterior urethra most often result from blunt trauma and almost always occur in the setting of pelvic fractures. Ninety percent of posterior urethral disruptions are associated with pelvic fractures, whereas 10% of pelvic fractures are associated with urethral injuries. The most common site of injury is just proximal to or at the urogenital diaphragm. Injuries occur at this site because of the prostate's fixation to the pubic symphysis by the puboprostatic ligaments. Frequently, the prostate and bladder are displaced superiorly by an expanding pelvic hematoma. Patients who present with a fractured pelvis accompanied by blood at the urethral meatus, a high-riding prostate, or voiding difficulties require radiographic evaluation. Catheterization of the urethra in this setting is contraindicated.

Retrograde urethrography demonstrates a complete posterior urethral laceration with extravasation of contrast medium into the perivesical or perineal space. With incomplete lacerations of the prostatomembranous urethra, there is extravasation of contrast material with some flow proximally into the bladder. This distinction may be difficult if cystography or intravenous urography had been previously performed and constitutes the rationale for evaluating the urinary tract in a caudad to cephalad orientation. Patients often present to the emergency department with an indwelling Foley catheter, which may or may not be draining urine. In this setting, retrograde urethrography should be performed around the indwelling catheter with a small feeding tube.

Treatment

Anterior urethral contusions generally require a short period of urethral catheterization until voiding is possible. Partial and complete lacerations of the anterior urethra may be treated by débridement and primary anastomosis or by placement of a suprapubic tube with delayed urethroplasty. Partial anterior urethral lacerations can also be stented under fluoroscopic control. A guidewire with an angiographic catheter is gently manipulated to negotiate the partial urethral injury. A urethral catheter with an end hole can then be placed coaxially over the guidewire to stent the injury.

The treatment of complete posterior urethral injuries is controversial. Some urologists prefer surgical placement of a suprapubic tube alone followed by delayed urethral reconstruction in 3 to 6 months. The advantage of this method is its simplicity, especially in unstable patients. Proponents of suprapubic tube placement with delayed urethroplasty cite the possibility of decreased incidence of impotence and reduced likelihood of infection of the pelvic hematoma. A second method of treatment involves manipulation of the urethra and bladder into continuity with realignment of the urethra over an indwelling urethral catheter. Dissection should be limited to the anterior aspects of the prostate to avoid further injury to the neurovascular bundle along the posterior lateral surface of the prostate, which controls erections. A suprapubic tube is also placed. The advantage of this procedure is that it reduces the need for future operative procedures to establish urinary continuity. The impotence and incontinence rates (25% and 2%, respectively) appear to related to the severity of the initial injury rather than the treatment method. Long-term urethral stricture disease and voiding dysfunction are common problems. Partial proximal urethral lacerations can be treated with either a suprapubic tube with delayed urethroplasty or gentle coaxial placement of an indwelling urethral catheter over a guidewire under fluoroscopic control.

A follow-up urethrogram with injection of contrast material through a small feeding tube along the indwelling catheter documents the resolution of urinary extravasation before catheter removal.

GENITAL INJURIES IN MALES

Serious injuries to the penis are unusual owing to its relative mobility. Penile injuries include fracture of the corporeal bodies, amputation, avulsion of the penile or scrotal skin, strangulation injuries, and penetrating injuries. Diagnosis is usually straightforward and is based on the history and physical examination. Fracture of the penis refers to rupture of the tunica albuginea surrounding the corpora cavernosa. This most often occurs during sexual intercourse and should be treated with surgical exploration and repair of the rupture site. Penetrating injuries to the erectile bodies are generally managed with surgical exploration, débridement, and closure of any corporeal defect. The possibility of concomitant urethral injury is assessed by urethrography. Penile amputation is a rare injury that is often self-induced. Repair with microsurgical techniques is sometimes possible. Avulsion of the penile skin is most often caused by farm or industrial machinery. The skin distal to the injury should be removed to within 2 to 3 mm of the coronal sulcus in order to avoid chronic lymphedema of the penile shaft. Once the skin is removed, split-thickness skin grafting of the penile shaft should be performed.

Injuries to the scrotum and testes can be caused by blunt trauma, penetrating trauma, or avulsion-type injuries. As in penile injuries, avulsion of the scrotal skin is most often due to accidents involving farm or industrial machinery. Treatment includes broad-spectrum antibiotics and tetanus prophylaxis followed by immediate surgical débridement and repair. Because of the elastic nature of the scrotal skin, this is frequently accomplished by primary closure. If the avulsion is complete, the testis should be placed in a subcutaneous thigh pouch and the scrotum later reconstructed with a pedicle thigh flap.

Trauma to the testicle generally results from blunt injury. These patients present with large scrotal hematomas, pain, and nausea and vomiting. The critical distinction that must be made is whether there is a fracture of the testicle with a hematocele or whether the blood is confined to the interstitial tissues in the scrotal wall. Ultrasonography usually determines whether the tunica of the testicle is intact. Rupture is best managed by open surgical repair consisting of débridement, closure of the defect in the tunica albuginea, and drainage. Patients with penetrating scrotal trauma through the tunica vaginalis should undergo surgical exploration. Without aggressive surgical management, convalescence is protracted and there is substantial morbidity. With an aggressive surgical approach, the risk of testicular loss is reduced to less than 5% and morbidity is minimized.

BENIGN PROSTATIC HYPERPLASIA

method of
DAVID A. RIVAS, M.D., and
MICHAEL B. CHANCELLOR, M.D.
Thomas Jefferson University
Philadelphia, Pennsylvania

Benign prostatic hyperplasia (BPH), primarily a disorder of men aged 40 years and over, is the most common benign tumor in men. BPH is a benign enlargement of any or all cellular prostate components, which can result in voiding dysfunction. Although advancing age and testicular function are required for the development of BPH, the specific biochemical factors that induce it are unknown.

It has been estimated that a 60-year-old man has a 50% probability of developing histologic evidence of BPH; the incidence rises to 100% in octogenarians. Despite the almost universal development of histologic BPH with age, a significantly smaller proportion of patients develop symptoms of bladder outlet obstruction or require therapy for relief of such obstruction. Only about 50% of men with histologically detectable BPH develop palpable enlargement of the prostate. Furthermore, only 50% of men with prostate enlargement develop clinical symptoms that necessitate treatment. Approximately 25% of all men will eventually require treatment for symptomatic relief of prostatism (clinical BPH) if they live to 80 years of age.

Prostate size is not the sole determinant of the development of symptoms of prostatism because other factors also play a role, such as detrusor muscle function and bladder neck and prostatic urethral tone, which are mediated by the autonomic nervous system.

PATHOGENESIS

The etiology and pathogenesis of BPH are incompletely understood. Nevertheless, the development of BPH is clearly related to aging and active testicular endocrine function. The role of testicular androgens is underscored by the fact that BPH does not develop in men castrated before puberty or in those with the genetic inability to produce androgens or active androgen receptors. Prostatic growth and functional integrity, with resultant changes in secretory and proliferative capacity, are dependent upon circulating androgen levels.

The hypothalamic-pituitary-testes-prostate axis creates the hormonal milieu for the development of BPH. The hypothalamus releases luteinizing hormone–releasing hormone (LHRH) in a pulsatile fashion, stimulating release of luteinizing hormone (LH) by the pituitary. Luteinizing hormone reaches the testes via the peripheral circulation, where it binds to surface receptors on Leydig cells, stimulating the biosynthesis of testosterone. Testosterone acts as a prehormone on the prostatic epithelial cell, where it is converted to dihydrotestosterone (DHT) by the enzyme 5-alpha-reductase. DHT binds to specific nuclear androgen receptors, promoting cell growth and proliferation. It has been shown that DHT levels in the prostate may remain at a normal level as men age, despite decreases in plasma testosterone levels.

Estrogens may also play a role in the pathogenesis of BPH. Most serum estrogen in men is derived from the peripheral conversion of testosterone to estrogens through the enzymatic pathway of aromatization. In addition, physiologic levels of estrogen increase the nuclear androgen receptor content of the prostate cells, which can contribute to the development of BPH.

Microscopically, hyperplasia is characterized by nodules of benign adenoma. The physiologic dysfunction associated with BPH may therefore be related to stromal mechanical obstruction and smooth muscular dynamic obstruction. Present pharmacologic therapy for the treatment of obstruction caused by BPH targets either the stromal or the muscular components.

Mechanical (Static) Obstruction

Mechanical or static obstruction is caused by the enlargement of the glands that surround the prostatic urethra, resulting in urethral compression. Pathologically, BPH develops as nodules of epithelial and stromal elements of the glands lining the proximal prostatic urethra. These nodules enlarge and coalesce within the anterior, posterior, and lateral walls of the prostate, forming lobular masses of various shapes and sizes. Because the anterior lobe is usually only minimally involved, BPH is often designated as bilobar (lateral lobe enlargement only) or trilobar (both lateral and posterior lobe enlargement). Some patients will have only posterior, median lobe hyperplasia, which may be obstructive. In these cases of BPH, the lateral lobes may be only minimally enlarged while the median lobe grows infravesically to obstruct the bladder neck. This explains why there is a variable correlation between rectally palpable prostatic size and the degree of obstruction. Treatment of the static component of BPH has in the past focused on the surgical removal of the mass of hyperplastic prostatic tissue and more recently on antiandrogen agents, which induce prostatic involution.

Smooth Muscle (Dynamic) Obstruction

The human prostate contains an abundance of alpha$_1$-adrenergic receptors that primarily govern its contractile properties. Stimulation of these receptors by norepinephrine and other alpha-active agents causes contraction of the smooth muscle and compression of the prostatic urethra, increasing the resistance to urinary flow.

The dynamic component of BPH is a result of the increased smooth muscle tone of the bladder neck, prostatic adenoma, and prostatic capsule. The smooth muscle tone in these areas changes in response to local and systemic adrenergic stimulation, mediated by such variables as emotion, temperature, and pain. Thus, the resulting symptoms vary in severity and frequency.

CLINICAL MANIFESTATIONS

Symptoms

The symptoms of BPH are highly variable: some men are asymptomatic while others suffer from a plethora of symptoms. These differences are generally related not only to the degree of urethral obstruction, but also to the secondary alteration of bladder function.

The size of the prostate does not always predict the type or severity of symptoms. Some men with large glands have minimal symptoms, whereas others with small glands may have numerous and/or severe clinical manifestations. This paradox is not completely understood but is due in part to the relative contributions of the dynamic and static components of obstruction.

In the early phases of BPH development, a minimal obstruction of the bladder outlet occurs. The detrusor mechanism of the bladder compensates for this with an increase in contractility, and the patient may have only minor symptoms. As resistance to urinary flow in the prostatic urethra increases, symptoms increase in intensity (Table 1). Certain symptoms are felt to be directly related to the degree of urethral obstruction; these include a decrease in the force and caliber of the urinary stream, hesitancy in voiding, inability to terminate micturition, a sensation of incomplete emptying, and occasionally urinary retention. Other symptoms are believed to reflect the changes in detrusor function caused by the obstruction. These irritative lower urinary tract symptoms include urgency, frequency, nocturia, and painful voiding.

As the detrusor compensates, connective tissue deposition increases within the bladder wall. Up to 50% of men with BPH develop uninhibited detrusor contractions, which can be demonstrated during urodynamic testing. These contractions are directly related to obstruction at the bladder neck and prostatic urethra, resulting in symptoms of urgency, frequency, or incontinence. After relief of bladder outlet obstruction, uninhibited bladder contractions may persist but usually resolve spontaneously.

The American Urological Association (AUA) Symptom Index is a recently developed and validated questionnaire that quantifies the severity of voiding symptoms and can be used to determine treatment outcome (Table 2). Although the AUA Symptom Index may indicate the degree of lower urinary tract functional impairment, the symptoms and the index that quantify these symptoms are unfortunately not specific for BPH. For example, the index has been used to monitor treatment effects in women with voiding symptoms. In a carefully monitored group of women with voiding dysfunction verified by video-urodynamic evaluation, the AUA Symptom Index scores rivaled those of men with moderate and significant BPH. Furthermore, the AUA Symptom Index scores in this study decreased significantly after appropriate therapy was instituted. It is important for all physicians to be aware of the fact that voiding symptoms are not specific in patients with BPH, and consequently, a specific set of symptoms should not be relied upon as the sole basis for treatment of patients with micturitional dysfunction.

Physical Signs

The most important physical sign of BPH is an enlarged, smooth, symmetrical prostate as determined by digital rectal examination. The gland may be soft or somewhat firm, and diffuse nodularity may be present. The nodules, however, lack the hard consistency associated with carcinoma. The AUA recommends that all men over the age of 50 have an annual digital rectal examination (DRE) and serum prostate-specific antigen (PSA) determination in order to rule out occult malignancy. Recent reports indicate that such screening should begin at age 40 if a patient is symptomatic or has a family history of prostatic adenocarcinoma.

Urinalysis may demonstrate white blood cells, bacteria, or sometimes microscopic hematuria. If obstruction has resulted in impairment of renal function, electrolyte abnormalities may occur, while the blood urea nitrogen (BUN) and serum creatinine levels may be elevated. An abdominal radiograph may reveal prostatic calculi.

TABLE 1. **Symptoms of Benign Prostatic Hyperplasia**

Irritative Symptoms	Obstructive Symptoms
Dysuria	Dribbling
Frequency	Hesitancy
Incontinence	Intermittency
Nocturia	Sensation of incomplete emptying
Urgency	Straining
	Weak stream

DIAGNOSTIC TESTS

A variety of additional diagnostic studies are employed in the evaluation of a patient with voiding symptoms and abnormal urinalysis results. Other conditions must be diagnosed and effectively treated prior to making the assumption that voiding symptoms emanate from a benign prostatic adenoma. These include prostate cancer, urethral stricture, urinary tract infection, urothelial malignancy, cystitis, abnormal detrusor function, and sensory abnormalities of the bladder. Ancillary diagnostic studies for these entities include intravenous urography, urethrography, urinary cytology, urine culture, urethral catheterization, cystometry, cystoscopy, and lumbar, suprapubic, and transrectal ultrasonography (TRUS).

Urodynamic Evaluation

Various physiologic parameters ensure an objective assessment of the effects of BPH (Table 3). The urinary flow rate and cystometrogram are both useful in this regard. Urinary flow rate determination is helpful in quantifying the efficiency of bladder emptying, measuring the rate of urine flow in milliliters per second using a urinary flowmeter. A low rate of flow may be caused by the prostatic urethral obstruction of BPH, but one must remember that bladder outlet obstruction can also be caused by a dysfunctional bladder neck, a dyssynergic external sphincter, or a scarred and stenotic urethra. Furthermore, diminished uroflow can be due to weak bladder muscle contractions or impaired detrusor contractility.

A more advanced urodynamic evaluation of the patient with prostatic obstruction is obtained with the cystometrogram. In this study, as the bladder is slowly filled with fluid, the volumes are noted at which the patient reports the sensations of bladder filling, distention, and the urge to urinate. In addition, the occurrence and force of bladder contractions are monitored. The cystometrogram is used to diagnose uninhibited detrusor contractions, involuntary bladder contractions at low bladder volumes, and poor bladder contractions resulting from muscle decompensation or neuropathic detrusor dysfunction. Patients with outlet obstruction secondary to BPH and detrusor instability (uninhibited bladder contractions) have symptoms of frequency, urgency, and often urge incontinence. Within 1 year of prostatectomy, these uninhibited contractions resolve in 70 to 80% of patients.

Cystoscopy

Cystoscopic examination is an effective method of evaluating the patient with BPH. The use of a small rigid or flexible cystoscope enables the physician to perform this examination in the office with only local anesthesia. Cystoscopy helps to determine the size of the prostate, the degree of obstruction, the secondary changes in the bladder caused by the obstruction, and the presence of an enlarged median lobe, which may not be rectally palpable. Frequently, cystoscopy aids in the selection of an open versus a transurethral approach to prostatectomy.

DIFFERENTIAL DIAGNOSIS

Statistically, most men with irritative and/or obstructive voiding symptoms have BPH. Such symptoms, however,

TABLE 2. **The American Urological Association Symptom Index**

	Not at All	Less than 1/5	Less than 1/2	About Half	More than Half	Almost Always
1. Over the past month, have you had a sensation of not emptying your bladder?	0	1	2	3	4	5
2. Over the past month, how often have you had to urinate again less than 2 hrs after you finished urinating?	0	1	2	3	4	5
3. Over the past month, how often have you found you stopped and started again several times when you urinated?	0	1	2	3	4	5
4. Over the past month, how often have you found it difficult to postpone urination?	0	1	2	3	4	5
5. Over the past month, how often have you had a weak stream?	0	1	2	3	4	5
6. Over the past month, how often have you had to push or strain to begin urination?	0	1	2	3	4	5
7. Over the past month, how many times did you get up at night to urinate?	0	1	2	3	4	5
Total Score:						

are caused by other conditions in about 10 to 20% of male patients. Bacterial cystitis, nonspecific cystitis (e.g., radiation or interstitial cystitis), papillary transitional cell carcinoma, carcinoma in situ, and bladder or ureteral calculi can all induce irritative symptoms suggestive of BPH. Obstructive symptoms can occur with a dyssynergic external sphincter mechanism, bladder calculi, bladder neck dysfunction, or urethral strictures. Strictures can develop not only after nonspecific or gonococcal urethritis, but also after urethral catheterization or cystoscopy. As the stricture narrows the urethral lumen, urinary flow is obstructed. Symptoms such as decreased force of the urinary stream and intermittency then become manifest.

Neurogenic vesical dysfunction is perhaps the most important entity that generates symptoms suggestive of BPH. Physicians should become familiar with the concept of neurologically mediated bladder disorders so that voiding irregularity in an older male patient is not summarily attributed to an enlarged prostate gland. Cerebrovascular accidents can affect the central micturition control centers in the brain, impairing the ability to inhibit spontaneous detrusor contractions; this results in symptoms of frequency, urgency, and urge incontinence. Prostatectomy in these patients may indeed relieve obstructive symptoms; however, irritative symptoms can persist and develop into troublesome incontinence.

TABLE 3. **Diagnosis of Benign Prostatic Hyperplasia**

Diagnostic Modality	Findings
History	Symptoms AUA Symptom Index
Physical Examination	Digital rectal examination to rule out cancer Palpable bladder
Laboratory Tests	Urinalysis and culture Serum prostate-specific antigen Serum creatinine
Urodynamic Evaluation	Urinary flow rate Postvoid residual urine volume Cystometrogram Renal radiographic imaging Transrectal prostate ultrasound Video-urodynamics (pressure/flow studies)

Functional bladder outlet obstruction can result from a number of neurologic lesions. Involvement of the central nervous system may affect voiding function, as in patients with myelodysplasia or spinal cord injury. Peripheral nervous injury, which can be caused by diseases, such as diabetes mellitus, or by trauma, such as radical pelvic surgery (e.g., abdominoperineal resection), can also induce such changes. In these conditions, the bladder muscle is hypotonic or even atonic and flaccid and unable to generate enough pressure to empty the bladder effectively.

In Parkinson's disease, the voluntary external sphincter may be the source of obstructive voiding symptoms. The bladder muscle and the urinary sphincters are under the control of the nervous system, in particular the parasympathetic (bladder muscle) nervous system, sympathetic nervous system (bladder neck, prostatic urethra), and the pudendal nerve (external striated sphincter). Neuropathic voiding dysfunction results from interference with bladder contraction (e.g., spinal cord injury) or sphincter function (e.g., multiple sclerosis, Parkinson's disease).

Men with neurologic impairment and symptoms of BPH require careful urodynamic assessment before decisions are made regarding prostatectomy and other treatments. This group of patients includes those with any disease process that affects nervous conduction, such as herniated intervertebral discs, multiple sclerosis, cerebrovascular accident, diabetes mellitus, Lyme disease, spinal cord injury, or neuromuscular disease, or with nervous injury caused by pelvic fracture or major abdominal or pelvic surgery. Prostatic resection in such patients without a thorough neuro-urologic evaluation can result in poor outcome and exacerbated symptoms of frequency and incontinence. Irritative voiding symptoms, in the absence of obstructive symptoms and any neurologic history, should alert the clinician to the presence of a disease process other than, or in addition to, BPH.

TREATMENT

The relative indications for the treatment of BPH include increased residual urine volume, detrusor instability, and decreased quality of life. Such symptoms do not mandate treatment for BPH, but several conditions absolutely indicate the need for therapy. These include recurrent febrile urinary tract infections, acute urinary retention, hydronephrosis, renal insufficiency, and gross hematuria. Although gross hematuria occurs uncommonly in men with BPH, treatment is required when it does occur. Bladder decompensation with overflow incontinence is also an indication for treatment, although detrusor contractility should be urodynamically documented prior to considering surgery. Impaired upper urinary tract function, a result of chronic bladder outlet obstruction, usually improves upon relief of the obstruction. The recovery of lower urinary tract function, however, depends upon the severity and duration of bladder decompensation.

Patient complaints and quality-of-life issues are the most common reasons for initiating treatment of men with BPH. As the less invasive approaches of medical management and minimally invasive procedures are further developed, patients will be likely to seek evaluation and treatment at earlier stages of the disease process.

It is important to remember that BPH is not necessarily a progressive disease. If men with symptomatic BPH are left untreated for up to 5 years, more than one-third will report a spontaneous improvement in symptoms. However, nearly one-half will report some degree of symptom progression. Thus, the decision to treat medically or surgically should be based on the general condition of the patient with consideration of his treatment preferences.

Treatment for benign prostatic hyperplasia can be broadly classified into surgical, minimally invasive, and medical therapy (Table 4). Surgical therapy for those with BPH includes open prostatectomy and transurethral resection of the prostate (TURP). TURP is considered the preferred treatment historically, if not the gold standard, for relief of symptoms attributed to an obstructing prostate gland. However, based on patient preference and risk/benefit analysis, the patient may also benefit from other less invasive treatment.

The minimally invasive therapies that are currently under investigation for the treatment of BPH include transurethral incision of the prostate (TUIP), transurethral dilatation of the prostate (TUDP) with a balloon catheter, the placement of prostatic stents, microwave prostatic hyperthermia, laser ablation of the prostate, and prostate cryotherapy. Pharmacologic therapy involves either androgen action antagonism or alpha-adrenergic blockade.

Surgical Treatment

An open prostatectomy is usually associated with less risk of morbidity and mortality for a patient with an extremely large prostate. Other indications for open prostatectomy include the presence of large bladder diverticula or calculi that can be corrected/removed at the time the bladder is exposed for the prostatectomy. The presence of a severe impassable urethral stricture or orthopedic conditions that obviate the lithotomy position, a prerequisite for endoscopic surgery, also indicate the need for an open procedure. Intraoperative hemorrhage, possibly requiring blood replacement, however, is greater with open prostatectomy.

Transurethral resection of the prostate (TURP) constitutes 95% of all prostatectomy procedures and has a low mortality rate (0.1%). The associated morbidity and postoperative complication rates are approximately 18%. Early postoperative complications include failure to void (3.9%), urinary retention caused by blood clot (3.3%), and genitourinary infections (2.3%). The most critical post-prostatectomy complication is stress urinary incontinence, which occurs in 1 to 1.5% of patients. With regard to sexual function, retrograde ejaculation is reported to occur in 65 to 75% of patients following TURP. Erectile dysfunction has been reported by 33% of patients in another study; 4 to 40% are reported for all the literature, but an impotence rate of 5 to 10% after TURP appears to be more accurate.

In general, the majority of patients enjoy durable symptomatic relief of symptoms after prostatic resection. Reoperation for recurrent obstruction has been required in approximately 15% of patients, although this may not be needed for many years. Recurrent obstruction may be caused by either regrowth of BPH with time or iatrogenic bladder neck and urethral stricture as a result of previous TURP. In such cases, a transurethral surgical approach is usually effective.

Minimally Invasive Therapy

Transurethral incision of the prostate (TUIP) is an alternative to formal prostatic resection in properly

TABLE 4. **Treatment Options for Benign Prostatic Hyperplasia**

Surgical	Minimally Invasive	Medical*
TURP	TUIP	Antiandrogen therapy
Open prostatectomy	Transurethral balloon dilatation	LHRH agonists
	Prostatic stent	Antiandrogen: Flutamide (Eulexin)
	Microwave hyperthermia	5-alpha-reductase inhibitor: Finasteride (Proscar)
	Laser ablation of the prostate	Selective alpha-adrenergic antagonists
	Cryotherapy	Terazosin (Hytrin), Doxazosin (Cardura), Prazosin (Minipress)

*Finasteride and terazosin are the only two pharmacologic agents approved by the FDA for the treatment of BPH.

Abbreviations: TURP = transurethral resection of the prostate; TUIP = transurethral incision of the prostate; LHRH = luteinizing hormone–releasing hormone.

selected patients, especially those with a minimally enlarged prostate (mass <30 grams). A single incision can be made at the 6 o'clock position of the prostatic urethra when viewed endoscopically. Alternatively, two incisions may be made, one at the 5-o'clock and one at the 7-o'clock position, extending from the ureteral orifice distally to the verumontanum.

In some cases, TUIP may be more advantageous than TURP, because it is technically easier to perform and is associated with a reduced incidence of bladder neck contracture, hemorrhage, and length of hospitalization. TUIP can be performed on an outpatient basis in properly selected patients. Occasional erectile dysfunction or retrograde ejaculation has been noted with TUIP, although to a significantly lesser extent than with TURP. The reoperation rate after 18 years was reported to be approximately 14%. TUIP, however, does not provide the opportunity to obtain histologic samples for evaluation, as does TURP; therefore, prostatic needle biopsy at the time of the procedure may be helpful to exclude an occult prostate malignancy not detected by digital rectal examination and serum prostate-specific antigen measurement. Clinical relevance of occult prostatic carcinoma is controversial.

Transurethral dilatation of the prostate (TUDP) entails the placement of a balloon catheter transurethrally to the level of the prostatic urethra and bladder neck by fluoroscopy, cystoscopy, or manual palpation. The balloon is inflated for 10 to 15 minutes to 75 to 120 French diameter (25–40 mm), depending on which of three FDA-approved dilatation systems is used. In theory, compression of the hyperplastic prostatic tissue increases the diameter of the prostatic urethra, thereby reducing the resistance to urinary flow. Such compressive forces, however, are not effective for large prostates (>50 grams), or those with prominent median lobes, which can act as a ball-valve against the bladder neck. In a recent randomized study, symptom scores improved significantly with TUDP, although they were not noticeably different from those obtained after cystoscopy. Thus, it appears that TUDP produces only moderate resolution of bladder outlet obstructive symptoms and may have only a temporary effect.

The use of a permanent intraurethral woven metal stent to maintain patency of the prostatic urethra in patients with intravesical prostatic obstruction is being investigated as a possible alterative to TURP. A specially designed deployment tool is used to endoscopically place the stent in the prostatic urethra from the bladder neck to the verumontanum. The stent must not protrude into the bladder proximally or extend into the verumontanum distally. Preliminary results have been encouraging. Results of prostate stent outcome rival those of TURP, but temporary irritative voiding symptoms are a major undesirable side effect.

Microwave hyperthermia has achieved favorable responses by reducing the mass of certain malignant solid tumors. It is currently being investigated as therapy for BPH. This modality is based on the principle that adenomatous tissue cannot dissipate heat to the same extent as normal tissue because of its aberrant blood supply. After the application of microwave hyperthermia, heat retention within the adenoma results in coagulation necrosis and subsequent shrinkage of the prostate. Microwave hyperthermia may be delivered via a transrectal or transurethral probe. The thermoequivalent dose that is delivered to the prostate is calibrated by thermosensors. Additional clinical trials are needed to fully assess the role of microwave hyperthermia for the treatment of BPH. In several reports, 30% of patients experienced temporary retention and a majority of patients developed irritative voiding symptoms after microwave hyperthermia.

Two methods for the delivery of laser energy are currently under investigation involving either direct tissue contact or free laser beam therapy. Direct contact involves focusing the energy of Nd:YAG laser light onto a sapphire tip of a conductive laser fiber. The intense heat generated at this point is endoscopically applied directly to the prostatic tissue, inducing immediate vaporization. At the terminus of the "contact" laser procedure, the obstruction has been relieved. This is in contrast to "free-beam" laser prostatectomy, in which Nd:YAG laser energy is projected onto the prostate gland. This application may be performed under direct endoscopic vision or with the assistance of ultrasound imaging. In either case, the laser energy penetrates the prostate, inducing coagulative necrosis of tissue. The depth of penetration is more uncertain than in cases of contact laser; therefore, critics caution against inadvertent injury to the rectum or sphincter mechanisms. Also troubling with regard to the free-beam technique is that, although the tissue has been irreparably damaged by the laser, time is required for the prostate to slough, relieving the obstruction. Therefore, after free-beam treatment, an indwelling urethral catheter must remain until adequate sloughing has occurred; this may require several weeks. Although laser therapy is only minimally invasive, complications have been reported, including erectile dysfunction and stress urinary incontinence, presumably from inadvertent damage to the urinary sphincter.

As with laser and microwave treatment, cryosurgery relies upon tissue necrosis to relieve outlet obstruction. Liquid nitrogen is applied through specially applied probes at sub-zero temperatures to induce cell lysis. This form of treatment is still in the very early stages of the investigational process. Historically, early attempts to treat BPH with cryotherapy were unsuccessful.

Medical Therapy

Current medical therapy for BPH includes the use of androgen deprivation therapy and selective alpha-adrenergic antagonists (see Table 4). Preliminary trials with anti-estrogen treatment are also under way, based on the demonstration of estrogen receptors on intraprostatic smooth muscle cells.

Androgen Deprivation Therapy

Androgen deprivation therapy for the treatment of BPH is based on the hypothesis that a critical level of androgen in the prostatic tissue is necessary to support hyperplasia. If this level is not maintained, prostatic size will decrease, reducing urinary outflow resistance.

Luteinizing hormone–releasing hormone (LHRH) agonists, when applied continuously, ultimately decrease the release of luteinizing hormone by the anterior pituitary, resulting in decreased androgen production. Dramatically reduced systemic testosterone levels effectively decrease prostatic cell growth, inducing involution of the gland. The decrease in prostatic size that occurs can effectively relieve infravesical prostatic obstruction. The side effects of LHRH agonists include those associated with castration, such as hot flashes (60%), impotence/loss of libido (100%), and gynecomastia (50%). Shortcomings of such treatment include the monetary expense, the requirement of chronic applications for ongoing effect, and the fact that serum PSA levels are decreased by LHRH therapy, reducing the utility of PSA for cancer screening.

Also used in androgen deprivation therapy are the antiandrogen flutamide* (Eulexin) and the 5-alpha-reductase inhibitor finasteride (Proscar). Flutamide is a nonsteroidal antiandrogen. Its mechanism of action is through competition with testosterone and dihydrotestosterone (DHT) for androgen receptor sites. Since flutamide does not possess any anti-gonadotropic or progestational activity, it does not depress plasma testosterone levels. There is some concern over a possible rebound increase in testosterone levels, due to compensation secondary to the androgen blockade, which may limit its usefulness as monotherapy.

In preliminary trials, flutamide achieved improvement in voiding symptom scores and flow rates similar to those with antiandrogen therapies. However, gynecomastia was experienced by 54% of the patients, and 49% experienced gastrointestinal side effects. Because of the high cost and incidence of effects encountered with flutamide, and the similar results with finasteride, which lacks significant side effects, it is unlikely that flutamide will be useful for BPH treatment.

Finasteride is a 5-alpha-reductase inhibitor that decreases plasma and tissue DHT to castration levels without lowering the plasma testosterone level. Necessary for the metabolism of testosterone to DHT, 5-alpha-reductase is found in high levels in the prostate. Finasteride addresses the mechanical component of BPH by decreasing the size of the prostate by approximately 25 to 30% over 6 months in preliminary studies. Although finasteride is more effective than other antiandrogen agents in the treatment of BPH, its side effect profile is extremely favorable. Fewer than 5% of patients reported decreased libido, ejaculatory disorders, or impotence.

*Not FDA approved for this indication.

Of special interest with finasteride is the recent discovery of two subtypes of 5-alpha-reductase inhibitors. Type 1 may be of clinical benefit for male pattern baldness and acne, while type 2 regulates BPH. The National Cancer Institute is also beginning a 10-year long-range study of finasteride versus placebo in men at increased risk of developing prostate carcinoma. It is important for the clinician using finasteride to know that the drug reduces PSA levels by 50%, and that PSA needs to be measured after 6 months. At the present time it is unclear whether decreasing PSA levels will limit its usefulness as a cancer screening tool.

Alpha-Adrenergic Antagonists

Given the distribution of $alpha_1$ receptors, selective $alpha_1$ antagonists have been used to promote relaxation of the bladder outlet without impairing the contractile properties of the bladder body. The relaxed state of the prostatic smooth muscle in the bladder outlet consequently decreases the resistance to urinary flow in the prostatic urethra.

$Alpha_1$ adrenergic antagonists can be either nonselective or selective. No hormonal manipulation occurs with alpha antagonist administration, obviating the side effects usually associated with medical therapy mediated by androgen suppression. Long-acting selective $alpha_1$ antagonists such as terazosin (Hytrin) and doxazosin* (Cardura) allow once-daily dosing for increased patient compliance.

Terazosin has been studied extensively and has recently gained FDA approval for the treatment of BPH symptoms. This application is based in part on three large-scale, placebo-controlled, multicenter phase III studies, results of which indicate that terazosin in 2-mg, 5-mg, and 10-mg daily doses elicited a 51%, 51%, and 69% improvement, respectively, in the total symptom score when compared with placebo.

In summary, $alpha_1$ adrenergic antagonists decrease the smooth muscle tone of the bladder neck and the prostate but do not decrease prostate size. Fifty to seventy percent of patients treated with $alpha_1$ adrenergic antagonists have noted improvement in AUA Symptom Index parameters, while 30 to 60% have demonstrated improvement in urinary flow rates; the degree of improvement is dose dependent. The treatment effect terminates if the drug is discontinued, therefore continuous effect requires continuous therapy.

The side effects of the selective $alpha_1$ antagonists are minimal. Those reported in terazosin and prazosin trials for the treatment of BPH include headache, asthenia, hypotension, and dysuria. Fewer than 10% of patients reported minimal sexual dysfunction with terazosin when compared to placebo. None of these adverse effects, however, necessitated adjustment of dosage or termination of the drug. In one trial, the additional complaint of fatigue was resolved by dosing at bedtime. This is in contrast to the side effects of the nonselective alpha-adrenergic antagonists,

*Not FDA approved for this indication.

such as phenoxybenzamine* (Dibenzyline), which are more significant and have included fatigue, dizziness, impaired ejaculation, nasal stuffiness, and decreased visual acuity.

Recent basic research has isolated at least three subtypes of the $alpha_1$ receptors with differential prostatic and vascular wall specificities. It may be possible in the near future to gain more potent and selective $alpha_1$ blockade of BPH without any adverse effects.

Combination Drug Therapy

Because of the different therapeutic profiles and side effects of $alpha_1$ antagonists and the 5-alpha-reductase inhibitor finasteride, a drug regimen using terazosin in combination with finasteride is currently under study to determine whether their concomitant use is more efficacious than either drug alone. The therapeutic effects of terazosin occur within a few days, while those of finasteride take approximately 3 to 6 months.

The diagnosis and treatment of BPH is undergoing dramatic changes. While approximately 400,000 TURPs were performed in 1988 in the United States for BPH, fewer than 180,000 were done in 1992. It is estimated that four to eight times that number of patients may seek active treatment in the near future with the availability of medical and minimally invasive therapies. Depending on a patient's symptoms, age, health, and personal preference, treatment may be surgical, minimally invasive, or medical.

PROSTATITIS

method of
JACKSON E. FOWLER, JR., M.D.
University of Mississippi Medical Center
Jackson, Mississippi

Prostatitis refers to a spectrum of real or imagined inflammatory disorders of the prostate manifested either by (1) the acute onset of severe irritative or obstructive voiding symptoms, fever, chills, and perineal or low back pain (acute prostatitis) or by (2) the complex of intermittent or chronic, ill-defined pelvic, perineal, testicular, or ejaculatory discomforts that may or may not be accompanied by irritative voiding symptoms (chronic prostatitis).

ACUTE PROSTATITIS

Acute prostatitis is an unusual disorder that is almost always caused by infection of the urine and prostate by aerobic gram-negative enteric bacteria (the Enterobacteriaceae and *Pseudomonas* species) and, rarely, *Enterococcus.* An extremely tender, enlarged, and indurated prostate is the characteristic physical finding. Pyuria (greater than five leukocytes per high-power [×400] microscopic field) is the rule.

*Not FDA approved for this indication.

Treatment

Hospitalization of the affected patient is usually advisable. Parenteral antibiotics should be administered immediately after urine and blood are obtained for culture. Intravenous ciprofloxacin* (Cipro), 200 mg every 12 hours, or ofloxacin (Floxin), 200 mg every 12 hours, is the treatment of choice. Combination therapy using gentamicin (Garamycin), 1.0 to 1.5 mg per kg of body weight every 12 hours, and ampicillin,* 1 gram every 6 hours, is a reasonable alternative. Hydration, analgesics, and stool softeners are helpful supportive measures. Acute urinary retention is not infrequent and is best managed by percutaneous cystostomy.

The response to treatment is typically rapid, and oral antimicrobial therapy using ciprofloxacin, 250 mg every 8 hours, or ofloxacin, 200 mg every 12 hours, can be instituted after 2 to 3 days. Since patients are at risk for chronic bacterial prostatitis, the treatment should be continued for 1 month. The therapeutic outcome is assessed by culture of the urine at 4 and 12 weeks after antimicrobial therapy is discontinued.

Patients who do not have a prompt response to appropriate treatment may have a prostatic abscess or a coexisting invasive renal infection. These possibilities should be investigated with computed tomography of the kidneys and prostate gland.

CHRONIC PROSTATITIS SYNDROMES

The chronic prostatitis syndromes are categorized by the presence or absence of objective evidence of prostatic inflammation and of culture-documented bacterial infection of the prostate (Table 1). Digital rectal examination of the prostate is generally unremarkable in patients with these syndromes. About 5% of men with chronic prostatitis have chronic bacterial prostatitis, about 65% have nonbacterial prostatitis, and about 30% have prostatodynia.

Chronic bacterial prostatitis is a well-defined infectious process that is caused by aerobic gram-negative enteric bacteria and, on occasion, *Enterococcus.* Most affected men have a history of frequent urinary tract infections caused by the same organism (persistent bacteriuria). In contrast, the etiology of nonbacterial prostatitis and prostatodynia is often obscure. Infec-

*Not FDA approved for this indication.

TABLE 1. **Clinical Classification of Chronic Prostatitis**

	Prostatic Inflammation	Prostatic Infection
Chronic bacterial prostatitis	+	+
Nonbacterial prostatitis	+	−
Prostatodynia	−	−

tion of the prostate by *Chlamydia trachomatis* or *Ureaplasma urealyticum* can be responsible for an occasional case of nonbacterial prostatitis, and spasticity of the external urinary sphincter can produce nonbacterial prostatitis and prostatodynia. Diseases of the bladder, anorectal disorders, neurologic disease and disorders of the pelvic viscera may also cause symptoms suggestive of prostatic inflammation. Such alternative etiologies for the symptomatology are more common in men with prostatodynia who, by definition, have no objective evidence of prostatic inflammation.

Differential Diagnosis

Inflammation of the prostate gland should be suspected if greater than 10 leukocytes per high power (×400) microscopic field are identified in the expressed prostatic fluid. Chronic bacterial prostatitis is generally associated with grossly purulent prostatic fluid, and sheets of leukocytes are visualized microscopically. The density of leukocytes in the expressed prostatic fluid is greater than 10 in men with nonbacterial prostatitis and less than 10 in men with prostatodynia. However, the density of prostatic fluid leukocytes in men with nonbacterial prostatitis and prostatodynia may be variable over time, and it can be difficult to differentiate the two disorders with any degree of certainty.

The possibility of prostatic infection is assessed by quantitative aerobic culture of the expressed prostatic fluid. If gram-negative enteric bacteria or *Enterococcus are not* isolated, the likelihood of chronic bacterial prostatitis is remote. However, expressed prostatic fluid is subject to contamination by the urine, and the urethral flora and pathogenic bacteria may be isolated from the prostatic fluid cultures of men without prostatic infection. To establish the diagnosis of chronic bacterial prostatitis with a high degree of certainty, quantitative aerobic culture of the first 10 mL of voided urine and the expressed prostatic fluid are performed to localize the infection to the prostate. Before the localization cultures are done, the patient is treated with nitrofurantoin (Macrodantin), 100 mg four times daily for 7 days, to clear pathogenic bacteria from the urethra and bladder urine. This treatment will not alter the bacteriology of the prostate and will amplify differences between the density of bacteria in the urine culture and prostatic fluid culture of men with bacterial prostatitis. As a general rule, a ten-fold increase in the density of pathogenic bacteria in the expressed prostatic fluid culture compared to the culture of the first voided urine is diagnostic of prostatic infection.

Treatment

Chronic Bacterial Prostatitis

Ciprofloxacin,* 250 mg three times daily, or ofloxacin, 200 mg twice daily, for 4 to 6 weeks is the treatment of choice for chronic bacterial prostatitis and will cure about 70% of the infections. Trimethoprim* (Proloprim or Trimpex*), 100 mg twice daily, and trimethoprim-sulfamethoxazole* (Bactrim, Septra), 160/800 mg twice daily, are less effective alternative treatments.

*Not FDA approved for this indication.

If the infection is not cured with 4 to 6 weeks of antimicrobial therapy, suppressive treatment is instituted to maintain a sterile urine. Suppressive therapy will not usually eradicate the prostatic infection, but most patients with chronic bacterial prostatitis are completely asymptomatic if the urine is uninfected. The nightly administration of ciprofloxacin,* 250 mg, ofloxacin,* 200 mg, trimethoprim, 50 mg, trimethoprim-sulfamethoxazole,* 40/200 mg, or nitrofurantoin,* 100 mg, is remarkably effective and well tolerated during long-term administration.

An extensive transurethral resection of the prostate may be curative in men with chronic bacterial prostatitis that is refractory to conventional treatment and is a reasonable consideration if there are coexisting prostatic calculi. Prostatic calculi can become secondarily infected and in most cases cannot be sterilized with antimicrobials. Surgical treatment, however, is not warranted if suppressive therapy is well tolerated and provides symptomatic relief.

Nonbacterial Prostatitis and Prostatodynia

The management of nonbacterial prostatitis and prostatodynia is by and large the same, because it may be difficult to differentiate the two conditions and because the disorders may have common etiologies. Oral doxycycline (Vibramycin), 100 mg twice daily for 7 days, is a reasonable initial treatment. However, chronic antimicrobial therapy is discouraged because evidence for an infectious etiology is limited at best and the erroneous concept of chronic infection is adopted by the patient. Urodynamic investigation is warranted to rule out spasticity of the external urinary sphincter if the symptoms persist or recur with any degree of regularity. Spasticity of the external sphincter is treated with terazosin* (Hytrin), an alpha-adrenergic blocker. Terazosin can produce symptomatic postural hypotension and should be administered at bedtime. The treatment is initiated at a dose of 1 mg and can be escalated over 4 weeks to a total dose of 10 mg. The drug is discontinued if there is no symptomatic relief.

Unrelenting symptomatology warrants a thorough investigation for extraprostatic disease. If irritative voiding symptoms predominate, interstitial cystitis or carcinoma in situ of the urinary bladder should be eliminated as diagnostic possibilities by cystoscopic examination. Magnetic resonance imaging will occasionally uncover unsuspected abnormalities of the seminal vesicles or the pelvic viscera. Neurologic evaluation is advisable if low back or groin discomfort is a major symptom, and evaluation for anorectal disease is advisable if perineal discomfort is a principal

*Not FDA approved for this indication.

complaint. Finally, men who appear emotionally unstable may benefit from psychiatric consultation.

When all conventional therapies prove ineffective and all relevant investigations are unrevealing, common sense and concern for the patient's frustrations are critical ingredients for successful management. Reassurance that the symptoms are not related to cancer or known sexual transmissible disorders and will not lead to impotence or infertility is rewarding.

ACUTE RENAL FAILURE

method of
GUILLERMO R. SAURINA, M.D., and
JOSEPH V. BONVENTRE, M.D., Ph.D.
Massachusetts General Hospital, Harvard Medical School and Harvard-MIT Division of Health Sciences and Technology
Boston, Massachusetts

Acute renal failure (ARF) is a clinical state characterized by rapid deterioration in renal function leading to accumulation of waste products of metabolism and abnormal fluid and electrolyte homeostasis. ARF develops in 2 to 5% of patients in tertiary care institutions and frequently is iatrogenic. Although potentially reversible in many cases, ARF has an associated mortality of 40 to 50%, and there has been little change in this mortality rate over the last four decades despite advances in therapy. To quote from the National Kidney and Urological Diseases Advisory Board 1990 Long Range Plan, "Acute renal failure is the most costly kidney or urologic condition requiring hospitalization."

ARF is defined by an increase in plasma creatinine concentration of at least 0.5 mg per dL if baseline is less than 3.0 mg per dL or 1.0 mg per dL if baseline is more than 3.0 over a period of days. Usually there is a proportional increase in blood urea nitrogen (BUN); however, since urea originates from catabolism of protein, hypercatabolic states, use of steroids, hyperalimentation, or increased absorption of protein owing to the presence of blood in the gastrointestinal tract can increase BUN out of proportion to increases in creatinine. Other states characterized by muscle damage and enhanced release of creatinine, such as crush injury with myoglobinuric acute tubular necrosis (ATN), can increase creatinine at a much greater rate than they can in BUN. ARF is classified as oliguric if urinary output is less than 400 mL per 24 hours or nonoliguric if urine output is greater than 400 mL per 24 hours. When there is intrinsic kidney injury, nonoliguric ARF has a better prognosis than oliguric ARF.

The causes of ARF can been classified into three categories—prerenal, intrinsic, and postrenal (Table 1)—and this classification is useful for diagnostic and therapeutic purposes. Prerenal ARF infers no functionally significant injury to the renal parenchymal tissue itself. There is deterioration in renal function because of decreased blood flow to the kidney as might arise from systemic hypotension, decreased intravascular volume, or renal artery stenosis. If prerenal ARF persists and/or worsens and if oxygen delivery to the tissue is impaired, then tubular necrosis can occur and pathologic findings of ATN will be seen if the kidney is examined histologically. Functionally, ATN is associated with impaired ability of the tubule to reabsorb sodium, excrete potassium and acid, and concentrate the urine. Prerenal ARF and ischemic ATN account for more than two-thirds of the cases of ARF, particularly when ARF develops in the hospital setting.

TABLE 1. **Causes of Acute Renal Failure**

Prerenal
- *Decreased effective intravascular volume*
  - Hypovolemia
    - Hemorrhage
    - Skin losses (e.g., burns, sweat)
    - Renal losses (e.g., diuretics, diabetes insipidus, salt-wasting nephropathy)
    - Gastrointestinal losses (e.g., diarrhea, vomiting, surgical drainage)
  - Volume redistribution without a decrease in total body water
    - Pancreatitis
    - Liver disease with ascites
    - Sepsis
    - Anaphylaxis
  - Cardiac dysfunction
- *Selective renal ischemia*
  - Renal artery stenosis
  - Surgical occlusion of renal artery

Intrinsic Renal
- *Glomerular*
  - Primary glomerulonephritis (e.g., membranoproliferative glomerulonephritis)
  - Glomerulonephritis secondary to systemic disease (e.g., postinfectious glomerulonephritis, systemic lupus erythematosus, Goodpasture's syndrome, Wegener's granulomatosis)
- *Tubulointerstitial*
  - Ischemia
  - Contrast agents
  - Nephrotoxins: aminoglycosides, other drugs, heavy metals
  - Pigments: hemoglobin, myoglobin (rhabdomyolysis)
  - Intratubular deposition (uric acid, myeloma)
  - Allergic interstitial nephritis: drug-induced
- *Vascular*
  - Malignant hypertension
  - Vasculitis
  - Microangiopathy
  - Embolism, thrombosis

Postrenal
- *Intrapelvic or intraureteral obstruction*
  - Calculi, blood clots, crystals, tumor, papillary necrosis
- *Extrinsic obstruction of ureter*
  - Retroperitoneal fibrosis, tumor
- *Bladder outflow obstruction*
  - Prostatic hypertrophy, calculi, blood clots, functional neuropathy
- *Urethral obstruction*
  - Phimosis, meatal stenosis, stricture

A large number of intrinsic kidney diseases can result in ARF. Any glomerular or interstitial renal disease whose onset is abrupt or that enters a state of rapid deterioration can result in ARF. A large number of cases of ARF are secondary to drug use and hence iatrogenic. Aminoglycosides are a major contributor to ARF. This class of antibiotic and other drugs and toxins cause tubular necrosis. Other drugs can cause ARF secondary to allergic interstitial nephritis. Atheroemboli lodging in the arterioles and glomeruli represent an important cause of ARF, especially in the patient with generalized atherosclerotic disease who has had an invasive procedure that can dislodge the atherosclerotic plaques.

Postrenal ARF results from any condition in which decreased renal function results from obstruction: a prominent example is prostatic hypertrophy. Other causes of postrenal ARF include retroperitoneal fibrosis and lymphoma that obstructs both ureters. When evaluating a patient, it is useful to categorize ARF as prerenal, intrinsic, or postrenal, as the therapeutic approach differs substantially for each.

DIAGNOSIS

History and Physical Examination

The diagnosis and categorization of ARF should start with a thorough history focusing on systemic diseases that can cause renal dysfunction, such as diabetes mellitus, hypertension, systemic lupus erythematosus; drug use (nonsteroidal anti-inflammatory agents, antibiotics, intravenous drug abuse); or recent surgery or invasive procedures with potential ischemia, hypotension, or exposure to contrast media. It is important to know the values of previous measures of renal function to evaluate how acute the process is. A history of hemoptysis may suggest a pulmonary-renal syndrome such as Goodpasture's syndrome or Wegener's granulomatosis. Finally, a history of prostatism, previous urinary tract obstruction or stones, or systemic signs or symptoms of malignancy help in the consideration of postrenal failure.

The physical examination can provide important additional clues to the diagnosis. Postural hypotension, tachycardia, sunken eyes, poor skin turgor, and flat neck veins all indicate volume depletion. Ascites/edema suggests the possibility of redistribution of body fluids with resultant intravascular depletion. A rash may be associated with allergic interstitial nephritis. Needle tracks are seen in patients with intravenous drug abuse. Retinopathy may provide evidence for severe diabetes mellitus or hypertension with end-organ vascular damage. Adenopathy is seen in lymphoma, metastatic disease, and acquired immune deficiency syndrome (AIDS). Nasal ulcers and otitis can be present in Wegener's granulomatosis. Hemoptysis may indicate Goodpasture's syndrome or Wegener's granulomatosis. Regurgitant murmurs suggest the possibility of endocarditis. Flank pain may indicate pyelonephritis, renal vein thrombosis, renal infarcts, or obstruction. Abdominal bruits can be present in patients with renal artery stenosis or an abdominal aortic aneurysm, which can interrupt blood flow to the kidneys. A percussible bladder or enlarged prostate may suggest obstruction.

Urinanalysis

Examination of the urine can provide a great deal of information regarding the cause of the ARF. Ideally, the specimen should be fresh, since blood cells and casts tend to deteriorate. A red color can be due to hematuria, myoglobinuria, porphyria, or drugs (rifampin, phenolphthalein). The urine can be blue-green in color in *Pseudomonas* infection or in a patient taking biliverdine, blue dyes, or amitriptyline. A white color suggests pyuria or chyluria. Hematuria is seen in trauma, stones, cystitis, tumors, intrinsic renal disease, and hematologic disorders of coagulation. It must be noted, however, that the most common cause of hematuria in women of reproductive age is menstruation. In hospitalized patients, blood in the urine is often due to trauma from urethral catheters. Hemoglobinuria in the absence of red blood cells can be secondary to hemolysis due to drugs, parasites, chemicals, incompatible blood transfusions, marching or running, paroxysmal nocturnal hemoglobinuria, or favism. Myoglobinuria can occur secondary to tissue damage, seizures, crush injuries, heat stroke, muscle diseases, and, in general, any cause of rhabdomyolysis.

In the absence of any urinary substances of high density, such as contrast material or glucose in high concentrations, a high specific gravity of greater than 1.020 suggests that the kidney is able to concentrate the urine and hence suggests that the ARF is prerenal. If tubular function and concentrating ability are impaired, as with intrinsic ARF or in patients on loop diuretics, the urine specific gravity is reflective of an isosthenuric state (approximately 1.010). Although urinary osmolarity usually correlates well with specific gravity, osmolality is less affected by large molecular weight urinary components such as contrast media, glucose, or protein. A high urine pH, especially in the setting of systemic acidosis, suggests an infection with urea-splitting organisms, as might occur with staghorn calculi with obstruction.

Nephrotic range proteinuria suggests glomerulonephritis as the cause of ARF, although atheroembolic disease can also result in significant proteinuria (3 to 4 grams per 24 hours) if there are emboli to the glomerular capillaries. If the dipstick test for protein is negative, the presence of proteins other than albumin can be detected by adding sulfosalicylic acid. Free light chains are excreted in diseases such as multiple myeloma, lymphoma, macroglobulinemia and amyloidosis in which there may be little reactivity of the urine with the dipstick but a strong positive response with sulfosalicylic acid. Glucose in the urine suggests diabetes mellitus, but it can also be secondary to tubular damage resulting in decreased reabsortion. Urinary ketones are seen in diabetes, starvation, severe liver damage, and fever.

A great deal of information can be obtained from analysis of the urinary sediment, which is obtained from 10 to 15 mL of urine centrifuged at approximately 2000 rpm for about 5 minutes. Dysmorphic red blood cells, which lose their halo when examined with phase contrast microscopy, usually derive from the kidney itself rather than from a postrenal source. Therefore, dysmorphic red blood cells suggest glomerulonephritis, severe hypertension, atheroemboli, papillary necrosis, toxins, disorders of coagulation, other renal diseases such as polycystic kidney disease, and systemic disorders affecting the kidney, such as systemic lupus erythematosus and tuberculosis. Red blood cell casts also imply renal hematuria and are suggestive of, but not diagnostic of, glomerulonephritis, as other renal pathologic processes such as trauma, renal infarction, severe pyelonephritis, interstitial nephritis, and severe hypertension can also generate red blood cell casts. White blood cells are found in the urinary sediment of patients with bladder infection, prostatitis, or renal parenchymal interstitial inflammation secondary to various inflammatory processes, such as those related to collagen vascular disease, urinary tract infections, or allergic interstitial nephritis. The presence of eosinophils suggests allergic interstitial nephritis or atheroemboli. The presence of white cell casts localizes the source of the white cells within the cast to the kidney and hence is useful in distinguishing intrinsic renal from postrenal processes. Renal tubular epithelial cells are the most sensitive indicator of tubular damage. Casts containing granular material of a coarse or fine nature, especially if they are muddy brown in appearance, or epithelial cells, are indicative of tubular damage. Calcium oxalate crystals are seen in ethylene glycol poisoning, and uric acid crystals may be present in acute urate nephropathy as might occur with tumor lysis resulting in a very large urate load to the kidney and intratubular obstruction. The presence of squamous epithelial cells in the specimen are indicative of contamination with vaginal flora.

Urinary Indices

The fractional excretion of sodium FE_{Na} represents the percent of the filtered sodium load that is excreted and is calculated as follows:

$$FE_{Na}(\%) = \{([Na_u]/[Na_p])/([Cr_u]/[Cr_p])\} \times 100,$$

where $[Na_u]$ and $[Na_p]$ are the urine and plasma sodium concentrations, respectively, and $[Cr_u]$ and $[Cr_p]$ the creatinine concentrations in the urine and plasma, respectively. If $FE_{Na}(\%)$ is less than 1%, the ARF is likely to be prerenal, because tubular function, as assessed by the ability to reabsorb sodium, is well preserved. A low FE_{Na}, however, can also be seen in other conditions in which tubular function is partially preserved even though the insult is intrinsic to the kidney or is postrenal, such as in early contrast media nephrotoxicity, acute interstitial nephritis, early obstruction, early myoglobinuric ARF, and acute glomerulonephritis. A $[Na_u]$ of less than 10 mEq per liter is most consistent with prerenal ARF, whereas a $[Na_u]$ of greater than 20 mEq per liter is most consistent with intrinsic causes of ARF or with postrenal causes. High urinary osmolality and urine/plasma creatinine ratios reflect good tubular function, whereas a urinary osmolality of less than 350 mOsm and a urine/creatinine ratio of less than 20 indicates tubular dysfunction and, hence, intrinsic renal or chronic postrenal ARF. Creatinine clearance must be interpreted with caution in patients with ARF because they are often not in a steady state and because serum creatinine is changing continuously. In addition, tubular secretion of creatinine is altered in ARF. Table 2 lists various indices that are useful in distinguishing among the three general categories of ARF: prerenal, intrinsic renal, and postrenal.

Additional Blood Tests

When the history does not suggest an obvious cause for ARF, additional blood tests may help in the differential diagnosis. An antineutrophil cytoplasmic antibody (ANCA) is present in the blood of patients with Wegener's granulomatosis. Anti–glomerular basement membrane antibodies are present in Goodpasture's syndrome. Low serum complement levels suggest postinfectious glomerulonephritis, systemic lupus erythematosus, or membranoproliferative glomerulonephritis.

Radiologic Studies

Ultrasound is a noninvasive way to evaluate the urinary tract for obstruction. In addition, it provides valuable information regarding kidney size that can provide insight into the chronicity of the renal failure in patients in whom sufficient information regarding past renal function is unavailable. Chronic renal disease frequently results in reduction in kidney size. The exceptions to this rule include multiple myeloma, diabetes mellitus, AIDS, amyloidosis, infiltrative lesions, polycystic kidney disease, and renal vein thrombosis, each of which can be associated with kidneys of normal size or even increased size. Asymmetric kidney size is seen in renal vascular disease. Ultrasound also helps to identify renal cysts or stones.

Other radiologic tests are useful in evaluating renal vascular disease in a patient believed to have prerenal ARF. While the renal radionucleotide scan is most helpful in establishing unilateral renal artery disease, it is less useful in distinguishing bilateral renal vascular disease from intrinsic renal parenchymal disease. Both kidneys are involved in ARF and so the renal scan is of limited value. Recently, magnetic resonance imaging has been successfully applied to the evaluation of renal vascular perfusion. This study is less invasive than renal arteriography, which carries with it the added risk of dislodging atherosclerotic plaques into the renal vascular bed and exposure to contrast media.

TABLE 2. **Diagnostic Indices***

	Prerenal	Intrinsic	Postrenal†
Urine sodium (mEq/L)	<10	>20	>20
Urine chloride (mEq/L)	<10	>20	>20
FE_{Na}	<1%	>2%	>2%
Urine osmolarity (mOsm)	>500	<350	<350
Urine/serum (creatinine)	>40	<20	<20

*While these indices are helpful, there are exceptions to these general guidelines that preclude a definitive diagnosis being made with this information only.

†Diagnostic indices in early obstruction can mimic prerenal azotemia.

Biopsy

A renal biopsy is generally not necessary to establish the diagnosis of ARF. In cases, however, when all other clinical and laboratory investigations have failed to identify the problem, and when a therapeutic decision depends on tissue diagnosis, a biopsy is indicated. If the patient is uremic, platelet count, prothrombin times, partial thromboblastin times, and bleeding time should be checked to minimize the chance of bleeding with the procedure.

THERAPY

General Aspects of Management

If the patient has prerenal azotemia, therapy should be directed toward enhancing renal perfusion, for example, by enhancing cardiac output or correcting an anatomic problem with percutaneous angioplasty or surgery to restore the patency of the lumen of the renal arteries. Postrenal causes of ARF should be approached by expeditious relief of the urinary tract obstruction. Drugs implicated in the generation of ARF should be discontinued. Those forms of glomerulonephritis that respond to therapy, such as Wegener's granulomatosis or Goodpasture's syndrome, should be treated as soon as the diagnosis is made and in some cases treated presumptively with steroids prior to the confirmation of the diagnosis as early treatment is critical. In most cases of ARF, however, there is no specific therapy currently available to hasten the recovery of the kidney. This is the case, for example, with postischemic ARF.

Fluid Management

The fluid status of the patient must be carefully evaluated, and in most cases, this can be done by physical examination. Under some circumstances, however, especially in patients with cardiopulmonary disease, invasive techniques are necessary to adequately assess systemic hemodynamic determinants of renal perfusion. The patient with prerenal ARF due to inadequate intravascular volume should be given crystalloid or colloid solutions. If the patient has oliguric ARF due to intrinsic parenchymal disease, it is important to avoid fluid overload. Careful records of fluid input and output should be kept along with daily weights. Intake should equal urinary output plus insensible losses, which are about 500 mL per 24 hours in afebrile patients, with marked increases in the febrile patient. The information one derives from input-output balances and daily weights has to be interpreted in the context of any third-space losses that occur, so that daily physical examination of the patient with specific attention to the cardiopulmonary examination is essential for drawing up daily fluid replacement orders. In the oliguric patient with severe ascites, extra precautions must be taken to avoid intravascular depletion and further decreases in effective arterial blood volume.

Diuretics. There is evidence that mortality and morbidity rates are lower in nonoliguric ARF than in oliguric ARF. This likely reflects the fact that patients with nonoliguric ARF as a group have less severe ARF. Nevertheless, it is often recommended that an attempt be made to enhance urine flow using a potent loop diuretic, such as furosemide, bumetamide, or mannitol, sometimes in combination with dopamine. While there is no consistent evidence that this therapy enhances patient survival, it is certainly the case that a patient with 1 to 2 liters of urine output per day is easier to manage, because most of the time obligate fluid inputs are greater than insensible losses as a result of necessary antibiotics or nutritional support. The effect of loop diuretics can be enhanced with concomitant use of a diuretic that acts in the distal nephron beyond the loop of Henle, such as metolazone or one of the thiazides. The usual starting dose of furosemide (Lasix) is 40 mg intravenously, with progressive increases to 80 to 200 mg if there is no response to the lower doses. In large cumulative doses, furosemide can cause hearing loss. Metolazone (Zaroxolyn), is given as 5 to 10 mg orally. Thiazides can be given orally or intravenously, 0.5 to 2.0 grams of chlorothiazide per day. Potassium-sparing diuretics, such as spironolactone (Aldactone), amiloride (Midamor), and triamterene (Dyrenium), should be avoided or used with extreme caution in ARF to avoid hyperkalemia.

Dopamine. When used in low doses (1 to 3 μg per kg per minute), dopamine increases renal blood flow and glomerular filtration rate and has been found to enhance urinary output in patients with ARF refractory to mannitol and furosemide. Hence, it is often administered along with diuretics to enhance urine output in patients with ARF. Dopamine has not been proved, however, to change the outcome of ARF.

Metabolic Abnormalities

Hyperkalemia. Hyperkalemia, a serious threat in ARF, results from decreased urinary excretion and redistribution from the intracellular compartment secondary to the acidosis usually associated with ARF. Potassium intake should be restricted. Severe hyperkalemia (plasma potassium levels higher than 7.0 mEq per liter or loss of P waves on the electrocardiogram) requires immediate treatment: 10 to 20 mL of a 10% solution of calcium gluconate infused over 10 minutes can protect the heart by reducing the threshold potential and decreasing the possibility of arrhythmias. This effect occurs within 5 to 10 minutes. Sodium bicarbonate (50 to 100 mL containing 50 to 100 mEq of bicarbonate) should be administered intravenously to treat the acidosis and hence promote potassium reuptake into cells (Table 3). This treatment should take effect rapidly. Glucose and insulin (250 mL of 20% glucose with 10 units of regular insulin), administered intravenously over 20 minutes, also promotes redistribution of potassium back into the intracellular compartment. This therapy reaches peak effect within 30 to 60 minutes. Sodium polystyrene sulfonate (Kayexalate), an ion exchange resin that binds potassium in exchange for sodium, effectively decreases total body potassium. Twenty-five to 50 grams are given orally every 2 to 4 hours with sorbitol to prevent constipation; alternatively, 50 to 100 grams can be given rectally. It should be noted, however, that sorbitol can cause intestinal necrosis. Kaliuretic diuretics, such as furosemide or the thiazides, also effectively decrease total body potassium when there is urinary output. Refractory cases of hyperkalemia should be treated with dialysis.

Acidosis. Metabolic acidosis in ARF occurs because of the decreased ability of the kidneys to excrete acid. Unless there is a high catabolic state, the acidosis of renal failure can be often treated with oral or intravenous sodium bicarbonate, especially if the patient is nonoliguric and can handle the sodium and volume load associated with this therapy. Severe acidosis that is not readily treatable is an indication for dialysis.

Hyperphosphatemia and Hypocalcemia. Hyperphosphatemia is due to impaired excretion of phosphates when the glomerular filtration rate falls below 25 to 30 mL per minute. In ARF caused by rhabdomyolysis, tumor lysis, or acute lymphoblastic leukemia, there is also excess liberation of phosphates from tissues. Hyperphosphatemia can lead to soft tissue calcification, especially when the calcium-phosphate product exceeds 70 when each is expressed as milligrams per deciliter. Hyperphosphatemia can cause hypocalcemia and cardiac conduction defects. Hyperphosphatemia is treated by decreasing intake and administering phosphate binders (e.g., calcium carbonate, calcium acetate, or aluminum hydroxide). Although aluminum-containing antacids can lead to aluminum accumulation with anemia, osteomalacia, and possibly dementia in patients on long-term therapy, these agents can be used for short-term therapy. Hypocalcemia is not usually symptomatic because acidosis helps to enhance ionized calcium levels. However, if acidosis is corrected rapidly without rec-

TABLE 3. **Treatment of Hyperkalemia**

Treatment		Onset
1. Antagonize membrane effect of hyperkalemia		
10% calcium chloride, 50 mL IV over 10 min		Onset: 2–5 min
2. Provoke intracellular shifts of potassium		
Sodium bicarbonate, 50–100 mL, containing 50–100 mEq IV		Onset: 10–20 min
Regular insulin, 10 units IV, with 250 mL of 20% glucose		Onset: 10–20 min
3. Promote potassium elimination		
Sodium polystyrene sulfonate	15–45 gm PO every 2–4 h	Onset: 1–2 h
Sodium polystyrene sulfonate	50–100 gm PR every 2–4 h	Onset: 30–60 min
IV diuresis: Furosemide, 40–200 mg		Onset: 15 min
Hemodialysis: Removes 30–40 mEq/h of potassium		
Peritoneal dialysis: Removes about 5 mEq/h of potassium		

ognition of the potential effects on ionized serum calcium levels, tetany can be precipitated.

Hyperuricemia. Uric acid levels are frequently elevated in patients with ARF; however, in most patients, no therapy is indicated if levels remain below 15 mg per dL. Very rarely, a gouty attack is precipitated, in which case the temporary use of colchicine or steroids is indicated. There is no evidence that elevation in serum uric acid levels has a detrimental effect on kidney recovery from ARF.

Hematologic Abnormalities

While patients with ARF without prior renal disease most often present with near normal hematocrits, several factors contribute to anemia in ARF. In the setting of frequent phlebotomies in the hospital, erythropoietin production decreases as kidney function decreases. Uremia reduces the survival time of the red blood cells, and there is an increased bleeding tendency because of platelet dysfunction. If bleeding is a problem, the platelet disorder can be corrected in the short term with 1-deamino-8-D-arginine vasopressin (DDAVP) administered intravenously at a dose of 0.3 μg per kg body weight. The hemostatic effect is seen approximately 1 hour after administration and persists for approximately 6 hours. Conjugated estrogens (e.g., Premarin) or cryoprecipitate can also help to counteract the platelet disorder of uremia. Premarin can be given at a dose of 10 to 50 mg per day. Blood transfusions are given if necessary, but their use is minimized to avoid sensitization in patients who may ultimately go on to end-stage renal disease and become candidates for renal transplant. If necessary, filtered leukocyte-free blood can be administered to this population of patients to minimize sensitization.

Cardiovascular Complications

Hypertension and pulmonary edema are frequently present in patients with ARF in the setting of volume overload. The best treatment is prevention. If the kidneys are refractory to diuretics, hypertension can be treated with vasodilators. Care should be taken not to decrease blood pressure too precipitously as the kidney is not able to autoregulate blood flow in the face of reductions in perfusion pressure, and hence rapid reductions in blood pressure can precipitate renal ischemia. Refractory pulmonary edema and difficult-to-manage hypertension are indications for dialysis. Cardiac arrhythmias in patients with ARF are generally caused by electrolyte disturbances, and therapy should be directed at correcting those abnormalities as described previously.

Infection

Many patients diagnosed with ARF die from infectious complications. Uremia leads to suppression of the body's natural defense mechanisms, and it is critical to appreciate this propensity for infection and to take steps to minimize the risk to patients. These steps include minimizing exposure to urinary catheters, prompt evaluation of leukocytosis, and judicious use of antibiotic therapy with dose adjustment for the level of renal function.

Nutrition

Several factors contribute to malnutrition in renal failure. There is poor intake due to the underlying disease and uremic toxins. Increased catabolism in ARF is due to multiple factors as a consequence of the underlying disease itself as well as to the uremic state. Dialysis can enhance the rate of protein breakdown as well as deplete water-soluble vitamins. Protein loss across the peritoneal membrane of patients on peritoneal dialysis can amount to several grams per day.

It remains controversial whether hyperalimentation alters the outcome in patients with ARF. Protein of high biologic value should be restricted to 0.5 to 0.7 grams per kg of body weight if the patient is not being dialyzed, and this amount should be increased in the hypercatabolic patient or once dialysis is initiated. If the patient is being fed parentally, 10 to 20 grams of essential amino acids per day are appropriate, with the addition of 10 to 20 grams of nonessential amino acids if the patient is undergoing dialysis.

A high caloric intake helps to minimize negative nitrogen balance in ARF. The patient should receive approximately 30 kcal per kg of body weight per day with this amount increased when the underlying disease results in a high catabolic state (e.g., trauma, burns, sepsis). The goal should be to maintain lean body weight. Because of the frequent need to decrease water intake, glucose is administered as a 20 to 70% solution of glucose monohydrate. When highly concentrated glucose solutions are administered, a central line should be used to prevent sclerosis in peripheral veins. Calories should also be given in the form of fat emulsions since the calorie value is twice that of glucose by weight and essential fatty acid deficiency is prevented with their use. Thirty to 40% of infused calories should be given as lipid emulsion. Patients on dialysis should be given vitamins, including folic acid, pyridoxine, and ascorbic acid. There are commercial preparations that contain all three.

TABLE 5. **Replacement Therapies**

Hemodialysis	
Advantages	Fast; relatively efficient; requires minimal patient effort/education; easy access for blood, medications; less risk of infection
Disadvantages	Requires machine and skilled personnel; risks for hypotension, bleeding, disequilibrium syndrome, hypoxia, complement activation, and reactions to membrane
Peritoneal Dialysis	
Advantages	No need for special machines; minimal anticoagulation; less cardiovascular stress; less fluid shifts; allows more independence for the patient
Disadvantages	More risk of infections; protein loss; hyperglycemia; avoid in patients with recent abdominal surgery
CAVHD or CVVHD	
Advantages	Because it is continuous, it is more physiologic with less fluid shifts and better control of volume and electrolytes; relatively simple to use
Disadvantages	Requires ICU setting, anticoagulation; less efficient than hemodialysis

Abbreviations: CAVHD = continuous arteriovenous hemodialysis; CVVHD = continuous venous-venous hemodialysis.

Dialysis and Hemofiltration

Indications for initiation of dialysis are listed in Table 4. There are various technical approaches to replacement therapy once the patient has progressed to the point at which conservative measures are no longer adequate. These approaches include hemodialysis (HD) and its variations—ultrafiltration, continuous arteriovenous hemodialysis (CAVHD), and continuous venous-venous hemodialysis (CVVHD)—and peritoneal dialysis (PD). The advantages and disadvantages of each mode of therapy are presented in Table 5.

Hemodialysis. All forms of hemodialysis require access to the vasculature, which can be temporary via the femoral, subclavian, or internal jugular veins, or more permanent, in the form of a fistula, Perma-Cath catheter, or graft. Hemodialysis offers the advantage of high-efficiency correction of fluid and electrolyte abnormalities and removal of waste products of metabolism. Its use is intermittent, and hence exposure to the dialysis membrane, extracorporeal circulation, and heparin are time limited. Other advantages include the fact that it requires minimal patient and nursing participation (other than that of the dialysis staff). Hemodialysis provides easy access for blood transfusions and medications, and confers less risk of infection than other modalities. Complications include hypotension, hypoxia, clotting, disequilibrium syndrome (attributed to central nervous system edema from rapid fluid shifts due to acute reduction in systemic osmolality), and problems related to vascular access.

TABLE 4. **Indications for Dialysis**

Fluid overload
Intractable acidosis
Hyperkalemia refractory to treatment
Symptomatic uremia (pericarditis, encephalopathy, neuropathy, bleeding)
Some overdoses/intoxications

Ultrafiltration. Ultrafiltration is similar technically to hemodialysis, but no dialysate is used. This allows for removal of large amounts of fluids due to the fact that patients tolerate hemodynamically high transmembrane pressure gradients. Since there is no dialysate on the non-blood side of the ultrafiltration membrane, there is much less change in the chemical composition of the blood during ultrafiltration than with hemodialysis. This results in fewer hemodynamic changes, and it is the ideal method when the primary indication for treatment is fluid overload. Frequently, the patient is treated first with ultrafiltration and then with hemodialysis if both fluid removal and dialysis are indicated.

Continuous Arteriovenous and Venovenous Hemofiltration. CAVHD and CVVHD provide continuous renal replacement in the setting of ARF. A small filter is used. In CAVHD, the patient's arterial pressure is sufficient to move the blood through the extracaporeal circuit, whereas in CVVHD, a pump is required. One advantage of these approaches is that they are a continuous form of therapy, which is generally better tolerated hemodynamically than intermittent hemodialysis, particularly if the patient has low blood pressure. In addition, these modalities allow for fine control of water and electrolyte balance, especially in the face of the various other disease processes that are operant in these patients. Disadvantages of these modalities include the need for continuous anticoagulation and for constant nursing care, which generally obligates the patient to be nonambulatory in an intensive care unit setting.

TABLE 6. **Adjustments for Some Commonly Prescribed Drugs in ARF**

Drugs That Do Not Require Adjustment

alprazolam (Xanax)	flurazepam (Dalmane)	metoprolol (Lopressor)
amiodarone (Cordarone)	furosemide (Lasix)	miconazole (Monistat)
amitriptyline (Elavil)	gemfibrozil (Lopid)	minoxidil (Loniten)
bromocriptine (Parlodel)	glipizide (Glucotrol)	nifedipine (Procardia)
carbidopa (Lodosyn)	griseofulvin (Gris-PEG)	nitroglycerin (Nitrostat)
cefoperazone (Cefobid)	haloperidol (Haldol)	pentobarbital (Nembutal)
ceftriaxone (Rocephin)	heparin	pentoxifylline (Trental)
chloramphenicol (Chloromycetin)	ibuprofen (Motrin, Advil)	phenytoin (Dilantin)
clindamycin (Cleocin)	indomethacin (Indocin)	piroxicam (Feldene)
clonazepam (Klonopin)	imipramine (Tofranil)	prazosin (Minipress)
clonidine (Catapres)	isosorbide (Isordil, Sorbitrate)	propranolol (Inderal)
diazepam (Valium)	isradipine (DynaCirc)	propafenone (Rythmol)
diazoxide (Hyperstat IV)	itraconazole (Sporanox)	rifampin (Rifadin)
dicloxacillin (Dynapen)	ketoconazole (Nizoral)	secobarbital (Seconal)
diphenhydramine (Benadryl)	labetalol (Trandate, Normodyne)	semisodium valproate (Depakote, Depakene)
diltiazem (Cardizem)	levodopa (Larodopa)	steroids
dipyridamole (Persantine)	lidocaine (Xylocaine)	streptokinase (Streptase)
dobutamine (Dobutrex)	lorazepam (Ativan)	sulindac (Clinoril)
esmolol (Brevibloc)	lovastatin (Mevacor)	theophylline (Theo-dur)
fluoxetine (Prozac)	metolazone (Zaroxolyn)	verapamil (Calan, Isoptin)

Dose Interval Adjustment for Some Commonly Prescribed Drugs

Drug	*Dose Interval:* GFR 10–50 mL/min EVERY ___ HRS	GFR <10 mL/min EVERY ___ HRS
acetazolamide* (Diamox)	12	—
acyclovir (Zovirax)	12	24
amantidine (Symmetrel)	48	96
amikacin (Amikan)	12	24–48
amphotericin (Fungizone)	24	24–36
cefazolin (Ancef, Kefzol)	12	24–48
ceftazidime (Fortaz, Tazidime, Tazicef)	12	24–48
cefotaxime (Claforan)	12	24–48
cefoxitin (Mefoxin)	12	24–48
cefuroxime (Zinacef, Kefurox)	12	24–48
cephalexin (Keflex)	6	8–12
chlorpropamide* (Diabinese)	24	—
ethacrynic acid* (Edecrin)	8–12	—
ethambutol (Myambutol)	24–36	48
digoxin (Lanoxin)	36	48
fluconazole (Diflucan)	24–48	48–72
gentamicin (Garamycin)	12	24–48
methyldopa (Aldomet)	12	24
pentamidine (Pentam 300)	24–36	48
procainamide (Pronestyl)	6–12	8–24
spironolactone* (Aldactone)	12–24	—
sulfamethoxazole (Gantanol)	18	24
tobramycin (Nebcin)	12	24–48

*Avoid if glomerular filtration rate (GFR) is less than 10 mL/min.

From Bennett WM, Aronoff GR, Golper TA, et al: Drug Prescribing in Renal Failure, Dosing Guidelines for Adults, 2nd ed. Philadelphia, American College of Physicians, 1991.

Peritoneal Dialysis. Peritoneal dialysis typically involves infusion of 1 to 2 liters of dialysate fluid into the peritoneal cavity. The dialysate contains 1.5, 2.5, or 4.25 grams per dL of glucose to provide an osmotic gradient across the peritoneal membrane. The fluid is left in the cavity for variable periods to allow dialysis to occur and is then drained. Peritoneal dialysis can be done as often as every hour, does not require machines or systemic anticoagulation, and produces less stress on the cardiovascular system. Complications include high risk for peritonitis, hyperglycemia, and protein loss. Peritoneal dialysis should be used with extreme caution or avoided in patients who have undergone abdominal surgery. Because of increased abdominal distention with decreased diaphragmatic mobility, pulmonary function may be further compromised in severe pulmonary disease.

Prevention

In many cases, ARF cannot be predicted and hence cannot be prevented. There are, however, a large number of patients at increased risk in whom close attention to fluid status, judicious use of diuretics, and avoidance of nephrotoxin exposure may prevent ARF. Risk factors include patients with pre-existing renal disease, volume depletion, diabetes, myeloma, liver disease, or vascular disease. Patients undergoing surgery, especially when the surgery results in hypotension or mechanical interruption of renal vascular perfusion, are particularly prone to ARF, as are patients with septicemia. It must be remembered that many commonly used drugs are cleared from the body by the kidney and hence have a prolonged half-life in ARF, and doses and/or dosing intervals of these agents must be modified (Table 6). Although there is a great deal of ongoing research to evaluate the role of potential mediators of ARF, such as endothelin, adhesion molecules, and leukocyte activation, which if blocked therapeutically might alter the natural history of the disease, at present there is no specific therapy once ARF is established.

CHRONIC RENAL FAILURE

method of
MICHAEL C. SMITH, M.D., and
MICHAEL J. DUNN, M.D.
Case Western Reserve University School of Medicine
Cleveland, Ohio

Chronic renal failure (CRF) is a major health problem in the United States. Currently, over 125,000 patients receive maintenance hemodialysis or peritoneal dialysis, and several thousand are the recipients of kidney transplants each year. The incidence of end-stage renal disease (ESRD) in the United States is 40,000 cases per year, and total expenditure for patients with ESRD exceeds 7 billion dollars. The most common causes of ESRD are shown in Table 1. Diabetes mellitus with diabetic nephropathy accounts for approximately 30% of all cases of ESRD. Arteriolar nephrosclerosis due to hypertension causes 25% of ESRD, whereas chronic glomerulonephritis (20%), polycystic kidney disease (15%), and chronic interstitial nephritis account for the remainder.

Renal failure is diagnosed by documenting a reduction in nephron mass. Because glomerular filtration rate (GFR) declines in proportion to the loss of nephrons, estimates of GFR, such as serum creatinine concentration or creatinine clearance, can be used to approximate the decrease in total renal mass. The blood urea nitrogen (BUN) concentration is less useful as a measure of renal function since it is dependent on factors other than GFR (e.g., dietary protein intake, extracellular fluid volume).

ACUTE VERSUS CHRONIC RENAL FAILURE

The initial task that often confronts the physician managing the patient with an increased serum creatinine concentration is to determine whether the decrease in renal function is acute or chronic. In the absence of documented progression of renal failure over months to years, several clinical, laboratory, and radiologic features help in making this important distinction. Patients with acute decrements in renal function often have an identifiable cause (e.g., hypotension, nephrotoxic drugs) preceding the decline in GFR and tend to be more symptomatic at any given level of renal function compared with their counterparts with CRF. If anemia is present in acute renal failure, it is usually mild, and serum calcium and phosphorus concentrations are often normal. On the other hand, moderate to severe anemia, hypocalcemia, and hyperphosphatemia are the rule in CRF. Finally, ultrasonographically documented renal size is normal or increased in patients with acute renal failure, whereas small kidneys are diagnostic of chronic renal disease.

TABLE 1. **Causes of End-Stage Renal Disease**

Disease	Prevalence
Diabetic nephropathy	30%
Hypertensive arteriolar nephrosclerosis	25%
Chronic glomerulonephritis	20%
Polycystic kidney disease	15%
Chronic interstitial nephritis	10%

ETIOLOGY

One of the common diagnostic problems encountered in office practice is to determine the etiology of a patient's CRF. A convenient approach to the differential diagnosis of chronic renal insufficiency is shown in Table 2. On the basis of several laboratory and clinical features, a generally reliable distinction can be made between glomerular disease on the one hand and chronic tubulointerstitial or vascular disease on the other. The presence of red blood cell casts on urinalysis, greater than 3.5 grams of proteinuria per 24 hours, or a systemic disease frequently associated with a glomerulopathy (e.g., diabetes, lupus erythematosus) strongly predicts glomerular disease on renal biopsy. In contrast, patients lacking these characteristics are likely to have chronic tubulointerstitial or vascular disease, especially if 24-hour protein excretion is less than 2 grams.

This clinical distinction is important and should be the first step in the algorithmic approach to the diagnosis of chronic renal disease. The various forms of nondiabetic glomerular disease can only be distinguished with certainty by renal biopsy, whereas chronic interstitial nephritis has similar histologic findings regardless of cause. The specific diagnosis of chronic tubulointerstitial disease, rather, is predicated on the knowledge of the common diseases associated with chronic interstitial injury (Table 2). A careful history with regard to analgesic ingestion, particularly nonsteroidal anti-inflammatory drugs (NSAIDs), should be obtained. In addition, in hypertensive patients, assessment of the duration of hypertension and control of blood pressure provide insight as to whether arteriolar nephrosclerosis is causally related to the chronic loss of renal function. Finally, renal ultrasonography supplies information with respect to renal size (chronicity), hydronephrosis, stone disease, and symmetry (atheromatous renal disease).

MANAGEMENT

The treatment of patients with established chronic renal insufficiency consists of several components. First, the physician must be able to identify and correct reversible causes of acute declines in GFR superimposed on chronic renal disease. Second, in the absence of specific therapeutic maneuvers to stabilize renal function, nonspecific measures should be employed to ameliorate the progression of renal disease. Third, the multiple clinical manifestations of progressive renal insufficiency must be recognized and treated. Finally, once ESRD occurs, the physician and patient should decide on the appropriate therapeutic modality.

TABLE 2. **Diagnosis of Chronic Renal Insufficiency**

Glomerular Disease	Tubulointerstitial or Vascular Disease
Diagnostic indices: red blood cell casts, >3.5 gm proteinuria or systemic disease associated with a glomerulopathy	Diagnostic indices: bland urinalysis, <2 gm proteinuria, no systemic disease associated with a glomerulopathy
Primary	Anatomic abnormalities
Focal glomerulosclerosis	Obstruction
Membranous nephropathy	Polycystic disease
Membranoproliferative glomerulonephritis	Hypertensive arteriolar nephrosclerosis
Secondary	Analgesic abuse
Diabetic nephropathy	Nephrolithiasis
Lupus nephritis	Idiopathic
Hereditary nephritis (Alport's syndrome)	Atherosclerosis
Amyloidosis	

Identification and Treatment of Reversible Decreases in Renal Function

Patients with chronic renal insufficiency of any etiology are susceptible to further acute decrements in renal function under a variety of circumstances. Table 3 lists some of the factors most commonly responsible for acute decreases in GFR in patients with preexisting CRF.

Volume Depletion

The normal kidney maintains renal blood flow (RBF) and GFR at relatively constant levels over a wide range of mean arterial pressure (80 to 180 mmHg). This phenomenon, known as autoregulation, is due to changes in vascular tone at the level of the afferent arteriole. Decreases in systemic blood pressure result in afferent arteriolar dilatation, whereas increments in arterial pressure cause afferent arteriolar constriction. Hence, RBF and GFR remain stable despite significant changes in systemic pressure. In the diseased kidney, however, renal autoregulation is impaired; the afferent arteriole is slightly dilated, possibly due to increased prostaglandin (PG) synthesis, and neither dilates nor constricts appropriately in response to variations in blood pressure. Consequently, degrees of volume depletion that would cause minimal or no change in BUN and creatinine in normal individuals can result in significant decrements in GFR in the patient with CRF.

Not only do patients with CRF tolerate volume depletion poorly, but they also are unable to decrease urinary sodium excretion appropriately (<30 mEq per liter) in the face of extrarenal sources of volume loss, thus exacerbating the salt depletion. The most common causes of volume depletion in patients with CRF include gastrointestinal losses (vomiting, diarrhea), excessive dietary sodium restriction (<80 mEq per day), and overzealous diuretic administration. Orthostatic changes in pulse and blood pressure, dry mucous membranes, and poor skin turgor are late signs of salt loss reflecting severe extracellular fluid volume depletion. More commonly, lesser degrees of volume depletion, often manifest only as a several-kilogram weight loss without orthostatic hypotension, are associated with a sharp increase in the BUN and creatinine.

Treatment of volume depletion in patients with chronic renal disease depends on the estimated volume deficit, the signs and symptoms, and the source of salt depletion. Patients with ongoing gastrointestinal losses or orthostatic hypotension frequently require hospitalization and parenteral rehydration. In contrast, lesser degrees of volume depletion can often be managed by increasing dietary salt intake or reducing diuretic dose, or both.

TABLE 3. **Reversible Causes of Renal Insufficiency in Chronic Renal Failure**

Volume depletion
Congestive heart failure
Urinary tract infection
Urinary tract obstruction
Accelerated hypertension
Nephrotoxic drugs
Aminoglycoside antibiotics
Nonsteroidal anti-inflammatory drugs
Contrast media
Ischemic nephropathy

Congestive Heart Failure

Impaired cardiac systolic function can reduce GFR further in patients with CRF not only by directly decreasing cardiac output, but also by stimulating sympathetic nervous activity and the renin-angiotensin-aldosterone system. These neurohumoral mechanisms further decrease RBF and GFR. In the setting of an already limited ability to excrete salt and water, an additional decrease in sodium excretion can quickly result in an increase in extracellular fluid volume and pulmonary edema.

Initial treatment of systolic dysfunction should consist of identifying and correcting obvious precipitating factors (e.g., ischemia, accelerated hypertension). Loop diuretics are the mainstay of therapy in patients with CRF and systolic dysfunction for several reasons. First, chronic diuretic therapy decreases afterload and increases cardiac output in patients with congestive heart failure. Second, the clinical and hemodynamic benefits of angiotensin-converting enzyme (ACE) inhibitors are attenuated with progressive renal insufficiency. Finally, thiazide diuretics are ineffective at a GFR below 30 mL per minute. If significant systolic dysfunction persists once therapy with loop diuretics has been optimized, ACE inhibitors can be cautiously added with frequent monitoring of renal function. Digitalis glycosides are rarely required. Not only are they of marginal therapeutic benefit, but they also can impair extrarenal potassium homeostasis in patients with CRF.

Urinary Tract Infection

Infection of the urinary tract rarely causes loss of renal function in the absence of anatomic abnormalities. However, in patients with urinary tract obstruction, polycystic kidney disease, or a neurogenic bladder, urinary infections can cause acute on chronic renal insufficiency. Hence, a careful urinalysis is indicated, even in asymptomatic patients, when abrupt changes in renal function occur in patients with CRF and anatomic abnormalities of the urinary tract.

Urinary Tract Obstruction

Acute reductions in GFR due to urinary tract obstruction in patients with CRF are generally seen in men with benign prostatic hypertrophy. Less common causes include neurogenic bladder due to diabetic autonomic neuropathy and bilateral upper tract obstruction. Renal ultrasonography to detect ureteral or pyelocalyceal dilation is the preferred method to exclude obstructive uropathy as a cause of a reversible decline in renal function in a patient with CRF.

Accelerated Hypertension

Pre-existing CRF is the most common cause of accelerated or malignant hypertension. In hypertensive patients with chronic renal disease, abrupt increases in arterial pressure can suddenly worsen renal function. Under these circumstances, the goal of therapy should be to smoothly decrease blood pressure to the 160 to 170/100 mmHg range over 24 to 48 hours; subsequently, arterial pressure should be reduced to normotensive levels over days to weeks. Although relatively rapid but transient decreases in blood pressure can transiently aggravate renal dysfunction because of impaired renal autoregulation, GFR often stabilizes or improves. Nevertheless, severe hypertension should be promptly treated because of its deleterious effect on cardiovascular morbidity and mortality.

Drugs

Patients with CRF are at increased risk of developing acute on chronic renal dysfunction due to aminoglycoside antibiotics. In most instances, increments in serum creatinine occur after at least 5 to 7 days of aminoglycoside therapy. While nephrotoxicity is most frequently associated with peak serum levels of 12 μg per mL or greater, further renal dysfunction can develop even in the face of "therapeutic" plasma concentrations. Risk factors that predispose to the development of aminoglycoside nephrotoxicity include prolonged therapy, elevated peak plasma aminoglycoside concentrations, liver disease, advanced age, and CRF. Hence, aminoglycosides should be given with caution to patients with underlying renal disease and only with careful monitoring of serum levels and renal function.

Nonsteroidal anti-inflammatory drugs do not appreciably alter the GFR in normal individuals. However, reversible acute renal failure has been reported with most NSAIDs in selected circumstances. Older patients receiving diuretics or patients with congestive heart failure, cirrhosis with ascites, nephrotic syndrome, or chronic renal insufficiency are at special risk for the development of worsening renal function due to NSAIDs. These clinical conditions are frequently associated with increased synthesis of angiotensin II, catecholamines, and antidiuretic hormone. Production of these vasoconstrictor compounds not only reduces RBF and GFR but also stimulates the synthesis of vasodilator PGs in the kidney. This increase in renal PG production attenuates the vasoconstrictive action of angiotensin II, catecholamines, and antidiuretic hormone. Therefore, in CRF associated with increased levels of vasoconstrictor compounds, interruption of PG synthesis by NSAIDs results in unopposed intrarenal vasoconstriction, a further decrease in GFR, and when severe, acute renal failure. Consequently, it is important to minimize the use of NSAIDs in patients with predisposing clinical conditions, especially CRF. If NSAIDs are required, sulindac (Clinoril) and piroxicam (Feldene) may be less nephrotoxic. Nevertheless, renal function should be carefully monitored, and if further renal dysfunction develops, the administration of NSAIDs should be discontinued.

Contrast Media

Radiocontrast agents are a frequent cause of nephrotoxicity in patients with chronic renal insufficiency. The risk of contrast media–induced renal failure with angiography, intravenous pyelography, digital subtraction angiography, or computed tomography is less than 1% in nondiabetic patients with normal renal function. However, the risk increases substantially in patients with pre-existing renal disease, especially diabetic nephropathy. Temporary or permanent dialysis may be necessary in as many as 15 to 20% of diabetic patients with serum creatinine concentrations greater than 5 mg per dL who undergo coronary or major vessel angiography. Contrast media–induced ARF generally occurs within 24 to 48 hours of the dye loading. The course of renal failure is characteristic, with peak serum creatinine concentration developing after 5 to 7 days and returning to baseline within 10 to 14 days. Recent studies suggest that administration of mannitol, maintenance of adequate hydration, and reduction of the amount of contrast media minimize the incidence of acute or chronic renal dysfunction, even in patients at highest risk.

Ischemic Nephropathy

Ischemic nephropathy can be defined as a clinically significant reduction in GFR due to atherosclerotic disease of the renal arteries. Although the natural history of ischemic nephropathy has not been well studied, most reports suggest that atherosclerotic renal disease is progressive. In patients treated medically and followed with serial angiograms over 5 to 7 years, progression of renal artery obstruction occurred in 40 to 45% of patients, and 10 to 15% progressed to total occlusion. Those most likely to develop progressive renal failure from ischemic nephropathy are older patients who demonstrate progressive azotemia in association with known renal artery disease, refractory hypertension, or generalized atherosclerosis. Patients with these features plus asymmetric kidneys (>2 cm difference in size) and significant increments in serum creatinine associated with antihypertensive therapy, especially ACE inhibitors, should be suspected of having atherosclerotic renal vascular disease. Definitive diagnosis requires renal angiography. However, because of the nephrotoxicity of contrast media in patients with preexisting renal disease and the morbidity and mortality associated with renal revascularization in patients with diffuse atherosclerosis, careful consideration should be given to the patient's suitability for revascularization before angiography is performed.

Slowing the Progression of Renal Disease

An important feature of chronic renal disease is the fact that once GFR is reduced to less than 25 to 30 mL per minute, regardless of etiology, inexorable progression to ESRD generally occurs. Numerous factors have been implicated in this progressive decline in renal function. Continued immunologic injury occurs in some diseases such as lupus nephritis or membranous glomerulopathy. In addition, some authorities have speculated that abnormalities of calcium and phosphorus metabolism, intraglomerular coagulation, or hyperlipidemia may account for the continued loss of nephron mass. While these factors may play significant roles in experimental models of renal insufficiency, their relevance to human renal disease remains unproved. On the other hand, three important factors play significant roles in the progression of human renal disease: systemic hypertension, dietary protein intake, and glycemic control in diabetic patients.

Control of Hypertension

Hypertension is an important manifestation of chronic renal disease and can occur even with mild decreases in GFR. With progression of CRF, the prevalence of hypertension increases, and elevated blood pressure is present in 80 to 90% of patients with ESRD. Control of systemic hypertension is imperative in hypertensive patients with CRF not only because of the well-known decrease in cardiovascular morbidity and mortality it confers, but also because reduction of blood pressure slows the rate of decline in GFR.

In both diabetic and nondiabetic kidney disease, renal function decreases more rapidly in hypertensive patients compared with their normotensive counterparts. The question of whether excellent blood pressure control ameliorates the progression of renal disease has been addressed by several prospective studies and is the subject of continued investigation. The available data support the belief that reduction of systolic blood pressure to 140 mmHg or less and of diastolic blood pressure to the 80 to 85 mmHg range retards the decline in GFR and should be a minimum goal in hypertensive patients with renal disease. Calcium channel antagonists and ACE inhibitors may be more renoprotective compared with conventional antihypertensive therapy. However, clinical trials to date do not indicate that one class of antihypertensive agents is clearly superior to others with regard to preservation of renal function.

Restriction of Dietary Protein

Until 1980, dietary protein was restricted when patients developed moderate to severe CRF (GFR 10–25 mL per minute) in order to minimize the signs and symptoms of uremia. Since then, data have accumulated to suggest that in patients with mild to moderate renal dysfunction (serum creatinine 2 to 4 mg per dL), dietary protein restriction to a level of 0.6 grams of protein per kg of body weight retards the rate of progression of renal disease. While the data regarding protein restriction are not as consistent as are those relative to reduction of blood pressure, beneficial effects have been reported in both diabetic and nondiabetic kidney disease. Further, no deleterious effects of such moderate dietary protein restriction have been reported. Hence, dietary protein restriction is an important therapeutic modality to slow the progression of renal disease, particularly in normotensive patients with CRF. It is unclear, however, whether the effects of protein restriction are additive to those of excellent blood pressure control.

Control of Blood Glucose

Only 30 to 40% of patients with insulin-dependent diabetes and 10 to 20% of those with non–insulin-dependent diabetes develop diabetic nephropathy. Risk factors include a genetic predisposition to hypertension, glomerular hyperfiltration (GFR >130 mL per minute), the development of microalbuminuria (excretion of more than 20 to 30 mg of albumin per 24 hours measured by radioimmunoassay), and poor glycemic control. Short-term studies have shown that excellent control of blood glucose lowers abnormally increased GFR and reduces microalbuminuria. More importantly, recent analyses of long-term studies in patients with insulin-dependent diabetes have demonstrated that excellent glycemic control (glycohemoglobin <7.5%) prevents the progression of incipient nephropathy (microalbuminuria) to overt nephropathy (dipstick-positive proteinuria) and retards the rate of decline in GFR in patients with overt nephropathy. Consequently, long-term glycemic control should be assessed by measurement of glycohemoglobin in patients with diabetic nephropathy, and doses of insulin or oral hypoglycemic agents should be adjusted to maintain glycohemoglobin levels below 7.5%.

Manifestations and Treatment of Chronic Renal Failure

Chronic progressive renal insufficiency results in multiple clinical manifestations that affect virtually every organ system in the body. Some of the more prominent manifestations are shown in Table 4. The clinical consequences of progressive CRF increase in severity and prevalence as GFR declines. Hypertension and fluid overload can occur even with mild renal insufficiency, whereas hyperkalemia, acidosis, calcium/phosphorus abnormalities, and anemia develop with moderate to severe renal failure. All are found in patients with ESRD.

Fluid Overload

Patients with CRF have a limited ability to excrete salt and water, not only because of a decrease in GFR but also due to the activation of salt-retaining neurohumoral stimuli (e.g., angiotensin II, aldosterone, sympathetic nervous system). Salt retention must be anticipated as GFR declines, and appropriate measures should be taken to avoid clinically apparent episodes of fluid overload. Patients with mild to moderate CRF should receive an 80- to 90-mEq sodium diet, particularly if they are hypertensive. With progressive renal failure, dietary salt restriction becomes insufficient to maintain sodium balance and diuretic therapy is necessary. Thiazide diuretics are ineffective at creatinine clearances less than 25 to 30 mL per minute. In moderate to severe renal failure (creatinine clearance 10 to 25 mL per minute), high doses of loop diuretics are required, often on a twice-daily basis. Patients with creatinine clearances of less than 10 mL per minute are frequently resistant to high doses of a loop diuretic and may require the addition of a thiazide diuretic to maintain adequate natriuresis.

Hypertension

Because abnormal salt metabolism is central to the pathogenesis of hypertension in patients with CRF, initial treatment logically begins with the restriction of dietary sodium to 80 to 90 mEq per day. In a few patients, blood pressure is adequately controlled with this maneuver alone; the majority, however, require additional pharmacologic therapy. Administration of a thiazide diuretic to hypertensive patients with mild CRF or a loop-blocking diuretic to those with creatinine clearances of less than 30 mL per minute controls blood pressure in one-third of patients. In those who do not achieve adequate control of blood pressure (i.e., ≤140/80–85 mmHg) with salt restriction or diuretic administration, further pharmacologic therapy is warranted. While no single class of antihypertensive agents has proved to be clearly superior, calcium channel antagonists, ACE inhibitors, and centrally acting sympatholytics (e.g., clonidine [Catapres]) are both effective and rational from a pathophysiologic standpoint. Calcium blockers and ACE inhibitors may be more renoprotective than conventional antihypertensive therapy. In addition, calcium channel antagonists are effective at extremes of dietary salt intake, whereas ACE inhibitors block the formation of angiotensin II, an important mediator of hypertension in patients with CRF. Finally, centrally acting sympatholytic agents inhibit the central sympathetic outflow that is often increased in hypertensive patients with chronic renal disease.

TABLE 4. **Manifestations of Chronic Renal Failure**

Electrolyte and acid-base	Cardiovascular
Hyperkalemia	Fluid overload
Metabolic acidosis	Hypertension
Endocrine	Hematologic
Calcium, phosphorus, vitamin D abnormalities	Anemia
	Platelet dysfunction
Gonadal dysfunction	Rheumatologic
Neurologic	Crystal-induced arthritis
Peripheral neuropathy	Amyloid deposition
Encephalopathy	

TABLE 5. **Renal and Extrarenal Factors That Impair Potassium Homeostasis**

- Decreased renal potassium excretion
  - Hypoaldosteronism
    - Idiopathic
    - Type IV renal tubular acidosis
    - Drugs
      - ACE inhibitors
      - Nonsteroidal anti-inflammatory drugs
      - Heparin
  - Potassium-sparing diuretics
- Redistribution from intracellular to extracellular fluid or decreased cellular uptake
  - Insulin deficiency
  - Acidosis
  - Nonselective beta blockade
  - Digitalis
- Increased intake
  - Diet
  - Salt substitutes

Hyperkalemia

In most patients with progressive renal insufficiency, potassium homeostasis is maintained until the creatinine clearance is 15 to 20 mL per minute. However, under certain circumstances, hyperkalemia can occur with less severe renal insufficiency. Table 5 lists the major renal and extrarenal factors that often further perturb potassium balance in patients with CRF. Drug-induced hypoaldosteronism (ACE inhibitors, NSAIDs, heparin) can contribute to the development of hyperkalemia in patients with moderate renal failure. Potassium-sparing diuretics should be used cautiously in patients with any degree of renal insufficiency and only with careful monitoring of the serum potassium concentration. Patients with diabetic nephropathy are especially prone to develop hyperkalemia because insulin deficiency impairs cellular uptake of potassium. Similarly, nonselective beta blockade and digitalis inhibit potassium translocation and predispose to hyperkalemia, particularly in patients with pre-existing constraints on potassium homeostasis. Excess dietary potassium intake is a major cause of hyperkalemia in patients with CRF and should be treated with potassium restriction. Salt substitutes should be avoided.

Hyperkalemia can be minimized in patients with CRF by limiting dietary potassium intake to 60 mEq per day and by recognizing the factors that often contribute to impaired potassium homeostasis. Serum potassium concentration should be monitored closely, particularly if drugs that interfere with potassium balance (see Table 5) are required. Occasionally, sodium polystyrene sulfonate (Kayexalate) is required to control hyperkalemia as the patient approaches ESRD.

Metabolic Acidosis

Chronic renal failure is associated with a progressive inability to excrete normal endogenously produced nonvolatile acid, amounting to approximately 1 mEq of hydrogen ion per kg of body weight per day. Serum bicarbonate often declines to 13 to 15 mEq per liter as moderate to severe renal failure develops. In general, no significant signs or symptoms are associated with this degree of acidosis. However, this progressively positive hydrogen ion balance is buffered, in part, by bone salts, results in osteopenia, and contributes to the development of renal osteodystrophy.

Although the development of metabolic acidosis can be minimized by dietary protein and phosphate restriction as CRF progresses, alkali therapy is ultimately necessary with development of moderate to severe renal insufficiency. Alkali can be given as sodium bicarbonate tablets (650 mg = 8 mEq of bicarbonate) or as Shohl's solution or Bicitra (1 mL = 1 mEq of bicarbonate). Ordinarily, it is advisable to begin with a dose of 20 mEq of bicarbonate twice daily and to titrate the dose upward until a serum bicarbonate concentration of 20 to 22 mEq per liter is achieved.

Calcium, Phosphorus, and Vitamin D Abnormalities

The development of CRF is accompanied by abnormalities in bone formation characterized by varying amounts of osteitis fibrosa cystica, osteomalacia, and osteoporosis. Hyperphosphatemia, due to a decreased GFR, and reduced renal synthesis of $1,25(OH)_2$ vitamin D_3 reduce serum levels of ionized calcium, thereby increasing parathyroid hormone (PTH) production. The increased circulating levels of PTH increase urinary excretion of phosphorus and enhance gastrointestinal and renal absorption of calcium. In addition, calcium is mobilized from bone. Consequently, serum calcium and phosphorus levels return toward normal at the expense of an elevated circulating level of PTH. As renal function declines further, this sequence of events is repeated. Ultimately, the increased levels of PTH result in osteitis fibrosa cystica, and a relative or absolute lack of $1,25(OH)_2$ vitamin D_3 causes osteomalacia. In patients with ESRD in the United States, secondary hyperparathyroidism and osteitis fibrosa cystica are the major manifestations of renal osteodystrophy.

In most patients with progressive CRF, frankly elevated serum phosphorus levels are not seen until the creatinine clearance decreases to 20 to 25 mL per minute. When an increase in the serum phosphorus level, with or without a decrease in serum calcium concentration, is noted, phosphate-binding antacids should be administered. In the past, these were primarily aluminum-containing antacids. However, recent evidence suggests that aluminum, although poorly absorbed, can accumulate and result in anemia, osteomalacia, and encephalopathy. Therefore, calcium carbonate or calcium acetate is preferred as a phosphate binder. Nevertheless, aluminum-containing antacids may be required until the serum phosphorus level is less than 7 mg per dL and the calcium-phosphorus product is less than 65 if calcium phosphate precipitation and metastatic calcification are to be prevented. The administration of calcium-containing phosphate binders to patients with hyperphosphatemia not only normalizes serum phosphorus levels but also ensures an adequate dietary supply of calcium. If the administration of calcium carbonate or calcium acetate in doses between 1 and 2 grams three times daily with meals does not normalize serum calcium levels, oral $1,25(OH)_2$ vitamin D_3 should be considered.

Anemia

Moderate to severe anemia occurs in over 95% of patients with chronic renal insufficiency. There is a significant inverse correlation between the hematocrit and the plasma creatinine concentration. The decrease in red blood cell mass results in multiple clinical manifestations, including fatigue, dyspnea, anorexia, insomnia, depression, and sexual dysfunction. The anemia of CRF is normochronic, normocytic, and hypoproliferative. Although shortened red blood cell survival and bone marrow suppression by uremic toxins contribute to the anemia in CRF, an absolute or relative deficiency of erythropoietin is the major pathophysiologic cause of anemia in chronic renal disease. Until recently, treatment for the anemia of CRF consisted of intermittent transfusions, adequate dialysis, administration of androgens, and supplementation with iron and folic acid. Within the last decade, however, recombinant human EPO (rHuEPO, epoetin alfa [Epogen, Procrit]) has proven particularly efficacious in the treatment of the anemia of chronic renal insufficiency.

Weekly subcutaneous administration of rHuEPO at a mean dose of 150 units per kg increases hematocrit to more than 30% in the majority of patients with CRF. An average dose of 75 units per kg is an effective maintenance dose once goal hematocrit has been achieved. Treatment of anemic patients with CRF with rHuEPO not only increases red blood cell mass and improves symptomatology but also improves cardiac performance and reduces left ventricular mass index. Patients with mild to moderate CRF as well as those with ESRD can develop worsening hypertension during treatment with rHuEPO. The hypertension associated with rHuEPO is multifactoral in origin and not solely the result of increased blood viscosity. Patients with CRF receiving rHuEPO should be monitored carefully for the development of hypertension and the need for intensified antihypertensive therapy.

Drug Dosage

As renal failure progresses, modification of drug dosage is often required because many pharmacologic agents are eliminated by the kidney. Antihypertensive drugs and diuretics are the most common classes of pharmacologic agents employed in patients with CRF. Although several are metabolized by the kidney, because treatment should be initiated at the lowest effective dose and subsequently titrated according to blood pressure or extracellular fluid volume, a priori dosage adjustments based on routes of metabolism are unnecessary. Guidelines for dosage modification for other pharmacologic agents can be found in several available review articles and in the Physicians' Desk Reference.

Diet

Dietary modifications in patients with CRF vary, depending on the level of renal function and on the presence or absence of hypertension. As previously noted, an 80- to 90-mEq sodium restriction is indicated and reasonable for patients with any level of renal dysfunction both to ameliorate hypertension and to minimize fluid overload. Dietary protein restriction to 0.6 grams per kg of body weight limits progression of renal disease in patients with mild to moderate renal failure and minimizes the signs and symptoms of uremia in those with severe renal insufficiency. This diet should provide 35 to 40 kcal per kg of body weight, chiefly from carbohydrate and polyunsaturated fats, restrict phosphorus intake to 600 to 800 mg per day, and limit daily potassium to 60 mEq. Because of its complexity and the need for ongoing supervision, dietary modification of this magnitude is best done under the auspices of a registered dietician. When ESRD supervenes, daily protein intake can be liberalized to 1 gram of protein per kg of body weight, but the sodium, phosphate, and potassium restrictions should be left in place.

Treatment Modalities in End-Stage Renal Disease

Three basic treatment options are available for patients when creatinine clearance declines to less than 5 to 10 mL per minute: hemodialysis, peritoneal dialysis, and renal transplantation. In general, vascular access for hemodialysis or peritoneal catheter insertion for peritoneal dialysis is performed in nondiabetic patients with progressive renal insufficiency when the creatinine clearance falls to approximately 10 mL per minute. Dialysis is then instituted when the patient develops uremic symptoms, electrolyte and acid base abnormalities unresponsive to medical therapy, fluid overload unresponsive to medical therapy, or a creatinine clearance of 5 mL per minute or less. In diabetic patients, access for dialysis is usually established when the creatinine clearance reaches 15 mL per minute, and dialysis is generally begun at a creatinine clearance of 10 mL per minute. Referral and evaluation for renal transplantation need not be delayed until the patient has begun dialysis. It is acceptable and, in fact, often preferable to refer the patient to a transplant center before dialysis is required. With careful planning on the part of the primary care physician, the nephrologist, and the transplant surgeon, transplantation can be performed before dialysis is even required.

The choice among treatment modalities for ESRD depends on several factors. Infants and children have high morbidity on long-term hemodialysis or peritoneal dialysis. Consequently, transplantation, especially from parents or siblings, improves growth and offers a more normal lifestyle. In contrast, patients older than 70 years of age have a higher complication rate and a greater mortality with transplantation. With few exceptions, these patients should be managed by hemodialysis or peritoneal dialysis. Additional factors that may influence the patient's decision regarding treatment modalities for ESRD include co-existent vascular disease, lifestyle considerations, economic factors, and work habits. Overall, mortality of patients undergoing either hemodialysis or peritoneal dialysis is approximately 8 to 10% per year. With regard to renal transplantation, 1-year allograft survival is 90% with kidneys from live related donors and 80 to 85% with cadaveric transplants. Patient mortality among cadaveric transplant recipients is quite similar to that of patients undergoing chronic dialysis. Hence, an improved quality of life for the transplant recipient is often the major consideration in recommending transplantation as opposed to dialysis. A successful transplant from a live related donor offers the best chances of prolonged survival for the patient with ESRD.

GENITOURINARY CANCER

method of
BRUCE A. LOWE, M.D.
Oregon Health Sciences University
Portland, Oregon

ADRENAL CANCER

Adrenal cortical carcinomas are rare neoplasms, arising in 1 of every 1.7 million individuals per year. Over 75% are functional and may produce multiple hormones and metabolites. Cushing's syndrome and virilization are the most common clinical presentations of functional adrenal tumors.

Diagnosis

Incidental diagnosis of adrenal tumors is steadily rising as a result of increased utilization of abdominal ultrasound and computed tomographic (CT) scanning for body imaging. The majority of adrenal malignancies are large (>6 cm); however, many smaller adrenal lesions are detected during abdominal imaging. All patients with adrenal masses should be evaluated for excess hormone production. This assessment includes measurement of serum levels of glucocorticoids and mineralocorticoids. Excessive urinary levels of 17-ketosteroids or dehydroepiandrosterone sulfate (DHEAS) suggest adrenal carcinoma.

Management

Any functional lesion, regardless of size, should be treated, usually by surgical exploration and removal of the adrenal or simple excision of the tumor. Lesions over 5 cm in diameter should be surgically excised regardless of functional status. Removal of malignant adrenal tumors requires total adrenalectomy and resection of adjacent involved structures such as the spleen and kidney. Functional atrophy of the contralateral uninvolved adrenal gland is common, and steroid replacement is often necessary following unilateral adrenalectomy. Nonfunctional adrenal masses smaller than 5 cm pose a clinical problem. A solid, nonfunctional tumor less than 5 cm in diameter should be imaged by magnetic resonance imaging (MRI). If the signal intensity of the tumor compared to normal liver is greater than 2:1, the lesion should be surgically removed; if less than 2:1, expectant management employing periodic CT scans every 6 months for 2 years is advisable. Enlarging lesions identified during follow-up are surgically removed. Cystic lesions undergo percutaneous needle puncture and are observed if clear fluid is found.

The only effective drug for disseminated tumors is mitotane (Lysodren), a derivative of the pesticide DDT. This drug palliates symptoms related to hormonal production but does not prolong survival. Serious gastrointestinal, neurologic, and dermatologic disorders are commonly seen following treatment with mitotane but usually resolve after discontinuation of therapy.

PHEOCHROMOCYTOMA

Pheochromocytomas can occur in any site where paraganglion chromaffin cells are located—from the mediastinum to the organs of Zuckerkandl located inferior to the origin of the inferior mesenteric artery. Rarely, these tumors are found in the bladder wall, but the majority are located in the adrenal glands. Nearly all pheochromocytomas are benign and functional, with slightly less than 10% being malignant.

Excessive production of catecholamines, such as norepinephrine, epinephrine, and dopamine, results in a clinical syndrome characterized by hypertension (sustained or paroxysmal) associated with severe headaches, flushing, palpitations, diaphoresis, and anxiety. Elevated urinary or serum levels of catecholamines confirm the diagnosis. Abdominopelvic CT or MRI will identify the location of the majority of these lesions. ^{131}I-meta-iodobenzylguanidine (MIBG) may localize lesions not seen on these imaging studies.

Management consists of surgical excision of the tumor. Preoperative and intraoperative control of blood pressure is critical. Manipulation of the primary tumor may trigger a severe hypertensive episode and cardiac instability. Preoperative use of alpha-adrenergic blockers can usually control the paroxysmal episodes these patients experience and allow restoration of circulating blood volume.

KIDNEY CANCER

A variety of neoplastic lesions, both benign and malignant, can arise from the renal parenchyma. Accurate diagnosis requires the procurement of tissue for histologic study, as the different renal tumors are indistinguishable by currently available imaging modalities.

Adenocarcinoma

Adenocarcinomas (renal cell cancers) are the most common renal neoplasms, with over 25,000 new cases and more than 10,000 deaths annually. These tumors can present at any age, but they are uncommon in adolescents and children. The peak incidence is between the fifth and seventh decades. Long thought to arise from proximal tubular cells, more recent studies employing immunohistochemical techniques have demonstrated that adenocarcinoma can originate from cells in the more distal nephron. The etiology is unclear, but there is a strong correlation with tobacco use, exposure to asbestos and certain heavy metals, and prolonged renal dialysis. Certain clinical disorders, such as von Hippel–Lindau syndrome, are frequently associated with renal cancer. These patients have multiple, small, bilateral tumors as opposed to the large solitary tumors noted with sporadic nonfamilial renal cancer. Cytogenetic studies demonstrate a consistent translocation of the short arm of chromosome 3 in patients with von Hippel–Lindau syndrome, while deletion of this same region has been noted in sporadic renal cell carcinoma. This region of chromosome 3 may contain one or more tumor suppressor genes whose loss leads to the development of cancer.

Presentation

Clinical presentation varies; the classic triad of gross hematuria, abdominal mass, and costovertebral pain is seen in fewer than 20% of cases and usually indicates advanced disease. Nonspecific symptoms such as weight loss, weakness, fever, night sweats, and abdominal fullness are more common. Hematuria occurs in over half of all patients. Paraneoplastic syndromes are common and include central and peripheral neuropathies, Cushing's syndrome, hypertension, polycythemia vera, hyperparathyroidism with hypercalcemia, and hepatic dysfunction. Incidental diagnosis of these tumors, occurring in nearly 20% of cases, continues to rise owing to the widespread use of imaging techniques for the evaluation of obscure complaints and in the management of a variety of conditions.

Diagnosis

Computerized tomography (CT) is the most sensitive and accurate method of detecting and staging renal masses and has largely replaced more traditional methods. Enhancement or increased density of a mass after intravenous contrast administration indicates increased vascularity and is a sign of malignancy, although not all adenocarcinomas will enhance and not all enhanced lesions are malignant. Any solid lesion noted by CT should be considered neoplastic until proved otherwise. Evaluation of both kidneys is important, as approximately 3 to 5% of renal tumors are bilateral and may be missed by cursory studies.

Historically, renal tumors were identified by nephrotomography during intravenous pyelography (IVP) and confirmed by angiography. Most renal tumors can be seen with these procedures, but they have been largely replaced by CT with its increased sensitivity. Staging by CT scanning is more accurate, allowing detection of perinephric adenopathy, adrenal or hepatic involvement, and contralateral renal masses. The IVP remains useful for the evaluation of gross or microscopic hematuria because of its superior ability to image the collecting system for the detection of urothelial carcinoma. Angiography is useful in differentiating indeterminate renal masses and in determining the extent of renal vein or vena caval involvement by tumor thrombus, which is present in 10% of cases. Angiographic embolization of the renal vessels can be used to make nephrectomy technically easier with massive tumors or to stop life-threatening hemorrhage in unresectable lesions.

Sonography frequently identifies many early-stage renal tumors. It is noninvasive, apparently harmless, and when high-quality hardware is combined with clinical experience is a very sensitive diagnostic tool. Though specificity is less than with CT, it is invaluable for differentiating solid tumors from cystic lesions. Doppler ultrasonography provides accurate high-resolution images of the retroperitoneum and can readily detect venous invasion and determine the extent of vena caval tumor thrombus.

Magnetic resonance imaging (MRI) provides high-quality images of the abdomen but is no more accurate than CT. In patients unable to tolerate intravenous contrast owing to renal insufficiency or hypersensitivity, gadolinium enhancement can help differentiate between neoplastic and hyperplastic lesions and is less toxic to the compromised kidney. MRI is superior to CT for vascular imaging and accurately demonstrates vena caval invasion. The increased cost of MRI compared to CT limits its routine use in the diagnosis of kidney cancer.

Needle aspiration of the renal mass for imaging purposes or to obtain tissue is controversial and in the CT era is of limited value. Results are unreliable owing to potential sampling errors, and there is a small but real possibility of renal injury. Needle biopsy can provide tissue for histopathologic study in the compromised patient with localized disease who is a poor candidate for surgical excision or in the patient with disseminated disease requiring diagnosis prior to initiation of systemic therapy. Seeding of the tumor along the needle track occurs more frequently than reported and represents a potential hazard to patient survival. Use of this procedure should be highly selective. Histologic confirmation may be necessary to identify secondary involvement of the kidney by other primary neoplasms or to identify less common renal tumors.

Staging

The Robson and the International Union Against Cancer (UICC) (TNM) classifications are the most widely used staging systems; however, the Robson system does not consider important parameters of disease extent used by most investigators. In the UICC system, the T parameter describes the primary tumor mass: T1 includes small lesions (<5 cm) that are confined to the kidney; T2 tumors are greater than 5 cm in diameter and are confined to the kidney; T3 tumors extend into the perinephric fat or exhibit vascular invasion; and T4 lesions extend beyond Gerota's fascia. N refers to nodal status, and M, to the presence of metastatic disease. Staging is prognostically important, as disease extent at presentation remains the most accurate predictor of long-term survival. Overall survival after diagnosis has stayed at 50% for over 10 years; 5-year survival ranges from 60 to 90% for organ-confined disease (T1 and T2) and 5 to 10% for metastatic disease. Regional nodal involvement conveys a poor prognosis with 5-year survival rates of 5 to 30%, and 10-year survival rates of 0 to 5%. Renal vein invasion appears to have little impact upon survival, while invasion into the vena cava reduces survival, especially if complete surgical excision is not possible. Supradiaphraghmatic extension of the tumor thrombus further reduces survival.

Management

Organ-Confined Disease. No effective chemotherapeutic agent has been found as yet, and although there have been advances in immunotherapy, long-term survival depends upon surgical excision. Radical nephrectomy is a relatively straightforward procedure that removes the kidney, perinephric fat, and the ipsilateral adrenal gland. Gerota's fascia is removed intact to prevent tumor spillage into the retroperitoneum. Concurrent excision of the regional lymph nodes has not been shown to improve survival, and many investigators do not routinely advocate lymphadenectomy. The surgical approach is not critical and is dependent upon the experience and personal preference of the surgeon. Small lesions can be excised using a flank approach; however, very large, upper pole lesions may require a thoracoabdominal incision to provide access through both the chest and the abdominal cavity.

Nephron-sparing techniques to preserve functional

renal tissue include tumor enucleation or partial nephrectomy and are used for managing small unilateral lesions. In selected patients, survival rates are similar to those for routine radical nephrectomy. Concerns about multifocality and microscopic local extension resulting in recurrence and reduced survival have limited widespread acceptance of these procedures for routine management. However, for the patient with bilateral involvement or disease involving a solitary kidney, nephron-sparing procedures can provide adequate disease control while preserving some degree of renal function. Occasionally, tumor extent will require removal of all renal tissue in order to eradicate the cancer. Although aggressive, this option combined with dialysis can result in substantial survival in selected patients.

Disseminated Disease. Cytotoxic chemotherapy is relatively ineffective in the management of adenocarcinomas of the kidney. Vinblastine (Velban) has shown the greatest activity against these tumors, but objective responses occur in only 10 to 12% of patients. Early reports indicated activity of medroxyprogesterone against renal cell cancer, but more recent studies indicate that fewer than 5% of patients will experience even a partial response. Cases of spontaneous remission and recent advances in molecular biology and immunology have led to the investigation of newer modalities in the management of these patients. Specific immunotherapy using tumor cell vaccines, autologous tumor extracts, and immune RNA has been inconsistent and disappointing. However, naturally occurring cytokines, such as the interferons and interleukins, are active against these tumors.

All classes of interferons are similar in activity and produce objective remission rates of 5 to 30% (mean 15%). The average duration of response is less than 2 years. Pulmonary metastases are the most responsive to immunotherapy and responses are more durable. Objective responses usually develop within 3 months; after that time it is unlikely that additional treatment will produce a response. Interferons are usually well tolerated, with the most commonly encountered side effects being flulike syndromes, fatigue, and gastrointestinal upset. Combining interferons with cytotoxic chemotherapeutic agents has met with little success. An observered in vitro synergy between 5-fluorouracil and interferon-alpha led to use of this combination in the treatment of metastasic disease. A slight increase in activity occurred with only mild toxicity. Combinations of different interferons have also failed to improve response rates. Adjuvant nephrectomy may improve the response to interferon, but results of studies in both Europe and the United States have been inconclusive.

Interleukins are naturally occurring lymphokines produced and secreted by T lymphocytes that modulate virtually all aspects of T cell immune response. Interleukin-2 (IL-2) alone produces response rates similar to those of the interferons, but responses are more durable, sometimes extending beyond 36 months. Combining IL-2 and lymphokine-activated killer (LAK) cells produces even better response rates. LAK cells are obtained by incubating peripheral venous lymphocytes isolated by plasmapheresis with IL-2 for 3 to 4 days; they are then reinfused into the patient. In highly selected patients, this combination results in a greater than 30% objective remission rate and in unselected patients, 20%. Toxicity can be significant and high costs limit more extensive use. Combining IL-2 and interferon-alpha gives response rates similar to those achieved with IL-2 and LAK cells, but with reduced toxicity. IL-2 can be given as a bolus intravenous injection, continuous intravenous infusion, or subcutaneous injection in an outpatient setting. Mild side effects include fevers, chills, malaise, nausea, vomiting, and diarrhea. Serious toxicity is due to a vascular leak syndrome, leading to hypotension, fluid retention, pulmonary edema, prerenal azotemia, and hepatic failure. Toxicity is lower when IL-2 is given by continuous infusion or subcutaneous injection. Treatment-related mortality is less than 2%. The effectiveness of IL-2 may be increased by excision of the primary tumor, but this has not been verified by prospective trials.

Other approaches to management currently being investigated include autolymphocyte therapy, incubation of peripheral lymphocytes with an autologous cytokine mixture of various interleukins, interferons, and tumor necrosis factor. These "activated" memory cells are then reinfused. Median survival in over 300 patients has been 21 months and 3-year survival, 29%. Another approach uses clonally expanded and activated tumor infiltrating lymphocytes harvested from fresh tumor tissue, which are then reinfused into the patient with IL-2. Early results are encouraging, but further investigation is required. Genetic transfer technology incorporating genetic material coding for tumor necrosis factor into lymphocytes harvested from fresh tumor tissues to enhance antitumor efficacy is also being investigated.

A variety of benign and malignant neoplasms arise in the kidney. Most are rare and have a variety of clinical manifestations. Radiographic appearance also varies, and preoperative diagnosis is often difficult. Management usually consists of simple excision or complete nephrectomy. The prognosis for malignant tumors of the kidney other than adenocarcinoma is generally poor.

Oncocytoma

The true incidence of oncocytomas is unknown, but many renal cell cancers exhibit oncocytic histologic features. Recent studies note that over 5% of lesions previously classified as adenocarcinomas were oncocytomas. The distinction is prognostically important, because the overwhelming majority of oncocytomas follow a benign course. Clinically, it is difficult to differentiate these lesions from adenocarcinomas by current imaging techniques. A characteristic central scar and an absence of necrosis and hypovascularity can be seen by CT or MRI, but these are inconsistent findings. Most clinicians advocate exploration rather than observation. Oncocytomas are usually asymptomatic and are discovered incidentally, although occasional patients present with flank mass, pain, and hematuria. Management consists of simple excision, and long-term follow-up is not necessary.

Angiomyolipoma

Only a small percentage of renal tumors are angiomyolipomas. These benign lesions occur as small, multiple, bilateral tumors or large, solitary, unilateral tumors. Small multifocal tumors are found in patients with hamartomatous lesions in various organs and are associated with tuberous sclerosis. In the patient without the stigmata of tuberous sclerosis, these tumors usually occur as large solitary unilateral renal masses. The benign nature of these lesions has been well documented, although there is a tendency for rapid growth and spontaneous hemorrhage. Clinical presentation is similar to that of other renal tumors. The lipomatous component of these tumors produces a characteristic appearance on CT scans that often provides the diagnosis. Angiographically, it is impossible to distinguish between angiomyolipomas and adenocarcinoma of the kidney. If the diagnosis is clearly demonstrated by CT scan, most patients can be followed nonoperatively. Tumors greater than 6 to 8 cm in diameter have an increased risk of spontaneous hemorrhage (nearly 40%) and require surgical excision. The multiplicity and frequency of these tumors in patients with tuberous sclerosis mandates that every effort be made to preserve renal tissue if surgical excision is required.

UROTHELIAL CANCERS

Transitional epithelium is present throughout the urinary collecting system from the ostia of the collecting tubules in the renal pelvic papilla to the midportion of the urethra. Tumors arising in this epithelium are usually transitional cell carcinomas (TCC). Approximately 95% of all bladder cancers are TCCs, with squamous cell carcinomas and adenocarcinomas accounting for the remaining 5%. Incidence is greatest in the sixth through eighth decades and there is a 3:1 male to female ratio due to the higher incidence of tobacco use and occupational exposure among men. Besides tobacco, other etiologic factors include occupational exposure to aniline dyes, aromatic amines, and volatile hydrocarbons. Chronic irritation and inflammation are associated with the development of squamous cell cancers. Areas in the Middle East and eastern Africa where schistosomiasis is common have an extraordinarily high incidence of squamous cell cancers of the bladder.

The most common presenting symptom of urothelial cancer is gross or microscopic hematuria. Nearly all patients with bladder cancer will have hematuria at some time during the course of their illness. Irritative voiding symptoms are also common and indicate involvement of the bladder neck or proximal urethra. Intraepithelial tumors, or carcinoma in situ, will often present with irritative symptoms in the absence of infection. Other laboratory studies are of little value. Cytopathologic analysis can detect tumor cells in the urine; however, sensitivity is low, with only 60% of low-grade tumors detectable, but 85 to 90% of high-grade tumors will have abnormal results. Flow cytometric analysis of cellular DNA content alone provides little diagnostic advantage over cytology, and combining the two studies improves sensitivity but decreases specificity while substantially increasing costs.

Upper Urinary Tract Tumors

Upper tract tumors are usually found when an intraluminal filling defect is noted on a contrast study of the urinary collecting system. In the presence of hematuria, any incomplete visualization of the urinary tract by excretory urography should be further investigated by endoscopic retrograde visualization of the ureter and renal pelvis. Occasionally, a CT scan will differentiate a noncalcified or slightly calcified stone and a soft tissue tumor. Improved instrumentation allows direct visualization of ureteral and renal pelvic lesions simultaneously with the ability to obtain tissue for diagnosis and treatment. Survival is dependent upon stage at diagnosis.

The difficulty of diagnosis, high recurrence rates, and the relatively thin ureteral-pelvic wall allowing for rapid extralumenal extension of tumors are reasons for aggressive initial management by surgical excision of the kidney and ureter. Currently available ureteroscopic instrumentation allows many superficial and isolated lesions to be managed by transluminal excision. Patient selection is critical to success. Larger, localized lesions can be removed by segmental ureterectomy. Very large, invasive, or multiple lesions can be effectively managed only by removal of the kidney, ureter, and a cuff of bladder wall surrounding the ureteral orifice.

Bladder Cancer

Although many bladder cancers can be detected by radiographic studies, a negative imaging study does not automatically rule out the presence of tumor, as fully a third of all bladder tumors are not visible by radiographic means. Only by careful endoscopic evaluation of the bladder can the presence of malignancy be determined accurately. Once the tumor is detected, an endoscopic resection is the next step in diagnosis and management. Accurate determination of stage at presentation is critical in selecting management.

Superficial Disease

Tumors confined to the bladder mucosa can be managed by simple transurethral resection alone. For lesions displaying multifocality, large size, high pathologic grade, associated carcinoma in situ, and prior history of bladder cancer, simple resection alone will result in a recurrence rate of over 80% within 2 years. Stage and grade migration with each recurrence will occur in 10 to 15% of patients. Intravesical treatment with a variety of agents is used to reduce this recurrence rate. The most effective agents currently available are nonspecific immunostimulants, such as Bacille Calmette-Guérin (TheraCys), and the chemotherapeutic agent mitomycin C (Mutamycin). These agents, administered by intravesical instillation weekly for 6 to 8 weeks, will reduce recurrence rates to less than 25% in 2 years.

Muscle Invasive Disease

Lesions invading the bladder muscle pose a significant threat to patient survival and require aggresive therapy. Standard treatment entails removal of the bladder, pelvic nodes, prostate, and in some patients the urethra. Even after extensive surgical excision, metastatic disease will develop in 20 to 30% of patients.

Removal of the bladder requires urinary diversion, which has traditionally been accomplished by isolating a segment of terminal ileum, anastomosing this to the ureters, and draining the system through a stoma to the anterior abdominal wall into an external collection device. The ileal conduit has significant impact upon body image, takes significant time to maintain, and requires expensive medical supplies. Continent diversion techniques were developed in an effort to overcome these disadvantages, but have been only partially successful. These pouches are constructed from a variety of bowel segments to create a continent internal reservoir drained by intermittent catheterization via a flush stoma to the anterior abdominal wall and, when successful, do not require external collection devices. One patient in five will require subsequent operative procedures to manage continence failure and pouch breakdown. When the urethra is preserved following cystectomy, a continent pouch can be anastomosed to the residual urethra as a neobladder. A neobladder empties by relaxation of the voluntary urethral sphincter and most do not require catheterization. Performing a nerve-sparing procedure in conjunction with construction of a neobladder can preserve erectile function while allowing relatively normal voiding. Nocturnal incontinence occurs in nearly all patients with neobladders. Similar neobladders can be constructed for female patients but require catheterization for drainage.

Disseminated Disease

Metastatic bladder cancer is managed by combination chemotherapy with cisplatin (Platinol), methotrexate, vinblastine, and doxorubicin (Adriamycin). A 50% response rate can be expected and is durable for many patients. Patients with a complete response can expect a median survival of nearly 3 years. The effectiveness of combination chemotherapy has led investigators to combine chemotherapy with radiation therapy and surgical excision in patents with localized disease in an effort to improve treatment results.

URETHRAL CANCER

Primary urethral cancers are very uncommon. Only 600 cases have been described in men and approximately 1200 in women. Although these tumors arise in women of all adult ages, more than 75% are reported during the sixth through ninth decades. Urethral cancer is more common among whites and appears to be related to chronic irritation. The majority of these tumors arise in the fossa navicularis in men and near the urethral meatus in women. Squamous cell cancers account for over half of cases, with transitional cell cancer and adenocarcinoma the next most common. Presentation usually consists of voiding dysfunction and bleeding in men; in women, irritative voiding symptoms and a vaginal mass are the usual manifestations.

Distal lesions are managed by surgical excision. Endoscopic electroresection or laser ablation can be used in small superficial lesions. Tumors with early invasion can be managed by a segmental urethrectomy; however, deeply invasive lesions require wide surgical excision. Lesions near the bladder neck can be managed by primary radiotherapy in women or by cystourethrectomy for large tumors that are poorly amenable to radiotherapy. Lymphatic drainage of the distal urethra is to the inguinal lymphatics, and this region needs to be evaluated in patients with invasive distal urethral tumors. Proximal urethral tumors will metastasize to the pelvic nodes. No long-term survivors with nodal metastasis have been reported, and the prognosis for patients with tumor extending into adjacent periurethral structures is also poor (10 to 17% at 5 years). Chemotherapy has little benefit, although bleomycin (Blenoxane) has showed some activity in squamous cell cancers. The M-VAC combination (methotrexate, vinblastine, doxorubicin, cisplatin) has been used with some success in transitional cell tumors of the urethra.

PROSTATE CANCER

Prostate cancer is the most common malignancy affecting men in the United States, with over 165,000 cases diagnosed annually and more than 35,000 deaths. There is a racial distribution with incidence being highest among men of northern European and African-American descent. There is a direct relationship between incidence and aging; however, this is the most common cancer in all adult males over age 40 years. Etiology is as yet unknown, but there is evidence of an association with high-fat diet. Approximately 55 to 60% of patients will present with clinically localized disease.

Staging systems vary around the world, but the most widely used system in this country is the American classification: A lesions are clinically undetectable and discovered incidentally, B lesions are palpable and confined to the prostate, C lesions are extraprostatic in extent, and D lesions represent disseminated disease. There are corresponding stages in the TNM system of the UICC. Survival is dependent upon stage at presentation, with disseminated disease associated with a high death rate. Mean survival for stage D cancer is approximately 4 years. Survival in patients with localized disease is less well defined.

Presentation

Clinical presentation is usually secondary to irritation or obstruction of the bladder outlet. Inflammation of the bladder neck is a cause of irritative voiding dysfunction, such as urinary frequency, urgency, dysuria, and incontinence. Obstruction of the bladder outlet by tumor growth is another common presentation, and hematuria is often seen with these tumors. Bone pain from tumor metastasis can occur with disseminated disease and is similar to the pain of arthritis but is more constant and intense. Unfortunately, symptomatic presentation is often a sign of advanced disease. In many patients, particularly those with localized disease, the tumor is discovered during a routine examination.

Diagnosis

Few physical findings are characteristic of prostate cancer. Digital rectal examination (DRE) identifies approximately 80% of patients with clinically significant disease. The normal prostate is the size of a walnut and has a consistency similar to that of the contracted thenar muscle. Any palpable nodules or increased firmness is abnormal and should be investigated. However, only 30% of suspicious lesions found by DRE will prove to be malignant.

The use of prostate-specific antigen (PSA) has been the most significant advance in prostate cancer diagnosis. PSA is an androgen-dependent serine protease produced by prostatic epithelial cells. Elevation of the serum PSA level is indicative of malignancy, yet it is important to realize that the test is not specific for cancer: PSA is also increased with benign prostatic hyperplasia, prostatitis, and trauma. However, the diagnostic accuracy of PSA increases as absolute value rises. In the presence of a normal digital rectal examination, prostate cancer will be detected in 2% of patients with PSA levels of less than 4 nanograms per mL, in fewer than 10% of those with PSA levels between 4 and 10 nanograms per mL, in fewer than 20% of those with PSA levels of 10 to 20 nanograms per mL, and in over 30% of those with PSA levels above 20 nanograms per mL.

Transrectal ultrasound (TRUS) examination of the prostate can assist in the diagnosis of prostate cancer. A neoplastic focus will characteristically appear as an area of decreased echogenicity, although many documented tumors appear normal on ultrasound examination. The overall accuracy is approximately 55 to 60%. Ultrasound-guided prostate biopsies are more accurate in detecting cancer and in determining tumor volume and extent than are digitally directed biopsies. The needles currently used are 18 gauge, spring loaded, and well tolerated by the patient. Rectal or urethral bleeding and bacteremia are complications of prostate biopsy.

Natural History

Even though prostate cancer is common, there is little consensus as to the natural history, impact upon survival, and proper management. Autopsy studies have shown that the clinical incidence is only a fraction of the actual prevalence: histologic evidence of malignancy was found in 30% of men at age 50 years and in 50% of those studied at age 80 years. Extrapolating this to the general population, it is estimated that nearly 10 million men are affected by prostate cancer. Tumors discovered at autopsy are labeled latent cancer, and the vast majority are microscopic. Obviously, only a small proportion of patients suffer any adverse consequences from their tumor. It is this discrepancy between clinical incidence and prevalence that is the source of much of the confusion regarding management of these patients.

It appears that tumor volume at diagnosis is the critical factor in determining the impact the tumor will have upon the individual patient. Current evidence indicates that prostate cancer originates as a small, well-differentiated malignant focus that over time increases in volume and becomes less differentiated. Studies indicate that a single transformed cell requires approximately 10 to 12 years to attain a volume of 1 mL and an additional 4 to 5 years to reach 4 mL. Only 10% of 1-mL tumors will have extraprostatic extention, while nearly a third of those attaining a volume of 4 mL will be unresectable. Subclinical tumors discovered at autopsy or during subtotal removal of the prostate for supposedly benign disease are classified as incidental cancers and are generally low-volume tumors, although a significant percentage will be more extensive. The probability of dissemination increases directly with histologic grade and volume. Given time, any prostatic malignancy can progress and eventually affect survival.

Screening

Screening will detect prostate cancer in approximately 3 to 4% of men over age 50 years. Given the high prevalence of latent tumor and the poor sensitivity of PSA levels, many screened patients will have cancers of such low volume that there is little threat to survival. In spite of the recognition that survival ultimately depends upon tumor volume, it is difficult to define this parameter short of prostatectomy. TRUS-directed biopsies of selected regions of the prostate gland provide some estimate of tumor volume. However, it is clear that many patients identified by screening programs will be subjected to unnecessary treatment, and conversely, many patients identified after presentation of clinical symptoms will have incurable disease. Many investigators are evaluating the value of screening programs in the management of these patients.

Management

The goal of management is to eradicate the disease. However, as noted, in many patients prostate cancer has no adverse impact upon the quality or length of life, and in these cases treatment is unnecessary and potentially a source of significant morbidity. Even the ability of treatment to increase survival has not been conclusively proved, although several studies indicate a survival advantage of treatment over observation in patients with clinically evident disease. Probably the best policy is to offer treatment to any patient whose potential survival exceeds the potential for the tumor to shorten that survival. Generally, any patient with a potential survival of greater than 10 years should be offered treatment.

Therapeutic options for the management of prostate cancer include surgical excision (i.e., radical prostatectomy), radiotherapy (both external beam or brachytherapy), androgen deprivation, and observation. Potentially curative treatments include surgical excision and radiotherapy, whereas androgen deprivation is used in the management of disseminated disease or for the relief of symptomatic local tumor. Observation is reserved for patients with limited survival potential or who choose not to undergo treatment.

Surgery

In radical prostatectomy, the entire prostate, the seminal vesicles, the ampulla of the vas deferentia, and the overlying fascia are removed. The procedure can be performed anteriorly through the retropubic approach or posteriorly through the perineum. Operative morbidity is low, with most centers reporting a mortality rate of less than 1% and a total significant complication rate of less than 10%. The complication of most concern to the majority of patients is loss of urinary continence. Two key components of urinary continence are recognized in the male: a passive sphincteric mechanism located in the region of the bladder neck and an active voluntary mechanism at the junction between the prostatic apex and the membranous urethra, the external sphincter. During prostatectomy, the bladder neck is disrupted and continence is dependent upon the integrity of the external sphincter. In the hands of an experienced surgeon, damage to this mechanism can be minimized. Most centers report that over 90% of patients maintain complete continence. Nearly all remaining patients experience varying degrees of stress incontinence or lose urine during moments of increased abdominal pressure. Dryness can be achieved with adult diapers, pads, condom catheters or penile clamps. However, severe incontinence requires placement of an artificial urinary sphincter or injection of collagen into the periurethral tissues.

Loss of erectile function can also result from prostatectomy. Sexual function in men is controlled by two separate neural pathways. The pudendal nerves control the tactile and orgasmic functions while the cavernosal nerves control the erectile response. The cavernosal nerves can be damaged by prostatectomy, causing loss of erections adequate for intercourse. However, procedures are available that preserve the cavernosal nerves during prostatectomy. When both cavernosal nerve bundles remain intact, erectile function will be preserved in most patients under 60 years of age. Older age, tumor volume, or inadvertent injury to one or both nerve bundles reduces the success of a nerve-sparing procedure. For organ-confined disease, radical prostatectomy effectively eradicates the tumor and results in long-term disease-free survival.

Radiotherapy

Radiation therapy is administered by exposing the patient to the beam of a linear accelerator or by implanting a radioisotope into the prostate gland. With external beam therapy, approximately 64 to 66 cGy are given over 6 weeks. Beyond this level, the risk of complications increase dramatically. The proximity of the rectum limits the possible dose. Clinical results of external beam radiotherapy are very similar to those of surgical excision; however, neither treatment modality has proven superiority and the choice of treatment depends on individual patient selection or risk factors. Viable tumor is often found in postirradiation biopsies, but there is controversy over the actual impact of this finding on a given patient.

Interstitial radiotherapy was the most common form of treatment during the 1970s and early 1980s, but relatively few patients presently undergo this treatment because several investigators have reported brachytherapy to be less efficacious than external beam radiotherapy. However, newer isotopes, such as palladium, and advanced techniques, such as percutaneous placement of the radioisotope, have renewed interest in this form of treatment. However, at present no long-term results are available and preliminary results from at least three studies indicate that treatment effectiveness has not improved. For the patient with localized prostate cancer requiring or desiring potentially curative therapy, external beam radiotherapy and surgical excision are the treatments of choice.

Several investigative trials are currently under way to evaluate the effect of alternative treatments on localized disease. Therapeutic modalities being studied include cryotherapy, hyperthermia, sonoablation, and laser-assisted prostatectomy. Of these, the most promising appears to be cryotherapy; however, if sonoablation becomes feasible it may be the best option. Cryotherapy uses supercooled probes to induce freezing injury of the prostate gland. Urethral and rectal warming probes protect these structures from injury. Small localized lesions can be eradicated by this technique. At this time, the procedure is considered acceptable for managing benign prostatic hyperplasia, but its potential role in the treatment of prostate cancer is unknown and its use in these patients is regarded as investigational.

Androgen Deprivation

Standard treatment for metastatic prostate cancer is androgen deprivation, achieved surgically by removal of the testicles (bilateral orchiectomy) or nonsurgically through interruption of testosterone production by the testis. Hormonal manipulation can be accomplished in a number of ways. The principal androgen for male reproductive function that affects prostate growth is testosterone. Production of testosterone by the testicular Leydig cells is stimulated by luteinizing hormone (LH) secreted by the pituitary under hypothalamic control, which in turn is regulated by testosterone through a negative feedback mechanism. Luteinizing hormone–releasing hormone (LHRH) agonists are believed to inhibit LH release through a deregulation mechanism after an initial dramatic rise in LH production. LHRH agonists are often combined with nonsteroidal antiandrogens during the first 1 to 2 weeks of therapy to prevent this "flare" phenomenon with exacerbation of symptomatic disease. The expense of these agents limits their use. Antiandrogens are competitive inhibitors of testosterone that bind with intracellular receptors. Although use of nonsteroidal receptors is theoretically appealing, application is limited by the fact that most cancers become refractory over a period of several months. Testosterone passively diffuses into the target cells and is metabolized by 5-alpha-reductase to dihydrotestosterone, which appears to be the active intracellular androgen. Finasteride (Proscar), a 5-alpha-reductase inhibitor, has the potential to inhibit prostatic growth with minimal side effects. Unfortunately, testosterone also binds with intracellular receptors, although with less affinity than dihydrotestosterone, which limits its use in prostate cancer. Estrogens, such as diethylstilbesterol, can suppress LH production and inhibit androgen activity on a cellular level. These agents are quite effective in achieving androgen deprivation and are very inexpensive, but the potential of estrogens to increase the risk of thromboembolic cardiovascular disease in males has limited their use in recent years. Combination therapy, usually orchiectomy or LHRH agonists with antiandrogens, directed at inhibiting testicular production of testosterone and blocking androgenic activity at the cellular level has been shown to increase mean survival in selected patient populations. Patients benefiting from such combination therapy are those with a potential for long-term survival—in general, younger individuals with minimal tumor burden.

Chemotherapy has been of limited use in the management of disseminated disease. No effective agent has been identified as yet. Recently, investigators have evaluated the ability of suramin to inhibit the growth of prostate cancer. Response rates of 50% have been reported, although nearly all responses were partial. Duration of response is limited and toxicity is severe and common.

PENILE CANCER

This is a relatively rare neoplasm in the United States, representing only 0.4 to 0.6% of all cancers, and its incidence has been stable for the past 25 years. The vast majority of these lesions are squamous cell cancers. Peak incidence is in the sixth decade of life; however, over one-fifth of patients are under 40 years of age. Prepubertal circumcision appears to substantially reduce the incidence of this cancer, which is associated with poor hygiene and the collection of smegma and other irritants beneath the foreskin. Patients may present with a large mass lesion of the penis in advanced cases or an irritated, inflamed, or discolored superficial lesion in early cases. Invasion of the deeper penile tissues with their rich supply of blood vessels and lymphatics can occur in larger lesions. Invasion into these structures is associated with a high incidence of inguinal lymph node involvement, which is often bilateral. The most common growth pattern is one of local progression with subsequent involvement of the regional lymphatics. Distant metastasis to the lungs, liver, bones, and central nervous system occur through hematogenous dissemination. Ultimate survival is dependent upon the stage at presentation. Treatment delays are common and can be attributed to both patient and physician. Nearly half of all patients had noted the presence of a penile lesion for more than 1 year before diagnosis. Many smaller early cancers are very similar to benign lesions and are treated as such. Failure to retract the penile foreskin during examination or during routine hygienic cleaning accounts for failure to diagnose the tumor in many patients. Overall survival at 5 years is 52%. In patients with no inguinal lymph node involvement, survival at 5 years is 66%, compared to 27% with nodal metastasis.

Management is dependent upon the stage at presentation. For early noninvasive lesions involving the foreskin, simple excision is adequate and very small lesions can be excised using a CO_2 laser to reduce scarring. More invasive lesions require a penectomy. Partial penectomy can be used for distal tumors leaving sufficient length to maintain sexual function; however, large or more proximal lesions will require total penectomy with perineal placement of the urethra for voiding. Inguinal node involvement is seen in at least 45% of patients at presentation, and another 10 to 15% of patients have lymphadenopathy related to inflammation rather than tumor. The timing of inguinal lymphadenectomy is controversial.

Treatment for disseminated disease has been unsatisfactory. Bleomycin, cisplatin, and methotrexate have the greatest activity, with nearly 50% of patients responding, but this is usually partial and of short duration. Adjuvant chemotherapy administered after surgical resection for patients with nodal involvement may be of value.

Sarcomas are the most common nonsquamous cell cancers of the penis. They can occur at any age and are usually located on the shaft. Patients usually present with gradually enlarging rubbery masses along the corporal bodies and occasionally will complain of painful erections, urinary retention, priapism, or a fungating mass. Kaposi's sarcoma is often associated with chronic immunosuppression as an opportunistic malignancy, particularly in patients with acquired immune deficiency syndrome (AIDS). Approximately

20% of AIDS-related Kaposi's sarcoma involves the genitalia, with the initial lesions arising on the penis in many patients. This malignancy appears as a reddish, smooth 2-mm to 1-cm nodule with well-defined margins.

Other malignancies that involve the penis only rarely include malignant melanoma, basal cell carcinoma, and lymphoma. Metastasis to the penis has been seen in a variety of tumors, but usually as a late manifestation of primary disease. Almost all of these secondary tumors arise from cancers of the urinary and gastrointestinal tracts.

TESTICULAR CANCER

Approximately 7000 new cases of testicular cancer are detected annually, with the vast majority being germ cell malignancies. Survival rates have steadily risen over the past three decades and currently are greater than 90% for all patients and 70 to 80% for those with disseminated disease. This remarkable success is due to a multimodal therapeutic approach that combines multiagent chemotherapy and surgical excision. A variety of germinal elements are expressed in testicular malignancy, all arising from subsequent differentiation of the basic germinal stem cells. This common cellular ancestry probably accounts for the relatively uniform response of these different histologic lesions to treatment. Historically, germ cell cancers are classified as seminomatous and nonseminomatous germ cell cancers (NSGCC).

Germ Cell Tumors

Seminoma

Seminomas, the most common of the germ cell cancers, probably arise from the seminiferous epithelium. The most common presentation is a palpable scrotal mass. Symptoms related to disseminated disease are uncommon causes for presentation. Only 20% of patients with seminoma have metastasis at initial diagnosis, and less than 5% have Stage III disease. Staging is straightforward: tumors confined to the testicle are classified as Stage I; disease with abdominal metastastic tumors less than 5 cm in diameter is considered Stage IIA and greater than 5 cm, Stage IIB. Extra-abdominal disease, such as pulmonary or CNS metastasis, is considered Stage III disease. Ureteral obstruction and bony metastasis are far more common with seminomas than with other germ cell tumors.

Diagnosis. Diagnosis is often made by physical examination. The presence of a solid, nontender mass that does not transilluminate should alert the physician to the possibility of cancer. Most patients self-discover the tumor on examination, although many describe an antecedent minor trauma. Trans-scrotal ultrasound is highly accurate and can differentiate malignant and benign cystic or inflammatory lesions in approximately 95% of patients. The rapid growth rate of these lesions mandates prompt exploration and excision. All potential testicular tumors are approached via the inguinal region with early control of the spermatic cord and vessels. Owing to the different lymphatic drainage pathways of the scrotum and testicle, violation of the scrotal fascial planes is considered inappropriate. Orchiectomy is required for all testicular tumors to establish the histologic diagnosis, excise the primary lesion, and predict the risk of further progression. Serum levels of beta-human chorionic gonadotropin (hCG-beta) and alpha-fetoprotein (AFP) should be obtained in all patients. Abnormally elevated levels of hCG-beta can be present in pure seminomas, although any level greater than 30 nanograms per mL is an indication of associated NSGCC elements. Elevation of the serum AFP levels does not occur with seminomas. Metastatic lesions can exhibit a different histology from the primary tumor, and NSGCC should be suspected whenever the AFP or hCG-beta levels are elevated.

Dissemination is almost invariably lymphatic, although seminomas can metastasize hematogenously. The ipsilateral retroperitoneal para-aortic and paracaval lymph nodes are the primary sites of dissemination. Extra-abdominal metastasis to the lungs or brain is less common at initial presentation. CT scans have replaced lymphangiograms owing to their greater accuracy (over 80%). Routine chest radiographs are usually adequate to evaluate the lungs. Approximately 2% of all seminomatous tumors are extragonadal in origin and can be found as primary lesions anywhere along the embryologic urogenital ridge, including the retroperitoneum and mediastinum.

Treatment. The marked radiosensitivity of seminomas was the basis for the classic differentiation of these tumors from the NSGCCs, which are relatively radioresistent. Historically, Stage I disease has been managed by irradiation of the retroperitoneal lymph nodes, but as long-term survival in these patients now approaches 99%, many investigators advocate observation instead. A number of studies employing surveillance for Stage I tumors have reported survival rates equal to those following radiotherapy. Approximately 20% of patients entered into surveillance protocols will subsequently develop metastatic disease and require adjuvant chemotherapy, reportedly without compromising survival. Stage II and III disease can be managed by radiation with acceptable results; however, these tumors are also highly susceptible to systemic chemotherapy, and treatment with cytotoxic agents will produce superior survival rates in advanced disease. Surgical excision is reserved for large lesions that fail to respond to systemic chemotherapy or radiation.

Nonseminomatous Germ Cell Cancer

These tumors vary histologically but share common patterns of dissemination, growth, and response to therapy. Histologic subtypes include embryonal cell carcinoma, yolk sac carcinoma, choriocarcinoma, and teratoma. Most primary tumors are composed of mixed germ cell elements.

Disseminated disease at presentation is more common (60%) in NSGCC than in seminoma, and a scrotal mass is the most common finding at presentation. Symptoms related to disseminated disease include abdominal mass, abdominal or back pain, and weight loss or anorexia. Serum tumor markers are elevated in the majority of patients with NSGCC. Elevation of serum hCG-beta is associated with embryonal cell carcinomas and choriocarcinomas, while alpha-fetoprotein is produced by yolk sac carcinomas. Detection of abnormal levels of either of these markers is strong evidence of germ cell malignancy, and persistent elevation after treatment is evidence of residual disease.

Management. Retroperitoneal lymph node dissection (RPLND) has been the traditional treatment option for the management of Stage I NSGCC. This procedure is highly effective in removing the primary landing sites of metastasis, and morbidity is low. However, infertility due to injury of the sympathetic nerves resulting in ejaculatory dysfunction can be as high as 40%. RPLND after orchiectomy in stage I lesions will achieve survival rates of nearly 100%. Given the staging accuracy of current diagnostic procedures, it has been realized that only 30% of patients with Stage I NSGCC will experience tumor relapse if untreated, usually in the retroperitoneal nodes. The proven effectiveness of chemotherapy in eradicating even bulky disease has led many centers to advocate surveillance rather than immediate treatment in Stage I disease. Since certain pathologic parameters, such as vascular, lymphatic, or cord invasion, have been associated with a high rate of relapse, exclusion of these patients from surveillance programs is recommended. A number of institutions report survival rates of nearly 100% in properly conducted surveillance protocols. Systemic chemotherapy given to Stage I patients also produces high survival rates. The excellent results reported by nearly all institutions using a surveillance program indicate that reserving chemotherapy for those patients experiencing relapse is the treatment of choice.

Dissemination to other sites represents Stage II or III disease, and initial management consists of systemic chemotherapy. The most effective agent against these tumors is cisplatin (Platinol), and most protocols include it with etoposide (VePesid), and bleomycin (Blenoxane), although some clinicians include vinblastine, cyclophosphamide (Cytoxan), or doxorubicin. Chemotherapy is very active and will completely eradicate all evidence of disease in 20 to 40% of patients, even those with large tumor masses. Residual tumors are surgically excised, and approximately 40% consist of fibrous scar only, 40% are teratomas, and 20% contain viable carcinoma. Ultimate survival is dependent upon tumor volume. In patients with minimal disease, even with pulmonary metastasis, ultimate survival is greater than 90%, and long-term survival is greater than 40% even in the face of massive metastatic disease. Surgical excision is reserved for patients with residual disease following chemotherapy. Radiation is seldom used in the management of NSGCC.

SCROTAL CANCER

It is widely acknowledged that squamous cell carcinoma of the scrotum is associated with exposure to carcinogens in chimney soot, paraffins, and grease. In 1775, Sir Percivall Pott noted a high incidence of scrotal cancer among the chimney sweeps of London. Repeated trauma and poor personal hygiene are also contributing factors. Fortunately, these tumors are rare in the United States and the incidence has steadily decreased over the past 50 years, but the disease remains more common in Europe, particularly England. Presentation is usually as a single lesion with the appearance of a wart or nodule. Within 6 months, central ulceration occurs with basal induration. Presentation for care usually occurs 8 to 12 months after appearance. Most of these tumors are found in men in their mid 50s. Nearly half of the patients will have inguinal nodal metastasis at presentation. Management consists of wide local excision with a 2-cm margin of uninvolved tissue in combination with removal of the inguinal lymph nodes. Local recurrence has been reported in 20 to 40% of patients. Radiation therapy and chemotherapy have been unsuccessful in controlling these cancers.

URETHRAL STRICTURE

method of
STEVEN SCHLOSSBERG, M.D., and
GERALD H. JORDAN, M.D.
Eastern Virginia Medical School
Norfolk, Virginia

A urethral stricture is a scar that results from tissue injury after local trauma or inflammatory disease. With healing, the scar contracts, decreasing the diameter of the lumen. Urethral strictures are classified as posterior or anterior (Fig. 1). Posterior urethral strictures involve the prostatic urethra and the membranous urethra. Prostatic urethral strictures usually occur after surgery for benign or malignant diseases of the prostate. Membranous urethral strictures are inevitably associated with pelvic fracture and attendant urethral distraction.

Anterior urethral strictures occur within the area of the urethra surrounded by the corpus spongiosum and can be localized to the bulbous urethra, the penile or pendulous urethra, or the fossa navicularis (glandular urethra). Anterior urethral strictures are commonly caused by blunt perineal trauma (occult or recognized), urethral infection (gonorrhea), or instrumentation (urethral catheterization or transurethral surgery). Currently available data do not appear to show any relationship between nonspecific urethritis (*Chlamydia* and *Ureaplasma urealyticum*) and the development of anterior urethral stricture.

Although many of the ensuing comments are applicable to all urethral strictures, the following discussion is mainly concerned with the diagnosis and treatment of anterior urethral strictures in males. Urethral strictures are extremely rare in women.

DIAGNOSIS

Symptoms are related to changes caused by obstruction of the flow of urine. Patients may notice a slow stream,

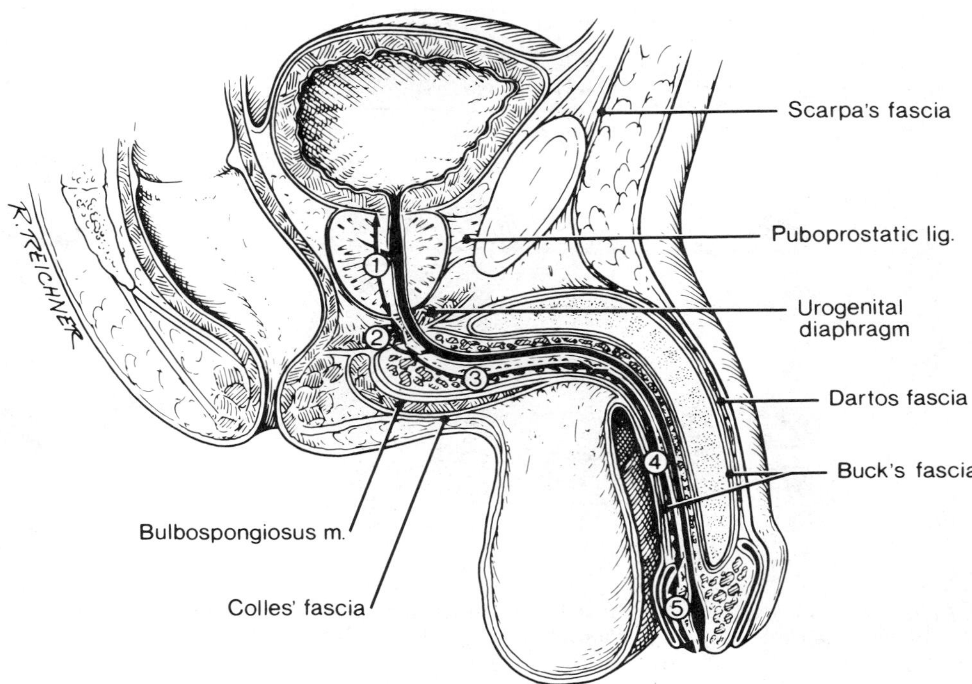

Figure 1. Cross-section of the pelvis demonstrating the anatomic divisions of the urethra. 1, Prostatic urethra; 2, Membranous urethra; 3, Bulbous urethra; 4, Pendulous portion of the penile urethra; 5, Fossa navicularis. (From Jordan GH: Urethral surgery and stricture disease. In Droller MJ [ed]: Surgical Management of Urologic Disease. Chicago, Mosby–Year Book, 1992.)

frequency, urgency, nocturia, dysuria, or occasional suprapubic pain. This constellation of symptoms may also suggest prostatic enlargement (bladder outlet obstruction) or prostatic inflammatory processes. Pyuria and recurrent urinary tract infections are common. Recurrent epididymitis in a young patient or the signs and symptoms of recurrent prostatitis should raise the possibility of an undiagnosed stricture. Additionally, in the patient presenting with Fournier's gangrene (rapidly progressive perineal and lower abdominal fasciitis), unsuspected urethral stricture with associated urinary extravasation, and undiagnosed perianal abscess must be excluded.

Although the presence of a stricture can be confirmed by the inability to pass a small catheter, the best diagnostic test is a dynamic retrograde urethrogram done with intravenous contrast material. A subsequent voiding cystourethrogram is helpful in determining the length of the stricture. To complete the evaluation, urethroscopy under local anesthesia is helpful. The length, depth, and density of the stricture can be determined from physical examination, the appearance on contrast studies, and the amount of elasticity noted at urethroscopy.

TREATMENT

Once the diagnosis is made, treatment depends on the "stage" or anatomy of the stricture (Figs. 2 and 3). Simple procedures can cure a stricture that involves only the urethral epithelium, while more complex strictures require open surgical repair. Despite its simplicity, this approach has not been widely practiced until recently. In the past, treatment of urethral strictures was based on the concept of the reconstructive ladder. The simplest treatment was always tried first, and when it failed for the third, fourth, or fifth time, a more complex procedure was attempted. In addition to complicating treatment in the long run, the "simple" treatment often produced more scarring, thereby increasing the stage of the stricture. Although reasonable in the era of more rudimentary reconstructive techniques, this approach is less acceptable today. With more accurate assessment of the stricture and better surgical techniques, the anatomy of the stricture should determine the appropriate treatment (Figs. 2 and 3). However, there is a place for the management rather than the cure of a urethral stricture in patients who are poor surgical candidates. As with many other diseases, the patient and physician should discuss the likelihood of success and the treatment-related morbidity that may be obtained with the different therapeutic options.

Urethral Dilation

Dilation is often the first treatment attempted. The goal is to stretch the scar without tearing healthy tissue and producing more trauma. If dilation causes significant bleeding, it has been too vigorous. A variety of different methods are available for dilating strictures. The initial caliber of the stricture and the experience of the physician often dictates the method chosen. For small-caliber strictures (less than 10 French), filiform and followers are often used initially. A small filiform, or guide, is passed through the stricture to allow safe passage of progressively larger followers, or dilators. Only woven (not metallic) followers should be used. With the advent of guidewire technology, a system is now available that uses a guidewire to traverse the stricture (sometimes passed with the aid of a flexible cystoscope) and a Teflon-coated polyethylene tapered dilator to enlarge the stricture. Our preferred treatment, if possible, is to use a balloon dilator that can be passed with the aid of a filiform, a guidewire, or a coudé (curved) tip.

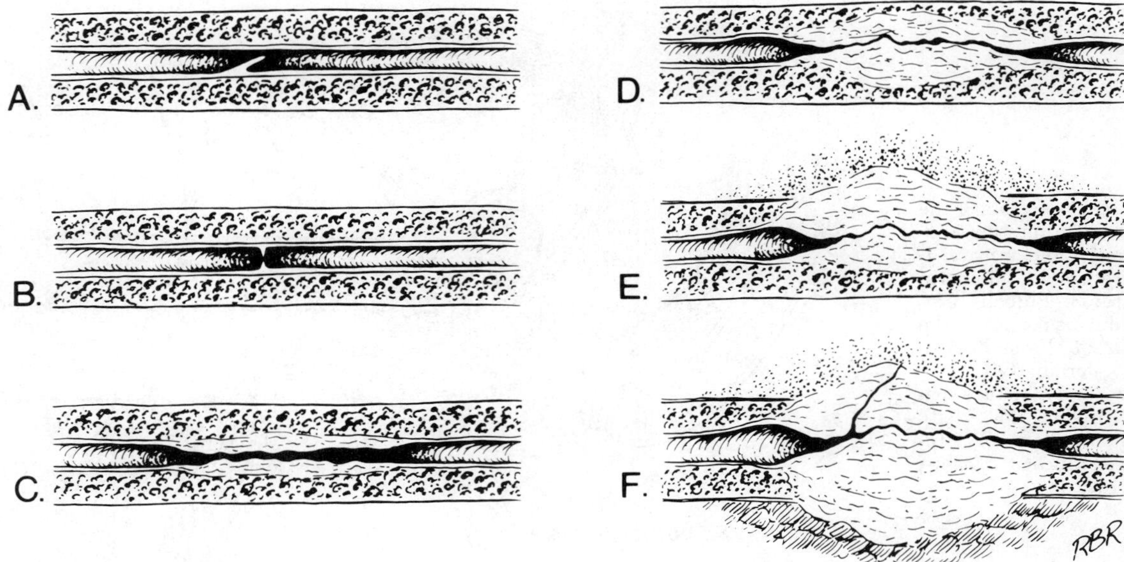

Figure 2. Classification of urethral stricture disease according to the anatomy of the stricture as described by Devine. (From Jordan GH: Problems in Urology, Vol. 1. Philadelphia, J.B. Lippincott, 1987.)

Since this provides radial dilation without the shearing forces generated by conventional dilators, there is less trauma and pain. Dilation should always be performed with intraurethral lidocaine jelly. Metal sounds or stiff coudé-tip catheters can also be used for larger strictures. Stretching of the scar ideally should be accomplished without tearing. Several sessions may be necessary to obtain a durable and sat-

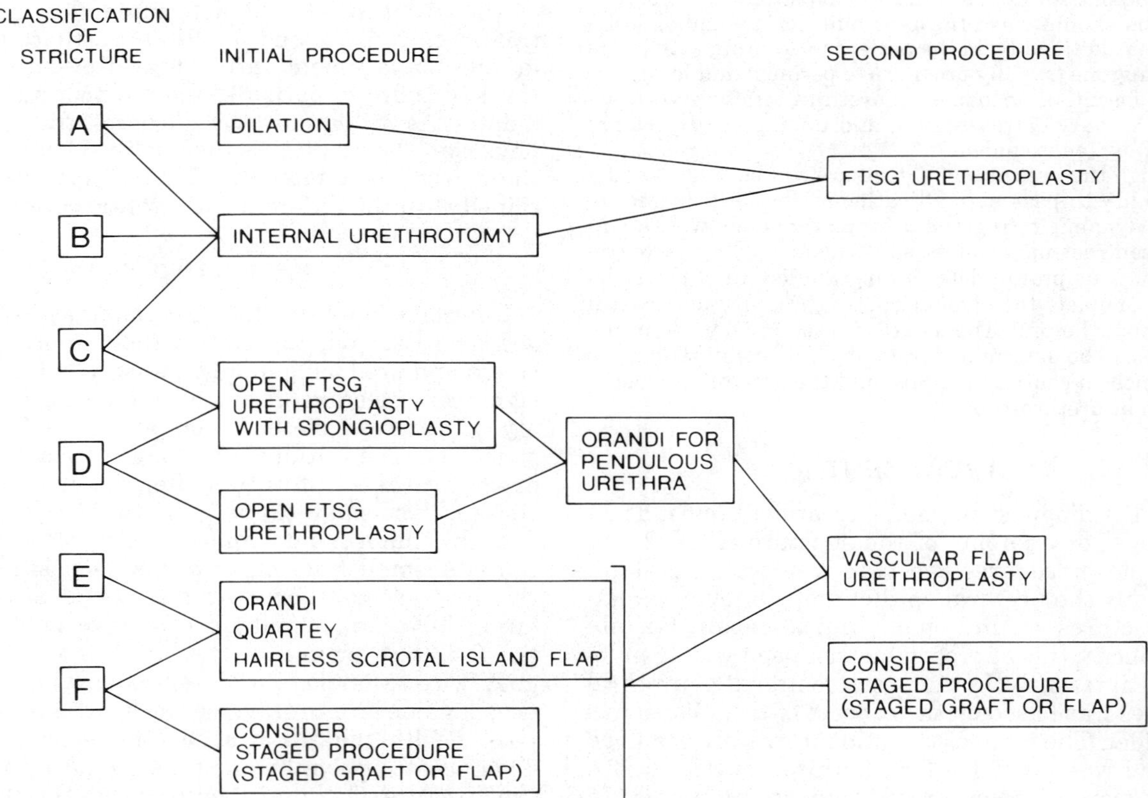

Figure 3. Flow chart of the approach to anterior urethral stricture disease as dictated by the anatomy. *Abbreviation*: FTSG = full-thickness skin graft. (From Jordan GH: Problems in Urology, Vol. 1. Philadelphia, J.B. Lippincott, 1987.)

isfactory luminal caliber (16–18 French). Although dilation may be curative for mucosal strictures, it is often used to manage the stricture, and if this is the case, twice a year is an acceptable frequency for repeat dilation.

Internal Urethrotomy

Transurethral incision of the scar is often attempted as initial therapy or as the next step after dilation for short strictures. Usually performed under general anesthesia or local anesthesia with heavy intravenous sedation, this procedure involves visualizing the stricture cystoscopically and cutting the scar until healthy tissue is seen, allowing the lumen to open to a 22- to 24-French diameter. A urethral catheter is left in place for a variable length of time. Some patients are placed on an intermittent catheterization program to keep the stricture open as the incision heals. The transurethral incision is usually made by the "cold-knife" technique. A specially designed attachment to an operative cystoscope allows the urologist to accomplish a precise and controlled incision. Recently, a variety of different laser techniques have been tried to improve the success over that of conventional internal urethrotomy, but the data suggest that a properly performed laser urethrotomy is no better than a standard approach and that a poorly performed laser procedure may yield disastrous complications. We currently do not see an advantage to laser urethrotomy.

Although internal urethrotomy may be curative (see Fig. 3), more often it is a form of management that yields a wider-caliber stricture. The practice of frequently repeated internal urethrotomy should be condemned except in patients who are not surgical candidates. For a short stricture (less than 1 cm), one or two attempts are reasonable. However, if this is not successful, there is a risk that a simple open repair (excision and primary anastomosis) may be converted into a more complex (flap or graft) repair.

Open Surgical Repair

The open repair of urethral strictures has evolved significantly over the last 40 years. Currently, almost any urethra can be reconstructed, often in a one-stage operation. The success rate of these procedures is usually in excess of 90% and in some situations 95%. A small subset of patients may require a staged approach. We have repaired urethras from the meatus to the external sphincter in one stage when there was sufficient healthy local tissue. Surgically, it is best to operate on a stable stricture. Therefore, in severe stricture disease requiring dilation every 3 to 4 weeks to prevent urinary retention, a suprapubic cystostomy tube may be needed to allow resolution of the urethral inflammation associated with repeated dilation.

The ideal operation consists of excision of the stricture and repair of the urethra without use of any foreign tissue. Since the corpus spongiosum has inherent elasticity and usually a good blood supply, short strictures (less than 2.5 cm) located from the penoscrotal junction to the membranous urethra can be repaired by excision of the stricture and primary anastomosis. This approach has been successful in 96% of cases. If local anatomy is not favorable, addition of tissue as either a graft or flap is needed.

Grafts are probably the most versatile tissue for urethral repair. The ideal graft source in urethral repair is penile skin, although bladder and buccal mucosa have been used. Hairless extragenital skin can be used, but it provides a much less reliable "take" and subsequent healing. Currently, grafts are most often used to repair short bulbar strictures where the bed of the graft may be the corpus spongiosum.

A better understanding of penile and scrotal blood supply has allowed reconstructive surgeons to generate reliable flaps to repair urethral strictures. In these procedures, the urethra is opened through the stricture into healthy urethra on either side. To compensate for the loss of circumference secondary to the scar, the urethra is patched with an island of skin carried on a vascular pedicle. The ideal donor site is an area of hairless penile skin. Penile island flaps based on a dartos pedicle (axial flaps) can be elevated from the ventral midline with either a longitudinal or a transverse orientation or on the dorsal aspect of the penis in a transverse fashion. Flaps measuring 15 cm in length and 2 cm in width can be mobilized and the penile skin closed primarily.

Although they are not universally accepted, we have found scrotal skin islands to be quite useful in some patients. Often, a hairless area of scrotal skin can be found and mobilized as an island flap in a similar fashion to a penile skin flap. At times, we have epilated scrotal tissue to enlarge a hairless area, but this is a tedious process that is performed with magnification and usually needs to be repeated at least once.

A staged repair may be necessary in a small subset of patients. This requires opening the stricture as described and placing a split-thickness skin graft next to the urethra. The urethra is left open and the patient voids through a perineal urethrostomy. Six months later, the urethra is closed. A staged repair is used in patients with a severe and/or long stricture who lack sufficient hairless tissue.

RENAL CALCULI

method of
DAVID A. LEVY, M.D., and
MARTIN I. RESNICK, M.D.
University Hospital of Cleveland
Cleveland, Ohio

Patients with symptomatic renal or ureteral calculi usually present with colicky type flank discomfort often radiating to the groin, microscopic hematuria, and associated nausea with or without vomiting. Following microscopic urinalysis, diagnostic films are obtained beginning with a plain film of the abdomen followed by an intravenous urogram. The films will often reveal the size of the stone as well as the level and degree of obstruction. Based on the size and position of the stone, one can then predict the likelihood of spontaneous passage, and from the patient's clinical condition a decision can be made whether to take a conservative or an interventional approach (Table 1).

MANAGEMENT

Stones 4 mm or less in their smallest diameter have an 80% chance of passing spontaneously. Stones located in the upper ureter at the time of presentation generally have a lower rate of spontaneous passage than those located in the lower ureter. Stones larger than 4 mm, particularly if located above the true pelvis, will often require intervention in the form of endoscopic manipulation/lithotripsy or placement of a ureteral stent, which will relieve the obstruction until a definitive procedure can be performed, such as extracorporeal shock wave lithotripsy or percutaneous nephrolithotomy.

If a patient presents with a fever and leukocytosis in the face of an obstructing calculus, prompt intravenous antibiotic therapy is mandatory as well as rapid decompression of the obstructed system, which can easily be achieved by placement of a percutaneous nephrostomy or a ureteral stent. This is a very effective way to drain the system and relieve the patient's discomfort with minimal manipulation and low morbidity. Once the patient defervesces, a decision on how to accomplish stone removal can be made electively.

If at the time of presentation the patient shows no sign of infection, the stone is small (less than 4 mm), and the patient can tolerate an oral diet, then expectant outpatient management with vigorous hydration and oral narcotics is acceptable. Oxycodone in combination with acetaminophen (Percocet, Tylox) or acetaminophen in combination with codeine administered in the form of two tablets every 4 to 6 hours will often provide adequate relief of pain while oral meperidine (Demerol) is seldom sufficient. Oral anti-inflammatory agents (ibuprofen) are also effective in relieving the pain associated with stone passage, and some believe that these agents assist in stone passage.* Conversely, if the patient shows signs of infection, cannot tolerate an oral diet, or has a stone that is unlikely to pass spontaneously, hospitalization with aggressive intravenous hydration is usually required. Antibiotics are administered depending on the presence of infection, and intramuscular or parenteral narcotics are warranted until the symptomatic stone can be treated.

Patients managed on an outpatient basis are instructed to maintain close contact with their physician in regard to changes in their condition, (development of fever, intractable vomiting, or pain). Additionally, they are instructed to strain all urine and to maintain adequate hydration. These patients are reevaluated with frequent plain films of the abdomen (every week) to monitor progression of the stone through the collecting system and renal ultrasound to assess for the development of associated hydronephrosis. In the event that complete ureteral obstruction develops, studies have shown that in the absence of infection the obstructed kidney will not incur permanent damage if the obstruction is relieved within 2 weeks.

Once a patient has passed a stone or it has been retrieved, a stone analysis is performed, and based on the chemical composition, appropriate therapy can be implemented. A full history is obtained regarding other illnesses and medications that may be associated with stone formation. A history of prior stones is detailed as is a family history for urolithiasis. A metabolic evaluation of the patient is also carried out consisting of a serum chemistry survey, a 24-hour urine test for uric acid, calcium, oxalate, citrate, creatinine, and volume. The stones generally fall into one of five major groups, pure calcium oxalate (33%), calcium oxalate and phosphate (34%), struvite (15%), uric acid (8%), and cystine (3%). All of these stone types except uric acid stones can be visualized on plain radiographs. Based on the chemical makeup of the stone, different therapeutic regimens have been developed.

Calcium-Based Stones

Calcium-based stones are the most common type of urinary tract calculi. The majority of these stones form secondary to either absorptive or renal hypercalciuria; however, they can form as a result of a variety of different metabolic defects. Therapy is aimed at identifying and correcting the defect as well as reducing urinary calcium. Primary hyperparathyroidism, absorptive and renal hypercalciuria, type I distal renal tubular acidosis as well as cancer metastatic to bone can all lead to excessively high urinary calcium levels and subsequent stone formation. Additionally, diets high in sodium and certain medications (e.g., diuretics, multivitamins, calcium channel blockers) can alter intestinal calcium absorption and/or renal tubular handling of filtered calcium loads, thereby increasing the risk of calcium-based stone formation. A thorough metabolic evaluation will often reveal the disorder.

Hyperparathyroidism, resulting in elevated serum parathyroid levels and a concomitant increase in serum calcium levels, causes an increase in the filtered load of calcium, placing the patient at risk for stone precipitation. Similarly, metastatic disease

*Not FDA approved for this indication.

TABLE 1. **Indications for Urgent Intervention**

Obstruction without infection for >2 weeks
Obstruction with associated infection
Deterioration in baseline renal function
Intractable pain and/or inability to tolerate an oral diet

TABLE 2. **Calcium Stone Disease Office Protocol**

1. Patient begins fasting at 6 P.M. and consumes two 300-ml glasses of distilled water during the fast.
2. Patient voids at 7 A.M. and then collects a 2-hour fasting urine for pH, calcium, magnesium, and creatinine.
   If pH is >5.3, measure pH of each void over next 3–5 days and if all are >5.3, consider renal tubular acidosis.
   If calcium/creatinine ratio is >0.11, a renal leak exists.
   If magnesium/calcium ratio is <33, the result indicates hypomagnesiumuria.
3. Fasting serum sample for creatinine, calcium, phosphorus, uric acid, and electrolytes is obtained at 9 A.M.
4. Patient resumes a normal diet for the next 24 hours including 1 gram of calcium, which can be supplied by 1 quart of milk.
5. 24-hour urine is collected the next day from 9 A.M. to 9 A.M. and is analyzed for volume, calcium, oxalate, citrate, and uric acid.
6. Creatinine clearance is calculated to ensure normal renal function.
7. Hyperabsorptive hypercalciuria is diagnosed if calcium excretion exceeds 4 mg/kg/day.
8. In the presence of hyperoxaluria, a primary intestinal disorder is sought.
9. If hyperuricosuria and hyperuricemia exist, consider a low purine diet and allopurinol.
10. If citrate is low (usually in association with elevated fasting pH), replace citrate.
11. If no abnormality exists (10% of patients), advise on high fluid intake to maintain 2000 mL of urine every 24 hours.

processes can be associated with liberation of calcium from osteoblastic bony lesions and hypercalciuria. Type I distal renal tubular acidosis, diagnosed on the basis of alkaline fasting urine pH as well as serum chemistry studies, is a condition in which the inability of the distal renal tubule to secrete H^+ ions against a gradient results in a severe metabolic acidosis which is buffered in part by bone. The resultant hypercalciuric/hypocitruric state coupled with a relatively alkaline urine favors calcium stone precipitation.

The ambulatory evaluation and categorization of patients with calcium-based stones is outlined in Tables 2 and 3 and the appropriate guidelines for therapy are listed in Table 4. Medical therapy for calcium-based stone disease is illustrated in Table 5.

Patients diagnosed with hyperoxaluria based on the 24-hour urine studies often have absorptive oxaluria secondary to inflammatory bowel disease or prior bowel surgery. The altered bowel function results in poor fat absorption and subsequent saponification of fats with calcium. This leaves oxalate unbound to calcium and available for absorption in excessive amounts. Patients may have primary oxaluria, but they usually present early in life and demonstrate nephrocalcinosis as well as elements of hepatic failure. Hyperoxaluria can also result from ingestion of foods high in oxalate. Treatment of the patient with absorptive hyperoxaluria is medical and is also illustrated in Table 4.

TABLE 3. **Differential Diagnosis of Hypercalciuria**

Classification	Serum Calcium	Fasting Ucalcium (mg/mL Creatinine)	24-Hour Urine Calcium (mg/kg/day)
Absorptive	Normal	<0.11	>4
Renal leak	Normal	>0.11	<4
Hyperparathyroid	High (>10.1)	>0.11	>4
Normocalciuria	Normal	<0.11	<4
Normal—control	Normal	<0.11	<4

TABLE 4. **Therapy for Calcium Stones**

Serum or Urinary Defect	Successful Therapy
Elevated PTH with hypercalcemia	Removal of abnormal parathyroid glands
Hypercalciuria, hyperabsorption	Neutral or cellulose phosphates
Hypercalciuria, renal leak	Thiazide diuretics
Relative hypercalciuria, magnesium deficit	Magnesium oxide or gluconate
Hyperuricemia and hyperuricosuria with calcium urolithiasis	Allopurinol
Intestinal hyperabsorption, hyperoxaluria	Low-oxalate diet plus citrate, magnesium gluconate

Abbreviation: PTH = parathyroid hormone.

Struvite Stones

Stones that develop as a result of infected urine are called struvite stones and most commonly are composed of a mixture of magnesium ammonium phosphate and carbonate apatite. These stones form only in an alkaline environment, as is created in the presence of urease-splitting bacteria. The bacteria involved metabolize urea to bicarbonate and ammonia, and ammonia complexes with free hydrogen ions to form ammonium, which becomes trapped in the renal tubules. The excessive levels of ammonium result in an elevated urinary pH, which leads to precipitation of magnesium-ammonium phosphate and carbonate apatite stones.

Struvite stones are more common in females than

TABLE 5. **Medications for Calcium Stone Disease**

Medication	
Neutral phosphate (Neutra-Phos)	Increases urinary calcium solubility Administered in 500 mg tid or qid Contraindicated in urinary infections or poor renal function May cause diarrhea
Cellulose phosphate (Calcibind)	Binds calcium in the intestine Administered 10–15 gm per day Contraindicated in urinary infections or poor renal function May cause diarrhea
Magnesium oxide (Maox); magnesium gluconate* (Magonate)	Increases urinary magnesium and decreases urinary calcium Administered 150 mg qid or 500 mg bid Contraindicated in urinary infections or poor renal function May cause diarrhea
Hydrochlorothiazide	Increases urinary magnesium and decreases urinary calcium Administered 25–50 mg bid Contraindicated in hypokalemia or when other diuretics are being used

*Not FDA approved for this indication.

in males (2:1) and tend to be soft stones that readily fragment when lithotripsy (ultrasound, extracorporeal, laser, electrohydraulic) is employed. These stones typically grow to fill the entire renal pelvis and infundibula; they are then termed staghorn calculi. If the patient is not rendered completely stone free with treatment, infection will persist despite antibiotic therapy and stone recurrence is inevitable. Stone removal can be accomplished by a variety of procedures or techniques, including open surgery, shock wave lithotripsy, and percutaneous procedures. Oftentimes multiple or combination procedures are required to eradicate stones. Urinary tract acidification accomplished with percutaneous administration of hemiacidrin (Renacidin) or Suby's solution G, both of which have a pH of 4, has been employed to dissolve stone fragments that may remain after primary therapy. After stone eradication, patients are maintained on oral antibiotics for extended periods (several months to years) and must have periodic urine cultures and x-rays to confirm the absence of infection and stones. All patients experiencing recurrent urinary tract infections or recurrent cystitis should have prompt treatment followed by imaging studies of the upper tracts to rule out the presence of infected stones.

Uric Acid Stones

Uric acid stones often form in the presence of an acidic urine containing a high concentration of urate for a given volume of urine, usually in a relatively dehydrated patient. Most patients have normal 24-hour excretion levels of uric acid. When pure, these stones are radiolucent. Most patients who form uric acid stones have low urinary volumes with persistently low pH (<5.5). Patients are evaluated by means of a 24-hour urine sample analysis, measurement of successive urine pH values over several days, and metabolic evaluations for contributory diseases such as disorders of purine metabolism and disorders that can lead to chronic metabolic acidosis, (chronic bowel disorders). Treatment involves increasing daily urinary output by means of increased fluid intake as well as alkalinization of the urine to maintain the urinary pH above 6.5. Maintaining a urinary pH above 6.5 allows for relatively quick dissolution of uric acid calculi and is the treatment of choice for a nonobstructing uric acid stone located in the kidney or ureter. If dissolution fails to occur, another form of intervention will be required.

Alkalinization of the urine is easily achieved with oral sodium-potassium citrate solutions or potassium citrate tablets in dosages of 15 to 20 mEq orally, three to four times per day. Allopurinol (Zyloprim) can also be used in dosages of 300 mg per day in patients with confirmed hyperuricosuria. Allopurinol is also helpful during attempts at stone dissolution but alkalinization alone is usually adequate for maintenance if the patient is not hyperuricosuric. Maintenance therapy in non-hyperuricosuric patients with 15 to 20 mEq potassium citrate only at bedtime is also beneficial.

Cystine Stones

Cystinuria is an inherited homozygous recessive disorder of dibasic amino acid transport across epithelial membranes. The defect manifests itself in the gastrointestinal tract as impaired absorption of amino acids and in the renal tubules as excessive excretion of the dibasic amino acids cystine, ornithine, arginine, and lysine. Patients heterozygous for the disorder usually excrete less than 250 mg of cystine per gram of urinary creatinine and do not develop stones. However, homozygous individuals usually secrete more than 600 mg of cystine in a 24-hour period. Cystine solubility in urine is highly pH dependent.

Alkalinization of the urine enhances cystine solubility, and if the urinary pH can be maintained above 7.8, cystine solubility will be increased two- to threefold. This is difficult to accomplish on a consistent basis but can be achieved with oral alkalinization in the form of 12.6 grams or more of sodium bicarbonate every 24 hours in divided doses, 60 to 80 mL of a balanced citrate solution per day in divided doses, or potassium citrate tablets. The citrate solutions are preferred because they also enhance calcium solubility and provide for a more constant elevation in urinary pH. Furthermore, high fluid intake to maintain a daily urine output of approximately 3 liters is important in preventing stone precipitation.

In patients who excrete more than 600 mg of cystine per day, hydration and alkalinization often do not suffice. These patients must be treated with chelating agents such as D-penicillamine (beta-beta-dimethylcysteine [Cuprimine]) or alpha-mercaptopropionylglycine (tiopronin [Thiola]), which contain a free sulfhydryl group and undergo thio-disulfide exchange which disrupts the cys-S-S-cys disulfide bond and acts to generate a more soluble cysteine-S-Thiola compound. Both agents are FDA-approved treatment modalities and can be administered orally; provided there is an appreciable decrease in excreted cystine, dissolution of an existing stone can occur. Cystine stone dissolution is a very slow process and these agents are more efficacious in prevention than in treatment. The dose of D-penicillamine is based on the known excreted amount of cystine in the urine. Every 250-mg increment in D-penicillamine can be expected to lower the excreted load of cystine by 75 to 100 mg per day. These medications have significant side effects, including gastrointestinal distress, dermatologic hypersensitivity, renal toxicity, and hematologic reactions, that can preclude their continued use in up to 50% of patients. Thiola is generally better tolerated.

Cystine stones tend to be quite hard and are difficult to eradicate with shock wave lithotripsy. To achieve stone-free status in a patient with a large cystine stone (>4 mm) usually requires intervention in the form of endoscopic or percutaneous extraction or laser lithotripsy. Due to the inherent metabolic defect, these patients tend to develop recurrent stones despite life-long alkalinization and chelation.

Overall, urinary tract stone disease is a challenging problem that requires patient cooperation and understanding of the disease process. People who develop stones are at increased risk for future stone development and should be followed by a physician at regular intervals. The potential for significant morbidity as well as loss of renal function exists in the patient with stone disease who is not appropriately treated.

Section 10

The Sexually Transmitted Diseases

CHANCROID

method of
D. W. CAMERON, M.D.
University of Ottawa at the Ottawa General Hospital
Ottawa, Ontario, Canada

Chancroid is a classic venereal disease, a bacterial sexually transmitted genital ulcer syndrome caused by the fastidious organism *Haemophilus ducreyi.* This infection is endemic in many urban centers worldwide and has appeared in United States cities since 1980 in sustained outbreaks. It has been strongly associated with prostitution, and more recently with illicit drug use. Concurrent syphilis and/or genital herpes is common. Chancroid is also an established promoter of sexual human immunodeficiency virus (HIV) transmission. Control of chancroid outbreaks has been achieved by partner follow-up and treatment of cases in identified core groups or reservoirs of infection. Reportage of chancroid cases is low, as the specific diagnosis requires microbiologic isolation of *H. ducreyi* from a genital lesion, and such specialized culture techniques are not generally available. Serodiagnostic tests have greater epidemiologic than clinical applications.

Clinical features include painful, friable suppurative ulceration, with common adjacent discrete lesions. In the female, genital lesions are often introital, especially at the fourchette. In the male, they are often subpreputial and have a predilection for the coronal sulcus and the frenulum. The ulcers are distinctive, painful lesions with undermining of the cutaneous border. Suppuration and friability are also characteristic. Suppurative inguinal lymphadenitis occurs in about 30%, which may spontaneously drain as buboes. Destructive ulcerative lesions with sequelae after cure are occasionally seen. Laboratory tests for HIV, syphilis, and herpes simplex virus should be performed, as well as a smear made of ulcer exudate to identify the characteristic gram-negative streptobacilli of *H. ducreyi.*

TABLE 1. **Antibiotic Therapy for Chancroid**

Recommended Regimens
Azithromycin (Zithromax), 1 gm orally in a single dose,
or
Ceftriaxone (Rocephin), 250 mg intramuscularly in a single dose,
or
Erythromycin base, 500 mg orally four times a day for 7 days.
Alternative Regimens
Amoxicillin, 500 mg, plus clavulinic acid (Augmentin), 125 mg, orally three times a day for 7 days,
or
Ciprofloxacin* (Cipro), 500 mg orally two times a day for 3 days.

*Ciprofloxacin is contraindicated for pregnant and lactating women, children, and adolescents under 18 years of age.
From Centers for Disease Control: 1993 Sexually Transmitted Diseases Treatment Guidelines. MMWR 42, 1993.

TREATMENT

Antibiotic therapies recommended by the Centers for Disease Control and Prevention in the *1993 Sexually Transmitted Diseases Treatment Guidelines* (Table 1) include azithromycin, ceftriaxone, and erythromycin. Alternatives include ciprofloxacin or amoxicillin plus clavulinic acid. Ciprofloxacin should not be used in children or in pregnancy. Trimethoprim-sulfamethoxazole (Bactrim, Septra), is no longer recommended, as antimicrobial resistance has appeared in several settings.

Single-dose therapies have been efficacious; however, longer term therapy may be needed for patients with concurrent HIV infection. All patients should be offered HIV and syphilis testing, to be repeated after 3 months if negative. A subjective response to therapy should be obvious within 3 days and a clinical response by 7 days; if not, noncompliance, antimicrobial resistance, coinfection, or misdiagnosis should be considered. Follow-up until complete cure is achieved is important, particularly with extensive lesions or in the relapse-prone HIV-infected patient. Fluctuant buboes respond best to needle aspiration through healthy skin; surgical incision is unnecessary. Cases should be reported, and partner follow-up for treatment is of value for disease control.

GONORRHEA

method of
CHARLES B. HICKS, M.D.*
Duke University Medical Center
Durham, North Carolina
(Formerly of Walter Reed Army Medical Center Washington, D.C.)

EPIDEMIOLOGY

Although its incidence has declined since a peak in the mid-1970s, gonorrhea is still responsible for over 1 million

*The views of the author do not necessarily reflect the position of the Army or the Department of Defense.

infections in the United States every year. It remains the most commonly reported infection in this country. Treatment of *Neisseria gonorrhoeae* became problematic during the 1960s and 1970s when increasing resistance to penicillin was detected. In response, the Centers for Disease Control and Prevention (CDC) in 1972 raised the recommended dose of penicillin to 4.8 million units to be administered in conjunction with probenecid. Although initially effective, even these large doses of penicillin proved insufficient with the emergence of plasmid-mediated, penicillinase-producing *N. gonorrhoeae* (PPNG) in 1976 and chromosomally mediated resistant *N. gonorrhoeae* (CMRNG) in 1983. Shortly thereafter, high-level resistance to tetracycline and spectinomycin (Trobicin) was also reported, although the latter remains rare in the United States.

In response to these reports of gonococcal resistance, the CDC implemented the Gonococcal Isolate Surveillance Project in 1986. This program regularly monitors antimicrobial susceptibility of gonococcal isolates from 26 publicly funded sexually transmitted disease (STD) clinics representing all areas of the United States. According to the most recently reported surveillance data, 32.4% of gonococcal isolates were resistant to penicillin or tetracycline. The proportion of isolates with high-level resistance to these antibiotics increased significantly over the period reported (1988 to 1991). During this same period, there were no documented clinical failures attributed to decreased susceptibility to ceftriaxone (Rocephin) or ciprofloxacin (Cipro).

CLINICAL MANIFESTATIONS

The vast majority of cases of gonorrhea are localized, urogenital infections. In men, these infections typically present as dysuria and urethral discharge and, in women, as dysuria or vaginal discharge depending on the predominant site of infection. Infections are more often symptomatic in men than in women. Less common sites of local involvement include the rectum and pharynx, both of which tend to be asymptomatic infections. More serious infections include pelvic inflammatory disease (PID), a term encompassing endometritis, salpingitis, and peritonitis, as well as disseminated gonococcal infection (DGI), which can include arthritis, tenosynovitis, dermatitis, and, rarely, hepatitis, myocarditis, endocarditis, and meningitis.

Diagnosis of gonorrhea almost always requires a culture from an infected site. Urethral infections in men can be diagnosed with reliability by Gram's stain, but cultures of urethral exudate will reveal a few additional cases not detected by Gram's stain alone, and thus, cultures should generally be done on all patients suspected of having gonorrhea. Patients whose symptoms subside after appropriate treatment do not need follow-up cultures; however, patients who remain symptomatic require complete re-evaluation, including appropriate smears and cultures. For men with suspected gonococcal urethritis, treatment decisions can be based on results of the Gram stain. For patients with other forms of gonorrhea, the sensitivity of smears is inadequate for decision-making, and they should be treated based on the presenting syndrome (as in the case of PID or DGI) or the results of culture. All cases of gonorrhea should be reported to appropriate public health authorities, and patients should be tested for other STDs such as syphilis and human immunodeficiency virus (HIV) infection. All sexual contacts of gonorrhea patients require evaluation and treatment, even if asymptomatic.

A significant proportion of patients with gonorrhea are co-infected with *Chlamydia trachomatis* or other pathogens that can cause urogenital infection. Because of the difficulty in diagnosing these pathogens, presumptive treatment directed at these potential infecting agents should be given to all patients with gonorrhea. Current therapies for gonorrhea do not adequately treat nongonococcal urogenital pathogens; thus, all patients with gonorrhea require a second antibiotic in addition to that directed at *N. gonorrhoeae.*

TREATMENT OF ADULTS

Uncomplicated Urogenital, Rectal, or Pharyngeal Infection

The CDC has recently revised its published STD Treatment Guidelines to reflect data accumulated on several newer antimicrobials shown to be effective against *N. gonorrhoeae.* While all of these drugs have efficacy rates of 95% or greater even against PPNG and CMRNG, some are unproven as treatment for pharyngeal infections. Appropriate treatments are listed in Table 1 in an approximate order of preference.

Ceftriaxone as a single intramuscular (IM) injection of 125 mg produces sustained drug levels that appear to be effective in curing incubating syphilis. None of the other treatments is likely to be similarly effective, although regimens used for presumptive treatment of *Chlamydia* will probably cure incubating syphilis as well. The advantage of ceftriaxone's increased activity against syphilis is offset by the need for intramuscular injection with its attendant discomfort to the patient and the requirement for a provider skilled in preparation and administration of IM medications. In settings in which these issues are not a major problem, ceftriaxone, 125 mg IM as a single dose, is the treatment of choice for uncomplicated gonorrhea, accompanied by a regimen for the presumptive treatment of coexistent *Chlamydia* (Table 2).

In situations in which oral antimicrobials are clearly preferred, cefixime (Suprax), 400 mg as a single dose, is recommended, but a number of other beta-lactams are probably equally effective. Cefixime

TABLE 1. **Treatment of Uncomplicated Adult Gonococcal Infections*†**

Preferred Regimens
Ceftriaxone (Rocephin), 125 mg IM as a single dose
or
Cefixime (Suprax), 400 mg orally as a single dose

Alternative Regimens for Patients Who Cannot Receive Beta-Lactam Antibiotics
Ciprofloxacin‡ (Cipro), 500 mg orally as a single dose
or
Ofloxacin‡ (Floxin), 400 mg orally as a single dose

Alternative Regimen for Patients Who Cannot Receive Beta-Lactam or Quinolone Antibiotics
Spectinomycin (Trobicin), 2 grams IM as a single dose

*Drugs are listed in order of preference.
†All regimens must also include presumptive treatment for *Chlamydia trachomatis* (see Table 2).
‡Quinolones are contraindicated in pregnant or nursing women and in children under the age of 16.

TABLE 2. **Presumptive Treatment Regimens for *Chlamydia* Infection in Patients with Gonorrhea***

Preferred Regimens
Doxycycline (Vibramycin), 100 mg orally twice daily for 7 days
or
Azithromycin (Zithromax), 1 gram orally as a single dose

Alternative Regimens
Ofloxacin† (Floxin), 300 mg orally twice daily for 7 days
or
Erythromycin base, 500 mg orally four times daily for 7 days

*Drugs are listed in order of preference.
†Quinolones are contraindicated in pregnant or nursing women and in children less than 16 years of age.

is preferred primarily because there is more experience with its use. For patients who cannot be given beta-lactam antibiotics, quinolones are suggested, with ciprofloxacin (Cipro), 500 mg, or ofloxacin (Floxin), 400 mg as a single oral dose, recommended. Quinolones are contraindicated in pregnant or nursing women and in children under the age of 16 because of the potential for damage to juvenile articular cartilage. Patients who cannot receive either beta-lactam antibiotics or quinolones should be treated with spectinomycin, 2 grams IM as a single dose. Spectinomycin is not effective in pharyngeal gonorrhea.

Pelvic Inflammatory Disease

Pelvic inflammatory disease (PID) is an infection of the female upper genital tract that sometimes also involves the peritoneum. It can be difficult to diagnose, and a discussion of appropriate diagnostic criteria for this syndrome is beyond the scope of this text. PID is almost invariably a polymicrobial infection in which *N. gonorrhoeae,* when present, is generally only one of several responsible pathogens. Accordingly, broad-spectrum treatment is needed in order to encompass all the potential pathogens. It is extremely important to identify those patients requiring hospitalization (Table 3) since the sequelae of undertreated PID are profound. Recommended regimens for PID are shown in Table 4.

Disseminated Gonococcal Infection

Most cases of disseminated gonococcal infection (DGI) present as tenosynovitis, arthritis, and a papulopustular rash. Rarely, disseminated infection can produce hepatitis, endocarditis, and meningitis. Most patients with DGI have little in the way of urogenital symptoms. Many cases are diagnosed presumptively based on the clinical presentation in a sexually active person, but efforts to recover the organism in culture from involved sites should be made. Initial treatment should be given in the hospital, and all patients treated for DGI need presumptive therapy for concurrent *C. trachomatis* infection. The treatment of choice is ceftriaxone, 1 gram IM or IV every 24 hours. Patients who cannot be given beta-lactam drugs should

TABLE 3. **Indications for Hospitalization in Pelvic Inflammatory Disease**

Uncertain diagnosis when surgical emergencies such as appendicitis and ectopic pregnancy cannot be excluded
Pelvic abscess is suspected
Pregnant patients
Adolescent patients
Severe symptoms or nausea and vomiting that preclude outpatient management
Inability to follow or tolerate an outpatient regimen
Incomplete clinical response to outpatient management
Outpatient follow-up within 72 hours of initiation of therapy cannot be ensured

be treated with spectinomycin, 2 grams every 12 hours. Parenteral therapy should be continued for 24 to 48 hours after clinical improvement begins, then either cefixime, 400 mg orally twice daily, or ciprofloxacin, 500 mg orally twice daily, should be given to complete a full week of therapy. If meningitis or endocarditis is suspected or diagnosed, longer duration therapy is required, and expert consultation is advised.

TREATMENT OF CHILDREN AND NEONATES

Neonatal Infections

Neonatal gonococcal infections are almost always the result of exposure to infected exudate from the mother during the birth process. Infection can occur in a wide variety of sites and can present as rhinitis, vaginitis, urethritis, arthritis, meningitis, or sepsis. The most common manifestation of peripartum exposure and infection, however, is gonococcal ophthalmia neonatorum. This infection is rare in the United

TABLE 4. **Treatment of Pelvic Inflammatory Disease**

Inpatient Regimens
Cefoxitin (Mefoxin), 2 grams intravenously every 6 hours, or cefotetan (Cefotan), 2 grams intravenously every 12 hours
plus
Doxycycline, 100 mg intravenously every 12 hours
or
Clindamycin (Cleocin), 900 mg intravenously every 8 hours
plus
Gentamicin, 2 mg/kg initial dose, followed by 1.5 mg/kg every 8 hours, adjusted for renal function

Outpatient Regimens
Cefoxitin, 2 grams IM, plus probenecid, 1 gram orally, in a single dose
plus
Doxycycline, 100 mg orally twice daily for 14 days
or
Ofloxacin‡, 400 mg orally twice daily for 14 days
plus
Clindamycin, 450 mg orally four times daily for 14 days

*Drugs are listed in order of preference.
†Inpatient regimens should be continued for at least 48 hours after the patient demonstrates substantial clinical improvement, after which doxycycline, 100 mg orally twice daily to complete a total of 14 days' therapy, should be given.
‡Quinolones are contraindicated in pregnant or nursing women and in children less than 16 years of age.

States due to the widespread use of ocular prophylaxis in newborns. Recommended treatment is ceftriaxone, 25 to 50 mg per kg IV or IM in a single dose, not to exceed a 125-mg total dose. Disseminated gonococcal infections in neonates are very rare in the United States. If gram-stained smears and/or cultures indicate that such an infection is present, recommended treatment is ceftriaxone, 25 to 50 mg per kg per day IV or IM in a single daily dose for 7 days. If meningitis is documented, treatment should be continued for a total of 10 to 14 days. Cases of neonatal DGI and gonococcal ophthalmia should be managed in conjunction with expert consultation.

Infants born to mothers with gonococcal infection are at high risk of infection and should be treated whether they are symptomatic or not. Recommended treatment is ceftriaxone, 25 to 50 mg per kg IV or IM as a single dose, not to exceed a 125-mg total dose.

Infections in Children

Gonorrhea occurring in preadolescent children after the neonatal period is almost always a consequence of child abuse. Diagnostic specimens should be obtained in conjunction with appropriate legal authorities so that information obtained through the medical evaluation can be used in legal proceedings if necessary. Children weighing more than 45 kg should receive the same treatment regimens as adults (see Table 1), except that quinolones should not be used in children under the age of 16. Children weighing less than 45 kg should receive ceftriaxone, 125 mg as a single IM injection, or alternatively, spectinomycin, 40 mg per kg (maximum 2 grams) as a single IM injection. Children with DGI should be treated with ceftriaxone, 50 mg per kg (maximum 1 gram) IM or IV in a single daily dose for 7 days. If meningitis is diagnosed, treatment should be given for 10 to 14 days at 50 mg per kg per day (maximum of 2 grams). Oral cephalosporins have not been adequately studied in children with gonorrhea, and their use is not recommended.

NONGONOCOCCAL URETHRITIS

method of
THOMAS M. HOOTON, M.D.
Harborview Medical Center
Seattle, Washington

Nongonococcal urethritis is caused by *Chlamydia trachomatis* in approximately 30 to 50% of cases and by *Ureaplasma urealyticum* in a smaller proportion. Sporadic cases of nongonococcal urethritis have been reported to be caused by other bacteria, and some cases are caused by *Trichomonas vaginalis* and herpes simplex virus. In at least 20 to 30% of cases, however, no cause can be identified, even with extensive culture efforts. In practice, the specific etiology of most cases of nongonococcal urethritis is often not determined because of the expense or unavailability of reliable diagnostic testing and because of difficulties in the interpretation of positive cultures for *U. urealyticum*. Newer sensitive nonculture assays for *C. trachomatis* using urine or urethral swab specimens should facilitate the diagnosis of this important pathogen.

Urethritis is manifested by urethral inflammation and may or may not be associated with dysuria, urethral discharge, or urethral pruritus. The clinical manifestations of nongonococcal urethritis overlap with those of gonococcal urethritis, and the two conditions cannot be definitively distinguished on clinical grounds. However, in general, the incubation period of nongonococcal urethritis is longer and the symptoms milder compared with gonorrhea. A presumptive diagnosis of nongonococcal urethritis is made in the absence of gram-negative diplococci on the gram-stained urethral swab specimen, but a negative urethral culture for *Neisseria gonorrhoeae* is required for a more definitive diagnosis. The clinical presentations of chlamydia-positive and chlamydia-negative nongonococcal urethritis are indistinguishable. Infection with *N. gonorrhoeae* and *C. trachomatis* may be asymptomatic, especially among persons named as sexual contacts of infected individuals.

Urethral inflammation is defined as the presence of an average of five or more polymorphonuclear leukocytes per 1000× (oil immersion) field in a Gram-stained urethral smear or 15 or more polymorphonuclear leukocytes in a 400× field in the spun sediment of a first-voided urine specimen. The leukocyte esterase test appears to be a sensitive marker for urethral inflammation and can be used to screen urine from asymptomatic males, but a diagnosis of urethritis should be confirmed with a urethral Gram stain. *C. trachomatis* can be present even though the leukocyte esterase test and urethral Gram stain are normal.

TREATMENT

Recommended regimens for nongonococcal urethritis are those with activity against *C. trachomatis* and include doxycycline, 100 mg orally twice daily, and erythromycin base, 500 mg orally four times daily for 7 days (Table 1). For those patients who are intolerant of the 7-day regimen of erythromycin, one of the erythromycin regimens listed in Table 1 can be used at half the respective dose four times daily for 14 days. Recent studies have demonstrated that a 1.0-gram single dose of azithromycin (Zithromax) is as effective and well tolerated as a conventional regimen of doxycycline for chlamydial and nonchlamydial nongonococcal urethritis. The obvious advantage of the azithromycin regimen is convenience to the pa-

TABLE 1. **Recommended Treatment Regimens for Nongonococcal Urethritis***

Drug	Dosage
Doxycycline	100 mg every 12 hours for 7 days
Erythromycin base	500 mg every 6 hours for 7 days
Erythromycin ethylsuccinate	800 mg every 6 hours for 7 days
Azithromycin (Zithromax)†	1.0 gram single dose
Ofloxacin (Floxin)†‡	300 mg every 12 hours for 7 days

*All regimens are effective against *Chlamydia trachomatis*.
†Considerably more expensive than the other regimens.
‡Quinolones are contraindicated in pregnancy and in children age 16 or less.

tient and assured compliance. It is possible, but not proved, that azithromycin treatment results in superior cure rates against *Chlamydia* in everyday practice given the poor compliance associated with multiple-day treatment regimens, especially in patients with mild or no symptoms. However, this potential advantage has to be weighed against the disadvantage of the considerably greater expense of azithromycin. Side effects with all of these drugs are primarily gastrointestinal.

Although all of the new fluoroquinolones are highly effective in single-dose regimens against *N. gonorrhoeae,* none will eradicate *C. trachomatis* reliably in such regimens. Ofloxacin (Floxin) is the only commercially available quinolone antibiotic that has acceptable activity against *C. trachomatis,* but a 7-day regimen is required. The approved regimen for chlamydial infection is 300 mg twice daily for 7 days (Table 1). This regimen also appears to be as effective as conventional regimens against nonchlamydial nongonococcal urethritis. None of the other new fluoroquinolones should be used when infection with *C. trachomatis* is thought to be possible.

Patients with nongonococcal urethritis should be considered for testing for other sexually transmitted diseases, especially syphilis and human immunodeficiency virus infection. Education about sexually transmitted diseases should be provided at the time of diagnosis. Sexual partners of men with nongonococcal urethritis should also be evaluated, tested, and treated given the potential for infectious sequelae in women. Patients treated for nongonococcal urethritis, regardless of whether *C. trachomatis* was initially isolated, do not require follow-up evaluation unless symptoms persist or recur or unless the patient was not compliant with the treatment regimen.

Men with persistent or recurrent symptoms following treatment for nongonococcal urethritis should be re-evaluated for objective evidence of urethritis. If post-treatment urethritis is documented and if reinfection or poor compliance in taking medications appears to be the reason for treatment failure, the patient should be re-treated with doxycycline or tetracycline for 7 days. If there is no apparent reason for treatment failure, the patient should be treated with erythromycin in one of the regimens previously outlined, since tetracycline-resistant *U. urealyticum* is known to cause some of these infections.

In men who have symptomatic persistent or recurrent nongonococcal urethritis following 1-week courses of doxycycline and erythromycin, *T. vaginalis* should be sought with a urethral swab culture (and treated if present), and a 3- (or more) week trial of erythromycin should be considered. If this fails, it is reasonable to discontinue further empiric therapeutic efforts with antibiotics. For anxious patients who desire further empiric treatment, several-week regimens of doxycycline, trimethoprim-sulfamethoxazole, ciprofloxacin (Cipro) or ofloxacin, clarithromycin (Biaxin) or azithromycin, nonsteroidal anti-inflammatory drugs, or other agents can be tried, although none have been systematically evaluated in this population, the cost can be quite substantial, and side effects are more likely. Although it appears that many of these men have evidence of prostatic inflammation, routine evaluation of prostatic secretions is not recommended, since such knowledge does not alter treatment recommendations. Likewise, routine cystourethroscopy does not appear to be helpful in patient management.

Although the natural history of persistent or recurrent nongonococcal urethritis has not been described, the condition appears to resolve in most men over a period of weeks or months, although it may recur several months later. There are no data to suggest that persistent urethritis has serious sequelae in men. It may be necessary to counsel the patient and his sexual partner together to alleviate undue anxiety. No consistent clinical or microbiologic abnormalities have been identified in the sex partners of men with persistent or recurrent nongonococcal urethritis; however, this issue has not been systematically studied.

GRANULOMA INGUINALE
(Donovanosis)

method of
NANCY J. ANDERSON, M.D.
Loma Linda University
Loma Linda, California

Granuloma inguinale is a chronic, slowly progressive, ulcerative anogenital infection caused by a gram-negative, obligate intracellular bacillus, *Calymmatobacterium granulomatis,* which is serologically related to *Klebsiella.* It is rare in the United States, and socioeconomic status and living conditions may be a major risk factor.

The incubation period ranges from several days to several months. The lesions begin as firm papules or vesiculopapules and later erode to a painless ulcer. Lymphadenopathy and systemic symptoms are uncommon. Four variants in morphology include

1. Nodular form, characterized by soft, red nodules that eventually ulcerate
2. Ulcerative or ulcerogranulomatous form, with a granulomatous ulcer that is nonindurated and hemorrhagic
3. Hypertrophic or verrucous form, which has an irregular surface and a granulomatous base
4. Sclerotic, or cicatricial, form, which presents as a bandlike scar of the genitalia

The differential diagnosis includes syphilis, chancroid, lymphogranuloma venereum, tuberculosis of the skin, squamous cell carcinoma, cutaneous amebiasis, and filariasis.

Diagnosis is made by demonstrating *C. granulomatis* by Wright or Giemsa stain of biopsy or crushed samples of granulation tissue taken from the periphery of a lesion. Donovan bodies are gram-negative bacilli that are seen as intracytoplasmic inclusions of mononuclear cells. No culture or reliable serologic testing is available for routine diagnosis.

TREATMENT

The treatment of choice is tetracycline, 500 mg four times a day for 14 to 21 days or until lesions are healed. If tetracycline fails, streptomycin should be used, 0.5 to 1.0 grams intramuscularly twice a day for 10 to 14 days. Alternatives include trimethoprim-sulfamethoxazole (Bactrim), 160 mg/800 mg two tablets twice a day for 10 to 14 days; chloramphenicol (Chloromycetin), 50 mg four times a day for 10 to 14 days; and gentamicin (Garamycin), 40 mg intramuscularly twice a day for 14 to 21 days. Pregnant women should be treated with erythromycin, 500 mg four times a day for 14 to 21 days.

In early cases, prognosis for complete healing is good. In late cases, irreparable tissue destruction may occur and reconstructive surgery may be required. Patients with granuloma inguinale (and their partners) should be screened for other sexually transmitted diseases.

LYMPHOGRANULOMA VENEREUM

method of
NANCY J. ANDERSON, M.D.
Loma Linda University
Loma Linda, California

Lymphogranuloma venereum (LGV) is an uncommon, systemic, sexually transmitted disease caused by the L1, L2, or L3 serotypes of *Chlamydia trachomatis.* The incubation period is highly variable and ranges from several days to several weeks. The disease is epidemic in parts of Asia, Africa, India, Southeast Asia, and the Caribbean but uncommon in the United States. In the United States, it is more commonly seen in Washington, D.C., and the southeastern states in lower socioeconomic groups. The age-specific rates are highest in the 20- to 40-year-old group.

The infection starts as a small, tender vesicle of the genitalia or perineum that rapidly ulcerates, becomes painful, then heals spontaneously in a few days. One to two weeks later, regional lymphadenitis and fever occur and can progress to buboes with multiple areas of suppuration and drainage. These areas often occur above and below Pauport's ligament, giving rise to the "groove" sign. If the rectum is involved, there is associated painful proctocolitis and rectal strictures. LGV is often accompanied by malaise, fever, myalgia, and arthralgia. Other dermatologic associations includes erythema nodosum, erythema multiforme, scarlatiniform exanthem, and urticaria.

Diagnosis is made by compatible clinical presentation and by implementing fixation titer, of which 1:64 is considered diagnostic. *C. trachomatis* can be identified by rapid diagnostic testing employing either an enzyme-linked immunosorbent assay or a direct fluorescent antibody method.

TREATMENT

The recommended treatment is tetracycline hydrochloride, 500 mg four times a day for 3 to 4 weeks, or doxycycline (Vibramycin), 100 mg twice a day for 3 to 4 weeks, or until all symptoms and signs have resolved. If lymphadenopathy fails to respond within 10 to 14 days or if a relapse occurs, an alternative regimen is either a 2- to 6-week course of sulfamethoxazole,* 1 gram four times a day, or a 2- to 6-week course of erythromycin, 500 mg four times a day. The latter treatment is preferred for pregnant women.

Fluctuant lymph nodes should be aspirated to prevent tissue breakdown and the formation of chronic draining sinuses. In patients with strictures and fistulas, reconstructive surgery may be necessary. With treatment, prognosis is excellent. Patients with LGV should be screened for other sexually transmitted diseases.

SYPHILIS

method of
ROBIN D. ISAACS, M.D.
Department of Veterans Affairs Medical Center
The University of Mississippi Medical Center
Jackson, Mississippi

Syphilis is a chronic, systemic infectious disease caused by the spirochete *Treponema pallidum* subsp. *pallidum.* During the past 6 years, syphilis has re-emerged as a major health problem in the United States, particularly in the inner cities and in association with illicit drug use. Although untreated syphilis is described as progressing through primary, secondary, latent, and tertiary stages, the natural history in an individual patient is variable and unpredictable. In order to make therapeutic decisions, the classification of syphilis is simplified into the following groupings:

1. *Early syphilis:* patients with primary and secondary syphilis and early latent syphilis of less than 1 year's duration.
2. *Late syphilis:* all other patients, including those patients with syphilis of unknown duration. This grouping is subdivided further into:
   a. *Neurosyphilis*
   b. *All other types,* including gummatous and cardiovascular syphilis and late latent syphilis of more than 1 year's duration.

DIAGNOSIS

As *T. pallidum* cannot be cultivated in vitro, diagnosis can be made only by direct visualization of the treponemes or indirectly by serologic studies. Darkfield or immunofluorescent microscopy is the diagnostic method of choice for examining chancres and moist lesions of secondary syphilis. Diagnosis of other stages of syphilis is reliant on serology because treponemes are not sufficiently abundant in other syphilitic lesions for routine microscopic identification.

The inability to diagnose syphilis by a single serologic test provides additional confusion. There are two types of serologic tests for syphilis: (1) nontreponemal tests (e.g., Venereal Diseases Research Laboratory [VDRL], rapid plasma reagin [RPR]), and (2) treponemal tests (e.g., the fluorescent treponemal antibody-absorbed [FTA-Abs], the microhemagglutination assay for antibody to *T. pallidum*

*Exceeds dosage recommended by the manufacturer.

[MHATP]). Nontreponemal tests are useful for screening purposes and for following disease activity because, in general, the titer falls after successful treatment. The diagnosis of syphilis must be confirmed by a treponemal test because false-positive results on nontreponemal tests are common. In contrast to nontreponemal tests, treponemal tests usually remain reactive for the life of the patient, even after successful treatment, and cannot be used as a marker of recent infection. A patient who has reactive nontreponemal and treponemal test results and has not previously received adequate treatment for syphilis should be evaluated and treated for the appropriate stage.

Patients with late syphilis need to be evaluated for symptomatic or asymptomatic neurosyphilis by a thorough clinical examination and a cerebrospinal fluid (CSF) examination. Although, ideally, all patients with late syphilis should receive a CSF examination, the decision to perform a lumbar puncture is often individualized (e.g., the yield is low in asymptomatic older patients). CSF examination, however, *should be performed* if nonpenicillin therapy is planned, if the patient is co-infected with HIV, or if the patient has neurologic signs or symptoms, has failed previous syphilis treatment, has a serum nontreponemal antibody titer of 1:32 or greater, or has other evidence of active syphilis. CSF examination is *not* recommended in patients with early syphilis because progression to symptomatic neurosyphilis is rare if an appropriate treatment regimen for early syphilis is prescribed.

The CSF should be analyzed for cell count, protein, and VDRL. A reactive CSF VDRL is specific for neurosyphilis, but neurosyphilis can be present even if the CSF VDRL is nonreactive. If the CSF VDRL is nonreactive, a CSF leukocyte count of more than 5 white cells per mm^3 and/or an elevated CSF protein may be indicators of neurosyphilis, and an appropriate treatment regimen should be administered. The CSF FTA-Abs is not recommended because it lacks specificity, but it can be useful in the setting of penicillin allergy because a nonreactive CSF FTA-Abs provides strong evidence against a diagnosis of neurosyphilis. Finally, some syphilitic patients have neurologic symptoms or signs compatible with a diagnosis of neurosyphilis but have normal results on CSF examination; these patients should be treated for neurosyphilis.

TREATMENT

The guidelines for the treatment of syphilis outlined in Table 1 are based on those published by the Centers for Disease Control and Prevention and are extrapolated from the clinical literature because no large prospective, randomized studies of any treatment regimen have been performed. Evaluation of nonpenicillin treatment regimens, in particular, has been extremely limited.

Penicillin is the drug of choice in all stages of syphilis. *All* patients with neurosyphilis and with syphilis during pregnancy require parenteral penicillin treatment; patients with a history of penicillin allergy should be skin tested and if reactive, should be desensitized prior to treatment with the appropriate penicillin regimen. Safe and effective protocols for oral penicillin desensitization are available, but it is best to refer such patients to specialist centers for management.

Either doxycycline or tetracycline can be used in penicillin-allergic nonpregnant patients without neurosyphilis. If follow-up cannot be guaranteed, strong consideration should be given to skin testing and, if necessary, desensitization prior to appropriate penicillin treatment. Doxycycline is preferred because it can be taken with meals and requires only twice-daily dosing. The role of newer agents (e.g., ceftriaxone* [Rocephin]) in the treatment of syphilis remains to be established, and standard regimens (see Table 1) should be used because they are well established, reliable, cheap, and easy to administer. Patients who cannot tolerate either a penicillin or a tetracycline regimen should be referred for specialist management.

Patients treated at any stage of syphilis, but most commonly with early syphilis, can develop a Jarisch-Herxheimer reaction. This is an acute febrile reaction that usually starts within a few hours of treatment and is often associated with myalgias and headache. No specific treatment is available, although antipyretics may ameliorate symptoms. Patients should be warned about the possibility of such a reaction and reassured that there are no long-term sequelae. Pregnant patients, in particular, need counseling because such reactions can precipitate premature labor; nevertheless, treatment for syphilis should be given promptly to pregnant patients because the risk of fetal infection is far greater than the risk posed by the reaction.

Neurosyphilis

Treatment of neurosyphilis requires high-dose continuous parenteral penicillin usually in the form of intravenous aqueous crystalline penicillin G (see Table 1). If patient compliance can be assured, a 10-day outpatient regimen consisting of both procaine penicillin, 2.4 million units intramuscularly daily, and probenecid (Benemid), 500 mg orally four times daily, is effective.

Treatment of Contacts

The standard antigonoccocal regimen employing ceftriaxone* (Rocephin) and doxycycline probably aborts incubating syphilis. In contrast, quinolone treatment is ineffective against incubating syphilis, and there are insufficient data with respect to the efficacy of newer azolide antimicrobials and single-dose oral cephalosporin regimens.

There is a significant risk of contracting syphilis after a single sexual exposure with a patient with early syphilis. Patients seen within 90 days of exposure should be evaluated and treated for syphilis. Patients who are seen more than 90 days after exposure should be evaluated and treatment planned if there is evidence of infection; if follow-up of the contact is problematic, treatment for early syphilis should be administered.

---

*Not FDA approved for this indication.

TABLE 1. **Suggested Treatment Regimens According to the Stage of Syphilis**

Stage of Infection	Regimens for Nonpenicillin-Allergic Patients	Regimens for Penicillin-Allergic Patients
Early syphilis*	Benzathine penicillin G, 2.4 million units IM, in one dose	Doxycycline, 100 mg PO twice daily for 2 weeks
Late latent syphilis, gummatous syphilis, and cardiovascular syphilis‡	Benzathine penicillin G, 2.4 million units IM, given 1 week apart for 3 weeks (total dose 7.2 million units)	Doxycycline, 100 mg PO twice daily for 4 weeks†
Neurosyphilis§	Aqueous crystalline penicillin G, 3 million units IV every 4 hours for 10 days‖	Penicillin desensitization
Syphilis in pregnancy§	Treat according to stage	Penicillin desensitization
Congenital syphilis§	Procaine penicillin, 50,000 units per kg IM once a day for 10–14 days *or* Aqueous crystalline penicillin G, 50,000 units per kg IV every 8–12 hours for 10–14 days	

*Primary and secondary syphilis and latent syphilis of <1 year's duration.
†Nonpenicillin regimens should be used only if neurosyphilis is excluded by CSF examination.
‡CSF examination is recommended in most patients with late syphilis (see text).
§Penicillin regimens must be used for patients with neurosyphilis or congenital syphilis and for pregnant patients with syphilis.
‖Intramuscular procaine penicillin can be administered as outpatient treatment in selected patients (see text).

Syphilis in Pregnancy

Pregnant women should be treated with a penicillin regimen appropriate for their stage of syphilis (see Table 1). Women with penicillin allergy should be skin tested and desensitized if necessary. Penicillin-based regimens are highly effective in preventing congenital infection. Monthly follow-up of the mother before delivery with nontreponemal serologic study is mandatory so that further treatment can be given if relapse or re-infection occurs; after delivery, follow-up is as for nonpregnant patients.

Congenital Syphilis

A full discussion of the management of congenital syphilis is beyond the scope of this article. Clinical assessment, diagnosis, and treatment of the neonate with potential congenital syphilis require consultation with physicians experienced in this area. All neonates born to mothers who had syphilis during pregnancy must be carefully examined for evidence of congenital infection. Penicillin is the only agent used for treatment of congenital syphilis (see Table 1). All neonates with confirmed congenital syphilis; those born to mothers who received no treatment, nonpenicillin treatment, or treatment for syphilis in the last month of gestation; and those neonates who cannot be followed after hospital discharge should receive appropriate treatment.

Older children occasionally present with congenital syphilis. They should be evaluated for neurosyphilis and treated with a regimen adequate for congenital syphilis, but the total penicillin dose should not exceed the adult dosage; children who are older than 8 years of age with penicillin allergy can be given doxycycline if no neurologic involvement is observed.

Follow-Up

It is important to follow all patients treated for syphilis for evidence of treatment response. This is evaluated by serial nontreponemal serologic testing, preferably performed at the same laboratory and using the same test. A four-fold reduction in the titer of a quantitative nontreponemal test is significant and is good evidence of response. Patients with early syphilis should have serologic testing repeated at 3 and 6 months; in the absence of evidence of reinfection, if the titer has not decreased significantly within 3 months in patients with primary or secondary disease or within 6 months in other patients with early syphilis, a CSF examination should be performed and the patient re-treated appropriately. Patients with late syphilis who do not have neurosyphilis should have serology repeated at 6 and 12 months; a small number of patients, generally those with initial low-titer nontreponemal antibody tests, may not show a significant change in titer. Ideally, all patients treated for syphilis should be assessed every 6 months until the nontreponemal antibody test is either nonreactive or of low titer and stable. Reassessment is required if the titer increases by four-fold, if a titer of 1:32 or greater fails to fall, or if the patient develops symptomatic syphilis; such patients need a CSF examination and appropriate treatment.

Patients with neurosyphilis require follow-up with serologic testing, and if the initial CSF test results was abnormal, by serial CSF examinations. The CSF white blood cell count generally responds first, and CSF examinations should be performed every 6 months until the white blood cell count has returned to normal. In general, the cell count will have fallen after 6 months and will have returned to normal by 2 years. Re-treatment should be strongly considered if the CSF parameters do not show normalization within 2 years.

Syphilis and Human Immunodeficiency Virus Co-Infection

Based on anecdotal case reports, concern has been expressed that the natural history of syphilis and its response to treatment may be altered in HIV-infected patients. In addition, serologic tests may be less sensitive in HIV co-infected patients. There is no conclusive evidence, however, that this is the case, and HIV-infected patients should be diagnosed and treated for syphilis according to the standard guidelines. It is prudent, however, to follow HIV co-infected patients closely to establish a therapeutic response. Serologic studies, therefore, should be assessed at least 1, 2, 3, 6, 9, and 12 months after treatment. In addition, it is advisable to perform CSF examinations as part of the initial diagnostic studies on all HIV co-infected patients and to treat for neurosyphilis if there are abnormal CSF parameters. Finally, if serologic studies are nonreactive in the clinical setting of possible syphilis, lesions should be biopsied to look for evidence of treponemal infection.

Section 11

Diseases of Allergy

ANAPHYLAXIS AND SERUM SICKNESS

method of
REBECCA B. RABY, M.D., and
MICHAEL S. BLAISS, M.D.
University of Tennessee, Memphis
Memphis, Tennessee

Anaphylaxis is a potentially fatal, acute systemic reaction resulting from the release of potent chemical mediators from tissue mast cells and peripheral blood basophils. It is estimated to occur in one of every 2700 hospitalized patients. Classic anaphylaxis is an immunologic reaction involving IgE in the release of chemical mediators. Anaphylactoid reactions have the same clinical manifestations as classic anaphylaxis but are not caused by the IgE-mediated release of chemical mediators from mast cells and basophils. Clinical symptoms of anaphylaxis can range from mild cutaneous manifestations such as generalized erythema, urticaria, and angioedema to life-threatening hypotension and cardiac arrhythmias. The most common causes are drugs, food and food additives, insect stings, and physical factors, such as exercise. In rare cases of anaphylaxis, an etiologic agent is never identified.

Serum sickness, as opposed to anaphylaxis, is an immune reaction triggered by circulating immune complexes involving IgG, IgM, or both with foreign antigens. Clinical symptoms classically occur 6 to 21 days after exposure to the antigen. Symptoms commonly seen in serum sickness are urticaria, fever, lymphadenopathy, and joint pain. True serum sickness is an infrequent event in humans today.

PATHOPHYSIOLOGY

Classic anaphylaxis is an IgE-mediated reaction to a foreign antigen, whether it is a protein, a polysaccharide, or a hapten. In susceptible persons, initial exposure to an antigen results in the production of specific IgE antibodies to that antigen. These antibodies bind to IgE receptors on the surface of mast cells and basophils. On re-exposure, the antigen can bind and cross-link the IgE antibodies on these cells. This leads to changes in the cell membrane with degranulation and release of chemical mediators, which include histamine, leukotrienes, prostaglandins, kallikrein, platelet-activating factor, and eosinophil and neutrophil chemotactic factors. These mediators produce the clinical symptoms of anaphylaxis by causing vasodilation, increased vascular permeability, and smooth muscle contraction.

Several mechanisms can lead to anaphylactoid reactions. One is the activation of the complement system, resulting in the formation of anaphylatoxins C3a and C5a. These proteins can directly trigger mast cell and basophil degranulation, releasing the same potent mediators. Blood products can induce this type of reaction. Another mechanism is the direct action of certain agents, such as hyperosmolar radiocontrast media and opiates, on mast cells and basophils with the release of mediators. This mechanism is independent of IgE and complement. Anaphylactoid reactions can also occur in situations in which the mechanism is not clearly understood; these reactions include systemic reactions initiated by exercise, aspirin, nonsteroidal anti-inflammatory drugs, and synthetic steroid hormones. Idiopathic anaphylaxis is a rare syndrome for which no triggering agent can be identified.

SIGNS AND SYMPTOMS

Anaphylaxis produces a spectrum of symptoms ranging from mild to fatal within minutes. The overwhelming majority of reactions occur within 1 hour of exposure to the inciting agent. In some persons, the onset of the symptoms may be delayed for several hours. Other persons may have a protracted or a biphasic anaphylactic reaction. A biphasic reaction occurs when symptoms reappear several hours after resolution of the immediate anaphylactic manifestations. The most commonly affected organ systems are the skin, gastrointestinal tract, respiratory tract, and cardiovascular system. The severity of an individual's response is dependent on rate, amount, and site of mediator release as well as any personal risk factors such as asthma, underlying cardiac disease, and use of beta blockers.

Skin manifestations are most commonly the first indications of anaphylaxis. These may include erythema, pruritus, urticaria, and angioedema. Swelling of the lips or tongue can impair ventilation, and swelling of the larynx, epiglottis, and surrounding tissue can cause upper airway obstruction with resultant stridor or suffocation. Gastrointestinal manifestations of anaphylaxis include nausea, vomiting, cramping abdominal pain, and diarrhea, which is often bloody. Respiratory symptoms include dyspnea, tachypnea, and wheezing. Hypotension and cardiac arrhythmias and arrest can also occur (Table 1).

When the aforementioned signs or symptoms of anaphylaxis occur within minutes of exposure to a known causative agent, it is usually not difficult to make the diagnosis of anaphylaxis. However, if the precipitating event is not known, the diagnosis could be confused with many other medical emergencies that clinically mimic anaphylaxis (Table 2). The condition most frequently mistaken for anaphylaxis is a vasodepressor (vasovagal) episode. These episodes are usually preceded by a stressful or frightening event and are characterized by sweating, pallor, hypotension, and bradycardia. These attacks can usually be distinguished from anaphylaxis by the lack of pruritus, urticaria, and bronchospasm. The distinction between anaphylaxis and a primary cardiac event may be difficult, especially if the event is preceded by what seems to be an anaphylaxis-inducing exposure (i.e., insect sting, drug or food ingestion, etc.). A complete cardiac evaluation and allergic work-up may be indicated.

Table 3 lists criteria that may aid the physician in making a diagnosis of anaphylaxis in people in whom the diag-

TABLE 1. **Clinical Manifestations of Anaphylaxis**

System/Structure	Symptoms
Skin	Erythema, general pruritus, urticaria, angioedema
Eye	Pruritus, conjunctival injection, lacrimation
Nose	Pruritus, congestion, sneezing, clear rhinorrhea
Upper airways	Sensation of narrowing airways, hoarseness, stridor, oropharyngeal or laryngeal edema, cough, complete obstruction
Lower airways	Dyspnea, tachypnea, use of accessory muscles, cyanosis, wheezing, respiratory arrest
Cardiovascular	Tachycardia, hypotension, arrhythmias, cardiac arrest
Gastrointestinal	Nausea, vomiting, cramping abdominal pain, diarrhea (often bloody)
Neurologic	Dizziness, weakness, syncope, seizures
Miscellaneous	Uterine contractions, intravascular coagulation, fibrinolysis

nosis may not be readily apparent. Measurement of serum levels of mast cell tryptase may help confirm an anaphylactic reaction. Unlike the plasma histamine level, which usually declines within 30 minutes of an anaphylactic reaction, mast cell tryptase level peaks 60 to 90 minutes after anaphylaxis and has an approximately 3-hour half-clearance time.

CAUSATIVE AGENTS

There are hundreds of agents that can cause anaphylactic reactions (Table 4). The most common offenders are medications, insect stings, and food substances. Penicillin remains one of the major medications that cause anaphylaxis. Deaths are more common when it is administered parenterally than orally. Of the people who have died from penicillin anaphylaxis, 75% had no history of previous reaction to penicillin. After injection (or ingestion), penicillin is metabolized into major and minor components or determinants. The minor determinant, which constitutes only 5% of the metabolites, is believed to be responsible for anaphylaxis in most persons sensitive to penicillin. Penicillin skin testing can be conducted by a trained allergist with these metabolites to confirm allergy in individuals whose history suggests the occurrence of a prior anaphylactic reaction. It is estimated that about 2 to 7% of patients allergic to penicillin (history and skin test are positive) are allergic to cephalosporins and therefore their use should be avoided.

Foods are another common cause of anaphylaxis. Legumes (peanuts, peas, soybeans, and beans), nuts, fish, shellfish, cow's milk, and eggs are the most common food allergens. Most anaphylactic reactions resulting from insect sting or bite are caused by an insect in the order Hymenoptera, which includes fire ants, hornets, yellow jackets, wasps, and honey bees. All patients with anaphylaxis caused by one of these insects should undergo venom skin testing by a trained allergist in order to document sensitivity. Of interest is the contribution of physical factors to anaphylactic or anaphylactoid reactions. Many of these factors are not well understood, but exercise, cold, heat, and sunlight have all been implicated as causative agents.

Rubber (latex) products have recently been involved in more and more anaphylactic reactions. Many reports have documented anaphylaxis during surgical and radiologic procedures that was caused by latex objects such as gloves and catheters. Three groups appear to be at high risk for anaphylaxis to latex: medical personnel, people with a history of pruritus from exposure to latex objects, and patients with spina bifida. In the last group, latex sensitization develops because of multiple surgical procedures. Skin testing and the radioallergosorbent test (RAST) are available in some medical centers to confirm the diagnosis.

TABLE 2. **Differential Diagnosis of Anaphylaxis**

Vasovagal response	Systemic mastocytosis
Primary cardiac event	Cold urticaria
Globus hystericus	Foreign body in trachea
Scombroid poisoning	Stroke
Hyperventilation	Medication overdose
Hereditary angioneurotic edema	Pheochromocytoma
Carcinoid	

TABLE 3. **Diagnosis of Anaphylaxis***

At least one of the following must be present: acute hypotension, bronchial obstruction, or upper airway obstruction (cardiac or respiratory arrest)
Presence of distinctive allergic symptoms and signs in other systems
Recent exposure to agents or activities known to be capable of inducing anaphylaxis
Evidence of IgE to an agent encountered just before onset of anaphylaxis
Absence of conditions that can mimic anaphylaxis
Elevated serum levels of mast cell tryptase
Elevated levels of other molecules associated with mast cell secretion: plasma and urinary histamine and metabolites, serum high–molecular-weight neutrophil chemotactic factor, and urinary PGD_2 metabolites

*Effective therapy of acute anaphylaxis requires accurate diagnosis based upon clinical criteria.

Abbreviation: PGD_2 = prostaglandin D_2.

From Sullivan TJ: Systemic anaphylaxis. *In* Lichtenstein LM, and Fauci AS (eds): Current Therapy in Allergy, Immunology, and Rheumatology–2. Philadelphia, BC Decker, 1988.

TREATMENT

Because acute anaphylaxis can be a life-threatening event, assessment and management must begin without delay (Table 5). This requires rapid evaluation of recent events, assessment of the severity of the clinical manifestations, rate of progression of symptoms, and a medical history, including known

TABLE 4. **Common Causes of Anaphylaxis**

Penicillin and derivatives	Blood products
Cephalosporins	Milk
Tetracycline	Eggs
Allergy extracts	Legumes
Human seminal plasma	Nuts
Streptokinase	Shellfish
L-asparaginase	Fish
Insulin	Stinging insects
Opiates	Cold
Aspirin	Exercise
Nonsteroidal anti-inflammatory agents	Heat
Radiocontrast media	Rubber (latex)

TABLE 5. **Management of Anaphylaxis**

1. Place patient in recumbent position with feet elevated
2. Secure and maintain airway, administer oxygen at 4–6 L/min
3. Epinephrine 1:1000, 0.01 mL/kg up to 0.30 mL SC; repeat every 15 minutes if necessary
4. Tourniquet above injection site and infiltrate site with additional epinephrine 1:1000, 0.01 mL/kg 0.10 to 0.20 mL SC
5. Administer diphenhydramine, 1–2 mg/kg IM or IV up to 50 mg every 4–6 h
6. Administer corticosteroids such as hydrocortisone, 5–10 mg/kg up to 500 mg IV every 4–6 h
7. Administer ranitidine, 12.5 mg to 50 mg IV every 6–8 h
8. Monitor vital signs frequently
9. If patient is hypotensive after epinephrine therapy, administer IV normal saline or colloids to replace intravascular fluid loss
10. If hypotension persists, administer norepinephrine bitartrate, 2–8 μg/min, or dopamine, 2–10 μg/kg/min, to maintain blood pressure
11. If hypotension is caused by beta-blockage, administer glucagon, 1–5 mg IV over 1 min, and begin continuous infusion 1–5 mg/h
12. Administer specific antiarrhythmic agents if indicated
13. For persistent bronchospasm, administer aminophylline, 6 mg/kg IV over 20 minutes, then continuous IV aminophylline drip at 0.9 mg/kg/h; monitor theophylline level; aerosolized beta$_2$-agonist as needed
14. Keep patient in observation for at least 6 to 8 h in case of a protracted course

Abbreviations: SC = subcutaneously; IM = intramuscularly; IV = intravenously.

allergies, present medications, and underlying health problems. Simultaneously, the ABCs of emergency management should be implemented: Is the patient's *a*irway patent or obstructed? Is it in potential danger of becoming obstructed in the near future? Is the patient ventilating (i.e., *b*reathing)? If so, the patient should immediately be given high-flow oxygen and placed in a recumbent position with feet elevated above the heart (Trendelenburg's position). Is the patient's *c*irculatory system compromised?

After initial rapid assessment, epinephrine should be administered. Many deaths from anaphylaxis could have been prevented if epinephrine was given at the first sign of symptoms. The recommended dose of epinephrine 1:1000 is 0.01 mL per kg, up to 0.30 mL administered subcutaneously, to be repeated every 15 minutes if indicated. If the inciting event was an injection (i.e., insect sting, drug injection), a tourniquet should be placed proximal to the site of injury. Epinephrine can be given subcutaneously near the injection site to help retard systemic absorption of the offending agent.

Although they are not effective in the acute management of anaphylaxis, H_1 antihistamines, H_2 antihistamines, and corticosteroids are commonly administered. H_1 antihistamines, such as diphenhydramine (Benadryl), 1 to 2 mg per kg intravenously or intramuscularly up to 50 mg every 4 to 6 hours, help control the pruritus and skin manifestations. The use of H_2 antihistamines, such as ranitidine (Zantac), in conjunction with H_1 antihistamines may be beneficial in treating hypotension. Corticosteroids, such as hydrocortisone, 5 to 10 mg per kg intravenously up to 500 mg every 4 to 6 hours, may prevent a protracted course of anaphylaxis and decrease the magnitude of late sequelae.

After these initial steps, the patient's response should be reassessed in order to determine the next course of therapy. Should the patient be hypotensive after subcutaneous epinephrine administration, treatment with volume expanders is indicated. The hypotension is a result of intravascular volume depletion secondary to increased capillary permeability as well as to vasodilation and decreased arteriolar tone. Normal saline or colloid may be used and administered at a rapid rate (in adults, as fast as 100 mL per minute). The patient's response, urine output, cardiovascular status, and age should be used as guidelines for the total amount of fluid to be given. Usually, a total of 3 liters can be given rapidly to an adult without ill effect. If hypotension persists, norepinephrine bitartrate, 2 to 8 μg per minute, or dopamine, 2 to 10 μg per kg per minute, should be administered to maintain blood pressure. The rate of infusion should be adjusted to maintain a systolic blood pressure of at least 80 to 100 mmHg.

Cardiac arrhythmias resulting from a combination of the chemical mediators, from hypoxia, from hypotension, and from the epinephrine itself can lead to cardiogenic shock. This condition necessitates the use of specific antiarrhythmic agents. Resistance to epinephrine may be seen in patients taking beta-blocking agents. In these situations, the use of glucagon, 1 to 5 mg intravenously over 1 minute and administered in a continuous drip, can partially overcome this resistance. Bronchospastic symptoms can be managed in a similar manner as those of status asthmaticus, with the use of beta-agonist aerosols and intravenous aminophylline therapy. Patients with severe anaphylaxis should be observed for at least 6 to 8 hours because of the possibility of a protracted or biphasic course.

PREVENTION

Prevention of recurrence of anaphylaxis is aimed at identifying the etiologic agent and educating the patient on its avoidance. If avoidance is not possible, however, other measures of prevention are available. In patients with a history of anaphylaxis in response to radiocontrast media, a premedication protocol is available (Table 6). Venom immunotherapy should be offered to all patients with documented Hymenoptera anaphylaxis. It has been shown to be effective in the prevention of anaphylaxis in more than 95% of treated patients. In patients with a positive history

TABLE 6. **Premedication for Radiocontrast Media Reactions**

1. Prednisone, 50 mg orally, 13, 7, and 1 h before the procedure
2. Diphenhydramine, 50 mg intramuscularly, 1 h before the procedure
3. Ephedrine, 25 mg orally, 1 hour before the procedure, unless the patient has underlying cardiovascular disease

and positive skin test responses to penicillin to whom penicillin or one of its derivatives must be administered, desensitization protocols are available.

Certain pharmaceutical agents should be avoided in patients with a history of anaphylaxis. Patients on beta-blocking agents and angiotensin-converting enzyme inhibitors who experience anaphylaxis may have profound hypotension and may not respond to epinephrine.

All patients with a history of anaphylaxis should wear a medical identification bracelet (Medic-Alert) to inform medical personnel of their known allergies. They should be equipped with and educated in the use of self-administered epinephrine such as EpiPen and Ana-Kit/Ana-Guard. If exposure to the anaphylactic agent occurs, patients should immediately use the epinephrine and promptly go to the nearest medical facility for evaluation.

SERUM SICKNESS

Serum sickness is a syndrome involving IgG, IgM, or both circulating immune complexes that was first described with the use of foreign antiserums. Today, the most common causes are medications (Table 7). The disease is usually milder in children and more severe in adults. As described in animal models, a few days after an antigen is present in excess in the circulation, antibodies (IgM and/or IgG) are produced that interact with the antigen, forming soluble circulating immune complexes. These complexes, if not removed from the circulation, are capable of migrating into vascular walls, where they may fix and activate complement. Monocytes and macrophages may be chemically attracted to these areas and contribute to tissue destruction as well. The resulting inflammation can lead to the vasculitis. Signs and symptoms of serum sickness are shown in Table 8. Cutaneous eruptions are seen in more than 90% of all patients and include urticaria, maculopapular or purpuric lesions, and erythema multiforme. A characteristic band of erythema on the plantar and palmar junctions of the feet and hands has been described. Nearly all patients have a mild fever, although it is higher in the more severe cases. Most patients have peripheral edema and arthritis or arthralgia. In the most severe cases, glomerulonephritis, peripheral neuritis, and rarely, Guillain-Barré syndrome may be present. Symptoms usually occur 7 to 21 days after exposure to the agent. In previously sensitized patients, the symptoms may occur as soon as 24 hours after re-exposure. Most serum sickness-type reactions are considered mild and resolve spontaneously within 2 to 3 weeks.

TABLE 7. **Common Causes of Serum Sickness**

Penicillin and derivatives	Phenylbutazone
Cephalosporins	Naproxen (Naprosyn)
Sulfonamides	Thiazides
Hydantoins	Propranolol
Blood products	Metronidazole

TABLE 8. **Symptoms of Serum Sickness**

Symptoms	Frequency (%)
Fever, malaise	100
Cutaneous eruptions	90
Arthralgia	50–75
Myalgia	25–50
Lymphadenopathy	10–20
Glomerulonephritis	Rare

From Younger RE: Anaphylaxis and serum sickness. *In* Rakel RE (ed): Conn's Current Therapy. Philadelphia, WB Saunders, 1992, pp 681–84.

If the patient is still receiving the offending antigen when serum sickness occurs, it should be discontinued immediately. Treatment is generally directed at symptomatic relief. Antihistamines relieve the pruritus, and nonsteroidal anti-inflammatory agents relieve the fever and arthralgias. If symptoms persist or worsen despite these measures, it may be necessary to administer corticosteroids. Prednisone, 1 to 2 mg per kg per day (maximal dose: 60 mg), tapering over 5 to 7 days and followed by a smaller daily morning dose for 1 week, usually provides good results. Shorter courses of corticosteroids may not be effective.

There is no definitive laboratory test for diagnosis of serum sickness. It is usually based on the history and clinical presentation. However, the erythrocyte sedimentation rate is usually mildly elevated, and there may be peripheral eosinophilia with leukocytosis or leukopenia, proteinuria, hematuria, decreased complement levels (CH50, C3, C4), and electrocardiographic changes. Circulating immune complexes may also be detected in some patients by using C1q binding assays or Raji cell immunoassays. Because serum sickness is a clinical syndrome with many similarities to other inflammatory diseases, re-evaluation of the diagnosis is indicated if the symptoms persist for longer than 3 weeks. In adults, other vasculitides are often confused with serum sickness, as is juvenile rheumatoid arthritis in children.

ASTHMA IN ADULTS AND ADOLESCENTS

method of
DEBORAH ORTEGA-CARR, M.D.
University of Wisconsin
Madison, Wisconsin

and

ROBERT K. BUSH, M.D.
William S. Middleton Veterans Affairs Hospital
Madison, Wisconsin

Asthma prevalence and morbidity have increased over the last decade. New insights into the pathophysiology of asthma have changed the definition of asthma as well as its modes of treatment. We now define asthma as a chronic disease characterized by airway hyperresponsiveness, recurrent and usually reversible airflow obstruction, and symptoms of wheezing and breathlessness. Each of these components must be addressed in the overall management of asthma, in both the acute and the chronic setting. The National Asthma Education Program (NAEP) has developed guidelines for asthma management that include patient education on the basic principles of the disease and effective methods of asthma monitoring. NAEP recommendations also stress reducing or avoiding asthma triggers, particularly through environmental allergen control. Furthermore, pharmacologic intervention, aimed at both obstruction and inflammation, is now felt to be essential for optimal control.

PRECIPITATING/AGGRAVATING FACTORS

Recent research has shown that asthma is a complex interaction of many cell processes and that the events that trigger or initiate these processes are multiple and varied. Two major triggers are allergens and viral infections. Although these two factors may be especially important in the pediatric population, they can provoke asthma symptoms in all age groups.

Allergens and Asthma

Allergens play a significant role in asthma pathogenesis in many patients. Up to 85% of asthma patients have positive skin test reactions to common aeroallergens. House dust mites are important in the development of allergic asthma; other pertinent indoor allergens include animal danders, particularly cat, and possibly insects, such as cockroaches. Fungal spores and pollens have also been associated with asthma exacerbations.

In patients with allergic asthma, inhalation of antigen first triggers immediate bronchoconstriction. In roughly half of the subjects with asthma, this challenge also provokes a delayed response 4 to 8 hours later, which is characterized by persistent airflow obstruction, airway inflammation, and bronchial hyper-responsiveness.

Viral Infections and Asthma

Viral infections also provoke and alter asthmatic responses. Viral respiratory illnesses may produce their effects by causing epithelial damage, producing specific IgE against respiratory viral antigens, and enhancing mediator release. Besides aggravating asthma, viral upper respiratory infections cause increased airway responsiveness that may persist for weeks beyond the infection, producing chronic symptoms of wheezing.

Additional Precipitating or Aggravating Factors

Other precipitating or aggravating factors include exposure to occupational chemicals (Table 1) and irritants such as cigarette smoke. Drugs that can precipitate an asthma attack include aspirin and cross-reactive nonsteroidal anti-inflammatory agents. The intensity of these reactions is variable and may be associated with naso-ocular symptoms. In certain subsets of asthma patients, particularly those with rhinosinusitis and nasal polyps, the prevalence of asthma sensitivity may approach 30 to 40%. The nonsteroidal anti-inflammatory agents that inhibit cyclo-oxygenase are most cross-reactive with aspirin; acetaminophen and salsalate, which are weak inhibitors of cyclo-oxygenase, are much less cross-reactive. Sulfiting agents, such as the bisulfites and metabisulfites of sodium and potassium, are antimicrobial agents and oxidants used as preservatives in various foods and medications. These agents can also precipitate attacks of asthma.

Strenuous exercise results in airway obstruction in nearly all asthmatics. The problem is clinically important in at least two-thirds of adolescents with asthma because it interferes with school and recreational activities. The mechanisms by which exercise causes bronchial obstruction are unknown, but a fall in temperature of the intrathoracic airway is a critical inciting event. Exercise-induced asthma usually begins after 6 to 10 minutes of exercise or after exercise is completed. In half of the patients, repetition of exercise within 1 hour elicits progressively smaller changes in peak expiratory flow and forced expiratory flow in 1 minute (FEV_1). Swimming and activities that involve brief intervals of strenuous activity interspersed with rest are best tolerated. The use of prophylactic drug therapy prior to exercise usually provides adequate protection for the patient. This prophylaxis usually consists of 2 puffs of a $beta_2$-agonist inhaler such as albuterol (Proventil, Ventolin) immediately prior to exercise. If patients continue to have symptoms during exercise, 2 puffs of cromolyn sodium (Intal) or nedocromil sodium (Tilade) can be added 15 minutes prior to exercise.

Any associated problems that may contribute to asthma symptoms should be identified. Coexistent illness, such as congestive heart failure with pulmonary edema, can also cause wheezing. Gastroesophageal reflux can induce cough and bronchospasm. Medications such as methylxanthines, in asthmatic patients, may decrease gastroesophageal sphincter tone and worsen gastroesophageal reflux, which in turn can provoke asthma.

TABLE 1. **Occupational Allergens**

Agriculture	Animal proteins: domestic animals, insects, ascarids Plant proteins: cereal grains, cottonseed, tobacco leaf
Food processing	Animal proteins: seafood Plant proteins: coffee dust, soy dust, cocoa dust, psyllium, flour Plant enzymes: papain, pectinase, flavorings
Woodworking (forestry, carpentry, wood manufacturing)	Wood dusts: boxwood, mahogany, oak, redwood, western red cedar (plicatic acid)
Animal handlers (laboratory workers, veterinarians, pet shop owners)	Animal proteins: dander, saliva, urine Avian proteins
Pharmaceutical industry	Drugs: antibiotics (penicillin), proteolytic enzymes (trypsin, pancreatin)
Manufacturing (automobile assembly, paint, foundry, polyurethane foam, plating, plastics including epoxy resins)	Chemicals: toluene diisocyanate, diphenylmethane diisocyanate, platinum, nickel phthalic anhydride, trimetallic anhydride, tetrachlorophthalic anhydride

Sinusitis and asthma frequently coexist, and several studies have reported a high (40 to 60%) incidence of sinusitis among patients with asthma. Also, patients with refractory asthma show relief of symptoms when the concurrent sinusitis is appropriately treated. The mechanisms by which sinusitis affects asthma are not yet clear but may involve the dripping of mediators from the sinuses to the lower airways or the presence of eosinophils acting as a common effector cell for both the upper and lower airways.

DIAGNOSIS/CLASSIFICATION

The diagnosis of asthma is based on the clinical history and examination, as well as the demonstration of reversible airflow obstruction. Clinical complaints include cough, wheezing, and chest tightness. The pattern of symptoms may also be helpful. Patients who cough or wheeze after certain exposures, or who wheeze with cold air or exercise, may be more likely to have asthma. In addition, patients whose symptoms interrupt their activity or their sleep often have more significant disease.

Airway reversibility is usually determined by pulmonary function testing. Baseline spirometry is performed; then the patient receives either nebulized isoproterenol or 2 puffs of a beta$_2$-agonist bronchodilator (albuterol, pirbuterol, terbutaline, or metaproterenol) by metered dose inhaler. An improvement in the FEV$_1$ of at least 15% is considered significant.

The methacholine inhalation challenge is employed as an additional diagnostic tool. This test is usually performed in a pulmonary function laboratory and should only be performed on individuals with normal baseline pulmonary function. A positive methacholine challenge, however, does not identify asthma specifically; rather, it merely indicates the presence of airway hyperresponsiveness, which can be present in other situations such as cigarette smoking, chronic obstructive pulmonary disease (COPD), and postviral infection. Other inhalation challenge methods include challenges with exercise or cold air. The diagnostic workup for asthma must include the clinical evaluation as well as these objective measures.

In the asthmatic patient with significant obstruction and airway inflammation (FEV$_1$ <70% of predicted), bronchodilator administration may not reveal a significant reversible component. In these patients, reversible airflow obstruction is best evaluated by pulmonary function testing before and after a short trial of oral corticosteroid, such as prednisone, 30 mg per day for 5 to 7 days, followed by prednisone, 10 mg per day for an additional 5 to 7 days.

TREATMENT

The NAEP has developed a clinical classification of asthmatic patients (Table 2) which we use to guide therapy. It is important to identify and avoid triggering agents, especially in allergic and occupational asthma. Dust mite control measures, especially in sleeping areas, can reduce symptoms. If it is impossible to remove a pet from the home, it should, at minimum, be kept from the bedroom at all times.

Medications to relieve symptoms of airflow obstruction as well as inflammation are vital for adequate control. Inhaled (beta$_2$-agonist) medications (Table 3) are the most effective bronchodilators and can quickly relieve airway obstruction. Anti-inflammatory agents include inhaled corticosteroids (Table 4), cromolyn sodium, and nedocromil sodium. These medications should be used in a stepwise fashion based on the NAEP guidelines. For a patient with mild asthma, therapy should consist of an inhaled (beta$_2$ agonist) as needed and pretreatment with 2 to 4 puffs of an inhaled beta$_2$ agonist (Proventil, Ventolin, Maxair, Brethaire) with or without 2 puffs of cromolyn sodium or nedocromil prior to exercise or contact with other triggers. Cromolyn or nedocromil may give additional protection from exercise- or allergen-induced bronchospasm.

For the patient with moderate asthma, chronic anti-inflammatory therapy (e.g., with an inhaled corticosteroid or inhaled cromolyn/nedocromil) is required. Inhaled corticosteroids have been shown both to relieve symptoms and to improve pulmonary function measurements and also to allow for decreased use of supplemental medication. Inhaled corticosteroids may be used at a dosage of 4 puffs twice a day, which may improve patient compliance. Inhaled beta$_2$ agonists should be continued on an as-needed basis for chronically symptomatic asthmatics. Should these measures not achieve optimal control, adding sustained-release theophylline (400 mg at bedtime or 200 to 300 mg bid) can be considered or, alternatively, using a long-acting beta$_2$ agonist such as salmeterol (Serevent) 2 puffs twice daily. Patients with acute symptoms or a marked change in status require a short course of oral corticosteroids followed by continuation of inhaled corticosteroids, possibly at a higher dose. A typical dosing schedule for a course of oral prednisone is 30 to 40 mg daily given in divided doses (two to three times a day) for 1 week, followed by 10 to 15 mg daily for an additional week.

Assessment by an asthma specialist should be considered if symptoms are not controlled by these measures, if pulmonary function tests continue to show marked variability, or if frequent courses of oral corticosteroids are required to control symptoms.

TABLE 2. **Classification of Asthma**

Mild	Moderate	Severe
<2 episodes per week	>1–2 episodes per week	Continuous symptoms Limited exercise and activity
Rare or absent nocturnal symptoms	Frequent nocturnal symptoms	Frequent exacerbations requiring excessive beta$_2$-agonist use
Normal FEV$_1$ between episodes	Exacerbations lasting >24 hours, FEV$_1$ 60–80% of baseline	Emergency room evaluations and hospitalizations Highly variable FEV$_1$ <60% of baseline

TABLE 3. **Beta$_2$ Agonists**

Drug	Trade Name	Dose	Special Characteristics
Metaproterenol	Alupent	2 puffs q 4–6 h as needed	Less β_2 selective than others, may have more systemic effects
Albuterol	Proventil, Ventolin	2 puffs q 4–6 h as needed	β_2 selective
Pirbuterol	Maxair	2 puffs q 4–6 h as needed	β_2 selective, may produce less muscle tremor in some patients
Terbutaline	Brethaire	2 puffs q 4–6 h as needed	β_2 selective, bronchodilator of choice in pregnancy
Salmeterol	Serevent	2 puffs bid	Slow onset, prolonged duration of action

Asthma specialists and particularly allergists may also be helpful in identifying allergic or environmental triggers.

Patients with severe asthma require high doses of inhaled corticosteroids (8 to 16 puffs per day). Despite this, these patients often receive frequent short courses of oral corticosteroids for repeated exacerbations and may even require prolonged courses of daily prednisone for control. The lowest effective dose of prednisone should be used in these circumstances, and alternate-day dosing with corticosteroids may produce fewer side effects. For patients with continued nocturnal symptoms, the addition of sustained-release theophylline (Uniphyl), 400 to 800 mg at supper, or the use of salmeteral, 2 puffs at bedtime, may offer additional relief. Peak serum concentrations of theophylline should be monitored and kept optimally in the 8 to 15 mg per liter range. Inhaled beta$_2$ agonists and theophylline are usually the most effective bronchodilators in asthma, and often both are required in severe asthma. For patients with severe asthma and COPD, ipratropium bromide (Atrovent) may also offer some benefit. High-potency inhaled corticosteroids (budesonide,* fluticasone*) are under investigation and show promise for asthma therapy.

Acute Asthma

An acute exacerbation of asthma is an urgent medical problem. The best strategy for management is early recognition, evaluation, and treatment to prevent deterioration and to abort further exacerbation and respiratory compromise. Each patient should have a "plan of action" to follow for acute asthma exacerbations.

*Investigational drug in the United States.

The intensity of the acute attack and its outcome are influenced by several factors, including the patient's age (with elderly having the greatest risk); the duration of the current episode; a history of previous life-threatening asthma exacerbations requiring hospitalization, intubation, and intensive care or of complications secondary to hypoxia; recent and frequent emergency room visits; and either systemic corticosteroid usage or recent withdrawal from corticosteroids.

The first line of therapy in this setting is repetitive inhalation of beta$_2$ agonists. Subcutaneous epinephrine (0.3 ml of 1:1000) may be administered on an emergency basis as well as repeated treatments with nebulized beta$_2$ agonists (as frequently as every 20 minutes for the first hour). Methylprednisolone, 1 to 2 mg per kg intravenously, should be administered if no immediate response is noted to beta$_2$-agonist therapy. As discussed previously, patients with acute exacerbations require 1 to 2 weeks of oral corticosteroids after discharge from the emergency room.

GENERAL CONSIDERATIONS

Asthma is a chronic disease with various presentations. Management must encompass modalities such as patient education, continued reassessment, and specific therapeutic intervention for successful long-term control.

Patient education should include the basic pathophysiology of asthma, identification and avoidance of specific triggers, and methods of objective monitoring with peak flow meters. Baseline values of peak flow measurement can be obtained over a 2-week period; then peak flow values are obtained during symptomatic episodes. These measurements can be helpful in the devising a "plan of action" for acute exacerba-

TABLE 4. **Anti-Inflammatory Medications**

Drug	Trade Name	Dose/Actuation (μg)	Recommended Adult Dosage
Beclomethasone dipropionate	Beclovent, Vanceril	42	2–4 puffs, 3–4 times daily
Flunisolide	Aerobid	250*	2–4 puffs, 2–4 times daily
Triamcinolone acetonide	Azmacort	100	2–4 puffs, 3–4 times daily
Cromolyn sodium	Intel	800	2 puffs, 4 times daily
Nedocromil sodium	Tilade	1750	2 puffs, 2–4 times daily

*Exceeds dosage recommended by the manufacturer.

tions. Patients may receive individual instructions on the adjustment of their medications (such as instituting a short course of prednisone, 30 mg per day for 5 to 7 days followed by 10 mg per day for 5 to 7 days) should peak flows fall to less than 70% of baseline with associated symptoms. Patients must also be instructed to contact a physician immediately for management of acute symptoms. Any emergency evaluation should be followed by a subsequent visit to the clinician's office for a re-evaluation of overall asthma control.

Patients with moderate to severe asthma require close follow-up and frequent assessment of pulmonary function. These patients should also receive influenza vaccine every fall (except egg-allergic patients).

Inhaler technique should be continually reviewed on follow-up visits in all patients. In addition, compliance must be reassessed and factors that may affect compliance (e.g., socioeconomic or psychosocial) should be discussed.

ASTHMA IN CHILDREN

method of
PAUL V. WILLIAMS, M.D., and
GAIL G. SHAPIRO, M.D.
University of Washington School of Medicine
Seattle, Washington

EPIDEMIOLOGY

Asthma is one of the most common chronic illnesses of childhood, affecting 5 to 10% of all children. Of the 12 million Americans who have asthma, 4 million are less than 18 years old. The prevalence of asthma is increasing: the percentage of the population with asthma increased 60% from 1979 to 1989. Asthma is the leading cause of time lost from school, amounting to 10 million lost days per year, and one of the most common reasons for visits to the physician.

Despite recent advances in the understanding of the pathophysiology of asthma and the development of a wide array of potent medications, hospitalizations for asthma have been increasing among children, up 56% from 1979 to 1989. The major factors contributing to this rise in morbidity are underdiagnosis and inappropriate treatment. Most exacerbations can be regarded as at least partial treatment failures, because they can be prevented if treatment is comprehensive and ongoing.

DEFINITION

There is no universally accepted definition of asthma. However, most authorities would agree that the following factors are present: chronic inflammation of the airways, variable airflow obstruction that is often at least partially reversible, and an increase in airway responsiveness to a variety of specific and nonspecific stimuli.

PATHOPHYSIOLOGY

The pathology of the airways in asthma consists of muscle spasm, airway edema, abnormal mucus production, and an inflammatory cell infiltrate.

The asthmatic response can have two phases: an immediate, or early phase, and a late phase. Not every patient will experience both phases with each exacerbation but instead may have an isolated early response, an early and late response, or an isolated late response.

The early response, as its name implies, occurs shortly after exposure, and consists primarily of bronchospasm and airway edema. This is a result of interaction between allergen and mast cells, resulting in degranulation of the mast cell and release of numerous mediators. Some of these mediators are chemotactic for eosinophils and neutrophils, which results in cellular infiltration into the airway epithelium. Macrophages, T helper cells, and their products are also involved in this process, promoting the development of inflammation. This inflammation leads to further airway narrowing, which manifests itself as the late response, resulting in an exacerbation of asthmatic symptoms 3 to 8 hours after the initial exposure.

The airway edema and bronchospasm of the early phase are usually responsive to bronchodilators, such as beta agonists, and can be blocked by use of the beta agonists cromolyn sodium (Intal) and nedocromil (Tilade) prior to exposure to allergens or other stimuli, such as exercise. The airway narrowing that occurs in the late phase is less responsive to bronchodilators but does improve with anti-inflammatory treatment and can be blocked by cromolyn or nedocromil given just before the initial exposure. It can also be blocked by systemic corticosteroids given 48 hours before exposure or inhaled corticosteroids given for 2 weeks before exposure.

The inflammation that occurs during the late phase also gives rise to increased bronchial hyper-responsiveness. This means that the airways of the asthmatic become more sensitive to both specific stimuli, such as allergens, and to nonspecific stimuli, such as exercise or cold air. This increased responsiveness is responsible for much of the chronicity of asthma, because it leads to airway narrowing and inflammation with further exposures, which leads to further increases in responsiveness, and so on.

DIAGNOSIS

The diagnosis of asthma can be straightforward, with wheezing, cough, and shortness of breath responsive to bronchodilators. While the symptoms can be much more subtle, a thorough history will usually provide the necessary clues to the diagnosis. Prolonged cough with viral upper respiratory infections, recurrent exacerbations of cough or chest tightness brought on by exercise or allergen exposure, or chronic cough at night should all be considered possible symptoms of asthma. It is also important to discern what triggers such symptoms in each patient. Common triggers of asthma in children include viral upper respiratory infections, allergens, exercise, and pollutants.

Since asthma symptoms are episodic, the physical examination is often normal. Auscultation of the chest may also be normal when the patient is mildly symptomatic. Signs of allergic disease or other triggers, such as otitis media or sinusitis, should be sought during the examination.

Laboratory tests can sometimes be helpful, but only in confirming the diagnosis, since normal results do not exclude the diagnosis of asthma. The complete blood count may show eosinophilia. A chest x-ray may demonstrate hyperinflation but is usually normal between episodes. A significant number of patients may have abnormalities on chest x-ray during episodes of status asthmaticus, including pneumothorax or atelectasis, and chest films should be obtained for hospitalized asthmatics. A smear of nasal mucus stained with Hansel's stain can be particularly helpful if large numbers of eosinophils or neutrophils and bacteria are present. The former indicates the likely presence of allergy, the latter, infectious rhinosinusitis, both of which are potent triggers of asthma.

Because the physical examination may be normal in symptomatic patients, and asthmatic patients frequently have poor recognition of symptoms and of the severity of their disease, objective measurements of airway obstruction and its response to treatment are critical in establishing a diagnosis. Although spirometry, including measurement of forced vital capacity (FVC), forced expiratory volume in 1 second (FEV_1) and forced expiratory flow (FEF_{25-75}), is more sensitive, reproducible, and informative, measurement of peak flow can be an inexpensive alternative.

When the history is suggestive but the physical examination and spirometry are normal, bronchoprovocation can be helpful in confirming the diagnosis of asthma. A number of pharmacologic and physiologic challenges can be used to provoke airway obstruction in asthmatic patients, including methacholine, histamine, exercise, and nonisotonic aerosols. Methacholine challenge is the most standardized test and is easy to administer in children who are old enough to perform adequate pulmonary function maneuvers. The diagnosis can be particularly difficult in children too young to perform such pulmonary function tests, and in these cases, examination at the time of symptoms or a trial of treatment with bronchodilators may be indicated.

Measurement of specific IgE, usually by allergy skin testing, is not used to diagnose asthma but can be helpful in identifying specific triggers of asthmatic symptoms. By age 5, most children with asthma have a significant allergic component to their disease. Avoidance of relevant environmental factors can favorably influence asthma control and possibly the ultimate outcome by promoting optimal lung growth and decreasing hyper-responsiveness.

CLASSIFICATION

Asthma can be classified according to etiology, such as intrinsic or extrinsic, or according to the pattern and severity of airflow obstruction. Etiologic classification is of limited usefulness in the management of asthma because of the overlap of triggers among groups. Classifying asthmatics according to the severity and pattern of their disease over the preceding year is helpful and correlates with the pathologic indices of airway inflammation. Asthma is classified as mild, moderate, or severe, which gives the clinician an indication of the severity and prognosis of the disease (Table 1). Although this classification is somewhat arbitrary, it provides a useful framework for treatment of the individual asthmatic.

MANAGEMENT

Management Goals

The goals for successful asthma management are listed in Table 2. Asthma is a chronic condition with acute exacerbations (attacks). The occurrence of frequent exacerbations during chronic treatment, however, should be considered a failure of the current treatment plan, and alterations are indicated. Prevention of exacerbations is one of the most important principles of therapy.

It is vital to a child's psychosocial growth and development to be able to maintain normal activities, including school attendance and play. It is also important that medication side effects do not interfere with these same functions or with school performance.

Longitudinal studies of adults with poorly controlled asthma have demonstrated the acquisition of a “fixed” component to their airway obstruction superimposed on the reversible component. Children may be at a particularly vulnerable stage because their disease involves the growing lung. Poor control of their asthma may have deleterious effects on lung growth.

The severity of an exacerbation of acute severe asthma is often underestimated by the patient, parents, and even physicians. This is largely because of failure to use objective measurements of assessment, and this may be more common in young children because of their inability to perform pulmonary function tests. Acute severe asthma that is not recognized and treated appropriately can be fatal. It is possible for any patient with asthma to have an acute severe exacerbation; however, factors have been identified that are associated with a higher risk of asthma mortality (Table 3).

Management Guidelines

According to the International Consensus Report on the Diagnosis and Management of Asthma, asthma management has six interrelated parts: (1) patient education to develop a partnership in asthma management, (2) assessment and monitoring of asthma severity with objective measurements of lung function when possible, (3) avoidance or control of asthma triggers, (4) medication plans for chronic management, (5) plans for managing exacerbations, and (6) regular follow-up care.

Patient Education. Initially, the patient or parent should be given information about the diagnosis and types of treatment available and should be instructed to avoid triggers of asthma and nonspecific irritants such as cigarette smoke. Written instructions should be provided on the use of medications, recognition of signs of trouble, instructions for handling acute episodes, and criteria for seeking emergency care.

Assessment and Monitoring of Lung Function. All asthma patients should have pulmonary function monitoring as a routine part of their follow-up. Patients on chronic medications who are of appropriate age and ability should be encouraged to perform home peak flow monitoring. This requires careful office instruction. The peak flow should be checked twice daily and the results recorded on a flow sheet. The peak flow results can be very helpful in monitoring the results of therapy and increased airway reactivity and early airway obstruction. Peak flow monitoring is particularly useful for both the patient and the physician during times of acute exacerbation at home. The patient should be instructed on a management protocol using the peak flow results. Such a protocol decreases the need for calls to the physician and involves the patient or parent directly in man-

TABLE 1. **Classification of Asthma Severity***

Asthma Severity	Clinical Features Before Treatment	Lung Function	Regular Medication Usually Required to Maintain Control
Mild	Intermittent, brief symptoms <1–2 times a week Nocturnal asthma symptoms <2 times a month Asymptomatic between exacerbations	Peak expiratory flow (PEF) >80% predicted at baseline PEF variability <20% PEF normal after bronchodilator	Intermittent inhaled short acting beta$_2$ agonist (taken as needed) only
Moderate	Exacerbations >1–2 times a week Nocturnal asthma symptoms >2 times a month Symptoms requiring inhaled beta$_2$ agonist almost daily	PEF 60–80% predicted at baseline PEF variability 20–30% PEF normal after bronchodilator	Daily inhaled anti-inflammatory agent Possibly a daily long-acting bronchodilator, especially for nocturnal symptoms
Severe	Frequent exacerbations Continuous symptoms Frequent nocturnal asthma symptoms Physical activities limited by asthma Hospitalization for asthma in previous year† Previous life-threatening exacerbation†	PEF <60% predicted at baseline PEF variability >30% PEF below normal despite optimal therapy	Daily inhaled anti-inflammatory agent at high doses Daily long-acting bronchodilator, especially for nocturnal symptoms Frequent use of systemic corticosteroids

*The characteristics noted in this table are general and may overlap because asthma is highly variable. Furthermore, an individual's classification may change over time.

One or more features may be present to be assigned a grade of severity.

An individual should usually be assigned to the most severe grade in which any feature occurs.

Once the minimum medication required to maintain control of asthma has been identified, then this medication requirement reflects the overall severity of the condition.

†The potential severity—related to a patient's past history (for example, a previous life-threatening exacerbation or a hospitalization for asthma in the previous year) as well as present status—should be considered at all times.

From International Consensus Report on Diagnosis and Management of Asthma, March 1992.

agement decisions (see Management of Exacerbations).

Avoidance or Control of Asthma Triggers. As mentioned, it is important to identify those factors that trigger an individual's asthma. If these can be avoided or controlled, then a significant amount of asthma morbidity may be prevented. Allergy testing, as mentioned, can be particularly useful in identifying triggers. If allergens cannot be avoided or avoidance is not sufficient to prevent exacerbations of asthma, specific immunotherapy has been found effective in decreasing the asthmatic response to allergic triggers.

Follow-up Care. Patients with asthma need regular supervision by a physician who is knowledgeable about the condition. In the initial stages of treatment, frequent follow-up visits are necessary to review peak flow and symptom records, control of environmental triggers, and inhaled medication technique. Consultation with an asthma specialist should be considered for any patient who has a life-threatening exacerbation, when signs and symptoms are atypical, when clinical problems such as sinusitis or nasal polyps complicate asthma, when additional testing is indicated, when the patient is not responding to optimal medications, or when the patient has moderate to severe asthma.

TABLE 2. **Goals for Successful Asthma Management**

Achieve and maintain control of symptoms
Prevent asthma exacerbations
Maintain pulmonary function as close to normal levels as possible
Maintain normal activity levels, including exercise
Avoid adverse effects from asthma medications
Prevent development of irreversible airway obstruction
Prevent asthma mortality

From International Consensus Report on Diagnosis and Management of Asthma, March 1992.

Medications (Table 4)

Medications used for the treatment of asthma can be broadly classified as anti-inflammatory medications or bronchodilators. Over the last several years, it has become increasingly evident that airway inflammation plays a major role in the pathophysiology of asthma. As a consequence, there has been a shift in pharmacologic therapy from the regular use of bronchodilators to the use of anti-inflammatory medications as the primary therapy for patients with moderate to severe asthma. Bronchodilators are now used as adjunctive medications.

Anti-Inflammatory Medications. *Cromolyn sodium* (Intal) is a nonsteroidal, topical anti-inflammatory drug that has been used for years for the treatment of asthma. The exact mechanism of action has not been elucidated, but cromolyn appears to have effects on the release of mediators from mast cells, a suppressive effect on other inflammatory cells, and

TABLE 3. **Factors Associated with Asthma Mortality**

Previous history of acute, life-threatening attacks
Hospitalization within the previous year
Psychosocial problems
History of intubation for asthma
Recent reductions or cessation of corticosteroids
Noncompliance
Low income, medically underserved, inner city populations

TABLE 4. **Dosages of Asthma Medications**

Medication	Dose
Beta$_2$ agonists	
Syrup/Tablets	
Metaproterenol (Metaprel)	0.07 mg/kg q 4 h
Albuterol (Proventil, Ventolin)	0.15 mg/kg q 4 h
Metered Dose Inhalers (MDI)	
(?) Bitolterol (Tornalate)	2–4 puffs q 6–8 h
All others	2–4 puffs q 4 h
Aerosol solutions	
Albuterol	0.15 mg/kg or 0.2 mL/kg q 4 h
Metaproterenol	0.1–0.3 mL q 4 h
Bitolterol	
Cromolyn (Intal)	
Spinhaler	20 mg qid
Aerosol solution	20 mg qid
MDI	2 mg (2 puffs) qid
Nedocromil (Tilade)	
MDI	2 puffs qid to start
Ipratropium bromide (Atrovent)	
MDI	2–4 puffs qid
Aerosol solution	
Corticosteroids	
Outpatient (prednisone, methylprednisolone)	1–2 mg/kg/d in divided doses for 3–5 d
Emergency department/hospital (Methylprednisolone IV)	2 mg/kg bolus, then 1 mg/kg/dose q 6 h for 1–2 d, then 1–2 mg/kg/d for 3–5 d

inhibition of certain neuronal reflexes. Although any patient can benefit from its use, it appears to be particularly useful in inhibiting the asthma associated with viral respiratory infections in infants and young children and in childhood allergic asthma. Like all anti-inflammatory medications, it must be used on a regular rather than an as-needed basis, and a 4- to 6-week trial may be necessary to determine its effectiveness. It can also be used prophylactically to block the early- and late-phase response to allergens and the acute response to exercise, cold air, or sulfur dioxide. Cromolyn is available as a solution for nebulizer use and in a metered dose inhaler (MDI). It is an extremely safe drug; no significant long-term side effects have been noted. As such, it should be considered one of the first-line anti-inflammatory drugs for asthma in children. The dose-response relationship of cromolyn remains to be determined, but the drug is usually started on a four-times-daily basis with a gradual decrease over the ensuing months in the frequency of use as the episodes of asthma become less frequent.

Nedocromil sodium (Tilade), a new anti-inflammatory pyranoquinaline, may be more effective than cromolyn in the treatment of nonallergic asthma in adults, although no direct comparisons have been done. It can also block acute bronchoconstriction when used prophylactically. No significant adverse effects have been noted, but nedocromil's role in childhood asthma awaits the outcome of clinical trials. Experience to date suggests that this drug may be similar to cromolyn in terms of therapeutic response.

Corticosteroids are the most potent anti-inflammatory drugs available for the treatment of asthma. Their effectiveness results from their ability to inhibit several different components of the inflammatory cascade, whereas most other anti-inflammatory medications have a more limited action. Corticosteroids can be administered parenterally, orally, or as aerosols. They should be used parenterally in any child who is sick enough to be hospitalized for asthma. Early use of oral corticosteroids in the treatment of acute exacerbations of asthma has been shown to prevent the progression of asthma exacerbations and to reduce the need for emergency department visits and hospitalizations. Oral corticosteroids are often given in "bursts" or "tapers" for the treatment of acute exacerbations. Neither the ideal dose nor the ideal duration has been well worked out, but it is important to give a sufficient amount (see Table 4) and to continue to treat until the patient is symptom free and the peak expiratory flow rate is over 80% of the patient's best (usually 5 to 7 days). It does not appear to matter how corticosteroids are tapered, if at all, but some authorities are reluctant to use high doses, often necessary at the outset of treatment, for the duration of treatment and prefer to taper the dose over the period of the burst rather than giving a constant daily dose. Chronic oral corticosteroid therapy is reserved for severe asthma that has failed all other forms of therapy. Patients who require frequent bursts of corticosteroids should have their asthma therapy programs reevaluated. The adverse effects of oral corticosteroid use are varied and widely known. In addition, fatal varicella has been reported among patients who were exposed to chicken pox while taking systemic corticosteroids, even in short bursts. If a patient is exposed to varicella while taking systemic corticosteroids, stopping the corticosteroid and using zoster immune globulin or acyclovir are considerations.

Inhaled corticosteroids are generally safe and effective for the chronic treatment of asthma and are more effective than cromolyn or nedocromil, especially at higher doses. While most reports show no negative effect of these drugs on growth and development when typical doses are used, a recent report suggests that even "moderate" doses in the range of 400 to 800 μg of beclomethasone* per day or its equivalent may have adverse effects on growth and cause adrenal suppression in children. It remains to be seen whether these findings are clinically significant, or perhaps reflect an effect of chronic asthma rather than inhaled corticosteroid use. Until this has been determined, inhaled corticosteroids are generally used in children only when nonsteroidal anti-inflammatory drugs have not been effective. High-dose inhaled corticosteroids (above 1600 to 2000 μg of beclomethasone* per day) have been associated with systemic effects. Local adverse effects from inhaled corticosteroids include oropharyngeal candidiasis, dysphonia, and occasional cough; these can be minimized by using spacer devices. Spacer devices should

*Exceeds dosage recommended by the manufacturer.

be used with MDIs in young children who are unable to coordinate their inspiration with actuation of the device.

Bronchodilators. *Beta$_2$ agonists* are the treatment of choice for the acute exacerbations of asthma and for pretreatment of exercise-induced asthma. These drugs relax airway smooth muscle, decrease vascular permeability, and inhibit mediator release to some degree. They block the early-phase response to allergy challenge and mitigate the late phase as well. Most of the available forms of beta$_2$ agonists have a limited duration of action (4 to 6 hours), but newer, long-acting inhaled beta$_2$ agonists may soon be available in the United States, although their exact role in the treatment of childhood asthma has yet to be determined. These newer agents diminish, but do not ablate, the late-phase response and questionably diminish airway hyperreactivity, and consequently, they are not replacements for anti-inflammatory treatment.

Beta$_2$ agonists are used intermittently in patients with chronic asthma to relieve acute episodes of bronchoconstriction. There is some evidence to suggest that the regular, scheduled use of these drugs may actually worsen the control of asthma, so they should only be used on an as-needed basis. Well-controlled asthma requires the minimal use of beta$_2$ agonists, so frequent use is a good indicator of poor control.

Aerosol or inhaled beta$_2$ agonists are equal to or better than the oral forms and cause fewer systemic adverse effects, such as tremor and cardiovascular and central nervous system stimulation. Sustained-release preparations of beta$_2$ agonists may be useful in some patients with nocturnal symptoms.

Theophylline (Tables 5 and 6) used to be the primary treatment for chronic asthma in the United States. However, since we now know that inflammation is responsible for chronic asthma, anti-inflammatory drugs have supplanted theophylline as primary treatment, and theophylline is now used adjunctively. The mechanism of action of theophylline is unknown. Sustained-release preparations have a prolonged duration of action and may be useful in the treatment of nocturnal symptoms. They may also be helpful in controlling frequent episodes of bronchoconstriction in patients whose asthma is not well-controlled with adequate doses of inhaled corticosteroids.

Theophylline can have significant adverse effects, and its metabolism can be altered by the concomitant use of many other medications (e.g., erythromycin, cimetidine, ciprofloxacin) or by febrile illnesses. It is therefore important to monitor theophylline levels closely in patients who have viral illnesses or are being treated with medications that are known to alter theophylline metabolism. The level should be maintained between 5 and 15 μg per mL and should be checked when therapy is started, every 6 to 12 months during chronic therapy, and whenever the patient manifests any signs of toxicity, which include insomnia, headache, gastrointestinal upset, seizures, arrhythmias, and coma. All patients on theophylline and/or their parents should be taught these signs of toxicity and what to do if they occur.

TABLE 5. **Oral Theophylline Dosage**

Age (Years)	Dose/24 h
<2	5–10 mg/kg
2–9	24 mg/kg
9–12	20 mg/kg
12–16	18 mg/kg
>16	13 mg/kg

TABLE 6. **Intravenous Aminophylline Dosage**

Loading Dose	If theophylline level is known, then every mg/kg of aminophylline will raise level 2 mg/mL. If theophylline level is unknown: 6 mg/kg if no previous theophylline 3 mg/kg if previous theophylline	
Infusion (aminophylline)	**Age**	**Dose**
	1–6 m	0.5 mg/kg/h
	6–12 m	1.0 mg/kg/h
	1–6 y	0.85 mg/kg/h
	7–16 y	0.65 mg/kg/h
	>16 y	0.45 mg/kg/h

Anticholinergics include atropine and ipratropium bromide (Atrovent). Atropine can be used as an aerosolized medication, and ipratropium bromide is available in an MDI and as an aerosol. These agents produce bronchodilatation by blocking intrinsic vagal tone to the airways and can reduce the bronchoconstriction due to inhaled irritants. They are less potent than beta$_2$ agonists and have a slower onset of action. They may prolong the duration of bronchodilatation when used concomitantly with beta$_2$ agonists, but their precise role in the treatment of children with asthma remains to be defined.

Antihistamines are weak bronchodilators, and newer agents, many of which are not available in the United States, have some anti-inflammatory properties. They are not as effective as other medications available for the treatment of asthma, and thus do not have a role in routine asthma management. They are mentioned here, however, to counteract the statements found in many package inserts that antihistamines should not be used in patients with asthma. Their use in patients with upper airway allergies is not contraindicated if the patient has asthma and they may have a beneficial effect on the asthma as well.

Stepwise Approach to Asthma Management (Fig. 1)

The selection of medications should be based on asthma severity and the patient's current therapy. This approach allows for individualized treatment and for changes in individual patients over time. It is important to remember the overall goals of asthma management when selecting and modifying treatment.

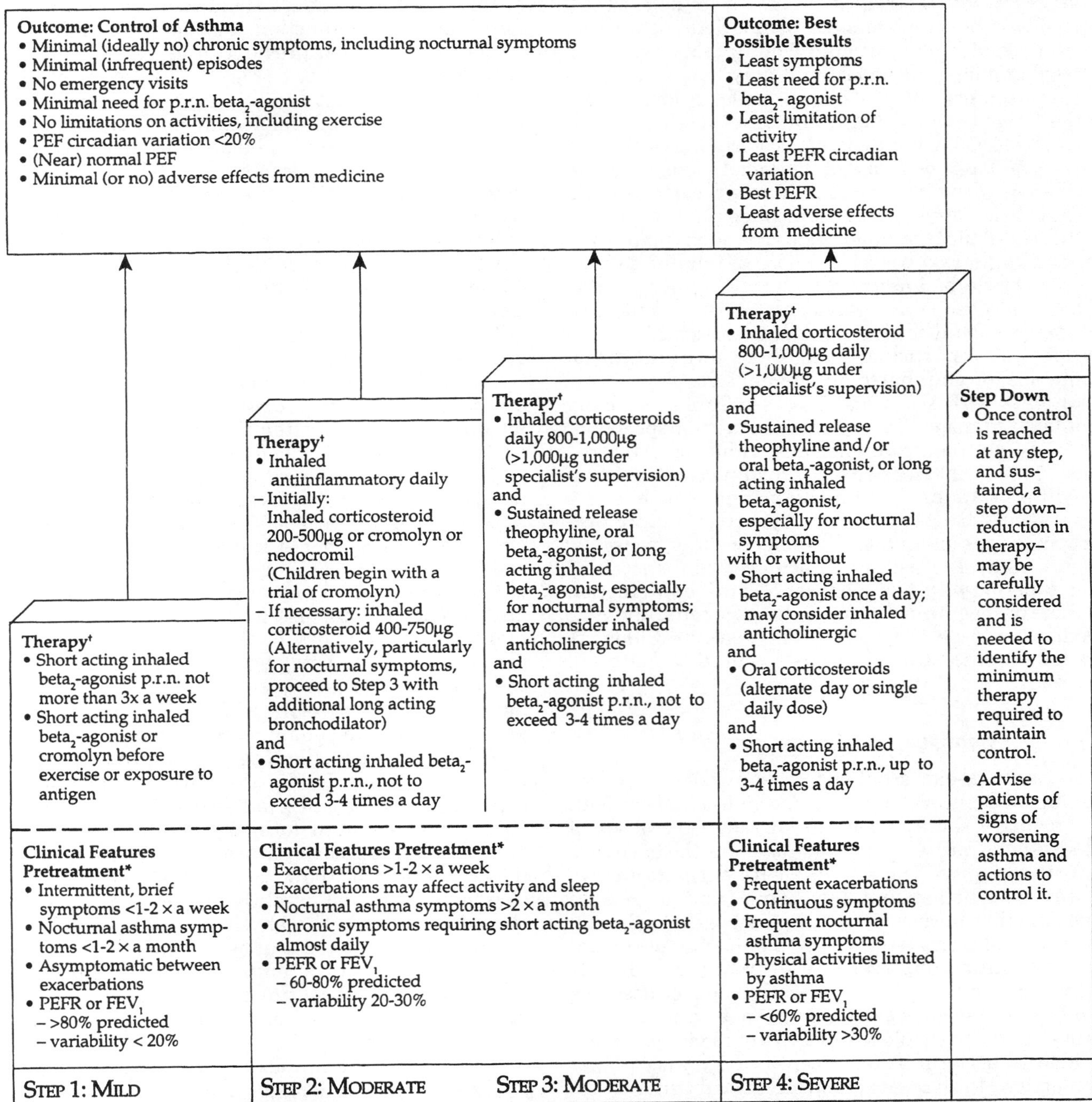

Figure 1. Management of chronic asthma: stepwise approach to asthma therapy. (From International Consensus Report of Diagnosis and Management of Asthma, United States Department of Health and Human Services, Public Health Service, National Institutes of Health, Publication No. 92-3091, March 1992.)

Patients with *mild asthma* (see Table 1) should be treated with $beta_2$ bronchodilators on an as-needed basis and before exercise. Alternatively, cromolyn can be used before exercise and should be used before allergen exposure.

Patients with *moderate asthma* (see Table 1) require regular anti-inflammatory treatment. In children, start with a trial of cromolyn or nedocromil. This should be supplemented with a $beta_2$ agonist on an as-needed basis. Patients who do not respond to inhaled cromolyn or nedocromil may be given a trial of nebulized cromolyn, which provides a larger dose to the lungs than the MDI. Failing that, they should be started on an inhaled corticosteroid at a dose of 200 to 500 μg per day of beclomethasone* or an equivalent dose of another inhaled corticosteroid such as triamcinolone or flunisolide. If the patient continues to have frequent exacerbations (more than one to two times a week), the dose of inhaled corticosteroid should be increased to 400 to 750 μg per day of beclomethasone or equivalent. At this point, consideration should be given to adding sustained-release theophylline, particularly if there are nocturnal symptoms, or an inhaled anticholinergic.

Patients with *severe asthma* (see Table 1) ideally should be managed in consultation with a specialist. They usually require higher dose inhaled corticosteroids (750 to 1200 μg per day), sustained-release theophylline or an inhaled anticholinergic or both, and a $beta_2$ agonist as needed. They may also require oral corticosteroids on an alternate-day or daily basis.

Once control of asthma is achieved and sustained over a period of a few months, a cautious reduction in therapy, beginning with the most potentially toxic agent, should be considered. The goal is to identify the lowest dose of medications required to maintain control.

Management of Exacerbations

In treating exacerbations, the physician should consider what works best for the individual patient. The primary therapy consists of repetitive doses of inhaled or nebulized $beta_2$ agonists and the early use of corticosteroids. The aim of treatment is to relieve airway obstruction and hypoxemia and to restore lung function to normal as soon as possible. Crucial to successful treatment is close monitoring of the patient's condition and response to treatment with serial measurement of lung function whenever possible. Symptoms and physical signs are not accurate indicators of airflow. Children over 5 years of age should be able to perform at least a peak flow with proper instruction. In younger children, auscultation of the lungs for a sense of the degree of air movement and observation of the chest for degree of retractions are often more useful than the presence or absence of wheezing. Pulse oximetry is not a substitute for lung function measurements, as a patient may have significant airway obstruction with normal oximetry. A low value, however, often indicates severe obstruction. Patients at high risk of fatal asthma (see Table 3) require intensive management and monitoring.

Full recovery from an asthma attack is usually gradual. It may take several days for lung function to return to normal and many weeks for airway reactivity to return to baseline. The increased treatment begun for exacerbations should continue until the patient's pulmonary function parameters have returned to normal or to their previous best.

Home Management (Fig. 2). Initiation of treatment at the earliest possible sign of deterioration is the key to successful management of exacerbations. Peak flow monitoring at home is particularly useful in this regard. In children too young to perform peak flow maneuvers, level of activity, presence of irritability, and degree of retractions may be helpful clues. As mentioned, a peak flow management protocol can allow the patient or parent to begin early treatment of asthma exacerbations, often without calling the physician.

A difference of more than 20% between A.M. and P.M. peak flow indicates increased airway hyperreactivity, and the patient should be instructed to increase the dose or frequency of anti-inflammatory medications. This is often the earliest sign of deterioration and may occur before symptoms are present.

If the patient is experiencing cough, chest tightness, wheezing or shortness of breath, and the peak flow result is between 50 and 80% of previous best levels, he or she should begin using a $beta_2$ agonist every 4 to 6 hours and increase the dose or frequency of the anti-inflammatory medication. If the peak flow after bronchodilator use is over 80% of best and remains so for 4 hours or more, the patient should continue to use a $beta_2$ agonist every 4 hours until the peak flow is consistently over 80%. If this requires 48 hours or more of frequent bronchodilator use, the physician should be contacted.

If the peak flow following a single treatment does not return to over 80%, the $beta_2$ agonist may be given in a dose of 2 to 4 puffs every 20 minutes for 1 hour, or a nebulized form of $beta_2$ agonist may be used. If this approach does not relieve symptoms or increase the peak flow to over 80%, the physician should be contacted urgently and oral corticosteroids should be started. The physician should also be contacted if the symptoms or peak flow do not remain normal for 4 hours after treatments. At this point, the patient should continue taking the regular $beta_2$ agonist every 3 to 4 hours with continued contact with the physician.

If the patient continues to have severe symptoms or the peak flow is less than 50% of best, oral corticosteroids should be started immediately, the $beta_2$ agonist should be repeated, and the patient should be seen immediately in the office or emergency department.

Emergency Department Management (Fig. 3). In the emergency department, initial assessment should include a history of the event, a history of asthma severity and treatment, physical examination

*Exceeds dosage recommended by the manufacturer.

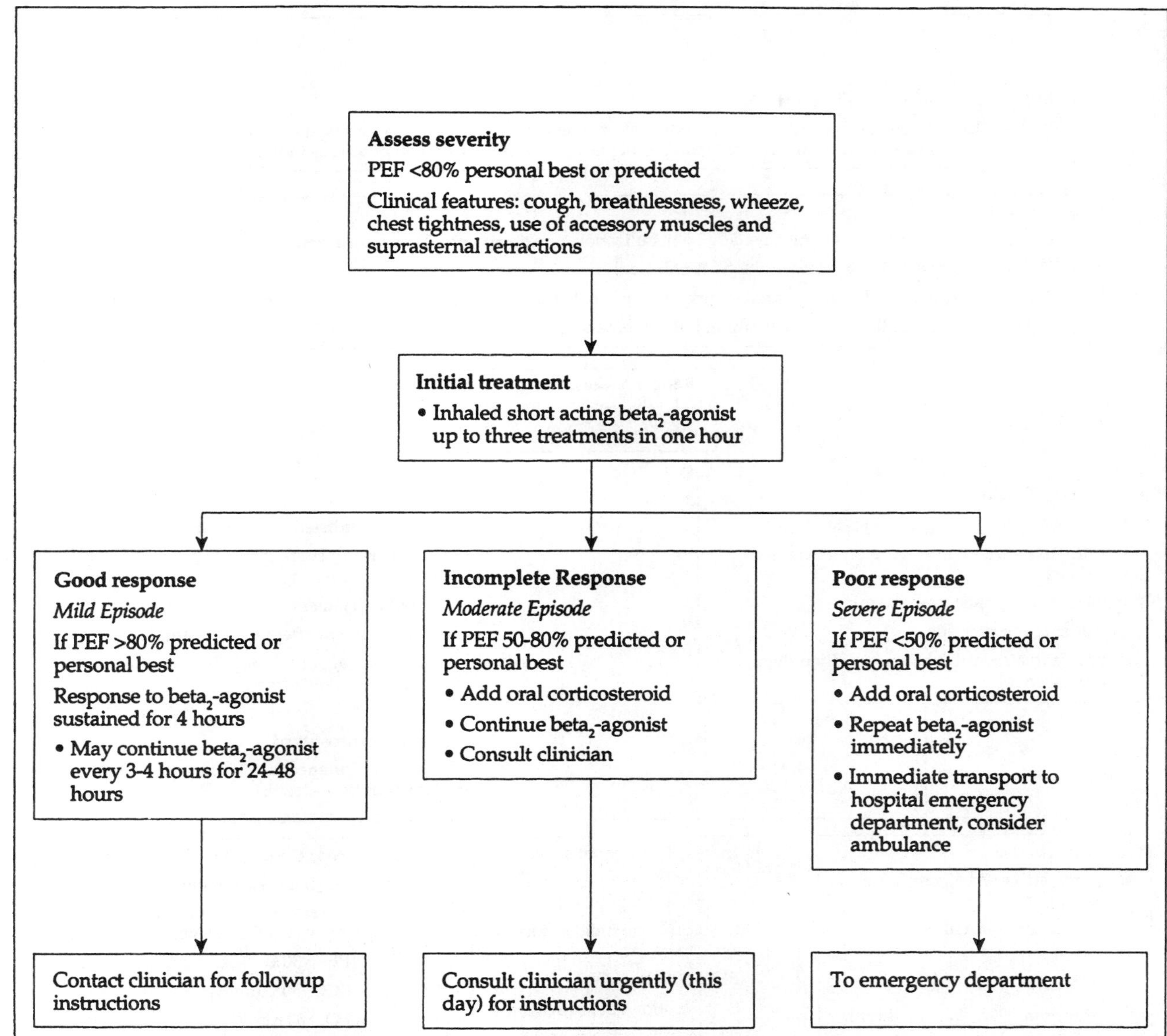

Figure 2. Management of exacerbation of asthma: home treatment. (From International Consensus Report of Diagnosis and Management of Asthma, United States Department of Health and Human Services, Public Health Service, National Institutes of Health, Publication No. 92-3091, March 1992.)

assessing air movement in the lungs; use of accessory muscles; tracheal symmetry; symmetry of breath sounds; vital signs including pulse, respiratory rate, and pulsus paradox; peak flow or spirometry; pulse oximetry; and blood gases in severe episodes.

The patient should be given a beta$_2$ agonist by nebulization every 20 minutes for 1 hour, oxygen to maintain O_2 saturation over 95%, and systemic corticosteroids if the episode is severe or if there has not been a response to oral corticosteroids. After this initial treatment, the patient should be reassessed with physical examination, peak flow or spirometry, O_2 saturation, and other tests as indicated.

Patients with peak flow of 50 to 70% of best and only moderate symptoms should continue treatment in the emergency room with a beta$_2$ agonist every hour* for another 1 to 3 hours. They may be discharged home if their physical examination is normal, peak flow is more than 70% of best and sustained for 1 hour after beta$_2$ agonist treatment, and O_2 saturation is over 95%.

Patients with a more severe episode (severe symptoms and peak flow of less than 50% of best) who do not immediately respond to the initial treatment or patients with a moderate episode who do not respond to additional treatments in the emergency room should be admitted to the hospital. Attention should always be given to precipitating factors such as ear infections, sinusitis, or pneumonia.

Hospital Management (Fig. 3). Patients with mild

*Exceeds dosage recommended by the manufacturer.

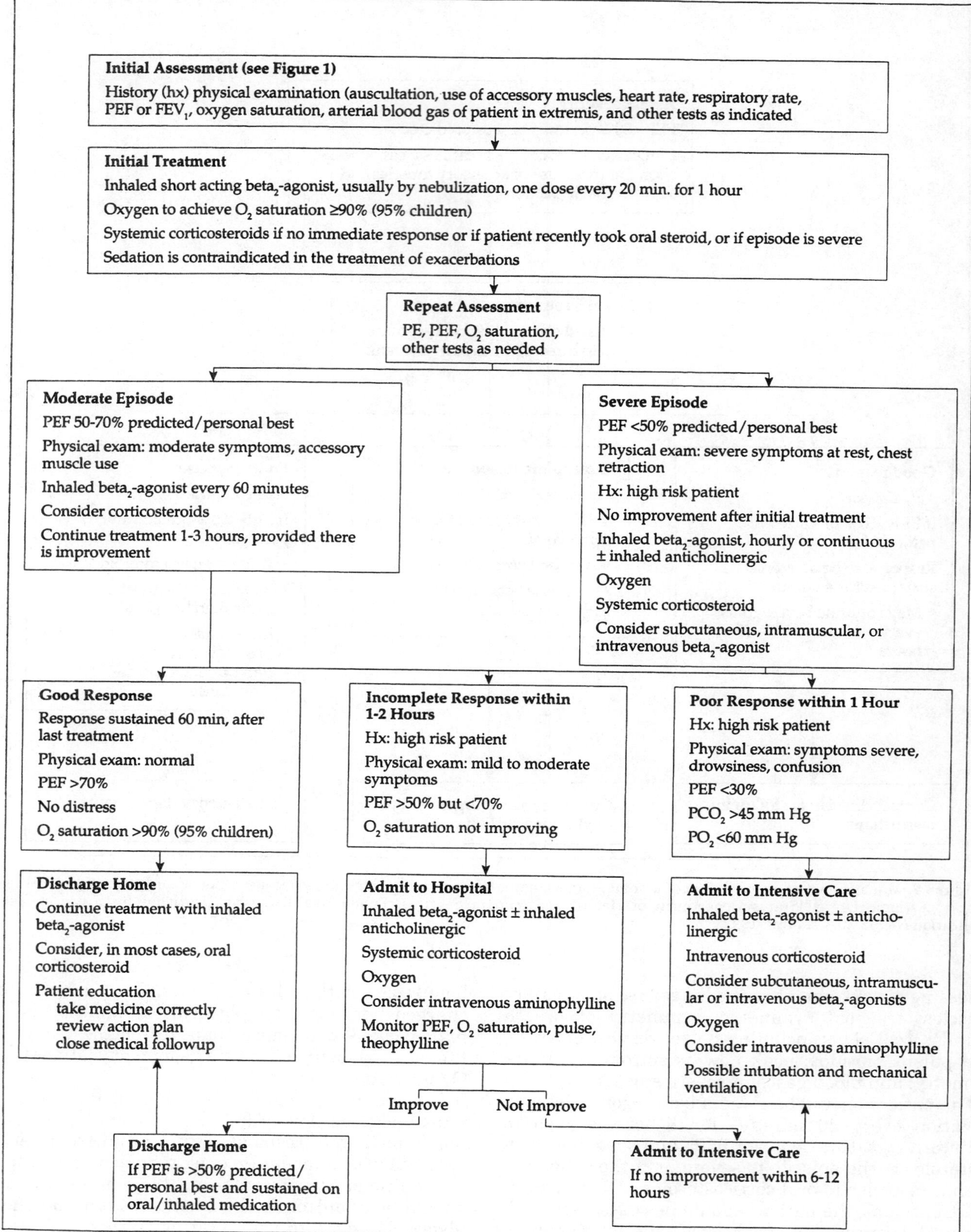

Figure 3. Management of exacerbation of asthma: hospital-based care. (From International Consensus Report of Diagnosis and Management of Asthma, United States Department of Health and Human Services, Public Health Service, National Institutes of Health, Publication No. 92-3091, March 1992.)

to moderate symptoms and peak flows between 50 and 70% of best should continue with nebulized $beta_2$ agonists every 1 to 4 hours, systemic corticosteroids, oxygen, and monitoring of peak flow or spirometry, oxygen saturation, and pulse. The use of systemic aminophylline should be considered. Patients with severe symptoms (peak flow $<30\%$, $PCO_2 >45$ mmHg, or $PO_2 <60$ mmHg) should be admitted to the intensive care unit (ICU) and treated with continuous nebulized $beta_2$-agonist medication at a dose of 0.45 mg per kg per hour.* Anticholinergics and intravenous aminophylline should be considered. Oxygen should be continued. Spirometry, oxygen saturation, serum electrolytes, and pulse should be monitored. Patients on the regular hospital unit who do not improve after 6 to 12 hours of treatment or who deteriorate should also be admitted to the ICU.

The patient can be discharged when the peak flow is more than 50% of best and symptoms are minimal and this improvement can be sustained on oral or inhaled medication. Patients should be discharged on a tapering dose of oral corticosteroids and regular anti-inflammatory and $beta_2$-agonist medication with a scheduled follow-up visit with the physician in 2 to 7 days.

Special Considerations

Exercise-Induced Asthma (EIA)

Approximately 90% of patients with asthma, 40% of patients with allergic rhinitis without asthma, and 10% of children without asthma or allergies experience bronchoconstriction after exercise. Symptoms include cough, chest tightness, wheezing, excessive shortness of breath, and even abdominal pain following exercise. Exercises vary with respect to their tendency to provoke bronchospasm, with running being the most asthmagenic. Prolonged periods of running are most likely to cause symptoms, while shorter periods of running (less than 5 minutes) with rest in between are usually better tolerated.

Playing with peers and participating in physical education and sports are important to the psychosocial development of children. EIA should be recognized and treated appropriately, so that children can participate fully in play and sports. Teachers and coaches need to be informed that pupils have EIA and educated about symptoms and treatment.

EIA is best treated with an inhaled $beta_2$ agonist 15 minutes before exercise. If this is not completely successful, then the addition of cromolyn 30 minutes before exercise may provide additional relief. Patients who do not respond to medications before exercise may need some sort of exercise modification.

Asthma in School

Children spend a great deal of their time in school, and teachers and other school personnel need to know that a student has asthma, what triggers it, and how it is treated. This requires that the physician and parent communicate with school personnel about the child's asthma, and this is best done by having an individual action plan on file for each student with asthma. This action plan should list peak flow values, medications, triggers, and plans for exacerbations. Children who are mature enough should be allowed to carry their own inhalers to use as indicated. The school environment should be examined for asthma triggers as well. Chalk dust, classroom pets, dust mites, and molds may all be problems in the school.

*Exceeds dosage recommended by the manufacturer.

ALLERGIC RHINITIS CAUSED BY INHALANT FACTORS

method of
JONATHAN CORREN, M.D., and
GARY S. RACHELEFSKY, M.D.
University of California, Los Angeles, School of Medicine
Allergy Research Foundation, Inc.
Los Angeles, California

Allergic rhinitis is the most common of all allergic diseases and has been estimated to affect up to 15% of the population in the United States. Although allergic rhinitis can develop at any age, two-thirds of patients report the onset of symptoms before age 30. Symptoms of nasal allergy vary widely, but in many cases are of sufficient severity to result in significant loss of time from school and the workplace. Allergic rhinitis is also strongly associated with chronic and recurrent sinusitis, otitis media, and bronchial asthma, and there is growing evidence that treatment of rhinitis may improve control of these other disorders.

DIAGNOSIS

Appropriate therapy for allergic rhinitis requires differentiation of this syndrome from other forms of chronic rhinitis (Table 1). A thorough history and physical examination are frequently all that is required to make an initial diagnosis and begin therapy.

History

Allergic rhinitis typically presents with symptoms of intermittent nasal congestion, clear rhinorrhea, sneezing, and itching of the nose, palate, and/or ears. A significant number of patients also report tearing, redness, and itching of the eyes, usually when nasal symptoms are most active.

TABLE 1. **Differential Diagnosis of Chronic Rhinitis**

Allergic rhinitis
Vasomotor rhinitis
Nonallergic rhinitis with eosinophilia
Rhinitis medicamentosa
Chronic sinusitis
Nasal polyps
Anatomic obstructive lesions (e.g., septal deviation, adenoidal hypertrophy)

Nasal and ocular pruritus are among the most helpful symptoms in differentiating allergic from other forms of chronic rhinitis. In severe cases, mucous membranes of the eustachian tubes, middle ears, and sinuses may become involved, causing ear fullness or popping, muffled hearing, and facial pressure. Significant postnasal drainage may result in sore throat and chronic cough. Malaise and fatigue may be prominent, usually in patients with florid nasal symptoms during the height of the pollen season.

In seasonal allergic rhinitis (pollinosis or hay fever), this constellation of symptoms occurs during a predictable, defined season, depending on which allergens the patient has become sensitized to. This temporal pattern is a key feature in distinguishing seasonal allergic from other forms of rhinitis. In perennial allergic rhinitis, however, aeroallergens are present in the environment throughout the year (e.g., house dust mite and animal proteins), causing symptoms to vary little between seasons and making differentiation from other types of rhinitis more difficult. Additionally, patients with perennial allergic rhinitis (particularly due to dust mites) tend to be more affected by persistent nasal congestion and rhinorrhea and less by ocular symptoms, making it difficult to discriminate allergic from nonallergic causes.

Physical Examination

Inspection of the face often reveals periorbital darkening, or "allergic shiners," due to chronic venous pooling. Children frequently rub their noses upward in response to itching (allergic salute), which may produce a persistent horizontal crease across the nose. The conjuntivae commonly appear mildly injected, with either watery or gelatinous exudate present. Both the allergic salute and the ocular findings are helpful in differentiating allergy from other causes of rhinitis.

Anterior rhinoscopy with a nasal speculum allows visualization of the anterior one-third of the nasal airway. Patients with allergic rhinitis typically have pale, swollen inferior and middle turbinates and clear discharge. Very red, irritated mucosa and thick, discolored secretions should raise suspicions regarding other causes of rhinitis. When severe mucosal edema is present, it may be helpful to spray the nose with a topical decongestant, such as oxymetazoline (Afrin), in order to visualize structures located more posteriorly. Better visualization of the nasal cavity may allow the examiner to detect a variety of obstructive abnormalities, including posterior deviation of the septum, septal spurs, and polyps.

Laboratory Testing

If the diagnosis has not been made from the history and physical findings, cytologic examination of nasal scrapings can be helpful. Significant eosinophilia in nasal secretions (greater than five eosinophils per high power field) is an excellent clue to the presence of allergy. While the detection of nasal eosinophilia is suggestive of allergic rhinitis, it is not diagnostic since eosinophils are also found in NARES (nonallergic rhinitis with eosinophilia). Large numbers of neutrophils without eosinophils should alert the clinician to the possibility of chronic bacterial rhinosinusitis.

Principal indications for allergy skin testing or in vitro measures of specific IgE (e.g., radioallergosorbent testing [RAST]) are determination of allergic sensitivities prior to institution of aggressive allergen avoidance measures or allergy immunotherapy. Assays for specific IgE are not necessary in patients who respond well to and tolerate empiric medical therapy for rhinitis. Skin or in vitro testing must be done in the context of the patient's geographic location and specific home environment in order to include all relevant allergens. Skin testing is the preferred method of investigation because of greater sensitivity, broader variety of available antigens, and lower cost. In most situations, prick or puncture tests are sufficient to assess specific sensitivities in allergic rhinitis, and intradermal testing should be reserved for special circumstances. In vitro allergy testing should be employed in patients who suffer from widespread dermatitis or dermatographism, who have poorly reactive skin (as seen in some young infants and elderly patients), who cannot withhold antihistamines, or who have recently taken astemizole (which suppresses responses for several weeks). Results often vary greatly among laboratories performing these assays, making interpretation difficult. Assessment of total serum IgE is an inadequate screening test, since many patients with normal or low levels of IgE may have strongly positive response to a small but highly relevant group of allergens on allergy skin or RAST testing.

TREATMENT

Allergen Avoidance Measures

Avoidance of aeroallergens is an effective, nonpharmacologic method for treating allergic rhinitis. These measures will ultimately limit long-term expense and potential adverse effects of medications. Since environmental control measures may be inconvenient and expensive to implement, allergy testing should be performed to confirm allergic sensitivities.

Outdoor Aeroallergens. For patients with strictly seasonal rhinitis caused by exposure to plant pollens, avoidance of outdoor activity during peak pollen hours (early afternoon) may be helpful. For patients who are allergic to grass pollen, wearing a surgical-type mask while mowing the lawn or gardening may help avert symptoms. Keeping the windows closed throughout the day is important, and use of an air conditioner prevents airborne pollen from entering the home. HEPA (high-efficiency particulate air) filters placed in the home also reduce indoor pollen counts.

Indoor Aeroallergens. For patients with perennial symptoms, the most common source of allergen sensitization is the house dust mite. Large reservoirs of these microscopic insects are usually found in bedding, mattresses, and carpeting. Down-filled pillows and comforters and wool blankets should be eliminated. Washing of all sheets, mattress pads, pillow cases, and blankets every 1 to 2 weeks in hot (>130° F) water effectively kills these organisms. Specially constructed mattress covers are available that act as a barrier between the interior of the mattress and the patient. Carpeting can be treated with a commercially prepared tannic acid spray, which denatures allergenic mite proteins. If these measures do not result in satisfactory improvement, patients can consider removing the carpeting from the bedroom, providing there are hardwood or linoleum floors underneath. Vacuuming with conventional vacuum cleaners does not significantly reduce mite numbers in carpeting and often increases the number of airborne mite allergen for short periods of time. Available acaricides have been demonstrated to provide only minimal benefit to mite allergic patients.

Domestic pets are an important source of allergen exposure in many atopic patients. The first and most important step in allergen avoidance is removal of the animal from the home environment. Since patients are often reluctant to do this, other less drastic methods of environmental control can be recommended. The animal should be kept out of the bedroom at all times and central air vents to the bedroom should be kept closed. Following removal of the pet from the bedroom, consideration should be given to removing upholstered furniture and carpeting. A HEPA filter reduces the quantity of airborne animal allergens. Finally, the pet should be washed every 1 to 2 weeks, preferably by someone other than the allergic patient. The patient should be informed that it may take several weeks to months for indoor levels of animal dander to return to low levels.

Indoor fungi, such as *Aspergillus* and *Penicillium* species, are usually found in homes that have experienced water damage. Leaky roofs and ceilings, flooded basements, damaged plumbing, and wet crawl spaces are common sites of mold growth within homes. The only effective way to reduce indoor levels of fungal spores is repair of water-damaged areas. For damp spaces where mold growth is a potential problem, a high-intensity heat lamp can be turned on for 1 to 2 hours. While most indoor plants do not elevate household levels of mold spores, wicker basket planters should be avoided.

Medications

Antihistamines. Antihistamines are frequently used as first-line therapy for patients with allergic rhinitis (Table 2). These medications effectively reduce rhinorrhea, sneezing, and nasal and ocular pruritus but have little effect on nasal congestion. Antihistamines are effective when taken occasionally for intermittent symptoms although they work best when administered before the onset of symptoms.

Patients often treat their symptoms with a variety of classic antihistamines which are available over the counter. These drugs have several possible central nervous system side effects, the most common of which is sedation. The sedative effect often attenuates with continued use over a period of 1 to 2 weeks, but if sedation persists, taking the antihistamine at bedtime only (e.g., chlorpheniramine, 4 to 8 mg) is clinically effective and significantly minimizes daytime sleepiness. An equally important adverse effect is prolongation of voluntary reaction time, the extent of which cannot be gauged by the degree of sedation. Classic antihistamines also have anticholinergic effects, including dryness of the mouth and eyes, blurred vision, and urinary retention. These drugs should be used cautiously in older patients, particularly elderly men, and should be strictly avoided in patients with histories of symptomatic prostatic hypertrophy, bladder neck obstruction, and narrow-angle glaucoma.

TABLE 2. **Commonly Used Antihistamines**

Antihistamine	Sedation	Dose
Diphenhydramine (Benadryl)	Strong	25–50 mg qid
Tripelennamine (PBZ)	Moderate	25–50 mg qid
Chlorpheniramine (Chlor-Trimeton)	Moderate	4 mg qid
Brompheniramine (Dimetane)	Moderate	4 mg qid
Clemastine (Tavist)	Mild	1.34–2.68 mg bid
Terfenadine (Seldane)	None	60 mg bid
Astemizole (Hismanal)	None	10 mg qd
Loratadine (Claritin)	None	10 mg qd

Newer antihistamines have clinical efficacy equal to or greater than that of the classic antihistamines but without central nervous system or anticholinergic side effects. Presently, all three of the currently available nonsedating antihistamines are approved for use in patients older than 12 years of age. Because of long drug half-lives, loratadine (Claritin) and astemizole (Hismanal) have the advantage of once-daily dosing. While loratadine has a relatively rapid onset of action, astemizole often requires several hours or longer to control symptoms. Terfenadine (Seldane) and astemizole have been noted to cause prolongation of the QT interval when taken in the following situations: larger than prescribed doses; with concomitant administration of ketoconazole, itraconazole, erythromycin, clarithromycin, or troleandomycin; and in patients with severe hepatic dysfunction. In association with QT interval prolongation, there have been rare reports of cardiovascular adverse events, including torsades de pointes, other ventricular arrhythmias, cardiac arrest, and death. Neither QT prolongation nor cardiovascular events have yet been linked to loratadine.

Decongestants. Alpha-adrenergic agonists are potent vasoconstrictors that are available in both topical and systemic forms. These medications significantly reduce nasal swelling and rhinorrhea but do not affect other symptoms of allergic rhinitis. Topical preparations include oxymetazoline (Afrin, Neo-Synephrine), and phenylephrine nasal sprays. In patients with severe nasal congestion, these medications enhance the penetration of other topical drugs, such as nasal cromolyn (Nasalcrom) and corticosteroids. Use should be limited to 3 to 5 days to avoid rebound nasal congestion and rhinitis medicamentosa.

Oral decongestants, such as pseudoephedrine and phenylpropanolamine, are also effective in relieving nasal blockage and do not cause rebound nasal swelling after prolonged periods of use. They are most often combined with antihistamines for treatment of allergic rhinitis (e.g., Drixoral) and are superior in clinical efficacy to either drug used alone. Oral decongestants frequently cause nervousness and insomnia and should not be taken during the evening hours in susceptible patients. While these drugs do not usually cause significant changes in blood pressure, they should be used with caution in patients with hypertension.

Cromolyn Sodium. Cromolyn sodium, given as a 4% topical nasal spray (Nasalcrom), appears to work by stabilizing mast cells and by direct anti-inflammatory effects on granulocytes. It is comparable to oral antihistamines in controlling symptoms of seasonal and perennial allergic rhinitis and is only partially effective in reducing nasal congestion. Nasal cromolyn needs to be used on a prophylactic basis, one spray per nostril three to four times per day. Cromolyn is not effective when taken on an as-needed basis. Except for mild, transient stinging, nasal cromolyn is well tolerated by most patients and is particularly useful in children who cannot tolerate classic antihistamines and decongestants.

Corticosteroids. Corticosteroid nasal sprays are an extremely effective form of therapy for allergic rhinitis. When started before allergen exposure, these medications reduce mast cell mediator release (e.g., histamine, prostaglandin D_2) and retard eosinophil influx into nasal tissue. They have been approved for use in seasonal and perennial rhinitis in patients over 6 years of age. Unlike many other available treatments for nasal allergy, topical corticosteroids are effective in controlling nasal congestion. While these drugs are most beneficial when used on a regular schedule, there is recent evidence suggesting that they may also be helpful when used on an as-needed basis. In addition to controlling allergic rhinitis, nasal corticosteroids appear to reduce lower airway symptoms in patients with concomitant bronchial asthma. Principal side effects include transient stinging, occasional mild epistaxis, nasal dryness, and pharyngeal irritation. Stinging and dryness may be lessened by switching from an aerosol to one of the aqueous preparations or by using a saline nasal spray before administering the corticosteroid. Epistaxis will usually resolve by stopping the spray for 2 to 3 days and applying a topical ointment, such as boric acid (Borofax), to the nasal septum. With long-term use, there do not appear to be any significant local effects on the nasal mucosa and septal perforations have been reported only on rare occasions.

The three available formulations, including beclomethasone (Vancenase, Beconase), triamcinolone (Nasacort), and flunisolide (Nasalide), are comparable in efficacy (Table 3). The most important difference among these products is the type of vehicle used. Vancenase and Beconase are available in both aerosol and aqueous preparations, while Nasacort is available as an aerosol only and Nasalide as a solution containing propylene and polyethylene glycol. Deciding among these preparations is largely a matter of individual patient choice, although the majority of patients in our experience prefer the aqueous or aerosol formulations over solutions containing glycol.

TABLE 3. **Intranasal Corticosteroids**

Preparation	Trade Name	Vehicle	Dose*
Beclomethasone	Vancenase, Beconase	Freon/alcohol	1–2 puffs bid
	Vancenase AQ, Beconase AQ	Aqueous	1–2 sprays bid
Flunisolide	Nasalide	Polyethylene glycol	2 sprays bid
Triamcinolone	Nasacort	Freon	2–4 puffs qd

*Dose per nostril.

In patients who have very severe nasal swelling, a 3- to 5-day course of oral corticosteroids (e.g., prednisone, 0.5 mg/kg in three divided doses) may be helpful prior to starting topical anti-inflammatory therapy. Because of the risk of severe complications (e.g., osteoporosis), long-term oral or injectable corticosteroid therapy should be avoided in allergic rhinitis.

Anticholinergic Agents. An aerosol preparation of ipratropium bromide* (Atrovent) has recently been demonstrated to reduce watery nasal secretions. An infant feeding nipple with an enlarged hole can be attached to the holder of the metered dose inhaler for nasal use. Ipratropium bromide has little effect on nasal congestion, sneezing, and pruritus, and is best used as a supplemental medication when rhinorrhea has not responded to other measures. An initial starting dose is 1 puff per nostril twice daily, which may be increased to 2 puffs per nostril three times daily, as tolerated. As might be expected, the principal side effect is mucosal dryness, which can be reduced by adjusting the dose. There appears to be no significant systemic absorption at the above doses given nasally.

Immunotherapy

Allergy immunotherapy (hyposensitization therapy) should be considered in patients who do not respond to allergen avoidance or medications, who have significant adverse side effects from medications, or who have difficulty adhering to a complex regimen of multiple drugs. Since immunotherapy has also been shown to be effective in allergic asthma, patients with concomitant rhinitis and asthma should be strongly considered as candidates for immunotherapy. Several placebo-controlled studies have documented efficacy with a variety of allergens, including dust mite, cat dander, and multiple grass, tree, and weed pollens. Approximately 80% of patients will experience symptomatic improvement after 1 to 2 years, and therapy should be continued for a total of 4 to 5 years. While the beneficial effects of hyposensitization persist for several years in some patients, in others it may be lost once the injections are stopped. These patients should be evaluated for the development of new sensitivities and may require immunotherapy on a long-term basis. Although the mechanisms by which immunotherapy works are still unclear, it has been documented to reduce mast cell mediator release, eosinophil infiltration, and circulating levels of specific IgE.

The success of immunotherapy depends on accu-

*Not FDA approved for this indication.

rate confirmation of allergic sensitivities with skin or in vitro testing and a history suggestive of clinical worsening after allergen exposure. The cumulative dose of extract is also important: low-dose immunotherapy has been shown to be no more effective than placebo. As the dose of extract is increased, local reactions are common and systemic reactions can occasionally occur. For this reason, it is important that immunotherapy be administered by practitioners who are skilled in adjusting the dose of immunotherapy and treating untoward reactions.

At present, effective allergy immunotherapy is available only by injection (subcutaneous route). Recent research has shown mixed results for other methods of extract delivery, including both the intranasal and oral routes.

ALLERGIC DRUG REACTIONS

method of
GILLIAN M. SHEPHERD, M.D.
New York Hospital—Cornell Medical Center
New York, New York

DIAGNOSIS

Patients frequently take multiple drugs, and it is often a challenge to determine whether an adverse reaction is due to a drug or a disease and, if a drug, which one. In most cases, a single drug is responsible.

First, one should consider the nature of the reaction. Drugs can cause a host of adverse reactions, only a small percentage of which are allergic. Allergy implies that various components of the immune system specifically overreact to the drug. This results in a limited number of signs and symptoms generally compatible with known immune mechanisms as noted in Table 1. Skin manifestations, primarily maculorpapular rashes are most common, followed by urticaria.

Second, one should consider the timing of the reaction relative to administration of the drug. When a drug is administered for the first time, allergic reactions generally do not occur for days, as it takes the immune system time to react to a new antigen. High intermittent dosing is the most sensitizing. Frequent courses are also a problem. Drugs given steadily for more than 3 months rarely cause later reactions. A drug started within days to weeks is usually the culprit, especially if the patient has had a prior course of the drug within a year. In some cases, rashes may appear several days after the drug is stopped, especially in the case of antibiotics given for 7 to 14 days.

Third, one has to consider the propensity of a drug to cause the reaction. This is largely due to the chemical structure of the native drug and its metabolic products. In general, antibiotics, particularly beta-lactam and sulfa drugs, induce reactions most frequently. Antiarrhythmics, anticonvulsants, and allopurinol are other common offenders.

TABLE 1. **Signs and Symptoms of Allergic Drug Reactions**

Reaction	Responsible Immune Mechanisms
Anaphylaxis	IgE antibody
Urticaria and angioedema	IgE antibody
Rash	Probably mediated by CD4-positive T cells
Fever	Release of cytokines (e.g., interleukin-1, tumor necrosis factor)
Immune complex reactions (rash, fever, arthralgias, myalgias, lymphadenopathy, nephritis, vasculitis)	IgG and IgM antibody
Cytopenias	IgG and IgM antibody

TREATMENT OF SPECIFIC REACTIONS

Anaphylaxis

In an anaphylactic reaction, a patient experiences some or all of the following signs and symptoms: anxiety, flushing, diffuse pruritus, urticaria and angioedema, diaphoresis, laryngeal obstruction, bronchospasm, nausea, vomiting, diarrhea, hypotension, and shock. Approximately 85% of reactions start within 1 hour of exposure, but in rare patients the reaction does not manifest until up to 3 hours afterward.

Specific treatment for anaphylaxis is outlined in Table 2. Drug administration should be stopped immediately. If the drug was given orally within 90 minutes, consideration should be given to inducing emesis with ipecac (15 to 30 mL of syrup followed by three to four glasses of water). There is a risk of aspiration if the patient loses consciousness or has significant respiratory symptoms. If the drug was given intramuscularly, the rate of absorption may be slowed by an injection of epinephrine (0.1 to 0.2 mL of 1:1000 [1 mg/mL]) at the site. If possible, a proximal tourniquet should be placed. Patients taking beta-adrenergic blocking drugs may have more severe symptoms and be more refractory to treatment. Additionally, use of epinephrine (an alpha and beta stimulant) can result in marked hypertension in these patients from unopposed alpha stimulation. The use of glucagon* has been recommended for patients on beta blockers with refractory anaphylaxis. After treatment and apparent resolution of symptoms, up to 20% of patients may have a recurrence up to 8 hours later. Therefore, all patients should be kept under observation for at least that long. Treatment with steroids does not seem to prevent this recurrence. Lesser symptoms, such as urticaria, may continue until the drug is completely eliminated (sometimes days to weeks). If there is a risk that the drug might subsequently be given in an emergency setting, the patient should be advised to avoid beta blockers and to wear a bracelet or necklace warning of the allergy.

Urticaria and Angioedema

This reaction can range from several scattered hives to systemic urticaria with diffuse angioedema.

*Not FDA approved for this indication.

TABLE 2. **Treatment of Anaphylaxis**

Drug	Dose	Route	Comments
Epinephrine (Adrenalin) 1:1000 (1 mg/mL)	0.3 mL for adults (0.01 mL/kg for children)	SC	Repeat in 15 minutes if necessary. **Do not give IV** if patient is alert, as fatal arrhythmia may develop.
	0.5 mL (0.5 mg) diluted to 10 mL with sodium chloride	IV or intracardiac	Give if patient is unconscious.
Diphenhydramine (Benadryl)	50 mg; repeat q 4–6 h	IV or IM	One to three doses usually sufficient.
Fluids: NaCl or 5% dextrose	1–2 L	IV	Corrects hypotension from intravascular volume depletion (from postcapillary venule dilation).
Methylprednisolone (SoluMedrol) or equivalent	60 mg once	IV	Does nothing for acute reaction but may blunt development of any later reactions.
Vasopressors, bronchodilators, O_2	As needed		
Glucagon	Start with 0.5 to 1.0 mg (0.5 to 1 unit)	IV preferable; or SC or IM	May help if patient is on beta-blocker drug.

Angioedema alone is a less common manifestation of an allergic drug reaction. The onset can range from minutes after administration to several days after the drug has been stopped. Most commonly, reactions occur from 1 to 7 days after exposure.

If symptoms occur within 1 hour of initial administration of drug, the patient should be treated for anaphylaxis and no more drug should be given. Treatment is otherwise symptomatic with antihistamines as outlined on Table 3. Antihistamines are competitive inhibitors of histamine receptors. Given after the reaction, they will not reverse existing urticaria but will block further development. Steroids are occasionally necessary for severe prolonged symptoms. They likewise will not reverse existing symptoms. Lip and tongue angioedema can sometimes be decreased by local application of epinephrine spray (Primatene Mist, Bronkaid Mist), especially if used in the first 15 minutes. If significant angioedema has occurred, it can take 2 to 3 days for extravasated fluid to be completely resorbed. Eyelid edema may appear worse after sleep due to increased hydrostatic pressure. This does not mean that the allergic reaction is progressing and further treatment is not needed. While symptoms persist, the patient should avoid aspirin and nonsteroidal anti-inflammatory drugs (NSAIDs) as they can sometimes cause marked flares. Rarely, when mild urticaria develops later, the drug may be continued under the direct supervision of an experienced physician, particularly if a limited course is required.

Rashes

A maculopapular morbilliform rash is the most frequent manifestation of drug allergy and typically occurs 7 to 10 days into treatment with a range of 2 days to several weeks. The rash can range from mild erythema to a severe exfoliative dermatitis. Penicillin, sulfas, barbiturates, allopurinol, gold, and chlorpromazine are the most common causes.

If the rash is mild, the drug can often be continued for another day with close observation, as some rashes do not progress with continued drug administration. If the drug is discontinued immediately, it will be difficult to restart it without risk of intensifying the rash. If the rash is obviously progressing or any vesiculation is seen, the drug must be discontinued because of the risk of an exfoliative dermatitis. All patients with morbilliform rashes should have a thorough examination for evidence of vesiculation or erosive changes of mucous membranes that might herald a bullous exfoliative rash. In these cases, the suspect drug should be stopped immediately and high-dose steroids (prednisone, 60 to 120 mg daily) started. The typical maculopapular rash usually starts to wane within 24 to 48 hours after the suspect drug is discontinued, but in the case of sulfa drugs, the rash may be prolonged. (See Sulfonamides for problems associated with their use in patients infected with the human immunodeficiency virus.)

TABLE 3. **Treatment of Urticaria and Angioedema**

Drug	Dose	Route	Comments
Diphenhydramine (Benadryl) or equivalent	25–50 mg q 6 h	PO, IM, or IV	For moderate to severe reactions
Doxepin* (Sinequan)	10–20 mg hs	PO	For milder reactions
Terfenadine (Seldane)	60 mg bid	PO	Weaker than diphenhydramine or doxepin but nonsedating
Loratadine† (Claritin)	10 mg daily	PO	Weaker than diphenhydramine or doxepin but nonsedating
Astemizole (Hismanal)	10 mg daily	PO	Weaker than diphenhydramine or doxepin but nonsedating
Prednisone	20–30 mg bid	PO	For severe reactions; taper pending symptoms

*Not FDA approved for this indication.
†Exceeds dosage recommended by the manufacturer.

A morbilliform rash occurs in 5 to 10% of patients taking ampicillin and amoxicillin, which is higher than the usual 2% incidence with other penicillins. This incidence approaches 60 to 100% in patients with concurrent Epstein-Barr infection or chronic lymphocytic leukemia. This rash is probably not immunologically mediated, and if the physician believes the rash to be morbilliform rather than urticarial, these patients should not be considered allergic to penicillin.

As most patients are only mildly symptomatic and the rash wanes after the drug is discontinued, specific treatment is often unnecessary. Antihistamines help pruritus but it is unclear whether they hasten clearance. Topical lubrication, menthol creams such as Sarna lotion and colloidal oatmeal baths (Aveeno) are often soothing. Hydrocortisone ointment may be needed. If the rash is severe, prednisone, 20 to 30 mg twice daily, can be added over several days.

Erythema multiforme (EM), the *Stevens-Johnson syndrome* (SJS) and *toxic epidermal necrolysis* (TEN) can also result from drug allergy. EM and SJS are generally considered part of the same spectrum. It is unclear whether TEN is a severe form of SJS or a separate entity. The mortality from TEN is high. The efficacy of steroids is unclear but they are given by most physicians at starting doses of 60 to 250 mg of prednisone. Patients with severe bullous-erosive disease should be treated in burn units for fluid management and infection prevention.

Contact dermatitis from drugs is rare as few drugs are administered topically. Reactions may be due to the vehicle rather than the drug. Treatment consists of avoidance and application of moderate-to-strong cortisone creams twice daily until the rash clears.

Fever

Drug fever results from activation of the immune system with release of endogenous pyrogens, such as interleukin-1 and tumor necrosis factor. A high index of suspicion must be maintained, as fever is often a manifestation of the underlying disease. There are no consistent associated signs and symptoms. Temperature patterns are variable with average peaks of 38 to 40° C; 50% of patients experience chills. Rashes and eosinophilia are associated in only 20% of cases. One clue may be a dissociation between the patient's good clinical status and the degree of fever. In one series, the following drugs (in order of frequency) were responsible for one half of the cases of drug fever: penicillin derivatives, methyldopa (Aldomet), quinidine, phenytoin, procainamide, and cephalothin.

If fever is due to a drug reaction, it will resolve in the majority of patients within 24 hours and in all within 48 hours of stopping the drug (assuming normal clearance). Conversely, if the fever has not abated within 48 hours after cessation, the drug is not responsible. If there is still a question, the suspect drug can be readministered with low risk of a serious reaction.

Immune Complex Reaction

An immune complex reaction consists of fever, myalgias, arthralgias, and occasionally frank arthritis, inflammation of serosal surfaces, glomerulonephritis, and lymphadenopathy. It classically presents 7 to 10 days into treatment but may occur earlier in a previously sensitized patient or rarely later. IgG and IgM antibodies form complexes with the drug in a ratio of slight antigen excess such that complexes can filter through basement membranes where they trigger a complement-dependent inflammatory reaction. Treatment is cessation of the drug. Removal of the antigen limits the complex formation and the clinical reaction wanes within a few days. In rare cases, the drug may be continued under experienced supervision as the reaction may be self-limited.

If necessary, steroids can be given. Prednisone, 1 mg per kg with a taper over 1 week is usually sufficient. Theoretically, antihistamines may hinder immune complex deposition in basement membranes by blocking vasodilatation from local histamine release. They should be used maximally (e.g., diphenhydramine, 25 mg, or hydroxyzine, 25 mg, every 6 hours).

Drug-Induced Immune Cytopenias

Drugs can induce immunologically mediated anemias, thrombocytopenias, and leukopenias by a variety of mechanisms, including direct binding to the cell or platelet membrane. If the drug is bound but the cell or platelet is not destroyed, it may be possible to continue treatment. Stopping the offending drug usually results in rapid resolution.

DRUG ALLERGIES

Multiple Drug Allergy

One to four percent of patients have a history of multiple drug allergy, primarily to antibiotics. Approximately 20% of patients with a history of a reaction to one antibiotic drug have a comparable reaction to an unrelated antibiotic. The mechanism is unknown. These patients are often difficult to manage and may benefit from consultation with an allergy specialist. Ideally, they should be given drugs to which they have not previously been exposed.

Penicillin

Twenty percent of hospital patients have a history of allergy to penicillin. When skin tested to penicillin, only 15% of hospitalized patients with a positive history will have a positive skin test. Sensitivity can be determined by skin testing with 0.02 mL (intradermal) injections of benzylpenicilloyl-polylysine (Pre-Pen) (major determinant) and penicillin G, 6000 units per mL (most important minor determinant), with a histamine control. These doses should be lowered 10- to 100-fold if the patient has a history of *any* reaction within 24 hours of penicillin administration. A wheal of 4 to 5 mm at 10 minutes is a positive reaction. The other minor determinants are not commercially available for skin testing. In our experience, a negative skin test to benzylpenicilloyl-polylysine and penicillin G is 99% predictive of the chance of developing an immediate reaction if given penicillin. Others have cited lower theoretical predictive values.

If the skin test is *positive,* the patient should be given another antibiotic or desensitized to penicillin. Desensitization can be done by the oral or intravenous route with the specific antibiotic to be given therapeutically. Because IgE specific to penicillin has been documented by skin testing, this is a potentially dangerous procedure that should be done in a monitored setting. Pretreatment with steroids and antihistamines is controversal as it may mask early warning signs of a reaction. A representative desensitization schedule is outlined in Table 4. If the skin test is *negative* the patient should receive a test dose of 1/100 to 1/1000 (depending on the severity of past history of reaction) of the full therapeutic dose (Table 4).

Cephalosporins

Confusion exists regarding the extent of cross-reactivity between cephalosporins and penicillins. Patients with a positive skin test to penicillin who are given cephalosporins have a 5% reaction rate with a very high frequency of anaphylaxis. In most cases, penicillin skin testing is not done and the decision to give cephalosporins is based only on history. In these cases, the reaction rate is 1 to 2%. This is expected, as only 15% of patients with a history of allergy to penicillin have a positive reaction to penicillin when skin tested. Of the 15% of the remaining patients who still have a positive skin test to penicillin, only 5% react if given a cephalosporin—hence the 1% rate in unselected patients. As with penicillin, these may be serious reactions. Note that a 2% allergic reaction rate is expected with beta-lactam drugs in general.

Ideally, all patients with a history of allergy to penicillin who need a cephalosporin would have a skin test for penicillin allergy, and if reacting positively, would receive an alternate drug or be *very gradually* test dosed to the drug. As this approach is time-consuming and expensive, if the patient has a past history that is vague or of a mild reaction, it may be sufficient to test dose as described previously. Patients who had a severe reaction should be skin tested to penicillin before receiving a cephalosporin. Some patients may develop antibodies to side chains of cephalosporins independent of any antibodies that cross-react with penicillin. Cephalosporin skin testing can be done using a 3 mg per mL solution but this is not standardized. It may be helpful if positive, but it is not predictive if negative. Carbapenems (e.g., imipenem) appear to cross-react with penicillin, whereas monobactams (e.g., aztreonam) do not.

Cefaclor (Ceclor), has been specifically associated with a reaction that typically occurs on day 10 to 14 and is characterized by urticaria, including erythema multiforme, and prominent arthralgias. Limited prospective trials suggest a reaction rate of 0.5%, but anecdotal evidence suggests that it might be higher. Symptoms usually last for 1 to 2 weeks but can persist for months. Treatment with steroids is often necessary (prednisone, 1 mg per kg on taper pending symptoms). It is unclear whether these patients can subsequently tolerate another beta-lactam antibiotic. To date, there are no reports of comparable reactions in patients given another beta-lactam drug; ideally, however, they should be given an alternate non–beta-lactam drug.

TABLE 4. **Desensitization and Test Dosing in Drug Allergy**

Sample Desensitization Protocol*	
Route	Oral or intravenous
Starting dose	1/100 of that which produced a positive skin test or 1/10,000 of the therapeutic dose
Increments	Double the dose every 15–20 min up to a cumulative dose that equals the therapeutic dose
Maintenance	Continue therapeutic doses at regular prescribed intervals
Test Dosing†	
Past history of severe reaction	Give 1/1000 of the therapeutic dose; observe for 1 h. If no reaction, increase to 1/100 of therapeutic dose and repeat as below.
Unknown or minimal past history	Give 1/100 of the therapeutic dose; observe for 1 h. If no reaction, proceed with full therapeutic dose.

*Use this protocol if the patient has documented IgE antibody to the drug.
†Use this protocol if the patient has a suspect past history or if skin testing is not available or is negative in the case of penicillin.

Sulfonamides

Approximately 50% (reported range 6 to 85%) of patients infected with the human immunodeficiency virus (HIV) develop rash and constitutional symptoms. The mechanism is unknown but may be due to a decreased ability to detoxify reactive metabolites. Reactions are less severe with lower doses and lower CD4 counts. Continuation of the sulfonamide despite the reaction has been associated with spontaneous resolution of symptoms in some cases, but in others there was progression.

Readministration to HIV-positive patients with a history of non–life threatening reactions has been successful in approximately 50% of cases; no severe reactions have occurred. Desensitization has been attempted with some success in patients who have had reactions with readministration. Multiple protocols have been used, all of which require days (versus hours with penicillin). An average one starts with 1/1000 of the therapeutic dose, which is increased twice daily over 2 weeks.

IgE-mediated reactions can occur with sulfonamides but are much less common. Many drugs are sulfonamide derivatives, and theoretically a patient sensitive to one group may react to others, although this has not been documented. Common sulfa derivatives are listed in Table 5.

Vancomycin

In the majority of patients rapid infusion (1 gram over 1 hour) results in pruritus and erythema of the face and upper trunk, often with hypotension (the red man's syndrome). This reaction is not immunologically mediated, and therefore the drug can be given again at a slower rate (1 gram over 2 hours or longer) with antihistamine prophylaxis (e.g., hydroxyzine or diphenhydramine, 50 mg).

Vancomycin can also cause true allergic reactions, most commonly rashes. If these patients receive vancomycin again, there is risk of an exfoliative dermatitis.

Protamine

As with vancomycin, rapid administration induces hypotension. There may be an IgE-mediated component, as the frequency of protamine reactions appears much higher in diabetic patients who have previous low-dose exposure via neutral protamine Hagedorn (NPH) insulin. Rare patients have received protamine again after an anaphylactic reaction with pretreatment with prednisone and diphenhydramine plus very slow infusion of the drug.

Quinolones

Rare cases of anaphylactoid reactions have been reported after the first dose of ciprofloxacin (Cipro). Otherwise the incidence of allergic reactions does not appear to exceed 1 to 2%. Cross-reactivity between various quinolones is likely. No specific testing is available, and therefore an alternate antibiotic should be used if a reaction has occurred.

TABLE 5. **Common Sulfa Derivatives**

Sulfonamide Antibiotics
Sulfamethoxazole (Bactrim, Septra)
Sulfisoxazole (Gantrisin, Pediazole)
Sulfacetamide (Sultrin cream, Blephamide eye drops)
Sulfadoxine (Fansidar)
Sulfasalazine (Azulfidine)
Sulfinpyrazone (Anturane)
Sulfonylurea Oral Hypoglycemics
Glyburide (Diabeta, Micronase)
Glipizide (Glucotrol)
Chlorpropamide (Diabinese)
Tolbutamide (Orinase)
Acetohexamide (Dymelor)
Tolazamide (Tolinase)
Diuretics
Thiazides (Hydrodiuril, Esidrix)
Antihypertensive
Diazoxide (Hyperstat)
Carbonic Anhydrase Inhibitor
Acetazolamide (Diamox)

Aspirin and Nonsteroidal Anti-Inflammatory Drugs

Aspirin can cause flaring of asthma, chronic rhinosinusitis, and nasal polyps in sensitive patients. Aspirin and nonsteroidal anti-inflammatory drugs (NSAIDs) can flare existing urticaria and angioedema. Rarely anaphylaxis can occur. The effects are not caused by IgE antibody and most likely result from inhibition of cyclo-oxygenase with a resultant change in the balance of prostaglandins and leukotrienes.

Treatment is avoidance. There is no clinically significant cross-reaction with sodium salicylate or acetaminophen. Desensitization with aspirin may be helpful for patients with chronic rhinosinusitus and nasal polyps but less so for asthma. Steroid requirements decrease and smell improves. This can be accomplished by incremental administration of aspirin twice a day starting with 30 mg and increasing the dose to a maintenance level of 650 mg twice a day.

If a patient with a history of reaction to aspirin or NSAIDs requires a NSAID for treatment, cautious test dosing can be done. The more potent inhibitors of cyclo-oxygenase (e.g., ibuprofen and indomethacin) have been responsible for most reactions. Alternate NSAIDs should be selected for test dosing.

Local Anesthetics

True IgE-mediated reactions are extremely rare. Past reactions may have been due to vasovagal or hyperventilation episodes or systemic effects of epinephrine (included with most local anesthetics for local vasoconstriction). Skin testing followed by incremental challenge shows that most patients can safely be given a local anesthetic. An alternate to the suspect drug can be selected from among the available local anesthetics listed in Table 6. Skin testing can be done with a 1:10 dilution prick test followed by a full-strength prick and then an intradermal injection pending the history. Skin testing should be done with epinephrine-free material or false positives may occur. Test dosing can be done with 0.2 mL subcutaneously. If there is no reaction, the patient should have no trouble with therapeutic doses (dental vials contain 1.8 mL).

Muscle Relaxants

There is a 0.7% incidence of anaphylaxis with general anesthesia, which may be due to muscle relaxants. The most commonly implicated are D-tubocurarine, alcuronium,* gallamine, succinylcholine, pancuronium, vecuronium, and atracurium. Although these drugs can cause nonspecific histamine release, an IgE mechanism is probably responsible

*Not available in the United States.

TABLE 6. **Classification of Local Anesthetics**

Group I
Benzoic acid esters
p-Aminobenzoic acid esters
Benzocaine
Procaine (Novocain)
Tetracaine (Pontocaine)
Benzoic acid esters lacking *p*-aminobenzoyl group
Cyclomethycaine (Surfacaine)*
Isobucaine (Kincaine)*
Piperocaine (Metycaine)*
Proparacaine (Ophthaine)
Group II
Bupivacaine (Marcaine)
Dibucaine (Nupercainal)
Dyclonine (Dyclone)
Diperodon (Diothane)*
Lidocaine (Xylocaine)
Mepivacaine (Carbocaine, Polocaine)
Oxethazaine (Oxaine)*
Pramoxine (Tronothane)
Prilocaine (Citanest)

*Not available in the United States.

for most reactions. These drugs share a quaternary ammonium structure and probably cross react. If a patient has reacted to one, the others should be avoided.

Angiotensin-Converting Enzyme Inhibitors

Angioedema occurs in approximately 0.1% of patients within hours to 1 week of administration and is not usually not severe. The reaction may be more common and more severe in patients with a history of idiopathic angioedema, and they should be switched to an alternate drug.

Cough occurs in 1.5 to 10% (range to 25%) of treated patients, generally within 1 to 2 months (range 1 day to 12 months) of exposure. The mechanism is unknown. It usually clears 4 to 6 days after the drug is stopped. With continued therapy, some patients will experience resolution or attenuation of the cough. Inhaled cromolyn* (Intal, 2 puffs q 6 h) may help.

Radiocontrast Media

Reactions to contrast media are not mediated by specific antibody. Fifteen to twenty percent of patients will experience a repeat reaction with readministration. This can be blocked in 91% of patients with prednisone, 50 mg orally, 13, 7, and 1 hour(s) before the procedure along with diphenhydramine (Benadryl), 50 mg parentally 1 hour before. The efficacy is improved if epinephrine 25 mg orally is added to this 1 hour before. The addition of an H_2 blocker (e.g., cimetidine*) is controversial; one study showed increased reactions in the cimetidine group. Patients who have reacted despite this regimen have only had mild to moderate reactions. The reaction is due in large part to the hyperosmolality of the media. Use of low-osmolar (nonionic) media is associated with a lower reaction rate but much greater expense. This should be used preferentially in patients with a history of severe past reactions or significant disease that would hamper resuscitation in anaphylaxis. High-risk patients should not be taking beta-adrenergic blockers. There is no association between reactivity to contrast media and iodine or shellfish allergy.

*Not FDA approved for this indication.

STINGING INSECT ALLERGY

method of
DOUGLAS K. SCHREIBER, M.D., and
J. ANDREW GRANT, M.D.
The University of Texas Medical Branch
Galveston, Texas

Stinging insects of the order Hymenoptera (bees, hornets, yellow jackets, wasps, fire ants) are widespread throughout the world. An estimated 0.4 to 4% of the general population are allergic to the venom of these insects. Approximately 50 to 150 people die each year in the United States as a result of insect sting anaphylaxis.

Hymenoptera venoms are complex mixtures of enzymes, biogenic amines, and peptides that have toxic effects on tissue. The usual reaction to a sting is local swelling, erythema at the site, pain, and itching; the symptoms are limited and resolve within 24 hours. Local application of cold compresses is ordinarily all that is needed. This "normal" reaction is due to the toxic properties of the venom and is not secondary to host immune response. If subjected to multiple stings, one can have a toxic reaction that mimics anaphylaxis. Toxic reactions are due to the pharmacologic effects of an overwhelming dose of venom and not to an IgE-mediated allergy. Children and the elderly are more likely to have toxic reactions than are younger adults. Having a toxic reaction does not predispose one to an allergic reaction if stung again at a later date.

The protein constituents of the venom are good allergens and can sensitize individuals, so that on subsequent exposure an allergic reaction may occur. As with any allergic reaction, there can be an immediate and a late phase. The immediate phase usually begins within a few minutes after the sting and peaks in 1 hour. The late phase usually starts 6 to 12 hours after the sting and can last 24 to 48 hours. The immediate reaction is more likely to be fatal than the late-phase one, although one should not underestimate the risk of late-phase reactions. Clinically, it is beneficial to separate allergic reactions to insect stings into two categories—large local reactions and systemic reactions. Systemic reactions can be further described as mild, moderate, and severe. Mild systemic reactions involve only the skin (urticaria or angioedema) at sites distant from the sting. Moderate systemic reactions involve the skin and other non–life-threatening symptoms such as mild asthma. Severe systemic reactions are life threatening and include symptoms such as shock, hypotension, upper airway edema, loss of consciousness, and severe respiratory distress. Large local reactions are characterized by erythema and edema that extend well beyond the site of the sting. These reactions peak in 48 to 72 hours and resolve slowly over the next week.

It is important to clarify the type of reaction because it

may predict the likely response to a sting in the future. Patients with insect venom allergy have a 50 to 60% chance of having a repeat reaction to a sting for as long as 10 years after the previous episode. Those with large local reactions seldom have systemic reactions to subsequent stings. Children with systemic reactions confined to the skin have a 10% chance of having anaphylaxis if stung again, and the systemic reactions are usually mild and rarely life threatening. However, adults with systemic reactions confined to the skin have a 10 to 40% chance of having anaphylaxis with another sting.

Factors that influence morbidity and mortality include age, location of sting, underlying medical conditions, and concomitant beta-blocker therapy. Adults are more likely to die from a systemic reaction to an insect sting than are children; the reason for this is unknown. The location of the sting is important for determining both treatment and the probability that a reaction will evolve into a life-threatening event. A sting on an extremity is less likely to cause anaphylaxis than one to the head or neck; moreover, a tourniquet can be applied to an extremity to decrease the severity of the reaction. Underlying medical conditions, such as coronary artery disease, asthma, and chronic obstructive pulmonary disease, increase the mortality of systemic reactions to insect stings. Concomitant beta-blocker therapy also increases mortality during allergic reactions. In the presence of beta-blockers, epinephrine and beta agonists are less effective therapy for the symptoms of anaphylaxis.

IMMUNOPATHOGENESIS

Insect venoms are complex mixtures of enzymes, biogenic amines, and peptides. The major enzymes are phospholipase A, hyaluronidase, and acid phosphatase. Phospholipase A can cause smooth muscle contraction, hypotension, increased vascular permeability, and histamine release from mast cells. Major peptides are melittin, apamin, and mast cell–degranulating peptide. Melittin can cause red blood cell lysis, local pain, and inflammation; increased capillary permeability; hypotension; smooth muscle contraction; and direct histamine release. These pharmacologic effects are responsible for the normal reaction to insect stings (erythema, edema, pain, itching).

The major allergens present in insect venoms vary depending on species. Antigens common to all honeybee and vespid venoms are phophoplipase A and hyaluronidase. Antigen 5 is present only in vespid venom and melittin, only in honeybee venom. A high degree of immunologic cross-reactivity exists between yellow jacket and hornet venom, a lesser degree with wasp venom, and very little with honeybee venom. Fire ant venom does not cross-react with any of the aforementioned. Compared with the other Hymenoptera venoms, fire ant venom is unusual in that it contains very little protein, only about 5%.

Allergic reactions to insect stings are classic IgE hypersensitivity reactions. Most patients who have had systemic or large local reactions have anti-venom IgE antibodies demonstrated by skin or radioallergosorbent testing (RAST). Cellular immunity is also believed to have an important influence in large local reactions. In some reported cases, patients have had a systemic reaction to a sting, but no venom-specific IgE antibodies could be detected.

DIAGNOSIS

In most cases of insect sting allergy, the diagnosis is obvious. One should document the location and number of stings, the rapidity of onset of the reaction, and the symptom complex. This information will aid in defining the patient's treatment. All patients with systemic allergic reactions to insect stings should undergo skin testing to insect venom. Skin testing differentiates between toxic reactions and IgE-mediated reactions, predicts sensitivity to other stinging insects, and is a less expensive and more reliable way of diagnosing insect venom allergy than are in vitro tests such as the radioallergosorbent test (RAST).

TREATMENT

Treating anaphylaxis from insect stings is similar to treating anaphylaxis from any cause. Early aggressive management is crucial. Immediate subcutaneous administration of epinephrine is the treatment of choice due to its rapid onset. The standard dosage for children 14 years and younger is 0.01 mL per kg up to a maximum of 0.3 mL of the 1:1000 dilution administered subcutaneously every 15 minutes as needed. For adults, the standard dosage is 0.3 to 0.5 mL of 1:1000 dilution given subcutaneously every 15 minutes as needed. Higher doses of epinephrine must be given with caution, especially in high-risk patients with underlying cardiovascular disease. One should also give an antihistamine to relieve cutaneous discomfort; intravenous or intramuscular diphenhydramine works quickly to make the patient more comfortable. Most authorities also recommend using an H_2 antagonist such as ranitidine (Zantac)*, 50 mg intramuscularly or intravenously every 6 to 8 hours, or by continuous infusion, 250 mg in 250 ml of 5% dextrose at a rate of 10.7 ml per hour; or cimetidine (Tagamet), 150 to 300 mg orally or intravenously (infuse over 15 to 20 minutes). Every patient should also receive at least one dose of steroids (methylprednisolone, 125 mg intravenously, or prednisone, 40 to 80 mg orally). Steroids help to prevent or decrease the severity of any late-phase reaction. Further therapy is supportive and depends on the organ systems affected. Intravenous fluids and pressor agents may be needed for hypotension. Aminophylline and beta agonists and oxygen may be needed for bronchospasm and hypoxia. Maintaining a patent airway is of paramount importance; one should not hesitate to perform tracheal intubation if laryngeal edema, stridor, or severe bronchospasm develops. Patients with systemic reactions should be observed for at least 12 hours so that any late-phase response may be treated.

Therapy for large local reactions consists of application of cold compresses, oral antihistamines, and oral analgesics. Oral steroids may also be given to patients with very large local reactions.

Before leaving the hospital or physician's office, every patient should be given a prescription for an injectable epinephrine device, either Ana-Kit or EpiPen. The Ana-Kit (Hollister-Stier Laboratories, Spokane, WA) contains 1.0 mL of 1:1000 epinephrine, four 2-mg chewable chlorpheniramine tablets, two sterile alcohol pads, and a tourniquet. EpiPen and EpiPen Jr (Center Laboratories, Port Washington,

*Not FDA approved for this indication.

NY) contain a 0.3 mL dose of 1:1000 epinephrine and a 0.15 mL dose of 1:1000 epinephrine, respectively. Patients should carry the device with them at all times and be instructed in its use in the event of an allergic reaction to a subsequent sting. They should also wear an identification bracelet or necklace describing their insect allergy. Finally, they should be referred to an allergist for skin testing and immunotherapy if indicated.

Avoidance

To avoid stings, one should not wear brightly colored clothing or flowers; exterminate known insect nests; not wear leather; not wear scented cosmetics, perfumes, or hair spray; keep insecticide available at all times; exercise caution near picnic areas, eaves, attics, trash containers; not walk outside with bare feet; and one should wear protective clothing such as a long-sleeved shirt, long pants, and gloves when gardening or doing other high-risk activities.

Immunotherapy

Venom immunotherapy is a useful means of preventing allergic reactions in venom-allergic patients and has been shown to be 98% effective in preventing anaphylaxis to re-sting challenge in venom-allergic patients. The exact mechanism of protection is unknown, but venom-specific IgG-blocking antibodies are found in the serum of these patients, and venom-specific IgE antibodies have been shown to decline after immunotherapy. Initiating venom immunotherapy in patients with venom allergy is a dangerous undertaking and should be done only in a controlled environment where trained personnel, equipment, and medications are readily available.

Venom immunotherapy should be reserved only for patients with a history of a systemic reaction to insect venom and proven venom-specific IgE documented by positive skin tests or RAST. Current recommendations about which patients should receive immunotherapy include any adult who has had a systemic reaction (mild, moderate, or severe) and children with moderate or severe systemic reactions. Children with a history of systemic reactions involving only the skin (urticaria, angioedema) do not need immunotherapy because fewer than 10% will have an anaphylactic to another sting. Patients with a history of a large local reaction do not need immunotherapy because they are at very low risk of an anaphylactic reaction to future stings.

Anaphylaxis is a frightening experience. The greatest value of venom immunotherapy is the peace of mind patients get from knowing that they are protected from a future allergic reaction.

Section 12

Diseases of the Skin

ACNE VULGARIS AND ROSACEA

method of
LARISA C. KELLEY, M.D., and
ROBERT S. STERN, M.D.
Massachusetts General Hospital
Boston, Massachusetts

ACNE

Acne is a disease of the pilosebaceous unit that characteristically arises around puberty and is distributed on the face, chest, and back. The predominant inciting factor is increased androgen. The typical clinical findings are papules, pustules, comedones, and nodules at different stages of development. Active lesions tend to continue into the late twenties; however, especially in females, it is not uncommon to have acne continue into the late thirties. The incidence is close to 100% when those with only occasional small lesions are included. Heredity plays a role in the severity of acne, as does gender. Men typically have more severe disease than women, but women are more likely to seek care for acne.

Pathogenesis

Acne is initiated by abnormal follicular keratinization and increased sebum production. The predominant follicular microbe is *Propionibacterium acnes,* which is found in abundance in acne lesions. *P. acnes* converts esterified sebum lipids to free fatty acids, thus helping to induce a localized inflammatory response. Androgens increase sebum production and sebaceous gland size. Women with irregular menses and acne should be suspected of possible androgen excess. Various exogenous agents can also provoke or exacerbate acne. These agents include cosmetics, occupational exposure, and drugs (corticosteroids, adrenocorticotropic hormone, antituberculous chemotherapeutics, halogens, anticonvulsants, and antidepressants).

Is it Acne?

Various pustular dermatoses can mimic acne. When treating acne patients, it is crucial to consider the differential diagnosis prior to initiating treatment, thus increasing the chance of implementing effective therapy.

In normal hosts, bacterial folliculitis is caused most commonly by *Staphylococcus aureus.* This condition appears as follicular papules and pustules (usually a hair is found protruding from the center of the lesion) and has a predilection for the scalp and extremities. Comedones are absent.

Pseudofolliculitis barbae consists of papules and pustules confined to the beard area. This entity is caused by penetration of hair into the skin rather than growth through the hair follicle and is most common in black males who have curly hair that exits at an acute angle; it is also caused by a close shave.

Pityrosporum folliculitis presents as follicular papules and pustules, usually pruritic, that are concentrated on the chest and back. Potassium hydroxide examination is positive, which differentiates it from bacterial folliculitis.

Eosinophilic pustular folliculitis is a generalized, intensely pruritic, follicular papular pustular disease seen most commonly in persons infected with human immunodeficiency virus. Pathologically, there is a dense eosinophilic infiltrate that also involves the pilosebaceous structure. Peripheral eosinophilia is also seen.

Clinical Presentation

The presentation of acne is protean. One must identify the predominant lesion type and institute therapy in accord with the clinical morphology. The most commonly seen lesions are comedones and inflammatory papules.

Comedones are typically the first lesions seen in acne. They are dilated pilosebaceous units with trapped keratinaceous material. Closed comedones, or whiteheads, are 1- to 2-mm white firm papules with a barely visible central pore. With time, the follicular orifice opens, revealing the keratinaceous debris, which, if oxidized, becomes black, producing open comedones, or blackheads.

Inflammatory lesions are caused by formation of free fatty acids within the dilated follicle that causes rupture of the follicular wall and thus inflammation in the surrounding dermis. The depth at which the inflammation takes place determines whether a superficial papule arises or a deeper, tender nodule develops.

Most patients develop multiple types of lesions. Treatment should be directed toward the types of lesions present in substantial numbers.

Comedonal Acne

Patients with predominantly comedonal lesions are best treated with a vitamin A acid, topical tretinoin

(Retin-A). Topical tretinoin manifests its comedolytic activity by decreasing follicular keratinocyte adhesion. In addition, topical tretinoin accelerates turnover of follicular and interfollicular keratinocytes. Topical tretinoin is available in a cream, gel, or liquid form. The cream is recommended for patients with dry sensitive skin, and the gel is recommended for oilier complexions. Both are dispensed in various concentrations. The concentration most often used is 0.05%. The most common adverse effect is dryness and irritation, which abates with continued use. If the drying effect is not tolerated with daily dosing, application every other or every third day may still be effectual treatment. It is advisable to council patients that the comedolytic effects of topical tretinoin are not expected until 4 to 6 weeks of treatment, and that the skin might initially appear worse before improvement is appreciated. Patients using topical tretinoin should be advised to avoid unprotected sun exposure and to use a sunscreen regularly.

Inflammatory Acne

Mild

Mild inflammatory acne consists of few, scattered, small (< 3 mm) erythematous facial papules without deep tender nodules or cysts. Comedones are also often present. This mild degree of acne usually responds to topical benzoyl peroxide or topical antibiotics. Benzoyl peroxide is available both by prescription and over the counter, and it is a highly effective topical agent for mild inflammatory acne. It is bacteriocidal against *P. acnes*. It should be used once or twice daily depending on patient tolerance. Topical antibiotics available by prescription, including erythromycin (EryDerm), and clindamycin (Cleocin T), are also effective for mild inflammatory acne.

All of the topical products are prepared in various vehicles. Lotions and creams tend to be less drying than solutions and gels. Gels tend to penetrate better into the follicle, and water-based gels are less drying than alcohol-based gels. The probability that topical preparations will substantially improve acne decreases as the number and size of inflammatory lesions increase. Patient preference and concern about side effects should be a key element in decision making.

Moderate to Severe

More extensive inflammatory acne includes larger, more numerous and tender nodular erythematous lesions. The back and chest are often involved, as well as the face.

Oral antibiotics typically used in acne have multiple actions. They decrease the number of *P. acnes* organisms, which, in turn, decreases the amount of bacterial lipases available to convert esterified follicular lipids to free fatty acids. They also have anti-inflammatory activity including inhibition of neutrophil chemotaxis and macrophage function. The tetracyclines (tetracycline, doxycycline, minocycline) and macrolides (erythromycin) are the most commonly used antibiotics. The usual starting dosages are 500 mg twice daily for tetracycline and erythromycin, and 50 to 100 mg twice daily for doxycycline and minocycline.

Patients are typically maintained on oral antibiotics until control of the inflammatory lesions is achieved. Response typically takes 6 to 12 weeks. At this time, the dose should be slowly tapered with the attempt to discontinue. Frequently, however, oral antibiotics are continued for years. There is individual variation in response to oral antibiotics. If there is not a noticeable response in 10 weeks, it is recommended to switch to another product or, if appropriate, increase the dosage.

It is recommended that topical agents, especially benzoyl peroxide or tretinoin, be used in conjunction with oral antibiotics in the hope that upon discontinuation of the oral antibiotics, maintenance can be achieved with topical therapy alone.

Side effects of oral antibiotics include allergic reaction; gastrointestinal upset; vaginal yeast infections; interaction with oral contraceptives; for tetracycline and doxycycline, photosensitivity; and rarely, for all tetracyclines, pseudotumor cerebri. Gram-negative folliculitis occasionally occurs with prolonged oral antibiotic therapy. This should be suspected when patients become resistant to antibiotic therapy or relapse follows initial improvement. A culture swab of a lesion will help confirm the diagnosis. Ampicillin is the treatment of choice.

Mixed Inflammatory and Comedonal Acne

Most patients have a mixture of comedones in addition to inflammatory lesions. Close examination of the lesion morphology is necessary to evaluate whether comedones are scattered within the inflammatory lesions. When mixed lesions are present, effective therapy is more often achieved when comedolytic preparations (e.g., topical tretinoin) are added to the above-mentioned anti-inflammatory regimen. A typical regimen for these patients is an oral antibiotic twice daily (tetracycline or erythromycin) with tretinoin cream at night, and if irritation is not a substantial problem, benzoyl peroxide may also be used.

Severe Scarring Acne (Acne Conglobata)

Patients with extensive deep nodules and interconnecting cysts must be treated very aggressively to avoid scarring. These patients should be given a 6- to 10-week trial of high-dose oral antibiotics. If no appreciable effect is obtained, oral isotretinoin (Accutane) is often indicated but only in reliable and well-informed patients. Isotretinoin is an oral vitamin A acid. Its mechanism of action is poorly understood. Its beneficial clinical effects are, however, well documented. They include a dramatic decrease in sebum production, and potent comedolytic and moderate anti-inflammatory properties. Prior to starting therapy with isotretinoin, patients should have extensive counseling regarding the potential adverse effects. The most noteworthy is a high risk of severe birth defects if these drugs are taken during pregnancy. Among the more frequently reported adverse effects are dryness of skin and mucous membranes, hypertriglyceridemia, myalgia, and pseudotumor cerebri. Long-term therapy or repeated courses are associated with an increased risk of hyperostosis. Laboratory evaluation must be performed prior to starting therapy and include beta-human chorionic gonadotropin, liver function tests, complete blood count, and measurement of triglyceride and cholesterol levels. Liver function tests and a lipid profile should be repeated at 2 to 3 and 4 to 6 weeks after starting therapy. In women, a highly effective means of birth control should be employed. Only physicians aware of this drug's risks and benefits should prescribe it.

Dosage varies with the extent of disease. With facial involvement, 0.5 mg to 1.0 mg per kg per day for 20 weeks is recommended. More severe facial and trunk involvement requires 1 mg per kg per day. Complete resolution, however, is not expected until a full course of therapy is finished. There often is a mild flare of disease when therapy is initiated. All concomitant topical and oral acne therapy should be discontinued when isotretinoin therapy is initiated.

Recalcitrant Acne

Patients with acne that does not respond to appropriate treatment, especially women with virilizing features or irregular menses, should be evaluated for androgen excess resulting from adrenal tumor, adrenocorticotropic hormone excess, polycystic ovarian disease, or hormonal therapy. Screening tests include free testosterone and dehydroepiandrosterone-sulfate. If these tests are unyielding and further work-up is clinically indicated, 17-hydroxyprogesterone, follicle-stimulating hormone, luteinizing hormone, and prolactin levels can be evaluated. If an abnormality is found, an endocrinologic evaluation should be undertaken.

Treatment for acne due to androgen excess should focus on amelioration of the underlying endocrine abnormality. Typical therapies are oral estrogens (usually as an oral contraceptive with 0.05 mg of estrogen), low-dose glucocorticoids (2.5 to 7.5 mg prednisone daily) or a mineralocorticoid androgen antagonist (spironolactone [Aldactone], 50 to 200 mg daily).

ROSACEA

Rosacea is a papular pustular skin disorder that shares clinical similarities with acne; however, it has several distinguishing features.

The lesions tend to be localized on the central face and forehead, and arise on skin that has prominent erythema and telangiectasias. Comedones are rare. Patients typically are older (30 to 60 years old), are descended from Celtic ancestry, and have a history of extensive sun exposure. Patients often flush and blush easily.

The disease evolves in phases. Initially facial flushing is the predominant finding. Gradually, increased telangiectasias, papules, and pustules arise within fixed erythematous patches. Occasionally, large granulomatous nodules occur, as well as overgrowth of the connective tissue and sebaceous glands, producing facial edema and a bulbous nose (rhinophyma). Ocular involvement is not rare and usually manifests as blepharitis or conjunctivitis, and, rarely, as keratitis.

Mild Rosacea

Mild rosacea consists of a facial blush and a few inflammatory lesions. The papules and pustules can be treated with topical preparations such as clindamycin and erythromycin. Lotion and cream preparations are preferable to solutions and gels because the erythematous skin is sensitive to drying agents. Topical metronidazole (MetroGel) has recently been shown to be equally effective. Unfortunately, minimal effect on erythema and telangiectasia is seen with topical antibiotics. Facial flushing is often made worse by tobacco smoke, alcoholic beverages, and hot spicy foods. Telangiectasias can be removed with the pulse dye or continuous wave lasers. Topical steroids should be avoided. They give mild symptomatic relief but exacerbate telangiectasias and may induced atrophy.

Moderate Rosacea

Moderate disease, which includes more prominent inflammatory lesions, is often treated with oral antibiotics. The best results have been obtained with oral tetracyclines (tetracycline, doxycycline and minocycline) and macrolides (erythromycin). Lower doses are typically required than with inflammatory acne. Dosing should be titrated with disease activity. Topical metronidazole is sometimes helpful.

Severe Rosacea and Rhinophyma

With more extensive involvement that is unresponsive to oral antibiotics, oral isotretinoin (Accutane) is sometimes thought to be helpful. Before initiating therapy, multiple antibiotics at full doses should be attempted. As mentioned earlier, it is crucial to select appropriate patients and properly counsel them about adverse effects. Dosages of isotretinoin are similar to those used for acne (0.5 to 1 mg per kg per day for 20 weeks).

Rhinophyma will decrease with isotretinoin therapy. This effect, however, is not permanent. Longer lasting treatments include surgical débridement, electrocautery, and CO_2 laser therapy.

HAIR DISORDERS

method of
DAVID A. WHITING, M.D.
Baylor University Medical Center
Dallas, Texas

An essential element in the diagnosis and management of alopecia is the time needed to listen to the patient's history and anxieties. An explanation of the hair growth cycle is often helpful: Hairs go through continuous cycles of growth and rest. The resting, or telogen, hair is eventually displaced by the new growing, or anagen, hair, which lies below. It is assumed, for convenience, that the average number of scalp hairs equals 100,000, comprising 90% anagen and 10% telogen hairs. If the average duration of the anagen phase is 1000 days and the telogen phase 100 days, then a daily loss of up to 100 hairs is normal. The average growth rate of the large, visible, or terminal scalp hairs is 0.35 mm per day, or 1 inch every 2½ months. Hair cycles and growth rate are affected by genetic factors, age, sex, race, and season, resulting in wide variations of normal. In the human scalp, growth cycles in individual hairs are not synchronized to ensure even hair coverage.

The investigation of alopecia starts with a careful examination of scalp hair, noting the pattern of hair loss and the length of affected hairs. The scalp itself, facial and body hair, as well as skin, nails, and teeth should also be checked. Simple pull tests in different areas of the scalp indicate whether hairs detach too easily and whether they break off or come out by the roots. Easily detachable hairs with depigmented, clubbed roots indicate telogen hairs, and more adherent hairs with pigmented roots and long white root sheaths indicate anagen hairs. Light microscopy is an easy office procedure to use to identify hair roots, fiber diameter, and most structural abnormalities of the hair shaft. Potassium hydroxide preparations of affected hair fragments can demonstrate fungal infections, which can be typed by fungal culture. Scalp biopsies are indicated for diagnostic purposes in all cases of cicatricial and unexplained noncicatricial alopecia. The new technique of horizontal sectioning of scalp biopsies supplements the diagnostic capability of vertical sectioning and has some value in the prediction of future hair regrowth. Laboratory tests should depend on clinical indications, but a basic work-up in the unexplained case should include a complete blood count, routine chemistry studies, serum iron, urinalysis, tests of thyroid function, and a serologic test for syphilis. Tests of androgenetic function are indicated in female-pattern alopecia if acne, hirsutism, menstrual disorders, deepening of the voice, and severe male type of alopecia with both temporal recession and vertical baldness are present.

The common causes of alopecia are listed in Table 1.

TABLE 1. **Common Causes of Alopecia**

Cause	Incidence (%)
Androgenetic alopecia	68.8
Diffuse alopecia	11.3
Alopecia areata	9.9
Cicatricial alopecia	4.9
Trichotillomania	1.3
Trauma, traction	1.1
Other (infections and infestations, hair shaft abnormalities, hereditary and congenital conditions)	2.7
	100.0

ANDROGENETIC ALOPECIA

Androgenetic alopecia affects both sexes and is of dominant inheritance. Scalp hairs on the vertex in these patients are unduly susceptible to the action of androgens and become progressively miniaturized. The hair is lost predominantly on the crown, with relative sparing of the back and sides of the scalp. In a young patient, the complaint of increased hair loss often precedes the appearance of alopecia. Telogen hairs are often more easily detached from the vertex than from the occipital area and sides of the scalp.

In men, the onset may be any time after puberty and is not infrequent by the age of 17 years. The sequence of hair loss usually starts with a typical male pattern of bitemporal recession, followed by vertex loss. The amount of progression through frontal and vertex loss is variable, influenced by genetic factors, and often intermittent rather than continuous. Male-pattern androgenetic alopecia is graded according to severity from Types I through VII on the Hamilton-Norwood scale (Table 2). It affects 50% of males aged 50 years.

In women, androgenetic alopecia may commence at any age after puberty but is not often clinically apparent in women younger than 25 years of age. The incidence figures lag behind those of men by approximately 1 decade. The hair loss usually appears over the frontal vertex region as a widened part line. Later, hair is lost more diffusely over the frontal and vertex regions, but an intact frontal hairline is preserved, without the marked bitemporal recession seen in men. Female-pattern androgenetic alopecia is graded as mild, moderate, or severe on the Ludwig scale and causes diffuse thinning of the vertex but not complete baldness.

TABLE 2. **Hamilton-Norwood Classification of Male-Pattern Androgenetic Alopecia**

Type I:	Full hair (e.g., normal prepubertal hair)
Type II:	Mild bitemporal recession (e.g., normal postpubertal hair)
Type III:	Deep bitemporal recession, possible midfrontal recession, possible vertex thinning
Type IV:	Increased frontotemporal recession, marked vertex thinning
Type V:	Marked frontotemporal and vertex thinning, becoming confluent
Type VI;	Large areas of frontotemporal and vertex alopecia, indefinite band of sparse hair in between
Type VII:	Complete confluence of frontotemporal and vertex areas of alopecia

Treatment

No treatment is required for Types I and II male-pattern androgenetic alopecia, nor is it helpful for Type III with bitemporal recession only. Topical 2% minoxidil (Rogaine) applied twice daily for a minimum of 1 year is indicated in Type III male-pattern androgenetic alopecia with midfrontal recession or vertex hair loss, or both, and in Types IV and V. The first observed effect from minoxidil is often a reduced rate of hair loss, usually after 6 to 8 weeks of treatment. Visible regrowth of hair, to be expected in approximately one-third of cases, may occur mostly on the vertex but rarely in the temples, after 3 to 9 months of treatment. The increasing hair growth rate may slow down and reach a plateau after 1 year, or it may continue to improve slowly over several years. Patients who respond best to this treatment are usually younger than 40 years of age, have a history of hair loss for less than 10 years, and have a bald area less than 10 cm in diameter. There is some evidence to suggest that minoxidil stops further hair loss in 80% of cases of male-pattern alopecia, and, therefore, it should be used for its preventive effects in young patients with early hair loss. If positive results are noted after 1 year of treatment, minoxidil should be continued twice daily indefinitely. No adverse systemic effects have been demonstrated, but local irritation may occur in a few cases. It has been shown that minoxidil has similar effects in female-pattern androgenetic alopecia, at least in mild and moderate cases.

If androgenetic alopecia in women is associated with undisputed evidence of androgenetic overactivity, then the source of the androgen excess must be identified and treated appropriately. Topical antiandrogens have not as yet been shown to produce consistent regrowth of hair in androgenetic alopecia. Estrogen-dominant oral contraceptives currently obtainable in the United States, such as ethynodiol diacetate with ethinyl estradiol (Demulen),* are similarly disappointing. Oral spironolactone (Aldactone),* in doses of 75 to 200 mg daily, is antiandrogenic and may be beneficial in some cases. Dexamethasone* in doses of 0.125 to 0.5 mg daily can be used to suppress adrenal overactivity. The side effects of and contraindications to systemic antiandrogens should be reviewed before initiating treatment. In view of the known effects of androgens in causing male androgenetic alopecia, there is considerable interest in finding a suitable topical or systemic antiandrogen that can be used safely and effectively in men. Such a drug should effectively block the action of dihydrotestosterone, the active androgen metabolite in the hair follicle, without affecting the action of testosterone itself and thereby preserving sexual function; the 5-alpha reductase inhibitor finasteride (Proscar),* which prevents the formation of dihydrotestosterone in the prostate gland, may be of future interest in this regard. However, use of this type of drug for such a condition is still experimental at this time.

*Not FDA approved for this indication.

TABLE 3. **Causes of Diffuse Alopecia**

Telogen effluvium	Malabsorption
Anagen effluvium	Renal failure
Drugs	Hepatic failure
Other chemicals	System disease
Thyroid disorder	Idiopathic global alopecia (chronic telogen effluvium)
Iron deficiency	Miscellaneous
Nutritional deficiencies	

If medical treatment fails or is not desired, the remaining alternatives are surgery with hair transplants, scalp reductions, or transposition of hair-bearing flaps, creative hairstyling, or hairpieces. The art of hair transplant surgery has improved considerably in recent times with the advent of minigrafts and micrografts.

DIFFUSE ALOPECIA

Diffuse alopecia is deceptive, because 40 to 50% of scalp hairs have to be lost before it becomes visible. Hairs can easily be detached from the back and sides of the scalp, as well as from the crown. The main causes of diffuse alopecia are listed in Table 3.

Telogen Effluvium

Telogen effluvium is a diffuse loss of normal club hairs from normal resting follicles. It is usually due to a premature interruption of growth in many anagen hairs, which then cycle through catagen into a telogen phase, so that the proportion of telogen hairs rises to 15% to 30% or more. When the resting phase ends 2 to 4 months later, new anagen hairs displace the club hairs, which loosen and fall out abruptly in large numbers from all over the scalp. A useful diagnostic marker of telogen effluvium in females is the presence of pronounced bitemporal recession, which is usually more severe than that seen in female pattern androgenetic alopecia. Causes of telogen effluvium are listed in Table 4.

Treatment

If a definite cause in the recent past can be identified and, if necessary, eliminated, an explanation of the mechanism involved and reassurances about impending regrowth should suffice. Follow-up is necessary, because a disappointing number of patients progress to a chronic form of telogen effluvium, presenting the clinical picture of idiopathic diffuse global alopecia. Minoxidil (Rogaine) applied twice daily may

TABLE 4. **Causes of Telogen Effluvium**

Childbirth	Crash diets
Febrile illnesses	Traction
Surgical operations	Severe emotional stress
Chronic systemic disease	Physiologic in newborn
Drugs: Antithyroids, anticoagulants, sodium valproate, beta blockers	

prolong anagen cycles in these patients and should be continued until the rate of hair loss returns to normal and hair regrowth is visible.

Anagen Effluvium

Anagen effluvium is characterized by the diffuse loss of anagen hairs from growing follicles. Arrested cell division in the hair bulb matrix leads to progressive narrowing of the hair shaft or to failure of hair formation. The weakened hairs easily fracture and their proximal ends are tapered (pencil pointing). The alopecia is severe and easily diagnosed, because it affects the 90% of scalp hairs that are normally in anagen. Anagen alopecia occurs within a few weeks, and if the inhibitory influence is removed, hairs will regrow promptly. Causes of anagen effluvium are listed in Table 5.

Treatment

The treatment of anagen effluvium lies in identifying the cause and treating or removing it, if possible.

Alopecia Due to Drugs and Chemicals

Alopecia due to drugs and chemicals is usually diffuse and confined to the scalp. Drug-related alopecia may be due to telogen or anagen effluvium, or it may be of a nonspecific dystrophic variety. In general, the only reliable way to confirm the diagnosis is to discontinue the suspected drug for a sufficient time to verify improvement and, later, if desirable and feasible, to rechallenge the patient with the same drug, unless the drug is known to cause alopecia. Fortunately, most of the alopecia caused by drugs is reversible. Many drugs can cause alopecia, including androgens, anticancer drugs, anticoagulants, anticonvulsants, antithyroid drugs, beta blockers, cholesterol reducers, gold, histamine H_2 receptor blockers, lithium, nonsteroidal anti-inflammatory drugs, oral contraceptives, retinoids and retinol, and tricyclic antidepressants.

Treatment

The treatment lies in identifying and eliminating the cause, if possible.

Other Causes of Diffuse Alopecia

Thyroid disorders, iron deficiency, nutritional deficiencies, malabsorption, renal failure, syphilis, collagen vascular diseases, carcinomatosis, and other miscellaneous underlying causes of alopecia require appropriate investigation and treatment.

TABLE 5. **Causes of Anagen Effluvium**

Cytostatic drugs	X-ray therapy
Endocrine diseases	Alopecia areata
Cicatricial alopecia	Trauma and pressure
Severe protein calorie malnutrition: Kwashiorkor, marasmus	Other toxic drugs: Retinoids, triparanol, thallium, thiourea, arsenic, gold, bismuth, borax, levodopa, colchicine

ALOPECIA AREATA

Alopecia areata can occur at any age and affects both sexes equally. An onset in early childhood is likely in the 20% of cases associated with atopy, in which a high incidence of alopecia totalis is present (75% in Japan). An onset in middle age is usual in the 5% of cases associated with organ-specific autoimmune diseases, which have a 10% incidence of alopecia totalis. The age of onset varies in the remaining 75% of cases not associated with any particular disease, which have a 6% incidence of alopecia totalis. Alopecia areata is characterized by the development of one or more circumscribed patches of hair loss associated with smooth, atrophic skin. Exclamation point–shaped hairs may be present in the active borders of the lesions. The disease may remain limited to a few patches, or it may progress to widespread mosaic forms, to horizontal or vertical wave forms of ophiasis, or to alopecia totalis or universalis. In doubtful cases, scalp biopsies may be diagnostic.

Treatment

Alopecia areata has an unpredictable course not easily altered by treatment. Localized patches in adults and older children are best treated with intralesional corticosteroid injections such as triamcinolone acetonide (Kenalog), 5 to 10 mg per mL. Medium-potency to high-potency topical corticosteroids, such as fluocinonide gel 0.05% (Lidex gel), are preferred for young children and for patients with widespread disease. The use of systemic steroids in alopecia areata is controversial, but prednisone, 20 to 40 mg daily for 1 to 2 months, can reverse rapid deterioration in widespread cases, although subsequent relapses are common. Minoxidil (Rogaine) has been tried with some success in alopecia areata, especially in cases with less than 75% hair loss. The drug should be continued until full regrowth occurs. Contact dermatitis can stimulate regrowth of hair and can be induced by short contact therapy for ½ to 1 hour daily with 0.25% to 1% anthralin (Drithrocreme),* a therapy suitable for children. Sensitization treatment with diphencyprone† should still be regarded as experimental. Oral cyclosporine (Sandimmune) therapy for alopecia areata, although effective, is experimental, expensive, and risky and has not been approved by the United States Food and Drug Administration for this indication.

CICATRICIAL ALOPECIA

Common causes of cicatricial alopecia are listed in Table 6. The scarring may be subtle or obvious. Always check the scalp for other changes, such as follic-

*Not FDA approved for this indication.
†Not available in the United States.

TABLE 6. **Causes of Cicatrical Alopecia**

Hereditary and Congenital	Aplasia cutis, epidermal nevi, epidermolysis bullosa
Infections	
bacterial	Acne keloidalis, dissecting cellulitis, folliculitis, syphilis
fungal	Favus, kerion, mycetoma
protozoal	Leishmaniasis
viral	Herpes zoster, varicella
Physical Injuries	Burns, mechanical trauma, radiodermatitis
Neoplasms	Angiosarcoma, basal cell epithelioma, lymphoma, melanoma, metastatic tumors, squamous cell carcinoma
Dermatoses	Cicatricial pemphigoid, dermatomyositis, folliculitis decalvans, lichen planopilaris, lupus erythematosus, neurotic excoriations, pseudopelade, scleroderma

ulitis, follicular plugging, absent follicular orifices, scaling, telangiectasia, and broken hairs. Look for associated lesions elsewhere on the skin and mucous membranes, including the mouth, ears, and nails, which may be useful in confirming the diagnosis of diseases such as lichen planus and lupus erythematosus. If disease activity is present, a specific diagnosis may be possible. In burned-out cases, the end result of scarring with permanent destruction of hair follicles may look much the same regardless of the cause. All cases of suspected cicatricial alopecia warrant a scalp biopsy, and special stains or immunofluorescence, or both, may be required.

Treatment

The treatment depends on the cause. Surgical treatment by excision, with scalp reduction or hair transplantation, may be suitable for nevoid lesions, tumors, and old scars. Infections can be treated appropriately. Folliculitis decalvans may respond to the long-term administration of antibiotics, such as tetracycline* and erythromycin,* or to trimethoprim/sulfamethoxazole (Bactrim, Septra)* or topical retinoic acid (Retin-A).*† Lichen planopilaris, lupus erythematosus, and pseudopelade can be treated with topical, intralesional, or oral corticosteroids or antimalarials.‡

TRICHOTILLOMANIA

Trichotillomania is an abnormal compulsion to pull out hair and is more common in females. It can lead to large areas of alopecia, which vary from a symmetric to a predominantly unilateral pattern. The scalp is usually unaffected and is neither atrophic and smooth nor inflamed and scaly. The hairs are broken off at different lengths.

*Not FDA approved for this indication.

†This use of retinoic acid is not listed in the manufacturer's official directive.

‡This use of antimalarials is not listed in the manufacturer's official directive.

Treatment

In children, underlying emotional problems are often identifiable, and the condition may be eliminated after these problems are resolved. Adults usually require psychiatric treatment.

TRACTION AND TRAUMA

Hair loss can result from many forms of physical and chemical trauma associated with overzealous hairstyling, from prolonged pressure on the scalp in motionless patients, from head rolling and habit tics, and from excoriations in pruritic dermatoses. The underlying cause requires identification and treatment.

INFECTIONS AND INFESTATIONS

Tinea Capitis

Tinea capitis causes patchy alopecia, especially in children. In the United States today, it is usually due to *Trichophyton tonsurans.* This endothrix infection weakens the hairs, which snap off against the skin surface, giving rise to characteristic black dots. A kerion should always be suspected in prepubertal children with persistent, boggy abscesses on the scalp resistant to antibiotics and associated with hair loss. The treatment of choice for tinea capitis or kerion is prolonged oral griseofulvin therapy, with oral ketaconazole (Nizoral) or itraconazole (Sporanox)* as alternatives in resistant cases.

Pediculosis Capitis

Head lice cause severe pruritus, and the resultant excoriations can cause alopecia. The most effective treatment is 1% premethrin creme rinse (Nix), although topical 1% lindane (Kwell) can be used.

CANCER OF THE SKIN

method of
IRA C. DAVIS, M.D., and
BARRY LESHIN, M.D.
Wake Forest University Medical Center
Winston-Salem, North Carolina

Basal cell (BCC) and squamous cell (SCC) carcinoma of the skin are the most common carcinomas in the white population. Seven hundred thousand new cancers are diagnosed annually in the United States. This incidence increases yearly. Basal cell carcinomas outnumber squamous cell carcinomas by a ratio of 5:1. Although the majority of skin cancers are on sun-exposed areas, a total body skin

*Not FDA approved for this indication.

examination is necessary for early detection of nonmelanoma skin cancers.

RISK FACTORS

Identification of multiple host and environmental factors aid the physician in identifying patients at increased risk for the development of nonmelanoma skin cancer. Skin cancers are more commonly found in older patients, and men are more often affected than women. A high index of suspicion is appropriate for patients who tan poorly, burn easily, or have prolonged erythema after sun exposure. Additional risk factors include freckling, fair skin; Celtic ancestry; red, blond, or light brown hair; and blue or light-colored eyes. Approximately 50% of patients with a previously diagnosed BCC or SCC will develop another skin cancer within 5 years after their initial diagnosis.

Environmental factors include exposure to ultraviolet light, ionizing radiation, cigarette smoking, and chemicals. Ultraviolet light consists of exposure to the sun or artificial sources such as tanning booths or psoralen and ultraviolet A photochemotherapy (PUVA). Ionizing radiation exposure includes childhood exposure for acne, tinea capitis, and other dermatoses. Cigarette smoking is associated with an increased risk in the development of squamous cell carcinoma. Exposure to chemicals, such as hydrocarbons and inorganic arsenic, or medications, such as topical mechlorethamine, predisposes patients to develop nonmelanoma skin cancer.

Certain medical conditions require vigilant skin examination for the possible development of nonmelanoma skin cancer. Immunosuppressed patients, especially transplant patients and individuals with chronic lymphocytic leukemia, are at greater risk for developing nonmelanoma skin cancer. Of particular concern in this patient population is the more common development of squamous cell carcinoma instead of basal cell carcinoma. Chronic ulcers, draining sinus tracts, and burn scars may develop aggressive forms of skin cancer within them.

DIAGNOSIS

The clinical appearance of the lesion forms the basis for the diagnosis of nonmelanoma skin cancer. In most cases, shave biopsy including the dermis is sufficient to confirm the clinical suspicion. Information gleaned from the biopsy includes the depth of tumor involvement, the presence of perineural tumor, and the histologic type. These histopathologic factors aid in the determination of proper treatment selection. Shave biopsies should never be performed on a lesion suspected of being malignant melanoma.

Other means of biopsy can be used. The use of a punch biopsy precludes the use of electrodesiccation and curettage for treatment of the lesion. If the diagnosis is certain and the clinical situation warrants it, excisional biopsy with an adequate margin of clinically noninvolved skin eliminates an additional patient visit and pathology laboratory charge, resulting in more cost-effective management of this increasingly common disease.

BASAL CELL CARCINOMA

BCC composes 80% of all skin cancers, 66 to 80% of which are found on the head and neck. The lesions are locally destructive and have a low propensity for metastasis. If they are ignored, these cancers can be associated with a high rate of patient morbidity.

Three clinical types of BCC are commonly described: noduloulcerative, superficial, and morpheaform. The noduloulcerative type is the most common representing 45% to 60% of lesions. Clinically, a pearly papule with overlying telangiectasia and central ulceration is noted. Superficial BCC manifests as an erythematous scaly macule or patch. Morpheaform (sclerosing) BCC appears as a white to yellow scarlike plaque.

Infiltrative and pigmented BCCs are two subtypes of noduloulcerative BCCs. Infiltrative BCC is usually diagnosed histologically and is more aggressive than the common noduloulcerative lesion. Pigmented BCC contains variable amounts of pigment and can clinically appear suspicious for melanoma.

SQUAMOUS CELL CARCINOMA

SCCs compose 10 to 15% of all skin cancers, 80% of which develop on sun-exposed areas of the head, neck, and extremities. These lesions have a higher propensity to metastasize (3 to 10%). Fewer than one out of five hundred patients die from their tumors. The clinical appearance of SCC is more variable. Commonly it appears as a hyperkeratotic papule, nodule, or plaque with possible ulceration. Less common aggressive histologic subtypes of SCC include spindle, adenosquamous, clear cell, and signet ring SCC.

TREATMENT

Treatment selection for SCC and BCC is based on a number of factors. Clinical factors considered include tumor type, size, distinctiveness of the tumor margins, and anatomic location. Anatomic locations prone to a high risk of recurrence with conventional treatment are the periauricular, periocular, scalp, and central face (nose, perioral, junction of the alanasolabial fold) areas. Histologic factors include tumor subtype, the presence of perineural space invasion of tumor, and the degree of differentiation for SCC. Common treatment modalities include electrodesiccation and curettage, excision, Mohs' micrographic surgery, cryosurgery, and radiotherapy. Photodynamic therapy and intralesional interferon are newer modalities currently under investigation.

Electrodesiccation and Curettage

Electrodesiccation and curettage entails removing the tumor with a curette, followed by electrodesiccation with an electrosurgical device. Commonly, two to three cycles are employed. This is a blind technique because no histologic confirmation of tumor clearance is obtained. The treatment is reserved for primary lesions only. Superficial and noduloulcerative BCCs and well-differentiated superficially invasive SCCs can be treated with this modality. Tumors in the head and neck area should be no larger than 1 cm. Tumors at sites for high risk of recurrence should not exceed 6 mm in diameter. All lesions should have a clinically distinct margin. The modality should not be used if involvement of the subcutaneous fat is noted. Furthermore, areas in which a firm surface to curette is not available, such as the periocular area and lip, should be avoided.

Postoperative care consists of second-intention

healing of the treatment site. Time to complete healing will depend on the wound size. A minimum of several weeks of wound care can be expected. Hypertrophic scars commonly develop on the trunk with use of this modality.

Excision

Excisional surgery provides a means to obtain histologic confirmation of complete tumor removal. Commonly, a margin of 3 to 4 mm of normal-appearing skin is obtained around the tumor. Tumors larger than 20 mm in diameter require margins of 6 mm. The specimen should include at least some subcutaneous fat. The specimen is submitted in formalin to the laboratory for pathologic examination. Suturing of the surgical defect results in decreased wound healing time and a superior cosmetic outcome when compared with electrodesiccation and curettage. Both primary BCCs and SCCs can be treated in this manner. Occasionally, a recurrent lesion can be re-excised if an adequate margin can be obtained. BCCs with an aggressive histologic pattern, such as infiltrative or morpheaform BCCs, can have clinically occult extension resulting in positive margins. For these tumors, Mohs' micrographic surgery or excision with frozen section control is the preferred treatment.

Suggested tumor margins on the head and neck may result in defects that require a flap or graft. If the anticipated defect cannot be closed primarily, treatment options include delay of closure until the tissue has been examined, or until excision with frozen section control or Mohs' micrographic surgery can be performed. If Mohs' micrographic surgery is available, excision and repair of the defect can be performed in a cost-effective, time-efficient manner.

Mohs' Micrographic Surgery

Mohs' micrographic surgery involves the surgical removal of the tumor and a small margin of normal-appearing skin. The process permits examination of 100% of the surgical margin. The dermatologic surgeon performs the excision and microscopic examination of the tissue. Positive areas for tumor are noted, and additional tissue is resected from those areas until a tumor-free margin is reached. The treatment is performed on an outpatient basis, frequently with immediate repair of the surgical defect after a tumor-free margin is obtained.

This method is the treatment of choice for recurrent nonmelanoma skin cancer because of its 96% cure rate. In addition, the treatment is used for primary lesions that exhibit aggressive histologic features, indistinct tumor margins, and perineural extension of tumor, as well as for lesions located in areas prone to a high risk of recurrence with conventional treatment. Because the method can preserve normal tissue, it is extremely valuable when tissue preservation and cosmesis is paramount. The method is also useful for treatment of incompletely excised lesions.

Cryosurgery

Cryosurgery uses liquid nitrogen, which destroys the tumor cells through freezing. In order to treat malignant lesions, a thermocouple must be placed just below the deep tumor margin in order to ensure adequate freezing of the tissue. This method is a blind technique as well because no tissue confirmation of cure is obtained. The subsequent surgical defect is allowed to heal by second intention. The method should be reserved for small (1 to 2 cm) superficially invasive lesions that do not involve bone or cartilage.

Radiotherapy

Radiation therapy is commonly reserved for patients who are poor surgical risks. Tumors selected for treatment should be restricted to head and neck lesions. Better results are obtained for tumors in which the clinical margin can be defined. Tumors smaller than 1 cm are best treated with surgical excision. The treatment should not be used in patients 50 years of age or younger because of the long-term sequelae of radiation treatment. Treatment requires multiple visits over a 2- to 6-week period.

Investigational Techniques

Intralesional interferon-alpha and 5-fluorouracil implants have been used in the treatment of primary SCCs and BCCs. These treatments are currently under investigation. Photodynamic therapy involves the use of a photosensitizing drug and light of a specific wavelength. To date, this method does not achieve the cure rate of conventional techniques but does allow for the treatment of multiple lesions in a single session.

PAPULOSQUAMOUS ERUPTIONS

method of
CARRIE D. ALSPAUGH, M.D., and
DARREL L. ELLIS, M.D.
Vanderbilt University Medical Center
Nashville, Tennessee

The papulosquamous eruptions comprise unrelated skin disorders characterized by papules and plaques, which are usually erythematous and scaly. Because topical glucocorticoids are a frequently used method of treatment for many of these disorders, they are discussed with a table of different types of glucocorticoids provided. The papulosquamous disorders are then addressed individually.

In children and especially infants, only low-potency glucocorticoids, such as 1% hydrocortisone, should be used, and they should be used for the shortest time possible. Only low-potency corticosteroids should be applied to the face, axilla, or groin in all age groups, with rare exception. As a rule, the lowest potency agent that is effective should be used for the least amount of time possible in all patients. The superpotent steroids should rarely be used longer than 2 weeks, owing to the likelihood of systemic absorption and the risk of local atrophy. In general, ointments are the most potent vehicles, followed by creams, gels, solutions, and lotions. A list of some of the topical corticosteroids and their potencies is included in Table 1.

SEBORRHEIC DERMATITIS

Diagnosis

Seborrheic dermatitis, a common disorder affecting both infants and adults, is characterized by erythema with an overlying white or yellowish greasy scale. It often involves the scalp, eyebrows, glabella, nasolabial folds, external ear canals, periauricular skin, central chest, and intertriginous areas (axilla and groin). Rarely, it presents as an exfoliative erythroderma. Pruritus is a frequent symptom. The least severe but most common form is seborrhea sicca, or dandruff, which presents as dry, fine desquamation of the scalp. Seborrheic dermatitis may be severe in patients with acquired immune deficiency syndrome (AIDS) and in patients with neurologic abnormalities such as parkinsonism. It may also occur in patients with acne vulgaris and rosacea.

The cause of seborrheic dermatitis is unknown. Increased sebum production is not always found but seems most closely linked with seborrheic dermatitis of infancy, a stage when the sebaceous glands are large, secreting high amounts of sebum. Increased numbers of, or sensitivity to, *Pityrosporum ovale,* a lipophilic yeast, has been postulated as another cause.

The differential diagnoses of seborrheic dermatitis should include psoriasis, atopic dermatitis, contact dermatitis, tinea corporis and tinea capitis, rosacea, and cutaneous candidiasis. In infants, two other disorders, histiocytosis X and Leiner's disease, should also be considered. Histiocytosis X, also known as Langerhans cell histiocytosis, is clinically characterized by seborrhea-like and possibly hemorrhagic skin lesions, as well as by hepatosplenomegaly. Leiner's disease, also known as erythroderma desquamativum, is typified by generalized erythema and scaling with anemia, emesis, diarrhea, and possibly, bacterial superinfection.

If there is any question about the diagnosis of seborrheic dermatitis, a skin biopsy and possibly fungal or bacterial cultures may be performed.

TABLE 1. **Topical Glucocorticoids and Their Potencies**

Generic Name	Brand Name
Super Potency	
Clobetasol propionate	Temovate, 0.05% cream and ointment
Betamethasone dipropionate	Diprolene, 0.05% cream and ointment
Diflorasone diacetate	Psorcon ointment, 0.05%
Halobetasol propionate	Ultravate, 0.05% cream and ointment
High Potency	
Amcinonide	Cyclocort ointment, 0.1%
Mometasone furoate	Elocon ointment, 0.1%
Halcinonide	Halog, 0.1% cream, ointment, and solution
Fluocinonide	Lidex, 0.05% cream, gel, ointment, and solution
Desoximetasone	Topicort, 0.025% cream and ointment; 0.05% gel
Intermediate Potency	
Amcinonide	Cyclocort, 0.1% cream and lotion
Betamethasone valerate	Valisone, 0.1% ointment, cream, and lotion
Triamcinolone acetonide	Aristocort and Kenalog, 0.1% and 0.025% ointment, cream, and lotion
Mometasone furoate	Elocon, 0.1% cream and lotion
Fluocinolone acetonide	Synalar, 0.025% ointment and 0.01% cream and solution
Hydrocortisone butyrate	Locoid, 0.1% cream, ointment, and solution
Hydrocortisone valerate	Westcort, 0.2% cream and ointment
Lowest Potency	
Hydrocortisone	Hytone, 1% and 2.5% cream, lotion, and ointment
Hydrocortisone acetate and pramoxine HCl 1%	Pramosone, 1% and 2.5% cream, lotion, and ointment

Therapy

Although in infants seborrheic dermatitis is usually a disease that is limited to the first few months of life, it is usually a chronic and recurrent disorder in adults. Therefore, the treatment goals are mainly to control inflammation and decrease the *Pityrosporum* population.

For seborrheic dermatitis in infants, routine care with a mild baby shampoo or mild soap and emollients should be performed. Additionally, scale may be removed with 3 to 5% salicylic acid in olive oil or a water-soluble base. Low-potency steroid preparations may be used once or twice daily for a few days, if necessary.

For seborrheic dermatitis of the scalp in adults, ketoconazole 2% (Nizoral) shampoo should be used twice weekly for 4 weeks and should be left on the scalp for 3 to 5 minutes at each application. It may then be used once weekly as a prophylactic agent. Other shampoos, such as those with pyrithione zinc (Head & Shoulders, Zincon), selenium sulfide (Selsun [2.5%], Selsun Blue [1%], Exsel [2.5%]), and chloroxine (Capitrol [2%]), may be used to decrease the load of *Pityrosporum* organisms. Also, shampoos with tar, sulfur, or salicylic acid may be used alone or in combination with other shampoos or topical steroids. These shampoos should be used at least every 3 days, and they should be lathered into wet hair and left on for 5 minutes before rinsing. Notably, shampoos with tar, selenium sulfide, and chloroxine may stain blond and gray hair. Intermediate-potency or, occasionally, higher potency steroid lotions or solutions may also be applied to the scalp one to two times daily and massaged in lightly.

Facial seborrheic dermatitis in adults may be treated with 2% ketoconazole cream (Nizoral) or a low-potency steroid cream twice daily. Seborrheic blepharitis should be treated with gentle daily débridement with a cotton-tipped applicator and baby shampoo. Topical steroids should not be used for blepharitis because they may induce glaucoma or cataracts.

Truncal seborrheic dermatitis also responds to anti-*Pityrosporum* agents, such as topical 2% ketoconazole cream, and to topical steroids applied twice daily. Intermediate-potency agents such as 0.1% triamcinolone cream may be used safely on the body in adults.

With seborrheic dermatitis of the groin, the area should be kept as dry as possible. One percent hydrocortisone cream and 2% miconazole cream (Monistat) or 1% clotrimazole cream (Lotrimin) may be used twice each day. Long-term use of steroids should be avoided in this anatomic area.

PSORIASIS

Psoriasis is a hyperproliferative epithelial disorder of unknown cause with a genetic predisposition and possible autosomal dominant inheritance. It is one of several disorders in which skin injury results in disease-specific lesions (Koebner's phenomenon). In addition to nonspecific physical trauma, infections, especially with streptococcal organisms and with human immunodeficiency virus type I; certain drugs, such as systemic corticosteroids, lithium, and beta-adrenergic blockers; and stress are all possible triggering factors. In general, systemic corticosteroids are not used to treat psoriasis because their withdrawal may trigger generalized pustular psoriasis, which may be life-threatening. There are several clinical variants, including psoriasis vulgaris (plaque type), guttate, pustular, and erythrodermic, each of which are described here along with their treatments.

The differential diagnosis of psoriasis should include eczema, pityriasis rubra pilaris, seborrheic dermatitis, syphilis, candidiasis, tinea, cutaneous T cell lymphoma, Paget's disease, pityriasis rosea, pityriasis lichenoides et varioliformis acuta, and in situ squamous cell carcinoma.

Psoriasis Vulgaris

This variant is characterized by erythematous plaques with overlying thick, mica-like scale located usually on the scalp, elbows, knees, and trunk. Nail changes including pitting, onycholysis, and yellowish brown spots under the nail plate, which are also known as oil drop spots, are common.

Topical steroids are the most common therapy for stable plaque stage psoriasis. Intermediate-potency steroid ointments are usually effective with twice-daily application, but sometimes high-potency or suprapotent steroids must be used for a short course (e.g., less than 2 weeks). Recalcitrant lesions may be occluded with plastic wrap and a low- to intermediate-potency steroid for up to 8 hours daily.

Topical tar and anthralin may be used as steroid-sparing agents for plaque-stage psoriasis. Tar preparations, such as Estar gel and MG217, may be applied to the plaques for 2 to 12 hours and then washed off. Short-contact anthralin therapy with 0.1% to 1% anthralin cream or ointment (Drithocreme, Anthra-Derm) applied only to the affected areas for 10 to 30 minutes and then washed off, can be effective. Both tar and anthralin may stain clothes or furniture. Anthralin may also stain normal skin red, purple, or brown and may cause an irritant dermatitis. Topical calcipotriene (Dovonex) 0.005% ointment used twice daily is a vitamin D analogue that regulates terminal differentiation of epidermal basal keratinocytes. It is a newer therapy that appears to be promising.

Widespread psoriasis vulgaris usually requires more than topical therapy. Ultraviolet light therapy with UVB alone or in combination with tar or anthralin may be quite effective. PUVA therapy, which is UVA treatment in combination with an oral photosensitizing agent (psoralen), may also be very effective. Both of these modalities should be administered by a physician who is familiar with these techniques, because of the risks of a sunburn-type reaction, nonmelanoma skin cancer, and ocular damage. If these methods fail, other systemic therapies that may be considered are methotrexate, etretinate, or less often, cyclosporine.

Guttate Psoriasis

Guttate (droplike) psoriasis presents as multiple, 0.5- to 1.5-cm, salmon-pink, scaly papules on the trunk and proximal extremities, usually in adolescents and young adults. Upper respiratory infections, especially streptococcal pharyngitis, frequently precede the onset or flare of guttate psoriasis. A 10-day course of penicillin VK or erythromycin (250 mg four times daily) may induce a dramatic remission. UVB therapy alone or in combination with tar may also be effective. If the involved area is more limited, intermediate-potency topical steroids may be used.

Generalized Pustular Psoriasis

Pustules arising on erythematous skin are disseminated on the trunk and extremities in generalized pustular psoriasis. The condition is also known as von Zumbusch's psoriasis. Fever, malaise, leukocytosis, and hypocalcemia may also be seen. Pustular psoriasis often follows the withdrawal of systemic glucocorticoids. It is a serious disorder, possibly life-threatening, and often requires hospitalization. Treatment consists of soaks, bland emollients, and management of hypocalcemia. Methotrexate or etretinate is the best initial therapy for pustular psoriasis.

Psoriatic Erythroderma

In psoriatic erythroderma, erythema is the most notable feature, usually with less prominent scaling. The entire body may be affected. Increased extrarenal water loss is a potential problem and must be monitored and treated as appropriate. It is also a potentially life-threatening disorder that often requires hospitalization. Frequent tub baths and lubrication with emollients and intermediate- to high-potency corticosteroid ointments are helpful. Antihistamines should be used to control pruritus. Methotrexate or etretinate is often required to control this disorder. Systemic steroids should not be used owing to the possibility of triggering a life-threatening generalized flare of pustular psoriasis.

PITYRIASIS RUBRA PILARIS

Diagnosis

Pityriasis rubra pilaris is a relatively rare disorder that is characterized by progressively enlarging orange-red, scaly plaques with sharp borders that enclose islands of normal skin. The palms and soles are remarkable for thick, yellow, hyperkeratotic lesions.

Therapy

The course of pityriasis rubra pilaris is usually chronic, but occasionally it may regress spontaneously. Systemic treatment with retinoids, such as isotretinoin (Accutane) and etretinate (Tegison), as well as the folic acid antagonist methotrexate, has been helpful.

PITYRIASIS ROSEA

Diagnosis

Pityriasis rosea usually begins with a single, red, scaly, 2- to 3-cm plaque (herald patch), which is followed by an eruption of 0.5- to 1.0-cm red, scaly papules on the trunk, neck, and proximal extremities. The pattern of the secondary lesions on the trunk has been described as similar to a fir tree. Pityriasis rosea has a peak incidence at between 10 and 35 years of age and usually occurs in the spring and fall. Pruritus may occur, but generally, the lesions are asymptomatic. The disorder usually lasts from 6 to 12 weeks. Its cause is unknown, although some favor a viral etiology. Secondary syphilis and guttate psoriasis must be considered in the differential diagnosis.

Therapy

Because of its asymptomatic nature and short course, pityriasis rosea often requires no therapy. Antihistamines and topical intermediate or low-potency steroids may be helpful for the associated pruritus. Ultraviolet radiation has been found helpful in more severe cases with pruritus.

LICHEN PLANUS

Diagnosis

The skin lesions of lichen planus are pruritic, tiny, flat-topped, violaceous, polygonal papules with a predilection for flexural surfaces. A fine network of white lines, called Wickham's striae, may be seen overlying the lesions. As with psoriasis, the Koebner phenomenon occurs in lichen planus with minor trauma. Hypertrophic lesions may occur, especially on the anterior lower legs. Pruritus is often severe in lichen planus. On the oral and genital mucosa, lichen planus may present as white plaques with a lacelike network or erosions.

Several drugs may induce lichenoid eruptions. Angiotensin-converting enzyme inhibitors, gold, antimalarials, phenothiazines, and thiazides are among the most common agents that produce lichenoid drug eruptions. Lichenoid eruptions may also be seen with chronic graft-versus-host reactions.

The diagnosis of lichen planus can usually be made on clinical findings, but a biopsy for histology and possibly for immunofluorescence may be confirmatory and is advisable for any long-standing mucosal lesion.

Therapy

Mild cases of lichen planus may be treated with topical antipruritic lotions (e.g., Prax, Sarna), low- to high-potency topical steroids, and oral antihistamines. For widespread or very symptomatic lichen planus, a 2- to 6-week course of oral corticosteroids, PUVA, oral retinoids, dapsone, and systemic cyclosporine have been reported to be helpful. For oral lesions, improvement has resulted from use of intermediate- to high-potency steroids in an adhesive base (e.g., Orabase) applied as often as six times daily, or 0.1% isotretinoin gel (Retin-A) applied daily.

PARAPSORIASIS

Diagnosis

Parapsoriasis can be categorized as two types: small plaque and large plaque. The lesions of both types are erythematous, scaly, usually asymptomatic, thin plaques. Lesions in the small-plaque type are less than 5 cm in diameter, and in the large-plaque type, they are usually between 5 and 10 cm in diameter. Some authorities consider large-plaque parapsoriasis to be either premalignant or an actual stage of cutaneous T cell lymphoma (i.e., mycosis fungoides).

Therapy

Lubrication and treatment with intermediate- to high-potency topical steroids may be used with both small- and large-plaque parapsoriasis. Because of the potential relationship with cutaneous T cell lymphoma, more aggressive therapy with topical nitrogen mustard or PUVA has also been advocated for the large-plaque variant.

CONNECTIVE TISSUE DISORDERS: SYSTEMIC LUPUS ERYTHEMATOSUS, DERMATOMYOSITIS AND OTHER MYOPATHIES, AND SCLERODERMA

method of
ROBERT G. LAHITA, M.D., PH.D.
Saint Luke's-Roosevelt Medical Center of Columbia University
New York, New York

SYSTEMIC LUPUS ERYTHEMATOSUS

The therapy for systemic lupus erythematosus (SLE) varies with disease activity and changes with time. Therapy for this disease can be simple for mild disease or complex for severe disease. Examples of this are the use of anti-inflammatory medications for mild disease and immunosuppressive agents for severe disease. The clinical manifestations of SLE typically vary with the extent and activity of the disease, and therapy should be individualized. All therapy for SLE should be based on an understanding of the pathogenesis, the organ system(s) involved, and the likely need for prolonged versus rapid resolution of the pathologic processes involved at any point in the illness. For example, impending severe organ damage of the kidneys or brain may require more aggressive therapy with immunosuppressive or cytotoxic agents, whereas the mere presence of anti-phospholipid antibodies, in the absence of coagulopathy, may simply require a daily aspirin. Generally, there are only two serologic tests that are of use in predicting severe organ damage. These are the anti-native DNA and total hemolytic complement (CH50).

Constitutional Symptoms

Malaise and fatigue are very disabling symptoms. Depression, anemia, and thyroid disease might complicate the malaise found in SLE and require treatment. Treatment of fatigue in SLE should be conservative. Bed rest by itself is often useful for patients with minor exacerbations. Aerobic conditioning should be used with care because exertional activity often results in worsened serologies. Low-grade fever (<38.8°C [102°F]) is commonly found in SLE patients (80%); however, in approximately 20% of patients a low-grade fever indicates infection. Because the most common cause of death in SLE is infection, this must be excluded in the febrile patient. Fevers of lupus should be treated with standard antipyretic agents. Vaccines are not contraindicated in patients with SLE; however, live vaccines should not be given to immunosuppressed patients or those with very active disease. Pneumococcal vaccine (Pneumovax 23) is exceptionally useful because SLE patients may be functionally asplenic.

Skin Manifestations

Only 40% of patients with lupus are sensitive to ultraviolet light and need to avoid direct exposure to sunlight. There are also a small number of patients who may be sensitive to fluorescent lights. Use of sunscreens, as well as protective clothing, should be encouraged in these patients. These sunscreens should have a protective factor of 15 or greater. Topical corticosteroids are useful for the treatment of skin eruptions from exposure to the sun. High-potency preparations (e.g., clobetasol 0.05% [Temovate], twice daily) may be required but should be avoided on the face because of the telangiectasias and atrophic changes that may result. Less potent agents like hydrocortisone (1%) may be used. Discoid skin lesions and other lesions that are refractory to topical corticosteroid therapy may be treated with intralesional injections. The concurrent use of antimalarial agents like hydroxychloroquine (Plaquenil), 200 mg orally twice daily, or chloroquine (Aralen), 250 mg once daily, is recommended. Glucose-6-phosphatase deficiency (G6PD) must be ruled out prior to initiation of therapy. Pre-use ophthalmologic exams followed by exams every 6 months are recommended with antimalarial agents to avoid retinal toxicity and corneal anesthesia. Dosage should not exceed 6 mg per kg per day after 3 months of therapy. Quinacrine (Atabrine) can also be a useful adjunct to antimalarial agents in patients with severe disease of the skin. Other skin lesions related to SLE, such as the livedo reticularis of the antiphospholipid syndrome, are not treated. Lupus profundus, a rare manifestation of SLE, may be treated with dapsone after an initial trial of antimalarial therapy.

Joint Manifestations

Arthritis can often be the presenting complaint, involves 95% of patients, and is mild, symmetrical, and polyarticular. Soft tissue deformities are found in 10 to 15% of patients, but fewer than 5% have erosions. Most joint pains can be managed with nonsteroidal anti-inflammatory drugs (NSAIDs). Several precautions are warranted. All NSAIDs should be used cautiously in patients with SLE because the efferent renal circulation may be compromised, resulting in decreased renal function. Several agents, such as sulindac (Clinoril), have sulfur nuclei to which patients may also be allergic. Some NSAIDs that can be used include naproxen (Naprosyn), 375 to 500 mg twice daily; nabumetone (Relafen), 1000 mg daily; etodolac (Lodine), 300 mg three times daily; and ibuprofen (Motrin), 2400 to 3200 mg per day. Hydroxychloroquine, 200 mg orally twice daily, may also be helpful. Low-dose prednisone (5 to 10 mg daily) is rarely used to control the arthropathy of SLE but can be tried in combination with other agents if the disease is particularly refractory. Monarthritis usually suggests infection, whereas refractory joint pain suggests aseptic necrosis, which is a result of steroid therapy or disease.

Pulmonary Manifestations

Pleuritis occurs in 33% of patients and is usually bilateral. A pulmonary infiltrate is more likely to be a reflection of infection. Pleuritis may be treated with anti-inflammatory drugs. NSAIDs may be used in conjunction with prednisone, 30 mg daily, until the pleuritis resolves. Acute lupus pneumonitis can be life-threatening and requires much larger doses of prednisone, 60 mg or more daily. Chronic interstitial fibrosis, a consequence of pneumonitis, in fewer than 5% of patients warrants a trial of prednisone (60 mg or more daily) for a period of 4 weeks. If improvement does not occur, then cytotoxic agents are warranted. Antiphospholipid antibodies are associated with pulmonary fibrosis, pulmonary hypertension, and pulmonary emboli. Only pulmonary emboli respond to anticoagulation in the usual manner.

Cardiac Manifestations

As many as one-third of patients with SLE have pericarditis. This manifestation can cause positional chest discomfort and, in rare cases, actual tamponade. Pericarditis usually responds to NSAIDs but, in rare cases, prednisone, 20 mg orally, is required. Tamponade usually requires immediate pericardiocentesis followed by high-dose (60 mg) prednisone. Myocarditis and vasculitis of the coronary arteries are rare and respond to high-dose prednisone. Antiphospholipid antibodies have been associated with valvular vegetation (Libman-Sacks syndrome), which can cause regurgitation or stenosis, or both, in patients of all ages. The mitral valve is most commonly affected, followed by the aortic valve. Pulmonary hypertension is common and is associated with antiphospholipid antibodies. Myocardial infarctions are common in young patients with SLE. These are the result of coronary stenosis from accelerated atherosclerosis, vasculitis, or coronary thrombosis secondary to vasculopathy. Long-term steroid therapy can cause lipid abnormalities, which predispose patients to coronary disease; however, such changes can occur with antiphospholipid syndrome for unknown reasons. SLE-associated renal hypertension can contribute to cardiac ischemia.

Lupus Renal Disease

Significant glomerulonephritis (GN) as defined by abnormal urinary sediment can occur in 70% or more patients with SLE. Fifty percent of SLE patients can develop proteinuria, while 25% develop nephrotic syndrome. Twenty percent of patients with nephritis develop end-stage renal disease within 10 years. Diffuse proliferative and membranoproliferative histology have the poorest prognoses. NSAIDs can decrease efferent renal blood flow in such patients and cause further worsening. It is important to consider early renal biopsy in order to differentiate active from inactive lesions. Active lesions predict continued injury to the glomerulus and merit cytotoxic therapy, whereas inactive lesions are irreversible and do not respond to therapy. It is very important to obtain immunofluorescence and electron microscopy on all biopsy sections, when possible.

Proliferative lesions may first be treated with prednisone, 60 mg orally per day for 4 to 8 weeks, with an expectation of decreased proteinuria or improvement of urine sediment. Pulse therapy, using 1 gram of methylprednisolone for 3 days each month, is an alternative therapy. The latter regimen may be followed for 2 months with concurrent modest doses (<30 mg) of oral steroids with careful observation. If improvement does not occur, cytotoxic therapy can be added or used alone (cyclophosphamide [Cytoxan],* 0.5 to 1 gram per mm^2). It can be given by intravenous push monthly for 4 to 6 months. After this course of therapy, repeat renal biopsy may be performed to assess its clinical efficacy. Renal biopsy may also be repeated to assess the rapidly progressive deterioration of renal function. Hydration is important to minimize the risks of bladder toxicity.

Side effects of Cytoxan include nausea, emesis, alopecia, cytopenia (dosage of the drug can be modulated with the nadir of the white blood cell count), hemorrhage, cystitis, ovarian failure, teratogenicity, opportunistic infection, and possible malignancy later in life. Bladder carcinoma is a long-term side effect of cyclophosphamide therapy and requires frequent cystoscopic assessment based on clinical follow-up.

Renal failure is often an inevitable effect of progressive lupus nephritis and may mandate dialysis. Dialysis often results in improvement of overall lupus activity. Transplantation of the kidney has been successful in SLE patients, and no evidence exists to indicate with certainty that SLE recurs in a transplanted kidney.

Central Nervous System Manifestations

Estimates of the central nervous system manifestations of SLE range from 35 to 75%. The peripheral nervous system is involved 8% of the time. Seizures, psychiatric manifestations, and cranial nerve abnormalities are very common. Standard epilepsy therapeutic agents such as phenytoin (Dilantin) and phenobarbital are used in the therapy of seizures. The seizures are usually grand mal in type, and large doses of corticosteroids (60 mg prednisone daily) or pulse therapy are used in conjunction with the antiseizure medication. Seizures can also result from hypertension, uremia, and even steroid therapy. Encephalitic manifestations and transverse myelitis are also

*Not FDA approved for this indication.

treated with high-dose steroids. Pulse cyclophosphamide is often used to control life-threatening situations. A differentiation must be made between the cerebritis of SLE and antiphospholipid-related cerebral thrombosis. The thrombosis should be treated with anticoagulation, as well as immunosuppression. An unusual form of central nervous system lupus is a demyelinating syndrome called lupoid sclerosis. This manifestation can be treated with high-dose oral steroids or pulse therapy. Psychiatric abnormalities and cognitive dysfunction are also commonly found in SLE patients, and these symptoms rarely require immunosuppression but should be treated with the usual psychiatric drugs.

Hematologic Manifestations

The anemia of chronic disease is most common in patients with SLE. Anemia occurs in 70 to 80% of SLE patients. Although 20 to 60% of SLE patients have a positive Coombs' test at some time during their illness, only 10% develop autoimmune hemolytic anemia. Leukopenia, which may be either granulocytopenia or lymphopenia, occurs in about 50% of SLE patients. Leukopenia is often a sign of active disease since antileukocyte antibodies may be at the core of such findings. Thrombocytopenia is observed in 14 to 45% of patients with SLE and is usually associated with antiphospholipid antibodies. Patients with hemolysis or profound leukopenia (less than 1000 cells per mm^3) respond to high-dose prednisone therapy (60 mg orally daily) for a period of 6 to 8 months with gradual tapering. Immunosuppressive therapy other than prednisone may confuse the issue because both cyclophosphamide and azathioprine (Imuran), can cause leukopenia. Patients with thrombocytopenia may respond to elevated doses of prednisone (60 mg orally daily). A gradual increase of platelets is observed; however, normal levels may not be achieved with prednisone alone. Alternative therapy includes splenectomy, danazol (Danocrine), 200 mg orally four times daily, or intravenous gamma globulin, 0.4 gram per kg daily for 5 days. In all cases, platelets will rise slowly over 7 days and drop over 4 weeks without additional therapy. Other, less popular means of treating SLE thrombocytopenia include the use of intravenous cyclophosphamide, dapsone, cyclosporine A (Sandimmune), and interferon-alpha.

Cryoglobulins may be a cause of digital infarction in SLE and be associated with profound vasculitis. Cryoglobulinemia usually responds to a single high dose of prednisone alone or in combination with plasmapheresis in severe cases.

Patients with SLE rarely have bleeding diatheses resulting from antibodies to clotting Factors (II, VIII, IX, XI, and XII most commonly). Corticosteroid therapy usually controls these symptoms. The most common coagulation abnormality in SLE is lupus anticoagulant (LAC), which is manifested by a variably prolonged partial thromboplastin time (PTT) and thrombosis. The effect is a procoagulant one. This procoagulant effect is often associated with thrombocytopenia, false-positive tests for syphilis, recurrent spontaneous abortions, and the presence of antiphospholipid antibodies such as anticardiolipin. Mild elevations of PTT without evidence of thrombosis are best treated with daily aspirin. If thrombotic events are associated with LAC, the patient should be treated with heparin and subsequently placed on warfarin (Coumadin). Use of immunosuppressives is additionally recommended in the presence of accompanying vasculitis or situations in which thrombosis continues despite anticoagulation.

Reproduction

Estrogens and androgens clearly play a role in the pathogenesis of SLE. Hormonal replacement therapy is used after menopause, although studies regarding the use of these agents do not exist. Oral contraceptives are to be avoided in premenopausal women with SLE because exacerbation of disease is believed to be directly related to the estrogen content of the agent. The role of progestational agents in women with SLE is unknown. Use of intrauterine devices should be avoided because of a high risk of infection. Barrier contraception is preferred in women with SLE. Pregnancy is deferred in SLE patients with active disease until the disease is quiescent. Pregnant SLE patients are to be considered high risk because fetal wastage and the phospholipid syndrome are commonly seen in patients with SLE who are pregnant. High-dose corticosteroids may be used in pregnant SLE patients who have active disease. Anticoagulation in pregnancy is limited to heparin use (usually 10,000 units subcutaneously twice daily) if the patient has thrombosis or a previous history of thrombosis during pregnancy. Pregnancy may worsen SLE in a variable percentage of patients (fewer than 25%), and this is especially true in patients with renal disease.

DERMATOMYOSITIS AND OTHER MYOPATHIES

Dermatomyositis and polymyositis are idiopathic inflammatory diseases of muscle. These diseases may be associated with specific autoantibodies to histidyl-tRNA synthetase and other muscle enzymes in about 50% of patients. The clinical presentation is symmetrical proximal muscle weakness developing over weeks to months, elevated serum creatine phosphokinase, and abnormal electromyograms (EMGs), usually showing mixed myopathic and neuropathic abnormalities. Muscle biopsy shows mononuclear cell infiltration. The blush discoloration around the eyes (heliotrope rash) and erythematous skin rashes are more common in dermatomyositis. One-third of patients have muscle pains and cramps, and these often occur with dysphagia. Polymyositis may accompany connective tissue diseases like SLE or vasculitis. Respiratory arrest is the most serious complication and should be expected in severe cases. Progressive interstitial pulmonary fibrosis can be seen (Velcro-like lungs). A cancer (usually gastrointestinal) can be found associated with dermatomyositis in 25% of patients who are older than 40 years of age. Other causes of myopathy to be considered include hypothyroidism, toxins (alcohol), inclusion body myositis (viral), and drugs (HMG coA reductase inhibitors, zidovudine, colchicine, penicillamine, clofibrate, and steroids). Eosinophilic myositis is rare and is associated with proximal weakness, myalgias, elevated serum enzymes, and an abnormal EMG. This disease can be focal but is more often associated with a generalized condition called eosinophilia-myalgia syndrome. Eosinophilia-myalgia has been associated with the ingestion of tryptophan.

Treatment of the inflammatory myopathies is largely empirical. Bed rest is important in the acute phase. Corticosteroids should be given in a dose of 1 to 2 mg per kg per day. Intravenous methylprednisolone may be substituted. Gradual improvement of strength lags behind the decrease of muscle enzymes. Once pain has subsided and the patient's strength has returned, the steroids can be gradually tapered at a rate of 10 mg per month. Other agents that might be helpful are azathioprine, 2 to 3 mg per kg per day, and methotrexate, 10 to 15 mg orally or 15 to 50 mg intravenously weekly. Hydroxychloroquine, 200 mg twice daily, can be useful in patients who have skin lesions. Cyclophosphamide, 2 mg per kg intravenously, may also be tried in refractory cases of dermatomyositis or polymyositis. Recent trials of intravenous immunoglobulin and cyclosporine indicate that these agents might have efficacy in a limited number of patients.

SCLERODERMA

Scleroderma is characterized by thickening and fibrosis of the skin. Besides the skin, there can also be forms that involve the gastrointestinal tract, kidneys, lungs, and heart. The cause and mechanisms of the disease are unknown. There is no known cure or effective therapy. Morbidity and mortality are related to visceral involvement, not skin involvement.

Cutaneous Manifestations and Raynaud's Phenomenon

In almost all cases, skin thickening begins in the fingers and hands. Transverse digital creases may disappear and hair growth usually disappears. The face and the neck are affected with decreased mobility, decreased gape, and so-called purse string lips. Dental hygiene may be a problem. Areas of hyperpigmentation or hypopigmentation can develop or be generalized, and the patient might look deeply tanned. Cytotoxic agents are ineffective. Several agents have been helpful in some patients. D-Penicillamine (Cuprimine), 750 to 1000 mg orally daily, has been shown to soften the skin in patients with early progressive skin disease. Urine and complete blood counts should be monitored weekly for the first 4 weeks and then monthly to avoid the membranoproliferative glomerulonephritis and thrombocytopenia observed with this drug. Low-dose corticosteroids (5 to 10 mg orally daily) for short periods may have palliative effects in patients with myalgias and arthralgias and may actually improve mobility. There is no treatment for the calcinosis of scleroderma. Raynaud's phenomenon is a typical clinical manifestation of scleroderma (95%). This clinical finding represents severe narrowing of digital arterial lumens. Normal cold or emotion related digital vasoconstriction is exacerbated when it occurs in conjunction with the intimal hyperplasia of scleroderma. Digital ischemia or infarction can occur. Patients should avoid cold exposure by wearing gloves or using hand warmers. Calcium channel blockers are useful in many patients and include nifedipine (Procardia), 10 mg three times per day, and diltiazem (Cardizem), 30 to 60 mg four times per day. Nitropaste may also be applied to digital ischemic areas four times daily to increase blood flow. More invasive procedures like surgical blocks are reserved for refractory vasospasm with severe ischemia.

Gastrointestinal Manifestations

Esophageal dysmotility is present in all forms of scleroderma and may be present in asymptomatic patients. Hypomotility of the entire gastrointestinal tract is the rule in this disease. Lower esophageal sphincter dysfunction and disordered peristalsis of the lower two-thirds of the esophagus result in pain, heartburn, and regurgitation. Antacids, elevation of the head of the bed, and avoidance of alcohol and nicotine help control symptoms. Treatment of patients with H_2 blockers like ranitidine (Zantac), 150 mg twice daily, or cimetidine (Tagamet), 300 mg three times daily, is useful. Special care should be used in administering H_2 blockers before bedtime, because a peak acid surge occurs at 2:00 A.M. Omeprazole (Prilosec) should be reserved for severe cases. Metoclopramide (Reglan), 5 to 10 mg three times daily, may be helpful for some patients.

Diarrhea and weight loss result from bacterial overgrowth and malabsorption in a hypomotile small bowel. Pseudo-obstruction can also occur. Antibiotics like metronidazole, tetracycline, or vancomycin are helpful in the management of this condition. Hyperalimentation has helped severely malnourished patients. Somatostatin analogues can help in cases of pseudo-obstruction.

Renal Manifestations

Malignant hypertension, rapidly progressive renal insufficiency, hyperreninemia, and microangiopathic hemolysis are all part of scleroderma renal disease. The pathogenesis is typically one of intimal proliferation with obliteration of the arterial flow. This aspect of the disease has been associated with Raynaud's syndrome. Blood pressure control is important to all patients with scleroderma. The hyperreninemic hypertension of scleroderma is best treated with angiotensin-converting enzyme inhibitors such as captopril (Capoten), enalapril (Vasotec), and lisinopril (Prinivil). Other useful agents are minoxidil (Loniten) and α-methyldopa (Aldomet). Immunosuppressive agents such as steroids and cytotoxic agents have no role in the treatment of scleroderma hypertension.

Pulmonary Manifestations

Pulmonary scleroderma is a leading cause of morbidity and mortality. Pulmonary fibrosis, vascular obliteration, and inflammation may be present. Pulmonary hypertension, reduced compliance and vital capacity, and diminished diffusion capacity for carbon monoxide (DLCO) are typical changes. High-dose corticosteroid therapy, 30 to 60 mg; colchicine, 0.6 mg per day; and NSAIDS may be tried early in the course of pulmonary disease. D-Penicillamine (250 mg three times daily) may be of some benefit in progressive pulmonary disease. Calcium channel blockers like nifedipine, diltiazem, and others may help reduce pulmonary vascular resistance, but this should be confirmed by pulmonary artery catheterization because long-term administration may have little effect.

Cardiac Manifestations

Myocardial fibrosis (patchy) can be found in approximately 80% of patients with scleroderma. Conduction disturbances may be found in 50% of patients. Pericardial thickening can occur but is of little consequence. Myocardial perfusion abnormalities respond to nifedipine and dipyridamole (Persantine), but clinical efficacy is lacking. Symptomatic pericarditis may respond to NSAIDs and glucocorticoids.

CUTANEOUS VASCULITIS

method of
ROBERT A. SWERLICK, M.D.
Emory University School of Medicine
Atlanta, Georgia

The most common form of cutaneous vasculitis is small vessel necrotizing vasculitis, which appears clinically with crops of palpable pupuric lesions. The initial lesions may be erythematous macules or urticarial plaques that rapidly become hemorrhagic and purpuric. A small but significant percentage of patients have atypical lesions characterized by pustules, bullae, plaques, or ulcerations. The lesions occur most frequently on the skin below the knees and, less commonly, on other dependent areas. Facial and mucous membrane lesions may be seen, particularly in patients with severe nausea and vomiting. Although it is much less common than typical small vessel vasculitis, cutaneous vasculitis may also involve larger muscular arteries. These lesions tend to clinically appear as deeper inflammatory nodules, with or without ulceration.

Histologic examination of cutaneous vasculitis most commonly demonstrates leukocytoclastic vasculitis. Immune complexes are trapped in small postcapillary venules, activate the complement cascade, and induce neutrophil influx and inflammatory mediator release. The inflammatory reaction results in vessel wall destruction, fibrin deposition, and erythrocyte extravasation. Fibrin, complement, and immunoglobulin deposition may also be seen on immunofluorescence examination, particularly of early lesions. When deeper vessels are involved, they are typically found in the subcutis and demonstrate infiltration of vessel walls with neutrophils associated with aneurysmal dilation or vessel wall destruction.

Differential diagnoses include both inflammatory and noninflammatory purpuras. Patients with disseminated intravascular coagulation or experiencing other hypercoagulable states may experience cutaneous infarction associated with intravascular coagulation and thrombosis. Patients with thrombocytopenia may present with noninflammatory dependent purpura that may simulate vasculitis. Additionally, other inflammatory skin conditions such as erythema multiforme that occur on dependent areas may exhibit varying amounts of purpura and may appear clinically similar to leukocytoclastic vasculitis.

EVALUATION

The critical elements of an evaluation of a patient with cutaneous vasculitis are confirmation of the diagnosis, identification of any treatable precipitating factors, and defining whether the vasculitis is limited to the skin or involves extracutaneous sites. Although cutaneous vasculitis can be diagnosed in many cases, it is prudent to obtain a biopsy to confirm the diagnosis histologically. Additionally, fresh-frozen tissue or tissue preserved in Michaelis's media can be examined for deposition of immunoglobulins or complement in dermal blood vessels. This may be useful to identify individuals with Henoch-Schönlein purpura, who demonstrate deposits of IgA in dermal blood vessels.

It is generally assumed that vasculitis results from an aberrant immune response to exogenous or endogenous antigens, although an inciting agent can only be identified in about half of cases of cutaneous vasculitis. In those individuals in whom agents can be identified, up to 60% are presumed to have drug-induced vasculitis, although patients are almost never rechallenged. The most commonly implicated medications are penicillins, diuretics, sulfonamides, nonsteroidal anti-inflammatory agents, and anticonvulsant agents.

Infection may be associated with cutaneous vasculitis in approximately 10% of reported cases. Acute necrotizing vasculitis may be seen in cases of bacterial endocarditis, meningococcal meningitis, or Rocky Mountain spotted fever. Chronic infections such as hepatitis B or chronic streptococcal infections have also been associated with cutaneous vasculitis.

Cutaneous vasculitis is a not uncommon manifestation of collagen vascular disease. The clinical course of patients with systemic lupus erythematosus, Sjögren's syndrome, or rheumatoid arthritis is not infrequently complicated by cutaneous vasculitis, with or without visceral involvement. It is essential to identify those individuals who have cutaneous vasculitis in association with visceral disease. The true incidence of systemic involvement in patients who present with cutaneous vasculitis is not certain and is difficult to define. Arthritis and arthralgias may be seen in up to 40% of patients, although those who have frank arthritis often have it in association with pre-existing rheumatologic disease. The actual incidence of renal involvement in patients with cutaneous vasculitis is also uncertain. Early studies suggested that the incidence of renal disease is as high as 63%, but more recent studies examining the incidence of significant renal disease in patients presenting to dermatologists in private practice suggest that the true incidence is less than 5%. However, renal disease may be completely asymptomatic and is the leading cause of end-organ failure in those affected with cutaneous vasculitis.

A subset of patients with malignancy may present with cutaneous vasculitis in association with other constitutional symptoms. Initial reports demonstrated an association of hairy cell leukemia with polyarteritis nodosa, but subsequent reports have demonstrated concurrent expression of small vessel cutaneous vasculitis associated with a variety of bone marrow dyscrasias, leukemias, and solid tumors. These patients tend to have a very poor prognosis.

The history and careful physical examination are crucial in determining the extent of the laboratory work-up necessary for evaluation of cutaneous vasculitis. A minimal laboratory screening evaluation should include a complete blood count with differential, as well as measurement of the platelet count, serum creatinine and blood urea nitrogen, liver enzymes and bilirubin, sedimentation rate, urinalysis, and stool for occult blood. Evaluation for renal disease is particularly important because renal disease may be completely asymptomatic.

Further tests should be dictated by the findings on the history or on the physical examination. Prominent pulmonary symptoms are not characteristic of cutaneous vasculitis, and should alert the examiner to the possibility of Wegener's granulomatosis or allergic granulomatosis. Neurologic findings or prominent gastrointestinal pain may suggest a diagnosis of polyarteritis nodosa, although Henoch-Schönlein purpura may be associated with prominent gastrointestinal symptoms in adults. Further testing may include serologic testing in the examination for rheumatoid factor, antinuclear antibodies, antineutrophil cytoplasm antibodies, complement levels, cryoglobulins, cryofibrinogens, anticardiolipin antibodies, serum protein electrophoresis, and hepatitis B antigen. Further diagnostic examinations may include chest x-ray study, arteriography, or biopsy of extracutaneous sites.

THERAPY

Most patients with cutaneous vasculitis have a self-limited disease with no extracutaneous manifestations. Be certain to identify any treatable causes, including any possible drug-induced etiology. It may be necessary to include a history for occult or illicit drug use. However, most patients have minimal to moderate symptoms associated with multiple crops of cutaneous lesions that develop and resolve over a period of a few weeks to a few months. Therapy should be supportive and directed toward symptoms. Mild burning or itching may benefit from antihistamines, and pain or arthralgias may benefit from nonsteroidal anti-inflammatory agents, although there is no evidence that either of these agents modify the course of the disease. Swelling may be improved by leg elevation or use of support hose, or both. A graded pressure stocking is preferable to antiembolism hose, and its usefulness alone or as an adjunct to any other therapy instituted should not be underestimated.

Certain patients have more severe cutaneous disease that, although limited to the skin, requires more aggressive therapy. After careful evaluation for extracutaneous disease or infection, a short course of oral corticosteroids may be extremely useful in controling severe cutaneous disease. When treating patients with non–life-threatening vasculitic syndromes, a short-acting oral preparation (prednisone or methylprednisolone [Solu-Medrol], 0.5 to 1 mg per kg per day) should be given as a single daily dose to minimize the chance of adrenal suppression. Systemic corticosteroids are extremely effective agents for patients with severely debilitating disease, but long-term use is limited by predictable toxicity. Long-term management of patients with persistent disease should be directed toward using alternate-day corticosteroid therapy, a steroid-sparing agent, or both.

Colchicine, 0.6 mg given once to three times daily, may be a very effective agent either alone or in conjunction with alternate-day corticosteroid therapy. Gastrointestinal intolerance, most commonly diarrhea, may limit colchicine's usefulness, although most patients tolerate up to 0.6 mg twice daily with minimal difficulty. Bone marrow toxicity has been reported, and it is prudent to monitor complete blood count and platelet counts during therapy.

Dapsone has also been shown to be useful in the management of subsets of individuals with cutaneous vasculitis. Patients with glucose-6-phosphate dehydrogenase (G6PD) deficiency do not tolerate dapsone, and individuals should be screened before use. Dapsone is generally used at doses of 100 to 200 mg daily, although higher doses can be used if tolerated. All patients develop some degree of hemolysis and methemoglobinemia, and patients with compromised cardiac or pulmonary function should be started on lower doses. Hemolysis may be alleviated to some degree by the daily administration of vitamin E (800 U per day). Methemoglobinemia associated with high-dose dapsone therapy may be monitored with venous blood and can be controlled by the administration of methylene blue tablets (Urolene Blue), 130 mg once to three times daily with meals. Dapsone may be associated with idiosyncratic reactions. These reactions include a flulike illness associated with elevated liver enzymes and potentially life-threatening neutropenia. These idiosyncratic reactions tend to occur early in the treatment course. Blood counts with differentials and liver function studies should be obtained on a biweekly basis for the first 2 to 3 months of therapy. Screening examinations should be obtained monthly for 2 to 3 months, and then every 3 to 4 months thereafter. High doses of dapsone may also be associated with a peripheral neuropathy.

The use of immunosuppressive agents for systemic vasculitis has been well described. Patients with life-threatening vasculitic syndromes such as Wegener's granulomatosis, polyarteritis nodosa, or allergic granulomatosis of Churg and Strauss are often treated with a combination of divided dose corticosteroids and immunosuppressive agents including cyclophosphamide (Cytoxan) or azathioprine (Imuran). Controlled studies have shown that treatment with these agents is lifesaving within this clinical context. However, despite the scattered anecdotal reports of their usefulness in skin-limited vasculitis, the use of these immunosuppressive agents in this type of vasculitis is of unproven benefit.

DISEASES OF THE NAILS

method of
ANTONELLA TOSTI, M.D., and
ANNA MARIA PELUSO, M.D.
University of Bologna
Bologna, Italy

The nail unit consists of four specialized epithelia: the nail matrix, the nail bed, the proximal nail fold, and the hyponichium. The nail matrix is a germinative epithelial structure that gives rise to a fully keratinized multilayered sheet of cornified cells—the nail plate. In longitudinal sections, the nail matrix consists of a proximal (dorsal) and a distal (ventral) region. Because the vertical axes of nail matrix cells are oriented diagonally and distally, proximal nail matrix keratinocytes produce the upper portion of the nail plate. The lower portion of the nail plate derives from distal nail matrix keratinocytes. Nail plate corneocytes are tightly connected by desmosomes and complex digitations.

The nail plate is a rectangular, translucent, and transparent structure that appears pink because of the vessels of the underlying nail bed. The proximal part of the nail plate of the fingernails, especially the thumbs, show a whitish, opaque, half moon–shaped area, the lunula, that corresponds to the visible portion of the distal nail matrix. The shape of the lunula determines the shape of the free edge of the plate. The nail plate is firmly attached to the nail bed, which partially contributes to nail formation along its length. The longitudinal orientation of the capillary vessels in the nail bed explains the linear pattern of the nail bed haemorrhages. Proximally and laterally the nail plate is surrounded by the nail folds. The horny layer of the proximal nail fold forms the cuticle, which intimately adheres to the underlying nail plate and prevents its separation from the proximal nail fold. Distally, the nail bed continues with the hyponichium, which marks the separation of the nail plate from the digit. The nail plate grows continuously and uniformly throughout life. Average nail growth is faster in fingernails (3 mm per month) than in toenails (1–1.5 mm per month). Replacement of a fingernail usually requires about 6 months, and replacement of a toenail requires 12 to 18 months. The peculiar kinetics of nail matrix keratinization explain why diseases of the proximal nail matrix result in nail plate surface abnormalities, whereas diseases of the distal matrix result in abnormalities of the ventral nail plate or the nail free edge, or both.

BRITTLE NAILS

Nail brittleness causes several clinical symptoms, including splitting, softening, lamellar exfoliation and onychorrhexis.

Brittle nails are a common complaint. They are often an idiopathic condition but can also be a symptom of a large number of dermatological nail disorders. Although brittle nails have been linked with many internal diseases, the high frequency of nail fragility in the general population makes it difficult to prove the validity of any such association. Environmental and occupational factors that produce progressive dehydration of the nail plate play an important role in the development of idiopathic nail brittleness. Management of brittle nails requires preventive and protective measures to avoid nail plate dehydration. Patients should wear cotton gloves under rubber gloves during household chores, avoid frequent handwashing, and keep their nails short. Nail varnishes may be protective, but the use of nail varnish removers should be restrained because it exacerbates brittleness.

Local therapies are useful in the treatment of nail brittleness. Application of hydrophilic petrolatum (Aquaphor) on wet nails at bedtime helps to retain the moisture in the nail plate. Frequent application of topical preparations containing hydrophilic substances, such as hyaluronic acid, alpha-hydroxy acids, and proteoglycans, may favor nail plate rehydration. An oral treatment with biotin,* 2.5 mg per day for several months, can be useful because it may improve the synthesis of the lipid molecules that produce binding between nail plate corneocytes.

ACUTE PARONYCHIA

Acute paronychia is usually caused by *Staphylococcus aureus,* although other bacteria and herpes simplex occasionally may be responsible. A minor trauma commonly precedes the development of the infection. The affected digit shows an acute inflammation with erythema, swelling, pus formation, and pain. Whenever possible, cultures should be taken. Treatment includes local medications with antiseptics, administration of systemic antibiotics, and incision and drainage of the abscess.

CHRONIC PARONYCHIA

Chronic paronychia is an inflammatory disorder of the proximal nail fold typically affecting patients whose hands are continually exposed to a wet environment and multiple microtraumas that favor cuticle damage. When the cuticle is damaged or lost, the epidermal barrier of the proximal nail fold is destroyed and the proximal nail fold is suddenly exposed to a large number of environmental hazards. Irritants and allergens may easily penetrate the proximal nail fold and produce a contact dermatitis that is responsible for the chronic inflammation. An immediate hypersensitivity reaction to food ingredients is commonly observed. Clinically, the proximal and lateral nail folds show mild erythema and swelling. The cuticle is lost, and the ventral portion of the

*Not FDA approved for this indication.

proximal nail fold becomes separated from the nail plate. With time, the nail fold retracts and becomes thickened and rounded. The nail plate frequently shows transverse grooves and discoloration of the lateral margins. Onychomadesis may be the result of a severe inflammatory exacerbation. The course of chronic paronychia is frequently interspersed with self-limited episodes of painful acute inflammation due to secondary *Candida* and bacterial infections.

Patients with chronic paronychia should avoid a wet environment, chronic microtrauma and contact with irritants or allergens.

High-potency topical steroids (clobetasol propionate 0.05% [Temovate ointment]) once a day at bedtime are an effective first-line therapy. If Candida is present, a topical imidazole derivative should be applied in the morning. Topical antifungals alone and systemic antifungals are not useful. In severe cases, systemic steroids (prednisone 20 mg per day) can be given for a few days to obtain a prompt reduction of inflammation and pain.

Acute exacerbations of chronic paronychia do not necessitate antibiotic treatment because they subside spontaneously in a few days. Complete recovery of the condition usually requires several weeks and treatment should be continued until the cuticle has regrown. Recurrences are frequent because the barrier function of the proximal nail fold may be impaired for months or even years after an episode of chronic paronychia.

ONYCHOLYSIS

Onycholysis is detachment of the nail plate from the nail bed. Starting from the central or lateral portion of the nail plate free margin, onycholysis progresses proximally and can even involve the whole nail. The onycholytic area looks whitish because of the presence of air under the detached nail plate. It may occasionally show a greenish or brown discoloration due to colonization of the onycholytic space by chromogenic bacteria (*Pseudomonas aeruginosa*), molds, or yeasts. Onycholysis may be idiopathic or represent a symptom of numerous diseases, such as psoriasis, onychomycosis, contact dermatitis, or drug reactions. The pathogenesis of idiopathic onycholysis is still unknown. A waterborne environment facilitates the development of this condition, which is much more frequent in housewives. We found Zaias's suggestion of using a hair-dryer to dry the subungual area after immersion in water very useful. The detached nails should be cut away, and this procedure should be repeated until the nail plate grows attached. A symptomatic treatment with a topical antiseptic solution (thymol 4% in chloroform) or a topical imidazole derivative can be prescribed.

ONYCHOMYCOSIS

The term onychomycosis describes fungal infection of the nail. Almost all cases of onychomycosis, however, result from a dermatophytic invasion of the nail, onychomycosis due to nondermatophytic fungi being exceedingly rare. *Candida* onychomycosis is a very uncommon condition that only occurs in chronic cutaneous candidiasis or human immunodeficiency virus infection. Even though molds can be occasionally isolated from dystrophic toenails, their role as primitive pathogens is still unclear, because molds most commonly colonize nails with pre-existent nail disorders, especially dermatophytic onychomycosis or traumatic dystrophies.

Except for superficial white onychomycosis, which can be treated with any topical antifungal after scraping of the affected area, treatment of onychomycosis always requires a systemic antifungal drug. Onychomycosis of the toenails is more difficult to cure and recurs more frequently than onychomycosis of the fingernails.

Unfortunately, most of the available antifungals can produce serious side effects especially in patients with impairment of their hepatic function. Although new topical antifungals, such as amorolfine 5% nail lacquer (Loceryl) and bifonazole 1% in 40% urea ointment, have been reported to be effective in a proportion of patients, further studies are needed for a final judgment. Until recently, oral treatment of onychomycosis had consisted of two antifungal drugs: griseofulvin and ketoconazole (Nizoral),* the latter being scarcely used because of its hepatotoxicity. Treating onychomycosis with griseofulvin (Grifulvin V), however, requires long-term administration of the drug (6 months for fingernails, up to 12 months for toenails), and high drug dosages (up to 2 grams per day). Toenail infections often fail to respond, and recurrences are frequent. In the last few years, three new systemic antimycotics have been introduced on the market: fluconazole (Diflucan),* itraconazole (Sporanox),* and terbinafine (Lamisil).†

All these drugs have been shown to reach the distal nail soon after starting the therapy and to persist in the nail plate for a long time (2 to 6 months) after interruption of treatment. The persistence of high post-treatment drug levels in the nail permits shorter therapies with less incidence of relapses and side effects.

Fluconazole and itraconazole are triazole derivatives with a broad-spectrum fungistatic activity. Fluconazole (Diflucan), 150 mg given once weekly or 100 mg every other day for 3 to 6 months, has been successfully tried in a limited number of patients. Itraconazole (Sporanox) is effective at dosages of 200 mg per day for 3 months. This agent may possibly work even when given for a shorter course of treatment or using intermittent therapy (400 mg daily for 1 week every month for 3 to 4 months).

Terbinafine (Lamisil) is an allylamine derivative with primary fungicidal properties against dermatophytes. This drug is probably more effective and safer than other antimycotics for long-term treatment of onychomycosis due to dermatophytes. Recommended

*Not FDA approved for this indication.
†Not available in the United States.

dosages are 250 mg per day for 2 months (fingernails) to 3 months (toenails). Preliminary studies, however, show that terbinafine may also be effective as a short-course treatment or used as intermittent therapy.

PSORIASIS

Because treatment of nail psoriasis is always disappointing, before starting a therapy the individual problems of every patient should be considered and, in particular, the degree of discomfort that results from the nail lesions. Reassuring the patients is probably the best approach for isolated nail pitting, oily patches, mild onycholysis, and splinter hemorrhages. However, diffuse onycholysis, subungual hyperkeratosis and severe nail plate surface abnormalities may require a therapeutic approach.

Local therapy of nail psoriasis is scarcely effective and only rarely induces a complete remission of the disease. Topical steroids or combinations of topical steroids with salicylic acid or retinoic acid, or both, are widely prescribed. Their efficacy is poor, even when they are applied with occlusive dressing after chemical or mechanical avulsion of the onycholytic nail plate. Long-term application of topical steroids may result in a marked atrophy of the soft tissues of the digits or even in focal resorption of the distal phalanges. Topical application of anthralin is also scarcely effective and poorly tolerated.

Topical cyclosporin A can be useful in selected cases. Because it is poorly absorbed, the drug is of little value in nail matrix psoriasis, but it can be effective in nail bed psoriasis, especially after nail plate avulsion.

In patients with pustular psoriasis, local treatment with topical antimetabolites (mercholorethamine, fluorouracil [Efudex]) is an option, even though results are variable. Possible side effects limit the use of these drugs in uncomplicated nail psoriasis.

Topical psoralens (e.g., Meladinin*) followed by ultraviolet A exposure are scarcely effective due to poor penetration of the UVA through the nail plate, especially when thickened. Topical psoralen plus ultraviolet A may be useful in pustular psoriasis when recurrent pustular lesions have produced destruction of the nail plate.

Intralesional injections of triamcinolone acetonide (Kenalog),* 2.5 mg per mL, have been proved effective in some cases of nail matrix psoriasis. However, routine use of this therapy is not recommended because of the pain caused by the injections, the local side effects (subungual hematoma, reversible atrophy and hypopigmentation on the injection site), and relapses of the nail abnormalities after discontinuation of the therapy.

Systemic treatment with steroids or cyclosporin A (Sandimmune)* can resolve the nail changes, but we recommend its use only when nail psoriasis is associated with widespread disease or psoriatic arthritis.

Retinoids are only of little value in the treatment of nail psoriasis. Administration of etretinate (Tigason) can even worsen the nail changes as a result of development of nail brittleness, pyogenic pseudogranuloma, and chronic paronychia. Oral photochemotherapy can improve crumbling of the nail plate and psoriatic involvement of the proximal nail fold. It is scarcely effective in nail pitting or in subungual hyperkeratosis. Superficial radiotherapy can have a beneficial effect on psoriatic nails, but it is not recommended because of its short-term results.

Pustular psoriasis of the nail unit usually fails to respond to conventional topical treatment. Retinoids, systemic steroids, PUVA, and cyclosporin can arrest the development of pustular lesions and avoid permanent scarring of the nail apparatus.

*Not FDA approved for this indication.

LICHEN PLANUS

Specific nail involvement occurs in about 10% of patients with lichen planus, and permanent damage of at least one nail occurs in approximately 4% of patients. Most commonly, the nail changes consist of thinning, longitudinal ridging, and distal splitting of the nail plate. The severity of the disease may vary in degree from nail to nail and within the same nail. Onycholysis and subungual hyperkeratosis can also be seen. Erythematous patches in the lunula are occasionally present. Definitive destruction of the nail matrix is responsible for pterygium and onychoatrophy.

Systemic steroids are effective in treating nail lichen planus and in preventing destruction of the nail matrix. Oral prednisone, 0.5 mg per kg every other day for 2 to 6 weeks, or intramuscular triamcinolone acetonide (Kenalog), 0.5 mg per kg every month for 2 to 3 months, usually produces recovery of the nail abnormalities. Intralesional injections of triamcinolone acetonide, 2.5 mg per mL, represent a possible, though painful, alternative when the disease is limited to a few fingernails. Mild relapses are frequently observed, but recurrences are usually responsive to therapy.

ALOPECIA AREATA (TWENTY-NAIL DYSTROPHY)

Alopecia areata has been associated with a large number of nail changes including diffuse or localized color changes, nail plate surface abnormalities, and onychomadesis. Most commonly alopecia areata of the nails produces a regular and superficial pitting that is due to focal involvement of the proximal nail matrix. A chronic and diffuse involvement of the nail apparatus causes twenty-nail dystrophy (trachyonychia), which may occasionally be the only symptom of the disease. The nail plate surface is opaque, lusterless, and rough due to excessive longitudinal striation. The nail changes do not necessarily involve all twenty nails and may occasionally be limited to a few digits. Trachyonychia is absolutely a benign condition that never causes nail scarring; the nail changes usually regress spontaneously in a few years. No treatment is recommended.

NAIL PIGMENTATION

The term melanonychia describes a brown-black discoloration of the nail plate. Longitudinal melanonychia may be caused by a focal activation of the nail matrix melanocytes or by nail matrix nevus or melanoma. Focal hyperactivity of the nail matrix melanocytes is usual in blacks and common in Japanese, but it is rare in whites. It may be seen in a large number of nail disorders or systemic conditions.

Patients with chronic adrenal insufficiency or with megaloblastic anemia due to vitamin B_{12} or folate deficiency may develop longitudinal pigmented bands in the fingernails and the toenails. Transverse or longitudinal melanonychia involving several fingernails and toenails can be a side effect of numerous drugs including cancer therapeutic agents and zidovudine. Differential diagnosis between benign longitudinal melanonychia and malignant melanoma may be impossible on a clinical basis. A light blue pigmentation of the lunulae can be a sign of Wilson's disease or of argyria. A grayish brown discoloration of the nails can occur after chronic exposure to topical preparations containing mercury. Nail pigmentation due to drugs or systemic disorders is usually reversible after discontinuation of the drug or resolution of the associated disease.

YELLOW NAIL SYNDROME

This term describes the association of slowly growing yellow nails with primary lymphoedema and respiratory tract involvement. Nails are pale yellow to yellow-green in color, thickened, opaque, and excessively curved from side to side. Onycholysis is frequent. The nail changes may improve spontaneously or after resolution of the associated systemic disease. Oral vitamin E*† at dosages of 600 to 1200 IU daily for 6 to 18 months induces a complete clearing of the nail changes in most patients. Although the mechanism of action of vitamin E in yellow nail syndrome is still unknown, antioxidant properties of α-tocoferol may account for its efficacy.

A 5% solution of vitamin E*‡ in dimethyl sulfoxide produced marked clinical improvement in a double-blind controlled study. The efficacy of topical vitamin E, however, still needs confirmation.

INGROWN NAILS

Ingrown nails which more commonly affect the great toe of young adults, are a common complaint. Hyperhidrosis, congenital malalignment, improper cutting of toenails, as well as unsatisfactory footwear all contribute to the development of this painful condition. The condition starts when spicules breaking off from the lateral edge of the nail plate penetrate into the tissues of the lateral nail fold. In this phase, the inflammatory reaction produces pain, redness, and swelling. Treatment is conservative and includes extraction of the embedded spicula and introduction of a package of nonabsorbent cotton (soaked in a disinfectant) under the corner of the nail to prevent further penetration of the lateral nail fold. This dressing should be replaced daily. In advanced stages, the lateral edge of the nail plate is enclosed in an overgrowth of granulation tissue that, with time, may become epithelialized. Although application of high-potency steroids or cryosurgery may reduce the granulation tissue, surgical or chemical (phenol) partial matricectomy is necessary in most cases.

*Not FDA approved for this indication.
†Exceeds dosage recommended by the manufacturer.
‡Not available in the United States.

WARTS

Periungual and subungual warts are usually difficult to treat and frequently recur. Routine treatments include cryosurgery, electrocautery and desiccation, CO_2 laser, and topical anti-wart solutions containing salicylic and lactic acids.

Intralesional injections of bleomycin (Blenoxane)* have been successfully used to treat viral warts for many years. The powder should be diluted to a concentration of 1 U per mL with saline. This solution can be stored at −20°C in glass for several months. Part of this solution should be further diluted to 0.1 to 0.5 U per mL and injected into multiple loci of the warts. Patients with vascular impairment and women of childbearing age should not be treated because the drug has been reported to produce Raynaud's disease and to be systemically absorbed.

A bifurcate vaccination needle can be used to introduce bleomycin (1 U per mL sterile saline solution) into warts using the multiple puncture technique suggested by Shelley†. After the administration of local anesthesia the bleomycin solution is dropped onto the wart, which is then punctured with a disposable bifurcated needle (Allergy Laboratory of OHIO Inc) approximately 40 times per 5 mm^2 area of the wart. No medications are required. Three weeks after treatment, the eschar can be pared away and the area examined for residual warts, which can be reinjected. This technique minimizes the amount of bleomycin introduced into the skin and avoids introduction of the drug into the dermis.

Topical immunotherapy with strong topical sensitizers (squaric acid dibutylester [SADBE],‡ diphencyprone) is an effective and painless modality of treatment for multiple warts. We use SADBE or diphencyprone 2% in acetone for sensitization. After 21 days, weekly applications are carried out with dilutions from 0.001% to 1.0% according to the patient's response. Complete cure usually requires 3 to 4 months.

*Not FDA approved for this indication.
†Shelley WB and Shelley ED: Intralesional bleomycin sulfate therapy for warts. Arch Dermatol *127*:234–6, 1991.
‡Not available in the United States.

MYXOID CYSTS

Myxoid cysts are common benign tumors of the nail unit, most frequently affecting elderly women. The cyst, which is usually located on the dorsal aspect of the distal phalanx, has a viscous, gelatinous content. Cysts localized in the proximal nail fold may compress the nail matrix and produce longitudinal depressions or grooves in the nail plate. The cysts frequently communicate with the distal phalangeal joint through a tract that pumps synovial fluid into the cysts.

Treatment of myxoid cysts include surgical excision, intralesional injections of triamcinolone acetonide (Kenalog, 3 to 5 mg per mL) or sclerosing agents (3% solution of sodium tetradecilsulfate [Sotradecol]*) after evacuation of the cyst content with a sterile needle. Cryosurgery is effective but painful and associated with considerable morbidity. Two 30-second freezes separated by 1 minute of thaw time are usually necessary. Before freezing, it is advisable to express the cyst content and ask the patient to remove rings.

Unfortunately recurrence rates are high with the use of any of the available treatments, and cysts frequently recur even after surgery if the tract leading from the cyst to the joint capsule is not dissected.

KELOIDS

method of
JOHN C. MURRAY, M.D.
Duke University Medical Center
Durham, North Carolina

Keloids are benign abnormal wound responses that develop in predisposed individuals. These patients may notice this abnormal connective tissue response following trauma, inflammation, surgery, or burns. The cause for this abnormal wound response remains unknown, because keloids may result from abundant deposition of collagen and glycoprotein. These fibrous growths create significant cosmetic and symptomatic problems. Multiple treatments for keloids have been attempted, and treatment responses are highly variable. Patients should be informed of the treatment limitations, and physicians should exercise particular care in choosing appropriate therapy for each lesion because no single treatment approach has been proved effective.

In order to determine appropriate therapy, it is essential to distinguish between hypertrophic scars and keloids. Hypertrophic scars tend to regress with time, and often these lesions may be treated with local measures such as intralesional corticosteroid injection, pressure devices, or topical therapy such as retinoic acid or Silastic gel sheeting. Hypertrophic scars tend to occur soon after local trauma and may subside or diminish within 1 to 2 years. In general, hypertrophic scars are limited to the wound boundary, and usually, the size of the hypertrophic scar is related to the extent of the wound or trauma. In general, surgical revision or excision of hypertrophic scars often improves the condition.

*Not available in the United States.

Keloids may be distinguished from hypertrophic scars, but sometimes this distinction is not always clear. Keloids may arise within 1 to 2 weeks following antecedent trauma or injury, but some keloids may appear after a delay of up to 1 to 2 years. In general, the clinical course of keloids is progressive and sustained without spontaneous resolution. Keloids may soften and flatten in elderly patients. In general, keloids extend beyond the site of the initial wound or trauma and tend to extend beyond this area. Disproportionately large fibrous growths may follow seemingly minor antecedent events. Keloids excised by surgery alone have a high frequency of recurrence; the best results have been reported with keloid excision followed by adjunct therapy.

TREATMENT

Corticosteroid Injection

An appropriate initial approach to keloids is intralesional corticosteroid injection. These injections may soften and flatten keloid bulk. Lesions rarely resolve completely, but patients often note symptomatic improvement with diminution in pain and pruritus. Patients' responses to intralesional corticosteroid injection are highly variable in terms of shrinkage of keloid bulk and pigment response. Test doses of triamcinolone acetonide may be varied from 10 mg per mL, 20 mg per mL, 30 mg per mL to 40 mg per mL. Trial injection volumes of 0.1 mL may identify the best response with least side effect. Side effects of these injections include skin atrophy, telangiectasia, and necrosis. Care must be exercised to inject the corticosteroid intralesionally and to avoid inadvertent deposition in surrounding dermis or subcutaneous tissue. The corticosteroid preparation is a suspension and should be well dispersed before injection.

Corticosteroid injection should be administered with Luer-Lok needle and syringe. A 25- or 30-gauge needle is generally used, but 30-gauge needles may be clogged with 40 mg per mL triamcinolone preparations. A dental syringe such as Intra-Lig Syringe (item #76–50 Miltex, NY) is a mechanical syringe that requires less effort to inject firm fibrous masses. Injections may be spaced 0.5 to 1.0 cm apart over the entire lesion so that the corticosteroid is injected into the center of bulk of the keloid mass. Subcutaneous lidocaine (Xylocaine) may be used for certain keloids, such as sternal keloids, to minimize patient discomfort. The treatment interval should be adjusted to patient response. In general, subsequent injections are less painful and the infiltration of corticosteroid is easier. Some patients report diminished effects after 3 to 4 weeks and should be treated at monthly intervals. Some patients may return every 2 to 3 months with satisfactory control of symptoms and lesion size.

Intralesional corticosteroid injection is often combined with cryotherapy. Keloids may be treated with a light frost for up to 5 seconds. After 15 to 20 minutes, local tissue edema and cellular change may facilitate ease of infiltration of the steroid injection. Cryotherapy alone has induced variable responses because hypopigmentation following cryotherapy has been a problem. When pigment effect is not a major consideration, aggressive cryotherapy (45-second freeze cycles, repeated every 3 to 4 weeks) flattens keloids.

Surgery

Surgical excision of keloids results in a high recurrence rate. Keloids to be excised should be selected carefully, and patients should be advised of the need of adjunct therapy to minimize the risk of recurrence. In general, significant symptomatic or disfiguring keloids that do not respond to corticosteroid injection or other conservative measures should be considered for surgical excision. Excision removes the keloidal mass, and patients must be willing to return for adjunctive therapy.

The surgical approach should be tailored to the size and location of the lesion. Small lesions with a base less than 1 cm may be excised and the wounds closed primarily. Keloids located in certain areas such as the posterior earlobe may be removed by shave excision and the base treated with adjunct therapy such as pressure therapy or intralesional corticosteroid injection. Larger lesions may be surgically excised, and the resultant defect may be repaired by using the epithelial surface as a flap. The overlying epithelium of the keloid may be used as a graft to cover the excised area in order to avoid another donor site that potentially could become another keloid.

During keloid excision, tissue trauma should be minimized, if at all possible. Any trauma, such as electrosurgical hemostasis, undermining, or suturing, may potentially exacerbate keloid formation. Keloid recurrence is more likely if the wound has dead space, foreign material, hematoma, infection, or wound tension. The surgeon should plan the excision so that skin edges can be joined with minimum tension. Keloidal remnants may remain in the wound edges in order to minimize tension. Such remnants do not increase the risk of recurrence. Such keloidal remnants may reduce tissue trauma during excision and may provide a better cosmetic result.

Laser surgery for removal of nuchal and earlobe keloids was reported with initial enthusiasm, but adjunct therapy with corticosteroid injection or other measures are necessary to minimize risk of recurrence. CO_2 laser surgical excision has a recurrence rate similar to that of scalpel excision without adjunct therapy. Lasers induce delayed healing times and modify wound healing by suppression of collagen synthesis. Further studies are needed to establish whether this modified wound healing has a clinical advantage over more conventional surgical techniques.

Adjuvant Therapy

Patients with keloids often describe significant symptoms such as pain and pruritus. For certain patients, oral antihistamines can provide significant relief of these symptoms. Keloids have an increased number of mast cells, and oral antihistamines may limit intense pruritus. Controlling this pruritus may help patients reduce local trauma from repeated rubbing. This local trauma may reduce mast cell mediators and other growth factors that may promote further keloid growth.

Oral medications have been used in keloid therapy. These medications, including penicillamine (Cuprimine, Depen),* methotrexate* and beta-aminopropionitile fumurate (BAPN)*† have been used to interfere with collagen synthesis and cross-linking. Experience with these medications is limited and remains experimental until further efficacy can be demonstrated. Colchicine* has been used to increase tissue collagenase activity and accelerate collagen degradation. When colchicine was combined with surgical excision, 32% of keloid lesions did not recur in 5-year follow-up.

Various pressure devices have been used to flatten keloids or to prevent recurrence after surgery. These devices include elastic garments tightly fitted to body sites, spring pressure earrings, and acrylic ear splints. The devices must exert 24 mm Hg pressure in order to exceed inherent capillary pressure and should be worn continuously for a minimum of 6 months. Removal for daily hygiene should not exceed 30 minutes per day. Although these devices test the limits of patients' compliance, they have been reported effective as an adjunct therapy.

For selected patients, radiation therapy may be considered with surgical excision. In general, radiation therapy is reserved for adult patients with significant symptoms or disability from their keloids. This therapy is not used for adolescents or young patients, as well as patients with keloids that can be managed by other techniques. A concern about the risk of postradiation neoplasm remains a deterrent for use of radiation therapy but none of the published reviews in the past 10 years cite such an occurrence. These reviews report good cosmetic results and relief of symptoms in 72% to 92% of patients. Various treatment regimens have been used such as electron beam or orthovoltage radiation. In general, radiation therapy is given immediately after surgery in three fractionated doses of 400 rads each. Radiation side effects include localized pruritus, paresthesias, and pain.

Another adjunctive therapy is the use of Silastic gel sheeting. This sheeting is made of polydimethyl siloxane polymer and has been reported to be useful in improving keloids and in preventing postoperative recurrence. The mechanism for improvement from Silastic gel sheeting is unknown, but release of silicon oil from the sheeting may account for this effect even though biopsy specimens of treated lesions have revealed no evidence of silicon absorption. Concerns about the potential deleterious effects of topical silicon may limit the use of this treatment.

Topical retinoids can soften and reduce keloid growth to a moderate extent. Patients may apply ret-

*Not FDA approved for this indication.
†Not available in the United States.

inoic acid cream* 0.1% once or twice daily to involved lesions. Patients have noted softening and shrinkage of the keloids with this therapy. Improvement with this treatment is modest in that a 20% reduction in total volume of treated keloids has been reported.

Unfortunately little consensus exists about appropriate therapy for keloids. Multiple therapies exist, and unsatisfactory results are common. It is essential that the physician emphasize the importance of prevention in that all efforts should be made to minimize or avoid stimuli that could promote an abnormal wound response in a predisposed individual. Physicians should select therapy after determining whether or not the lesion is a keloid and should counsel the patient about the possible outcomes with each treatment.

WARTS
(Verruca Vulgaris)

method of
MORRISA BASKIN, M.D.
University of Washington
Seattle, Washington

Warts (verrucae) are caused by infection with the DNA-containing human papillomavirus (HPV). Warts are common in children and young adults, with an incidence approaching 10%. Breaks in the skin, moisture, and maceration facilitate transmission of the virus. Autoinoculation is common so that new lesions may develop on adjacent surfaces in a so-called kissing fashion.

There are several morphologic subtypes of verruca. Common warts are keratotic, well-defined verrucous papules occurring typically on the hands, feet, elbows, and knees. Plantar warts on the sole of the foot are flat owing to constant pressure pushing them inward. Flat warts (verruca plana) are flesh-colored or light pink, flat-topped papules occurring most commonly on the face of children. Venereal warts or condylomata acuminata occur in moist anogenital regions. Condylomata can be pink cauliflower-like exophytic growths, or they may appear as individual discrete pink papules. Anogenital warts are usually, but not exclusively, transmitted by sexual contact.

More than 60 HPV types have been identified using DNA hybridization. There are important clinical considerations concerning HPV typing because genital tract carcinoma and dysplasia have been linked with HPV infection. HPV types 16, 18, 31, 34, 35, 39, and 48 are strongly associated with genital and cervical carcinoma.

PRINCIPLES OF THERAPY

The majority of warts are benign epithelial tumors that will spontaneously regress in 3 months to 5 years. Warts should be treated because they are contagious and have the potential for rapid proliferative growth. Plantar warts may be painful and interfere with normal ambulation. All condylomata need to be treated because of their oncogenic potential. The ideal goals of treatment should be destruction of the wart, with minimal pain and morbidity and no recurrence. Unfortunately, none of the many treatments available fulfill these goals. A conservative nonscarring approach with avoidance of undue pain and trauma should be used for children with nongenital warts.

Available treatments are either destructive or immunologic (Table 1). Destructive methods are successful because verrucae are limited to the epidermis. However, if the wart is not totally destroyed, recurrences are common. Because the cell-mediated immune response is responsible for the eradication of the virus, immunologic methods would seem to hold the most promise, but these are not yet uniformly successful.

*Not FDA approved for this indication.

Cryotherapy

Freezing with liquid nitrogen is one of the most common therapies and can be used for all types of warts. After first paring the wart of excess keratin, the wart is frozen with a hand-held unit (Cry-Ac or Cryogun) or cotton-tipped applicator. A 2- or 3-mm margin of normal skin surrounding the wart is also frozen to reduce recurrences. The length and number of freeze-thaw cycles depends on the size and thickness of the verruca. Flat warts typically require a 5- to 20-second freeze, whereas plantar warts may need a 1-minute freeze-thaw cycle. A red halo develops around the wart after freezing, and a blister or hemorrhagic blister may develop in 1 or 2 days. Throbbing pain after freezing typically subsides in 15 to 30 minutes. Small warts may respond to a single treatment, but for large warts, recurrences can be reduced if the warts are treated again in 2 or 3 weeks. Side effects of cryotherapy include hypopigmentation, hyperpigmentation, and scarring (rarely). Prolonged parasthesias can develop if warts are located over nerves, such as the lateral digits. Freezing is contraindicated in patients with a history of cold urticaria, cryoglobulinemia, or Raynaud's disease (especially when warts are on the fingers).

Surgery

After local anesthesia, warts can be debulked or destroyed with electrodesiccation and curettage, or

TABLE 1. **Methods of Wart Treatment**

Destructive	Immunologic
Cryotherapy	Dinitrochlorobenzene*
Surgery	Squaric acid*
Laser	Diphenylcyclopropenone*
Keratolytics	Interferons
Trichloracetic acid	
Podophyllin	
5-Fluorouracil (Efudex)*	
Bleomycin (Blenoxane)*	
Cantharidin (Cantharone)	
Tretinoin (Retin-A)*	

*Not FDA approved for this indication.
Modified from Bolton RA: Nongenital warts: classification and treatment options. Am Fam Phys *43*(6):2049–2056, 1991. Published by the American Academy of Family Physicians.

cold surgical steel. Recurrences around the surgical site can be problematic. Side effects of surgery include infection and scarring. Scarring can be a significant problem, especially for warts located over joints. Some studies have shown no difference in success rates between conventional surgical techniques and the carbon dioxide laser, whereas others have shown an advantage (higher success rates) for electrocautery over laser for treatment of perianal condylomata.

Laser

The CO_2 laser has been used as a successful therapeutic modality for both verrucae and genital warts. The CO_2 laser can be used for surgical debulking of large warts, especially condylomata, or for treatment of warts recalcitrant to other modalities. Cure rates range from 50 to 90%, whereas recurrences can be up to 10%. The advantages of the CO_2 laser are a bloodless surgical field and potentially decreased postoperative pain because of sealing of nerves. Disadvantages include scarring (both atrophic and hypertrophic), high cost, temporary loss of function of the treated area, and potentially prolonged healing time. Treatment of periungual warts may lead to permanent nail dystrophy. Additionally, intact HPV DNA has been recovered from the CO_2 laser plume after treatment of warts.

Keratolytics

The use of topical salicylic acid in liquid, gel, or plasters has the advantage of home therapy and may be preferred by children who cannot tolerate painful procedures. The warts are first soaked in warm water for about 5 to 10 minutes, dried, and then the salicylic acid preparation is applied under tape occlusion. After 8 to 10 hours, the tape is removed and a pumice stone or nail file is used to remove excess keratin. The process is repeated every day or every other day for many weeks. Irritation of the surrounding normal skin may occur. Keratolytics can be effective therapy, but patient compliance is important because the process is prolonged.

Trichloracetic Acid

Trichloracetic acid in concentrations from 15 to 85% produces tissue sloughing and is used primarily for genital warts but occasionally for verrucae as well. The penetration of trichloracetic acid is difficult to control, and if it penetrates into the dermis, ulcerations, scar tissue, prolonged healing, and prolonged patient discomfort may result. There have been few controlled published studies comparing TCA with other treatment modalities.

Podophyllin and Podophyllotoxin

Podophyllin, a crude resin extract from the May apple plant, has been used to treat anogenital warts for nearly 50 years. The best results are achieved when it is applied to moist condylomata that have been present for less than 6 months. The number of applications of podophyllin varies greatly. Typically, three or more treatment sessions are needed. Recurrences with podophyllin therapy vary from 20 to 70%. Local side effects include burning, inflammation, erythema, and occasionally, necrosis and scarring. Some of the irritation can be minimized by protecting the surrounding skin with an inert cream or paste, and washing the podophyllin off in 4 to 6 hours. Allergy to benzoin, which is frequently used in compounding podophyllin, can develop. Systemic side effects may occur, especially if the medicine is used on a large surface area for prolonged periods of time. Systemic side effects may include nausea, vomiting, fever, confusion, coma, leukopenia, thrombocytopenia, and renal failure. Rare deaths have been reported. Podophyllin is contraindicated in pregnancy, because it is teratogenic and toxic to the fetus.

Podophyllotoxin is one of the most biologically active lignans in podophyllin resin. Podophyllotoxin (Condylox) can be used successfully for penile and vulvar and vaginal warts. Condylox is applied twice a day for 3 days in a row, and this cycle is repeated each week for 4 weeks. Mild local side effects include burning, stinging, erythema, and erosions. Systemic absorption at usual doses of Condylox is uncommon. Advantages of Podophyllotoxin are that it is applied by the patient, and it has a better safety profile as compared with podophyllin.

Bleomycin

Bleomycin* has been successfully used to treat warts for over 10 years. Bleomycin has antitumor, antibacterial, and antiviral activity. Success rates with intralesional bleomycin have ranged from 65% to 100%. Bleomycin sulfate is injected at a concentration of 0.5 to 1.0 U per mL with a 30-gauge needle directly into the warts to achieve blanching. Warts smaller than 5 mm receive approximately 0.2 mL, whereas warts larger than 1 cm may require approximately 1.0 mL. The total volume of bleomycin injected at one visit is limited to 2.0 to 3.0 mL. If necessary, warts may be retreated at 2- to 4-week intervals. Moderate pain with injection occurs, and local pain, erythema, and swelling may be present for 24 to 72 hours. The pain of injection can be reduced by using bleomycin reconstituted in 1% lidocaine. During the first week after injection, the warts become black and an eschar develops. Pigmentary changes and scarring are rare. Serious but uncommon side effects include Raynaud's phenomenon in fingers injected with bleomycin and permanent nail dystrophy if the nail matrix is inadvertently infiltrated. Nail changes and Raynaud's phenomenon have not been reported when bleomycin is injected with the bifurcated needle puncture technique. A drop of bleomycin sulfate solution is dropped onto the wart and then a bifurcated beveled vaccination

*Not FDA approved for this indication.

needle is used to rapidly puncture the wart. Bleomycin is widely used for treatment of warts in Japan and Canada, but it is currently not FDA approved for this indication.

5-Fluorouracil

5-Fluorouracil (5-FU), a fluorinated pyrimidine antimetabolite, has been used successfully for years for the treatment of genital warts, but it is not FDA approved for this indication. Papillary condylomata respond better than flat lesions. Periodic application of 5% 5-FU cream (Efudex)* is as effective as daily application, but it is tolerated better. In general, the cream needs to be applied for prolonged periods, usually 10 weeks, for a favorable response to occur. In addition to being used for therapy of resistant condylomata, 5-FU can be used after surgery or laser treatment to prevent recurrences. The main limitation with 5-FU is the high rate of irritation. Irritant dermatitis, mucosal erosion, and ulceration are common and can be severe. 5-FU should not be used in pregnancy.

Interferons

Interferons have antiviral, antiproliferative, and immunomodulatory properties. Thus far, genital warts respond more favorably than nongenital warts. Systemic interferon is more effective than placebo for condylomata, but the number of complete responses is low and systemic side effects are common. Intralesional interferon-alpha is FDA approved for the treatment of genital warts. Recombinant interferon alpha-2B (Intron A) is injected intralesionally with 1 million IU per lesion, up to 5 million IU per treatment session, 3 times a week for 3 weeks. Human leukocyte–derived interferon-alpha n 3 (Alferon N) is injected with 250,000 IU per wart twice a week for 8 weeks with a maximum dose per treatment session of 2.5 million IU. Intralesional injection is typically accompanied by transient burning or stinging. Mild flulike symptoms consisting of fever, myalgias, and headache may occur in up to 50% of patients. Advantages of intralesional interferon are that warts disappear without scarring, and treatment is generally well tolerated. Disadvantages are that the number of complete resolutions of lesions is low and recurrences are common.

Immunotherapy

An allergic contact dermatitis develops in topical immunotherapy and stimulates the patient's cell-mediated immune response. First, the patient is sensitized to a chemical, and the antecubital fossae is used for warts located on the hands while the popliteal fossae is the site of sensitization for warts located on the feet. Approximately 3 weeks after sensitization, a lower concentration of the sensitizing agent is applied to each of the warts and covered with tape occlusion. Every 2 to 3 weeks the chemical is re-applied until gradually the warts become dry and brown. At present, three chemicals are used for immunotherapy, including dinitrochlorobenzene (DNCB), diphenylcyclopropenone (DCP), and squaric acid dibutylester. Dinitrochlorobenzene is positive in the Ames test of mutagenicity. Pruritus and erythema at the sites of treatment can occur with topical immunotherapy. Less common, but more serious, side effects include a blistering eruption or lymphangitis.

*Not FDA approved for this indication.

NEVI

method of
RONALD J. BARR, M.D.
University of California, Irvine
Irvine, California

Melanocytic nevi represent benign proliferations of melanocytes, which are the melanin-producing cells in the skin. For the most part, nevi are important because they are related to malignant melanoma. Approximately 30 to 50% of malignant melanomas appear to arise in pre-existing nevi. Also, studies have shown that the risk for developing malignant melanoma is proportional to the number of melanocytic nevi one has, even if these nevi are clinically normal. Ultraviolet light exposure appears to be important in the development of nevi as well as malignant melanoma, and it may be responsible for some nevi evolving into malignant melanoma. There are various types of melanocytic nevi. The most important are acquired melanocytic nevi, dysplastic nevi (atypical nevi), and congenital melanocytic nevi. Other variants include common and cellular blue nevi, Spitz nevi, pigmented spindle cell nevi and deep penetrating nevi. The latter three nevi derive their importance primarily because of their histologic similarity to malignant melanoma.

ACQUIRED MELANOCYTIC NEVI INCLUDING ATYPICAL NEVI

These lesions represent the most common variants of nevi. The average adult has approximately 20 acquired nevi. Most develop within the first 4 years of life and have a predilection for sun-exposed skin. Conventionally, acquired nevi are divided into junctional, intradermal, and compound variants. Junctional nevi exhibit a proliferation of nevus cells at the junction between the epidermis and the dermis, intradermal nevi contain nevus cells predominantly within the dermis, and compound nevi contain nevus cells in both locations. Junctional nevi are flat; whereas intradermal and compound nevi are elevated. All of these lesions usually measure less than 6 mm in diameter, and are symmetrical and uniform in color. Junctional nevi have a tendency to be darker brown than the others.

In recent years, much attention has been given to

clinically atypical nevi because some may represent precursors to malignant melanoma. These lesions have been referred to as dysplastic nevi, atypical nevi, atypical moles, and a variety of other terms, many of which refer to histologic abnormalities or atypia. For purposes of this discussion, these lesions are referred to simply as atypical nevi. Although some experts believe that these lesions are distinct from acquired nevi, there is considerable evidence that they are present on a spectrum with normal acquired nevi at one end and malignant melanoma at the other. Atypical nevi have macular or papular components, or both, and irregular borders. They are usually larger than common nevi and exhibit color variation, ranging from tan to dark brown, often on a pink background. There is a definite relationship between the presence of atypical nevi and malignant melanoma, either as precursor lesions, or less likely, as cutaneous markers for melanoma. All patients with atypical nevi are at some increased risk for developing melanoma. Those with a few atypical nevi without any family history of melanoma are at only slightly greater risk than the general population. However, for those individuals with multiple atypical nevi and a family history of atypical nevi with accompanying melanomas (classical familial melanoma syndrome or dysplastic nevus syndrome), the lifetime risk may be as high as 100%. Therefore, it is imperative that prognostication for atypical nevi be based on a clinicopathologic correlation. Single or a few atypical nevi are extremely common and probably occur in approximately between 30% and 50% of the adult population.

Histologically, atypical nevi are characterized by cytologic atypia, an abnormal pattern of distribution of nevus cells, and a host inflammatory response. Although it is controversial, the degree of atypia may be graded from mild to severe. The NIH Consensus Conference on the Diagnosis and Treatment of Early Malignant Melanoma (January, 1992) suggested that these lesions be called nevi with architectural atypia, with a statement as to the presence and degree of melanocytic atypia. Because this is rather cumbersome terminology, many pathologists continue to use terms such as dysplastic nevus, atypical nevus, atypical mole, Clark's nevus, and atypical melanocytic proliferation. It is imperative, therefore, that the pathologist communicate with the clinician regarding specific terminology and its clinical implications. Minimal atypia is probably of no major concern and is an extremely common finding. Moderate atypia or worse is probably significant insofar as it makes sense that these nevi do have a greater chance of becoming malignant melanoma compared with normal nevi. Some nevi with severe atypia probably represent melanoma in situ or perhaps even melanoma with invasion.

Treatment of Acquired Nevi Including Atypical Nevi

Nevi showing any clinical or histologic atypia should be completely excised. Even if a lesion shows no clinical evidence of atypia, if the patient is concerned about it because of possible changes in sensation or growth, complete excision is suggested. Complete excision can take the form of a punch excision, a deep shave (tangential excision), or a small ellipse. Shave excision is the least effective.

Initial excisional biopsy is recommended for atypical nevi, and appropriate clinical margins of 2 mm are suggested. This is based on a study showing that clinically atypical nevi did not extend beyond 2 mm of their clinically apparent margins. Once the lesions have been removed and histologically examined, additional therapy may or may not be indicated. For those lesions exhibiting no more than moderate atypia, complete excision is probably adequate; ie, pathologic examination reveals that no residual nevus cells are present at the histologic margins and that clinically the lesion was removed with 2-mm margins with no remaining nevus identifiable. For nevi exhibiting moderate atypia that are at the histologic margin, conservative re-excision may be indicated. For those nevi exhibiting severe atypia, it is suggested that 5- to 10-mm margins be used. A 5-mm margin is appropriate for melanoma in situ, and a 10-mm margin for superficially invasive malignant melanoma. Margins are still controversial, and narrower margins may be adequate.

Probably the only type of nevi that can be removed in part (usually shave removal) are those typical skin tag–appearing intradermal nevi or those removed purely for cosmetic purposes. Obviously, if the clinician is dealing with a pigmented lesion that is not an apparent melanocytic nevus, incisional biopsies may be appropriate. Thus, complete excision for atypical nevi is primarily recommended for the following reasons:

1. It is possible that a more significant component has been left in the patient, even though the pathology may show no atypia.
2. Even if the risk of melanoma arising within a clinically normal nevus showing minimal atypia may be no greater than a melanoma arising within normal skin, if it does occur, litigation could follow.

Excisions (punch, shave, ellipse) are performed in the conventional fashion under sterile technique, usually using lidocaine with or without epinephrine as the local anesthetic. Punch biopsies measuring 4 mm or larger and elliptical excisions are closed with appropriate suturing. For shave excisions, electrodesiccation or chemical hemostasis with 20% aluminum chloride can be used. In the past, Monsel's solution (ferric subsulfate) was often used for hemostasis, but in pigmented lesions, this may create histologic problems due to residual brown iron pigment.

Generally speaking, a nevus that is identified by the clinician as atypical or that is brought to the clinician's attention because of change in size or sensation, should not be observed but removed. For those individuals who have a disorder that falls into the category of classic dysplastic nevus syndrome and who have a high risk of malignant melanoma and numerous atypical nevi, removal of all nevi is not obligatory nor practical. Instead, these patients should have any suspicious nevi removed at the initial visit and be carefully followed subsequently. Ideally, follow-up should include the use of clinical photographs or more sophisticated imaging equipment. Any lesions that do exhibit change are then excised. Follow-up periods differ from one medical center to another. Family members also must be followed appropriately.

CONGENITAL MELANOCYTIC NEVI

The term congenital melanocytic nevus is used as a specific clinicopathologic entity. These lesions are present at birth and are most often considerably larger than conventional acquired nevi. Giant pigmented nevi (giant hairy nevi, garment nevi) are terms usually reserved for lesions measuring more than 20 cm in greatest diameter. These lesions do have a higher risk for malignant degeneration than do conventional acquired nevi. Approximately 5% of these lesions may eventuate into malignant melanoma. For these large nevi, treatment is controversial. There are some that advocate complete excision, but this may result in considerable deformity. Also, in some situations, excision is impossible. Even with so-called complete excision, it is frequently difficult to remove all of the nevus cells because some may extend deep into subcutaneous tissues. Some variants are even associated with involvement of the meninges. For the giant forms, the decision to completely excise should weigh the possibility of deforming surgery against the risk of malignant melanoma. Cosmetic modalities such as laser therapy and dermabrasion have been used, but they are only cosmetic and do not appreciably decrease the risk of malignant degeneration. It has been stated that approximately 60% of congenital nevi that do eventuate into malignant melanomas do so in the first decade of life. This further complicates therapeutic decisions. Additionally, careful clinical follow-up may not always detect foci of evolving melanoma because melanoma can arise in deeper tissues that are not clinically apparent. Smaller congenital nevi also exist, and some may be no larger than 1 to 2 cm. It seems prudent to remove small congenital nevi that can be removed easily. In our institution, easily removable usually means without significant deformity and without the use of general anesthesia.

OTHER NEVI

Simple, or common blue, nevi occur most frequently on the head and distal extremities. As the name implies, they are usually clinically blue in color. Cellular blue nevi are very closely related to, and, as the name implies, are much more cellular and usually larger than common blue nevi. They often present on the buttocks and sacral area. Both types of blue nevi are benign, but the cellular type occasionally can be confused with malignant melanoma. Conservative excision is appropriate because these lesions could recur. Very rare cases of malignant degeneration have also been described.

Spitz nevi, unfortunately previously referred to as juvenile melanoma, are unusual variants of melanocytic nevi. Histologically, they may be confused with malignant melanoma but are benign. The lesion is most common in children but can occur in adults. Often, the lesions are elevated, dome shaped, and may be pink to flesh colored rather than pigmented. Complete conservative excision is usually recommended because these lesions may recur. If lesions are located in cosmetically sensitive areas such as the face, partial shave excision can be considered. Pigmented spindle cell nevi are also variants that histologically and clinically may be confused with melanoma. The lesions are frequently jet black and are seen most commonly on the thighs of young women. Complete conservative excision is recommended. Deep penetrating nevi share some features with pigmented spindle cell nevus. These lesions may be heavily pigmented and are frequently seen on the face of young adults and in women, in particular. Histologically, many have been confused with malignant melanoma. These are benign lesions, and conservative excision is curative.

It is important to remember that, at times, histologic diagnoses of nevi may not be straightforward, and borderline and controversial lesions do exist. In those particular situations, a wider margin may be prudent to cover the possibility of more aggressive behavior of the tumor.

MALIGNANT MELANOMA

method of
ELISA B. RUSH, M.D., and
ALLAN W. SILBERMAN, M.D., PH.D.
Cedars-Sinai Medical Center
Los Angeles, California

Malignant melanoma currently accounts for approximately 1% of all cancer deaths. However, the worldwide incidence of melanoma is increasing at a faster rate than any other neoplasm, with the exception of lung cancer in women. In the United States alone, the incidence has tripled in the last forty years and has nearly doubled in the last decade. An estimated 32,000 Americans will develop melanoma in 1993, of whom 6800 will succumb to their disease. Based on current projections, by the year 2000, 1 in every 90 whites will eventually develop melanoma.

Melanoma can affect all ethnic and racial groups; however, the typical melanoma patient has a fair complexion and a tendency to sunburn rather than tan, even after a brief exposure to sunlight. Although there is no conclusive evidence that exposure to sunlight is causally related to the development of melanoma, lesions are most commonly found on sun-exposed areas of the body. Other epidemiologic risk factors include the occurrence of a previous melanoma and an afflicted first-degree relative. Patients with the dysplastic nevus syndrome, an autosomal dominant disorder characterized by the presence of many large, irregularly shaped nevi, are also at increased risk for developing melanoma.

SIGNS AND SYMPTOMS

Benign skin lesions can usually be differentiated from malignant ones by each of the following properties, which can be remembered using the mnemonic ABCD: (1) Assymetry. Pigment assymetry is more frequently found in malignant lesions. (2) Border irregularity. Well-circumscribed lesions are more likely to be benign. (3) Color variation. Lesions with any combination of brown, black, gray, or red hues are more likely to be malignant than lesions of uniform color. (4) Diameter. Lesions larger than 5 to 10 mm in diameter or lesions that have increased in size are more likely to be malignant. Although melanomas may have a variety of clinical appearances, the common denominator is their changing nature. Any pigmented lesion that undergoes a change in size, configuration, or color should be considered a melanoma, and an excisional biopsy should be performed.

TYPES OF CUTANEOUS MELANOMA

There are four pathologic types of cutaneous melanoma each with a characteristic growth pattern. (1) Superficial spreading melanoma is the most common type, accounting for 70% of all cases. This type typically arises from a preexisting nevus and expands in a radial fashion before it enters a vertical growth phase. (2) Nodular melanoma, a more aggressive tumor, accounts for approximately 15 to 30% of cases. This lesion arises de novo from normal skin and has no radial growth phase. It is found more commonly in males. (3) Lentigo maligna melanoma accounts for less than 10% of cases. This type of lesion is found more commonly in females and the elderly population. The lesions are typically large and flat, follow an indolent growth course, and rarely metastasize. (4) Acral lentiginous melanoma also accounts for less than 10% of lesions, but occurs in a higher proportion (35 to 60%) of nonwhite patients.

BIOPSY TECHNIQUE

An excisional biopsy, when possible, or an incisional biopsy should be performed on every suspicious skin lesion. Care must be taken to ensure that the full thickness of the lesion is included in the biopsy specimen because staging, treatment, and prognosis depend on accurate assessment of depth and level of infiltration of the lesion. A shave biopsy should not be performed because this technique fragments the lesion preventing accurate assessment of the depth and thickness of the melanoma.

STAGING SYSTEMS

Microstaging is an integral part of the staging and clinical management of melanoma. Two methods have been used. The Breslow microstaging method measures the thickness of the lesion in millimeters using an ocular micrometer. The total vertical height of the melanoma is measured from the granular layer to the area of deepest penetration. If the lesion is ulcerated, measurements are made from the surface of the ulcer to the deepest part of the lesion. The Clark method assesses the level of penetration into the various skin layers (Table 1).

Although the tumor thickness and the level of invasion can predict the risk for metastases, data from several institutions have demonstrated that tumor thickness is a more accurate and reproducible prognostic parameter than interpreting the level of invasion. Significant regression of the tumor invalidates the prognostic value of these microstaging methods. Clinical staging criteria can be found in Table 2.

TABLE 1. **Clark Classification System of Microstaging**

Level I: Confined to the epidermis (in situ)
Level II: Invasion into the papillary dermis
Level III: Penetration to the papillary-reticular interface
Level IV: Invasion into the reticular dermis
Level V: Penetration into subcutaneous fat

PROGNOSIS

Many factors are known to predict risk in patients with melanoma including Breslow depth, Clark level, anatomic location, gender, tumor ulceration, and growth pattern. Multifactorial analysis in Stage I and II patients demonstrates that tumor thickness is the single most important prognostic factor. Other important risk factors include the presence of ulceration and anatomic location, with extremity lesions having a better prognosis than those on the trunk or head and neck. Multifactorial analysis of Stage III patients shows that the number of metastatic nodes, the anatomic site of the primary lesion, and tumor ulceration are the dominant prognostic variables. Patients with primary lesions less than 0.76 mm have a 10-year survival rate of greater than 90%. However, the presence of positive nodes lowers the survival rate to 13 to 40%. There are virtually no survivors with Stage IV disease.

TREATMENT

The treatment of Stage I cutaneous melanoma (i.e., local disease not clinically involving the regional lymph nodes) is wide excision of the lesion. Current recommendations are that surgical margins should be proportional to the depth of the lesion with 0.5- to 1.0-cm margins for in situ lesions; 1.0-cm margins for 1.0-mm lesions; 2- to 3-cm margins for 1.0 to 2.0 mm lesions; and 3 to 4 cm for lesions greater than 2.0 mm. The excision should include the underlying subcutaneous fat up to and including the deep fascia. Surgeons often select margins wide enough to constitute adequate excision but modest enough to allow primary closure. Sensible compromise is obviously required for lesions on the face and extremities. Skin grafts are advisable when primary closure would

TABLE 2. **Clinical Staging System Adopted by the American Joint Committee on Cancer**

Stage	Criteria
IA	Localized melanoma <0.75 mm or Clark level II
IB	Localized melanoma 0.76 to 1.5 mm or level III
IIA	Localized melanoma 1.5 to 4 mm or level IV
IIB	Localized melanoma >4 mm or level V
III	Limited nodal metastases involving only one regional lymph node basin, or fewer than 5 in-transit metastases without nodal metastases
IV	Advanced regional metastases or any patient with distant metastases

compromise appropriate margins. It remains controversial whether prophylactic regional lymph node dissection (PRLND) should be considered in patients who have primary malignant melanoma and clinically negative regional lymph nodes. The advocates of this method point out correctly that surgery is the only effective therapy for regional lymph node disease; moreover, in several retrospective studies, a survival advantage of as much as 25% has been demonstrated in patients with clinically negative but pathologically positive lymph nodes. The opponents of PRLND point to the randomized, prospective, multi-institutional study by the WHO Melanoma Group, which failed to demonstrate any survival advantage in patients who have prophylactic lymph node dissection.

However, besides the potential but inconclusively demonstrated survival advantage, there are two other reasons for performing PRLND. First, clinically negative nodes that are found to be histologically positive for micrometastatic disease provide important prognostic information. In addition, patients found to have histologically positive nodes become eligible for experimental adjuvant protocols.

The treatment for patients with clinically positive regional lymph nodes without evidence of distant metastatic disease (Stage III and some Stage IV patients) would include wide excision of the primary lesion and therapeutic lymphadenectomy. These patients would be candidates for experimental adjuvant protocols after surgery. At present, no adjuvant therapy, including chemotherapy, immunotherapy, hormonal therapy or any combination thereof, has been proved effective.

The most common sites of metastatic melanoma include skin and subcutaneous tissue, distant lymph nodes, and visceral spread to lung, liver, and brain. At present, after 20 years of experimentation, dacarbazine (DTIC) is the only agent approved by the FDA for treatment of metastatic melanoma, and no combination of chemotherapeutic agents has been shown to be more effective than DTIC alone. DTIC therapy is associated with a response rate of 15 to 25%, with only 5% of patients achieving a complete response.

Current research in melanoma is focused on finding effective systemic therapy. Avenues of current work include combination chemotherapy including tamoxifen (Nolvadex),* high-dose chemotherapy with autologous bone marrow support; use of biologic agents, including the interferons,* interleukin-2,* and tumor necrosis factor,*† and active and passive specific immunotherapy.

---

*Not FDA approved for this indication.
†Investigational drug in the United States.

PREMALIGNANT LESIONS

method of
CHRISTINE M. HAYES, M.D., and
DUANE C. WHITAKER, M.D.
University of Iowa Hospitals and Clinics
Iowa City, Iowa

Recognition and treatment of premalignant lesions is important because of the preventive benefit this therapy provides for all patients.

A history of excessive sun exposure, arsenic ingestion, topical tars, or a family history of melanoma or other skin cancers may predispose patients to the development of malignancy. Patients with scars from thermal injury or chronic ulcers are at increased risk for the development of squamous cell carcinoma in the region of these nonhealing ulcers.

The physical examination of the skin should include sun-protected areas as well as sun-exposed areas. Good lighting is essential, and lesions are often felt more easily than seen, so it is important for the examiner to run his or her fingers over the skin while performing this examination. Patient education regarding sun protection and self-examination of pigmented lesions is important in the prevention of malignancy.

When the diagnosis is uncertain regarding benign or malignant skin disease, a biopsy may be necessary. A shave biopsy is adequate for actinic keratoses, Bowen's disease, basal cell carcinoma, or squamous cell carcinoma. Pigmented lesions require a full-thickness biopsy, extending to and including the subcutis. This is best obtained with an incisional, excisional, or punch biopsy.

ACTINIC KERATOSIS

The most common premalignant cutaneous lesions are actinic keratoses (AK), which are also called solar keratoses. AKs are caused by solar radiation and appear as discrete, erythematous, tan or brown, scaling macules, approximately 2 to 6 mm in diameter. They are most commonly found on the sun-exposed surfaces of the face, neck, trunk, arms and dorsa of hands. AKs are common in fair-skinned, middle-aged, and elderly persons who have had excessive sun exposure. The rate of progression to invasive squamous cell carcinoma is uncertain but may range from 1% to 10%.

There are numerous treatment modalities for AKs, most causing superficial destruction of the abnormal cells in the epidermis. Cryotherapy is often used for individual lesions; however, if numerous AKs are present, topical agents such as 5-fluorouracil (5-FU) and dermabrasion or chemical peels are employed.

Liquid nitrogen cryotherapy is an effective and efficient method of AK removal. AKs may be frozen with a cotton swab or spray device. A bulky cotton swab applicator is dipped into liquid nitrogen and then pressed against the AK for several seconds. Because nitrogen vaporizes at room temperature, the swab must be frequently redipped and applied briefly in 2 to 4 cycles for a total of 5 to 15 seconds. The length of freeze depends on the size, thickness of the lesion, its anatomic location, and risk to underlying structures. A spray device that dispenses liquid nitrogen must be used carefully because this method applies cryogen very rapidly.

Following cryotherapy, a blister may form at the site and the patient should be instructed about proper wound care. Healing usually occurs within a week. If an AK does not resolve after treatment, a second cryotherapy cycle can be considered but recalcitrant lesions should be biopsied to identify possible squamous cell carcinoma.

The chemotherapeutic agent 5-FU is available in a topical cream (Efudex), 1% and 5%. This is a mainstay of therapy in patients with extensive AKs. The standard method employs application of cream to the affected areas twice daily for 3 to 4 weeks. Some clinicians begin with 1% 5-FU on the face, and if a vigorous reaction is not seen, the strength is increased to 5%. Care must be taken to avoid applying the cream to the eyes and mouth. The 5% cream is used on the arms, hands, and trunk. This approach will treat all clinically apparent lesions and unmask inapparent lesions as well. Patients must be cautioned that this treatment causes marked skin erythema and tenderness, and the skin may be painful during treatment. Some patients may also require topical steroids for discomfort associated with topical 5-FU therapy. Excellent results with long remissions are often seen. Topical tretinoin cream (Retin A)* has been shown to be effective in the treatment of AKs when used in conjunction with 5-FU.

Recently, application of 5-FU on a weekly basis has been shown to be efficacious in the eradication of AK. Five percent 5-FU is applied 1 day each week, morning and evening, for 6 to 9 weeks. Patients noted mild erythema and tenderness, and were relatively comfortable. This course is better tolerated and is successful in achieving AK-free remissions. This approach is also useful in patients who previously used the conventional method and cannot tolerate the severe local reaction.

A 10% masoprocol cream (Actinex) has recently been introduced as a topical agent for numerous AKs. It is applied twice daily for 2 to 4 weeks, and promising results have been reported. The symptoms of redness, irritation, itching, and burning did occur, although perhaps less than with topical 5-FU. Approximately 10% of patients experience a contact dermatitis due to this product. At the present time, clinicians have many more patient-years experience with 5-FU, and additional clinical trials with masoprocol are necessary to establish its efficacy.

BOWEN'S DISEASE

Bowen's disease (BD) is epidermal squamous cell carcinoma in situ. Clinically, BD appears as a sharply defined red macule or patch, which may have overlying scale or crust. BD is more common in older men, most frequently on sun-exposed surfaces, but it can be seen in either sex on sun-protected skin as well. Histologically, the dysplasia is full thickness throughout the epidermis, with an intact dermal-epidermal junction. If the lesion invades the dermis, it has become invasive squamous cell carcinoma.

BD can be caused by solar radiation and chronic ingestion of inorganic arsenic (historically via patent medicines such as Fowler's solution and asiatic pills). Clinicians should be aware that arsenic ingestion causes BD in sun-protected areas, multiple keratoses of the palms and soles (arsenical keratoses), and visceral malignancies, most commonly affecting the pulmonary and the genitourinary tracts.

Many treatment options exist for BD and range from surgical excision to topical 5-FU. However, the therapeutic decision should be modified to fit the clinical and histopathologic features of the lesion, its anatomic location, and the general health of the patient. Surgical excision is often the best form of treatment for small, well-defined lesions. Mohs' micrographic surgery offers the option of complete margin control with tissue preservation and is recommended for tumors that are large, have indistinct margins, or are in critical anatomic sites.

Other treatments, such as cryotherapy, curettage and fulguration, and shave excision, may be suitable for use on the trunk and proximal extremities. These methods, however, may be ineffective if anaplastic cells extend down the hair follicles. In such cases, surgical treatment is preferable.

ERYTHROPLASIA OF QUEYRAT

Erythroplasia of Queyrat is squamous cell carcinoma in situ of the glans penis or coronal sulcus. Clinically, a red, velvety, moist plaque is seen. Single or multiple lesions may be present. Erythroplasia of Queyrat is more common in uncircumcised males, aged 50 and older. The transition to invasive squamous cell carcinoma occurs with a higher frequency than in BD, and the cancers are more aggressive with earlier metastasis.

Treatment modalities include surgical excision, Mohs' micrographic surgery, CO_2 laser ablation and topical 5-FU. Uncircumcised males should be considered for therapeutic circumcision. Close follow-up is required to evaluate clearance of the lesion.

KERATOACANTHOMA

Keratoacanthoma is a firm, flesh-colored, solitary nodule with a central, keratin-filled crater. The classic history is rapid growth over a number of weeks. Strictly speaking, keratocanthoma is not a premalignant lesion but may be indistinguishable from squamous cell carcinoma. A true keratocanthoma may resolve spontaneously. Biopsy must include full-thickness dermis for adequate tissue evaluation be-

*Not FDA approved for this indication.

cause the architectural features of the lesion are a key to its diagnosis.

Treatment options include surgical excision, Mohs' micrographic surgery, and in selected instances, intralesional chemotherapeutic agents or watchful waiting. Multiple eruptive keratoacanthomas may require administration of systemic retinoid therapy.

CONGENITAL NEVOCYTIC NEVI

Congenital nevocytic nevi (CN) are pigmented nevi that are present at birth. With maturation, they may begin as light brown lesions, darken, and develop dense hair growth. They range in size from small (1 cm or less) to giant CN (larger than 20 cm), which are the bathing trunk/garment variety. Because controlled, prospective studies have not been conducted, quantification of melanoma risk in CN is difficult to establish. However, most authorities quote a lifetime risk of melanoma at 1% in small lesions and 10% or more in giant CN.

For small and medium-sized CN, treatment options include watchful waiting and surgical excision near the onset of puberty. The giant nevi can involve the trunk and extremities. Evaluation of such lesions should include permanent photographs for the medical record and biopsy of suspicious areas. Serial excision with grafting or tissue expansion has been undertaken in these patients, but any decision regarding surgery must be arrived at on an individual basis.

DYSPLASTIC NEVI

Dysplastic nevi (DN) are pigmented lesions that differ in appearance from common, acquired nevi. Common nevi are uniform in color (tan to brown) with regular borders and are 2 to 6 mm in size. DN have variegated color, with tan, brown, and pink shades. The borders are irregular compared with the sharp demarcation of common nevi. The size is larger, being 5 to 12 mm in diameter. They may be few in number or many. Histologically, they have unique cytologic and architectural features.

Families have been reported with atypical moles and multiple melanomas, and these lesions with a familial association have been called the dysplastic nevus syndrome. The gene is inherited in an autosomal dominant fashion, but sporadic cases are seen frequently. The number of DN varies, but there may be more than 100. DN patients with familial melanoma and many DN are at greater risk, whereas those with no family history and only a few DN are at lower risk for the development of melanoma.

Close monitoring is necessary for a DN patient with many atypical moles and a family history of melanoma. Examinations are recommended at 6- to 12-month intervals. Total body photographs are useful to identify changing lesions, and surgical excision of new, changing, or markedly irregular lesions is warranted. DN patients without a family history may require biopsy of a characteristic lesion to exclude malignant melanoma, yearly examinations, and total body photographs.

All patients should practice sun-avoidance behaviors, including use of protective clothing and sunscreens, avoiding sun from 10 A.M. to 3 P.M., as well as closely following their own pigmented lesions for changes. The ABCDs of pigmented lesions are a simple way to remember these features and include

A Asymmetry
B Border irregularity
C Color variation
D Diameter over 6 mm (the size of a pencil eraser)

These criteria are helpful in distinguishing DN and malignant melanoma.

LENTIGO MALIGNA

Lentigo maligna is melanoma in situ, commonly located on sun-exposed areas of the face or scalp of elderly persons. Clinically, lentigo maligna is a tan to brown macule that may show progressive peripheral extension over many years. Perhaps 5% or more of lentigno maligna lesions become invasive melanoma, although it is difficult to establish reliable figures. Irregular pigmentation or induration suggests malignant progression. A full-thickness biopsy is required to establish the diagnosis. Complete surgical excision is the recommended treatment, with the margin determined by depth of invasion.

VERRUCA/CONDYLOMA ACUMINATUM

Verruca vulgaris and condyloma acuminatum are caused by human papillomavirus. Human papillomavirus has been found in digital squamous cell carcinoma, so periungual verruca vulgaris may play a premalignant role. Biopsy is indicated for periungual or genital warts that are atypical in presentation or resistant to therapy. Human papillomavirus types 16 and 18 have oncogenic potential and cause condyloma acuminatum, cervical dysplasia, and neoplasia in women. Therefore, cervical examination is important in patients with condyloma acuminatum and their partners.

BOWENOID PAPULOSIS

Bowenoid papulosis (BP) is a term used for genital lesions that clinically resemble verruca vulgaris but histologically appear identical to BD. Clinically, red to brown macules or verrucous papules are present on the glans or shaft of the penis, or the labial or perineal area in women. BP tends to appear in late adolescence or early adulthood. BP is caused by human papillomavirus, and transition to cervical dysplasia in female patients with BP and partners of male patients with BP has been reported. Invasive squamous cell carcinoma in sites of BP and spontaneous resolution of BP lesions have been reported, so the clinical course and therefore neoplastic potential of BP is variable.

Treatment options for BP include surgical excision, cryotherapy, topical podophyllum, and CO_2 laser ablation. Cryotherapy technique is performed, as described earlier. These methods are preferable to topical podophyllum because the lesions may be resistant to this form of therapy. In addition, podophyllum should not be used in pregnant women or on internal mucous membranes due to its neurotoxicity. If podophyllum is used, a 25% solution is applied for 2 to 6 hours and requires retreatment every 3 to 4 weeks until the condition resolves. However, because of the high malignant potential of the condition, close follow-up and biopsy of unresponsive lesions is recommended.

ORAL/LABIAL LESIONS

Oral leukoplakia is a term used for a whitish, adherent thickening of the epithelium of oral mucous membranes. It is seen more commonly in men over the age of 40. The differential diagnosis for oral leukoplakia is extensive and includes bite line, benign and precancerous leukoplakia, lupus erythematosus, squamous cell carcinoma, and rare lesions such as white sponge nevus, among others. Candidal plaques should scrape off with a tongue depressor. When evaluating leukoplakia, it is often difficult to differentiate between a premalignant lesion and cancer, and a biopsy may be required.

The treatment for benign leukoplakia is close monitoring and the discontinuation of offending agents such as poor-fitting dentures, chewing tobacco, cigarettes, cigars, and pipes. Because squamous cell carcinoma is a risk, persistent or progressive leukoplakia may require surgical excision.

Erythroplakia is a term used for red plaques found on the oral mucosa. Common locations include the floor of the mouth, soft palate, buccal mucosa, or under the tongue. These lesions require biopsy because 90% are carcinoma in situ or invasive squamous cell carcinoma. Treatment is best delivered by an oncologic head and neck surgeon.

Actinic cheilitis is sun-induced premalignancy of the lips. This condition most commonly affects the lower lip and is seen in men more frequently than women. Lip squamous cell carcinoma has a greater risk of metastases than other cutaneous squamous cell carcinoma and provides additional rationale for ablative treatment of actinic cheilitis. Cryotherapy can be employed for individual actinic lip lesions. Diffuse lip involvement can be treated with CO_2 laser ablation with excellent results. For severe disease, surgical vermilionectomy may be appropriate. Prior to any treatment, biopsy is indicated to identify possible invasion.

SPECIAL CONSIDERATIONS

Particular attention must be given to certain patient populations. These populations include organ transplant recipients and other immunocompromised individuals, as well as patients with previous exposure to ionizing radiation. Immunocompromised patients are at increased risk for viral infections including human papillomavirus, and they develop premalignant lesions and cutaneous malignancies at a higher rate. Metastasis from skin cancers is also a significant risk in this population.

Patients with a history of cutaneous radiation therapy are at higher risk to develop aggressive basal cell carcinoma and squamous cell carcinoma, which are often difficult to detect clinically. Examinations at frequent, regular intervals and early biopsy of suspicious lesions is indicated for these patient populations. These patient populations present diagnostic and therapeutic dilemmas, and it may be helpful to follow them jointly with a skin cancer specialist.

BACTERIAL DISEASES OF THE SKIN

method of
RICHARD F. EDLICH, M.D., PH.D.,
SHERRY T. SUTTON, PHARM.D., and
DIETER H. M. GRÖESCHEL, M.D., PH.D.
University of Virginia
Charlottesville, Virginia

When considering common bacterial diseases of the skin, rather distinct clinical responses to a variety of bacterial infections have been identified. In these cases, it is the specific site of infection and the attendant inflammatory responses that provide the characteristic clinical picture.

IMPETIGO

There are two classic forms of impetigo: the nonbullous and the bullous forms. Nonbullous impetigo is the most common pediatric skin infection; however, it can occur at any age. It starts in a traumatized area (a scratch or insect bite). It occurs primarily in exposed anatomic sites, such as the face and extremities. In adults, individuals living in close quarters, as well as those with an increased risk of bruising, are especially prone to nonbullous impetigo. This form of impetigo is usually noted in the summer in temperate climates, and it may be endemic year-round in warm climates. Factors implicated in this disease include warm ambient temperature, humidity, crowding, skin bruising, and poor hygiene.

The typical lesion usually begins as an erythematous papule that becomes a unilocular vesicle measuring less than 0.5 mm in diameter, situated between the stratum corneum and stratum granulosum and often located near the opening of a hair follicle. When the subcorneal vesicle becomes pustular, it ruptures, releasing a yellow, cloudy fluid and leaving a weeping bed. The seropurulent fluid dries, forming a yellow, golden crust that is the hallmark of the disease process.

Our clinical studies have been supported by a grant from the Texaco Foundation, White Plains, New York.

These lesions rarely elicit pain, and usually are not accompanied by fever or systemic signs (malaise or anorexia). Its asymptomatic nature accounts for the frequent delay in seeking medical attention. Without treatment, the condition often remains stable or becomes slowly progressive over a period of weeks. Occasionally, it may progress to ulcer formation. Regional lymphadenitis, cellulitis, and septicemia become evident in a small percentage of patients, who always seek treatment for these complications rather the primary problem, nonbullous impetigo. When a nephritogenic strain of group A streptococci is present, acute glomerulonephritis may follow. Postinfectious glomerulonephritis may occur in a sporadic form or in outbreaks. Although 95% of such patients with nephritis recover, progressive renal failure occasionally is encountered. The average time between the onset of impetigo and the development of nephritis is 20 days. Treatment of nonbullous impetigo probably does not decrease the chance of an individual's developing acute glomerulonephritis, but the successful treatment of these lesions may prevent spread to others and thereby reduce the general incidence of glomerulonephritis.

Nonbullous impetigo is caused by *Staphylococcus aureus*, group A streptococci, or both. Because it is difficult to distinguish on clinical examination between a streptococcal or staphylococcal cause, Gram's stain and culture of the vesicle fluid or weeping bed are recommended. *S. aureus* is the sole pathogen recovered most often. *S. aureus* alone or in combination with group A streptococci is found in over 80% of the patients. *S. aureus* is encountered at all ages, whereas group A streptococci are not frequently observed before the age of 1 and 2 years but are noted in older children.

Treatment of this condition must include intervention against the pathogen and improvements in the hygiene and living conditions of the patient. A fundamental tenet in the treatment of impetigo is to debride the crust (scab) from the wound surface. This scab is an accumulation of extravasated blood proteins, including fibrin, that surround the bacteria and protect them from host defenses as well as from topical and systemic antibiotics. The scab also serves as a culture medium that encourages bacterial growth to concentrations greater than 10^8 bacteria per gram of tissue. Disruption and removal of the crust are accomplished by aggressive wound cleansing. The lesions are scrubbed with a coarse mesh gauze sponge (Type VIII) soaked in a soap to prevent reaccumulation of crusts. The pain encountered in this mechanical scrub can be lessened considerably by the use of a non-toxic surfactant, poloxamer 188 (Shur-Clens), as the wound cleanser. Wound cleansing must be complemented by antibiotic treatment.

If the lesions are not widespread, topical mupirocin, applied three times daily, is the treatment of choice. A beta-lactamase–resistant antibiotic drug is indicated if there is widespread disease. Erythromycin should not be used if there is widespread erythromycin resistance in the community. Impetigo should respond to these treatments in 7 days. If the results of treatment are not satisfactory, antibiotic resistance of the pathogen or poor patient compliance should be suspected, necessitating reculturing the wound. If poor compliance is confirmed, daily intramuscular ceftriaxone should be implemented.

Because this condition is commonly found under conditions of poor hygiene and overcrowding, improvements in the patient's living conditions, personal hygiene, and general health are an integral part of our treatment regimen. The patient should shower twice daily with soap, using a clean washcloth and towel. The patient should be instructed to use only his or her towels and washcloths, which are not to be used by other family members. Daily washing of the patient's own clothing and bed linen is also advised. Reduction in minor skin trauma through control of biting insects appears to be important in preventing infection. Efforts are also made to identify the source of infection, focusing on members of the immediate family or friends who are simultaneously ill with a skin pyoderma.

Bullous impetigo is the less common form of impetigo. It occurs in infants and is characterized by rapid progression of vesicles to the formation of bullae measuring larger than 5 mm in diameter in previously untraumatized skin. These lesions frequently occur in the axilla, with satellite lesions soon appearing that may cover large portions of the body. The bullae are flaccid and transparent. In the newborn, this disease is so extensive that it is called pemphigus neonatorum. This type of infection is highly contagious, leading to epidemics in the nursery. When the large intraepidermal blebs rupture, the seropurulent discharge dries, forming a thin crust. As the lesions spread peripherally by autoinoculation, central healing of the denuded vesicles usually occurs without scarring. Cellulitis and lymphangitis are rarely encountered.

Bullous impetigo is caused exclusively by staphylococci and is seldom superinfected by streptococci. The bacteriocin produced by this strain of staphylococcus inhibits the growth of streptococci and may account for their absence. This organism also produces an exfoliative toxin that may cause the bulla formation. Treatment of this condition must include meticulous wound care complemented by the intravenous administration of a beta-lactamase–resistant penicillin (oxacillin [Bactocill, Prostaphlin] or nafcillin [Nafcil, Unipen]).

FOLLICULITIS

Folliculitis is a pyoderma located within a hair follicle. *S. aureus* is the most frequent pathogen. Less common pathogens are coliform bacteria and streptococci. This infection is classified according to its depth of penetration as either superficial or deep. The superficial type is a form of impetigo (Bockhardt's impetigo) in which the pustule is located at the opening of the hair follicle, often surrounded by a rim of erythema. Rupture of a pustule leads to crust formation and, in some cases, to the development of another superficial follicular abscess. The lesions usually heal within several days and only rarely persist to become furuncles. The location of the superficial folliculitis varies according to the age of the patient. The infection appears often in the scalp of children. In the adult, the scalp, beard, or an extremity may be involved.

This superficial folliculitis may extend beyond the confines of the hair follicles, resulting in several types of deep folliculitis. A furuncle or boil is the most common skin lesion of deep folliculitis. It occurs particularly in regions subject to friction and perspiration (face, neck, axillae, and buttocks). Chronic carriers of *S. aureus* are especially prone to this disease. The systemic host factors that predispose an individual to furuncles include obesity, blood dyscrasia, defects in neutrophil function, immune globulin deficiency states, and treatments with corticosteroids and cytotoxic agents. The infection in a furuncle spreads along multiple tracts into the subcutaneous tissue. It starts as a tender red nodule, usually located at the nape of the neck, in the axilla, or on the buttock. As the nodule enlarges, it becomes tender and fluctuant, and eventually ruptures, discharging creamy, yellow pus and a core of necrotic debris from multiple draining sinuses with interconnecting tracts. Keratin plugs filling dilated follicular infundibula are characteristic features of furuncles. Accumulation of keratin may be due to overproduction, possibly stimulated by sweat or sebum or the result of decreased shedding of keratin. Carbuncles are aggregates of interconnecting furuncles that drain through multiple openings of the skin. A carbuncle is a larger, more serious inflammatory lesion with a deeper base. The involved area is red and indurated, and multiple pustules soon appear on the surface, eventually draining externally around multiple hair follicles. Sycosis barbae (barber's itch), a less common form of deep folliculitis, occurs in the bearded area of the face. If the condition is left untreated, it may progress to the deep chronic cicatricial form of sycosis barbae called lupoid sycosis.

Acne keloidalis is a chronic folliculitis of the posterior neck and occipital scalp of young black men. It is exhibited clinically by follicular papules that coalesce into firm plaques and nodules. Hair can be seen perforating the papules. In-grown hairs are not seen. Successful treatment of this condition involves complete removal of the scarred skin with its hair follicles.

In most cases, superficial and deep folliculitis are minor problems. After the lesions rupture, the redness and edema disappear in several days. Recurrence of these lesions does, however, occur in some patients over a period that may last several years. Bacteremia is a rare but clinically significant consequence of this type of pyoderma. Folliculitis around the lips and nose may spread to the cavernous sinus via the emissary veins.

Treatment

Treatment of folliculitis must include searching for and avoiding any predisposing factors that encourage its development. Plucking hair (e.g., eyebrows, upper lips) should be discouraged. Shaving should be performed with razors with recessed blades or electric clippers that avoid nicking the injured skin. The skin should be kept dry, providing a climate that is not conducive to bacterial growth. Frictional forces from surfaces such as a tight collar should be avoided.

Treatment of a small, isolated pyoderma of a hair follicle can be initiated with warm skin compresses until the lesion ruptures. In these cases, antimicrobial therapy is not needed. When the pyoderma involves multiple hair follicles, surgical intervention complemented by antimicrobial prophylaxis is recommended. Because the skin around a carbuncle is exquisitely sensitive, a regional nerve block of the site with a local anesthetic (1% lidocaine) is recommended. In skin that is not easily susceptible to this anesthetic technique, infiltration anesthesia via a No. 27 needle through the skin around the carbuncle is necessary. Surgical drainage of the carbuncle must be accomplished with an incision that will heal with the most aesthetically pleasing scar. This goal can be accomplished by designing the incision so that its long axis is perpendicular to the dynamic tensions of the skin. The ultimate appearance of the planned incision can be predicted by rather simple practical measurements. At the ends of the planned incision, mark points A and B, and then mark points C and D to be perpendicular to and equidistant from points A and B (Fig. 1). Measure first the distance between points A and B and then the distance between C and D, both before and after flexion or extension of the neck or contraction of the muscles of facial expression. The dynamic skin tensions will be in the direction of the greatest changes in dimension. If the long axis of the incision is perpendicular to the direction of dynamic skin tensions, it will heal with a narrow scar that does not interfere with function and has an aesthetically pleasing appearance.

After deepening the incision into the pyoderma, the necrotic debris and exudate must then be evacuated using 0.9% saline irrigation delivered to the infected site under low pressure (Asepto syringe, 1 pound per square inch). Undermining the skin edges may be necessary to open and expose subcutaneous tracts of the carbuncle. The wound is then packed with a 1-inch-wide gauze pack (Type 1). One day after surgery, the gauze is removed to permit cleansing with 0.9% saline that is again delivered to the wound using an Asepto syringe, after which the wound is packed with sterile gauze. Daily wound care is repeated until the cavity becomes filled with granulation tissue and the wound edges close by contraction. Without this meticulous care, wound repair may be accomplished by epithelial cells that migrate into the interstices of the wound, resulting in epithelialized sinus tracts. These sinusoidal tracts provide a moist environment for the growth of bacteria that may lead to the development of recurrent pyoderma.

Immediately before surgical intervention, antibiotic treatment is initiated with either a beta-lactamase–resistant antibiotic (cloxacillin [Tegopen] or di-

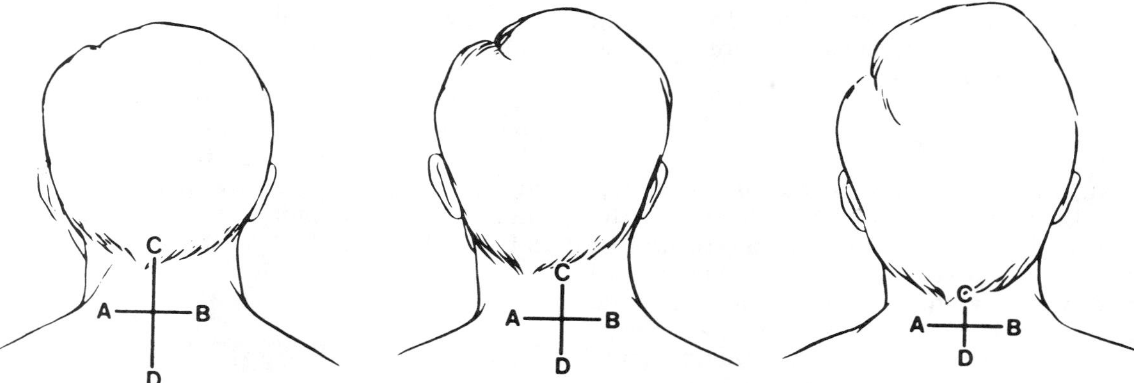

Figure 1. As the neck flexes (left) and extends (right), the distance between points C and D changes considerably, whereas the distance between points A and B remains relatively unchanged. Incisions for drainage of carbuncles located in the posterior neck should be placed in the direction of points A and B, which are perpendicular to the dynamic skin tensions.

cloxacillin [Dynapen], 25 to 50 mg per kg of body weight per day in four divided doses given orally every 6 hours) or a cephalosporin (cephalexin [Keflex] or cephradine [Velosef], same dose as for cloxacillin) if not contraindicated in patients who are allergic to penicillin. If a cephalosporin is contraindicated, clindamycin (Cleocin) or a quinolone may be used. Antimicrobial therapy should be continued until the inflammation has disappeared. The antimicrobial sensitivity of the pathogen must be checked to ensure that this antibiotic regimen is indeed appropriate.

Management of patients with recurrent episodes of carbuncles is a challenging problem. In addition to treatment of the localized infection, careful evaluation for any predisposing systemic illnesses or local factors is essential. Pyogenic infections in other family members or friends must be considered. The following skin care measures must be initiated in an effort to reduce the numbers of *S. aureus* on the patient's clothes and bed linen. Local use of antibiotic ointment containing mupirocin* in the nasal vestibule has been suggested to reduce the nasal carriage of *S. aureus* and thereby limit the dispersal of these bacteria to other regions of the body. Thrice-daily treatment must be continued for at least 3 months, because recurrence of carbuncles is very frequent after short courses of topical antibiotic treatment. Draining lesions should be covered with sterile dressings to prevent autoinoculation. After each dressing change, the dressings should be wrapped in a plastic bag and promptly disposed of after removal. Although immunization with staphylococcal vaccines of various types would also appear to be reasonable in such cases, it has not been successful in the prevention of recurrent infections.

Surgery occasionally is warranted as prophylaxis against recurrent infections. The indication for surgery is the presence of epithelialized tracts that are sequelae of wound repair of the drained carbuncle. These tracts extend deep into the subcutaneous tissue and harbor prodigious numbers of bacteria. Their serpiginous course can be traced by passing a probe coated with methylene blue dye through their orifices on the surface of the skin. The staining of the tracts with the blue dye facilitates their identification when wide surgical excision of the scarred tissue is accomplished.

The development of epithelialized sinus tracts after drainage is also encountered in hidradenitis suppurativa. This is an extremely troublesome infection of blocked hair follicles occurring in the axillary, perianal, and genital regions. Use of antiperspirants appears to predispose an individual to its development. After repeated applications, they form an occlusive cover over the skin that blocks the hair follicles. Initial lesions appear as small red nodules at the site of obstructed hair follicles. When the nodules become fluctuant and drain, they form irregular sinus tracts that predispose the patient to further infections. In the presence of these blind-ended sinuses, radical excision of the involved tissue is necessary.

CELLULITIS

Cellulitis is an acute inflammatory reaction involving the skin and underlying subcutaneous tissue. It usually starts as erysipelas and may advance to lymphangitis, lymphadenitis, or gangrene. Erysipelas is a superficial, acute, expanding infection of the skin, usually of the face and head, characterized by its reddened, brawny, edematous appearance.

Periorbital cellulitis is a distinct clinical entity that is usually secondary to an infection of a contiguous structure (e.g., paranasal sinusitis, osteomyelitis, conjunctivitis, dental infections). Infected thrombi are sometimes evident in associated lymphatics and veins that may extend posteriorly from the orbital cellulitis to involve the cavernous sinus. Inflammatory exudate accumulates within the bony orbit, resulting in proptosis and painful ophthalmoplegia. The diagnosis of periorbital cellulitis is made when an abscess cavity is noted on computed tomography or when pus is drained from the orbit or subperiosteal space at the time of surgery. Immediate treat-

*Not FDA approved for this indication.

ment of this condition may prevent life-threatening complications, such as cavernous sinus thrombosis, meningitis, and brain abscess.

Treatment

In general, antimicrobial prophylaxis is the cornerstone of treatment of cellulitis. The selection of the appropriate antibiotic is based on the results of Gram's stain, which are confirmed by the culture and antibiotic sensitivity tests. Cellulitis occurring in the absence of a break in the skin is usually due to *Streptococcus pyogenes* (Group A streptococci) and should be treated with penicillin G, 1 to 2 million units intravenously every 2 to 3 hours. Patients allergic to penicillin may be treated with cefazolin (Ancef, Kefzol), 75 to 80 mg per kg of body weight per day, given intravenously in four divided doses. Because of the cross-sensitivity in penicillin-allergic and cephalosporin-allergic patients, one might prefer to use vancomycin (Vancocin). In patients between the ages of 3 and 24 months with cellulitis in whom Gram's stain reveals gram-negative rods, *Haemophilus influenzae* should be suspected as the pathogen, and ampicillin,* 200 to 250 mg per kg of body weight per day, should be administered intravenously in six divided doses. With the recent emergence of beta-lactamase–producing, ampicillin-resistant strains, a cephalosporin (cefuroxime or cefotaxime) is very useful in these cases. In the penicillin-allergic patient, trimethoprim-sulfamethoxazole is a useful alternative agent. When Gram's stain reveals a mixture of gram-positive and gram-negative organisms, a combination of a cephalosporin, an aminoglycoside, and clindamycin should be used. As an alternative, imipenem may be used as a single agent. For the penicillin-allergic patient, vancomycin may be used with an aminoglycoside and clindamycin. A prompt response to antimicrobial therapy is usually seen within 72 hours. In conjunction with antimicrobial treatment, immobilization and elevation of the injured extremity are mandatory. Cool, sterile saline soaks decrease the local pain and are particularly helpful in the presence of bullae. In periorbital cellulitis, it is important to determine the primary site of infection so that the appropriate surgical therapy can be instituted. For example, pus-filled maxillary sinuses should be subjected to immediate drainage.

Cellulitis occasionally progresses to gangrene, after the vessels of the skin thrombose. The occurrence of gangrene usually indicates the presence of a mixed bacterial infection. The location of these gangrenous changes has led physicians to coin a variety of names for this clinical entity, such as necrotizing fasciitis and Fournier's gangrene. Regardless of the terminology, each is an infection of the subcutaneous tissue that results in thrombosis of the vessels to the skin. The cornerstone of treatment of gangrene is immediate débridement in conjunction with appropriate antibiotic therapy. Patients with gangrene of the skin are often hypermetabolic and require considerable nutritional support. If this requirement is left unsatisfied, the caloric demand leads to weight loss and impaired resistance to infection. The nutritional needs of these patients must be calculated and supplied by the enteral route, if possible. If enteral feeding is impossible, intravenous alimentation techniques must be employed to achieve caloric and nitrogen balance.

*Exceeds dosage recommended by the manufacturer.

VIRAL DISEASES OF THE SKIN

method of
ROBERT S. PURVIS, M.D., and
LUKE LEWIS, M.D.
Texas Tech University Health Sciences Center
Lubbock, Texas

HERPES SIMPLEX VIRUS

Mucocutaneous Herpes

Herpes simplex infections are among the most common infections in humans. These are caused by *Herpesvirus hominis,* or herpes simplex virus (HSV), which has two major antigenic types. Type 1 (HSV 1) causes most facial or oral infections, whereas Type 2 (HSV 2) causes most genital infections. Whether they are oral or genital, the infections are lifelong and are characterized by periods of latency and reactivation.

Clinical Manifestations

Primary Infections. Primary HSV infections follow transmission of the virus to a susceptible individual about 2 days to 2 weeks after exposure. Because these viruses do not survive for long periods in the environment, and the virus cannot easily penetrate intact skin, spread is mostly person-to-person via mucosal secretions. Contacts of patients with herpes infections may also become inoculated with the virus through traumatized keratinized skin. This is a particular hazard of workers in the health care field.

Most primary HSV 1 infections are asymptomatic and occur during childhood. Gingivostomatitis is the most common symptomatic infection and is characterized by fever, malaise, pain on eating and drinking, and foul breath. The gums are tender and may bleed easily. Vesicles may be present on the buccal mucosa, tongue, palate, oropharynx, nose, or chin. The vesicles on mucosal surfaces rapidly ulcerate, whereas those on the skin pustulate and become crusted over several days. Tender cervical lymphadenopathy is present. Primary infections generally resolve within 3 weeks in immunocompetent patients, whereas immunocompromised patients may have a protracted course.

Primary genital herpes infections are most commonly due to HSV 2. These infections are more often symptomatic than orolabial herpes infections and usually affect young adults. Fever and malaise, along with pain of the affected area, occur after an incubation period of about 2 to 7 days. The pain is followed by grouped red papules, which mature to vesicles, pustules, and crusts. Ruptured vesicles or pustules may form shallow ulcers prior to crusting. Common sites in men are the shaft, prepuce, and glans of the penis, as well as the pubic triangle and scrotum. In women, the vulva, vagina, cervix, and perineum may be involved. Homosexual men may develop painful perianal lesions or proctitis. In both sexes, bilateral tender inguinal lymphadenopathy is present. As with primary orolabial infections, a 2- to 3-week course is common for primary genital infection in immunocompetent patients.

The clinical presentation of primary herpetic infections is the same regardless of the type of infecting herpes simplex virus. Besides orolabial and genital locations, primary herpes simplex infections may involve any external site. The eye is a fairly common site of infection, in which case the involvement is usually unilateral. Blepharitis, with vesicles on and around the lids, is present, along with conjunctivitis. Photophobia, edema, and tearing are the rule. Herpetic infection of the extremities or torso is characterized by the findings of grouped vesicles, pain, and regional lymphadenopathy.

Recurrent Infections. Following primary infection, the herpes simplex virus travels to, and becomes latent in, the sensory nerve ganglion serving the affected site. There, the virion persists without lysis of the neuronal host cells. Reactivation of the viral genome leads to recurrences in the general region of the initial infection. Recurrences may be triggered by emotional stress, sunlight, concurrent infections, and in women, menstruation. In some patients, no precipitating cause can be identified.

Recurrent orolabial herpes simplex episodes occur in about one-third to one-half of infected patients. These fever blisters or cold sores may be preceded by pain or paresthesia of the area affected. Grouped papules occur, which mature into vesicles and crusts. Recurrent infections are usually mild and resolve in 1 week without treatment. Genital herpes is recurrent in three-fourths or more of those infected. Subsequent recurrences are less severe than the initial infection and heal in about 1 week. Patients with significant compromise of cell-mediated immunity may have a longer course. Grouped lesions on an erythematous base evolve from papules to vesicles to ulcers and crusts. A prodrome of pain or paresthesia often alerts the patient to an impending outbreak.

Complications

Both primary HSV infection and recurrences may be accompanied by complications. Keratitis with corneal ulceration may occur in patients with ocular herpes, resulting in epithelial opacities and blindness. Patients with primary or recurrent ocular herpes should be referred for prompt ophthalmologic evaluation. Painful urethral lesions may result in urinary retention in either sex. Sacral radiculoneuropathy may also cause urinary retention, as well as paresthesias and constipation. Systemic dissemination or encephalitis may complicate primary infection, especially in immunocompromised patients. The mortality rate for encephalitis is very high. Kaposi's varicelliform eruption, or eczema herpeticum, is a widespread cutaneous infection with herpes simplex virus in a patient with a predisposing inflammatory skin disease, the most common of which is atopic dermatitis. It may occur with either primary or recurrent disease. The typical target or iris lesions of erythema multiforme may either accompany or follow HSV infections. This is most likely an immunologic response to an HSV antigen.

Diagnosis

Most cases of herpes simplex infection can be diagnosed clinically with the finding of grouped vesicles on an erythematous base. The identification of multinucleated giant cells on a Wright- or Giemsa-stained scraping from a vesicle base (Tzanck smear) implicates either HSV or varicella zoster virus infection as the causative agent. However, this test is difficult to interpret for the infrequent examiner. The standard in diagnosis is viral culture, which takes from 1 to 14 days for growth and identification. The best results are obtained from aspiration of fluid from an unruptured vesicle. Swabs from ulcers may also yield a positive culture. New in-office diagnostic kits offer results within minutes. Knowledge of the type of virus responsible has prognostic significance because genital infections due to HSV 1 tend to recur less frequently than those due to HSV 2.

Treatment

Acyclovir (Zovirax), a purine analogue preferentially taken up by virus-infected cells, is useful in the treatment of both primary and recurrent herpes simplex infections. If severe gingivostomatitis is present or in immunocompromised patients with severe infection, the intravenous form at a dose of 5 mg per kg over 1 hour every 8 hours for 7 to 10 days should be given. The oral form* may be given for less severe primary infections at a dose of 200 mg 5 times daily for 7 to 10 days. Adequate hydration should be maintained with both oral and intravenous routes of administration.

Mild recurrences require no treatment in many cases; however, some patients find treatment necessary. Acyclovir 200 mg orally five times daily for 5 days hastens healing time. Genital herpes responds to acyclovir better than does orolabial herpes outbreaks. Some patients find that they can abort outbreaks by taking this medication at the appearance of the very first prodromal symptom. Therefore, such patients should have medication on hand at all times. Selected patients prefer acyclovir ointment over the oral medication. It is used topically five or six times daily.

Patients who have frequent recurrent genital disease may be candidates for suppression of their disease with oral acyclovir. An adequate dosage is 400

*Not FDA approved for this indication.

mg twice a day for most patients, but the lowest effective daily dose should be used.

Foscarnet (Foscavir), though not FDA approved for herpes simplex infections, may be considered for use in immunocompromised patients with acyclovir-resistant strains of herpesvirus.

Prevention

The high titer of virus present during an acute outbreak of either orolabial or genital herpes makes transmission very likely if intimate contact occurs. However, asymptomatic virus shedding is probably responsible for most infections. Regular use of latex condoms with spermicide may reduce, but does not eliminate, the risk of asymptomatic transmission in patients with genital herpes. Counseling regarding the infectious and incurable nature of the disease, as well as modes of transmission and treatment, may help patients deal more effectively with this socially calamitous disease.

VARICELLA ZOSTER VIRUS

Varicella

(see the article entitled Varicella [Chickenpox])

Herpes Zoster

Herpes zoster is a painful skin eruption caused by reactivation of a latent infection with the varicella zoster virus. Factors triggering reactivation include advancing age, immunosuppression, surgery, trauma, and possibly, stress.

Clinical Manifestations

The clinical course often begins days to weeks before the eruption with prodromal pain, pruritus, or paresthesia in the area affected. Conversely, there may be no prodrome. The rash begins with one or more erythematous macules that quickly progress to vesicles, which are typically distributed unilaterally within a dermatome or perhaps two adjacent dermatomes. Thoracic dermatomes are most frequently affected, followed by the dermatome of the ophthalmic division of the trigeminal nerve. Lesions may number from a few to several hundred. Within several days the vesicles become pustules, or they may rupture to form ulcers. Next, crusts form, which often progress to atrophic scars.

Pain may range from none to excruciating, may exist as a continuation of the prodrome, or may begin 1 or more days following the onset of the eruption. The pain may subside with healing of the skin lesions, or it may persist as post-herpetic neuralgia months to years after cutaneous healing has taken place. Post-herpetic neuralgia occurs more commonly in patients over 50 years of age. The pain of post-herpetic neuralgia may be mildly annoying to severe enough to lead the patient to consider suicide.

Diagnosis

The diagnosis of herpes zoster usually is straightforward once the unilateral dermatomal vesicular rash has appeared, but prodromal pain has been mistaken for pain from myocardial disease, aortic aneurysm, or an acute abdomen. The presence of multinucleated giant cells on Tzanck smear establishes a herpetic viral origin and rules out other vesicular conditions such as contact dermatitis. A viral culture is the most readily available method of distinguishing herpes zoster from zosteriform herpes simplex, which may have an identical appearance.

Complications

Complications of herpes zoster include cutaneous or visceral dissemination (pneumonitis, hepatitis, carditis, pancreatitis, esophagitis, enterocolitis, cystitis, synovitis, meningoencephalitis) and cranial and motor neuropathies. Approximately 50% of patients with ophthalmic zoster experience ocular complications such as conjunctivitis, scleritis, keratitis, uveitis, and rarely, acute retinal necrosis. Complications of zoster in the normal host with nonophthalmic zoster are rare. Patients who have documented recurrent zoster or who have multidermatomal involvement at the time of presentation should be evaluated for an underlying immunodeficiency, especially AIDS. When sacral dermatomes are involved, or when the eruption is recurrent, herpes simplex should be suspected and viral culture performed.

Treatment

The treatment of herpes zoster depends on the patient's age and immune status, as well as the duration of illness prior to diagnosis. The treatment of choice in the immunocompromised patient is intravenous acyclovir (Zovirax), 10 mg per kg every 8 hours until lesions are fully crusted. Such treatment has been shown to shorten the period of viral shedding and new vesicle formation, accelerate healing, and shorten the duration of pain in the acute phase. The major side effect of crystalluria and renal damage can be avoided or treated with hydration. In the less severely immunocompromised patient or one who refuses hospitalization, oral acyclovir at a dose of 800 mg five times daily until full crusting occurs (usually 7 to 10 days) is an alternative. This regimen is recommended also for the immunocompetent adult over the age of 50 years because it has been shown to decrease healing time, viral shedding, and acute pain. Some studies have shown a reduction in post-herpetic neuralgia with acyclovir as well. In the immunocompetent adult under the age of 50 years, in whom the complications of zoster are infrequent and pain and post-herpetic neuralgia are generally not as severe, the benefits of acyclovir are less evident and must be weighed against its cost, which is substantial. Regardless of age, patients with ophthalmic zoster should be treated with acyclovir and referred to an ophthalmologist for consideration of adjunctive topical therapy.

Intravenous vidarabine (Vira A), in doses of 10 mg per kg per day, is effective in treating zoster and in immunocompromised patients. However, it is less effective, more difficult to administer, and more toxic than acyclovir.

Interferon-alpha* at a dosage of 1 to 2 times 10^6 IU per kg intramuscularly for 7 days has been shown to reduce new vesicle formation, cutaneous and visceral dissemination, and visceral and central nervous system complications as well as post-herpetic neuralgia. Its use cannot be routinely recommended, however, because of its toxicity and cost.

In general, antiviral therapy for herpes zoster is less effective the longer the delay in initiating therapy. In fact, most investigational studies evaluating antiviral agents for zoster exclude patients whose rash has been present for over 72 hours.

During the acute phase of herpes zoster, the application of cool compresses with Burow's solution may help provide some soothing relief and help dry the lesions. Analgesics such as acetaminophen with codeine help to reduce the pain to tolerable levels in most patients. More potent analgesics or nerve blocks are rarely needed for acute neuralgia. It is important to counsel patients that they should avoid physical contact with anyone who has not had chicken pox until their lesions are fully crusted.

The prevention of post-herpetic neuralgia is difficult. Like the studies performed with acyclovir, studies using systemic steroids during the acute phase have shown variable results in preventing post-herpetic neuralgia. A popular regimen begins with daily doses of oral prednisone* of 60 mg for 1 week, followed by 30 mg for the second week, and 15 mg for the third and final week. Intramuscular triamcinolone acetonide,† 80 mg given on presentation, may be repeated in 5 days if there is persisting acute neuralgia. Such therapy may decrease acute neuralgia as well as possibly reducing subsequent post-herpetic neuralgia. We recommend the use of systemic steroids in patients over 50 years of age unless the patients are immunocompromised or brittle diabetics, or unless the agents are otherwise contraindicated. With a short course of steroids, the side effects are minimal and the potential risk of provoking dissemination is negligible.

Once the condition is established, post-herpetic neuralgia may be especially difficult to manage, because there is no extremely effective therapy. Topical treatment with capsaicin 0.025% cream (Zostrix) or 0.075% cream (Zostrix-HP) applied three to four times a day may help, but the initial burning associated with its application is often not tolerated and several weeks of therapy are required before a therapeutic effect is reached. A eutectic mixture of lidocaine and prilocaine (EMLA)* has been reported to be helpful in post-herpetic neuralgia, but in addition to its expense, it is cumbersome to use because it must be applied under occlusion every 12 hours.

Oral systemic therapy for post-herpetic neuralgia includes the use of tricyclic antidepressants, phenothiazines, anticonvulsants, and narcotic analgesics.

*Not FDA approved for this indication.
†Exceeds dose recommended by the manufacturer.

The most popular drug is amitriptyline (Elavil),* started at a dose of 25 mg every night and increasing to 50 mg three times daily, as necessary. Amitriptyline may be combined with perphenazine (Trilafon),* 2 to 4 mg three times a day; fluphenazine hydrochloride (Permitil),* 1 mg three to four times a day; or thioridazine (Mellaril),* 25 mg four times a day. The combined use of carbamazepine (Tegretol),* 600 to 800 mg per day, or phenytoin sodium (Dilantin),* 300 to 400 mg per day, with nortriptyline (Aventyl, Pamelor),* 50 to 100 mg per day, has also been shown to be of some benefit, as have combinations of carbamazepine* at up to 1000 mg per day and clomipramine (Anafranil)* at up to 75 mg per day.

Intramuscular triamcinolone acetonide,*† 80 mg, repeated in 4 or 5 days if the response is unsatisfactory, has been shown to reduce established post-herpetic neuralgia in some cases, as have daily intralesional (subcutaneous) infiltrations of triamcinolone acetonide* at a concentration of 2 mg per mL with a total volume per treatment of no more than 15 mL for up to 2 weeks. Although narcotic analgesics should not be the mainstay of treatment for post-herpetic neuralgia, they may be useful adjuncts for breakthrough pain because they often do provide temporary pain relief. A record of narcotic use is also helpful in quantifying pain so that concomitant therapy may be adjusted accordingly.

Transcutaneous electrical stimulation may also be helpful in relieving post-herpetic neuralgia. Neurosurgical intervention is sometimes necessary in patients with intractable pain.

CYTOMEGALOVIRUS

Cytomegalic Inclusion Disease

Cytomegalovirus, the most common viral infection of the newborn, usually appears as a subclinical infection. Symptomatic neonates may have jaundice, hepatosplenomegaly, interstitial pneumonitis, chorioretinitis, convulsions, cerebral calcifications, and microcephaly. Petechiae and purpura may be seen secondary to thrombocytopenia. A generalized maculopapular eruption may occur and, occasionally, a bluish red papulonodular eruption (so-called blueberry muffin baby) can be seen. Some infants die; survivors often have neurologic impairment.

Symptomatic infection may also occur in adults. For instance, a transient rubelliform rash may occur in the face of a mononucleosis-like illness. A more serious illness occurs in immunocompromised patients.

High-dose acyclovir and interferon-alpha* may be useful in prophylaxis of cytomegalovirus infection, whereas ganciclovir (Cytovene) and foscarnet (Foscavir) have shown some benefit in patients actually infected with cytomegalovirus.

*Not FDA approved for this indication.
†Exceeds dosage recommended by the manufacturer.

HERPESVIRUS 6

Roseola Infantum (Exanthema Subitum)

Roseola infantum, caused by human herpesvirus 6, most commonly affects babies between 6 and 36 months of age. Clinically, it is characterized by high fever, which lasts approximately 4 days, after which time the fever suddenly drops and there appears a morbilliform erythematous eruption consisting of rose-colored discrete macules on the neck, trunk, buttock, and at times, the face and extremities. No treatment is required because the rash fades spontaneously within 1 to 2 days.

PARVOVIRUS B19

Erythema Infectiosum (Fifth Disease)

This exanthem, caused by infection with parvovirus B19, is characterized by the sudden development of erythema over the malar areas and lateral face giving a so-called slapped cheek appearance. There may also be a lacelike erythema of the shoulder girdle. The disease usually requires no treatment, but adults may develop pruritus and polyarthritis that lasts beyond the usual 7-day course. Aplastic anemia may complicate some cases, especially in patients with hemolytic disease, such as sickle cell anemia.

COXSACKIEVIRUS

Hand-Foot-Mouth Disease

This viral disease may be caused by several strains of the coxsackievirus, most commonly type A16. Typical findings include sparsely distributed papules and vesicles on the hands, feet, buttocks, and oral mucosa. Each vesicle usually sits on an erythematous areola. In adults, pain may be severe and interfere with oral intake. The disease usually runs a 5- to 7-day course. Diagnosis is determined either by the clinical presentation, viral culture of the lesions, or rising antibody titers. Treatment is symptomatic. Swishing diphenhydramine (Benadryl) elixir or an oral anesthetic solution in the mouth may temporarily alleviate mouth discomfort in patients with painful oral lesions.

POXVIRUS

Molluscum Contagiosum

Molluscum contagiosum is a poxvirus infection of the skin that is most commonly found in children, in whom the lesions are often widespread. However, the condition also occurs as a sexually transmitted disease in the genital region of adults. Infection is spread mainly through contact, although infectivity is low.

Clinically, molluscum contagiosum presents as one or more umbilicated dome-shaped flesh-colored papules, which can occur on almost any part of the body. Lesions are often larger and more widespread in patients with acquired immune deficiency syndrome.

Diagnosis may be made by incising one of the papules, smearing the contents between two glass slides, staining (Wright, Giemsa, or Gram's stain), and visualizing the oval, smooth-walled homogeneous molluscum bodies under low power of a microscope.

In the immunocompetent host, individual lesions usually last for about 2 months but new lesions continue to appear from 6 months to 2 years. The lesions generally heal without scarring.

Because molluscum contagiosum is a self-limited, harmless infection that heals without scarring, treatment is not absolutely necessary. However, the lesions are unsightly and most patients, or parents of patients, demand their removal. The best method is by curettage with either no anesthesia or local anesthesia with ethyl chloride spray, EMLA cream,* or lidocaine.* Light cryotherapy is probably the next best alternative. Light electrodesiccation is also effective and may be the treatment of choice for eyelid lesions. Application of a minute drop of a vesicant such as cantharidin (Cantharone)* under occlusion for 24 hours is the treatment of choice for most children, who will not tolerate more painful methods, but it cannot be used around the eyes. Patients treated with destructive methods or cantharidin should be followed-up at weekly intervals and retreated until no new lesions appear. Topical tretinoin (Retin-A)* is painless but ineffective. Anecdotal reports have described some cures resulting from the administration of oral griseofulvin, given for 4 to 6 weeks. Molluscum infection in acquired immune deficiency syndrome is especially difficult to eradicate, but improvement has been noted with initiation of zidovudine (Retrovir).

Orf

Orf is caused by human contact with sheep infected with sheep pox. The virus affects the skin by first causing the formation of a solitary painless papule, which becomes targetoid with a red center surrounded successively with a white ring and then a red halo. It next turns into a red weeping nodule, which becomes papillomatous and then flattens to form a dry crust with eventual healing with a slight scar. Lesions occur most commonly on the fingers, hands, wrists, and face. Mild swelling, fever, pain, or lymphadenitis may accompany the lesions. No treatment is required for this self-limited disease unless the patient is immunosuppressed, in which case surgical excision is warranted. Lesions usually heal within 5 to 6 weeks, and the resulting immunity is lifelong.

PARAVACCINIA VIRUS

Milker's Nodules

Milker's nodules are caused by infection with paravaccinia virus. They are transmitted from cows, in

---

*Not FDA approved for this indication.

which the lesions commonly occur on the teats or udder. Human lesions are usually confined to the hands and forearms, and usually number from one to four. Initial erythematous macules progress to papules to targetoid papulovesicles, each with a red center surrounded by a white ring and red halo. Next, the lesions weep and erode, and eventuate to crusted nodules, which are about 1 cm in diameter. Finally, papillomatous elevations develop and the lesions darken and slough. No treatment is needed for milker's nodules because they usually regress spontaneously in about 6 weeks.

PARASITIC INFECTIONS OF THE SKIN

method of
KEN HASHIMOTO, M.D., and
HARRY H. SHARATA, M.D., PH.D.
Wayne State University School of Medicine
Detroit, Michigan

SCABIES

Scabies used to occur in an epidemic every 8 to 12 years. Today, it is a common perennial disease caused by a mite, *Sarcoptes scabiei* var *hominis* (Mégnin, 1880). The infestation is usually related to poor hygiene but also seen in nursing homes, hospital wards, and schools. It can be transmitted by promiscuous sexual contact, as well as through a contaminated sofa, carpet, bedding, and clothing, where the mites can survive for as long as 3 days detached from the host. The female mite measures 0.4 × 0.3 mm and the male about half this size. They prefer nonhairy soft parts of the body such as interdigital webs, genitalia, intergluteal folds, axillae, flexor surface of the wrists, and lower abdomen. In infants, palms and soles are predilection sites. The female mite lives in a subcorneal mite burrow, which is a few millimeters long and often attached to a vesicle at the blind end. To demonstrate the mite, prick this vesicle with a blade, smear on a glass slide, add a drop of 25% KOH, wait for 10 minutes, and cover with a coverslip. A gentle heating may help dissolve keratin and release the mite. A chain of dark brown feces (scybala) or egg shells with or without larva are diagnostic even if the mite is missed. Superficial shave biopsy demonstrates the tissue reaction typical of an insect bite (i.e., patchy lymphocytic infiltrations with eosinophils). In immunosuppressed, debilitated, or institutionalized patients, the infestation can be severe and chronic. In Norwegian scabies, numerous mites infest hands, feet, genitalia, and auricles. Hyperkeratosis and crusting are predominant, and the clinical picture is different from that of ordinary scabies. In patients with acquired immune deficiency syndrome, scabies is generalized and exaggerated.

Treatment

The mainstay of scabies treatment is still gamma benzene hexachloride or lindane (Kwell), which has a high cure rate (>95%). Total body application of 1% lotion or cream after a bath or shower is recommended. Hydration of keratin by a cool bath facilitates the uniform penetration of 1% lindane (Kwell). The application should include the entire body, from neck to toes. Although the head is usually spared in adults, it may be involved in infants and children; if clinical signs indicate, it should also be treated. The medication should be left on the skin overnight and washed off with soap the next morning. Ulcerated or infected areas should be avoided until the patient is re-treated. Systemic or topical antibiotics, or both, covering staphylococci and streptococci should be prescribed, and hydroxyzine hydrochloride (Atarax) or hydroxyzine pamoate (Vistaril) tablets or syrup given at bedtime should be added for pruritic patients. Most patients benefit from topical corticosteroid creams or ointments such as 0.1% mometasone furoate (Elocon) for general use and 0.05% betamethasone dipropionate (Diprosone or Diprolene AF) for problem spots. Lindane 1% (Kwell) should be applied again after 1 week, particularly in severe cases, because no matter how carefully it was applied, some lesions may be missed. Family members may or may not have symptoms because the pruritus is mainly due to hypersensitivity to the mites and their scybala, and sometimes it takes a month to develop symptoms. Therefore, asymptomatic family members should be treated and furniture and beds should be sprayed with gamma benzene hexachloride spray (R&C Spray).* Patients' underwear should be washed with hot water. Continuous pruritus after two or three treatments may not be caused by persistent mites but may be an allergic reaction to dead mites and their products. In some patients, particularly infants, pruritic nodules persist on extremities for several months or longer. Prurigo-like large nodules may be seen on the scrotum in adults. Because these lesions last so long and persist after the pruritus has already subsided, the preceding episode of scabies is often forgotten and other differential diagnoses such as lymphoma and histiocytic proliferations are considered. The biopsy specimen demonstrates immunophenotypes compatible with benign indeterminate cell histiocytosis. These lesions are best treated with a focal application of superpotent corticosteroid ointments, such as 0.05% clobetasol propionate (Temovate) ointment or 0.05% halobetasol propionate (Ultravate) ointment twice a day, or intralesional injection of 0.2 mL of triamcinolone acetonide suspension (10 mg/mL) (Kenalog 10).

Side effects of Kwell range from headache to convulsions. However, these complications are extremely rare in our routine treatment of scabies. Excoriated skin or skin of abnormal keratinization such as in psoriasis, atopic dermatitis, and ichthyosis lacks the normal skin barrier, and absorption of the drug is tremendously increased. Small infants have a relatively large skin surface area to body volume ratio, and their skin barrier is immature. Pregnant women,

*Not available in the United States.

nursing mothers, and seizure-prone patients may be advised about potential side effects, although our experience does not preclude the use of 1% lindane (Kwell) in these situations. A short application (6 hours) on a dry skin may be the option.

Permethrin (Elimite) 5% cream paralyzes the mite by disturbing polarization of the nerve cell membrane. It is not as effective as lindane (Kwell), although it may be safer for infants. It may temporarily enhance pruritus and cause a mild burning and stinging sensation. The method of application is the same as that for 1% lindane (Kwell).

Crotamiton (Eurax) 10% cream or lotion is antipruritic as well as scabicidal. This is the least effective among chemical scabicides; however, it has been used for a long time without many reported side effects. The application method is similar to that used for 1% lindane (Kwell) but it should be repeated in 3 to 5 days without washing.*

Precipitated sulfur 6% in petrolatum is the safest choice for premature infants, pregnant women, and nursing mothers. The ointment should be applied daily for 3 consecutive days and washed only after the fourth day. The entire body should be treated. Sulfur dermatitis may be treated with mometasone furoate (Elocon) cream twice a day.

Animal scabies mites such as *Notoedres cati* may cause pruritic inflammatory papules, often on the flexor surface of forearms and frontal trunk, where the contact with pets is common. Fingerwebs and genitalia are spared, and no mite burrow is found because they do not lay eggs in the human skin. The auricles, forehead, and other parts of the suspected animal should be examined for alopecia caused by scratching, papules, and crusting. The infested animal should be treated or eliminated in severe cases.

PEDICULOSIS

Pediculosis capitis (head louse infestation) is caused by *Pediculus humanus* var *capitis*. This is most commonly seen among schoolgirls and is transmitted through shared brushes and combs. The posterior and lateral areas of the scalp show many excoriations and broken papules. These lesions may extend down to the nape and even to the upper shoulder, which is covered by long hair. The hairs are spread and examined under good illumination with a 10× hand lens. This examination reveals white-reflecting nits firmly cemented to the hairs. Wood's light facilitates the identification of nits. Eggs are first laid at the base of the hair shaft and move distally with hair growth. The duration of infestation can be estimated by the position of nits and the average growth of human scalp hair (1 cm per month). Adult lice are found on the hair shaft, and they resemble small flakes of dandruff but cannot be flipped off. Pediculosis capitis is rare among blacks because short, curled hairs are resistant to head lice.

Phthirus pubis (crab louse) is a broad, crablike organism that infests the hairs of apocrine gland–rich areas such as genitalia, axilla, eyebrow, and eyelashes. They are transmitted by sexual contact. Eggs or nits are first laid at the base of hair and move more distally as hair grows. Firmly attached nits are best examined on a cut or extracted hair under the microscope. The adult louse can be identified with 10× hand lens as a whitish moving object of 0.8 to 1.2 mm. Nits hatch in 1 week and become adult lice in 13 to 16 days. The female louse lays 1 to 4 eggs a day and lives for a month but dies within a few days if separated from the host. Intense pruritus, secondary infection, and eczematization are usual presenting symptoms. Bruiselike blue patches (maculae caeruleae) may be found on the trunk.

Pediculosis corporis is caused by body lice (*Pediculus humanus* var *corporis*), which are longer than head or pubic lice. This is mostly seen among people who live with poor hygiene, for example, the homeless, refugees living in a refugee camp, and prisoners. Clinical pictures vary from papuloerythematous eruptions to urticarial lesions. In severe cases, the body surface is covered with bloody streaks and crusts due to deep excoriations. The lice and eggs are found not on the skin but in the seams of clothing. Body lice can be a vector for typhus (*Rickettsia prowazekii*), louse-borne relapsing fever (*Borrelia recurrentis*), and trench fever (*Rochalimaea quintana*).

Treatment

Head lice and pubic lice can be treated with 1% lindane (Kwell) shampoo, which should be applied to dry hair thoroughly for 5 to 10 minutes; water is then added to form a good lather and to rinse. This treatment may be repeated after 1 week. Nits should be removed with nit comb or tweezers. Permethrin 1% (Nix), which is available over the counter with nit comb, should be applied in a similar manner. Pyrethrins (RID) can be used in a similar fashion but should be repeated after 1 week because of its poor ovicidal effect. Eyelash involvement can be treated by petrolatum applied to eyelashes 3 to 5 times daily for 1 week, or by physostigmine (Eserine), 0.25% ophthalmic ointment* applied similarly 3 to 5 times daily for 3 days. As many nits as possible should be removed with fine tweezers. Chemical pediculocides should not be used on the eyelashes because they irritate the eyes.

The elimination of body lice is accomplished by cleaning the patient's clothing. Hot washer and hot dryer cycles kill the lice, but heavily infested underwear should be packed in a plastic bag and incinerated. Cleaning of the environment including bedding is essential. Pruritus should be treated with corticosteroid ointments such as mometasone furoate (Elocon) and antihistamines such as hydroxyzine hydrochloride (Atarax). Secondary infection should be treated with oral antibiotics that cover staphylococci and streptococci.

*Exceeds dosage recommended by the manufacturer.

*Not FDA approved for this indication.

LEISHMANIASIS

Interest in this disease was rekindled with U.S. troop involvement in the Middle East. In Old World leishmaniasis, localized cutaneous disease may be exhibited as a small papule or plaque with central scaling 2 to 4 weeks after a sandfly bite, usually on exposed skin such as the face. The initial papular eruption at the bite site enlarges slowly with central ulceration. Peripheral satellite papules (as caused by *Leishmania major*) or diffuse cutaneous nodules resembling lepromatous leprosy (as caused by *L. aethiopica*) may develop. In New World leishmaniasis, *L. mexicana* complex (Mexico, Texas, Central America) may cause an ulcerated nodule at the bite site that eventually heals with a depressed scar. *L. braziliensis* complex (Brazil and Bolivia), on the other hand, may evolve from the initial nodule to destruction of the mouth, nose, pharynx, and larynx.

Visceral leishmaniasis, or kala-azar, occurs when the parasite invades bone marrow and viscera, and the condition is fatal if it is left untreated. This fulminant category is caused by *L. donovani* in India and Africa, *L. infantum* in the Mediterranean basin, and *L. donovani chagasi* in Central and South America.

The diagnosis of cutaneous leishmaniasis requires demonstration of amastigotes by direct microscopic examination of exudate from an incised papule or from the edge of an ulcerated lesion. After Giemsa staining, the parasites appear as eosinophilic inclusions in the cytoplasm of tissue macrophages. Alternatively, the parasites may be cultured in Novy-MacNeal-Nicolle medium. Promastigotes may be detected as early as several days or as late as 4 weeks in culture. Leishmania (Montenegro) intradermal test with phenolized suspension of promastigotes is highly sensitive and specific for both New and Old World leishmaniases. It is useful in the diagnosis of leishmania-poor lesions such as in late-stage mucocutaneous leishmaniasis, but it may produce false-negative results in anergic cases of visceral disease.

Treatment

The treatment of choice for both New and Old World leishmaniasis is pentavalent antimonials. Sodium stibogluconate (Pentostam*) and meglumine antimonate* are available from the Centers for Disease Control and Prevention (CDC) and should be given as 20 mg antimony per kg per day intravenously or intramuscularly for 3 to 4 weeks for adult and pediatric patients. Adverse reactions to the pentavalent antimonials are rare and include pain at the site of intramuscular injection, gastrointestinal symptoms, and reversible EKG changes with Q-T prolongation.

Second-line drugs include amphotericin B, 0.25 to 1 mg per kg by slow intravenous injection given daily or every other day for up to 8 weeks; pentamidine isethionate, 2 to 4 mg per kg daily or every other day intravenously for up to 15 doses; and ketoconazole, 400 mg orally daily for 4 weeks.

*Investigational drug in the United States.

TRYPANOSOMIASIS

African Trypanosomiasis

African trypanosomiasis (sleeping sickness) is caused by *Trypanosoma gambiense* and *Trypanosoma rhodesiense,* which are transmitted by the bite of the tsetse fly in equatorial Africa. A painful nodule (chancre) appears in 4 to 10 days at the bite site, accompanied by regional lymphadenopathy. After 2 weeks, the initial lesion disappears and ensuing parasitemia causes fevers; symmetrical adenopathy; transient edema of eyelids, palms, and soles; and generalized pruritic eruptions with erythematous annular plaques. Posterior cervical lymphadenopathy (Winterbottom's sign) is prominent. Cardiac and central nervous system involvement lead to death. History of travel to an endemic area and the finding of the trypanosome on peripheral blood smear or by immunologic assay (enzyme-linked immunosorbent assay [ELISA] and indirect hemagglutination) help confirm the diagnosis.

Treatment

Treatment is usually with suramin* (available from CDC); a 100- to 200-mg intravenous test dose is given, followed by 1 gram given intravenously on days 1, 3, 7, 14, and 21. The pediatric dose is 20 mg per kg on days 1, 3, 7, 14, and 21. Pentamidine isethionate (Pentam 300) is an alternative. In patients with late disease and CNS involvement melarsoprol (Arsobal)* (available from CDC) or eflornithine (Ornidyl) is advocated; both are associated with serious toxicities.

South American Trypanosomiasis

South American trypanosomiasis (Chagas' disease) is caused by *Trypanosoma cruzi* after a reduviid bug (kissing bug) bite on the face of a sleeping victim. A boardlike induration (chagoma) develops at the bite site, with periorbital edema (if the bite was conjunctival) and regional adenopathy. Parasitic invasion of the gut and heart occurs as the chagoma clears with a scar in 1 to 4 months; this leads to end-organ insufficiency with progressive heart failure, megacolon, and megaesophagus. The diagnosis of Chagas' disease requires demonstration of trypanosomes in the peripheral blood smear.

Treatment

Treatment is with nifurtimox* (Lampit) (available from CDC) or benznidazole,† 5 to 7 mg per kg per day for 30 to 120 days. Anorexia, vomiting, weight loss,

*Investigational drug in the United States.
†Not available in the United States.

paresthesia, and polyneuritis may occur with nifurtimox, whereas benznidazole may cause allergic dermatitis, dose-dependent polyneuropathy, and gastrointestinal disturbances.

AMEBIASIS

Entamoeba histolytica invades the skin as a result of direct inoculation of the skin with infected material from the bowel following heterosexual and homosexual intercourse. This is particularly true for patients with acquired immune deficiency syndrome, in whom cell-mediated immunity is diminished and the disease may be fatal. A nonspecific ulcerated granuloma develops at the site and must be distinguished from epithelioma, syphilis, and other infectious granulomas. Trophozoites may be found at the edge of an ulcer or on biopsy.

Treatment

The treatment of choice for cutaneous and intestinal disease is metronidazole, 750 mg orally or intravenously three times a day for 10 days, or dehydroemetine* (Mebadin) (available from CDC), 1 to 1.5 mg per kg per day (maximum 90 mg per day) intramuscularly for up to 5 days. The side effects of metronidazole are arrhythmias, precordial pain, muscle weakness, and gastrointestinal disturbances.

HELMINTHIC INFECTIONS

Roundworm Infections

Enterobius vermicularis is the most common worldwide helminthic infection, with a prevalence of 30% in children and 16% in adults. The worm is spread via the fecal-oral route with ingestion of embryonated eggs. After completion of the life cycle (2 to 8 weeks) in the cecum, the gravid female worm emerges from the host's anus to lay a fresh crop of eggs in the perineal and perianal areas. This usually occurs at night and is accompanied by severe pruritus and irritability. The larvae hatch after several hours. Demonstration of the worm on clothing or bedding or of eggs on the involved skin leads to the correct diagnosis. A loop of cellophane tape may be pressed against the skin and subsequently placed upon a drop of toluene on a microscope slide to detect the characteristic oval eggs.

Treatment

Treatment with mebendazole (Vermox), 100 mg as a single oral dose with re-administration after 2 weeks, is curative in adults and children. All family members should be examined and treated if eggs are found. Alternative treatment is oral pyrantel (Antiminth), 11 mg per kg up to 1 gram, as a single oral dose, repeated in 2 weeks. Both treatments are well tolerated.

*Investigational drug in the United States.

Cutaneous Larva Migrans (Creeping Eruption)

This refers to intensely pruritic migratory eruptions on the buttocks, hands, and feet after contact with soil, commonly on the beach, contaminated with dog or cat feces that contain hookworm ova. Eggs in the feces hatch infective *Ancylostoma* (hookworm) larvae, which can penetrate intact human skin and begin wandering in the lower epidermis. Migratory burrows forming geographic linear tracts, urticarial bands with intense pruritus, excoriation, and secondary bacterial infection may persist for weeks to years. *Strongyloides stercoralis* and *Gnathostoma spinigerum* may also cause larva migrans.

The diagnosis of larva migrans is clinical and is based on the patient's history and the distinctive appearance of the migrating tracts (1 to 2 cm per day for *Ancylostoma;* up to 10 cm per day for *Strongyloides stercoralis*).

Treatment

Treatment is best accomplished by topical application of 10% aqueous suspension of thiabendazole (Mintezol), applied four times a day to the tracts and surrounding normal skin, and with oral thiabendazole, 25 mg per kg twice daily for 2 days. Thiabendazole can be associated with nausea, vomiting, and vertigo. Albendazole (Zentel),* 400 mg given as a single oral dose, is an alternative.

Gnathostomiasis may require surgical removal of the parasites.

CUTANEOUS SCHISTOSOMIASIS

Cercarial dermatitis, or swimmer's itch, occurs in the Great Lakes of North America and in other parts of the world where swimmers come in contact with water harboring infected snails and waterfowl. Cercariae of approximately 20 species have been implicated as the cause of swimmer's itch. The cercariae are attracted to the water surface and adhere to the skin of bathers as they emerge from the water. The patient experiences an itching, prickling sensation within minutes as the cercariae penetrate exposed skin. Evanescent diffuse erythematous macules appear and are subsequently replaced by erythematous papules and vesicles in 10 to 15 hours. The covered areas are usually spared.

To avoid epidemics, destruction of infected snails by addition of copper sulfate and sodium pentachlorphenate to affected lakes is required. The patients may be treated symptomatically with oral antihistamines until the eruption spontaneously resolves.

So-called seabather's eruption is a closely related cercarial dermatitis occurring in saltwater beaches off the Atlantic or Gulf Coasts. The eruption is confined to the swimming trunk area and consists of pruritic crusted papules that occur within hours of bathing and resolve within several days. The pruritus may be controlled with oral antihistamines until the lesions resolve spontaneously.

*Investigational drug in the United States.

CUTANEOUS MYIASIS

Myiasis occurs when eggs are deposited by botflies and blowflies in open wounds or discharging orifices (such as nostrils), and larvae infest the skin. As the larvae burrow and develop in the skin over a period of weeks to months, crawling, itching sensations may be experienced by the patient. Groups of furuncle-like lesions with a central opening or a serous discharge may be seen.

Treatment

Treatment consists of incising the lesion and removing the larvae with forceps. Other treatments include the application of petroleum jelly to bring the larvae to the surface or pork fat or bacon, which attracts the feeding larvae. Some patients have required psychiatric counseling after larval extraction.

Current drug information for rare parasites is available from the Centers for Disease Control and Prevention at 1-404-639-3670.

SUPERFICIAL FUNGAL INFECTIONS OF THE SKIN

method of
EDGAR B. SMITH, M.D.
University of Texas Medical Branch
Galveston, Texas

The superficial fungal infections, dermatophytosis, candidiasis, and tinea versicolor, are common and are frequent causes of both self-treatment with over-the-counter agents and visits to physicians. All of these conditions are due to organisms that invade the outermost layer of the epidermis, the stratum corneum, and produce varying degrees of inflammation in the underlying cutaneous structures. Although these infections often have typical clinical features, they may be simulated by other inflammatory skin diseases. Therefore, mycologic confirmation with potassium hydroxide preparation or culture, or both, always should be sought to ensure most effective management.

DERMATOPHYTOSIS

The dermatophytes are a class of fungi that live in the stratum corneum of humans or animals and in soil. Although there are many species, most infections in the United States are due to five species: *Trichophyton rubrum, Trichophyton tonsurans, Trichophyton mentagrophytes, Microsporum canis,* and *Epidermophyton floccosum.* Clinical manifestations of the infection vary somewhat with the causative organism but more with the site of infection and the host inflammatory response.

Dermatophytosis of the scalp, tinea capitis, is the most common fungal infection of children and is most commonly due to *Trichophyton tonsurans.* This organism invades the hair shaft and produces spores within the hair (endothrix infection). It does not produce fluorescence on Wood's light examination. Clinical findings can vary from slight scaling suggestive of seborrheic dermatitis to classic ringworm with scaling patches or plaques with broken hairs to kerion formation with marked edema and the presence of exudate. It is common to find infection in other family members, and examination and treatment of all in the household are recommended. In Europe and in some cities of the United States, the most common cause of scalp infections is *Microsporum canis,* which normally infects dogs and cats. This organism is more likely to produce classic scalp ringworm and does cause fluorescence of hairs on Wood's light examination. Dermatophytosis of the scalp should be treated with oral ultramicronized griseofulvin (Gris-Peg, Fulvicin, Grisactin), 10 to 15 mg per kg per day in either a single dose or divided doses for 6 to 8 weeks. Patients who cannot tolerate griseofulvin or fail to respond should be treated with oral ketoconazole (Nizoral), 200 mg per day for the same length of time. Topical therapy is not effective, but frequent washing with povidone-iodine (Betadine), selenium sulfide (Selsun, Exsel), or ketoconazole (Nizoral) shampoos reduces the spread of infectious spores.

Dermatophytosis of nonhairy skin, or tinea corporis, is characterized by scaling patches or plaques with sharp margins. Infections due to *Microsporum canis* frequently result in multiple lesions and tend to be more inflammatory. Chronic infections, which can be extensive, are most commonly due to *Trichophyton rubrum.* Tinea cruris (infection of the inguinal folds) occurs frequently in athletes or those who work outdoors in hot humid climates and is commonly due to *Trichophyton rubrum* or *Epidermophyton floccosum.* Tinea cruris and solitary lesions respond well to topical treatment with any of the imidazoles (clotrimazole [Clotrimazole, Mycelex], miconazole [Micatin, Monistat], econazole [Spectazole], ketoconazole [Nizoral], oxiconazole [Oxistat], sulconazole [Exelderm]), the allylamines (naftifine [Naftin], terbinafine [Lamisil]), or ciclopirox olamine (Loprox). Oral griseofulvin, ultramicronized, 500 mg two times a day for 4 to 6 weeks, is the treatment of choice for extensive infections or those due to multiple inoculations. Griseofulvin-resistant infections due to *Trichophyton rubrum* are a growing problem, and oral ketoconazole, 200–400 mg per day, should be given. Infections resistant to both griseofulvin and ketoconazole have responded to topical naftifine or terbinafine, and the new oral triazole, itraconazole (Sporonox), although it has not yet approved by the FDA for this indication, has been reported to be effective.

The most common dermatophyte infections in adults are those of the feet and nails. There are three variants of tinea pedis: the interdigital type, with scaling and itching of the webs between the toes; the inflammatory type, with vesicles involving the toes or the instep (most commonly due to *Trichophyton mentagrophytes*); and the plantar hyperkeratotic variety (like the interdigital type, usually due to *Trichophyton rubrum*), with slight redness and itching but marked thickening and scaling of the skin of the sole.

Dermatophytes do not commonly cause infections of the hands, but when they do, they produce chronic disease of the palmar skin and are usually unilateral. The common toeweb infections and the inflammatory form usually responds well to topical treatment for 4 to 6 weeks with the imidazole, allylamine, or ciclopirox creams mentioned earlier. Recurrences are common and require either intermittent therapy or prophylactic use of an antifungal powder (tolnaftate [Tinactin] or undecylenic acid [Desenex]). Chronic infections should be treated with either oral griseofulvin or ketoconazole. The topical allylamines naftifine and terbinafine are often effective in the more resistant infections.

Dermatophytosis of the nails (onychomycosis, or tinea unguium) is common (especially toenail infections) and often responds poorly to treatment. The most common form is distal subungual onychomycosis, which is usually due to *Trichophyton rubrum* and is characterized by separation of the nail from the nail bed, subungual scaling and thickening, and white to brown discoloration of the nail. Infections of the fingernails respond reasonably well (60% to 70%) to oral ultramicronized griseofulvin, 500 mg two times a day for 6 to 8 months, but the cure rate for toenails is poor even with up to 24 months of therapy and avulsion of the nails. The author currently recommends frequent clipping and filing of the infected nail, with application of a topical allylamine (naftifine or terbinafine) twice daily after bathing or following brief soaking in warm water. Published studies suggest that the new triazoles itraconazole and fluconazole (Diflucan) and the not yet available oral form of terbinafine may be more effective than available agents, but optimal dosing schedules have not been determined. The less frequent superficial white onychomycosis due to *Trichophyton mentagrophytes* is exhibited as white spots on the dorsum of the nail plate. The condition responds well to any of the topical antifungal agents. Proximal subungual onychomycosis, with whitish discoloration of the proximal nail, occurs most frequently in persons who have human immunodeficiency virus disease or who are otherwise immunosuppressed, and the condition usually clears with correction of the immune problem and use of oral griseofulvin.

CANDIDIASIS

Cutaneous candidiasis is usually due to *Candida albicans,* a yeast normally found in the gastrointestinal tract. The most common forms of infection involve the inguinal folds, perineum, and perianal and vaginal areas and are characterized by redness, superficial erosions, and itching or pain in the skin folds. Typically, satellite papules, pustules, or scaling macules occur around the borders of the larger patches. Other skin folds can be involved. Although candidiasis is a common cause of disease of the inguinal folds in healthy athletes and those whose work produces excessive sweating, predisposing factors such as obesity, diabetes, immunosuppression, oral contraceptives, and treatment with antibiotics or systemic steroids are frequently noted in the patient's history. Cutaneous candidiasis usually responds well to topical treatment with any of the imidazoles, or with nystatin (Mycostatin) or ciclopirox olamine (Loprox) creams, applied twice daily for 2 weeks. Allylamines are almost as effective as the imidazoles. Extensive or refractory disease should be treated with oral ketoconazole, 200 mg per day, or the newer triazoles (itraconazole or fluconazole). Predisposing causes should be corrected, if possible.

TINEA VERSICOLOR

Tinea versicolor is due to the lipophilic yeast *Malassezia furfur,* which is normally found in small quantities on the skin. Overgrowth of this organism produces discrete and confluent, slightly scaly patches or plaques on the upper trunk and proximal part of the arms. It occurs most frequently in young adults and is much more common in the summer and in hot, humid climates. As the name suggests, the involved skin can be slightly erythematous, slightly hyperpigmented, or more commonly, hypopigmented. The treatment of choice is selenium sulfide, 2.5% suspension, applied with water to the scalp, neck, upper trunk, and extremities for 10 minutes daily for 1 week. Patients should be warned that the pigmentary changes will persist for weeks to months. Topical antifungal creams are effective, but the extensive skin involvement makes their cost prohibitive. Alternative treatments include the use of ketoconazole shampoo in the same way, or in very extensive or resistant cases, oral ketoconazole, 400 mg in a single dose, or 200 mg per day for 10 days.

DISEASES OF THE MOUTH

method of
CARL M. ALLEN, D.D.S., M.S.D.
The Ohio State University College of Dentistry
Columbus, Ohio

A wide variety of disease processes other than dental caries and periodontal disease affect the oral region. These diseases may be classified based on the etiopathogenesis of the disease (e.g., viral, neoplastic), the clinical form of the lesions (e.g., plaque, vesicle, ulcer), or the anatomic region that is affected (e.g., lips, buccal mucosa). The clinical form and anatomic region are particularly useful for the clinician who is confronted by an unknown lesion. An accurate diagnosis is the most important aspect of patient management, because treatment is predicated on diagnosis. In this chapter, the lesions that tend to preferentially affect certain oral mucosal sites are listed according to their frequency; space limitations prohibit discussion of rare entities.

GENERALIZED ORAL INVOLVEMENT

Xerostomia

Xerostomia is the subjective feeling of a dry mouth. In most instances, this is caused by any of a variety of medications (antihypertensives, antihistamines, psychoactive drugs), and withdrawal or substitution of the medication may be helpful. A smaller number of patients may have xerostomia secondary to autoimmune destruction of the salivary gland tissue (Sjögren's syndrome) or due to radiation therapy of the head and neck region. Such patients may develop a number of problems. The mucosa is not as well lubricated and becomes susceptible to traumatic ulceration. The dry environment predisposes the individual to the erythematous or angular cheilitis forms of oral candidiasis. If the patient has natural teeth, a marked increase in dental caries is noted.

A number of over-the-counter artificial saliva substitutes, both in liquid and gel form, are available to help manage the symptoms of dryness. Oral ulcerations should be managed conservatively using a protective hydroxypropyl methylcellulose protective medication (Zilactin), applied as often as necessary. Oral candidiasis can be treated with any of several antifungal medications, although those with high sucrose content, such as nystatin pastilles (Mycostatin Oral Pastilles), should probably be avoided in dentulous patients because these agents could contribute to caries activity. A prescription-strength topical fluoride preparation, such as 0.4% stannous fluoride gel (Gel-Kam), should be used daily by patients who have natural teeth in order to prevent dental decay. Application of the topical fluoride is best performed at night after brushing the teeth and before retiring. Several drops of the fluoride gel should be placed on the toothbrush and gently massaged onto the surfaces of the teeth next to the gum tissue.

LIPS

Common Conditions

Fordyce Granules

Fordyce granules, a variation of normal anatomy, are heterotopic sebaceous glands seen in over 80% of adults. They present as 1-mm yellow-white submucosal dots distributed on the lateral upper lip and the buccal mucosa. No treatment is indicated due to the completely benign nature of the condition.

Angular Cheilitis

Angular cheilitis is characterized by inflammation of the corners of the mouth, accompanied by fissuring and sometimes scaling. Previously, this condition was thought to be due to B vitamin deficiency, but the vast majority of these lesions are now thought to be caused by a low-grade infection of *Candida albicans,* with or without *Staphylococcus aureus.*

These lesions can be easily treated with a topical antifungal agent such as nystatin-triamcinolone cream (Mycolog Cream). Another alternative is clioquinol-hydrocortisone cream (Vioform HC), which is both antifungal and antibacterial but must be used externally. Either medication should be applied three to four times daily for at least 1 week. With recurrence, a careful search for an intraoral source of infection may be indicated, and the possibility of human immunodeficiency virus (HIV) infection may need to be ruled out. Angular cheilitis with associated intraoral candidiasis requires treatment. Topical agents include clotrimazole troches (Mycelex Oral Troches) and nystatin pastilles (Mycostatin Oral Pastilles), each dissolved in the mouth 4 to 5 times daily for 7 to 10 days. Systemic therapy with fluconazole (Diflucan) may be more convenient for some patients, because it is given orally, 200 mg the first day, followed by 100 mg daily for the next 6 days.

Herpes Labialis (Fever Blisters, Cold Sores)

Recurrent herpes labialis affects approximately 25% of the population. Reactivation of the virus is usually triggered by sun (ultraviolet light) exposure. A cluster of vesicles develops on the vermilion zone of the lip or on perioral skin, rupturing within 1–3 days and leaving a crusted area that resolves after a few more days.

No therapy exists for this condition, and treatment results may be difficult to interpret due to strong placebo effect in some instances. High sun protection factor (SPF) sun-blocking agents have been shown to significantly reduce the frequency of episodes which are triggered by exposure to ultraviolet light. Low-dose acyclovir (Zovirax) may prevent attacks if it is taken continuously (600 mg per day), but attacks resume as usual once the medication is stopped. Systemic acyclovir,* 200 mg five times each day given during the prodromal phase, has been shown to reduce lesion formation in a subset of individuals affected by this condition. Topical acyclovir ointment has been shown to have no benefit in double-blind, placebo-controlled trials in immunocompetent patients.

Melanotic Macule

This solitary lesion usually develops on the vermilion zone of the lips, but it may be seen intraorally. The lesion presents as a 1- to 5-mm macule that exhibits a uniform, well-demarcated brown to black color.

If the patient indicates that the lesion has been present for several years and that no change in size or color has been observed, then no treatment is indicated unless the patient is concerned about cosmetic appearance. If changes have developed in the lesion recently, then excisional biopsy is indicated to rule out the possibility of an early melanoma.

Actinic Keratosis (Cheilitis)

Actinic keratosis is a premalignant process affecting the lower vermilion zone of the lip of fair-skinned

*Exceeds dosage recommended by the manufacturer.

adults who have had chronic sun exposure. The lesions have a scaly texture and ill-defined margins.

Excision, by either scalpel or laser, or cryosurgery is indicated for treatment. Excision is often accomplished by vermilionectomy, in which the entire vermilion zone is removed as a strip for histopathologic examination. The labial mucosa is then advanced over the resulting defect. Topical chemotherapy with fluorouracil (Efudex) has been used, but dysplastic epithelial cells have been shown to persist histologically. All patients with sun-damaged lips should be advised to use a sunscreen with high SPF applied particularly to the lower lip when sun exposure is anticipated.

Uncommon Conditions

Squamous Cell Carcinoma

This malignancy affects the lower vermilion zone, typically arising in a pre-existing actinic keratosis. Such lesions usually have a relatively slow, steady growth, with a roughened or ulcerated surface. The diagnosis should be established by biopsy. Wide surgical excision, obtaining at least a 1 cm margin of normal tissue, is usually adequate treatment because these lesions are rather indolent and do not metastasize until relatively late in their course.

Reactive Cheilitis

Occasionally, patients may present with a complaint of fissured, painful lips. Evaluation of the problem should include a history of onset, duration, and use of medications and cosmetics. Lipstick and artificially flavored cinnamon products may produce a contact cheilitis. Isotretinoin (Accutane) often causes exfoliative cheilitis. Solitary chronic lip fissures, which usually occur in the winter months, may respond to topical antibiotic preparations, with surgical excision reserved for resistant lesions. Many cases of reactive cheilitis appear to be factitial, although patients may be reluctant to admit their habit of licking and nibbling at the vermilion zone. Constant moistening of the lips also predisposes the individual to a superimposed candidal infection, which exacerbates the inflammatory symptoms.

Telangiectasias

Superficial dilated blood vessels may be seen on the vermilion zone of the lips as an isolated finding or, if multiple, as a component of either hereditary hemorrhagic telangiectasia or CREST (*c*alcinosis, *R*aynaud's phenomenon, *e*sophageal dysfunction, *s*clerodactyly, and *t*elangiectasias) syndrome. Patients should be evaluated to distinguish between these two entities, because their prognoses are different. Treatment of the telangiectatic lesions can be performed by laser excision, cryotherapy, or electrodesiccation.

LABIAL MUCOSA

Common Conditions

Mucocele

The mucocele represents a collection of extravasated mucin within the submucosal connective tissue caused by the disruption of a minor salivary gland duct by minor trauma. Most mucoceles develop on the lower labial mucosa, appearing suddenly as a painless, soft, bluish, circumscribed swelling. A cycle of swelling, breaking, and swelling again is typical.

Usually, surgical excision of the mucous deposit and the associated gland is necessary for resolution of the problem.

Varix

The varix, similar to varicose veins of the leg, is seen on the labial mucosa, lips, buccal mucosa and tongue of patients over the age of 50 years. Patients usually describe the gradual onset of a painless purplish or bluish nodule.

Generally, no treatment is indicated. If the lesion is a cosmetic problem or if it occurs in areas likely to be traumatized, the varix may be treated by surgical excision or cryotherapy.

Aphthous Ulcer (Canker Sore)

This condition is perhaps one of the most misdiagnosed, mismanaged, and misunderstood of all oral diseases. Most authorities now believe that aphthous ulcers are immunologically induced. There have been no convincing scientific data linking the process to viral infection. Furthermore, studies suggesting that the lesions are associated with certain foods or vitamin deficiencies have not been able to be duplicated. There may be several mechanisms that initiate the abnormal immune response leading to focal destruction of the oral mucosa. The lesions are typically recurrent, ranging from 1 to 24 episodes per year. The most common form of aphthous ulcer is the minor aphthous ulcer, presenting as a 1- to 10-mm ulceration with an erythematous periphery and smooth borders. From one to five ulcers may develop simultaneously. Aphthous ulcers are located on movable mucosa, not mucosa bound to periosteum, a situation directly opposite to what is seen in recurrent intraoral herpes. Usually, the patient reports pain that seems out of proportion to the size of the lesion. With no treatment, minor aphthae heal within 5 to 10 days. Patients with frequent attacks should be questioned regarding ocular complaints or genital ulcerations in order to rule out Behçet's syndrome. Infrequently, aphthous-like oral ulcerations may be seen as a manifestation of Crohn's disease or celiac sprue as well.

Topical application of a relatively strong corticosteroid such as fluocinonide (Lidex Gel) is most effective in controlling the lesions. For optimum response, small amounts of the medication should be applied often (four to five times daily) and as early in the course of the lesion as possible.

Uncommon Conditions

Major Aphthous Ulcers

Major aphthae are debilitating oral lesions that resemble minor aphthae, except they are much larger (ranging up to 3 cm in diameter), and they persist for periods of up to 6 weeks before healing. Topical application of fluocinonide (Lidex Gel) or betamethasone dipropionate (Diprolene Gel) usually controls this process. If the lesions are in the posterior segments of the mouth, betamethasone syrup (Celestone Syrup) used as a mouth rinse and swallowed (10 mL after meals and at bedtime for 7 to 10 days) often provides relief.

Herpetiform Aphthous Ulcers

These lesions resemble primary herpetic gingivostomatitis, and they can be distinguished from that condition by their history of recurrence. Herpetiform aphthae are most effectively treated with one of the topical corticosteroid preparations or rinses described earlier.

Angioedema

Angioedema is thought to occur due to localized release of histamine from mast cells. Most cases are sporadic and harmless. The lips are most frequently affected, followed by the tongue. A tingling sensation usually precedes the sudden onset of rather dramatic, nontender swelling. The overlying skin appears normal, and the patient is otherwise asymptomatic; these features should help distinguish this condition from cellulitis associated with a dentoalveolar abscess. With no treatment, the condition resolves in 24 to 48 hours; however, oral antihistamine therapy seems to speed resolution. Attacks are commonly recurrent, and the precipitating factor is often difficult to identify. A rare hereditary form, caused by a deficiency of C1 esterase inhibitor, can be life-threatening if the laryngeal tissues are involved. With persistent swelling, biopsy may be indicated to rule out relatively rare conditions such as orofacial granulomatosis (cheilitis granulomatosa, Melkersson-Rosenthal syndrome).

BUCCAL MUCOSA

Common Conditions

Linea Alba

The oral linea alba merely represents a mild thickening of the epithelium along the plane of occlusion in dentate patients. The extent to which it is evident varies tremendously from patient to patient. No treatment is indicated for this completely benign condition.

Leukoedema

Leukoedema is considered a variation of normal. Clinically, it has a whitish, filmy, almost opalescent appearance, usually affecting the buccal mucosa. Stretching the mucosa causes the white appearance to greatly diminish or disappear completely. The surface epithelial cells histologically are edematous but otherwise normal, and no treatment is necessary for this benign condition.

Cheek-Chewing

Cheek-chewing is a harmless chronic habit. Although the anterior buccal mucosa is the most common site, the labial mucosa and lateral tongue may also be affected. A white, ragged alteration of the mucosa is seen clinically. Actual ulceration is uncommon, because only the outer layers of the epithelium (which have no nerve fibers) are nibbled. The patient usually admits to the habit if questioned. This habit is completely benign and requires no further management once it has been identified.

Fibroma (Irritation Fibroma, Focal Fibrous Hyperplasia)

The fibroma represents an accumulation of dense collagenous connective tissue at a site of irritation. For this reason, most of these lesions are found on the buccal mucosa. Clinically the lesion appears as a sessile, dome-shaped, smooth-surfaced nodule. Patients may complain because they bite the lesion inadvertently.

Because this lesion cannot be definitively differentiated clinically from a wide array of other neoplasms, excisional biopsy is generally indicated. Recurrence is uncommon.

Lichen Planus

Lichen planus is an immunologically mediated condition of unknown cause that affects adults. The oral lesions present in two patterns: reticular and erosive. The reticular pattern is most common, and it is usually seen bilaterally on the posterior buccal mucosa, presenting as fine, white, interlacing lines or papules. The gingivae and the tongue may also be affected. The erosive form of the condition is symptomatic due the presence of ulcerations. These ulcerations usually have a central yellow-white area of fibrin surrounded by an erythematous halo and radiating white striae.

Reticular lichen planus requires no treatment. In 25% of these cases, candidiasis is present and it should be treated with an antifungal agent. Erosive lichen planus can usually be managed effectively with the more potent topical corticosteroids such as fluocinonide (Lidex Gel) or betamethasone dipropionate (Diprolene Gel). Application of a thin film of medication, four to five times a day, to the lesional areas often resolves the ulcers within a few days. Other conditions, such as epithelial dysplasia, lichenoid amalgam reactions, lichenoid drug reactions, and lupus erythematosus, may mimic lichen planus clinically; therefore, biopsy is warranted if classic clinical features are not present. Malignant transformation of reticular lichen planus is not thought to be likely, although the possibility of erosive lichen planus being premalignant has not been ruled out. Affected patients should be reevaluated periodically for evidence of significant mucosal change, with re-biopsy performed, if necessary.

Uncommon Conditions

Verrucous Carcinoma

This relatively low-grade malignancy of surface epithelial origin may arise after decades of smokeless tobacco abuse. It appears as a diffuse, white, rough-surfaced, spreading plaquelike lesion affecting the buccal mucosa, palate, or alveolar process in an elderly patient.

Treatment is complete surgical excision, via scalpel or laser, with evaluation of the lesional tissue histopathologically, because 25% of verrucous carcinomas may contain foci of routine squamous cell carcinoma. The prognosis is generally good because this lesion does not metastasize.

Oral Mucosal Cinnamon Reaction

This condition affects the buccal mucosa, the lateral tongue, and gingivae. The lesions appear as diffuse areas of mucosal erythema with varying degrees of superimposed white plaques and, less commonly, ulceration. Such lesions may be mistaken clinically for lichen planus, candidiasis, leukoplakia, or erythroplakia. Discontinuing the artificially flavored cinnamon product (usually chewing gum) results in resolution of the lesions within 1 week. The diagnosis can be confirmed by challenging the oral mucosa with the offending agent, although patients are often reluctant to do so after their lesions clear.

HARD PALATE

Common Conditions

Torus

Palatal tori are common developmental lesions representing a benign accumulation of dense bone in the midline posterior hard palate region. The diagnosis can be made clinically, because no other condition presents as a bony hard midline palatal mass. No treatment is necessary for this benign process, although denture construction may be hampered. Removal of the torus by an oral surgeon would be recommended in that situation.

Denture Stomatitis

Denture stomatitis is almost invariably associated with a maxillary removable denture that is worn 24 hours per day. The palatal mucosa directly beneath the denture appears red, although it is asymptomatic. The redness is confined to the denture-bearing mucosa.

In many cases, simply having the patient remove the denture at night may resolve the palatal erythema. If the patient has a complete upper denture, it can be soaked in a mild sodium hypochlorite solution (Clorox) (1 teaspoon in 8 ounces of water) each night for a week in order to disinfect it. (Important: Do not place chrome-cobalt metal frameworks in Clorox; severe corrosion will result and ruin the denture.) Because denture stomatitis is a benign and asymptomatic condition, treatment need not be a top priority.

Inflammatory Papillary Hyperplasia (IPH, Denture Papillomatosis)

This condition is seen almost exclusively in patients who wear ill-fitting complete upper dentures. The lesions appear as multiple, erythematous, 1- to 2-mm papules that are usually confined to the palatal vault area. These papules are composed of dense fibrous connective tissue that has accumulated secondary to chronic irritation in the superficial mucosa.

Treatment of this benign process is somewhat controversial. Some prosthodontists prefer to have these lesions surgically removed prior to constructing a new denture, although this procedure may not be necessary in every case.

Nicotine Stomatitis

Nicotine stomatitis is a benign condition that affects the posterior palate and represents a tissue reaction to heat, usually due to pipe smoking. A diffuse white appearance is seen, representing reactive hyperkeratosis, and scattered on this background are variable numbers of erythematous papules, representing the inflamed orifices of minor salivary glands.

Nicotine stomatitis is a benign condition requiring no treatment. If the patient discontinues smoking, the palatal mucosa returns to normal in a short period of time, usually no more than 1 week.

Uncommon Conditions

Recurrent Intraoral Herpes

This condition is much less common than aphthous ulcerations, a condition with which it is frequently confused. Recurrent intraoral herpes affects only the hard palate and the attached gingiva (the paler, firm gum tissue directly adjacent to the teeth). Most patients experience mild symptoms, and may give a history of recurrent episodes. Lesions are seen as a cluster of 1- to 2-mm shallow ulcerations that heal within 1 week. Generally, no treatment is necessary, although the patient should be cautioned that virus is being shed from the lesion.

Salivary Gland Tumors

The posterior hard palate/anterior soft palate region is the most common site for the development of intraoral salivary gland neoplasia. This type of lesion presents as a slowly growing, rubbery firm, nontender mass that may or may not be ulcerated. The clinical appearance does not distinguish benign from malignant tumors, so a biopsy should be obtained. The biopsy should include a margin of normal adjacent tissue. Approximately 50% of these tumors are pleomorphic adenomas, whereas the remainder represent mucoepidermoid carcinoma, polymorphous low-grade adenocarcinoma, adenoid cystic carcinoma, or acinic cell carcinoma. Complete excision is recommended for the pleomorphic adenoma, including overlying mucosa and underlying periosteum. The malignancies should be treated with a much more aggressive surgical approach, depending on the histologic type, the extent of bone involvement, and the size of the lesion. Adjunctive radiation therapy may be indicated for adenoid cystic carcinoma and high-grade mucoepidermoid carcinoma.

SOFT PALATE/TONSILLAR PILLARS

Common Conditions

Papilloma

The squamous papilloma is the most common benign epithelial neoplasm that affects the oral mucosa, typically presenting as a solitary exophytic growth with numerous finger-like or frondlike projections on its surface. The soft palate/tonsillar pillar region is the most common site for the papilloma, and its color may range from pink to white.

Excisional biopsy, including the base of the lesion, should be performed. For those lesions of the posterior soft palate, periodic observation may be appropriate, particularly if the patient is experiencing no symptoms and the lesion is clinically characteristic.

Uncommon Conditions

Pemphigus Vulgaris

Pemphigus vulgaris is an immunologically mediated condition characterized by the formation of vesicles and bullae secondary to attack of desmosomal complexes of the surface epithelium by autoantibodies. The condition usually is first seen intraorally, with painful, erosive lesions distributed diffusely on the oral mucosa. The soft palate is a primary site of involvement. Diagnosis should be established by light microscopy with direct and indirect immunofluorescence studies. Systemic immunosuppressive therapy is necessary to control this condition, and this has been addressed in other areas of the text.

TONGUE

Common Conditions

Coated and Hairy Tongue

These conditions represent the accumulation of excess keratin on the filiform papillae of the dorsal tongue, resulting in the formation of elongated, filamentous strands that superficially resemble hairs. Contrary to what has been described in numerous textbooks, this condition is not caused by an overgrowth of yeast.

No treatment is required, but if the patient is concerned about the appearance of the tongue, gentle daily débridement with a tongue scraper or the edge of a spoon assists in removing the accumulations of dead keratinized cells.

Fissured Tongue

This is essentially a variation of normal that usually develops sometime after the first decade of life. The patient may be concerned about the appearance of the tongue, but no symptoms are associated with the condition. The extent and pattern of fissuring can vary, and no treatment is indicated.

Benign Migratory Glossitis (Erythema Migrans, Geographic Tongue)

This condition of unknown etiology is seen in about 2% of the population. Most patients are asymptomatic, with lesions being detected on routine examination. The dorsal lateral tongue exhibits one or more well-demarcated zones of papillary atrophy, which are surrounded at least partially by slightly raised, yellow-white, linear serpentine borders. The lesions typically resolve in one area and move to another, appearing in various stages of resolution and activity concurrently.

Because this is a benign condition, treatment is usually unnecessary. About 5% of patients complain of sensitivity to hot or spicy foods when their lesions are active, but usually they do not require treatment. With severe symptoms, topical fluocinonide (Lidex Gel), applied as a thin film to the lesions several times daily, seems to reduce the discomfort.

Traumatic Ulcer

The traumatic ulcer occurs most frequently on the lateral tongue, buccal mucosa, and overlying bony prominences such as tori and exostoses. Most of these lesions are associated with relatively little pain. Clinically, the traumatic ulcer presents as a defect covered by creamy white fibrin. Although most of these lesions heal within a week or so, some tend to persist, developing a rolled margin and peripheral induration.

Often, no treatment is required due to the minimal degree of discomfort and the rapid healing time. If the patient complains of tenderness when eating salty or acidic foods, a protective medication such as hydroxypropyl methylcellulose (Zilactin) can be applied as needed. Topical corticosteroids should probably not be used, because they may delay healing in this situation. If an ulcer has been present for longer than 2 weeks, with or without previous treatment, a biopsy is mandatory to rule out malignancy. A possible exception to this rule might be those ulcers overlying tori, because they are notoriously difficult to resolve.

Burning Tongue Syndrome (Idiopathic Glossopyrosis)

This condition seems to affect postmenopausal women predominantly. The patient often reports the rather sudden onset of a sensation that feels like the tongue has been scalded. Symptoms are usually localized to the anterior tongue, although the labial mucosa and anterior hard palate may also be affected. Clinically, the mucosa appears normal. If mucosal erythema is identified, a variety of conditions should be ruled out, including candidiasis, anemia, local trauma, and erythema migrans. A culture for *C. albicans* and a complete blood count should be performed. If the work-up shows no evidence of these conditions, then a diagnosis of burning tongue syndrome can be made. Because there is no medically proven therapy, no specific treatment exists. The numerous suggested treatments seen in the literature have generally not been examined in controlled trials, and their efficacy is typically no more than that of placebo effect. Reassuring patients that this is a harmless condition that is nothing more than a nuisance and that the condition often resolves spontaneously after a period of months or years is usually sufficient.

Uncommon Conditions

Squamous Cell Carcinoma

The lateral/ventral tongue is one of the most common sites for squamous cell carcinoma. In the early stages, the lesion is relatively asymptomatic, which underscores the importance of a thorough oral mucosal examination on a regular basis. Slight thickening or nodularity within a white or red plaque frequently heralds the onset of invasion. As the lesion grows, the surface becomes ulcerated and symptoms of pain and tenderness develop. On palpation, squamous cell carcinomas are usually firm and show infiltrative borders. Biopsy is mandatory because other chronic ulcerative processes such as chronic traumatic ulcer, deep fungal infections, mycobacterial infections, Wegener's granulomatosis, and other malignancies may have a similar clinical presentation.

Treatment consists of wide surgical resection or radical radiation therapy, or both, depending on a number of factors. Prognosis is directly related to the tumor stage, although, in general, these patients do poorly because their lesions are not diagnosed until the later stages.

Hairy Leukoplakia

This is an HIV-related lesion that is significant in that it often heralds a rapid decline in the patient's immune status. The lesion affects the lateral borders of the tongue, usually bilaterally, appearing as white plaques with vertical streaks. Sometimes the degree of keratinization may be so great as to produce hairlike projections, hence the name. Because this is otherwise a benign condition, no treatment is necessary. Because hairy leukoplakia is caused by Epstein-Barr virus, medications used against other herpesviruses, such as acyclovir (Zovirax) and dihydroxypropoxymethylguanine (DHPG, ganciclovir [Cytovene]),* may produce transient resolution.

Herpes in the Immunocompromised Host

With an immunocompromised host, the normal rules governing the location of the lesions of recurrent herpes are not applicable. The virus is not contained by the host, as in the normal individual, and the result is the formation of large, shallow, painful ulcerations with slightly elevated, serpentine or scalloped margins. The diagnosis should be established by exfoliative cytology or viral culture, and treatment should be instituted immediately with systemic acyclovir, orally or intravenously, depending on the severity of the clinical infection.

Macroglossia

Macroglossia is the term used to describe enlargement of the tongue. Among the more frequent causes of macroglossia are hemangiomas and lymphangiomas. Hemangiomas are usually present at birth or develop shortly thereafter, with the tongue being the most common site. These lesions are typically red or purple in color. If no compromise in function of the involved tissue is seen, treatment should be delayed until the child is older than 6 years of age, because many of these lesions regress spontaneously. For those lesions that do not regress, argon laser excision is the optimal therapy. Other methods of management include cryotherapy and sclerosing agents.

Lymphangiomas affecting the oral tissues often exhibit a characteristic so-called frog-egg or tapioca-pudding surface morphology due to the dilated lymphatic vessels that are close to the surface. Treatment is surgical excision, although the decision to treat may depend on the size and site of the lesion. Recurrence rates as high as 40% have been reported in some series of cases.

Other causes of macroglossia are much less common and include amyloidosis as well as benign and malignant tumors. Biopsy would be indicated to establish a diagnosis prior to treatment planning.

FLOOR OF THE MOUTH

Common Conditions

Leukoplakia

Leukoplakia is a clinical term that should be applied only to those white patches of the oral mucosa that cannot be wiped off and cannot be diagnosed as any other condition clinically. These premalignant lesions are usually diagnosed in the sixth and seventh decade of life. Clinically, the condition appears as a well-defined white plaque that may show varying degrees of redness. The most worrisome sites of involvement include areas prone to cancer development, such as the lateral tongue, floor of the mouth, and the tonsillar pillar region.

Ideally, treatment is complete removal with microscopic evaluation of the excised specimen. Cryotherapy and laser excision may be used, but tissue may be rendered unsuitable for histopathologic examination. More concern should be given leukoplakias found in nonsmokers, in high-risk areas for oral cancer, in lesions with a red component, in multifocal lesions, or those found in younger patients. If complete excision has been accomplished, 30% of leukoplakias recur nevertheless, so careful follow-up with re-biopsy is indicated.

Sialolithiasis

Salivary duct stones may appear with symptoms or may be discovered on routine examination. The classic presentation is sudden painful unilateral swelling of the involved salivary gland occurring at mealtime. Most stones involve the submandibular gland, and these can be palpated as a hard submucosal mass in the floor of the mouth. Treatment usually involves surgical removal of the stone with repositioning of the salivary duct opening proximally. Sialography

*Not FDA approved for this indication.

should then be performed to assess the function of the gland, and if it appears abnormal, then it should probably be removed in order to prevent subsequent episodes of chronic recurrent sialadenitis.

Uncommon Conditions

Erythroplakia

This premalignant lesion represents the nonkeratinized version of leukoplakia. Erythroplakia appears as a well-demarcated, velvety red plaque that is typically asymptomatic. Dysplastic changes are much more likely to be seen, and treatment should consist of complete removal by the most expedient means.

Squamous Cell Carcinoma

The clinical appearance of squamous cell carcinoma at this site is similar to that of the lateral tongue, as is treatment.

ALVEOLAR PROCESS/GINGIVA

Common Conditions

Mandibular Tori/Exostoses

These benign developmental lesions consist of dense, viable bone. Mandibular tori are located on the lingual surface of the mandible in the premolar region, whereas exostoses occur on the alveolar process in other sites. Radiographic evaluation of any asymmetric bony swelling is indicated, and the exostosis should appear as a well-defined radiopacity. Generally, no treatment is necessary unless the bony outgrowths interfere with denture construction, in which case surgical removal is indicated.

Amalgam Tattoo

The amalgam tattoo is produced by the iatrogenic implantation of dental amalgam into the oral soft tissues. Amalgam tattoos are usually macular and range in color from gray to blue to black or brown. Periapical radiographs often show the fine radiopaque metallic particles.

No treatment is necessary if the diagnosis can be made definitively from the radiograph. If no radiopacity is seen, then biopsy is generally indicated to rule out a relatively rare oral melanocytic process such as nevus or melanoma.

Dental Sinus Tract (Parulis)

This lesion represents a proliferation of granulation tissue at the drainage site of a sinus tract originating from the apical root portion of a nonvital tooth. Clinically, the parulis appears as an erythematous papule on the alveolar mucosa. Symptoms of pain may wax and wane. Treatment consists of either extraction or endodontic therapy for the offending tooth, and the prognosis is good.

Acute Necrotizing Ulcerative Gingivitis (Trench Mouth, Vincent's Infection)

Acute necrotizing ulcerative gingivitis is a disease produced by bacteria that are normal inhabitants of the oral microflora. The condition occurs in the third or fourth decade of life and is associated with poor oral hygiene, poor diet, and stress. College students are especially vulnerable during final examinations, and the condition may be seen in HIV-positive patients as well. Patients invariably present with a complaint of painful, foul-smelling gingivae. Examination shows punched-out ulcerations of the interdental papillae. Acute necrotizing ulcerative gingivitis is frequently confused with primary herpes, which also is associated with pain and ulceration, but the punched-out interdental papillae are not seen in herpes infection.

Débridement, often requiring topical or local anesthesia, or both, is very important. This should be combined with systemic antibiotic therapy, such as tetracycline, 250 mg every 6 hours, or potassium penicillin V, 500 mg every 6 hours. HIV-infected patients should also use chlorhexidine (Peridex) mouth rinse twice daily to prevent recurrence of acute necrotizing ulcerative gingivitis. For non-HIV patients, the prognosis is reasonably good, assuming that they improve their diet and oral hygiene status.

Primary Herpetic Gingivostomatitis

This condition is caused by the initial exposure of the patient to herpes simplex virus, usually Type I. Most of these infections occur during childhood, but occasionally an individual escapes contact with the virus until adulthood. Patients present with fever, cervical lymphadenopathy, malaise, and oropharyngeal pain. Examination of the oral mucosa reveals multiple shallow ulcerations distributed diffusely throughout the mouth, although the gingivae are often markedly affected. The gingival involvement is different than that of acute necrotizing ulcerative gingivitis, in that the interdental papillae do not show the punched-out ulcerations with the herpetic infection.

Patients should be managed symptomatically with analgesics, antipyretics, and topical anesthetics as indicated. Dehydration is sometimes a problem if oral pain prevents intake of fluids. Having the patient rinse with 5 mL of viscous lidocaine (Xylocaine Viscous) or dyclonine HCl (Dyclone) prior to meals provides temporary relief. Systemic or topical acyclovir (Zovirax) has not been shown to have a significant impact on the course of this disease in an immunocompetent patient.

Inflammatory Fibrous Hyperplasia (Denture Epulis, Epulis Fissuratum, Denture Fibroma)

This condition is caused by low-grade irritation from an ill-fitting denture. Clinically, the lesions are seen as smooth-surfaced sessile masses, that appear to arise from the mucosa of the alveolar process or vestibule. Sometimes, a groove or fissure runs lengthwise across the lesion, corresponding to the denture flange. Ulceration of the surface may be seen.

Surgical excision of the lesion is indicated prior to construction of new dentures. If the lesion is removed and the patient continues to wear the old denture, then inflammatory fibrous hyperplasia will recur, but this is a completely benign process that does not undergo malignant transformation.

Uncommon Conditions

Pyogenic Granuloma, Peripheral Giant Cell Granuloma, and Peripheral Ossifying Fibroma

These benign gingival lesions are probably initiated by chronic irritation in most instances. Although they are histologically distinctive, their clinical appearance and biologic behavior are similar. All lesions appear present as sessile, dome-shaped masses that are present mainly on the gingiva (although pyogenic granuloma may be seen on any surface). They range from pink to reddish purple in color, and they are often ulcerated. Excisional biopsy is recommended in order to rule out the less likely possibility of metastatic neoplasm, which may clinically appear very similar. A recurrence rate of 15% can be expected for each of these lesions.

Generalized Gingival Hyperplasia

This condition usually develops as a side effect of medication: phenytoin (Dilantin), calcium channel blocking agents, or cyclosporine (Sandimmune). Only 30% to 50% of patients receiving one of these drugs show the diffuse gingival enlargement, and this is usually related to the level of oral hygiene of the patient. If the drug cannot be discontinued or substituted, then periodic periodontal surgery with reinforcement of oral hygiene instruction can usually control the problem. Rarely, such enlargement may be associated with any of several genetic syndromes. These patients typically require periodic surgical reduction of the gingival tissues by a periodontist. Generalized gingival hyperplasia may also be a manifestation of myelomonocytic leukemia, although these patients usually complain of other signs and symptoms related to their leukemic state. Biopsy and appropriate hematologic evaluation are necessary to establish a diagnosis.

Desquamative Gingivitis

This is a descriptive term for a reaction pattern that affects the gingival tissues of adults. Patients complain of red, tender gingival mucosa that has a tendency to slough with minor manipulation. Vesicles may sometimes be reported. This condition must be biopsied for light microscopic evaluation as well as direct immunofluorescence studies, because it invariably represents one of several distinct entities: erosive lichen planus, cicatricial pemphigoid, linear IgA disease, pemphigus vulgaris, or chronic ulcerative stomatitis. Once the definitive diagnosis is established, the patient can be managed appropriately.

STASIS ULCERS

method of
JOHN R. BARTHOLOMEW, M.D., and
CARMEN FONSECA, M.D.
Cleveland Clinic Foundation
Cleveland, Ohio

Leg ulcers, although fairly common, can present a difficult diagnostic problem to the practicing physician. Although most leg ulcers are caused by venous or arterial insufficiency, the list of causes also includes hematologic disorders, infections, vasculitis, metabolic disorders (diabetes mellitus), tumors, and a number of miscellaneous causes (Table 1). Differentiation of leg ulcers is important since treatment can vary.

DIAGNOSIS

Venous stasis ulcers are the most common type encountered by the physician, afflicting between 500,000 and 600,000 people in the United States. The diagnosis of stasis ulcers can be made on the basis of a carefully taken patient history and physical examination. There is often a history of recurrent deep vein thrombosis, and sometimes, varicose veins may be obvious on physical examination. Patients with venous ulcers usually have stasis pigmentation and edema in the area of the ulcer prior to its appearance. In addition, venous stasis ulcers are classically located near the medial malleolus, although they can occur laterally and posteriorly. These ulcers usually appear as a single lesion. Patients may complain of pruritus on the leg or skin and around the ulcer. Stasis ulcers are usually only mildly painful; however, if they are associated with trauma or cellulitis, this situation can change. The base of a stasis ulcer usually weeps and contains extensive granulation tissue, which is pink-red in appearance.

The use of routine laboratory tests in the diagnosis of venous stasis ulcers is generally not needed, unless the diagnosis is in doubt. A routine blood count, urinalysis, blood glucose, and chemistry profile helps in excluding other causes for the ulcer. A small biopsy at the edge of the ulcer may also be helpful for definitive diagnosis if this remains in doubt. Noninvasive vascular laboratory examinations can provide information on the state of the patient's arterial and venous systems. Patients occasionally

TABLE 1. **Classification of Leg Ulcers**

Vascular	**Metabolic**
Arterial	Diabetes mellitus
Venous	Gout
Lymphatic	Porphyria
Vasculitis	**Tumors**
Systemic lupus erythematosus	Basal cell
Atrophie blanche	Squamous cell
Scleroderma	Kaposi's sarcoma
	Melanoma
Hematologic	**Miscellaneous**
Sickle cell	Drugs
Thalassemia	Burns
Leukemia	Insect bites
Dysproteinemias	Frostbite
Infections	Factitial
Fungal	
Bacterial	
Syphilis	

present with a mixed arterial and venous ulcer. In this setting, it is important to know both their arterial and venous status.

TREATMENT

Many new methods have evolved over the last few years for the treatment of venous stasis ulcers. Although there may be many advantages to some of these newer treatments, certain basic principles must be followed to ensure proper wound healing. These principles rely on the promotion of venous return, prevention of leg edema, and gently débriding and cleansing the ulcer.

Historically, the Unna boot and wet-to-dry compression dressings have been our mainstays of treatment for venous stasis ulcers. These two methods employ the basic principles mentioned earlier.

The wet-to-dry compression dressing, using a normal saline or 3% boric acid solution as the base, keeps the ulcer clean and débrides it with frequent dressing changes. The leg must be washed first. We prefer a mild soap and warm water. The leg is then rinsed and dried, especially between the toes. It is advisable to apply a moisturizing cream to the legs and feet, but not between the toes or on the ulcer itself. A 4- × 3-inch dressing is then applied with the appropriate solution. If the ulcer has excess drainage or appears infected, we use boric acid. If the ulcer base is moist and granulating in well, we prefer to use normal saline. To avoid the use of tape, a compression liner stocking is applied over the dressing. A knee-high compression stocking providing 30 to 40 mmHg of pressure or an Ace bandage is then put over the liner. The dressing is changed every 8 hours. This method is our most commonly used approach.

The Unna boot also acts as a compression bandage containing a combination of gelatin, zinc oxide, calamine, and glycerin. It requires a great deal of skill and time to apply and is changed every 5 to 7 days. If there is excessive drainage, dermatitis, or infection is present, the Unna boot should not be applied. It has definite advantages, however, because it facilitates ambulatory treatment, places no responsibility on the patient for dressing changes, is more convenient for elderly or arthritic patients who cannot apply a compression dressing, and is ideal for patients with a suspected factitial component to their ulcer. Because of the time involved, however, we no longer use this as our method of choice.

Benzoyl peroxide (BPO)* is occasionally used in our clinic to stimulate granulation tissue in our stasis ulcers. This method is more difficult to use. We follow the steps outlined with the saline dressing but modify it somewhat. A thin film of petroleum jelly is applied around the base of the ulcer to protect it from the benzoyl peroxide. We then cut a piece of terry cloth to the exact size of the ulcer and moisten it with normal saline. One or two drops of benzoyl peroxide are applied to the cloth, and it is set inside the ulcer. A piece of plastic wrap is placed over the ulcer, and then a 4- × 3-inch dressing put over this. An Ace wrap or compression hose is then put in place.

*Not FDA approved for this indication.

A number of new synthetic occlusive dressings are available and include Duoderm, Op-site, Vigilon, and Tegaderm. These dressings are reported to influence wound healing; however, we have not found them to be advantageous and do not routinely use any of these products.

The surgical management of stasis ulcers includes split-thickness and full-thickness skin grafting. These methods are reserved for extensive ulcerations, whenever it will shorten the healing time, when the patient does not respond to conservative treatment, and in those patients who are unable to care for their ulcers by the above-mentioned methods. Other surgical approaches seldom used in our practice include ligation and stripping of varicose veins and ligation of incompetent perforating veins. Postoperatively the basic principles of compression must be adhered to.

A number of medications have been tried as adjunctive treatment of venous stasis ulcers. Antibiotics, given either topically or systemically, are generally not necessary unless there is an infection. We find that topical antibiotics often sensitize the patient's ulcer and impede healing. More recently, pentoxifylline (Trental),* a hemorrheologic agent used in the treatment of arterial disease, has been tried. It is believed to improve perfusion and transport by reducing the viscosity of blood and inhibits platelet aggregation and neutrophil activation. We have used this agent occasionally with varying degrees of success. Other agents that have been reported to help in the treatment of venous stasis ulcers include a steroid preparation (stanozolol), silver sulfadiazine* in a 1% cream (Silvadene), and platelet-derived wound healing formula (PPWHF); however, we have no experience with stanozolol (Winstrol)* and have not found Silvadene or PDWHF very helpful.

PRESSURE ULCER

method of
JOSEPH A. WITKOWSKI, M.D., and
LAWRENCE C. PARISH, M.D.
University of Pennsylvania School of Medicine
Philadelphia, Pennsylvania

A pressure ulcer is a localized loss of skin that may include the subcutaneous tissue and fascia. It results from vascular occlusion caused by pressure or shear force injury. The skin of a person lying on a bed or sitting on a chair is subjected to two types of stress: pressure and shear. Although pressure is applied vertically to the skin surface, shear stress is applied tangientially to the skin surface. Shear stress occurs when the skin moves across the deeper fixed layers of tissue.

PRESSURE ULCER PATHWAY

The pressure ulcer pathway consists of a series of cutaneous events that occur in a stepwise fashion. In some

*Not FDA approved for this indication.

instances, when pressure sites are subjected to extremes of pressure for prolonged periods of time, some of the preliminary phases may not be seen. The first sign of pressure on a bony prominence is erythema that blanches on finger pressure. Nonblanchable erythema represents a more profound change in the skin. Decubitus dermatitis is the result of unrelieved pressure on nonblanchable erythema often complicated by friction. Continued pressure results in a superficial and deep ulcer. The eschar/gangrene is the result of shear stress on normal skin or sustained pressure on the site of nonblanchable erythema.

DIAGNOSIS

The diagnosis of a pressure ulcer is made clinically. The lesions occur over bony prominences. In the bed-confined patient, the sacrum, trochanters, and heels are most commonly involved. In the patient confined to a chair, the ischeal tuberosities are most often affected.

The extent of tissue injury is quantified by using the following classification: Stage 1 is nonblanchable erythema, Stage 2 is an ulceration resulting from loss of epidermis and dermis, Stage 3 is a loss of tissue into the subcutaneous fat, and Stage 4 is an ulcer that extends into tendon, bone, or joint capsule.

Evaluation of a pressure ulcer requires visual, tactile, and olfactory examination. Only the gloved hand can determine whether there is undermining of the ulcer edges and the nature of the structures in the ulcer base. The diagnosis of anaerobic colonization or infection can often be made by the characteristic odor. The eschar/gangrene is not staged until after débridement.

ETIOLOGY

Although many factors contribute to the formation of pressure ulcers, a consensus exists that application of an external load beyond some pressure-time threshold is the prime causal event. Duration of pressure is increased by inactivity, immobility, and lack of sensory perception. Tissue tolerance to pressure is decreased by both extrinsic and intrinsic modifiers. Extrinsic modifiers are friction, moisture, and shear injury. Intrinsic modifiers are age, anatomic defects, edema, fever, hypotension, malnutrition, and vasoconstriction. When tissue tolerance to pressure is exceeded the effect of pressure is seen on the skin.

IDENTIFY THE HIGH-RISK PATIENT

Any patient who is inactive, immobile or immobilized, insensate, unconscious, aged, edematous, hypotensive, or malnourished or who has increased interface moisture or a healed pressure ulcer is at high risk for developing a pressure ulcer.

The time of greatest risk is during the first 10 days of hospitalization. Pressure changes occurring after this critical period are usually associated with deterioration of the clinical status of the patient.

PREVENTION

Although repositioning the patient every 2 hours while in bed is the standard of care, the positioning schedule should be determined by the level of risk and response of the skin to pressure. Observe the rule of 30. Do not raise the head of the bed more than 30 degrees from horizontal for long periods of time. In the side-lying position, the hips and shoulders should be tilted 30 degrees away from the supine position. Pillows and foam wedges are used to maintain the position. Keep the patient's heels off the mattress by placing a pillow under the legs or place the feet in boots that suspend the heels. Use a cradle over the feet to keep the bed clothes off the feet. Separate the knees and ankles with a pillow. Use lifting devices or lift sheets for position changes and transfers. Avoid the effects of incontinence by timely linen changes, or insert a Foley catheter and apply a rectal pouch. Consider the use of a support surface.

SELECTING A SUPPORT SURFACE

Selecting a support surface depends on the goal of therapy, whether it be prevention, treatment, or comfort. Support surfaces vary greatly in complexity and cost. They are classified as nonpowered, static and powered, or dynamic. Air, foam, water, or gel mattress overlays and mattresses are the nonpowered surfaces. They are indicated when one sleep surface is involved, and the patient can be positioned off the ulcer. Always check nonpowered overlays for bottoming-out by placing the hand between the overlay and the bed mattress. At least one inch of support surface should be present between the fingers and the patient's bony surface. If a patient bottoms out, more air should be added to an air overlay, or a static mattress or powered system is necessary.

Alternating pressure overlays and mattresses; low air-loss overlays, mattresses, and beds; and air-fluidized beds are the powered surfaces. A powered system is indicated when multiple sleep surfaces are involved. Alternating pressure air overlays must have tubes with a diameter large enough to lift the body off the underlying bed mattress. A 6-inch diameter is usually adequate. When the interface environment requires modification because of increased sweating, wound exudate, or occasional incontinence, a low air-loss overlay, mattress, or bed, or an air-fluidized bed, is indicated. Continuous head elevation greater than 30 degrees from the horizontal can be provided by a low air-loss mattress or bed. Patients with severe pulmonary disease should be placed on a bed providing oscillation to mobilize pulmonary secretions and promote ventilation. Pulsating systems are indicated to improve capillary circulation.

MEDICAL MANAGEMENT

The primary concern in the management of a pressure ulcer is the treatment of the disease that immobilized the patient. Adequate dietary intake should be maintained or instituted. This may require assisted feeding, or enteral or parenteral nutrition. At least 30 to 35 calories per kg per day, which includes 1.25 to 1.50 grams of protein per kg per day, is necessary. Malnourished persons require 500 mg to 1 gram of ascorbic acid (vitamin C) daily. A plasma protein level of 6 grams per dL and a hemoglobin level above 10 grams per dL are optimal. A transthyretin (pre-albumin) level less than 10 mg per dL indicates a need for nutritional therapy. Although analgesics may be required, pain relief can often be accomplished by covering the ulcer with an occlusive dressing and placing the patient on a support surface. Spasticity occurring in patients with neurologic disease or cord injury can be alleviated by diazepam, 2 to 10 mg given three or four times daily, or dantrolene sodium (Dantrium), 25 to 100 mg two, three, or four times daily. Pentoxifylline (Trental), 400 mg orally three times daily, is often helpful in treatment of heel ulcers in patients with occlusive peripheral vascular disease. Because all ulcers are colonized by a variety of bacteria, routine cultures provide no useful information. Infection is diagnosed clinically by the presence of an ulcer with an advancing indurated red border that is warm and usually tender. It is filled with necrotic debris and a purulent exudate. A foul odor, crepitus, and a thin sanguinous exudate suggest anaerobic infection. Systemic signs such as temperature elevation, leukocytosis, and an elevated sedimentation rate are present. The infected ulcer requires aerobic and sometimes anaerobic cultures from the ulcer and the blood. Material for anaerobic culture is obtained by curettage, biopsy, aspiration, or swabbing under the lip of the ulcer. Until bacteriologic confirmation is obtained, therapy should be initiated with a parenteral cephalosporin such as ceftazidime (Fortaz), 1 gram every 12 hours intravenously, or a quinolone such as ciprofloxacin (Cipro), 500 mg every 12 hours intravenously or orally. If anaerobic infection is suspected, metronidazole (Flagyl), 1 gram given every 12 hours orally, may be added to the regimen. An infectious disease consultation is indicated for serious infections.

LOCAL MANAGEMENT

Early Phases

No treatment other than pressure relief is necessary for blanchable erythema. The bright red form of nonblanchable erythema is treated with 2% nitroglycerin ointment. One-half to one inch of the ointment is placed on the lesion and occluded with an impermeable plastic wrap. To prevent development of tolerance, it is applied for 12 hours daily. The deep red or purple nonblanchable erythema is covered with a thin hydrocolloid dressing for protection. Cool Burow's solution compresses followed by a fluorinated steroid ointment or gel every 8 hours are used to treat decubitus dermatitis (erythema, scaling, vesicles, or bullae). After the vesicles break and the skin is still red, the area is treated with Burow's solution compresses followed by application of silver sulfadiazine (Silvadene) cream every 8 hours. Large erosions on dermatitic skin are covered with a hydrogel dressing. After the dermatitis clears, the large erosions are covered with hydrocolloid dressings.

Débridement

Ulcers with a large amount of necrotic material and debris are débrided surgically at the bedside. This is performed in a staged fashion over several days with forceps, scissors, or scalpel. Excising only necrotic material and debris minimizes pain. When necessary, local anesthesia can be administered by applying the eutectic mixture of lidocaine and prilocaine (Emla cream) to the ulcer and covering it with an impermeable plastic wrap for 1 hour. Brisk bleeding is avoided. Mild bleeding is controlled by applying an absorbable gelatin sponge, a calcium alginate dressing, or pressure. (Remember to turn the air-fluidized bed off for 15 to 20 minutes after having the patient lay on the ulcer.) Although surgical débridement is essential, it may cause transient bacteremia. This can be prevented by systemic antibiotic coverage. Should underlying bone be exposed, it is appropriate to perform an x-ray study to rule out osteomyelitis. Soft bone at the base of the ulcer is débrided and sent for culture and sensitivity studies.

Uninfected ulcers with a small amount of necrosis are débrided autolytically by covering with a hydrocolloid dressing. Autolytic débridement occurs only if the ulcer is exudative. Infected ulcers with a small amount of necrosis are débrided by applying an osmotic débriding agent such as a magnesium sulfate paste on the ulcer. Magnesium sulfate paste consists of dried magnesium sulfate 38.0%, phenol 0.5%, and anhydrous glycerol 61.5%. This mixture is spread on a soft piece of gauze cut to fit the ulcer or slightly larger if the ulcer has undermined edges. The gauze is placed on the ulcer bed and tucked under the overhanging edges. After the ulcer is rimmed with zinc oxide paste to protect the surrounding skin, it is covered with a dry dressing. Repeat applications are made every 8 hours after cleansing with normal saline solution.

Clean Ulcers

Clean ulcers are managed by cleaning with normal saline solution and covering the ulcer with a hydrocolloid dressing. Because of the large quantity of wound exudate produced early in treatment, initial therapy with a hydrocolloid dressing often requires the concomitant use of a hydrocolloid paste in the ulcer. This helps to absorb the fluid and extends the life of the dressing. Dead space under undermined edges and in deep ulcers is filled with hydrocolloid paste before the ulcer is covered with a hydrocolloid dressing. A calcium alginate pad or rope may be used in a manner similar to the hydrocolloid paste under a hydrocolloid dressing.

Eschar/Gangrene

If the eschar is separating from the surrounding skin or there is underlying fluctuation or the surrounding skin is red, indurated, and tender, and the patient is febrile, the eschar is exised. An eschar that is tightly adherent to the surrounding skin is scarified. After rimming with zinc oxide paste, an osmotic débriding agent (magnesium sulfate paste or hypertonic saline gel [Hypergel]) is spread on a gauze pad cut to fit over the eschar and its margin. This is placed on the eschar, and the lesion is covered with an impermeable plastic wrap. Repeat applications are made every 8 hours after cleansing with normal saline solution. After separation is complete, the eschar is excised.

Surgical Management

Whether to treat medically or employ a plastic surgical repair depends on the goal of therapy. In some instances, the goal may be to create a clean stable ulcer that can be easily managed and not pose a threat to the patient's life. In others, the goal may be to cover the ulcer. The factors of importance in deciding which course of action to take are the life expectancy of the patient, the potential and motivation for rehabilitation, the nature of the underlying disease, the suitability of the patient for surgery, and the ulcer itself. The young patient with a spinal cord injury is often a suitable candidate for surgical repair. The geriatric patient, on the other hand, is often too debilitated to undergo surgery.

ATOPIC DERMATITIS

method of
BERNICE R. KRAFCHIK, M.B., CH.B.
University of Toronto
Toronto, Ontario, Canada

Atopic dermatitis (AD) is a genetically determined chronic, relapsing disorder, characterized by a specific skin eruption and xerosis and an ability to overproduce IgE antibodies in response to common environmental antigens. In 1933, Wise and Sulzberger used the term AD, and in 1935 Hill and Sulzberger characterized the clinical entity.

Eczema (Gr., ekzein [to boil over]) often refers to the infantile form of AD and is used loosely by both physicians and the general public. Dermatologists use the word eczema as a descriptive term implying erythema, scaling, vesicles, and crusts. One may find eczematous lesions in conditions other than AD (scabies, autosensitization reactions, and tinea pedis).

The chronic form of AD is characterized by lichenification, which is thickening of the skin with an increase in normal skin markings. This reaction is pathognomonic of AD.

Atopic dermatitis is a major cause of morbidity in children in the Western world. In children with AD born after 1970, the incidence has increased to 9% to 12%. There is a strong family history of associated atopic diseases in families of patients with AD. These include asthma, hay fever, and urticaria.

AD is usually the first manifestation of atopic disease and appears in 85% of patients during the first year of life. In 95 percent of patients, the disease develops by 5 years of age. Hill and Sulzberger characterized three distinct clinical phases of AD, in which both the site and the morphology of the lesions change with age. These phases may overlap or be separated by a period of remission: (1) the infantile phase occurs up to 2 years of age; (2) the childhood phase occurs from age 2 to puberty; and (3) the adult phase occurs from puberty onward.

The characteristic and most important symptom and the major cause of morbidity in AD is pruritus, which may be unbearable and often interferes with normal sleep.

In infants, the eruption characteristically starts on the cheeks and scalp but often involves the lateral aspects of the extensors of the lower legs, and other areas may also be involved. The diaper area is often spared. The lesions are usually symmetrical, ill-defined, scaly, erythematous patches with areas of crusting. Xerosis is a major feature and is most helpful in establishing the diagnosis. The hair is often dry, and the scalp scaly. Lymphadenopathy may be marked.

In the childhood phase, the flexural areas are the sites of predilection. The antecubital and popliteal areas are most commonly affected, with the neck, flexures of the wrists and ankles, and buttock-thigh crease also commonly involved. These areas are particularly prone to sweating. The lesions are ill-defined erythematous, scaly plaques, often with excoriations.

At puberty, the clinical features once again involve the face, neck, and body diffusely, with erythema, more scaling, and less exudation. Xerosis and lichenification persist. Atopic dermatitis lesions do not scar. The disordered pigmentation disappears after weeks to months.

There are many associated features of the disease that may be helpful in making the diagnosis. The Dennie-Morgan fold is a double line found under the lower eyelid of patients with AD and may be present at birth or soon thereafter. Loss and thinning of the outer eyebrows, which is known as Hertog's sign, occurs frequently in children with AD who rub their eyebrows. Other signs are hyperlinear palms and ichthyosis.

Atopic dermatitis is a disease of exacerbations and remissions. Most patients tend to improve with age. Those patients with persistent disease are not as severely affected as they were in infancy and have much longer periods of remission between exacerbations of the AD.

MANAGEMENT

General Measures

It is important to establish a good relationship with the parents, explaining the nature of the disease and that treatment cannot provide a cure but good control. This is the most important information that the physician can communicate to the parents, so that they do not have unrealistic expectations. A distraught, guilt-ridden mother with a sleepless child who is unable to stop scratching needs a great deal of reassurance. It is important to discuss the psychological impact of the disease, emphasizing that although this disease is not caused by stress (as is often believed), the condition itself is stressful and may cause problems in family relationships. There is a strong tendency for the child with a chronic pruritic problem to become manipulative.

Clothing is important. Cotton should be worn all year, and in winter, layering cotton clothing provides good insulation. Cotton socks and tights are available. Nylon and wool are irritating to the skin of patients with AD.

It is important to allow the child as much freedom as possible. If swimming is part of the school program or a summer activity, it is helpful to use a barrier of petrolatum after the initial shower and before entering a chlorinated pool. Unfortunately, other activities such as running, soccer, and hockey often make the children hot and sweaty, thus promoting itch. Nevertheless, for their own psychological well-being, it is probably advisable to allow them to participate in sports activities.

In the summer months, patients improve in the

sun but find the heat exacerbates the pruritus. Thus, a sunny environment with a breeze is most helpful.

Parents should be warned that extreme fluctuations in temperature as well as fever may produce a flare in the condition. Many patients find that extreme cold exacerbates their AD. A clinical observation in many patients with AD is that change in environment or climate, or both (e.g., hospitalization or vacation), may improve the clinical condition.

Patients should be monitored for growth retardation from topical steroid use. This is unusual in the majority of children and may be associated with the disease process itself.

Specific Measures

Role of Food

Since the 1930s, food has been incriminated in causing AD, particularly in infants and young children. It is well known that skin testing produces both false-positive and false-negative reactions, and in vitro testing of specific antibodies in the serum against known antigens (RAST) has not provided better information.

There are two important issues regarding the role of food in AD. Does long-term breast-feeding protect against the development of AD? Does the elimination of certain foods in established AD help the existing dermatitis? A large retrospective study performed by Kramer and Moroz has not confirmed that continued breast-feeding prevents the development of AD, although other studies have shown the opposite.

Sampson and associates have shown clearing of lesions of AD in a small percentage of patients with specific food withdrawal and exacerbation on reintroduction. The original testing by Sampson was performed by double-blind challenge. It should be stressed that only a small proportion of the patients studied improved on food avoidance, and there were no cures. For many years, soy milk has been advocated as being much less antigenic than cow milk, but this also has not been confirmed.

The controversial question of the role of food in causing or exacerbating the lesions of AD has not been fully answered. If parents believe that a specific food is causing a problem for their child, that food should be withdrawn. However, the elimination of vital foods has led to malnutrition in some instances, and one should be cautious about dietary advice. Compliance to restricted diets is usually poor.

Topical Treatment

At present, until the basic defect is recognized the mainstay of management is to treat the inflammation, dryness, and itch. The inflammation is best treated with corticosteroid ointments. Potent corticosteroids should never be used on the face. Hydrocortisone 1% ointment three times a day is very effective on the facial area. This should be used until improvement occurs, and then it should be withdrawn. Ointment bases are more effective than creams because they are better absorbed and act as emollients for the dry skin, although cream bases should be used in very humid weather. When dermatitis on the body is severe, a mid-potency corticosteroid ointment, such as betamethasone valerate (Valisone) 0.1% or 0.01%, is applied three times a day to the affected areas until improvement is noticed. As soon as the dermatitis resolves, either a milder corticosteroid ointment (hydrocortisone 1% ointment applied three times a day), or a lubricating ointment may be used instead of the stronger corticosteroids. In all normal areas and once the dermatitis is in remission, emollients should be substituted for steroid ointments. When the scalp is involved, application of a corticosteroid lotion or cream (three times a day) and a bland or tar shampoo daily is helpful.

Various emollients are available, some containing urea. Parents should be warned only to apply urea products when the skin is moist because a burning sensation may otherwise occur. Urea-containing products may be too strong to use on the face.

The dryness is best treated with a bathing regimen using agents such as nonperfumed bath oils or oilated oatmeal to soothe the skin. Bathing should only take 5 minutes to avoid dehydration. Showers are contraindicated because of their drying effect. After bathing, the child should be left moist, and the noninflamed normal areas of skin should be covered with a lubricating ointment such as petroleum jelly or 10% urea in Eucerin after applying corticosteroids to the inflamed areas. A humidifier in the child's room is beneficial. A mild detergent, such as Ivory Snow, should be used to wash the child's clothes. Bleach and fabric softeners, as well as perfumed products, are also to be avoided because they cause dryness and irritation.

Soaps may be eliminated completely because the oils contain cleansing agents, or a mild soap that is nonperfumed, such as Dove or Lowila, may be used.

Tar preparations when prescribed as liquor carbonis detergens (LCD) 5% to 10%, combined with a corticosteroid, are of great benefit particularly in treating nummular patches.

Antihistamines, such as hydroxyzine hydrochloride (Atarax), in an appropriate dosage may alleviate the incessant itch and allow the patient some peaceful hours of sleep. In a child over 9 months of age, hydroxyzine hydrochloride, 10 mg three times a day, should be administered because the side effects are minimal and the lack of response is usually the result insufficient dosage. The combination of H_1 and H_2 antihistamines does not appear to be more useful. Less sedating antihistamines such as terfenadine (Seldane)* and astemizole (Hismanal)* have been used, but they do not appear to be as useful as traditional antihistamines.

Oral antibiotics may be useful in treating recalcitrant lesions. They are of obvious value in patients with infected lesions but should only be used to treat clinical infection. Although antibacterial scrubs may reduce the staphylococcal colony count, they are very irritating and their use is not advised.

Widespread Kaposi's varicelliform eruption responds extremely well to treatment with acyclovir (Zovirax).* The mortality from this disease has declined since the elimination of vaccination and the advent of acyclovir. The dose is 10 to 15 mg per kg per day for children and 200 mg five times per day for adults.

Systemic corticosteroids control severe exacerbations, but in view of the multiple side effects and an unwanted rebound flare when they are discontinued, they are rarely indicated. In the occasional case in which they are used as a last resort, a 2-week tapering dose should be used. Prednisone is given as 1 mg per kg per day for 4 days, 0.75 mg per kg for 4 days, and 0.5 mg per kg for 4 days, after which the medication is stopped. It should be stressed that continued use of systemic steroids is unwarranted and dangerous.

New agents are being tested as our understanding of the disease increases. Oral ketotifen (Zaditen)† has been effective in a dose of 1 mg two times a day for children and 2 mg two times a day for adults. Oral evening primrose oil,* a source of essential fatty acids, was found to produce an improvement in adults with AD, but this finding has not been verified. Interferon-gamma (Actimmune)* has been used in a trial with some success. Light in the form of ultraviolet A and ultraviolet B has been used with success. The addition of psoralen with ultraviolet A has led to long-term improvement.

ERYTHEMA MULTIFORME

method of
SYLVIA L. BRICE, M.D.
University of Colorado Health Sciences Center
Denver, Colorado

Erythema multiforme (EM) is an acute, self-limited cutaneous or mucocutaneous disorder. Two subsets of EM have been defined. EM minor (Hebra's disease) is the more common, and generally milder form, whereas EM major, also known as Stevens-Johnson syndrome, is the less common but more serious form. Because EM minor and EM major differ in many of their clinical features as well as their management, each will be discussed separately.

ERYTHEMA MULTIFORME MINOR

Clinical Features

EM minor is characterized by the development of symmetrically distributed, fixed, red lesions. Some lesions evolve concentric zones of color to form target or iris lesions, the hallmark of EM. Almost all patients develop lesions on the upper extremities, especially the dorsal aspects of the hands and forearms, and the elbows. Lesions on the trunk, face, and lower extremities are also commonly seen. Oral mucosal lesions occur in about 25% of patients. The duration of EM minor is from 1 to 4 weeks.

TABLE 1. **Treatment of Erythema Multiforme Minor**

Topical antipruritic agents
Topical anesthetics and antacids for oral involvement
Oral antihistamines
In recurrent disease:
Sun protective measures
Oral acyclovir
Eliminate immunosuppressive agents

By far, the most common precipitating factor in EM minor is an antecedent herpes simplex virus infection, although drugs may be implicated in a small minority of cases. In herpes-associated EM, the EM lesions typically develop within 2 days to 3 weeks of an episode of HSV (either Type 1 or 2). EM minor may be recurrent, or even continuous, with one episode immediately following another. In these cases, an association with HSV is highly suspect, even if clinical reactivation of the virus is not appreciated. EM minor is thought to be the result of a cell-mediated immune response.

The differential diagnosis of EM minor includes urticaria, non-EM drug eruptions, viral exanthems, lupus erythematosus, bullous pemphigoid, dermatitis herpetiformis, vasculitis, Sweet's syndrome, and Kawasaki disease. A skin biopsy for routine histopathology is recommended to confirm the diagnosis of EM, especially if the disease is recurrent, so that appropriate treatment may be initiated.

Therapy

In many cases of EM minor, symptomatic care may be all that is needed (Table 1). For itching, topical antipruritic agents such as calamine lotion, Sarna lotion, or pramoxine HCl (Prax lotion or cream) may be helpful, in addition to oral antihistamines, including diphenhydramine (Benadryl) or hydroxyzine (Atarax), 25 to 50 mg orally every 6 to 8 hours. Topical steroids are of limited benefit and are not routinely recommended. Although systemic steroids may initially appear to improve the condition, their use has been associated with the development of frequently recurring, or continuous, EM minor. Thus, they are not recommended.

For oral lesions, topical anesthetics may provide temporary relief. Possibilities include diphenhydramine HCl elixir (Benadryl),* 12.5 mg per 5 mL, 2% viscous lidocaine (Xylocaine), and dyclonine HCl solution (Dyclone), 0.5% or 1%. Mixing any of the above-mentioned medications with an equal volume of an aluminum-silicate solution (e.g., Kaopectate)* may help by more effectively coating the lesions with the active agent. Liquid antacids may be soothing used alone or in combination with an anesthetic

*Not FDA approved for this indication.
†Not yet approved for use in the United States.

*Not FDA approved for this indication.

agent. All these medications are used in a swish-and-spit method or applied directly to individual lesions. Very frequent use in patients with extensive mucosal disruption may result in loss of the gag reflex or some systemic absorption, but this has not proved to be a problem with judicial application. If significant secondary infection and painful lymphadenopathy develop, oral antibiotics (erythromycin, penicillin, or a cephalosporin) may be initiated.

In frequently recurrent EM minor, factors important in reactivation of herpes simplex virus (e.g., ultraviolet light) should be considered. Routine use of sunscreens is advised. In some cases, minimizing outdoor activities between 10 A.M. and 3 P.M. may be necessary. Oral acyclovir (Zovirax),* in chronic suppressive doses (400 mg twice daily or 200 mg every 8 hours), is recommended in patients with 6 or more episodes of EM per year. Once control of the disease is achieved, the dose of acyclovir may be tapered to the lowest level needed (usually not less than 400 mg per day). As in other situations in which chronic acyclovir is used, a drug holiday every 12 months is recommended to assess the continued need for therapy. Not all patients respond immediately to acyclovir, and it should be continued for at least 6 months before it is considered a treatment failure. Doubling the dose of acyclovir (800 mg twice daily) may also be considered if the patient fails to respond. Topical acyclovir has not been found to be effective.

When there is a clear-cut association with HSV infection and a well-defined interval between the onset of the HSV and subsequent development of EM, a short course of acyclovir (200 mg five times daily for 5 days)* initiated at the earliest evidence of the HSV may be effective in preventing the EM. However, most patients require the chronic suppressive regimen for optimal response.

In patients who deny any history of clinical HSV (even in the remote past), testing serum for HSV antibodies may be considered prior to initiating therapy. Seronegative individuals are unlikely to benefit from acyclovir therapy, and thus may be spared the expense of the medication.

In some cases of frequently recurring or continuous EM minor, the patient is currently being treated, or was recently treated, with systemic steroids or another immunosuppressive agent. In these cases, it is recommended that the immunosuppressive agent be discontinued and acyclovir be initiated. This approach may result in a temporary worsening of the disease but is ultimately successful in most patients.

In patients with frequent and debilitating disease who fail to respond to acyclovir, anecdotal reports have suggested that diaminodiphenylsulfone (dapsone),* 100 to 150 mg orally per day, and cimetidine (Tagamet),* 400 mg orally three times per day, are alternate agents to consider. Appropriate laboratory screening before and during therapy is essential for patients who are started on diaminodiphenylsulfone.

*Not FDA approved for this indication.

ERYTHEMA MULTIFORME MAJOR

Clinical Features

Unlike EM minor, EM major, or Stevens-Johnson syndrome, characteristically begins with a prodrome of an upper respiratory infection. Several days later, skin lesions that initially resemble those seen in EM minor develop abruptly. However, these lesions may rapidly progress to form blisters, with large areas of denuded skin. Mucosal lesions are often severe, with two or more mucosal sites involved. The mouth and conjunctivae are most commonly affected, but the genital mucosa may also be involved. The duration of EM major is at least 3 weeks and more often 6 to 8 weeks.

Although EM major may be precipitated by infectious agents, including HSV and *Mycoplasma pneumoniae,* antecedent drug exposure is much more likely. Nonsteroidal anti-inflammatory agents, sulfonamides, penicillins, and anticonvulsants are most commonly implicated. EM major is thought to be the result of toxic cutaneous injury.

The differential diagnosis of EM major includes pemphigus vulgaris, staphylococcal scalded skin syndrome, and acute graft-versus-host disease. The clinical history and a skin biopsy will usually differentiate between these entities. Testing serum for pemphigus antibodies may be useful, if this diagnosis is entertained. Toxic epidermal necrolysis (TEN) is considered by some authorities to be a severe form of EM major. Whether this is an appropriate classification has not been established. However, the recommendations for treatment of severe EM major and TEN are the same.

Therapy

Elimination and subsequent avoidance of the causative drug or treatment of the underlying infection is imperative (Table 2). In general, it is best to discontinue all unnecessary drugs. In the patient with sulfonamide-induced EM, it is important not to inadvertently initiate other sulfa-containing agents, or agents containing compounds that cross-react with sulfa (e.g., certain eye drops, topical dressings, diuretics).

Depending on the extent of cutaneous involvement,

TABLE 2. **Treatment of Erythema Multiforme Major**

Eliminate causative drug or treat precipitating infection
Admit to a burn unit, depending on extent of cutaneous involvement
Monitor for secondary infection, initiate antibiotics as indicated
Skin grafting or synthetic wound dressings
Monitor and replace fluids and electrolytes
High caloric replacement
Pulmonary hygiene
Ophthalmologic consultation
H_2-blocking agents, antacids
Pain control
Topical anesthetics for oral involvement
Avoid systemic steroids or other immunosuppressive agents

management in a burn unit may be advised. Careful attention to secondary infection and the potential development of sepsis is critical. Skin grafting or synthetic wound dressings may provide protection from bacterial infection. Periodic cultures of involved cutaneous sites and blood should be performed and systemic antibiotics initiated as indicated. Monitoring and replacement of fluids and electrolytes, high caloric replacement (2200 kcal per square meter per day), and good pulmonary hygiene (suctioning, postural drainage, incentive spirometry) are also important. Pain management is needed, especially early in the course of disease.

When conjunctival involvement is present, prompt ophthalmologic consultation is strongly advised to minimize long-term sequelae. For oral mucosal lesions, treatment as described for EM minor may be initiated. In addition, H_2-blocking agents and antacids are recommended to avoid gastrointestinal ulceration.

The use of systemic steroids in the management of EM major remains controversial. However, no benefit with the use of these agents has been proved, whereas an increased number of complications, including overwhelming sepsis, has been reported.

BULLOUS DISEASES

method of
GRANT J. ANHALT, M.D.
Johns Hopkins University
Baltimore, Maryland

PEMPHIGUS

There are three distinctive diseases that share the term pemphigus. These are pemphigus vulgaris, pemphigus foliaceus, and paraneoplastic pemphigus. Although each is a distinct autoimmune disease, they share the presence of intraepidermal blister formation caused by a disruption of normal epithelial cell-to-cell adhesion and IgG autoantibodies against epithelial adhesion proteins that have been proved to cause cell detachment in vivo.

Pemphigus Vulgaris

Pemphigus vulgaris is a blistering disease of mucous membranes and skin, and is a potentially life-threatening illness. The disease is associated with painful, fragile blisters and erosions that appear first in the mouth and later on the cutaneous surface of the head and neck area, upper chest, and back. Without adequate therapeutic intervention, painful lesions of the oropharynx lead to decreased oral intake of fluid and nutrients, and persistent loss of cutaneous surface causes fluid and electrolyte imbalance, debilitation, sepsis, and death. The diagnosis is established by the following criteria: (1) clinical lesions, as described; (2) the demonstration of loss of adhesion in the epidermis, with intraepidermal blister formation and loss of cell-to-cell cohesion (acantholysis), (3) demonstration of IgG autoantibodies bound to the cell surface of the affected epithelium, and (4) demonstration of circulating antibodies in the serum that are specific for the cell surface of stratified squamous epithelium. It is clearly established that affected patients have IgG autoantibodies directed against 130-kilodalton glycoprotein present on the surface of only stratified squamous epithelium that belongs to the cadherin family of cell adhesion molecules. Autoantibodies are produced in the bone marrow, circulate in the serum, and bind to the epithelium, causing loss of normal cell-to-cell adhesion, resulting in intraepithelial blister formation. It has been proved that these autoantibodies are pathogenic in the disease, and passive transfer of human pemphigus vulgaris autoantibodies into neonatal mice will reproduce blistering skin lesions. This is a disease primarily of middle age, with a peak incidence in the forties and fifties. There is a proven immunogenetic predisposition for certain racial groups, and the disease is more common in Jews of Eastern European origin. However, all races and ethnic groups are affected by pemphigus vulgaris to some degree.

Prior to the introduction of an effective therapy with oral corticosteroids in the 1950s, the disease had a dismal natural course, with a 50% mortality rate at 2 years and 100% mortality rate by 5 years after the onset of the disease. The mortality rate now is estimated at about 5%, and death is almost invariably due to the complications of immunosuppressive therapy. This disease is rare enough so as to render large-scale controlled treatment trials impractical. Therefore, treatment recommendations are based on information gleaned from uncontrolled small series, case reports, and the personal experience and biases of the author.

Long-term therapy for pemphigus vulgaris must be directed toward reducing autoantibody synthesis, because as long as significant levels of antiepithelial antibodies are present, the disease will persist. Therefore, topical treatments are of secondary importance, and sustained improvement occurs only with treatment of the hematopoietic system. Remissions are rare, and most individuals require therapy for life. Those that have resistant disease or are intolerant of corticosteroids should receive a second, steroid-sparing agent. In decreasing order of efficacy, these agents are cyclophosphamide, azathioprine, chlorambucil, methotrexate, and gold.

Oral corticosteroids remain the first line of treatment for all cases of pemphigus vulgaris. Some individuals with pemphigus vulgaris respond rapidly and completely to treatment with moderate doses of oral corticosteroids, others are rather refractory. About one-half of patients respond to oral corticosteroids alone (prednisone 1.0 mg per kg per day, tapered slowly over 6 to 9 months). Almost all individuals treated with prednisone require every-other-day maintenance indefinitely to control their disease. Prior to the widespread availability of effective second agents, it had been standard practice to use very large doses of corticosteroids in refractory cases. Typically, an individual would be treated initially with 60 or 80 mg of prednisone per day. If there was not a rapid response to therapy, the dose of corticosteroids would be doubled and often doubled once again. Under this regimen, patients would be treated with several hundred milligrams of prednisone per day, often with devastating or fatal complications. With the advent of effective immunosuppressive agents, it is generally not necessary to use such massive doses of corticosteroids.

Cyclophosphamide (Cytoxan), is an extremely effective agent in the treatment of pemphigus vulgaris, but it is also very toxic. It is very effective in reducing autoantibody synthesis, and has a preferential cytotoxic affect on proliferative plasma cells. It is generally reserved for patients who have the most therapy-resistant forms of pemphigus vulgaris in a dose of 1 to 2 mg per kg per day or by intermittent intravenous pulse. Major side effects include a predictable leukopenia, toxic effects of urinary metabolites causing hemorrhagic cystitis, and an increased lifetime risk of malignancy. The precise risk of lymphoma, leukemia, or bladder carcinoma secondary to treatment with cyclophosphamide has not been established for patients with pemphigus vulgaris, but in patients treated with similar doses for Wegener's granulomatosis, the lifetime risk may approach 5% to 10%. In addition, treatment with cyclophosphamide may produce sterility in patients with childbearing potential. Chlorambucil (Leukeran) is a useful alternative to cyclophosphamide if a patient has developed hemorrhagic cystitis due to cyclophosphamide therapy but still requires an alkylating agent to reduce antibody synthesis. Major potential problems of chlorambucil include its carcinogenic potential, and prolonged and unpredictable neutropenia.

Azathioprine (Imuran) is more widely used for the control of corticosteroid-resistant pemphigus. It is less toxic than cyclophosphamide but is also slightly less effective. It is preferentially used under several circumstances: (1) In young individuals, it is more desirable to use a less toxic agent to reduce the lifetime risk of malignancy and potential for sterility. (2) If a patient cannot be monitored closely by complete blood counts and urinalysis or is not compliant. (3) If the patient is intolerant of cyclophosphamide due to profound leukopenia, thrombocytopenia, or hemorrhagic cystitis. Azathioprine, however, must be used in adequate doses for proper effect. Initial doses of 2 to 3 mg per kg per day are usually required to produce reduction of antibody synthesis. Again, it should be used in conjunction with a low dose of oral corticosteroids.

Methotrexate was used for the treatment of pemphigus before other agents were available. It is a less effective but generally well-tolerated therapy for patients who cannot use alkylating agents or azathioprine.

Intramuscular gold has also been reported widely to be effective in management of both pemphigus vulgaris and pemphigus foliaceus. Response to this therapy has not been generally recognized, and the drug is not uniformly beneficial in everyone's experience. The incidence of allergic phenomena, such as nephritis and cutaneous or pulmonary hypersensitivity reactions, is very high and approaches 25%. Therefore, gold is being used with much less enthusiasm now than it has been in the past. The side effects appear to be the same whether one administers gold by mouth or intramuscularly.

Plasmapheresis has been used with mixed results in the therapy of pemphigus. If plasmapheresis alone is used, it can produce a short-term decrease in circulating autoantibody levels with subsequent clinical improvement. However, it must be recognized that the autoantibodies are under feedback inhibition control. If one simply removes the end-product, the B cells that produce the antibody are actually stimulated to produce more, and a rebound flare with worsening of the disease will occur several weeks after plasmapheresis has been discontinued. Therefore, it is best to reserve plasmapheresis as an adjunct to therapy and to use it in conjunction with an alkylating agent. It is recommended to use a short course of intensive pheresis (5 to 6 pheresis, ~3 liters per run). At the same time, an oral alkylating agent, such as cyclophosphamide, 1.5 mg per kg per day, with prednisone, 0.75 mg per kg per day, is begun. After the plasmapheresis has been discontinued, the loss of circulating antibody from the serum causes a preferential stimulation of the B cells producing the autoantibody. As they proliferate, they are preferentially destroyed by the cyclophosphamide. The patients who are treated with this combination of plasmapheresis and an alkylating agent sometimes go into prolonged disease-free remissions after 1 to 2 years of therapy.

Cyclosporine (Sandimmune) has been used with benefit in some cases of pemphigus vulgaris, but it is not generally accepted to be particularly effective. The high incidence of nephrotoxicity also limits its usefulness.

Finally, treatment should always be adjusted according to the disease activity that is clinically apparent, without being unduly influenced by autoantibody titers as estimated by indirect immunofluorescence. The antibody titers generally are high when the disease is active and are low or undetectable when the disease is in remission. If a patient is in apparent clinical remission but has persistent low titers, that should not prevent planned reductions of drug dosages. The indirect immunofluorescent titer is most useful during maintenance if a patient develops a flare of disease activity. In this circumstance, a low or negative antibody titer would be reassuring that the flare may be self-limited and may not require increased drug dosages. On the contrary, a high titer raises more concern and prompts earlier intervention.

Pemphigus Foliaceus

Pemphigus foliaceus is another autoimmune disorder in which IgG autoantibodies are directed against a cell adhesion molecule of the epidermis, but there are very distinct clinical and immunopathologic differences that distinguish it from pemphigus vulgaris. Unlike pemphigus vulgaris, lesions in pemphigus foliaceus occur only on cornified epidermis, and lesions of mucosal surfaces are extremely rare. In pemphigus foliaceus, IgG autoantibodies are directed against a separate cadherin of stratified squamous epithelium called desmoglein I, with an estimated molecular weight of 165 kilodaltons. Binding of IgG to this cadherin molecule produces acantholysis in only superficial levels of cornified epithelium. Therefore, pemphigus foliaceus is diagnosed by the following criteria: (1) superficial crusting erosions of the head and neck, central chest and back, or proximal extremities in the absence of mucosal lesions; (2) histologic examination showing acantholysis (cell-to-cell detachment) occurring only through more well-differentiated upper levels of the epidermis; (3) the demonstration of IgG autoantibodies on the cell surface of affected epithelium; and (4) demonstration of IgG autoantibodies in the serum that bind specifically to the cell surface of stratified squamous epithelium.

The mortality rate for pemphigus foliaceus is very low. This may due to the superficial nature of the cutaneous lesions and the absence of mucosal involvement. Most patients experience some morbidity from the disease, but one is not compelled to be as aggressive in treatment of pemphigus foliaceus. Some individuals, however, do have very aggressive disease and develop erythrodermic and exfoliative disease. These patients have severe morbidity, discomfort, and debilitation, and require more intensive intervention.

Most cases of pemphigus foliaceus can be controlled by oral corticosteroids alone. A starting dose of 0.5 to 1.0 mg per kg per day, with a slow taper over a period of 6 months and the use of an alternate-day steroid regimen, is usually effective. Topical or intralesional steroids are somewhat effective in limited cases of pemphigus foliaceus. The list of drugs that are useful as second or steroid sparing agents is identical to that in pemphigus vulgaris, with the possible addition of antimalarials such as hydroxychloroquine (Plaquenil), 200 mg twice daily. The necessity of using an immunosuppressive agent, such as cyclophosphamide, azathioprine, or other agents such as gold or methotrexate in management of this disease is less frequent than in pemphigus vulgaris. Efficacy and toxicities of these therapies have already been outlined.

Paraneoplastic Pemphigus

Paraneoplastic pemphigus is a more recently described mucocutaneous autoimmune disease associated with neoplasia. Most individuals with paraneoplastic pemphigus have non-Hodgkin's lymphomas, chronic lymphocytic leukemia, Castleman's tumors, thymoma, or Waldenström's macroglobulinemia. The most common characteristics of this syndrome are painful erosions of the mucous membranes of the mouth and vermilion of the lips. These oral erosions tend to be painful, debilitating, and very resistant to therapy. In addition, individuals develop very polymorphic cutaneous lesions, consisting of acantholytic blisters, lichenoid lesions, and lesions resembling those of erythema multiforme. Patients with paraneoplastic pemphigus also have IgG autoantibodies that bind to the cell surface of squamous epithelia; however, unlike pemphigus vulgaris or foliaceus, these autoantibodies bind to epithelia other than just stratified squamous epithelia. As seen by indirect immunofluorescence, they bind to transitional epithelium of urinary bladder, respiratory epithelium, and intestinal epithelium. This difference is due to the known specificity of these autoantibodies. The antibodies recognize desmoplakins I and II, which are components of all of the desmosomes of all epithelia. In addition, there is variable reactivity with additional antigens such as the bullous pemphigoid 230 antigen and two other uncharacterized proteins. Patients with malignant neoplasms have a rather poor prognosis. Although there have been reports of long-term survivors, in personal experience with a series of 33 cases, 30 of 33 patients with malignancies died from complications of treatment or from the syndrome. In individual cases, death was attributed to multiple factors including sepsis, gastrointestinal bleeding, multiorgan failure, and respiratory failure.

Individuals with benign tumors such as thymoma or Castleman's tumors should have them surgically excised. The majority of patients that are freed of tumor burden will either improve substantially or clear completely within a year of surgery.

In patients with malignant neoplasms, there is no clear therapy that is effective at the present time. Oral corticosteroids in a dose of approximately 1 mg per kg per day will produce partial improvement, but not complete resolution of lesions. Cutaneous lesions respond more quickly to therapy, the stomatitis being generally quite refractory to any form of therapy. Aside from corticosteroids, many other agents have been tried in individual cases on an anecdotal basis and none of these have really stood out as particularly effective in the treatment. Methods that have been tried and have generally failed include immunosuppression with cyclophosphamide or azathioprine, gold, dapsone, cyclosporine, and plasmapheresis.

PEMPHIGOID

The term pemphigoid applies to cutaneous diseases that are characterized clinically (1) by the presence of large, tense blisters; (2) by subepidermal blister formation with an inflammatory infiltrate usually rich in eosinophils; and (3) by the deposition of IgG and complement components along the basement membrane zone of affected skin or mucous membrane.

Bullous Pemphigoid

Bullous pemphigoid is an acquired blistering disease of the elderly. It is characterized histologically by subepidermal bullae and immunopathologically by in vivo deposition of autoantibodies and complement components along the epidermal basement membrane zone. Approximately one-half of these patients also have circulating autoantibodies directed against the basement membrane zone of stratified squamous epithelium. Because of these characteristics, bullous pemphigoid is believed to be an autoimmune disease in which the cutaneous lesions may result as a consequence of these anti–basement membrane zone antibodies.

Generalized bullous pemphigoid requires systemic therapy, using agents similar to those effective in pemphigus vulgaris but in lower doses and for shorter periods of time. Patients with localized bullous pemphigoid have responded well to therapy with topical or intralesional steroids alone (such as triamcinolone suspension, 10 mg per mL). Systemic corticosteroids are the mainstay of therapy in generalized bullous pemphigoid; the most widely used preparation is prednisone. Some individuals prefer a nongeneric brand of prednisone to ensure reliable absorption; others rely on intramuscular triamcinolone (Kenalog), 40 to 60 mg monthly, if compliance is a problem. Most series show that the majority of patients with generalized disease were controlled with 40 to 80 mg daily of prednisone, and only rarely was it necessary to exceed 80 mg daily. The severity of disease, age of the patient, and presence of underlying diseases, especially diabetes mellitus, tuberculosis, and hypertension, must be considered in determining the dose of corticosteroids. Mild disease, which has been arbitrarily defined as presence of 20 lesions or less, usually responds to lower doses of prednisone (less than 0.5 mg per kg per day) than does moderate (20 to 40 lesions) or severe disease (greater than 60 lesions). Healing of existing lesions and cessation of new blister formation reflects a response to therapy. Once the disease is under control, the prednisone dose should be tapered slowly and eventually changed to an every-other-day regimen to minimize steroid side effects.

A minority of patients may not respond to corticosteroids, or they may require a high maintenance dose of the drugs. These patients may benefit from the addition of an immunosuppressive agent. The most frequently used agents are azathioprine and cyclophosphamide. My personal preference is to use azathioprine as the first immunosuppressive agent in bullous pemphigoid. It is easy to administer; does not produce significant leukopenia and, therefore, does not require as close observation as other agents; and is generally well tolerated. In addition, it has some anti-inflammatory effects that are useful in bullous pemphigoid and are not found with other immunosuppressive drugs. Azathioprine is effective at doses of 1 to 2 mg per kg per day in bullous pemphigoid.

Experience with cyclophosphamide in bullous pemphigoid is more limited, but it has also been shown to have steroid-sparing effects. It is reserved for patients who have unusually aggressive disease and have failed to respond to other agents.

Methotrexate (7.5 to 15 mg weekly) has also been used in a limited number of patients with success but is usually less effective than other immunosuppressives. Dapsone or sulfapyridine may be useful in management of patients in whom corticosteroids are contraindicated or not tolerated. In my personal experience, only about 10% to 15% of patients show a convincing response to sulfone therapy.

Corticosteroid pulse therapy, in which patients are given 1 gram of methylprednisolone intravenously for 3 consecutive days, can also be successful in initial control of patients with severe bullous pemphigoid. Plasmapheresis has also been used in treating patients with bullous pemphigoid, but it has only temporary beneficial effects. In fact, there is some evidence that the concomitant use of plasmapheresis may increase the chance of death from infectious complications, so it is generally not used. Finally, cyclosporine has proved beneficial in the treatment of some bullous pemphigoid patients, but its inherent nephrotoxicity and cost render it an infrequently used drug. Further studies are needed to determine the role of this agent in the treatment of bullous pemphigoid.

Finally, there have been reports of the effectiveness of a combination of oral erythromycin or tetracycline (2 grams per day) and niacinamide (1500 to 2500 mg per day) in the treatment of bullous pemphigoid. Anecdotal reports have confirmed this report, but I have generally found it to be ineffective. It could be attempted in patients with limited disease who likely would not tolerate oral steroids well, but its usefulness will have to be determined by larger studies.

Cicatricial Pemphigoid

Cicatricial pemphigoid is predominantly a disease of the elderly, with a peak incidence between 60 and 80 years of age. Lesions can arise on any mucosal surface covered by stratified squamous epithelium, including the nasopharynx and oropharynx, conjunctiva, esophagus, larynx, urethra, and anal mucosa. Morbidity and mortality is due to the scarring that recurrent lesions produces. The major criteria distinguishing bullous pemphigoid from cicatricial pemphigoid is the presence of scarring secondary to the blistering, and that in bullous pemphigoid, cornified epithelium is the primary tissue involved, whereas in cicatricial pemphigoid, mucosal epithelium is primarily affected.

Clinically, lesions present as smooth bordered erosions with distinct margins. The gingivae are commonly involved, and cicatricial pemphigoid is one cause of desquamative gingivitis. The conjunctival epithelium is affected in about two-thirds of cases of cicatricial pemphigoid, and it is cause for considerable concern. In the conjunctiva, erosions are rare, and signs of active disease include a violaceous inflammatory infiltrate, superficial fine fibrotic bands, shrinkage of the conjunctival fornices, and entropion. Lesions of the laryngeal, esophageal, and genital mucosae consist of smooth-bordered erosions, with eventual stricture formation. Skin lesions occur in more than 20% of patients and are usually transient. When the lesions are present, they consist of small intact blisters or erosions, usually in the head and neck area.

The diagnosis is established by three criteria: (1) scarring blisters and/or erosions, as described; (2) subepithelial blistering on histologic examination, with an intact basal cell layer and variable inflammatory infiltrate; and (3) direct immunofluorescence of perilesional epithelium showing IgG and complement components along the basement membrane zone. In mucosal cicatricial pemphigoid, the indirect immunofluorescence for circulating antibodies is highly unreliable and is negative in the majority of cases. It is important to obtain positive direct immunofluorescence results, even if it requires repeat biopsies, because the clinical and histologic features can be closely mimicked by erosive lichen planus, and a syndrome indistinguishable from cicatricial pemphigoid also occurs in about 10% to 15% of patients with linear IgA dermatosis and epidermolysis bullosa acquisita.

Treatment is dictated by the organs involved and the anticipated morbidity. This disease is not highly steroid responsive, and it is progressive. Spontaneous remissions are rare. So, for example, if only the oropharynx and nasopharynx are affected, anticipated morbidity is minimal, and treatment should be limited to topical steroids such as fluocinonide gel (Lidex), intralesional steroid injections with triamcinolone, 10 mg per mL, or occasional short bursts of oral corticosteroids. This approach provides palliation but does not halt progression of the disease. If only the gingivae are involved, topical therapy with occlusion can be delivered by application of a flexible dental tray (similar to the disposable molds used to deliver fluoride treatments to the teeth), in which a medium-potency topical steroid such as betamethasone valerate (Valisone) ointment is applied. This can be used twice or thrice daily to provide convenient topical therapy of the attached gingiva.

A different situation exists if the eyes, esophagus, or larynx are involved. In such cases, the anticipated morbidity includes blindness and asphyxiation, and aggressive systemic therapy is warranted. Systemic steroids alone will not adequately control progression; most other therapies only slow the scarring process. The treatment of choice is oral cyclophosphamide, given in a regimen that has been confirmed to be effective in double-blinded studies. Initial therapy requires combined use of prednisone, 1.0 mg per kg per day, with tapering discontinuation within 6 months. Cyclophosphamide is started at the same time but is maintained for a period of 18 to 24 months at a dose of 1 to 2 mg per kg per day (until the white blood count is depressed to 3000 to 4000 per mm^3). About three-quarters of the patients treated with this regimen tolerate the drug, and at the end of this period, most of these patients will have complete clinical remissions that will persist after all drugs are withdrawn. To date, this cyclophosphamide regimen is the only treatment that provides the potential for a cure of this disease. Chlorambucil (Leukeran), 4 to 6 mg per day, is used as an alternative agent if cyclophosphamide is not tolerated.

Occasionally, patients respond to oral dapsone, in doses of 100 to 150 mg per day. Those that respond well do so quickly, but unfortunately in our experience, these patients are a minority. Azathioprine is an alternative for patients that cannot tolerate cyclophosphamide, and it has fewer acute toxicities. The use of cyclosporine is not recommended owing to the chronicity of the disease. It is important to recognize that treatment with any agent other than cyclophosphamide or chlorambucil may suppress symptoms, but scarring will progress and eventual morbidity or mortality will not be avoided.

EPIDERMOLYSIS BULLOSA ACQUISITA

Epidermolysis bullosa acquisita is an unwieldly name applied to a distinct subepidermal blistering disorder. The clinical spectrum of this disease is rather varied, but it primarily presents as an adult-onset acquired mechanobullous disease with skin fragility, blistering, and scarring on extensor surfaces. Another variant is an inflammatory form with blisters that heal with milia and scarring, and this form most closely resembles bullous pemphigoid. This disease is associated with autoantibodies bound to the basement membrane zone, and subepidermal blister formation. It is distinguished from bullous pemphigoid by autoantibodies that bind to molecules of Type VII collagen in the very upper dermis. This causes a subepidermal blister that forms through the upper dermis, in contrast to bullous pemphigoid, in which the blister forms in the basement membrane zone at the level of the lamina lucida. Epidermolysis bullosa acquisita can most readily be distinguished from bullous pemphigoid by specialized immunofluorescent studies on split skin. Approximately 10 to 15% of patients have a variant of epidermolysis bullosa acquisita in which mucosal lesions with scarring predominate. This variant can very closely mimic the clinical phenotype of cicatricial pemphigoid.

Some cases of epidermolysis bullosa acquisita are quickly responsive to standard therapies, and some are resistant. The list of effective medications in this disease is similar to that for bullous pemphigoid. The disease is chronic and prolonged, and indefinite treatment is usually required. Oral corticosteroids, such as prednisone, 0.5 to 1 mg per kg per day, is the initial treatment of choice. This can be tapered over a period of several months, and some fortunate patients respond very well. Dapsone, 100 to 200 mg daily, has been shown to have significant benefit in individual patients, and it is often used as a second agent for its steroid-sparing effects in this disease. Other agents such as azathioprine, methotrexate, cyclophosphamide, and gold have also been used with variable effects. Plasmapheresis has been employed but its benefits are not obvious. For debilitating and refractory cases of epidermolysis bullosa acquisita, cyclosporine has been shown to be an effective therapy. However, control of the blistering process requires high doses of cyclosporine (6 to 9 mg per kg per day), and the disease recurs on discontinuation of the drug. Therefore, the toxicity of cyclosporine may outweigh the benefits.

DERMATITIS HERPETIFORMIS

Dermatitis herpetiformis is possibly the most pruritic cutaneous bullous disease. Individuals present with excoriations distributed in a symmetrical manner over the shoulders and scapulae, elbows and knees, and also on the sacrum and forehead. The condition usually presents in young adulthood and is linked to HLA haplotypes B8 and DR3. All patients have an asymptomatic gluten-sensitive enteropathy associated with the skin disease. Diagnosis is established by histology and direct immunofluorescence of the skin that show clusters of neutrophils in the dermal papillary tips, co-localizing with a granular deposition of IgA. There is no significant morbidity associated with this disease other than occasional suicides due to the intense pruritus, and a 100-fold increased risk for intestinal lymphoma, presumably due to the occult gluten-sensitive enteropathy. The risk for intestinal lymphoma in the general population is approximately 0.03%, and in individuals with dermatitis herpetiformis, it is estimated at 3%.

The primary treatment for this disease is oral dapsone (diaminodiphenylsulfone). The response to dapsone is so rapid and reproducible that in the past it was regarded as a therapeutic test to confirm the diagnosis. One must first be certain that an individual to be treated has adequate levels of glucose-6-phosphate dehydrogenase (G6PD). In the presence of a G6PD deficiency, rapid and dangerous hemolysis could occur. Dapsone is started first with a trial dose of 25 mg orally daily for 1 week. After this, a complete blood count is obtained, and if no significant hemolysis has occurred, full doses of dapsone can be started. The dosage requirement for dapsone varies widely from patient to patient. Initial therapy usually requires as little as 100 to a maximum of 200 mg of dapsone per day. Beyond 200 mg orally daily, unacceptable levels of anemia and neurologic toxicity can occur. In general, once the disease is controlled, the dose of dapsone may be decreased slowly over the following months, and some individuals can be maintained with very low doses such as 50 mg once or twice weekly for the long term. Unpredictable side effects of dapsone include rare development of agranulocytosis or pancytopenia. Long-term dapsone therapy, usually with higher doses (≥200 mg orally daily) have been associated with a mixed motor and sensory neuropathy that is not necessarily reversible after discontinuation of the drug. Therapy with dapsone does not reverse the coexistent gluten sensitive enteropathy and does not decrease an individual's lifetime risk for developing intestinal lymphoma.

If an individual is intolerant of dapsone, sulfapyridine therapy is an acceptable alternative agent, used in a dose of 2 to 4 grams daily in divided daily doses. One must be cautious to maintain generous oral intake of fluids to avoid crystallization of the drug in the urinary tract. In the United States, it is currently difficult to obtain sulfapyridine, because it is not generally available by prescription. It can, however, be obtained on an individual basis from Jacobus Pharmaceutical Company, 37 Cleveland Lane, P.O. Box 5290, Princeton, New Jersey 08540.

Curiously, dermatitis herpetiformis has a minimal response to topical steroids, anti-inflammatory agents, and oral corticosteroids.

Because of the associated gluten-sensitive enteropathy, there has been much speculation and debate about the role of gluten in the pathogenesis of the cutaneous lesions and the role of a gluten-free diet in inducing remission of the cutaneous disease. The following observations seem to be generally accepted: First, any diet instituted for therapy must incorporate complete and absolute avoidance of gluten in all forms. Ingestion of even small amounts of gluten will completely reverse any benefits. In North America, absolute avoidance of gluten requires very careful patient education, and long-term compliance is very difficult. Second, a response to gluten avoidance takes a very long time. Typically, one will not see any variation in disease activity for 1 to 3 years after institution of complete abstinence from gluten ingestion. Most individuals will be able to reduce their dapsone requirement significantly, but only a minority of patients will be able to discontinue dapsone or sulfapyridine use completely. Third, there is recent evidence that gluten elimination will reduce an individual's risk of intestinal lymphoma to baseline (0.03%), but with incomplete elimination of gluten from the diet, the risk will remain elevated by 100-fold. Therefore, gluten-free diets are strongly encouraged in those individuals who are concerned about the risk of intestinal lymphoma, those who require large doses of dapsone, and those in whom long-term neurologic toxicity is anticipated.

LINEAR IGA DERMATOSES

This is another subepidermal blistering disorder that is associated with the presence of linear deposits of IgA along the basement membrane zone. This disease occurs in all age groups, and may actually represent more than one autoimmune disease that has similar clinical presentations. Most commonly, the disease appears in childhood with tense pruritic blisters on the trunk and extremities, and it is frequently referred to as chronic bullous disease of childhood. The disorder can also start in adult life with blistering eruption on the skin. Again, a small percentage of patients with this disorder may have a clinical phenotype that is essentially identical to cicatricial pemphigoid.

Linear IgA dermatitis is diagnosed by (1) the presence of pruritic blisters on the skin or mucous membranes, (2) subepidermal blister formation on histologic examination, and (3) the deposition of linear deposits of IgA along the basement membrane zone. Circulating IgA autoantibodies against the skin are rarely detectable in the blood. There is no association of linear IgA with gluten-sensitive enteropathy and no increased risk for intestinal lymphoma, in contrast to dermatitis herpetiformis. This disorder is distinguished immunopathologically from dermatitis herpetiformis by *linear* deposition of IgA in contrast to *granular* deposition of IgA.

The treatment for linear IgA dermatitis usually requires some combination of oral corticosteroids and dapsone. Use of oral dapsone in doses similar to those used in dermatitis herpetiformis usually results in incomplete resolution of lesions, in contrast to the dramatic effect produced in dermatitis herpetiformis. Linear IgA dermatitis is somewhat sensitive to oral corticosteroids (unlike dermatitis herpetiformis), and one must often use a small dose of prednisone (20 to 40 mg daily) and a moderate dose of dapsone (100 mg daily) for adequate control. If dapsone is not tolerated, or the patient is G6PD deficient, sulfapyridine is an acceptable alternative. There is very limited experience with other immunosuppressive agents in this disease, so that the benefit of other steroid-sparing agents cannot be adequately evaluated.

CONTACT DERMATITIS

method of
DANIEL J. HOGAN, M.D.
Bay Pines Veterans Administration Medical Center
Bay Pines, Florida
University of South Florida
Tampa, Florida

and

PHILIP D. SHENEFELT, M.D.
University of South Florida
James A. Haley Veterans Administration Medical Center
Tampa, Florida

Contact dermatitis is typically manifested by erythema, edema, and vesiculation of the skin due to direct exposure of the involved areas to an external agent. Vesicles and edema in the epidermis are always present histologically and are frequently present grossly in acute severe allergic contact dermatitis, such as poison ivy dermatitis. Vesicles are typically deep seated on the palms, where the morphologic pattern termed dyshidrosis or pompholyx may be induced by both irritants and allergens. Typically there is a relatively sharp demarcation between involved and uninvolved skin where areas not exposed to the irritant or allergen are typically free of dermatitis. However, severe dermatitis may produce nonspecific hyperreactivity of the entire integument, and dermatitis may spread to areas not directly exposed to the irritant or allergen. Allergens in particular may be airborne and produce airborne contact dermatitis typically maximal on the face, particularly the eye lids. Ingestion of nickel in foods has been associated with flaring of pompholyx in European studies. Intravenous administration of gentamicin in those with contact allergy to neomycin has caused cases of systemic contact dermatitis. A similar form of dermatitis may arise in those with contact allergy to ethylenediamine who are treated with aminophylline.

Secondary lesions seen in contact dermatitis include excoriations of pruritic skin and secondary bacterial infections, usually staphylococcal, often appearing as yellow crusts in areas of dermatitis.

Chronic contact dermatitis is usually manifested by lichenification or thickening of the skin from chronic inflammation and scratching and hyperpigmentation or hypopigmentation of the skin, which is most noticeable in dark-skinned individuals.

Irritants directly damage the skin with consequent inflammation. Allergens mediate inflammation through specific immunologic mechanisms. Some inflammatory pathways are common for both irritant and allergic contact dermatitis. Almost any substance may be a cutaneous irritant depending on the duration of exposure to the substance and the concentration of the substance. Allergens induce a specific T cell mediated sensitivity whereby severe inflammation may be produced by exposures to minute concentrates of allergens. Over 2800 substances have been identified as contact allergens. Potent sensitizers such as poison ivy are able to sensitize the majority of healthy individuals. Some substances sensitize only a small minority of exposed individuals.

Accurate diagnosis is the key to proper management of contact dermatitis. If the agent(s) causing dermatitis can be identified by history or patch testing and if the patient can avoid these agents the chances for recovery are maximized. If contact with the causative allergen or irritant continues, the risk of chronic disabling dermatitis increases, with permanent impairment of the ability to work and perform activities of daily living. Even with the most expert evaluation individuals with contact dermatitis may have persistent dermatitis.

It is necessary to obtain a thorough history in evaluating individuals with contact dermatitis. Crucial items about which the patient should be queried directly include exact nature of work; whether or not other workers are similarly affected; changes in work procedure; chemical exposure; protective measures used at work; agents used to cleanse the skin; hobbies, particularly gardening and exposure to plants; use of personal care products, including those used by spouse or other household members; family history of atopy, particularly atopic dermatitis; previous treatment, including over-the-counter medications; and treatment recommended by other physicians and health care workers.

The patch test is the standardized diagnostic procedure of choice for identifying allergy to chemicals that commonly cause allergic contact dermatitis. Patch testing is particularly indicated for identifying causes of allergic contact dermatitis due to workplace exposures and personal care products. It is crucial that physicians performing patch testing relate the relevance of positive reactions to the patient's dermatitis.

Patient education is very important in the management of contact dermatitis. The better informed the patient is about the causes of his or her contact dermatitis and the measures they can take to avoid these causes, the better the prognosis for clearing his or her dermatitis and remaining clear. A pamphlet on measures to protect the skin from cutaneous irritants is of particular help for patients with dermatitis affecting the hand. Such pamphlets may be obtained from the American Academy of Dermatology. Patients who are tested and found to be allergic to one or more chemicals should be given all the known names and trade names of the chemical(s) and should be instructed on where they may be exposed to this allergen at home and at work.

Occasionally, skin biopsies are indicated to differentiate contact dermatitis from psoriasis; KOH preparations are used to exclude fungal infections and bacterial cultures to confirm primary or secondary pyoderma in the patient with contact dermatitis.

Inappropriate diagnostic tests include occlusive patch testing to irritant concentrations of materials. Radioallergosorbent (RAST) tests are not helpful in the diagnosis of contact dermatitis, although they may be helpful in certain cases of contact urticaria.

TREATMENT

Severe, acute, widespread allergic contact dermatitis usually requires treatment with systemic corticosteroids. Prednisone can be given in an initial dose of 40 to 60 mg a day in adults. Systemic corticosteroids are particularly indicated for severe flares of hand dermatitis and allergic contact dermatitis involving the face or, in men, the genital areas. Systemic corticosteroids should be tapered over a 2- to 3-week period. Systemic corticosteroid courses of less than 2 weeks' duration are inadequate to maintain suppression of dermatitis until the allergen is desquamated from the skin. Systemic antibiotics are helpful in dermatitis with secondary bacterial infection. Sedating antihistamines such as hydroxyzine (Atarax), 25 mg three times a day, are helpful in the symptomatic treatment of pruritus. They are particularly helpful at nighttime, when their side effect of sedation may be a benefit rather than a detriment.

Topical corticosteroids are the most frequently prescribed medication for contact dermatitis (Table 1). Topical corticosteroid creams and ointments are more effective in the treatment of allergic dermatitis than irritant contact dermatitis. Potent class I topical corticosteroids are indicated for 2- to 3-week courses for episodes of allergic contact dermatitis that are not so widespread that systemic corticosteroids are indicated.

Cool compresses with saline or aluminum subacetate are helpful in drying acute vesicular plaques. These compresses should be discontinued promptly when sufficient drying of the vesicles occurs because excessive drying could then produce irritant contact dermatitis. Colloidal oatmeal in lukewarm baths is helpful for widespread contact dermatitis. Topical antibiotic ointments and creams should be used with caution because of the problem of sensitization to these products, particularly when they are applied to otitis externa, perineal and perianal dermatitis, stasis dermatitis, and leg ulcers. Neosporin and bacitracin are the two most frequently identified causes of allergic contact dermatitis to topical antibiotics.

Bland emollients such as Neutrogena hand cream or Aquaphor are important in the management of contact dermatitis, particularly irritant contact dermatitis and chronic dermatitis, because of their effect in helping to restore normal barrier function and protection to the skin.

TABLE 1. **Topical Corticosteroid Potency Ranking***

Group	Brand Name	Generic Name
I	Temovate 0.05%	Clobetasol propionate
	Diprolene 0.05%	Betamethasone dipropionate
	Psorcon 0.05%	Diflorasone diacetate
	Ultravate 0.05%	Halobetasol propionate
II	Cyclocort 0.1%	Amcinonide
	Elocon 0.1%	Mometasone furoate
	Florone 0.05%	Diflorisone diacetate
	Halog 0.1%	Halcinonide
	Lidex 0.05%	Fluocinonide
	Maxiflor 0.05%	Diflorasone diacetate
	Topicort 0.25%	Desoximetasone
III	Valisone 0.1%	Betamethasone valerate
IV	Kenalog, Aristocort 0.1%	Triamcinolone acetonide
	Cordran 0.05%	Flurandrenolide
	Elocon 0.1%	Mometasone furoate
	Synalar 0.025%	Fluocinolone acetonide
	Topicort LP 0.05%	Desoximetasone
V	Locoid 0.1%	Hydrocortisone butyrate
	Tridesilon 0.05%	Desonide
	Westcort 0.2%	Hydrocortisone valerate
VI	Aclovate 0.05	Alclometasone dipropionate
VII	Hytone 1.0%	Hydrocortisone
	Miscellaneous	Dexamethasone, fluorometholone, prednisolone, and methylprednisolone

*Group I is the superpotent category. Group VII is the least potent. Within Group I, Temovate is most potent. In general, ointment formulations are more potent than cream formulations, which are more potent than lotion formulations. Occluded formulations are the most potent.

Ultraviolet light treatment with ultraviolet B is occasionally indicated in cases of chronic contact dermatitis. Photochemotherapy is indicated in cases of severe chronic hand dermatitis unresponsive to topical therapy.

THE SPECIFIC DERMATOSES OF PREGNANCY

method of
S. A. VAUGHAN JONES, M.D., and
M. M. BLACK, M.D.
St. Thomas' Hospital
London, England

The specific dermatoses of pregnancy have led to much confusion in the past resulting from poorly defined classification and misleading terminology. Table 1 proposes an up-to-date classification.

PEMPHIGOID GESTATIONIS

Pemphigoid gestationis (PG) is a pruritic bullous disorder occurring in pregnancy and the puerperium, and it is also associated with choriocarcinoma, trophoblastic tumors, and hydatidiform mole. Its inci-

TABLE 1. **Dermatoses of Pregnancy**

New Classification	Previous Terminology
Pemphigoid gestationis	Herpes gestationis Toxemic rash of pregnancy Late-onset prurigo of pregnancy
Polymorphic eruption of pregnancy (PEP)	Pruritic urticarial papules and plaques of pregnancy (PUPPP) Toxic erythema of pregnancy Erythema multiforme of pregnancy
Prurigo of pregnancy	Prurigo gestationis of Besnier Early onset prurigo of pregnancy
Pruritic folliculitis of pregnancy	

dence is 1 in 60,000 pregnancies, arising in the second and third trimester of pregnancy with a tendency to recur in subsequent pregnancies at an earlier stage. Clinically, it is characterized by grouped lesions consisting of urticarial papules and polycyclic wheals. Eighty-seven percent of patients first develop lesions in the umbilicus. Later, the lesions spread to thighs, palms, and soles but rarely involve the face or oral mucosa. Target lesions, vesicles, and large, tense bullae subsequently develop, the clinical features of which closely resemble bullous pemphigoid.

Histologic tests show subepidermal bullae with spongiosis and a perivascular lymphohistiocytic infiltrate rich in eosinophils. Using conventional indirect immunofluorescence, only 25% of patients have circulating anti–basement membrane zone antibodies. However, using more sensitive techniques, all patients demonstrate circulating anti-IgG1 complement-binding antibodies. Using chemically split skin, the antigens that recognize these antibodies localize to the epidermal aspect of the lamina lucida.

Direct immunofluorescence of perilesional skin demonstrates linear deposition of C3 and IgG at the basement membrane zone. These C3 deposits signify the presence of an avid complement-binding IgG autoantibody directed against an antigen in epidermal basement membrane with cross-reactivity to the amniotic epithelial membrane in the placenta.

The PG antigen has been identified as a 180 kilodalton epidermal protein. Abnormal expression of MHC Class II HLA-DR3 antigens in the placentas of PG patients produces an allogenic reaction to the fetoplacental unit, triggering an autoantibody response similar to that seen in bullous pemphigoid. IgG1 autoantibodies bind complement, and tissue damage results from immune complex deposition and complement activation in the skin.

The relationship to pregnancy and oral contraceptives suggests that PG is hormonally modulated. Patients with PG are also known to have a high incidence of antibodies against their partner's HLA antigens.

Although IgG1 antibodies cross the placenta, the fetus remains relatively protected from this immunologic activity by the placenta. The placenta absorbs and deposits IgG1 onto its basement membrane, preventing IgG1 transfer into the fetal circulation. This explains the increased frequency of placental insufficiency, low birth weight, and prematurity in patients with PG, although the rate of fetal mortality is not increased. A transient vesiculobullous rash has been reported in fewer than 5% of infants born to mothers with PG, and this rash resolves rapidly within a few weeks.

Treatment

In mild cases, treatment with sedating antihistamines such as chlorpheniramine maleate, 4 mg every 6 hours, or promethazine hydrochloride (Phenergan), 10 to 20 mg every 8 hours and 25 to 50 mg at night, can be helpful, although regular long-term use is not recommended in pregnancy by the manufacturers. Furthermore, Phenergan should be avoided during the final 2 weeks of pregnancy and chlorpheniramine avoided during the third trimester because both agents can lead to irritability or sedation in the newborn. Their safety has not been fully established, and use should be restricted to cases in which the benefit outweighs any potential risk. All the newer nonsedating antihistamines, including astemizole (Hismanal), loratadine (Claritin), and terfenadine (Seldane) are contraindicated in pregnancy because no formal trials for their use have been carried out. Moderately potent topical corticosteroids such as Betnovate-C (betamethasone [Valisone] 0.1% and clioquinol [Vioform] 3%) are also effective. The use of clobetasol propionate 0.05% (Temovate) should be restricted to short-term use only, although it can be extremely effective in severe cases. As with bullous pemphigoid, systemic treatment is inevitably required and corticosteroids remain the mainstay of treatment. A dose of 20 to 40 mg of prednisone usually prevents new lesions from developing and relieves symptoms within a few days. Treatment can then be reduced fairly rapidly to a maintenance dose of 10 mg. Later, this should be increased again in anticipation of a postpartum flare, which commonly occurs. Administration of low-dose systemic steroids in the latter stages of pregnancy does not give rise to an increase in congenital abnormalities, although gestational diabetes or hypertension may develop. Fetal adrenal insufficiency can also result, but the perinatal mortality rate is not increased in PG patients treated with systemic steroids.

Plasmapheresis, although successful, has limited use owing to inconvenience and expense. Gold, methotrexate, and dapsone have produced disappointing results, and all three are contraindicated in pregnancy. Both gold and methotrexate are teratogenic, and dapsone can cause hemolytic disease of the newborn. A recent report suggests that treatment by reversible chemical oophorectomy using the luteinizing hormone–releasing hormone analogue goserelin (Zoladex) is successful in difficult or persistent cases, although its use is *contraindicated in pregnancy.* This can be a particularly useful therapy in postpartum

PG in which the rash persists for a long time. One patient with PG troubled by persistent premenstrual flares went into remission within 6 months of initiating treatment with goserelin, enabling systemic steroids to be discontinued.* The disadvantage of this treatment is that it requires a monthly subcutaneous injection into the anterior abdominal wall, at a dose of 3.6 mg every 28 days, with or without local anesthetic. Goserelin† has a reversible effect on fertility with ovarian function, which returns to normal on cessation of treatment.

POLYMORPHIC ERUPTION OF PREGNANCY

Polymorphic eruption of pregnancy (PEP, previously termed PUPPP) is the most common gestational dermatosis, with an incidence of 1 in 160 pregnancies. It may arise from damage to connective tissue within striae. Seventy-six percent of affected patients are primagravida, and the rash develops in the third trimester or the postpartum period. In contrast to PG, when PEP recurs, the second eruption is less severe than the first. There is no association with autoimmune disease or any hormonal influence, and fetal prognosis is normal.

Lesions begin on the lower abdomen with umbilical sparing, and they usually appear within striae. Urticarial papules develop that coalesce to produce plaques, vesicles, target lesions, and polycyclic wheals. Lesions are confined to abdomen, buttocks, and proximal limbs.

Histologic testing demonstrates variable features, including dermal edema, scanty eosinophils, and a perivascular lymphohistiocytic infiltrate. Direct and indirect immunofluorescence, and immunoelectron microscopy are characteristically negative.

Circulating immune complexes are reduced in the acute eruption. This has led to one theory suggesting that PEP may result from extravasation of small immune complexes through dilated upper dermal blood vessels, and the initiation of an inflammatory reaction in a perivascular distribution.

Treatment

As PEP is self-limiting and often resolves after delivery without sequelae, symptomatic treatment alone is required. Moderately potent topical corticosteroids such as fluclorolone acetonide 0.025% (Topilar)‡ or betamethasone 0.1% and fusidic acid 2% (Fucibet)‡ are more effective in relieving pruritus than antihistamines. The eruption rarely lasts longer than 6 weeks but can be severe for 1 week or so when a short course of oral prednisone, 20 to 40 mg, may be required, with gradual dosage reduction thereafter.

PRURIGO OF PREGNANCY

This condition affects one in 300 pregnancies, usually in the third trimester, and can persist for several months postpartum. The lesions are grouped, excoriated papules on the extensor surfaces of the limbs, abdomen, and shoulders. Papular dermatitis (previously described with elevated urinary human chorionic gonadotropin levels and a high fetal mortality rate) is now regarded as part of this clinical entity. Patients with prurigo of pregnancy generally have features of underlying atopy, with prurigo resulting from excoriation. The evidence of a high fetal mortality rate has now been refuted. Treatment is entirely symptomatic, with antihistamines and usage restrictions during pregnancy, as noted earlier.

PRURITIC FOLLICULITIS OF PREGNANCY

This eruption is common and thought to be a hormonally induced form of acne. The clinical appearances are of follicular erythematous papules similar to the monomorphic acne seen in patients taking corticosteroids or progestogenic steroids. Topical applications of 10% benzoyl peroxide and 1% hydrocortisone cream have proved effective in relieving symptoms.

PRURITUS ANI AND VULVAE

method of
MARILYNNE McKAY, M.D.
Emory University
Atlanta, Georgia

The most common causes of acute-onset perineal itching are candidal infection, irritant and contact dermatitis, urinary tract infection, hemorrhoids, pinworms, and condylomata. Fecal contamination of the anus can be extremely irritating, as can overcleansing; contact dermatitis may develop after application of medications such as neomycin, benzocaine, or those containing preservatives such as ethylenediamine. Cleanliness, the use of bland emollients, and treatment of infection or infestation generally resolves itching of the perineum that has been present for a few days to a few weeks.

Diagnostic tests should specifically rule out infection, and the female examination should include a vaginal smear for candida, trichomonas, and bacterial vaginosis (BV, *Gardnerella* spp). Even though BV is not typically itchy, the characteristic odor may cause patients to overcleanse or douche with irritating solutions. Culture of the vagina for candida is often helpful, and anal culture should be considered in both sexes. Risk factors for Candida infection include use of antibiotics for sinusitis, urinary tract infections, or acne; steroids or other immunosuppressants; human immunodeficiency virus (HIV) infection; and estrogen therapy (oral contraceptives, estrogen replacement). Estrogen deficiency–induced itching may be important in perimenopausal women, because dry mucosal epithelium is easily irritated. Systemic disorders associated with itching include diabetes, uremia, and hepatitis.

Evaluation of chronic perineal itching is different from that of recent onset, because the likelihood of discovering an underlying cause is significantly diminished when itching has persisted for months. In these cases, repeated episodes of itching and scratching cause local thickening of the

*Garvey MP, Handfield-Jones SE, and Black MM: Pemphigoid gestationis—response to chemical oophorectomy with goserelin. Clin Exp Derm *17*:443–445, 1992.

†Not FDA approved for this indication.

‡Not available in the United States.

skin called lichen simplex chronicus (LSC). LSC is recognized by a leathery scaly texture with accentuation of skin lines. Irritable nerve endings in LSC lesions trigger an itch-scratch-itch cycle, which typically continues long after the initial insult has resolved. LSC is secondary to rubbing and scratching and this condition must be treated separately from the usual primary causes of acute perineal itching. Lichen sclerosus is an entirely different condition that may itch or burn; this dermatosis typically presents with thin, pale, friable skin around the anus or vulva, or both.

Biopsy may be necessary to differentiate LSC from other genital dermatoses such as psoriasis, lichen planus, or lichen sclerosus, as well as to rule out malignancies such as intraepithelial neoplasia (carcinoma-in-situ) or extramammary Paget's disease. A 3- to 4-mm punch biopsy should be performed in the thickest area(s) of any lesions (plaques, scarring, thickening). Acetowhitening (application of vinegar or 3 to 5% acetic acid for 1 to 2 minutes) can be used to highlight thickened areas if there is a history of genital warts (human papillomavirus infection). If human papillomavirus infection is found on the vulva, colposcopy of the vagina and cervix is recommended; if it appears on the anus, proctoscopy. Multifocal lesions, typical of human papillomavirus–associated intraepithelial neoplasia, should be biopsied.

THERAPY

As mentioned earlier, the etiology of acute-onset perineal itching is most likely to be discovered by diagnostic testing. Therapy for infections should reduce itching within a few days, but *Candida* may be especially recalcitrant. Women with a tendency for recurrent candidiasis may need to use vaginal creams such as clotrimazole (Gyne-Lotrimin) or terconazole (Terazol) once a week for several months. One percent hydrocortisone cream is effective for relatively mild itching, especially when mixed with pramoxine (Pramosone, Zone-A Forte), a mild anesthetic.

Proper cleansing is the single most important factor in management of perineal itching. After each bowel movement or possible soiling, the patient should cleanse gently with Tucks pads, Balneol, or Cetaphil lotions, or a mild soap (Neutrogena, Purpose) followed by cool water rinses. Plain white unscented toilet tissue is recommended, but Tucks cloth pads are probably better. The patient should be advised to pat the skin gently, because rubbing can be irritating. Tight or occlusive garments should be avoided; these include plastic-backed panty shields which can contribute to maceration—perfumes in these products can be irritating as well. Use of cotton underwear and the avoidance of fabric softeners are often helpful.

There is some debate over whether spicy or caffeine-containing foods contribute to pruritus ani; probably the best course is to advise the patient to adopt a bland diet at first and then add back one or two items a week to determine whether symptoms exacerbate. Some patients already realize that certain foods worsen their problem. Food allergens are another possible factor, and a trial elimination of milk, tomatoes, corn, and nuts should be considered.

Older patients who complain of burning or stinging rather than itching (and who usually have little skin change as a result) may actually have a cutaneous dysesthesia. Low-dose tricyclic antidepressants* like amitriptyline (Elavil) or nortriptyline (Pamelor) are especially effective. Begin with 10 to 20 mg at bedtime and increase by 10 mg weekly to a dose of 30 to 50 mg. It may take 4 to 6 weeks to reach an adequate therapeutic dose. Once improvement has been maintained for a month or two, the dosage can gradually be tapered.

For lichen simplex chronicus, the mainstay is topical steroid therapy. Caution has been advised in using fluorinated topical steroid preparations in intertriginous areas; side effects include skin thinning, striae formation, rebound erythema, and burning. On the other hand, nonfluorinated Class VII preparations like hydrocortisone are unlikely to be effective in severely thickened LSC. Short-term application of a high-potency Class I steroid such as betamethasone dipropionate 0.05% (Diprolene ointment) can be extremely effective: I prescribe applications twice daily for 3 to 4 weeks, then once daily for 3 to 4 weeks. Evaluation of the patient at 6 to 8 weeks almost always reveals significant improvement, sometimes for the first time in years. At this point, the potency or frequency, or both, of application should be decreased, using only the strength necessary to control symptoms. Triamcinolone acetonide 0.1% (Kenalog, Aristocort) may be used as a short-term stepdown level to maintenance therapy with 1% hydrocortisone. Fluorinated steroids are recommended only for use in patients with LSC or severe lichen sclerosus; they are contraindicated for erythema and burning, both of which can be worsened by their use. Overuse of potent topical steroids on vulvar skin causes steroid rebound dermatitis; perianal skin is more likely to develop thinning and telangiectasia.

It often takes 3 or 4 weeks for a topical steroid to begin to affect well-established LSC, and itching typically flares from time to time during the healing process. The patient must be told that this does not mean that the medication is not working, especially if symptom-free intervals indicate that treatment is progressing satisfactorily. Patient anxiety is often a significant factor in episodic itching, and reassurance is an important part of therapy.

URTICARIA

method of
JERE D. GUIN, M.D.
University of Arkansas
Little Rock, Arkansas

Urticaria represents a complex of conditions that are characterized by whealing. Angioedema is a deeper form of swelling that may or may not be associated with hives. The approach to treatment is deter-

*Not FDA approved for this indication

mined by the form of urticaria present. Classifications vary in complexity, but the conditions affecting most patients fit into the category of acute, chronic, physical or contact urticaria, or urticarial vasculitis.

EVALUATION

Acute and chronic urticarias may or may not be associated with dermographism or angioedema, and they are distinguished by having more or less than a certain duration, usually 6 to 8 weeks. Physical urticarias are easily recognized by their location, pattern, history, and frequently, by a characteristic lesion, such as the linear whealing in dermographism, or the 3- to 5-mm wheals with a large flare seen in cholinergic urticaria. Often, these conditions can be confirmed by relatively simple tests. Contact urticaria is common, but it often goes unrecognized because it is not presented for medical treatment.

Urticarial vasculitis is a special case. It represents an immune complex vasculitis involving complement consumption. A diligent search for an underlying problem is indicated in patients with this condition (especially for hepatitis B and C, infectious mononucleosis, and rheumatologic diseases), and its treatment is very different from that of most other conditions appearing as urticaria. Lesions often persist for 1 to 3 days, leaving a discolored, scaly, or purpuric mark; frequently, the lesions burn or sting rather than itch. Other symptoms found include arthralgias, gastrointestinal complaints, fever, adenopathy, erythema multiforme–like lesions, and neuralgic disorders. Laboratory abnormalities include an elevated erythrocyte sedimentation rate and a depressed complement level in most patients and a histologic appearance of vasculitis in a high percentage of patients. The latter may be the most reliable laboratory criterion, but no one finding is absolute.

The history in acute and chronic urticaria should concentrate especially on medications being taken, and in cases of the chronic type, the physician should tactfully and empathetically look for emotional stress. One should also identify previous therapy and vasodilating influences. Treatment of chronic urticaria is both challenging and time consuming, but it should not be considered hopeless. Searches for a specific cause are indicated, although as few as 10% may be positive if one eliminates emotional causes and physical urticarias, in patients in whom the cause is obvious and the eruption is identifiable. A more aggressive approach is probably indicated for persons who are unresponsive to treatment. A history of a prior urticarial reaction to penicillin indicates the need for a trial of avoidance of dairy products, which may be contaminated with penicillin. Internal disease, parasitic infestation, malignancy, or a focus of infection may rarely be found as an underlying cause in a specific patient, but work-ups for problems should be ordered on a case-by-case basis, because extensive testing for routine screening has been shown not to be cost effective. In the author's experience, when a cause for chronic urticaria is found, it is most commonly a drug and often occurs after a totally negative history on a number of earlier occasions.

In chronic urticaria, certain dietary ingredients, although not obvious to the patient, may represent a source of aggravation. Use of a printed questionnaire in taking the history allows the patient to mark the various foods containing salicylates, benzoates, and azo dyes (especially FD&C Yellow No. 5). In patients who demonstrate an immediate skin test reaction to yeast, it may also help to look for foods containing yeast and perhaps tyramine; this can also be accomplished with the same printed form. Such dietary factors probably do not represent a source of allergy but are probably pharmacologically aggravating.

Identifying the presence (or absence) of emotional stress can also be helpful in chronic urticaria. This requires tact and empathy on the part of the physician, and it is best done personally in a quiet environment, where an unhurried and sympathetic attitude to the patient's plight demonstrates genuine care and concern for what is often an impressively stressful situation. Formal psychological testing may help prove that stress is present, but this is not usually necessary. Developing a relationship of trust and understanding is helpful in another way. Compliance with the routine required of patients with chronic urticaria is difficult at best, and the patient is much more likely to be compliant if the physician is perceived as being genuinely involved.

ACUTE URTICARIA

It is obvious that a known cause should be eliminated whenever possible. Although diet can be important as a source of allergy in acute urticaria, patients with acute urticaria due to food allergy are not often a problem because the patient generally identifies the offending food. Treatment of adults with oral cyproheptadine (Periactin), 4 mg four times daily, or hydroxyzine (Atarax), 10 to 25 mg three or four times daily, is helpful in controlling symptoms. Intramuscular or intravenous diphenhydramine (Benadryl), 50 mg, can be helpful in severe reactions. In patients in whom a known cause can be found and eliminated (as in an urticarial drug reaction), one might consider a course of oral corticosteroid therapy for those without contraindications. The initial dosage depends on the severity of the condition, but a typical course might comprise an initial dose of 30 to 40 mg of prednisone by mouth daily after breakfast, tapered over a 10- to 14-day period.

Severe laryngeal edema or other life-threatening situations may require subcutaneous or intramuscular administration of 0.3 to 0.5 mL of 1:1000 epinephrine. Intravenous use, which is limited to severe anaphylaxis with signs of shock, requires dilution to 1:10,000 concentration, administering 1 mg at a time and repeating the dosage if no response is obtained. Maintenance of the airway may require intubation or even tracheostomy, and maintaining an intravenous saline drip has been recommended for patients with severe reactions.

CHRONIC URTICARIA

Adults are typically treated with oral cyproheptadine (Periactin), 4 mg four times daily, or hydroxyzine (Atarax), 10 to 25 mg three or four times daily, or both, with drowsiness being a limiting factor. For persons who are extremely sensitive to the sedative effect or who are intolerant to anticholinergic effects of antihistamines, terfenadine (Seldane), 60 mg twice daily; astemizole (Hismanal), 10 mg daily; or loratadine (Claritin), 10 mg daily, by mouth can often be substituted. With the first two drugs, one must exclude persons with hepatic disease and those who are on treatment with macrolide antibiotics (e.g., erythromycin), ketoconazole (Nizoral), or itraconazole (Sporanox). Unresponsive patients sometimes improve with either oral doxepin (Sinequan) or amitriptyline (Elavil), 10 mg three times daily, but an effective dose may be a bit higher. These agents are much better antihistamines than most other tricyclic antidepressants; so for patients who already are taking another such medication, it may be helpful to substitute doxepin. Addition of an H_2 blocker theoretically should reduce the effect of histamine on blood vessels but may adversely affect mast cells, which form histamine and other inflammatory mediators. This may explain the conflicting reports on the effectiveness of such treatment in chronic urticaria.

The calcium channel blocker nifedipine (Procardia)* reportedly helps some resistant cases. Treatment is started with a single dose, increasing to 10 mg three times daily, avoiding H_2 blockers and monitoring for hypotension.

Elimination of vasodilating factors such as heat, exercise, and alcohol, and the avoidance of nonspecific histamine-releasing agents such as opiates are indicated. Exposure to salicylates and certain azo dyes, especially FD&C Yellow No. 5 (tartrazine), tends to aggravate the problem, especially in more severe cases and at higher levels of challenge. FD&C yellow No. 6, found in many antihistamines, can also be a problem. Diet lists of foods high in salicylate content are available, and foods and drugs that contain tartrazine must by law be labeled as containing FD&C Yellow No. 5. Patients demonstrating an immediate skin test reaction to yeast are said to be more likely to benefit from a yeast-free diet because many foods containing yeast are high in tyramine as well.

URTICARIAL VASCULITIS

Urticarial vasculitis is frequently associated with an underlying cause, including medications, hepatitis B, mononucleosis, and a variety of rheumatologic conditions. There are uncontrolled reports of benefit with oral colchicine, 0.6 mg twice daily; dapsone (Avlosulfon), 100 mg daily; indomethacin (Indocin), 75 to 200 mg daily in divided doses; or hydroxychloroquine (Plaquenil), 200 mg twice daily. The author has seen good results with colchicine. The minimum effective dose of prednisone is likely to be high, so another agent would seem preferable for initial treatment.

*Not FDA approved for this indication.

PHYSICAL URTICARIAS

Dermographism can usually be adequately controlled with low doses of cyproheptadine or hydroxyzine, along with avoidance of unnecessary trauma and vasodilating factors, especially heat. For an adult, one might start with cyproheptadine, 2 to 4 mg four times daily, or hydroxyzine, 10 mg three or four times daily by mouth, and adjust the dosage to the patient's response. In some cases, 2 to 4 mg daily of oral cyproheptadine is adequate for maintenance. Treatment is directed toward preventing the response to injury. The duration of the eruption is short, so one cannot wait until the eruption appears to treat it. Effectiveness of treatment can be measured by controlled stroking of skin of the upper back.

Some cases of cold urticaria may require a serologic test for syphilis and a test for cryoproteins to rule out symptomatic cold urticaria, but the most common cause is essential acquired cold urticaria, which can be treated in adults with avoidance of cold and the administration of oral cyproheptadine (Periactin), 4 mg four times daily. When a patient is known to have an IgE-mediated urticaria, elimination of exposure (in the case of penicillin allergy, avoidance of dairy products) is sometimes associated with clearing. Control here can be measured with change in response to a 5-minute application of an ice cube in a plastic bag.

Recommended treatment for cholinergic urticaria involves administration of oral hydroxyzine, 25 mg three times daily and avoidance of sweating. Aquagenic pruritus reportedly improves with antihistamines and doses of ultraviolet B radiation (UVB) sufficient to cause erythema, and graduated exposure to ultraviolet A radiation (UVA), UVB, and psoralen with UVA light (PUVA) plus antihistamines raises the threshold in at least some patients with solar urticaria.

Acute treatment of hereditary angioedema sometimes requires maintenance of an airway and intravascular volume. Long-term treatment is with oral anabolic steroid therapy, especially danazol (Danocrine), 200 mg twice or three times daily, tapered to 200 mg daily or alternate days according to the patient's response. An alternative drug is stanozolol (Winstrol), 2 mg three times daily initially, reduced to 2 mg daily. The maintenance dose is individualized, but there is a high incidence of flares when less than 2 mg is administered daily. About 50% of women treated with 2 mg daily have an androgenic effect; 20% will show this effect at 0.5 mg daily, a dose that is not adequate to prevent episodes in most patients. Both drugs alter menses but are not effective as contraceptives, so birth control is required in sexually active females. Patients with delayed pressure urticaria and nonhereditary angioedema associated with lymphoproliferative disease may also respond to this treatment approach, but those with acquired angioedema without lymphoproliferative disease (with antibodies to C1INH) may not respond, and corticosteroids have been recommended.

CONTACT URTICARIA

Contact urticaria may be immunologic or nonimmunologic, but treatment of the latter in most cases is not a problem, because most patients do well by avoiding the offending substance. The mediators for contact urticaria vary, and antihistamines are helpful for some agents but not others. Nonsteroidal anti-inflammatory agents benefit nonimmunologic contact urticaria from several mediators, but have less effect on nonimmunologic contact urticaria from cinnamaldehyde. Antihistamines do not markedly reduce nonimmunologic contact urticaria from these three mediators but may reduce severity of the condition from many other mediators.

Immunologic contact urticaria to latex gloves and other rubber objects has become a widespread problem in health care workers and their patients. Contact with many protein materials and certain medications can cause whealing, eczema, and even anaphylaxis requiring immediate treatment as with acute urticaria.

Contact urticaria comprises a diverse group of immediate "urticarial" reactions, and it includes reactions following exposure to certain plants and animals, such as nettles, jellyfish, and caterpillars. Pretreatment with topical corticosteroid also helps in prevention but does not totally eliminate the reaction. For most patients with contact urticaria, avoidance of the cause is the most important treatment.

PIGMENTARY DISORDERS

method of
MARVIN RAPAPORT, M.D.
University of California, Los Angeles
Los Angeles, California

HYPERPIGMENTATION

No matter what the cause of hyperpigmentation, whether it be endogenous or exogenous, the darker pigment is usually noted on the sun-exposed areas of the body. Sun exposure induces the immediate pigment darkening of the readily available melanocytes in the epidermis, also induces pigmentation at a later date, and furthermore, has been demonstrated to induce new melanocytes at distant unexposed areas. Pigmentation occurs from exposure to the sun, artificial sources of ultraviolet B (UVB) (280 to 320 nanometers) and ultraviolet A (UVA) radiation (320 to 400 nanometers), fluorescent lights, and infra-red lights.

Prolonged exposures to ultraviolet radiation lead to hyperpigmentation and severe photoaging. Furthermore, formation of keratoses, basal cell carcinomas, squamous cell carcinomas, and melanomas has been demonstrated in association with sun-induced hyperpigmentations. The skin damage and hyperpigmentation proportionately increase with humidity, altitude, and wind. Therefore, certain areas of the United States and the rest of the world carry a greater risk of sun exposure. There is some evidence that acute burns may have worrisome sequelae years later, whereas protective pigmentation produced by low-dose exposure offers some protection against tumors and aging.

Treatment

Sunscreening agents are available that protect against UVB and UVA rays. PABA, PABA-esters, benzophenone, salicylates, cinnamates, and oxybenzones are available as chemical protective agents that absorb ultraviolet light. Physical protection is afforded by the use of titanium dixoide and zinc oxide, as well as specially made clothing, fabricated by the swelling of cotton fibers. In treating any hyperpigmentation disorder, adequate sun protection is necessary. A sun protection factor (SPF) of 2 yields minimal protection, and an SPF of 15 or higher offers maximum protection. Animal studies have demonstrated that protection with sunscreens helps avoid hyperpigmentation. There are some further data that demonstrate that after damage has occurred, protection with sunscreening agents might indeed reverse some of the aging process and hyperpigmentation.

Sunscreening agents such as Sundown, Presun, Eclipse, and Supershade, as well as products from numerous cosmetic houses, offer well-tested effective protection.

Periorbital Hyperpigmentation

One very common hyperpigmentation complaint is the presence of dark circles under the eyes, or periorbital pigmentation. Its cause has been ascribed to aging, tiredness, diet, nervousness, and cosmetic usage. Biopsies have shown increased melanin formation, and it appears that this entity has a genetic basis. It is often seen in darkly pigmented individuals, especially of Mediterranean background. It can be seen in individuals as early as puberty.

Treatment

Specific therapy is not helpful, and avoidance of surgical procedures is recommended. Changes in eating or sleeping habits have not been effective. At times, the topical use of tretinoin (Retin-A)* cream, .05%, has been somewhat effective in lightening the color.

Systemic Hyperpigmentation

Table 1 lists various causes and clinical patterns associated with hyperpigmentation.

Treatment

Often, these problems are difficult to treat. However, correction of the underlying problem and cessa-

*Not FDA approved for this indication.

TABLE 1. **Causes and Clinical Patterns of Systemic Hyperpigmentation**

Cause	Pattern
Drugs	
Antimalarials	Photodistribution
Amiodarone (Cordarone)	Photodistribution
Minocycline (Minocin)	Extremities and acne scars
Phenothiazines	Photodistribution
Zidovudine (Retrovir)	Nail bed
Bleomycin (Blenoxane)	Trunk
Cyclophosphamide (Cytoxan)	Photodistribution
Metals	
Mercury	Generalized
Gold	Photodistribution
Silver	Photodistribution and mucosa
Metabolic/Endocrine Disorders	
Pellagra	Photodistribution
Addison's disease	Generalized
Acanthosis nigricans	Neck, axilla, groin
Scleroderma	Extremities

tion of the causative drug or chemical helps alleviate the pigment disorder.

Melasma (Chloasma)

Melasma is an acquired form of hyperpigmentation seen as a mottled pattern over the bridge of the nose, the cheeks, the upper lip, and the forehead. Pregnancy, oral contraceptives, and heredity are among the etiologies of this endogenous or exogenous, estrogen- or progesterone-induced entity.

Treatment

The best chance for resolution of this disorder is the cessation of oral contraceptives, and continual usage of sunscreening agents and the depigmenting preparations. Dermabrasion, liquid nitrogen, and face peels are to be avoided. The sunscreening agents protecting against the UVA range offer the best protection.

Depigmenting creams with hydroquinone (2 to 4%) are the most commonly used agents. Eldoquin, Melanex, and Eldoquin Forte are good products. A preparation containing hydroquinone (1 to 3%), retinoic acid (0.01 to 0.1%), and triamcinolone cream (0.025%) has been used for the past 20 years with fairly good results. Most recently, the alphahydroxy acids, namely glycolic acid and pyruvic acid, have been applied daily to the face. Also, as a peeling agent at a 70% concentration, glycolic acid is used in a series of 6 to 10 treatments.

Hyperpigmentation Streaks

Pigmentary demarcation lines are seen in individuals of pigmented races. The most frequent lines run along the upper extremities and as transpectoral extensions. Dorsal skin is more deeply pigmented than ventral skin.

Pigmented streaks also are seen coursing down nails from the base to the tip of the nail. These also are invariably seen in pigmented peoples, and they are normal and benign. When a new band appears along one nail in lighter skinned individuals, there is always a suspicion of melanoma at the base of the nail. Postinflammatory streaks and patches can occur after contact dermatitis, phytophotodermatitis, lichen planus, eczema, and psoriasis.

Treatment

Biopsy of suspicious nail lesions is indicated.

Lentigines

Lentigines, or liver spots, typically appear on the dorsum of the hands and on the cheeks often years after youthful sun exposures. They are worrisome to the patient because of concerns about the presence of tumor. They are invariably sun induced and remain benign, but on a rare occasion, a malignant transformation can occur to form a lentigo maligna melanoma.

Treatment

The hydroquinone creams have used with only limited success. Superficial and minimal spraying of liquid nitrogen can help peel this pigmented process. Also, light swabbing with various acids, such as trichloroacetic acid (20 to 35%),* may also be effective. Care should be used to avoid scarring.

Carotenoderma

The ingestion of large amounts of yellow vegetables such as carrots can cause a yellow staining of the skin, or carotenoderma. The ingestion of beta carotene and canthaxanthin also can give this jaundice-like look to the skin (sclera is normal here). It has been suggested that the carotenoids protect against sun exposure, and they have been used for treatment of erythropoietic protoporphyria.

Some tanning preparations capitalize on the staining ability of certain chemicals to give a yellowish-orange "tan" to the skin when applied externally. These chemicals, usually hydroxyacetones, are shed in the keratin layer.

Treatment

No treatment is necessary, because the stain fades when ingestion of the offending food or agent stops.

HYPOPIGMENTATION

Commonly, hypopigmentation, or leukoderma, occurs as the aftermath of a prior inflammatory process affecting the skin. Usually, with time, the color returns, although in darkly pigmented individuals, this might not always occur.

Vitiligo

Vitiligo is an idiopathic, acquired, loss of pigmentation of the skin that affects about 1% of the popu-

*Not FDA approved for this indication.

lation. Often, there is a familial pattern, with 10% of the cases having a family member affected by the disease. On rare occasions, it has been associated with autoimmune and endocrine disorders such as pernicious anemia, alopecia areata, hyperthryoidism, hypothyroidism, and myasthenia gravis. Industrial exposure to certain agents such as phenols, quinones, and thiols can cause depigmentation. These chemicals act by killing the melanocytes, resulting in permanent depigmentation.

Treatment

The easiest and least problematic therapy is cosmetic. Numerous preparations such as Covermark, Walnut Stain, and Vita Dye serve a useful purpose in camouflaging the disfiguring depigmentation, especially when it occurs on the face and hands.

Sometimes improvement occurs with the usage of high-potency topical corticosteroids. Clobetasol propionate (Temovate)* and diflorasone diacetate (Psorcon)* creams have been used on a twice-daily basis. The best results appear to occur in facial lesions of Asian and black patients. Long-term usage of steroids should be avoided. Autografts have been used in small areas of leukoderma and vitiligo, and have provided pigment spreading.

When the problem is more widespread, psoralens and UV radiation are used. When smaller areas are involved, topical psoralen therapy may be useful, but great care must be exercised to avoid excessive exposure to the sun or too much ultraviolet A radiation. A 1% solution of 8-methoxypsoralen is diluted with 50% ethanol, giving a final concentration of 0.1%. It is painted on the vitiliginous areas between 1 and 2 hours before sunlight or UVA exposure. Cautious exposure of 30 seconds to 1 minute of noon sunlight, with 30-second increases on a daily basis, is the best way to start. If artificial UVA is available, then 0.1 to 0.3 joule per cm^2 should be the initiating dose. Slow incremental increases three times a week might be needed for up to 4 to 6 months.

Larger areas of vitiligo require the use of systemic psoralen therapy, 0.5 mg per kg, ingested 2 hours before light therapy. This combination of psoralens and UVA is called PUVA. It is best to use artificial ultraviolet A rather than sunlight. Care must be taken to protect the eyes for the entire day when therapy is given. Prior to initiating the treatment, an antinuclear antibody test and an eye examination should be performed. Those patients who are pregnant, have photosensitive dermatoses, or have histories of skin cancers or cataracts should not be treated with this method.

Repigmentation is usually apparent after 3 months of therapy. If no response is evident after 20 treatments, then the oral psoralen therapy should be discontinued. Total body depigmentation is a final alternative in order to obtain even coloration. Monobenzone (Benoquin) is applied for 3 days. If no irritation occurs, then the patient can reapply the medication on a twice-daily basis. Depigmentation usually begins after several weeks. Folic acid,* 2 mg twice a day; vitamin C,* 500 mg twice a day; and vitamin B_{12},* 1 mL or 100 mg intramuscularly every 2 weeks have been demonstrated to repigment patients with vitiligo. Further studies are needed to corroborate this treatment.

*Not FDA approved for this indication.

IDIOPATHIC GUTTATE HYPOMELANOSIS

Idiopathic guttate hypomelanosis is an acquired leukoderma characterized by multiple well-circumscribed macules usually measuring 2 to 8 mm in diameter. The lesions are off white, tend to increase with age, and are found on the extensor surfaces of the arms and legs. It is believed that sunlight is a causative factor. Interlesional steriods—e.g., triamcinolone (Kenalog,* 3 mg, per 1 mL)—have been injected, and some repigmentation has been noted. In addition, lightly touching the lesions with liquid nitrogen has also met with some success in repigmentation.

TINEA VERSICOLOR

Tinea versicolor is a superficial fungus infection that commonly occurs on the chest, back, and upper arms in younger individuals. A potassium hydroxide mount shows typical hyphae and spores of *Malassezia furfur.* Often, individuals with eczema have similar leukodermic areas on their upper arms, but these areas have indistinct borders and should be differentiated from this fungus infection.

Treatment

Tinea versicolor responds to selenium sulfide (Selsun) shampoo applied for 30 minutes on five consecutive nights. If the area is not extensive, then topical antifungal agents such as clotrimazole (Lotrimin, Mycelex), ciclopirox (Loprox), and econazole (Spectazole) are very effective. These preparations should be applied twice daily for at least 3 to 4 weeks. Tinver, a sodium thiosulfate preparation, can be applied on a once-a-day basis for about a month. Recently, it has been demonstrated that ketoconazole (Nizoral),* 200 mg daily for 3 days, can also suppress this disease process. Care should also be taken to evaluate liver function if it is known that therapy will be prolonged.

OCCUPATIONAL DERMATOSES

method of
JAMES S. TAYLOR, M.D.
Cleveland Clinic Foundation
Cleveland, Ohio

Occupational skin disorders are the second most common cause of all reported work illnesses, despite

*Not FDA approved for this indication.

the fact that they are almost fully preventable. No industry, whatever its size, scope, or location, is immune to their occurrence. Occupational skin diseases are produced from old chemicals in processes both old and new, new chemicals in new processes, and a wide variety of biologic, mechanical, and physical agents. The major categories of work-related skin disorders are contact dermatitis (allergic, irritant, and photosensitivity), acne and follicular eruptions, and pigmentary abnormalities. Accurate diagnosis is imperative in patients with putative occupational skin disorders. Diagnostic procedures in addition to history and physical examination include skin scrapings for fungi, viruses, parasites, and fiberglass; cultures for microorganisms; skin biopsy; and tests for allergy (patch, photopatch, or prick). Physicians treating these conditions should have some knowledge of their individual state's workers' compensation regulations.

CONTACT DERMATITIS

In this category are most occupational dermatoses. They may be caused by a number of the hundreds of thousands of chemicals used in industry. About 80% of cases of contact dermatitis are produced by irritants, 20% from allergens, and a small percentage, which are often overlooked, from photosensitivity. Most affected are the hands, but any part of the body may be involved. High-risk occupations include those dealing with wet work and chemical exposure, such as food processing, homemaking, cosmetology, health care, metal working, and chemical manufacturing.

Treatment of Acute Contact Dermatitis

1. Avoid contact with the offending agent. This may require several days away from work or temporary transfer to another job.
2. Avoid contact with potential aggravating factors such as excessive soap and water, alcohol, thimerosal, and sensitizers, such as topically applied antihistamines, antibiotics (neomycin or nitrofurazone), and anesthetics ("caine" preparations). Other contributing factors to be avoided are heat, friction, and radiant energy.
3. Apply cool, wet compresses to weeping and blistered areas for 15 minutes, two to three times daily. Isotonic saline solution may be used. With commercial preparations of Burow's solution (Bluboro powder or Domeboro powder or tablets), 1 packet or tablet per 500 mL (pint) of water makes approximately a 1:40 dilution. Make certain the mixture is completely dissolved before it is applied. A soft cloth such as Kerlix gauze; an old, clean thin white handkerchief; or a towel is immersed in the solution. The cloth is wrung slightly and applied to the affected area of the skin. When the cloth begins to dry, remove it completely and resoak it in the solution before reapplying. Do not pour the solution directly on the dressing; a fresh solution should be prepared before each treatment.

   As an alternative, the patient may soak the affected part, such as a hand or a foot, directly in the solution for the same period of time.

   For severe, generalized involvement, especially with secondary infection, hospitalization may be necessary. Compresses may be applied to all affected areas of the body, and in some cases, baths with use of an agent such as with Aveeno Oilated Bath may be preferable.

   Treatment should be continued for no more than a few days (usually 3 to 4) to avoid excessive drying of the skin.
4. Immediately following the compresses, soaks, or baths, apply a topical corticosteroid spray (triamcinolone acetonide [Kenalog] spray or betamethasone diproprionate [Diprosone] aerosol). A 2- or 3-second spray to each affected area is sufficient with the container held at a distance of 6 inches from the skin. One of the many topical corticosteroid creams such as betamethasone valerate (Valisone), triamcinolone (Kenalog), or fluocinolone acetonide (Synalar) may be used when the acute dermatitis is not extensively vesicular. Avoid ointments in the acute stages.
5. Do not apply fluorinated topical corticosteroids to the face for more than 2 weeks; prolonged use may produce severe steroid rosacea.
6. Oral antihistamines such as cyproheptadine (Periactin), hydroxyzine (Atarax), or diphenhydramine (Benadryl) help relieve itching. It is imperative that workers be warned not to drive or operate dangerous machinery while taking these antihistamines.
7. Systemic use of corticosteroids is indicated in patients with severe, localized dermatitis, such as a vesiculobullous eruption of the hands or feet, or with severe, generalized dermatitis. An injection of 1 mL of triamcinolone acetonide suspension (Kenalog-40 injection) may be given, or oral corticosteroids such as prednisone (Deltasone), 30 to 60 mg daily in two or three divided doses, is begun initially and tapered over 10 to 30 days.

Treatment of Subacute and Chronic Contact Dermatitis

1. Avoid the same elements as outlined in items 1, 2, and 5 in the previous section.
2. Do not use compresses or soak.
3. Use a topical corticosteroid cream or ointment two to three times daily and continue treatment for 2 to 3 weeks after the skin appears normal.
4. Administer oral antihistamines as in item 6 in the previous section.
5. The author wishes to emphasize that frequently recurring cases of acute contact dermatitis should be considered chronic, and frequent use (more than once every 3 months) of short courses of systemic corticosteroids should be avoided. In these patients, a tireless search for precipitating and aggravating factors is necessary (see Ancillary Measures later).

Treatment of Secondarily Infected Contact Dermatitis

In the author's experience, this is a rare condition. A low-grade bacterial infection such as that from a coagulase-positive *Staphylococcus* may occur. In patients with this condition, compresses or soaks with povidone-iodine (Betadine solution) are helpful. Bacterial cultures should be made, and antibiotic therapy such as erythromycin stearate (Erythrocin), 250 mg three to four times daily for 10 days, is initiated. As the infection resolves, topical corticosteroid therapy may be reinstituted. Acute cellulitis with accompanying chills, fever, and lymphangitis requires more aggressive and closely supervised antibiotic therapy; hospitalization may be necessary.

ANCILLARY MEASURES FOR DIAGNOSIS AND TREATMENT

Resources to Identify Causative Agent(s)

It is imperative that the causative agent(s) be identified in every patient. Unless this is accomplished, treatment may be doomed to failure and the patient will experience recurrences of the dermatosis. A careful job description and work history should be obtained to determine all the patient's past and present industrial contacts. Inquiry into exposures from second jobs, hobbies, and household contacts is essential, as is the presence of predisposing factors such as atopy, prior skin disease or use of harsh cleansers or solvents to clean the skin. In this regard, the author has found it most helpful to consult standard texts on occupational and contact dermatitis. In addition, two other resources are helpful:

1. Division of Technical Services, National Institute for Occupational Safety and Health, United States Public Health Service, 4676 Columbia Parkway, Cincinnati, Ohio, 45226, AC, 800-356-4674.
2. The patient's employer (with the consent of the patient), such as the plant manager, the industrial research department, the plant physician, the nurse, the safety officer, the industrial hygienist, the toxicologist, or the personnel manager.

Together, these resources may provide lists of chemicals contacted in various occupations (material safety data sheets should be requested), information on cutaneous and systemic toxicity of chemicals, suggested patch-testing concentrations, and information on sources of products and processes containing a particular chemical. Knowledge of chemicals used is extremely important, because a worker may be exposed to the same chemical at home and at work (e.g., rubber, metal, chromates, dyes, plastic resins), or at several sources at work.

Diagnostic Patch Testing

Patch testing, when properly performed and correctly interpreted, is unquestionably of great value in identifying the causative agent(s) of allergic contact dermatitis. Initial testing is usually conducted with the most frequent contact allergens (nickel, chromates, rubber, medicaments, preservatives, dyes, and resins). Other materials, found at home or work may also have to be tested *in appropriate concentrations* to distinguish occupational and nonoccupational factors. Patch testing should be employed only by physicians experienced with this technique. Pre-employment patch testing generally should be avoided. The same recommendations and precautions apply to photopatch testing, which is used to diagnose photoallergic contact dermatitis.

Preventive Measures

It is impossible to separate treatment from prevention. Personal protective measures such as gloves, masks, and clothing may be required when they can be worn safely. Barrier or protective creams should be used only as a last resort and should not be applied to inflamed skin. Environmental controls such as good housekeeping, local exhaust ventilation, process isolation, engineering controls, and removal of physical and chemical hazards are the most important preventive measures.

FIBERGLASS DERMATITIS

This special form of pruritic papular, eczematous, and occasionally, purpuric dermatitis is produced by mechanical irritation from glass fibers. Body folds and areas of tight-fitting clothing are common sites of involvement. Hardening usually occurs after several weeks of exposure.

Treatment

1. Limit further exposure to fiberglass by environmental control.
2. Wear loose-fitting clothing, which is changed daily.
3. Clean skin frequently.
4. Use topical corticosteroid creams (see Contact Dermatitis earlier).
5. Lightly apply a thin coating of talcum powder.
6. Workers with dermographism or urticaria should not work with fiberglass.

OIL ACNE

Today most cutting fluids are synthetic or semisynthetic types that typically cause contact dematitis (for treatment, see Contact Dermatitis in this section). However, exposure to insoluble, straight cutting fluids may produce folliculitis (so-called oil boils) in areas uncommon for acne vulgaris, usually the extremities.

Treatment

1. Avoid contact with oils and grease.
2. Daily changes of work clothing.
3. Cleanse the skin frequently with soap and water.
4. Avoid cleansing the skin with fabric waste, which is intended only for cleaning machines and tools.

5. Use local acne medications (benzoyl peroxide 5% gel [Panoxyl 5] or tretinoin cream 0.025% to 0.1% [Retin-A]).
6. Bacterial culture and appropriate oral antibiotics (e.g., tetracycline, 250 mg four times daily, or minocycline, 100 mg two times daily) are indicated in severe cases.

CHLORACNE

This extremely refractory form of industrial acne is produced by exposure to various polyhalogenated aromatic compounds, such as naphthalenes, biphenyls, dibenzofurans, and phenol and aniline herbicide intermediates.

Treatment

1. Chemical exposure should be absolutely avoided through a totally enclosed manufacturing process.
2. Possible systemic toxicity should be appraised, including liver, kidney, neurologic, and porphyrin studies.
3. Work clothing should be laundered at work.
4. Double locker rooms (clean and dirty) with adequate shower facilities should be provided.
5. Barrier creams should not be used.
6. Optimal control is obtained by preventing formation of the toxic chloracnegen by altering the chemical synthesis pathway.
7. Isotretinoin (Accutane), 0.5 to 1 mg/kg/day, may be indicated in severe cases for a course of up to 20 weeks. This drug should be administered only by those experienced in its use and in strict accordance with current prescribing instructions. It is a potent teratogen with other potentially significant side effects.

PIGMENTATION DISORDERS

Staining

A number of chemicals stain the skin by direct external contact. The stain usually responds to attempts at cleansing, avoidance of chemical exposure, and the passage of time.

Hyperpigmentation

Exposure to tar, pitch, and chemicals such as psoralens in combination with ultraviolet light may produce increased pigmentation of the skin. Protective clothing and sunscreens may be helpful. Hydroquinone (Eldopaque-Forte), applied twice daily for up to 3 months, may reduce the pigmentation. In resistant cases, tretinoin cream 0.025% (Retin-A), initially applied once every 3 days, increasing to once daily as tolerated for up to 3 months, may help.

Hypopigmentation

Exposure to paratertiary butyl phenol or catechol, or paratertiary amyl phenol (found in some germicidal disinfectants, oils, plastics, paints, or resins) and certain other chemicals may produce occupational leukoderma. Treatment involves avoiding chemical exposure and using dihydroxyacetone containing stains for the skin (Vitadye, Dy-O-Derm). Photochemotherapy with oral psoralen (8-methoxypsoralen [Oxsoralen-Ultra]) and psoralen plus ultraviolet A (PUVA) may occasionally be effective in the treatment of this form of leukoderma.

OTHER OCCUPATIONAL DERMATOSES

Microbial infections (sporotrichosis), granulomatous reactions (foreign bodies), ulcerations (chrome), neoplasms (tar, pitch), and repeated mechanical trauma (calluses, blisters, and vibration white finger) may occasionally occur. In addition, patients with tight-building syndrome and alleged multiple chemical sensitivity syndrome may present with nonspecific skin complaints that are difficult to evaluate. There is a wide spectrum of other occupational dermatoses, and therapy depends on their cause. The hallmarks for the successful treatment of occupational dermatoses are identifying the causative agent(s), prescribing therapy early, and preventing further exposure.

SUNBURN AND OTHER DERMATOSES INDUCED BY SUNLIGHT

method of
HENRY W. LIM, M.D.
New York Veterans Affairs Medical Center
New York University School of Medicine
New York, New York

Electromagnetic radiation emitted by the sun is classified according to its wavelength (Table 1). Ultraviolet (UV) C radiation is absorbed in the atmosphere and does not reach the surface of the earth; it is present only in artificial light sources used primarily as germicidal lamps. By far the most common side effects of sun exposure are from acute and chronic exposure to UVB; these range from sunburn to skin cancers to induction of photodermatoses (Table 2). It is clear that atmospheric ozone depletion further increases the intensity of UVB on the surface of the earth. UVA may potentiate the photocarcinogenic effect of UVB and is responsible for the development of photoallergy and phototoxicity. In addition, UV and visible light may induce the development of idiopathic photodermatoses (e.g., polymorphous light eruption, solar urticaria, chronic actinic dermatitis) and may exacerbate other conditions, such as lupus erythematosus.

SUNBURN

Sunburn results from acute exposure to UVB, and to a lesser extent, to the shorter wavelength UVA

TABLE 1. **Classification of Electromagnetic Radiation From the Sun**

Type	Wavelength Range (nm)	Major Biologic Effects
UVC	200–290	Germicidal
UVB	290–320	Sunburn, skin cancers, photodermatoses
UVA II	320–340	Photodermatoses; potentiates effects of UVB
UVA I	340–400	Photodermatoses
Visible	400–760	Illumination

(e.g., UVA II). It consists of immediate darkening of pigment on exposed sites, which occurs during and immediately after exposure; this is followed by erythema and edema, peaking at 24 hours. It resolves with tanning and desquamation. In severe cases, blisters and erosions may develop.

Treatment

Sunburn with mild to moderate erythema, edema, and tenderness should be treated with cool water compresses (10 minutes three times daily), and topical corticosteroids (hydrocortisone cream 1% [Hytone] twice daily to face and intertriginous areas, triamcinolone acetonide cream 0.1% [Kenalog] twice daily to body) to reduce the inflammation. Because prostaglandins have been implicated as one of the mediators of UVB-induced erythema, aspirin or one of the nonsteroidal anti-inflammatory agents is the preferred analgesic agent; administration should be started as soon as possible to obtain the full therapeutic effect.

Should blisters develop, blister fluid should be drained without removing the blister roof. Blisters and erosions should be treated with compresses soaked in normal saline or Burow's solution (Domeboro, Bluboro), followed by a topical antibiotic such as polymyxin-bacitracin ointment (Polysporin), or silver sulfadiazine cream 1% (Silvadene) twice daily. Systemic corticosteroids (prednisone, 40 to 60 mg per day, tapered over a 5- to 10-day period) should be reserved only for the most severe cases.

TABLE 2. **Dermatoses Induced by Sunlight**

Dermatosis	Etiology
Sunburn	Acute UVB
Photoaging, actinic keratoses, skin cancers	Chronic UV
Photoallergy	Photoallergens + UVA
Phototoxicity	Phototoxic agents + UVA
Polymorphous light eruption	Idiopathic; UVB, UVA, visible light
Solar urticaria	Idiopathic; UVB, UVA, visible light
Chronic actinic dermatitis	Idiopathic; UVB, UVA, visible light
Porphyrias	Porphyrins + 400–410 nm light
Lupus erythematosus (photoexacerbation)	Autoimmune; UVB, UVA

The following measures should be taken to minimize the acute as well as the chronic (see later) effects of sunlight. Sun exposure between the hours of 10 A.M. and 2 P.M. should be avoided, because this is the time when the irradiance is most intense. Protective clothing, including hats, should be worn. For those individuals with exquisite photosensitivity, clothing is available that is manufactured using specifically designed materials that minimize the transmission of sunlight. Individuals with fair skin who always burn and never tan should use sunscreens with a sun protective factor (SPF) of 15 or above, whereas those who are able and have the desire to tan may use sunscreens of lower SPF. Because UVA may potentiate the deleterious effects of UVB, broad-spectrum sunscreens that protect against UVA and UVB are recommended. These broad-spectrum sunscreens contain benzophenones, avobenzone (Parsol 1789), and micronized titanium dioxide. Repeated applications of a sunscreen are necessary following contact with water. It should be emphasized that sunburn occurs not only from direct sunlight but also from sunlight reflected from surfaces such as snow, sand, and water.

PHOTOAGING, ACTINIC KERATOSES, AND SKIN CANCERS

These conditions are the result of chronic exposure to the sun.

Photoaging

Photoaging is dryness and wrinkling on sun-exposed areas. Topical tretinoin (Retin-A) cream is now used to improve the fine, but not the coarse, wrinkling associated with photoaging. The therapy is initiated by using the 0.025% tretinoin cream once every other night or once a night; the concentration is increased every few months, the limitation being the development of tretinoin-induced cutaneous irritation. In patients who can tolerate it, a maximal concentration of 0.1% may be reached. Patients with photoaging should be educated on sun avoidance and the use of sunscreens to prevent further photodamage.

Actinic Keratoses

Actinic keratoses are rough, skin-colored to erythematous flat spots on sun-exposed areas such as the forehead, nose, and dorsum of hands. They are asymptomatic and are usually multiple. They are considered precancerous and can rarely evolve into squamous cell carcinoma. Cryotherapy and electrodesiccation are two very effective therapeutic modalities. In patients with numerous lesions, these modalities may be combined with topical application of 1% or 5% 5-fluorouracil cream or solution (Fluoroplex or Efudex, twice daily for 2 to 3 weeks). Patients should be warned that treated areas will be inflamed and tender. This reaction usually occurs within 1 week of the initiation of therapy, and it may take 2 weeks following the completion of therapy to resolve. Triamcinolone cream 0.1% (Kenalog) may be used twice a day concurrently with 5-fluorouracil to minimize the inflammation.

Skin Cancers

Squamous cell carcinoma, basal cell carcinoma, and melanoma are associated with chronic sun exposure. They are discussed in detail elsewhere in this textbook.

PHOTOALLERGY AND PHOTOTOXICITY

The clinical manifestations of photoallergy and phototoxicity are erythema, blisters, erosions, hyperpigmentation, and thickening of the skin in sun-exposed areas. Photoallergy is a type of a delayed hypersensitivity reaction in which the combined presence of photoallergens and UV light is required for the sensitization and elicitation. It occurs only in sensitized individuals. Sunscreen ingredients and fragrances are some of the most common photoallergens (Table 3). In contrast, phototoxicity can be elicited in all individuals exposed to adequate doses of phototoxic agents and appropriate radiation. Medications lead the list of the most common exogenous phototoxic agents (Table 4).

Avoidance of the offending photosensitizers and of sun exposure are essential in the management of photoallergy and phototoxicity. The action spectrum of these two disorders is in the UVA range. Because para-aminobenzoic acid (PABA) is a poor UVA sunscreen, broad-spectrum sunscreens are recommended for these patients. Otherwise, treatment is identical to that outlined above for sunburn.

POLYMORPHOUS LIGHT ERUPTION

This is the most common idiopathic photodermatosis, occurring in 10 to 20% of healthy individuals. Patients present with erythematous macules or urticarial papules that appear within hours to days of sun exposure. Treatment modalities include sun avoidance; sunscreens; hydroxychloroquine (Plaquenil), 200 to 400 mg daily during spring and summer months; UVB phototherapy; or 8-methoxypsoralen plus UVA (PUVA).

TABLE 3. **Common Photoallergens**

Property	Photoallergen
Antibacterial agents	Halogenated salicylanilides
Fragrance	Musk ambrette
Psychotropic medications	Phenothiazines
Sunscreens	Benzophenones Cinnamates p-Aminobenzoic acid (PABA) PABA esters (Padimate O, Padimate A)

TABLE 4. **Common Phototoxic Agents**

Property	Phototoxic Agent
Antibacterials	Ciprofloxacin Nalidixic acid Tetracyclines
Antihistamine	Diphenhydramine
Antimalarials	Chloroquine Quinine
Antimitotics	5-Fluorouracil Vinblastine
Antipsoriatics	Psoralens Tar
Cardiac medications	Amiodarone Nifedipine Quinidine
Diuretics	Furosemide Thiazides
Dyes	Eosin Methylene blue Rose bengal
Hypoglycemics	Tolbutamide Chlorpropamide
Nonsteroidals	Ketoprofen Naproxen Piroxicam
Psychotropics	Chlorpromazine Desipramine Imipramine

SOLAR URTICARIA

Patients with this condition present with urticaria following sun exposure. The action spectrum can be in the UVB, UVA, or visible range. The cause is unknown. In addition to avoidance of the sun, other treatment modalities include antihistamines, desensitization by repeated exposure to UV of the appropriate wavelengths, and PUVA.

CHRONIC ACTINIC DERMATITIS

This idiopathic photodermatosis occurs most commonly in elderly men, appearing as chronic photosensitivity to a broad-spectrum radiation. As a result, patients present with erythema to markedly thickened skin on sun-exposed areas. Association with HIV infection has been reported. Aside from photoprotection, treatment modalities include psoralen and UVA (PUVA) photochemotherapy, azathioprine (Imuran, 50 to 150 mg per day), hydroxychloroquine sulfate (Plaquenil, 200 to 400 mg per day), and for recalcitrant cases, cyclosporine (Sandimmune, 3 to 5 mg per kg per day).

PORPHYRIAS

Porphyrias are examples of phototoxicity induced by endogenous phototoxic agents. Because of enzymatic defects in the heme biosynthetic pathway, patients with porphyrias have elevated levels of porphyrins in their plasma, erythrocytes, urine, and feces. The most common type of porphyria is porphyria cutanea tarda, associated with a deficiency in uroporphyrinogen decarboxylase. Patients present with skin fragility, blisters, and erosion on sun-exposed areas, especially the dorsum of the hands. These patients may also have sclerodermoid skin changes, as well as periorbital mottled hyperpigmentation and hypertrichosis. Association of porphyria cutanea tarda with human immunodeficiency virus (HIV) infection is now well recognized. Treatment modalities include repeated phlebotomies or low-dose hydroxychloroquine (Plaquenil), 200 mg twice weekly. There are several other less common types of porphyrias. A good screening method is the determination of plasma and erythrocyte porphyrin levels, which is available commercially. Because the action spectrum in porphyrias is in the range of 400 to 410 nm (Soret band), only physical blockers (clothing or sunblocks containing titanium dioxide or zinc oxide) can afford adequate photoprotection for these patients.

LUPUS ERYTHEMATOSUS

Sun exposure frequently exacerbates the cutaneous manifestations of lupus erythematosus, consisting of erythema, edema, and fine scaling on exposed areas. Frequently, discoid lesions (atrophic patches with hyperpigmentation and hypopigmentation, telangiectasia, follicular plugging, and fine scales) also appear on sun-exposed areas. The action spectrum is in the UVB and UVA range. Treatment of cutaneous manifestations of lupus erythematosus consists of sunscreens, as well as topical and intralesional corticosteroids. In severe cases, systemic corticosteroids (Prednisone, 20 to 60 mg daily), or antimalarials (hydroxychloroquine [Plaquenil], 200 to 400 mg daily) may be used.

Section 13

The Nervous System

BRAIN ABSCESS

method of
GLENN E. MATHISEN, M.D.
UCLA School of Medicine
Los Angeles County-Olive View Medical Center
Los Angeles, California

A brain abscess is a focal, suppurative intracerebral infection the diagnosis and management of which continues to remain a challenge. Although modern diagnostic strategies have considerably improved the outlook for patients with this condition, the morbidity and expense associated with the condition remain considerable. The increasing numbers of immunocompromised individuals have served to alter the epidemiology and clinical presentation of the condition; patients may have infection with exotic organisms (e.g., fungi) that were once uncommon.

The pathology of brain abscess represents a continuum from very early brain infection, with localized cerebral inflammation (cerebritis), to the full-blown brain abscess—a focal collection of pus surrounded by a connective tissue capsule. Brain abscesses may be classified by the route of entry of the pathogen into the brain substance; such a classification helps predict the likely location and microbiology of the abscess (Table 1). Brain abscess is frequently secondary to focal cranial infection (otitis, mastoiditis, dental abscess, paranasal sinusitis) through subsequent seeding of the brain substance via venous channels. Intracerebral abscess secondary to metastatic spread from a distant focus is another important route of infection; bacteremia from an extracranial source (e.g., lung abscess, intra-abdominal abscess) may lodge in the brain substance itself. Direct inoculation of an organism into cerebral tissue may occur during neurosurgical cases or following penetrating cranial trauma. Finally, it should be recognized that 10% to 30% of cerebral abscesses have no obvious source; a previously healthy individual may present with a brain abscess, and thorough investigation of the case reveals no predisposing factors.

CLINICAL PRESENTATION AND DIAGNOSIS

The symptoms and clinical presentation of brain abscess are influenced by a number of factors, including location, size, virulence of infecting organism, and underlying systemic conditions. Headache is the most common symptom and is present in over 90% of patients who are able to give an accurate history. Other signs of more serious central nervous system disease, such as drowsiness, stupor, and obtundation, may also be seen; rapid diagnosis and definitive therapy are especially important in these cases because they suggest elevated intracranial pressure, which may lead to cerebral herniation. Other neurologic symptoms depend on the location of the abscess; they may be relatively subtle and detected only on careful neurologic examination. A common misconception is the frequency of fever in patients with brain abscess; fever may be seen in only 50% of patients; focal neurologic findings (hemiparesis, hemisensory deficits, aphasia, ataxia) often overshadow signs of infection. Papilledema is seen in up to 25% of cases; its absence does not rule serious intracranial hypertension. Clinical differentiation of brain abscesses from meningitis may be difficult. In general, meningitis has a much more acute onset (within 24 hours), whereas brain abscess may have a more subacute or chronic evolution. Recognition of a focal cranial inflammatory process (dental abscess, chronic otitis media, sinusitis) should be carefully sought and may uncover the source of a serious intracranial infection. Laboratory findings in patients with brain abscess tend to be nonspecific. Although leukocytosis is commonly seen, it rarely exceeds 20,000 cells per mm^3 and the peripheral leukocyte count is often normal. Performance of a lumbar puncture in a patient with a brain abscess rarely gives any useful information and is contraindicated in patients with significant mass lesions owing to the risk of intracerebral herniation. Cerebrospinal fluid (CSF) findings are nonspecific and tend to show a CSF pleocytosis, elevated total protein, and a normal CSF glucose. CSF cultures are usually negative and generally of little help in identifying the underlying microbial pathogen in a patient with a cerebral abscess.

The availability of computed tomography (CT) scanning has revolutionized the diagnosis and management of brain abscess; all patients with suspected brain abscess should undergo CT or magnetic resonance imaging (MRI) scanning. The use of intravenous iodinated contrast material is helpful and may allow detection of areas of cerebritis not visualized with a noncontrast scan. Focal cerebritis or early brain abscess generally shows a focal, contrast-enhancing lesion on CT scan; more advanced lesions show the classic ring-enhancing lesion found in the relatively mature abscess. The greater sensitivity of MRI scanning may allow earlier detection of areas of cerebritis; however, it is not clear that this technology offers a clear advantage over CT scanning in the diagnosis and management of intracerebral abscess.

CLINICAL MANAGEMENT

The clinical management of brain abscess involves a team approach, which requires collaboration between the internist, neurologist, and neurosurgeon. Although rare cases may be managed with antibiotics alone, most patients require surgical intervention at some stage of the infection, and neurosurgery consultation should be obtained as early as possible. Antimicrobial therapy should be started promptly with an empiric regimen based on the likely source of the infection (see Table 1). Attempts to define the microbiology of the abscess (e.g., needle aspiration) are important but should not delay institution of antimicro-

TABLE 1. **Brain Abscess: Microbiology and Antimicrobial Therapy**

Source of Abscess	Site of Abscess	Microbial Flora	Antimicrobial Therapy*†
1. Paranasal sinus	Frontal lobe	*Streptococcus* spp (aerobic or anaerobic), *Fusobacterium, Bacteroides, Haemophilus* spp	Penicillin + metronidazole
2. Otitis media	Temporal lobe, cerebellum	*Streptococcus* spp, *Bacteroides fragilis,* Enterobacteriaceae, Pseudomonadaceae	Penicillin + metronidazole + 3rd-generation cephalosporin
3. Metastatic spread	Multiple cerebral lesions common, especially in middle cerebral artery distribution, but any lobe can be involved	Depends on source Urinary tract Enterobacteriaceae, Pseudomonadaceae Intra-abdominal *Streptococcus* spp, anaerobes, Enterobacteriaceae Lung abscess *Streptococcus* spp, *Fusobacterium, Actinomyces, Nocardia*	Depends on site Penicillin + metronidazole Add 3rd-generation cephalosporin for potential gram-negative source
4. Penetrating trauma	Depends on site of wound	*Staphylococcus aureus, Clostridium* spp, *Bacillus* spp	Nafcillin + penicillin + metronidazole
5. Post-neurosurgery	Depends on surgical site	*Staphylococcus epidermidis*	Vancomycin

*Suggested antimicrobial therapy for initial empiric treatment. Antibiotic selection will vary depending on clinical situation and culture results.
†Recommended antibiotic dosages: dosage for 70 kg patient; dosing may need adjustment in patients with underlying renal or liver disease.

Penicillin:	2–4 million units IV q 4 h
Metronidazole:	500 mg IV q 6 h
Cefotaxime:	1–2 gm IV q 4–8 h (maximum dose of 12 gm per day)
Ceftazidime:	1–2 gm IV q 4–8 h (maximum dose of 6 gm per day)
Nafcillin:	2 gm IV q 4 h
Vancomycin:	1 gm IV q 12 h

bial therapy. Indeed, positive cultures (or Gram's stain) may be obtained at surgery despite several days of antimicrobial therapy.

Brain abscess secondary to a dental or sinus infection is likely to contain microaerophilic streptococci (e.g., viridans streptococci) and oral anaerobic species (fusobacteria, *Bacteroides* spp, *Actinomyces* spp). Combination therapy with penicillin and metronidazole (Flagyl) is recommended in this situation; penicillin is active against the microaerophilic streptococci, whereas metronidazole has excellent activity against strict anaerobes. A special advantage of metronidazole is its excellent central nervous system (CNS) penetration and its activity against beta-lactamase–producing anaerobes. Cerebral abscess secondary to an otogenic focus may contain gram-negative facultative aerobes (Enterobacteriaceae, Pseudomonadaceae) as part of a mixed microbial flora; addition of an agent with activity against these organisms (e.g., ceftazidime [Fortaz]) is wise until cultures are available. Although gram-negative facultative aerobes are less common in brain abscess, they may be seen following gram-negative bacteremia from an underlying focus such as a urinary tract infection or intra-abdominal abscess. In these situations, addition of a third-generation cephalosporin (e.g., cefotaxime [Claforan], ceftazidime) to the standard regimen is recommended until cultures are available. Aminoglycosides have poor CNS penetration and should not be used as sole therapy for serious gram-negative intracerebral infection. Chloramphenicol, which provides coverage against streptococci, anaerobes, and some gram-negative facultative anaerobes, was once the drug of choice for intracerebral abscess and still may be useful in selected situations; however, most specialists are reluctant to use it because of the potential for adverse hematologic side effects. The role of quinolones in the management of intracerebral abscess remains unclear; at the present time there are little clinical data concerning their use in this situation.

Brain abscess due to *Staphylococcus aureus* may be seen following staphylococcal bacteremia or penetrating intracerebral trauma; high-dose antimicrobial therapy with a semisynthetic penicillin (e.g., oxacillin, nafcillin) active against *Staphylococcus aureus* should be started in this situation. Vancomycin can be used in patients with a penicillin allergy and is the drug of choice in brain abscess following neurosurgical procedures where *Staphylococcus epidermidis* (frequently resistant to nafcillin) is a frequent pathogen.

Although there is no clear guideline, most patients require a prolonged (4- to 6-week) course of parenteral antibiotics. This is especially important for patients who have not had surgical drainage or excision of the abscess.

Surgical intervention is frequently required to determine the microbiology of an intracerebral abscess. Knowledge of the specific pathogens present is extremely valuable in allowing the physician to design the least toxic and most directed antimicrobial regimen. The availability of CT-guided stereotactic equipment has made attempts at surgical drainage and aspiration much safer and more precise. The proper role of surgical drainage versus excision of the abscess is controversial and depends on the individual case; modern sterotactic equipment allows early and repeated needle aspiration and may abrogate the need for a more aggressive surgical approach. Surgical excision is especially appropriate in patients with exotic organisms (e.g., fungi) or multiloculated abscesses, which may prove difficult to drain by aspiration alone. The issues surrounding these decisions are complex and must be made in consultation with a neurosurgeon. In certain cases, nonoperative management of brain abscess may be appropriate. This could be the best option in patients with small (<2.5 cm), multiple, deep-seated abscesses the location of which may preclude a surgical approach. Whatever the course of therapy, therapeutic decisions must be guided by frequent clinical evaluation and weekly CT scans to follow resolution of the lesions.

Adjunctive therapy with corticosteroids may be lifesaving in certain situations (intracranial hypertension with impending herniation) but is generally avoided because of potentially deleterious effects. There is some evidence to suggest that corticosteroids may impair antibiotic penetration into affected areas and could hinder sterilization of an abscess. In immunocompromised patients, a reduction in steroid dosage may improve host immune response and allow more rapid containment of the infection. Antiseizure medications are generally not started unless the patient has experienced a seizure; however, many surgeons recommend them for a period of time following a neurosurgical procedure.

The mortality from brain abscess—once over 50%—has improved over the past several decades and is now less than 10%. Patient outcome is dependent on early and aggressive diagnosis and therapy; individuals who are obtunded and comatose at the time of presentation tend to do poorly and are more likely to die or be left with significant neurologic deficits.

BRAIN ABSCESS IN ACQUIRED IMMUNE DEFICIENCY SYNDROME AND IMMUNOCOMPROMISED PATIENTS

The increasing number of immunocompromised patients (including acquired immune deficiency syndrome [AIDS] patients) has broadened the number of pathogens that can be seen in brain abscess. Patients receiving steroids (or with underlying defects in cell-mediated immunity) are at risk for infection with opportunistic pathogens such as *Nocardia* spp, fungi (*Aspergillus* spp, *Candida* spp, *Mucor* spp), mycobacteria, and parasites (*Toxoplasma gondii*). Aggressive measures to identify the pathogen are paramount since therapy may require prolonged courses of toxic drugs that may have only marginal efficacy.

Cerebral mass lesions in AIDS patients are particularly challenging because of the considerable morbidity and mortality seen in these patients if they are not treated promptly with efficacious therapy. The possibility of underlying human immunodeficiency virus (HIV) infection should be considered in all patients with a cerebral mass lesion; attempts to identify potential HIV risk factors and an aggressive approach to HIV testing are important because the differential diagnosis and primary therapy are often different in this patient population. The most common cause of intracerebral mass lesions in AIDS patients is toxoplasmosis (Table 2); initial empiric therapy with pyrimethamine and sulfadiazine (with concomitant folinic acid) should be given. Cryptococcomas may be seen and can be diagnosed with a serum or CSF cryptococcal antigen titer. Patients who fail to respond to therapy may require surgical intervention to rule out underlying lymphoma or infection with one of a host of less common pathogens, such as tuberculosis or *Nocardia*. Again, early involvement of the neurology and neurosurgery services is important to plan an approach to these potentially life-threatening infections.

TABLE 2. **Focal CNS Lesions in AIDS Patients**

Common
Toxoplasma gondii
Primary CNS lymphoma
Less common
Cryptococcus neoformans
Mycobacterium tuberculosis
Mycobacterium avium—intracellulare complex
Progressive multifocal leukoencephalopathy
Nocardia asteroides
Listeria monocytogenes
Salmonella spp
Aspergillus spp
Bacterial brain abscess

ALZHEIMER'S DISEASE

method of
ALAN LERNER, M.D.,
PETER HEDERA, M.D., and
PETER WHITEHOUSE, M.D., PH.D.
Case Western Reserve University
Cleveland, Ohio

Dementia is a clinical syndrome characterized by loss of function in multiple cognitive abilities in an individual with a previously normal intellectual level and clear consciousness. The term *dementia* does not imply a specific underlying cause, progressive course, or irreversibility. Causes of dementia associated with neuronal death, often with specific pathologic stigmata but without typical signs of diseases of known cause, are termed *degenerative dementias*. Alzheimer's disease (AD) is the prototypical degenerative dementia and the most frequent single cause of dementia in North America and western Europe, accounting for approximately 60% of all cases of dementia and affecting 5 to 10% of individuals over age 65.

The etiology of AD is unknown, but a number of risk factors other than age have been defined. Individuals with trisomy 21 are at particular risk, especially after age 35. Familial forms of AD have been associated with markers on chromosomes 21, 19, and 14. Current attention is focused on apolipoprotein E, especially the $\epsilon 4$ isotype. Both familial late-onset and sporadic AD have been associated with the presence of one or more $\epsilon 4$ alleles. Other possible risk factors include female gender, family history of dementia or Down's syndrome, head trauma, thyroid disease, myocardial infarction, and low educational level. Epidemiologic studies have indicated that cigarette smoking may be a mild protective factor.

Clinical features of AD are variable but include progressive loss of memory and other cognitive functions over time. Initially, loss of short-term memory is more prominent than deficits in remote recall. Language deficits often result in functional communication difficulties due to underlying impairments in verbal fluency, speech content, comprehension, and naming. Visuospatial dysfunction, presenting with difficulties estimating distances, recognizing objects, or spatial dyscoordination, may be a presenting feature. Executive functions such as planning, concept formation, set shifting, and problem solving are frequently impaired. AD patients, particularly in the middle stages of the illness, may have behavioral disturbances, including depression, delusions, hallucinations, anxiety, agitation, wandering, and insomnia. Smaller numbers of patients may have other neurologic signs, such as extrapyramidal rigidity, seizures, myoclonus, or gait disorder, particularly in the more advanced stages.

Every patient with suspected dementia should undergo a complete evaluation for diagnosis of specific disorders associated with dementia (Table 1). Evaluation should include a detailed history from the patient and a collateral source who is familiar with the patient. Information regarding approximate date and mode of onset, specific symptomatology, and course is particularly important. Medical history should be explored for evidence of systemic or neurologic conditions associated with dementia. A family history is essential, because several dementias can be inherited. Occasionally, home or occupational exposure to toxic substances may be relevant. The history should also include an assessment of the functional impact of the disease on patient and family life, including activities of daily living.

Physical examination should include general medical examination, neurologic examination, and mental status testing. The physical examination may help uncover signs of systemic illness contributing to cognitive dysfunction. The elementary neurologic examination in AD is frequently normal initially. Early signs of dysfunction in the extrapyramidal, cerebellar, or motor system, or in the peripheral and cranial nerves, may indicate other neurologic illnesses presenting with dementia.

Mental status testing should include evaluation of short- and long-term memory, language, visuospatial skills, praxis, planning, attention, and judgment. The use of standardized short instruments, such as the Mini Mental State Examination or the Blessed Information-Memory-Concentration Test, helps confirm the clinical impression of dementia. The presence of psychiatric features, such as change in personality, hallucinations, delusions, affective disorder, anxiety, agitation, and sleep disturbance, should be sought.

Ancillary laboratory studies are an important part of the diagnostic evaluation (Table 2). This includes complete blood cell count, metabolic screen, thyroid function testing, vitamin B_{12} and folate levels, tests for neurosyphilis, urinalysis, electrocardiogram, and chest x-ray study. Structural brain imaging, either computed tomography or magnetic resonance imaging, is indicated in all patients with dementia, and may reveal other causes for dementia, such as stroke, neoplasm, hydrocephalus, or subdural hematoma. Other studies such as human immunodeficiency virus (HIV) testing, lumbar puncture, and electroencephalography are used in cases where other illnesses are being considered, such as acquired immune deficiency syndrome (AIDS), seizures, or chronic meningitis.

Neuropsychological referral is useful in identifying subtle cognitive abnormalities in cases of suspected early dementia and in helping differentiate dementia from normal aging or possible coexistent depression. It may also help establish a baseline for longitudinal follow-up in doubtful or atypical cases.

TABLE 1. **Conditions Causing Dementia**

Degenerative dementias
Vascular dementias
Metabolic, nutritional, toxins, drugs
Depression and other psychiatric disorders
Neoplasms
Infections and central nervous system inflammatory diseases
Normal pressure hydrocephalus
Post trauma
Miscellaneous

TABLE 2. **Diagnostic Testing of the Demented Patient**

Standard tests	Other potentially useful tests
Screening metabolic panel	Formal psychiatric assessment
Complete blood count and differential	Neuropsychology battery
Urinalysis	Electroencephalography
Thyroid function tests	Lumbar puncture
Syphilis serology (FTA and VDRL)	HIV titer
Vitamin B_{12} and folate levels	Serologic testing for vasculitis
CT or MRI scan	Heavy metal screening
Electrocardiogram	Angiography
Chest x-ray	Brain biopsy
	Apolipoprotein E isotyping

Abbreviations: FTA = fluorescent treponemal antibody; VDRL = Veneral Disease Research Laboratory (test); CT = computed tomography; MRI = magnetic resonance imaging; HIV = human immunodeficiency virus.

PHARMACOLOGIC THERAPY

Lack of understanding of fundamental pathologic processes in AD limits our current therapeutic options. Recent progress in basic research has opened some rational approaches for treatment of AD, focusing on symptomatic relief of cognitive and behavioral symptoms. Recent clinical trials have also explored the feasibility of slowing disease progression.

Symptomatic Treatment of Cognitive Symptoms

Cholinergic Approach

Based on the well-established deficit of acetylcholine in AD and its role in memory process, cholinergic agents have been extensively tested in AD, and tacrine (tetrahydroaminoacridine or THA, Cognex), a long-acting, reversible cholinesterase inhibitor, has been approved for the treatment of mild to moderate AD. The initial dosage is 10 mg four times a day, increasing by 40-mg increments every 6 weeks to a maximum daily dose of 160 mg. Serum alanine aminotransferase (ALT) levels should be measured weekly during the first 18 weeks of therapy and when going to higher doses of tacrine, because reversible hepatotoxicity may occur. At higher doses, parasympathetic side effects, such as bradycardia, sweating, nausea, vomiting, and delirium, may occur. Cholinergic innervation can theoretically also be enhanced by administration of acetylcholine precursors (e.g., lecithin), nicotinic and muscarinic agonists, and irreversible cholinesterase inhibitors; the latter two groups are currently being tested in clinical trials.

Other Agents

Information about deficits in other neurotransmitter systems in AD has resulted in the development of new therapeutic strategies. Agents affecting neuropeptide systems, such as opiate antagonists, captopril, vasopressin, and desmopressin, have not met theoretical expectations. A putative role of serotonin in the cognitive and behavioral disturbances in AD led to the testing of several serotonin receptor subtype agonists and antagonists as well as serotonin re-uptake blockers, but results are inconclusive. Nootropics are a poorly defined group of various nonspecific compounds with possible effects on neuronal metabolism. The most thoroughly studied members of this family are piracetam,* aniracetam, and oxiracetam. They have a generally good safety profile, but clinical usage has failed to demonstrate a consistent positive effect in AD. Hydergine (1 to 3 mg three times daily), a combination of four ergoloid mesylates, was approved years ago for treatment of ill-defined categories of cognitive dysfunction in aging. Controlled studies have not shown a marked effect, but some patients report subjective improvement, especially in mood. Hydergine is generally well tolerated and, unlike other ergot derivatives, it lacks vasoconstrictor properties. Positive response to treatment, if it occurs, should be evident within 3 months of therapy.

Treatment Enhancing Viability of Neurons and Slowing Disease Progression

This newly developing approach targets prevention of neuronal loss. Acetyl-L-carnitine showed some promise in long-term trials and has been claimed to slow disease progression, particularly in younger patients. Intracellular influx of calcium can initiate cell death through activation of lytic enzymes, and testing of calcium channel blockers is underway. Selegiline (Eldepryl), a selective MAO-B inhibitor approved for the treatment of Parkinson's disease, may show some benefit in improving memory and behavior in AD. This agent and vitamin E are currently under study to determine whether they slow disease progression. Other attempts at transforming basic research models to clinical practice, such as nerve growth factor administration or drugs to prevent amyloid accumulation, have not yet reached clinical application. Another remaining issue is how to design clinical trials that can differentiate prolonged symptomatic benefit from slowing of disease progression (Table 3).

Pharmacologic Treatment of Behavioral Symptoms

Behavioral symptomatology in AD, such as depression, agitation, delusions and hallucinations, sleep disturbances, and wandering, can be a significant burden for caregivers and patients. They appear in the majority of the patients with AD at some point during the illness and are the most common reason for institutionalization. The presence of these symptoms does not always represent disease progression. They can be a manifestation of physical illness (e.g., urinary tract infection), a side effect of other medications, or secondary to changes in familiar environment and routine. A thorough analysis of these possible causes should be undertaken before planning a psychopharmacologic intervention, as the latter can be associated with adverse or paradoxical effects outweighing the desired benefit. Hallucinations or delusions ought not be treated indiscriminately, but only when they are stressful for the patient or have an unbearable impact on the caregiver.

General principles of psychopharmacologic usage should apply: definition of a target symptom, use of the lowest possible initial dose, careful titration, and monitoring of side effects. Because symptom intensity may fluctuate, dose reduction after positive response and even discontinuation of therapy are often possible.

Depression occurs in up to 30% of AD patients. Successful treatment of depression can positively influence cognitive deficit, because depression can present with symptoms of dementia. AD-associated

TABLE 3. **Medications Used in Alzheimer's Disease**

- Cognitive symptoms
  - Tacrine (Cognex)
- Behavioral symptoms
  - Depression
    - Nortriptyline (Pamelor)
    - Fluoxetine (Prozac)
    - Sertraline (Zoloft)
    - Trazodone (Desyrel)
  - Agitation and psychotic symptoms
    - Neuroleptics: Haloperidol (Haldol), Thioridazine (Mellaril), Loxapine (Loxitane), Chlorpromazine (Thorazine)
    - Non-neuroleptics: Trazodone (Desyrel), Carbamazepine (Tegretol)
  - Anxiety
    - Oxazepam (Serax)
    - Alprazolam (Xamax)
    - Low-dose neuroleptics
  - Insomnia
    - Chloral hydrate
    - Trazodone
    - Benzodiazepines

*Investigational drug in the United States.

depression is treated with a similar spectrum of anti-depressants as major depression, because there is no firm evidence of a different etiologic mechanism for major depression and depression in AD. Choice of initial therapy depends partly on side effects, with an emphasis on avoiding excessive anticholinergic activity that can result in increased confusion, orthostasis, or dry mucous membranes. Nortriptyline (Pamelor), 10 to 50 mg daily, and desipramine (Norpramin), 25 to 75 mg daily, have minimal anticholinergic effects. They can be safely used in a geriatric population with monitoring of blood levels. Fluoxetine (Prozac), 5 to 20 mg daily; trazodone (Desyrel), 50 to 150 mg daily; sertraline (Zoloft), 25 to 100 mg daily; and paroxetine (Paxil), 10 to 40 mg daily, are new agents with a low incidence of anticholinergic side effects.

Neuroleptics have been the medication of choice for treatment of agitation and psychotic symptomatology. No particular neuroleptic has been demonstrated to have superior efficacy; their relative indications are based on their potential for side effects, such as extrapyramidal symptoms, akathisia, increased confusion, falling, or hypotension. Mild extrapyramidal dysfunction is commonly found in AD and can increase even after small doses of neuroleptics. Low doses of haloperidol (Haldol) up to 3 mg per day in divided doses usually do not cause significant extrapyramidal symptoms. Thioridazine (Mellaril) has a relatively high anticholinergic effect and should not be used in doses greater than 75 mg per day. Intermediate-potency neuroleptics such as loxapine (Loxitane) starting at 5 mg a day may be useful. Non-neuroleptic agents used for treating agitation and psychotic-like symptoms include trazodone (Desyrel) up to 150 mg per day and carbamazepine (Tegretol) 100 to 300 mg per day.

Anxiety is common in AD, often associated with minor depression. Benzodiazepines with short to intermediate half-lives are preferred by some. Cautious use of these agents will limit their potential for sedation, risk of falling, and paradoxical agitation. Oxazepam (Serax), 10 to 30 mg up to three times a day, and alprazolam (Xanax), 0.125 to 0.5 mg two or three times daily (which also has a mild antidepressant action), are effective anxiolytics in this population. Low-dose neuroleptics may also be effective in these patients.

Sleep disturbances are frequent in AD. An active routine minimizing daytime naps and reduction of liquid intake before bedtime may be sufficient. Chloral hydrate up to 1000 mg as needed, trazodone (50 to 100 mg at bedtime), or low doses of benzodiazepines are the safest hypnotic medications in AD patients.

BEHAVIORAL THERAPY

Management of problem behaviors often entails use of nonpharmacologic methods of behavior modification. Clinically, the first goal is to focus on elucidating the scope and impact of the problem behavior. The circumstances under which the behaviors manifest help identify precipitating factors and suggest specific behavioral interventions (Table 4). Mace and Rabins' book, *The Thirty-Six Hour Day,* and other information regarding behavioral management should be recommended to caregivers. The overall caregiving burden should also be addressed and alternative care options, such as day or respite care, discussed. Families often benefit from referral to local community social service agencies, support groups, and the Alzheimer's Association (telephone number: 1-800-272-3900).

OTHER ASPECTS OF AD PATIENT CARE

Comprehensive management of AD includes assessment of activities of daily living, home safety, and practical care issues. These evaluations often benefit from the input of nurses and social workers in addition to medical evaluation. A summary conference attended by the patient, family, and clinical staff is effective in providing an integrated diagnostic and prognostic view. When the diagnosis is made early in the course, the patient can participate in legal, financial, and long-term care planning. With progression of the illness, families frequently desire information about nursing home placement. This must be an individualized decision involving cultural, socioeconomic, legal, and medical elements. Advanced directives regarding treatment should be discussed as appropriate. Referral to research programs should be offered if available.

Reassessment should be planned at regular intervals or when a significant change in functioning occurs. AD patients are especially vulnerable to conditions or medications that can cause excess disability; that is, more cognitive disability than can be explained by the primary illness itself. Appropriate di-

TABLE 4. **Principles of Behavior Management—The Six Rs**

Reassess:	When change is observed or when an intervention no longer works.
Restrict:	Prevent a behavior from occurring or stop a behavior from continuing. This is the most common method and usually the fastest way to ensure safety, but can be unnecessarily restrictive when no one is at risk.
Reconsider:	Ask: From the patient's point of view, is this a reasonable behavior? For example, if the patient does not recognize the proper context, the patient's actions may seem inappropriate to us.
Rechannel:	Find a way for the patient to continue acting in a way that is not disruptive or dangerous.
Redirect:	Divert behavior that is leading toward an outburst: use distraction or offer a substitute behavior.
Reassure:	Reassure the patient that he/she is safe and that you will see that he/she are not embarrassed or lost. Reassure the patient that you recognize his/her feelings after a catastrophic reaction.

Adapted from Whitehouse P (ed): Dementia. Contemporary Neurology Series, Volume 40. Philadelphia, F. A. Davis, 1993, p 406.

agnosis and treatment of intercurrent medical and psychiatric disorders will ensure that the patient functions as well as possible throughout the illness.

PARENCHYMATOUS BRAIN HEMORRHAGE

method of
CHIN-SANG CHUNG, M.D., and
LOUIS R. CAPLAN, M.D.
Tufts New England Medical Center Hospitals
Boston, Massachusetts

Intracerebral hemorrhage (ICH) is a major cause of morbidity and death and accounts for approximately 10 to 15% of all strokes in western countries. There is a higher incidence of ICH in populations such as African Americans and individuals of Asian ancestry, who have a higher frequency of hypertension. Hypertension is the most common cause of spontaneous ICH. Bleeding is usually from deep penetrating arteries of the circle of Willis, especially lenticulostriate, thalamogeniculate, and thalamoperforating branches and perforating branches from the vertebrobasilar system. Hypertension-induced pathologic changes in these arteries include fibrinoid necrosis and microaneurysm formation, changes that predispose the individual to bleeding. An acute increase in blood pressure and blood flow can precipitate ICH, even in the absence of pre-existing severe hypertension. Hypertensive hemorrhages have a definite predilection for certain regions and are distributed approximately as follows: putamen, 40%; lobar, 22%; thalamus, 15%; pons, 8%; cerebellum, 8%; caudate, 7%.

INITIAL EVALUATION AND MANAGEMENT

Prompt and careful management of patients with ICH may be lifesaving and is important even in those who will later undergo surgical drainage of their hematomas. Adequate airway and respiratory support should be established as needed. Blood gases should be measured in all patients with reduced alertness to determine oxygen and carbon dioxide levels. Endotracheal intubation is performed for patients presenting in coma, for those who are unable to protect their airways, and for those who display an inadequate ventilatory effort. Blood pressure should be determined. Wide swings in blood pressure, especially hypertension, are common in the initial period following ICH. Intravenous sodium nitroprusside (Nipride) with concomitant intra-arterial pressure monitoring is an effective method of controlling such elevations. Labetalol (Trandate) is also an excellent antihypertensive drug to use. Continuous cardiac monitoring for arrhythmias is also important. Hypotension from cardiac or other etiologies can be devastating due to the impact on cerebral perfusion pressure. During the initial evaluation, blood samples for basic laboratory studies including complete blood chemistry (CBC), chemistries, coagulation studies, toxicology screen, and arterial blood gases are obtained.

Computed tomography (CT) is an essential tool in diagnosis, management, and follow-up of ICH. It accurately documents the size and location of the hematoma, the presence and extent of mass effect, and the presence of hydrocephalus and intraventricular hemorrhage. We perform CT scanning immediately in patients suspected of having an ICH. Follow-up CTs are ordered to monitor changes in the effective size of the lesion and ventricular system, and to detect important pressure shifts.

If the clinical syndrome and CT findings are those of a typical hypertensive hemorrhage in the basal ganglia, caudate nucleus, thalamus, pons, or cerebellum, we do not perform angiography. If the hemorrhage is in an atypical location for hypertensive ICH or the patient is young and not hypertensive, we pursue angiography to exclude an arteriovenous malformation (AVM), aneurysm, vasculitis, or tumor, because the presence of any of these lesions would affect treatment. In patients who have ICH after cocaine use, there is a high frequency of vascular malformations and aneurysms, so we do perform angiography in cocaine-related ICH. We routinely order coagulation tests, such as prothrombin time, partial thromboplastin time, bleeding time, and platelet count. If the patient is not fully alert, arterial blood gases are drawn to detect hypoventilation.

Any management scheme designed to treat patients with ICH must control local tissue pressure and intracranial pressure (ICP). Six key factors should be considered in selecting the treatment modalities: (1) size and (2) location of the hematomas; (3) presence of significantly increased intracranial pressure (ICP); (4) etiology of ICH; (5) lesion age, that is, time since onset; and (6) clinical course, that is, whether the patient is improving, stable, or worsening.

The available medical and surgical treatment modalities are outlined in Table 1. They should not be considered competitive. A combined approach using both medical and surgical modalities will most often yield satisfactory results.

SIZE OF HEMATOMA AND TREATMENT OPTIONS

Most studies correlate mortality with the size of the lesion. Indications for surgical removal of ICH are either neurologic deterioration or uncontrollable elevation in ICP in otherwise salvageable patients. Prognosis for survival and ultimate recovery is largely dependent on the level of consciousness at the time of presentation, the size and location of the hematoma, and the age and clinical condition of the patient.

Small hematomas resolve gradually and leave slitlike scars. Recovery is usually good unless they are located in vital regions such as the thalamus and brain stem. Surgical drainage is unnecessary in small lesions that are less than 2 cm in diameter. Treatment should be limited to control of blood pressure and other etiologic factors that could cause recurrence. There is no evidence that surgical drainage of

TABLE 1. **Treatment of Intracerebral Hemorrhage**

Medical
Medical Decompression for Increased Intracranial Pressure
Intubation and mechanical hyperventilation
Dexamethasone (Decadron), 4 mg q 6 h
Mannitol, 0.5–1 gm per kg q 4 h IV
Glycerol, 1–1.5 oz PO q 6 h
Furosemide (Lasix),* 40 mg (4 mg per min) IV
Control of Hypertension
Labetalol (Trandate, Normodyne) 10 mg IV, followed by 10-mg doses as needed
Trimethaphan camsylate (Arfonad), 0.5–1 mg per min IV by drip
Nitroprusside sodium (Nipride), 15–200 μg per min
Hydralazine hydrochloride (Apresoline), 50–100 mg bid PO
Reversal of Bleeding Diathesis
Fresh-frozen plasma
Antihemophilic factor
Phytonadione (vitamin K, aquaMEPHYTON) 20–40 mg IV
Platelet transfusion
Fresh blood transfusion
Surgical
Drainage of hematoma—stereotactic drainage or surgical evacuation
Ventricular drainage or shunt
Removal of bleeding AVM or tumor
Repair of aneurysm

*Not FDA approved for this indication.

small hematomas will reduce long-term morbidity in patients with ICH. Hematomas over 3 cm in their widest diameter have a higher mortality and a more delayed recovery rate than do smaller lesions. Thus, the larger the lesion is on CT, the more logical its drainage would be. Well-localized round or oval hematomas are easier to drain than lesions that are slitlike or that extend longitudinally along white matter fiber tracts. Massive hemorrhages usually increase ICP rapidly and cause fatal, irreversible cerebral and brain stem damage even before physicians can treat the patient. Treatment of these massive lesions is seldom, if ever, effective. Survival, when it occurs, is usually vegetative.

LOCATION OF HEMATOMA AS TREATMENT DETERMINANT

Some ICH locations, such as the cerebellum, cerebral lobes, and right putamen, are more accessible to surgical drainage. Cerebellar hemorrhages are usually drained through a posterior fossa surgical approach because they can compress the caudal brain stem and lead to respiratory arrest without preceding gradual deterioration of neurologic function or alertness. Removal of cerebellar lesions usually leaves little serious disability. If the cerebellar hematoma is larger than 3 cm in diameter, we advise surgical decompression in most circumstances. Lobar hemorrhages are relatively close to the brain surface and can usually be drained through a cortical incision. Putaminal hemorrhages can be drained through an incision into the lateral ganglionic lesion through the insula. Large left basal ganglionic hemorrhages usually leave patients aphasic and dependent, so treatment should be less aggressive than for right-sided lesions. Caudate hemorrhages usually drain themselves spontaneously and early into the adjacent lateral ventricles, and rarely require surgical intervention. In thalamic hemorrhage, direct surgical drainage is seldom useful. Thalamic hemorrhages, however, sometimes require ventricular drainage to relieve obstructive hydrocephalus caused by associated intraventricular hemorrhage. Brain stem hemorrhages, especially those in the pons, are relatively inaccessible to drainage and are usually considered nonsurgical lesions because surgical damage to the thalamus or pons is more likely to cause severe disability or death.

INCREASED INTRACRANIAL PRESSURE

Death from ICH is usually due to the consequences of increased ICP. The addition of extra mass in the form of hematoma, surrounding edema, and dilated ventricles increases ICP. Pressure increases maximally in the region of the hematoma and can cause shifts or herniation of tissues through dural compartments and fatal brain stem compression. Increased ICP causes decreased responsiveness and hypoventilation and, in turn, hypoventilation causes low arterial oxygen tension and high carbon dioxide tension, which lead to vasodilation and a further increase in ICP and also compromise cerebral blood flow.

ICP can be monitored by clinical signs or CT changes, or by direct pressure measurements requiring a surgically placed intracranial monitor. It has not been our practice to advise placement of ICP monitors unless the clinical situation is unusual or a surgical procedure is going to be performed and the monitor can be incidentally placed at the same time.

We raise the head of the bed for the patient with ICH because gravity facilitates venous return and thereby reduces ICP. Following head elevation, cerebral perfusion pressure (CPP) may fall. Head elevation is frequently associated with reductions in mean arterial pressure, thereby reducing CPP. Reduction in arterial pressure following head elevation is more common in patients with reduced intravascular volume or compromised cardiac status. The goal, with respect to head positioning, is to maintain CPP above 75 torr. In the presence of inadequate CPP, the head is positioned to maximize cardiac filling and to minimize elevation of ICP.

When deterioration is rapid and urgent measures are needed, intubation with forced mechanical hyperventilation is the most effective and rapid means of reducing ICP; it takes effect in 2 to 30 minutes, with a mean of 8 minutes. Return of ICP to previous levels frequently occurs within an hour. Maximal vasoconstriction appears to occur at a $PaCO_2$ of 20 torr. Below this level, cerebral hypoxia can occur as a result of intense vasoconstriction. The goal, then, is to maintain $PaCO_2$ in the range of 25 to 30 mmHg.

Osmotic agents are routinely used for ICH patients who deteriorate or have uncontrolled elevations in ICP. Mannitol is the agent of choice for a number of theoretical and practical reasons. Mannitol acts by establishing an osmotic gradient between the vascular space and brain, resulting in the exit of interstitial fluid. Additionally, mannitol may reduce CSF production and improve brain microcirculation by reducing blood viscosity. Mannitol is infused intravenously in bolus doses of 0.5 to 1 gram per kg every 4 to 6 hours or 0.25 gram per kg every 2 to 3 hours. Supplemental furosemide (Lasix)* can potentiate and prolong the effect of mannitol on ICP. If the situation is less urgent, glycerol* in doses of 1 to 1.5 ounces can be given orally or in nasogastric tubing every 4 to 6 hours. Glycerol is often effective in controlling increased ICP, and it can be effective and tolerated for longer periods than mannitol. Because osmotic agents can cause rapid but usually temporary increases in intravascular volume, the patient should be monitored carefully for congestive heart failure or pulmonary edema. Frequent monitoring of serum electrolytes and osmolality is also mandatory because osmotherapy can cause hypernatremia and serum hyperosmolality, particularly in diabetic patients, and because hyponatremia also can be caused by diuretic or osmotic agents or inappropriate antidiuretic hormone release.

The adrenocorticosteroids are often used in patients with ICH, although they have not been proved effective. Usually dexamethasone (Decadron) is given in doses of 4 mg every 6 hours. Although some advocate so-called megadose levels of steroids, there is little evidence that they are more effective, and we believe that they probably increase the risk of steroid therapy. Steroids do not work immediately.

Barbiturates should be considered when other methods of reducing ICP have failed. Although it is not clear whether barbiturate therapy improves neurologic outcome, certain patients do respond favorably to barbiturates.

These medical decompressive measures may suffice to pull the patient through the critical first 24 to 72 hours and may obviate the need for surgery. They are also adjuncts to surgical treatment and probably reduce the mortality associated with operations in patients with increased ICP. If patients do not improve and become more alert after the previously described treatment, or if they deteriorate, surgical drainage should be considered. We would like to re-emphasize the crucial role of monitoring the patient's progress in the therapeutic decision.

TREATMENT RELATED TO SPECIFIC ETIOLOGIES

Hypertension

Control of arterial hypertension is important in stemming the bleeding and in preventing subsequent episodes of ICH. During the acute phase, control of systemic blood pressure (BP) helps stop intracerebral bleeding but must be done cautiously. In some patients with increased ICP, systemic BP is further increased to ensure adequate perfusion of the brain. Increased ICP causes increased venous pressure, so elevated arterial pressure is needed to overcome the increased venous pressure in order to perfuse the tissues. Overzealous lowering of BP can lead to underperfusion and clinical deterioration. BP should be lowered quickly but not to hypotensive levels, and patients must be watched carefully during the treatment. Neurologic signs and level of alertness should be monitored as the BP is lowered. If the patient worsens, we allow the BP to rise if the findings are sensitive to changes in arterial pressure and perfusion.

*Not FDA approved for this indication.

If the BP is extremely high, we begin a drip of trimethaphan camsylate (Arfonad), using an intravenous drip delivering 0.5 to 1 mg per minute of the drug while titrating BP. Labetalol (Trandate, Normodyne), is an excellent drug for BP control. We begin with 10 mg intravenously and then give doses of 10 or 20 mg as needed. Labetalol acts on adrenergic receptors and has little effect on intravascular volume or cardiac rate or output.

Alternatively, nitroprusside sodium (Nipride) can be given by intravenous drip in a dosage of 15 to 200 μg per minute, again titrating the arterial pressure. We attempt to reduce the systolic BP to 120 to 150 mmHg and the diastolic pressure to 80 to 90 mmHg. Hydralazine hydrochloride (Apresoline), 50 to 100 mg orally twice daily, is then frequently used to maintain the lower BP levels.

Bleeding Diathesis

Advances in medical therapy for occlusive vascular disease have increased the incidence of ICH. Anticoagulant use has become an important iatrogenic cause of ICH. Anticoagulant-associated hemorrhages progress more slowly and are more commonly lobar and cerebellar than hypertensive ICH. Mortality is high. Hypoprothrombinemia should be reversed immediately by using phytonadione (AquaMEPHYTON) (vitamin K), 20 to 40 mg intravenously. The incidence of major hemorrhage with thrombolytic therapy is much higher than with anticoagulant therapy. The mortality rate of patients with ICH from thrombolytic therapy approaches 50%.

Hemorrhage due to hemophilia or deficiency of other coagulant factors can be treated with infusion of fresh-frozen plasma or antihemophilic factor. Thrombocytopenia-related ICH is treated by platelet transfusion or infusion of fresh blood.

Drugs

Cocaine, phencyclidine (PCP), amphetamines, and phenylpropanolamine have effects on catecholamine metabolism and release, and can cause sudden blood pressure elevations and ICH. Amphetamines and the intravenous use of drugs prepared for oral use, such as methylphenidate (Ritalin),* pentazocine (Talwin),*

*Not FDA approved for this indication.

and tripelennamine (Pyribenzamine),* can cause a cerebral vasculitis and ICH. Arteriography may show focal narrowing and beading of small intracranial surface arteries. Medical control of increased ICP is usually sufficient to allow survival. Cessation of drug abuse is essential.

Bleeding Lesions (Arteriovenous Malformations, Aneurysms, and Tumors)

Arteriovenous malformations (AVMs) and aneurysms pose a different problem from those already considered, that of potentially serious rebleeding. Tumors require treatment unrelated to the propensity for rebleeding. The identification of these lesions by computed tomography (CT), magnetic resonance imaging (MRI), or angiography is essential for optimal treatment. MRI is especially helpful for recognizing cavernous angiomas. AVMs should be suspected in young patients with superficial hemorrhages in the absence of hypertension, drugs, or trauma. Primary intraventricular hemorrhages are also commonly caused by vascular malformations in or adjacent to the ventricular system. Preceding headache, seizures, and abnormal cranial calcifications are clues to the presence of these lesions. Often, enhanced CT or MRI shows abnormal vessels. When operating on hematomas caused by AVMs, ideally, surgeons would like to remove the AVM while also draining the hematoma. Aneurysms can cause meningocerebral hemorrhages; hematomas are usually contiguous to the brain base, and associated subarachnoid bleeding is seen on CT. Tumors are also often identifiable on CT. The presence of prior neurologic signs and a known primary tumor, such as bronchogenic carcinoma, melanoma, renal cell carcinoma, or choriocarcinoma, should raise the suspicion of this etiology. If hematomas require surgical drainage, it would be optimal to remove the tumor at the same time.

Amyloid Angiopathy

Cerebral amyloid angiopathy occurs secondary to the deposition of amyloid in the media and adventitia of small- and medium-sized arteries located near the surface of the cerebral cortex. It is a frequent cause of lobar ICH in nonhypertensive patients older than 65 years and characteristically causes multiple and recurrent lobar hemorrhages. Some cerebellar hematomas are also due to amyloid angiopathy. Hematomas tend to bleed or ooze even after surgical drainage because of the fragility of the blood vessels. Suspicion of cerebral amyloid angiopathy should deter surgery unless the situation is life-threatening.

AGE OF HEMATOMA AND TIMING OF SURGERY

When surgical drainage is under consideration, the age of the hematoma should be another important factor used to determine the timing of surgery. Soft or nearly liquid blood is much easier to drain than a firm clot. Early in the course of the ICH, during the first 24 to 36 hours, blood is still semiliquid and can usually be removed by suction through a small incision. Later, hematomas solidify and become technically more difficult to drain, requiring a wider incision. After 7 to 10 days, blood begins to be absorbed and again the lesion becomes softer. Thus, ideally, for technical reasons, drainage should be done either very early or after 7 to 10 days. In general, if the patient has survived the first week, improvement usually occurs as edema subsides, so there seems little argument for late drainage, except for concurrent removal of structural bleeding lesions such as AVMs or tumors.

MONITORING OF CLINICAL COURSE

Perhaps the most important factor to consider is whether the patient is improving, stable, or worsening. Patients who deteriorate and show a decrease in level of consciousness to severe lethargy or stupor have a poor outlook for recovery. Thus, careful monitoring of the patient's neurologic signs and state of alertness is critical if the physician is to respond quickly to the need for decompressive intervention. Nothing can substitute for frequent and careful examination by a physician experienced in central nervous system disease. As ICP begins to rise, the patient usually complains of headache and vomits. In posterior fossa ICH, the neck becomes stiff. Further rises in ICP cause a progressive decline in the level of consciousness. Lethargy is followed by agitation and delirium, and finally, stupor and coma as pressure rises to critical levels. In putaminal or ganglionic ICH, an increase in the effective size of the lesion due to continued bleeding or edema causes fixed conjugate deviation of the eyes to the side of the hematoma. Compression of the contralateral hemisphere and brain stem causes an ipsilateral extensor plantar reflex, and later bilateral conjugate gaze palsy and third cranial nerve dysfunction in the form of an ipsilateral fixed or dilated pupil. When these signs develop while the patient is under observation, in our experience the hematoma invariably proves fatal unless decompression measures are quickly instituted. Papilledema is not a very helpful sign because it is often absent. Worsening neurologic signs and a decreasing level of alertness are ominous prognostic signs and warrant urgent intervention. In deteriorating patients with accessible lesions, surgery should not be delayed if medical decompression is not beneficial.

Recent advances in neuroimaging techniques have made it possible to drain hematomas percutaneously using stereotactic surgery. A burr hole is made, and the drainage instrument is guided stereotactically, using CT or MRI, to the core of the hematoma, which is then evacuated. Fibrinolytic agents also can be instilled to soften and lyse the clot. As yet, there is too

*Not FDA approved for this indication.

little experience to allow comparison of open versus stereotactic drainage of hematomas.

CT and MRI findings also can document the development of significant pressure. Compression of the ipsilateral lateral ventricle, dilatation of the contralateral lateral ventricle because of compression of the foramen of Monro, symmetrical hydrocephalus, shift of the midline, and compression of the rostral brain stem cisterns are helpful signs to note. Deviation of the proximal cisternal segment of the anterior choroidal artery or posterior cerebral arteries, and shift of the anterior cerebral artery to the opposite side, are also helpful angiographic signs of herniation. When a monitor is in place, elevation of the ICP above 20 mmHg is worrisome. Pupillary dilatation often occurs if ICP exceeds 28 mmHg.

We use phenytoin sodium (Dilantin), 500 mg intravenously, if seizures occur and continue this drug orally in doses of 300 mg a day, but we do not use anticonvulsants prophylactically. Higher doses of phenytoin or other anticonvulsants are used if seizures are not controlled.

ISCHEMIC CEREBROVASCULAR DISEASE

method of
DIANE H. SOLOMON, M.D., and
DAVID G. SHERMAN, M.D.
University of Texas Health Science Center
San Antonio, Texas

EVALUATION AND DIFFERENTIAL DIAGNOSIS

Ischemic stroke is caused by a spectrum of disease states, each of which must be identified in each patient in order to optimize treatment. Acute evaluation of the stroke patient begins with assessment of the blood pressure with prevention of hypotension and assurance of adequate oxygenation. The patient is carefully examined for evidence of predisposing disease with special attention to regularity of pulse, the funduscopic examination, the presence of bruits, and abnormalities of the cardiac examination. The neurologic examination is focused on the patient's level of consciousness and whether the pattern of signs is consistent with an anterior (i.e., carotid) or posterior (i.e., vertebrobasilar) lesion. If anterior, cortical findings may indicate a larger lesion with the potential for more serious sequelae, including herniation, than are seen with subcortical infarcts. Metabolic derangements, such as hyperglycemia and hypokalemia, are corrected, and an emergent computed tomography (CT) scan is obtained. Although severe headache at onset and decreased level of consciousness are hallmarks for intracerebral hemorrhage, a bleed cannot be excluded clinically. Subdural hematomas and tumors may also mimic transient ischemic attacks (TIAs) and ischemic strokes, and will usually be identified on CT.

Because preventive treatment for ischemic stroke is specific for stroke etiology, further evaluation is required to determine the cause of stroke in a given individual. The four major etiologic categories of stroke (Table 1) may overlap, presenting a clinical challenge that is invaluably assisted by selected tests. Carotid ultrasound, or Doppler examination, is generally performed to screen for carotid atherosclerosis. This test is warranted even in those patients with a lacuna presumed to be due to small-vessel disease, because lacunae may sometimes be the result of vessel-to-vessel emboli from the carotids, especially if the lacuna is greater than 1.5 cm in size. Another noninvasive imaging study of the vessels, magnetic resonance angiography, is now in wide use. It has the advantage of visualizing intracranial disease, but similar to carotid ultrasound, it cannot differentiate a high-grade carotid stenosis from complete occlusion. An angiogram serves as the gold standard on patients with 70% or greater carotid stenosis on the symptomatic side, or if vasculitis, carotid dissection, or sinus venous thrombosis is suspected. A 1% risk of stroke with angiogram justifies the use of non-invasive screening techniques.

A transthoracic echocardiogram is recommended for patients with clinical evidence or a history of heart disease and brain ischemia. Patients less than 40 years old with stroke of undetermined cause and older patients without evidence of cerebrovascular atherosclerosis should be screened. Transesophageal echocardiography is more sensitive than routine precordial echocardiography for detection of

TABLE 1. **Mechanisms of Ischemia**

I.	Large-artery atherosclerosis	60%
	Hemodynamic (flow) compromise	
	Arteriogenic emboli	
	Intracranial atherosclerosis	
II.	Penetrating-artery disease	20%
	Hypertension	
	Diabetes mellitus	
III.	Cardiogenic embolism	15%
	Atrial fibrillation	
	Mitral or aortic valve disease	
	Left ventricular hypokinesis	
	Paradoxical emboli	
	Myxoma	
	Atrial septal aneurysm	
IV.	Unusual	5%
	Drug induced (cocaine, amphetamines)	
	Vasculitis	
	Dissection (trauma, fibromuscular dysplasia, syphilis, Marfans)	
	Sinus venous thrombosis	
	Migraine	
	Moya moya	
	Hematologic	

TABLE 2. **Transthoracic Versus Transesophageal Echocardiography in Stroke**

Detected as Well or Better by Transthoracic Echocardiography	Detected Better by Transesophageal Echocardiography
Left ventricular thrombus	Mitral valve vegetations
Aortic stenosis	Infective endocarditis
Aortic valve vegetations	Nonbacterial thrombotic carditis
Mitral stenosis	Atrial septal aneurysm
Mitral annulus calcification	Atrial septal defect
Myxomatous mitral valvulopathy with prolapse	Patent foramen ovale
	Atrial myxoma
	Atrial thrombus
	Atrial appendage thrombus
	Aortic arch atheroma/thrombi

abnormalities of the interatrial septum, atrial thrombi associated with atrial fibrillation, and mitral valve vegetations, but it does not visualize the left ventricle, other mitral valve disease, or the aortic valve as well (Table 2). Because of the invasiveness of transesophageal echocardiography, it is reserved for those patients with suspected left atrial disease and an unhelpful transthoracic echocardiogram.

In addition to routine blood work, a serologic test for syphilis, sedimentation rate, and triglyceride profile are obtained. A young patient without obvious cause for stroke is screened for collagen vascular disease and a prothrombotic state, including anticardiolipin antibody. If there are abnormalities on routine screening, laboratory tests such as hemoglobin, hematocrit, platelet count, prothrombin time and partial thromboplastin time, anticardiolipin antibody, and hemoglobin electrophoresis (especially in blacks) are indicated. When a personal or family history of thrombosis is present, antithrombin III, protein C, and protein S antigens are also obtained (Table 3).

ACUTE TREATMENT

As yet, there is no proven treatment for acute ischemic stroke. Several clinical trials are currently under way to study the effectiveness of thrombolytic and other agents. Aspirin is usually given after the CT scan has established the absence of hemorrhage, but its benefit has not been studied in this setting. The value of subcutaneous heparin for deep venous thrombosis prophylaxis is well established in debilitated patients, and a potential benefit for stroke reduction is being studied. The traditional use of intravenous heparin for acute noncardioembolic stroke is not supported by recent well-designed, but small, clinical trials. The Consensus Conference of Antithrombotic Therapy for Cerebrovascular Disorders recently published its conclusion that anticoagulants are either of no value or are harmful to patients with completed strokes.

Heparin is used by some clinicians for the subset of crescendo TIA and progressing stroke based on a theoretical belief that there is ongoing thrombosis in these disorders and heparin will prevent the formation of a larger thrombus. This may be within the range of acceptable care, considering that there is now little else to offer outside of research protocols, but many would argue heparin adds further risk for more serious impairment. If the decision to use heparin in this subgroup of patients is made, a baseline prothrombin time, partial thromboplastin time (PTT), complete blood count, and platelet count are obtained and carefully followed with the goal to achieve a PTT ratio of 1.5 to 2 times baseline. There is a 5% incidence of thrombocytopenia associated with heparin use, in addition to a bleeding rate of 2% to 4%. The risk of intracerebral hemorrhage is particularly increased in cardioembolic strokes, severe hypertension, and large strokes. If the patient's neurologic status has changed since the initial imaging study, a CT is repeated to rule out spontaneous hemorrhagic transformation prior to beginning heparin.

TABLE 3. **Hematologic Mechanisms of Ischemic Stroke**

Anticardiolipin antibody
Sickle cell anemia
Protein C and S, antithrombin III
Increased fibrinogen
Polycythemia
Myelogenous leukemia
Hypercoaguable states
Post partum, birth control pills

SECONDARY PREVENTION

Antiplatelet Agents

Aspirin

Aspirin is the mainstay of preventive treatment following minor ischemic stroke or TIA. By blocking the rate-limiting enzyme cyclooxygenase, aspirin inactivates the arachidonic acid pathway of platelet aggregation for the life of the platelet. Aspirin reduces the risk of stroke by approximately 22%, according to meta-analysis of multiple clinical trials of antiplatelet therapy.

There has been debate in the past over the effectiveness of aspirin in women. Recent trials have confirmed the utility of aspirin in women, and it is now generally recognized that earlier studies did not randomize enough women to show a benefit, considering their lower event rate.

The optimal dose of aspirin remains controversial. Doses as low as 30 mg have been shown to be beneficial, but no studies have directly compared low-dose to high-dose aspirin to determine which is more effective. The United Kingdom TIA trial found no significant difference in effectiveness between 300 mg (medium dose) and 1200 mg (high dose), but did show a dose-related increase in gastrointestinal hemorrhage. Platelet aggregation studies suggest that about 20% of patients treated with daily low doses of aspirin have less than optimal inhibition of platelet aggregation, but at higher doses improvement of inhibition is achieved. In an effort to decrease the risk of gastrotoxicity without jeopardizing effectiveness, we recommend 325 mg per day (Table 4).

Ticlopidine

Ticlopidine (Ticlid) is a recently available antiplatelet agent that inhibits the adenosine diphosphate pathway to prevent platelet aggregation. It has been compared to aspirin in one well-designed study and has been found to be more effective in preventing stroke. The Ticlopidine Aspirin Stroke Study (TASS) randomized 3069 patients with TIA or minor ischemic stroke to ticlopidine or aspirin. Over 3 years, stroke recurred at rates of 13% in patients taking 1300 mg per day aspirin and 10% in patients taking 500 mg per day ticlopidine for a relative risk reduction of 21%, an absolute ischemic stroke risk reduction of 1% per year with ticlopidine therapy as compared with aspirin. The Canadian American Ticlopidine Study (CATS) showed ticlopidine to be

TABLE 4. **Pharmaceutical Antithrombotic Therapy in Stroke**

Clinical Situation	Recommended Therapy	Reasonable Options
Chronic secondary prevention		
TIA or stroke*	ASA 325 mg per day	ASA 75–1300 mg per day, ticlopidine 250 mg bid
TIA or stroke during ASA	Ticlopidine (Ticlid) 250 mg bid	ASA 75–1300 mg per day, warfarin to INR 2-3
Atrial fibrillation		
Primary prevention†	ASA or warfarin (Coumadin)	Warfarin to INR 1.5–4, ASA 325 mg per day
Secondary prevention	Warfarin to INR 2-3	Warfarin to INR 1.5–4, ASA 325 mg per day
Acute brain ischemia		
Acute noncardioembolic stroke or TIA	ASA 325 mg per day plus low-dose SC heparin‡	ASA 75–1300 mg per day with low-dose SC heparin, no acute antithrombotic Rx
Progressing stroke or crescendo TIA	IV heparin (PTT ratio 1.5–2.0)	ASA 325–1300 mg per day
Acute cardioembolic stroke		
Large stroke	Delay anticoagulation for 5–14 days	ASA 325–1300 mg per day with low-dose SC heparin
TIA or small stroke	IV heparin after CT scan at 72 h§	Warfarin-delayed anticoagulation, ASA 325–1300 mg per day

Abbreviations: DVT = deep venous thrombosis; TIA = transient ischemic attack.
*Carotid artery endarterectomy for TIA or minor stroke associated with 70 to 99% ipsilateral stenosis unless contraindicated.
†See risk factors for thromboembolism for identification of high-risk subgroups.
‡Low-dose SC heparin for DVT prophylaxis; potential reduction of recurrent stroke under study.
§Patients with nonvalvular atrial fibrillation may have a lower risk of early recurrence and warrant special consideration.
ASA = acetylsalicylic acid (aspirin); bid = twice daily; INR = international normalized ratio; SC = subcutaneous; IV = intravenous.

more effective than placebo in preventing stroke in survivors of major disabling stroke. Aspirin has not been tested in this high-risk group.

Common minor side effects that occur with ticlopidine include diarrhea (10%) and rash (5%). More serious is a 2% idiosyncratic incidence of neutropenia, which may present during the first 3 months of therapy. There is also a 9% increase in all cholesterol fractions, but because follow-up has been limited to 3 years, any long-term effect is unknown. Ticlopidine has no advantage over aspirin in preventing myocardial infarction, but the gastrotoxicity with ticlopidine was less than with 1300 mg of aspirin.

Ticlopidine is given in 250-mg increments twice daily. If diarrhea or rash becomes a problem, the dose can sometimes be reduced and successfully slowly titrated to the recommended dose. A complete blood count (CBC) and differential must be checked every 2 weeks for the first 3 months, and if the absolute neutrophil count falls below 1000 cells per mm^3, the drug is discontinued. The neutropenia is reversible, generally correcting within 3 weeks.

Ticlopidine is used for so-called aspirin failures (those with recurrent stroke or TIA while compliant with aspirin), those unable to tolerate aspirin, and in patients with a history of peptic ulcer. Ticlopidine is the only established effective therapy following major stroke, although it is likely aspirin works in this setting. Ticlopidine may be chosen as first-line therapy, especially during the first year following TIA or completed stroke when the relative risk reduction is greatest compared with aspirin and placebo. Ticlopidine should not be prescribed to patients unable or unwilling to have biweekly CBC monitoring.

Anticoagulation

Preventive therapy with long-term anticoagulation for noncardioembolic ischemic stroke has not been proved to be beneficial when compared to antiplatelet agents in three small, recent randomized trials. The small number of stroke events in these trials and the multiple methodologic problems of earlier studies make the results inconclusive, but the lack of a proven benefit combined with a 1% to 4% yearly incidence of serious bleeding in the elderly argues strongly against using warfarin as initial therapy. Patients with TIA or stroke while taking aspirin are treated with ticlopidine as a validated alternative rather than warfarin. Anticoagulation is sometimes empirically used as third-line therapy for aspirin and ticlopidine failures, and it is also sometimes preferentially used in high-risk patients with severe symptomatic inoperable carotid or vertebrobasilar stenosis, but these practices remain unsupported by adequate clinical studies.

Surgical Treatment

The North American Symptomatic Carotid Endarterectomy Trial (NASCET) and European Carotid Surgery Trial compared surgery followed by medication with best medical therapy. Carotid endarterectomy was associated with a 15% absolute reduction in stroke and vascular death, with a complication rate of only 2% at these carefully selected centers. Based on these results, surgical candidates with 70% to 99% symptomatic carotid stenosis are recommended for surgery, taking into consideration the success rate of the available surgical center. Guidelines for medical management versus surgery in patients with 30% to 69% symptomatic stenosis are pending the second part of the NASCET trial, which is currently ongoing. Optimal management of asymptomatic carotid stenosis is unclear, but is currently being assessed.

CARDIOEMBOLIC STROKE

The increased sensitivity in identifying cardiac thrombi achieved using transesophageal echocardiography in selected patients suggests cardiogenic embolism is a more common potential cause of stroke than previously recognized. Antithrombotic therapies are highly effective for prophylaxis of cardiogenic embolism and are tailored to the specific cardiac disorder.

Five recent, large clinical trials evaluating primary therapy for patients with nonrheumatic atrial fibrillation have established a 5% per year overall stroke rate in this subgroup. Even in the absence of rheumatic heart disease, atrial fibrillation is the most common source of cardiogenic embolism, particularly in elderly women. These five trials in aggregate showed a mean stroke reduction of 70% with warfarin, but the risk of bleeding and the need for frequent monitoring associated with warfarin have discouraged its use in some patients (especially the elderly, the group at highest risk for stroke).

The Stroke Prevention in Atrial Fibrillation (SPAF) I and II studies have shown the effectiveness of aspirin for stroke prevention in low-risk patients. Patients younger than 75 years old without hypertension, recent heart failure, or prior thromboembolism had an ischemic stroke and systemic embolism rate of 0.5% per year in SPAF II. Considering all patients in this age group, there was a relative risk reduction of 0.7% per year with warfarin as compared with aspirin. Unfortunately, neither aspirin, 325 mg, nor warfarin anticoagulation adjusted to an international normalized ratio (INR) of 1.5 to 4 adequately provided protection for patients older than 75 years old, considering both ischemic and hemorrhagic strokes. At present, chronic anticoagulation with warfarin (INR 2–3) is recommended for atrial fibrillation patients with one or more risk factors for thromboembolism (Table 5). Aspirin and fixed-dose warfarin in combination are being compared with adjusted-dose warfarin (INR 2–3) in SPAF III as a possible alternative for high-risk patients.

Antithrombotic treatment of acute cardioembolic stroke raises some special concerns, particularly regarding the increased risk of hemorrhage into these infarcts. Spontaneous hemorrhagic transformation occurs in up to 40% of cardioembolic strokes and is especially likely in large infarcts. Hemorrhage is rare within the initial 12 hours following stroke so that the clinician should not be reassured if blood is not seen on the initial CT scan. The neurologic examination is a poor indicator of hemorrhagic transformation as well, because the degree of spontaneous bleeding that generally occurs does not affect clinical status. If such a patient is taking anticoagulants, however, there is the potential for massive bleeding and clinical devastation. The key dilemma regarding the timing of anticoagulation, that is the risk of recurrent emboli versus the risk of hemorrhage, depends on the cardiac source and the size of the infarct. Overall, the risk of recurrent emboli is about 10% during the first 2 weeks so that in most cases, the risk of serious bleeding with anticoagulation outweighs the risk of recurrent emboli. Seventy-five percent of infarcts destined to undergo hemorrhagic transformation will do so between 12 and 48 hours, mandating delay of anticoagulation by at least 48 hours, pending a repeat CT scan clear of blood (with the exception that patients with TIA or very small strokes can sometimes be anticoagulated sooner). Large infarcts, defined as involving greater than 30% of the affected cerebral hemisphere, warrant delay of anticoagulation for 5 to 14 days.

TABLE 5. **Predictors of Thromboembolic Risk in Atrial Fibrillation***

History of hypertension
Prior stroke/TIA
Diabetes
Recent heart failure (within 3 months)

*Based on the Stroke Prevention in Atrial Fibrillation (SPAF) I placebo data set.

REHABILITATION OF HEMIPLEGIA

method of
SUSAN J. GARRISON, M.D.
Baylor College of Medicine
Houston, Texas

Hemiplegia is a functional diagnosis. It refers to the loss of voluntary muscular movement of one side of the body. The cause of hemiplegia can be a multitude of factors, including cerebrovascular accident, arteriovenous malformation bleed, brain tumor, subdural hematoma, and traumatic brain injury.

The etiology of hemiplegia determines the prognosis for recovery, as well as the pattern of recovery. Typically, the recovery from a middle cerebrovascular accident is proximal to distal, and the arm independent of the leg. This does not necessarily occur in other etiologies, especially in those in which significant brain edema is present or surgical intervention has occurred. In such instances, there may be no discernible pattern. Therefore, sequential neurologic examinations become paramount in rehabilitative management. A diagram of rehabilitation for hemiplegia resulting from stroke is shown in Figure 1.

CANDIDATES

The appropriate candidate for rehabilitation is one who is capable of learning new information and is able to use it. There is a role, however, for caregiver training for a patient who has specific functional deficits that may improve over time but currently is unsafe when alone due to cognitive problems. The frail elderly patient often fits this category. Inability to follow verbal commands is not a valid reason for exclusion from rehabilitation; the patient may be capable of learning from visual cues such as demonstrations. Studies have shown that certain factors may indicate poor outcome from stroke rehabilitation (Table 1). At the time the information listed was compiled, the patient's ability to return home, rather than functional outcome, was used as

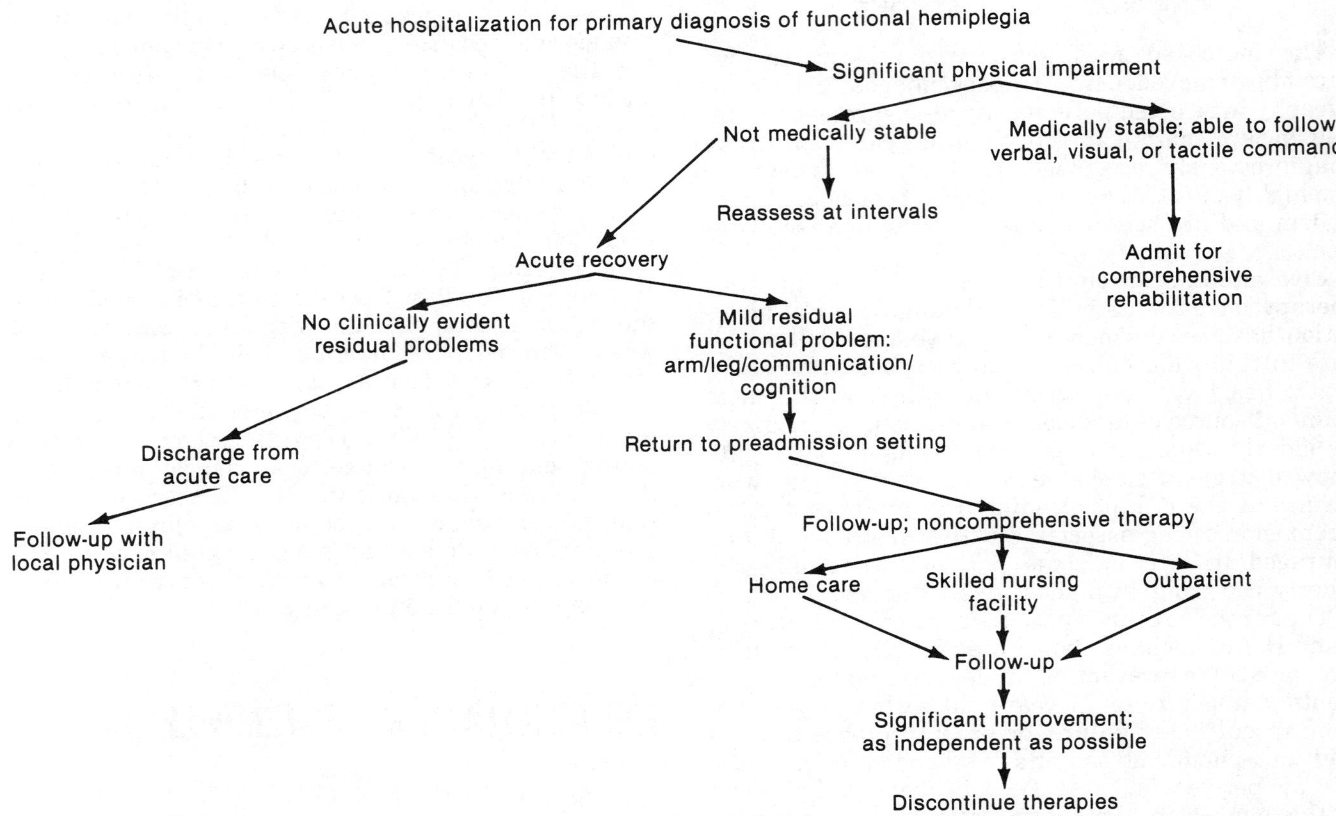

Figure 1. Flow diagram for rehabilitation of hemiplegia. (Adapted from Garrison SJ: Geriatric Stroke Rehabilitation, Rehabilitation of the Aging and Elderly Patient. Baltimore, MD, Williams & Wilkins, 1994.)

an indicator for success. Fortunately, the factors as cited do not apply to all hemiplegics. The ability to learn and apply new information as an adult is influenced by many things, including past educational experiences.

INTERDISCIPLINARY TEAM APPROACH

The interdisciplinary team approach is typically used for hemiplegic rehabilitation. As compared with a multidisciplinary team, this team is more focused on specific patient goals agreed on by the team, with input from the patient and family. Good communication is essential for this process to work smoothly. In many teams, the physician is the leader, but a designated team member may serve as the case manager, who is responsible for keeping the team on track in working toward the team goals. These goals include not only physical activities, such as independence in mobility and activities of daily living with adaptive devices, but also communication skills, psychosocial adjustment, and compliance with medical regimens. The team works to attain the patient's goals; however, this presumes that the patient is aware of achievable goals in his or her situation. Part of the team's responsibility is to educate the patient and family in what goals are appropriate so that the patient can make his or her own decisions, with input from rehabilitation professionals.

TABLE 1. **Prognostic Indicators of Poor Outcome (from Stroke Rehabilitation)**

Advanced age	Severe memory problems
Inability to understand commands	Urinary/bowel incontinence
Medical/surgical instability	Visual/spatial deficits
Previous stroke	

Adapted from Jongblood L: Prediction of function after stroke; a critical review. Stroke *17*:765–776, 1986. Reproduced with permission from the American Heart Association.

FUNCTIONAL EVALUATION

The functional evaluation involves assessment and documentation of the patient's physical and cognitive abilities. The team approach is valuable here due to the complexity of this process. In most cases, the cause of the hemiplegia may superimpose medical problems, such as generalized deconditioning, cardiovascular impairment, or decreased visual fields that even further impair abilities. If the hemiplegia is due to traumatic injury, there may also be musculoskeletal problems such as fractures. Any patient who has paralyzed or severely weakened upper and lower limbs on the same side of the body may experience difficulty in mobility, including bed positioning, transferring from bed to chair or wheelchair, as well as to the toilet, and ambulating, including on uneven ground and stair climbing. This patient may also have problems in performing self-care activities such as grooming, feeding, dressing, and toileting, known as activities of daily living. Over the years, many functional evaluation scales have been developed. The one most commonly used today in stroke and other diagnoses seen in medical rehabilitation is the Functional Independence Measure. Six areas, including self-care, sphincter management, mobility, locomotion, communication, and social cognition, are scored into seven levels by trained individuals at the time of rehabilitation admission and again at discharge. Results are compared regionally and nationally.

PATIENT AND FAMILY EDUCATION

Information regarding the cause of hemiplegia, medical problems, and expected treatment must be available to the patient and significant others, and repeated as often as necessary. Booklets, videos, and interaction with recovering hemiplegics assist those involved in accepting the situation. It is difficult to overeducate the patient about current needs, future rehabilitation plans, and goals. As the patient progresses through rehabilitation, support groups are helpful for recognition of similar problems and solutions. Caregivers should also be educated.

REHABILITATIVE TREATMENT

Typical rehabilitation of hemiplegia involves teaching the patient to use compensatory skills for lost functional abilities, while natural recovery occurs over time. This presumes that the patient is capable of learning as well as retaining new information, usually instructions, in the use of equipment, in addition to understanding, attempting, practicing, and successfully integrating new physical skills. Anything that may interfere with learning, such as illness, poor attention span, inability to see or hear normally, or psychosocial problems, usually does interfere at some time during the rehabilitative process. A well-functioning team can often identify these issues so that they may be addressed, if at all possible.

The typical time frame and treatment is indicated in Table 2. These are only suggestions; however, they can be modified to be useful in most situations. Such a comprehensive approach is not feasible unless there is a knowledgeable interdisciplinary team, committed to individualized patient care. This type of planning will be integrated into future treatment plans, termed *critical,* or *clinical, pathways.* Further refinement must be undertaken, however, to make this approach to rehabilitation feasible.

TABLE 2. **Rehabilitative Interventions and Suggested Time Frames**

Day 1–3 Post Event (Bedside)
Avoid positioning on affected extremities
Relieve common pressure areas, such as heels and sacral area
Document reflexes, tone, and muscular strength
Begin PROM and AAROM, daily by OT/PT or nursing
Dangle out of bed
Sit in chair
Document bowel/bladder function
Identify communication deficits
Implement dietary modification
Assess social situation
Day 3–5 (to Therapy Department)
Send to PT/OT department by wheelchair
Use wheelchair cushion; avoid donut cushion
Check ambulation potential in parallel bars
Baseline evaluations by PT/OT
Provide upper extremity sling
Remove Foley catheter; begin timed voiding
Day 7–10 (Acute Inpatient Rehabilitation)
Transfer activities (wheelchair to mat; wheelchair to bed)
Pre-gait activities
Admission to acute rehab unit
ADL practice—A.M. care and dressing
Psychological evaluation
Strategies for communication
Swallowing addressed by speech/dietary
Learing independence at wheelchair level
2–3 Weeks (Acute Inpatient Rehabilitation)
Upgrade gait—assistive device/AFO
Team family conference regarding prognosis and discharge planning
Therapeutic home evaluation
Upgrade from bedside commode to bathroom
3–6 Weeks
Family member/caretaker learns home program
Self-medications taught
Independent in dressing, grooming
Independent in wheelchair transfers and mobility
Bathroom and kitchen evaluations complete
Upgrade diet
Communication needs addressed
10–12 Weeks (Outpatient Physician Office Follow-Up)
Review functional abilities
Discuss safety issues (falls)
Renew/adjust outpatient therapy orders
Renew medications
Obtain follow-up with other physicians, as indicated
Assess need for further patient/family counseling

Abbreviations: PT = physical therapy; OT = occupational therapy; PROM = passive range of motions; AAROM = active assist range of motion; AFO = ankle foot orthosis; ADL = activities of daily living.

Adapted with permission from Garrison SJ: Stroke. *In* Garrison SJ (ed): Handbook of Physical Medicine and Rehabilitation Basics. Philadelphia, J. B. Lippincott, 1994.

COGNITIVE ISSUES AND DEPRESSION

Regardless of the etiology of the hemiplegia, the hemisphere as well as the area of the brain affected results in typical functional behaviors (Table 3). Awareness of these characteristics can greatly aid the team in teaching compensatory strategies, taking advantage of the hemiplegic's cognitive abilities, and minimizing methods that may result in patient confusion. Specific examples are presented in Table 4.

Depression can also negatively affect patient participation in rehabilitation. While it is normal to grieve over the loss of independence in body function, it is abnormal to cry constantly, change eating patterns drastically, or sleep too much or not at all. It is most common to see depression develop in the patient whose left hemisphere has been affected. The emotional response to hemiplegia, however, depends on a variety of factors in each case, including previous psychological traits, current physical health, social support, and many others. Patients may be unreliable in assessing their own degree of depression; family input as well as professional opinion may be required.

PHYSICAL THERAPY

Physical therapy for hemiplegia generally focuses on mobility issues and strengthening of major muscle groups, both those affected and those unaffected by

TABLE 3. **Characteristics of Right and Left Hemiplegic Patients**

Right Hemiplegic (Left Brain Injured)	Left Hemiplegic (Right Brain Injured)
Communication impairment	Visual-motor-perceptual problems; left side neglect
Learns from demonstration	Loss of visual-spatial memory
Can learn from mistakes	Overestimates abilities; impulsive
May require supervision due to communication problems	Requires supervision due to lack of insight/judgment; denies disabilities

Reprinted from Garrison SJ: Learning after stroke; left versus right brain injury. Topics in Geriatric Rehabilitation, *6*(3):45–52. With permission of Aspen Publishers, 1991.

the hemiplegia. All patients want to walk, but the focus is first mobility, even at the wheelchair level, while functional muscular recovery occurs. Typically, bed mobility, then static (supported) and dynamic (unsupported) sitting are taught and practiced. Use of overhead trapeze bed attachments is discouraged; patients typically strain their shoulders, and can easily be taught bed mobility without this device.

Application of the principles of typical recovery of hemiplegia due to stroke (proximal to distal muscle groups) indicates that the patient may be able to transfer to a wheelchair independently long before being able to ambulate with a gait-assistive device.

The typical progression of voluntary muscle function recovery allows use of a plastic ankle foot orthosis to provide enough stability at the ankle for ambulation. Hyperextension of the affected knee can be decreased by setting the ankle foot orthosis into approximately 5 degrees of dorsiflexion at the ankle, due to the center of gravity effect. Unfortunately, there is as yet no appropriate external bracing available to control absent or weak hip musculature. Therefore, the hemiplegic patient who does not have good proximal muscle strength in the lower limb, despite good to normal muscle strength below the knee, will not be a safe ambulator and, due to energy requirements, will eventually resort to wheelchair mobility. Double-upright, short leg metal braces are only indicated in specific cases of severe spasticity, where a plastic ankle foot orthosis creates sustained clonus at the ankle.

Types of Therapies

Traditional physical therapy involves the use of passive range of motion of hemiplegic limbs, with strengthening exercises as recovery occurs. Many other therapies have evolved, such as the neurophysiologic and developmentally based techniques by Brunnstrom, Rood, Bobath, Kabat, Knott, and Voss.

TABLE 4. **Teaching Approach and Rationale**

Learning Activity	Right Hemiplegia (Left Brain Injury)	Left Hemiplegia (Right Brain Injury)	Rationale
Transferring from wheelchair to mat	Present material as a unit, then break into separate parts and review	Present material in small steps, then sequence logically	Right hemisphere can synthesize; left hemisphere uses sequential logistic learning
Eating a meal	Present material from the left side	Present material from the right side	The unaffected hemisphere directs attention to the opposite side
Donning clothing	Use actual setting for teaching task	Simulate setting to ensure a quiet, distraction-free environment	Right hemisphere is reality-oriented; left hemisphere is easily alerted and habituates, causing short attention span and easy distractibility
Receiving feedback on efforts	Use facial expression frequently	Omit use of facial expression	Facial recognition is a right hemispheric function
Donning upper limb sling	Minimize speech	Verbal instructions should be simple and brief	Speech is a left hemisphere function; verbalization decreases attention span in right brain injury
Gait sequencing with assistive device	Employ prolonged therapy sessions	Encourage verbal self-cueing	Right hemisphere can remain alert over long periods; the linguistic mode may compensate for cognitive deficits
Performing bathroom transfers	Allow patient to observe others performing a learning task	Minimize instructional time spent in therapy department	Right hemisphere learns from observation; left hemisphere is easily distracted

Adapted from Shah M, Avidan R, Sine RD: Self-care training: Hemiplegia, lateralized stroke program, parkinsonism, arthritis, and spinal cord dsyfunction. *In* Sine RD, Liss SE, Roush RE, et al. (eds): Basic Rehabilitation Techniques. Rockville, MD, Aspen Publishers, 1988.

Most of these therapies incorporate use of cutaneous reflexes, proprioceptive stimuli, or specific task-appropriate postures to facilitate voluntary motor movements and to modify tone.

Usually, the best therapy technique involves a combination of the above-mentioned approaches, and it should be individualized based on that specific patient's response at any given time. Lack of response to a particular technique does not indicate that it will never be appropriate for the patient; the timing is important. A therapeutic approach not currently helpful may be beneficial at a later date.

Modalities typically are used for discomfort or lack of range of motion in the affected upper limb, particularly the shoulder, wrist, and hand. Application of superficial heat should be avoided, due to the risk of burns in insensate areas and the possible presence of cognitive impairment. Deep-heating apparati, such as ultrasound, can be used safely. Edematous hands and wrists typically respond best to ice, for analgesia, followed by aggressive passive range of motion and appropriate positioning. Avoid contrast baths because they may increase edema.

Occupational Therapy

Occupational therapy addresses issues of independence in activities of daily living, such as grooming, feeding, dressing, and toileting. After evaluation, patients are taught compensatory skills for lost abilities, using devices such as reachers, toilet aides, and long shoehorns or button fasteners, or both. Bathroom and kitchen evaluations and training demonstrate areas for further activities.

In recent years, emphasis on teaching one-handed activities has diminished; the patient is encouraged to integrate the use of the involved hand as an assist. This avoids a learned nonuse phenomenon of the affected hand. As the patient gains strength and independence in skills, and motor recovery in the affected upper limb occurs, more use of the arm is expected. At first, the hand may only be used as an assist, but as fine motor abilities improve over time, additional two-handed activities are emphasized.

Both physical therapy and occupational therapy may employ functional electrical stimulation (FES), a type of biofeedback used to improve sensation of muscle contraction and resultant joint motion in hemiplegic limbs. Physical therapy predominately uses FES in the anterior tibialis muscle to improve ankle dorsiflexion during gait. Occupational therapy uses FES at the affected shoulder to assist in increased movement and possibly to decrease shoulder subluxation. Functional electrical stimulation also may assist in wrist extension.

Speech Therapy

The role of speech therapy is to facilitate a form of communication that allows the patient to be more independent. It is usually the left brain–injured, right-hemiplegic patient who exhibits difficulty with speech. Devices such as communication boards may not be useful for the patient who does not have full use of both upper limbs or has a visual field deficit. Speech pathologists may also screen for decreased auditory acuity and recommend further evaluation or devices through audiologists. Co-treatment, in which the speech pathologist works in the gym with physical and/or occupational therapists, may improve the ability of the patient to cooperate with therapists in the treatment plan through enhancing communication.

Equipment Needs

Specialists in physical and occupational therapy may work together to make recommendations for an appropriate wheelchair for patients currently unable to ambulate for long distances. A typical wheelchair for a hemiplegic patient is a lightweight, adult, hemi-height (usually 18 to 21 inches from seat to floor) folding wheelchair with removable desk armrests and removable, swing-away footrests, with heel loops. Tubeless pneumatic tires allow ease of propulsion over uneven ground as well as infrequent maintenance. A lapboard may be used for the nonambulatory patient who has difficulty maintaining good sitting posture or requires support of the affected arm, for example, to assist in positioning management of shoulder subluxation. The lower-than-standard seat height allows the patient to propel the chair independently after practice, using the unaffected arm and leg.

The use of a sling for reduction of shoulder subluxation in the affected upper limb has always been controversial; there is no one best design, and the sling itself reinforces the internally rotated flexed elbow and wrist position of the arm. If an ambulatory patient has a dependent arm with little or no muscular movement or tone, a sling should be used when the patient is ambulating to prevent injury to the affected arm and the development of dependent edema. When the patient is sitting, the elbow can be supported by an arm rest or pillow. The sling should not be worn at all in bed due to the poor positioning of the arm that it creates. As tone and muscular recovery occur in the shoulder, subluxation decreases. When the patient stands, typically proximal tone reduces the subluxation. If, however, the hemiplegic patient has more distal than proximal tone, a sling may be required when standing, until the proximal tone improves, if ever.

Once sufficient motor recovery has occurred in the proximal muscles of the affected lower limb and ambulation with a gait-assistive device is possible, the wheelchair should be used only for long distances. An ambulatory hemiplegic patient should sit in a regular chair instead of a wheelchair. Electric mobility devices, such as wheelchairs and scooters, are not indicated for these types of patients who have normal use of their unaffected limbs.

Usually, the ambulatory hemiplegic patient benefits from sequential use of one-handed gait devices, from more to least stable. Typically, a hemi-walker (pyramid cane), then wide-based quad cane, then a narrow-based quad cane, and finally, a single-point cane may be used. Some patients who have some use of their affected hand may use a rolling-gait device, such as a rolling walker or a grocery cart, in the therapy gym for training purposes. This is rarely used independently for gait.

COMPLICATIONS

The etiology of the hemiplegia will, of course, predispose the patient to certain complications. Any previous medical or surgical problems may also influence the rehabilitation outcome. For example, a patient with osteoarthritis affecting the knees may experience increased discomfort in the nonhemiplegic knee when weight-bearing activities must be accomplished by reliance on that knee. In general, the patient who is hemiplegic as a result of a middle cerebrovascular accident is at risk for a second stroke, seizures, deep venous thrombosis and subsequent pulmonary embolus, and shoulder-hand syndrome, a type of reflex sympathetic dystrophy.

SWALLOWING

Difficulty with swallowing is not specific to the side of the brain injury. The swallowing process, which is not a reflex, is not related to the gag reflex; a positive gag response simply means that the patient can regurgitate stomach contents and may then aspirate. If swallowing problems are suspected by a history of cough or by poor voluntary swallow (silent aspiration can occur without coughing), a swallowing attempt using regular foods should be assessed. If indicated by poor voluntary swallowing, trained personnel such as speech pathologists may participate with the radiologist in a modified barium swallow procedure. Appropriate dietary modification is then indicated in an effort to improve nutrition and prevent aspiration pneumonia.

SPASTICITY

Antispasticity medications including baclofen (Lioresal) and dantrolene (Dantrium) may be indicated. Diazepam (Valium) is not indicated due to the possibility of depression. Baclofen, although frequently used, is not approved for spasticity of cerebral origin and may interfere with cognition. Dantrolene, working at the skeletal muscle level, requires follow-up of liver enzymes, specifically serum glutamic-oxaloacetic transaminase (SGOT) and serum glutamic-pyruvic transaminase (SGPT). In severe cases, motor point blocks of specific muscles, using phenol or Botox,* for example, may be indicated. Less permanent measures include the use of biofeedback and tone-inhibitive orthotic devices, such as hand splints and plastic ankle braces with customized indentations in appropriate areas, to minimize tone problems. Use of these devices always puts the patient at risk of skin breakdown at pressure points; frequent skin checks are necessary.

*Investigational drug in the United States.

PROGNOSIS/PREDICTIVE OUTCOMES

The hemiplegic patient will experience functional recovery determined by the etiology of the hemiplegia. A patient whose recovery is slow will typically continue a prolonged recovery period. Conversely, a patient who rapidly regains function will usually continue this pattern. Recovery may cease at any time, however, with residual functional deficits despite continued physical and occupational therapy. Communication deficits, including speech, reading, and writing, may improve over a long time period. Any patient who has experienced a hemorrhagic brain lesion is at greater risk for increased tone that may impair muscular recovery.

EPILEPSY IN ADOLESCENTS AND ADULTS

method of
THOMAS R. BROWNE, M.D.
Boston University School of Medicine
Boston Department of Veterans Affairs Medical Center
Boston, Massachusetts

Epilepsy is a common disease, with a prevalence estimated at 6 to 34 per 1000 population. Hughlings Jackson put forth the modern definition of a seizure in 1870: "an occasional, excessive, and disorderly discharge of nerve tissue." The points to note are that there is an excessive rate of firing of brain cells, that this firing occurs occasionally (i.e., the firing begins and ends abruptly), and that the usual methods of controlling neuronal discharge break down.

APPROACH TO THE PATIENT WITH EPILEPSY

Determine Type of Epileptic Seizure

The first step in managing a patient who may have epilepsy is establishing definitively whether or not the patient has epilepsy. If a patient who does not have epilepsy is given the diagnosis of epilepsy, he or she is unnecessarily subjected to many inconveniences, including medication that may produce serious side effects, expensive laboratory tests, loss of a driver's license, and possible loss of employment.

If a patient has epilepsy, it is crucial to determine accurately which type(s) of epileptic seizure the patient has, in order that he or she be given correct therapy. The diagnosis of seizure type should be made according to the International Classification of Epileptic Seizures (Table 1). Persons not familiar with this diagnostic system should consult a textbook on epilepsy. An incorrect seizure diagnosis often results in the patient's being given medication that will not control the seizure disorder and that may cause serious side effects.

TABLE 1. **International Classification of Epileptic Seizures**

Partial (Focal, Local) Seizures
Simple partial seizures (consciousness not impaired)
With motor signs
With sensory symptoms
With autonomic symptoms or signs
With psychic symptoms
Complex partial seizures (temporal lobe or psychomotor seizures) (consciousness usually impaired)
Simple partial onset followed by impairment of consciousness
With simple partial features (see first section of table) followed by impaired consciousness
With automatisms
With impairment of consciousness at onset
With impairment of consciousness only
With automatisms
Partial seizures evolving to secondarily generalized seizures (tonic-clonic, tonic, or clonic)
Simple partial seizures (A) evolving to generalized seizures
Complex partial seizures (B) evolving to generalized seizures
Simple partial seizures evolving to complex partial seizures evolving to generalized seizures

Generalized Seizures (convulsive or nonconvulsive)
Absence (petit mal) seizures
Myoclonic seizures
Clonic seizures
Tonic seizures
Tonic-clonic (grand mal) seizures
Atonic seizures

The best way to diagnose which type of seizure a patient has is to actually observe a seizure, although the physician usually does not have the opportunity to do so. Often, the most important differential diagnostic information is contained in the history gathered from the patient, reliable observers, or both. The physician must elicit the exact details of events before, during, and after the patient's seizures.

The electroencephalogram (EEG) is a helpful diagnostic tool in the investigation of a seizure disorder. It confirms the presence of abnormal electrical activity, gives information regarding the type of seizure disorder, and discloses the location of the seizure focus. There are instances in which the routine EEG is normal in spite of the fact that the patient has seizures or is suspected of having them. Under these circumstances, the study is repeated after the patient is deprived of sleep for an entire night, and special (e.g., temporal or nasopharyngeal) leads may also be employed. This procedure is helpful in bringing out the abnormality in many cases, especially if discharges arise from the temporal lobe.

If the history unequivocally points to a seizure disorder, the patient should be treated despite a so-called normal waking and sleep-deprived EEG. The usual EEG study samples only about an hour of time and is normal in a significant percentage of patients with epilepsy. In cases in which it is not certain if the patient has epilepsy or in which it is not certain which type of seizure a patient has despite a careful history, physical examination, and routine waking and sleep-deprived EEG, the diagnosis often can be established by prolonged monitoring of the EEG.

THERAPY

Treat Underlying Causes and Precipitating Factors

Epilepsy is a symptom, not a disease. A seizure can be a symptom of old or recent cerebral trauma, a brain tumor, a brain abscess, encephalitis, meningitis, a metabolic disturbance, drug intoxication, drug withdrawal, and many other disease processes. It is imperative that the underlying cause of a patient's seizures be identified and treated so that a reversible cerebral disease process is not overlooked and so that seizure control can be facilitated.

Determining the cause of a patient's seizure disorder involves a combination of history taking, physical examination, and laboratory tests. The history should include questions regarding family history of epilepsy, birth complications, febrile convulsions, middle ear infections and sinus infections (which may erode through bone and cause cerebral focus), head trauma, alcohol or drug abuse, and symptoms of malignancy. The physical examination should be directed toward uncovering evidence of past or recent head trauma, infections of the ears and sinuses, congenital abnormalities (e.g., hemiatrophy, stigmata of tuberous sclerosis), focal or diffuse neurologic abnormalities, stigmata of alcohol or drug abuse, and signs of malignancy. Usually, the following laboratory tests should be performed in evaluating the cause of a newly diagnosed seizure disorder: metabolic screen, EEG recording in waking and sleep states, and magnetic resonance imaging (preferred) or computed tomographic (acceptable) scan. A lumbar puncture (for opening pressure, cell counts, protein, glucose, cytology, culture, and serology) should be performed if infection or malignancy is suspected.

In addition to determining the underlying cause(s) of a patient's seizure disorder, it is also important to identify and manage factors that precipitate seizures in a given individual, such as anxiety, sleep deprivation, and alcohol withdrawal. Management of such precipitating factors reduces seizure frequency as well as the patient's need for medication.

Identify and Deal with Psychological and Social Problems

Seizures are a relatively rare phenomenon for most patients. The psychosocial consequences of having epilepsy, however, are present all the time. Loss of one's driver's license, employment, self-esteem, and position in peer groups are all potential problems and may cause more suffering than the seizures themselves. Furthermore, the anxiety associated with these psychosocial consequences of epilepsy may precipitate seizures in some patients. One must anticipate that the patient will experience psychosocial problems as a consequence of having epilepsy. Also, one must be prepared to assist the patient by carefully explaining the nature of the medical problems and the effect the problems will have on driving and employment by providing emotional support, by giving the patient an opportunity to talk through his or her problems, and by referring the patient to various resources available to assist the patient with epilepsy (e.g., social workers, epilepsy societies, vocational counselors).

Begin Monotherapy with Drug of Choice

Once the exact type of seizure has been determined, the physician should initiate monotherapy (single-drug therapy) with the drug that has shown the best combination of high efficacy and low toxicity in comparative studies of drugs for the patient's seizure type. If a patient has more than one type of seizure, therapy should begin with the drug of choice for the combination of seizure types present (see later).

The single-drug approach for initial treatment is based on a growing body of evidence indicating that monotherapy with an appropriately selected drug pushed to the adequate dosing rate will control seizures in a majority of patients and that polytherapy (more than one drug therapy) exposes the patient to several unnecessary risks. Monotherapy for simple partial, complex partial, and tonic-clonic seizures with carbamazepine or phenytoin using the guidelines outlined here results in satisfactory long-term seizure control in 70% to 90% of patients. Monotherapy for absence seizures with ethosuximide, valproic acid, or clonazepam results in satisfactory long-term seizure control in 50% to 90% of patients and complete seizure control in 50% of patients. Factors that appear to be associated with failure of modern monotherapy include persistent noncompliance, drug allergy, large or progressive brain lesions, partial seizures, more than one type of seizure, neuropsychiatric handicaps, and high pretreatment seizure frequency.

The risks of unnecessary polytherapy are many. Chronic toxicity is associated with the use of any antiepileptic drug. Polytherapy may include barbiturates, which are associated with a high risk for cognitive and behavioral toxicity. Other risks of unnecessary polytherapy include drug allergy, drug interactions, exacerbation of seizures, and the inability to evaluate the effectiveness of individual antiepileptic drugs.

Push the First Drug Tried

The first drug tried for a seizure disorder is usually among the least toxic drugs available, and the physician must be certain that he or she has obtained the maximum possible therapeutic effect from the first drug before adding other drugs. Therapy usually begins with a so-called average dose of antiepileptic drug. If the seizures are controlled with this average dose and there are no serious side effects, no further changes are necessary. If the seizures are not controlled with this dose and there is no serious drug toxicity, the dose of the drug should be systematically increased until the seizures are controlled or until side effects preclude further dosage increase.

The drug plasma concentration should be determined if a patient's seizures are not controlled by an average or high drug dosage. There are many correctable causes of lower than expected drug plasma concentration, including inadequate dosing rate, noncompliance, poor absorption, drug interactions, generic drug substitution, pregnancy, and patient error. It would be a serious error to substitute or to add a more toxic drug because the patient has a low plasma concentration of the first drug. A drug cannot be said to be ineffective until it is documented that the seizures are not controlled with a high therapeutic plasma concentration of the drug unless drug toxicity precludes reaching such concentrations.

The therapeutic range of drug plasma concentrations represents values applicable to average patients. Some patients require higher drug plasma concentrations than the therapeutic range for good seizure control. If a patient has a high therapeutic plasma concentration of a nontoxic drug, poor seizure control, and no drug side effects, the best approach usually is to increase the dose of the first drug rather than add a more toxic second drug.

Add Additional Drugs

If the first drug is pushed to its maximum tolerated dose and seizures still are not controlled, a second antiepileptic drug should be added. In general, it is best to add the second drug and continue administration of the first drug (at least temporarily) because (1) the first drug will provide protection while the plasma concentration of the second drug is being built up, (2) discontinuing the first drug may result in withdrawal activation of the seizure disorder, and (3) there is evidence that two antiepileptic drugs in combination may control seizures in some patients when either drug alone does not.

When a therapeutic plasma concentration of the second drug is obtained, the physician should consider tapering the patient off the first drug because of the many hazards of chronic polytherapy. The decision to taper the patient off the first drug must be individualized and should take into consideration the antiepileptic effect of the first drug when it is given alone, the side effects of the first drug, and the psychosocial consequences to the patient of having a seizure if withdrawal of the first drug results in loss of complete seizure control. The adverse effects of antiepileptic drugs on behavior and cognition are so great that one should attempt to minimize the number of these drugs given to children. In adults, the hazards of polytherapy must be weighed against the risk of loss of job, driver's license, or both if withdrawal of the first drug results in a recurrence of seizures. If it is elected to withdraw the first drug, the withdrawal should be done slowly (discussed in detail later).

A third drug should not be added until it is documented that seizures cannot be controlled with maximum tolerated doses of the first two drugs tried. It is usually better to add a third drug (at least temporarily) than to substitute the third drug for the first or second drug for reasons similar to those cited earlier for adding rather than substituting the second drug. After a therapeutic serum concentration of the third drug is reached, the physician may elect to withdraw one of the first two drugs using the guidelines outlined earlier.

Duration of Therapy

Uncontrolled seizures and seizures due to a progressive neurologic illness (e.g., astrocytoma) are indications for continuing antiepileptic drug therapy indefinitely. Antiepileptic drug therapy usually should be maintained for a minimum of 2 to 5 years after diagnosis of epilepsy, even if the patient has no further seizures. When a patient has been free of seizures for 2 to 5 years on antiepileptic drug therapy, the need for continued therapy can be re-evaluated. Risk factors have been identified that help evaluate the likelihood of seizures recurring after medication has been discontinued.

Patients who continue to have an abnormal EEG (spikes, sharp waves, paroxysmal activity, or nonparoxysmal abnormalities) have a 50% chance of seizure recurrence if antiepileptic medication is discontinued. Other risk factors include (1) the occurrence of many generalized seizures before control with medication, (2) long duration between onset of therapy and seizure control, (3) presence of a known structural lesion or neurologic deficit, (4) mental retardation, (5) onset of seizures before 2 years of age, (6) adult onset of complex partial seizures, and (7) more than one seizure type.

Each decision must be made on an individual basis. A history of seizure frequency and risk factors must be obtained. A routine EEG is mandatory, and a long-term EEG recording is sometimes desirable. The probability of recurrent seizures, the consequences of having another seizure, and the benefits of living without medication must be discussed with the patient, and the judgment must be weighted by the needs of the individual.

If it is elected to discontinue antiepileptic therapy, medication should be withdrawn slowly. Elimination of one pill per day every five elimination half-lives is probably the optimal regimen. More rapid tapering of therapy may precipitate seizures, and more prolonged withdrawal probably does not reduce the risk of seizure recurrence.

Antiepileptic Drug Therapy During Pregnancy

Infants born to women with epilepsy who are taking no medication have an increased risk of malformations, including cleft lip and palate, cardiac anomalies, microcephaly, and digit abnormalities in varying combinations (fetal epilepsy syndrome).

Many antiepileptic drugs appear to increase the risk of fetal epilepsy syndrome, and this risk may be dose dependent. Lowering of body stores of folic acid may be part of the mechanism of production of fetal epilepsy syndrome. Women of childbearing potential should be advised of these risks. Women with epilepsy, whether they are receiving medication or not, should take supplemental folic acid (e.g., 4 mg per day) and should have normal plasma and red blood cell folic acid levels *before* becoming pregnant. If possible, antiepileptic drugs should be discontinued during pregnancy. If not, the lowest effective dose of the least teratogenic drug should be administered. Unfortunately, the relative teratogenicity of antiepileptic drugs in humans has never been established definitively. Any combination of two antiepileptic drugs appears to be much more teratogenic than any single-drug regimen, thus a strong argument for monotherapy. There are some controversial data that phenobarbital may have less teratogenic risk than alternative agents. Carbamazepine and valproic acid may possess greater risk than alternative agents because of the increased risk of spina bifida with these two drugs.

The dosing rate necessary to maintain a given plasma concentration increases because of increased volume of distribution, increased biotransformation, and decreased absorption. Antiepileptic drugs may lower maternal vitamin K level and may increase the risk of neonatal hemorrhage because of depression of vitamin K–dependent clotting factors. The mother who is taking antiepileptic drugs should be given vitamin K (20 mg per day orally) during the last month of pregnancy, and the infant should be given vitamin K (1 mg intramuscularly) at birth.

ANTIEPILEPTIC DRUGS OF FIRST CHOICE FOR SIMPLE PARTIAL, COMPLEX PARTIAL (PSYCHOMOTOR, TEMPORAL LOBE), AND TONIC-CLONIC (GRAND MAL) SEIZURES
(Table 2)

Simple partial, complex partial (psychomotor, temporal lobe), and tonic-clonic (grand mal) seizures are the most common types of seizure disorders in adolescents and adults (Table 2). Note that tonic-clonic seizures may be focal (partial seizures secondarily generalized) or generalized (primarily generalized) in onset (see Table 1). Carbamazepine (Tegretol), phenobarbital, phenytoin (Dilantin), primidone (Mysoline), and valproic acid (Depakote) (which is not yet Food and Drug Administration [FDA] approved for these indications) are the drugs that have been employed as initial therapy for partial and tonic-clonic seizures. These five drugs have been compared in two large Veterans Administration Cooperative Studies. Primidone was inferior to the other four drugs for all seizure types because of a significantly higher incidence of intolerable toxicity.

Carbamazepine and phenytoin are the two drugs of choice for partial seizures and partial seizures secondarily generalized based on the following data: (1) carbamazepine and phenytoin have fewer side effects than phenobarbital or valproic acid regardless of seizure type, (2) carbamazepine and phenytoin are more effective than phenobarbital or valproic acid for complex partial seizures, and (3) there were no statistically significant differences in efficacy or toxicity when carbamazepine was compared with phenytoin.

Three new drugs have been approved by the FDA for partial and tonic-clonic seizures: felbamate (Fel-

TABLE 2. **Antiepileptic Drugs of Choice**

Seizure Type	Drug(s) of First Choice*	Drugs of Second Choice*	Alternative Drugs*
Partial (simple, complex, secondarily generalized tonic-clonic)	Carbamazepine Phenytoin	Gabapentin Lamotrigine‡	Felbamate Phenobarbital Primidone Valproic acid
Primarily generalized tonic-clonic	Phenytoin Valproic acid†	Carbamazepine Valproic acid	Phenobarbital Primidone
Absence	Ethosuximide Valproic acid†	Valproic acid	Clonazepam

*Listed alphabetically within groups.
†Used if combination of absence and tonic-clonic seizures present.
‡Investigational drug in the United States.

batol), gabapentin (Neurontin), and lamotrigine (Lamictal).* Only felbamate is approved as initial therapy for these seizure types; all three drugs are approved for use when first-choice drugs fail. There are no published studies on the long-term efficacy and safety of any of these three drugs as initial monotherapy. The Veterans Administration Cooperative Studies have established that initial monotherapy with carbamazepine or phenytoin will produce a satisfactory long-term result in approximately 80% of patients. At this time, it is the author's practice not to use any of these three drugs as initial therapy.

For primarily generalized tonic-clonic seizures, carbamazepine, phenytoin, and valproic acid appear to be equally effective. Valproic acid has efficacy against absence and myoclonic seizures (sometimes associated with primarily generalized tonic-clonic seizures), whereas carbamazepine and phenytoin do not. Absence seizures may worsen in some patients taking carbamazepine or phenobarbital. Valproic acid is the drug of first choice for persons with primarily generalized tonic-clonic plus absence and/or myoclonic seizures.

SECOND-CHOICE DRUGS FOR SIMPLE PARTIAL, COMPLEX PARTIAL, AND TONIC-CLONIC SEIZURES

There are no definitive published trials establishing the drug of second choice for patients failing a trial with a first-choice drug (carbamazepine or phenytoin). Probably the most common practice is to add or substitute (see earlier) the other first-choice drug based on results of initial therapy studies.

Three older drugs (phenobarbital, primidone, valproic acid) and three new drugs (felbamate, gabapentin, lamotrigine) have been used as alternative drugs in patients failing to respond to carbamazepine or phenytoin, or both. These six drugs appear to be approximately equally effective (a good response in one-third of patients refractory to carbamazepine and phenytoin) based on indirect comparisons. Gabapentin and lamotrigine appear to be less toxic than the other four drugs, again based on indirect comparisons. Gabapentin has no drug interactions with other antiepileptic drugs, and lamotrigine has clinically significant drug interactions only with carbamazepine and valproic acid. The other four drugs have clinically significant drug interactions with several antiepileptic drugs. These observations indicate that gabapentin or lamotrigine should be used first when one is selecting a second-choice drug.

*Investigational drug in the United States.

DETAILS OF DRUGS USED FOR SIMPLE PARTIAL, COMPLEX PARTIAL, AND TONIC-CLONIC SEIZURES (LISTED ALPHABETICALLY)

Mechanism of Action of Antiepileptic Drugs

Antiepileptic drugs are divided into six types, depending on their mechanism of action. Type I drugs (carbamazepine, phenytoin) prevent activation of the sodium channel and block sustained repetitive firing of axons. Type II drugs (clonazepam, phenobarbital, primidone, valproic acid) prevent activation of sodium channels and enhance chloride (inhibitory ion) conductance into neurons. Type III drugs inhibit T calcium currents, which appear to be the generators of the three-per-second discharges characteristic of absence seizures (ethosuximide). Type IV drugs block presynaptic release of excitatory neurotransmitters (lamotrigine). Type V drugs enhance chloride conductance and inhibit N-methyl-D-aspartase (NMDA, excitatory) responses (felbamate). Type VI drugs function by an unknown mechanism (gabapentin). These differences in mechanism suggest that rational drug combinations (rational polytherapy) of drugs may be more effective than random selection of drug combinations. As noted earlier, however, there are no hard data on the relative efficacy and safety of the various possible drug combinations.

Carbamazepine (Tegretol)

Advantages

Carbamazepine was found to be one of the two best drugs in the Veterans Administration Cooperative Studies. It is relatively nonsedating (sedation is mild and similar to that of phenytoin) and does not have the cosmetic side effects of phenytoin.

Disadvantages

A loading dose of carbamazepine cannot be administered by any route. The drug must be given in divided doses and must be started at a low dose, and the dosage must be built up over time. There is an increased risk of spina bifida in infants born to mothers taking carbamazepine during pregnancy.

Pharmacokinetics (Table 3)

Approximately 75% to 85% of an orally administered dose of brand name Tegretol, 200-mg tablets, is slowly absorbed after oral administration. The bioavailability of generic carbamazepines is usually less than that of Tegretol. Carbamazepine is 70% to 80% protein bound. Carbamazepine is metabolized by the liver into 32 or more metabolites, some of which (especially epoxide) possess antiepileptic activity. Carbamazepine biotransformation exhibits time-dependent pharmacokinetics (self-induction), which means that the serum concentration may fall unexpectedly during the first 4 months of administration when self-induction occurs.

Usual Adult Dosage

The initial dosage is 200 mg twice daily, increased at weekly intervals by adding up to 200 mg per day using a three- or four-times daily regimen until the best response is obtained. The dosage generally should not exceed 1000 mg daily in children 12 to 15 years of age or 1200 mg daily in patients older than 15 years of age. Doses up to 1600 mg daily have been used in adults in rare instances. The maintenance dosage is adjusted to the minimum effective level, usually 800 to 1200 mg daily.

Tegretol OROS* (should be FDA approved in 1994) is a constant-release carbamazepine preparation using osmotic pump tablet technology. Twice-daily dosing with the OROS formulation produces mean plasma concentrations similar to those obtained with three-times-daily administration of standard carbamazepine tablets with less peak to trough variability. This reduces the toxicity associated with high peak values and the breakthrough seizures associated with low trough values. This author believes that the OROS formulation is the carbamazepine formulation of choice.

Toxicity

Local toxicity consists of gastric irritability (usually managed by taking the drug after meals). Dose-related toxicity includes diplopia or blurred vision, dizziness, drowsiness, ataxia, headache, tremor, dystonia, chorea, depression, irritability, psychosis, convulsions, water retention (inappropriate antidiuretic-hormone–like syndrome), congestive heart failure, and cardiac arrhythmias.

Idiosyncratic toxicities are rash (common) and, more rarely, anemia, agranulocytosis, leukopenia, thrombocytopenia; hypersensitivity syndrome (der-

*Investigational drug in the United States.

TABLE 3. **Pharmacokinetics of Antiepileptic Drugs***

Drugs	Indications	Starting Dose (mg per day)	Maintenance Dose (mg per day)	Elimination Half-Life (h)	Time to Steady-State Plasma Concentration (days)	Therapeutic Range of Plasma Concentration (μg/mL)
Carbamazepine (Tegretol)	T-C, CP, SP	400	600–1200	14–27	3–4	4–12
Clonazepam (Klonopin)	A/R, AT, M	1.5	1.5–20	20–40	—	—
Ethosuximide (Zarontin)	A	500	500–1500	20–60	7–10	40–120
Felbamate (Felbatol)	T-C/R, CP/R	1200	2400–3600	20–23†	—	—
Gabapentin (Neurontin)	T-C/R, CP/R	300	900–3600	5–7	—	—
Lamotrigine‡ (Lamictal)	T-C/R, CP/R	100	300–500	12–50 (monotherapy) 7–23 (polytherapy)	—	—
Phenobarbital	T-C/R, CP/R, SP/R	90	90–240	46–136	12–21	10–40
Phenytoin (Dilantin)	T-C, CP	300	300–500	10–34	7–12	10–20
Primidone (Mysoline)	T-C/R, CP/R, SP/R	125	750–1500	6–18	4–7	5–12
Valproic acid (Depakene, Depakote)	A	1000	1000–4000	6–15	1–2	40–150

Abbreviations: A = absence; AT = atonic; CP = complex partial; SP = simple partial; M = myoclonic; /R = refractory to first-choice drugs; T-C = tonic-clonic.
*All values are for adults.
†Less in the presence of other antiepileptic drugs.
‡Investigational drug in the United States.

matitis, eosinophilia, lymphadenopathy, splenomegaly); and cholestatic and hepatocellular jaundice. The rate of fatal idiosyncratic reactions with carbamazepine is estimated currently at 1 in 100,000 to 200,000 patients. Although this factor is a matter of concern, this risk is in a range similar to other commonly used drugs, such as penicillin.

Drug Interactions

Adding carbamazepine may increase the plasma concentration of phenytoin and lower the plasma concentrations of felbamate, lamotrigine, oral contraceptives, theophylline, and valproic acid. Propoxyphene, erythromycin, chloramphenicol, isoniazid, verapamil, and cimetidine may elevate the plasma carbamazepine concentration, whereas phenobarbital, phenytoin, felbamate, and primidone may lower the plasma carbamazepine concentration.

Disease States

Carbamazepine may precipitate or enhance congestive heart failure. Its use should be avoided in this setting or in cases in which major arrhythmias are a concern. Plasma levels and potential toxicity need to be closely watched if the drug is used in patients with renal or hepatic disease.

Pregnancy

In common with several other antiepileptic drugs, there is a 2% to 3% increase in fetal epilepsy syndrome in infants born to mothers taking carbamazepine. In addition, there is a 1% risk of spina bifida (vs. 1 in 1500 in the normal population).

Felbamate (Felbatol)

Advantages

Felbamate is sometimes effective when first-choice drugs have failed. It has no serious toxicity, and there is no need to monitor laboratory values with its use.

Disadvantages

There are significant drug interactions between felbamate and other antiepileptic drugs. Other antiepileptic drugs must be discontinued because of drug interactions, with the risk of worsening seizures in some patients. There are significant nuisance side effects (nausea, headache, drowsiness, sleep disturbance) in some patients. Three-times-daily dosing is required, and felbamate cannot be given as a loading dose. Parenteral administration of felbamate is not possible. Last, felbamate is more expensive than the older drugs.

Pharmacokinetics

Felbamate is well absorbed by the oral route. Felbamate is 22% to 25% protein bound, and its binding extent is not concentration dependent. The elimination half-life of felbamate is 20 to 23 hours when taken alone but less when taken with most other antiepileptic drugs. Approximately half of a dose of felbamate is excreted unchanged in the urine. The remaining half is excreted as metabolites formed by the liver. The therapeutic range of felbamate serum concentration has not been established.

Usual Adult Dosage

Because of drug interactions, the best efficacy and safety results for refractory partial or tonic-clonic seizures are obtained if other drugs are slowly removed when felbamate is added. This is accomplished by initiating felbamate at 1200 mg per day in three or four divided doses. Reduce concomitant antiepileptic drug (AED) dosage by one-third at the initiation of felbamate therapy. At week 2, increase felbamate dosage to 2400 mg per day while reducing the dosage of other AEDs up to an additional one-third of their original dosage. At week 3, increase felbamate dosage up to 3600 mg per day and continue to reduce the dosage of other AEDs as clinically indicated.

If the physician does not wish to discontinue concomitant AEDs, the dosage of other AEDs should be decreased by 20% when felbamate therapy is initiated. Further reduction in concomitant AED dosage may be necessary to minimize side effects due to drug interactions. Increase the dosage of felbamate by 1200-mg-per-day increments at weekly intervals to 3600 mg per day.

Toxicity

Local toxicity includes nausea, anorexia, dyspepsia, constipation, diarrhea, and abdominal pain. Dose-related toxicity includes nausea, vomiting, anorexia, weight loss, fatigue, somnolence, headache, insomnia, nightmares, and dizziness. Reduction of concomitant AEDs may decrease these side effects. No long-term toxicity is known. Rash (rare) is an idiosyncratic toxicity.

Drug Interactions

Addition of felbamate increases the plasma concentration of phenytoin, valproic acid, and carbamazepine epoxide (the active carbamazepine metabolite) and reduces the plasma concentration of carbamazepine. Carbamazepine and phenytoin reduce the plasma concentration of felbamate.

Pregnancy

There are no adequate studies on felbamate in pregnant women.

Gabapentin (Neurontin)

Advantages

Gabapentin is sometimes effective when first-choice drugs have failed. It has no serious toxicity, minimal dose-dependent toxicity, and no drug interactions. There is no need to monitor laboratory values.

Disadvantages

A three-times-daily dosing is required, and gabapentin cannot be given as loading dose. Parenteral administration is not possible. Gabapentin is more expensive than older drugs.

Pharmacokinetics (Table 3)

Gabapentin has a bioavailability of approximately 60%. Gabapentin is less than 3% protein bound. The drug is eliminated by renal excretion as unchanged gabapentin. Gabapentin is not appreciably metabolized in humans. The gabapentin elimination half-life is 5 to 7 hours and is not affected by dose or other drugs. A therapeutic range for gabapentin plasma concentration has not been established.

Usual Adult Dosage

Considerable experience indicates that daily doses of 900 to 1800 mg are effective and well tolerated when gabapentin is used as add-on therapy for refractory partial or tonic-clonic seizures. Lesser experience indicates that higher doses up to 3600 mg per day are usually well tolerated and produce better seizure control in some patients. The initial dose is 300 mg at bedtime. The dosage may be increased to 300 mg twice daily on day 2 and 300 mg three times daily on day 3. Further increases may be increments of 300 or 400 mg per day as needed, with a three-times-daily regimen. The maximum time between doses should not exceed 12 hours.

Toxicity

To date, all reported studies of gabapentin have addressed add-on therapy. No unique side effects have been identified as presumably due to gabapentin. The following common dose-related side effects of antiepileptic drugs were increased in frequency or severity in some patients when gabapentin was added: drowsiness and fatigue, dizziness, ataxia, and diplopia. No idiosyncratic or long-term toxicity has been demonstrated. There are no known drug interactions.

Disease States

The clearance of gabapentin is reduced in patients with reduced renal function, including the elderly. Consult the package insert for dosage instructions when renal function is reduced.

Pregnancy

There are no adequate studies on gabapentin in pregnant women.

Lamotrigine (Lamictal)*

Advantages

Lamotrigine is sometimes effective when first-choice drugs have failed. It has minimal dose-dependent toxicity, and there is no need to monitor laboratory values. Dosing is twice daily.

Disadvantages

Rash with Steven-Johnson syndrome is an occasional side effect. Lamotrigine cannot be given as a loading dose, and parenteral administration is not possible. There are some modest drug interactions, and lamotrigine is more expensive than older drugs.

Pharmacokinetics

Table 3 details the pharmacokinetics of lamotrigine. Lamotrigine is rapidly and completely absorbed following oral administration. Protein binding is 55%. Lamotrigine undergoes hepatic metabolism and is excreted primarily as the 2-*N*-glucuronide metabolite. The elimination half-life of lamotrigine is 30 hours when taken alone, and this value does not change with chronic administration. Co-administration with carbamazepine or phenytoin reduces the elimination half-life to 15 hours. A therapeutic range for lamotrigine plasma concentration has not been established.

Usual Adult Dosage

The maintenance dose of lamotrigine was 300 to 500 mg per day in clinical trials. Consult package insert after FDA approval.

Toxicity

To date, all reported studies of lamotrigine have addressed add-on therapy. No unique side effects have been identified as presumably due to lamotrigine. The following common side effects of antiepileptic drugs were increased in frequency or severity in some patients when lamotrigine was added: drowsiness, dizziness, headache, ataxia, tremor, and nausea. Rash is an idiosyncratic toxicity (occasionally with Stevens-Johnson syndrome). No long-term toxicity has been reported.

Drug Interactions

Lamotrigine increases the plasma concentration of carbamazepine epoxide. Carbamazepine and phenytoin reduce the plasma concentration of lamotrigine. Lamotrigine does not affect the plasma concentration of carbamazepine, phenobarbital, phenytoin, primidone, or valproic acid. Valproic acid dramatically increases plasma concentration of lamotrigine.

Pregnancy

There are no adequate studies on lamotrigine in pregnant women.

Phenobarbital

Advantages

Serious toxicity is rare with phenobarbital. Parenteral administration is possible, and a loading dose may be given by the oral or intravenous route. Phenobarbital is inexpensive and need be taken only once a day by many adults.

Disadvantages

Phenobarbital is less effective than phenytoin or carbamazepine. It causes disabling sedation, irritability, and impairment of higher intellectual function in a high percentage of patients.

---

*Investigational drug in the United States.

Pharmacokinetics (Table 3)

Phenobarbital is absorbed slowly (over 6 to 18 hours) but completely from the small intestine. The drug is 40% to 60% protein bound. Approximately one-third of an administered dose of phenobarbital is excreted unchanged in the urine, and two-thirds is excreted as metabolites created by hepatic biotransformation. Phenobarbital exhibits linear (non-concentration-dependent) pharmacokinetics.

Usual Adult Dosage

Phenobarbital is given in doses of 1 to 3 mg per kg per day. Phenobarbital's long elimination half-life (approximately 4 days) allows for the drug to be given only once daily (usually at bedtime) unless the toxicity associated with attainment of peak serum concentration causes the patient difficulty. In this case, the drug can be given in two divided doses. Because of its 4-day elimination half-life, it takes 14 to 21 days for attainment of the steady-state phenobarbital serum concentration after a change in the dosing rate.

Toxicity

Dose-related toxicity includes sedation and slowed mentation as well as ataxia. Rash is a common idiosyncratic toxicity, and agranulocytosis, aplastic anemia, and hepatitis are very rare. Long-term toxicity includes folic acid, vitamin K, and vitamin D deficiency.

Drug Interactions

The phenobarbital plasma concentration is increased after the addition of valproic acid. Phenobarbital may lower the plasma concentrations of carbamazepine, valproic acid, bishydroxycoumarin* warfarin, theophylline, and cimetidine.

Disease States

The risk of phenobarbital intoxication must be monitored carefully in patients with renal and hepatic disease.

Pregnancy

Available reports are conflicting as to whether phenobarbital is or is not teratogenic when it is taken alone. Phenobarbital in combination with other antiepileptic drugs appears to increase the risk of teratogenesis.

Phenytoin (Dilantin)

Advantages

Phenytoin was one of two best drugs studied in Veterans Administration Cooperative Studies. It is relatively nonsedating (sedation is mild and similar to that of carbamazepine), and serious toxicity is rare. Parenteral administration of phenytoin is possible, and a loading dose may be given by the oral, intramuscular, or intravenous route. Phenytoin need be taken only once a day by many adults and is inexpensive.

*Not available in the United States.

Disadvantages

Use of phenytoin may result in reversible gingival hyperplasia and other cosmetic side effects (hirsutism, acne, coarsening of facial features; not conclusively proven to be due to phenytoin).

Pharmacokinetics (Table 3)

Approximately 85% of an orally administered dose of phenytoin, 100-mg extended-release Kapseals, is absorbed slowly over a period of 24 hours. Intramuscular phenytoin is slowly and erratically absorbed. Phenytoin is 69% to 96% protein bound and is biotransformed by the liver. Phenytoin has concentration-dependent (nonlinear) pharmacokinetics that have the following consequences: (1) plasma concentration increases (or decreases) faster than the dosing rate when the dosing rate is increased (or decreased); (2) the time to reach steady state after a change in the dosing rate may vary from 5 to 28 days; and (3) the plasma concentration at one dosing rate does not directly predict the plasma concentration at another dosing rate.

Usual Adult Dosage

The usual dose of phenytoin is 4 to 5 mg per kg using 100-mg capsules, an extended-release formulation that may be administered once daily in many adults. The daily dosage is usually given at bedtime to minimize side effects associated with peak plasma concentration. The following persons should receive Dilantin Kapseals in two divided doses daily: (1) persons who have unacceptable toxicity associated with peak plasma concentration with once-daily administration, (2) children (children have shorter phenytoin elimination half-lives than adults), and (3) persons not obtaining complete seizure control with once-daily administration (seizures may occur at the time of trough plasma concentration). Persons receiving a prompt-release phenytoin preparation (i.e., a preparation that is not an extended-release preparation; all current generic phenytoin products) should use a twice-daily or three-times-daily regimen. Phenytoin is available in 30- and 100-mg capsules and 50-mg tablets. Note that the only extended-release form of phenytoin is brand name Dilantin, 100-mg capsules. A syrup for oral dosage and a parenteral form are also available. Because of phenytoin's concentration-dependent pharmacokinetics, this author uses two special rules for titrating dosage: (1) Daily dosing rates should be changed by only 30 or 50 mg when the phenytoin plasma concentration is 10 μg per mL or higher; (2) one should wait 28 days before assessing the full effect of a change in dosing rate.

*Intramuscular Administration and Fosphenytoin**

Standard injectable sodium phenytoin is poorly soluble in water. When injected into muscle, it is slowly

*Investigational drug in the United States.

and unpredictably absorbed and may cause local tissue damage. Fosphenytoin is a water-soluble phosphate ester of phenytoin that is rapidly and predictably absorbed by the intramuscular route and causes minimal local tissue damage. Once in the circulation, fosphenytoin is cleaved by alkaline phosphatase in red blood cells and liver to yield phenytoin. Fosphenytoin by the intramuscular route may be used in place of oral or intravenous phenytoin for short-term maintenance dosing or for administration of a loading dose. See package insert after FDA approval.

Toxicity

Local toxicity includes gastric distress with early treatment (can often be alleviated by taking medication with meals). Dose-related toxicity consists of cerebellar signs (ataxia, limb movement, dysarthria, nystagmus), encephalopathy, changes in mental state ranging form dysphoria and mild confusion to coma, choreiform movements, and increased seizure frequency. Idiosyncratic toxicity commonly includes rash (usually morbilliform and appearing within the first 12 weeks of therapy). Very rarely, agranulocytosis, thrombocytopenia, and aplastic anemia; Stevens–Johnson syndrome; hepatitis; nephritis; lymphoma-like syndrome; thyroiditis; systemic lupus erythematosus; and hyperglycemia are seen. Gingival hyperplasia occurs in approximately 20% of patients taking long-term phenytoin. The gingival hyperplasia can be treated with good oral hygiene or, rarely, gingivectomy. The gingival hyperplasia usually resolves within a few months if phenytoin is discontinued. Hirsutism, acne, and coarsening of facial features have all been attributed to phenytoin, but definitive scientific evidence for a cause-and-effect relationship with phenytoin has never been published for any of these. The following laboratory abnormalities (usually asymptomatic) have been associated with long-term phenytoin administration: decreased levels of folic acid, vitamin K, vitamin D, and immunoglobulin A; decreased bone density; decreased motor nerve conduction velocity; and increased plasma alkaline phosphatase levels.

Drug Interactions

The addition of phenytoin may decrease the plasma concentrations of carbamazepine, valproic acid, felbamate, lamotrigine,* methadone, theophylline, bishydroxycoumarin,† and oral contraceptives. The following drugs may raise the plasma concentration of phenytoin: carbamazepine, felbamate, cimetidine, bishydroxy coumarin,† chloramphenicol, isoniazid, and disulfiram. The following drugs may lower the plasma concentration of phenytoin: rifampin, antacids, and valproic acid (free phenytoin plasma concentration is unchanged).

Disease States

Phenytoin intoxication is not likely in patients with renal disease, but relatively high concentrations of unbound drug are present and may need to be specifically determined at times. There is some risk of phenytoin intoxication in hepatic dysfunction.

Pregnancy

In common with several other antiepileptic drugs, there is a 2% to 3% increased risk of fetal epilepsy syndrome in infants born to mothers taking phenytoin.

Primidone (Mysoline)

Advantages

Serious toxicity is rare with primidone.

Disadvantages

Primidone is less effective than phenytoin or carbamazepine. A high incidence of toxicity is seen at the time of initiation of therapy (nausea, dizziness, ataxia, somnolence). Primidone causes disabling sedation, irritability, and/or impairment of higher intellectual function during chronic administration in a high percentage of patients. Parenteral administration of primidone is not possible, and a loading dose cannot be administered by the oral or intravenous route. The drug is administered in a thrice-daily regimen.

Pharmacokinetics (Table 3)

Primidone is rapidly absorbed from the gastrointestinal tract. Protein binding is minimal. Biotransformation of primidone leads to the formation of two metabolites, phenobarbital and phenylethymalonamide. Each has antiepileptic activity along with primidone per se. The rate of conversion to phenobarbital is enhanced by concurrent use of inducing drugs such as phenytoin. When primidone is given as monotherapy, the derived phenobarbital concentration may be less than the serum concentration of primidone. Concurrent use of inducing drugs often provides serum concentrations of primidone that are one-third those of the metabolically derived phenobarbital. Concurrent use of primidone and phenobarbital should be avoided to prevent phenobarbital toxicity (this is further enhanced if a third drug with metabolic induction qualities is employed).

Usual Adult Dosage

Special care is needed with the initiation of therapy, particularly in patients who are starting drug treatment for the first time. Previous treatment with phenobarbital (which should be discontinued if primidone is to be used) allows for a smooth introduction of this drug. The patient should take the initial dose of primidone at bedtime, and no more than 125 mg should be given (50-mg tablets are available for initiation, and it is often best to begin with a dose of this size). Patients need to be forewarned about side effects such as dizziness, nausea, sedation, and ataxia. Thirty percent of individuals are unable to tolerate this drug and discontinue it during the first 3 months

*Investigational drug in the United States.
†Not available in the United States.

of administration. Dosage adjustments are made with the goal of attaining plasma concentrations at not greater than 15 μg per mL (2 hours after ingestion). Fifty- and 250-mg tablets and a suspension are available.

Toxicity

Dose-related toxicity includes sedation and ataxia. Idiosyncratic toxicity commonly includes rash and, very rarely, leukopenia and thrombocytopenia, agranulocytosis and aplastic anemia, lymphadenopathy, hepatitis, and lupus erythematosis.

Side Effects

Prolonged therapy may be associated with folic acid, vitamin D, and vitamin K deficiency.

Drug Interactions

Valproic acid and isoniazid may increase the plasma concentrations of primidone. Carbamazepine and phenytoin increase the plasma concentration of the phenobarbital-derived form of primidone. Primidone decreases the plasma concentration of carbamazepine and valproic acid.

Disease States

The risk of primidone toxicity is enhanced in instances of renal disease. Its effect in patients with hepatic disease is less clear.

Pregnancy

There are no adequate studies in pregnant women.

Valproic Acid (Depakene, Depakote)

See antiepileptic drugs.

Other Drugs for Partial and Tonic-Clonic Seizures

An occasional patient whose seizures cannot be controlled with first-line or second-line drugs may respond to ethotoin (Peganone), methsuximide, clorazepate dipotassium, phenacemide, or mephenytoin. In particular, ethotoin should be considered for patients who have had a good therapeutic response to phenytoin but were forced to discontinue the drug because of toxicity.

ANTIEPILEPTIC DRUGS OF CHOICE FOR ABSENCE SEIZURES

Ethosuximide, valproic acid, and clonazepam are the three drugs used to treat absence seizures (see Table 2). These three drugs have been shown to have equal efficacy against absence seizures in definitive, double-blind studies. The selection among these agents is based on weighing advantages and disadvantages other than efficacy.

Ethosuximide (Zarontin)

Advantages and Disadvantages

Ethosuximide is the drug of first choice for patients with only absence seizures because it is extremely effective and most patients experience little or no side effects during chronic administration. The common side effects of ethosuximide—gastrointestinal upset and drowsiness—tend to occur early in therapy and then diminish as tolerance develops. The drug seldom causes behavioral or cognitive disturbances. About 1 to 7% of patients taking ethosuximide develop leukopenia, which is reversible if detected early.

Pharmacokinetics (see Table 3)

Ethosuximide is readily and almost completely absorbed in the alimentary tract. There is little or no binding to serum proteins. The drug is transformed in the liver to either a ketone or an alcohol metabolite, which is then excreted with or without glucuronide conjugation.

Usual Adult Dosage

The initial dose is 500 mg per day. The dosage thereafter is individualized according to seizure control and plasma concentration. The daily dosage may be increased by 250 mg every 4 to 7 days until seizure control is achieved. The optimal dosage is usually 15 to 30 mg per kg per day. Ethosuximide may be administered in a twice-daily regimen unless toxicity associated with peak plasma concentration produces unacceptable toxicity, in which case a three-times-daily or four-times-daily regimen should be employed. Ethosuximide is available as a 250-mg capsule or as a syrup.

Toxicity

Local toxicity includes gastric irritation, anorexia, nausea, and vomiting. Dose-related toxicity includes drowsiness, dizziness, and headache. Idiosyncratic toxicity commonly includes rash and leukopenia and, very rarely, pancytopenia, agranulocytosis, aplastic anemia, psychosis, lupus erythematosus, and parkinsonian changes.

Drug Interactions

There are no known drug interactions of clinical significance.

Disease States

Renal and hepatic disorders do not appear to pose major problems for enhanced toxicity of ethosuximide.

Pregnancy

There are no adequate studies on ethosuximide in pregnant women.

Valproic Acid (Depakene, Depakote)

Advantages and Disadvantages

Valproic acid is extremely effective in controlling both absence seizures and tonic-clonic seizures. Valproic acid seldom causes leukopenia. Despite these possible advantages of valproic acid, ethosuximide remains the drug of first choice for patients with only absence seizures because (1) the risk of serious hepatotoxicity as a result of valproic acid administration appears to be greater than the risk of serious bone marrow depression as a result of ethosuximide administration; (2) the common side effects of valproic acid (gastrointestinal upset, weight gain, drowsiness, tremor) are more severe and persistent than with ethosuximide; (3) the longer elimination half-life of ethosuximide allows for more constant blood levels with less frequent administration; (4) valproic acid is much more expensive than ethosuximide; (5) valproic acid produces more clinically significant drug interactions with other antiepileptic drugs than ethosuximide; and (6) the onset of an antiabsence effect is sooner with ethosuximide than with valproic acid. In patients with both absence and tonic-clonic seizures, valproic acid is the drug of choice because it has efficacy against tonic-clonic seizures and ethosuximide does not.

Pharmacokinetics (see Table 3)

Valproic acid is rapidly and completely absorbed after oral administration, with a slight delay in absorption if taken after meals. The drug is approximately 90% protein bound. Protein binding varies with drug plasma concentration, and the free fraction increases with increasing plasma concentration. Primary metabolism is by hepatic hydroxylation and conjugation with glucuronide. Valproic acid also appears in the bowel and undergoes enterohepatic circulation. Beta- and omega-oxidation may also take place. Excretion as glucuronide in the urine follows, with minor amounts lost in feces and expired air.

Usual Adult Dose

Therapy is started at 15 mg per kg per day and is gradually increased by 5 to 10 mg per kg per day every week until therapeutic success is achieved, until a maximum dose of 60 mg per kg per day is reached, or until the plasma concentration exceeds 150 μg per mL. Valproic acid (Depakene) is available in 250- and 500-mg tablets and as a syrup. It is also available as enteric-coated divalproex sodium, a stable coordinate compound (Depakote), which is available in 125- and 500-mg tablets. The absorption of this enteric-coated formulation is delayed by about 1 hour, with a peak concentration reached in 3 to 4 hours. Depakene must be administered in three or more divided doses per day. Depakote can usually can be administered twice daily and produces fewer gastrointestinal side effects in many patients.

Toxicity

Local toxicity includes anorexia, nausea, and indigestion. These symptoms may be reduced with the enteric-coated preparation. Dose-related toxicities are action tremor (40% of adults, less frequent in children), elevated plasma transaminases (usually transient but may be a harbinger of serious hepatic disease), and hyperammonemia. Idiosyncratic toxicity includes hepatic necrosis, thrombocytopenia, pancreatitis (0.5%), stupor and coma, so-called worsened behaviors, and depression. The risk of hepatic fatality is greatest in children younger than 11 years of age and in persons taking valproic acid in combination with other antiepileptic drugs. Long-term toxicities are weight gain (20%), hair loss (4%), and platelet dysfunction.

Drug Interactions

Valproic acid raises the plasma concentration of lamotrigine and phenobarbital. Phenytoin, phenobarbital, and carbamazepine lower the plasma concentration of valproic acid. Felbamate increases the plasma concentrations of valproic acid.

Disease States

The use of valproic acid is best avoided in the presence of liver disease. Because of possible effects of valproic acid on hemostasis (thrombocytopenia, platelet dysfunction), persons taking valproic acid who are about to undergo surgery should have a through hemostasis evaluation.

Pregnancy

In common with several other antiepileptic drugs, valproic acid may increase the risk of fetal epilepsy syndrome. In addition, there is a 2% risk of spina bifida in infants born to mothers taking valproic acid (vs. 1 in 1500 in the normal population).

Clonazepam (Klonopin)

Clonazepam is the third-choice drug for absence seizures because disabling side effects (drowsiness, ataxia, behavior disturbance), and development of tolerance to the antiepileptic effect of the drug are more common with clonazepam than with ethosuximide or valproic acid.

Pharmacokinetics (see Table 3)

Clonazepam appears to be well absorbed by the alimentary tract. It is 47% protein bound. Extensive biotransformations take place, and less than 0.5% is recovered from the urine as clonazepam.

Usual Adult Dose

The usual dose in adults is 1.5 mg per day in three doses initially. An increase of 0.5 to 1 mg is made at 3- to 4-day intervals until seizure control is attained or a maximum dose of 20 mg per day is reached. A clear correlation between plasma clonazepam concentration and seizure control has not been established. Approximately one-third of patients receiving clonazepam develop tolerance to the antiepileptic effect of the drug after 1 to 6 months of administration. In some patients, the antiepileptic effect of clonazepam can be restored by increasing the dosing rate. The drug should be withdrawn very slowly to avoid withdrawal seizures. Tablets sizes include 0.5, 1.0, and 2.0 mg.

Toxicity

Dose-related toxicity includes drowsiness, ataxia, behavioral change (irritability, depression, psychosis), dysarthria, and diplopia. Idiosyncratic toxicity commonly includes skin rash and, very rarely, hair loss, anemia, leukopenia, and thrombocytopenia.

Drug Interactions

Phenobarbital may lower the clonazepam plasma concentration. Concurrent use of amphetamines and methylphenidate may cause central nervous system depression and respiratory irregularities. Depressant effects may also be enhanced by alcohol, antianxiety and antipsychotic drugs, antidepressants, and other antiepileptic drugs. Concurrent use of valproic acid has, in some individuals, been associated with the development of absence status.

Disease States

Renal disease is unlikely to affect the elimination of clonazepam, but liver disease may require a decrease in dosage.

Pregnancy

There are no adequate studies on clonazepam in pregnant women.

GENERIC ANTIEPILEPTIC DRUGS

The American Academy of Neurology has reviewed the complex and controversial topic of generic antiepileptic drugs. They recommend that for two drugs, carbamazepine and phenytoin, patients should remain on the same preparation made by the same manufacturer because of theoretical and documented risks of therapeutic inequivalence when switching among different manufacturers' preparations. For the other antiepileptic drugs, there are no generic preparations or the generic preparations appear to be performing adequately.

MEDICALLY INTRACTABLE EPILEPSY

Many cases of so-called intractable epilepsy are due to improper diagnosis of seizure type, resulting in the use of improper antiepileptic drugs, failure to push the drugs used to the maximal dosage, or failure to use all available antiepileptic drugs. There are some patients, however, who continue to have seizures despite a proper seizure diagnosis and maximal therapy with conventional antiepileptic drugs. Patients with partial seizures should be considered for cortical resection procedures. The efficacy and safety of such procedures in properly selected patients are well proved. In patients whose seizures are not controlled with conventional drugs and who are not candidates for cortical resection procedures, there are four therapeutic options: (1) less commonly used antiepileptic drugs, (2) experimental drugs, (3) experimental surgical procedures, and (4) behavioral therapies. Such therapies usually are available only at specialized epilepsy centers.

STATUS EPILEPTICUS

Definition

Status epilepticus is defined as seizures (of any type) occurring so frequently that the patient does not fully recover from one seizure before having another. Tonic-clonic status epilepticus is the most common and dangerous type. The mortality rate for patients with tonic-clonic status epilepticus is 6% to 20%, and permanent brain damage may result from metabolic exhaustion of neurons.

Management of Tonic-Clonic Status Epilepticus (Table 4)

Maintain Vital Functions

The patient should be positioned to avoid aspiration, suffocation, or falls. A soft plastic oral airway should be taped in place if it is possible to do so without forcing the teeth apart. Forcing an airway between clenched teeth may result in dental injury and aspiration of teeth. Wooden tongue blades may cause injuries from splinters and cuts. Metal spoons may injure teeth. Intubation may be necessary to maintain respirations. A large intravenous catheter should be placed for administration of medication and fluids. Metabolic acidosis often is present and should be corrected promptly with sodium bicarbonate.

TABLE 4. **Treatment Protocol for Tonic-Clonic Status Epilepticus**

0–5 min	Assess cardiorespiratory function, obtain history, perform neurologic and physical examinations. Confirm seizure diagnosis by observing one seizure or ongoing seizure activity. Draw blood for drug levels, glucose, metabolic screen, complete blood count, and toxic screen. Insert oral airway (if possible), and administer oxygen (if necessary and available). Call EEG technician, but do not delay treatment for EEG unless EEG is needed to establish diagnosis.
5–9 min	Start IV infusion. Administer 100 mg thiamine followed by 50 mL of 50% glucose by direct IV push. Administer 5–10 mg of diazepam at 5 mg per min now or at any time during first 180 min if (1) frequent seizures prevent performing above procedures or (2) seizure activity has been ongoing for more than 2 min.
10–40 min	Administer phenytoin loading dose of 14 mg per kg at a rate no faster than 50 mg per min. Administer an additional 4–6 mg per kg of phenytoin if no complications occur during initial infusion.
60 min	If seizures persist, administer phenobarbital 10 mg per kg at a rate of 60–100 mg per min IV.
120 min	If seizures persist, administer phenobarbital 10 mg per kg at a rate of 60–100 mg per min IV.
180 min	If seizures persist, barbiturate coma or general anesthesia (paraldehyde 0.1–0.15 mL per kg IM or per rectum [diluted with 7 mL mineral oil] if barbiturate coma is present or general anesthesia not available).

Abbreviation: EEG = electroencephalogram.

Identify and Treat Precipitation Factors

The majority of cases of tonic-clonic status epilepticus do not occur randomly or as a result of a massive new cerebral lesion. Rather, there is a specific precipitating factor that causes a patient with a known seizure disorder to develop status epilepticus at a specific time. The most frequent causes of tonic-clonic status epilepticus are withdrawal from antiepileptic drugs and fever. Other precipitating factors include (1) withdrawal from alcohol or sedative drugs, (2) metabolic disorder (hypocalcemia, hyponatremia, hypoglycemia, hepatic or renal failure), (3) sleep deprivation, (4) acute new brain insult (meningitis, encephalitis, cerebrovascular accident, or trauma), (5) diagnostic procedures, and (6) drug intoxication (e.g., cocaine, tricyclics, or isoniazid). The precipitating factors in a case of status epilepticus must always be vigorously sought and treated to facilitate seizure control and to be certain that any reversible cause of cerebral dysfunction is treated before it results in irreversible cerebral damage.

Role of Electroencephalography

If available, EEG monitoring confirms the diagnosis of status epilepticus and the presence or absence of proxysmal activity after treatment. This is useful information. *Treatment should not be delayed because of EEG procedures,* however, unless the EEG is needed to establish the diagnosis of status epilepticus.

Loading Dose

Administer a loading dose of a long-acting antiepileptic drug (phenytoin or phenobarbital). To quickly control tonic-clonic status epilepticus and prevent its recurrence, one must immediately obtain a high therapeutic plasma concentration of a long-acting antiepileptic drug (phenytoin or phenobarbital in most cases) and then maintain the plasma concentration in the therapeutic range. An intravenous loading dose of drug must be given in order to avoid the otherwise long delay in achieving a therapeutic steady-state plasma concentration of drug if the drug is given in its usual maintenance dosage. The usual loading dose of phenytoin is 14 mg per kg intravenously at a rate no faster than 50 mg per minute followed by the first maintenance dose of 100 mg in 6 hours. Alternatively, a loading dose of 18 mg per kg at a rate no faster than 50 mg per minute may be administered followed by a first maintenance dose in 24 hours. The advantages of the larger loading dose are (1) anecdotal evidence suggests that the larger dose may be more effective, possibly because high plasma concentrations of phenytoin inhibit calcium conductance (needed to sustain status epilepticus), and (2) the time to the first maintenance dose is increased. The usual loading dose of phenobarbital is 6 to 20 mg per kg intravenously at a rate no faster than 60 mg per minute.

Fosphenytoin*

Fosphenytoin may be substituted for injectable sodium phenytoin in the treatment of status epilepticus. Infusion of fosphenytoin at a rate of 150 mg per minute has been shown (1) to produce free phenytoin plasma concentrations equivalent in time and amount to those produced by infusion of sodium phenytoin at 50 mg per minute and (2) to have efficacy for status epilepticus similar to sodium phenytoin infused at 50 mg per minute. Advantages of fosphenytoin are that (1) it dissolves readily in any standard intravenous solution and (2) it has less local toxicity. See package insert after FDA approval for details of dosage and administration.

Diazepam (Valium)

Intravenous diazepam has a relatively brief duration of action (30 to 120 minutes), is not a definitive therapy for status epilepticus, and can cause life-threatening cardiorespiratory depression. Intravenous diazepam, however, transiently produces high plasma and brain concentrations of the drug and often brings about immediate (but temporary) control of status epilepticus. Intravenous diazepam is indicated for tonic-clonic status epilepticus (1) if generalized tonic-clonic activity has been going on without interruption for more than a few minutes and (2) if a tonic-clonic seizure occurs in a post-ictal patient who is being evaluated and is receiving a loading dose of a long-acting antiepileptic drug.

*Investigational drug in the United States.

EPILEPSY IN INFANTS AND CHILDREN

method of
HARRIET KANG, M.D.
Montefiore Medical Center
Albert Einstein College of Medicine
Bronx, New York

Children may have any of the types of seizures to which adults are susceptible, although the specific causes differ in frequency. The prevalence of seizures, both acute symptomatic and unprovoked recurrent (epilepsy), is greater in infants and children than in adults. The management of pediatric seizure disorders requires knowledge of not only drug treatment of the seizures but also recognition of the developmental, familial, and social effects of both the epilepsy and its treatment. Some epileptic syndromes may be found only at specific ages and developmental states. The prognostic outlook in some settings is excellent for seizure control, remission, and neurodevelopmental outcome. Other syndromes present the most difficult challenges for seizure management.

EVALUATION OF NEW-ONSET SEIZURES

The acute diagnostic evaluation for new-onset seizures is directed toward finding any acute, treatable provocation. Children are more likely than adults to have seizures as a symptomatic response to a variety of acute conditions, ranging from metabolic or systemic illnesses (including fever) to otherwise mild head trauma (impact seizures). For the child who presents acutely with a seizure or in a post-ictal state, the evaluation should cover the following possibilities.

Status Epilepticus

If the patient has exhibited ongoing convulsive activity for 30 minutes, or repetitive seizures with onset while still post-ictal, initiate the protocol for status epilepticus (see previous section). For initial treatment, lorazepam (Ativan)* may be given at a dosage of 0.1 mg per kg, repeated once if needed. Diazepam (Valium) 0.3 mg per kg is equally effective but has a much shorter duration of action, so that a second drug must then be given to prevent seizure recurrence. Transient apnea may occur with intravenous administration, and respiratory support should be available.

Phenytoin (Dilantin) 20 mg per kg may be used initially if the child's respiratory and cardiovascular status is not compromised. This drug has less effect on the examination than the benzodiazepines, and it allows better assessment of changes in mental status. Children are less likely than adults to develop hypotension or arrhythmias during administration, but the patient's blood pressure and heart rate should be monitored during infusion.

Phenobarbital is used if status epilepticus persists; it may also be given initially for neonatal seizures or febrile status. There is a high risk of apnea if it is used in combination with a benzodiazepine, and the patient who has already received lorazepam or diazepam should be intubated before being given phenobarbital. The initial dose for children is 10 mg per kg, but neonates require 20 mg per kg. If status continues after this dose is repeated, then further options (including general anesthesia or barbiturate coma) require intensive specialized neurologic and systemic support.

Acute Cause or Provocation

The immediate history and examination should seek any evidence of an acute precipitant. Signs and symptoms of infection (particularly meningitis), intoxication or poisoning, fluid and electrolyte disturbances, and trauma should be sought; the possibility of occult trauma (child abuse) should not be overlooked. Focal seizures or signs suggest a structural etiology. Fever is the most common cause of new-onset seizures in otherwise normal children, and it may also precipitate seizures in patients with known epilepsy. A prior history of neurologic insult or impairment (such as mental retardation or cerebral palsy) supports a more remote symptomatic etiology. Seizures due to electrolyte or metabolic disturbances will be relatively refractory to treatment unless the underlying abnormality is corrected.

Risk of Recurrence

Single brief seizures do not in themselves cause neurologic damage. The need for prolonged antiepileptic drug treatment is based on an assessment of risk of injury or adverse effect should seizures recur versus the risks and side effects of medication over a prolonged period of time. Two-thirds of children who present with a first unprovoked seizure will not have a second, with even better outcomes for children who are neurologically and developmentally normal and who have normal neurodiagnostic studies. Given the potential cognitive and other side effects of current antiepileptic drugs, most children should not be placed on continuing drug therapy until after a second seizure.

Seizure Type for Recurrent Seizures

The choice of a maintenance antiepileptic drug is based on many factors, but the most significant is the seizure type, whether of partial (focal) or generalized onset. The classification of epileptic seizures is summarized in Table 1 in the chapter on Epilepsy in Adolescents and Adults.

A Specific Epileptic Syndrome

An epileptic syndrome is defined by a combination of features, including seizure type, etiology, age of onset, associated neurologic findings, electroencephalographic (EEG) characteristics, response to treatment, and prognosis for remission. Although the major factor in choosing a specific drug treatment is the seizure type, recognition of an age-related or developmental epileptic syndrome also influences the choice of treatment. The early diagnosis of a benign syndrome also allows a more reassuring discussion with the family regarding the absence of concurrent neurologic disease, the likelihood of complete seizure control, and in many cases, the excellent outlook for discontinuing medication in the future. Some of the more common syndromes are discussed in the following section.

EPILEPTIC SYNDROMES IN INFANCY AND CHILDHOOD

Febrile Seizures

The most common provocation for a seizure in childhood is fever in an infant or preschool-aged child. Approximately 3% of children in the United States have a seizure with fever in this setting. Clas-

*Not FDA approved for this indication.

sically, the child's first febrile seizure occurs between the ages of 6 months and 5 years. Seizures attributable solely to fever may recur up to about age 7. There is often a family history of febrile seizures. The seizures themselves are usually brief, single, generalized tonic or clonic events. Atypical features (focal seizures, duration greater than 10 minutes, or multiple seizures within a day) or onset outside the usual age range may occur, but they should raise the possibility of other etiology or an underlying seizure diathesis; fever also lowers the seizure threshold in patients with known epilepsy.

Simple febrile seizures are those without atypical features. The risk for later unprovoked or epileptic seizures in children with simple febrile seizures does not significantly differ from the risk for children without febrile seizures; atypical features raise the risk of the development of epilepsy later in life, but there is no evidence that maintenance antiepileptic treatment reduces this risk. Children who have had a febrile seizure have about a one-third risk of having a second; subsequent seizures carry a 50% risk of recurrence. A higher recurrence risk in younger children reflects the longer remaining period of age susceptibility.

Because children with febrile seizures are usually otherwise neurologically and developmentally normal, any benefit of treatment must be carefully weighed against the risks and adverse effects of medications. In the past, many children were treated with phenobarbital, but this drug produces behavioral and cognitive side effects that most parents and pediatricians find unacceptable in a condition that is self-limited. Valproic acid (Depakene) is effective in preventing recurrence but carries an increased risk of hepatotoxicity in younger children, particularly those under 2 years of age. More recently, a number of centers in Europe and North America have presented studies demonstrating the effectiveness of rectally administered diazepam (Valium) in preventing recurrent febrile seizures. Diazepam is given at the onset of fever at a dosage of 0.2 to 0.3 mg per kg using the parenteral solution. For some children, the first sign of fever is the seizure itself, but even in this setting, rectal diazepam may help those who are prone to prolonged or multiple seizures. Dosing may be repeated at 12-hour intervals, but aggressive antipyretic treatment may obviate the need for this. Many families opt for nontreatment, given the benign nature of the seizures in most cases. In any case, parents need to learn basic first aid for seizures, including avoidance of potentially injurious maneuvers (such as the common myth of putting a hard object in the mouth).

Neonatal Seizures

The clinical characteristics of this epileptic syndrome result from the anatomic and physiologic immaturity of premature and full-term infants. Although generalized seizures may occur, neonates are much more likely to have focal or multifocal seizures (which do not imply a focal lesion) or subtle manifestations, such as lip-smacking or other motor automatisms. Neonatal seizures are rarely idiopathic, and their presence mandates an investigation for underlying infectious, metabolic, or structural etiologies. If the cause is a transient or reversible metabolic condition (such as hypoglycemia, hypocalcemia, hypomagnesemia, pyridoxine dependency, or some inborn errors of metabolism), the prognosis is excellent and long-term treatment is not indicated. Severe hypoxia and ischemia, cerebrovascular events, and brain malformations carry a more guarded prognosis, although acute seizures provoked by these may again not require prolonged treatment. Management is complicated by the fact that neonates may have electrographic seizures without clinical manifestations, as well as clinical seizure-like phenomena without EEG correlation. The extent to which aggressive therapy should be pursued in these cases is an area of controversy.

Antiepileptic drug management for neonatal seizures is complicated by the unique pharmacokinetic features of newborns. Drug half-lives may be initially prolonged, unless metabolism has been induced by prenatal exposure. After hepatic induction, however, per kilogram dosage requirements are higher than for adults because of wider distribution and a higher liver to body mass ratio. Gastrointestinal absorption tends to be poorer, however. Concurrent systemic disorders may affect hepatic or renal disposition. Fortunately, most laboratories can now perform drug assays on small samples if they are forewarned.

The mainstay of neonatal anticonvulsant treatment is phenobarbital, with a loading dose of 20 mg per kg. A useful rule of thumb in neonates is that each 1 mg per kg bolus dose raises the phenobarbital level by 1 mg per L. Following induction, the maintenance requirement is usually 5 to 10 mg per kg per day, but levels should be followed to ensure an appropriate rate of metabolism or to adjust the dosage, if necessary. Treatment with phenobarbital produces or enhances behavioral depression and hypotonia. Diazepam (Valium)* and lorazepam (Ativan)* may be useful in acute management of neonatal seizures or status if respiratory support is available. Phenytoin (Dilantin) may also be useful but requires secure intravenous access; the parenteral solution is caustic and may cause severe tissue injury if extravasated. Dilantin also has poor gastrointestinal absorption in newborns and young infants, so that conversion from intravenous to oral use is not available; most neonates do not require prolonged use, however.

Infantile Spasms

Infantile spasms are unique seizures that occur only in infants and very young children, most cases beginning before 1 year of age and remitting even without effective treatment by 2 years of age. The significance of the syndrome is its association with

*Not FDA approved for this indication.

underlying neurologic abnormalities, including mental retardation in the vast majority (90% or more). Most cases are symptomatic of severe early neurologic insults, brain malformations, or genetic disorders such as tuberous sclerosis, and even successful treatment of the seizures does not affect the long-term outcome. Many of these children go on to have other types of seizures, including the Lennox-Gastaut syndrome. In about a third of the cases, no clear etiology can be identified and the neurodevelopmental outlook is slightly better.

The infantile spasms most commonly consist of abrupt, briefly sustained flexion of the head and neck with extension or elevation of the arms and legs, occurring in clusters at intervals of 5 to 15 seconds. Variations include different combinations of flexor and extensor components, which may sometimes be asymmetrical, and manifestations can be subtle (e.g., eye deviations, slight head nods). Clusters are more likely to occur during so-called twilight states (on going to sleep or waking up). Because the physician usually does not witness the seizures at initial presentation, home videotaping by the parents is often helpful. The EEG may also be diagnostic, because the syndrome has a high correlation with an inter-ictal background pattern of very high amplitude chaotic electrical activity with multifocal spikes (hypsarrhythmia). Because of the grossly abnormal EEG and the abnormal mental status, some consider this syndrome to be an epileptic encephalopathy that is progressive if it does not respond to treatment.

Infantile spasms are classically refractory to treatment with most of the conventional anticonvulsants. Valproate (Depakene) and the benzodiazepines may be helpful in some cases, although each has associated risks. Infantile spasms appear to be most responsive to treatment with adrenocorticotropic hormone, although the mechanism of action is unknown. Adrenocorticotropic hormone must be given by injection and often produces steroid-related side effects, including behavioral changes, weight gain, blood pressure elevation, glucose and electrolyte disturbances, and gastrointestinal effects (including gastrointestinal bleeding). Specific dosage regimens vary by center or consultant, but generally fall into high-dose and low-dose protocols. My colleagues and I use a high-dose protocol of 100 to 150 units per M^2* given daily for 30 days, followed by a 1-week taper. Because the duration of treatment is limited, long-term side effects of prolonged immunosuppression and growth retardation are not seen. Some rapid responders cease having spasms after the first dose and have normalization of the EEG within a day or two. On the other hand, lack of response within 2 weeks should usually terminate the trial. Parents can usually be trained to give the injections, with monitoring for side effects through a combination of visiting nurse services and office check-ups. A select group of children with focal brain lesions may be candidates for surgery.

*Exceeds dosage recommended by the manufacturer.

Lennox-Gastaut Syndrome

This epileptic syndrome, like infantile spasms, is characterized by relatively refractory seizures in children who are mentally retarded and neurologically impaired. The patients usually have several different types of generalized and focal seizures, including pure tonic or clonic, myoclonic, and atonic seizures, and if the seizures are poorly controlled, they are at high risk for seizure-related injury. Although the onset of the characteristic features is generally between 2 and 10 years, the condition is chronic; patients with Lennox-Gastaut syndrome form a substantial portion of the refractory population followed in adult epilepsy programs. The etiologies vary and are similar to those found with infantile spasms. Patients with uncontrolled seizures may show a deterioration in behavior and cognitive function, even if the cause is a focal structural lesion, and this syndrome, like infantile spasms, may be a progressive epileptic encephalopathy.

The EEG in this syndrome is also highly characteristic, showing generalized spike-wave complexes occurring at a frequency of 2.5 per second or less (slow spike-wave pattern). In areas where the complexes are visible, the background activity is usually slow and disorganized. Asymmetrical or focal epileptiform features may be seen, particularly in those patients with underlying focal structural abnormalities.

Because these patients have a combination of partial and generalized features to their epilepsy, valproate (Depakene, Depakote) is usually the most effective single antiepileptic agent. Optimal seizure control may require levels well above the usual therapeutic range, pushing the limits of valproate-induced tremor and platelet depression. Drugs of choice for partial seizures, such as carbamazepine (Tegretol) and phenytoin (Dilantin), may be used in combination with valproate if partial seizures are persistent, but these drugs can worsen minor motor and absence seizures in some patients. Clonazepam (Klonopin) and other benzodiazepines are sometimes helpful, but behavioral effects and the development of tolerance limit the use of this class of drugs as chronic therapy. The novel new anticonvulsant felbamate (Felbatol), approved in 1993, has been shown to be helpful in this syndrome. Felbamate, which is approved for use in children over age 2 years as well as adults, has relatively few cognitive and behavioral side effects. It has metabolic interactions with other anticonvulsants, whose dosages must be reduced and levels monitored to avoid toxicity. Felbamate is usually titrated to a dosage of 45 mg per kg per day over 2 weeks but is titrated more slowly if side effects such as nausea, insomnia, or dizziness appear. Despite treatment, most patients with the Lennox-Gastaut syndrome do not achieve seizure-free status.

Benign Rolandic Epilepsy

In contrast to the syndromes discussed earlier, the identification of benign Rolandic epilepsy allows giving early reassurance to families as to the excellent prognosis for seizure control, developmental outcome, and eventual seizure remission. This syndrome, which has a number of synonyms, including benign focal epilepsy with centrotemporal spikes, usually begins at 4 to 10 years of age in children who are otherwise neurologically normal. The seizures begin with focal clonic jerks in the mouth and face, causing dysarthria or anarthria but not a true aphasia, and with maintenance of consciousness if awake. Seizures are more likely to occur with sleep or sleep deprivation. There may be spread to involvement of the arm, and secondary generalization may occur during sleep. The EEG, which should be performed after sleep deprivation, shows a characteristic high-amplitude spike-wave complex over one or independently both centrotemporal regions, increasing in frequency with drowsiness and sleep. Virtually all of the affected children have cessation of seizures and normalization of the EEG at some point during adolescence. Because this syndrome responds to treatment with most anticonvulsant agents (excluding ethosuximide), the choice of drug is primarily based on minimizing the risk of medication toxicity. Carbamazepine (Tegretol) is an effective drug of first choice in most cases. There is even some support for nontreatment because of the benign and self-limited seizure course.

Absence Epilepsy

Absence seizures are brief episodes of unresponsiveness and motor arrest, generally lasting less than 10 seconds, with either an aura or post-ictal depression. Although rhythmic blinking or subtle clonic movements may be present, automatisms and significant alterations in posture or tone are uncommon and atypical. Absence seizures are classically associated on the EEG with generalized bilaterally synchronous three-per-second spike-wave discharges. Although absence seizures may be present in a number of mixed seizure syndromes (including Lennox-Gastaut syndrome), the syndrome of childhood absence epilepsy usually has an onset between 4 and 10 years of age, occurring in otherwise neurologically normal children who may have a family history of absence or generalized epilepsy. These children may have hundreds of brief seizures daily, and seizures can be readily provoked by hyperventilation in the examining room. The disorder is inherited as an autosomal dominant trait with variable penetrance. The syndrome of juvenile absence epilepsy cannot be clearly differentiated from childhood absence by age, although onset is usually later in the age range; these children tend to have less frequent absences but a higher incidence of generalized tonic-clonic seizures and a lower chance for spontaneous remission in adolescence.

Although the seizures themselves are benign, the frequency with which they occur can cause poor academic performance and raise the risk of injury during other activities. Fortunately, the absence seizures almost always respond to treatment with ethosuximide (Zarontin) or valproate (Depakene, Depakote); valproate is also effective against generalized tonic-clonic seizures if they are also present (ethosuximide is not). Both drugs also eradicate the spike-wave abnormality on the EEG, so that a normal EEG on treatment does not necessarily indicate remission with age. For children with pure absence seizures, the prospects for outgrowing the disorder are excellent.

DISCONTINUING ANTIEPILEPTIC THERAPY

In discussing epilepsy prognosis with families, it is important to remember that even in the absence of a benign syndromic diagnosis, the outlook for spontaneous remission of epilepsy in childhood is good. Studies have shown that two-thirds of children who achieve control on treatment for 2 years can be withdrawn from medication without recurrence. Even patients with higher recurrence risks may merit an attempt at withdrawal, particularly adolescent females approaching reproductive potential. Persisting EEG abnormalities may influence the risk of recurrence but should not in themselves exclude withdrawal. For most drugs, a phased taper in 25% dosage steps over a period of 1 to 2 months is safe; the risk of recurrence is highest during and shortly after the taper, with almost half of recurrences occurring during the first 6 months. If seizures do recur, treatment can be reinitiated, and in most cases, another trial of withdrawal can be considered after 2 more years of seizure control.

GILLES DE LA TOURETTE SYNDROME

method of
GERALD ERENBERG, M.D.
Cleveland Clinic Foundation
Cleveland, Ohio

Once considered rare, Gilles de la Tourette syndrome (GTS) is now being recognized with increased frequency. The exact incidence is not known, but it is estimated to occur in 1 out of every 2500 persons. Several factors have contributed to the increased recognition of this disorder. In the past, it was assumed that GTS occurred only in a severe form, but it is now known that this is a spectrum disorder. The combination of motor and vocal tics can occur in individuals in a mild, moderate, or severe form. Another factor contributing to misdiagnosis in the past has been the idea that coprolalia is an inevitable part of this disorder and was required for diagnosis. Coprolalia occurs in only a minority of persons with GTS, and the diagnosis of GTS can be made without coprolalia being present. Finally, an aggressive campaign by the Tourette Syndrome Association has helped educate the public as well as the medical community about this disorder.

This disorder is named for Gilles de la Tourette, who first described this syndrome in 1885. In spite of ever-intensifying interest and research work on this disorder, no biologic marker has yet been discovered. It has long been assumed that the locus of abnormality is within the central nervous system, and specifically involves the basal ganglia. The disorder is considered one of neurotransmitter dysfunction, and much attention has been focused on dopamine. It is likely that other neurotransmitters are also involved, and some evidence of abnormalities of the endogenous opioid system has been discovered.

Gilles de la Tourette syndrome is now considered to be a genetic disorder, although the exact gene site has not yet been discovered. Eighty percent of cases of GTS are believed to have a genetic cause, but the gene may manifest itself in a number of different ways. The gene can lead to various types of tic disorders, or even to a purely behavioral disorder without tics. Tic disorders are divided by duration as well as complexity. The most common form is the acute simple tic of childhood, which is a single motor or vocal tic beginning in childhood and lasting for less than 1 year. Chronic simple tic disorder is the diagnosis made in those persons who exhibit a single motor or vocal tic beginning in childhood but lasting for longer than 1 year. Tics that change form over time and wax and wane in intensity can be limited to either motor tics or vocal tics. Chronic motor tic disorder and chronic vocal tic disorder are now assumed to be variations on how the gene for GTS may manifest. The classic disorder begins in childhood, lasts for more than 1 year, and consists of a changing pattern of motor and vocal tics that vary in intensity over time. It is now believed that the gene may also lead only to a behavioral disorder in the form of an obsessive compulsive disorder. The gene is more likely to express as a tic disorder in males and as a behavioral disorder in females. Within families, the form and severity of the disorder varies from individual to individual, and it is thought that the exact manner in which the gene manifests itself may be due to individual environmental experiences.

DIAGNOSIS

Because of the lack of a biologic marker, the diagnosis of GTS is based on criteria listed in the American Psychiatric Association's Diagnostic and Statistical Manual (DSM). The current edition (DSM-IV) lists the criteria for diagnosis as follows: (1) both multiple motor and one or more vocal tics have been present at some time during the illness, although not necessarily concurrently; (2) the tics occur many times a day (usually in bouts), nearly every day, or intermittently throughout a period of more than 1 year, and during this period, there was never a tic-free period of more than 3 consecutive months; (3) the disturbance causes marked distress or significant impairment in social, occupational, or other important areas of functioning; (4) the onset is before the age of 18 years; (5) the disturbance is not due to the direct physiologic effects of a substance (e.g., stimulants) or a general medical condition (e.g., Huntington's disease or postviral encephalitis).

GTS does not cause an abnormality on any of the currently available clinical diagnostic tests. In the future, tests such as positron emission tomography scans or volumetric measurements of the basal ganglia on magnetic resonance imaging scans may allow an objective diagnosis. The diagnosis of tics is based on clinical observation. Tics must be differentiated from other movement disturbances, including myoclonus, tremor, dystonia, chorea, athetosis, hemiballismus, spasms, dyskinesias, and mannerisms. Specific neurologic disorders potentially mistaken for tics include myoclonic seizures, subacute sclerosing panencephalitis, Wilson's disease, posthemiplegic chorea, cerebral palsy, Lesch-Nyhan syndrome, heavy metal poisoning, torsion dystonia, reaction to psychoactive drugs, and Sydenham's chorea.

In actuality, however, the diagnosis of GTS is generally not difficult. The typical story is of an otherwise healthy person, with the onset of tics between the ages of 4 and 10 years. The initial tic is usually transient, and the child may not be brought to medical attention until the tic returns, often in a different or more severe form. Many patients have initially been evaluated for specific phenomena, such as being seen by an ophthalmologist because of eye blinking or an allergist because of recurrent sniffing or throat clearing. Evaluation should include developmental, behavioral, and academic histories as well as a complete medical history to determine whether any medical event might have led to an encephalopathic process. There should be documentation of the age of onset of the involuntary movements, their pattern of waxing and waning, and their exact form. Physical examination should be completely normal except for the presence of tics, although tics may be suppressed during an office visit. Even so, the history is reliable if the description fits the expectations of a tic disorder.

Because all clinical test results are normal in persons with tic disorders, laboratory testing is only ordered when other causes for involuntary movements must be considered, such as an encephalogram for a person suspected of myoclonic seizures or screening for copper metabolism abnormalities for the patient who possibly has Wilson's disease.

ASSOCIATED CONDITIONS

GTS is now recognized as a complex neurologic and psychiatric disorder that often is exhibited as a combination of tics and specific behavior patterns. More than 50% of children diagnosed with GTS have various forms of behavioral or learning difficulties along with their tic symptoms, and the associated conditions often last into adulthood. Emotional and behavioral problems were initially considered a cause of GTS, but it is now accepted that these are an integral part rather than a cause of GTS. The associated problems often cause more difficulties in everyday life than do the tics. Complex relationships exist between emotions and tics, even in persons whose day-to-day behavior is not out of the ordinary. For patients with GTS, the severity of the tics at any given time often seems to be a barometer of the person's positive or negative emotional state.

The most common associated behavioral difficulties include attention deficit hyperactivity disorder, manifesting as short attention span, distractibility, impulsiveness, and motor restlessness. When present, these behaviors usually precede the onset of tics. Many children, therefore, have already been seen for medical intervention because of their behavior problems, even before evidencing tics. The other commonly occurring behavior pattern is the presence of obsessive-compulsive traits in different degrees of severity. To a lesser degree, persons with GTS also have high incidences of problems with anxiety, fearfulness, emotional lability, and low frustration tolerance. These behavioral patterns are considered part of the disorder, and there may be further complications due to the emotional reactions to the burden of the tic disorder.

Children with GTS often have difficulty in school because their tics can be disruptive, and some people mistakenly believe that their movements or noises are voluntary. Children with attention difficulties may perform poorly because of their inability to concentrate, their becoming easily distracted, and their poor organizational skills. In addition, however, many have true underlying learning disabilities as well. Although Intelligence Quotients are in the normal range for persons with GTS, many score low on tests that require visuo-spatial and visuo-motor skills, and many have difficulties with handwriting and timed tests.

TREATMENT

No cure currently exists for GTS. All medical treatments are symptomatic, and there is no evidence that early treatment alters the natural course of the disorder. Many nonpharmacologic therapies have been attempted without success, including psychotherapy, hypnotherapy, psychoanalysis, lobotomy, thalamotomy, and shock therapy. Behavior therapy, including biofeedback, has occasionally been reported to be of some help. There is no evidence, however, that this is of sustained benefit for the usual person with GTS. Unfortunately, assessment of any treatment program is difficult because the condition spontaneously worsens and improves with or without active treatment.

In the past, simply making the diagnosis of GTS was a major accomplishment that satisfied the person's and family's desire to simply know what was the problem. As the community has become more knowledgeable about GTS, there is a hope and expectation that treatment is available to help with the symptoms of this disorder when they reach a level of intensity that causes problems with success in daily life. The issue for persons with GTS is the quality of their life, because the disorder, although chronic, does not lead to any physical deterioration and does not shorten life span.

COPING AND ADAPTING

Persons with GTS react to the diagnosis based on their individual personalities, their abilities to cope with uncertainty and stress, and the availability of social and medical support. The manner in which families having children with GTS respond to the diagnosis greatly influences how the children feel about themselves and how others learn to adapt to the new reality. Some families initially react with relief that a name has been found for the child's problem; others react with anger and disbelief.

Rather than allowing persons with GTS and their families to regress and become isolated, health care professionals need to help them adapt to the disorder and to deal with the anxiety, shame, anger, and guilt that may be engendered. Physicians, as well as mental health professionals and community support groups, need to listen patiently to the bitterness and frustration that may be expressed.

EDUCATION

Persons with GTS, as well as their families and the medical and educational community, can be helped greatly through publications and services available from the Tourette Syndrome Association, an active public support group with national and regional offices (Tourette Syndrome Association, 42–40 Bell Blvd., Bayside, NY 11361). Information on GTS must be provided to patients and their families as well as to others who play a meaningful role in their lives. Information should be made available to employers, school personnel, neighbors, and all others who may be involved in the patient's everyday life. These persons must help in fostering feelings of self-worth and self-esteem by showing that the person is accepted and respected even with the disorder.

Parents of children with GTS are frequently confronted with the comment from others that the involved child simply needs more discipline. Punishment for the motor and vocal tics is inappropriate because these tics are totally involuntary. Other than these, however, any unacceptable behavior in a family, school, or neighborhood environment, such as that revolving around the person's tendency to become angry quickly, have a low frustration tolerance, or have frequent temper tantrums, must be controlled. The individual must be guided toward an acceptable pattern of behavior so that he or she can continue to develop normally, both socially and emotionally.

As persons with GTS become older, many learn to adopt covering-up mechanisms for their tics by disguising a facial movement as a yawn, by transforming head jerking into a body-stretching movement, or by making coughing or sniffing noises that appear to be an allergic symptom by placing a handkerchief to the nose or hand over the mouth. Others learn to suppress their tics for as long as possible while they are with other people and then excuse themselves to enter a private area where they can release their pent-up tics.

PHARMACOLOGIC TREATMENT OF MOTOR AND VOCAL TICS

There is no such thing as a GTS medication. Instead, there are a variety of different medications available that have the ability to diminish, but not eliminate, specific aspects of the GTS disorder. Because the use of pharmacotherapy does not eliminate the disorder, lead to a cure, or alter the long-term prognosis, the decision to use medication at all is based on the impact that GTS is having on the individual person. In my experience, less than 50% of persons with GTS ever require treatment with medication. Pharmacotherapy is indicated, however, when the symptoms are interfering with success in school or in the work place, or are compromising normal social development. Because there is great variability in the ability of individuals to deal with the tics, the ultimate decision about whether or not to use pharmacotherapy must be made jointly through extensive discussion among the individual, his or her family, and the medical care provider.

Haloperidol (Haldol), a dopamine-blocking agent discovered more than 30 years ago, has traditionally been the most widely used medication to reduce the tics in GTS patients. Experience indicates that haloperidol reduces tics in 70% of treated patients, but over 50% of those who receive this medication complain of side effects. Only 25% of patients report significant improvement without any side effects. Because therapeutic and excessive doses are so close, the total dose is best kept at an amount that decreases symptoms by approximately 75%. Persons with GTS are often very sensitive to haloperidol, and treatment is begun with extremely low dosages. I usually recommend beginning treatment with 0.25 mg taken once each day. The dosage is increased by 0.25 mg a day on a weekly basis until the tics are significantly decreased or the patient begins to exhibit side effects. The dosage of haloperidol is divided into a twice-a-day or three-times-a-day program, and it is unusual for a dosage of over 10 mg a day to be required or tolerated.

The potential side effects of all neuroleptics are similar. The most common are tiredness and increased appetite. Other side effects can include depression and even school or work phobia. Symptoms of parkinsonism may occur along with cholinergic symptoms. It is usually unnecessary to counteract the side effects with anticholinergic drugs, but individual patients may benefit by being placed on concomitant treatment with low doses of anticholinergic medications such as trihexyphenidyl (Artane) at doses of 0.5 to 1 mg taken twice daily. Although the possibility of tardive dyskinesia must be considered, experience has indicated that this rarely, if ever, seems to occur permanently in persons treated with neuroleptics for GTS.

Other neuroleptic drugs are able to block dopamine receptors and may cause fewer side effects or a better clinical effect in individual patients. The most widely used alternatives include pimozide (Orap) and fluphenazine (Prolixin).* Possible side effects are exactly the same as those with haloperidol. Pimozide (Orap) has been the most widely used alternative. I begin treatment with 1 mg daily, and increases of 1 mg per day are made on a weekly basis. The maximum dose generally recommended is 10 mg per day for children and 20 mg per day for adults. Pimozide has been shown to potentially increase the QT interval on electrocardiographic recordings, and periodic electrocardiograms are recommended when this medication is used. In my experience, however, this has never become a clinical problem. Because of how pimozide entered the clinical market, the Food and Drug Administration (FDA) has mandated that pimozide only be used if the patient has failed a treatment trial with haloperidol.

Even when tics are treated with medication, the typical pattern of waxing and waning symptoms continues. Because of this, it is unwise to maintain a fixed dosage of medication. When the individual's tics have lessened considerably for 3 months, I generally recommend that a program of decreasing dosage be attempted. At other times, however, it will be necessary to temporarily increase the dosage above the usual baseline because of a worsening of symptoms.

*Not FDA approved for this indication.

It is also not known whether continuous therapy is better than intermittent therapy. There is no clear benefit to drug holidays, but medication should be discontinued when possible in patients whose symptoms have lessened.

Problems with neuroleptic agents have led to a search for better medications to treat tic disorders. In addition, the neuroleptic agents generally do not alter the associated behavioral aspects of this disorder. A better medication would decrease tics with equal efficacy as do the neuroleptics, cause fewer side effects, not lead to tardive dyskinesia, and alter the behavior patterns as well as the tic frequency. Clonidine (Catapres)* is an alpha-adrenergic agonist originally placed on the market for the treatment of hypertension. It is relatively free of serious side effects, and it does not lead to tardive dyskinesia. In various studies, clonidine has also been found to potentially improve attention span, decrease impulsiveness, decrease anxiety, and help a person deal with obsessive compulsive tendencies. Sedation is the most common side effect, whereas orthostatic hypotension and dizziness can occur at higher doses.

Clonidine is usually my first drug of choice for children with GTS because their tic problem is often accompanied by behavioral difficulties. Unfortunately, however, clonidine does not appear to be as potent an anti-tic medication as the neuroleptic agents. The reported effectiveness of clonidine* has varied greatly from study to study. In my practice, approximately 30% of patients treated with clonidine have sufficient relief of symptoms that this becomes their ongoing treatment program. Improvement with clonidine may take up to 2 months to occur, and this may make interpretation of the treatment results difficult because of the natural waxing and waning of the GTS symptoms. The initial dosage is 0.05 mg, taken once each day and increased by 0.05 mg per day on a weekly basis until improvement or side effects occur. A typical dosage for children is 0.05 mg taken three times per day. There is individual tolerance, however, and a dosage of up to 0.5 mg per day can be reached in individual patients.

A third type of medication used for the control of tics has been clonazepam (Klonopin).* This drug has been less extensively studied, but there are individual patients who respond to treatment with clonazepam. The initial dosage is 0.5 mg taken daily, and this is increased by 0.5 mg per day on a weekly basis until a clinical effect is observed or until the patient reaches a point of discomfort.

Experience has also shown that individual patients may respond to nonstandard medications. Such medications include calcium channel blockers, opioid antagonists, and neurotransmitter depleters, such as tetrabenazine,† which is currently unavailable except on an experimental basis. The final point to make is that patients may be treated with combinations of medications. Combinations may include anti-tic medications, such as using both haloperidol and cloni-

*Not FDA approved for this indication.
†Not available in the United States.

dine.* Also, an anti-tic medication may be used along with a behavior-altering medication.

Pharmacologic Treatment of the Behavioral Accompaniments of Gilles de la Tourette Syndrome

Treatment of Attention Deficit Hyperactivity Disorder

As mentioned earlier, the majority of children presenting with GTS have accompanying symptoms of attention deficit hyperactivity disorder (ADHD). Because these symptoms generally occur before the onset of the tics, many have already been treated with psychostimulant medications, such as methylphenidate (Ritalin), pemoline (Cylert), or dextroamphetamine (Dexedrine). After tics were sometimes noted to begin while patients were receiving such treatment, a concern arose that the treatment itself was the cause of the tic disorder. Although the findings remain somewhat controversial, the majority of persons active in the field of GTS have now concluded that the onset of tics is coincidental with and not due to treatment with psychostimulants. Some persons being treated with psychostimulants, however, may experience an increase in tic activity with the use of such medications. If tics occur in a person receiving stimulant medication, I generally recommend that the first course of action be to discontinue the stimulants. In the usual case, the tic activity continues even without such treatment.

As a precaution, I generally next treat the ADHD with alternative medications not in the stimulant category. Clonidine,* as previously mentioned, is one such treatment alternative. It carries the advantage of being able to suppress tics as well as to modify the problems with restlessness and inattentiveness. If unsuccessful, treatment can be attempted with one of the tricyclic antidepressants. These agents have long been used in the treatment of ADHD. They are much less likely to bring out tics, although some anecdotal experience has indicated that some persons also react to this class of medication with an increased frequency of involuntary actions. The most commonly used tricyclic antidepressants are imipramine (Tofranil),* desipramine (Norpramin),* and nortriptyline (Pamelor).* There is little evidence to indicate that one is better than the other, and the clinician can use whichever of these agents with which he or she has had the most experience.

The most serious potential complication with the use of tricyclic agents has been the possibility of prolongation of the QT interval on the electrocardiogram, and there have also been reports of sudden and unexplained death in persons receiving desipramine. For this reason, it is suggested that an electrocardiogram be performed prior to treatment with such agents, and repeat studies should be performed periodically as the dosage is increased. I generally begin treatment using 10 mg twice per day, and the dosage is similar for each of the agents. The dosage in children can be raised to a daily dosage of 3 mg per kg per day, although the ultimate dose is influenced by the individual's reactions as well as by periodic blood level testing. In addition to influencing restlessness and attention span, the tricyclic agents are also capable of decreasing anxiety and stabilizing mood. Several weeks are required before the ultimate effect is seen, and there are patients who will develop tolerance to the medication after they have been successfully treated for several months. Other potential side effects include tiredness, constipation, orthostatic hypotension, dryness of the mouth, and flushing of the skin.

If the symptoms of ADHD cannot be controlled by either clonidine or one of the tricyclic antidepressants, I next restart or initiate a trial of treatment with one of the psychostimulants. I generally prefer to use methylphenidate because the dosage can be closely titrated, and because it need not be taken on an everyday basis to be effective. Many of the children have relief of their symptoms in the school setting and do not require medication on non-school days. The initial dosage is 5 mg taken two or three times per day, and the maximum dosage that I generally use is 20 mg three times per day. There is little evidence that a dosage of more than 60 mg per day leads to any further improvement than do the lower dosages.

Treatment of Obsessive-Compulsive Disorder

It is now recognized that many of the phenomena previously diagnosed as tics are actually obsessive compulsive patterns. The need to touch or tap as well as to perform certain patterns in a ritualistic manner is now recognized as being part of the obsessive-compulsive disorder (OCD) spectrum. Obsessive-compulsive traits are often present at or near the time of the onset of the tics, but they tend to become more prominent in the adolescent and early adult years. For many persons, therefore, their difficulties with obsessive-compulsive tendencies begin to predominate as the major cause of disability at a time when their tics are actually beginning to become less noticeable.

I generally begin treatment with clonidine* because of the previously mentioned possibility that this medication can also help control tics and the attentional difficulties. Recently, more powerful medications have become available for controlling these symptoms. These medications share a mechanism of action wherein they function as selective serotonin reuptake inhibitors. One such medication is clomipramine (Anafranil), a tricyclic agent that has all the attributes of other such agents, except that it is also capable of inhibiting obsessive compulsive traits. Fluoxetine (Prozac)* was the first nontricyclic agent marketed that had a serotoninergic action. Subsequently, two other agents have become available.

*Not FDA approved for this indication.

*Not FDA approved for this indication.

These are sertraline (Zoloft)* and paroxetine (Paxil).* Clomipramine shares all the potential side effects of the other tricyclic agents, including sedation. Fluoxetine,* sertraline,* and paroxetine* have a different side effect profile. These agents can lead to decreased appetite and weight, insomnia, and heightened excitability and agitation. Fluoxetine* carries with it the potential of interfering with the metabolism of other medications. All OCD medications are long acting.

I generally begin treatment for OCD with fluoxetine.* The initial dosage for children in 10 mg taken each morning, and the adult dosage for instituting treatment is generally 20 mg each morning. There is a lag before the optimal response is noted, and medication must be used for 4 to 8 weeks before final decisions are reached. A dosage of up to 80 mg per day can be used in adults. If the obsessive compulsive symptoms are responding to medication but there are problems with excitability or insomnia, I often add either a dosage of clonidine* or a small dosage of clomipramine to be taken at bedtime. Others have found that the use of trazodone (Desyrel)* in a small dosage at bedtime can also be helpful. When treatment is initiated with clomipramine, the initial dosage is 25 mg at bedtime. This can be increased weekly until a dosage of 150 to 250 mg per day is reached for adults. The medication can be taken on a once-a-day or twice-a-day basis, and the maximum dosage for children is approximately 3 mg per kg per day. The maximum dosage, however, is generally that which can be tolerated comfortably or which places the blood level in the desired range. The anti-OCD medications can be used with the anti-tic drugs, although often a smaller dose of such anti-tic medications is used.

HEADACHE

method of
EGILIUS L. H. SPIERINGS, M.D., PH.D.
Brigham and Women's Hospital
Harvard Medical School
Boston, Massachusetts

The head is the focus of pain more often than any other part of the body. Seventy to 80% of the population, men and women alike, experience pain in the head, or headache. Fifty percent of the population experience headache at least once per month, 15% at least once per week, and 5% daily.

Headaches can be of different intensities and, for the sake of simplicity, are generally divided into three categories—mild, moderate, and severe. Moderate and severe headaches occur twice as frequently in women than in men, owing to the menstrual cycle in women. Moderate headaches occur in 13% of men and 23% of women, and severe headaches occur in 6% and 12%, respectively. The prevalence of migraine lies in between those of moderate and severe headaches, and the incidence is 9% for men and 16% for women.

The high frequency of occurrence makes headache a common report in medical practice. It occurs as an acute, subacute, or chronic condition. The acute headache is generally severe in intensity, and often patients with this condition present in the emergency department. Patients with subacute and chronic headaches, on the other hand, are presented in the office.

The diagnostic considerations depend, to a great extent, on the presentation of the headache. Whatever the presentation, however, headache is *always* a valid complaint. It should *always* be investigated seriously and never be considered merely a product of the imagination.

ACUTE HEADACHE

Headache not caused by trauma accounts for 1% to 2% of visits to the emergency department. Men and women are equally represented here, and 80% of the patients are between 15 and 54 years old. Muscle-contraction headache is the most common diagnosis (32%), followed by migraine (22%), and upper respiratory infection (12%). The following diagnoses each account for 5% or less of nontraumatic headache in the emergency department: sinusitis, hypertension, gastroenteritis, cerebral tumor, and cervical degeneration. Apart from cerebral tumor, the neurologic causes of headache—that is, subarachnoid hemorrhage, meningitis, temporal arteritis, and subdural hematoma—each account for less than 1%.

The combination of fever and meningeal irritation should raise suspicion of meningitis, either viral or bacterial. Lumbar puncture should be performed once cerebral involvement (encephalitis, cerebral abscess) has been excluded by neurologic examination and neurodiagnostic imaging. Meningeal irritation without fever should lead to suspicion of subarachnoid hemorrhage, for which computed tomography should be performed; if findings are negative, it should be followed by lumbar puncture. Cerebral tumor is a cause of subacute headache but may be associated with acute headache when it is complicated by hemorrhage.

Temporal arteritis and subdural hematoma are diagnoses that should be considered in patients over the age of 60. These conditions present themselves with subacute headache. Temporal arteritis is generally associated with a significantly elevated sedimentation rate of 50 mm or higher. Therefore, it is important to determine the sedimentation rate in *all* patients over the age of 60 who present with headache. Muscle-contraction headache and migraine are chronic headache conditions. Hence, if diagnosed in acute headache, there must be a previous history of similar headaches.

MENINGITIS

The incidence of meningitis is estimated at 10 to 20 cases per 100,000 population per year. Children younger than 5 years of age are affected most frequently and account for 70% of all cases. In about half of these patients, the meningitis is caused by a bacterial infection. In most of the remaining cases, it is viral in origin.

Meningitis is an acute condition that develops over hours or days. It may or may not be preceded by a respiratory or gastrointestinal illness, either bacterial or viral. Severe bilateral headache associated with photophobia, nausea, and vomiting is its main presentation. When it is bacterial in nature, altered sensorium with drowsiness, disorientation,

---

*Not FDA approved for this indication.

and confusion is also common. Fever is present in 80% of cases, and in 80% signs of meningeal irritation are found. The diagnosis is made through lumbar puncture and spinal fluid analysis, which should be performed in *every* suspected case. The treatment of bacterial meningitis is with antibiotics, while that of viral meningitis is symptomatic only.

SUBARACHNOID HEMORRHAGE

The incidence of subarachnoid hemorrhage is estimated at 10 to 15 cases per 100,000 population per year. In 75% of patients, the hemorrhage originates from a ruptured aneurysm, and in the remainder it is caused by an arteriovenous malformation or bleeding disorder. Two thirds of the patients are between 40 and 60 years old. Women are affected slightly more frequently than are men, possibly because of the higher prevalence of hypertension in women. Sometimes, the hemorrhage is precipitated by activities such as lifting, straining, intercourse, or emotional excitement. It can, however, also occur during sleep, probably owing to the increase in blood pressure that occurs during rapid eye movement (REM) sleep.

Headache of *hyperacute* onset is the characteristic presentation of subarachnoid hemorrhage and is the key feature in diagnosing the condition. The patient should be asked explicitly how fast the headache came about in terms of seconds, minutes, or hours. The headache of subarachnoid hemorrhage comes about in a matter of seconds, like a blow on the head or neck. If this is the history that is obtained, the diagnostic process should be pursued to the point of lumbar puncture. The lumbar puncture, however, should *always* be preceded by computed tomography and be performed only when the results of tomography are negative.

TREATMENT

Generally, for the treatment of acute headache, parenterally administered medications are used. Prochlorperazine maleate (Compazine),* given slowly intravenously in a dose of 10 mg, is most effective, with an efficacy of 88% in providing complete or partial relief. Second is chlorpromazine hydrochloride (Thorazine),* also given intravenously, with an efficacy of 80%. Chlorpromazine* is given in intravenous boluses of 12.5 mg, and repeated, if necessary, twice at intervals of 20 minutes with a maximum of 37.5 mg. Adverse effects that can occur with either prochlorperazine* or chlorpromazine* (both of which are phenothiazines) are drowsiness, hypotension, and dystonia.

Next in line is metoclopramide hydrochloride (Reglan),* either alone or in combination with dihydroergotamine mesylate (D.H.E. 45).* Metoclopramide,* when given in a dose of 10 mg intravenously, has an efficacy of 67% in providing effective pain relief. Adding dihydroergotamine,* in a dose of 1 mg intravenously, increases the efficacy to 70%. Dihydroergotamine* alone, in a dose of 1 or 2 mg intravenously, has an efficacy of only 37%.

Dihydroergotamine* should *never* be given without prior administration of an antinausea medication because it is very potent in causing nausea and vomiting. When given alone, the occurrence of these adverse affects may, to a great extent, reduce the beneficial effect of the medication.

*Not FDA approved for this indication.

Of the narcotic medications, butorphanol tartrate (Stadol),* 2 mg intramuscularly, has an efficacy of 64%. The combination of meperidine hydrochloride (Demerol)* and hydroxyzine pamoate (Vistaril),* 100 and 50 mg intramuscularly, respectively, has an efficacy of 59%. A nonsteroidal anti-inflammatory analgesic that is available for parenteral administration, ketorolac tromethamine (Toradol),* 60 mg intramuscularly, has an efficacy of 57%. More effective is the new antimigraine medication, sumatriptan succinate (Imitrex).* The efficacy of this medication, in a dose of 6 mg subcutaneously, is 70% in decreasing the intensity of moderate and severe headaches to no or mild headache.

Subacute Headache

The patient with subacute headache complains of headache of recent onset. Subacute headaches develop over the course of days or weeks, as opposed to acute headaches, which develop over hours or days. Cerebral tumor, temporal arteritis, and subdural hematoma are diagnoses to consider here.

Cerebral tumor is especially a concern in children with subacute headache. In adults, the tumors are usually located in a hemisphere, giving rise to neurologic symptoms early in the course of the illness. In children, on the other hand, they are often located in the posterior fossa, where they easily obstruct the spinal fluid flow, giving rise to headache without neurologic symptoms.

Particulars in the history that in children should raise suspicion of cerebral tumor as the cause of headache are as follows: (1) headache on awakening in the morning, (2) being awoken by headache at night, (3) persistence of headache in high intensity, and (4) change in nature or frequency of the headache. From the general history, a change in behavior and/or school performance can be added to this list.

In the evaluation of headache in childhood, the neurologic examination is very important and should include evaluation of visual acuity and fundi. In children with headache due to cerebral tumor, 55% show abnormalities on the examination within 2 weeks of headache onset. Within 2 months, this is the case in 85% of the children, and after half a year, *all* children with headache due to cerebral tumor have abnormalities on the neurologic examination.

Cerebral Tumor

The cerebral tumors are categorized as primary, secondary, or metastatic. Metastatic tumors reach the brain through hematogenic seeding, most notoriously from lung or breast cancer. By the time the cerebral metastasis occurs, the primary tumor is generally

*Not FDA approved for this indication.

known. With lung cancer in particular, however, a cerebral metastasis may be the first manifestation of the illness.

The incidence of primary cerebral tumors is estimated at 5 to 10 cases per 100,000 population per year. Most of those affected are between the ages of 50 and 70. In about half, the tumor originates from the glial cells of the brain and is thus termed a glioma. In 60% of patients, the glioma is a so-called malignant glioma or glioma multiforme. This is a very malignant tumor that entails a short duration of illness and often leads to death within half a year. Its initial manifestation is generally not headache but neurologic symptoms or seizure.

The other gliomas, that is, astrocytoma and oligodendroglioma, have a much less disastrous course but are still malignant. They grow slowly but invasively, generally leading to death within 3 to 5 years. They generally also present themselves with neurologic symptoms or seizure, but the symptoms progress very slowly and can be very subtle.

The cerebral tumor that comes next to glioma in frequency of occurrence is meningioma. This is basically a benign tumor that originates from the dura mater. It occurs three times more frequently in women than it does in men. It is often localized over the cerebral hemisphere and manifests itself through headache or seizure. Nonfocal neurologic symptoms, such as lack of perseverance, irritability, emotional lability, and memory impairment, generally occur before focal symptoms develop.

The headache that is caused by meningioma is localized to the side of the tumor but not necessarily limited to its exact location. It may be intermittent or continuous, but it is usually progressive over weeks or months. It is very easily mistaken for muscle-contraction or migraine headache. The localization of the headache is *always* to the same side, and its gradually progressive nature should raise suspicion.

When a cerebral tumor leads to increased intracranial pressure because of its size, induction of edema, or obstruction of spinal fluid flow, generalized headache develops independent of the location of the tumor. Vomiting, which is typically explosive and without or with minimal nausea, may also occur as well as a decrease in the level of consciousness. On neurologic examination, the increased intracranial pressure is evident from congested optic disks (papilledema).

Temporal Arteritis

Temporal arteritis is a condition that affects the elastic arteries, in particular those of the head (cranial arteritis). Histologically, it is characterized by necrosis of the media with formation of granulomatous tissue and giant cells (giant cell arteritis). The cause of the condition is unknown but probably involves the production of (auto)antibodies against elastine.

Temporal arteritis almost exclusively occurs over the age of 60 and equally affects men and women. It is a relatively rare condition, the incidence of which increases with age. The symptoms can be divided into those specific for the arteries involved and those reflecting the systemic, inflammatory nature of the condition. The systemic symptoms include general malaise, generalized weakness, easy fatigability, lack of appetite, weight loss, and low-grade fever.

Headache is probably the most common of the specific symptoms of temporal arteritis. This is due to the preference of the condition for the arteries of the head, and in particular, the temporal arteries. The headache is often severe in intensity and described as a deep, burning pain, sometimes with a throbbing quality. It is caused by dilation of the larger extracranial arteries, the lumens of which are narrowed by swelling of the vessel wall. In addition, the vessel wall is very sensitive to stretch due to the inflammatory process affecting the arteries. Ischemia of the scalp is another factor that contributes to the headache of temporal arteritis.

On physical examination, usually very little is found in terms of specific abnormalities. Routine laboratory testing generally reveals a strongly elevated sedimentation rate, slight anemia, and a slightly elevated alkaline phosphatase level. The sedimentation rate is generally increased to between 50 and 100 mm but may also be normal. This means that in case of strong clinical suspicion, even in a patient with a normal sedimentation rate, a biopsy of the temporal artery should be performed.

In 30% of cases, temporal arteritis affects the ophthalmic arteries, leading to partial or complete blindness due to retinal ischemia. It is because of this potential complication that the condition, once diagnosed, should be treated as soon as possible. Treatment consists of corticosteroids, which generally have a positive effect on the course of the illness. Otherwise, the condition is self-limiting, and the symptoms gradually disappear over the course of several months. Nonsteroidal anti-inflammatory analgesics are often effective in relieving the symptoms of temporal arteritis, such as the headache, but they do *not* reduce the potential risk of blindness.

Subdural Hematoma

Subdural hematoma is the result of head injury. In the elderly, however, the injury may be minimal and is easily forgotten. In addition, confusion and impairment of memory are common symptoms of the condition, making it difficult to obtain an accurate history. The cause of the hematoma is rupture of a so-called bridging vein due to trauma of the head. However, it is almost never associated with fracture of the skull, indicating the generally mild nature of the injury.

Apart from infants, subdural hematoma predominantly occurs over the age of 50 years. Its incidence, like that of temporal arteritis, increases with age. The condition is more common in men than in women. Headache is most frequently its presenting symptom, but headache may also be absent. It is generally mild in intensity, present continuously, and localized to the side of the hematoma. Mental symptoms, in particular confusion and disorientation, are also common presenting symptoms of the condition, as is drowsiness. Focal neurologic symptoms or signs are much less common, and papilledema is hardly ever present.

Subdural hematoma can be treated medically or surgically. Medical treatment consists of corticosteroids, which, in the very old patient, may be preferred over surgical treatment. Surgical treatment consists of evacuation of the hematoma and is associated with the general risks of surgery. Also, in the very old patient, the brain may not expand after evacuation of the hematoma, resulting in a subdural space filled with air. Generally, patients improve with either treatment, but the improvement may be slow and only partial.

Chronic Headache

The adjective chronic describes a condition of long duration or frequent occurrence. The patient with chronic headache complains of headache of long duration. This means that the headache has been present, either intermittently or continuously, for months, years, or sometimes decades.

The patient with chronic headache is generally between 20 and 50 years old, because these are the years of highest headache prevalence. The prevalence of headache sharply increases during the second decade of life and remains stable until the age of 50. After 50, it gradually decreases with the advancement of age. The patient is also more likely to be a woman than a man because of the fact that headache in women is more intense than in men. Men and women suffer from headache with equal frequency, but headaches of moderate and severe intensity are twice as common in women as they are in men.

In general, chronic headache relates to an abnormal functioning of extracranial tissues, in particular muscles and arteries. Muscle contraction causes pain by accumulation of waste products in the muscles when the contraction is prolonged. The waste products, in turn, irritate the nerve fibers in the muscles. Arterial vasodilation causes pain by stretching of the nerve fibers that coil around the blood vessels.

The two most common chronic headache conditions, that is, muscle-contraction headache and migraine, are not well defined. Their distinction is, in most cases, relatively arbitrary and generally of little or no relevance to treatment. They both involve muscle contraction and arterial vasodilation, often in combination, as their mechanisms.

Clinically, muscle-contraction headache and migraine fall on a continuum that is schematically shown in Figure 1. The episodic form of muscle-contraction headache stands on one side of the continuum and migraine on the other. In between are chronic muscle-contraction headache and muscle-contraction vascular headache. The latter condition is also referred to as chronic muscle-contraction headache with coexisting migraine, mixed, or combined headache. Patients with chronic headache may present with symptoms anywhere on the continuum and can, in the course of time, move along it, as indicated by the arrows in Figure 1.

Muscle-Contraction Headache

Muscle-contraction headache is a condition involving mild to moderate headaches of diffuse location and pressing quality. The headaches usually come about during the day, often in the afternoon, and gradually build up in intensity as the day progresses. They generally lack associated symptoms such as photophobia or nausea because of the relatively low intensity of the pain.

Muscle-contraction headache is categorized as episodic or chronic, depending on the frequency of occurrence of the headaches. In chronic muscle-contraction headache, the headaches occur daily or almost daily. Chronic muscle-contraction headache is more often secondary than primary, that is, it generally develops out of episodic muscle-contraction headache. When the chronic muscle-contraction headache is primary, there is often a precipitating physical event, such as a whiplash injury of the neck or a flulike illness. Sometimes, the precipitating event is meningitis, subarachnoid hemorrhage, or myelography, with the meningeal irritation initiating the contraction of the craniocervical muscles.

The most common cause of progression of episodic into chronic muscle-contraction headache is treatment of the headaches with analgesics. Analgesics, whether over-the-counter or prescription, only address the symptom of headache and neglect the underlying mechanisms. As a result, the underlying mechanisms progress over time and the headaches gradually increase in frequency.

Frequent use of analgesics also decreases the efficacy of preventive treatments, that is, treatments aimed at decreasing the frequency, intensity, and duration of the headaches. This negative effect of frequent analgesic use extends to all, pharmacologic and nonpharmacologic, preventive treatments of headache. Therefore, it is important that with frequently occurring headaches, even when these headaches are mild in intensity, accurate information is obtained on the intake of analgesics, both over-the-counter *and* prescription. The information needs to include the number of tablets taken per day and the number of days per week or month that the medications are taken. When analgesics are taken more often than 1 or 2 days per week, they need to be discontinued as the first step of treatment.

Discontinuation of analgesics is often followed by improvement of the headaches, even without the prescription of preventive treatment. The analgesics are generally best discontinued abruptly rather than tapered. Abrupt discontinuation is, however, often followed by initial worsening of the headaches for 2 or 3 days. Corticosteroids can be used to mitigate the

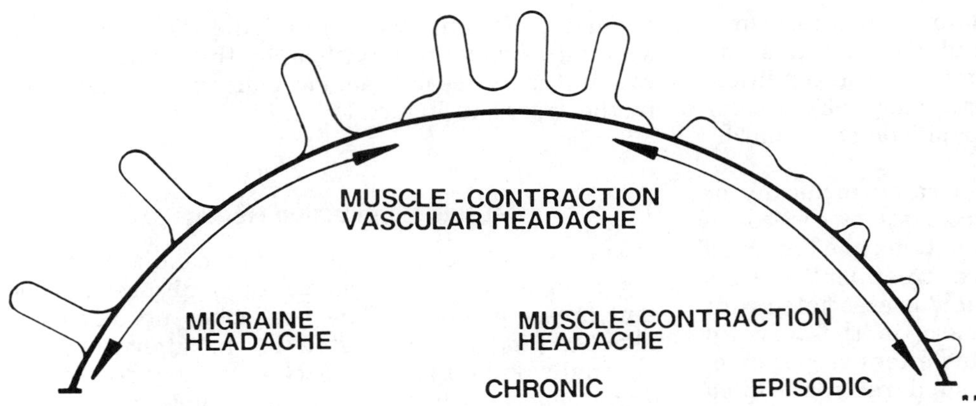

Figure 1. The continuum of muscle-contraction headache and migraine, covering episodic and chronic muscle-contraction headache *(right),* muscle-contraction vascular headache *(center),* and migraine *(left).*

withdrawal headache, for example, prednisone* 60 mg the first day, 40 mg the second day, and 20 mg the third.

Treatment

The two medications that have been shown to be effective in the preventive treatment of chronic muscle-contraction headache are amitriptyline hydrochloride (Elavil)* and doxepin hydrochloride (Sinequan).* The medications are best prescribed once daily at bedtime because they cause sedation. The doses used for the treatment of headache are lower than those for depression and range from 25 to 75 mg per day. Apart from sedation, the medications cause dry mouth, constipation, and weight gain. They are particularly helpful in patients who also have problems falling asleep or sleeping through the night.

Treatments other than medications that relax the craniocervical muscles and prevent muscle-contraction headache are physical and relaxation therapy. The simplest form of physical therapy is to have the patient use a heating pad daily for the neck and shoulder muscles. This is an effective way of decreasing the tightness of the muscles, provided it is applied regularly, preferably daily. Exercises can be added to the daily use of the heating pad in order to stretch and strengthen the muscles. More formal physical therapy modalities for the neck and shoulder muscles include massage, ultrasound, and traction. Injection of the muscles, for example, the trapezius muscles, with a local anesthetic can further help to relax them.

Relaxation therapies that can be used are autogenic and biofeedback training. In autogenic training, suggestions of warmth and heaviness are used to relax successive parts of the body. Biofeedback training makes use of providing information on the state of contraction of the muscles, thereby enabling the patient to relax the muscles more effectively. The relaxation therapies, however, are only effective when practiced regularly, preferably daily, as with the preventive medications, which have to be taken daily.

*Not FDA approved for this indication.

Migraine

Migraine is a condition of moderate to severe headaches. The headaches are often localized, usually to the temple or behind the eye, or both, and are sharp or throbbing in nature. They are generally associated with other symptoms, such as photophobia and phonophobia, as well as nausea and vomiting. The headaches are often present on awakening in the morning or awaken the patient out of sleep at night. They last from several hours to a few days and occur at greatly varying frequency. When they occur frequently, that is, more than once or twice per month, they are often interspersed with muscle-contraction headaches. The headache condition may subsequently develop into a muscle-contraction vascular headache (see earlier).

In women, migraine headache often occurs in relation to the menstrual cycle, that is, with menstruation and ovulation. The decrease in estrogen level that occurs at these times of the menstrual cycle is probably the cause. Stress is also a common precipitating factor, and typically the migraine headache occurs *after* the stressful event.

Other important precipitating factors of migraine are the vasoactive agents, which can be either vasodilator or vasoconstrictor in nature. Examples of vasodilator agents that can bring on a migraine headache are alcohol and sodium nitrite. Sodium nitrite is a food additive used to preserve meat and is present in cured-meat products. Vasoconstrictor agents that can bring on a migraine headache are caffeine and the sympathomimetic amines, tyramine, and phenylethylamine.

Caffeine brings on headache on withdrawal (so-called weekend migraine) when consumed in a quantity of more than 200 to 300 mg per day, which is the equivalent of two cups of coffee. Tyramine and phenylethylamine are chemicals that are present in dietary products, such as aged cheese, red wine, and dark chocolate. They act on the sympathetic nerve fibers and release from them the neurotransmitter substances, noradrenaline, and adrenaline. These neurotransmitter substances cause vasoconstriction, and the headache occurs as a result of the rebound vasodilation following the vasoconstriction.

In classic migraine or migraine with aura, the headache is preceded by transient focal neurologic symptoms, generally known as aura symptoms. These aura symptoms are sensory in nature, either visual or somatosensory; occasionally, however, a speech disturbance occurs. The visual disturbance typical of migraine is the scintillating scotoma, also called teichopsia or fortification spectra.

The scintillating scotoma generally starts near the center of vision as a small spot surrounded by bright, often flickering, and sometimes colorful zigzag lines. After slight enlargement, the circle of zigzag lines opens up on the inside to take the form of a horseshoe, which gradually further expands into the periphery of the visual field. Vision is usually not only obscured by the zigzag lines but also by a band of dimness, which lies against the inside of the horseshoe (Fig. 2).

From its onset near the center of vision to its disappearance in the periphery of the visual field, the scintillating scotoma lasts from 10 to 30 minutes, with an average of 20 minutes. This is also the approximate duration of the somatosensory disturbance, which typically presents itself in the form of digitolingual paresthesias. The paresthesias consist of a feeling of numbness or pins-and-needles, which start in the fingers of one hand. They gradually extend up into the arm, ultimately to involve the face, especially the nose and mouth area, on the same side.

The somatosensory disturbance follows the visual disturbance but can also occur alone, although this is less common. The headache follows the visual and/or somatosensory disturbance immediately or with an interval of, for example, 1 hour. The headache is often unilateral in location and can be on the same side as the visual or somatosensory disturbance, or can be on the opposite side.

Treatment

The treatments of migraine, as of headaches in general, can be divided into those that are abortive and those that are preventive. Abortive treatment is *always* indicated when headaches are moderate or severe in intensity, which is generally the case in migraine.

For the abortive treatment of migraine, analgesic and vasoconstrictor medications are most effective. When these medications are taken by mouth, as is often the case, their absorption has to be considered. It has been shown that the absorption of oral medications is impaired during the migraine headache due to a dysfunction of the gastrointestinal tract. This dysfunction consists of atony and dilation of the stomach with closure of the pyloric sphincter, as is shown in Figure 3. The dysfunction is probably due to the increased activity of the sympathetic nervous system that occurs secondary to the pain.

The gastrointestinal dysfunction of migraine can be addressed with metoclopramide hydrochloride (Reglan),* which is an antinausea medication with gastrokinetic properties. Metoclopramide stimulates the gastrointestinal tract and, thereby, corrects the impaired absorption of oral medications during the migraine headache. It can be taken by mouth in a

*Not FDA approved for this indication.

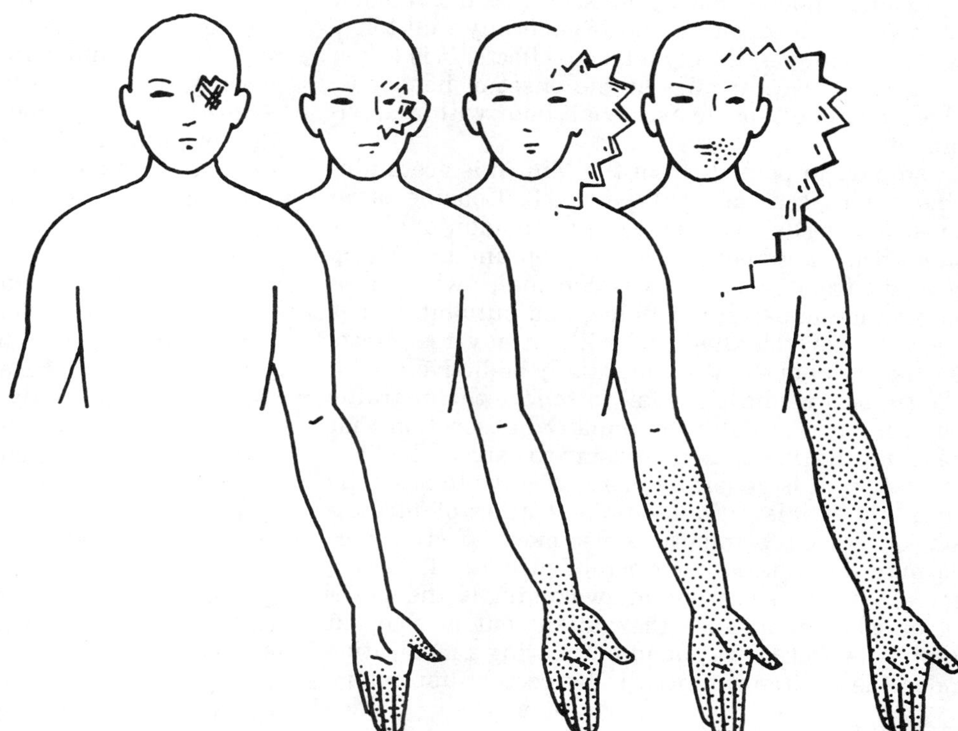

Figure 2. The two most typical aura symptoms of migraine, the scintillating scotoma *(above)* and digitolingual paresthesias *(below)*, shown from left to right in their successive stages of development.

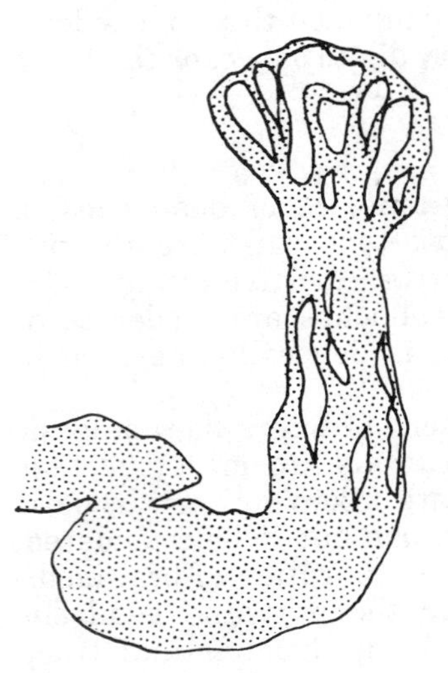

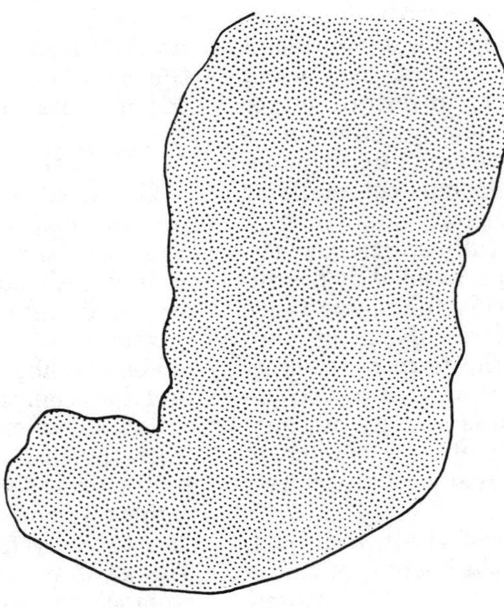

Figure 3. The stomach during the migraine headache *(right)* and between headaches *(left)*, showing dilation and atony with closure of the pyloric sphincter during the headache.

dose of 10 mg but also needs to be taken early in the onset of the headache for it to be absorbed. It generally does not cause drowsiness or any other adverse effects and, therefore, can be taken early in the onset of the headache. Medications for the headache can be taken 15 minutes after the metoclopramide* and is more effective when used in this way.

A useful oral medication for the abortive treatment of migraine is Midrin, which is a combination of isometheptene mucate, dichloralphenazone, and acetaminophen. Isometheptene is an indirectly acting sympathomimetic with vasoconstrictor properties, and dichloralphenazone is a muscle relaxant. It is not a very potent medication and is generally well tolerated, producing few if any adverse effects. It is taken in a dose of two capsules at the onset of headache, followed by one capsule every half hour with a maximum of six.

A step up in potency from the Midrin is acetaminophen* with codeine or Tylenol #3. Codeine often causes nausea as an adverse effect, an additional reason for prior treatment with metoclopramide.* A step up again from Tylenol #3 is Fiorinal,* which is a combination of aspirin, caffeine, and butalbital. It is generally well tolerated and without adverse effects but, like Tylenol #3, it is potentially addictive.

When oral medications fail to relieve the migraine headache, it is usually the impaired absorption that is at fault. Rather than increasing the strength of the medication, it is generally more effective to alter the route of administration. Administration of medications other than by mouth is also more effective once the migraine has already established itself, for example, when it is present on awakening in the morning or when it awakes the patient out of sleep at night. An effective way of administering a medication under these circumstances is by rectal suppository. The suppositories that can be used for this purpose are indomethacin (Indocin) and ergotamine tartrate and caffeine (Cafergot).

Indomethacin is a potent anti-inflammatory analgesic with a mild constrictor effect on the cerebral and extracranial arteries. It is available as a 50-mg suppository, one of which can be taken every half-hour with a maximum dosage of four. The medication can cause gastric and rectal irritation as adverse effects, as well as mild orthostatic hypotension.

The Cafergot suppository contains 2 mg ergotamine tartrate in combination with 100 mg caffeine to improve its absorption. Ergotamine is a very potent vasoconstrictor and is, therefore, contraindicated in hypertension and coronary artery disease. In a dose of 1 mg, that is, one-half of a Cafergot suppository, it relieves the migraine headache within 3 hours in 73% of patients. Nausea and vomiting are common adverse effects of ergotamine use and, therefore, it is important to administer the medication with care. I usually advise patients to take one third of a suppository, which can be repeated, if necessary, every half to 1 hour with a maximum dosage of two.

Ergotamine is a long-acting medication, and its vasoconstrictor effect has been shown to last at least 3 days. This means that the medication should not be used more frequently than once per week. If used more frequently, the wearing off of the effect of the medication is followed by rebound vasodilation and headache indistinguishable from migraine. A cycle is thus created in which the occurrence of headache and intake of ergotamine gradually increase over time, ultimately leading to what is often referred to as migraine status. This is an intractable condition in which headaches occur frequently and that requires daily or almost daily intake of ergotamine. The only way this condition can be treated is by total discontinuation of the use of ergotamine, for which hospitalization may be required. A dramatic reduction in

*Not FDA approved for this indication.

the frequency of occurrence of the migraine headaches usually follows once the withdrawal has been accomplished.

Another route of administering a medication other than by mouth is by injection. An abortive antimigraine medication that is available for administration by subcutaneous injection is sumatriptan succinate (Imitrex). It is marketed in a prefilled syringe, which contains 6 mg of the medication. It is supplied with an autoinjector device for easy administration by the patient.

The efficacy of sumatriptan is 70% in decreasing the intensity of moderate and severe headaches to no or mild headache. The medication can be repeated after 1 hour, but this has been shown *not* to increase its efficacy. Because the duration of action of the medication is relatively short, the headache may recur. If this is the case, the headache usually recurs between 8 and 12 hours after the injection. The injection can be repeated at this point, or a longer acting medication, such as the Cafergot suppository, can be administered. Adverse effects of sumatriptan are a hot, tight, or tingling sensation, generally in the upper chest, anterior neck, and face, and lightheadedness. The medication is, like ergotamine, a potent vasoconstrictor and, therefore, is contraindicated in patients with hypertension and coronary artery disease.

When migraine headaches occur frequently, that is, more than twice per month, preventive treatment may be indicated. Preventive treatment may also be indicated when the headaches are intense or prolonged, and when abortive treatment is ineffective. The medications that have been shown to be effective in the preventive treatment of migraine are methysergide maleate (Sansert); the beta blockers that lack partial agonist activity, amitriptyline hydrochloride (Elavil),* and verapamil hydrochloride (Isoptin).*

Methysergide is available in 2-mg tablets. Treatment is usually initiated with a dose of one tablet twice daily, after which the dose is increased to one tablet four times per day. The medication is given in divided doses because of its relatively short duration of action. It is taken with the meals and at bedtime with some food because it can cause nausea and indigestion. With long-term use, methysergide can cause retroperitoneal, pleuropulmonary, or endocardial fibrosis. The medication should, therefore, not be taken for longer than 4 to 6 months, after which it should be discontinued for 2 to 4 weeks. It is contraindicated in hypertension, vascular disease, valvular heart disease, chronic pulmonary disease, collagen disease, and fibrotic conditions.

The beta blockers that lack partial agonist activity are atenolol (Tenormin),* metoprolol tartrate (Lopressor),* nadolol (Corgard),* propranolol hydrochloride (Inderal), and timolol maleate (Blocadren). Of these medications, propranolol is the most commonly used, generally in doses ranging from 80 to 160 mg per day. When use is made of the long-acting capsule, the medication can be given once daily. Adverse effects of propranolol are fatigue, depression, insomnia, and impotence. The medication is contraindicated in patients with sinus bradycardia, atrioventricular block, congestive heart failure, obstructive pulmonary disease, and diabetes mellitus.

*Not FDA approved for this indication.

The other beta blockers are generally better tolerated than propranolol but still often cause fatique. Atenolol and metoprolol are cardioselective and, therefore, can be used with care in patients with obstructive pulmonary disease, such as asthma. The dose of the beta blockers should be increased gradually while the effect on the headaches is monitored. The pulse rate can be reduced, if necessary, to 50 or 60 beats per minute.

Amitriptyline* is best prescribed once daily at bedtime because it causes sedation. Treatment is usually initiated with a dose of 25 mg and gradually increased until dryness of the mouth occurs. The medication is particularly helpful in patients who also have problems falling asleep or sleeping through the night. Apart from sedation and dry mouth, amitriptyline causes constipation and weight gain as adverse effects. The medication is contraindicated in patients with glaucoma, prostate hypertrophy, epilepsy, and cardiac arrhythmias.

Verapamil* can be given twice daily when the slow-release tablet is used. Treatment is usually initiated with a dose of 240 mg per day, after which it is increased to 480 mg per day. Verapamil is generally well tolerated, with constipation as its most common adverse effect. The medication has been shown to cause infertility in men. It is contraindicated in patients with atrioventricular block and sick sinus syndrome, as it slows down atrioventricular conduction.

Of the preventive medications described earlier, the beta blockers are probably the most effective and also the best tolerated. Verapamil is probably the least effective, and amitriptyline* falls somewhere in between. A beta blocker should always be tried first to manage the migraine condition preventively with a single medication. The medications can also be combined, however, and a good combination is that of a beta blocker with amitriptyline. Special care should be taken when a beta blocker is combined with methysergide (peripheral vasoconstriction) or with verapamil (bradycardia).

Cluster Headache

Cluster headache is a chronic headache condition related to migraine but is much less common. Its prevalence in the general population is estimated at 70 per 100,000, with a male-to-female ratio of 14 to 1. The headaches of cluster headache last from ½ to 2 hours and occur once or twice per 24 hours. They have a tendency to occur during the early night, awakening the patient out of sleep 1 or 2 hours after retiring. In 85% of the patients, the headaches occur in episodes that last from ½ to 2 months, separated by remissions of ½ to 1 year. In the remaining 15% of

*Not FDA approved for this indication.

patients, the headaches occur for longer than 1 year without remission. In this case, the condition is referred to as chronic, as opposed to episodic, cluster headache. The pain of cluster headache is always unilateral and, in 90% of patients, *always* affects the same side of the head. It is usually located in and around the eye, in the forehead, temple, or in the face. In these areas autonomic symptoms often occur, such as reddening and tearing of the eye, edematous swelling and drooping of the upper eye lid, narrowing of the pupil, increased sweating over the forehead, and stuffiness and running of the nose. These symptoms are *not,* however, pathognomonic for cluster headache, and their presence is *not* required for the diagnosis. Systemic symptoms, such as nausea and vomiting, are rare in cluster headache.

Apart from instructing the patient to avoid alcohol and daytime napping during the episodes, treatment of cluster headache is pharmacologic in nature. The pharmacologic treatment can be either abortive or preventive, although generally both are applied with emphasis on preventive treatment. Four medications, that is, methysergide maleate (Sansert), verapamil hydrochloride (Isoptin),* prednisone,* and lithium carbonate,* are effective in the preventive treatment of cluster headache. The three medications that are effective in aborting the headaches of cluster headache are ergotamine tartrate, oxygen, and sumatriptan succinate (Imitrex).*

Ergotamine is most effective in cluster headache when taken as a sublingual tablet that contains 2 mg of the medication (Ergomar). It aborts at least 7 out of 10 headaches in 70% of patients, mostly within 10 to 12 minutes of treatment. The most common adverse effects of the medication are nausea, leg cramps, and a bad taste in the mouth. The medication is contraindicated in patients with hypertension and coronary artery disease.

Inhalation of 100% oxygen is somewhat more effective than ergotamine use. It is inhaled through a face mask at a rate of 8 to 10 L per minute for 15 minutes at the onset of headache. It aborts at least 7 out of 10 headaches in 82% of patients, in more than half within 6 minutes of treatment. There are no adverse effects or contraindications to the use of oxygen.

Sumatriptan, in a dose of 6 mg subcutaneously, aborts 74% of headaches within 15 minutes of treatment. A hot, tight, or tingling sensation, generally in the upper chest, anterior neck, and face, and lightheadedness are its most common adverse effects. Like ergotamine, the medication is contraindicated in patients with hypertension and coronary artery disease.

Methysergide, in a dose of 8 mg per day, has an efficacy of 53% in episodic and 7% in chronic cluster headache. Efficacy is determined as a reduction in headache frequency of at least 75%. Verapamil* has an efficacy of 73% in episodic and 60% in chronic cluster headache. The daily dose of verapamil to obtain this effect ranges from 240 to 600 mg in episodic and from 240 to 1200 mg (sustained-release tablets) in chronic cluster headache. With the use of doses greater than 480 mg per day, an echocardiogram should be performed to exclude heart muscle disease. It is also recommended that an electrocardiogram be performed several days after every dose increase to determine the effect of the medication on atrioventricular conduction.

*Not FDA approved for this indication.

When prednisone* is used as a preventive treatment, it is usually given in a course of 3 or 4 weeks. The initial dose is 40 to 60 mg per day, which is maintained for 3 to 5 days. Subsequently the dose is gradually decreased in steps of 5 mg per 2 days. The efficacy of prednisone is 77% in episodic and 40% in chronic cluster headache. Adverse effects are insomnia, fluid retention, mood changes, and gastritis. The medication is contraindicated in patients with hypertension, diabetes mellitus, infections, peptic ulcer disease, and diverticulosis.

Lithium* is particularly effective in patients with chronic cluster headache, in which it has an efficacy of 87%. The therapeutic dose is generally between 600 and 1200 mg per day. Lithium* is contraindicated in the presence of electrolyte imbalance or when sodium restriction and diuretic therapy are required. In the latter cases, lithium intoxication easily develops due to the increased tubular reabsorption of the medication, leading to symptoms ranging from tremor to convulsions.

Common adverse effects of lithium are gastrointestinal symptoms, such as nausea, abdominal discomfort, and diarrhea. The symptoms often respond rapidly, however, to a slight lowering of the dose of the medication. The maintenance dose of lithium in the treatment of cluster headache does *not* depend on the serum level of the medication. It is, however, advisable to keep the serum level below 1.5 mEq per liter and to determine it regularly, together with the serum electrolyte levels, and kidney and thyroid functions.

Paroxysmal Hemicrania

Paroxysmal hemicrania is a variant of cluster headache that is rare but easy to diagnose and treat. It consists of severe unilateral headaches that are similar to cluster headache but are shorter in duration and occur more frequently. The headaches last from 10 to 30 minutes and occur 5 to 15 times per 24 hours. They often occur with clockwork regularity, every 2 hours during the day and at night. The headaches occur in episodes with remissions or daily for years; that is, they are chronic. They are totally relieved by preventive treatment with indomethacin (Indocin).* The dose generally required is 25 mg four times per day or 75 mg of the sustained-release formulation twice daily. The beneficial effect is usually apparent within 2 to 5 days of treatment. Indomethacin is contraindicated in patients with peptic ulcer disease and bleeding disorders.

*Not FDA approved for this indication.

EPISODIC VERTIGO

method of
CAROL A. FOSTER, M.D., and
ROBERT W. BALOH, M.D.*
University of California, Los Angeles School of Medicine
Los Angeles, California

Dizziness is a nonspecific term used by patients to describe a sensation of altered orientation in space. Vertigo is a special form of dizziness associated with disease of the vestibular system. Reflexes providing postural and ocular responses to head motion are mediated through pathways involving the paired vestibular nuclei in the brain stem. These nuclei receive and transmit neural impulses from the labyrinths, the visual system, and the somatosensory system of the neck and limbs, and communicate with the cerebellum, thalamus, and cortex. Damage involving any of these pathways may give rise to vertigo. The word vertigo is derived from the Latin word *vertere,* meaning to spin, and it is frequently used to describe the sensation of spinning. Other illusions of movement, such as tilting or linear displacement, may also result from vestibular lesions.

Vertigo may be associated with other symptoms and signs that assist in the diagnosis and localization of disease. Most syndromes that cause vertigo, however, share several common features. Nausea and vomiting commonly accompany severe vertigo and are the focus of most symptomatic treatments. Postural instability and gait imbalance are often present acutely and can predispose the patient to damaging falls. Oscillopsia, the visual illusion of movement and blurring of the stationary environment, can occur either during head movement, as a result of damaged vestibular reflexes controlling eye movements, or when the head is still owing to nystagmus.

TREATMENT

Treatment of vertigo can be divided into three general categories: specific, symptomatic, and rehabilitative. Specific therapies are those directed at the underlying cause of vertigo and have the potential for eliminating vertigo. Symptomatic therapy is used to control troublesome symptoms during the acute stage and may also be used when a specific treatment does not exist. Rehabilitation is appropriate when damage to the vestibular system is expected to persist and is used to reduce symptoms of dizziness, gait imbalance, and oscillopsia.

Specific Therapy for Vertigo Syndromes

Motion Sickness

Unaccustomed exposure to prolonged motion can cause marked autonomic symptoms in susceptible persons. Typically, these include perspiration, nausea, vomiting, increased salivation, yawning, and malaise. The syndrome is worsened when there is a conflict between visual cues and vestibular cues about self-motion. For example, reading or sitting in an enclosed space while in motion in a boat or car gives the visual system the miscue that the environment is stationary, while the vestibular system receives strong self-motion cues. This mismatch can be reduced by viewing the environment—the horizon from aboard ship or the road while driving—so that self-movement can be accurately perceived. For susceptible persons, use of a vestibular suppressant with moderate sedating action helps prevent the development of symptoms by diminishing the sensation of motion detected by the inner ear. For short exposures, dimenhydrinate (Dramamine) is usually effective (Table 1). For longer trips, transdermal scopolamine (Transderm Scōp) has proved effective, but the patch must be in place for several hours before exposure to motion. Most people are able to acclimate to motion within a few days of continuous exposure.

Benign Positional Vertigo

Patients with benign positional vertigo develop brief episodes of vertigo following position change, typically when turning over in bed, lifting the head after bending over, or extending the neck to look up. The syndrome is believed to be due to the presence of otoconial debris within the posterior semicircular canal; this debris causes gravity-dependent movement of the cupula. It can follow any form of injury to the inner ear and is particularly common following head trauma, viral neurolabyrinthitis, or prolonged bed rest. The physical examination is usually completely normal. Rapidly moving the patient from the sitting to the head-hanging position (the Dix–Hallpike maneuver), however, induces a torsional, upbeat nystagmus when the affected ear is down. The nystagmus appears after a brief latency, lasts for less than 1 minute, and fatigues with repeated positioning. A positioning maneuver is used to move the debris along the posterior canal and out its opening, effectively curing the syndrome (Fig. 1). The maneuver can be reapplied several times in succession until the positional nystagmus disappears. Patients are cautioned to keep the head elevated at least 30 degrees above the horizontal for 48 hours following the procedure.

Acute Peripheral Vestibulopathy

An acute episode of severe vertigo with nystagmus, nausea, and vomiting that gradually resolves over days to weeks can result from a number of different causes. Viral involvement of the vestibular nerve and inner ear is the most common cause. Findings and specific therapies for several syndromes are listed in Table 2. Symptomatic treatment is usually necessary to control acute vertigo and nausea as the work-up progresses, and vestibular rehabilitation is often needed to speed recovery.

*Dr. Foster is supported by grant NINCD DC 01404, and Dr. Baloh is supported by grants NIA AG 09693 and NINCD DC 01404.

TABLE 1. **Antivertiginous Drugs**

Drug	Dosage	Action: Sedative	Action: Antimetic	Major Side Effects	Precautions
ANTIHISTAMINE					
Meclizine (Antivert, Bonine)	Oral: 25 mg qd–qid	±	+	–	Asthma, glaucoma, prostate enlargement
Dimenhydrinate (Dramamine)	Oral: 50 mg q 4–6 h	+	+	–	Same as above
Promethazine* (Phenergan)	Oral: 25 mg q 6 h Supp: 50 mg q 12 h IM: 25 mg q 4–6 h	+ +	+	Extrapyramidal	Same as above
ANTICHOLINERGIC					
Scopolamine (Transderm-Scōp)	Patch: 0.5 mg q 3 days	±	+	Mental status changes	Glaucoma, tachyarrhythmias, prostate enlargement
PHENOTHIAZINE					
Prochlorperazine* (Compazine)	Oral: 5–10 mg q 6 h Supp: 25 mg q 12 h IM: 5–10 mg q 6 h	+	+ + +	Tardive dyskinesia, dystonia, parkinsonism	Known hypersensitivity
BENZODIAZEPINE					
Diazepam* (Valium)	Oral: 2, 5, 10 mg PO bid–qid IM: 5–10 mg q 4–6 h IV: 5–10 mg (slow) q 4 h	+ + +	+	Respiratory depression, drug dependency	Glaucoma
BUTYROPHENONE					
Droperidol (Inapsine)	IM or IV: 2.5–5 mg q 12 h	+ + +	+ +	Extrapyramidal	Known hypersensitivity

*Not FDA approved for this indication.

Relapsing Vestibulopathy

Common syndromes resulting in recurrent episodes of vertigo are listed in Table 3. Key factors in the differential diagnosis include the duration of typical vertigo attacks (minutes vs. hours), and the presence or absence of hearing loss and abnormalities on electronystagmography. Symptomatic therapy can be used during acute, severe attacks of vertigo, but it is less effective when used daily because of the long-term, chronic nature of these conditions. Treatment aimed at relieving the underlying disorder is critical.

Chronic Vestibulopathy

Processes that result in slow loss of vestibular function, or that involve both labyrinths simultaneously, do not usually result in attacks of severe vertigo. Such syndromes may result in recurrent, transient sensations of mild vertigo, nonspecific dizziness, or progressive gait imbalance. Associated symptoms and signs are necessary for diagnosis in these cases. Slowly growing tumors of the eighth nerve or cerebellopontine angle (acoustic neuroma) are usually associated with progressive hearing loss and can cause facial weakness or central signs; magnetic resonance imaging and brain stem auditory evoked response testing are diagnostic, and surgical consultation is indicated. Exposure to ototoxic drugs (particularly aminoglycosides) can result in bilateral vestibular damage, which causes gait imbalance and oscillopsia. Therapy includes discontinuation of the drug and the implementation of a vestibular rehabilitation program.

Drugs Used for Symptomatic Therapy

Normally, the vestibular nuclei receive a balanced, tonic input from the vestibular receptors in the inner ears. Any asymmetry in this tonic firing rate causes vertigo. Antivertiginous drugs are believed to act by suppressing the firing rate of primary afferent neurons and by decreasing transmission of impulses from primary to secondary vestibular neurons, thereby decreasing the imbalance resulting from a vestibular lesion. Commonly used drugs and their dosages are listed in Table 1. The effectiveness of these drugs has been determined empirically, and it is often difficult to predict which drug or combination of drugs will be most effective in any given patient.

A drug or drug combination should be chosen based on the known effects of each drug and on the severity and time course of the patient's symptoms. Acute, severe vertigo with nystagmus is an extremely distressing symptom, and sedation is useful during the early phase of treatment (i.e., diazepam,* droperidol*). Side effects can be serious, and parenteral treatment should be reserved for settings in which emergency resuscitation equipment is available. When nausea and vomiting are prominent, a potent antiemetic such as prochlorperazine can be combined with an antivertiginous medication. Severe, infrequent vertigo spells associated with nausea can be managed on an outpatient basis with promethazine, taken orally or as a suppository at the onset of symptoms.

Chronic, frequently recurrent vertigo is a different therapeutic problem, because the patient must attempt to carry on normal activities and because sedation is undesirable. Milder antivertiginous medications, such as meclizine, 25 mg every 6 hours, can be used for less severe vertigo. These drugs are gen-

*Not FDA approved for this indication.

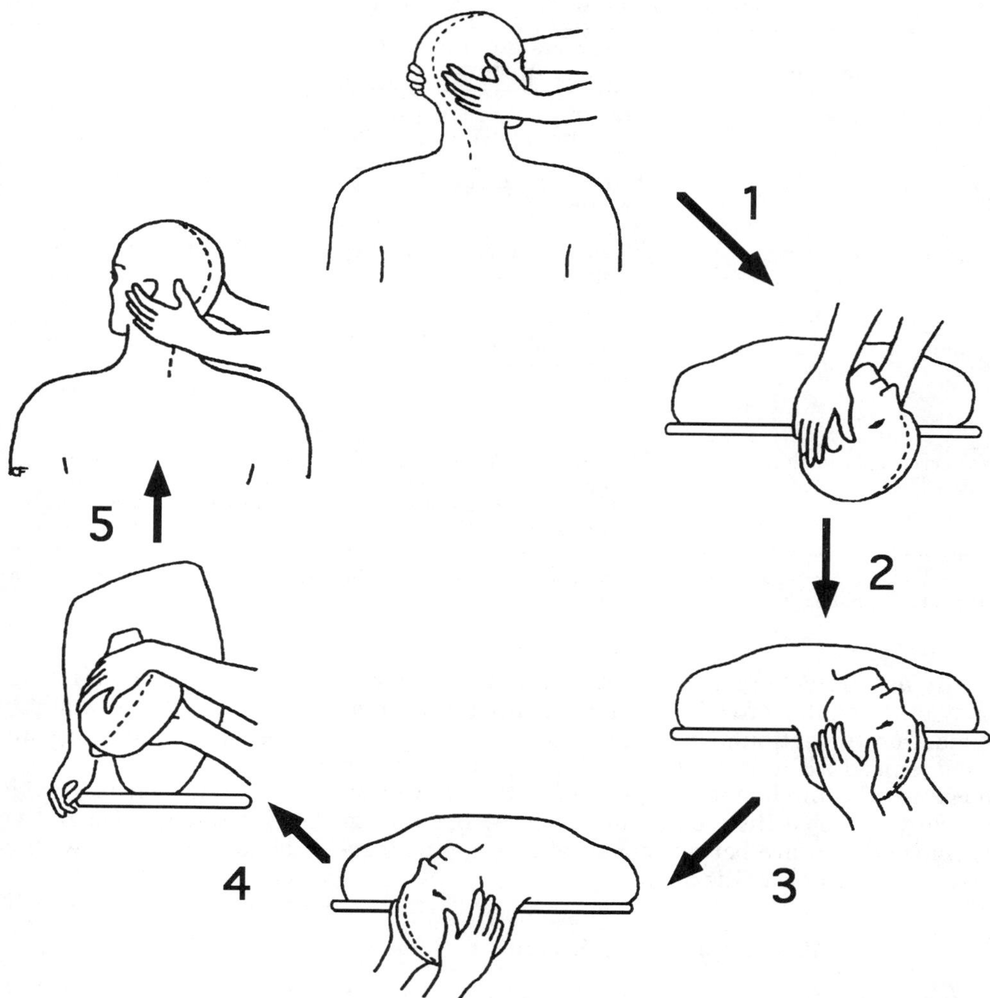

Figure 1. Treatment maneuver for benign positional vertigo affecting the right ear. The procedure can be reversed for treating the left ear. (1) The patient is seated upright, with the head facing the operator, who is standing on the right. The patient should grasp the forearm of the operator with both hands for stability. The patient is then rapidly moved into the supine position, allowing the head to extend just beyond the end of the examining table, with the right ear downward. This position is maintained until the nystagmus ceases. (2) The operator moves to the head of the table, repositioning the hands as shown. (3) The head is quickly rotated toward the left, stopping with the right ear upward. This position is maintained for 30 seconds. (4) The patient rolls onto the left side, while the examiner rapidly rotates the head leftward until the nose is directed toward the floor. This position is then held for 30 seconds. (5) The patient is rapidly lifted into the sitting position, and now faces left. The entire sequence should be repeated until no nystagmus can be elicited.

TABLE 2. **Diagnosis and Management of Common Causes of Acute Peripheral Vestibulopathy**

Syndrome	Vertigo History	Examination	Treatment
Bacterial labyrinthitis	Abrupt onset; history of ear infection, or headache and fever	Profound hearing loss, nystagmus, otitis media, or meningitis	Antibiotics based on culture results; surgical débridement; vestibular rehabilitation
Stroke	Abrupt onset, age >50 yr, prior history vascular disease, other neurologic symptoms	Signs of brain stem or cerebellar infarct; nystagmus, unilateral hearing loss, MRI changes	Supportive measures; vestibular rehabilitation
Trauma and labyrinthine concussion	Abrupt onset following head trauma ± other neurologic symptoms	Nystagmus, hearing impairment, hemotympanum, ± facial weakness, temporal bone fracture on CT	Surgical consult if seventh nerve injured; vestibular rehabilitation
Viral neurolabyrinthitis	Develops over hours, resolves over days, prior flulike illness	Nystagmus, vomiting, ± high-frequency hearing loss	Consider steroids (methylprednisolone sodium succinate [Solu-Medrol* dosepak]); vestibular rehabilitation

Abbreviations: MRI = magnetic resonance imaging; CT = computed tomography.
*Not FDA approved for this indication.

TABLE 3. **Diagnosis and Management of Common Causes of Relapsing Vestibulopathy**

Syndrome	Vertigo Duration and History	Examination	Treatment
Autoimmune disease	Hours; rapidly progressing bilateral hearing loss	Hearing loss, ± inflammatory process in eye, joints, other organs ± elevated ESR	Steroids: Prednisone 100 mg* qd; Solu-Medrol 1 g* qd
Meniere's syndrome	Hours; aural fullness, tinnitus, hearing loss	Low-frequency hearing loss during attacks, ENG abnormal	1 g sodium diet; diuretics; surgery if vertigo is uncontrolled
Migraine-associated vertigo	Minutes to hours; past history of aura or unilateral throbbing headache	Normal, ± ENG abnormalities	Migraine prophylaxis: Acetazolamide 250 mg bid; propranolol LA, 80–160 mg qd; imiprimine 50–100 mg qd
Syphilis	Similar to Meniere's; history of sexually transmitted disease or congenital infection	Bilateral progressive hearing loss, ENG abnormalities, signs of congenital syphilis	Penicillin and steroids: benzathine penicillin 2.4 million units IM q week × 6 week; prednisone 60 mg qod × 3 months
Vertebrobasilar insufficiency and TIA	Minutes; abrupt onset, age >50 yr, prior history vascular disease, other neurologic symptoms	Normal between attacks; nystagmus, ataxia, other neurologic signs during attack	Antiplatelet therapy—aspirin 325 mg qd; ticlopidine 250 mg bid

Abbreviations: TIA = transient ischemic attack; ESR = erythrocyte sedimentation rate; ENG = electronystagmography.
*Not FDA approved for this indication.

erally not indicated for long-term, daily use, because they tend to interfere with the normal process of compensation to vestibular disorders. Diazepam* can be used episodically, but prolonged usage on a daily basis results in chemical dependency. Rehabilitation therapy or a specific treatment aimed at the underlying condition are better choices of therapy for persistent symptoms of dizziness.

Vestibular Rehabilitation

When the vestibular system has been permanently damaged, the initial state of imbalance at the level of the brain stem nuclei results in acute vertigo. Gradually, the patient adapts to this imbalance through a process of compensation, which requires intact vision and depth perception, normal proprioception in the neck and limbs, and intact sensation in the lower extremities. Central pathways are also integral to compensation, and damage to these areas results in a less effective recovery.

Clinicians have long been aware that vestibular compensation occurs more rapidly and is more complete if the patient begins exercising as soon as possible after a vestibular lesion. Controlled studies in primates have supported this general clinical observation. Baboons whose hind limbs were restrained by plaster casts after onset of a unilateral vestibular lesion showed markedly delayed recovery of balance compared with lesioned animals that had been allowed normal motor exploration. Visual experience is also necessary; lesioned animals kept in the light compensated faster than those kept in darkness. Compensation is accelerated by stimulant drugs and is slowed by sedation. For these reasons, vestibular exercise programs should be instituted as soon as possible after an injury to the vestibular system has been identified, and the use of sedating drugs and vestibular suppressants should be limited to the acute stage.

*Not FDA approved for this indication.

In addition to vertigo, vestibular lesions interfere with reflexes controlling eye movement during active head motion and with postural righting reflexes. This can result in symptoms of oscillopsia caused by head movements and in a tendency to veer or fall to the side when gaiting. These symptoms and the associated dizziness can be improved by active exercises designed to speed compensation. Vestibular exercises should begin as soon as the acute stage of nausea and vomiting has ended and the underlying disease process has begun to subside. Many of the exercises result in dizziness. This sensation is a necessary stimulus for compensation; antivertiginous medications should be avoided during this period to maximize the beneficial effect. Exercises should be performed at least twice daily for several minutes, but they may be performed as often as the patient can tolerate.

While nystagmus is present, attempts should be made to focus the eyes and to move and hold them in the direction that provokes the most dizziness. Once the nystagmus diminishes to the point that a target can be held visually in all directions, the patient should begin eye-head coordination exercises. A useful exercise involves staring at a visual target while oscillating the head from side to side, or up and down. The speed of the head movements can be gradually increased, as long as the target can be kept in good focus. Target changes, using combined eye and head movements to jump quickly back and forth between two widely separated visual targets, are also useful. Blinking during these fast head turns can help reduce symptoms of dizziness or visual blurring.

Attempts should be made by the patient to stand and walk while nystagmus is still present. It may be necessary for the patient to walk in contact with a wall or with the aid of an assistant in the early stages. Slow, supported turns should be made initially. As improvement occurs, head movements should be added while the patient stands and walks—at first slow, side-to-side or up-and-down movements, then fast head turns in all directions. Learning to combine fast head turns with brief eye closure or blinks during gaiting turns can increase stability and decrease dizziness.

Compensation requires from 2 to 6 months. Dizziness that persists beyond this time indicates either the presence of an ongoing, recurrent vestibular illness or poor compensation. The patient's history should be reviewed, and any vestibular suppressants should be discontinued. Evidence of central involvement or impairment of vision, proprioception, or sensation should be evaluated. If all areas are normal, no evidence of active disease is present, and no medications are in use, a program of habituation to dizziness should be instituted. All movements that provoke dizziness should be identified, and they should then be repeated as often as possible to maximize the symptom. This will gradually result in habituation to the provoking stimulus.

MENIERE'S DISEASE

method of
HAMED SAJJADI, M.D., and
MICHAEL M. PAPARELLA, M.D.
Minnesota Ear, Head and Neck Clinic
Minneapolis, Minnesota

In 1861, Prosper Ménière first described the pathologic condition in peripheral end organs, endolymphatic hydrops, that causes episodes of vertigo and fluctuating sensorineural hearing loss, tinnitus, and aural fullness. This condition is more common in adults 20 to 60 years of age. It is seen in children as young as 4 years of age and in older adults in their nineties, equally in the right or left ear, and in each sex (although Meyerhoff in 1981 indicated a female-to-male ratio of 1.3:1). In 1978, Stahle in Sweden estimated Meniere's disease to be four times more common than otosclerosis. Proportionate figures would suggest that 2.4 million people in the United States suffer from this disease.

The incidence of bilateral Meniere's disease is approximately one in three patients, and about 78% of patients with unilateral Meniere's disease demonstrate some sensorineural hearing loss in the contralateral ear as time progresses. Half of the patients with unilateral disease demonstrate a peak audiometric configuration typical of Meniere's disease, in which the hearing is worse in the low and in the high frequencies and is better in the range of 1000 to 2000 Hz. Other audiometric patterns commonly seen include low-frequency hearing loss (in early Meniere's disease) and a flat sensorineural hearing loss (in advanced Meniere's disease). Some patients may progress to complete sensorineural deafness in the affected ear.

This work was supported in part by the International Hearing Foundation.

Usually the major triad of symptoms (episodic vertigo, fluctuating hearing loss, and aural pressure) occurs together, but in many patients, either just vestibular or just auditory symptoms may be present months or years before other symptoms develop. Aural pressure seems to be the most persistent of symptoms in different variations of Meniere's disease. Episodic vertigo is suffered by 96.2% of patients. One in four report vertiginous attacks of less than an hour, half lasting 1 to 2 hours, and the rest for 2 hours or more, up to a day or so at a time. In 87.7% of patients, there is fluctuating sensorineural hearing loss, and 91.1% of patients report tinnitus. Fifty-six percent of patients report the hearing of loud sounds as a painful experience, and 43.6% have diplacusis. Aural pressure in one or both ears is related by 74.1% of patients.

PATHOGENESIS

The main underlying problem in Meniere's disease appears to be dysfunctional absorption of endolymph in the endolymphatic sac. Once a known etiologic factor is determined, the condition is called Meniere's syndrome. Cases of Meniere's disease are most likely cases of multifactorially inherited predisposition. Up to 20% of patients with Meniere's disease report the same diagnosis in family members. A characteristic displacement, anteriorly and medially, of the lateral sinus has been described in these patients, indicating possibly that the developmental anomaly has led to pressure in the area of the endolymphatic sac.

DIAGNOSIS

In its classic form, a diagnosis of Meniere's disease is usually not difficult to establish. A detailed history, a complete neurotologic and neurologic assessment, and a physical examination are needed to make the diagnosis. The classic symptoms include episodic, disabling vertigo (often associated with vegetative symptoms such as nausea and vomiting), with fluctuating sensorineural hearing loss, a roaring unilateral tinnitus, and pressure or fullness in or near the affected ear. Patients are frequently well between attacks of vertigo, but the pressure and fullness in the ear may continue between attacks indefinitely. Positional changes precipitating vertigo are also commonly seen in patients with Meniere's disease.

The acute, disabling vertiginous episodes are usually short lived (a matter of minutes to less than an hour), but at times they may be prolonged (for several minutes or hours, or even for a day or two). There is no loss of consciousness during an attack, and the patient has no neurologic deficit, such as paresthesia, diplopia, weakness or paralysis, or dysarthria. Because of the nystagmus during vertiginous attacks, however, vision may seem blurred. In rare cases, vertiginous attacks may be so explosive and severe that the patient falls violently to the ground. Such so-called drop attacks have been called utricular crises or falling spells of Tumarkin.

Hearing acuity is always decreased during a definite spell and may remain decreased or may improve dramatically once the spell is finished. This paradoxical improvement in hearing after an acute attack is sometimes called Lermoyez's syndrome.

In the acute phase, for diagnostic purposes, a complete history taking and physical examination are sufficient. Once the patient is treated for the acute phase, further diagnostic testing, such as audiography, tympanography and acoustic reflex testing, electronystagmography, electro-

TABLE 1. **Differential Diagnosis of Meniere's Disease**

Peripheral Etiologies	
Etiopathic postural vertigo	Otosclerosis
Benign paroxysmal positional vertigo	Paget's disease
	Latent congenital neurosyphilis
Benign paroxysmal vertigo of childhood	Cogan's syndrome
	Ototoxicity
Vestibular neuronitis	Intermittent tubotympanitis
Labyrinthitis	Barotrauma with sudden hearing loss
Labyrinthine fistula	
Herpes zoster oticus	Intralabyrinthine hemorrhage
Traumatic labyrinthine concussion or fracture of the temporal bone	
Central Causes	
Vertebrobasilar ischemia	Hereditary ataxia
Multiple sclerosis	Vestibular epilepsy
Tumors of the cerebellopontine angle (vestibular schwannomas, meningiomas)	Postural imbalance of the elderly
	Vascular accidents in cerebral and cerebellar cortex

cochleography, and auditory brain stem response audiometry, is performed on all patients suspected of having Meniere's disease. Posturography and magnetic resonance imaging with gadolonium contrast of the cerebellopontine angle of the brain are reserved for selected cases of suspected central or retrocochlear pathologic conditions. The differential diagnosis of Meniere's disease includes central causes of episodic vertigo, including presyncopal lightheadedness, cerebellar brain stem strokes or hemorrhages, vertebral basilar transient ischemic attacks, and in rare cases, Arnold-Chiari malformation. Metabolic toxicities, such as arsenic poisoning and hyperventilation syndrome with epileptic seizures, also may be associated with episodic vertigo. Toxicities of prescription drugs, such as tranquilizers, antihypertensives, aminoglycoside antibiotics, and anticonvulsants, are also well-known causes of disorientation, presyncopal lightheadedness, and disequilibrium and a variety of complaints of dizziness without true vertigo. Peripheral causes of vertigo, other than Meniere's disease, also have to be evaluated (Table 1).

TREATMENT

For the severely disabled individual in an acute phase, diazepam (Valium)* 10 mg orally or 5 mg intramuscularly may be sufficient to control the initial symptoms. Trimethobenzamide hydrochloride (Tigan)* capsules, 250 mg orally every 8 hours in adults, or 100 mg every 8 hours in children, can also be given to control nausea and vomiting. If there is excessive nausea, this medication should be given in the intramuscular form, 200 mg every 12 hours, to control nausea and vomiting. Vestibular sedatives such as meclizine (Antivert) containing H_1 blocking agents can be used in both the acute and chronic phases; usual for the acute phase is a 50-mg loading dose, followed by 25 mg every 8 hours to control vertigo. Once the vertigo is controlled, 3 or 4 days after the acute episode, the medication can be gradually withdrawn or tapered. For patients suspected of also having an autoimmune inner ear phenomenon, a high-dose trial of steroids can also be attempted, 1 mg per kg orally in the emergency room, followed by a similar dose for the next 7 days given in divided dosage every day, then gradually tapered off over the next 7 days.

*Not FDA approved for this indication.

For a patient with an established diagnosis of Meniere's disease, once an acute attack starts the patient is given either meclizine or dimenhydrinate (Dramamine) (25 mg every 8 hours for the next 3 or 4 days); once the symptoms have subsided, the patient is gradually taken off this medication. As mentioned earlier, antiemetic medications also are used for these patients. The mainstay of therapy for patients with Meniere's disease is dietary control, mainly maintaining a low-salt diet (no more than 2000 mg per day). Also, patients are encouraged to completely stop all consumption of tobacco, caffeine, alcohol, and chocolate because these items have been associated with exacerbations of symptoms. A low-fat diet is also recommended for these patients. Vestibular exercises have been shown to improve adaptation in the vestibular balance system. For patients who fail to control symptoms with diet, an intermittent use of vestibular suppressants and diuretic therapies is also instituted: hydrochlorothiazide* (25 mg) and triamterene (Dyrenium)* 50 mg, one tablet per day on a long-term basis.

More than 80% of patients who present with Meniere's disease are controlled on a regimen that includes diet modification, vestibular sedatives and suppressants, and diuretic therapy. The remaining patients who are not controlled on this regimen may require more aggressive intervention, such as the use of ototoxic drugs or surgical treatment, or both. The use of vestibulotoxic drugs is a rather destructive procedure, is highly controversial, and is best reserved for patients who are not candidates for surgical therapy. Streptomycin is the most commonly used agent for this condition.

Because the incidence of bilaterality in this disease is as high as 30 to 40% in many studies, it is best to avoid destructive procedures as much as possible. Destructive procedures include vestibular neurectomy, labyrinthectomy, and instillation of vestibulotoxic drugs such as streptomycin into the labyrinth during a surgical procedure. Nondestructive procedures include mainly the endolymphatic sac-enhancing procedure. We prefer the endolymphatic sac-enhancing procedure as the first surgical treatment of choice in patients who have failed medical therapy. Endolymphatic sac enhancement has a 76.6% chance of controlling vertigo for a period of 5 years or more, a 30% chance of improvement in hearing, and a 30% chance of stabilization of hearing. The endolymphatic sac-enhancement procedure has only a 2% chance of total loss of hearing or worsening of sensorineural hearing. It can also be performed in elderly patients (as old as 90 years) and in children, and in patients with bilateral illness.

Ten percent of patients who have undergone endo-

*Not FDA approved for this indication.

lymphatic sac-enhancement surgery show no improvement and continue to deteriorate, demonstrating progression of the disease. We find that these patients are best managed with a vestibular neurectomy, using a retrolabyrinthine, retrosigmoid combined approach. Even with excellent attempts to preserve hearing and an uneventful surgical procedure, 20% of patients undergoing vestibular neurectomy may show significant loss of sensorineural function in the affected ear up to several months after the procedure. Labyrinthectomy in various forms is generally avoided for patients with Meniere's disease because these patients may develop bilateral disease. Furthermore, studies have shown that endolymphatic sac–enhancement surgery has helped improve hearing in one in three patients, even though their hearing was extremely poor preoperatively.

Medical therapy is the mainstay for patients with Meniere's disease. Ten to 20% of patients fail all sorts of medical therapy, including diuretic therapy, and may require surgical therapy. Nondestructive surgical therapy, such as endolymphatic sac–enhancement surgery, is the current first choice for therapy for such patients. Destructive procedures, such as vestibular neurectomy and labyrinthectomy, are reserved for patients who have failed endolymphatic sac–enhancement surgery.

VIRAL MENINGITIS AND ENCEPHALITIS

method of
ROBERT L. KNOBLER, M.D., PH.D.
Thomas Jefferson University
Philadelphia, Pennsylvania

VIRAL MENINGITIS

Viral meningitis, which is one form of aseptic meningitis, is usually a benign, self-limited illness, although it is now recognized that this condition may also be among the first clinical manifestations of acquired immune deficiency syndrome and seeding of the nervous system with human immunodeficiency virus-1 (HIV-1). In its benign form, it is typically characterized by the meningeal sign of neck stiffness, in association with headache and fever. In some patients, the headache may be severe, and is usually the most frequent clinical finding. The fever may range from low grade to high, and it is usually accompanied by a sense of malaise. Photophobia and pain on movement of the eyes are also common findings. Typically, the mental status is intact and focal neurologic signs are absent. Examination of the cerebrospinal fluid (CSF) characteristically shows a lymphocytic pleocytosis and normal sugar, without evidence of bacterial infection.

In this clinical presentation, the principal role of the physician is to rule out problems requiring different treatment strategies (Table 1), which include bacterial, fungal, or other treatable infections and disorders, as well as to determine whether or not there is direct involvement of the central nervous system. Additional goals are to comfort the patient with supportive care through the use of analgesics, hydration, frequent follow-up observations, and reassurance.

TABLE 1. **Differential Diagnosis of Viral (Aseptic) Meningitis**

Viral meningitis (self-limited course, agent rarely identified)
Infection with HIV-1
Infection with nonviral microbial organisms
Bacterial infections (including tuberculosis, syphilis, leptospirosis, Lyme disease)
Fungal infections (including cryptococcosis)
Parasitic infections
Parameningeal infections (e.g., sinus infection, otitis media)
Be wary of a sterile CSF due to partial treatment with antibiotics
Noninfectious conditions
Drug reaction
Malignant disease (e.g., meningeal carcinomatosis from lung, breast, melanoma, and other sources)
Chemical irritants
Vasculitis (e.g., systemic lupus erythematosus, Behçet's disease, Vogt–Koyanagi–Harada's disease, and Mollaret's recurrent meningitis)
Subarachnoid hemorrhage

In some cases, particularly when the initial examination of the CSF occurs during the first 2 days of viral meningitis, a neutrophilic or mixed cellular pleocytosis may be found. Although this will be replaced by the more characteristic lymphocytic pleocytosis of viral meningitis within hours, there should be a high index of suspicion for bacterial infection as the source of the symptoms and findings under these circumstances. In this context, antibiotic treatment should be considered, at least for the period until the results of the cultures are available or a repeat of the lumbar puncture can be performed, especially if the patient is worsening clinically.

The CSF glucose is usually in the normal range in aseptic meningitis. A low CSF glucose is suggestive of other processes, such as tuberculous meningitis, fungal meningitis, meningeal carcinomatosis, lymphoma, or sarcoidosis. Therefore, suspicion of these conditions and clues of their presence should be sought in the face of this finding. Characteristically, the CSF pleocytosis of aseptic meningitis may last to some degree for up to 2 months, despite clinical improvement. Nevertheless, the lumbar puncture should be repeated within 1 week of the initial diagnostic tap to assess progress. If clinical symptoms worsen early on, however, or persist beyond 1 week, the lumbar puncture should be repeated sooner and an infectious disease specialist should be consulted.

It is important to note that the syndrome of aseptic meningitis is now recognized as one that may be caused by a variety of processes. As previously stated, infection with HIV-1, infection with nonviral microbial organisms, parameningeal infections, and noninfectious conditions, such as drugs, malignant disease (meningeal carcinomatosis), chemical irritants, vasculitis, and subarachnoid hemorrhage, can all cause aseptic meningitis. A detailed history, careful examination of the CSF, and follow-up of the patient help exclude these conditions.

VIRAL ENCEPHALITIS

The clinical diagnosis of viral encephalitis is indicative of the presence of a central nervous system infection caused by a virus, which involves infection of the substance of the brain rather than being limited to the surrounding meninges, as in viral meningitis. As such, a change in level of consciousness and mental status, the new onset of seizures, or other focal neurologic findings will be present, in addition to the possibility of fever, headache, and meningeal signs.

Efforts at clinical diagnosis are important because of the possibility that this represents a manifestation of HIV-1 infection, or that there is a specific therapeutic agent available for treatment, such as acyclovir for herpes simplex encephalitis. Early diagnosis and treatment are important because of the risk of residual neurologic sequelae, such as hemiplegia and/or seizures, and of death.

The clinical features of viral encephalitis are further evaluated by laboratory studies, which help to further distinguish this diagnosis from other possible disorders. These tests include neuroimaging studies such as computed tomography, magnetic resonance imaging, electroencephalography, and if no contraindication is present, such as a focal mass lesion or focal swelling (edema), examination of the CSF.

The CSF is evaluated for protein and sugar content; for cells, in the search for pleocytosis; and finally, for cultures. As in the case of aseptic meningitis, it may be necessary to repeat the lumbar puncture in 24 to 48 hours to refine the diagnostic considerations. In addition to the CSF, swabs of the throat, stool, and any skin lesions should be cultured for viral, bacterial, and fungal growth, and also should be processed for Gram's stain, acid-fast stain, and cryptococcal antigen.

Serum and CSF samples should be evaluated for acute and convalescent titers of viral antibodies to search for a specific rise directed against the causative virus, which is infrequently identified. The antibody rise in the convalescent period, however, if detected, is often too late to help treat the acute phase illness and may reflect a secondary infection. Nevertheless, virus identification may have clinical importance in identifying an epidemic. Particular attention should also be directed toward such diseases as Lyme disease, syphilis, rickettsiosis, and HIV-1–related diseases, which have prognostic significance.

It is very rare that a virus is actually isolated from any source, and the virus so isolated may not be the actual causative agent. Therefore, there is a great need to develop alternative measures of diagnosis, and the polymerase chain reaction, as a method to detect viral genetic material, is showing great promise for further development in use on cells in the CSF as well as in brain biopsy specimens.

TABLE 2. **Viral Encephalitides**

Sporadic Encephalitis
Herpes simplex
Rabies
Epstein–Barr virus and cytomegalovirus
Lymphocytic choriomeningitis virus
Other viruses
Epidemic Encephalitis
Arboviruses (arthropod borne–eastern, western, and Venezuelan equine encephalitides); usually occur in summer and early fall
Enteroviruses also occur in summer and early fall
Mumps tends to occur in spring
Exanthems (e.g., measles, varicella) and other viruses
Post-Infectious Encephalitis
Following exanthems (e.g., measles, varicella, rubella)
Following other virus infections

Important clinical information includes where the patient lives; the time of the year; travel history; recent exposure to insects, animals, or infected individuals; and the immunization record of the individual and those to whom he or she has been exposed. As indicated in Table 2, there are sporadic, epidemic, and post-infectious forms of encephalitis. Furthermore, there are conditions that clinically resemble viral encephalitis, although they are separate diagnostic entities. Because of the requirement for different forms of treatment for these conditions, they must be considered (Table 3). These conditions would include, but would not be limited to, bacterial abscess, Lyme disease, neoplasm, parameningeal infection, sarcoid, syphilis, toxoplasmosis, tuberculoma, vasculitis, and recurrent or relapsing encephalitis.

Sporadic encephalitis is most commonly caused by herpes simplex virus, which produces a focal encephalitis, as detected by clinical signs and diagnostic tests, although there are also other causes. Typically, herpes encephalitic lesions are in the orbital-frontal or medial temporal regions of the brain. They are often characterized as a necrotizing encephalitis with many red blood cells in the CSF. Of great significance is the fact that there is an effective treatment available (Table 4). The recommended dose is acyclovir (Zovirax), 10 mg per kg infused intravenously over 1 hour, every 8 hours for 10 days; a total of 30 mg per kg per day in adults. The dosage may have to be adjusted in the presence of impaired renal function.

TABLE 3. **Differential Diagnosis of Viral Encephalitis**

Cerebral abscess
Cerebral neoplasm
Primary glioma
Primary lymphoma
Cerebral vasculitis
Lyme disease
Parameningeal infection
Recurrent or relapsing encephalitis
Sarcoidosis
Syphilis
Tuberculoma
Toxoplasmosis
Vasculitis

A longer course of therapy may be required in certain cases.

At present, there is debate regarding the necessity of brain biopsy when the diagnosis of herpes simplex encephalitis is suspected. A biopsy is considered more likely to confirm the diagnosis of herpes simplex encephalitis than examination of the CSF alone. More important, a biopsy also helps rule out whether another disorder that may be treatable with different therapy is present. These disorders include conditions such as subdural empyema, cerebral abscess, and septic emboli. The decision to go ahead with a biopsy should be based on the clinical presentation, with the support of both a detailed neurologic examination and a magnetic resonance imaging study supporting the location to be biopsied.

If increased intracranial pressure is present, then appropriate treatment with elevated head position and intubation with hyperventilation; dexamethasone (Decadron), 10 mg every 6 hours by any route; and mannitol should be considered and used prior to the procedure. Other supportive measures to be considered include the use of anticonvulsants in those with seizures or suspected seizure disorder, as well as proper fluid and nutritional balance, frequent checks of electrolyte levels and renal function, and careful monitoring of skin breakdown.

Epidemics of encephalitis are associated with the agents listed in Table 2, most commonly arboviruses. Although no specific treatment exists for most of these viruses, supportive treatment (Table 4) is very important because the prognosis is generally favorable, even in patients who may initially be in a coma. A specific diagnosis may be established by serology and is important in directing public health measures such as mosquito control.

Post-infectious encephalitis does not actually reflect direct, late effects of viral replication on neural cells as the cause of neurologic damage. Instead, it represents indirect, immunopathologic responses elicited by the virus. A number of synonyms exist for this syndrome, including parainfectious encephalitis, acute disseminated encephalomyelitis, and allergic encephalomyelitis.

Post-infectious encephalitis typically occurs within the 2-week period after recovery from an infection, such as a childhood exanthem. The spinal cord, optic nerves, and peripheral nervous system are frequently involved. Patients often have headache, fever, nausea, vomiting, and focal neurologic signs. Neuroimaging usually demonstrates multifocal white matter lesions, which may be hemorrhagic in severe cases.

Immunotherapy (Table 5), with a 6-hour infusion of either intravenous corticotropin (ACTH), 100 units in 250 mL of 5% dextrose, daily for 10 days, or intravenous methylprednisolone (Solu-Medrol), 1 gram in 250 mL of 5% dextrose, daily for 5 to 7 days, followed by 2 days of dosing with adenocorticotropic hormone, 100 units per day, infused over 6 hours in 250 mL of dextrose 5% in water, to stimulate the adrenal gland. Although the benefit of either of these therapies has not been proved in large, controlled trials, they have worked effectively in the clinical setting over the past 27 years. If either the adenocorticotropic hormone or steroid protocol is used, antacids and histamine receptor (H_2) antagonists should be administered concomitantly, and blood pressure, electrolyte levels, and serum glucose must be closely monitored for the duration of treatment.

TABLE 4. **Treatment of Viral Encephalitis**

Specific Therapies
Acyclovir (Zovirax): herpes simplex, herpes zoster, possibly other herpes viruses (10 mg per kg infused IV over 1 h, every 8 h for 10 days; a total of 30 mg per kg per day in adults; see text for details)
Amantadine (Symmetrel): Possibly for influenza
Zidovudine (azidothymidine AZT [Retrovir]): acute retroviral encephalitis
Supportive Therapies
Close observation, usually in the intensive care unit with infectious precautions, although the patient is not usually contagious
Management of increased intracranial pressure (see text for details)
Careful monitoring of fluid and electrolyte status
Anticonvulsants for observed or suspected seizures, after biopsy, or if the electroencephalogram suggests marked cerebral irritability

TABLE 5. **Treatment of Postinfectious Encephalitis**

Immunotherapy
Intravenous infusion of ACTH, 100 units in 250 mL of 5% dextrose, over 6 h daily for 10 days, or methylprednisolone (Solu-Medrol), 1 gm in 250 mL of 5% dextrose, over 6 h daily for 5–7 days, followed by 2 days of dosing with adenocorticotropic hormone (see text for details)

REYE'S SYNDROME

method of
RICHARD H. HAAS, M.B., B.CH.
University of California, San Diego Medical Center
San Diego, California

First described in 1963, Reye's syndrome (RS) is an acute, life-threatening metabolic disorder, the hallmarks of which are hepatic dysfunction and progressive encephalopathy. A preceding viral infection (often varicella or influenza B) is followed in the recovery period by pernicious vomiting and increasing obtundation. Diagnostic criteria are listed in Table 1. Reye's syndrome is predominantly a disorder of children. The Centers for Disease Control reported an annual incidence in the United States of 0.31 to 0.88 per 100,000 children between 1970 and 1979. In the United Kingdom between 1990 and 1991, the median age of disease onset was 10 months, compared with 15 months in the preceding decade. There is a bimodal distribution of cases, with the highest frequencies before the age of 4 years and between 10 and 14 years.

Since 1981 the incidence has fallen worldwide for un-

TABLE 1. **Diagnostic Criteria for Reye's Syndrome (Based on Centers for Disease Control and Prevention Guidelines)**

1. Acute unexplained noninflammatory encephalopathy with alteration of consciousness.
2. Hepatic dysfunction with one or more of the following: serum transaminase greater than threefold elevated, hyperammonemia, characteristic microvesicular fatty infiltration of the liver.
3. Commonly associated features include normal or minimally elevated plasma bilirubin, prolonged prothrombin time, lactic acidemia, hypoglycemia (particularly in younger children), and elevated creatine phosphokinase.

known reasons, although increasing identification of inborn errors of metabolism previously classified as RS (Table 2) and a decreased use of salicylate in children following its association with RS may be factors. Mortality remains at 30%. Early diagnosis, hypertonic glucose infusion, and aggressive management of intracranial pressure in an intensive care unit are essential for the best outcome.

In recent years, inherited metabolic disorders, and particularly fat metabolism defects, have been increasingly identified as causes of RS and RS-like disorders. In 1991, of the 25 cases of RS reported to the British Reye's Syndrome Surveillance Scheme, 48% were reclassified as inherited metabolic disorders, and this is considered an underestimate. Medium-chain acyl-CoA dehydrogenase deficiency was the most common, followed by organic acidurias and urea cycle defects. Every patient with RS should be evaluated for the group of inborn errors listed in Table 2. The diagnostic samples listed in Table 3 should be collected in the acute illness in every case for subsequent study because autopsy samples are often inadequate for diagnosis. DNA testing for the common mutation responsible for medium chain acyl-CoA dehydrogenase deficiency can be rapidly performed from a blood sample. In patients with these disorders, recurrent RS is a risk, follow-up care in a metabolic clinic is indicated, and autosomal recessive inheritance poses a risk of metabolic decompensation for siblings. Acute treatment for inborn errors causing RS is similar to that for RS (Table 4), with the addition of specific measures for inborn errors, which may include protein restriction, intravenous arginine and benzoate or phenylacetate (urea cycle defects), aggressive management of acidosis, and hemodialysis.

TABLE 3. **Tests Needed to Diagnose Reye's Syndrome and Inherited Metabolic Disease (Should be Collected During the Acute Illness)**

Infection screen: Complete blood count and differential: lumbar puncture; cultures of blood, urine, and CSF
Cardiorespiratory status: blood gases, bicarbonate, and pH
Hepatorenal status: hepatic and renal function tests, blood glucose, serum ammonia, amylase, uric acid and creatine phosphokinase, prothrombin and partial thromboplastin times
Toxin screen: Urine toxicology screen
Metabolic disease: Blood lactic acid; plasma quantitative amino acids; urine quantitative amino and organic acids; plasma and urine carnitine and esters; blood for DNA studies; skin biopsy for fibroblast culture, consideration of liver and possible muscle biopsy for histology; electron microscopy, include a frozen sample for metabolic and DNA studies

TREATMENT

Treatment of RS should always be carried out in a hospital intensive care unit, where close observation is possible, because rapid deterioration is common. The most important early treatment is administration of intravenous hypertonic glucose and electrolyte solutions containing 10% to 15% glucose at 80% of maintenance (1300 mL per M^2 per 24 hours). Frequent monitoring of blood glucose and osmolality is advisable, with optimal blood glucose levels at 150 to 175 mg/dL and osmolality less than 320 milliosmoles. Early hypertonic glucose treatment may prevent disease progression. Neomycin should be given orally, by nasogastric tube, or rectally in hyperammonemic children at 25 mg per kg every 6 hours. Protection against the mitochondrial toxicity of elevated free fatty acids and the secondary carnitine deficiency of many inborn errors of metabolism form the rationale for the use of intravenous levocarnitine (Carnitor), which should be given at a dosage of 50 mg per kg per dose every 6 hours.

Aggressive intervention is necessary in any child entering stage III, corresponding roughly to a Glasgow coma score of 8 (Glasgow coma scoring may not be appropriate for metabolic encephalopathies). Treatment at this stage includes endotracheal intubation, sedation and paralysis, the placement of cen-

TABLE 2. **Inborn Errors Associated with Reye's Syndrome (Younger Age of Onset, Recurrent Disease, and Positive Family History May Be a Clue)**

Disorder or Defect	Clinical and Biochemical Features
Fatty acid oxidation disorders	Hypoglycemia, hypoketonuria, abnormal urinary organic acids, carnitine abnormalities, abnormal fibroblast enzyme assay, positive DNA analysis in MCAD
Organic acid disorders	Metabolic acidosis, marked ketosis, abnormal urinary organic acids, lactic acidemia and hyperammonemia, carnitine abnormalities, abnormal fibroblast enzyme assay
Urea cycle defects	Marked hyperammonemia, respiratory alkalosis, abnormal plasma and urine amino acids (i.e., orotic aciduria, ↑ glutamine, ± citrullinemia)
Oxidative metabolic defects	Preceding psychomotor delay and/or motor deficit, lactic acidosis, abnormal plasma and urine amino or organic acids, ± metabolic and mitochondrial myopathy, abnormal brain magnetic resonance imaging, tissue enzyme and DNA studies may be abnormal

Abbreviation: MCAD = medium chain acyl-CoA dehydrogenase deficiency.

TABLE 4. **Stages and Treatment of Reye's Syndrome**

Stage	Features	Treatment
Stage I	Vomiting, lethargy, responds to verbal stimuli	D_{10-15} glucose with electrolytes IV at 80% of maintenance; vitamin K_1 1 mg IV, monitor blood glucose, ammonia, gases, electrolytes q 6 h, neomycin (50 mg per kg q 6 h if hyperammonemic)
Stage II	Combative, confused, delirium, appropriate responses to pain stimuli	As stage I; ICU mandatory, cooling blanket, careful I/O fluid measurement, sedation, D_{15} IV glucose and electrolytes, IV L-carnitine 50 mg per kg q 6 h
Stage III	Coma, decorticate posturing, intact pupillary and oculocephalic reflexes, hyperventilation	As stage II stat plus intubation; ICP monitoring, hyperventilation (CO_2 25–30 mmHg), IV mannitol 0.25 g per kg per dose as needed to maintain CPP >50 mmHg, keep serum osmolality at 310–320 mOsm; intermittent IV pentobarbital 3–5 mg per kg for poorly controlled peaks of ICP; EEG monitoring; consider plasmapheresis
Stage IV	Coma, decerebrate posturing; pupils sluggish, loss of oculovestibular reflexes, EEG delta or burst suppression	As stage III; consider pentobarbital coma if ICP is uncontrollable and blood pressure is adequate
Stage V	Coma, flaccid, no response to pain, fixed pupils, absent brain stem reflexes, absent respiration, EEG low-voltage delta, burst suppression becoming isoelectric	Same as for stage IV

Abbreviations: ICU = intensive care unit; CPP = cerebral perfusion pressure; I/O = intake and output; ICP = intracranial pressure; EEG = electroencephalogram.

tral venous and arterial lines, and urinary catheterization. Good oxygenation should be maintained at all times. Nursing care plays an important part in the management of increased intracranial pressure (ICP). The head should be elevated to 30 degrees and held in the midline. Careful chest physical therapy with cautious suctioning and the avoidance of mucus plugs helps avoid peaks of ICP. Table 4 details a treatment regimen linked to the clinical stages of RS. ICP control with sedation, mannitol, and hyperventilation requires the use of an intracranial catheter or bolt to record ICP, and such monitoring is advisable in patients in stage III who do not rapidly respond to treatment. The cerebral perfusion pressure is the difference between the mean arterial blood pressure and the ICP. It should be maintained above 50 mmHg. There is no convincing evidence that use of barbiturate coma improves the outcome in RS. There are grounds for expecting mitochondrial toxins such as barbiturates to be detrimental, and so the use of barbiturate coma, which is often complicated by hypotension, should be reserved for children with otherwise uncontrollable ICP. Small doses of short-acting barbiturates can be used to control peaks in ICP without resorting to barbiturate coma, and hypothermia may be helpful. Plasmapheresis and exchange transfusion have been used with reported success in shortening the severity and duration of RS.

Complications of RS require prompt treatment. Any question of sepsis warrants intravenous antibiotic treatment (i.e., cefotaxime [Claforan], 25 mg per kg every 6 hours until culture results are available). Hypoglycemia may require bolus treatments of 25% glucose intravenously at 2 mL per kg. Patients who are ventilated and paralyzed generally require dopamine pressor support. Perfusion should be maintained, avoiding high central venous pressures (in excess of 6 cm H_2O) in order to avoid increasing ICP by reducing cerebral venous return. Hypotension, however, must be avoided because even a brief fall in systemic blood pressure may dangerously reduce the cerebral perfusion pressure. Volume expanders, such as 5% albumin or Plasmanate, may be needed but should be used cautiously, while monitoring central venous pressure.

Seizures must be rapidly controlled because ICP rises with seizure activity. Seizure activity may be a symptom of hypoglycemia. Immediate control may be achieved with lorazepam (Ativan), 0.05 to 0.1 mg per kg as a stat dose. Phenytoin (Dilantin) is the preferred maintenance anticonvulsant, given as a slow intravenous loading dose (over 30 minutes) of 20 mg per kg. The maintenance dose, which depends on blood levels (aim for 15 to 25 μg per mL), should be repeated every 12 hours but is generally 5 to 10 mg per kg per day divided into an every-6-hour schedule. In paralyzed patients, electroencephalographic monitoring is needed to detect electrographic seizure activity.

Intravenous calcium may be needed for hypocalcemia and phosphate supplementation for hypophosphatemia. Coagulopathies that are unresponsive to vitamin K_1 require intravenous fresh-frozen plasma 10 to 15 mL per kg per 24 hours. Platelet transfusion may be needed for thrombocytopenia. Marked, persistent, or increasing blood ammonia levels (>400 μM at any time or >250 μM at 24 hours) are suggestive of a urea cycle defect and should be treated acutely with intravenous arginine and sodium benzoate and phenylacetate. With such treatment, if a rapid fall in blood ammonia does not occur, hemodialysis is indicated.

OUTCOME

Despite the falling incidence of RS in the last decade, the mortality remains high, averaging 30%. In 1980, case fatality rates in stages I through III totaled 39%, compared with 46% in stage IV and 62% in stage V. Infants with onset in the first year and those children with high blood ammonia levels have the worst prognosis. Fortunately, most survivors recover fully, but learning disabilities and language impairments persist in some. Mental retardation, persistent seizures, and motor disability can occur, usually in children with a severe clinical course in the acute illness.

MULTIPLE SCLEROSIS

method of
ROBERT M. HERNDON, M.D.
Multiple Sclerosis Clinic
Legacy Good Samaritan Hospital
Portland, Oregon

Multiple sclerosis (MS) is a disease of the white matter of the nervous system that is disseminated in time and location. Onset is usually between the ages of 15 and 55, peaking at 27 to 29 years of age. Childhood cases and cases beginning after age 55 are uncommon. The etiology is unknown. The most widely held theory is that it is an autoimmune disease, probably induced by viral infection. There is a substantial north-south gradient in disease distribution in North America, in Europe, and probably also in the Southern Hemisphere, with a considerably higher incidence at the higher latitudes, which suggests an environmental factor in its causation, though a possible alternative explanation is that the distribution relates to the distribution of individuals with a northern European genetic background. Prevalence can exceed 100 in 100,000 in high-risk areas. It is the most common crippling neurologic disease developing in the young-adult age group. As with most autoimmune diseases, it is more common in women, who compose two-thirds of the cases.

DIAGNOSIS

Multiple sclerosis is a clinical diagnosis. There is no single test or combination of tests that will unequivocally diagnose the disease. Misdiagnosis of other diseases as MS is common, and nearly 10% of patients referred to MS clinics do not have the disease. The *sine qua non* of diagnosis is the occurrence of lesions in the white matter of the central nervous system disseminated in time and location. MS is not the only disease that produces these lesions, so the caveat that there be no better explanation is included as a qualification. Although the presence of high-signal lesions on magnetic resonance imaging (MRI) scan is important in the diagnosis, reliance on MRI in the absence of typical signs and symptoms has led to many instances of misdiagnosis.

Systemic diseases, such as disseminated lupus erythematosus, polyarteritis nodosa, Sjögren's syndrome, and even complicated migraine can produce central nervous system signs and symptoms resembling MS, and also can produce MRI changes that may be mistaken for those of MS. Ancillary studies, including MRI of the brain or spinal cord, spinal fluid examination, and evoked potential testing, may be helpful, but the diagnosis fundamentally remains a clinical diagnosis. The diagnostic criteria in current use for research protocols, although not strictly applicable to many clinical situations, are instructive. These criteria were developed at a meeting of investigators working on MS held in 1983 and are listed in Table 1.

Since the advent of MRI, overinterpretation and misinterpretation of MRIs have replaced posterior fossa and craniocervical junction lesions as the most common causes of misdiagnosis. Some conditions that may be misdiagnosed as MS are listed in Table 2. Duration of diagnosis is not an excuse for accepting the diagnosis uncritically. The author has examined patients who have carried an erroneous diagnosis of MS for decades because no one took the trouble to look critically at the basis for the diagnosis. Many older patients who carry the diagnosis have never had an MRI or lumbar puncture, and if the disease course or features are at all atypical, they deserve a thorough evaluation.

INFORMING THE PATIENT

When the diagnosis is suspected, it is useful to find out what the patient's concerns are and to discuss them realistically. Many patients, particularly if they know someone with MS or have a family member with it, are already very concerned about the diagnosis. Understanding the patient's concerns is the first step in dealing with these concerns. Most patients have heard of the disease, and many will know someone seriously affected by the disease. Once the diagnosis is clear, it is essential that the patient be informed. Because treatment is available, even though it is not appropriate for all patients, it is important that patients be made aware of their diagnosis and of their treatment options. When informing a patient, I usually allow a half-hour to inform the patient and answer questions. It is best if a spouse, close friend, or relative is with the patient because the patient may remember little other than the diagnosis. I explain that MS is a highly variable disease and that many patients with MS do very well; 60% of patients are still ambulatory after 20 years with the disease. I take the time to explain what I know about their disease, what I know of the prognosis, and what therapeutic options are available. I then set up another appointment in a week or so because both patients and family members need to adjust to and accept the diagnosis and, as they do so, they will think of many additional questions. Dealing with patient and family questions and concerns up front prevents many unnecessary phone calls and visits.

I provide patients with reading materials and a list of recommended books, such as Rosner and Ross' *Multiple Sclerosis* (Simon and Schuster), Scheinberg's *Multiple Sclerosis, a Guide for Patients and their Families* (Raven Press), or Burnfield's *Multiple Sclerosis, a Personal Exploration* (Souvenir Press). There are numerous books on MS, many of which contain a great deal of misinformation, and many patients will go to the local library or bookstore and find one. A little guidance helps keep patients out of the hands of the charlatans. I also will cite the National Multiple Sclerosis Society as a resource and suggest patients contact the local chapter. If they inquire about alternative approaches or the latest fad treatment, I refer them to *Sibley's Therapeutic Claims in Multiple Sclerosis* (Demos Publications), which discusses almost all of the standard and alternative therapies that have gained currency, ranging from colostrum to snake venom. This volume is extremely valuable in helping patients deal with treatment fads,

TABLE 1. **Washington (Poser) Criteria for the Diagnosis of Multiple Sclerosis**

Category	Attacks	Clinical		Paraclinical	CSF OB/IgG
Clinically definite					
CD-MS A1	2	2			
CD-MS A2	2	1	and	1	
Laboratory-supported definite					
LSD-MS B1	2	1	or	1	+
LSD-MS B2	1	2			+
LSD-MS B3	1	1	and	1	+
Clinically probable					
CP-MS C1	2	1			
CP-MS C2	1	2			
CP-MS C3	1	1	and	1	
Laboratory-supported probable					
LSP-MS D1	2				+

Abbreviations: CD = clinically definite; LSD = laboratory-supported definite; CP = clinically probable; LSP = laboratory-supported probable; CSF = cerebrospinal fluid; OB = oligoclonal bands.

From Poser CM, Paty DW, Scheinberg L, et al.: New diagnostic criteria for multiple sclerosis: Guidelines for research protocols. Anna. Neurol. *13*:227–231, 1983.

quack cures, and the large volume of misinformation appearing in the tabloids and the news media.

TREATMENT

The first step in planning therapy is classifying the disease and assessing its severity. Some typical disease patterns are shown in Figure 1. Exacerbations and remissions are generally typical of disease in the younger age group. Disease that has its onset later in life, particularly after age 40, is more likely to be either progressive from onset or to begin with one or two attacks with partial recovery, followed by steady progression. In exacerbating-remitting patients, the frequency of attacks usually declines as the patients get older, but in some a progressive pattern develops.

Benign cases in which the diagnosis is based on two or three attacks occurring years apart with little or no residual signs or symptoms may need no treatment. Exacerbating and remitting disease, characterized by more frequent attacks or progressive disease, requires more active treatment, and acute progressive disease with rapid deterioration requires very aggressive therapy. Treatment of MS is changing rapidly with the introduction of interferon-beta (Betaseron) in 1993, new information on the effects of high-dose steroids on the disease, and several new products in therapeutic trials.

Treatment of MS is divided into (1) treatment directed at controlling the disease process and (2) symptomatic treatment. Treatment directed at controlling the disease process is intended to alter the immunologic process that leads to demyelination and inhibition of remyelination. This is further divided into (1) treatment of acute attacks, (2) prevention of attacks, and (3) slowing progression. Symptomatic treatment is directed at management of a variety of symptoms, such as spasticity, pain, neurogenic bladder, and imbalance.

Treatment of the Acute Attack

We frequently do not treat mild acute attacks, consisting of minor paresthesias, slight weakness, or incoordination or other symptoms that do not significantly interfere with normal activities. These attacks often subside in 1 to 2 weeks without treatment. For attacks that produce significant discomfort or disability, I use high-dose methylprednisolone (Solu-Medrol) given intravenously in a dose of 1 gram over 30 to 60 minutes. I usually prescribe a 3-day course of 1 gram daily but will extend it to 5 to 10 days if the attack continues to progress or is slow in improving. I follow this with a prednisone taper beginning at 100 mg every morning and decreasing the dose by 20 mg every third day. The rate of taper varies greatly among individual physicians, but in our hands this schedule appears to minimize recurrence of disease activity during the taper. If the patient has a history of peptic ulcer or is subject to upper gastrointestinal system problems, I usually start ranitidine (Zantac) 150 mg every day to minimize the risk of gastrointestinal complications.

The prednisone taper reduces the frequency of early recurrence of symptoms. There is good evidence from the optic neuritis treatment trial that a course of methylprednisolone followed by a prednisone taper prolongs the time to the next demyelinating event in optic neuritis. This is particularly true in patients with multiple MRI high-signal areas, and thus I believe it applies to MS as well as to cases in which optic neuritis is the initial clinical manifestation.

TABLE 2. **Disorders Misdiagnosed as Multiple Sclerosis**

Premature vascular disease
Complicated migraine (hemiplegic migraine, ophthalmoplegic migraine)
Subacute combined degeneration
Lyme disease
Craniocervical junction and high cervical tumors
Vasculitis (periarteritis, giant cell arteritis, etc.)
Sjögren's syndrome
Disseminated lupus erythematosus
Behçets disease
Central nervous system lymphoma
Moya moya disease

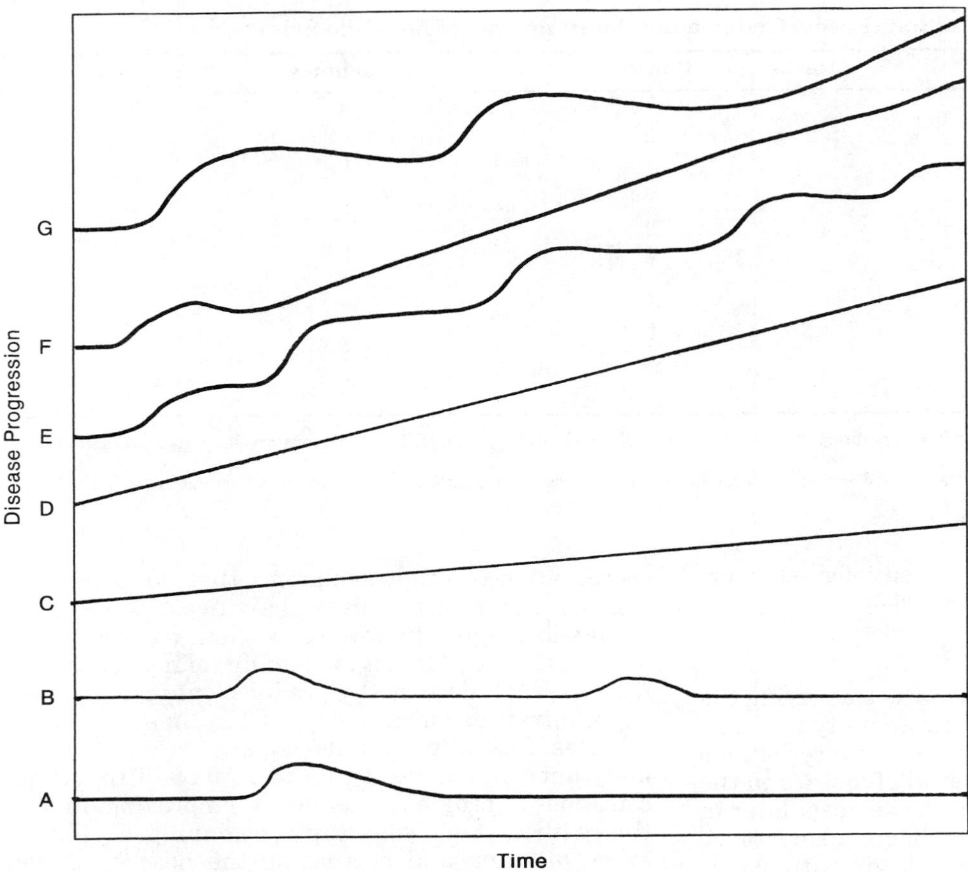

Figure 1. The varied courses of multiple sclerosis. A = Single demyelinating event such as optic neuritis or demyelinating transverse myelitis without recurrence; B = benign multiple sclerosis; C = multiple sclerosis which is slowly progressive from onset; D = more rapidly but steadily progressive disease; E = intermittently progressive disease without clear remissions; F = single attack followed by progressive disease; G = progressive course beginning after more than one discrete attack.

There is also evidence that lower doses of steroids do not prolong the time to the next attack and may shorten it. For this reason, oral prednisone in doses of 60 to 100 mg per day, previously used as the principal therapy for optic neuritis, is no longer recommended for optic neuritis, and I rarely use it for any type of acute attack of MS.

Prevention of Acute Attacks

The only treatment that has been demonstrated, in a controlled trial, to reduce the frequency and severity of acute attacks of MS is interferon-beta b1b, (Betaseron). This is the first new drug approved for treatment of MS since the introduction of steroids. Interferon-beta is a genetically engineered version of human interferon-beta that differs from natural interferon-beta in that it is not glycosylated and has a single amino acid substitution in the chain to prevent incorrect cross-linking. It has been shown to decrease the number of acute attacks of MS by about one-third and to decrease the average severity of attacks so that attacks classified as moderate or severe were reduced by more than 50%. It also caused a dramatic reduction in the appearance of new lesions on MRI. Studies have thus far failed to show a significant effect on progression of disability. Other interferon-beta products are under study, and additional results should be available in the coming year. Testing of interferon-beta in more advanced MS and in progressive MS is currently in the planning stage.

At the present time, I recommend interferon-beta for patients with moderate to severe exacerbating and remitting, or exacerbating progressive, MS. It is administered by subcutaneous injection every other day in a dose of 8.3 million international units because it is new, extremely expensive, and does have unpleasant side effects of influenza-like muscle and joint aching, headache, and fatigue. In addition, the injection sites become reddened and indurated, and may remain visible for a month or more. Frequency of injection is based on limited information and the way in which this drug is used is likely to change over time.

Interferon-beta is not a cure. It reduces the number of new attacks, which can be difficult for either a patient or physician to detect in an individual case. As a result, many patients will be disappointed in their response to treatment, and many may be unwilling to continue using it. Side effects generally decrease over time and are rarely a problem after the first few months; however, the side effects were sufficiently severe that the drop-out rate due to side effects was 7% to 8% in the clinical trial. In addition, depression, although infrequent, is a known and potentially serious side effect, which requires prompt treatment if it occurs. Some decrease in white blood cell count and liver abnormalities also are seen and may necessitate dose reduction or discontinuation of the drug.

I consider interferon-beta a significant advance, but it will probably be a number of years before its role in treatment, the best dosing schedule, and criteria for use are fully defined. We still do not know whether treatment needs to be continued for life or, as suggested by an earlier intrathecal interferon trial, treatment for a few years will have long-term benefits. Its value in progressive disease remains to be established.

Copolymer-1

Copolymer-1 (COP-1) is a synthetic random polymer, designed to resemble myelin basic protein, that has undergone clinical trial in MS and, although not yet approved by the Food and Drug Administration (FDA), is available through the treatment investigational new drug (IND) process. Studies indicate that it reduces the number of acute attacks and slows progression of the disease, and has an effectiveness similar to that of interferon-beta. It is given by subcutaneous injection twice daily. Side effects consist mainly of local redness and irritation at the injection site. For the present, this drug is available only through clinics that have the treatment IND. Because the drug has not received formal approval, the costs are not covered by medical insurance, and it is expensive. Patients interested in exploring this treatment must be referred to a clinic that is involved in the program to receive the drug.

Pulse Methylprednisolone

I use intermittent high-dose methylprednisolone in very severe exacerbating remitting MS and find that it reduces the number and severity of acute attacks. I usually prescribe 1 gram of methylprednisolone intravenously daily for 3 days, followed by 1 gram once a month for 6 months to 2 years. I try to spread out the interval between pulses to 6 weeks after 12 months of treatment if the patient is doing well and continue to lengthen the period between doses if the patient continues to do well. Another approach is to give high doses of methylprednisolone for 3 to 7 days and then repeat this every 3 to 12 months, as needed. This treatment appears to decrease relapses and slow progression in most patients. There is presently no study that definitely demonstrates the effectiveness of this treatment, but evidence from the optic neuritis treatment trial strongly suggests that methylprednisolone can prolong the time between attacks. Trials are in progress that should demonstrate the effectiveness of this therapy. Although relatively safe, I recommend this treatment only in persons with very active relapsing-remitting disease or those with fairly rapidly progressive MS.

The side effects of prolonged continuous use of steroids are well known and include worsening of existing or latent diabetes, hypertension, weight gain, acne, moon facies, osteoporosis, buffalo hump, and mood changes, with occasional mania. Use of pulse Solu-Medrol rarely causes these problems. Transient hyperglycemia may be seen but is uncommon. Aseptic necrosis of the femoral or humoral head occurs but fortunately is rare.

PROGRESSIVE MULTIPLE SCLEROSIS

Immunosuppressant Drugs

Immunosuppressant drugs used in MS include cyclophosphamide (Cytoxan), azathioprine (Imuran), methotrexate (Rheumatrex), and cyclosporin A (Sandimmune). The use of these drugs carries considerable risks, and they should not be used casually. The latter, cyclosporin A, although slowing disease progression, is sufficiently toxic, particularly to the kidney, that I do not use it.

Azathioprine is an immunosuppressant antimetabolite that has been used widely to treat aggressive MS. It appears to reduce the frequency and severity of attacks and the overall rate of progression, but its effects are sufficiently limited that they have been demonstrated convincingly only through meta-analysis of a number of studies. Many patients cannot take it because of gastrointestinal side effects or skin rash. Its use is declining, and it is being replaced largely by interferon-beta; azathioprine has the advantage of being much cheaper, but it is also less effective. I continue to use it in a limited number of patients who do not tolerate or cannot afford interferon-beta. I use 50 mg twice daily, although higher doses are used by some. It is necessary to monitor the white blood cell count and liver function frequently, particularly early in the course of treatment. Intravenous methylprednisolone can be used when necessary to treat acute attacks in patients on azathioprine without apparent undue risk.

Cyclophosphamide is an alkylating agent used in chemotherapy of malignancies that is also immunosuppressant. I reserve cyclophosphamide for very aggressive disease that has not responded to less aggressive measures. I use the Harvard protocol.* This consists of intravenous cyclophosphamide in a dose of 150 mg every 6 hours and adrenocorticotropic hormone given until the white blood cell count drops to 4000, usually after 10 to 14 days. This course of therapy halts disease progression in most patients for 1 to 2 years and produces significant improvement in some. When the MS starts to progress again, they can be treated again. More recently, monthly injections of cyclophosphamide have been shown to prolong the response to the drug. The drug works best in relatively young patients with aggressive, exacerbating progressive disease.

The major problem with cyclophosphamide and the reason it is reserved for more severe cases is that, following treatment, the white blood cell count, which continues to go down for several days, may go below 1000 for a short period, leaving the patient at high risk for infection. Most patients lose their hair following the treatment, although it does grow back. Nausea and vomiting during therapy can usually be con-

*See Houser SL, Dawson DM, Lehrick JR, et al: Intensive immunosuppression in progressive multiple sclerosis: A randomized, three-arm study of high-dose intravenous cyclophosphamide, plasma exchange and ACTH. N Engl J Med *308*:173, 1983

trolled with metoclopramide (Reglan) or droperidol (Inapsine). Long-term use of cyclophosphamide increases the risk of cancer, but this risk is minimal when the drug is used in this intermittent fashion.

Methotrexate

Methotrexate is an immunosuppressive drug that has been used in rheumatoid arthritis and in leukemias, and shows considerable promise for the treatment of progressive MS. Preliminary information on a recent trial suggests that it will significantly slow the pace of progressive disease. The dose is 7.5 mg (three 2.5-mg tablets) once a week. Before embarking on methotrexate therapy, it is essential to become familiar with the toxic effects of the compound, and patients must be informed of the risks and side effects. Indigestion, nausea, and vomiting are fairly common, but can usually be controlled with antacids; however, antiemetics such as metoclopramide or droperidol may be needed. Patients on methotrexate must avoid alcohol, which increases the risk of hepatotoxicity, and precautions must be taken to avoid drugs that will affect its absorption or metabolism. Complete blood count, serum glutamic-oxaloacetic transaminase, and serum glutamic-pyruvic transaminase assays should be performed monthly, and folic acid, 1 mg daily, should be given to prevent anemia.

SYMPTOMATIC TREATMENT

Despite the availability of disease-specific therapy for some patients with MS, symptom management will probably continue to have a greater impact on patient well-being than disease treatment for some time to come. Appropriate attention to symptomatic therapy can significantly improve the quality of life of most MS patients, and often is crucial to continued employment or independence.

Spasticity

Spasticity is a frequent and troublesome symptom in MS, but it also plays a role in maintaining function. Spasticity often provides the extensor strength for bearing weight, allowing the patient to transfer, or even to walk, despite significant pyramidal system weakness. Thus, effective drug therapy for spasticity can increase weakness, and a balance between weakness and spasticity must be found.

Physical therapy is essential in the management of spasticity. Patients and caregivers need to be instructed in stretching and strengthening exercises to maintain function and to prevent contractures. Hip and knee contractures are extremely common and are easier to prevent than to treat after they have occurred. Daily range-of-motion exercises usually prevent contracture. If the muscles are too tight to permit exercise, other measures need to be instituted before fixed contracture occurs.

Baclofen (Lioresal) has proved to be the most effective drug for the treatment of spasticity. The appropriate dose is enough but not too much. Some patients receive considerable relief from as little as 5 mg taken once or twice daily and become weak when taking 10 mg per dose, whereas others require much higher doses and do well with doses at or exceeding the manufacturer's recommended limit of 20 mg four times daily. We start baclofen in a dose of about 10 mg administered twice daily and increased by 10 mg per day until the spasticity is adequately relieved or weakness occurs. When weakness occurs, the dose should be decreased until the appropriate balance between spasticity and weakness is achieved.

Diazepam (Valium) is an effective muscle relaxant that may be used alone or in combination with baclofen when results with baclofen alone are unsatisfactory. We usually start at a dosage of 2 to 5 mg twice daily and increase gradually. It is much more sedative than baclofen, is habituating, may interfere with cognitive function, and with prolonged use can cause depression. I use it in patients who cannot tolerate baclofen or as an adjunct to baclofen therapy, particularly in patients who have a high level of anxiety in addition to their spasticity.

Dantrolene sodium (Dantrium) has a very limited role in the therapy of spasticity in MS patients in my experience. It is generally less effective than baclofen or diazepam; carries a greater risk of toxicity, particularly liver toxicity; and generally causes more weakness relative to its antispastic effect. It can be useful in bedridden patients with flexor spasms in whom the weakness does not interfere with function.

For spasticity that cannot be adequately controlled with oral medication, intrathecal baclofen is an increasingly useful option. Using a Medtronics pump and a catheter, baclofen can be administered intrathecally in doses sufficient to relieve spasticity without producing significant sedation. Patients in whom spasticity cannot be adequately controlled on oral medication should be referred to a center with experience in managing spasticity using this technique.

More drastic measures previously used for intractable spasticity are rarely, if ever, needed at the present time. These destructive procedures, which include ethanol block of lumbar nerve roots, dorsal rhizotomy, and Bischoff's myelotomy, are reserved for bedridden patients without sphincter control. Even then, there are usually better alternatives. Considerable attention is needed to prevent decubitus ulcers in patients with impaired sensation that is either a direct result of MS or a result of destructive treatment aimed at relieving spasticity.

Bladder Dysfunction

Partial bladder denervation leading to urinary urgency, frequency, and incontinence is frequent in MS. Neurogenic bladder problems can be divided into failure to store and failure to empty. The most frequent problem is failure to store with a small spastic bladder. This can be diagnosed by having the patient void, then catheterizing and measuring the residual volume. If the patient has a residual less than 100 mL, the use of oxybutynin (Ditropan), 2.5 to 5 mg 2 to 4 times a day, will often relieve the problem.

Failure to empty may represent either a large, flaccid bladder with overflow incontinence or dyssynergia. A large, flaccid bladder can usually be adequately managed with intermittent catheterization. Dyssynergia due to simultaneous contraction of the sphincters and detrusor represents a more difficult management problem. The increased pressure may lead to reflux with recurring pyelonephritis. Management requires involvement of a knowledgeable urologist.

In the absence of a clear MS attack, an abrupt change in bladder function is most frequently due to infection, and urinalysis and culture should be the first step in assessment. If infection is not present, a neurogenic bladder should be suspected and further evaluation is indicated.

Bowel Dysfunction

Constipation is a frequent and troubling occurrence in patients with MS. Bowel motility is decreased, both because of altered autonomic function and decreased physical activity. This is further aggravated in many patients by decreased fluid intake, which is a common response in patients with neurogenic bladder. It is normally best to manage the bowel with stool softeners such as docusate sodium (Colace), in a dose of 50 to 200 mg per day, and bulk laxatives such as bran or Perdiem. Increased fluid intake is also helpful but is difficult for patients with bladder problems. Administration of over-the-counter preparations, such as glycerin suppositories or Therevac-SB, a gelatin ampule of soft soap, glycerine, and stool softeners, often solves the problem. If these measures prove inadequate, bisacodyl (Dulcolax) may be useful. Bisacodyl tablets usually work overnight, and the suppositories work within 1 to 2 hours.

Painful injury in severely paraparetic MS patients frequently results in ileus. Patients with vertebral compression fractures and lower extremity fractures are predisposed to ileus, and narcotics used to control pain often aggravate the problem. Severe constipation should not be ignored, because obstipation with rupture of the bowel has been known to occur in patients with MS.

Fatigue

Fatigue is so universal in MS patients that we consider absence of significant fatigue grounds for a thorough re-evaluation of the diagnosis. Fatigue may be severe enough to interfere significantly with work performance, particularly in the afternoon. Fatigued patients often have trouble with complex mental tasks. Thus, many working MS patients plan their day so that all difficult decision making is done early and the afternoons are used for routine work.

Because fatigue is not externally visible, it is especially troublesome. Affected patients may be labeled as lazy by employers or family members who do not understand that there is a disease-related reason for reduced work performance. Family members often do not understand failure to participate in family activities or help with household chores in the evening after work, or why the patient with MS must stop to rest frequently during the day.

There are a number of different types of fatigue in MS, and it is important to determine the causes of fatigue in order to treat it effectively. Types of fatigue seen in MS include normal fatigue, fatigue related to depression, fatigue of handicap, nerve fiber fatigue, and profound lassitude.

Normal Fatigue

People with MS are subject to the same factors that cause fatigue as everyone else. This does not normally present a problem and is a cause for complaint only in those few patients who consistently try to do too much. This type of fatigue is occasionally a problem in young, ambitious MS patients with type A personalities who decide they must succeed in life as quickly as possible because they have been diagnosed as having a chronic illness that may disable them in a few years. There is little that can be offered beyond counseling for these individuals.

Fatigue Due to Depression

Loss of energy and fatigue are usual manifestations of depression. The chronically depressed person finds it difficult to get through a day's activities. In people with MS who have a pseudobulbar affective exaggeration, apparent mood often fluctuates rapidly and uncontrollably, and may not reflect internal mood. There may be a marked disparity between the patient's outward appearance and inward feelings. In these people, the underlying depression will go unrecognized if you do not listen to the patient. It is particularly important that evaluation of fatigue in people with MS rule out depression as the cause. If depression is present, treatment with antidepressant medication usually improves the patient's energy level.

Fatigue of Handicap

Handicap fatigue is an under-recognized cause of fatigue in MS. It is the fatigue resulting from increased use of functioning muscles to compensate for muscles that are weakened, that are spastic, and that fail to relax normally during movements or are paralyzed. A person with a weak leg who needs a cane or a crutch, for instance, will fatigue the muscles of his or her arms and opposite leg while walking. The increased effort necessary to accomplish normal tasks under these circumstances is often under-rated, both by the person with MS and his or her family and coworkers. Even tasks as simple as bathing or dressing become major obstacles in the presence of significant disability and can be extremely fatiguing. Compensatory techniques can often be found to help individuals accomplish their tasks more efficiently and with less energy expenditure. Referral to a physical or occupational therapist, depending on the problem area, is frequently in order. The increased energy expenditure needed to overcome spasticity may be helped by physical therapy and by the use of muscle relaxants. There is a true energy cost to spasticity, and measurements of oxygen consumption indicate that walking may require twice the normal energy expenditure.

Nerve Fiber Fatigue

Nerve fiber fatigue is a unique feature of demyelinating diseases. Demyelinated nerve fibers are able to conduct, but the safety margin for conduction is very small, the fibers fatigue rapidly, and conduction fails. Such nerve fibers are also very temperature sensitive and fail to conduct with even minor elevations in body temperature. Elevated body temperature, as might occur with a cold or the flu, or even a hot bath or sitting in the sun, interferes with nerve conduction and results in increased neurologic symptoms, such as weakness, numbness, incoordination, and general fatigue. These symptoms, because they are due to failure of nerve conduction, cannot be overcome by increased effort. Thus, a person with MS who can perform certain tasks when rested may be unable to perform the same tasks when he or she is even modestly fatigued. This is often most evident in walking, in which the legs just cannot perform after walking a limited distance, and the person cannot walk until he or she has rested. A good example of this is Uhthoff's phenomenon. Following optic neuritis, many patients lose vision during exercise or in very bright light. The effect is transient but may be disturbing.

Profound Lassitude

Some MS patients experience periods of severe fatigue and lassitude, during which they find it extremely difficult to do anything. Even getting out of bed or getting dressed seems to require too much effort. These bouts may accompany acute attacks of the disease, but they can occur in the absence of new focal neurologic symptoms. They can last up to several weeks, during which these individuals can do very little and may even have great difficulty caring for themselves, even though they are not physically weak. A short course of methylprednisolone may be helpful in this situation, but many cases do not respond to any known treatment. Fortunately, most episodes are self-limited.

Pain

The view often expressed in the literature that MS is a painless disease is wrong. Pain is a problem in a significant number of MS patients. Pain in MS can be divided into (1) pain secondary to abnormal stress on muscles and joints, secondary to weakness and spasticity, and (2) pain of neurogenic origin.

Pain secondary to abnormal stress ranges from mild muscular aches and pains to fairly severe pain secondary to joint trauma. The knee and ankle are particularly susceptible to trauma secondary to leg weakness and spasticity. If there is severe weakness of ankle dorsiflexors along with spasticity, both the ankle and the knee are at risk because the tight heel cords throw the knee into hyperextension. An ankle-foot orthosis is often very helpful.

The milder pain problems, and particularly musculoskeletal pain, can usually be managed with nonsteroidal anti-inflammatory drugs and measures to relieve the pressure on overstressed muscles and joints. Pain from knee hyperextension can often be relieved by an ankle-foot orthosis, which reduces the tendency to hyperextend that is produced by tight heel cords.

Tic douloureux is a fairly common problem in MS. In the majority of patients, carbamazepine (Tegretol), pushed to tolerance controls the pain. If that fails I add phenytoin (Dilantin) and maintain the levels of both drugs in the high therapeutic range. If this does not control the pain, perphenazine-amitriptyline HCl (Triavil) may be useful in temporizing, but referral to a neurosurgeon for surgical intervention, such as glycerol injection, is indicated.

Chronic dysesthetic pain, though uncommon, is a very troublesome and often intractable symptom. Narcotic analgesics do not work. They produce temporary relief, but the dose required escalates rapidly and, in the end, does not control the pain. If the pain is intermittent and has a shooting or electric shock–like quality, it may respond to carbamazepine (Tegretol) alone or in combination with phenytoin. For pain with a burning dysesthetic quality, there is no satisfactory drug therapy. Perphenazine-amitriptyline HCl usually produces some relief and may be used with carbamazepine. If the pain is confined to the legs and lumbar region, intrathecal morphine or baclofen using a Medtronics pump may provide relief.

Cognitive and Emotional Aspects

Cognitive and emotional changes are experienced by many MS patients. They may be subtle, but in many patients with well-established disease measurable changes in cognitive function are noted, and many also have disturbances in the emotional sphere. There are several relatively simple measures that can help in the management of these problems, although, at present, little can be done to improve function in those with serious cognitive impairment.

Depression

Depression is common in patients with MS, and hypomanic episodes are fairly common. Such episodes may occur spontaneously or follow steroid administration. These affective disorders should be distinguished from the problems of exaggerated or inappropriate affective display described later. There is evidence of an increased incidence of both depression and of true bipolar disease in MS patients and in relatives of MS patients, although the reasons for this are unknown. Bipolar disease usually responds to traditional treatment with lithium carbonate or with carbamazepine (Tegretol). We treat hypomanic episodes occurring during steroid treatment with carbamazepine in a dose of 300 to 800 mg daily. The carbamazepine dose can usually be increased faster than is usual, because hypomanic patients appear to tolerate the side effects better than most other patients. We usually begin with 100 mg every 8 hours and increase to 200 mg every 8 hours the following day. This works more rapidly than lithium and can be easily introduced if sleeplessness and other signs of mania occur during steroid treatment. If carbamazepine does not work satisfactorily or cannot be used because of toxic side effects, lithium carbonate usually proves to be effective.

Some situational depression is often associated with MS, but the incidence of depression is significantly higher in MS than it is in a number of comparably serious diseases. Both tricyclic antidepressants and fluoxetine (Prozac) are generally effective in the management of depression in MS. The required dose for the tricyclics is much less than that traditionally required for the treatment of depression. I begin with 10 to 25 mg of amitriptyline (Elavil), or imipramine (Tofranil), which would rarely be effective in a standard endogenous depression. A dose of 10 to 50 mg at bedtime is generally adequate. The higher doses traditionally used to treat depression are rarely required. Fluoxetine also works well and in refractory patients can be combined with tricyclics.

Pathologic Laughing and Weeping

Lability of affective display, including its more extreme form, pathologic laughing and weeping, occurs with increasing frequency as MS progresses. The laughter or weeping may bear little relationship to the internal affective state of the patient. This dissociation between internal affective state and affective expression often goes unrecognized and seriously disrupts the patient's emotional communication. Such disruption of emotional communication is frequently socially disabling. Such patients are unable to modulate affective expression, so that even relatively mild emotional stimuli bring on an affective display that is exaggerated in intensity and that may be inappropriate in relation to the patient's feelings or internal affective state. In milder cases, an exaggeration of the appropriate affective display is all that is seen.

These disorders of affective display are often described inaccurately as emotional lability. It is extremely difficult for the spouse, or indeed the physician, to recognize depression in someone who is laughing. From infancy, we learn to believe facial expression, and if the facial expression does not accurately reflect what the person is saying, we believe the expression. Thus, this problem can have devastating effects on interpersonal relations.

Both pathologic laughing and weeping, and lability of affective display, are responsive to treatment in the majority of cases. Amitriptyline or imipramine in a dose of 10 to 50 mg at bedtime is effective in reducing lability of affective display in 80 to 90% of patients. The effect is more rapid than in the treatment of depression. There is a reduction in the extreme emotional expression so that the affective display is more consonant with the internal affective state.

Inability to Focus Attention

The ability to focus attention is an active process in which the nervous system shuts off extraneous input. In many MS patients, this ability is impaired. As a result, they have a great deal of difficulty with concentration in a distracting environment. The active filtering process needed to maintain the focus of attention is disrupted. This problem frequently interferes with work performance and often causes irritability. Appropriate modification of the work place often results in improved job performance.

Patients who have difficulty focusing their attention are intolerant of noisy environments and family situations with young children in which the television is often on and multiple simultaneous conversations are taking place. The removal of as much of the distraction as possible, or providing a quiet room where the patient can do one thing at a time without distraction, often greatly improves the patient's temper and his or her ability to cope with the frustrations of the disease much better.

Another closely related problem is the need to compensate for deficits in normally automatic functions. Patients with gait difficulty may have to concentrate on walking. Imagine, if you will, what it would be like if you had to think about every step you took. Patients with disturbed gait may be unable to walk and carry on a conversation at the same time, because they need to concentrate on their walking to maintain balance.

A FEW PATIENT MANAGEMENT PRINCIPLES

1. Listen to your patient. He or she will tell you what the problems are.
2. Manage the patient's symptoms. Despite the institution of therapy, which will alter the course of the illness, specific therapy is only a small part of the overall management of the patient. Symptom management remains important.
3. *Physical aids,* such as canes, ankle-foot orthoses, crutches, and wheelchairs, *are tools* to allow handicapped individuals to continue to do what they could not or would not do without them. It is better for patients to go shopping in a wheelchair than to become isolated at home. It is better to use a cane for balance than to fall or stay at home for fear of falling.
4. Make appropriate use of consultants, physiatrists, physical and occupational therapists, clinical psychologists, and speech therapists. All have a role and can assist you in improving your patient's well-being.

MYASTHENIA GRAVIS

method of
DONALD B. SANDERS, M.D.
Duke University Medical School
Durham, North Carolina

Myasthenia gravis (MG) usually results from an acquired immunologic abnormality, although rarely there is a genetic abnormality at the neuromuscular junction. The prevalence of MG in the United States is estimated at 14 per 100,000 population, approximately 36,000 cases. As the population has grown older, the average age at onset has increased. The onset of symptoms is now usually after age 50, and males are more often affected than females.

CLINICAL PRESENTATION

Most patients with MG have eyelid ptosis or diplopia as their first symptom, and almost all have one or both of these symptoms within 2 years after onset. Difficulty chewing, swallowing, or talking is also common. Occasionally, the first symptoms may be due to weakness of single muscle groups, such as neck or finger extensors or hip flexors.

Weakness in MG varies during the day, usually being least in the morning and becoming worse as the day progresses, especially after prolonged use of affected muscles. Ocular symptoms typically become worse while reading, watching television, or driving, especially in bright sunlight. Jaw muscle weakness typically becomes worse during prolonged chewing.

In most patients, symptoms fluctuate over the short term but become progressively severe. Periods of spontaneous improvement are common, especially early in the disease. Maximum weakness occurs during the first year in two thirds of patients. Weakness remains limited to ocular muscles in about 10% of patients (ocular myasthenia). Myasthenic symptoms are made worse by systemic illness (especially viral respiratory infections), hypothyroidism or hyperthyroidism, pregnancy, the menstrual cycle, drugs that affect neuromuscular transmission, and elevated body temperature. After many years without effective treatment, weakness may become fixed with atrophy of involved muscles. The unusual distribution and fluctuating weakness of MG often suggest psychiatric illness. Conversely, ptosis and diplopia suggest intracranial pathology.

PHYSICAL FINDINGS

Patients with known or suspected MG should be examined in a way that will detect variable weakness in specific muscle groups, with particular attention to the ocular and oropharyngeal muscles. Strength should be assessed before and after sustained muscle activity and again after a brief rest.

Most patients with MG have weakness of ocular muscles and eye closure. Weakness is most frequent and usually most severe in the medial rectus muscles. The pupillary responses are normal. Ptosis is usually asymmetrical and varies during sustained activity. To compensate for ptosis, the frontalis muscle may be chronically contracted.

Oropharyngeal muscle weakness causes changes in the voice, difficulty chewing and swallowing, inadequate maintenance of the upper airway, and altered facial appearance. The voice becomes nasal, especially after prolonged talking, and liquids may escape through the nose when swallowing. Weakness of the laryngeal muscles causes hoarseness and difficulty producing a high-pitched "eeeee" sound. Difficulty chewing and swallowing produces frequent choking, clearing of the throat, or coughing after eating.

If jaw closure is weak, the examiner may able to force the jaw open against resistance, which is not possible normally. The patient may have to hold the jaw closed, frequently with the thumb under the chin, the middle finger curled under the bottom lip, and the index finger extended up the cheek. Facial muscle weakness may make the patient appear sad or depressed.

Any trunk or limb muscle can be affected. Neck flexors are usually weaker than neck extensors, and the deltoids, triceps, and extensors of the wrist and fingers are frequently weaker than other limb muscles.

PATHOPHYSIOLOGY OF MYASTHENIA GRAVIS

In acquired MG, the postsynaptic muscle membrane is distorted and simplified, having lost its normal folded shape. The concentration of acetylcholine receptor (AChR) on the muscle end-plate membrane is reduced, and antibodies are attached to this membrane. Acetylcholine is released normally from the nerve, but its effect on the muscle is reduced. The postjunctional membrane is less sensitive to applied acetylcholine, and there is a reduced probability that any nerve impulse will cause a muscle action potential.

Antibodies to AChR are found in the serum of three fourths of patients with acquired generalized myasthenia and one half of those with ocular myasthenia. The serum concentration of AChR antibody varies widely among patients with similar degrees of weakness and does not predict the severity of disease in individual patients. Approximately 10% of patients who do not have binding antibodies do have antibodies that modulate the turnover of AChR in tissue culture. AChR binding antibodies may be slightly increased in systemic lupus erythematosus, inflammatory neuropathy, amyotrophic lateral sclerosis, thymoma without MG, and in normal relatives of patients with MG. Elevated AChR antibodies in patients with compatible clinical features confirm the diagnosis of MG, but normal antibody concentrations do not exclude this diagnosis.

THYMUS IN MYASTHENIA GRAVIS

Ten percent of patients with MG have a thymic tumor and 70% have hyperplastic changes in the thymus (germinal centers) that indicate immunologic activity. The thymus contains all the elements necessary for the pathogenesis of MG: myoid cells that express the AChR antigen, antigen-presenting cells, and immunocompetent T cells. Although surgical removal of the thymus is followed by improvement in most patients, the role of the thymus in the pathogenesis of MG is not clear. Most thymic tumors in MG are benign, well-differentiated, and encapsulated, and can be completely removed surgically.

DIAGNOSTIC PROCEDURES

Edrophonium Chloride (Tensilon) Test

Weakness from abnormal neuromuscular transmission improves after intravenous administration of edrophonium chloride (Tensilon). This test is most reliable when the patient has ptosis, ocular muscle weakness, or nasal speech. Improved strength after edrophonium chloride may also be seen in motor neuron disease and in lesions of the oculomotor nerves. The best dose of edrophonium chloride differs among patients and cannot be determined in advance. Administration of 10 mg in fractional doses is recommended: 2 mg is injected initially and the response is monitored for 60 seconds. Subsequent injections of 3 and 5 mg are then given. If improvement is seen within 60 seconds after any dose, no further injections are necessary. The total dose in children is 0.15 mg per kg. An Ambu bag should be handy when giving edrophonium chloride because some people are supersensitive to even small amounts.

Blinded administration of edrophonium chloride has questionable value and is not necessary when there is a well-defined end point, such as relief of ptosis. Some patients who do not respond to edrophonium chloride may respond to intramuscular neostigmine, which has a longer duration of action. This is particularly useful in infants and children whose response to edrophonium chloride may be too brief for adequate observation. In some patients, a therapeutic trial of oral pyridostigmine (Mestinon) for several days may produce improvement that cannot be appreciated after a single dose of edrophonium chloride or neostigmine.

Electromyography

Characteristically, the amplitude of the muscle response falls during trains of low-frequency nerve stimulation in MG. This decrementing response is seen more often in proximal or facial muscles than in hand muscles and is seen in some muscle in about three fourths of patients. The single-fiber electromyogram is the most sensitive clinical test of neuromuscular transmission and shows an abnormality in some muscles in almost all patients with MG. Patients with mild or purely ocular muscle weakness may have an abnormal single-fiber electromyogram test only in facial muscles. If either test demonstrates abnormal neuromuscular transmission, other disease of nerve or muscle must be excluded before diagnosing MG.

TREATMENT OF ACQUIRED, AUTOIMMUNE MG

No single treatment is ideal for all patients with MG. Each patient needs an individual treatment plan, which may need to be changed from time to time.

Cholinesterase Inhibitors (Table 1)

Cholinesterase (ChE) inhibitors improve muscle weakness but do not modify the evolution of the disease, which usually progresses without more definitive treatment. Pyridostigmine bromide (Mestinon) and neostigmine bromide (Prostigmin) are the ChE inhibitors that are used clinically; the former is usually preferred because of its longer duration of action.

The optimal dose and schedule vary among patients and in the same patient from time to time. The beginning dose of pyridostigmine is usually 30 mg every 4 to 6 hours. Doses and dosing intervals should be modified to determine the least amount that gives maximum improvement for the longest time. Patients should not modify doses more than 15 mg or dose intervals by more than 1 hour without discussing this with their physician. The response varies among muscles, and thus the schedule should be adjusted to produce the best response in the muscles that are of greatest concern in each patient. In patients with oropharyngeal weakness, doses should be timed to produce optimal strength during meals. In 80% of patients, the best dosage is between 30 and 120 mg every 4 hours.

If the patient is strong enough, it may be sufficient and preferable to give pyridostigmine only during daytime hours; however, if there is respiratory compromise or the patient is too weak on awakening in the morning, it may be necessary to give the medication also during the night. Under these circumstances the use of timed-release pyridostigmine tablets (Mestinon Timespan) is sometimes advisable: one half, three quarter, or one tablet may be sufficient for the whole night. Because of variable absorption of this preparation, it is preferable to use regular pyridostigmine during the day.

Patients who take these medications chronically should periodically reduce the dose to determine the minimal necessary amount. Many patients who have taken ChE inhibitors for years can, with encouragement, discontinue them or markedly reduce the dose without becoming weaker.

Side effects of ChE inhibitors include queasiness, nausea, vomiting, abdominal cramping, and loose stools or frank diarrhea. Taking food with the medication minimizes these symptoms. ChE inhibitors also increase bronchial and oral secretions, which may be a serious problem for patients with impaired swallowing or breathing. Anticholinergic drugs suppress most side effects, but in so doing may mask the

TABLE 1. **Cholinesterase Inhibitors**

Drug	Equivalent Doses (mg)*		Available Forms
	Oral	*Parenteral*	
Neostigmine bromide (Prostigmin)	15		15-mg tablets
Neostigmine methylsulfate (Prostigmin Injectable)		0.5	0.25 mg per mL 0.5 mg per mL 1.0 mg per mL
Pyridostigmine bromide			
(Mestinon, Mestinon syrup,	60		60-mg tablets, 60 mg per 5 mL
Mestinon Injectable,		2.0	5 mg per mL
Mestinon Timespan)	90–180		180-mg tablets

*These values are approximations only. Appropriate doses should be determined for each patient based on the clinical response.

signs of impending overdose. Bradycardia is seen almost exclusively after parenteral administration of edrophonium chloride or neostigmine, and may be prevented by giving 0.6 to 1.2 mg intravenous atropine sulfate first. Loperamide hydrochloride (Imodium), propantheline bromide (Pro-Banthine), glycopyrrolate (Robinul), or diphenoxylate hydrochloride with atropine (Lomotil) may be used to treat the gastrointestinal side effects of oral ChE inhibitors. These drugs should be used cautiously, because some may produce weakness when taken in high doses.

It is usually not possible to maintain a schedule that produces the optimal response at the time of peak drug effect without incurring some weakness before and after this time. If the dose is increased (or the interval shortened) to eliminate all weakness, there is a danger of producing an overdose at the time of peak effect. Patients and physicians also tend to increase the dose of these medications beyond the level at which improvement is seen, with consequent overdosing. To avoid this problem, the level should be kept low enough that definite improvement is seen 30 to 45 minutes after each dose and the effect of each dose can be seen to wear off before the next is given.

Pyridostigmine is available as a syrup for children or for administration by nasogastric tube in patients with impaired swallowing. Neostigmine and pyridostigmine can be administered intranasally or by nebulizer in patients who have irregular absorption of oral medications or cannot swallow them.

Thymectomy

Thymectomy is recommended for most patients with MG that begins before age 60. The maximal improvement usually occurs 2 to 5 years after surgery, but this is unpredictable. Although the best response to thymectomy occurs in young people early in the course of their disease, improvement can occur even after 30 years of symptoms. In my experience, patients with disease onset after the age of 60 rarely show substantial improvement from thymectomy.

The preferred surgical approach is transthoracic; the sternum is split, and the anterior mediastinum explored. Transcervical and endoscopic approaches have less postoperative morbidity, but do not allow sufficient exposure for total thymic removal. The operative morbidity from transthoracic thymectomy is very low when patients are optimally prepared with plasma exchange or immunosuppression, if necessary, and skilled postoperative management is provided. Extubation is usually accomplished within hours after surgery, and patients may be discharged home as early as the third or fourth postoperative day.

Repeat thymectomy provides significant improvement in some patients with chronic, refractory disease and should be considered when there is concern that all thymic tissue was not removed at prior surgery and when a good response to the original surgery was followed by later relapse.

Corticosteroids (Tables 2 and 3)

Marked improvement or complete relief of symptoms occurs in more than 75% of patients treated with prednisone, and some improvement occurs in most of the rest. The severity of disease does not predict the ultimate improvement. Patients with thymoma usually have an excellent response to prednisone before or after removal of the tumor.

The most predictable response to prednisone occurs when treatment begins with a daily dose of 60 mg per day. This dose is given until sustained improvement occurs, which is usually within 2 weeks. The dose is then changed to 100 mg every other day. This dose is gradually decreased over many months to the lowest dose necessary to maintain improvement, which is usually less than 20 mg every other day. The rate of decrease must be individualized: Patients who have a prompt, complete response to prednisone can reduce the alternate-day dose by 20 mg each month until the dose is 60 mg, then by 10 mg each month until the dose is 20 mg every other day, then by 5 mg every 3 months to a minimal dose of 10 mg every other day. Most patients who respond well to prednisone become weak if the drug is discontinued or reduced too rapidly. I usually do not reduce the dose to less than 10 mg every other day unless the patient is taking other immunosuppression.

About one third of patients become weaker temporarily after starting prednisone, usually within the first 7 to 10 days, and this may last for up to 6 days. This worsening can usually be managed with ChE inhibitors. In patients with oropharyngeal weakness or respiratory insufficiency, plasma exchange is used before beginning prednisone to prevent or reduce the severity of these exacerbations. These patients should be hospitalized to start treatment. Once improvement begins, further exacerbations are unusual and treatment can be continued on an outpatient basis.

This prednisone regimen is used for both generalized and purely ocular myasthenia. An alternative approach in treating ocular myasthenia is to begin with 20 mg of prednisone per day and increase the dose 10 mg every week until improvement begins (Table 3). The dose is then kept constant until maximum improvement is achieved, and then tapered over 4 to 6 months to a maintenance dose of 5 to 10 mg every other day.

The major disadvantage of chronic corticosteroid therapy is its side effects. The severity and frequency of these increase when high daily doses are continued

TABLE 2. **High-Dose Daily Prednisone Regimen**

1. If there is oropharyngeal weakness or respiratory compromise, plasma exchange until definite improvement occurs.
2. Prednisone, 60 mg per day, with Mestinon, if necessary.
3. Maintain dose until definite improvement has been present for at least 3 days.
4. Begin 100 mg prednisone every other day.
5. Reduce Mestinon dose as tolerated. Discontinue if possible.
6. Reduce prednisone *slowly* to minimum necessary dose.

TABLE 3. **Incrementing-Dose Prednisone Regimen**

1. Begin 20 mg per day prednisone (with Mestinon, if necessary).
2. Increase dose by 10 mg per day every week to a maximum of 60 mg per day or until definite improvement occurs.
3. After definite improvement has been present for at least 3 days, change to an alternate-day dose that is slightly less than twice the daily dose. Continue this dose until maximum improvement occurs.
4. Reduce Mestinon dose as tolerated. Discontinue, if possible.
5. Reduce prednisone *slowly* to minimum necessary dose.

for more than 1 month. Most side effects resolve as the prednisone dose is reduced and become minimal at doses less than 20 mg every other day. Side effects can be minimized by a low-fat, low-sodium diet and supplemental calcium. Postmenopausal women should also take supplementary vitamin D. Patients with peptic ulcer disease or symptoms of gastritis need H_2 antagonists. Prednisone should not be given in patients with untreated tuberculosis.

Immunosuppressive Drugs

Azathioprine (Imuran) produces sustained improvement in most patients with acquired MG, but the effect may be delayed by 4 to 8 months. The initial dose is 50 mg per day, which is increased by 50 mg per day every 3 days to a total of 150 to 200 mg per day. Improvement persists as long as treatment continues, but weakness recurs after several months if it is discontinued or the dose is reduced below therapeutic levels. Patients who fail corticosteroids may respond to azathioprine, and the reverse is also true. Some respond better to treatment with both drugs together than to either alone. Because the response to azathioprine is delayed, both drugs may be started simultaneously with the intent of rapidly tapering prednisone when azathioprine becomes effective.

A severe allergic reaction, with flulike symptoms and rash, may occur within 2 weeks after starting azathioprine; the occurrence of this reaction requires that the drug be stopped. Approximately one third of patients have mild dose-related side effects that clear after the dose is reduced and do not require stopping treatment. Gastrointestinal irritation can be minimized by giving divided doses after meals or by dose reduction. Leukopenia and even pancytopenia can occur any time during treatment. The blood count should be checked every 2 weeks during the first month, monthly for 6 months, and every 3 to 6 months thereafter. If the peripheral white blood count falls below 3500 cells per mm^3, the dose should be temporarily reduced and then gradually increased after the white blood count rises above 3500 cells per mm^3. Counts below 1000 WBC per mm^3 require that the drug be temporarily discontinued. Serum transaminase concentrations may be slightly elevated, but clinical liver toxicity is rare. Treatment is discontinued if transaminase concentrations exceed twice the upper limit of normal and is restarted at lower doses when these values have returned to normal. Rare cases of azathioprine-induced pancreatitis are reported, but the cost effectiveness of monitoring serum amylase concentrations is not established. Azathioprine is potentially mutagenic, and females of childbearing age should practice adequate contraception while taking it.

Cyclosporine (Sandimmune) is used in MG patients who cannot take azathioprine or who have not responded satisfactorily to it. Treatment begins with 5 to 6 mg per kg per day, in two divided doses taken 12 hours apart. Serum concentrations of cyclosporine and creatinine should be measured monthly, and the dose adjusted to produce a trough serum cyclosporine concentration of 75 to 150 ng/mL and a serum creatinine concentration less than 150% of pretreatment values. The dose necessary to maintain these values becomes less after tissue saturation is achieved. Ten to twenty mg prednisone is usually given every other day with cyclosporine to maximize the response.

Improvement usually begins 1 to 2 months after starting cyclosporine and persists as long as therapeutic doses are given. Maximum improvement is usually seen within 6 months after starting treatment. Thereafter, the dose is gradually reduced to the least amount that maintains improvement.

Renal toxicity and hypertension, the important adverse reactions of cyclosporine, are usually avoided or managed using this approach. Many drugs interfere with cyclosporine metabolism and should be avoided or used with caution.

Cyclophosphamide (Cytoxan) has been used intravenously and orally for the treatment of MG. The intravenous dose is 200 mg per day for 5 days, and the oral dose is 150 to 200 mg per day to a total of 5 to 10 grams. More than half of patients become asymptomatic after 1 year. Alopecia is the rule. Leukopenia, nausea, vomiting, anorexia, and discoloration of the nails and skin occur less frequently.

All immunosuppressive treatment carries an increased risk of infection. The long-term risk of malignancy is not established, but there are no reports of an increased incidence of malignancy in patients with MG receiving treatment with immunosuppressive agents.

Plasma Exchange (Plasmapheresis)

Plasma exchange is used as a short-term intervention for patients with sudden worsening of myasthenic symptoms for any reason, to rapidly improve strength before surgery, and as a chronic intermittent treatment in patients who are refractory to all other treatments. The need for plasma exchange and its frequency of use are determined by the clinical response in the individual patient.

Almost all patients with acquired MG improve temporarily following plasma exchange. A typical protocol is to remove 2 to 3 liters of plasma three times a week until improvement levels off, which usually occurs after five to six exchanges. Improvement usually begins within 48 hours of the first exchange and usually lasts for weeks or months. Weakness returns thereafter in the absence of thymectomy or immunosuppressive therapy. Most patients who respond to the first plasma exchange will respond again to subsequent courses. Repeated exchanges do not have a cumulative benefit.

Adverse reactions to plasma exchange include transitory cardiac arrhythmias, nausea, lightheadedness, chills, visual obscurations, and pedal edema. Thromboses, thrombophlebitis, and subacute bacterial endocarditis may occur when arteriovenous shunts or grafts are placed for vascular access. Severe bacterial and systemic cytomegalovirus infections have been reported in patients receiving concurrent immunosuppressive therapy.

Intravenous Immune Globulin (Table 4)

Improvement occurs in most patients with MG who receive high doses of intravenous human immune globulin (IV-IG), usually beginning within 1 week and lasting for several weeks or, at most, a few months. The indications for IV-IG are similar to those for plasma exchange. Side effects include headaches, chills, and fever, which can be reduced by giving acetaminophen (Tylenol) or aspirin with diphenhydramine (Benadryl) before each infusion. Renal failure has occurred in patients with impaired renal function receiving IV-IG. Aseptic meningitis has also been reported.

Patients with selective IgA deficiency may have an anaphylactic reaction to the IgA in immune globulin preparations. To prevent this problem, patients can be screened with serum immunoglobulin determinations before receiving IV-IG.

Miscellaneous Treatments

Splenectomy, splenic radiation, and total body irradiation have been used in a small number of patients in whom all other forms of immunotherapy have failed. 3,4-Diaminopyridine* produces significant improvement in some patients with acquired MG and congenital myasthenia, but it is not commercially available. Ephedrine can be useful in patients with congenital myasthenia and in patients with acquired myasthenia in whom ChE inhibitors alone are not effective.

*Investigational drug in the United States.

TABLE 4. **High-Dose Intravenous Immune Globulin Regimen**

1. Exclude IgA deficiency with serum immunoelectrophoresis.
2. Premedicate with diphenhydramine hydrochloride (Benadryl) and acetaminophen (Tylenol).
3. Total dose per course: 2 gm human immune globulin per kg (400 mg per kg per day for 5 days, or 1000 mg per kg per day for 2 days).
4. Infusion rate: 0.01 to 0.02 mg per kg per min for 30 min, then 0.08 mg per kg per min.

Selection of Treatment

Treatment must be determined individually for each patient. This is my approach to the patient with suspected MG:

1. Confirm the diagnosis: Rule out genetic myasthenia and Lambert–Eaton myasthenic syndrome. Measure serum AChR antibodies: If the initial measurement is normal and it was performed within 6 months after onset, repeat after 3 to 6 months.
2. Exclude or treat underlying disease, especially hyperthyroidism.
3. Chest computed tomography: If thymoma is present, it usually should be removed surgically (details follow).
4. Begin administration of ChE inhibitors: Adjust dose to lowest amount that produces maximum benefit. If this approach does not produce a satisfactory response, treat as indicated in the following section.

Ocular Myasthenia

If the response to ChE inhibitors is unsatisfactory, prednisone is given, either in incrementing or high daily doses. If weakness develops in muscles other than the ocular or periocular muscles, treat as for generalized disease.

Generalized Myasthenia, Onset Before Age 60

Thymectomy is recommended for all patients. High-dose daily prednisone or plasma exchange is used before surgery in patients with oropharyngeal or respiratory muscle weakness to minimize the risks of surgery. If disabling weakness recurs or persists after thymectomy, or if there is not sustained improvement 12 months after surgery, immunosuppression with high-dose daily prednisone, azathioprine, or cyclosporine is recommended.

Generalized Myasthenia, Onset After Age 60

If the response to ChE inhibitors is unsatisfactory, azathioprine is begun in patients who can tolerate the delayed response. If treatment with azathioprine is unsatisfactory, high-dose daily prednisone is added or cyclosporine is substituted for azathioprine. High-dose daily prednisone is given, with or without plasma exchange, in patients who need a rapid response. Azathioprine or cyclosporine is added to prednisone if the response to prednisone alone is not satisfactory or unacceptable weakness develops as the prednisone dose is reduced.

Generalized Myasthenia with Onset in Childhood

Myasthenia gravis that begins in childhood may be autoimmune or a form of genetic myasthenia, which does not respond to immunotherapy. Almost one half of patients with autoimmune MG that begins before puberty do not have detectable AChR antibodies. In children with seronegative MG, plasma exchange or IV-IG may be given as a therapeutic trial: Those who clearly improve have autoimmune disease and are candidates for thymectomy or immunotherapy. Failure to improve does not exclude autoimmune MG. Patients who can be managed with ChE inhibitors alone should avoid other therapies. If unacceptable weakness persists despite optimal treatment with these medications, I recommend thymectomy. Many children with acquired MG improve so well after thymectomy that they do not require further therapy. Removal of the thymus in infants or children has no deleterious effects on subsequent immunologic development. If thymectomy does not produce a satisfactory response or if weakness persists after adolescence, treatment is the same as for adults.

Thymoma

Surgical removal of the tumor and all thymus tissue is indicated in virtually all patients with thymoma. The patients are pretreated with high-dose daily prednisone, with or without plasma exchange, until maximal improvement is attained. Postoperative radiation is used if tumor resection is incomplete or if the tumor has spread beyond the thymic capsule. Medical treatment is then the same as for patients without thymoma. Elderly patients with small tumors who are not good candidates for surgery because of other health problems may be managed medically while monitoring tumor size radiologically.

Treatment of Associated Diseases

Concomitant diseases and their treatment may have significant effects on myasthenic symptoms. Both hypothyroidism and hyperthyroidism adversely affect myasthenic weakness and should be treated vigorously. Intercurrent infections require immediate attention because they exacerbate MG and can be life-threatening in patients who are immunosuppressed.

Drugs that compromise neuromuscular transmission make myasthenic patients weaker. Neuromuscular blocking agents such as D-tubocurarine and pancuronium have exaggerated and prolonged effects in MG. Some antibiotics, particularly aminoglycosides, antiarrhythmics (quinine, quinidine, and procainamide), and beta-adrenergic blocking drugs, compromise neuromuscular transmission and increase weakness in MG. Iodinated contrast agents produce transitory worsening in patients with MG. Many other drugs increase myasthenic weakness in some patients, and all patients with MG should be observed for clinical worsening after any new medication is started.

D-Penicillamine should not be used in MG (see later discussion). If corticosteroids are needed to treat concomitant illness, the potential adverse and beneficial effects on MG must be anticipated. Annual immunization against influenza is recommended for all patients with MG, and immunization against pneumococcus is recommended before starting prednisone or other immunosuppressive drugs.

Special Situations

Seronegative Myasthenia Gravis

Twenty-five percent of patients with acquired immune-mediated MG do not have detectable serum antibodies against AChR antibody. In seronegative patients, the diagnosis is based on the clinical presentation, the response to ChE inhibitors, and electromyographic findings. Genetic myasthenia must be excluded when seronegative MG begins in childhood. The treatment of seronegative, acquired MG is the same as for seropositive patients.

Myasthenic or Cholinergic Crisis

Myasthenic crisis is respiratory failure from disease. Respiratory failure of any cause is a medical emergency and requires prompt intubation and ventilatory support. If myasthenic crisis occurs in a patients who previously had well-compensated respiratory function, a precipitating event, such as infection, surgery, or rapid tapering of immunosuppression, can usually be defined.

Cholinergic crisis is respiratory failure from overdosage of ChE inhibitors. Although it should be easy to determine if a patient is weak because of too little or too much medication, in practice this is often difficult. The use of edrophonium chloride to make this distinction in crisis is dangerous unless the patient is intubated and ventilated, in which case observation after discontinuing ChE inhibitors provides the same information. It also is easier to monitor the course of the disease when the patient is not taking ChE inhibitors. These medications can be resumed later at low doses and increased as needed.

Respiratory insufficiency from weakness of the diaphragm or chest muscles produces symptomatic air hunger, restlessness, tachycardia, and rapid, shallow breathing. Respiratory assistance is needed when the patient cannot maintain an inspiratory force of more than -20 cmH_2O, a tidal volume of 4 to 5 mL per kg body weight, and a maximum breathing capacity three times the tidal volume, or when the forced vital capacity is less than 15 mL per kg body weight. Weakness of upper airway muscles may produce acute respiratory insufficiency and is usually marked by noisy breathing or frank stridor. The patient in crisis should be intubated and hospitalized on an intensive care unit. Low-pressure, high-compliance endotracheal tubes may be tolerated for long periods of time and usually obviate the need for tracheostomy. A volume-controlled respirator set to provide tidal volumes of 400 to 500 mL and automatic sighing every 10 to 15 minutes is preferred. Assisted respiration is used when the patient's own respiratory efforts can trigger the respirator. An oxygen-enriched atmosphere is necessary only when arterial blood oxygen values fall below 70 mmHg. The inspired gas must be humidified to at least 80% at 37° C (98.6° F) to prevent drying of the tracheobronchial tree. Tracheal secretions should be removed periodically using aseptic aspiration techniques. When respiratory strength improves, weaning from the respirator should be started for 2 or 3 minutes at a time and increased as tolerated. At this point ChE inhibitors can be restarted and the dose adjusted to provide optimal strength of oropharyngeal and respiratory muscles. Extubation should be considered when the patient has an inspiratory pressure greater than -20 cmH_2O and an expiratory pressure greater than 35 to 40 cmH_2O. The tidal volume should exceed 5 mL per kg, which usually corresponds to a vital capacity of at least 1000 mL. If the patient complains of fatigue or shortness of breath, extubation should be deferred, even if these values and the results of blood gas measurements are normal.

Myasthenia Gravis in Pregnancy

MG frequently improves during pregnancy, but it may show no change and occasionally becomes worse. ChE inhibitors and prednisone may be used during pregnancy, but cytotoxic drugs should be avoided because of their potential mutagenic effects. Intravenous ChE inhibitors should not be given during pregnancy because they may produce uterine contractions that could induce abortion or premature labor.

Delivery should be performed at a hospital familiar with the management of MG and neonatal myasthenia. Labor and delivery are usually normal, and cesarean section is necessary only when there is an obstetric indication. Regional anesthesia is preferred for delivery or cesarean section. Magnesium sulfate should not be used for preeclampsia because of its neuromuscular blocking effects; barbiturates are usually adequate. Breast-feeding produces no problems despite the theoretical risk of passage of maternal AChR antibodies via the colostrum. Postpartum exacerbations are common and should be anticipated.

Transitory Neonatal Myasthenia

A transitory form of MG affects 10 to 20% of newborns whose mothers have immune-mediated MG. Affected newborns are hypotonic and feed poorly during the first 3 days. Symptoms usually last less than 2 weeks but may continue for as long as 12 weeks. Myasthenia does not recur later on. The diagnosis is established by the edrophonium chloride test or repetitive nerve stimulation. Affected newborns require symptomatic treatment with ChE inhibitors if swallowing or breathing is impaired. Plasma exchange should be considered in those with respiratory weakness.

Surgical Management of the Myasthenic Patient

The stress of surgery and drugs used perioperatively may cause worsening of myasthenic weakness. Anesthetic agents, neuromuscular blockers, and antibiotics should be used with caution during or after surgery because of their potential effects on MG. Local or spinal anesthesia is generally preferred over inhalation agents when feasible, and neuromuscular blocking agents should be used sparingly, if at all. Assisted respiration should be continued after general anesthesia until the patient is awake and demonstrates adequate respiratory function.

Genetic Myasthenic Syndromes

Genetic forms of myasthenia are a heterogeneous group of disorders caused by several different abnormalities of neuromuscular transmission and are not immune mediated. Symptoms are typically present at birth or early childhood, but can be delayed until young adult life. Ocular muscle weakness is usually the most prominent feature, but more widespread weakness is seen in many patients. Abnormal neuromuscular transmission is confirmed by the response to edrophonium chloride and characteristic electromyographic findings. Cholinesterase inhibitors improve limb muscle weakness in many forms of genetic myasthenia. Ocular muscle weakness is less responsive. The weakness in some children responds to 3,4-diaminopyridine,* but this drug is not commercially available in the United States.

Penicillamine-Induced Myasthenia Gravis

Patients treated with D-penicillamine for rheumatoid arthritis, Wilson's disease, or cystinuria may develop a myasthenic syndrome. Penicillamine-induced myasthenia is usually mild and often restricted to the ocular muscles. The diagnosis is established by the response to edrophonium chloride, characteristic electromyographic abnormalities, and elevated serum AChR antibodies. It is likely that D-penicillamine stimulates or enhances an immunologic reaction against the neuromuscular junction. The myasthenic response induced by D-penicillamine usually remits within 1 year after the drug is stopped. ChE inhibitors usually relieve the symptoms. If myasthenic symptoms persist after D-penicillamine is stopped, the patient should be treated for acquired MG.

TRIGEMINAL NEURALGIA

method of
NICHOLAS M. BARBARO, M.D.
University of California, San Francisco
San Francisco, California

Trigeminal neuralgia is a condition characterized by episodic lancinating facial pain confined to a division of the trigeminal nerve. The pain has an electrical quality, and is frequently triggered by particular activities, such as talking, chewing, or brushing the teeth. Patients often describe specific trigger zones on the face, which may or may not be within the region of pain. Patients may report that the pain began following dental procedures, but a careful history will often disclose that the patient was actually seeing the dentist for pain, which was thought to originate from the teeth. The condition is somewhat more common in women and is more common in the elderly. The onset of trigeminal neuralgia before the age of 40 should raise the question of an associated diagnosis, such as multiple sclerosis, posterior fossa vascular malformation, or tumor. The presence of a significant sensory abnormality or other cranial nerve deficit on examination is rare and should also increase the suspicion of an associated diagnosis. All patients with a new onset of trigeminal pain should be evaluated with mag-

*Investigational drug in the United States.

netic resonance imaging, including special attention to the cerebellopontine angle.

Most patients with so-called idiopathic trigeminal neuralgia have compression of their trigeminal nerve by a blood vessel where the nerve enters the brain stem. Approximately 10% of patients have no such pathology and their syndrome is truly idiopathic.

MEDICAL THERAPY

In assessing the response to medical (and surgical) treatment, one must remember that trigeminal neuralgia is characterized by episodic pain and that spontaneous remissions lasting up to several months can occur without a change in therapy. Approximately 80% of patients can be effectively managed with medical therapy alone, usually carbamazepine (Tegretol). In fact, response to this drug is considered by many to be an important diagnostic indicator that the condition in question is actually trigeminal neuralgia. Carbamazepine dosages are titrated to the clinical response rather than a specific blood level. Patients are typically started on 200 mg twice daily and increased gradually until side effects develop or until effective pain relief is achieved. Most physicians use 1200 mg per day as a maximum dose. Patients on carbamazepine should have periodic (more frequent at the onset of therapy) blood counts and liver function tests. Other side effects that may limit the use of carbamazepine include drowsiness, confusion, ataxia, and allergic responses.

Alternative drugs that are not as effective as carbamazepine include phenytoin (Dilantin), which is usually given at 100 mg three times daily and increased until pain relief or side effects develop. Baclofen (Lioresal) may be effective as an adjunct to carbamazepine or by itself. It is usually begun at 10 or 20 mg per day and increased gradually until side effects such as sedation limit its use. Other anticonvulsant medications, such as clonazepam (Klonopin) and valproic acid, may be effective, but most patients who fail to respond to carbamazepine do not obtain long-lasting relief from these other drugs.

SURGICAL THERAPY

Surgical therapy is reserved for patients who fail to achieve adequate pain relief from medical therapy. Procedures can be divided into two classes: percutaneous and open approaches. Percutaneous approaches include radiofrequency neurotomy (rhizolysis), glycerol injection, and balloon compression techniques. These all have the advantage of being less invasive, requiring minimal hospitalization, and having minimal morbidity and mortality. They are also less likely to give permanent relief of pain and are usually associated with at least a partial sensory deficit. Along with this is the possibility of corneal sensory loss and painful paresthesias, which may be as debilitating as the original pain. The main open approach is microvascular decompression, which requires posterior fossa craniotomy and carries a slightly higher risk of serious neurologic morbidity. It has the highest so-called cure rate and is less likely to give permanent trigeminal sensory deficit. Typically, percutaneous approaches are recommended for elderly or medically debilitated patients, patients with multiple sclerosis, or those who fail to obtain relief from the open approach. Younger and healthier patients should be encouraged to consider the open approach.

PERCUTANEOUS RADIOFREQUENCY RHIZOLYSIS

This technique is designed to produce a thermal injury to a specific portion of the trigeminal nerve. A needle is advanced under fluoroscopic guidance through the face and into the foramen ovale at the skull base. Patients are usually under sedation, but then are allowed to awaken and report the effects of electrical stimulation. The tip of the radiofrequency needle is manipulated until the patient reports paresthesias in the appropriate location. Then the patient is placed under a brief general anesthetic, and a radiofrequency lesion is produced. The surgeon has the option of re-examining the patient and producing additional lesions. Patients are usually sent home the same day. Trigeminal sensory loss is usually slight and is not unpleasant for the patient. At least 80% of patients report significant pain relief with this technique. As many as 40% have a recurrence of pain, which may respond to reinstitution of medical therapy or may require additional surgical treatment.

PERCUTANEOUS GLYCEROL RHIZOLYSIS

This technique is similar to that used for rhizolysis, except that instead of a thermal injury, a chemical injury is produced by bathing the trigeminal ganglion in anhydrous glycerol. The resultant sensory loss is mild but is not as specific to the painful region as that produced by the radiofrequency technique. Although the early experience with this approach reported a smaller incidence of corneal sensory loss than for radiofrequency lesioning, subsequent experience with larger numbers of patients showed that the incidence is nearly equal. This technique produces approximately the same success and recurrence rate as radiofrequency lesioning. The only specific syndrome for which glycerol injection should be recommended over other percutaneous procedures is that of neuralgia in the first trigeminal division in a patient who is not a candidate for an open approach.

PERCUTANEOUS BALLOON COMPRESSION

This approach is newer than the other percutaneous approaches. A catheter with an inflatable balloon is inserted into the foramen ovale, and the trigeminal nerve is compressed by inflating the balloon. Results appear to be similar to other percutaneous approaches, but larger numbers of patients must be followed over longer periods before it can be adequately evaluated.

MICROVASCULAR DECOMPRESSION

Most cases of trigeminal neuralgia are associated with compression of the proximal nerve by an artery in the posterior fossa. Unfortunately, radiographic studies do not provide the necessary resolution to distinguish these cases from those with no such compression. When such compression is relieved by moving the vessel away from the nerve and preventing it from migrating back (typically with a piece of Teflon felt), patients experience relief of their pain with no associated sensory loss. When no such compression is identified, the nerve can be partially cut (rhizotomy), and the results are similar to those of percutaneous techniques. This procedure has the highest success rate (approximately 90%) and lowest recurrence rate of any of the surgical procedures used to treat trigeminal neuralgia. Because it requires posterior fossa craniectomy, however, this procedure has a small incidence of serious neurologic morbidity.

OVERALL RESULTS OF TREATMENT

The main indicator of success of medical and surgical therapy for trigeminal neuralgia is having made the correct diagnosis. Patients with other (atypical) facial pains may respond to medical treatment but usually not to the same extent as those with more typical syndromes. Likewise, such patients do not respond well to surgical techniques and may actually experience worsening of their symptoms if their pain originated as a result of nerve injury. Patients with atypical features, or patients who do not respond in the expected way to standard medical therapy, should be evaluated in a multidisciplinary pain center.

OPTIC NEURITIS

method of
MICHAEL WALL, M.D.
University of Iowa College of Medicine
Iowa City, Iowa

Optic neuritis is a clinical syndrome of visual loss due to immunologic inflammation of optic nerve myelin. Patients develop progressive optic nerve dysfunction with loss of visual acuity and color vision, a relative afferent pupillary defect, and characteristic visual field defects. It is usually accompanied by pain, especially with eye movements. Patients spontaneously recover over a period of weeks. The term optic neuritis is *not* used when the etiology is toxic, traumatic, ischemic, infectious, or congenital.

The age of onset is usually between 20 and 50, with a mean age of 30 years. About three fourths of patients are women. It is well known that optic neuritis is associated with multiple sclerosis. The acute pathologic response is inflammatory with perivascular cuffing and infiltration of plasma cells and T cells. This results in plaques located in the optic nerve. Because optic neuritis is a clinical diagnosis, there is potential for diagnostic error.

SYMPTOMS

Characteristically, patients develop unilateral visual loss that is gradually progressive, usually over days to a week. The visual loss ranges from minimal to severe. In over 90% of patients, it is preceded or accompanied by an orbital ache and twinges of pain with eye movements. Patients sometimes report worsening of their symptoms whenever their body temperature is elevated (Uhthoff's phenomenon).

SIGNS

Visual loss involving the central visual field is a cardinal finding of acute optic neuritis. This takes the form of acuity loss on the Snellen test, color vision deficits, and central scotomas. Other visual field defects, however, such as arcuate defects, altitudinal defects (defects lining up on the horizontal meridian), other nerve fiber bundle defects, and patchy generalized loss, are also common. The optic disc initially appears normal in 65%; in these cases the term retrobulbar optic neuritis is often used. The disc is edematous in 35%, and this is sometimes called papillitis. Relative afferent pupillary defects are the rule and diminish with time but seldom completely resolve.

DIFFERENTIAL DIAGNOSIS

Patients with acute optic neuritis should have a characteristic clinical course and fall in the appropriate age group. Unilateral disk edema in a patient over age 50 is usually ischemic optic neuropathy; unlike optic neuritis, there is generally not much improvement in vision as the disk edema resolves. Expanding masses affecting the optic nerve cause relentlessly progressive visual loss over weeks to months. Children with a process similar to optic neuritis often have a macular star, that is, the retina and optic nerve head are both involved (neuroretinitis); a history of an antecedent viral illness is often obtained. Neuroretinitis is not associated with multiple sclerosis. Inflammation of the optic nerve can occur with systemic infectious or inflammatory processes, such as sarcoidosis, Lyme disease, systemic lupus erythematosuis, and syphilis. Ethmoid and sphenoid sinus mucoceles, chromophobe adenomas, and other tumors can masquerade as optic neuritis. These patients are identified clinically by the progressive character of their visual loss.

LABORATORY FINDINGS

The cerebrospinal fluid may show findings typical of multiple sclerosis (mononuclear pleocytosis with a white blood cell count of less than 40, presence of oligoclonal banding, and elevation of myelin basic protein). The major positive peak of the visual evoked potential is characteristically abnormally prolonged, but this test is seldom necessary. Magnetic resonance imaging (MRI) scans of the orbit, performed with surface coils and special sequencing, sometimes show evidence of plaques in the optic nerve. Brain MRI may show high signal intensity lesions on the T2-weighted images in the cerebral white matter. This pattern is not diagnostic of optic neuritis or multiple sclerosis.

EVALUATION

If the patient has a typical presentation, diagnostic studies are unlikely to yield useful information. A complete blood count, erythrocyte sedimentation rate, Venereal Disease Research Laboratory test, fluorescent treponemal antibody absorption test, and chest roentgenogram can be performed to evaluate for other inflammatory disorders but may be delayed several weeks and not performed if the patient recovers appropriately. Neuroimaging of the orbit is performed if there is no improvement by 3 weeks to be sure there is no compressive etiology. Because of data from the Optic Neuritis Treatment Trial, I obtain brain MRI imaging to evaluate the risk of multiple sclerosis and to decide whether to give a 3-day course of intravenous methylprednisolone followed by 11 days of treatment with oral prednisone (see below).

TREATMENT

The definitive treatment study for acute optic neuritis is a national collaborative study, the Optic Neuritis Treatment Trial. To be included in this multicenter study, the patient had to be between the ages of 18 and 46, have a history compatible with acute optic neuritis, and have visual symptoms lasting 8 days or less. In addition, they were required to have a relative afferent pupillary defect and visual field defect in the affected eye. Patients (n = 497) were randomized to three groups: (1) oral prednisone, 1 mg per kg per day for 14 days; (2) hospitalization and intravenous methylprednisolone, 1 gram per day for 3 days, followed by oral prednisone, 1 mg per kg per day for 11 days; and (3) oral placebo. There were no serious side effects in any of the three groups.

This trial demonstrated vision recovered slightly faster in the intravenous group compared with the other two groups, but there was no significant difference in visual outcome in the three groups at 1 year. The group treated with oral prednisone alone (no intravenous methylprednisolone), however, had a higher rate of recurrences of optic neuritis than the other two groups. Therefore, *oral* prednisone alone should *not* be used to treat acute optic neuritis.

More important, at 2 years of follow-up the patients in the trial treated with *intravenous methylprednisolone, 1 gram per day for 3 days—250 mg intravenously every 6 hours—followed by oral prednisone, 1 mg per kg per day for 11 days* had a 50% reduction in the rate of development of multiple sclerosis. The beneficial effect was greatest in the group with abnormal brain MRI scans and lessened after 2 years.*

Other Immunologic Treatments

If the optic neuritis patient has multiple sclerosis, use of interferon-beta-1b (Betaseron) should be considered. A double-blind, multicenter trial using 8 million international units of interferon-beta-1b, subcutaneously every other day, has also shown a reduction in the rate of recurrences of relapsing-remitting multiple sclerosis by about 50%. The treatment is well tolerated but the cost, at present, is high. Other immunosuppressives, occasionally used for multiple sclerosis, have no place now in the treatment of acute optic neuritis.

Symptomatic Treatment

Symptomatic treatment begins with patient education. Results from studies vary, but patients with optic neuritis have about a 50% risk of developing multiple sclerosis. Once a definite diagnosis of optic neuritis is made, a neurologist should explain the natural history of multiple sclerosis to the patient and emphasize the importance of diagnosis because the rate of recurrence can be decreased. Patients' anxiety is lessened when they realize that about one third of multiple sclerosis patients have a benign form of the disease (another one third have mild to moderate disability). The National Multiple Sclerosis Society is an excellent source for current information.

Patients should be warned that symptoms can be worsened by heat. For example, taking a hot bath or shower, exercising, or even smoking a cigarette can induce enough elevation in temperature in the region of the optic nerve to cause blurring of vision. Eye pain is usually alleviated by the course of intravenous methylprednisolone and oral prednisone. The pain can also be treated with nonsteroidal anti-inflammatory agents.

Patients may complain of visual distortions as objects approach them, such as misperceived veering of oncoming tennis balls, called the Pulfrich pendulum phenomenon. It is due to relatively delayed conduction through one optic nerve. These patients can be fitted with a neutral-density contact lens over the good eye to alleviate this type of distortion. Some patients with the optic neuropathy of multiple sclerosis see better in dim light than bright light. This may be due to cross-talk between neurons with damaged myelin. Dimming room lights or tinting of patient's spectacles may improve vision.

Potassium channel blockers to improve conduction in the damaged nerve are under investigation. Both 4-aminopyridine* and digoxin reportedly improve symptoms and nerve conduction (lessen the delay on a visual evoked response). They appear to work best in patients with temperature-sensitive symptoms.

COURSE

The typical course of acute optic neuritis worsens over about 1 week and then stabilizes for days. This is followed by steady improvement that is rapid for the first 6 weeks; surprisingly, the improvement may continue for 1 year (at a much slower rate). Less than 1% of patients with acute optic neuritis will worsen when their 2-week course of steroids is stopped. A similar percentage of patients not treated with steroids, however, will also worsen between 2 and 4 weeks. This likely represents a second attack. Because this phenomenon is so uncommon and can occur when a disease simulating acute optic neuritis is

*See Beck RW, Cleary PA, Anderson MA, et al: A randomized, controlled trial of corticosteroids in the treatment of acute optic neuritis. N Engl J Med *329*:1764–1769, 1993.

*Investigational drug in the United States.

treated with a short course of glucocorticoids, the diagnosis should be reconsidered and the patient should be restudied.

Because of outcomes such as this, it is important to follow patients with acute optic neuritis whether or not they are treated. Patients should have weekly formal visual field examinations (perimetry), visual acuity, pupil testing, color vision testing, and ophthalmoscopy until they begin improving. If patients worsen after tapering steroids or do not start improving by 1 month after onset, other diagnoses should be entertained.

The data from the optic neuritis treatment trial have revolutionized our approach to acute optic neuritis. Year 2 of a 5-year follow-up has been completed. All physicians treating optic neuritis should keep abreast of the information generated from this very well-run and informative treatment trial.

GLAUCOMA

method of
EDWARD J. ROCKWOOD, M.D.
Cleveland Clinic Foundation
Cleveland, Ohio

Glaucoma is an ocular disease in which elevated intraocular pressure is the greatest risk factor for visual loss. Untreated, progressive optic nerve damage and visual field loss occur. Optic nerve disease is manifested as progressive cupping or focal notching and thinning of the rim of the intraocular portion of the optic nerve. Central visual acuity may be preserved until late in the disease.

The ciliary body of the eye produces aqueous humor, which circulates from the posterior chamber into the anterior chamber and exits through the trabecular meshwork. In most glaucomas there is an abnormality of the trabecular meshwork, which causes a secondary elevation of intraocular pressure. The rate at which visual loss occurs is greater with increasing intraocular pressure. Some patients, however, manifest intermittent intraocular pressure elevation, and some patients have normal tension glaucoma with progressive glaucomatous visual loss despite normal or high-normal intraocular pressures. The incidence of glaucoma increases with age, and the risk of glaucomatous visual loss from elevated intraocular pressure is increased in patients with a family history of visual loss from glaucoma, patients with African American heritage, diabetes mellitus, and myopia (nearsightedness). Many of the glaucomas are inherited.

TYPES OF GLAUCOMA

The glaucomas can be divided into three groups: the open-angle, angle-closure, and developmental (congenital) glaucomas. Primary open-angle glaucoma is the most common type of glaucoma. In primary open-angle glaucoma, there is elevated intraocular pressure with evidence of glaucomatous visual loss without associated ocular findings. Secondary open-angle glaucoma can occur after ocular trauma, intraocular bleeding, in association with intraocular inflammation, after ocular surgery, or may be associated with pigment dispersion from the iris into the anterior segment or a condition known as pseudoexfoliation, in which proteinaceous deposits are released in the anterior segment of the eye.

Primary angle-closure glaucoma may have an acute onset but more typically occurs on a chronic basis. Secondary angle-closure can also occur after intraocular inflammation, after ocular surgery, or after ocular trauma.

Primary infantile (congenital) glaucoma is rare and may be manifest within the first few days to 2 years of life. These children may develop an enlarged globe with tearing, blepharospasm, photophobia, and haziness of the cornea. Developmental glaucoma may be associated with congenital cataracts, aniridia, or some of the phakomatoses. Children with juvenile rheumatoid arthritis can develop a secondary (inflammatory) glaucoma.

SYMPTOMS

Acute glaucomas may present with ocular pain, headache, blurred vision, and the appearance of halos around lights. More commonly, however, glaucoma is painless and may not become symptomatic until advanced, permanent visual loss occurs. The patient with early to moderate glaucomatous visual loss may complain of narrowed peripheral vision or note that portions of objects seem to disappear in the field of view. Cataract, another common ocular disease, often causes glare, blurring of vision, and difficulty reading fine print or road signs. Macular degeneration, also a common disorder in the elderly, may cause visual distortion and poor central visual acuity with retention of good peripheral vision.

OPHTHALMOLOGIC EXAMINATION

Intraocular pressure was historically measured with the Schiøtz tonometer, a hand-held metallic device that is placed on the supine patient's eye. Goldmann applanation tonometry is quicker, easier, more accurate, and probably less traumatic to the globe. It is usually attached directly to the ophthalmologist's slit lamp. Normal intraocular pressure is usually 10 to 21 mmHg. Not all patients with mild to moderate intraocular pressure elevation, however, develop glaucomatous visual loss and require treatment.

Peripheral visual field loss is detected either by manual Goldmann perimetry or one of a number of automated perimeters, which are used to outline the size and depth of defects (scotomas) in the visual field.

Optic nerve examination confirms the presence and extent of glaucomatous visual loss. Some ocular disorders can cause optic nerve damage, which mimics glaucomatous visual loss.

GENERAL ASPECTS OF GLAUCOMA THERAPY

Glaucoma can be managed with any one or a combination of medical, laser, or surgical therapeutic approaches. Traditionally, the open-angle glaucomas are managed with medication first, with laser or surgical treatment reserved for medically uncontrolled glaucoma. The high cost of medication, noncompliance, and growing evidence that early surgical therapy may be preferred in at least some patients have led ophthalmologists to begin to question the traditional approach.

The primary angle-closure glaucomas require early laser iridectomy. In some patients, this procedure may be curative; however, in others, additional medical or surgical therapy may be required to control intraocular pressure. Early retinal laser photocoagulation is required in addition to glaucoma management of the patient with neovascular glaucoma, a secondary complication of diabetes and diabetic retinopathy. Primary infantile glaucoma is managed surgically with medications used only to temporize.

Medical Therapy

Medical therapy for glaucoma can be used on an acute or chronic basis (Table 1). Glaucoma medications usually either decrease aqueous humor production or increase aqueous humor outflow or do both.

Beta-Adrenergic Antagonists

Carteolol (Ocupress), levobunolol (Betagan), metipranolol (OptiPranolol), and timolol (Timoptic) are nonselective beta-adrenergic antagonists. Betaxolol (Betoptic) is predominantly $beta_1$-receptor selective and has a lower efficacy than the noncardioselective agents. These agents are usually well tolerated with few local, ocular side effects. The nonselective beta-adrenergic antagonists can exacerbate shortness of breath in patients with asthma and chronic obstructive lung disease. In these patients, betaxolol is preferred. All of the beta-adrenergic antagonists should be avoided in patients with severe respiratory disease, such as corticosteroid-dependent asthma or end-stage chronic obstructive lung disease.

Each of the beta-adrenergic antagonists can beneficially reduce systemic blood pressure in hypertensive patients and have beneficial effects in patients with angina or tachyarrhythmias. Both selective and nonselective beta-adrenergic antagonists should be avoided in patients with Grade 2 or Grade 3 heart block, congestive heart failure, pulmonary edema, and other forms of severe ventricular dysfunction. Healthy patients may note that they have decreased exercise tolerance. Depression, fatigue, confusion, and impotence any occur with beta-adrenergic antagonists.

Adrenergic Agonists

For years, topical epinephrine was the most commonly prescribed ocular adrenergic agonist. Frequent problems with red eye, chronic conjunctivitis, and allergies have limited its usefulness. Epinephrine may also cause pupillary dilation, photophobia, blurred vision, and in some patients, an increased risk for angle-closure glaucoma. Epinephrine can cause hy-

TABLE 1. **Glaucoma Medications**

Medication Class	Generic Name	Brand Name	Strength	Dosage
Beta-adrenergic antagonists				
Nonselective	Timolol maleate	Timoptic	0.25%, 0.5%	qd, bid
	Levobunolol hydrochloride	Betagan	0.25%, 0.5%	qd, bid
	Metipranolol	OptiPranolol	0.3%	qd, bid
	Carteolol hydrochloride	Ocupress	1%	qd, bid
Selective	Betaxolol hydrochloride	Betoptic	0.25%, 0.5%	qd, bid
Adrenergic agonists	Epinephrine hydrochloride	Epifrin	0.25%, 0.5%, 1%, 2%	qd, bid
		Glaucon	1%, 2%	qd, bid
	Epinephryl borate	Epinal	0.5%, 1%, 2%	qd, bid
		Eppy/N	1%, 2%	qd, bid
	Epinephrine bitartrate	Epitrate	2%	qd, bid
	Dipivefrin	Propine	0.1%	qd, bid
$Alpha_2$-adrenergic agonist	Apraclonidine hydrochloride	Iopidine	1%	Before and after laser
Parasympathomimetic (miotic)				
Cholinergic agents	Pilocarpine hydrochloride	Isopto Carpine	0.25% to 10%	bid to qid
		Pilocar	0.5%, 1%, 2%, 3%, 4%, 6%	bid to qid
		Other generic	0.5%, 1%, 2%, 3%, 4%, 6%	bid to qid
		Pilopine-HS gel	4%	qd at bedtime
		Ocusert-Pilo	20 or 40 μg/h	Weekly
	Pilocarpine nitrate	Pilagan	1%, 2%, 4%	bid to qid
	Carbachol	Isoptocarbachol	0.75%, 1.5%, 3.0%	bid to tid
Cholinesterase inhibitors	Echothiophate iodide	Phospholine iodide	0.03%, 0.06%, 0.125%, 0.25%	qd, bid
	Demecarium bromide	Humorsol	0.125%, 0.25%, 0.5%	qd, bid
	Physostigmine	Eserine ointment	0.25%	*
		Isopto Eserine	0.25%, 0.5%	qd, bid
Carbonic anhydrase inhibitors	Acetazolamide	Diamox	125 mg, 250 mg	bid to qid
		Diamox Sequel	500 mg	qd, bid
	Acetazolamide parenteral	Diamox	500 mg	†
	Dichlorphenamide	Daranide	50 mg	bid, tid
	Methazolamide	Neptazane	25 mg, 50 mg	bid, tid
Osmotic agents	Glycerin	Osmoglyn	50% solution	4 to 7 oz‡
	Isosorbide	Ismotic	45% solution	4 to 7 oz‡
	Mannitol parenteral	Osmitrol	5–25% solution	2 gm per kg body wt‡

*Used after cataract surgery.
†Usually up to 1 gm per day.
‡Should not be used chronically or repeatedly.

pertension, cardiac tachyarrhythmias, nervousness, anxiety, headache, and tremor. Dipivefrin (Propine), an epinephrine prodrug formulation, is probably less likely to cause systemic effects. Local ocular side effects, however, are similar to those of epinephrine.

Selective Alpha$_2$-Receptor Agonists

Apraclonidine (Iopidine) was previously approved for use in conjunction with ophthalmic laser procedures. Late in 1993, it was approved for widespread use in patients with glaucoma. Apraclonidine does not have the potential for severe systemic hypotension, which is seen with clonidine. There are few systemic side effects of apraclonidine. Local ocular effects include conjunctival blanching, pupillary dilation, lid retraction, and local ocular allergic reaction. Tachyphylaxis to this agent is reported.

Cholinergic (Parasympathomimetic) Agents

Pilocarpine and carbachol are the most commonly prescribed agents in this group. They are effective but often poorly tolerated. Local ocular effects include miosis (pupillary constriction), dim vision, ciliary spasm, brow ache, ocular ache, and decreased visual acuity in patients with cataracts. Young, nearsighted patients may experience substantially increased nearsightedness. Retinal detachment has been reported after cholinergic therapy.

The stronger cholinergic agents, ecothiophate iodide (Phospholine Iodide) and demecarium bromide (Humorsol) are known to cause cataract formation and are not used in patients who have had previous cataract surgery. They are irreversible cholinesterase inhibitors, and can potentiate and extend the effect of succinylcholine administered during general anesthesia. The irreversible cholinesterase inhibitors should be discontinued about 6 weeks prior to elective general anesthesia.

Carbonic Anhydrase Inhibitors

At present these agents are marketed in oral and intravenous forms. They have traditionally been used after the institution of maximum tolerated topical ocular medical therapy for glaucoma. Oral carbonic anhydrase inhibitors are used to chronically lower intraocular pressure, and both oral and intravenous agents can provide substantial acute reduction of intraocular pressure in emergent situations.

Frequent and sometimes severe side effects limit their usefulness. Paresthesias, dysesthesias, anorexia, weight loss, fatigue, confusion, depression, and urolithiasis can occur. Most patients on chronic oral carbonic anhydrase inhibitor therapy have a mild metabolic alkalosis, which is of no clinical significance. This can be a greater problem in patients with acid-base abnormalities or renal insufficiency. Concurrent use with high-dose acetylsalicylic acid may potentiate the metabolic acidosis. The potassium-depleting effects of acetazolamide (Diamox) are usually minor, but they can be substantial in patients on non–potassium-sparing diuretic therapy. Acetazolamide is metabolized in the kidney and methazolamide (Neptazane) is metabolized in the liver. Topical carbonic anhydrase inhibitor therapy offers promise of reducing or eliminating some, if not many, of the systemic effects of the oral agents.

Osmotic Agents

Intravenous mannitol, oral glycerine, and oral isosorbide are used for rapid, acute intraocular pressure reduction. Intravenous therapy is advantageous in the severely nauseated patient. Mannitol and isosorbide are excreted from the kidney nonmetabolized; however, glycerine can cause severe hyperglycemia in diabetes mellitus. These agents should never be used chronically. Systemic effects include severe headache, dizziness, nausea, vomiting, and cardiovascular collapse from severe fluid shifts within the body.

Anticholinergic (Parasympatholytic) Agents

Atropine, homatropine, scopolamine, and cyclopentolate can benefit the patient with traumatic, inflammatory, or postoperative glaucoma. Cholinergic therapy can exacerbate intraocular inflammation, and anticholinergic therapy is preferred. Anticholinergic agents are frequently used after glaucoma surgery. They cause visual blurring and pupillary dilation. Angle-closure glaucoma can be precipitated by ocular or systemic anticholinergic therapy.

Topical Corticosteroid Agents

Topical ocular corticosteroid therapy can cause severe intraocular pressure elevation, particularly in patients with primary open-angle glaucoma. These drugs should be prescribed only under the direction of an ophthalmologist. These agents, however, are required for the management of glaucoma associated with intraocular inflammatory disease, after recent ocular trauma without infection, and after recent ocular surgery.

Surgical Therapy

Laser therapy for glaucoma can delay or prevent the need for incisional surgery in some patients. The choice between laser and incisional surgery can be affected by the amount of intraocular pressure lowering required, type of glaucoma, degree of visual loss, life expectancy, and general health.

Laser Trabeculoplasty

Argon laser trabeculoplasty is an outpatient procedure performed under topical anesthesia with delivery of laser energy through a contact lens with gonioprism. A series of 50-micron burns are placed on the junction of the anterior and middle trabecular meshwork over 180 degrees or 360 degrees in one or both eyes. Typically, patients respond within 6 weeks, and there may be as much as one third reduction of intraocular pressure. In patients with medically uncontrolled glaucoma, laser trabeculoplasty may improve intraocular pressure control, but usually with continuation of medication.

Side effects of argon laser trabeculoplasty include

mild transient iritis; mild ocular pain; temporary visual blurring, usually lasting minutes; and post-laser intraocular pressure elevation. Rarely, the intraocular pressure elevation is substantial and prolonged, and may require incisional surgery.

Laser Peripheral Iridectomy

Prior to laser therapy, surgical iridectomy was required in patients with acute and chronic primary angle-closure glaucoma. Laser iridectomy is required early in the course of angle-closure glaucoma, irrespective of the need for medical management. Laser iridectomy is most commonly performed, using either the argon or the neodymium: yttrium aluminum garnet laser.

Glaucoma Filtering Surgery

Glaucoma-filtering surgery involves the creation of a fistula through the corneoscleral limbus and is either full-thickness or is performed as a guarded procedure with partial flap closure over the fistula. Trabeculectomy, a guarded filter, is the most commonly performed glaucoma-filtering procedure. Primary trabeculectomies have a high rate of success; however, the success rate is reduced in patients with previous ocular incisional surgery, including cataract surgery, severe ocular trauma, active intraocular inflammation, and anterior segment neovascularization, seen in some patients with proliferative diabetic retinopathy. Intraoperative and postoperative antimetabolite therapy has improved the chance for successful filtration in these eyes. Mitomycin c (Mutamycin) is used at the time of surgery. Fluorouracil (Adrucil) can be used intraoperatively or administered as postoperative subconjunctival injections. Each is known to inhibit fibroblastic proliferation and to reduce fibrosis at the fistula site.

For more recalcitrant glaucoma, various valves (setons) may be implanted to facilitate aqueous drainage. The most successful forms combine a tube, which is inserted into the anterior or posterior chamber, connected to an aqueous reservoir, which is sutured on the extraocular scleral surface.

Cyclodestructive Surgery

If severe conjunctival scarring precludes filtering surgery, or if ocular visual potential is poor, cyclodestructive surgery may be performed. Diathermy, cryotherapy, or laser photoablation may be used to destroy the ciliary epithelium to cause decreased aqueous production.

Cyclocryotherapy was more traditionally performed; however, laser cycloablation usually causes less pain and ocular inflammation.

EFFECTS OF SYSTEMIC MEDICATION ON GLAUCOMA

Many systemic decongestants, antihistamines, and anticholinergic agents have written warnings regarding the use of these agents by patients with glaucoma. Most patients with glaucoma have an open-angle mechanism and are not at risk for a systemic-medication–induced angle-closure event. With improved ophthalmologic care and early diagnosis, most patients with angle-closure glaucoma after a laser iridectomy can take these medications.

Caffeine probably has a slight effect of increasing intraocular pressure but is generally of no consequence. Excessive water imbibing can elevate intraocular pressure; however, glaucoma patients should not be encouraged to dehydrate themselves. Ethanol lowers intraocular pressure.

Prolonged systemic corticosteroid therapy poses the greatest risk to patients with glaucoma. Corticosteroid-induced glaucoma typically begins after 2 weeks of therapy. Patients with glaucoma who are placed on systemic corticosteroid therapy may require closer ophthalmologic monitoring.

IDIOPATHIC FACIAL PARALYSIS
(Bell's Palsy)

method of
BRUCE J. GANTZ, M.D., and
PETER C. WEBER, M.D.
University of Iowa Hospital and Clinics
Iowa City, Iowa

Idiopathic facial nerve paralysis (Bell's palsy) is an acute, unilateral, peripheral facial paralysis that is considered a diagnosis of exclusion. Although the cause remains elusive, histopathologic, radiographic, and clinical evidence suggest the pathophysiology is due to edema of the nerve within the confines of the temporal bone fallopian canal. This edema, in turn, inhibits axoplasmic flow and nerve impulse propagation. The most common site of the conduction block is at the narrowest portion of the fallopian canal at its entrance, meatal foramen, and labyrinthine segments. This article highlights the epidemiology, clinical presentation, evaluation, and treatment protocols of Bell's palsy at our institution.

EPIDEMIOLOGY

The prevalence of Bell's palsy is approximately 30 cases per 100,000 individuals, thus making it the most common cause of unilateral facial paralysis. There appears to be no sex predilection, and the ages range from infant to elderly, with the fifth and sixth decades of life most common. Right- and left-side facial palsy occurs equally. Recurrence may be uni- or contralateral in up to 10% of patients, but should alert the physician to perform a rigorous examination to rule out other etiologies. Pregnancy triples the risk, while hypertension and diabetes mellitus are only associated with a small increase in incidence. Roughly 10% have a familial orientation, and 70% relate an upper respiratory tract infection preceding the onset.

Recovery begins within 3 weeks for 85% of the patients, with full recovery occurring in 6 months. Only 4 to 6% of patients will experience severe deformity with minimal return of facial movement. Ten to 15% of patients will be troubled with asymmetrical movement, mass movement of all branches when closing the eye, or movement of the mouth. Some cases may demonstrate total inability to close the eye. Identification of this poor recovery group must be accomplished within 2 weeks of the onset of complete paralysis. Delay beyond 2 weeks renders surgical intervention in severe injury situations ineffective.

EVALUATION

A detailed history is mandatory for any patient presenting with facial paralysis. Date of onset, duration of associated symptoms, and other precipitating factors are important to document. Many patients report an antecedent viral illness 7 to 10 days prior to the onset of paralysis. Description of otalgia associated with skin and auricular blebs or blisters is not Bell's palsy, but rather herpes zoster oticus (Ramsay Hunt syndrome), which is treated best with intravenous antiviral agents (acyclovir). The facial paralysis in Bell's palsy may be abrupt or worsen over 2 to 3 days, but is not slowly progressive over weeks to months. Patients with Bell's palsy *do not* complain of facial twitching, decreased hearing, otorrhea, severe otalgia, or balance dysfunction. It is equally important to rule out recent trauma, tick bites, or current ear infections.

Physical examination should confirm a facial paralysis of all branches. If the forehead is intact, a central etiology is of concern, whereas involvement of a single branch indicates a tumor or trauma. The middle ear, tympanic membrane, and external canal should be normal. No aural or oral vesicular lesions should be seen. The parotid gland is palpated bimanually to ensure against a deep lobe tumor. All other cranial nerves should function normally, including cranial nerve V, even though patients may complain of a vague facial numbness.

Audiometric evaluation is necessary for every patient. Unilateral hearing loss or acoustic reflex decay is suggestive of a cerebellar pontine angle tumor and an indication for further retrocochlear evaluation. If vestibular complaints are present, an electronystagmogram is performed.

Radiographic studies are important in patients with facial paralysis. It is not necessary, however, to obtain expensive imaging studies on all patients with acute facial paralysis immediately. Imaging studies are obtained immediately if the signs and symptoms are not compatible with Bell's palsy or if no return of facial motion is observed at 5 to 6 months. Both high-resolution computed tomography and magnetic resonance imaging with gadolinium are useful. The computed tomography scan will allow better visualization of the fallopian canal and associated temporal bone structures. The magnetic resonance imaging scan can demonstrate inflammatory changes associated with Bell's Palsy as well as tumors.

Topognostic testing (stapedial reflex, Schirmer's tearing test, and salivatory testing) have currently been replaced by more objective and accurate electrical diagnostic testing.

ELECTRODIAGNOSIS

Electroneurography (ENoG) and electromyography (EMG) are the two electrical diagnostic tests used most often to assess facial paralysis. ENoG can estimate the amount of severe nerve fiber degeneration from a minor

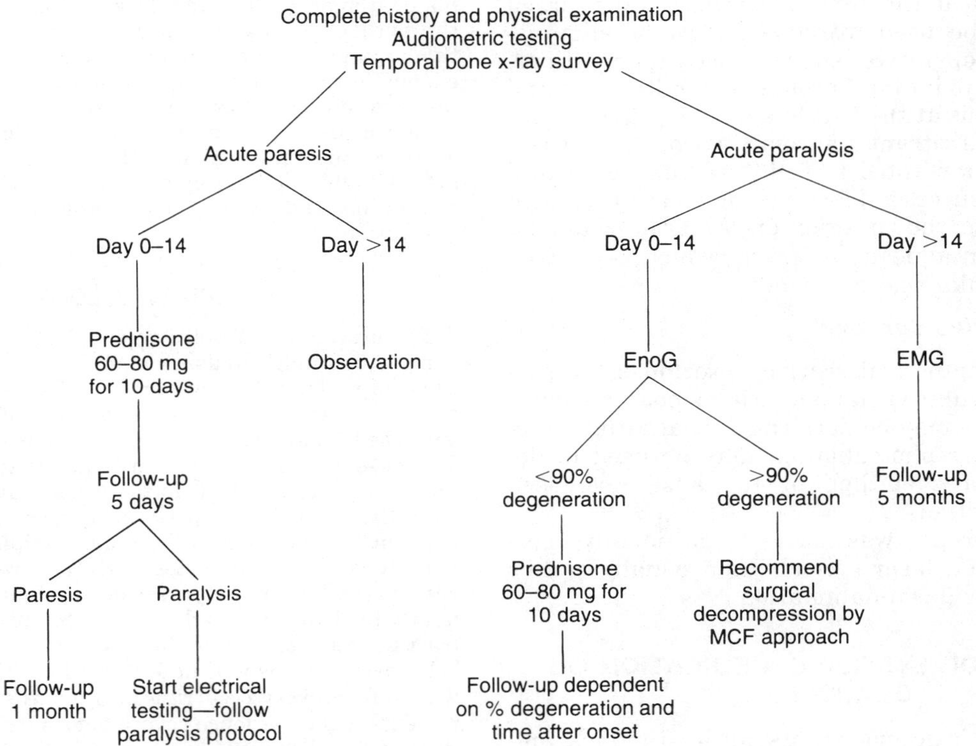

Figure 1. Acute facial paralysis flow chart.
ENoG = Electroneurography; EMG = electromyography; MCF = middle cranial fossa.

injury or conduction block, such as neuropraxia. It takes approximately 3 days for wallerian degeneration to occur following severe injury, therefore ENoG is not performed until after 3 days following total paralysis. Electrical testing is not employed if a patient exhibits paresis, because the presence of even minimal voluntary motion after 3 days indicates minor injury, with full recovery to be expected.

ENoG uses an evoked electrical stimulus to activate the facial nerve as it exits the temporal bone at the stylomastoid foramen. Resulting facial movement generates a compound muscle action potential (CMAP) that can be measured with surface electrodes. The amplitude of the CMAP biphasic response correlates with the number of remaining stimulatable fibers. The CMAP from the paralyzed side can be compared with the CMAP of the normal side. A percentage of functioning or degenerated nerve fibers can then be calculated. Degeneration of greater than or equal to 90% of the fibers indicates poor recovery in greater than 50% of patients. Conversely, if 90% degeneration is not obtained by 3 weeks, a good prognosis is indicated. In addition to the percent of degeneration, the time course to get to 90% degeneration is important. Patients reaching 90% degeneration within 5 days have a far worse prognosis than those who exhibit 90% degeneration in 2 to 3 weeks.

If the ENoG demonstrates 100% degeneration and no CMAP is discernible, then voluntary EMG testing is recommended. EMG measures voluntary motor activity: The patient is asked to make forceful contractions and the single motor unit action potentials are recorded. Because all nerve fibers must depolarize synchronously to generate a CMAP, no response may be seen on ENoG, even when polyphasic potentials (a sign of regenerating nerve fibers) are noted on EMG. ENoG is also not of benefit in long-standing facial paralysis (>3 weeks) because of polyphasic potentials when degeneration and regeneration are occurring. ENoG is not a useful diagnostic test for tumors for similar reasons.

TREATMENT PROTOCOLS

The management of patients with idiopathic facial paralysis depends on a number of variables. An overview of our treatment protocol is seen in the flowchart in Figure 1. This chart is a general guide. Alterations may be made on an individual basis depending on specific circumstances.

Patients presenting with so-called paresis and seen within the initial week of onset are treated with oral steroids. Prednisone is usually prescribed at 60 to 80 mg per day for 10 days without taper. Patients are re-evaluated within 5 days to assess the progress of the disease. Although patients presenting 7 to 14 days after the onset of paresis with stable motor function may improve without steroids, steroids are usually prescribed, because studies do not always demonstrate equal results with or without steroid therapy. Patients presenting more than 14 days after onset are only followed with intermittent examinations. If during the course of treatment complete paralysis ensues, the patient is managed according to the acute paralysis protocol (Fig. 1).

Patients presenting with complete paralysis within the first 14 days are started on oral prednisone, 60 to 80 mg per day. ENoG is obtained on the third day after the onset of paralysis. If degeneration is less than 90%, steroids are continued for a full 10 days. ENoG testing is then repeated every other day until 2 weeks have elapsed from the date of onset of total paralysis. If more than 90% neural degeneration is appreciated, then surgical decompression of the internal auditory canal, labyrinthine segment, and tympanic portion of the facial nerve via a middle cranial fossa approach is recommended. Decompression is only considered if more than 90% degeneration occurs within 2 weeks following the onset of complete paralysis. Surgical decompression and its timing are still controversial, but our data support Professor Ugo Fisch's observation that after 21 days of paralysis, surgical decompression is of little benefit, but before 14 days, the benefits outweigh the risks.

If ENoG demonstrates 100% degeneration, EMG is performed to confirm that complete wallerian degeneration has occurred. EMG testing is also performed if patients present after 3 weeks from the onset of paralysis. EMG testing will demonstrate nerve regeneration with polyphasic potentials.

Preventive eye care is mandatory for all patients with Bell's palsy. Failure to keep the eye moist (with drops during the day and ointment/moisture chamber at night) may result in corneal abrasions and ulcers.

Bell's palsy invariably demonstrates some improvement by 6 months. If no movement is identified 6 months after the onset of paralysis, the original diagnosis of Bell's palsy is incorrect and another etiology is explored.

PARKINSON'S DISEASE

method of
WILLIAM J. WEINER, M.D., and
LISA M. SHULMAN, M.D.
University of Miami School of Medicine
Miami, Florida

There are many etiologies for the akinetic rigid syndrome, or parkinsonism (Table 1). Parkinsonism is a symptom complex consisting of resting tremor, cogwheel rigidity, bradykinesia and akinesia, and impaired postural reflexes. Parkinson's disease is the most commonly occurring akinetic rigid syndrome. Although our concepts of the clinical entity Parkinson's disease have been modified over the years, the original James Parkinson monograph, "An Essay on the Shaking Palsy," published in 1817, remains a remarkable description of the major features of this disease. Parkinson's description of the "involuntary tremulous motion with lessened muscular power, in parts not in action and even when supported; with a propensity to bend the trunk forward and to pass from a walking to a running pace and of the hand failing to answer with exactness to the dictates of the will" is easily recognized in current descriptive terms as resting tremor, gait disturbance, and bradykinesia. In addition to these major features of Parkinson's disease that James Parkinson described, he also noted the speech disturbance, problems with constipation,

This work supported in part by a grant from the National Parkinson Foundation.

TABLE 1. **Parkinsonism**

Idiopathic (Lewy body) Parkinson's disease
Postencephalitic parkinsonism
Encephalitis lethargica
Other encephalitides, including syphilis
Drug- or toxin-induced parkinsonism
Neuroleptics, antiemetics
MPTP
Manganese
Parkinsonism in other degenerative diseases
Olivopontocerebellar degeneration }
Shy–Drager syndrome } Multiple-system atrophies
Striatonigral degeneration }
Pallidal degenerations
Progressive supranuclear palsy
Wilson's disease
Acquired hepatocerebral degeneration
Machado–Joseph–Azorean disease
Alzheimer's disease
Creutzfeldt–Jakob disease
Cortical-basal ganglionic degeneration
Pick's disease
Parkinson-dementia-ALS complex of Guam
Rigid variant of Huntington's disease
Hallervorden-Spatz disease
Calcification of the basal ganglia (idiopathic and symptomatic)
Rare variants of other neurodegenerative and neurometabolic disorders (e.g., Gaucher's disease, GM_1 gangliosidosis; Chédiak-Higashi syndrome; chorea-acanthocytosis syndrome; neuronal intranuclear inclusion disease; familial depression; alveolar hypoventilation and parkinsonism)
Parkinsonism due to other known triggers
Postanoxia, carbon-monoxide intoxication, cyanide poisoning, carbon disulfide, methanol, ethanol
Punch drunk syndrome
Hydrocephalus (normal pressure and high pressure)
Space-occupying lesions; tumors, arteriovenous malformations
Multiple cerebral infarcts (atherosclerotic parkinsonism, including Binswanger's disease and amyloid angiopathy)

Abbreviations: MPTP = N-methyl phenyl tetrahydropyridine.
Reprinted with permission from Weiner WJ, and Lang AE: Movement Disorders: A Comprehensive Survey. Mount Kisco, NY, Futura Publishing, 1989, p 118.

the tendency to fall, the progressive nature of the disorder, sleep disturbances, and the influence of sensory input on transient fluctuations and signs of the disorder itself.

It was Charcot in the latter part of the nineteenth century who named the disease after Parkinson and who himself added rigidity to the features that had already been described by Parkinson. It was not until the beginning of the twentieth century that the substantia nigra lesion associated with these clinical features became known, and it was not until the 1960s that the role of the nigral striatal dopaminergic pathway became integrated into the clinical picture of parkinsonism. The loss of the dopaminergic input to the striatum as the dopaminergic nigral neurons die is the major biochemical feature of Parkinson's disease. The current symptomatic therapy of Parkinson's disease is linked entirely to these basic facts. The pharmacotherapeutic agents that are available to treat this disorder are attempts to replace and enhance the dopamine deficiency by replacement strategies, interference with the catabolism of the remaining dopamine, or through the use of dopamine receptor activation.

Despite intensive recent interest and research, the etiology of Parkinson's disease remains unknown. There is no known environmental toxin that has been demonstrated to induce Parkinson's disease and, except in a rare family, there is no definite evidence of a genetic factor.

DIAGNOSIS

There currently is no biologic marker to confirm the diagnosis of Parkinson's disease. The diagnosis of Parkinson's disease remains a clinical judgment based on the history and neurologic examination of the patient. The major signs that are present on examination that help confirm the presence of parkinsonism include *t*remor, *r*igidity, *a*kinesia, and *p*ostural reflex impairment (TRAP). All major signs of the disorder do not have to be present to make the diagnosis. A patient who presents with a characteristic unilateral resting tremor and mild cogwheel rigidity in the same extremity can easily be recognized as having parkinsonism. When the patient presents with unilateral cogwheel rigidity and bradykinesia, however, the diagnosis is often delayed.

The typical history that is elicited from patients with Parkinson's disease includes the recent onset of resting tremor; some mild difficulty using the involved hand to button shirts or blouses; difficulty performing finger movements that require dexterity; dragging of the involved leg; feeling of loss of power in the affected limb; diminished natural arm swing during ambulation; uncomfortable sensations of tightness, stiffness, and achiness in the affected limb; altered handwriting (micrographia); diminished spontaneity of facial expression (masked face); bent-over flexed posture (simian posture); and decreased spontaneous blinking (reptilian stare). With the exception of the appearance of tremor, which is usually a dramatic occurrence for most patients with Parkinson's disease, the rest of the history reflects the very insidious and mildly progressive nature of the illness. Parkinsonism usually develops between 50 and 70 years of age. The most common age at which symptoms begin is 60.

Once the typical history and characteristic findings are elicited on neurologic examination, the remainder of the time spent with the patient should be directed at establishing that there are no unusual or specific etiologic factors that might account for the presentation of parkinsonism. In particular, there should be no historical features that suggest another diagnosis (e.g., unusually young age of onset, history of encephalitis, exposure to neuroleptics, reserpine-containing antihypertensives, metoclopramide, or toxic exposures, including N-methyl phenyl tetrahydropyridine, manganese, or carbon monoxide). In addition, the physician should note whether or not there are any unusual features on the examination in association with the parkinsonism that bring to mind one of the Parkinson plus syndromes. These unusual features might include impairment of voluntary eye movements (progressive supranuclear palsy), a moderate kinetic tremor in the upper extremities (olivopontocerebellar degeneration), and autonomic features such as orthostasis, diaphoresis, and impotence, suggesting multiple system atrophy. In the vast majority of patients who present with parkinsonism, there are no unusual historical features, nor are there any unusual neurologic examination findings, and the diagnosis of idiopathic Parkinson's disease can be made with confidence. It is sobering to note that in a report from England, neurologists who were well trained in movement disorders evaluated patients that they had clinically diagnosed with Parkinson's disease and followed them until their deaths. At autopsy, the clinical diagnosis of these patients was confirmed in only 75% to 80% of the patients. In other words, in 20% to 25% of patients in whom the diagnosis of Parkinson's disease is made on clinical grounds, the diagnosis may be in error.

Accurate diagnosis is important not only for therapy but

also for prognosis. The initial diagnosis of Parkinson's disease in the mildly affected patient is often followed by questions regarding what the outlook for the future is for that particular patient. There is really no accurate way to be certain what the rate of progression will be in any given patient with Parkinson's disease. Some patients will have considerable difficulty with the activities of daily living and will be obviously unable to continue in their occupations 4 to 5 years into their illness, whereas other patients who look exactly the same at the onset of their disease will do well for 10 years. Accurate diagnosis is also important because if one discovers the etiology of the parkinsonism, the progression and response to therapy might be markedly different. Patients with drug-induced parkinsonism have a much different response to therapy than patients with postencephalitic parkinsonism. By the same token, patients with one of the multiple system atrophies have a much worse prognosis than patients with idiopathic Parkinson's disease.

PHARMACOTHERAPY

Levodopa

The degeneration of the neurons of the zona compacta of the substantia nigra with resulting destruction of the nigral striatal pathway results in striatal dopamine loss. It is this loss of dopaminergic input to the striatum that is responsible for the major motor symptoms of Parkinson's disease. The dopamine loss in the striatum is more pronounced in the putamen than in the caudate. The concentration of dopamine metabolites, including homovanillic acid and dihydroxyphenylacidic acid, is also decreased in the striatum. Levodopa therapy for the treatment of Parkinson's disease is a precursor loading replacement therapy. The precursor of dopamine levodopa is administered in large quantities, enters the brain, and is decarboxylated to dopamine. It is the replenishing of the missing dopamine in the caudate and putamen that is responsible for the dramatic reversal of the motor symptoms of Parkinson's disease.

Since the introduction of high-dose levodopa therapy in 1968 and 1969, levodopa has been recognized as the most important and significant pharmacotherapeutic tool in the treatment of Parkinson's disease. Levodopa therapy is so effective in the early treatment of Parkinson's disease that patients often are able to remember their first experience with levodopa. Statements like "it was a miracle drug" and "it returned me to normal behavior and normal motor activity" are not at all uncommon. In fact, when a patient with parkinsonism gives a history that he or she has never been able to recognize, even in the beginning, the positive effect of levodopa administration, the diagnosis of idiopathic Parkinson's disease should be questioned. As a corollary to this statement, a patient with parkinsonism should receive at least 1000 to 1500 mg of levodopa per day for 7 to 10 days in combination with decarboxylase inhibitors before reaching the conclusion that the patient is levodopa unresponsive. The importance of stating that the patient is unresponsive to levodopa is that it is a good clinical rule that such a patient does not have Parkinson's disease.

When levodopa (Larodopa) is administered alone, a very large amount is required in order to overcome the peripheral decarboxylase systems. In the late 1960s and early 1970s, a common effective dose of levodopa was 4 to 6 grams per day. Levodopa is absorbed from the small bowel by an aromatic amino acid active transport system. The half-life of levodopa is relatively short (1 to 3 hours), and peak plasma levels usually occur 90 minutes post-ingestion. Many factors, including the pH of the gastric contents, the rate of gastric emptying, and the time of exposure to the degradative enzymes in the intestinal flora, affect the rate of absorption. Once absorbed, more than 95% of the compound is decarboxylated to dopamine outside the central nervous system and, therefore, is unable to cross the blood-brain barrier. Hence enormous quantities of levodopa, 4 to 6 grams per day, are required in order to treat Parkinson's disease. When these enormous quantities of levodopa are used, nausea and vomiting are quite frequent. Since the 1970s, peripheral decarboxylase inhibitors, carbidopa and benserazide, have been used in combination with levodopa. Use of peripheral decarboxylase inhibitors (PDI) has enabled the treating physician to reduce the amount of levodopa administered. This has been a very significant advance in the treatment of Parkinson's disease patients. The lower dose of levodopa in combination with the PDI allows a significant and successful therapeutic response but markedly reduces problems related to anorexia, nausea, and vomiting.

The introduction of a combination carbidopa/levodopa tablet (Sinemet) in the United States and the introduction of benserazide/levodopa (Madopar or Prolopa)* in Europe and Canada has become the standard of care for patients who require dopaminergic therapy. The combination of levodopa and the PDI allows the treatment of most Parkinson's disease patients to progress without the uncomfortable gastrointestinal side effects described. Carbidopa/levodopa comes in fixed ratio combinations, 10–1 ratios (Sinemet 10–100 and 25–250), and 4–1 ratios (Sinemet 25–100). In those few patients (about 10%) who still experience nausea and vomiting with the use of the fixed ratio carbidopa/levodopa preparations, it is possible to administer additional PDI in the form of carbidopa (Lodosyn) in order to increase the amount of PDI that is being administered. In these patients, if an additional 100 to 150 mg of carbidopa is administered along with their levodopa/carbidopa dosage, much of the nausea and vomiting can be eliminated. In those few patients who still experience gastrointestinal distress, including nausea, vomiting, and bloating with the administration of Sinemet that is not relieved by increased carbidopa administration, the use of a peripheral dopamine receptor antagonist such as domperidone is in order. Domperidone (Motil-

*Not available in the United States.

ium)* is not available in the United States but can be readily obtained through Canadian pharmacies. Domperidone 10 to 20 mg three times each day can be very effective in alleviating this side effect.

Another peripheral side effect of the administration of PDI/levodopa is orthostatic hypotension. Orthostatic hypotension in association with the administration of PDI/levodopa appears to be the result of both peripheral and central mechanisms. The degree of orthostatic hypotension seen in these patients is usually mild and is often not symptomatic when using PDI/levodopa alone. Orthostatic hypotension, however, can be more of a problem with the use of dopamine-receptor agonists, as will be discussed later. When orthostatic hypotension occurs, it may be a levodopa dose-limiting problem. Instruction in gradual postural adjustments, full-length elastic stockings, increased dietary sodium intake, and the use of fludrocortisone for more intractable cases may all be beneficial. If orthostatic hypotension becomes a persistent unmanageable problem, the diagnosis of multiple system atrophy should be entertained. There has been a question throughout the years of whether or not PDI/levodopa enhances cardiac arrhythmias. There does not appear to be much evidence, however, to suggest that PDI/levodopa can cause or worsen cardiac arrhythmias.

It is the long-term side effects induced by the administration of levodopa that have proved to be the major obstacle in using this drug to treat Parkinson's disease. These problems result from the central side effects of levodopa (Table 2). Levodopa-induced dyskinesias are abnormal involuntary movements, usually of a choreic nature. Lingual, facial, and buccal regions; neck; trunk; extremities; and occasionally, thoracic and abdominal musculature may all be involved. In some patients, dystonia or myoclonus may be the predominant dyskinesia. Levodopa-induced dyskinesias are probably the most common central side effect observed with the chronic administration of levodopa. Between 75% and 80% of parkinsonian patients treated with levodopa for 5 years will develop dyskinetic movements.

The most common temporal pattern for the appearance of dyskinesia is peak-dose dyskinesia. Peak-dose dyskinesias occur at the time of maximum clinical benefit with regard to levodopa improvement of parkinsonian features. Another temporal sequence for the appearance of hyperkinetic dyskinesias is disphasic dyskinesia, in which the dyskinetic movements appear shortly after levodopa is taken, improve when maximal benefit in terms of antiparkinsonian benefit is reached, and reappear when the effect of levodopa is wearing off. The pathophysiologic mechanisms underlying both peak-dose dyskinesia and disphasic dyskinesia remain unknown. From a therapeutic standpoint, however, it is clear that in the parkinsonian patient with levodopa-induced dyskinesias, a discontinuation or reduction in the dose of levodopa will ameliorate the involuntary movements. Unfortunately, the reduction in levodopa administration not only alleviates the dyskinetic movements but also worsens the overall motor symptoms of Parkinson's disease. Most patients with Parkinson's disease prefer to tolerate choreoathetosis rather than be undermedicated and experience increased akinesia and rigidity.

It is often possible to ameliorate levodopa-induced dyskinesias by reducing the dosage of levodopa and adding a dopamine receptor agonist such as bromocriptine (Parlodel) or pergolide (Permax). Other therapeutic maneuvers that attempt to alleviate levodopa-induced dyskinesias include simplifying the patient's overall medication regimen. If a patient is experiencing dyskinesias and is taking levodopa/carbidopa, a dopamine agonist, amantadine, selegiline, and anticholinergics, it is often possible to ameliorate the dyskinesia by slowly reducing the anticholinergics, amantadine, and selegiline, while leaving the most powerful therapeutic agents with regard to helping the patient's parkinsonism, namely, the levodopa and dopamine receptor agonists, intact.

Dystonic postures involving the lower extremities, the hands, and the face are all observed in the spectrum of levodopa-induced movement disorders. Blepharospasm and oral mandibular dystonia have been described in this setting. In addition, painful dystonic postures of the lower extremity, particularly the feet, occur in up to one third of parkinsonian patients being treated with levodopa. These painful dystonias may occur in a peak dose pattern or in a random distribution. Early morning dystonia is a foot dystonia that occurs when the patient first awakens, usually before the first dose of levodopa is taken. It is experienced by patients when they are also experiencing increased parkinsonian symptomatology and, therefore, is often referred to as a low-levodopa-level dystonia. The use of Sinemet CR can be effective in this situation. The administration of one Sinemet CR tablet prior to bedtime, or half a Sinemet CR tablet prior to bedtime and a half-tablet during the night, when many of these patients reawaken, may result in significant improvement. The idea is to raise the early morning level of levodopa. The use of Sinemet CR in this clinical situation is often spectacular.

Levodopa-induced myoclonus occurs primarily in the lower extremities as a nocturnal event. The onset of levodopa-induced myoclonus may coincide with the presence of levodopa-induced psychiatric side effects. Levodopa-induced akathisia is estimated to occur in 25% of patients treated with chronic levodopa. Akathisia is a subjective feeling of restlessness and the need to move. Akathisia itself is not a movement disorder. Levodopa-induced akathisia is often experi-

*Investigational drug in the United States.

TABLE 2. **Levodopa-Induced Central Side Effects**

Dyskinesias: chorea, dystonia, ballismus, myoclonus
Motor fluctuations: end-of-dose failure, on/off phenomenon
Psychiatric: vivid dreaming, nocturnal vocalization, nonthreatening vivid hallucinations, psychosis
Akathisia

enced independent of the current state of levodopa-induced improvement in parkinsonian motor disability. Treatment for levodopa-induced akathisia is difficult.

Although it is true that patients, almost without exception, would rather be hyperkinetic and able to move than hypokinetic, rigid, and dependent on others, levodopa-induced dyskinesias can be a significant side effect. Dyskinesias can become severe enough to interfere with the activities of daily living, interfering with swallowing, speaking, walking, and dressing.

Fluctuating levels of motor performance are often seen in patients with Parkinson's disease who are receiving long-term levodopa therapy. Fluctuating motor performance was seen prior to the levodopa era usually in two settings: (1) the striking episodes of kinesia paradoxica in which a totally disabled and immobile parkinsonian patient under severe emotional stress is able to rise, walk, or run out of danger only to return to the immobile state once danger has passed; (2) freezing, which is a sudden, short-lived interruption of a specific motor act. Other types of motor fluctuations have been seen only since the introduction of levodopa therapy.

The two most common examples of levodopa-related motor fluctuations are end-of-dose failure or end-of-dose wearing-off phenomenon and the on/off phenomenon. When patients first begin therapy with carbidopa/levodopa there is a definite honeymoon period during which time a dosing schedule of three or four tablets per day entirely controls the motor manifestations of Parkinson's disease. As time progresses, usually within 1 to 3 years, patients begin to note that the dose of medication does not seem to last until it is time to take the next dose (wearing-off phenomenon), and they may become very akinetic in the morning before the first dose of medication (morning akinesia). With the passage of time, the length of good or on time that each dose of carbidopa/levodopa induces becomes shorter, and the length of time that it takes for carbidopa/levodopa to kick in becomes longer. As the dosage of carbidopa/levodopa is increased and the length of time between dosages is shortened, the patient begins to cycle between a mobile state that may have associated dyskinesia and an off state. These changes in motor status may begin to appear randomly with no obvious relation to dosage timing. Sudden, rapid, often unpredictable fluctuations between these two extremes have been termed the on/off phenomenon. Clinically, this phenomenon can be striking. The patient may degenerate from moderate to severe generalized dyskinesias of a choreiform nature to an akinetic rigid state, with the patient being unable to walk, in a matter of minutes.

Motor fluctuations can be disabling to patients. The predictable problem of wearing off of the dose can be managed from the patient's standpoint if the patient knows that at the end of 2 to 3 hours that he or she will experience a half-hour to 1 hour of down, or off, time. His or her social life and activities of daily living can be adjusted. But if the patient begins to experience the on/off phenomenon, then the patient never knows when in a short period of time he or she is likely to become completely disabled and immobile. Turning off in this fashion for a parkinsonian patient who is shopping, walking across the street, or trying to engage in other social activities can be devastating.

There are several available therapeutic choices that often are of help in treating motor fluctuations. Carbidopa/levodopa can be given in smaller, more frequent dosages throughout the day. This approach usually improves end-of-dose akinesia for a period of time. The difficulty that often arises in this setting, however, is that the smaller dosages of carbidopa/levodopa are not capable of producing an equivalent improvement in the patient's parkinsonian symptoms. Larger doses administered with greater frequency often induce dyskinesias and psychiatric side effects.

Levodopa competes for absorption from the gastrointestinal tract with other large neutral amino acids. It has been known for some time that high-protein meals interfere with the absorption of levodopa and may produce an erratic response to the administration of levodopa. Some patients report that a high-protein meal eradicates the effect of a carbidopa/levodopa dose. A restricted protein diet has been introduced for patients with Parkinson's disease who are experiencing motor fluctuations. Breakfast and lunch should consist of low-protein foods, and the required dietary protein for adequate nutrition is administered at dinnertime. Therefore, there will be less interference with the absorption of levodopa during the day and a smoother motor response may be observed. In some patients, the institution of a restricted protein diet effectively ameliorates their motor fluctuations.

The introduction of Sinemet CR, the controlled-release form of Sinemet, has also been beneficial for patients with motor fluctuations. The use of Sinemet CR is based on the hypothesis that the maintenance of stable levodopa blood levels will result in the amelioration of these fluctuations. Sinemet CR is available in a fixed ratio of 50 mg carbidopa and 200 mg of levodopa, or 25 mg carbidopa and 100 mg levodopa. It is prepared as a slow-eroding matrix tablet that provides for slower and more protracted absorption of levodopa as compared with regular levodopa preparations. The use of Sinemet CR results in a lower dosing frequency throughout the day and often is valuable in ameliorating fluctuating motor responses. Sinemet CR is also of great value in alleviating nocturnal akinesia, bradykinesia, and gait difficulties. All of these nocturnal problems can contribute to the patient's inability to sleep. In addition, Sinemet CR is useful for relieving early morning akinesia and foot dystonia.

Sinemet CR is less bioavailable than regular Sinemet because of the characteristics of the matrix tablet. If a patient is to be changed from regular carbidopa/levodopa to Sinemet CR, an additional 30% levodopa will have to be administered in the form of

CR. In other words, if a patient was receiving carbidopa/levodopa 25/250 four times per day, the appropriate dosage of Sinemet CR would be 6½ CR tablets per day or 1300 mg of levodopa. Although Sinemet CR has been shown repeatedly to increase the amount of on time and decrease the amount of off time, there are motor side effects associated with the use of Sinemet CR. Late afternoon and evening dyskinesias are often potentiated with the use of CR due to accumulation and elevation of levodopa blood levels later in the day. Also, the slower onset of action of Sinemet CR is often commented on by patients. In fact when Sinemet CR is used for the total treatment of the parkinsonian patient, it is often advisable to use a half of a 25/100 carbidopa/levodopa tablet in the morning in association with the initial CR dose in order to serve as a booster of early morning motor function.

Additional approaches to the treatment of motor fluctuations include the introduction of dopamine-receptor agonists such as bromocriptine (Parlodel) or pergolide (Permax). The use of dopamine-receptor agonists in these circumstances is often effective in alleviating motor fluctuations. The dosage of the dopamine-receptor agonist has to be titrated against the dosage of levodopa in order to prevent the occurrence of dopaminergic side effects, such as dyskinesias and psychiatric symptoms. Selegiline (Eldepryl), an MAO-B inhibitor, is often useful in this same setting to improve motor fluctuations in the patient with Parkinson's disease who is failing on conventional carbidopa/levodopa therapy. In addition, amantadine, which has been available to treat patients with Parkinson's disease for many years, may be surprisingly effective in this same setting. In the most severe patients with motor fluctuations, in whom these various pharmacologic manipulations are ineffective, the use of liquid carbidopa/levodopa preparations or the use of a gastrojejunostomy to directly instill carbidopa/levodopa preparations can be employed.

Levodopa-Induced Psychiatric Side Effects

Another major complication of chronic levodopa treatment is the induction of altered behavioral states (Table 3). These states include disturbed sleep rhythms, vivid dreaming, nightmares, nonthreatening visual hallucinations, and overt psychosis. Psychiatric side effects usually occur following chronic use of levodopa (usually after 3 to 5 years). The appearance of levodopa-induced psychiatric side effects can represent a severe dose-limiting problem in the administration of levodopa. Levodopa-induced psychiatric effects can be ameliorated or ended by lowering the dose or stopping the administration of levodopa altogether. Obviously, if this is required, the motor disability from Parkinson's disease will be markedly increased. It may take up to 2 to 3 weeks for the mental status to return to normal after levodopa dosage is lowered or stopped.

TABLE 3. **Dopaminergic-Induced Psychiatric Side Effects**

Vivid dreams
Nocturnal vocalization
Nonthreatening visual hallucinations
Paranoia
Psychosis

Vivid dreams, nightmares, and nocturnal vocalizations are more often reported by the bed partner of the patient than the patient himself or herself. Occasionally, patients do complain of very frightening nightmares, but more often, it is the spouse who reports that during the night the patient was thrashing about in bed screaming, yelling, and kicking. One of the most common psychiatric side effects of the administration of levodopa is the appearance of nonthreatening visual hallucinations. These hallucinations are often of people and animals, and are common at dusk, when shadows become more apparent indoors. At first appearance, they will often frighten and upset the patient, and the patient may respond to the hallucination as if it is real, alarming the family. After a short period of time, however, the patient seems to become accustomed to the hallucinations. Hallucinations are often benign, meaning that the patient is aware that he or she is experiencing a hallucination. With the passage of time, however, if the levodopa dosage is maintained, the patient may become increasingly delusional, paranoid, and psychotic. The importance of the appearance of the hallucinosis in these patients is to alert the treating physician that alterations in the patient's pharmacotherapy should be undertaken.

Treatment of levodopa-induced psychiatric effects, other than reduction in levodopa dosage, is problematic. In the past, thioridazine (Mellaril) has often been tried in this setting in an attempt to block the levodopa-induced hallucinations and/or psychosis, and not to interfere markedly with the levodopa-induced motor benefit. This use of Mellaril, however, is often only effective for a very short time because invariably Mellaril increases the severity of parkinsonian symptoms.

The use of the atypical neuroleptic clozapine (Clozaril)* has been reported to block levodopa-induced psychosis without worsening the motor symptomatology of Parkinson's disease. In fact, there have been some suggestions that clozapine will actually help some of the symptoms of Parkinson's disease (tremor, motor fluctuations, dyskinesias). Therefore, the use of clozapine in Parkinson's disease patients has been increasing with very good results. Parkinson's disease patients are extremely sensitive to clozapine, and the dosage administered has to be extremely small. The usual starting dosage is 6.25 to 12.5 mg (¼ to ½ tablet) at bedtime. The dosage can then be advanced by 6.25 to 12.5 mg per week up to 50 to 100 mg per day, depending on the patient's response. The most important side effects of this drug include its hematologic effects (1% of patients started on this

*Not FDA approved for this indication.

medication develop agranulocytosis). Complete blood counts are mandatory in order to prescribe the medication. Other side effects that are particularly severe and dose limiting in Parkinson's disease patients include excessive sedation and increased salivation.

Dopamine Receptor Agonists

Dopamine receptor agonists directly stimulate the dopamine receptors in the striatum. Because levodopa preparations require enzymatic decarboxylation to dopamine to be effective, the fact that the dopamine receptor agonist directly stimulates the dopamine receptor and bypasses the degenerating presymptomatic dopamine neuron raised the potential theoretical advantage that dopamine receptor agonists might be more efficacious in treating Parkinson's disease and might induce less side effects than levodopa. Although the dopamine receptor agonists play an important role in the management of moderate to advanced Parkinson's disease, they unfortunately have not proved more efficacious than levodopa and are associated with considerable side effects of their own. Monotherapy with dopamine receptor agonists in early Parkinson's disease generally is not effective. The most important use of the dopamine receptor agonists is in conjunction with levodopa administration. Even in this setting, the efficacy of the agonist tends to diminish with time. On the other hand, there is some evidence to suggest that switching from one agonist to another can be beneficial for deteriorating Parkinson's disease patients. Adverse effects of the agonists include worsening of dyskinesias, hallucinations, psychosis, nausea, vomiting, and orthostatic hypotension.

At present, there are only two agonists available in the United States, bromocriptine (Parlodel) and pergolide (Permax). Efficacy and tolerability of these two drugs appear to be similar, although it is clear that some patients who cannot tolerate one can tolerate the other. On a cost basis, pergolide is more economical. Both drugs must be started at low dosage, usually administered at dinnertime and gradually titrated upward. The starting dosage of bromocriptine is 1.25 mg, increasing in increments of 1.25 mg every 5 to 7 days. The usual dose range at which patients begin to show some therapeutic response is 10 to 20 mg per day. The initial dosage of pergolide is 0.125 mg, increased incrementally by 0.125 mg every 5 to 7 days. The usual dosage at which patients begin to show therapeutic response to pergolide is 0.75 to 1 mg per day. In many patients, however, the dosage of pergolide can be advanced to 3 to 4 mg per day with time and with increased benefit.

Selegiline (Eldepryl)

Selegiline is a selective inhibitor of monoamine oxidase type B. Monoamine oxidase (MAO) is one of the catabolic enzymes for dopamine. Inhibition of this enzyme system may prolong the action of dopamine, which may, of course, be of benefit in dopamine deficiency syndromes such as Parkinson's disease. In fact, selegiline has been demonstrated to be effective in treating the wearing-off phenomenon seen in patients who are taking levodopa. The recommended dosage of selegiline is 5 mg twice a day taken at breakfast and lunch to avoid any alerting side effects that might affect sleep. At this dosage of selegiline, the relative selectivity for MAO-B avoids the MAO type A inhibitor tyramine pressor effects.

There has been considerable recent attention as to whether or not selegiline in this dosage can exert a neuroprotective effect in Parkinson's disease. Clinical trials employing selegiline in the early treatment of Parkinson's disease indicated a delay in the need for patients to receive levodopa. Unfortunately, considerable confusion has arisen about whether or not the effect of selegiline in the treatment of early Parkinson's disease patients is neuroprotective or symptomatic. There is considerable evidence to suggest that a mild symptomatic effect was exerted by selegiline in these early patients and that no true neuroprotection exists. Further research is being carried out with agents of this type to try to clarify this issue.

Amantadine (Symmetrel)

Amantadine has both mild anticholinergic effects and mild dopaminergic effects. Amantadine can be useful in the treatment of early Parkinson's disease to relieve symptoms such as mild bradykinesia and tremor prior to the initiation of levodopa therapy. Amantadine is also useful on occasion in patients who are experiencing motor fluctuations later in the course of their Parkinson's disease. Amantadine's beneficial effects are said to last for only 2 to 3 months. In many patients, however, attempts to withdraw amantadine after 1 to 2 years or longer reveal that amantadine's effects are more persistent than is commonly believed. Amantadine is usually benign when administered to patients with Parkinson's disease. Adverse reactions include confusion, hallucinations, livedo reticularis, and mild peripheral edema. Amantadine should be initiated in a dosage of 100 mg daily and advanced to no more than 200 to 300 mg per day. Amantadine is contraindicated in patients with compromised renal function.

Anticholinergics

Anticholinergic agents were the first pharmacologic agents to be used in Parkinson's disease. The mechanism of action of the anticholinergic agents is believed to be the restoration of a more normal cholinergic dopaminergic balance in the striatum. Commonly used anticholinergics include trihexyphenidyl (Artane), benztropine (Cogentin), and ethopropazine (Parsidol). Parsidol is not available in the United States. The anticholinergics are particularly useful for tremor reduction. Side effects of the anticholinergics include mild memory impairment, confusion, dry mouth, urinary retention, constipation, and visual disturbances. Anticholinergics must be administered with caution in the very elderly parkinsonian patient, because elderly patients are more susceptible to the anticholinergic side effects. These agents can prove useful for tremor reduction in all age groups.

COMMON THERAPEUTIC ISSUES IN THE MANAGEMENT OF PARKINSON'S DISEASE

Does the Early Parkinson's Disease Patient Require Treatment?

When the diagnosis of Parkinson's disease is first made, the patient may have very few symptoms that interfere with daily function. In such a patient, the question about whether or not they require treatment revolves around whether or not the concept of neuroprotective therapy is valid. If there is a so-called neuroprotective therapy, then it would be wise to institute such a treatment at the earliest possible time in an attempt to delay or slow progression of Parkinson's disease. Unfortunately, at this time there is a great deal of confusion regarding whether or not selegiline is a neuroprotective agent. Selegiline has been shown to delay the need for the initiation of Sinemet therapy, but there is evidence that this effect may be related to its mild symptomatic effect in early Parkinson's disease. Other drugs that may be beneficial to the early mildly symptomatic patient include amantadine and the anticholinergics. Anticholinergics, amantadine, or selegiline may control mild symptoms and delay the need for the initiation of levodopa therapy.

When Should Levodopa Be Initiated?

The timing of the initiation of levodopa therapy in the early Parkinson's patient has generated a great deal of controversy. The two opposing view points include initiating therapy early or late in the evolving symptomatology of the parkinson patient. When members of both camps are brought together, however, it is clear that the initiation of levodopa therapy is triggered by the feeling on the part of both the physician and the patient that the patient's symptoms are becoming too intrusive on the patient's lifestyle. The initiation of levodopa therapy may be triggered by events as diverse as an altered golf or tennis game, difficulty sewing, difficulty walking, difficulty getting out of chairs, or difficulty functioning in a business situation.

Carbidopa/levodopa (Sinemet) should be initiated at a dosage of 25 mg carbidopa/100 mg levodopa, one tablet three times daily. This dosage is usually effective in controlling early to moderate symptomatology and is usually well tolerated. The dosage of Sinemet should be advanced prudently and should be guided by the patient's symptoms. There has been considerable recent interest in the use of Sinemet CR 50/200 to treat the initial symptoms of Parkinson's disease. There is some theoretical reason to believe that a more controlled and stable release of Sinemet to the brain might be beneficial in preventing long-term side effects of levodopa administration. This has not been proved at this point, however, and the use of Sinemet CR in the early treatment of Parkinson's disease is not as economical as the use of regular Sinemet.

What Is the Role of Dopamine Receptor Agonists and Selegiline in the Management of Parkinson's Disease?

Early to moderate Parkinson's disease can be extremely well managed with carbidopa/levodopa. As the patient's disease progresses, motor fluctuations, drug-induced dyskinesias, or psychiatric manifestations may begin to appear. The dopamine receptor agonists are best used in this setting when the failure of carbidopa/levodopa begins to be observed by the patient or the physician. In these circumstances, the dopamine receptor agonist should be introduced gradually and titrated upward slowly, without any alteration in the carbidopa/levodopa dose. When and if there are increased dopaminergic side effects, the carbidopa/levodopa dose should then be adjusted downward gradually. This same strategy can be used for introducing selegiline in the same clinical setting of failure of carbidopa/levodopa. Selegiline and the dopamine receptor agonists can be used together but should not be introduced simultaneously to avoid confusion concerning what is happening therapeutically.

OTHER THERAPEUTIC MEASURES

Although the pharmacotherapy of Parkinson's disease can result in marked improvement in the patient's motor status with gratifying improvement in the performance of activities of daily living, with the passage of time and progression of the disease many patients require additional support measures. Physical therapy and occupational therapy can be valuable to the parkinson patient. Physical therapy training including passive range-of-motion and stretching exercises to keep the joints mobile is useful. In addition, gait training is often of value in helping the patient overcome difficulties due to freezing that can develop in the disease. Therapists can be helpful in arranging to have the patient's house outfitted with safety equipment such as handrails, elevated toilet seats, and hospital beds. Therapists are often able to assist the patient to become more independent with the activities of daily living by providing specific tools and aids for compromised manual dexterity.

In recent years the nonmotor manifestations of Parkinson's disease have received increasing attention. These problems can often be as distressing to the patient as his or her motor disability. This type of problem includes gastrointestinal dysfunction, including sialorrhea, constipation, and dysphagia. It also includes sexual dysfunction, particularly impotence in men, and urinary frequency and urgency in both men and women. Transient sensory phenomena that are associated with Parkinson's disease have only recently begun to be recognized. These include parasthesias, burning, tingling, and the most newly described sensory phenomenon, internal tremor. Internal tremor is the sensation of tremor felt by the patient in whom no observable tremor is seen. This sensation of internal tremor can be troublesome to patients. In addition, akathisia, or the feeling of a need to move, is often seen in these patients when they are treated with dopaminergic agents.

Seborrheic dermatitis is a common finding in patients with Parkinson's disease, and the condition can be both annoying and embarrassing to the patient. Several different topical agents are available to treat this condition, including selenium sulfide (Selsun shampoo), fluocinolone (Synalar), and ketoconazole cream (Nizoral). Additional nonmotor manifestations of Parkinson's disease include the common complaint of mild visual blurring or diplopia when attempting to read. This is related to difficulty with convergence. No effective therapy is available for this problem other than making sure that anticholinergics that might have been prescribed are minimized or discontinued.

Finally, the question of depression and anxiety in patients with Parkinson's disease has been re-examined. There seems to be an increased incidence of both anxiety and depression in patients with Parkinson's disease compared with age-matched controls. Whether or not anxiety and depression are part of the central biochemical dysfunction seen in Parkinson's disease or whether they relate to the development of motor impairments that lead to handicaps is still being ascertained. Treatment of anxiety and depression in this setting is no different than that in other clinical settings.

There are a number of patient support groups, including the National Parkinson Foundation (Miami), the American Parkinson Disease Association (New York), the Parkinson Disease Foundation (New York), and the United Parkinson Foundation (Chicago), which serve as valuable resource centers. These nationally based foundations can provide patients with information concerning their disease, information regarding clinical research, and information regarding local support groups.

PERIPHERAL NEUROPATHIES*

method of
S. H. SUBRAMONY, M.D., and
V. VEDANARAYANAN, M.D.
University of Mississippi Medical Center
Jackson, Mississippi

The peripheral nerves are subject to a variety of pathologic processes. Anatomically, peripheral nerves are composed of the processes of neurons within or close to the central nervous system extending out into the various parts of the body. At each spinal segmental level, the ventral roots, carrying motor axons, and the dorsal roots, carrying sensory axons, join to form mixed spinal nerves. In the cervical, brachial, and lumbosacral areas, the mixed spinal nerves form the plexuses from which the major anatomically defined limb nerves emanate. Each peripheral nerve trunk is composed of a large number of myelinated and unmyelinated fibers of varying diameter. In general, large myelinated fibers include the efferent motor axons to skeletal muscles and afferent sensory fibers subserving proprioceptive function. The small myelinated fibers primarily subserve nociceptive afferent function. Unmyelinated fibers include efferent autonomic fibers supplying structures such as blood vessels and sweat glands, as well as afferents carrying nociceptive information. Thus, lesions in peripheral nerves tend to cause motor, sensory, and autonomic disturbances in the distribution of affected nerves. Most peripheral nerve lesions involve all types of nerve fibers more or less equally. Preferential involvement of large or small fibers, however, can occur in some polyneuropathies. For example, some diabetics may have preferential large fiber loss with significant proprioceptive impairment and sensory ataxia, but no loss of pain and temperature sensation. Patients with amyloidosis have preferential small fiber involvement with autonomic deficits and pain and temperature loss but little motor or reflex loss.

The definitive therapy of peripheral nerve diseases is to identify and eliminate the causative factors. Other therapies include rehabilitation of neurologic deficits related to the neuropathies and treatment of symptoms related to the neuropathies. Classification systems that facilitate etiologic diagnosis are listed in Table 1. In the following sections, we elaborate our approach to these problems.

MONONEUROPATHIES

Trauma is the most common cause of mononeuropathies. Mononeuropathies and focal neuropathies, however, can occur in nontraumatic settings.

TABLE 1. **Classification of Peripheral Nerve Diseases**

Based on Pattern of Nerve Involvement
Mononeuropathy (affliction of large, anatomically defined single nerves) and *mononeuropathy multiplex* (affliction of several anatomically defined nerves), e.g., traumatic lesions, carpal tunnel syndrome
Polyneuropathy (generalized affliction of nerves with no restriction to anatomically defined nerves), e.g., diabetic and uremic neuropathy
Based on Tempo of Evolution
Acute polyneuropathies (rapid evolution of neuropathic symptoms), e.g., Guillain-Barré syndrome, toxic neuropathies, porphyria
Chronic polyneuropathies, e.g., diabetic neuropathy, uremic neuropathy, etc.

*S.H.S. would like to thank Mrs. Trissy Crosswhite for her patience in the preparation of this manuscript.

Entrapment Neuropathies

Carpal tunnel syndrome (CTS) is the most common entrapment seen in clinical practice. Patients, often women in their 40s, complain of hand paresthesias, typically with nocturnal exacerbation. It should be pointed out that pain related to CTS often extends into the forearm and elbow area, and occasionally into the shoulder. Hand pain alone is an uncommon manifestation of CTS. Sensory and motor deficits in the median nerve distribution occur late. Provocative maneuvers, such as Tinel's sign and Phalen's sign, are not reliable and lack specifity and sensitivity. Very often, CTS is misdiagnosed as cervical radiculopathy, thoracic outlet syndrome, or a variety of other disorders. The danger of not diagnosing CTS in its early stages is the later occurrence of wasting, atrophy, and weakness of the thenar muscles, leading to hand dysfunction. Electromyography and nerve conduction studies are excellent tools to document CTS, though in a very small proportion of patients with early CTS these tests may be normal as well. When encountering a patient with CTS, one should rule out underlying predisposing factors, especially hypothyroidism, diabetes, and rheumatoid arthritis. Previous trauma to the wrist and repetitive hand motion are other risk factors. Weight reduction and adequate control of hypothyroidism or diabetes alone may reverse early and mild CTS. If these treatments do not reverse the symptoms, carpal tunnel release by an experienced hand surgeon becomes mandatory.

Other entrapment neuropathies commonly seen include ulnar nerve lesions at the elbow and entrapment of the lateral cutaneous nerve of the thigh under the ilio-inguinal ligament (meralgia paresthetica). The latter leads to paresthesias and sensory loss in the anterior lateral aspect of the thigh. Weight reduction helps this situation. The value of surgery has not been clearly established. Ulnar nerve lesions at the elbow are difficult to localize with electromyographic studies, and the entrapment often occurs in different areas, including the retrocondylar groove and the cubital tunnel. Progressive ulnar neuropathies in this area need surgical correction. Common compression neuropathies seen in clinical practice include radial nerve compression in the spiral groove, leading to wrist drop, and peroneal nerve compression at the fibular head, leading to foot drop. These conditions can be readily documented as such by electromyography and usually resolve spontaneously. Acute ulnar nerve compression may also occur at the elbow. One should be aware that acute ulnar compressive neuropathies at the elbow as well as peroneal palsies located at the fibular head can be iatrogenic, resulting from faulty positioning of limbs during surgery or intensive care, and adequate preventive measures need to be taken.

Miscellaneous Mononeuropathies

Other rarer mononeuropathies encountered in clinical practice include neuralgic amyotrophy, which is characterized by painful paralysis of the shoulder girdle or other brachial plexus innervated muscles, often following a nonspecific viral infection. If this diagnosis is established after excluding compression in the cervical area, adequate control of pain with drugs, including narcotics, for short periods of time is all that is needed. This disorder has an excellent prognosis, with nearly 90% recovery over a period of about 3 years. The brachial plexus can also be involved by either tumor infiltration or following radiation. The important function of the clinician is to make an accurate diagnosis because tumor infiltration needs to be treated with radiation therapy. There is no acceptable treatment for radiation plexopathy.

POLYNEUROPATHIES

The term polyneuropathy is used to describe a clinical syndrome that appears to involve all the nerves in the body in a generalized fashion due to a generalized metabolic, toxic, or genetic error. Even though the term indicates that all the nerves are involved, this is not strictly true, because most polyneuropathies have a specific pattern of involvement. This is related to the fact that many polyneuropathies behave as distal axonopathies.

Their pathology involves a so-called dying-back phenomenon, in which the axons degenerate from the tip backward toward the cell body. Much of the synthetic apparatus of the neuron resides in the cell body; proteins, transmitters, and a variety of other substances that are made in the soma have to be transported to the entire length of the axon by axoplasmic transport. Therefore, the very ends of the axons appear to be metabolically vulnerable and, in situations that lead to polyneuropathies, axons appear to die backward. The largest and longest axons in the body are the earliest to degenerate. Such axons subserve sensory and motor function distally in the feet. This explains the typical clinical syndrome of polyneuropathy, which often begins with sensory dysfunction, both positive (paresthesias, dysesthesias, burning pain) as well as negative (numbness and sensory loss), in the feet. The sensory dysfunction ascends up the lower extremities in a symmetrical fashion and is soon associated with motor dysfunction.

The earliest muscles to be involved are the intrinsic foot muscles with inability to move the toes. Subsequently, a bilaterally symmetrical foot drop develops. By the time the motor and sensory dysfunction in the lower extremities reaches the lower one third of the thigh, sensory loss and motor dysfunction appear in the hands. This is associated with reflex loss beginning with the ankle reflex, subsequently the knee reflex, and finally, when the disorder becomes more severe, the upper extremity reflexes. This is the typical clinical syndrome of glove-and-stocking pattern sensory loss and motor dysfunction in polyneuropathies.

There are variations in the theme of polyneuropathy, with some being relatively purely sensory and others being predominantly motor in their nature.

There is also considerable variability in the severity of this syndrome. The vast majority of patients with polyneuropathy have mild to moderate disability involving lower extremity muscles and often the intrinsic hand muscles. In others, polyneuropathies can be so severe as to lead to ventilatory failure. The severity of the polyneuropathy is often related to its etiology. When faced with the syndrome of polyneuropathy, the clinician has to elucidate the etiology accurately so that appropriate treatment can be applied. Two factors, in my experience, seem to be important in the probability of uncovering an etiology for polyneuropathies. The younger the age of the patient, the more likely that one will uncover a cause for it. The more disabling the polyneuropathy, the more likely one will be able to determine its cause. A mild polyneuropathy in an elderly person often has no apparent cause.

Table 2 is a classification of polyneuropathies that is clinically based, and it also details a diagnostic approach to these patients.

Acute Polyneuropathies

In this situation, a patient who has previously been in good health rapidly develops sensory loss as well as severe motor dysfunction over a period of a few days to a few weeks. The prototype of an acute polyneuropathy is Guillain-Barré syndrome (GBS). GBS is often preceded within the previous 2 to 3 weeks by nonspecific infectious illness or occasionally by surgery. The disorder often begins with sensory symptoms such as paresthesias in the feet, but these sensory features are soon overshadowed by muscle weakness.

Muscle weakness can have an ascending or descending pattern in GBS. This is related to the fact that the pathogenesis of this polyneuropathy involves a primary affliction of the myelin sheaths rather than the axons. The patient usually begins with lower extremity weakness, often evolving into bilateral foot drop, and then will lose his or her ability to walk. Within a few days there are problems with upper extremity motor function, extending into the shoulder girdle muscles. In about 50% of these patients, a variety of cranial nerve deficits appear, including facial weakness, oculomotor weakness, and pharyngeal palsy with resultant dyphagia.

The muscle weakness is relatively symmetrical, and in about 20% of these patients, especially in those in whom there is involvement of the shoulder girdle muscles and bulbar muscles, respiratory failure develops. The patient loses all deep tendon reflexes. There is mild but definite sensory loss in the majority of patients. Typically, the illness does not progress beyond 4 weeks. Sphincter control is relatively preserved, although many patients can go through a short phase of urinary retention. When one encounters an acutely paraplegic or quadriplegic patient, it is essential to rule out spinal cord compression in a very expedient fashion.

The clinical signs that distinguish GBS from acute spinal cord compression include the lack of a sensory level, the relative sparing of sphincters, and the lack of upper motor neuron signs, such as hyperreflexia and Babinski signs. None of these may be absolute,

TABLE 2. **Classification of and Diagnostic Approach to Polyneuropathies**

	Clinical Clues	Laboratory Studies
Acute Polyneuropathies		
Guillain-Barré syndrome	Ascending areflexic paralysis, previous "viral" syndrome	Cerebrospinal fluid electromyogram
Arsenic*	Hyperkeratosis, previous GI syndrome	LFT; blood counts; urine, hair, nail and aresenic levels
Porphyria	Family history, change in urine color, abdominal pain, psychiatric manifestations	24 h urine for porphyrin metabolites
Solvent toxicity*	History of exposure (glue sniffing)	Nerve biopsy
Vasculitis*	Systemic organ disease	ESR, chest roentgenogram, nerve biopsy, mesenteric angiogram
Chronic Polyneuropathies		
Metabolic disease	Diabetes, renal failure, hypothyroidism	Blood sugar, BUN, creatinine, T_3, T_4, TSH
Toxic exposure	History of alcohol, drugs (vinca alkaloids, cisplatin, B_6, amiodarone, Antabuse), industrial toxins	Urine for lead, thallium, LFT
Nutritional deficiency	Alcohol abuse, malabsorption, weight loss	Hematocrit, serum proteins, B_{12}, folate levels
Immune mediated or possibly immune predicted	Lupus erythematosus, Sjögren's syndrome, rheumatoid arthritis, myeloma, sarcoid	ANA, rheumatoid factor, serum/urine IEP, skeletal survey, EMG-NCS, chest roentgenogram
Infectious	HIV, leprosy, Lyme disease	Nerve biopsy, Lyme antibody, HIV
Paraneoplastic	Lung and ovarian cancer	Pelvic exam, chest roentgenogram
Genetic	High arched feet, family history, young onset	Electromyogram

Abbreviations: LFT = liver function test; ESR = erythrocyte sedimentation rate: BUN = blood urea nitrogren; T_3 = triiodothyronine; T_4 = thyroxine; TSH = thyroid stimulating hormone; ANA = antinuclear antibody; IEP = immuno-electrophoresis; EMG-NCS = electromyogram and nerve conduction studies; GI = gastrointestinal; HIV = human immunodeficiency virus.

*May be chronic or subacute depending on tempo of exposure and disease.

however, and if suspicion exists spinal imaging needs to be performed. In addition, other causes of an acute polyneuropathy need to be ruled out diligently in any person suspected of having GBS (see later).

The treatment of GBS revolves around supportive care of patients who have varying degrees of quadriplegia, including respiratory failure and dysphagia. Specific therapies are directed at the immunologic mechanisms responsible for the disease. The more rapid the evolution of weakness, the more likely it is that the patient will need ventilatory support. The patient needs to be monitored for evolution of dysphagia and difficulty with handling secretions as well as progressive respiratory failure. Such monitoring includes repeated neurologic evaluation of the patients, assessing the need for frequent suctioning, including blind endotracheal suctioning, and serial measurements of pulmonary mechanics. Vital capacity and negative inspiratory force, which can be measured at the bedside, are valuable tools.

The frequency with which patients are monitored depends on the severity of the illness and rate of progression at that time. Thus, patients who already are nonambulatory and have proximal upper extremity muscle weakness with or without mild bulbar symptoms need very frequent monitoring several times during the day and night. A vital capacity below 20 mL per kg, a negative inspiratory force that goes below -30 cmH_2O, and inability of the patient to keep the pharynx clear of secretions, as well as the need for blind endotrachial suctioning, are all indications for transfer of the patient to an intensive care setting. Further fall in pulmonary mechanics, such as a vital capacity of 15 to 18 mL per kg, a negative inspiratory force less than -25 to 22 cmH_2O, and inability to protect the airway are also indications for endotracheal intubation. It is essential that these patients be electively intubated and not in the setting of code blue, which indicates frank respiratory failure with hypercapnia, hypoxia, confusion, and other central nervous system effects.

In patients with severe illness, supportive care includes care of the skin to prevent trophic ulceration; prophylaxis for venous thrombosis in the legs, using either subcutaneous heparin or pneumatic boots; care of nutrition with, if necessary, a Dobbhoff tube; and monitoring for infection with frequent chest roentgenograms, urinalysis, and blood studies. Cardiac and blood pressure monitoring are essential in severely involved patients, since autonomic dysfunction is frequently associated with GBS.

The prognosis for GBS is excellent, with 80% of patients making a complete recovery and about 20% having mild to moderate residual dysfunction. The mortality rate for this disease, however, remains at about 2 to 3%, and causes of death include infections, pulmonary embolism, and dysautonomia. Need for communication by the patient is an integral part of general care. Communication boards or electronic equipment that would facilitate communication should be used. Ability to indicate needs by these patients, especially those who have been intubated, greatly improves their comfort and allays anxiety.

The specific treatment for GBS is undergoing evolution. Over the last 7 years plasma exchange has become the treatment of choice for GBS. Exchanges are performed at the rate of 3 to 3.5 L per session every other day for a total of three to five exchanges. Such therapy reduces the time spent on a ventilator and the number of days spent in the hospital, and quickens the recovery of motor function. It prevents many patients from reaching a point of ventilatory support. Equally good results may be obtained by a simpler procedure involving the infusion of immunoglobulins intravenously at a rate of 400 mg per kg per day for a total of 5 days. This therapy needs further confirmation of its usefulness.

Other illnesses can give rise to acute polyneuropathies. It is important to recognize them and differentiate them from GBS because they need other types of specific therapies rather than plasma exchange or immunoglobulin infusion. Acute arsenic poisoning gives rise to a peripheral nerve syndrome that is identical to GBS, with rapid evolution of ascending paralysis, elevation of cerebrospinal fluid protein and, in the early stages, electrodiagnostic abnormalities that are very similar. The diagnosis of arsenical neuropathy should be suspected if there is other evidence of systemic toxicity, such as abnormal liver function tests and abnormal bone marrow function, indicated by a leukopenia or thrombocytopenia. The diagnosis can be further substantiated by measuring 24-hour urinary levels of arsenic, although this may not be elevated for long periods of time after a single acute exposure because of the short half-life of arsenic. Other tissues that are useful for measurement of arsenic include hair and nails, which retain arsenic for long periods of time after exposure.

The treatment of acute arsenical intoxication includes all the supportive care pointed out for GBS.

The role of chelation therapy either with British anti-Lewisite or with D-penicillamine is unclear. Only small series of patients have been treated, but none in a prospective randomized study. British anti-Lewisite may be given in a dose of 2.5 mg per kg of body weight four times a day for 2 days, two times a day for a third day, and once a day for 10 days. An alternative is to administer D-penicillamine in a dose of 250 mg four times a day and to measure 24-hour urine levels for arsenic every 24 hours for the next 72 hours. If penicillamine increases the urinary arsenic level, the treatment is continued until the arsenic level in urine falls below 25 μg per 24 hours. Recovery from arsenical neuropathy takes a long time because of the severe axonal degeneration associated with the condition.

Still another cause of an acute rapidly evolving polyneuropathy is that related to inborn errors of porphyrin metabolism. The most common porphyria that causes an acute polyneuropathy is acute intermittent porphyria, which is related to the deficiency of an enzyme, porphobilinogen deaminase. The genetic defect is dominantly inherited, and there may be a positive family history in other members of the family with similar attacks of neuropathy. In the basal state many of these patients do not have any symptoms. On exposure to pharmacologic agents, however, or other precipitating factors that induce liver enzymes, the porphyrin metabolites, preceding the level of the block, increase in amount, resulting in a porphyric attack.

The exact pathogenesis of porphyric neuropathy is not clear. Acute attacks of polyneuropathy often occur in combination with evidence of autonomic dysfunction, such as hypertension, abdominal cramping, and also central nervous system dysfunction, such as confusional state and psychosis. The neuropathy resembles GBS.

It is best to prevent attacks of acute porphyric neuropathy. Patients identified as having the enzyme defect should avoid all drugs that are known to precipitate such attacks, and an appropriate textbook should be consulted for a list of such drugs. In the case of new drugs, sufficient information often does not exist. Any drug that is known to induce hepatic P450 enzyme systems should be avoided. In addition, low intake of carbohydrates is also known to precipitate attacks, and patients should be encouraged to eat a high-carbohydrate diet. Acute attacks of porphyric neuropathy are treated with glucose infusion at the dose of 500 gm per 24 hours. In addition, intravenous infusion of hemin (Panhematin), at a dose of 2 to 5 mg per kg per day for 3 to 14 days is often useful in producing rapid remission of symptoms, presumably by suppressing the enzymes that have been induced during the attack. Drugs that are useful for treating pain and anxiety include chlorpromazine, meperidine, and morphine.

Acute polyneuropathy can occur in patients who are admitted to critical care units for other reasons, such as sepsis, making weaning from the ventilator more difficult. In a proportion of such individuals, electrodiagnostic studies and sural nerve morphology suggest the presence of an axonal neuropathy that is distinct from GBS and the label critical illness polyneuropathy has been applied to this syndrome. The pathogenesis of this syndrome is unclear and seems to involve the length of stay in the intensive care unit, and perhaps may also be related to elevations of blood glucose and lowering of serum albumin during such critical care. It is important to identify this and to distinguish it from GBS, because it will not respond to plasma exchange and there is no known treatment. It is also important to note that some individuals in critical care units develop a primary muscle disease, such as rhabdomyolysis with myoglobinuria or a myopathy of uncertain etiology, and again it is important to recognize this because such a myopathy may have a better prognosis with quicker recovery than an axonal-degeneration type of neuropathy.

Chronic Polyneuropathies

When confronted with a patient who has the clinical syndrome of a chronic or subacute polyneuropathy, two important tasks need to be accomplished. First, one should be certain that the syndrome is, indeed, a polyneuropathy. Illnesses that can mimic a polyneuropathy include multiple lumbosacral radiculopathies caused by discogenic compression or lumbar canal stenosis, and cervical myelopathy caused by spondylotic disease of the cervical spine. An adequate physical examination and judicious use of laboratory tests, such as imaging and particularly electromyography, are useful in making the diagnosis of peripheral polyneuropathy. The second task of the clinician is to establish an etiology for the polyneuropathy. This often can be a daunting task. Important causes of a polyneuropathy have been listed in Table 2.

Diabetic Polyneuropathy

Diabetes is one of the most common causes of polyneuropathies in clinical practice. The most common peripheral nerve syndrome caused by diabetes is a distal symmetrical polyneuropathy, which is indistinguishable from many other causes of polyneuropathy. The prevalence of symptomatic diabetic neuropathy is related to the duration of the diabetes. About 50% of diabetics with duration of diabetes for 25 years have symptomatic polyneuropathy. In most of the patients diabetic neuropathy remains a mild to moderate illness, although disabling sensory symptoms, such as pain and burning, may be found. The treatment of such diabetic polyneuropathy at the moment remains strict control of hyperglycemia. Studies have shown that peripheral nerve function improves with stricter control of blood glucose by using continuous infusion methods than can be achieved with routine types of therapy. Other groups of drugs haven been tried in diabetic polyneuropathy based on current hypotheses of the pathogenesis of diabetic neuropathy. Based on studies showing reduction in myo-inositol levels in nerves of animal models of diabetic polyneuropathy and studies demonstrating accumulation of sugar alcohols such as sorbitol from activity of aldose reductase, myo-inositol supplementation and drugs capable of inhibiting aldose reductase such as tolrestat (Alredase)* have been tried in diabetic polyneuropathy. Small studies have not revealed any significant beneficial effect of such modalities of treatment.

Diabetes can affect the peripheral nervous system in several other ways. Diabetics may be more prone to entrapment neuropathies, and such superimposed lesions need to be recognized and treated with appropriate surgery. Another not uncommon clinical situation is one in which the patient presents with rapid evolution of pain and profound muscle weakness involving the proximal lower extremity muscles, often bilateral but nevertheless asymmetrical. Initially, the pain is severe and often nocturnal in character. As the pain gets somewhat better, the patient notices progressive weakness, particularly involving the thigh muscles, such as the quadriceps and iliopsoas. Although the term femoral neuropathy has been used

*Investigational drug in the United States.

to describe such an illness, in our experience this illness has never been confined to the distribution of the femoral nerve, but primarily seems to involve muscles in the distribution of the lumbar plexus. The important task is to recognize that this is a complication of diabetes and to exclude other causes of a similar nerve lesion, such as compression or infiltration of the same nerve roots, either at the level of the lumbosacral spine or at the level of the lumbar plexus. Adequate control of pain needs to be achieved. Strict diabetes control needs to be instituted. The patient can be reassured that this illness usually has a good prognosis, with nearly complete recovery occurring over a period of a year or more. This entity has been variously described in the literature as diabetic proximal neuropathy and diabetic amyotrophy.

Occasionally, patients with diabetes present with pain, sensory loss, and discomfort in the distribution of a truncal intercostal nerve. These patients often are determined to have intra-abdominal pathology before it is recognized that the problem may be along the intercostal nerves. Electromyography may be useful in establishing this diagnosis, and the term diabetic truncal neuropathy has been used to describe this entity.

Finally, autonomic symptoms may predominate in patients with diabetic neuropathy. The symptoms and signs include sexual dysfunction, orthostatic hypotension (OH), and a variety of gastrointestinal disturbances. OH may respond to physical measures, such as elastic stockings, high fluid intake, and occasionally, medications such as fludrocortisone (Florinef), 0.1 mg one to two times per day. Impaired gastric motility may respond to metoclopramide (Reglan), 10 mg 30 minutes before meals.

Uremic Neuropathy

Peripheral neuropathy is commonplace in patients with renal failure and probably occurs in nearly 100% of patients on chronic hemodialysis or peritoneal dialysis. The pathogenesis of uremic polyneuropathy is unclear and may be related to retention of a variety of toxic molecules termed middle molecules. Reversal of the metabolic abnormalities, either with peritoneal dialysis or with repeated hemodialysis, reverses many of the symptoms of uremic neuropathy and prevents their progression. Renal transplantation reverses uremic polyneuropathy even better than dialysis.

Alcoholic Neuropathy

Clinically it is not possible to distinguish alcoholic polyneuropathy from other types of distal symmetrical polyneuropathies without the history of alcohol intake and nutritional deficiency. It is believed that much of the neuropathy in alcoholism is related to deficiency of a variety of vitamins, particularly the B group. Treatment of alcoholic polyneuropathy includes strict abstinence and the improvement of nutritional status, including supplementation with the entire group of B vitamins, including vitamins B_1, B_6, and B_{12}. Folic acid supplementation may also be needed.

Toxic Neuropathies

Barring alcohol, the most common examples of toxic neuropathies are drug-induced neuropathies. A careful drug history is very important in the evaluation of patients with polyneuropathy. Although it is recognized that several drugs may be related to polyneuropathies, the common drugs that are involved include certain cancer chemotherapeutic agents (vinca alkaloids, cisplatin [Platinol], and taxol), certain antibiotics (especially isoniazid), some of the newer cardiac active drugs (amiodarone and perhexiline maleate),* gold when used in the treatment of rheumatoid arthritis, Antabuse used in the treatment of alcoholism, recreational use of nitrous oxide, and megadose use (doses exceeding 50 to 200 mg per day) of vitamin B_6.

Other drug-induced neuropathies include those related to nitrofurantoin, metronidazole, colchicine, and phenytoin. Toxic neuropathies due to industrial or accidental exposure include those related to hexacarbon solvents such as n-hexane, acrylamide, and metals such as arsenic, thallium, and lead. In each of these instances, it is important to identify the offending toxic agent, using a detailed history and, when applicable, appropriate laboratory measures, and to eliminate the toxic agent so that the peripheral nervous system can recover. Most toxic neuropathies are primarily axonal in type and take a long time to resolve once the offending agent is removed. Isoniazid neuropathy can be prevented by coadministering pyridoxine 10 mg with each daily dose of isoniazid.

Immunologically Mediated Polyneuropathies

Many autoimmune disorders, readily recognized by internists and other primary care physicians, are associated with polyneuropathy as a complication. These disorders include lupus erythematosus, rheumatoid arthritis, and Sjögren's syndrome. Sarcoidosis may also be associated with a polyneuropathy. The treatment of these polyneuropathies is that of the underlying autoimmune disease and should be directed to the appropriate specialty.

It has become increasingly recognized that a variety of peripheral nerve syndromes of a subacute or chronic nature can be related to autoimmune mechanisms directed solely against the peripheral nervous system. An example of a presumed autoimmune disease of the peripheral nervous system is GBS. A more chronic disorder of the peripheral nervous system that is believed to have autoimmune pathogenesis is known as chronic demyelinating inflammatory polyneuropathy (CDIP). This is an important polyneuropathy to be recognized because it is eminently treata-

*Not available in the United States.

ble. CDIP should be considered whenever a patient has a disabling polyneuropathy that does not appear to have any other cause on routine laboratory evaluation. The clinical recognition of CDIP is straightforward if adequate laboratory support is available.

The illness resembles GBS in many respects. It evolves in the form often of ascending paralysis and is predominantly motor with more modest sensory loss. There is usually generalized areflexia, just like in GBS. The spinal fluid protein shows a similar abnormality with normal cell count. Electrodiagnostic testing reveals similar abnormalities, including severe slowing of conduction velocities and the presence of conduction blocks because the pathogenesis of this neuropathy also involves primary demyelination. CDIP differs from GBS in two important respects. The evolution of this illness is slower, and therefore, these patients often do not look that ill in the acute phase of the illness. On the other hand, spontaneous recovery does not occur in CDIP. Left untreated, patients with CDIP will gradually progress, and significant mortality and morbidity is associated with this illness. Accurate diagnosis depends on the recognition of the clinical syndrome and is supported by electrodiagnostic tests. A nerve biopsy occasionally helps. The treatment of choice for CDIP is the use of high-dose steroids. Prednisone is begun in a dose of 60 to 100 mg every day and continued for 8 to 12 weeks as the patient is monitored for improvement in muscle strength. Once this goal is achieved, a gradual tapering is begun. In my experience, the best results are achieved with an extremely slow tapering of prednisone at a rate of not more than 5 mg per week. This is begun with even-day doses until an alternate-day regimen is achieved in many patients. At any level of prednisone, if symptoms recur the previous higher level of prednisone is used for a longer period of time.

Patients who are unresponsive to prednisone may be treated with other immunosuppressive regimens. Experience with such regimens is anecdotal, and my preference is to start with azathioprine (Imuran), at a dose of 2 mg per kg per day. It should be pointed out that the beneficial effects of azathioprine may take several months to appear. Both prednisone and azathioprine have numerous side effects that need careful monitoring. It has also been shown that CDIP responds to plasma exchange. Certainly patients who are severely weak with CDIP may be subjected to plasma exchange as an initial approach; similarly, some patients may benefit from repeated courses of plasma exchange at periodic intervals to keep them functional. Intravenous immunoglobin infusion may also help patients with CDIP.

A syndrome indistinguishable from CDIP can be triggered by many underlying illnesses. It is assumed that these underlying illnesses trigger immune mechanisms responsible for the CDIP. Therefore, any time one encounters a patient with the syndrome of CDIP, it is essential that such underlying disorders be ruled out. These include malignancy such as bronchogenic carcinoma, asymptomatic human immunodeficiency virus infection, and a monoclonal gammopathy.

The presence of a monoclonal gammopathy related to a variety of illnesses can be associated with a polyneuropathy. It is believed that, at least in some instances, the monoclonal protein may be directed against peripheral nerve antigenic determinants and induce the neuropathy via autoimmune mechanisms. The causes of such monoclonal gammopathies that can be related to polyneuropathy include multiple myeloma, isolated plasmacytoma, Waldenström's macroglobulinemia, the Poems (polyneuropathy organomegaly, endocrinopathy, monoclonal gammopathy, and skin changes) syndrome, and the so-called monoclonal gammopathy of undetermined significance. The polyneuropathy associated with monoclonal gammopathies may present with a variety of features, including a syndrome that closely resembles CDIP, a syndrome of pure sensory neuropathy, and a syndrome of mild to moderate sensory and motor neuropathy indistinguishable from other garden-variety neuropathies. In addition, a proportion of patients with monoclonal gammopathies and polyneuropathy have secondary amyloidosis as the pathogenic mechanism.

The method of choice for detecting monoclonal proteins in the setting of a polyneuropathy includes immunofixation electrophoresis rather than the routine serum protein electrophoresis. It is also important to search the urine for monoclonal protein using similar techniques. Finally, if a gammopathy is suspected, it is important to obtain a metastatic skeletal survey, looking for either isolated plasmacytoma or osteosclerotic multiple myeloma, which appears to be particularly associated with polyneuropathies. Isolated suspicious bone lesions should be biopsied. Bone marrow examination is also needed. The treatment of neuropathies associated with such gammopathies includes suppression of the monoclonal protein using a variety of chemotherapeutic agents. There is anecdotal evidence that some of these patients will improve by eliminating the monoclonal protein via plasma exchange.

Recently, a syndrome of progressive muscle weakness, often of an asymmetrical nature, often beginning in the upper extremities, and often in the absence of sensory loss, has been recognized. Such a syndrome has been associated with the presence of an electrophysiologic phenomenon known as conduction block along the peripheral nerves, which can be detected using careful nerve conduction studies. This illness often superficially resembles amyotrophic lateral sclerosis, but the distinction is made by detecting conduction blocks using nerve conduction studies. The illness may have an immune basis and has often been linked to the presence in the blood of a variety of antibodies, particularly antibodies against peripheral nerve gangliosides known as anti-GM_1 antibodies. Routine immunosuppression with steroids often is not helpful; treatment with cyclophosphamide or immunoglobulin infusion may be beneficial in patients with multifocal motor neuropathy conduction blocks.

Finally, vasculitis related to any cause can result in significant involvement of the peripheral nervous system. The basis for peripheral nerve damage in vasculitis is probably multiple nerve infarctions and, therefore, is strictly a mononeuropathy multiplex rather than a polyneuropathy. In its end stage, however, mononeuropathy multiplex can resemble a severe polyneuropathy. The underlying causes of vasculitis in this situation include systemic necrotizing vasculitis, such as polyarteritis nodosa and Wegener's granulomatosis, as well as other collagen disorders, such as rheumatoid arthritis and lupus erythematosus. In an occasional patient, vasculitis may be limited to the peripheral nervous system. It should not be forgotten that peripheral nerve involvement may be the earliest sign of vasculitis, and when the peripheral nervous system is involved nerve biopsy is a very useful technique for establishing the diagnosis of vasculitis.

The treatment of mononeuropathy multiplex related to vasculitis is that of the underlying systemic vasculitis. We use large-dose steroids (prednisone 100 mg per day, often in combination with cyclophosphamide at 2 mg per kg). With especially aggressive disease, an initial course of high-dose intravenous methylprednisolone (Solu-Medrol) may be given for several days. The prognosis of vasculitic neuropathy is often related to underlying systemic complications of vasculitis.

Inherited Neuropathies

A variety of gene abnormalities can result in polyneuropathies. Most of these are uncommon and include porphyria, amyloidosis, a variety of neuropathies, such as pure sensory neuropathy and Dejerine–Sottas polyneuropathy, as well as Refsum's disease. The most common type of familial neuropathy in clinical practice is Charcot-Marie-Tooth disease (CMT). The CMT phenotype is characterized by the onset of a very slowly progressive polyneuropathy, often in the second or the third decade, with gradual evolution of bilateral foot drop, followed subsequently by hand-muscle wasting and weakness. Sensory complaints tend to be uncommon with CMT; however, sensory loss can be readily documented, particularly involving proprioceptive function, and follows the typical stocking-and-glove pattern.

The progression of this disorder tends to be almost imperceptible; only a small proportion of patients with CMT eventually lose ambulation. A significant proportion, however, will need assistive devices for continued ambulation, such as appropriately fitted ankle-foot orthoses, canes, or walkers. A genetically determined polyneuropathy, especially CMT, should be considered in any patient whose polyneuropathy has its onset during childhood or young adulthood.

In the majority of patients with CMT, as described earlier, the pattern of inheritance is autosomal dominant. Therefore, one is able to identify other persons in the family, particularly one of the parents, as being affected. The disorder, however, often tends to have extreme variability in its clinical expression in the same family. Thus, one rarely encounters severe neuropathy in some members of the family, whereas others are often asymptomatic. The occurrence of skeletal deformities, such as high-arched feet and kyphoscoliosis, can be a clue to the presence of genetic neuropathy, but occurs only in about 60% of these patients. One variety of CMT (CMT-type I) is characterized by severe slowing of nerve conduction velocities, and this may be another clue. In fact, nerve conduction studies are excellent tools to document the expression of the abnormal gene in asymptomatic individuals. The importance of recognizing familial neuropathy is that one is able to avoid an expensive laboratory work-up to uncover the causation of such a neuropathy.

In another variety of CMT (CMT-type II), the clinical phenotype is very similar; however, the nerve conduction velocities are either not slowed at all or only minimally slowed. Both of these disorders are dominantly inherited. Occasionally, the same CMT phenotype can be inherited in other ways, including autosomal recessive and sex linked. In addition to the genetic heterogeneity of this syndrome suggested by the various inheritance patterns, emerging evidence suggests genetic heterogeneity, even among a clinically homogeneous group of patients such as those with CMT-type I.

At least two different gene-locus abnormalities can give rise to an identical CMT-type I clinical picture and electrophysiologic findings. One of these is the result of a duplication in the short arm of chromosome 17 in the region that codes for PMP 22 gene. This duplication can be directly detected and is useful in making a diagnosis of CMT-type 1 when there is lack of a convincing family history. Ethical considerations regarding prenatal testing in a relatively benign disorder such as CMT have not been addressed.

At the moment there is no specific treatment for inherited neuropathies of the CMT type. The patients need rehabilitative efforts depending on the degree of their disability.

Infectious Neuropathies

Both human immunodeficiency virus (HIV) infection and Lyme disease can affect the peripheral nervous system. A variety of peripheral nerve syndromes can occur in the setting of HIV infection. Demyelinating polyneuropathies that clinically and physiologically resemble GBS as well as CIDP have been associated with HIV infection. These usually occur early in the course of HIV infection, when the patients are otherwise asymptomatic. Such demyelinating neuropathies in the setting of HIV infection can be treated in a manner similar to GBS and CDIP in HIV-I-seronegative patients. There may be concerns regarding the use of long-term corticosteroids, however, in patients with HIV-I infection. A vasculitic mononeuropathy multiplex can occur in HIV-infected patients usually during the phase of AIDS-related complex. Because of limited experience, the ideal way to treat such vasculitic neuropathy in the setting of HIV infection is unclear. During full-blown HIV infection, a more garden-variety, distally symmetrical, predominantly sensory polyneuropathy occurs. The cause of this disorder is unknown. It may be related to direct HIV infection in the nervous system or to a variety of other factors, including nutritional deficiency and the use of a variety of drugs in patients with such severe illness. Finally, patients in the late stage of an HIV infection (acquired immune deficiency syndrome) can present with a subacutely evolving cauda equina syndrome that is asymmetrical, painful, and predominantly motor. There is often bowel and bladder incontinence. This has been related to a cytomegalovirus polyradiculitis. The spinal fluid reveals polymorphonuclear leukocytosis, low glucose, and elevated protein. Other tissues, such as retina, blood, and urine, can reveal evidence of cytomegalovirus. The antiviral drug, ganciclovir, may be effective in stabilizing and improving cytomegalovirus polyradiculitis.

Lyme disease is a multisystem disease caused by a tick-borne spirochete, *Borrelia burgdorferi*. Peripheral nerve lesions can occur both during the early disseminated stage (stage II) as well as during late stages of infection (stage III). During stage II, peripheral nerve involvement takes the form of cranial nerve lesions, especially seventh nerve palsy, which closely resembles Bell's palsy. Headache and meningismus often accompany such cranial neuropathies, and there is usually cerebrospinal fluid pleocytosis. In about 40% of patients with stage II infection, a peripheral radicular neuritis develops. This is a painful illness, characterized by radicular pain, paresthesias, and spinal pain, followed by asymmetrical muscle weakness, usually more common in the lower extremities than in the upper extremities. An occasional patient will develop a syndrome indistinguishable from GBS. Again, cerebrospinal fluid mononuclear pleocytosis is a common finding. In late stages of infection, a mild symmetrical polyneuropathy occurs, and often paresthesias in the extremities are troublesome complaints. The diagnosis can be established by estimating IgM and IgG antibodies to *B. burgdorferi* using a variety of immunologic techniques such as the enzyme-linked immunosorbent assay. Cerebrospinal fluid antibodies also become positive. In Lyme disease with such neurologic involvement, the treatment choices include penicillin G 20 to 24 million units per day for 10 to 14 days intraveneously or intravenous ceftriaxone at 2 grams per day for 2 to 4 weeks. Other regimens, including cefotaxime and doxycycline, have been described as well.

POLYNEUROPATHIES IN CHILDREN

In contrast to adults, polyneuropathies in children are rare and in a majority of instances are secondary to an identifiable etiology. The presentation of several metabolic neuropathies occurs in early childhood, and often the symptoms relating to involvement of the brain and other organ systems overshadow the neuropathy. The peripheral nerves are involved in several lysosomal disorders, such as metachromatic leukodystrophy, Krabbe's disease, gangliosidosis, and peroxisomal disorders. The peripheral nerves are involved in certain organic acidurias and other central nervous system disorders. In addition, inherited neuropathies, although symptomatic later in life, can present early with progressive motor difficulties. Acquired neuropathies do occur and can present acutely or in a subacute or chronic fashion.

Acute Polyneuropathies in Childhood

GBS is the most common cause of polyneuropathy presenting acutely in children. The clinical course is more rapid in children than in adults, and the recovery of function is more rapid and complete than in adults. The recovery is good despite very advanced changes in electrodiagnostic studies. An acute spinal cord syndrome needs to be excluded in all cases who are paraplegic or quadriplegic. Rarely, tick paralysis may mimic this disorder, and the diagnosis of tick paralysis is established by finding the female tick in the child with its proboscis attached to the skin, and by documenting rapid recovery of strength after the tick has been removed.

Management of GBS is similar to managing adults with this condition. Intravenous immunoglobulin infusions are preferred over plasmapheresis due to the ease of administration. Intravenous immunoglobulin at 400 mg per kg is administered for 5 consecutive days. Some neurologists use 1 gram per kg of intravenous immunoglobulin for 2 consecutive days. The principles of monitoring pulmonary function and management of respiratory failure are similar to those in adults. Autonomic dysfunction is common, and children need to be monitored for rapid changes in cardiovascular function.

Acute porphyric attack can be precipitated in childhood in those who have hepatic porphyria. An acute polyneuropathy can occur, resulting in motor paralysis. Acute arsenic poisoning rarely occurs in children, and the diagnosis is established by measuring arsenic in the urine, hair, or nails. Mees' lines are rarely seen in children. Rarely, an acute axonal neuropathy occurs in children with critical illness, such as fulminant sepsis and respiratory failure.

Chronic Polyneuropathies in Childhood

The chronic polyneuropathies in children are underdiagnosed because of difficulty in obtaining a detailed examination of the peripheral nervous system. Loss of muscle bulk, weakness, and reflex abnormalities lead to suspicion of polyneuropathy. In the interpretation of electrophysiologic data, age-dependent changes in amplitude and conduction velocities need to be taken into consideration.

Involvement of the peripheral nervous system occurs with several inherited disorders of the nervous system in children. Demyelinating polyneuropathy is seen in metachromatic leukodystrophy, Krabbe's disease, adrenoleukodystrophy, and Cockayne's syndrome. Type I CMT disease can be detected in children by electrodiagnostic tests and rarely may be symptomatic, presenting with motor weakness and difficulty with motor activities.

Metachromatic leukodystrophy is an autosomal recessive disorder that usually presents in childhood. Although the manifestation of the central white matter dominates the clinical picture, involvement of peripheral nerves can be be seen as absence of distal tendon reflexes, and electrophysiologic data show evidence of a demyelinating sensorimotor polyneuropathy. Krabbe's disease presents in the first year of life, and often the encephalopathy and upper motor neuron dysfunction dominate the clinical picture. The disorder is inherited in an autosomal recessive fashion, and the diagnosis is established by measurement of galactocerebrosidase activity in leukocytes or fibroblasts. Adrenoleukodystrophy is an X-linked recessive disorder and presents in childhood. The changes from involvement of the central white matter dominate the clinical picture.

An axonal polyneuropathy is seen in neuraxonal dystrophy, giant axonal neuropathy, Rett syndrome, orotic aciduria, xeroderma pigmentosum, and Lowe's syndrome.

Acquired Polyneuropathies

These are rare and occur secondary to toxic or autoimmune injury and rarely secondary to nutritional disturbances. An axonal polyneuropathy results from exposure to drugs such as vincristine, cisplatin, taxol, nalidixic acid, nitrofurantoin, phenytoin, and a high dose of pyridoxine. Rarely, a slowly progressing axonal polyneuropathy is seen as a result of heavy metal intoxication, such as arsenic, antimony, or lead. An axonal polyneuropathy resulting from glue sniffing can be seen in adolescents.

An acquired chronic demyelinating polyneuropathy can rarely be seen in children. The diagnosis is established based on electrodiagnostic findings and is confirmed by finding evidence of repeated bouts of demyelination and remyelination in the nerve biopsy. The children with this disorder are treated with prednisone. Episodes of acute worsening are treated with intravenous immunoglobulin infusion or plasmapheresis. The long-term prognosis is better in children than in adults.

Mononeuropathies are rare in children. Trauma is the most common etiology. Children with chronic renal failure are prone to develop median nerve entrapments at the wrist. Multiple mononeuropathies are seen in some children with systemic vasculitic disorders, such as polyarteritis nodosa or Churg-Strauss syndrome. Brachial plexus injury involving the upper and middle trunk are seen as a result of birth injury in large newborns.

TREATMENT OF PAIN IN PERIPHERAL POLYNEUROPATHIES

A variety of painful and unpleasant positive sensory symptomatologies occurs in patients with polyneuropathies. These include paresthesias and unpleasant dysesthesias, such as burning and tingling, as well as sharp, lancinating and stabbing pains. Often, there is exaggeration of the response to otherwise innocuous stimuli in patients with peripheral nerve lesions. In a typical patient with polyneuropathy, such symptoms are most troublesome in the distal lower extremities. Other features include the interpretation of a nonpainful stimulus as being painful and the perception of a normally noxious stimulus as being more painful than it should be.

In general, we treat the pain associated with peripheral polyneuropathy only if it is incapacitating. The specific treatment for the polyneuropathy involved will usually eventually relieve the pain as well. In patients who require it, pharmacotherapy may be tried with the full understanding that some degree of trial and error is involved in finding the right agent. For sharp, burning, diffuse pain, we use tricyclic antidepressants, starting with amitriptyline, doxepin, or trazodone. The dosage employed varies from 75 to 150 mg per day. If there is a significant lancinating component to the pain, an anticonvulsant such as carbamazepine may be the drug of first choice; alternatively, diphenylhydantoin may be used. The carbamazepine (Tegretol) dose ranges up to 800 mg per day, and the phenytoin (Dilantin) dose ranges up to 300 to 400 mg per day. It should be pointed out that in elderly patients with peripheral polyneuropathies, the added central nervous system balance difficulties created by these anticonvulsants may be particularly troublesome. Topical capsaicin (Zostrix) used as a cream containing 0.025% or 0.075% of the active agent is being reported to be effective in the treatment of painful dyesthesias. Finally, in an occasional patient, we have found temporary use of a transcutaneous electrical nerve stimulator to be useful in controlling pain without the side effects noted with pharmacotherapy.

REHABILITATION IN PATIENTS WITH PERIPHERAL POLYNEUROPATHIES

Patients with significant neurologic deficits related to peripheral polyneuropathies can receive considerable benefit from a good physical medicine and rehabilitation consultation. Physical and occupational therapists can advise patients regarding exercising muscles that are still functional for optimal performance stretching, and other methods for keeping physically fit. Patients can be equipped with the right type of rehabilitative devices such as ankle-foot orthoses, canes, and walkers with the help of physical therapists. In more severely disabled patients, a variety of other devices may be helpful, such as raised toilet seats, shower benches, deltoid assists, and modifications in the home and at the work place that can be suggested by specialists in physical medicine and rehabilitation.

ACUTE HEAD INJURIES IN ADULTS

method of
J. PAUL MUIZELAAR, M.D., PH.D.
Medical College of Virginia
Richmond, Virginia

Head injuries pose a major health problem in industrialized countries, both because of premature death and disability, as well as sheer numbers. Trauma is the leading cause of death in the male population between 4 and 30 years of age, and many die primarily because of brain injury. It is estimated that 500,000 new cases of head or brain injury with loss of consciousness and post-traumatic amnesia occur each year in the United States, and many more patients seek medical attention for more trivial injuries. There is a wide range in severity of traumatic brain injury, but this is commonly reduced into four categories: trivial, mild, moderate, and severe. Each requires its own clinical and radiologic assessment and its own treatment (Table 1).

TREATMENT

Trivial Injuries

Although the definition of trivial injuries includes radiologic criteria (i.e., absence of skull fracture or intracranial contusion or hematoma), it is generally not necessary to obtain skull roentgenograms or a cerebral computed tomography (CT) scan in these patients. Patients in whom it is justified to obtain skull roentgenograms are those with extensive hematomas or contusions, or both, of the forehead or scalp, and those with orbital or retromastoid hematomas. These patients should not be left unobserved the first 6 hours after their injury; after that period, they will not have to be awakened for checking. These patients can return to work immediately, and follow-up is scheduled on an as-needed basis only. If a patient later returns complaining of headache, one needs to distinguish between tension headaches and vasomotor headaches. After trivial head injuries, tension headaches are more common, and they can best be treated with diazepam (Valium),* 2 mg three times a day for 5 days. Vascular headaches, which are often accompanied by complaints of orthostatic dizziness, photophobia, and difficulty in concentrating, are eminently amenable to treatment with a combination of phenobarbital,* 40 mg; ergotamine tartrate, 0.6 mg; and belladonna alkaloids, 0.2 mg (Bellergal-S), two tablets twice daily. Chronic subdural hematomas may occur after trivial head injuries and may remain without neurologic symptoms for a long time. They usually occur only in the elderly, in alcoholics, or in patients using coumadin derivatives; therefore, later CT scans need to be obtained if the patient is in one of these risk groups. If a chronic subdural hematoma has developed, it is best treated by drainage through multiple burr holes made under local anesthesia, with extensive flushing of the hematoma with warm normal saline solution.

*Not FDA approved for this indication.

TABLE 1. **Categories of Head Injury Severity**

Trivial	No loss of consciousness or post-traumatic amnesia; no skull fracture, cerebral contusion, or intracranial hematoma
Mild	Loss of consciousness and/or post-traumatic amnesia with a combined duration of less than 30 min; no skull fracture, cerebral contusion, or intracranial hematoma
Moderate	Loss of consciousness or post-traumatic amnesia, or both, for 30 min to 24 h; or skull fracture; no intracranial contusion or hematoma
Severe	Loss of consciousness or post-traumatic amnesia, or both, for more than 24 h; or cerebral contusion, laceration, or intracranial hematoma

Scalp lacerations can be flushed with povidone-iodine (Betadine) solution, cleaned, and closed in one layer with interrupted 3–0 silk sutures. Cutting the ends fairly long will facilitate stitch removal later. The patient can shower his or her head 2 days later, and stitches can be removed on the fifth day.

Mild Injuries

For all patients with a mild head injury, a series of skull roentgenograms should be obtained. If these are normal, no CT scan needs to be obtained unless the patient is in a high-risk group for intracranial bleeding. The patient should be observed in the emergency room until 3 to 6 hours after injury and then can be sent home. Reliable relatives or friends should be instructed to ascertain every 1 to 2 hours that the patient is fully oriented for the first 24 hours, waking the patient up as necessary. If no reliable person is available to carry out this order, or in case of alcohol intoxication, it is often necessary to admit the patient to the hospital overnight.

Further management is similar to that outlined under the section on trivial injuries. With loss of consciousness, however, vascular headaches are more common than tension headaches. The patient may have complaints that give the impression of being neurasthenic; however, on neuropsychological testing, considerable deficits are sometimes found months after the injury. This may have important legal consequences, and the physician should be alert to these sequelae.

Moderate Injuries

If the patient is in this category solely because of a skull fracture, a CT scan should be obtained. The patient with a normal scan is admitted or transferred to a hospital with capacities for neurosurgery, and hourly checks of pupillary status and consciousness are carried out. Moreover, at this time an intravenous line is inserted in order to have immediate access for emergent administration of 500 mL 20% mannitol solution, in case of rapid deterioration. With a strong suspicion of epidural hematoma (skull fracture with ipsilateral unresponsive pupil and lucid interval), any surgeon can perform a temporal craniectomy,

*Not FDA approved for this indication.

with chisel and hammer if necessary. Remember, irreparable brain damage may occur in 10 to 15 minutes, whereas even large skull deficits can easily be dealt with later, with most satisfactory cosmetic results.

If a patient in this category has prolonged unconsciousness, a CT scan is obtained, irrespective of whether the patient has regained consciousness or not at the time of being first seen. By definition of the category of moderate injuries, this CT scan is normal (except for possible skull fracture); otherwise, the patient will be in the severe category. Whether the patient needs to be intubated before the CT scan depends to some extent on the level of coma. Any patient not able to follow simple commands such as "stick out your tongue" or "hold up your thumb" is considered to be in coma (unless the cause is aphasia), the depth of which is further assessed with the Glasgow coma scale (GCS) (Table 2). In general, intubation and ventilation are necessary, as is insertion of an intra-arterial catheter and a Foley catheter. Ample intravenous fluids are administered; use of fluid restriction to prevent cerebral edema is probably detrimental. Assuming there are no other injuries necessitating blood transfusion or colloid solution administration, the patient is given 2 mL per kg per hour of glucose 2.5% half-normal saline for the first 24 hours. For sedation one can use 10 mg of morphine intravenously every 3 hours, as needed. In case of extreme restlessness or for diagnostic procedures, complete paralysis can easily be obtained by injection of 5 to 10 mg pancuronium bromide (Pavulon). After 24 hours, a decision is made as to which category the patient belongs: If the patient follows commands or is localizing briskly bilaterally, and with eye opening, then ventilatory support is quickly tapered and the patient is extubated. During this period, monitoring of intracranial pressure is not necessary; in patients with moderately severe injuries, intracranial pressure (ICP) problems seldom occur, and they develop usually only after 24 hours in patients in prolonged coma but with normal CT scans.

TABLE 2. **The Glasgow Coma Scale**

Verbal Response	
None	1
Incomprehensible sounds	2
Inappropriate words	3
Confused	4
Oriented	5
Eye Opening	
None	1
To pain	2
To speech	3
Spontaneously	4
Motor Response	
None	1
Abnormal extension	2
Abnormal flexion	3
Withdraws	4
Localizes	5
Obeys	6

Severe Injuries

The primary goal in the treatment of severe head injuries is the prevention of so-called secondary insults: inadequate cerebral perfusion, high ICP, cerebral distortion, seizures, or hypoventilation. In all these conditions, the brain—whole or in part—is inadequately supplied with oxygen. Prevention of secondary insults begins at the scene of the accident. By far, the most important issue here is to secure the airway and ventilation. In the 1970s in Paris, France, a switch was made to intubation of all comatose head-injured patients at the scene of the accident; the result was an immediate, dramatic reduction of mortality. Therefore, we favor intubation by the rescue squad personnel of patients with GCS of 7 or below (see Table 2). (Incidentally, the rescue squad personnel also should be able to use the GCS.) If intubation is not possible, an oropharyngeal airway should be used, and the patient should be force-ventilated with a face mask. Also, an intravenous line should be inserted, and ample fluid administration is in order. Whether any medication should be given by a rescue squad is controversial. Seizures may be treated by slow intravenous injection of 10 mg of diazepam (Valium). If the patient has a unilaterally wide pupil, 300 mL of mannitol 20% can be administered. Although it is possible that very early administration of corticosteroids is beneficial, we do not favor this until more definite data are available. The efficacy of other drugs, such as oxygen radical scavengers (polyethylene glycol superoxide dismutase,* Dismutec), and inhibitors of lipid peroxydation (mesylate camsylate,† Freedox), is under investigation in phase III trials, and results will be available by the end of 1994.

Stabilization and Diagnosis

Once in the emergency room, the comatose patient is first intubated (if this has not yet been done). At the same time, an intra-arterial catheter is placed for measuring blood pressure and blood gases. At least 50% of all patients with severe head injuries have multiple injuries, and the treatment of the hypoxia and/or shock which could develop is given priority over the brain injury. At the same time, a lateral cervical spine film is obtained; C7 must be visualized, because in 10% of these patients there is also a fracture or dislocation of the spine. A large-bore, multiple-port intravenous access is secured. We prefer a jugular catheter, but a subclavian line is satisfactory. Once ventilation and blood pressure are adequate, the GCS is determined, and pupil width and responsiveness to light are assessed. Oculovestibular responses (ice water test and doll's eye signs) are tested in cases of more severe injuries if the corneal reflex is absent. A full CT scan is obtained, which obviates the need for obtaining emergency skull roentgenograms.

In case the patient needs to undergo emergency laparotomy or thoracotomy, it is wise to obtain a two-

*Not FDA approved for this indication.
†Investigational drug in the United States.

cut cerebral CT scan. If there is a surgical lesion, this can be dealt with simultaneously with the other operation. If there is no intracranial surgical lesion, an intracranial pressure monitor (ventricular catheter, subarachnoid screw, or intraparenchymal pressure device [Camino]) can be employed for intraoperative ICP monitoring.

Surgery

Our indication for surgery is the removal of all hematomas that cause a shift greater than 5 mm of the midline structures. It should be performed as early as possible, not only for epidural hematomas, but also for subdural hematomas. It has been shown that the prognosis is much better in cases in which subdural hematomas are removed within 4 hours after injury than in cases in which this could not be accomplished within this period. Intracerebral hematomas are also evacuated. The indication for removal of contusions is less firm. We tend not to remove these lesions unless ICP cannot be controlled under 20 mmHg with medical measures. Before acute surgery and often even before CT scanning, in cases of suspicion of a surgical lesion, the patient is given 500 mL of mannitol 20% intravenously.

Medical Therapy

The main purpose of the medical treatment of the severely head-injured patient is to keep the brain well oxygenated. The simplest way to monitor this is by continuously measuring the oxygen saturation of venous blood in the jugular bulb with a fiberoptic catheter. The catheters used are similar to the ones used for umbilical venous monitoring in neonates (Oxymetrics, Abbott) and are inserted into the jugular vein in the middle of the neck, and then retrogradely positioned in the jugular bulb (confirmation with roentgenograms is necessary). The aim is to keep saturation above 50%; if it falls below this level, this means that parts of the brain apparently cannot extract enough oxygen to maintain oxidative metabolism. The correlation between poor outcome and the occurrence of a jugular bulb desaturation lasting longer than 15 minutes is very strong, and becomes even stronger in case of repeated episodes of desaturation. Thus, when a desaturation occurs, the instrument is calibrated first (sufficient light intensity), and if it is found to be in order, the cause of the desaturation is determined as follows: high ICP, low blood pressure, too vigorous hyperventilation, low arterial oxygenation, anemia, or seizures (of course, some of these causes may have already been noticed earlier from other types of monitoring).

Cerebral Perfusion Management

We aim to maintain cerebral perfusion pressure (mean arterial blood pressure minus ICP) above 70 mmHg, first by keeping ICP below 20 mmHg, and secondly by keeping mean arterial blood pressure above 90 or more if ICP cannot be controlled sufficiently. Mean arterial blood pressure is maintained by adequate fluid administration: normal saline (plus potassium and magnesium added as needed) 1.5 mL per kg per hour plus a colloid 500 to 1000 mL per day. For administration for more than 24 to 48 hours, 10% plasma protein fraction (human albumin or plasmanate) is the colloid of choice. If mean arterial blood pressure needs to be raised in order to maintain cerebral perfusion pressure above 70 mmHg, we prefer to use phenylephrine (Neo-Synephrine) 80 mg in 500 mL of normal saline, but dopamine (Dopastat), epinephrine, or dobutamine (Dobutrex) also appear to be efficacious.

Intracranial Pressure Monitoring and Management

ICP should be monitored in almost all patients with abnormal admission CT scans and in those patients with normal CT scans whose GCS remains 7 or below after 24 hours. We prefer to use a catheter monitor with the transducer in the tip (Camino monitor) so that if intraventricular placement turns out to be impossible, one can still obtain reliable intraparenchymal readings.

A clear relationship has been established between outcome and percentage of time with ICP above 20 mmHg, thus we try our hardest to keep ICP below that value. We use a stepwise treatment plan (Table 3) to accomplish this. First, we use sedation with morphine, 10 mg intravenous push. Obviously the patient would be on a respirator, so there is no fear of respiratory depression.

Next, we try to determine which position of the head results in the greatest cerebral perfusion pressure: In most cases, this is with the head 20 to 30 degrees upward, but occasionally raising the head above the heart leads to a virtual blood pressure drop at the level of the brain, leading to compensatory vasodilation and then increased ICP. Therefore, the best possible position needs to be re-assessed time and again, even in the same patient, and in case one has a jugular bulb oxygen saturation monitor in place, the head position resulting in the highest saturation can be maintained.

Ventricular drainage can be used either intermittently (open stopcock only when ICP is above 20 mmHg, drain a few drops, and close again) or continuously (drainage level 20 mmHg or 32 cm above level of ear); either has some theoretical advantages over the other, but in practice, they appear to be equally effective.

In the past, it was often advocated to use sedation

TABLE 3. **Consecutive Steps to Keep Intracranial Pressure Below 20 mmHg**

Sedation: Morphine, 10 mg IV
Head inclination between +30° and −20°
Ventricular drainage
Paralysis
Mannitol 20%, 0.25–1 gm per kg IV
Hyperventilation
Artificial coma with etomidate (Amidate), 0.5–1 mg per kg IV push, followed by 0.25–1 mg per kg per h maintenance dose

and paralysis as the first steps for ICP control. The reason to use paralysis only after ventricular drainage has failed to control ICP is because it has been shown that paralysis leads to an increased incidence of pulmonary infections and sepsis.

Osmotic agents, such as mannitol, are often effective both in decreasing ICP and in increasing cerebral blood flow independently from one another, so that jugular venous oxygen saturation will be improved either way. Because of the rebound effect, one should probably use these agents as little as possible. One can administer mannitol 20% solution, 0.25 grams per kg (approximately 100 mL), repeatedly. The extra fluid excretion by the kidneys must be matched with extra fluid administration, but despite this measure, blood osmolality will increase. Once osmolality has reached 320 milliosmoles, mannitol cannot be used until osmolality has decreased again; otherwise, irreversible renal failure may ensue. In patients on kidney dialysis, a 30% sorbitol solution can be used, as this is entirely metabolized by the liver and not excreted by the kidneys, as are the other hyperosmolar agents. Parenthetically, the effectiveness of sorbitol in anuric patients proves that most of the effect of the other hyperosmolar agents is not via dehydration of the patient and bolsters the case for fluid replacement with the use of those agents.

Hyperventilation is usually very effective in lowering ICP, but it is low on our list, nevertheless. *Preventive* hyperventilation has been shown to adversely affect outcome, *prolonged* hyperventilation (more than 20 hours) becomes counterproductive, and *short, deep* hyperventilation can lead to dangerously low levels of cerebral blood flow. Such ischemia would be revealed by a further decrease in jugular oxygen saturation, and therefore hyperventilation should ideally be used only when jugular bulb monitoring is employed.

Artificial coma is the last resort and is only very occasionally associated with a favorable outcome. Because barbiturates tend to decrease the blood pressure, even when cerebral venous pressure or pulmonary artery wedge pressure is normal (or high), we now use etomidate (Amidate)* to induce such coma. To induce and maintain a totally isoelectric electrocardiogram, one usually needs 0.25 to 1 gram per kg push and 0.25 to 1 gram per kg per hour maintenance intravenously. Because the prolonged use of etomidate can lead to adrenocortical insufficiency, steroid supplementation is administered after 48 hours of etomidate use and is tapered once the etomidate is discontinued. Adrenocortical function tests should then determine whether or not further steroid supplementation is necessary.

Nursing

With several recent papers indicating that induced moderate hypothermia (to 32° to 33° C [89.6° to 91.4° F]) might improve outcome after severe head injury, we believe that until this is proved at least any fever should be avoided, and with the usual medications (acetaminophen) and nursing measures (cooling blankets) we try to maintain rectal temperature at 36° to 37° C (96.8° to 98.6° F). The most common secondary complications in comatose head-injured patients are pulmonary problems (atelectasis, pneumonia, infiltrates) and infection. Pulmonary care should consist of frequent suctioning, chest percussion, and postural drainage. In this respect, we have found the Rotorest kinetic beds to be a helpful adjunct.

We are not in favor of preventive administration of antibiotics. Frequent temperature measurements, daily white blood cell counts, and culturing of urine, sputum, and CSF (in case of a ventricular drain), however, should be performed to begin treatment as early as possible with the appropriate antibiotics in case of infection. It has been shown that early nutritional support by total parenteral nutrition rather than enteral feeding helps prevent infections as well as improves overall outcome. Therefore, total parental nutrition should be instituted by 48 hours after injury with amino acid and dextrose solutions, multivitamins, trace elements, and lipid emulsions.

Last but not least, close nursing observation of the patient is of paramount importance. The detection of early neurologic changes, such as pupillary size or reactions and changes in coma scale parameters and ICP levels, may allow the institution of treatment in time to avoid the permanent detrimental effect of these events.

*Not FDA approved for this indication.

ACUTE HEAD INJURIES IN CHILDREN

method of
BRUCE MATHERN, M.D., and
JOHN D. WARD, M.D.
Medical College of Virginia
Richmond, Virginia

Trauma is the leading cause of death in the pediatric population, and, among those who die, the majority have an associated head injury. Additionally, there are numerous minor, non–life-threatening pediatric head injuries that require evaluation and possible treatment. The purpose of this review is (1) to describe the initial evaluation and treatment of the severely head-injured child, (2) to give a scheme for the management of elevated intracranial pressure (ICP), and (3) to describe a method for the evaluation and treatment of minor head injury in children.

BASIC PRINCIPLES

There are several basic concepts or principles that aid in the understanding of the treatment of these children.

1. Primary versus secondary injury: At the time of injury, there are areas in the brain where anatomic and physiologic damage occurs that is beyond repair. These primary injuries include contusions and lacerations of brain tissue, hemorrhage, and neuronal injury. If the damage is of significant magnitude, it will be immediately fatal. Most patients survive the initial injury. There are areas of the

brain, however, that are not irreparably damaged, but are at high risk for injury due to secondary factors. These factors include hypoxia, ischemia, elevated ICP, infection, and seizures. It is these factors that most treatment protocols attempt to prevent or control.

2. Intracranial pressure and compensation mechanisms: The Monroe–Kellie Doctrine states that the cranium and its contents can be thought of as a closed space with a fixed volume and that brain tissue is noncompressible. If a mass lesion is added or brain swelling occurs, the system can initially compensate by decreasing the size of the vascular or cereberospinal compartments. Once this compensation is exhausted, small increases in the size of the mass will lead to significant increases in intracranial pressure. Clinically this idea is important for two reasons. First, all patients who are unconscious due to head injury should be considered in an uncompensated state of increased intracranial pressure until proved otherwise. Secondly, this concept shows the importance of serial neurologic examinations and how quickly deterioration can occur.

3. Age and outcome: As a general rule, excluding the very young, children have a better outcome from head injury than adults with similar injuries. It is for this reason that an aggressive approach is taken with children.

EVALUATION AND TREATMENT OF THE SEVERELY HEAD-INJURED CHILD

As in any trauma situation, management of the patient begins at the scene. This includes securing an adequate airway, appropriate fluid resuscitation and maintaining hemodynamic stability, stabilizing the spine, and identifying and treating immediate life-threatening injuries.

On admission to the emergency room, a detailed survey of the child is undertaken to look for occult injuries, such as fractures or lacerations. Then, the severity of the neurologic injury is determined. This is best performed with the use of the Glasgow coma score (GCS). If the child has a GCS of 8 or less, an aggressive multidisciplinary trauma evaluation is performed. The airway is assessed, and if it was not previously secured, the patient is intubated. All unconscious patients are intubated, even if they appear to be respirating well. Second, adequate intravenous access is obtained, preferably with central venous lines. Once intravenous access has been obtained, a full set of blood tests should be taken, including hematology, chemistry, coagulation, blood gas, drug screen, and urinalysis. Fluids are used as needed to maintain the blood pressure such that there is good tissue perfusion. There is no place for fluid restriction. This will be different for each age group. Concurrent with the placement of intravenous lines, lateral cervical spine, chest, and pelvic roentgenograms are performed. The cervical spine film should provide a view down to and include the C7–T1 junction.

At this point, an abbreviated neurologic examination should be performed consisting of (1) GCS after resuscitation (this may need to be modified in a child under 2 years of age), (2) pupillary function, and (3) motor function. The purpose of this examination is to determine the extent of injury and the presence of a focal lesion, and to provide a baseline for subsequent or previous examinations. If the initial examination is suspicious for a mass lesion (asymmetrical examination, dilated pupil or deterioration from previous examination), mannitol (1 gram per kg) is given rapidly intravenously and the patient is hyperventilated to a $PaCO_2$ of 35 ± 2 mmHg.

After stabilizing the patient, the next highest priority is the identification of intracranial mass lesions. The radiographic test of choice is computed tomography (CT) scanning because it is fast and readily available. CT scans are required in any child who (1) has a GCS score of 13 or less, (2) is lethargic, (3) has had a seizure, (4) has a focal neurologic deficit, and/or (5) has a deteriorating neurologic examination. Skull radiographs are not necessary and add little to the evaluation of a child with this level of injury.

If the child has a life-threatening injury requiring emergency surgery prior to CT scanning, a neurosurgeon should accompany the patient to the operating room. In the operating room, a ventriculostomy is placed to obtain ICP measurements and to perform an air ventriculogram to look for a shift indicating a mass lesion. If a mass lesion is found, concurrent surgery is performed to evacuate the lesion. If no mass lesion is found by ventriculography, the patient receives a CT scan as soon as possible after surgery.

Once the evaluation in the emergency room is complete, the child is admitted to a pediatric intensive care unit for continued interdisciplinary care. All children with a GCS score of 8 or less should have ICP monitoring. A ventriculostomy provides the advantage of reliable ICP measurement as well as the ability to treat elevated ICP by cerebrospinal fluid drainage. Occasionally, however, because of small ventricular size, it is necessary to place a fiberoptic ICP monitor into the brain tissue for ICP monitoring (even though this monitor does not provide for cerebrospinal fluid drainage). An arterial line and central line (if not inserted earlier) are placed for continuous hemodynamic monitoring.

The treatment of elevated ICP is done in a stair-step fashion (Table 1). This allows for graded levels of care depending on the severity of the ICP elevation. Level 1 is sedation and paralysis using morphine (2 to 4 mg intravenously per hour) and vecuronium (Norcuron) (2 to 10 mg intravenously per hour). Because the patient is paralyzed, CO_2 control is also part of level 1, and we maintain mild hyperventilation with $PaCO_2$ 35 ± 2 mmHg. Level 2 is the use of CSF drainage if the ICP is greater than 20 mmHg for 5 minutes. The ventriculostomy is set to drain to a pressure of 10 mmHg and is opened for 2 to 3 minutes, as prolonged drainage may result in ventriculostomy failure. Level 3 is the use of mannitol (0.5 to 1.0 gram per kg intravenous push) for ICP greater than 20 mmHg for 5 minutes and when CSF drainage fails to control the ICP. An attempt should be made to use the lowest dose of mannitol that controls ICP to prevent complications and keep serum osmolarity below 320. Each dose of mannitol is followed by a fluid bolus of 0.50 to 0.25 normal saline sufficient to maintain fluid and electrolyte balance.

TABLE 1. **Management Algorithm for Raised Intracranial Pressure**

Treatment Objective: To minimize time that ICP is above 20 mmHg while maintaining CPP above 70 mmHg

Level 1 Sedation, Paralysis, and Mild Hyperventilation
- If ICP is >20 mmHg for 5 min
  - Morphine 4 mg IV every hour or continuous infusion at 2–4 mg per h
  - Vecuronium 2–10 mg IV as a continuous infusion, titrate to maintain paralysis
  - Mild hyperventilation to maintain $PaCO_2$ of 35 ± 2 mmHg

Level 2 CSF Drainage
- If ICP is >20 mmHg for 5 min and does not respond to Level 1
  - Drain ventriculostomy for 2–3 min to an ICP of 10 mmHg

Level 3 Mannitol
- If ICP is >20 mmHg for 5 min and does not respond to Level 2
  - Give mannitol 0.5–1.0 gm per kg IV push
  - Continue mannitol therapy until serum osmolarity reaches 320 mOsm

Level 4 Hypothermia, Hypertension, and Hyperventilation
- If ICP is >25 mmHg for 5 min and does not respond to Level 3 or if CPP is ~50 mmHg
  - Begin controlled hypothermia to maintain a core temperature at 92°–94° F
  - Check daily surveillance cultures
  - Induce hypertension with phenylephrine to maintain SBP >180 mmHg in patients without parenchymal contusions or 160 mmHg in patients with contusions
  - Begin more aggressive hyperventilation to maintain $PaCO_2$ of 30 ± 2 mmHg

Level 5 Hypnotics
- If ICP is >25 mmHg for 5 min and does not respond to Level 4
  - Repeat CT scan
  - Give etomidate 40 mg IV push and start a continuous infusion at 40 mg per h; titrate dose to burst suppression by EEG
  - Monitor renal function; give stress-dose corticosteroids
  - If ICP does not respond to etomidate or if long-term (>2 days) hypnotic therapy is anticipated, start phenobarbital 2 gm IV over 1 h and give 200 mg per h to titrate serum level to 75–85 mg per dL

Definitions: ICP = intracranial pressure; CPP = cerebral perfusion pressure; CSF = cerebrospinal fluid; SBP = systolic blood pressure; EEG = electroencephalogram.

The main goal is to prevent a decrease in intervascular volume. Serum electrolytes and osmolarity are checked 30 to 60 minutes after each mannitol dose. Level 4 is reached when ICP is greater than 25 mmHg for more than 5 minutes and is unable to be controlled by mannitol or if cerebral perfusion pressure is less than 70 mmHg. The first intervention at this level is to control hypothermia to a core temperature of 33.3° to 34.4° C (92° to 94° F) to decrease metabolic demand. In cooled patients, we check daily surveillance cultures including blood, urine, sputum, and cerebrospinal fluid, as well as ordering a daily chest roentgenogram. If cerebral perfusion pressure is 70 mmHg or less, then hypertensive therapy is initiated. Phenylephrine as a continuous infusion is used to maintain cerebral perfusion pressure greater than 70 mmHg. The last intervention on level 4 is aggressive hyperventilation, maintaining a $PaCO_2$ of 30 ± 2 mmHg. Level 5 consists of the use of hypnotic medications to induce metabolic coma. Any child who reaches level 5 should have a repeat CT scan to detect mass lesions prior to being placed in pharmacologic coma. Etomidate (Amidate) (40 mg intravenously) is used as an initial agent because of its rapid onset of burst suppression and minimal hemodynamic effects. It does carry the risks of hyperosmolar renal failure and adrenal suppression with chronic use. Therefore, if long-term (2- to 3-day) hypnotic treatment is required, then phenobarbital is begun to maintain a serum level of 75 to 85 mg/dL. Great care should be taken to avoid hypotension associated with high-dose phenobarbital therapy, and aggressive pressor treatment is often required to maintain cerebral perfusion pressure. Once the ICP is under good control, the therapies are removed in reverse order; if there is a transient elevation of ICP, the last level removed is reinstated. When ICP has not required treatment for a 24-hour period, the ventriculostomy is removed.

Children with severe head injuries frequently require long-term intensive care unit admissions and should have multisystem intensive care unit management. Nutrition, either enteral or parenteral, should be started within 24 hours after injury. Aggressive pulmonary toilet should be performed to prevent pneumonia. Systemic infections should be detected and treated early with broad-spectrum antibiotics. Seizure prophylaxis is routinely used by giving phenytoin (Dilantin), 15 mg per kg loading dose and 5 mg per kg as maintenance, to maintain a serum level between 10 and 20 grams per dL. If there is any question of seizure activity, an electroencephalogram should be obtained. Routine CT scans should be performed on days 1, 3, and 5 after injury to detect any delayed intracranial pathology. CT scans should be obtained urgently whenever the patient has a deterioration in a previously stable neurologic examination or when ICP becomes difficult to control.

EVALUATION OF THE MILD AND MODERATELY HEAD-INJURED CHILD

A far more common problem is the evaluation of a child who has suffered from a minor blow to the head. The vast majority of these children recover completely with little intervention. The mild and moderately head-injured child can harbor significant intracranial pathology, however, with few signs on examination. Therefore, an aggressive approach should be taken with these children with the liberal use of CT scanning in the emergency department. Any child that has had a significant blow to the head and is not entirely neurologically normal should have a head CT scan.

If the head CT is normal and the child's examination returns to normal, it is reasonable to discharge the patient home with proper observation. If the head CT is normal and there are persistent neurologic findings, including decreased level of consciousness,

TABLE 2. **Criteria for Hospital Admission Following Head Injury**

Alteration of consciousness
Focal neurologic deficits
Post-traumatic seizures
Persistent vomiting
Severe headache
Memory deficit
Skull fracture
Circumstances of head injury cannot be obtained

the child should be admitted for observation. Any child with acute intracranial pathology (contusion, small subdural hematoma) not requiring surgery should be admitted to a pediatric intensive care unit for at least 24 hours of observation. It is also reasonable to admit a child with a linear or basilar skull fracture, who is otherwise normal, for 24 to 48 hours of observation. If signs of meningitis develop, the patient needs an aggressive work-up including lumbar puncture. When deciding whether a child should be admitted, several factors should be kept in mind: (1) If there is any question, err on the side of admission, (2) be sure that a responsible person will be home with the child if the patient is not admitted, (3) be sure that the responsible person has a clear idea of what to check for and when to return the patient to the hospital if problems develop, (4) ascertain that the child does not live so far away that help will not be available should the child's clinical condition change, and (5) be certain that there is no evidence of possible child abuse (Table 2).

As a rule, children have a better outcome after a head injury than an adult. This is only true, however, if appropriate aggressive diagnosis and treatment of this problem is provided. If handled properly, many children can have an excellent outcome from what initially appeared to be a devastating injury. It is incumbent on all those who treat children with head injury to be cognizant of what constitutes appropriate care.

BRAIN TUMORS

method of
LISA M. DeANGELIS, M.D.
Memorial Sloan-Kettering Cancer Center
Cornell University Medical College
New York, New York

The term brain tumor encompasses several neoplasms, including primary brain tumors such as gliomas, metastatic tumors, and tumors that arise within the cranial vault but do not originate from nervous system tissue, such as primary central nervous system lymphomas. As a group, brain tumors are a relatively uncommon neoplasm compared with lung, breast, or colon cancers. The incidence of primary brain tumors, however, has been steadily rising, particularly in the elderly population. In addition, there is evidence to suggest a rising incidence of metastatic brain tumors because patients with systemic cancer survive longer with advances in oncologic treatment. In adults the most common primary brain tumor that comes to clinical attention is glioma. Meningiomas may be more common in autopsy studies, but many are asymptomatic. In the United States, brain metastases are as common as all primary brain tumors combined and are twice as common as gliomas.

CLINICAL PRESENTATION

Parenchymal brain tumors of any type produce symptoms and signs that reflect the location and mass effect of the tumor. Headache is seen in at least half of patients. Symptoms of increased intracranial pressure with nausea and vomiting are less common but are seen early in tumors arising in the posterior fossa, such as medulloblastomas, or in those that obstruct the ventricular system, such as intravenous ventricular ependymomas. Personality change and somnolence are common and may develop insidiously. Lateralizing signs, including hemiparesis, aphasia, and visual field deficits, are also seen in more than half of patients. Seizures are a presenting symptom in 15 to 20% of patients with gliomas or metastatic tumors, but are an uncommon feature of primary central nervous system lymphomas and are rarely seen with posterior fossa neoplasms. When these neurologic symptoms develop in a patient, neuroradiologic investigation is warranted, and the best initial test is a contrast enhanced magnetic resonance scan. If a magnetic resonance (MR) scan is unavailable, a computed tomography (CT) scan can be used but may miss posterior fossa masses or low-grade neoplasms.

BRAIN METASTASES

Brain metastases are found at autopsy in approximately 15% of patients with cancer. The majority of brain metastases are clinically symptomatic and diagnosed prior to death, but approximately 10 to 15% of all brain metastases are asymptomatic. The most common tumors that give rise to brain metastases are lung, breast, and melanoma. Certain neoplasms, such as melanoma and choriocarcinoma, have a predilection for metastasizing to the brain, and approximately 75% of patients with these tumors have brain metastases in autopsy series. Other tumors, such as prostate cancer or systemic lymphomas, rarely produce parenchymal brain lesions, although dural and leptomeningeal metastases, respectively, are seen fairly frequently. In both CT scan and autopsy studies, half of patients with brain metastases have a single lesion. An additional 20% have only two metastases and only 10% have greater than five lesions. This suggests that a significant proportion of patients may be candidates for local treatment of their metastatic disease.

On CT or MR scan, most brain metastases appear as ring-enhancing lesions surrounded by edema of the white matter. The amount of edema can be highly variable and contributes to the total mass effect of the metastasis; corticosteroids ameliorate neurologic symptoms often within 24 hours by reducing peritumoral edema. The lesions usually occur at the hemispheric gray-white matter junction; however, they may occur in any location within the brain. The diagnosis of brain metastasis is usually inferred in a patient with known systemic cancer who develops contrast-enhancing cerebral lesions. The diagnosis is correct in at least 90% of patients, but other processes may be indistinguishable radiographically. Brain abscess, primary brain tumors, and occasionally vascular disease can also occur in cancer patients and can be difficult to differentiate from metastatic tumors. In a prospective study of patients with single brain metastases, all of whom had a diagnostic biopsy, 11% had lesions other than metastatic brain tumors. Biopsy should be considered in those patients with unusual lesions or in those whose primary tumor rarely metastasizes to the brain, such as prostate cancer.

The mainstay of treatment for brain metastases is cranial radiotherapy (RT). In large series of patients with metastatic brain disease from a variety of primary tumors, the median survival is 4 to 6 months after a course of whole-brain radiation. Occasionally, patients may have prolonged survival, but only 10% survive for 1 year or longer. Most patients die from progressive systemic tumor while their cerebral disease is in remission or under control. A wide range of radiation doses and fractionation schedules have been studied for the treatment of brain metastases. All appear to have equal efficacy, and most patients receive 300 cGy whole-brain RT in 10 daily fractions for a total dose of 3000 cGy. This schedule is widely used because it combines effective palliation with a rapid schedule, which permits the patient to return home as soon as possible. More rapid administration of radiotherapy using very high daily fractions (>400 cGy per day) is associated with a higher incidence of acute radiation toxicity, manifested by headache, nausea, and vomiting. Rarely, these regimens may precipitate cerebral herniation in patients with elevated intracranial pressure from their brain metastases.

Alternatively, patients who may be expected to have prolonged survival, such as patients with no evidence of systemic cancer, should be treated with a more protracted RT regimen, using daily fractions of approximately 200 cGy. The lower daily fractionation scheme reduces the risk of late toxic effects, particularly dementia, in patients who are likely to have a good response to treatment. Focused irradiation using stereotactic radiosurgery or brachytherapy may be used for patients with one or possibly two lesions. These techniques offer the benefit of highly localized RT and are more appropriate for the treatment of recurrent focal disease. They can safely be administered after whole-brain RT. They cannot be used to treat any areas of microscopic disease not detected by CT and MR scan, which is the rationale for whole-brain radiation in patients with metastatic brain tumors.

Surgery is reserved for the few patients who require diagnostic confirmation of metastatic disease and for those with single surgically accessible lesions. Two randomized prospective studies comparing whole-brain RT with resection followed by RT have now established the therapeutic role of extirpation in the treatment of single brain metastases. Patients had significantly longer survival (10 months vs. 4 to 6 months), improved neurologic function throughout their survival, and approximately 30% survived for at least 1 year. Patients with uncontrolled widely disseminated systemic disease did not fare better when surgery was added to RT. Therefore, surgical resection should be considered in any patient with a single brain metastasis seen on MR scan who has no or limited evidence of active systemic cancer.

Chemotherapy is not routinely administered to patients for brain metastases. It has no role as adjuvant therapy after cranial irradiation or following surgical resection for most patients. It is not used routinely because most patients with brain metastases have primary malignancies that are not usually chemosensitive, such as lung cancer. There are some patients, however, with particular neoplasms whose brain metastases may respond to systemic chemotherapy. Brain metastases from small cell lung cancer, germ cell tumors, and breast cancer may all respond to chemotherapy tailored to the primary tumor, for example, using standard doxorubicin-based regimens for breast cancer. For these primary tumors, chemotherapy may be used as the initial treatment, particularly when it will be administered anyway for treatment of systemic disease. In many cases, RT may be required after completion of chemotherapy.

Recurrent brain metastases are particularly difficult to treat. Recurrence after RT may be treated with a second course of RT, provided there was a reasonable response and remission was achieved after the first course. Stereotactic radiosurgery or interstitial brachytherapy may be considered for patients with a single or few sites of relapse. Surgery is also an appropriate consideration for focal recurrences. Chemotherapy may be used for recurrent brain metastases when further surgery or RT is no longer an option.

PRIMARY BRAIN TUMORS

Primary brain tumors encompass a wide range of different neoplasms, but the most common is glioma. In the United States, approximately 14,000 patients are diagnosed with gliomas each year. The glial tumors arise from astrocytes or oligodendrocytes. The astrocytic tumors are pathologically graded using a three-tiered system: astrocytoma, anaplastic astrocytoma, and glioblastoma multiforme. The oligodendrogliomas are divided into low-grade tumors and anaplastic oligodendrogliomas. Other grading systems have been used, but none have been found superior, and these straightforward systems have the greatest clinical utility. The pathologic grade of the tumor is an important prognostic factor that is inversely related to survival. Patients in a better clinical condition, younger patients, and those with little residual tumor following surgical resection also have longer survival.

Astrocytoma

Low-grade gliomas or astrocytomas usually occur in young adults. Typically, they are associated with a seizure in an otherwise neurologically normal patient. On CT and MR scans, a nonenhancing mass is evident, which may appear hypodense on CT or hyperintense on T2-weighted MR images. CT scan may miss the tumor, and MR imaging is essential for the accurate diagnosis of this tumor and to plan a surgical approach to the lesion. Most astrocytomas eventually undergo malignant transformation into high-grade gliomas, although this event may take several years. This is usually accompanied by clinical deterioration and the development of enhancement on CT and MR scans. These changes warrant a biopsy or resection for pathologic confirmation and to debulk the mass, if possible.

Complete surgical removal is the treatment of choice and may be curative, but is rarely possible. Partial resection can often be achieved, but even in patients in whom debulking is not possible, stereotactic biopsy can afford pathologic confirmation of the diagnosis. The timing of subsequent postoperative therapy, particularly RT, is controversial. Although retrospective data suggest that immediate radiation may afford longer survival, many of these lesions may lie quiescent for years without causing progressive neurologic problems. In addition, the morbidity associated with cranial irradiation, particularly memory impairment, may be significant in a disease associated with a median survival of 5 years. Therefore, we often defer cranial RT until the patient develops progressive neurologic dysfunction or tumor growth on MR scans. At present, a randomized prospective trial examining the value of high-dose versus moderate-dose early RT in low-grade gliomas is being conducted and will provide some information regarding the best therapeutic approach in the immediate postoperative period. Once a low-grade tumor becomes malignant, RT should be given if it was not already administered, and chemotherapy should be added to the regimen. Chemotherapy has no established adjuvant role in the treatment of astrocytomas. It may be used for recurrent low-grade astrocytoma after surgery and radiotherapy have already been administered.

Malignant Gliomas

The anaplastic astrocytoma and glioblastoma multiforme occur primarily in the sixth and seventh decades of life. Both usually appear as single contrast-enhancing masses on CT and MR scans. They typically involve the hemispheric white matter and may involve the corpus callosum, presenting as a bilateral lesion. In approximately 5% of patients, the disease is multifocal at diagnosis and may be confused with metastatic brain disease. These tumors incite edema formation in the surrounding white matter, and symptoms and signs may improve dramatically, often within 24 hours, with the administration of corticosteroids.

The treatment of both the anaplastic astrocytoma and the glioblastoma multiforme is identical. Surgery is the first step, and every effort should be made to obtain a complete resection, which can be safely accomplished in most patients with hemispheric lesions. Extirpation, as opposed to partial resection or biopsy, is associated with more accurate diagnosis in heterogeneous tumors, longer survival, improved neurologic function in the postoperative period, and fewer acute and subacute RT complications. Except for patients with bilateral or midline disease, most patients can safely undergo an extensive debulking procedure, which usually improves their neurologic condition and enables the subsequent medical therapy to be more effective.

Surgery is followed by involved-field RT to a total tumor dose of 5000 to 6000 cGy. Adjuvant chemotherapy, usually including a nitrosourea, is administered after radiation. There have been numerous clinical trials examining single and multiple chemotherapeutic agents, but none have proved superior to carmustine (BCNU) 200 mg per M^2 intravenously over 1 to 2 hours every 8 weeks to a cumulative dose of 1500 mg per M^2. The benefits of adjuvant chemotherapy are modest. The addition of chemotherapy to cranial irradiation does not improve the median survival of patients with malignant gliomas but does offer prolonged survival for a subgroup of 25% of these patients. Because this subgroup can not be identified at diagnosis, and nitrosoureas are well tolerated and do not require hospitalization for administration, we generally treat all patients with adjuvant chemotherapy. With this treatment, the median survival is 3 years for patients with an anaplastic astrocytoma and 1 year for those with a glioblastoma multiforme. Acutely, carmustine can cause nausea and vomiting, although this can be managed and usually eliminated with appropriate antiemetic agents, especially ondansetron (Zofran). Nitrosoureas cause cumulative myelosuppression, which may delay or limit subsequent courses of therapy. Pulmonary fibrosis can occur but is unusual in patients without underlying pulmonary disease.

New techniques using highly focused irradiation with stereotactic radiosurgery or brachytherapy are being employed with increasing frequency in the treatment of patients with malignant gliomas. Both techniques deliver high doses of radiation to a well-defined region, which is designed to deliver additional RT to the tumor bed while sparing the normal surrounding brain tissue. The role of these techniques remains to be defined. A randomized prospective study examining the efficacy of adding brachytherapy with temporary ^{125}I seed implants at initial diagnosis to external-beam RT and standard chemotherapy will be completed this year and should clarify this issue. Frequently, these techniques are used at relapse for tumors with defined margins not involving critical structures. On average, they increase survival about 10 months from the time of recurrence. Both techniques can cause focal radionecrosis, which may not appear for several months after therapy; the radionecrosis can mimic tumor recurrence both clinically and radiographically and, particularly after brachytherapy, may require surgical removal to improve survival, to improve the patient's neurologic function, and to reduce cerebral edema. In addition to the new focal RT techniques, a second surgical resection can also prolong survival an average of 6 months after recurrence. Other chemotherapeutic agents, such as procarbazine (Matulane),* high-dose tamoxifen (Nolvadex),* or intra-arterial cisplatin 3 (Platinol),* may also be beneficial.

Oligodendrogliomas

Low-grade oligodendrogliomas often have an identical clinical presentation to the astrocytoma; that is, seizures in an otherwise neurologically normal patient. Calcification that is often difficult to appreciate on MR imaging may be apparent on noncontrast CT scan. The tumor is best visualized, however, on MR scan, particularly the T2-weighted images, because the lesion is often nonenhancing. Therapy of low-grade lesions is identical to that for low-grade astrocytomas. Surgical resection should be performed, if possible. Patients who are neurologically normal may often be followed for years without requiring further treatment after subtotal resection or even biopsy for tissue diagnosis. Patients with progressive neurologic dysfunction or poorly controlled seizures usually require additional therapy. Focal radiation can be effective and improve local control, and is often considered first-line therapy. Recent evidence, however, suggests that chemotherapy using procarbazine, lomustine, and vincristine (Oncovin)* (PCV) may cause tumor regression, even without RT. Chemotherapy is an attractive alternative to RT since patients do not develop the memory and cognitive impairment associated with cranial irradiation.

Malignant oligodendrogliomas are treated in an identical fashion to malignant astrocytomas. Surgical removal followed by 6000 cGy focal RT and chemotherapy is the initial treatment in all patients. The specific effectiveness of PCV chemotherapy for oligodendroglial tumors was first demonstrated in patients with recurrent malignant oligodendrogliomas in whom the response rate was much higher than that typically seen in patients with anaplastic astrocytomas. Most investigators would include PCV as part of the initial treatment. Recurrence may be treated with repeat surgery, interstitial brachytherapy or stereotactic radiosurgery, chemotherapy, or a combination of these modalities, depending on the size and location of the recurrent tumor. If chemotherapy had not been administered initially, PCV would be the first choice; otherwise, an alternative consideration may be melphalan* or thiotepa,* although the patient may have limited bone marrow reserve to tolerate a prolonged therapeutic regimen. Some investigators are currently studying autologous bone marrow transplantation after high-dose chemotherapy for malignant oligodendrogliomas.

*Not FDA approved for this indication.

Meningiomas

Meningiomas are benign neoplasms that arise from the dural surface and produce neurologic symptoms by compressing the underlying brain tissue. They are slow-growing neoplasms and may be present for many years before producing neurologic symptoms. They can be found at autopsy in asymptomatic patients, and they are occasionally discovered when a CT or MR scan is performed for another purpose. Asymptomatic meningiomas do not necessarily require treatment, particularly in an elderly patient.

Meningiomas may be associated with seizures, progressive hemiparesis, personality change, and cranial nerve dysfunction, depending on the location of the tumor. The most common sites for meningiomas are the parasagittal region, the convexity, and the sphenoid bone; they may also occur in the spinal canal. When patients present with cerebral symptoms, a CT or MR scan is usually the first test obtained. On CT scan or T1-weighted pre-gadolinium MR images, meningiomas appear isodense or isointense to normal brain tissue. After contrast administration, diffuse and prominent enhancement is seen. There may be some edema of the underlying brain tissue, but this is usually modest. The tumors are frequently calcified, which is best appreciated on CT scan, and there may be hyperostosis of the underlying bone. The lesions are always adjacent to a dural surface, except for the rare intraventricular meningiomas, and usually the extra-axial nature of the tumor can be clearly identified, particularly on MR scan.

The definitive treatment for meningiomas is surgical resection. Complete removal is associated with a high cure rate, approximately 70% at 15 years, and incomplete removal is commonly associated with recurrent growth. The ability to achieve a complete resection is dependent on the location of the tumor, with convexity lesions having a high rate of complete removal (96%) and sphenoid lesions a low rate (only 28%). Radiation therapy is used only for the rare malignant meningioma and may be used in patients with multiple recurrences when a second resection is no longer an option. Multiple recurrences of a meningioma that is impossible to resect are a particularly difficult problem. Stereotactic radiosurgery is beneficial for some patients, but requires a fairly well-circumscribed tumor. Although 75% of meningiomas have progesterone receptors, in preliminary studies mifepristone (RU-486)* has had only a modest effect,

*Not available in the United States.

usually only maintaining stable disease. Chemotherapy has no role in the treatment of meningiomas.

Primary Central Nervous System Lymphoma

Primary central nervous system lymphoma (PCNSL) has been considered a rare disease, but its incidence has been steadily rising since the mid-1970s. Although it occurs frequently in patients with acquired immune deficiency syndrome or other types of immunosuppression, it also develops in apparently immunocompetent individuals, and it is in this population that the most dramatic epidemiologic change is being seen. The cause of this increased incidence is unknown.

PCNSL has a characteristic radiographic appearance. The lesion is frequently hyperdense on CT scan prior to contrast administration or hyperintense on pre-gadolinium T1-weighted MR images. After contrast, PCNSL has a dense and diffuse enhancement pattern without any central necrosis, which distinguishes PCNSL from either malignant gliomas or metastatic brain tumors. PCNSL may be multifocal in 20% to 45% of patients and typically occurs in periventricular regions. Lymphomatous involvement of the eye may accompany PCNSL in about 15% of patients, and leptomeningeal infiltration is present in virtually 100% at autopsy.

PCNSL is uniquely sensitive to corticosteroids. Corticosteroids are often given to patients immediately after intracranial mass lesions are demonstrated on CT and MR scans. In most situations, steroids decrease perilesional edema and improve the patient's neurologic condition (see later). Corticosteroids, however, function as a chemotherapeutic agent in PCNSL, causing the lesion to shrink and occasionally disappear completely. Marked reduction in the lesion can occur within days of beginning steroids or may evolve over weeks. Once tumor regression has occurred, the opportunity for histologic confirmation has been lost, and plans for definitive therapy are compromised. The diagnosis of PCNSL must be established pathologically, since other CNS processes, such as multiple sclerosis or sarcoidosis, can also appear as contrast-enhancing lesions, which regress with steroid administration.

Unlike other primary brain tumors, surgical extirpation has no therapeutic role in PCNSL. Diagnosis can be established by stereotactic biopsy, but resection does not improve survival and may produce significant neurologic deficits because the lesions involve deep structures. Definitive treatment should consist of chemotherapy and cranial irradiation. A number of Phase II studies have demonstrated the chemosensitivity of PCNSL and strongly suggest that adding chemotherapy to cranial irradiation is superior to RT alone. Most effective chemotherapeutic regimens include high-dose methotrexate* in combination with high-dose cytarabine* or coupled with blood-brain barrier disruption and procarbazine and

*Not FDA approved for this indication.

cyclophosphamide. Standard systemic lymphoma regimens have not proved effective, likely because those agents do not penetrate the blood-brain barrier.

SUPPORTIVE CARE

Most patients with brain tumors of any type require symptom management using anticonvulsants or corticosteroids independent of definitive treatment for their neoplasm. Corticosteroids are used in almost every patient with a central nervous system tumor. Apart from the consideration of a primary central nervous system lymphoma (see earlier discussion), most patients are begun on steroids immediately after a diagnosis of an intracranial mass lesion has been made on CT or MR scan. For patients with symptoms of increased intracranial pressure, such as headache, nausea, or vomiting, or for those with progressive lateralizing signs, institution of corticosteroids often produces dramatic clinical improvement within 24 hours. This improvement may be sustained for weeks, but symptoms will gradually reappear unless definitive therapy is instituted.

Dexamethasone* has been the corticosteroid of choice because it has little mineralocorticoid activity. The usual starting dose is 16 mg per day, but this can be adjusted according to the patient's needs. Higher doses may be necessary, particularly during the perioperative period after craniotomy or biopsy. More important, the lowest dose that controls symptoms should be used because chronic corticosteroid administration is associated with significant morbidity. After completion of surgery and RT or other definitive treatment, most patients with gliomas or brain metastases can be safely tapered off steroids. Patients with low-grade neoplasms may never need steroids, even if they receive cranial irradiation. In addition to reducing brain tumor symptoms, steroids can also ameliorate symptoms due to acute radiation toxicity, such as headache and nausea.

Common steroid-associated complications that develop in brain tumor patients include hyperglycemia, frequently requiring insulin; steroid myopathy; weight gain; insomnia; and hyperfragility of the skin. In addition, chronic steroid use can predispose to the development of *Pneumocystis carinii* pneumonia (PCP). Patients taking corticosteroids for longer than 2 to 3 weeks should receive concurrent prophylaxis with trimethoprim-sulfamethoxazole* for 3 consecutive days each week or monthly aerosolized pentamidine* for those with sulfa allergies. PCP prophylaxis should continue for 1 month after stopping corticosteroids.

Anticonvulsants are routinely administered to brain tumor patients who have had a seizure. Many physicians, however, give prophylactic anticonvulsants to all patients with a brain tumor. Although no prospective data are available, retrospective studies suggest that prophylactic anticonvulsants are not protective and are associated with additional toxicity. Also, compliance appears to be poor because most

*Not FDA spproved for this indication.

patients had subtherapeutic levels when tested. Consequently, we do not recommend prophylactic anticonvulsants for brain tumor patients, except possibly those with brain metastases from malignant melanoma, which are associated with an unusually high incidence (50%) of seizures because of their hemorrhagic nature.

Section 14

The Locomotor System

RHEUMATOID ARTHRITIS

method of
MARC D. COHEN, M.D.
Mayo Clinic Jacksonville
Jacksonville, Florida

Rheumatoid arthritis (RA) is a chronic systemic disease of unknown etiology characterized by inflammation, most commonly involving the synovium of the peripheral joints. The course of RA is variable, and the treatment must be commensurate with the aggressiveness of the disease. No curative treatment is available, but almost all patients benefit from a combined therapeutic program involving medical, rehabilitative, and sometimes surgical expertise. Patient education, suppression of inflammation in articular and extra-articular sites, preservation of joint function, and prevention of deformities are important features of any RA treatment plan.

DIAGNOSIS

In its earliest phases RA may be a difficult diagnosis to establish. Fatigue, malaise, and nonspecific musculoskeletal symptoms may be presenting features. Synovitis most often develops gradually, although an acute onset with a more explosive course can be seen. Symmetrical involvement of peripheral joints with a chronic disease pattern characterized by exacerbations and remissions is most typical. The American College of Rheumatology has defined criteria for the diagnosis of RA (Table 1). Although these are potentially helpful in establishing a diagnosis, failure to meet these criteria, particularly during the early phases of the disease, does not exclude the diagnosis.

MANAGEMENT

Once the diagnosis has been established, patient and family education is critical. Frank discussions between the physician and the patient are important to provide specific points of information, emotional support, and even vocational and sexual counseling. The benefits and risks of drug therapy, physical medicine modalities, and the importance of sufficient rest, good nutrition, and available community social services should also be taught. Many patients require continual help in coping with their disease. Medical management must be individualized. Certain medications are helpful in controlling the signs and symptoms of the disease without producing dramatic effects on the underlying disease progression, whereas others have potentially more effect on the disease and in certain patients may cause frank remission. Many patients require more than one medication to minimize inflammation and prevent structural damage.

Nonsteroidal Anti-Inflammatory Drugs (NSAIDs)

NSAIDs attempt to suppress inflammation through the inhibition of prostaglandin synthesis. Although these drugs are often effective, they are not considered truly disease-modifying and may not be sufficient if used alone for the treatment of RA. Responses to each drug tend to be idiosyncratic, so drug selection remains empirical. To evaluate a response, most NSAIDs should be given for 3 to 4 weeks at an adequate dosage. The list of commonly prescribed NSAIDs is summarized in Table 2.

Side effects from NSAIDs include dyspepsia and nausea, and gastritis, gastric ulceration, and frank gastrointestinal bleeding may occur. Some patients taking NSAIDs benefit from supplemental gastric protection medications; misoprostol is probably more protective than H_2 blockers or sucralfate (Carafate). Patients with pre-existing renal dysfunction, including those taking diuretics concurrently, have hypertension, or are taking other medications that reduce renal blood flow, may be at increased risk for NSAID-induced renal insufficiency. The development of a nephrotic syndrome or acute interstitial nephritis is less common. NSAIDs may also cause edema. Reversible elevations of liver transaminase levels can occur, and platelet dysfunction may also be expected. NSAIDs may aggravate asthma. Central nervous system reactions including headaches, dizziness, and confusion have been reported. Most of these reactions can be related to the antagonism of specific prostaglandin production and are generally reversible with discontinuation of the drug.

Salicylates remain effective in the treatment of RA because of their low cost and their analgesic and anti-inflammatory properties. Acetylsalicylic acid (aspirin) has anti-inflammatory effects in dosages ranging from 3 to 6 grams daily but has analgesic properties at lower doses. Blood levels of between 15 and 25 mg/dL are usually required to provide the anti-inflammatory effects, and maintenance of constant serum drug levels requires dosage intervals of between 4 and 6 hours. The dosage and schedule necessary to achieve therapeutic levels can be difficult to achieve, and measurement of serum salicylate levels are usually necessary to direct schedules and monitor compliance. Because of first-order kinetics, a small increase in dose may cause a large increase in the serum salicylate level.

Plain aspirin and the other NSAIDs should be taken with food or antacids to provide some gastric

TABLE 1. **1988 Revised ACR Criteria for Classification of Rheumatoid Arthritis (RA)***

Criteria	Definition
1. Morning stiffness	Morning stiffness in and around the joints lasting at least 1 hour before maximal improvement
2. Arthritis of three or more joint areas	At least three joint areas have simultaneously had soft tissue swelling or fluid (not bony overgrowth alone) observed by a physician. The 14 possible joint areas are (right or left) PIP, MCP, wrist, elbow, knee, ankle, and MTP joints
3. Arthritis of hand joints	At least one joint area swollen as above in wrist, MCP, or PIP joint
4. Symmetrical arthritis	Simultaneous involvement of the same joint areas (as in 2) on both sides of the body (bilateral involvement of PIP, MCP, or MTP joints is acceptable without absolute symmetry)
5. Rheumatoid nodules	Subcutaneous nodules over bony prominences or extensor surfaces, or in juxta-articular regions, observed by a physician
6. Serum rheumatoid factor	Demonstration of abnormal amounts of serum rheumatoid factor by any method that has been positive in less than 5% of normal control subjects
7. Radiographic changes	Radiographic changes typical of RA on posteroanterior hand and wrist radiographs, which must include erosions or unequivocal bony decalcification localized to or most marked adjacent to the involved joints (osteoarthritis changes alone do not qualify)

Abbreviations: PIP, proximal interphalangeal; MCP, metacarpophalangeal; MTP, metatarsophalangeal.
*For classification purposes, RA said to be present if at least four of the above seven criteria have been met. Criteria 1 through 4 must be present for at least 6 weeks. Patients with two clinical diagnoses are not excluded.

protection. Buffered aspirin tablets attempt to reduce gastric irritation and enteric-coated tablets may also be better tolerated, but serum salicylate levels should be monitored when these medications are used because of variable absorption. Nonacetylated salicylates may cause less gastrointestinal bleeding and less platelet function inhibition, but they are weaker anti-inflammatory agents and therefore may be less effective. Tinnitus and deafness can be early indications of salicylate toxicity in adults. Central nervous system symptoms such as headaches, vertigo, and irritability may also be found with high serum levels,

TABLE 2. **Nonsteroidal Anti-Inflammatory Drugs**

	Usual Dosage/Day for RA	Comments	Dosage Range (mg/day)
Nonsalicylates (Trade Name)			
Ibuprofen (Motrin, Rufen, Advil, Nuprin), 200, 400, 600, 800 mg	800 mg tid	—	1600–3200
Naproxen (Naprosyn), 250, 375, 500 mg	500 mg bid	—	500–1000
Indomethacin (Indocin SR), 25, 50, 75 mg,	75 mg bid	Headaches; dizziness	100–150
50-mg suppository; 25 mg per 5 mL oral suspension	50 mg tid		
Tolmetin (Tolectin), 200, 400 mg	400 mg tid	—	600–1800
Fenoprofen (Nalfon), 200, 300, 600 mg	600 mg qid	Renal failure	200–2400
Meclofenamate (Meclomen), 50, 100 mg	100 mg qid	Diarrhea	200–400
Piroxicam (Feldene), 10, 20 mg	20 mg qd	Long half-life	20
Sulindac (Clinoril), 150, 200 mg	200 mg bid	—	300–400
Ketoprofen (Orudis), 50, 75 mg	75 mg tid	—	150–300
Diclofenac (Voltaren), 50, 75 mg	75 mg bid	Hepatic toxicity	100–200
Flurbiprofen (Ansaid), 100 mg	100 mg tid	—	200–300
Etodolac (Lodine), 200, 300 mg	300 mg tid	—	900–1200
Nabumetone (Relafen), 500, 750 mg	1500 mg qd	—	1000–2000
Oxaprozin (Daypro), 600 mg	1200 mg qd	—	1200–1800
			Recommended Dosage (mg/day)
Salicylates (Trade Name)			
Acetylsalicylic acid (Aspirin)			3600 (900 qid)
Enteric-coated aspirin (Ecotrin)			3600 (900 qid)
Aspirin-dialminate (Bufferin)			3600 (900 qid)
Aspirin–magnesium aluminum hydroxide (Ascriptin)			3600 (900 qid)
Sustained-release aspirin (Bayer Timed-Release Aspirin)			3600 (1200 tid)
Matrix-formulation aspirin (ZORprin)			3200 (1600 bid)
Microencapsulated aspirin (Measurin, Easprin)			3900 (1950 bid)
Salicylates, Nonacetylated (Trade Name)			
Choline salicylate (Arthropan)			40 ml (10 mL qid)
Choline magnesium trisalicylate (Trilisate)			3000 mg (1500 bid)
Salicylsalicylic acid (Disalcid)			3000 mg (1000 tid)
Diflunisal (Dolobid)			1000 mg (500 bid)

particularly in elderly patients. True aspirin allergy is uncommon and usually results in a hypersensitivity reaction. Platelet adhesiveness and aggregation are inhibited by small amounts of aspirin and are irreversible for the life of platelet, generally approaching 10 days. This effect may be potentially important before and after surgical procedures.

NSAIDs differ in their potency, toxicity, and plasma half-lives. Cost, toleration, and compliance are important issues and should be considered for each patient. NSAIDs are rarely used in combination because of their potential side effects. They should also be avoided with concurrent anticoagulants. NSAIDs must be used sparingly, if at all, during pregnancy or nursing.

Corticosteroids

Corticosteroids are potent and very effective anti-inflammatory drugs. They often have beneficial effects on symptoms related to RA. They are generally thought not to alter the course of RA, and the potential benefit must be weighed against the potential toxicity in each patient. Small doses of corticosteroids may be used as an adjunct to other medications including NSAIDs and disease-modifying medications. Low-dose corticosteroids, less than 7.5 mg of prednisone or its equivalent, are often effective in treating sustained, debilitating synovitis, particularly synovitis involving many joints. The more aggressive disease with systemic symptoms such as fever, weight loss, vasculitis, or serositis may require higher doses that produce more toxicity. Toxicity from corticosteroids clearly is dependent on both dosage and duration of therapy. Even low-dose corticosteroids have toxic effects including cutaneous changes, osteoporosis, gastrointestinal side effects, and fluid retention. Moderate doses may be associated with these side effects as well as accelerated cataract formation, insomnia, psychosis, glucose intolerance, centripetal obesity, avascular necrosis of bone, increased risk of infection, aggravation of hypertension, muscle weakness, glaucoma, and hyperlipidemia. When these agents are used in patients with RA, small dosages must be used, and frequent attempts to lower the dosage should be made. Potentially life-threatening complications such as rheumatoid vasculitis, particularly if manifested by end-organ ischemia, may justify the use of higher doses of corticosteroids.

After 6 weeks of chronic use, corticosteroids must be tapered very gradually. Patients taking corticosteroids regularly need larger doses parenterally before, during, and after surgery. One acceptable regimen is to administer 100 mg of hydrocortisone sodium succinate or cortisone acetate intramuscularly immediately before the induction of anesthesia, an additional dose intravenously during surgery, and another dose intravenously on the first postoperative day. As an oral drug, prednisone is considered the standard corticosteroid. Five milligrams of prednisone is equivalent to 20 mg of hydrocortisone, 4 mg of methylprednisolone (Medrol), and 0.75 mg of dexamethasone (Decadron). To reduce any tendency toward steroid-induced osteoporosis, supplemental calcium, 1000 mg premenopausally and 1500 mg postmenopausally, is often recommended. The addition of estrogen, if practical, should also be considered. Supplemental vitamin D, 50,000 units once or twice per week, may also be helpful in some patients to prevent accelerated osteoporosis and to lower the risk of fracture.

Intra-articular corticosteroids may be effective in relieving swelling, synovial fluid accumulation, and inflammation in a specific joint. Aseptic technique should be used, and injection with 0.5 to 2 mL of a long-acting crystalline suspension of a corticosteroid such as triamcinolone hexacetonide (Aristospan), betamethasone (Celestone Soluspan), or prednisolone tebutate (Hydeltra-TBA Suspension) is popular. Relief of symptoms may vary and ranges from days to months. Frequent intra-articular injections, particularly more than three injections in a single joint per year, should probably be avoided because of possible acceleration of cartilage damage. A post-injection synovitis has been reported infrequently, presumably as a result of leukocyte phagocytosis of steroid crystals, but this usually subsides within 48 hours. Synovial fluid removed from affected joints should be analyzed particularly for the possibility of infection. Obviously, joints in which infection is suspected should not be injected with corticosteroids. Injection of corticosteroids may cause local skin and subcutaneous atrophy, and the procedure must be done carefully to ensure that the medication is placed in the joint space.

Disease-Modifying Drugs

These drugs attempt to control inflammation through interaction with the immune system. Controversy remains about how effective these medications are in inhibiting disease progression, but most rheumatologists believe that these drugs are essential in the treatment of aggressive RA, particularly because of their ability to preserve joint function and to improve overall prognosis. These drugs are being used earlier in the course of RA therapy. They have few local anti-inflammatory or analgesic effects, and anti-inflammatory drugs should be continued during their administration. Regular evaluation of response is imperative, and improvement is demonstrated by reductions in morning stiffness and palpable synovitis and improvement in hematologic evidence of disease activity. These drugs are all associated with considerable potential toxicity, and careful monitoring is mandatory. The potential benefits and toxicities of each of the available drugs are important in making the initial choice. (Some of the important features of these medications are summarized in Tables 3 and 4.) Fortunately, lack of response or development of toxicity to one drug does not preclude a beneficial response from another. No clinical or laboratory feature of RA predicts response to any of the potentially remittive agents.

TABLE 3. **Disease-Modifying Antirheumatic Drugs***

Medications	Dosage	Comments
Gold sodium thiomalate (Myochrysine)	50 mg/wk IM	Nitritoid reactions may be seen
Aurothioglucose (Solganal)	50 mg/wk IM	—
Auranofin (Ridaura)	3 mg bid PO	Used in early disease; may not be as effective as IM gold
Hydroxychloroquine (Plaquenil)	200–400 mg/day qd	Used in milder disease
Penicillamine (Cuprimine, Depen)	250–750 mg/day qd	—
Sulfasalazine (Azulfidine)	1000–1500 mg bid	Used in milder disease
Methotrexate (Rheumatrex)	7.5–20 mg/wk	Used first in more severe disease
Azathioprine (Imuran)	1.5–2.5 mg/kg/day PO qd	Effective in refractory rheumatoid arthritis
Cyclophosphamide (Cytoxan)	1–2 mg/kg/day PO 500–750 mg/m²/month IV	Usually used in rheumatoid vasculitis

*Complete drug information must be read before these medications are used.

Gold

Gold salts are effective in the treatment of RA and may limit the progression of bony erosions. Approximately two-thirds of patients with RA show some therapeutic benefit; however, many patients cannot tolerate the drug because of its potential toxicity. Parenteral gold salts (Solganal, Myochrysine) require intramuscular injection, and test doses of 10 mg are generally recommended. If the initial dose is tolerated, 50 mg is usually administered weekly. Response is usually not seen until a significant cumulative dose has been administered, usually greater than 500 mg and often more than 1000 mg. If a significant response occurs, the frequency of the 50-mg injections can be reduced slowly. If a relapse occurs, the preceding shorter dosage interval can be repeated, although re-initiation of the drug is not always successful. Patients who respond without adverse effects are often maintained for prolonged periods of time, often indefinitely, on monthly gold injections of 50 mg. If no improvement occurs after a cumulative dosage of more than 1000 mg, the drug is generally discontinued and considered a failure. Oral gold is also available but may not be as effective as parenteral gold. The initial dose of the oral medication is usually 3 mg twice daily. Serum gold levels do not correlate with drug efficacy.

Gold toxicity often occurs, and some adverse reactions are reported in a third to a half of all those who receive the drugs. Side effects that require discontinuation of medication are less common.

Dermatitis is the most common side effect of gold salts. The rash is highly variable but is often associated with pruritus. Dermatitis may also be associated with eosinophilia. Stomatitis may also occur and may be painless. These mucocutaneous side effects require withholding gold salts until the lesions clear, and occasionally therapy may then be carefully reinstituted at a lower dose.

Renal toxicity is usually manifested by proteinuria with nephritis; frank nephrosis is fortunately less common. If the proteinuria is mild, less than 500 to 1000 mg per 24 hours, gold may be cautiously continued. Proteinuria greater than 1 to 1.5 grams per 24 hours mandates cessation of the medication. The proteinuria is usually slowly reversible. Urinalyses must be obtained before each gold injection. Nephropathy is less common in patients treated with oral gold.

Hematologic disorders including thrombocytopenia, agranulocytosis, and aplastic anemia are the most potentially serious side effects of gold therapy but are fortunately rare. These effects are not dose related. These potential abnormalities require a complete blood count before each gold injection.

Nitritoid reactions of flushing, dizziness, shortness of breath, and even syncope have been reported with the administration of gold salts, particularly gold thiomalate (Myochrysine). Oral gold more commonly causes gastrointestinal side effects including diar-

TABLE 4. **Toxic Side Effects of Disease-Modifying Antirheumatic Drugs**

Toxic Effect	Azathioprine (50–150 mg/day)	Methotrexate (7.5–35 mg/week)	Cyclophosphamide (50–150 mg/day)
Marrow suppression	+ +	+	+ +
Nausea	+	+	+ +
Oral ulceration	+	+	+
Hair loss	+	+	+ +
Interstitial pneumonitis	+	+ +	+
Susceptibility to infection	+	+	+ + +
Azoospermia	0	0	+ +
Anovulation	0	0	+ +
Carcinogenicity	+	0	+ + +
Liver fibrosis	0	+ +	0

0 = none; + = mild; + + = moderate; + + + = marked.

rhea, abdominal pain, and nausea. Gold salts may also cause a variety of other adverse reactions including colitis, pulmonary infiltrates, and cholestatic jaundice. Patients with a severe toxic reaction such as exfoliative dermatitis, significant cytopenias, or severe nephropathy should not receive more gold, but patients with less severe toxicity may be able to tolerate lower doses of the drug.

Methotrexate

Methotrexate has been found to be efficacious in the treatment of RA. It is available as an oral or intramuscular medication. Initial dosage ranges from 7.5 to 15 mg per week. This medication works relatively quickly, and if no response has been observed after 12 to 16 weeks of therapy, the drug may be discontinued. If the patient does respond, the dosage should be tapered to the smallest effective maintenance dose. Methotrexate is administered weekly, usually in two or three divided doses separated by 8 to 12 hours because this schedule may reduce toxicity. Although usually well tolerated, methotrexate has many side effects including bone marrow suppression, hepatotoxicity, stomatitis, nausea, and pulmonary reactions. Regular monitoring of complete blood counts and liver function tests is mandatory, usually at 2- to 4-week intervals, particularly initially. Increases in liver transaminase concentrations may require cessation of the drug, particularly when they are three to four times normal, but transaminase elevations may not correlate with permanent liver damage. Prolonged use of methotrexate has been associated with hepatic fibrosis, but this is fortunately rare. The potential use of liver biopsy in monitoring patients on long-term methotrexate remains controversial, but early routine liver biopsy is usually not recommended. Other medications associated with liver toxicity including alcohol should probably be avoided. Supplemental use of folic acid (1 mg of folic acid daily) may reduce methotrexate toxicity. Medications affecting methotrexate metabolism or transport such as sulfa antibiotics should be used with great care, and other conditions associated with liver toxicity including diabetes and obesity warrant more careful use and perhaps lower doses of methotrexate. Pulmonary reactions of cough, dyspnea, and infiltrates may require discontinuation of the medication and treatment with corticosteroids.

Hydroxychloroquine

Hydroxychloroquine (Plaquenil) was developed as an antimalarial agent but has been found to be effective in some patients with RA. The drug is administered orally, generally at a dosage of 200 to 400 mg per day. This drug is slow acting, and months are generally required to show improvement. Six months is an adequate trial of this medication. Toxicity is perhaps less common than with gold, although hydroxychloroquine can be deposited in the eye. Early retinal lesions can be visualized before symptoms appear, and every patient must have an ophthalmologic examination at 6- to 9-month intervals, including visual field and color vision testing. The drug must be discontinued if there is any visual impairment or change in ophthalmologic test results. Other common side effects include gastrointestinal intolerance and skin rash. The drug should be avoided in patients with porphyria, glucose-6-phosphatase deficiency, or significant renal dysfunction. Other complications include neuropathy, hematologic alterations, dizziness, and psychological changes. In patients with extremely aggressive disease, this agent has been combined with other disease-modifying drugs such as methotrexate or gold.

Penicillamine

Penicillamine (Cuprimine, Depen) is another medication that is effective in patients with RA. It is a slow-acting oral drug and is generally begun in low dosages of 125 to 250 mg daily. Increases in dosage should not be made more frequently than every 2 to 3 months. Toxicity seems to increase with higher doses. Doses of 750 to 1000 mg are considered maximal. Responders generally demonstrate improvement within 6 months of initiation of therapy. Although toxicity is relatively common, patients who improve without toxicity can be maintained on this medication indefinitely.

Dermatitis is the most common side effect. The rash is highly variable and may appear soon after initiation of therapy; it often resolves with discontinuation of the drug. The rash may not recur if the drug is restarted. Rashes occurring after months of therapy may be slower to resolve and generally prohibit re-administration of the drug. Stomatitis is also not uncommon. Changes in taste perception often occur during the initial weeks of penicillamine therapy but tend to disappear even with continuation of the drug.

Proteinuria may also occur, and urinalyses should generally be performed at monthly intervals. With protein excretion of less than 1 gram in 24 hours, the drug can often be continued, but the dosage of penicillamine should not be increased if proteinuria exists. When proteinuria exceeds 2 grams per 24 hours, the drug should be discontinued. Renal toxicity may persist up to 1 year even after discontinuation of the drug.

Hematologic toxicity is the most serious side effect. Complete blood counts must be obtained monthly. Hematologic toxic effects include leukopenia, agranulocytosis, aplastic anemia, and, perhaps most commonly, thrombocytopenia. These reactions are usually reversible when the drug is discontinued.

Other toxicities include the development of other autoimmune syndromes such as myasthenia gravis, polymyositis, systemic lupus erythematosus, and Goodpasture's syndrome. These demand discontinuation of the drug. Other uncommon adverse reactions include cholestatic jaundice, yellowing or wrinkling of the skin, and gastrointestinal intolerance. An allergy to penicillin does not preclude the use of penicillamine.

Sulfasalazine

Sulfasalazine (Azulfidine) has more recently been recognized as being effective in the treatment of RA. Its onset of action is probably somewhat faster than that of gold or hydroxychloroquine. Doses of 500 to 1000 mg per day are usually used initially, the dosage then being increased to a total dose of 2 to 3 grams per day. Side effects include neutropenia, which requires monitoring of blood counts; intestinal symptoms such as nausea, anorexia, and dyspepsia; and central nervous system reactions such as headache, fever, and lightheadedness. Less common adverse effects include skin rash, abnormal liver function test results, and pulmonary infiltrates. Side effects with sulfasalazine are probably less common than those seen with other disease-modifying drugs for RA, and the most common side effects are probably dose-related so that slight reductions in dosage may allow continuation of the drug. Sulfasalazine may be particularly effective in patients with early RA and may also be used in the future as part of a combined medical therapy. The drug cannot be used in patients with sulfa allergy.

Azathioprine

Azathioprine (Imuran) in doses of between 1 and 2.5 mg per kg per day has been used to treat RA with some effectiveness. The initial dosage is usually 50 mg per day. Even in responders it is a slow-acting drug, and often 3 months are required for demonstration of efficacy. Side effects include bone marrow suppression and hepatic toxicity, and complete blood counts, liver function tests, and urinalyses should be performed probably biweekly. Leukopenia in particular may require reductions in dose. The risk of malignancy, particularly malignancy of the hematopoietic system, is increased in patients receiving immunosuppressive drugs like azathioprine. This drug is usually reserved for patients who have failed to respond to therapy with other potential remittive agents. Even if the disease has been controlled for several months, the lowest dose of this agent necessary to control the disease should be used. Chronic use of this medication will render the patient immunosuppressed and susceptible to common and uncommon infections.

Cyclophosphamide

Cyclophosphamide (Cytoxan) is another cytotoxic agent that is most often reserved for the most relentless or severe cases of RA. It may be the agent of choice for rheumatoid vasculitis. The dosage is 1 to 2 mg per kg per day orally. Leukopenia may limit the amount of drug that can be given. In addition to bone marrow suppression, an increased risk of malignancy, and renal or hepatic toxicity, cyclophosphamide has several other severe side effects including alopecia, sterility, hemorrhagic cystitis, and an increased incidence of bladder carcinoma. Obviously, although this medication is effective in controlling severe rheumatoid disease, it must be used with great care and must be very closely monitored. The use of larger doses, particularly intravenous doses given at less frequent intervals, has not been established as efficacious in patients with RA. The chronic dosage usually is adjusted to maintain a white blood cell count of close to 3000 per cubic millimeter. This represents a compromise between an adequate dose and a more serious predisposition to serious infection.

EXPERIMENTAL THERAPIES

Several experimental therapies are generally available at selected medical centers for patients who are unresponsive to more conventional medications. Monoclonal antibodies against T lymphocyte antigens and receptors, immunomodulary drugs directed against interleukins, and antibodies directed at integrins have been tried or have generated interest as being of potential benefit in RA. Other medications such as gamma interferon and cyclosporine (Sandimmune), have also been used with some success in some patients with RA. These agents should be used with great care because clear evidence of their usefulness and safety has not been established. Fish oil supplements have been used and may be helpful in providing anti-inflammatory effects. Studies have not demonstrated any advantage with diet or vitamin supplements beyond basic and balanced nutritional principles. Combinations of medications and modalities have not been completely studied, although further work in this regard is ongoing at selected centers.

PREGNANCY IN RHEUMATOID ARTHRITIS

Pregnancy tends to ameliorate some of the inflammatory symptoms of RA. None of the NSAIDs are particularly recommended for use during pregnancy or lactation. Gold salts, penicillamine, and hydroxychloroquine should probably be discontinued during pregnancy. Immunosuppressive agents must not be used during pregnancy. Even a simple drug such as aspirin, if taken until the time of delivery, has been reported to prolong gestation and labor and increase perinatal maternal bleeding in certain patients. Minimizing all medications is generally recommended.

SURGERY

Surgical procedures may be important in the management of patients with RA who have severely affected or damaged joints. Joint replacements can be performed for virtually any affected joints; however, hip and knee replacements are the most successful. Orthopedic surgery on rheumatoid joints requires special attention and expertise. For severe wrist and hand involvement, a combination of tendon repositioning and joint fusion may be necessary. Finger joint prostheses should be reserved for carefully selected patients. Synovectomy, particularly of the wrists or knees, might be helpful if involvement is limited to a small number of joints and traditional therapies have been ineffective. This procedure should probably be viewed as temporizing. Rupture of the extensor tendons, particularly of the fingers, generally requires surgical repair. Carpal tunnel syndrome that does not respond to local injection may require surgical release. Subluxation of the C1–2 vertebrae can cause cervical myelopathy or brain stem effects, and vigorous movements of the neck should be avoided in patients with severe rheumatoid arthritis. Subluxation fortunately rarely requires surgical fixation. Corrective surgical procedures should have specific goals, usually including pain relief, correction of deformity, and sometimes functional improvement. This latter goal is clearly the most difficult to achieve.

PHYSICAL AND OCCUPATIONAL THERAPY

Occupational and physical therapy techniques may be beneficial in the treatment of RA. Sufficient exercise to maintain joint mobility and periarticular muscle strength without causing pain or fatigue must be defined and then encouraged. Home programs can be developed. Splinting may be very helpful in resting individual joints and preventing deformities. Occupational therapists can provide information about making any necessary modifications in activities of daily living. Assistive devices may be extremely helpful, and instruction in the use of these products can be obtained. General cardiovascular conditioning programs, particularly for patients with less severe RA, often include swimming, cycling, or walking. Exercise programs specifically developed for patients with RA have been devised and may be available in some communities. A combined approach including the services of a physical therapist, occupational therapist, and even a psychosocial professional is often helpful in defining a regimen of regular, active exercise, the principles of joint protection, maintenance of muscle strength, the usefulness of various assistive devices, and avoidance of activities detrimental to the patient.

DISEASE ASSOCIATIONS

Several disease associations are important in patients with RA. Sicca syndrome requires topical and local treatment. Pain and swelling in the popliteal fossa and calf may represent a Baker's cyst, which often responds to an intra-articular steroid injection of the knee. Felty's syndrome is defined by RA, splenomegaly, and granulocytopenia, but other hematologic abnormalities, recurrent infections, and leg ulcerations are also common. These patients must be treated carefully, and rheumatologic expertise may be required. In patients with RA the development of rheumatoid vasculitis is a poor prognostic sign. There is a significant mortality rate, particularly if severe tissue necrosis, neuropathy, or severe constitutional features develop. Extremely aggressive therapy is warranted, and hospitalization is often required. The pulmonary manifestations of RA often require particular therapeutic interventions as well. Systemic symptoms such as fatigue generally correlate with disease activity, but the potential contribution of depression, medication toxicity, stress, and coexisting medical issues need to be analyzed.

RA is a chronic disease that can result in significant disability and pain and affect every aspect of the patient's life. The extent and aggressiveness of this disease are extremely variable. In each patient the disease must be correctly diagnosed and treatment initiated based on demonstrated manifestations of the disease. The initial therapeutic approach attempts to treat the patient's symptoms. If symptoms persist, if radiographic evidence of cartilage or bony destruction become manifest, or if extra-articular manifestations develop, potentially remittive medications are usually warranted. These medications require careful monitoring to gauge their potential benefits and toxicities, and patients must be fully informed and must interact with the physician about these therapeutic choices. This chronic disease requires chronic therapy, and even when remittive drugs are effective, antiinflammatory drugs, joint injections, and even surgical treatments are often necessary concurrently. When patients have persistent inflammatory disease despite attempts at remission or if severe extra-articular manifestations such as serositis, scleritis, and vasculitis occur, use of even more aggressive immunosuppressive or experimental approaches should be considered. Realistic therapeutic goals must be understood if a satisfactory outcome is to be reached.

JUVENILE RHEUMATOID ARTHRITIS

method of
CHARLES H. SPENCER, M.D.
La Rabida Children's Hospital and Research Center, University of Chicago
Chicago, Illinois

Juvenile rheumatoid arthritis (JRA) is chronic synovitis of childhood of unknown cause. The physician should diagnose JRA only if a child has the features of one of the three subtypes of JRA (systemic, polyarticular, pauciarticular) and does not have features of other diseases that may mimic JRA (e.g., psoriatic arthritis, systemic lupus erythematosis, Lyme disease, leukemia). The diagnosis of JRA rests less on laboratory tests and more on the presence of day-in, day-out swelling and limitation of motion in one or more joints for at least 6 weeks.

The treatment program should have several goals: (1) to stifle the symptoms and signs of JRA; (2) to suppress the joint or other problems sufficiently to allow the disease's natural tendency toward remission to express itself; (3) to prevent long-term joint damage and disability; and (4) to provide a family-centered, community-based team program that cares for the child's and family's needs.

BASIC PROGRAM

Once the diagnosis has been established, the rheumatologist and the primary physician consider the drug therapy alternatives and make the necessary referrals to team members and consultants (Table 1). Usually the physician starts the child initially on a nonsteroidal anti-inflammatory drug (NSAID) and discusses the risks of the disease versus the risks and benefits of the treatment with the child and his or her family. The physician monitors the child's progress every 1 to 3 months by means of outpatient visits. Children with severe disease may have to be seen more often. At each visit it is important to ask how long the morning stiffness lasts and whether new or continuing joint pains and swellings are a problem. Are there problems with activities of daily living (ADL), sleep, or school activities, or any drug side effects or compliance difficulties? The physician should also use global assessments of the child's status: Is the child better than, the same as, or worse than at the last visit? The physician and team members should ask about any recent weight loss or gain.

At each visit the physician should perform an especially thorough physical examination because rheumatic diseases and the drugs used to treat them may affect multiple organ systems. The emphasis should be on examination of the joints, muscles, skin, and eyes. At each visit the physician should note any changes in joint swelling, limitation, pain, or tenderness from previous visits. The physician should determine a joint count—i.e., the number of joints active at the time of that visit—and should follow this outcome measure from visit to visit. (Note: An active joint is a joint with swelling or a joint that is limited by pain, tenderness, or swelling.)

To follow disease activity and monitor the child for drug side effects, the physician should order certain laboratory tests regularly. For the child who is being treated with a NSAID, the physician should order a complete blood count (CBC), serum glutamic-oxaloacetic transaminase (SGOT), serum glutamate pyruvate transaminase (SGPT), and urinalysis every 3 to 4 months. Measurements of erythrocyte sedimentation rate (ESR) or quantitative C-reactive protein (CRP) should be performed every 1 to 3 months. To monitor the child for joint destruction, the physician should evaluate radiographs of selected joints obtained every 6 to 12 months.

To anticipate rather than react to clinical problems, the team should review each child's status every 6 to 12 months. This review should include recent complaints, global assessments, drug history, radiographs, joint counts, ESRs, progress in school work, physical and occupational therapists' evaluations, and opinions of other team members. The team completes the full team assessment, formulates new treatment plans, and shares this review with the child and family.

DRUG THERAPY

Nonsteroidal Anti-inflammatory Drugs

The current philosophy of drug therapy for children with JRA is to use the least amount of the mildest medication needed to suppress the disease and help the arthritis go into remission (Table 2). Unlike the chance for remission in adult rheumatoid arthritis, there is an excellent chance of permanent remission in JRA within 5 to 15 years of disease onset. Children who have pauciarticular JRA often take only two to three NSAIDs during the entire course of the disease, whereas children with polyarticular JRA may require multiple NSAIDs and several remittive drugs as well.

TABLE 1. **Members of Team Program for Juvenile Rheumatoid Arthritis**

Primary Team Members	Secondary Team Members
Primary physician	Ophthalmologist
Pediatric rheumatologist	Orthopedist
Nurse specialist	Dentist
Occupational therapist	Oral surgeon
Physical therapist	Orthodontist
Nutritionist	
Physiatrist	

TABLE 2. **Drug Therapy for JRA**

NSAIDs	Corticosteroids	Remittive
Naproxen	Oral prednisone	Hydroxychloroquine
Tolmetin	Intra-articular steroids	Sulfasalazine
Ibuprofen		Methotrexate
Aspirin	Methylprednisolone (intravenous)	Azathioprine
Indomethacin		Combination of two drugs
Nabumetone		Experimental drugs

The first-line drugs for mild arthritis are NSAIDs. There is no evidence that one NSAID is better than another. Each NSAID may cause significant gastrointestinal toxicity. Two NSAIDs are seldom taken together owing to their additive side effects. Aspirin used to be the NSAID of choice, but this is no longer true because of the risk of Reye's syndrome. Most pediatric rheumatologists in the United States use not aspirin but naproxen, tolmetin, or ibuprofen as their initial NSAID. Aspirin can be used in teenagers, particularly slow-release aspirin products (e.g., ZORprin).

Naproxen (Naprosyn) is an excellent first-line drug that is approved by the Food and Drug Administration (FDA). The dosage is 10 to 20 mg per kg per day in two divided doses. The drug should always be administered with food. Naprosyn suspension is useful for younger children (125 mg per 5 mL). The drug is available for older children in 250-mg, 375-mg, and 500-mg tablets and is now available in generic forms. The arthritis physician should monitor the patient closely for gastrointestinal toxicity. Naproxen may also cause a pseudoporphyria-like rash, particularly on the face.

Tolmetin (Tolectin) is also an excellent NSAID and has a dosing schedule of three or four times a day. The dose is 15 to 30 mg per kg per day. Tablets are available in 200-mg, 400-mg, and 600-mg doses. For young children, a parent may cut a tablet into pieces and mix the piece with an agreeable substance such as applesauce or with cheese.

Ibuprofen (Motrin, Advil, Rufen, Nuprin) also is an excellent NSAID and is noteworthy for its wide availability at reasonable prices in the generic form. This drug is available in liquid form (Liquid Advil, Pediaprofen). The dose is 20 to 40 mg per kg per day, three or four times a day.

Nabumetone (Relafen)* is a new NSAID for teenagers that appears to be as effective as other NSAIDs

*This drug has not been approved by the FDA for this indication in children under 14 years old.

and has fewer gastrointestinal side effects (500 mg twice a day). Indomethacin* (Indocin, 1 to 2 mg per kg per day) can control the fevers of systemic JRA and effectively treat spondyloarthropathy in teenagers. Children who take indomethacin should be monitored for headaches, gastrointestinal problems, and nephritis.

CRISIS INTERVENTIONS

Occasionally the child with arthritis experiences a significant flare-up of disease in which control of fever, joint pain, swelling, stiffness, or other problems is inadequate. The interventions mentioned in this section should stifle such flare-ups without causing significant side effects (Table 3).

Mild flare-ups can be treated by increasing the NSAID dose or switching to another NSAID. Indomethacin is often effective in treating children with systemic JRA who have high fever or pericarditis. The classic crisis drug for moderate to severe flare-ups is prednisone. Prednisone (1 to 2 mg per kg per day) can be used for flare-ups of systemic JRA (e.g., fever, polyarthritis, pericarditis) and is effective for a flare-up of severe arthritis in a child with polyarthritis (1 mg per kg per day in divided doses). The physician maintains this high dose for 2 to 4 weeks and then consolidates it into a single daily dose and slowly decreases the dose to a maintenance level. There may be a gradual onset of the drug effect of prednisone, and it may expose the child to significant steroid side effects. Another option is an oral "pulse" given for a moderate JRA flare. The prednisone dose of 0.5 to 1 mg per kg per day is taken for 4 to 7 days. The physician then tapers the steroids over a period of 1 to 2 weeks.

Intravenous methylprednisolone (Solu-Medrol) pulses are effective in treating severe flare-ups of JRA and can be administered in the hospital or at home. Three daily doses of methylprednisolone (30 mg per kg per dose to a maximum of 1 gram) often produce an impressive therapeutic effect within 24 hours of the first dose. This aggressive treatment can be effective in treating painful polyarthritis, high fevers, or pericarditis. This regimen often buys some time for fine tuning with oral medications (e.g., NSAIDs, remittive drugs) and may allow lower doses and lead to fewer potential side effects with these drugs. If a remittive drug is not already being used, the physician should consider prescribing one to provide better long-term control of disease.

Intra-articular injections of corticosteroids may decrease disease activity in one or several troublesome joints without producing the systemic effects of oral or intravenous medications. This treatment is particularly useful in the child with pauciarticular JRA who has knee arthritis with a flexion contracture of 20 to 30 degrees. Injection of a triamcinolone preparation (e.g., Aristospan) in combination with serial casting, a home physical therapy program, and regular physical therapy check-ups has an excellent chance of decreasing the disease activity and contracture of the joint. Unlike joint injection in adults, joint injection in children is a major undertaking that often requires intravenous sedation (e.g., midazolam [Versed 1 to 2 mg] and meperidine [Demerol, 0.5 to 1 mg per kg]) and careful monitoring. Care must be taken not to inject the steroid subcutaneously because skin atrophy can occur. Any one joint should not be injected more than twice a year. Despite these concerns, these joint injections are often worth the risks.

*This drug has not been approved by the FDA for this indication in children under 14 years old.

TABLE 3. **Crisis Intervention Drug Therapy for JRA**

NSAID—begin new drug or increase dose of current NSAID
Indomethacin—1–2 mg per kg per day
Oral prednisone—*full dose*, used over 1–2 months (1–2 mg per kg per day); *oral pulse*, low to moderate dose used over 1–2 weeks (0.5–1 mg per kg per day)
Intravenous methylprednisolone—one to three single daily doses given over 1–3 days (30 mg per kg per dose up to 1 gram); also weekly dose for 2–4 months in combination with remittive drug
Intra-articular corticosteroids—2–40 mg depending on joint size

REMITTIVE THERAPY

Fewer than 50% of children with JRA have uncontrolled arthritis while taking NSAIDs or do not tolerate these drugs. They may need aggressive remittive therapy (Table 2). Indications for remittive therapy for JRA include (1) poor clinical response to NSAIDs over at least 2 months or significant NSAID toxicity; (2) uncontrolled arthritis and systemic disease; (3) joint damage noted on radiographs or magnetic resonance imaging scans; and (4) prednisone dependence or toxicity.

Remittive drugs should not be used lightly. Each drug has significant potential benefits and toxicities. The team should exclude poor compliance and psychosocial problems as contributors to a child's difficult clinical course; if present, these problems should be addressed. The remittive drug is given in combination with the NSAID. The critical issue is the need to prevent joint damage. Physicians are rarely too aggressive but rather are often reluctant to use remittive drugs. It is not uncommon to evaluate a referred child who already has joint damage but has never received remittive therapy.

The child's response to the remittive drug is often partial—i.e., the child improves but continues to have active arthritis. However, it is likely that even a partial response will suppress the arthritis for 2 to 4 years. At that time, another remittive drug is likely to be available that may be effective for several more years, and so on, until the disease eventually burns out. The question at that point will be whether the child has damaged joints and functional loss.

If a child is not doing well on NSAIDs, it may be possible to use an intermediate remittive drug. Hydroxychloroquine (Plaquenil)* is a good anti-inflam-

*This drug has not been approved by the FDA for this indication.

matory drug with low toxicity for a child with mild to moderate arthritis. The initial dose is 6 to 7 mg per kg per day. The dose should be reduced to 5 mg per kg per day after 2 to 3 months. An ophthalmologist should examine the child every 4 to 6 months to evaluate color vision and peripheral field vision. Sulfasalazine (Azulfidine* [30 mg per kg per day]) is now gaining acceptance as an intermediate remittive drug comparable to hydroxychloroquine.

Oral methotrexate (Methotrexate, Rheumatrex)* is the best remittive drug for JRA. This drug can push JRA into a less active clinical state or even into remission. Methotrexate's most impressive effect on JRA is its ability to reverse radiographic joint damage. Its onset of action (2 to 4 weeks) is faster than that of gold shots (1 to 2 months), and it appears to be less toxic. Methotrexate is used in a weekly dosage schedule, the usual maximum dose being 10 mg per square meter of body surface per week.

The initial dose should be low (e.g., 2.5 mg). The physician should slowly increase the dose by 2.5 to 5.0 mg per month up to a maintenance dose while monitoring the child closely for side effects. A dose of over 20 mg per week is occasionally needed for a child with severe arthritis who has a partial response. If the child does not respond well to methotrexate, it is useful to check a 1-hour post-dose methotrexate level because some children do not have good gastrointestinal absorption of methotrexate. The drug level should be 0.6 to 0.8 mg/dL. If the methotrexate level is low, the dose may be increased or the route of administration changed to subcutaneous or intramuscular. If compliance is poor, a change to a methotrexate injection may help.

Potential problems with toxicity include hematologic (decreasing hemoglobin, white cell count, platelets), hepatic (increasing transaminase levels), gastrointestinal (nausea, abdominal pain), and pulmonary (nonspecific pneumonitis) abnormalities. In practice, these problems often occur at the onset of methotrexate therapy. Thus it is important to monitor side effects by checking the CBC, ESR, SGOT, and SGPT weekly for 8 weeks, every 2 weeks for 8 weeks, and then monthly until the child is off methotrexate. The team should keep track of the child's cumulative dose. The physician should also order a 24-hour post-dose methotrexate level, which may identify the child who retains an unhealthy high level of methotrexate.

The major toxic effect of methotrexate is liver damage. The drug may cause an acute chemical hepatitis. It is prudent to withhold the drug if the transaminase levels are greater than 200 international units per mL and restart it when the enzymes are less than 50 international units per mL. Methotrexate can occasionally cause chronic liver damage with potential fibrosis and cirrhosis. Judging from recent experience in the pediatric rheumatology community, this risk of chronic liver disease in these children may be much less than was originally feared. The physician should monitor the transaminase levels monthly and examine the liver for enlargement and the bumpy, knobby texture typical of a cirrhotic liver process. Once the total cumulative dose is greater than 2.5 grams, it is prudent to review the child's liver status and the indications for a liver biopsy with a gastroenterologist.

*This drug has not been approved by the FDA for this indication.

After the child with JRA has been on methotrexate for 1 to 2 years, the physician should start to consider how long to use the drug and what new remittive drug or drug combination to use next. Generally, the duration of methotrexate therapy is 2 to 4 years, depending on effectiveness, toxicity, and total dose. Children whose disease remits can be slowly tapered off the drug, whereas those with a partial response are often continued on the drug. The maximum duration of therapy is not known.

Gold given in weekly intramuscular injections (Myochrysine, Solganol) is the classic remittive agent for arthritis. A test dose of 2.5 to 5 mg is administered initially. The dose is increased in two steps to a dose of 1 mg per kg per week (maximum of 50 mg per dose). This dose of gold is administered weekly for a minimum of 20 weeks or more, gradually tapering off to monthly gold shots. Laboratory tests (CBC, ESR, urinalysis, blood chemistries) are performed before each injection to check for bone marrow suppression, nephritis, and other side effects. Addition of an equal volume of 1% lidocaine to the gold shot reduces the pain of the injection for the child.

Penicillamine (Cuprimine)* is an effective remittive drug but is currently out of favor owing to its significant side effects. Azathioprine (Imuran)* can be an effective alternative to methotrexate, but it has more potential long-term side effects. Weekly intravenous methylprednisolone* is currently being used as a remittive drug in several centers with some success, but it remains experimental.

Various combinations of remittive drugs may be tried if a child's disease is unrelenting despite use of single remittive drugs. The risk/benefit ratios of these combinations are not yet known. The combinations of methotrexate and hydroxychloroquine and of methotrexate and intravenous methylprednisolone both have been beneficial in selected cases. Azathioprine with intravenous methylprednisolone also suppresses severe JRA well. Low-dose cyclosporine* (Sandimmune), 3 to 5 mg per kg per day, may be the next remittive drug for JRA. At present, experience with this drug in the United States is limited, the renal toxicity is of concern, and its use remains experimental.

TEAM APPROACH

Care of the chronically ill child is best provided by a family-centered, community-based team of professionals (Table 1). The physician should consider team referrals early in the course of disease, e.g., to the nurse specialist. The nurse specialist is often the coordinator of the rheumatology program. She performs many important tasks such as screening phone calls,

*This drug has not been approved by the FDA for this indication.

following up on a child's laboratory and other needed appointments, organizing clinic visits, calling in prescriptions, educating the patient and family, performing play therapy with the patient, and organizing JRA parent activities. The nurse specialist is invaluable as the main team contact person who is usually more available to parents than is the physician. The nurse should watch for school difficulties such as decreased writing endurance due to painful fingers, tardiness to class due to difficulty in walking or climbing stairs, wrist pain while carrying books, and inability to keep up in physical education classes. If phone calls to the school do not solve the problem, the nurse often advises the parents to request an individual education plan (IEP) at school.

The occupational therapist (OT) evaluates and follows upper extremity range of motion, muscle strength, fine motor abilities, and ADL evaluations. The OT teaches the child and family a home exercise program and modifies it as necessary. Some of the problems that the OT may address include loss of wrist extension, swan neck and boutonniere finger deformities, splinting, and school problems due to upper extremity joint problems. The OT often fabricates night extension splints or ring finger splints to preserve range of motion and prevent deformities.

The physical therapist (PT) evaluates and monitors hip, knee, ankle, subtalar, and back joint involvement as well as muscle strength. The PT teaches the family and patient a home therapy program of daily exercises and evaluates the child's problems regularly on an outpatient basis. Substantial physical therapy involvement is often crucial with certain clinical problems, e.g., knee flexion contractures, severe hip disease, ankle and subtalar problems, back arthritis, gait patterns, and leg length discrepancies.

The social worker should get to know the child and family and discuss problems such as grieving, stress, denial, school adjustments, and other issues as they come up in clinic visits. The social worker can also help the team understand what a family might be going through at any particular time. The social worker can advise families about their eligibility for different state and federal programs and can provide counseling or an outside counseling referral. The value of an aggressive mental health professional in the clinic cannot be overemphasized.

Because children with JRA rarely complain of eye symptoms when iritis is beginning, the ophthalmologist must perform a slit lamp examination to monitor the child for iridocyclitis regularly every 4 to 6 months (see Academy of Pediatrics guidelines).* When mild iritis is present, the ophthalmologist often prescribes dilating eye drops (e.g., atropine) with or without steroid drops. For the occasional child with severe iritis, it may be necessary to consult a specialist in uveitis. This specialist may prescribe steroid injections, prednisone, cyclosporine, or immunosuppressive drugs. In the child with pauciarticular JRA, the eye problems may be a greater risk to the child's future than arthritis.

It is our hope that the child with JRA never has to see an orthopedist. Yet for some patients who develop severe JRA, the orthopedist can be very helpful in evaluating and treating severe hip or knee disease, soft tissue contractures, cervical spine arthritis, wrist arthritis, finger deformities, and severely damaged joints requiring joint replacements. The pediatric rheumatologist, physiatrist, occupational and physical therapists, and orthopedist often work together to solve difficult rehabilitation problems in JRA.

The child with JRA also may develop temporomandibular joint (TMJ) disease. This type of arthritis is often insidious in onset and course, because it has few symptoms, and it needs close monitoring with early referral to dentists for TMJ problems and to an oral surgeon or orthodontist for micrognathia. Some arthritis drugs, e.g., aspirin or methotrexate, can predispose the child to tooth decay.

Teenagers may need help in making a successful transition to an adult medical care system and adulthood. In coordination with school efforts, the team can assist the teenager in setting and achieving realistic educational and vocational goals as well as in planning for adequate health insurance coverage for the young adult years. The team can assist the teenager by providing good sex education and counseling, avoiding pregnancy, and identifying an adult physician for future medical care.

The entire team strives to provide comprehensive, multidisciplinary, aggressive medical care during the child's childhood and teenage years that will aid the transition of the teenager into adulthood with no significant disability. In the last 2 decades, this team program has permitted 75% of all children with JRA to obtain this goal. It is our current objective in the 1990s to target the 25% who have major problems with JRA. With an aggressive team program and better medications, the outcome of these special children with severe JRA should continue to improve.

*Pediatrics 92(2):295–296, 1993.

ANKYLOSING SPONDYLITIS

method of
GLEN T. D. THOMSON, M.D.,
SAMUEL M. STEINFELD, B.Sc., BMR(PT),
and RON GALL, BMR(PT)
St. Boniface Hospital, University of Manitoba
Sports Physiotherapy Center, Pan Am Sports Medicine Center
Winnipeg, Manitoba, Canada

Ankylosing spondylitis (AS) is an inflammatory systemic disease that affects predominantly the spine and sacroiliac joints. AS is a member of a larger family of disorders known as the spondyloarthropathies (SpA), which include both post-infectious "reactive arthritis" and arthropathies asso-

The support of the Arthritis Society of Canada is gratefully acknowledged.

TABLE 1. **Spondyloarthropathy Family**

Predominant axial joint arthritis
AS
AS associated with ulcerative colitis or Crohn's disease
AS associated with psoriasis
Predominant peripheral joint arthritis
Reactive arthritis following dysentery (*Salmonella, Shigella, Yersinia, Campylobacter*)
Reactive arthritis following venereal infection (*Chlamydia, Ureaplasma*)
Base (*B*27, *A*rthritis, *S*acroiliitis, *E*nthesitis) (same clinical disease as reactive arthritis but no antecedent clinical infection)

Abbreviation: AS, ankylosing spondylitis.

ciated with inflammatory bowel disease and psoriasis (Table 1). Many clinical and laboratory features overlap the specific disease designations in the SpA (Table 2). HLA-B27 transgenic rat research has demonstrated this interaction of host genetic type, microbial infection, and gut inflammation in the etiopathogenesis of SpA.

AS affects between 0.1 and 0.2% of the white population and is recognized more frequently in men (3:1). The incidence of AS follows the frequency of HLA-B27 in the population. Even though more than 90% of AS patients have the HLA-B27 phenotype, only 1 of 2% of those with HLA-B27 develop AS. This increases tenfold if a first degree relative has AS.

CLINICAL FEATURES AND COURSE

AS usually begins insidiously in the individual's late teens or early twenties as alternating or bilateral buttock pain or thoracolumbar pain. The patient awakes at night because of back pain. The morning stiffness improves with exercise and with nonsteroidal anti-inflammatory drugs (NSAIDs) but not with analgesics alone. It is unusual for peripheral joint arthritis to be present at the onset except in adolescent patients. The presence of extra-articular features of SpA or a positive family history of SpA may raise the index of suspicion of AS (Table 2).

TABLE 2. **Features of Spondyloarthropathy Family**

Clinical Features
Axial arthritis or sacroiliitis: low back, alternating buttock, or thoracolumbar junction pain lasting more than 3 months
Oligoarthritis: high frequency of lower limb, asymmetrical involvement (but not exclusively)
Enthesitis: plantar fasciitis, Achilles enthesitis
Dactylitis: "sausage" digit
Ocular inflammation: iritis, conjunctivitis (in reactive arthritis)
Mucocutaneous inflammation: psoriasis, balanitis, keratoderma blennorrhagica
Bowel inflammation: Crohn's disease, ulcerative colitis, or subclinical inflammation on ileocolonoscopy
Urologic inflammation: sterile urethritis, sterile prostatitis
Family history: AS, reactive arthritis or Reiter's syndrome, psoriasis, Crohn's disease, or ulcerative colitis
Infectious history: antecedent nongonococcal venereal infection or dysenteric infection within previous 6 weeks
Laboratory Features
Seronegative: negative tests for rheumatoid factor and antinuclear antibody
HLA-B27: present in more than 90% of cases of idiopathic AS but in only 50 to 75% of patients in whom antecedent infection or associated disease (psoriasis, Crohn's disease, ulcerative colitis) is present
Radiologic sacroiliitis: spectrum of changes from joint line erosions (earliest) to joint space "pseudo-widening" and reactive sclerosis, culminating in complete joint ankylosis

There is a spectrum of severity in AS from asymptomatic radiologic sacroiliitis to complete ankylosis of the axial skeleton (bamboo spine). Peripheral joint arthritis complicates 10% of cases of AS and is usually confined to girdle joints (hips and shoulders). Individuals in whom there is an early age of onset, hip arthritis, and failure to respond to medication have a worse long-term prognosis.

Arthritis of the costotransverse and costospinal joints may lead to restriction of chest expansion, although there is minimal impairment of breathing in nonsmokers. Arthritis of the costosternal, manubriosternal, sternoclavicular, and acromioclavicular joints is also frequent.

Iritis can occur in up to 30% of AS patients at some point in their lives. The iritis is primarily associated with the HLA-B27 phenotype, not the AS.

Among the less frequent manifestations of AS are aortic insufficiency and cardiac conduction defects. Upper lobe pulmonary fibrosis may occur and may be complicated by infections such as aspergillosis. Cauda equina syndrome with saddle anesthesia and characteristic diverticula on myelography is a late manifestation of AS, as is secondary amyloidosis.

Many patients remain functional and continue to work despite chronic pain and physical limitations. Prolonged inflammatory back pain and consequent inactivity will result in additional mechanical back pain. The typical alteration of posture results in muscle imbalances, such as lengthening of antigravity muscles and shortening of their antagonists, resulting in joint contracture.

The longevity of patients with AS is reduced by systemic complications such as amyloidosis. Fractures of the cervical spine due to minor trauma may lead to spinal cord damage, quadriplegia, and death.

INVESTIGATIONS

Laboratory tests are nonspecific. The erythrocyte sedimentation rate (ESR) is elevated in 75% of patients, especially those with peripheral joint arthritis. Other acute phase reactants, such as C-reactive protein, are elevated, and the serum IgA may be mildly to moderately elevated. The rheumatoid factor and antinuclear antibody test are negative. HLA-B27 typing is costly and is seldom helpful because of the high frequency (10%) of well individuals with HLA-B27 in typical white populations.

Plain radiographs of the sacroiliac joints or other spinal joints are usually normal for several years after the onset of symptoms. Nuclear medicine scans are more sensitive to early change but are not specific. Computed tomography (CT) and magnetic resonance imaging (MRI) may demonstrate early erosive changes of the sacroiliac joints and are the most definitive (albeit costly) early investigations.

MANAGEMENT

The goals of therapy are (1) to reduce pain and stiffness and (2) to maintain good posture and range of motion. The physiotherapy program (Table 3) is facilitated by NSAID therapy (Table 4). Phenylbutazone was commonly used in the past but has been abandoned because of rare but life-threatening hematologic side effects. Salicylates are not of much therapeutic benefit in AS or other SpA.

TABLE 3. **Physiotherapy Programs**

1. Education*
   The disease
   Posture, body mechanics, resting and sleeping positions
   Modification of activity and exercise during exacerbation
   Appropriate sporting activities (e.g., swimming)
   Proper use of heat and ice
2. Prevention of contractures
   Specific stretching and strengthening exercises
3. Reduction of pain and inflammation
   Ultrasound, electrical stimulation, acupuncture
4. Maintenance or improvement of range of motion
   Manual therapy techniques (e.g., passive joint mobilization and muscle stretching)

*Additional educational materials available from The Arthritis Foundation, The Ankylosing Spondylitis Association, and The Arthritis Society (Canada).

Use of second-line drugs in refractory cases should be considered with the help of a rheumatologist (Table 5). Sulfasalazine (Azulfidine), 1 gram orally twice daily for 3 months, may improve symptoms. Increasing the dose to 3 grams per day for an additional 3 months may be necessary if the response is suboptimal. The dose at which the patient becomes asymptomatic should be maintained for an additional 3 to 4 months. If the patient remains asymptomatic, tapering the dose by 500 mg every 4 months to a dose of 1 gram per day may be desirable.

Methotrexate (Rheumatrex) in oral doses of 7.5 to 15 mg per week may also be helpful in treating patients with refractory AS. Gold therapy (Myochrysine, Ridaura) or hydroxychloroquine (Plaquenil) has been used in patients with refractory peripheral joint arthritis.

Refractory peripheral joint monarthritis, sacroiliitis, and enthesitis may respond to corticosteroid injection. When no bony changes are evident on radiographs, cervical spine restriction of range of motion may be improved by aggressive physiotherapy and a short course of systemic corticosteroids: prednisone, 0.5 mg per kg per day given orally for a week followed by a rapid taper during the following week, or intramuscular methylprednisolone acetate (Depo-Medrol) 2 mg per kg. Pulsed intravenous corticosteroids (methylprednisolone sodium succinate [Solu-Medrol], 1 gram given intravenously daily for one to three doses) may provide short-term benefit to patients with refractory systemic AS. Systemic daily oral corticosteroids should not be used as long-term therapy for AS.

Analgesics and muscle relaxants can be used as adjunctive therapy for AS, particularly in patients who are disturbed by night pain. Amitriptyline (Elavil), 10 to 50 mg orally at bedtime, may also be helpful in encouraging sleep and relieving pain.

TABLE 4. **NSAID Therapy**

Choose a nonsalicylate NSAID: indomethacin (Indocin), naproxen (Naprosyn), diclofenac (Voltaren), tenoxicam (Mobiflex),* piroxicam (Feldene), ketoprofen (Orudis), sulindac (Clinoril), tolmetin (Tolectin), flurbiprofen (Ansaid), ibuprofen (Motrin, Advil), fenoprofen (Nalfon)
Prescribe full dose
Do *not* use combinations of NSAIDs
Use time-release formulations or suppository to treat night pain and morning stiffness
Trial period for a NSAID is 2 to 3 weeks minimum
Switch to another NSAID if previous response is suboptimal
Add cytoprotective agent if there is a high risk for ulcer
Allow reduction or cessation of therapy after several months to determine efficacy of current NSAID
Educate patient about the benefits and potential risks of NSAIDs

*Not available in the United States.

TABLE 5. **Indications for Second-Line Therapy in AS**

1. Failure to achieve control of peripheral joint arthritis
2. Failure to achieve control of axial symptoms with NSAIDs
   IF
   a. Early disease is present (within 5 years of onset) *or*
   b. Increased ESR, C-reactive protein, or serum IgA is present *or*
   c. Axial symptoms with minimal or no radiologic ankylosis and/or positive bone scan

COMPLICATIONS

Iritis

Immediate referral to an ophthalmologist is warranted to confirm the diagnosis and begin therapy with topical corticosteroids and mydriatic or cycloplegic eyedrops. Refractory cases may require systemic corticosteroids.

Suspected Spinal Fracture

Plain radiographs may not immediately reveal a fracture. Tomography, CT, MRI, or bone scan may be necessary to rule out a fracture. Referral to a spinal trauma specialist is advisable.

Total Hip Replacement

There is an increased risk of heterotopic ossification in AS patients. Postoperative radiation should be considered as prophylaxis.

ASSOCIATED DISEASES

Inflammatory Bowel Disease

Treatment of the bowel disease medically or surgically will not influence the course of AS. NSAIDs may exacerbate bowel inflammation, but NSAIDs absorbed in the proximal gut may be better tolerated than slow-release or enteric preparations.

An acute self-limited peripheral joint arthritis is seen in 5% of Crohn's disease patients. NSAIDs or intra-articular injections are sufficient to relieve the symptoms. Successful treatment of the underlying bowel disease terminates the acute arthritis.

Psoriasis

The activity of the skin disease does not influence the course of AS. Sulfasalazine (Azulfidine) therapy sometimes results in significant skin improvement.

Psoriatic arthritis of the peripheral joints can be initially treated with NSAIDs. Methotrexate in refractory cases may cause improvement in both the joint and the skin disease.

Reactive Arthritis

Post-dysenteric and post-venereal reactive arthritis may be a self-limited disease of less than 6 months duration or may become a chronic arthritis characterized by a waxing and waning course. The presence of Reiter's triad (conjunctivitis, urethritis, and arthritis) at onset is more frequent in post-venereal reactive arthritis. Acute flares usually respond to the same NSAIDs used for AS. A 3-month course of tetracycline, 250 mg orally four times per day, or minocycline (Minocin), 100 mg orally twice a day, may be successful in treating refractory cases of post-venereal reactive arthritis. Sulfasalazine in the same doses used for AS may be helpful in patients with chronic reactive arthritis.

TEMPOROMANDIBULAR DISORDERS

method of
CHARLES C. ALLING III, D.D.S., M.S., D.SC.(HON)
Brookwood Medical Center
Birmingham, Alabama

Temporomandibular disorders are frequently and often inaccurately referred to as TMJ (temporomandibular joint) disorders, syndromes, or dysfunctions. The confusion in terms has resulted in dentists, physicians, and other health professionals embracing a concept that "TMJ" is a disease entity; this has resulted in both a profusion of treatments based on *symptoms* of chronic pain in all areas above the neck and in a few practitioners' even espousing the idea that TMJ is the cause of disorders in distant anatomic areas, e.g., the gastrointestinal tract, spinal column, neurologic speech center, central nervous system, cardiovascular system, and urologic system. To emphasize that the temporomandibular joint is merely a portion of the musculoskeletal system, I refer to it as the TM joint, not the TMJ.

TM disorders are often several clinical problems involving either the TM joint or the major and minor muscles of mastication. The patients' complaints may include facial pain, pain in muscular areas, earaches, headaches, limitation of mandibular movements, TM joint sounds, and TM joint pains. TM disorders, which occur in the musculoskeletal system, may be either augmented by or mistaken for diseases and disorders of the psychogenic controls of the vascular and nervous systems and occult inflammatory and neoplastic lesions of the nasoantral and dentoalveolar structures. The trend in the medical and dental professions has been to avoid determining precise diagnoses for TM joint and facial myofascial pains and instead to create nomenclatures for all-encompassing syndromes and disorders. These have been referred to as Costen's syndrome, TMJ syndrome (or disorder), TMJ, TMJ pain dysfunction syndrome, myofascial pain dysfunction syndrome, TM disorders, and craniomandibular disorders.

It is likely that many patients who cannot cope with facial myofascial pains and TM joint disorders are biologically different from other individuals who have similar lifestyles, personalities, emotional stresses, and medical backgrounds but who either do not suffer or are able to cope. Facial myofascial pains and TM joint disorders are a subset of chronic pain categories that afflict patients. For example, it is possible that when the ultimate therapies for tension (muscle contraction) and migraine (vascular instability) headaches are established, the treatment for the great majority of facial myofascial pains will likewise be found.

Patients who cannot cope with chronic pain are not well understood by many physicians and dentists and may be subjected to surgical procedures and other therapies that are directed at symptoms and not causes and that may do harm. In time, chronic pain that is influenced by subtle disturbances of the brain, biochemistry, and general physiology on a molecular biologic level will be clearly identified. For the present, it is important for patients with facial myofascial and TM joint pains that physicians and dentists identify and treat discrete somatic maladies and the overwhelming influences of the psyche.

PREVALENCE

Epidemiologic studies of cross-sections of specific populations revealed that 33% have at least one painful symptom in the craniomandibular area and that 75% have at least one TM joint sign, such as TM joint noise, that may be interpreted as TM joint dysfunction. The majority of patients with facial pain, which includes the TM joints and masticatory and facial myofascial disorders, are between 15 and 45 years of age. Of patients seeking care, women predominate. Significantly, among individuals not seeking care, the signs and symptoms are about equal between the genders.

ETIOLOGY

For clinical accuracy in defining the cause, establishing a diagnosis, and developing a prudent, logical treatment plan, the complaints, symptoms, history, and physical findings of the patient should point to the facial pain complaints and TM joint disorders as having a cause in one of several major systems or categories: psychogenic, musculoskeletal and TM joint, vascular, neurologic, and occult pathology in the oral cavity or the nasal and sinal areas. As a rule, there are overlapping and reinforcing etiologic factors.

The TM joint may be implicated as the cause of disorders in the oral and maxillofacial region when in fact it is injured by other factors. The delicate TM joint is a stress-bearing structure with a complex movement; the complex movement is possible owing to the meniscus that divides the joint space into superior and inferior compartments. A patient, often a woman in the second or third decade of life who is subjected to psychosocial stresses, may unwittingly introduce unusual stresses and relationships into the TM joint by abnormal and noxious habits of posturing the mandible, for example, by clenching the teeth in full or modified occlusion. An unusual TM joint movement may result that may be painful. The movement may feature a subluxation (clicking) or dislocation (closed lock) position of the disk. A treatment regimen may ensue that features a variety of somatic treatments, including adjusting the occlusion, inserting splints between the teeth, and even surgery to the TM joint itself.

Somatoform Pain Disorders

Somatoform pain disorders, manifested in the facial tissues, are identified if there are no physical or functional causes and if contributing psychogenic and psychological factors are present. The pain may be manifested in tensions and trigger points in the major and minor muscles of mastication and in the cervical muscles. The resultant abnormal muscle activity may produce a disorder within the TM joint. The patient and physician may focus on the TM joint disorder as a priority rather than on the true cause: that is, the psyche of the patient. Treatment with somatic therapies, including surgery, of a noisy, abnormally functioning, and possibly painful TM joint in many social settings is more acceptable to the patient than undergoing behavior modification treatment. For many physicians who treat TM disorders, a comfortable treatment focus may be on the muscular pain and the TM joint dysfunction rather than on recognizing the anxieties and depressions of the patient. One clinician after another may subject the patient to a favorite treatment procedure that has relieved pain in other patients. Patients with facial pain with a psychosomatic cause may pressure clinicians to provide somatic treatments even when the probability of restoration of function is minimal. The attempts at treatment may become a series of worsening failures and mutilations when the primary problem is undiagnosed as a psychogenic pain disorder. The problem is fueled when a clinician does not appreciate the power of a patient's mind over the body, and the patient is unwilling to discuss or admit to having a somatoform pain disorder.

Musculoskeletal Disorders

Musculoskeletal disorders may be either the etiologic factor or, as in the case of psychogenic maladies, secondary manifestations of facial pain. Trigger points may arise in musculature secondary to mandibular abusive posture habits, trauma, or as a factor of psychogenic stress. The major muscles of mastication (the masseter, temporalis, and internal and external pterygoid muscles) may have pain trigger points within the muscles, and the trigger points may produce referred pain. As a representative masticatory muscle, trigger points in the temporalis muscle may, for example, refer pain to the TM joint or the maxillary teeth in the form of a temporal headache. As a representative cervical muscle, trigger points in the sternocleidomastoid muscle may, for example, produce referred pain in the form of an earache, a frontal headache, or pain to the eye and cheek. The clinical diagnosis of various referred myofascial pains from the sternocleidomastoid muscle are labeled atypical facial neuralgia, myofascial pain dysfunction syndrome, tension headache, and cervicocephalalgia.

The TM joint has a unique design. Most of the freely movable joints have articular surfaces of hyaline cartilage that function directly against one another or with an incomplete intervening cartilaginous meniscus. The TM joint meniscus comprises all the tissues between the mandibular condyle and the temporal bone articular fossa and eminence; the meniscus has an avascular disk that is positioned around the superior and anterior curve of the condyle and extends anteriorly below the temporal articular crest. In healthy TM joints, the anterior attachment of the disk is to the sphenomeniscus muscle (the superior head of the external pterygoid muscle), the posterior is to fibers of the bilaminar zone, and the lateral and medial attachments are to poles of the condyle. The thinnest and most compact part of the disk is its central zone, and this is positioned, when the mouth is either in the rest position or closed in a full intercuspal position of the dental arches, between the posterior incline of the articular eminence and the anterior-superior surface of the condyle. As the mandible moves, embrasures of varying dimensions are created between the condyle and the temporal bone. The volume of the flexible disk is adequate to fill the potential superior and inferior TM joint spaces during all functional positions of the condyle and thus to provide stabilization for the mandible relative to the temporal bone. If there is laxity of the posterior, medial, or lateral attachments of the disk or if there is a muscular dysfunction at the anterior attachment, there is a disharmonious movement between the condyle and the disk, and a subluxation of the disk occurs, producing a clicking sound. It is noted that TM joint sounds occur as either transient or permanent physiologic variations of normal in the majority of individuals. If the greatest bulk of the disk is positioned anterior to the condyle, the disk is dislocated, and a block, expressed as a closed lock, of the mandible occurs. By inspection of mandibular movements and by auscultation, a diagnosis is possible of the painful and painless disk subluxations and dislocations. Other disk problems include perforations, which may be a normal physiologic finding in some individuals; degenerative changes associated with TM joint arthritis; and fractures or tears of the disk following acute trauma.

Inspection, palpation, and auscultation of the TM joints identify anterior subluxations and dislocations of the disks. Anterior subluxations of the disks usually occur during the opening movements of the mandible or may also occur as a reciprocal click on the closing movements. Dislocations of the disks (not the mandible) usually occur at about a 25-mm opening as measured between the incisal edges of the anterior teeth when a definite blocking movement is reported by the patient and is observed by the physician. Definitive subcategories of pathologic functions of the disk are established by clinical evaluations that indicate the type of treatment, usually splint therapy. After an accurate diagnosis is established, a series of clinical tests is performed to establish the probability of responsiveness to nonsurgical therapy. In rare instances, surgery may be indicated if there is more of a painful medial than an anterior displacement of the disk; then open TM joint surgery is performed to reposition and stabilize the disk.

Psychogenic stress, facial skeletal deformities, trauma, and deflective occlusal relationships are more likely to produce disk movement discoordination in women. This may be explained in part by the fact that many women may have less stable and sturdy musculoskeletal systems compared with men. Any definitive treatment, as discussed later, should include preoperative, intraoperative, and postoperative physical therapy to stabilize the TM joint.

Vascular Disorders

Vascular disorders and abnormalities may produce painful sensations to the face by referral from intracranial vessels, temporal arteritis, and migraine and migrainous instabilities of the carotid systems. Emotional stress is a frequent precipitant of migrainous attacks, although no evidence is apparent that migraine patients are subjected to greater stress than nonmigraine subjects. Migraine headaches usually are clearly identified and are not mistakenly labeled TM joint disorders.

Two recurring disorders of vascular origin have been labeled as being TMJ. Patients with lower half headaches that affect the facial tissues, usually with periorbital manifestations, have been referred for treatment with a transfer diagnosis of TMJ. As with chronic facial myofascial pain problems, there may be a dysfunctioning of the TM joint, often including the signs of disk subluxation (clicking), and this finding may be mistaken for the cause of a lower half headache. The other unusual manifestation that erroneously may be thought to originate in the TM joint is neurovascular odontalgia (atypical odontalgia). The closed, confined spaces of the dental pulp chambers in each individual tooth are rich in nociceptors, and stimulation from changes in the vascular system may be manifested as toothaches. The resultant unusual posturing of the mandible, which produces TM joint signs and symptoms, may give the clinician the impression that the TM joint is awry, producing the malocclusion and hence the toothaches. Neurovascular odontalgia often has been successfully treated by physicians specializing in neurology.

Neurologic Disorders

Neurologic disorders are usually clearly identified by the patient in the area of distribution of the affected nerve. Pains are characteristically of short duration but of great intensity. The second and third cervical nerves innervate areas at the angle of the mandible. Pain of cardiac muscle ischemia can be referred to both angles of the mandible, but more frequently it is referred to the left; the only complaint of an ischemic heart attack may be a complaint of pain in the mandibular area. It is rare but not surprising that patients are referred with TMJ, but the final diagnosis is commensurate with variations of major and minor trigeminal neuralgias, central cranial lesions, or cardiac ischemia.

Occult Pathology

Occult pathology of the dentition and nasal and sinal passages may result in a diagnosis of TMJ and in the provision of a variety of intraoral procedures or the placement of devices on the occlusal surfaces of teeth. Occult pathology of teeth includes impacted teeth destroying contiguous tissues, teeth with scarcely detectible cracks, pulp stones, and other anomalies. The pain is often diffuse along the applicable branch of the trigeminal nerve, and it may be referred to a distant site while the pathologic tooth is relatively pain free. Pathology in the sinal or nasal passages may be manifested as pain in dentition or as pain referred to a distant site.

TREATMENT

The management of TM joint disorders, as a portion of the locomotor system, must include a precise diagnosis. The human face is the most expressive portion of the body, and the TM joint, masticator muscles, and muscles of facial expression are key portions. At the onset of the evaluation, the patient is asked to point with one finger to the area of pain. If the pain is psychogenic in origin, the patient may insist on pointing to bilateral areas rather than to a single area, pointing to widely diverse locations, or waving fingers in the air around the face and cranium. If pain is vascular in origin, the patient may point to the area around the eyes; if neurologic, along a branch of a trigeminal nerve or the second or third cervical nerve; if locomotor, that is, if the problem is actually a TM joint or a muscle problem, he or she may point to the involved muscle or the TM joint. Occult pathology results in a wide variety of indications.

Physical evaluation includes inspection, palpation, auscultation, and percussion, as indicated, of the TM joint and cervical spine; the facial, cervical, and masticatory muscles; intraoral structures; movements of the TM joint as recorded by mandibular excursions; the cranial and cervical nerves; and the vascular structures. Assuming, as often occurs, that the history and physical examination reveal a strong psychogenic element underlying the TM joint and muscle pain, a prudent, rational treatment would be centered on referral to a psychiatrist or psychologist. If the history and physical examinations reveal a neurologic or vascular etiology of the patient's complaints, definitive care would be centered on referral to a general medical practitioner or a neurologist who specializes in managing headaches.

In the facial musculoskeletal system, the factors of stress, trauma, iatrogenesis, and malocclusion predispose the TM joints and masticator and facial expression musculature to myofascial dysfunctions. Initiating factors of TM joint dysfunctions, especially in women, are repetitive loading traumas to the TM joint. The initiating trauma may be caused by sustained, repetitive loading of the TM joints by clenching, bruxism, stress and anxiety, or medications. Perpetuating factors that sustain the TM joint and muscle disorders include social, emotional, and cognitive difficulties. There may be a social gain for the patient in having pain that attracts and holds attention. An emotional perpetuating factor may be depression, seen in many chronic pain patients. Cognitive factors of confusion and misunderstanding are often seen in chronic pain patients because of the varied and opposing diagnoses and recommendations for therapy. Often these patients have an unrealistic expectation that the physician can provide complete and immediate pain relief.

Imaging should not substitute for responsible clinical evaluation but may be indicated to confirm or enhance the clinical findings. In general, imaging studies should be ordered when the results of the imaging have the probability, not a mere possibility, of altering the treatment plan; unfortunately, nonmedical reasons may prevail and dictate the ordering of imaging: a routine of the practice, medical-legal considerations, and documentation for insurance companies. For osseous abnormalities of the TM joint, transpharyngeal, panoramic, and transorbital radiographs with the usual equipment in outpatient dental clinics provide surveys and, in some cases, final diagnostic views of the TM joint osseous structures. Definitive views of the TM joint osseous structures are obtained with either computed tomography or polycyclic tomograms corrected for the long axis of the mandibular condyle. For soft tissue imaging, TM joint arthrography uses radiopaque materials in the superior and inferior potential TM joint spaces to outline the position of the meniscus. Arthrography demonstrates a perforation, which may be a normal physiologic change, of the TM joint disk portion of the meniscus. Magnetic resonance imaging displays the soft tissues of the TM joint and confirms the location of the disk, which is usually already ascertained by history and physical evaluation.

Arthroscopy is confined by most currently used procedures to delivering clear images only of the superior joint space, and it should be noted that degenerative arthritic and other pathologic changes, often associated with the mandibular condyle, occur in the inferior joint space. The flushing of fluids through the superior joint space that accompanies an arthroscopic examination results in increased joint mobility; this phenomenon has been observed in the past with the injection of anesthetics, antibiotics, and other solutions, including radiopaque media, when performing arthrographic examinations.

The treatment plan includes controlling pain, decreasing adverse loading, restoring function, and restoring the normal activities of life. Nonsurgical therapy, such as behavior modification, physical therapy, and use of short-term intraoral splint devices, is indicated first instead of instituting a nonreversible change in the occlusal relationships or performing TM joint surgery. The success rate in studies that have included up to 10 years' follow-up of nonsurgical therapy ranged between 85.5% and more than 90%. If there has been no structural change in the TM joint, which may require surgery to correct, the usual patient with TM joint and muscle pain can be treated by an integrated program that includes patient education, behavior modification, physical therapy, palliative home care, and pharmacotherapy. Some patients require occlusal therapy as a form of physical therapy, and a few patients are benefited by surgery.

Patient Education

Patient education is a fundamental aspect of care. The responsible physician should tailor a one-on-one conference with the patient to ensure that the patient understands the applicable anatomy, physiology, and pathology. One of the key items to be learned by the patient is that the relationship of the mandible to the maxilla in health is the rest position with a separation of the maxillary and mandibular teeth. This position relieves most pains in the TM joint and muscles. A patient who has been thoroughly indoctrinated by a dentist striving for perfect occlusion in the fully *closed position* of the mandible to the maxilla may be initially frustrated by the information on the physiologic desirability of the *rest position* of the mandible and the muscles of mastication. For a receptive patient who wishes to be rid of facial myofascial pain and TM joint dysfunction, the use of visual aids helps to illustrate how the rest position is the normal healthy relationship of the mandible to the maxilla and that full, closed occlusion is not; the patient needs to understand that the rest position both removes internal compressive strains in the TM joint space and relaxes muscle that may be laden with painful trigger points.

Behavior Modification

Behavior modification may be necessary through stress management and counseling programs. These may embrace biofeedback, progressive relaxation, and changes in lifestyle. This type of treatment may be administered by a psychiatrist or a psychologist informed about TM joint and muscle disabilities. Chronic pain patients are often laden with anxieties, depressions, and anger associated with the chronicity of their disorder. Somatic direct treatments to the dentition or to the TM joints should await stabilization of the patient's condition under the care of a mental health professional who is informed about TM joint and muscle disabilities. In many cases, no somatic direct treatments to the dentition or in the TM joints is necessary after behavior modification treatments.

Physical Therapy

Physical therapy alters sensory inputs and strengthens coordinated muscle activity and is especially indicated for female patients who may have loose, unstable TM joints. For patients who are to undergo intraoral treatments or TM joint surgery, physical therapy ideally should be prescribed from the preoperative through the postoperative phases of treatment. One objective of physical therapy is to obtain mandibular posture training, with the mandible in the correct anatomic rest position without contact of the dentition except when swallowing. Exercise therapy of mandibular movements to establish coordinated muscle functions, isotonic exercises designed to increase range of motion, and isometric exercises directed toward strengthening the muscle are goals and modalities in most physical therapy regimens. In many cases, no direct somatic care of the teeth or the TM joints is necessary after physical therapy.

Palliative Self-Care

Palliative self-care, in combination with physical therapy, may consist of the application of thermal packs to the TM joint and muscle areas, modification of abusive habits, avoidance of functions that strain the TM joint and muscles, control of clenching, and practicing prescribed mandibular exercises calculated to strengthen muscle groups.

Pharmacotherapy

Pharmacotherapy for patients with chronic TM joint and muscle pains and disabilities should be adjunctive to patient education, physical therapy, palliative self-care, and behavior modification procedures. When used as a part of a comprehensive management program, pharmacotherapy can be a powerful catalyst for the comfort and rehabilitation of the patient. The medications should be prescribed for a short term and should be discontinued as physical therapy, palliative self-care, and behavior modification become effective. The agents used in various circumstances include non-narcotic analgesics, low-dose antidepressants, anti-inflammatory drugs, occasionally corticosteroids, and, for specific short-term goals, narcotic analgesics.

Interocclusal Splints

Interocclusal splints are effective in reducing pain in TM joints and muscle and for repositioning most of the subluxated TM joint disks. There are many varieties of splints designed to either stabilize the mandible in the rest position or reposition the mandible in relation to the maxilla, thus altering the relationships within the TM joint space. Splints should be used for short prescribed periods of time lest they cause irreversible changes in the relationships of the maxillary and mandibular dental arches.

Occlusal Therapy

Occlusal therapy, which irreversibly alters the occluding surfaces of the dental arches, should follow, when indicated, successful management of a patient's facial myofascial pain and TM joint disorder. The maxillomandibular relationship, neuromuscular activity, and psychosocial problems should be normal or under control before occlusal therapy is initiated.

Orthognathic Surgery

Orthognathic surgery, like occlusal therapy, should await normalization of a painful and malfunctioning TM joint and muscles. Abnormal facial skeletal relationships may have been the inciting cause of TM joint and muscle pain, but the painful episode should be resolved and under control before orthognathic surgery is instituted. Orthognathic surgery to alleviate ongoing chronic and acute TM joint and muscle pains and dysfunctions is not indicated.

Temporomandibular Joint Surgery

Decisions about TM joint surgery for a painful TM joint and muscles caused by an internal joint derangement should be based on the following considerations: (1) one is assured that effective behavioral therapy has been given to the patient and that the patient has a sound psyche; (2) positive evidence exists that the cause of the myofascial and TM joint pain is related to the disk displacement or other joint disorder; (3) appropriate imaging documentation of TM joint disk displacement or other pathology exists; (4) disabling pain or dysfunction is present and is believed to have a somatic TM joint etiology; (5) prior nonsurgical treatments that included sound physical and possible interocclusal splint therapies have been done; (6) control of oral parafunctional habits or conditions that would adversely affect the outcome of the surgery has been achieved; and (7) informed consent and request for surgery have been provided by the patient.

The surgical approaches are numerous and may be grouped into arthroscopic procedures and open surgical procedures of the TM joint. Arthroscopic surgery, using both mechanical and laser modalities, has a high success rate in managing persistent, nonreducing displaced TM disks; in revising procedures following earlier surgery by removing intracapsular fibrosis; in biopsies; and in débridement and lavage. Interestingly, distention of the joint space, usually *only the superior joint space,* with the lavaging flood of fluid that commonly accompanies arthroscopic procedures, is beneficial in freeing adhesions and increasing joint mobility even when, inexplicably, the pathologic changes, as with most arthritides, are found to be on the mandibular condyle in the inferior joint space.

OTHER TEMPOROMANDIBULAR JOINT MALADIES

The TM joint is subject to the usual array of arthritides and joint maladies. These include degenerative, rheumatoid, psoriatic, infectious, systemic lupus erythematosus–induced, and traumatic arthritides; synovial chondromatosis; neuropathic joint disease; and other maladies, including neoplasms and hemarthrosis secondary to hemophilia. In this group, the degenerative arthritides have pathogeneses that are unique to the TM joint. There is a monarticular reversible degenerative TM joint arthritis that occurs in young women in the first 10 to 20 years after the menarche. The disease goes through four stages and, after 18 to 48 months, resolves with a normally functioning joint. The painful episodes are managed with patient (and sponsor, if indicated) education; interocclusal splints to relieve TM joint intracapsular pressures; physical therapy; and antidepressant, if indicated, and anti-inflammatory medications. In some patients, arthroscopic TM joint procedures are beneficial in relieving painful episodes. Irreversible TM joint degenerative arthritis occurs in the elderly, as with other joints.

The oral and maxillofacial manifestations of TM joint rheumatoid arthritis include a progressive apertognathism (anterior open bite) and usually are bilateral in the TM joints. The systemic general management of the TM joint is the same as for other joints. The onset of a fibrous ankylosis may require surgical intervention; in some cases, after the disease becomes quiescent, orthognathic surgical correction or TM joint reconstruction may be considered.

Infectious arthritides of the TM joint may result in an ankylosis that is treated by surgical TM joint reconstruction following the cessation of the disease.

A variant of traumatic arthritis is an acute hypertranslation of the TM joint, a so-called whiplash injury of the TM joint. In the twentieth century, millions of patients have been treated for maxillofacial fractures and injuries incurred in violent accidents, altercations, and warfare; however, only in the past 20 years have TM disorders and so-called TM joint whiplash injury been diagnosed as incurred by the trauma. In many cases, patient awareness of a clicking or other actual internal derangement of a TM joint and a history of an episode of trauma may be combined with a hope of the benefits of legal recourse. Individuals with either a normal or abnormal TM joint clicking sound who experience myofascial facial pains may be diagnosed by a physician as having either a TM disorder or one of the synonymous disorders. The individual with the preceding combination of symptoms and a diagnostic label may seek legal recourse by citing as the cause acute trauma; general anesthetic intubation; or intraoral, transoral, or pharyngeal surgical procedures. In the area of imaginative legal gamesmanship, it is helpful to recall the words of the orthopedic surgeon H. M. Frost: "In my time, I have seen for diagnosis and/or treatment more than 10,000 patients with unresolved liability from a real or imagined injury. Yet in the same period, I have seen only three patients desiring help or advice for such injury after the liability was closed."*

*Mahan PE, Alling CC: Facial Pain, 3rd ed. Philadelphia, Lea & Febiger, 1991, p. 103.

FIBROMYALGIA, TENDINITIS, AND BURSITIS

method of
JEFFREY M. THOMPSON, M.D.
Mayo Clinic
Rochester, Minnesota

FIBROMYALGIA AND OTHER MUSCLE PAIN SYNDROMES

Muscle pain is one of the most common reasons for patients to see their doctor. In a general internal medicine practice 30% of the patients with a complaint of pain met the criteria for a localized muscle pain syndrome (myofascial pain), and 11% of the general population in northern England report the presence of chronic widespread pain. Fibromyalgia is the third most common diagnosis reported by rheumatologists. It is surprising that such a common disorder remains such an enigma.

Although many names and definitions have been used to describe chronic muscle pain (nonarticular rheumatism, myofibrositis, nonrestorative sleep syndrome, chronic myalgia), the three most commonly used terms at present are fibromyalgia, myofascial pain, and fibrositis. Fibrositis is a misnomer and should no longer be used because inflammation has never been shown to be present in these disorders. Myofascial pain is a localized or regional muscle pain problem, whereas fibromyalgia is more generalized and has systemic features. There is much debate about the relationship between the two. I find it useful to use the term tension myalgia to describe the spectrum of chronic muscle pain syndromes (see treatment section subsequently).

Diagnosis

The American College of Rheumatology in 1990 developed criteria for the classification of fibromyalgia. Emphasis was placed on widespread pain (both sides of the body, above and below the waist) of 3 months' or longer duration and tenderness at 11 of 18 points. Previous requirements of disturbed sleep, generalized fatigue, and other constitutional symptoms have been dropped from the official definition but are often cited as characteristic features of fibromyalgia. Myofascial pain is defined as chronic muscle pain involving one or a few muscles. The major diagnostic features are referred pain on palpation of tender points (trigger points), ropey muscle (or taut band), and a twitch response in the band of muscle when it is "snapped" by the examining finger.

It is not uncommon for patients to complain of various neurologic symptoms such as paresthesias in the upper extremities, "numbness," and "weakness." These complaints usually do not fit with any specific nerve root distribution, and electrodiagnostic studies are negative. Psychological stress almost always makes the pain worse and in some cases is a major factor.

I believe the distinction between myofascial pain and fibromyalgia is somewhat artificial because it is based largely on the number of sites involved. A clinically useful paradigm is to consider a spectrum of muscle pain from localized tension myalgia (myofascial pain) to regional tension myalgia to generalized tension myalgia (fibromyalgia). As the pain becomes more generalized, elements of chronic pain syndrome become more important, accounting for many of the constitutional symptoms described earlier.

The differential diagnosis is long (Table 1) but is easily sorted out by physical examination and a few simple laboratory tests. I usually obtain a complete blood count; determinations of sedimentation rate, rheumatoid factor, and antinuclear antibody; thyroid studies; and muscle enzymes. On examination patients often move stiffly, have reduced range of motion of the affected areas, and demonstrate co-con-

TABLE 1. **Partial Differential Diagnosis of Muscle Pain Syndromes**

Polymyalgia rheumatica
Hypothyroidism
Bursitis, tendinitis
Prodromal phase of a connective tissue disease
Polymyositis
Metabolic myopathy
Hyperparathyroidism
Parkinson's disease
Osteopenia, osteomalacia
Primary Sjögren's syndrome
Enthesopathies

traction of agonist-antagonist pairs with movement. A simple test for co-contraction is to ask the patient to elevate the arms overhead and watch for a "shuddering" movement rather than the normal smooth motion, especially when the arms are lowered.

Etiology

The cause of these muscle pain syndromes is unknown. Most recent theories focus on a very localized process within the muscle involving depletion of adenosine triphosphate (ATP), local ischemia, and release of substances that sensitize nociceptive nerve fibers. These changes may be initiated by muscle trauma (overuse, poor posture). There have been no consistent histologic findings. It makes sense that sleep disturbance might be a perpetuating factor, but its role as a causative factor is unclear. Studies have shown that alpha waves intrude into stage 4 (non-REM) sleep, but this is a very nonspecific finding and is not seen in all patients. Often there is an element of motor dysfunction with prominent co-contraction, increased resting tone, and shortened muscles, but these findings have been difficult to quantitate.

Treatment

There are several approaches to treatment of the various muscle pain syndromes but very little evidence to support them. Aerobic exercise has been shown to be more effective than a general flexibility program. Amitriptyline (Elavil)* in low doses has been shown to be effective in short-term trials, as has cyclobenzaprine (Flexeril). I find that a combination approach involving reassurance, elimination of contributing factors, physical therapy, conditioning, and medications is most effective.

Reassurance and Education

Providing a definite diagnosis to patients with chronic muscle pain and spending some time educating them about what it means and what they can do about it relieves much of the anxiety that often accompanies and perpetuates these disorders. The term tension myalgia is useful in patient education. "Myalgia" refers to the most characteristic finding—muscle pain. The word tension has two connotations. First, it suggests that a major characteristic in these patients is muscle under tension, from poor posture, habitual contraction, or overuse. Second, the word tension suggests that psychological tension or stress may play a major role and may contribute to the muscular tension. When presented in this context, patients are more willing to acknowledge the role of psychological factors in their pain disorder and are more likely to accept suggestions about stress management and other psychological interventions.

Elimination of Contributing Factors

The literature on myofascial disorders lists many "perpetuating factors" that must be addressed to ensure successful treatment. The most important are motor dysfunction, sleep disturbance, psychological stress, and anatomic variations (short leg).

Physical Therapy

The goals of physical therapy are to decrease pain, promote muscle relaxation, return muscles to their normal resting length, and promote normal neuromuscular functioning. A short (5-day) intense (twice daily) course of physical therapy is initiated. It includes hot packs, massage, high-intensity galvanic stimulation, posture training, stretching exercises, and, if muscle dysfunction is a problem, surface electromyographic biofeedback. After this week of intensive therapy the patient continues with a home program.

Conditioning

Part of the home program is graduated aerobic exercise. Pain usually diminishes as the level of fitness improves. The patient must be able to avoid co-contraction during exercise, however, or more muscle pain may result.

Medications

If disturbance of sleep is a problem, a low-dose tricyclic medication should be considered. Amitriptyline (Elavil),* starting at 10 mg each evening and increasing to 25 to 50 mg, or cyclobenzaprine (Flexeril), 10 mg each evening, has been shown to be effective. Anti-inflammatory agents (including corticosteroids) and analgesics generally are not useful.

Other Approaches

Other recommended treatments include the use of spray and stretch with vapocoolant sprays or trigger point injections. These methods are most useful for the most localized muscle pain disorders. If the pain is generalized and chronic pain behaviors predominate, an organized pain management approach may be necessary. The overall goal of any treatment approach should be to teach the patient to manage the muscle pain disorder without relying on (or overusing) health care professionals.

TENDINITIS AND BURSITIS

Tendinitis and bursitis are often the result of excessive repetitive loads and are commonly referred to as overuse injuries. Less common are traumatic causes of tendinitis and bursitis. These injuries frequently occur in athletes and laborers but are also seen in sedentary individuals owing to repetitive postural stresses.

General Principles of Treatment

The general approach to treatment of these disorders is simple. The first objective is to decrease the stresses on the injured tissue and in the process de-

*This drug has not been approved by the Food and Drug Administration (FDA) for this indication.

*This drug has not been approved by the FDA for this indication.

crease the pain. Relative rest is important to allow the tissue to heal. Measures are then employed to decrease inflammation and swelling. During this time pain-free range of motion (ROM) is attained or maintained. When full pain-free ROM is accomplished, a gradual return to activity or strengthening can begin.

Tendinitis or Bursitis of the Shoulder

Many soft tissue problems can cause pain around the shoulder (Table 2). The most common situation is the middle-aged patient who reports a gradual onset of pain in the anterior shoulder or the deltoid insertion area, especially when raising the arm above shoulder level or with internal rotation (putting on a coat). There is tenderness over the insertion of the supraspinatus tendon and the impingement test is positive. Resisted contraction of the supraspinatus ("empty can test") often reproduces the pain. Internal rotation is limited, and there is a painful arc on abduction of the arm. If tenderness is more diffuse the term periarthritis is sometimes used, and if motion is severely limited (with or without the pain) it is termed frozen shoulder. Some clinicians believe that there is a progression from impingement to frozen shoulder and that the problem will resolve in about 2 years no matter what is done. Certainly shoulder pain problems can be frustrating for both the patient and the physician.

The initial approach to supraspinatus tendinitis with impingement is to decrease the pain by using ice and avoiding impingement (no overhead activities). Nonsteroidal anti-inflammatory drugs (NSAIDs) are sometimes useful. If ROM is limited, gentle pain-free ROM exercises are used; one technique is relaxed supine ROM using a cane in the other hand to assist the movements of the affected arm. Strengthening of the rotator cuff can begin using resisted internal and external rotation of the arm with the elbow at the side when the patient can do so without pain. It is important also to strengthen the scapular stabilizers.

If the area of tenderness is well localized, an injection of betamethasone (Celestone Soluspan) and bupivacaine (Marcaine) in a 1:4 ratio into the subacromial space can help speed recovery. Injections alone are often unsuccessful and are best used in conjunction with an exercise program.

Greater Trochanteric Bursitis

Isolated greater trochanteric bursitis is rare and is usually associated with direct trauma in the area. More often, pain in the area of the greater trochanter is associated with pain within the bodies of muscles that attach there (piriformis, gluteus medius and minimus). The pain is often referred along the iliotibial band down along the lateral thigh to the knee. In as many as 50% of patients with a complaint of "sciatica" or "radicular pain" the pain can be reproduced by deep palpation of the hip abductors or external rotators or the iliotibial band.

Injection of the trochanteric bursa is often very effective in obtaining relief of the localized pain (ice massage is also often effective), but without the addition of prolonged gentle stretch of the piriformis, gluteal muscles, and iliotibial band the relief is often short-lived. Use of a cane on the nonsymptomatic side immediately reduces the stress on the muscles mentioned, thereby reducing pain.

TABLE 2. **Causes of Shoulder Pain**

Supraspinatus impingement
Subacromial bursitis
Anterior instability
Acromioclavicular degenerative joint disease
Periarthritis
Rotator cuff tear
Aseptic necrosis of the head of the humerus

"Tennis Elbow"

Lateral epicondylitis is usually secondary to repetitive forceful movements of the wrist and forearm such as flexion and extension, pronation and supination, or power grip. Tenderness over the condyle or just distal to it along with pain on resisted extension of the long finger are typical findings. Injection is seldom necessary, and many clinicians believe that it is contraindicated. Ice massage, avoidance of overuse (perhaps with the use of a volar-based wrist splint), prolonged gentle stretch of the wrist extensors, and a short course of a NSAID are usually successful. For pain that does not respond to these measures, eight to ten sessions of ultrasound (or phonophoresis) followed by stretching can be tried. Once the patient is asymptomatic it is important to stress very gradual return to activity. Counterpressure straps around the proximal forearm help (it is thought) by dissipating the force of extensor pull on the epicondyle.

Heel Pain

Heel pain is usually localized to one of two areas—the insertion of the Achilles tendon or the plantar surface of the heel. The former pain is usually due to Achilles tendinitis or bursitis and is associated with tenderness, occasional fusiform swelling, and "squeaking" of the tendon as it glides through an inflamed synovial sheath. The latter is usually due to plantar fasciitis and is associated with tenderness at the origin of the plantar fascia and severe pain with the first step on arising. Both are overuse injuries and can be associated with overpronation.

Treatment is accomplished with relative rest, ice, NSAIDs, and stretching (of the hamstrings, heel cord, and longitudinal arch). A counterpressure strap for Achilles tendinitis is available and is often helpful. In plantar fasciitis strengthening of the intrinsic muscles of the foot is important, and if pronation is a problem orthotics may be necessary to achieve a cure.

OSTEOARTHRITIS

method of
RICHARD B. TOMPKINS, M.D.
Mayo Clinic
Rochester, Minnesota

Osteoarthritis is the most common form of arthritis. It involves the synovial joints and is characterized by focal loss of cartilage, hypertrophic reaction at the margins of joints, and sclerosis with cyst formation in the subchondral bone. It has a predilection for the distal interphalangeal joints, proximal interphalangeal joints, and carpometacarpal joints of the hands, knees, and hips, and the facet joints of the spine. It is more common in women except in the hips, where it is more common in men. There is no marker for the disease, which is strongly age-related, and there is no clear correlation between pathology, radiographic findings, and symptoms.

Changes in the cartilage are characterized by cartilage degeneration, regeneration, microfractures with fibrillation, fissures, and loss. The changes in bone are secondary to the changes in cartilage, and synovial inflammation can be seen.

As seen in Table 1, osteoarthritis can be idiopathic or secondary to a variety of joint problems. Symptoms consist of joint pain, stiffness and gelling, swelling, decreased mobility, instability, and deformity. Initially the pain is aggravated by use and is relieved by rest, but as the disease progresses rest pain can occur. Particularly in the hip and knee, pain can be referred away from the involved joint. In contrast to rheumatoid arthritis, the stiffness and gelling with rest usually clear quickly when the joint is used. When the facet joints and intervertebral disks of the cervical or lumbar spine are involved, neurologic symptoms secondary to compression can occur including radicular pain, long tract symptoms secondary to compression of the cervical spine, and cauda equina symptoms secondary to involvement of the lumbar spine.

Diagnostic radiographs show narrowing, often asymmetrical, of the involved joints, osteophytes at the margins of the joints, and subchondral bone cysts and sclerosis. Frequently there is no correlation between the radiologic findings and symptoms.

Some combination of tenderness, effusion, inflammation, deformity, and decreased function is found on examination of the peripheral joints. When the spine is involved, there is usually decreased motion. Neurologic findings depend on the structure being compressed and may consist of spasticity with upper motor neuron signs when the cervical cord is compressed, weakness with decreased reflexes and sphincteric disturbances when the cauda equina is compressed, and weakness with decreased reflexes when radicular symptoms are present.

Synovial fluid examination characteristically shows low total white blood cell counts (less than 2000 per mL) and a predominance of mononuclear cells. Calcium pyrophosphate dihydrate crystals are found in chondrocalcinosis and occasionally other calcium crystals are seen as well. In some of the unusual causes of secondary osteoarthritis, abnormalities in peripheral blood and urine examinations are found, but in the more common forms of the disease these examinations are normal.

Management of osteoarthritis consists of physical therapy, occupational therapy, and pharmacotherapy. Physical therapy and occupational therapy are used to maintain or improve range of motion, maintain or increase muscle strength, and relieve both pain and stiffness. Canes or crutches can be used to relieve weight bearing in osteoarthritis of the lower extremities, and orthotics can be used to manage problems in the feet and ankles. Anti-inflammatory medications or simple analgesics such as acetaminophen are commonly used, but narcotics should be avoided. Intra-articular corticosteroid injections can be helpful, but repeated injections of any single joint should be avoided. Surgery can consist of arthroscopy, osteotomy, fusion, or arthroplasty. For joints with severe involvement such as knees and hips, arthroplasty is the preferred treatment.

TABLE 1. **Classification of Osteoarthritis**

Primary or idiopathic
Secondary
Post-inflammatory (e.g., rheumatoid arthritis)
Post-traumatic
Metabolic (e.g., ochronosis, hemochromatosis, acromegaly)
Anatomic (congenital dislocation of hip, aseptic necrosis)
Neurogenic (diabetic neuropathy, syringomyelia)

POLYMYALGIA RHEUMATICA AND GIANT CELL ARTERITIS

method of
STEVEN A. LAUTER, M.D.
Washington University School of Medicine
St. Louis, Missouri

Polymyalgia rheumatica is a syndrome of the elderly, characterized by aching and stiffness of the neck, shoulders, and pelvic girdle. There is no known cause, and the disease occurs about two to three times as often in women. Criteria for diagnosis included in most definitions are the presence of constitutional symptoms such as low-grade fever, weight loss, fatigue, disease duration of greater than 1 month, and an elevated erythrocyte sedimentation rate (ESR) of greater than 50 mm per hour. Some practitioners also include a rapid response to corticosteroids. The differential diagnosis includes other inflammatory and noninflammatory rheumatic diseases (seronegative rheumatoid arthritis, polymyositis, and fibromyalgia), malignant neoplasms, and occult infections such as subacute bacterial endocarditis.

Giant cell arteritis is a form of a large- or medium-size vessel vasculitis that occurs in the same age group as polymyalgia rheumatica. Symptoms may be systemic or local. Systemic symptoms include anorexia and weight loss, fever (sometimes high), night sweats, depression, and myalgias as seen in polymyalgia rheumatica. Localized symptoms are most often secondary to involvement of the branches of the carotid arteries. These include headache, jaw claudication, scalp tenderness, and visual disturbances. Occasionally other large-size vessels such as the branches of the aotic arch or the abdominal aorta may be involved, leading to either peripheral claudication or aneurysms. The diagnosis is verified by temporal artery biopsy.

Polymyalgia rheumatica and giant cell arteritis are believed to be part of a spectrum of the same underlying disorder. Giant cell arteritis occurs in almost 20% of patients who have polymyalgia, and the great majority have symptoms suggesting giant cell arteritis.

TREATMENT

The goal of therapy in patients with polymyalgia rheumatica is to abolish the symptoms and not overlook the possibility of occult giant cell arteritis. If the disease is mild and of brief duration, aspirin or nonsteroidal anti-inflammatory agents may be tried for 7 to 14 days. This approach is successful in only a minority of patients. Most rheumatologists, including myself, favor corticosteroid treatment using 7.5 to 15 mg of prednisone per day. The response to prednisone therapy is more rapid, and patients often obtain dramatic symptomatic relief within a few days, with the ESR falling to a near-normal range within 1 to 2 weeks. At this point the dose of prednisone can be tapered slowly while closely monitoring the patient's clinical status as well as the ESR. Any deviation from the outcome just mentioned should make one suspicious of the original diagnosis. A reasonable approach is to taper the dose of prednisone by 1 to 2.5 mg every 2 weeks until a dose of 5 mg per day is reached and then taper further by 1 mg per month.

The duration of therapy in patients with polymyalgia rheumatica is variable and should be weighed against the risk of corticosteroid treatment in an age group that is more prone to its adverse effects such as osteopenia, cataracts, and peptic ulcer disease. In some patients corticosteroid therapy can be stopped after 1 to 2 years. Many patients, however, require treatment with low doses of 2.5 to 5 mg of prednisone for more than 4 years. Relapses may occur during the tapering of corticosteroids or after therapy has been discontinued. These exacerbations may be lessened by very slow tapering or by the addition of a nonsteroidal anti-inflammatory drug for brief periods while the doctor carefully monitors the patient's clinical state as well as the ESR. An exacerbation may be controlled by raising the dose of prednisone by as little as 1 to 2 mg.

There is little disagreement about the treatment of giant cell arteritis. Once the diagnosis is strongly suspected on the basis of clinical symptoms of headache, jaw claudication, decreased vision, temporal artery tenderness, and a markedly elevated ESR, therapy should be instituted. Prednisone in a dosage of 60 mg, given in a single morning or divided (two to three times per day), should be initiated. Therapy should not be delayed until temporal artery biopsy is performed because treatment is not expected to alter the histologic appearance for at least 1 to 2 weeks or longer. Temporal artery biopsy is performed as an outpatient procedure under a local anesthetic. Skip lesions are known to occur, so it is important to instruct the surgeon to obtain at least 3 cm of artery and it is necessary for the pathologist to prepare multiple sections. Complications of the procedure are rare. If the diagnosis is strongly suspected and the initial biopsy is negative, consideration should be given to a biopsy of the contralateral side. If involvement of larger vessels is suspected, angiography should be performed.

Therapy for giant cell arteritis is begun with high doses of corticosteroids to prevent complications such as blindness. High doses are recommended for at least 1 month or until symptoms abate and the ESR has decreased to normal. Consideration should be given to adding 1.5 grams of calcium per day and 50,000 units of vitamin D weekly in an attempt to counteract corticosteroid-induced osteoporosis. The dose can be tapered by 5 to 10 mg monthly if symptoms are absent and the ESR remains near normal. Relapses are less frequent than in polymyalgia rheumatica but may occur, requiring an increase in the dose of prednisone. The patient should be made alert to this possibility. In some patients steroids can be completely stopped in 1 or 2 years, but, as in patients with polymyalgia rheumatica, some may require ongoing corticosteroid therapy for a number of years. Alternate-day therapy is generally not effective, and patients often experience increased symptoms on the day they are not taking the corticosteroids.

The question often asked in the management of these syndromes is whether a temporal artery biopsy should be performed routinely in patients with polymyalgia rheumatica alone. Several studies have demonstrated that the risk of blindness in patients with polymyalgia rheumatica and no symptoms of giant cell arteritis is extremely low, probably less than 2%. It appears clinically justified to treat these patients with 10 to 15 mg of prednisone per day, stressing repeated clinical observation and frequent measurement of the ESR.

OSTEOMYELITIS

method of
JOSE H. SALGADO, M.D., M.P.H., and
RICHARD N. GREENBERG, M.D.
University of Kentucky College of Medicine
Lexington, Kentucky

The treatment of osteomyelitis should be scientific (not empirical). Treatment should be based on several important criteria: the age of the patient, adequate circulation at the site of infection, presence of necrotic tissue, presence of a foreign body at the site of infection, allergies to medication, and the results of cultures. In addition, treatment is influenced by the patient's signs and symptoms and by whether the infection is acute or chronic. Recent advances have dramatically improved the therapy of osteomyelitis for some patients.

PATHOPHYSIOLOGY

The bones of neonates and infants up to 18 months of age contain numerous transphyseal vessels. In this type of circulation, infection can occur on both sides of the metaphysis and can lead to destruction of the epiphysis and the metaphysis. Neonatal osteomyelitis can be subtle but very destructive, involving numerous bones. The most common pathogens at this time are *Staphylococcus aureus, Haemophilus influenzae* type B, Enterobacteriaceae, and streptococci (groups A and B, and pneumococci).

In children, infection caused by hematogenous spread of organisms most often involves rapidly growing bone (long bones) and tends to start just beneath the metaphysis, where the nutrient arterioles bend. Infection tends to spread through the cortex and may collect under a sturdy periosteum, where it is confined by a fibrous capsule (Brodie's abscess). Any significant collection of purulent material can eventually lead to an ineffective blood supply and avascular bone. Hence, early treatment of children with osteomyelitis provides better long-term results than treatment after the development of purulent material in the periosteum, with subsequent sequestrum (devitalized bone) or involucrum (new periosteal bone). *Staphylococcus aureus* causes osteomyelitis in children of all ages. *Pseudomonas aeruginosa* is generally the cause of osteomyelitis in children older than 9 years.

In adults, because the periosteum is firmly attached to bone, subperiosteal abscesses form infrequently; instead, adults develop chronic suppurative and necrotic lesions with sequestrum and avascular bone. Patients older than 50 years of age may develop osteomyelitis as a result of a contiguous focus of infection (infected surgical wound or a soft tissue infection) or vascular insufficiency.

Osteomyelitis can be classified on the basis of pathogenesis as hematogenous, secondary to contiguous focus of infection, or secondary to peripheral vascular disease. In addition, osteomyelitis can be considered acute or chronic. The symptoms of acute osteomyelitis are typically fever and bone pain; on the other hand, chronic osteomyelitis is often indolent, with periodic exacerbations characterized by sinus tract drainage and associated bony sequestra. A distinction between the two categories of osteomyelitis is sometimes difficult to establish. A classification based on anatomic staging and host factors has been proposed by Mader and Cierney and is found in the 1993 edition of *Conn's Current Therapy.*

SPECIAL CONSIDERATIONS

In addition to age, other important predispositions to osteomyelitis include the presence of diabetes mellitus, sickle cell disease, or severe peripheral vascular disease; the presence of a prosthesis or metal device; immunologic status, a long illness, and a history of fracture, surgery, or trauma; the specific location (e.g., spine, hip, foot); and hematogenous or nonhematogenous origin.

Diabetics often develop foot infections that require a combination of antibiotics because of the presence of multiple organisms: *S. aureus,* Enterobacteriaceae (i.e., aerobic gram-negative rods), *Corynebacterium,* and anaerobic bacteria. These infections heal with adequate débridement and appropriate antibiotics as long as there is adequate circulation. Amputation rather than antimicrobial treatment is indicated when circulation to the infected bone is compromised and inadequate. Circulation to the infected site must be verified either by physical examination or by special vascular studies. Diabetics also often "hide" infection because they have an increased threshold for pain. Hence, not only a detailed examination (especially in paraplegics) but also a scanning procedure (discussed later) may be required to find occult osteomyelitis. Any cellulitis or draining skin lesions in a diabetic patient should be considered to involve the underlying bone until proved otherwise.

Osteomyelitis in a patient with sickle cell disease is frequently associated with hematogenous spread of the organisms. The infection usually occurs in the diaphysis of long bones and is caused by *Salmonella* species, other aerobic gram-negative rods, or *S. aureus.* An important problem in treating these patients is distinguishing between infection and infarction. A negative bone scan suggests the presence of infarction. Osteomyelitis is more likely to cause elevations in temperature, white blood cell count, and erythrocyte sedimentation rate; in addition, the results of a bone scan will be positive. Blood, stool, and bone cultures should be taken and may reveal *Salmonella* species infection. Once cultures have been taken, presumptive treatment should include coverage for *Salmonella* species (e.g., ampicillin, trimethoprim-sulfamethoxazole, ciprofloxacin, or another effective quinolone antibiotic).

The clinical picture of patients with significant peripheral vascular disease can suggest osteomyelitis, even though in actuality these patients have bone infarction caused by significant vascular trauma and interruption of the arterial blood supply. This condition occurs especially often after vascular surgery. Cultures of affected bone (and bone biopsy whenever possible) are needed to rule out infection. Patients with osteomyelitis must be evaluated for adequate circulation to the infected bone.

Patients with a metal apparatus or prosthesis at the infection site cannot be considered curable unless treatment eventually includes removal of the foreign object and sterilization of the site (proved by culture) before the prosthesis is reintroduced. Often the condition of these patients is too severe to permit removal of the foreign object; treatment is then directed toward suppression of the infection. Suppressive treatment is often achieved with oral antibiotics rather than parenteral antibiotics. Regardless of whether treatment is given for cure or suppression, cultures identifying the pathogen are necessary for successful therapy. Suppressive treatment always includes the inherent risk of bacteremia, and patients should be instructed to seek attention if symptoms such as fever, dizziness, and nausea occur. Bacteremia in the presence of an infected appliance demands removal of the foreign object.

Immunologically compromised patients can harbor unusual pathogens. Culturing must be extensive, and consideration must be given to the possibility of finding unusual bacterial and fungal species. One such fungal pathogen, *Sporothrix schenckii,* often infects joints or may appear as a cellulitis but actually has invaded the underlying bone. Sporotrichosis is associated with contamination of wounds through gardening or other contact with the soil. Other fungal pathogens include *Blastomyces dermatitidis, Histoplasma capsulatum, Cryptococcus neoformans, Candida* species, *Mucor* species, and *Coccidioides immitis.*

Location of the lesion often suggests a pathogen and influences the presumptive treatment. Osteomyelitis of the spine is occasionally seen after hematogenous dissemination of uropathogens (*Escherichia coli, Klebsiella* species), *S. aureus,* group B streptococci, or *Mycobacterium tuberculosis.* The spine is the most frequent site of tuberculous osteomyelitis in adults, whereas the metaphysis of long bones is the most frequent site in children (followed by the hip and the knee). *Mycobacterium tuberculosis* is the most common pathogen involving the ribs. Rarely, other mycobacteria are bone pathogens. Infection of the foot after a nail puncture is frequently caused by *Pseudomonas aeruginosa,* presumably introduced from the host's own skin flora. Anaerobic osteomyelitis (especially *Bacteroides* species) may occur in the long bones and in the skull and facial bones in association with previous fractures, diabetes, sinusitis, or human bites.

Bone infections related to trauma (open fractures) may be caused by pathogens from the host's own flora or by those introduced by the contaminating elements. Human bites can lead to osteomyelitis involving mouth flora, including anaerobic organisms. Cat bites can introduce *Pasteurella multocida* (a common organism in the oral secretions of cats) or *Rochalimaea* species. *Rochalimaea* infection is most often found in patients with acquired immune deficiency syndrome (AIDS). Dog bites may introduce aerobic gram-negative rods including *Capnocytophaga* (DF-2 organisms or dysgonic fermenters: slow-growing, gram-negative rods commonly found in the oral secretions of dogs) as well as anaerobic organisms.

Hematogenous osteomyelitis in children is nearly always caused by *S. aureus.* This organism also is common in bone infections related to indwelling catheters (e.g., in hemodialysis patients) or intravenous infections (e.g., drug addicts). Drug addicts sometimes develop osteomyelitis caused by gram-negative rods (especially *P. aeruginosa*) and *Candida* species.

Nonhematogenous osteomyelitis either is a result of contiguous spread of pathogens from nearby infected soft tissue (e.g., decubital ulcers) or is related to trauma. These patients may not exhibit systemic signs unless the infection becomes bacteremic as well. Surgical wound infection after midsternotomy may lead to sternal osteomyelitis; the bacteria most frequently found are *S. aureus, Staphylococcus epidermidis,* and *P. aeruginosa.*

Vertebral osteomyelitis is generally acquired after bacteremia originating from infections of the skin, intravenous drug abuse, urinary tract infections, and endocarditis. The patient complains of dull back pain and progressive paraplegia caused by an epidural abscess. The etiologic diagnosis is made by blood cultures or isolation of pathogens from a needle biopsy of the vertebral body or disk space. *S. aureus* and Enterobacteriaceae are more frequently isolated, but tuberculosis, salmonellosis, brucellosis, candidiasis, or other fungi can also involve the spine. Magnetic nuclear resonance imaging (MRI) is extremely helpful in evaluating the extent of infection in vertebral osteomyelitis. MRI is more precise than computed tomography (CT) scans and may preclude a myelogram.

PATIENT EVALUATION

The patient's history may provide clues about the types of pathogens present. These clues include nail puncture (*P. aeruginosa*); exposure to plants (*S. schenckii*) or sea water (atypical mycobacteria, *Vibrio* species, and *Aeromonas* species); recent skin infection (*S. aureus*); human bite (anaerobes); hemodialysis (*S. aureus*); drug addiction (*Staphylococcus* species, *Pseudomonas* species); dental work or periodontal disease (mouth flora); animal bite or exposure (*Pasteurella multocida,* DF-2 organisms, *Rochalimaea* species and *Brucella* species); and exposure to tuberculosis.

The duration of the infection is particularly important in children. It seems that if acute osteomyelitis is treated early (within 1 week of the onset of symptoms), shorter courses of antibiotics (3 to 4 weeks instead of 6 weeks) without surgical débridement may be effective. Thus, the duration of chills, sweating, fever, malaise, and pain; inability to flex or move the involved area; joint pain; redness or erythema of skin; swelling of soft tissue; or muscle spasms should be assessed.

Chronic infections are often characterized by drainage or open sinus tracts, and prior pathogens tend to be the current ones. A foul odor from sinus tract drainage is highly suggestive of the presence of anaerobes. Unusual pathogens may be present in immunologically compromised patients or in those who have recently traveled to tropical areas. Any metal or prosthetic devices should be identified.

Identification of a history of drug allergies is essential. Any recent surgery or joint aspirations (or injections) should be noted.

It is important to realize that neonates may have no signs or symptoms except for fever, vomiting, diarrhea, or all three.

Physical examination should identify the area involved (e.g., tenderness to palpation, swelling, redness, and warmth over the infected bone). A draining sinus with a feculent odor indicates the presence of anaerobic pathogens. In children especially there may be only an inability to move the adjacent joint. Systemic signs include not only fever, chills, and malaise but also evidence of an underlying disease (periodontal disease, sinusitis, signs of diabetes mellitus, or signs of decreased peripheral circulation such as decreased pulses and lack of nail bed filling).

LABORATORY EVALUATION

Laboratory evaluation includes a white blood cell count with differential count and a Westergren erythrocyte sedimentation rate. These test results are followed during treatment and should return to normal or pre-infection values if the osteomyelitis is cured or suppressed. Other blood tests used for particular patients may include a sickle cell preparation or determination of blood glucose level. A skin test for tuberculosis is indicated in any patient with spine or rib osteomyelitis or an infection that does not appear to have an easily identified bacterial pathogen as a cause.

IMAGING

Radiographic films, radionuclide scans, computed tomography, and magnetic resonance imaging are used to locate the infection and to observe for spread of infection. Because these procedures can be expensive (Table 1), judgment and restraint are required to order only the tests that are indi-

TABLE 1. **Cost of Radiographic and Scanning Procedures***

Procedure	Cost (U.S.$)
Radiograph (foot)	$57
Radiograph (spine)	$73
Three-phase bone scan	$313
Total body scan	$375
CT scan of lumbar spine (with contrast)	$517
^{111}In-labeled leukocyte scan, total body scan	$639
Total body gallium scan	$650
MRI scan of lumbar spine (with contrast)	$800

*1994, University of Kentucky Medical Center. Does not include physician charge.

cated. Radiographic films should be obtained of the area or areas in which osteomyelitis is suspected based on the history or physical examination. The first radiographic sign of osteomyelitis is soft tissue swelling (there may be no such evidence for up to 14 days). Later, bone destruction and periosteal elevation occur.

A technetium-99m bone scan is specific for increased osteoblastic activity or bone formation (it is not diagnostic for infected bone because it can be positive in areas of trauma, tumor, synovitis, arthritis, or noninfected inflammatory processes). It is positive as early as 3 days after the onset of symptoms and is helpful in locating the osteomyelitis when the radiograph appears normal. The scan can miss infected avascular areas. This test is unnecessary if the involved area is known. Our review of 30 studies evaluating ^{99m}Tc three-phase bone scans in 1460 patients with suspected bone infections found a combined sensitivity of 547/591 (93%) but a low specificity of 553/869 (64%).

Although the ^{67}Ga citrate scan may be more specific for infection, it is less sensitive than the ^{99m}Tc scan, and its resolution is not as good in small bones. A large amount of purulent material and active phagocytosis at the infected site are required to produce a positive scan. A review of 15 papers evaluating ^{67}Ga citrate scans in the diagnosis of osteomyelitis found an overall sensitivity of 209/257 (81%) and a specificity of 188/272 (69%). This scan is unnecessary if the involved area has been identified.

The ^{111}In-labeled leukocyte scan uses the labeling of the host's own leukocytes, which are then reinjected into the patient and accumulate in areas of infection. The scan is specific for osteomyelitis when the infection occurs in areas of increased bone remodeling. We reviewed 22 published studies evaluating ^{111}In-labeled leukocyte scans in a total of 1199 patients with suspected osteomyelitis and found a sensitivity of 498/586 (85%) and a specificity of 549/613 (85%). The false-positive results were primarily caused by the presence of rheumatoid arthritis, healing fractures, noninfected prostheses, and metastatic carcinoma.

When infection is extensive or near vital organs, CT scan or MRI is helpful. These expensive studies are of special value in following vertebral osteomyelitis and infection involving the skull, pelvic area, or hips. Both modalities can delineate the depth and extent of bone involvement. MRI has the best resolution. We reviewed 14 studies in which MRI was used in the diagnosis of possible osteomyelitis; the overall sensitivity was 245/261 (94%) and the specificity was 154/174 (89%).

Two experimental imaging modalities appear promising: the ^{99}Tc-HMPAO-labeled leukocyte scan has a reported sensitivity of 91/103 (88%) and a specificity of 71/86 (83%), and labeled antigranulocyte antibodies have a reported sensitivity of 172/193 (89%) and a specificity of 118/136 (87%).

When radiographic results are normal and bone infection is still a consideration, the current practice is to obtain a whole-body three-phase bone scan or gallium scan in neonates and children and a ^{99m}Tc bone scan, an MRI, or a CT scan in adults.

It is not possible at this time to claim with certainty that positive scans indicate a need for continued treatment of an infection. Treatment should end at 6 weeks if the clinical condition has completely healed, or when the patient's condition has returned to baseline with no further radiographic evidence of bony destruction. Scans at this time can be misleading and are unnecessary. It is preferable to follow the patient clinically and to re-treat him or her if symptoms recur or to continue treatment if the infection has not totally healed.

ISOLATION OF THE PATHOGEN

Blood cultures (up to three sets, each drawn at a different time) show the pathogen in most cases of acute hematogenous osteomyelitis but rarely in cases of chronic osteomyelitis (less than 5%). Bone cultures identify the pathogen in nearly all cases of acute osteomyelitis and in at least 60% of chronic infections.

Treatment should never start until after at least one set of blood cultures (aerobic and anaerobic) has been taken. Furthermore, an aspirated sample from the infected bone should be obtained with a 16- or 18-gauge needle (with an inner stylet if possible) before treatment is begun. Because acute hematogenous osteomyelitis can be associated with potential life-threatening complications, every effort should be made to obtain blood and bone material for culture quickly so that presumptive treatment with antibiotics can begin. In contrast, patients with chronic osteomyelitis need not be treated until surgical débridement and gathering of material for bone cultures has been performed. Treatment for these patients can begin in the operating room once material for cultures has been obtained.

If bone aspiration is attempted, the needle should enter through an uninvolved area of skin that has been prepared with an iodine-containing disinfectant (iodine disinfectants work quickly, whereas alcohol requires several minutes to sterilize). Lidocaine can be used only to anesthetize the skin; it should not be injected along the periosteum because it can retard bacterial growth in culture. Specimens from infected bone should be analyzed for Gram's stain and for aerobic, anaerobic, mycobacterial, and fungal cultures. Even if only a few drops of serous-sanguineous material are obtained, they should be sent to the pathology laboratory for, at least, culture and Gram's stain. When patients are immunocompromised (including those with human immunodeficiency virus infection) or are suspected of harboring fungal pathogens, bone should also be stained for fungal pathogens. In addition, these stains must include a silver stain if *Rochalimaea* species are suspected.

Transport of the material to the laboratory is critical, and one should consult the laboratory personnel for the best transport method available in the hospital. If transport medium is not available, one should leave the material in the syringe and send it to the laboratory as quickly as possible.

Deep wound cultures or cultures taken from sinus tracts are misleading and a waste of money. Skin-colonizing organisms may mislead the physician, and the true pathogens may not be recovered.

Stool and urine cultures for *Salmonella* species are indicated for patients with sickle cell disease.

TREATMENT

Basic Concepts

Treatment of osteomyelitis requires removal of necrotic, avascular, infected bone and relatively long-term antibiotic treatment. Amputation may be necessary if an inadequate blood supply cannot be improved. Surgery is not necessary for every patient because children and neonates treated early for acute hematogenous osteomyelitis are often cured with appropriate antibiotic treatment alone.

Chronic osteomyelitis requires surgical débridement for cure. The type of surgery is determined by the extent of the infection and may include removing a metal appliance or prosthesis or immobilizing bone.

For infected knee arthroplasties, resection arthroplasty is much more efficient than débridement alone in controlling the infection. If a foreign object must remain in place to stabilize a fracture or maintain a joint, antimicrobial treatment should be designed to suppress the infection and allow the patient to be discharged from the hospital. Suppressive treatment is usually provided by an oral antibiotic given for several months and is restarted if symptoms recur. An occasional patient may require nearly lifelong daily administration of antibiotics to suppress infection in a prosthetic joint. If all foreign objects can be removed from the bone, a cure is attempted. For patients with large or multiloculated cavities in long bones or with long bone infections for which bone grafting can be used, the Ilizarov procedure should be considered. This radical and relatively painful procedure has succeeded in eradicating debilitating chronic osteomyelitis that is refractory to all other treatments.

Initial Treatment

Choice of antibiotic depends on which pathogen is present. Empirical treatment does not exist. Once cultures have been taken, it is important to select the appropriate treatment on the basis of the patient's evaluation. If the patient is acutely ill (possibly bacteremic), an initial combination of antimicrobials such as vancomycin, an aminoglycoside (e.g., gentamicin, tobramycin, or amikacin), and metronidazole in an adult or cefotaxime and an aminoglycoside in a child can be used. This coverage is extensive (and potentially toxic) but may be necessary in a severely ill individual with acute hematogenous osteomyelitis. The regimen is changed to appropriate (cost-effective) and safer drugs as soon as the culture reports are available.

Treatment Guidelines

Parenteral or oral antibiotics, or both, are preferable to local application of antibiotics alone. One can determine whether the choice (a parenteral or oral antibiotic) is appropriate by obtaining serum bactericidal levels against isolated pathogens. Serum bactericidal activity is the only true laboratory measure of an antibiotic's effectiveness in osteomyelitis. In adults, trough (just before the next dose) serum bactericidal (i.e., not serum bacteriostatic) levels should exist at 1:2 dilutions or higher of serum in patients with acute bone disease and at 1:4 dilutions or higher serum with chronic bone disease. In children, peak (30 minutes after dosing) serum bactericidal levels should exist at 1:8 dilutions or higher except for streptococci, which should be at 1:32 dilutions or higher.

Children who respond after only 2 weeks of intravenous treatment may be switched to an effective oral antibiotic for an additional 3 to 4 weeks. Treatment for cure requires a total of 6 or more weeks of antibiotic therapy except in cases of vertebral osteomyelitis, mycobacterial disease, or fungal disease. Vertebral osteomyelitis therapy continues for up to 6 months and is stopped only when radiographs and computed tomography or MRI show no further disease and the Westergren erythrocyte sedimentation rate has returned to baseline. Mycobacterial disease is usually treated initially with four drugs: isoniazid (isoniazid use requires pyridoxine as well), rifampin, pyrazinamide, and ethambutol. Treatment should continue until the possibility of multidrug-resistant tuberculosis is ruled out. If *M. tuberculosis* is not drug resistant, isoniazid, rifampin, and pyrazinamide are continued for 2 months, followed by isoniazid and rifampin for an additional 4 months. If the patient is unable to take both isoniazid and rifampin, alternative drugs must be used and continued for up to 18 months. Two effective drugs should always be used to treat active tuberculosis. Fungal therapy requires amphotericin B or perhaps a new imidazole derivative (ketoconazole, fluconazole, or itraconazole); the treatment plan should be discussed with an infectious disease specialist.

Antibiotics for Specific Organisms

For osteomyelitis caused by *Staphylococcus* species, an appropriate initial choice is oxacillin or nafcillin (vancomycin for methicillin-resistant staphylococci or for the patient with penicillin allergy) (Table 2). No oral agent can be relied on to provide consistently adequate serum bactericidal levels against staphylococci. Once the patient has shown clinical improvement and has been treated with parenteral antimicrobials for several weeks, oral regimens may be tried. Patients treated with oral agents must be carefully observed for signs of treatment failure and must have adequate serum bactericidal levels. Oral agents with antistaphylococcal activity include cloxacillin, dicloxacillin, and clindamycin. These agents could be combined with rifampin, which has been shown to enhance nafcillin activity in chronic staphylococcal osteomyelitis. Rifampin should not be used alone because patients rapidly develop resistance to it. Currently available quinolone antibiotics are rarely effective treatment for staphylococcal osteomyelitis. We use them only as a last resort because we have found them frequently ineffective. When quinolone antibiotics are used, great care must be taken to observe and evaluate the patient frequently.

Osteomyelitis caused by *Streptococcus* species is treated with penicillin; Penicillin-allergic patients may receive vancomycin, a first-generation cephalosporin, a long-acting cephalosporin (ceftriaxone, cefonicid), or clindamycin. Currently available quinolones are ineffective.

Osteomyelitis caused by *Haemophilus* species (a consideration in children) is treated with ampicillin, cefotaxime, trimethoprim-sulfamethoxazole (co-trimoxazole), a quinolone, cefuroxime, or ceftriaxone.

Bone infections caused by Enterobacteriaceae (e.g., *E. coli*, *Klebsiella* species, *Proteus* species) are treated with ampicillin (if the pathogen is sensitive), a third-

TABLE 2. **Antibiotic Preferences for Osteomyelitis***

Organism	Drug	Children (mg/kg)	Daily Dose Adults	Hours Between Doses	Route of Administration	Wholesale Daily Price (U.S.$)‡
Methicillin-sensitive *Staphylococcus aureus*	Nafcillin (Nafcil) (oxacillin [Bactocill])	50–100	8 grams†	6	IV	$68.06
	Cefazolin (Ancef)	40–100	6 grams	8	IV	$20.35
	Clindamycin (Cleocin)	20–40	2.7 grams	8	IV	$18.60
Methicillin-resistant *S. aureus* and other staphylococci	Vancomycin (Vancocin)	15–40	2 grams	12	IV	$21.87
Streptococcus species	Penicillin	100,000–200,000 U 100–300	15–20 million U	4–6	IV	$15.02
Enterobacteriaceae (*Escherichia coli, Proteus* species, *Klebsiella* species)	Ampicillin	100–300†	8 grams	6	IV	$18.72
	Aztreonam (Azactam)	—	6 grams	8	IV	$82.76
	Cefotaxime (Claforan)	50–200	6 grams	8	IV	$57.70
	Aminoglycosides‖					
	Ciprofloxacin (Cipro)	—	1.5 grams	12	PO	$10.32
Pseudomonas species	Aminoglycosides with aztreonam§	—	8 grams (aztreonam)	6	IV	$110.34
	Aminoglycosides with ceftazidime	30–100	6 grams (ceftazidime)	8	IV	$90.06
	Aminoglycosides with piperacillin	—	16–18 grams (piperacillin)	4	IV	$79.30
Salmonella species (ampicillin-sensitive, ampicillin-resistant)	Ampicillin	100–300	8 grams	6	IV	$18.72
	Trimethoprim-sulfamethoxazole (Bactrim, Septra)	10/50	480/2400–640/3200 mg†	6–12	IV	$48.62
	Ciprofloxacin	—	1.5 grams	12	PO	$10.32
Haemophilus species (ampicillin-sensitive, ampicillin-resistant)	Ampicillin	100–300	8 grams	6	IV	$18.72
	Cefotaxime	50–200	6 grams	8	IV	$57.70
	Trimethoprim-sulfamethoxazole	10/50	480/2400–640/3200 mg†	8–12	IV	$48.62
	Aztreonam	—	6 grams	8	IV	$82.72
Anaerobes	Metronidazole (Flagyl)¶	15–35	1.5–2 grams	8–6	PO or IV	$0.30 or $23.43
	Clindamycin	25–40†	2.7 grams	8	IV	$18.60
	Ampicillin/Sulbactam (UnaSyn)	110/55	12/4 grams	6	IV	$52.25

*The drug listed is the first choice. Other drugs are options if reason exists to choose an alternative agent. Daily dose assumes normal renal function.
†May exceed manufacturer's recommended dose.
‡Wholesale prices according to the Red Book, 1993.
§In severe *Pseudomonas* infections (potential for bacteremia is present), the combination of an aminoglycoside and a beta-lactam agent should be used. Aztreonam, the most specific beta-lactam for *Pseudomonas* species, is preferred.
‖The most cost-effective aminoglycoside is gentamicin, followed by netilmicin. Tobramycin and amikacin are least cost effective. Aminoglycosides could be used initially until sensitivities are known but should be discontinued if the Enterobacteriaceae species are sensitive to less toxic agents.
¶Safety and efficacy in children have not been established.

generation cephalosporin (cefotaxime), a monobactam (aztreonam), an aminoglycoside (gentamicin), or a quinolone. *Pseudomonas* infections of bone require an aminoglycoside (gentamicin) and a beta-lactam antibiotic such as ceftazidime or aztreonam. Ciprofloxacin is always ineffective if the minimal inhibitory concentration of the *Pseudomonas* species is equal to or greater than 1 μg per mL. We have not found the current quinolone antibiotics effective in the treatment of *Pseudomonas* osteomyelitis.

Anaerobic osteomyelitis is treated with metronidazole; this agent can be given orally (over 80% absorption). Other choices include intravenous clindamycin, piperacillin, cefoxitin, cefotetan, or other agents with adequate anaerobic coverage.

Overall, the best antibiotic is the least toxic agent with adequate serum bactericidal activity.

Treatment with Oral Agents

A combination of the oral agents ciprofloxacin and metronidazole should be excellent for osteomyelitis caused by Enterobacteriaceae and anaerobes. After adequate débridement, these drugs may be reasonable for treatment of osteomyelitis of the foot. However, such coverage is *inadequate* for elimination of *Pseudomonas* species, *S. aureus,* or *Streptococcus* species. At this time, oral therapy is possible if the patient can receive oral medication, is able to absorb drugs via the gastrointestinal tract, and has an anaerobic pathogen (metronidazole) and/or an Enterobacteriaceae organism (ciprofloxacin or a comparable quinolone). Oral treatment is also indicated for suppressive therapy for an infected prosthesis. The combination of rifampin and ofloxacin was successful in

74% of patients with *Staphylococcus*-infected orthopedic implants when given for up to 9 months.

Local Treatment with Beads, Cement, and Flaps

Local administration of antibiotics to bone is currently being studied. Antibiotic-impregnated polymethyl methacrylate beads placed in open bone cavities after débridement have yielded good results in animal models. In vitro studies also suggest that local delivery of an appropriate antibiotic is possible. If beads are to be used, the antibiotic must remain active against the pathogen once the bone has been prepared with the polymethyl methacrylate. The use of aminoglycosides in impregnated beads has been studied most thoroughly; these agents are stable and active against sensitive aerobic, gram-negative rods and staphylococci. Aminoglycosides cannot be used for streptococci or anaerobic infections. Beads need to be removed or replaced after 2 to 3 weeks because a dense fibrous tissue starts to surround them. There is also a real concern that these beads could act as foreign bodies and could harbor pathogens (resistant to antibiotics in the beads), thus prolonging the infection. Not enough data are available to recommend treatment with beads alone; however, beads plus systemic antibiotics help to deliver antibiotic to both vascular and avascular areas of infection.

Use of antibiotic-impregnated cement cannot be recommended if its purpose is to deliver antibiotic to an infected area. In theory, the cement could be used as prophylaxis in sterile areas. The use of such cement to prevent infection (rather than systemic antibiotic prophylaxis) is debatable. In uncontrolled trials, the use of antibiotic-impregnated cement has been reported to contribute to successful revision of infected arthroplasties. The primary advantage of antibiotic-impregnated beads and cement is that high local concentrations of antibiotics in bone can be achieved for a short period; serum levels remain nearly negligible, and systemic toxicity is unusual.

Local administration to bone of appropriate antibiotics by means of a drug pump is investigational.

For certain patients (e.g., those with long bone infections), antibiotic beads and microvascular muscle grafting may assist in clearing the infection before bone grafting can be performed. Bone grafts may form the nidus for sequestered bacteria if the wound is not sterile. It is not clear whether hyperbaric oxygen treatment assists in the resolution of osteomyelitis. Hyperbaric oxygen treatment does speed soft tissue healing in areas with vascular compromise.

COMMON SPORTS INJURIES

method of
M. PATRICE EIFF, M.D., and
WILLIAM L. TOFFLER, M.D.
Oregon Health Sciences University
Portland, Oregon

Sports injuries comprise a significant portion of the musculoskeletal problems seen by primary care physicians. With the increasing popularity of sport and exercise in the United States today, physicians need to be prepared to provide care for injuries ranging from prevention to rehabilitation. Sports injuries can result from either acute traumatic injury or chronic overuse.

TRAUMATIC INJURIES

Traumatic sports injuries are those resulting from a specific episode of trauma, either acute or subacute. Traumatic injury to the bone usually results in a fracture or, less commonly, periosteal injury. Traumatic injury to a joint and its surrounding supporting structures may lead to instability such as subluxation or dislocation. A sprain is a stretch or tear of a ligament, and a strain is a stretch or tear of a musculotendinous unit. The classification of sprains and strains is presented in Table 1. Other traumatic sports injuries include contusions, hematomas, abrasions, and lacerations secondary to direct force applied to soft tissues. Most acute sports injuries involve the shoulder, knee, ankle, hand, and wrist. The RICE treatment guidelines should be used for the acute management of traumatic injuries (Table 2).

Shoulder Dislocation

The most common type of shoulder dislocation is an anterior dislocation, usually the result of forced external rotation and abduction of the shoulder. The athlete with a dislocated shoulder has severe pain, resists moving the injured arm, and may have experienced a "popping" sensation. On examination, the athlete is unable to rotate or abduct the arm. The dislocated shoulder may have a sharp square contour compared with the smooth rounded outline of the uninjured shoulder. Radiographs reveal an anterior and slightly inferior displacement of the humerus out of the glenoid fossa.

Prompt reduction before significant muscle spasm

TABLE 1. **Classification of Sprains and Strains**

Grade 1.	Minimal tear or stretching of fibers. Mild swelling, pain, and disability. No muscle weakness or joint instability
Grade 2.	Partial tear of fibers. Moderate amount of swelling, pain, and disability. Partial weakness on muscle contraction or partial joint instability
Grade 3.	Complete tear. Severe pain, swelling, and disability. Extremely weak on muscle testing or definite joint instability

TABLE 2. **Acute Injury Management**

Rest	Helps minimize further injury. Usually necessary for 24 to 48 hours
Ice	Reduces pain, swelling, and spasm. Ice should be applied for 20 minutes every 1 to 2 hours for first 48 hours
Compression	Reduces swelling. An elastic wrap with a foam or felt pad directly over the area of maximal swelling is best
Elevation	Improves fluid drainage and adds to the benefits of ice and compression. Extremities should be higher than cardiac level

or joint swelling develops yields a higher success rate. In athletes with a first-time dislocation, the arm is placed in a sling for 3 to 4 weeks, but in those with chronic recurrent dislocation, immobilization may not be necessary. Rehabilitation has been shown to reduce the rate of recurrence of anterior shoulder dislocations. Goals of shoulder rehabilitation include restoration of full shoulder abduction and strengthening of the rotator cuff muscles, especially those involved with internal and external rotation of the shoulder.

Acromioclavicular Separation

Acromioclavicular (AC) separation, also known as shoulder separation, may occur following a direct blow to the lateral aspect of the shoulder or a fall on an outstretched arm. AC separations are classified as Grade 1, 2, or 3 based on the degree of coracoclavicular ligament injury. Symptoms of an AC separation include immediate pain near the AC joint that becomes worse with arm movement. On examination, the area over the AC joint is found to be tender, and the clavicle may be riding above the level of the acromion. Pulling down on the arm elicits more pain, and swelling and ecchymosis are present in more severe cases. In Grade 2 (partial tear) or Grade 3 (complete tear) injuries, an anteroposterior view of both shoulders will show elevation of the distal clavicle when compared with the opposite side. Treatment of Grade 1 injuries begins with shoulder strengthening exercises when pain allows, which is usually 2 to 7 days following the injury. A Grade 2 injury requires a 10 to 14 day period of immobilization followed by beginning strengthening exercises. Orthopedic consultation should be obtained for a Grade 3 AC separation.

Knee Ligament Injuries

The most common knee ligament injuries are the anterior cruciate ligament (ACL) injuries and collateral ligament injuries. The most common mechanism of an ACL injury is a hyperextension deceleration force on the knee with or without rotation. Immediate pain and moderate to severe swelling within 4 hours after injury are highly suggestive of an ACL injury. A positive Lachman's test confirms the diagnosis. A radiograph of the knee is necessary to rule out a tibial plateau fracture. Athletes with mild laxity and a firm end point on ligament testing can usually be managed with a functional rehabilitation program. Those with marked joint laxity or complaints of giving way on twisting or pivoting motions should be referred to an orthopedic surgeon for possible arthroscopic repair.

The usual mechanism of injury of a collateral ligament tear of the knee is a direct blow to either the medial or lateral side of the knee with the foot planted. The medial collateral ligament (MCL) is most often injured. Ligament stability should be assessed with varus and valgus joint stressing. Early functional knee rehabilitation has been shown to be an effective treatment for Grades 1 and 2 and isolated Grade 3 collateral ligament sprains. The rehabilitation program for collateral ligament injuries emphasizes quadriceps muscle strengthening and hamstring stretching.

Meniscal Injuries

Acute meniscal tears most often occur following a twisting motion of the knee, usually when the athlete is running or cutting. Tears of the medial meniscus are twice as common as lateral tears. Symptoms of a meniscal tear are immediate knee pain, swelling within 12 to 24 hours after the injury, and locking or clicking. Examination findings include joint line tenderness and a painful pop or click with knee motion. Meniscal injury without an associated ligamentous injury can be managed initially with symptomatic treatment and knee rehabilitation. If there is no improvement with this regimen, arthroscopy should be considered for diagnosis and treatment.

Ankle Sprains

Ankle sprains are one of the most common injuries in any sport. The majority of all ankle sprains involve the lateral ligaments following an inversion injury. Common symptoms include immediate pain, a sensation of a pop, swelling, and decreased range of motion. Laxity detected during the anterior drawer and inversion stress test indicates a tear of the anteriotalofibular ligament and calcaneofibular ligament, respectively. Ankle radiographs should be obtained in Grade 2 and 3 injuries to rule out associated fractures or ankle instability as shown by widening of the ankle mortise. Early mobilization of ankle sprains has been shown to be an effective treatment for all injuries regardless of severity. A 24- to 48-hour period of RICE followed by early weight bearing and rehabilitation will return the athlete to activity sooner. An effective ankle rehabilitation program emphasizes range of motion, stretching and strengthening of the calf muscles, and proprioception training. Use of functional bracing such as a lace-up support or an Aircast brace provides increased stability of the ankle during rehabilitation and may prevent reinjury.

Hand and Wrist Injuries

Most traumatic hand and wrist injuries result from a direct blow or fall on an outstretched hand. Finger sprains are common minor injuries and are usually treated successfully with "buddy" taping to an adjacent finger for 2 to 4 weeks. Dislocations without fracture can be managed similarly. Gamekeeper's thumb or skier's thumb, a sprain of the ulnar collateral ligament, results from forced abduction of the thumb. Symptoms include pain and swelling over the ligament and decreased pinch strength if severe. Ligament stressing following radiograph to rule out an associated avulsion fracture is essential to identify complete ligament tears. Complete tears of the ulnar collateral ligament, as demonstrated by marked laxity in full extension, may require surgical repair. Grade 1 and 2 injuries are best treated with a thumb spica cast or splint protection for 4 to 6 weeks. Wrist sprains are common following hyperextension or hyperflexion of the wrist. Radiographs should be obtained to rule out a fracture or scapholunate dislocation. Point tenderness over the anatomic snuffbox following a fall on an outstretched hand may indicate a scaphoid fracture even if the initial films are negative. Repeat films in 10 to 14 days are necessary if a fracture is suspected. Most simple sprains can be managed with splinting and rehabilitation exercises. Persistent pain and swelling for more than 6 to 8 weeks warrant further radiographic evaluation or orthopedic consultation.

OVERUSE INJURIES

Overuse injuries result from microtrauma to soft tissues secondary to repetitive motion or activity. Biomechanical factors such as malalignment or muscle imbalance, poor training techniques, and faulty equipment predispose the athlete to these injuries. Overuse syndromes most commonly involve the musculotendinous unit and result in tendinitis or tenosynovitis. Repetitive mechanical trauma to a joint may result in synovitis or arthritis, and repetitive overuse stress on bones results in periostitis or stress fractures. Overuse injuries are classified according to grades (Table 3). Treatment plans for overuse injuries attempt to control inflammation and restore normal function and mobility through modification of activity and an appropriate rehabilitation program.

TABLE 3. **Guide to Overuse Injuries**

Grades	History	Physical Examination	Treatment
1	"Soreness" or pain, usually hours after activity	Generalized tenderness	Ice
2	Pain late in activity or just after activity	Localized pain	Ice Decrease activity by 25%
3	Pain early or in middle of activity	Point tenderness Erythema Swelling	Ice Decrease activity by 50% NSAID*
4	Pain at rest	Grade 3 signs plus decreased range of motion Impaired function	Ice Rest NSAID

*Nonsteroidal anti-inflammatory drug.

Shoulder Impingement Syndrome

Shoulder impingement syndrome, also known as swimmer's shoulder, is a painful arc syndrome caused by impingement of the supraspinatus and biceps tendon. Following repetitive overhead motion, the supraspinatus and biceps tendons are subjected to repeated microtrauma, causing inflammation. The athlete with shoulder impingement complains of anterior shoulder pain and decreased abduction. Tenderness over the coracoacromial ligament or biceps tendon and pain elicited with forward flexion past 180 degrees suggest impingement. Control of inflammation with ice massage and nonsteroidal anti-inflammatory medications is useful when symptoms of impingement are most prominent. Rehabilitation exercises include stretching of the rotator cuff muscles, strengthening of internal and external rotators, and weighted shoulder flexibility exercises.

Tennis Elbow

Lateral epicondylitis, better known as tennis elbow, is a periostitis at the attachment of the extensor carpi radialis brevis tendon to the lateral epicondyle and is a common overuse syndrome in any activity that requires gripping. Dull, aching, lateral elbow pain is characteristic, and rest from the offending activity usually relieves the symptoms. On examination, point tenderness is found over the lateral epicondyle, and pain is elicited by shaking hands. Ice massage alternated with friction massage helps to control inflammation. Steroid injection in the area of the lateral epicondyle should be considered as a first-line treatment to control inflammation. Use of a counterforce brace placed just distal to the lateral epicondyle may reduce the amount of friction over the epicondyle and may diminish pain. Improved backhand technique and a slightly larger grip size can also be useful. A rehabilitation program emphasizing stretching and strengthening exercises of the forearm extensors and flexors can help prevent this problem from recurring.

Patellofemoral Pain Syndrome

Patellofemoral pain syndrome, the most frequent knee problem in runners, comprises a number of conditions all characterized by peripatellar pain. Risk factors for this condition include excessive mileage, rapid change in the training routine, and improper running shoes. Patellofemoral pain also results from a biomechanical abnormality of the hips, knees, ankles, or feet. This syndrome is characterized by peripatellar aching that often becomes worse with descending stairs, squatting, or maintaining prolonged flexion. Examination begins with a search for biomechanical factors that may aggravate symptoms. Often the knee examination is entirely normal despite the presence of continued symptoms. Treatment of this condition focuses on correction of any biomechanical abnormality combined with a functional rehabilitation program. Modification of activity to include decreased mileage or pace for the runner or avoidance of activities requiring excessive flexion is often useful. The rehabilitation program emphasizes hamstring stretching and quadriceps muscle strengthening. Icing the knee before and after exercise and using nonsteroidal anti-inflammatory medications allow a quicker return to activity.

Plantar Fasciitis

Plantar fasciitis, an inflammation of the plantar fascia at its insertion on the base of the calcaneus, is the most common cause of heel pain in runners. Predisposing factors include flat feet, hyperpronation, and tight calf muscles. The pain associated with plantar fasciitis is usually localized to the base of the heel at the point of the insertion of the fascia into the calcaneus. The pain is worse in the morning and is sometimes relieved with activity. The presence of a heel spur on foot radiographs is indicative of a more chronic problem and is not a useful aid in the diagnosis or management of this condition. Ice massage, nonsteroidal anti-inflammatory medications, and decreased activity help to alleviate inflammatory symptoms. Proper shoe wear with excellent heel support and arch support or orthotics help in treatment and prevention. Rehabilitation exercises emphasize calf muscle stretching and strengthening of the foot muscles. Successful treatment of plantar fasciitis often takes up to 8 weeks.

Section 15

Obstetrics and Gynecology

ANTEPARTUM CARE

method of
CARL V. SMITH, M.D.
University of Nebraska College of Medicine
Omaha, Nebraska

PRECONCEPTION COUNSELING

Preconception counseling is perhaps the most neglected area in all of health care. Primary care physicians who are evaluating patients for illnesses unrelated to pregnancy may not remember to consider the effects of chronic disease and medical therapy on pregnancy. The converse is also true. Similarly, health care maintenance may be overlooked.

All women of childbearing age who have the potential to become pregnant should undergo preconception counseling. A complete review of systems and a physical examination frequently identify areas of potential concern. In general, the following components serve as a framework with which to conduct a preconception counseling session: family history, genetic history, current medication use, substance abuse, nutrition, environmental factors, and obstetric history.

A family history of medical diseases should be elicited from every pregnant patient. In many instances, the family history (e.g., of hypertension or atherosclerotic heart disease) will not affect the current pregnancy. However, diseases such as diabetes mellitus may adversely affect maternal and fetal well-being. Therefore, screening selected patients for diabetes prior to conception may reduce the incidence of poor diabetic control at conception. Poor control is associated with higher rates of fetal malformations and perinatal morbidity and mortality.

Genetic diseases may also complicate pregnancy. When a genetic disorder is uncovered, consideration should be given to referring the patient to a genetic counselor for more specific information. Factors important to the patient undergoing preconception counseling include the risk of recurrence, the availability and reliability of prenatal diagnosis, and the clinical and social significance of the particular disorder. Specifically, prenatal diagnosis may alter the obstetric or neonatal management. Only in this way can the morbidity and mortality associated with genetic disorders be reduced.

A complete medical history is important to allow the clinician to understand the interaction between pregnancy and the medical disease. Of critical importance is the need to obtain optimal control of the medical problem. Patients with diabetes mellitus benefit from tight preconception diabetic control, which substantially reduces the incidence of complications. Timing of pregnancy is also very important for patients with chronic medical disease. Diseases such as chronic hypertension, renal disease, and systemic lupus erythematosus are of much less concern when they are either controlled or inactive at the time of conception. Last, and perhaps most important, medical therapy may affect the pregnancy. For example, medical treatment of hypertension with angiotensin-converting enzyme (ACE) inhibitors is contraindicated. Some patients may require anticoagulation with warfarin (Coumadin), which is not recommended during pregnancy. In many cases the most appropriate choice is to change the medical therapy to one that poses a lower risk to the pregnancy (e.g., heparin). The average patient takes three or four over-the-counter medications during pregnancy. The best time to alert patients that indiscriminate use of over-the-counter substances to relieve minor aches and pains during pregnancy is neither needed nor appropriate is prior to conception.

Alcohol and tobacco use remain active problems for society in general. Although the clinician frequently becomes frustrated with a patient who does not seek or heed advice, it is our experience that patients are more likely to be successful in stopping substance abuse when they are contemplating pregnancy. They may be personally unwilling to suffer withdrawal symptoms from nicotine and alcohol but may do so to benefit the fetus. Intensive education with or without the use of nicotine substitutes may be appropriate. The safety of these alternative sources of nicotine for pregnant patients is largely unknown. The chronic abuser of narcotics and cocaine presents special problems for health care providers. Identification of these patients preconceptually may offer health care providers the opportunity to enroll them in treatment programs prior to the time of pregnancy. Unfortunately, most patients who abuse drugs do not seek early prenatal care.

A detailed social and work history is important in the preconception examination. A surprising number of women work in hazardous areas and may be exposed to dangerous chemicals. When helping patients plan for pregnancy, it is important to inquire about their daily life. In some instances, training for different job opportunities may be the most appropriate solution to the problem. In many others, the use of protective devices may reduce the overall risk to both the patient and her as yet unconceived fetus.

Last, a detailed obstetric history is important. A

prior history of an uncomplicated pregnancy and delivery usually enables the physician to reassure the patient that the subsequent pregnancy outcome will probably be similar. When pregnancies have been complicated, medical therapy may be initiated prior to delivery to improve the outcome. Patients with a history of severe preeclampsia or severe chronic hypertension may benefit from low-dose aspirin (60 to 80 mg per day) to reduce the incidence of severe or superimposed preeclampsia. Similarly, patients with multiple pregnancy losses secondary to lupus anticoagulant or anticardiolipin antibodies may also benefit from low-dose aspirin with or without low-dose corticosteroids.

Obstetric care has largely failed to reduce the incidence of preterm birth in this country. Identification of the patient at risk for preterm birth allows the patient to be enrolled in intensive prenatal and preconception education programs. Lifestyle changes such as reducing physical activity and abandoning the use of tobacco and alcohol may reduce the risk of recurrent premature birth.

FIRST PRENATAL VISIT

Establishing the Estimated Date of Delivery

Confirming an accurate estimated date of delivery (EDD) is an important goal in the management of normal and high-risk pregnancies. Subsequent recommendations for management depend on the gestational age of the fetus. The most accurate single predictor of the EDD is the patient's last menstrual period. To be used to calculate an EDD the last menstrual period should have been part of a regular menstrual history, have been normal and on time, and not preceded by the recent use (within 3 months) of oral contraceptives. When a last menstrual period does not meet these criteria, it cannot be used to predict the estimated date of delivery, and confirmation with ultrasound is advised.

History

A complete medical history and review of systems is essential. Ideally, this information is already available from a preconception counseling visit. If it is available, it should be updated.

Obstetric History

Prior pregnancy outcomes should be carefully documented and should include the number and duration of all pregnancies, the presence of medical or obstetric complications, the route of delivery, the estimated gestational age at delivery, complications of pregnancy, and any neonatal malformations. In patients who were delivered by Cesarean section, documentation of the direction of the uterine scar is important. In most instances, copies of previous prenatal and operative records should be requested and added to the patient's medical record. This information then permits counseling about the optimal method of delivery and establishes whether the patient is a candidate for vaginal birth after Cesarean.

Physical Examination

A complete history and physical examination should be performed at the first prenatal visit. The patient's height, weight (both present and prepregnant), and vital signs should be recorded. The general physical examination should include examination of the head, neck, breasts, lungs, heart, and abdomen. During the pelvic examination uterine size should be carefully documented in weeks gestation equivalent (prior to 20 weeks). The presence of fetal heart tones should be sought and recorded. During first-trimester examinations fetal heart tones may be heard as early as 10 weeks with the aid of Doppler ultrasound. The cervix should be examined with the goal of detecting any lesions, dilation, or effacement. When the cervix is markedly shortened (less than 3 cm), cervical incompetence and subsequent premature labor should be suspected. Last, some assessment of the adequacy of the maternal pelvis should be obtained. In a normal pelvis the ischial spines are blunt, the obstetric conjugate is greater than 11.5 cm, and the subpubic angle measures greater than 90 degrees.

Laboratory Tests

Table 1 lists the routine laboratory tests obtained throughout pregnancy. In certain high-risk groups, additional evaluations may be required. For example, black patients should undergo sickle cell screening, and glucose-6-phosphate dehydrogenase testing should be considered. If the sickle cell screening test is positive, hemoglobin electrophoresis is necessary to determine the carrier status for sickle cell anemia.

TABLE 1. **Prenatal Laboratory Tests**

First prenatal visit in all patients
Complete blood count with platelets
Blood type and Rh
Indirect Coombs' test (antibody screen)
Serologic test for syphilis (VDRL or RPR)
Rubella titer
Hepatitis B surface antigen
Cervical cytology
First prenatal visit in selected patients
Tuberculin skin test
Cervical cultures for chlamydia, gonorrhea
Diabetes screening
Sickle cell testing
Glucose-6-phosphate dehydrogenase testing
16 weeks—Maternal serum alpha-fetoprotein (AFP) or triple screen (estriol, AFP, human chorionic gonadotropin)
28 weeks gestation
Antibody screen
Administer Rh_o (D) immune globulin (RhoGAM) (300 μg) if infant is Rh-negative
Diabetes screening
Hemoglobin
36 weeks in selected patients
Hemoglobin or complete blood count
Cervical cultures

If the mother is a carrier, determination of the sickle cell carrier status of the father of the baby is necessary to predict the risk of sickle cell anemia in the infant. Additional testing in selected high-risk groups of patients includes tuberculin skin testing, screening for diabetes mellitus, and screening for *Chlamydia trachomatis*. Diabetes screening is recommended for all pregnant patients. Patients who have risk factors for the development of gestational diabetes should undergo testing at the first prenatal visit. These risk factors include a prior stillbirth, a prior macrosomic infant, gestational diabetes in a previous pregnancy, and a family history of diabetes and obesity. If the test results are negative, a repeat screen is indicated between 24 and 28 weeks of gestation. In Rh-negative patients, administration of Rh immune globulin is indicated following a repeat antibody screen at 28 weeks.

At approximately 36 weeks' gestation consideration should be given to repeating the patient's complete blood count (CBC) or hemoglobin level. In certain patients, serologic testing for syphilis and cervical cultures for gonorrhea or *Chlamydia* may be indicated.

Subsequent Prenatal Visits

The optimal frequency of prenatal visits remains controversial. Most clinicians recommend monthly visits until 28 weeks. Biweekly visits are advised between 28 and 36 weeks and weekly visits after 36 weeks. At each of these prenatal visits ongoing risk assessment should be performed. The patients should be questioned about appetite, weight gain, the presence of abdominal pain, vaginal fluid leakage, or vaginal bleeding. Evidence of uterine contractions or abdominal pain should be sought. The estimated gestational age should be determined by the most accurate means. Weight, blood pressure, fundal height, and fetal heart tones are measured, and a urinalysis for protein glucose levels is also performed. Leopold's maneuvers are needed in the latter part of the third trimester to detect the presence of an abnormal fetal lie.

Prenatal Diagnosis of Fetal Conditions

Through use of the previously mentioned mechanisms, the risk of fetal abnormalities should already have been identified. The most common reason for prenatal diagnosis is advanced maternal age. Mothers beyond the age of 35 are offered genetic counseling and prenatal diagnosis for fetal karyotype determination. At age 35 the approximate risk of Down's syndrome in a live-born child is 1 in 365. The total risk of chromosomal abnormalities is approximately twice that of Down's syndrome. Inborn errors of metabolism such as Tay-Sachs disease may also be detected prenatally. Patients of Jewish ancestry should be offered carrier detection prior to pregnancy. If this has not been done, screening the father of the baby is the most reasonable approach. Screening of pregnant patients for Tay-Sachs disease is more difficult because of the effects of pregnancy. If the father of the baby is not a carrier of Tay-Sachs disease, additional evaluation is unnecessary. If paternity is in question, or if the father of the baby is a carrier, prenatal diagnosis is appropriate. The list of diseases amenable to prenatal diagnosis changes rapidly. Fetuses known to be at risk for any disorder should be evaluated by a genetic counselor to determine whether prenatal diagnosis is possible.

Another common situation requiring prenatal evaluation of the fetus is an abnormality of the maternal serum alpha-fetoprotein (MSAFP) levels. It is currently recommended that all gravidas be offered MSAFP screening between 16 and 20 weeks of pregnancy. This screening should be done by a laboratory that has sufficient numbers of patients to be proficient at this technology. Patients with a single MSAFP elevation at 16 weeks are generally encouraged to undergo repeat screening. A second abnormal result requires additional evaluation.

A patient with two elevated MSAFP levels should then undergo an ultrasound evaluation to search for major malformations, the presence of fetal life, and the presence of a multiple gestation. If the ultrasound evaluation supports the patient's estimated date of delivery, counseling should be offered in regard to prenatal diagnosis. An amniocentesis with analysis of amniotic fluid alpha-fetoprotein level can then be performed. A normal amniotic fluid alpha-fetoprotein level is reassuring, and additional testing is not recommended. If the amniotic alpha-fetoprotein level is elevated, the laboratory should be instructed to determine the acetylcholinesterase level. Acetylcholinesterase is an enzyme that is relatively specific for fetal neural tissue but may also be elevated in fetuses with ventral abdominal wall defects. Table 2 lists common reasons for elevated MSAFP levels.

Newer antenatal screening tests are being advocated. The most popular is the so-called triple screen. The triple screen consists of MSAFP, an unconjugated plasma estriol determination, and a human chorionic gonadotropin (hCG) determination. This triple screen combines the results of these laboratory

TABLE 2. **Associations with Elevated Maternal Serum Alpha-fetoprotein (MSAFP)**

Fetal malformations
Meningomyelocele
Anencephaly
Gastroschisis
Encephalocoele
Omphalocoele
Renal disease
Cystic hygroma
Fetal conditions
Multiple gestation
Fetal death
Recent amniocentesis
Rhesus isoimmunization
Maternal conditions
Inaccurate dating
Ovarian germ cell malignancies

tests with maternal age and weight and estimates the risk of Down's syndrome in the fetus. In most screening programs, if the triple screen report indicates that the patient's risk of having a fetus with Down's syndrome exceeds that of a 35-year-old, prenatal diagnosis with amniocentesis is then offered. A repeat triple screen is not recommended when the patient is being analyzed for the risk of Down's syndrome in the fetus. Independent of the triple screen, the MSAFP is determined as part of a risk assessment for neural tube defects. The MSAFP may be repeated as outlined previously even when it has been determined as part of the triple screen.

Chorionic Villus Sampling

Chorionic villus sampling (CVS) is, in essence, a biopsy of the placenta. The rapidly dividing trophoblastic cells may permit rapid karyotype determination within several hours of obtaining this specimen. To reduce the incidence of placental mosaicism, most laboratories establish cell growth in tissue culture and do not use the direct method unless a rapid diagnosis is essential. Typically, CVS is performed at 10 to 13 weeks of pregnancy. Earlier performance of CVS, although technically possible, may be associated with an increase in incidence of limb reduction defects. The approximate pregnancy-related loss rate with CVS approaches 1 to 2% and is similar to that of amniocentesis. A problem unique to CVS is placental mosaicism. It has been recognized that the placenta may contain different cell lines that would otherwise indicate mosaicism. When direct fetal blood sampling or amniocentesis has been performed, karyotypes have been normal. This infrequent complication may delay determination of a normal karyotype. In addition, patients at risk for having a fetus with a neural tube defect should undergo amniocentesis because the amniotic cavity is not entered in CVS and alpha-fetoprotein levels cannot be determined.

The advantages of CVS include earlier diagnosis, which increases the therapeutic options available to the patient. The disadvantages of CVS are placental mosaicism, the inability to assess the amniotic fluid alpha-fetoprotein level, and the reduced availability of this procedure.

Amniocentesis

Genetic amniocentesis has typically been performed at approximately 16 weeks for a variety of indications. Table 3 lists the most commonly accepted indications for genetic amniocentesis. In general, amniocentesis is performed under real-time ultrasound guidance. Amniotic fluid is removed, amniocytes are maintained in tissue culture, and a karyotype is performed. The time required to obtain a result varies among laboratories, but in general it takes 7 to 14 days. Amniocentesis is associated with a pregnancy loss rate of approximately 1 of 200 and an overall 1% complication rate including bleeding and ruptured membranes. As part of our routine, the amniotic fluid alpha-fetoprotein level is determined in every patient undergoing genetic amniocentesis regardless of the indication for testing. Amniocentesis may also be of benefit in analyzing the metabolic byproducts that may be elevated in certain fetal conditions. In pregnancies at risk for these disorders, genetic counseling is recommended.

TABLE 3. **Indications for Genetic Amniocentesis**

Maternal age ≥35 years at delivery
Elevated MSAFP
Low MSAFP
Abnormal triple screen
Sex determination in families at risk for X-linked disorder
Abnormal fetal anatomy seen on ultrasound
Prior child with neural tube defect
Prior child with chromosome abnormality
Metabolic disorders for which prenatal diagnosis is possible

Abbreviations: MSAFP = maternal alpha-fetoprotein.

There is increasing evidence about the risks of early amniocentesis (14 weeks or earlier). It appears that the procedure is technically feasible, but limitations of the early procedure include failure of the cell culture to grow, lack of normative data for amniotic fluid alpha-fetoprotein, occasional false-positive acetylcholinesterase activity, and lack of data regarding complications.

Ultrasound

Ultrasound has significantly changed the modern practice of obstetrics. The value of routine ultrasound examination in all pregnancies remains controversial. The current recommendations are that it be used for specific indications. There is no definitive evidence that ultrasound poses any particular risks to mother or fetus. It should be emphasized that diagnostic ultrasound is of relatively low intensity and pulsed rather than continuous. Indications for ultrasound evaluation include, but are not limited to, the diagnosis of early pregnancy, suspicion of intrauterine growth retardation, as an aid to the performance of genetic amniocentesis, diagnosis of fetal malformations, evaluation of placental location, estimation of fetal weight, and confirmation of the estimated date of delivery.

The accuracy of the ultrasound estimated date of delivery varies with gestational age. A first-trimester ultrasound measurement of the fetal crown-rump length is accurate to within 5 days of the date of delivery. Examinations in the second trimester may be associated with a 2-week measurement error. In the third trimester of pregnancy this error may exceed 4 weeks.

A basic ultrasound examination, except in emergent situations, should consist of the images listed in Table 4. In addition, documentation of the images obtained is critical for later review as well as for medicolegal concerns. Exceptions to this rule of documentation include ultrasound assessment of fetal position in advanced labor and antepartum assessment of fetal well-being (e.g., amniotic fluid volume assessment and biophysical profile scoring).

TABLE 4. **Components of Basic Ultrasound Examination**

First Trimester
Location of gestational sac
Presence and measurement of crown-rump length
Fetal number and viability
Evaluation of uterus and adnexa
Second and Third Trimesters
Fetal lie, number, presentation
Estimation of amniotic fluid volume
Placental location
Gestational age assessment
Biparietal diameter, head and abdominal circumferences, femur length
Assessment of fetal growth
Evaluation of uterus and adnexa
Fetal anatomic survey
Cerebral ventricles
Cerebellum and cisterna magna
Spine
Four-chamber view of the fetal heart
Stomach
Cord insertion
Renal fossa
Urinary bladder

A detailed ultrasound examination is frequently called a targeted ultrasound examination (formerly called a Level II or Level III ultrasound) and is indicated for the diagnosis of specific fetal malformations. It is indicated in patients with elevated MSAFP levels and when certain fetal malformations are suspected. These more detailed ultrasound evaluations are best performed in centers experienced with advanced ultrasound.

COMPLICATIONS OF PREGNANCY

Hypertension

Approximately 10% of all pregnancies are complicated by hypertension. Preeclampsia is defined as a blood pressure elevation of 140/90 or greater measured on two separate occasions at least 6 hours apart. Additional hypertensive criteria for a diagnosis of preeclampsia include a 30-mm increase in systolic or a 15-mm increase in diastolic blood pressures over baseline levels. Proteinuria should be present for a diagnosis of preeclampsia to be made. The treatment for preeclampsia at term is delivery, generally under anticonvulsant prophylaxis with parenteral magnesium sulfate. The most common dose is a 4-gram bolus followed by a 2-gram per hour continuous infusion. Evidence of toxicity includes absent or diminished deep tendon reflexes, inadequate urinary output (less than 25 mL per hour), or serum levels above 8 mg per dL. Patients prior to term with mild preeclampsia require bedrest with close observation, assessment of fetal well-being, creatinine clearance, and additional laboratory assessment. In most instances, hospitalization and close observation are recommended. Additional outpatient care of these patients may be appropriate if they remain hemodynamically stable and there is no laboratory evidence of severe or worsening disease. Deterioration of blood pressure, declining renal function, and the presence of fetal compromise are additional indications for delivery regardless of gestational age.

Criteria for a diagnosis of severe preeclampsia include sustained elevated blood pressure (in excess of 160/110), 4 to 5 grams of proteinuria per 24 hours, the appearance of subjective symptoms including headache and epigastric pain, and significant abnormalities of liver or renal function. Severe preeclampsia is an indication for delivery regardless of gestational age.

A variant of severe preeclampsia is being recognized with increasing frequency. This syndrome consists of hemolysis, elevated liver enzymes, and low platelet counts. It has been given the eponym HELLP syndrome. Many of these patients do not have significantly elevated blood pressure but still have severe preeclampsia. Therefore, the presence of the HELLP syndrome requires delivery.

Chronic hypertension is said to exist when hypertension is known to occur prior to pregnancy. In addition, the appearance of hypertension prior to 20 completed weeks of pregnancy may indicate chronic hypertension. The level of blood pressure control needed in patients with this disorder is controversial. In general, it is recommended that blood pressure not exceed 140/90 mm Hg. Table 5 lists the most commonly used antihypertensive medications and their dosages for use during pregnancy. The most commonly used are methyldopa (Aldomet) and hydralazine (Apresoline). These drugs have been used extensively in obstetrics and appear to be safe. Antihypertensives that are contraindicated in pregnancy include diuretics and angiotensin-converting enzyme (ACE) inhibitors. Fetuses whose mothers have chronic hypertension are at risk for intrauterine growth retardation, and serial ultrasound examinations are recommended to ensure normal fetal growth. These patients may also be at risk for the development of superimposed preeclampsia, abruptio placentae, and fetal death. These patients should undergo antepartum fetal surveillance no later than 32 weeks of pregnancy.

Diabetes Mellitus

Diabetes mellitus is another common complication of pregnancy. It occurs as frequently as hypertension. It is currently recommended that all patients undergo diabetes screening during pregnancy. As outlined previously, those patients at high risk for the disease should undergo screening at initial presentation. Diabetes screening is accomplished by administering 50 grams of carbohydrate and performing a blood sugar determination 1 hour later. A value of less than 140 mg per dL is considered normal. Values in excess of that level require additional evaluation with a 3-hour glucose tolerance test (GTT). The upper limits of normal for plasma glucose values in the 3-hour GTT are fasting, 105 mg per dL; 1 hour; 190 mg per dL, 2 hours, 165 mg per dL; and 3 hours, 145 mg

TABLE 5. **Commonly Used Oral Antihypertensives**

Drug	Site of Action	Dose
Methyldopa (Aldomet)	Centrally acting	250 mg bid–500 mg qid
Hydralazine (Apresoline)	Peripheral vasodilator	10 mg tid–50 mg qid
Nifedipine (Procardia)	Calcium channel blocker	90–120 mg/day
Labetalol (Trandate)	Beta blocker	100–300 mg bid
Atenolol (Tenormin)	Beta blocker	25–50 mg/day

per dL. A diagnosis of gestational diabetes is made when two or more of these values are abnormal. Some authors have reported an increased complication rate when only one of the four values is abnormal. Insufficient data exist at present to make recommendations about a diagnosis of gestational diabetes when only one value is abnormal.

Patients with gestational diabetes should be placed on a diet based on 30 to 35 kcal per kg of ideal body weight. This restores normal glucose values in approximately 85% of patients. Serial assessment of glucose levels should reveal fasting blood sugar levels of less than 100 mg per dL and 2-hour postprandial blood sugar levels of less than 120 mg per dL. Failure to achieve these levels requires consideration of insulin therapy.

Patients with diabetes prior to the onset of pregnancy benefit from tight periconceptual glucose control. In most instances this can be achieved with a mixture of intermediate and long-acting insulin given twice daily. In patients with poor control of diabetes the administration of long-acting (ultralente) insulin once or twice a day with regular insulin doses at mealtime may result in improved diabetic control.

The majority of patients with diabetes mellitus can be managed at home. The use of a reflectance meter permits home glucose monitoring in the fasting and 2-hour postprandial states and has increased our ability to care for these patients at home. Hospitalization of insulin-requiring diabetics is necessary when reasonable outpatient glucose control is not possible. In these instances, it is our practice to admit patients for continuous intravenous insulin administration. The continuous intravenous insulin infusion is administered in a sliding scale (Table 6). At the end of a 24-hour period of acceptable glucose control, a 24-hour daily insulin requirement is calculated.

TABLE 6. **Sliding Scale for Intravenous Insulin**

Capillary Blood Glucose (mg/dL)	Insulin (Units/hour)*
0–60	0
61–80	0.3
81–110	0.8
111–140	1.2
141–160	1.5
161–200	2.0
201–250	3.0
251–300	4.0

*For the hour during the three major meals the insulin infusion rate is increased by two steps.

This 24-hour insulin requirement is then divided as follows: two-thirds of the daily total insulin dose is administered in the morning and one-third in the evening. The morning dose is distributed as NPH insulin (two-thirds) and regular insulin (one-third). The evening dose is composed of half NPH and half regular. The patients are then candidates for discharge with close follow-up.

Patients with pre-existing diabetes benefit from close ultrasound evaluation. Fetal echocardiography is recommended at 20 weeks to rule out congenital heart disease. Maternal serum alpha-fetoprotein screening and targeted ultrasound imaging between 16 and 20 weeks are also recommended.

Antepartum assessment of fetal well-being should begin no later than 32 weeks of pregnancy. Patients who have long-standing insulin-requiring diabetes with vascular complications need evaluation earlier in pregnancy. Patients in whom diabetic control is excellent may be permitted to continue until term with reassuring fetal surveillance. In general, prior to elective delivery, ascertainment of fetal maturity is required. Lung maturity of fetuses in diabetic pregnancies mandates the presence of phosphatidyl glycerol (PG) in the amniotic fluid. The majority of patients with diabetes can be expected to deliver vaginally. Prostaglandin E_2 (dinoprostone [Prostin E2]), cervical ripening, and induction of labor are appropriate methods of management. Cesarean section should be reserved for traditional obstetric indications.

Preterm Delivery

The incidence of premature birth has remained unchanged in the last 20 years. Our success in treating this condition has been hampered by inconsistencies in diagnostic criteria for premature labor, lack of properly designed randomized clinical trials regarding prevention of premature birth, and an inability to discover the cause of premaure labor. Despite this, there are well-recognized risk factors for the development of premature labor. Table 7 lists the more common associations with premature labor.

Numerous risk-screening programs have been developed and none appear to have substantial advantages. Once a patient has been identified as high-risk, she needs to undergo an extensive educational program. The purpose of this educational program is to help the patient understand her role in the development of premature labor. Self-destructive behavior such as smoking, drug use, and alcohol abuse should

TABLE 7. **Risk Factors for Preterm Labor**

Prepregnancy
Incompetent cervix
Diethylstilbestrol exposure
Uterine anomaly
Tobacco or substance abuse
Two or more second-trimester abortions
Three or more first-trimester abortions
Prior history of preterm labor or delivery
Prior cone biopsy of cervix
Pregnancy conditions
Low socioeconomic class
Age <17, >35
Multiple gestation
Hydramnios
Pyelonephritis
Abdominal surgery during current pregnancy

be discouraged. Most important, patients should be taught to palpate uterine contractions themselves. Written material is essential to a successful preterm birth prevention program. This written information should outline the subtle signs and symptoms of premature labor that may not be obvious to patients or health care providers. The patient should be instructed when to call, who to call, and when to present to the hospital. Currently, 60% of women are not candidates for tocolytic therapy when they come to the Labor and Delivery department. In many instances it is because preterm labor is too far advanced.

The use of home uterine activity monitoring (HUAM) is intensely controversial. The American College of Obstetricians and Gynecologists has recommended that this technology be considered experimental until additional prospective clinical trials have demonstrated its effectiveness. It is clear from the published studies of HUAM that the daily health care provider contact is perhaps the most important element. This contact is usually a nurse who reinforces good behavior and seeks information about uterine activity and symptoms that indicate premature labor. Most HUAM companies provide monitoring and telephone hook-ups so that the frequency of uterine contractions can be identified. If uterine activity is thought to be excessive, the patient may then be given tocolytics.

Isoimmunization

All pregnant patients should undergo blood type and antibody screening at the initial visit. This antibody screening is usually performed using an indirect Coombs' test. This test seeks to identify which antibodies are present in the maternal serum. The fetus is at risk when these maternal antibodies are of the IgG class, which can cross the placenta. With the widespread use of Rh_o (D) immune globulin, the incidence of sensitization to the D antigen appears to be decreasing. Consequently, more pregnancies are being complicated by sensitization to other red cell antigens. These red cell antigens may be part of the Rh system (CcEe) or other antigen systems.

When these antibodies are identified, it is important to determine their immunoglobulin class. If IgM antibodies are present, the risk to the fetus is negligible. If IgG antibodies are present, it is sometimes helpful to determine the phenotype of the father of the baby. If paternity is certain and if the paternal phenotype (i.e., antigen status) is negative for the red cell antigen in question, the risks to the fetus are low. If the fetus is at risk, referral to a high-risk perinatal center may be helpful in determining the need for additional treatment.

Additional studies that may be recommended by the tertiary referral center include amniocentesis to determine the level of bilirubin in the amniotic fluid. Alternatively, the use of fetal blood sampling (cordocentesis) is helpful in determining not only whether the infant has the red cell antigen but also whether or not the child is anemic. In fetuses with severe disease, intrauterine transfusion may be appropriate.

Practitioners need to be aware of the indications for Rh_o (D) immune globulin (RhoGAM). Table 8 lists the indications and amounts of immune globulin required. It is also important to remember that the administration of Rh_o (D) immune globulin will not prevent the development of isoimmunization to other red cell antigens.

Antepartum Fetal Surveillance

Pregnancies at risk for antepartum fetal death benefit from antepartum fetal surveillance. The most common indication for this surveillance in most centers is a postdate pregnancy. Table 9 lists the indications as well as the approximate gestational age at which testing is recommended. At our institution the principal method of fetal surveillance is a nonstress test combined with the amniotic fluid index. A reactive nonstress test and a normal amount of amniotic fluid volume are considered reassuring, and tests are repeated at intervals of 3 to 7 days depending on the

TABLE 8. **Indications for Rh_o (D) Immune Globulin (RhoGAM)**

	Dose (μg)
First Trimester	
Spontaneous abortion	50
Induced abortion	50
Chorionic villus sampling	300
Ectopic pregnancy	300
Second Trimester	
Rh-negative	300
Genetic amniocentesis	300
Third Trimester	
Maternal trauma	300 or more
External cephalic version	300 or more
Amniocentesis	300 or more
Delivery of a Rh-positive infant	300 or more
After fetal death	300 or more

Note: When the amount of fetomaternal hemorrhage is uncertain but could be excessive, a quantitative Kleihauer-Belke test is advised. The laboratory will report the amount of fetal blood likely to have entered the maternal circulation. A 300-μg ampule of Rh_o (D) immune globulin will protect against 30 mL of whole blood or 15 mL of fetal cells.

TABLE 9. **Indications for Antenatal Fetal Surveillance**

Indication	Estimated Gestational Age (week)
Post dates	41
Diabetes	
Class A	36
Class B or greater	26–32
Hypertension	26–32
Suspected intrauterine growth retardation	At diagnosis
Decreased fetal movement	At diagnosis

indication for testing. Term infants with persistently nonreactive nonstress tests or decreased amounts of amniotic fluid volume should be evaluated for delivery. Preterm patients with nonreactive nonstress tests are generally evaluated with the fetal biophysical profile. This multi-parameter test includes assessment of fetal heart rate reactivity, amniotic fluid volume, fetal breathing, fetal movement, and fetal tone. Scores of 0, 2, and 4 are considered abnormal and require evaluation for delivery. A score of 6 is considered indeterminate and requires repeat testing within 12 to 24 hours. Biophysical profile scores of 8 or 10 are considered normal, and the pregnancy may safely be permitted to continue.

Because fetal sleep states and prematurity may affect the frequency with which a reactive nonstress test is encountered, additional testing is always required prior to the delivery of a preterm infant for suspected fetal compromise.

CONCLUSION

Perinatal outcome may be improved by careful preconception counseling and thoughtful prenatal care. The appropriate use of laboratory tests, ultrasound, and prenatal diagnosis is also of critical importance. The perfect baby is an elusive goal but one worthy of attempt.

ECTOPIC PREGNANCY

method of
MARILYN R. RICHARDSON, M.D.
Permanente Medical Association of Texas
University of Texas Health Science Center at Dallas
Dallas, Texas

The incidence of ectopic pregnancy, wherein implantation of the fertilized ovum occurs in an extrauterine location, has increased by approximately 11% per year during the past 25 years. Most recent estimates place the occurrence at more than 120,000 cases in the United States in 1990. However, our facility in the diagnosis and management of this entity has increased in parallel during the same time frame, leading to a substantial reduction in morbidity and mortality. One surgeon trained in the 1940s relates how symptoms of hypovolemic shock constituted the primary diagnostic measure of an ectopic pregnancy, which was followed by surgery for an acute abdomen. Currently, the ability to quantitate the beta-subunit of human chorionic gonadotropin (hCG-beta), technical advances in ultrasound, and the widespread use of operative laparoscopy have led to earlier diagnosis and decreased the necessity for ablative surgery. These improvements are reflected in a reduction of the average length of hospital stay from greater than 7.2 days to 1.4 days.

ETIOLOGY

Most ectopic implantations (97%) occur in the fallopian tube, which is thought to have sustained damage from previous pelvic inflammatory disease. Additionally, increased risk is associated with previous pelvic surgery (including tubal ligation), prior use of intrauterine contraceptive devices, and treatment for infertility. Cervical, ovarian, and intra-abdominal implantations occur rarely. Although these account for less than 5% of all ectopic pregnancies, the mortality associated with them is disproportionately higher (20%).

DIAGNOSIS

A female of reproductive age who reports a missed or abnormal menstrual period or unpredicted vaginal bleeding should have as a first-line assessment a qualitative hCG-beta, which is sensitive enough to detect levels of 25 mIU per milliliter, performed on either urine or serum. A history of any of the risk factors listed previously raises the index of suspicion for ectopic pregnancy should the hCG be positive. A past history of treatment for gonorrhea or *Chlamydia* infection (without symptoms) is important because subclinical salpingitis may have occurred. Pelvic pain is reported frequently, and pelvic examination may elicit tenderness or demonstrate a mass.

A positive qualitative hCG-beta should then be quantitated in serum, and if it is found to be greater than 6000 mIU per milliliter, it should be associated with a finding on transabdominal ultrasound (TAUS) that is consistent with early uterine gestation equivalent to 6 postmenstrual weeks. The enhanced resolution afforded by transvaginal ultrasound (TVUS) transducers allows recognition of this appearance at hCG levels of 1500 to 2000 mIU per milliliter, or 35 postmenstrual days, and has therefore reduced the gestational age at which the diagnosis of ectopic pregnancy can be established and therapy initiated. The absence of intrauterine markings in the presence of an extrauterine mass when hCG exceeds these "discriminatory zones" indicates a greater than 97% probability of ectopic pregnancy. Lower levels of hCG warrant further study. The quantity of hCG in serum doubles every 36 hours in a normal pregnancy. Therefore, serial determinations of hCG, if increasing, provide reassurance of the probability of a normal uterine gestation. The absence of an appropriate increase further heightens the suspicion of ectopic implantation, and this absence is associated with approximately 85% of nonviable intrauterine and ectopic pregnancies. A serum progesterone level of less than 15 ng per milliliter is present in the great majority of abnormal pregnancies (intrauterine or extrauterine) and may provide some guidance. When the quantity of hCG has exceeded the level at which visualization by ultrasound should occur, and if the size of the suspected ectopic gestation is less than 3.5 cm, medical rather than surgical therapy may be considered. A simple uterine curettage can serve as the final diagnostic step to visualize the presence of chorionic villi (by flotation of the tissue obtained in saline) to rule out intrauterine gestation.

Often the greatest diagnostic dilemma is the differentiation of an ectopic pregnancy from a nonviable intrauterine gestation. The regression observed during the period of observation required for elucidation may be from either an intrauterine or extrauterine location. However, few clinicians at this time are willing simply to observe the regression of a pregnancy *known* to be ectopic. For the most part, purposeful observation has been limited to institutional protocols.

MANAGEMENT

Surgical Therapy

Therapy until recently consisted of surgical procedures designed first to confirm the diagnosis of "suspected" ectopic pregnancy because our armamentarium did not allow noninvasive extraoperative confirmation. Culdocentesis was traditionally used, and is still used by some, to determine the presence or absence of hemoperitoneum. The withdrawal of nonclotted blood from the cul-de-sac dictated immediate laparotomy. Because hemoperitoneum can be caused by other factors, such as a ruptured corpus luteum, retrograde menstruation, or incomplete abortion, and because intra-abdominal hemorrhage can frequently be controlled with laparoscopy, many clinicians have abandoned this diagnostic procedure. The choice of procedure (laparoscopy or laparotomy) depends on (1) the surgical skill of the clinician, (2) the level of hemodynamic stability, (3) the amount of tubal damage, if present, and (4) the desire to preserve fertility. The products of conception may be expressed from the distal end of the tube or evacuated through a tubal incision. The tube itself may be partially or completely excised. Intra-abdominal (nontubal, nonovarian) pregnancies are not often amenable to laparoscopic techniques because these pregnancies have frequently progressed much further and are larger than tubal pregnancies, necessitating laparotomy.

More than 50% of women achieve a subsequent intrauterine pregnancy within 2 years following the more conservative surgical procedures. However, in some women, fertility remains impaired.

Medical Therapy

Methotrexate (MTX), a folinic acid inhibitor, can be administered by peritoneal instillation, by injection into the gestation, or intramuscularly. Early systemic protocols required multiple injections over a 7-day period with citrovorum factor (leucovorin calcium) (in the same fashion as for choriocarcinoma). However, most centers have found a single injection of MTX equally effective, which leads to a marked reduction in side effects. Hemoglobin, hematocrit, platelet function, and liver function should be established as normal prior to injection. A 15% decrease in the quantity of hCG is anticipated by the fourth day after injection. If this does not occur, a second injection is administered, and hCG levels are allowed to fall until they are absent. Although some degree of pelvic discomfort and vaginal bleeding may occur, in our experience only a few cases have warranted operative intervention. In general, an 80 to 90% success rate can be anticipated. Moreover, hysterosalpingography has demonstrated tubal patency in 70 to 90% of patients. Side effects are minimal, localized to the oral cavity or gastrointestinal tract, and are, for the most part, easily tolerated.

In addition, MTX has been used postoperatively for residual trophoblastic activity and is reportedly successful in the treatment of cervical implantation as well.

Early detection utilizing the most current diagnostic technology is the key to unlocking the use of conservative laparoscopic surgical procedures. The likelihood of successful nonsurgical therapy is also enhanced by early diagnosis. The resultant decreases in hospitalization, medical expense, recuperative time, and lost productivity rest to a large extent on education of those women who are at increased risk of development of ectopic pregnancy.

VAGINAL BLEEDING IN LATE PREGNANCY

method of
JEFFREY C. KING, M.D.
Georgetown University School of Medicine
Washington, D.C.

The occurrence of vaginal bleeding during the second and third trimesters of pregnancy is almost always unexpected and should result in prompt communication between the patient and her physician. Vaginal bleeding in late pregnancy complicates approximately 3 to 4% of all pregnancies. Not only is the health of the parturient placed at risk, but also the rates of premature delivery and perinatal mortality rate are at least quadrupled. The development of significant vaginal bleeding in late pregnancy converts a previously normal pregnancy into a high-risk pregnancy that warrants immediate evaluation, hospitalization for observation, fetal assessment, stabilization with crystalloids or blood products, and preparation for possible delivery. The national standard of care requires appropriate preparation for care of the newborn, who may be premature, anemic, or hypoxic as a result of the bleeding episode or the delivery itself. A neonatologist or pediatrician available for consultation or management of the newborn plus an appropriate nursery setting for neonatal care is essential. Consideration must be given to arranging for maternal transport of the stable obstetric patient to a regional perinatal center if the current facilities are assessed as inadequate.

Although the rate of maternal mortality has been reduced by the availability of crossmatched blood and blood products, deaths resulting from antepartum hemorrhage continue to be listed in most maternal mortality reports. Of the antepartum causes of significant bleeding in late pregnancy, clinical evidence of abruptio placentae is found in 31% of cases, and placenta previa is identified in 22% of cases. The cause of bleeding in the remaining 47% of cases is usually classified as undetermined. The term significant is used in reference to vaginal bleeding in late pregnancy to differentiate it from show or bloody show, which occurs near the onset of labor in most parturients.

GENERAL APPROACH

When notified by or about the bleeding patient, the care provider must quickly obtain historical information about the estimated date of confinement, the amount and color of blood loss, any associated pain or recent trauma, therapeutic or recreational drug usage, and prior episodes of bleeding or other complications during the current pregnancy. Generally, the patient should be sent to the hospital for evaluation and assessment. Standing guidelines for the preliminary assessment of patients with vaginal bleeding in late pregnancy may be helpful so that evaluation can begin as soon as the patient arrives at the hospital. These guidelines should include the following items: prohibition against digital or speculum examination, initiation of continuous electronic monitoring to record fetal heart rate and uterine activity, documentation of maternal vital signs every 5 to 10 minutes, establishment of venous access with a large-bore intracath, and collection of blood samples for various baseline laboratory studies. These studies should include a complete blood count, platelet count, fibrinogen level, and a Kleihauer-Betke test for evidence of fetomaternal transfusion. Quantification of fibrin split products has been suggested, but because they are identified in up to 15% of normal pregnancies, a positive result may be misleading. A blood specimen should be sent to the blood bank for at least blood typing and screening. This process usually allows blood to become available for emergency transfusion within 30 minutes. If blood loss is estimated to be heavy or continuous, two to four units of packed red blood cells should be crossmatched and kept available at all times. If the blood bank is unable to provide sufficient blood products promptly on request owing to staffing, lack of product availability, or presence of maternal antibody, consideration of maternal transport is warranted. Uncrossmatched type O, Rh-negative blood should be available within the blood bank and may be used for transfusion in an extreme emergency.

A blood sample can be obtained in a tube without anticoagulant and retained on the patient's unit. This specimen can be observed for clot formation, which should occur within 8 minutes. If the specimen does not clot or the clot undergoes prompt lysis, more extensive testing of the maternal coagulation mechanism is indicated. Additional laboratory tests that should be considered include serum or urine toxicology studies for illicit drugs, particularly cocaine, which has been associated with abruptio placentae.

During the physical examination, the physician should pay particular attention to ongoing bleeding, maternal and fetal heart rates, and uterine tone and size (fundal height measurement should be documented and marked to help identify concealed hemorrhage). The physician needs hourly urine output information provided by means of a Foley catheter if shock is suspected or is a likely development. Ultrasound evaluation of the gravid uterus is indicated to help guide patient management, but it should not delay the initial approach outlined previously. Ultrasound evaluation can provide valuable information about the estimated gestational age, fetal weight and viability, placental implantation site and integrity, and possible fetal anomalies, and the effacement and dilation of the cervix may be estimated in some situations. Translabial ultrasound scanning may provide valuable clues to the anatomic relationship between the placenta and cervix when the use of a transvaginal ultrasound transducer is thought to be risky. The use of color-flow Doppler ultrasound may be diagnostic during the evaluation for possible vasa previa.

DIFFERENTIAL DIAGNOSIS

Abruptio Placentae. Abruptio placentae is defined as premature separation of a normally implanted placenta prior to the third stage of labor; it complicates about 1% of all pregnancies. Although it is mild in 66% and moderate in 19% of cases, abruptio placentae is classified as severe in about 15% of cases. The overall perinatal loss associated with abruptio placentae is more than 30%. The risk of recurrence of abruptio placentae in a subsequent pregnancy is 5 to 15%.

Placenta Previa. Placenta previa is defined as implantation of the placenta in the lower uterine segment in advance of the fetal presenting part. It is often classified by the relationship of the placental margin to the internal cervical os. Placenta previa complicates about 0.5% of all pregnancies, and perinatal loss occurs in less than 20% of cases, primarily due to prematurity.

Vasa Previa. Vasa previa is a rare condition complicating approximately 1 of 3000 pregnancies, during which the fetal umbilical vein or artery inserts into the membranes and passes across the internal cervical os in advance of the fetal presenting part before inserting into the placenta. Vasa previa places the fetus at great risk because of the speed of exsanguination that can occur if a fetal vessel is torn during spontaneous or artificial rupture of membranes.

Other Causes. The most common "other" cause of bleeding in late pregnancy is bloody show, characterized by the vaginal discharge of dark blood mixed with copious mucus. This occurs as the mucus plug is expelled from the cervix either remote from or during early labor.

Severe vaginitis or cervicitis, particularly that due to *Trichomonas,* may cause bleeding but usually results in only mild pink staining.

Endocervical polyp(s) may bleed as a result of coital injury, although this bleeding is usually limited.

Vulvar or vaginal varicose veins may develop owing to elevated venous pressure below the level of the uterus. These veins may rupture spontaneously, leading to significant maternal blood loss.

Abdominal or pelvic trauma, coital or otherwise, is an uncommon but potentially serious cause of bleeding that may result in maternal or fetal morbidity or mortality.

Invasive cervical cancer is uncommon in the reproductive age group but must be ruled out after the more common causes have been considered.

Rupture of a uterine scar from a prior cesarean delivery, myomectomy, or metroplasty must be considered when appropriate clinical circumstances are present.

RESUSCITATION AND OTHER EVALUATION

The attending physician must consider all potential explanations for vaginal bleeding in late pregnancy. Each diagnosis has a variety of specific clinical features that must be compared with the signs and symptoms elicited from the patient. Although an exhaustive discussion of specific clinical features is beyond the scope of this article, painless bleeding suggests placenta previa and painful or tetanic uterine contractions are associated with abruptio placentae.

Close attention should be paid to the maternal and fetal vital signs, the amount of ongoing blood loss, and maternal urine output. The general aims are to maintain the hematocrit above 30% and a urinary output of at least 30 mL per hour. Prompt transfusion with packed red blood cells is indicated when the estimated blood loss exceeds 800 to 1000 mL. Identification of intrauterine fetal demise should result in a complete assessment of the maternal coagulation status, as should spontaneous bleeding from a mucous membrane or from an intravenous puncture site.

Continuous electronic monitoring allows assessment of placental function and uterine response to the various causes. The fetal heart tracing should be watched for evidence of nonreassuring patterns including alterations of variability, periodic and nonperiodic changes, and a wandering or unstable baseline. The uterine tracing may provide important information about the frequency, intensity, and duration of uterine contractions. In addition, changes in baseline uterine tone may be assessed.

The primary intent of the clinical evaluation is to identify the most likely cause of vaginal bleeding in late pregnancy and to reduce as much as possible maternal or fetal morbidity or mortality. The attending physician should use a variety of symptoms, physical signs, and personal clinical experience to guide the management and ultimate outcome. After a thorough ultrasound evaluation of the fetus and placenta, amniocentesis may be considered to assess fetal pulmonary maturity in selected cases or to evaluate hemorrhage concealed within the amniotic sac.

Digital or speculum examination is generally contraindicated, particularly when ultrasound confirms evidence of total or even partial placenta previa. If a low-lying placenta or marginal previa is diagnosed and the patient is in labor or has progressive vaginal bleeding, a double set-up digital examination may be performed after preparations have been made to proceed with immediate cesarean delivery when indicated.

If ultrasound rules out placenta previa, a careful speculum or digital examination may then be performed to evaluate the genital tract for lesions, tumors, or injury. It is critically important to remember that a normal ultrasound assessment of the placental attachment site does not rule out an abruptio placentae.

Because fetomaternal bleeding may occur as a result of vaginal bleeding in late pregnancy, it is necessary that all Rh-negative, unsensitized mothers be given the appropriate intramuscular dose of Rh_o (D) immune globulin (RhoGAM, Gamulin, HypRho-D). Each vial contains 300 μg of Rh_o (D) immune globulin and will protect against sensitization following exposure to 30 mL of Rh-positive fetal whole blood or 15 mL of Rh-positive fetal packed red blood cells. The Kleihauer-Betke stain of a peripherally obtained maternal blood sample can assist in the volume calculation of fetomaternal transfusion. Sufficiency of protection can be documented by confirming a positive indirect Coomb's test 48 hours following the injection.

MANAGEMENT

Abruptio Placentae

Treatment of suspected abruptio placentae depends on the clinical severity, fetal health and tolerance, and gestational age. In general, once abruptio placentae begins, delivery is necessary in the relatively near future. However, with mild abruption, irregular contractions, and an apparently healthy although immature fetus, carefully monitored conservative treatment, including blood transfusion as necessary, is reasonable. Tocolysis of uterine contractions may be considered.

With moderate degrees of placental separation, blood or blood product administration is necessary. Tocolysis may be cautiously attempted in the presence of suspected fetal immaturity. However, if progressive separation develops or tocolysis fails, prompt delivery is necessary.

Delivery should be performed regardless of fetal status if severe abruptio placentae is present. If the fetus is alive and of appropriate age (more than 25 to 26 weeks' gestation), prompt cesarean delivery is indicated. If fetal demise has already occurred, vaginal delivery should be the goal. With moderate or severe placental separation, physiologic support with crystalloids plus blood or blood products is necessary to maintain cerebral and renal perfusion or to correct coagulation defects.

Continuous electronic monitoring is necessary to assess fetal tolerance. If nonreassuring fetal heart rate tracings develop, prompt delivery by the most expeditious route is indicated. Invasive hemodynamic monitoring should be used when ongoing hemorrhage or oliguria becomes unresponsive to standard measures.

Heparin or fibrinolytic therapy is contraindicated for management of this condition. Hypogastric or uterine artery ligation or even hysterectomy may become necessary owing to postpartum hemorrhage.

Placenta Previa

Therapy is dependent on the extent of placenta previa, the amount of bleeding, fetal tolerance, and gestational age. In general, placenta previa results in recurrent episodes of painless vaginal bleeding. The amount of bleeding in any particular episode is unpredictable and may range from light spotting to profuse hemorrhage. When symptomatic placenta previa is confirmed after 36 weeks' gestation, treatment should consist of immediate blood replacement followed by cesarean delivery.

Management at less then 36 weeks' gestation requires clinical judgment balanced against the probability of fetal lung maturity. Transfusion and tocolysis may be attempted in pregnancies of less than 34 weeks as long as blood replacement maintains the hematocrit above 30% and there is no evidence of coagulopathy.

Vaginal delivery is generally reserved for the subset of patients with marginal placenta previa or a low-lying placenta confirmed at a double set-up examination. These patients must have the fetal head in the pelvis along with a favorable cervix for rupture of membranes followed by cautious induction of labor.

Approximately 15% of patients who have had a prior cesarean delivery and whose present pregnancy is complicated by placenta previa develop placenta accreta. This complication of pregnancy often results in a need for emergency hysterectomy owing to uncontrolled postpartum hemorrhage or failure of the lower segment to contract following removal of the placenta.

Vasa Previa

Therapy of suspected or documented cases is immediate cesarean delivery if the fetus is alive. Although color-flow Doppler ultrasound may be diagnostic, there is seldom time for this testing procedure before fetal demise occurs from a ruptured fetal vessel. Whenever late or severe variable decelerations, a sinusoidal heart rate pattern, or a changing fetal heart rate baseline is identified, the possibility of vasa previa should be given consideration. An Apt test may help in the evaluation of any vaginal blood loss to determine whether the bleeding is fetal in origin. This test involves mixing equal volumes of blood with 0.25% NaOH. Fetal blood containing fetal hemoglobin remains pink, whereas the adult hemoglobin present in maternal blood undergoes denaturation, resulting in a light brown color.

Uterine Rupture

Treatment usually requires cesarean delivery of the fetus regardless of gestational age. Following delivery, the uterine defect can be assessed, and an ultimate management decision can be made. Débridement back to healthy tissue can often lead to satisfactory repair with closure requiring multiple layers. Occasionally, hysterectomy can be both necessary and lifesaving.

Other Causes

This group of patients usually does not have excess fetal or maternal morbidity or mortality with the exception of those with invasive cervical cancer. Therefore, these conditions should be managed expectantly.

HYPERTENSIVE DISORDERS OF PREGNANCY

method of
MARSHALL D. LINDHEIMER, M.D., and
ADRIAN I. KATZ, M.D.
Pritzker School of Medicine, University of Chicago
Chicago, Illinois

Hypertension is a worrisome complication of pregnancy, affecting 5 to 10% of all gestations. This contribution focuses on preeclampsia, a specific disorder of pregnancy responsible for most of the reported morbidity of the hypertensive complications of gestation, and a leading cause of both maternal death and fetal demise.

Supported by grants from the National Institutes of Health, American Heart Association, and the Mother's Aid Fund of Chicago Lying-in Hospital.

DETECTION AND CLASSIFICATIONS OF HYPERTENSION IN PREGNANCY

There is still controversy about the measurement of blood pressure in pregnancy, including which Korotkoff sound (fourth = muffling, or fifth = disappearance) represents more accurately the diastolic levels. The World Health Organization and many national societies suggest the fourth Korotkoff sound (K-IV), but we concur with the recommendations of the National High Blood Pressure Education Program (NHBPEP) that K-V be taken to measure diastolic levels because K-IV substantially overestimates intra-arterial pressure and appears to be more difficult to determine accurately. Also, because blood pressure measurement of gravidas positioned on their sides is impractical in an outpatient setting, quiet sitting remains the preferred approach. If the patient is hospitalized and blood pressure is measured with the subject in the lateral recumbent position (virtually a tradition in obstetric wards), care must be taken to ensure that the cuff is at the level of the heart, because the tendency by many to hold the arm higher leads to an underestimation of both systolic and diastolic levels.

The Working Group Report on High Blood Pressure in Pregnancy, published by the NHBPEP in 1990, retained the definition of high blood pressure in pregnancy currently contained in most texts—namely, increments in systolic and diastolic values of more than 30 and 15 mmHg, respectively, or a blood pressure of at least 140/90 mmHg. However, because blood pressure normally decreases in pregnancy, women with diastolic levels exceeding 75 mmHg during the second or 85 mmHg during the third trimester also require careful scrutiny.

A source of confusion is the existence of many terms used in classifying the hypertensive disorders of pregnancy. For example, the disease we define below as preeclampsia appears elsewhere in the literature under a variety of terms including toxemia, gestosis, pregnancy-induced hypertension (PIH), and pregnancy-associated hypertension. Furthermore, many of the proposed classifications are complex and overly detailed, and the same term may have different definitions in different reports. We use the scheme developed in 1972 by a committee of the American College of Obstetricians and Gynecologists (and endorsed in the NHBPEP report), which is concise but accurately separates the more benign from the serious disorders. In it the hypertensive disorders of pregnancy are divided into only four categories: (1) chronic hypertension (of whatever cause); (2) preeclampsia-eclampsia; (3) preeclampsia superimposed on chronic hypertension; and (4) transient or late hypertension.

Chronic Hypertension. Almost half the incidence of high blood pressure occurring during pregnancy is due to essential hypertension. Diagnosis is most certain when hypertension is present prior to gestation, but women with high blood pressure discovered prior to gestational week 20 or persisting after the puerperium are included here. Gestations are usually uneventful provided the blood pressure elevation is mild and evidence of maternal end-organ damage is absent. These women, however, have a higher incidence of superimposed preeclampsia, the complication responsible for most of the morbidity associated with their gestations (see subsequent discussion).

There are unusual instances of pregnancy in women with secondary causes of hypertension, some of whom do poorly. For instance, Cushing's syndrome may be exacerbated after conception, and the prognosis for the fetus is poor. Pheochromocytoma is particularly lethal, especially when undiagnosed; it is fortunately rare, but has a propensity to present in gestation. When detected, the disease can be managed pharmacologically until delivery, after which an operable tumor can be resected. Thus, it is prudent to screen for catecholamine excess at the slightest suspicion. Two collagen disorders, scleroderma and periarteritis nodosa, are associated with poor maternal and fetal outcomes. On the other hand, pregnancy may reduce blood pressure in women with renal artery stenosis and ameliorate potassium loss in patients with primary hyperaldosteronism.

Preeclampsia-Eclampsia. Preeclampsia, especially if *superimposed on chronic hypertension* (category 3), is a serious complication of pregnancy that may imperil both the mother and the unborn child. Preeclampsia occurs primarily in nulliparous women, mainly after midpregnancy, and most frequently near term. It is characterized by hypertension, increased urinary protein excretion (at least 300 mg per day, or at least 2+), and edema. Other signs include abnormal liver function and coagulation abnormalities, primarily thrombocytopenia. Preeclampsia may rapidly progress to a dramatic and life-threatening convulsive phase termed eclampsia, which is often preceded by ominous premonitory symptoms and signs including hemoconcentration, hyperreflexia, visual disturbances, severe headaches, and epigastric or right upper quadrant pain (Table 1), but the eclamptic fit has been known to occur suddenly without warning in a seemingly asymptomatic patient who appears to have only mildly elevated pressures. *This is why preeclampsia, regardless of apparent severity, always presents a potential danger to mother and fetus.*

There is an ominous variant of preeclampsia that may have a deceptively benign presentation. The patient manifests only minimal (if any) increments in blood pressure, small declines in platelet counts, modest increments in liver enzymes, and little or no alterations in renal function, prompting the practitioner to consider temporization. However, this form of preeclampsia may rapidly become life-threatening because it develops (often within 24 hours) into a syndrome characterized by hemolysis (due to a microangiopathic hemolytic anemia), marked changes in coagulation and liver function (platelet counts plunge to as low as 100×10^3 per cubic millimeter, and transaminase and lactic acid dehydrogenase levels increase to as much as and even beyond 1000 IU within 24 hours). This preeclampsia variant is termed the HELLP syndrome (hemolysis, elevated liver enzymes, low platelet counts). It is an emergency requiring prompt termination of the pregnancy, in which case postpartum recovery is usually rapid. In some instances, however, the disease has occurred in the puerperium, and more rarely, the severe thrombocytopenia has persisted, leading to plasma exchange, although the need for and efficacy of the latter approach remain to be determined. Preeclampsia tends to regress rapidly postpartum, although in severe cases the blood pressure may take 2 to 3 weeks to return to normal. There is also a rare entity termed late postpartum eclampsia, characterized by hypertension, edema, proteinuria, and convulsions within the first 10 days of the puerperium.

TABLE 1. **Ominous Signs and Symptoms in Women with Preeclampsia**

Preeclampsia is always potentially dangerous but particularly ominous may be:
- Blood pressure ≥160 mmHg systolic or ≥110 mmHg diastolic
- Proteinuria of new onset at a rate ≥2 gm per 24 h or ≥100 mg per dL in a random urine sample
- Increasing serum creatinine levels (especially >2 mg per dL [177 μmol per liter], unless known to be elevated previously)
- Platelet count <100,000 per microliter, or evidence of microangiopathic hemolytic anemia (e.g., schistocytes, or increased lactic acid dehydrogenase and direct bilirubin levels)
- Upper abdominal pain, especially epigastric and right upper quadrant pain
- Headache, visual disturbances, or other cerebral signs
- Cardiac decompensation (e.g., pulmonary edema). Usually associated with underlying heart pathology or chronic hypertension
- Retinal hemorrhages, exudates, or papilledema (these are extremely rare in the absence of other indicators of severity and, when present, almost always indicate underlying chronic hypertension)

The presence of intrauterine growth retardation and decreasing urine volumes also require added vigilance.

Modified from Cunningham FG, Lindheimer MD: Hypertension in pregnancy. N Engl J Med 326:927–932, 1992.

Superimposed preeclampsia may be difficult to distinguish clinically from an exacerbation of a renal disorder (such as chronic glomerulonephritis) or acceleration of chronic essential hypertension, both of which can manifest high blood pressure, proteinuria, and edema. Superimposed preeclampsia is distinguished from the "pure" form of the disease only by its tendency to occur earlier in the second half of gestation; it is often more severe because of the preexisting hypertension.

Transient Hypertension. Transient hypertension in pregnancy develops after midgestation or shortly after delivery and is characterized by mild elevations of blood pressure and usually a benign gestational outcome. The hypertension regresses postpartum but frequently recurs in subsequent pregnancies (this entity occurring in a nullipara is obviously a retrospective diagnosis). Transient hypertension of pregnancy is believed by some to predict essential hypertension later in life.

ETIOLOGY AND PATHOPHYSIOLOGY OF PREECLAMPSIA

Preeclampsia, especially the severe variety, is characterized by reduced cardiac output, the increased blood pressure being due to markedly increased peripheral resistance. The hypertension, often labile, is characterized at times by reversal of normal circadian blood pressure patterns, the highest values occurring at night. There is also a reversal of the normal hemodynamic adaptations of pregnancy (namely, decreases in peripheral vascular resistance and reduced pressor responses to infused angiotensin [AII]), because preeclamptics manifest exaggerated pressure responses to AII many weeks before the disease becomes clinically manifest. This striking increase in pressor responsiveness may be due to up-regulation of vascular receptors to AII because circulating levels of this peptide actually decrease.

The cause of the altered vascular responses is not known, current research focusing on factors that may increase vessel reactivity such as endothelial cell damage resulting in decreases in relaxing factors or increments in endothelin release. This damage has been postulated to be caused by circulating "toxic" factors, cytokines, or excess lipid peroxides. Other theories implicate prostanoids, calcium metabolism, natriuretic factors, and aberrations in hormone levels and action including those of insulin and parathyroid hormone.

There is a renal lesion in preeclampsia (termed glomerular endotheliosis) that may be responsible for the increased protein excretion as well as decrements in both glomerular filtration rate (GFR) and the clearance of uric acid. Plasma values of creatinine and uric acid, however, may still be

TABLE 2. **Laboratory Evaluation of Women Who Develop Hypertension After Midgestation**

Test	Rationale
Hemoglobin and hematocrit	Hemoconcentration favors diagnosis of preeclampsia and is an indicator of severity. Decreased values, however, may occur when hemolysis accompanies the disease
Blood smear	Signs of microangiopathic hemolytic anemia (e.g., schistocytes) favor the diagnosis of preeclampsia and may be present when blood pressure is only mildly elevated
Platelet count	Decreased levels are associated with severe preeclampsia
Serum creatinine	Abnormal or rising levels, especially if associated with oliguria, suggest severe preeclampsia
Serum uric acid	Aids in the differential diagnosis of preeclampsia and is an indicator of disease severity
Oxaloacetic transaminase	Abnormal levels suggest severe preeclampsia with liver involvement
Lactate dehydrogenase	Elevated levels are associated with both hemolysis and liver involvement and suggest severe preeclampsia
Serum albumin	May be decreased even in the absence of heavy proteinuria and may relate to "capillary leak" or liver involvement in preeclampsia
Urinalysis	Do quantitative measurement of protein excretion if dipstick is 1+ or greater. Excretion of ≥300 mg/24 h suggests development of preeclampsia

Modified from the Consensus Report, National High Blood Pressure Education Program Working Group Report on High Blood Pressure in Pregnancy. Am J Obstet Gynecol 163:1689–1712, 1990.

lower in preeclamptics than in nonpregnant women because GFR and urate clearance are markedly increased early in normal pregnancy. Thus, plasma creatinine and uric acid levels of 0.9 and 5 mg per dL, respectively, are abnormal in gravid subjects. Finally, the ability to excrete sodium may be reduced, leading to salt and water retention, but severe disease may occur even in the absence of edema. Most of the fluid retained is in the interstitial space, but even when they are edematous, preeclamptics have decreased intravascular volumes and manifest hemoconcentration.

CAN PREECLAMPSIA BE PREVENTED?

Discovery of a way to prevent preeclampsia would revolutionize prenatal care and save countless maternal and fetal lives. In the past, sodium restriction and prophylactic diuretics were popular. However, there is no evidence that limitation of dietary sodium modifies the incidence or severity of preeclampsia, and current nutritional recommendations for gravidas stress adequate salt rations. Also, a meta-analysis of randomized studies of over 7000 women found that the incidence of proteinuric hypertension (presumably preeclampsia) was similar among women who received prophylactic diuretics compared to untreated controls. Two approaches, suggested more recently, include low-dose aspirin (60 to 100 mg per day starting after gestational week 12), and supplemental dietary calcium (approx 2 grams per day) throughout pregnancy. The former therapy is predicated on the hypothesis that these doses of aspirin inhibit thromboxane but spare prostacyclin production. Despite two favorable meta-analyses of a number of limited trials, the results of several very large multicenter randomized trials (one of which includes over 8000 patients) have been disappointing (although the results from a large number of high-risk patients remain to be reported). One should await the results of the latter studies before prescribing these drugs. Calcium supplementation is based on the observation that preeclamptic women are hypocalciuric, and on the hypothesis that low dietary calcium intake is associated with hypertension in general. Again, one should await the results of a large multicenter trial in progress, which should be concluded by mid or late 1995.

THERAPY

Managing Preeclampsia

If one suspects preeclampsia it is always prudent to consider hospitalization, although a well-informed patient may be managed while resting at home (monitoring services that save hospitalization costs are appearing worldwide). Such aggressive approaches will diminish the incidence of convulsions, reduce diagnostic error, and improve fetal outcome. Near term, induction of labor is the treatment of choice, but earlier in pregnancy one may carefully try to temporize.

TABLE 3. **Guidelines for Treating Severe Hypertension Near Term or During Labor**

Control of Blood Pressure

The degree to which blood pressure should be decreased is disputed. The Working Group's "consensus" report recommends maintaining levels between 90 and 105 mmHg (see text)

Drug Therapy

1. Hydralazine administered intravenously is the drug of choice. Start with low doses (5 mg intravenous bolus), then administer 5–10 mg every 20–30 min to avoid precipitous decreases. Side effects include tachycardia and headache. Neonatal thrombocytopenia has been reported.
2. Diazoxide is recommended by the NHBPEP for the occasional patient whose hypertension is refractory to hydralazine. Use 30-mg miniboluses because precipitous hypotension may result with higher doses. Side effects include arrest of labor and neonatal hypoglycemia.
3. There is also considerable experience with labetalol, and many use this agent instead of diazoxide as a second-line drug (see also Table 4).
4. Favorable results have also been reported with calcium channel blockers. However, if magnesium sulfate is being infused, the magnesium ion may potentiate the effect of the calcium channel blockers, resulting in precipitous and severe hypotension.
5. Refrain from using nitroprusside because fetal cyanide poisoning has been reported in animal models. However, in the final analysis, maternal well-being will dictate choice of therapy.

The Working Group retained parenteral magnesium sulfate as the drug of choice for preventing impending eclamptic convulsions. A loading dose of 4–6 gm $MgSO_4$ (infused over 10 min; never a bolus) is followed by infusion of a sustaining solution (24 gm $MgSO_4$ in 1 liter of 5% dextrose in water) delivered at a rate of 1–2 gm/h, which aims to maintain plasma levels at 5–9 mg/dL (2.1–3.5 mM/L). Therapy should continue for 12–24 h into the puerperium because one-third of patients with eclampsia have convulsions after childbirth.

Modified from Lindheimer MD, Katz AI: Hypertension in pregnancy. N Engl J Med *313*:675–680, 1985; and Cunningham FG and Lindheimer MD: Hypertension in pregnancy. N Engl J Med *326*:927–932, 1992.

TABLE 4. **Antihypertensive Drugs Used to Treat Chronic Hypertension in Pregnancy**

Alpha$_2$-adrenergic receptor agonists	Methyldopa (Aldomet) is the most extensively used drug in this group, its safety and efficacy supported in randomized trials and in a 7.5-yr follow-up study of children born to treated mothers. *Methyldopa is the drug of choice recommended by the Working Group.*
Beta-adrenergic receptor antagonists	These drugs, especially atenolol (Tenormin) and metoprolol (Lopressor), appear safe and efficacious in late pregnancy, but fetal growth retardation has been noted when treatment was started in early or midgestation. Fetal bradycardia can occur, and animal studies suggest that the fetus' ability to tolerate hypoxic stress may be compromised.
Alpha- and beta-adrenergic receptor antagonists	Labetalol (Normodyne) appears as effective as methyldopa, but there is little or no follow-up information on children born to mothers treated with labetalol, and there is concern about maternal hepatotoxicity.
Arteriolar vasodilators	Hydralazine is used frequently as adjunctive therapy with methyldopa and beta-adrenergic receptor antagonists. Rarely, neonatal thrombocytopenia has been reported. Trials with calcium channel blockers look promising. Experience with minoxidil (Loniten) is limited; this drug is not recommended.
Converting enzyme inhibitors	Captopril (Capoten) causes fetal death in various animal species, and several converting enzyme inhibitors have been associated with renal failure in the newborn when administered to humans. *Do not use in pregnancy.*
Diuretics	Many authorities discourage their use, but others continue these medications if they were prescribed before gestation or if a chronic hypertensive appears to be quite salt-sensitive. *The latter views have been endorsed by the Working Group.*

Modified from Lindheimer MD, Katz AI: Hypertension in pregnancy. N Engl J Med *313*:675–680, 1985; and Cunningham FG and Lindheimer MD: Hypertension in pregnancy. N Engl J Med *326*:927–932, 1992.

Delivery is indicated, however, regardless of gestational age or fetal size, if severe hypertension cannot be controlled within 24 to 48 hours, at the appearance of any of the "ominous" signs or symptoms described in Table 1 (especially thrombocytopenia, liver dysfunction, progressive decrements in renal function, headache, epigastric pain, or hyperreflexia), or evidence of fetal jeopardy. Table 2 suggests the laboratory tests that aid in monitoring women who develop hypertension after midpregnancy.

There is some controversy about the best approach to use when blood pressure increases rapidly near term, often during delivery. Table 3 summarizes our recommendations, reflecting also the conclusions of the NHBPEP consensus report. They cautioned against administering diuretics to preeclamptics and indicated that diastolic pressures of 105 mmHg or more should be treated (although some current texts list this figure as 110 mmHg or higher). Certain circumstances, however, may prompt treatment at lower levels, such as a very young gravida whose recent diastolic levels were 70 mmHg or lower. Table 4 summarizes the antihypertensive agents currently used in such urgent situations. Parenteral hydralazine remains the agent of choice owing to its record of safety in obstetric populations. Given cautiously it is successful in most cases, and surprisingly low doses are required to control even striking levels of hypertension.

There is also controversy about the prevention or management of eclamptic convulsions, reflecting in part our ignorance of their genesis. The NHBPEP report recommended parenteral magnesium (we use 4 grams of magnesium sulfate given over 15 minutes as a loading dose, with 1 to 2 grams per hour given intravenously as maintenance; see standard obstetric texts for precautions), recognizing that its success has been documented only in uncontrolled series and that definitive trials are needed. In 1994, a large randomized study sponsored by the World Health Organization, which compares magnesium, a benzodiazepine, and phenytoin in eclamptic women was in progress.

Finally, detailed consideration of anesthetic choices and the role of invasive monitoring is beyond the scope of this contribution but is discussed in major obstetric texts. In brief, although epidural analgesia for labor is favored by many anesthesiologists, the tendencey of this approach to provoke hypotension and the fact that intravascular volume is decreased in preeclampsia lead some obstetricians to prefer general anesthesia. Considering certain characteristics of severe preeclampsia such as hemoconcentration, the use of epidural analgesia requires caution and the presence of an experienced obstetric anesthesiologist (a view endorsed by the American College of Obstetricians and Gynecologists). Finally, we believe that only a small minority of women require invasive monitoring, most cases being manageable with standard clinical acumen. In this respect, even when oliguria is present, and as long as creatinine levels are stable, fluid replacement during delivery should be restricted to 75 to 100 mL per hour.

Managing Chronic Hypertension in Pregnancy

Most "chronic" hypertension occurring in gestation is of the essential variety and is mild in nature, so that over 85% of such women have uncomplicated pregnancies. In a minority, however, there is increased morbidity, which includes fetal growth retardation, abruption, acute renal failure, cardiac decompensation, or cerebral accidents. Most of the latter cases appear to occur in older gravidas (over 30 years old) whose hypertension has been present for many years and who may have evidence of end-organ damage. Also, extremely obese women with chronic hypertension are at special risk for cardiac decompensation near term, especially if volume overloading occurs during labor. In such patients echocardiographic evaluation may be warranted during gestation to evaluate ventricular compliance and performance.

Antihypertensive treatment is indicated during gestation when diastolic levels are 100 mmHg or higher but at lower levels if risk factors are present (e.g., renal parenchymal disease, end-organ damage). Table 4 summarizes the clinical experience with a variety of agents. The NHBPEP report recommends methyldopa as the drug of choice, given its long record of use during gestation and evidence of safety from a 7.5-year follow-up study of infants whose mothers were treated with this agent during gestation. Few other drugs have been tested as thoroughly in gravid populations, and when trials of other drugs have been reported their efficacy only paralleled that of methyldopa. The consensus document noted that diuretics taken before conception could be continued in pregnancy and could be prescribed to pregnant women whose high blood pressure appears to be overly salt-sensitive.

Finally, we note that although a diastolic pressure of 100 mmHg has been recommended as the level that requires beginning antihypertensive therapy, some authorities, mainly outside the United States, have suggested that treatment of mild hypertension (90 to 100 mmHg) may prevent superimposed preeclampsia and may decrease the number of hospital days and the number of preterm births. We do not prescribe drugs to pregnant women who have only mild hypertension, but this is clearly an area that needs investigation.

OBSTETRIC ANESTHESIA

method of
BRADLEY E. SMITH, M.D.
Vanderbilt University Medical Center
Nashville, Tennessee

The "consumer movement," which has encouraged a healthy new emphasis on full participation by the parents in the birth process, has also accelerated acceptance of regional obstetric anesthesia and has led to the long-awaited demise of the routine use of heavy medication and general anesthesia in obstetrics in the United States. Nonetheless, anesthesia still probably accounts for 7% of maternal mortality in obstetric patients in the United States. Aspiration of vomitus may still cause one-fourth of obstetric anesthesia deaths. Obstructed airway, inability to intubate the trachea, laryngospasm, anoxia, overdose of anesthetic, and chronic hypoventilation all result in maternal and fetal mortality and morbidity. Regional anesthesia also presents the possibility of serious complications; these include convulsions, "total spinal block," and hypotension with epidural block. "Spinal" anesthesia, although effective and safer than epidural anesthesia, is fast losing popularity, largely because it has not been possible to maintain it for long periods during labor and because of fear of "spinal headache." The decision about which pain relief method to use should consider not only the obstetric situation but also the abilities of the anesthetist actually present to administer the anesthetic. Poorly qualified or inexperienced anesthesia personnel must not be asked to perform difficult and potentially hazardous types of anesthesia, thus exposing two lives to serious complications.

CHOICE OF MANAGEMENT OF ANESTHESIA IN NORMAL PREGNANCIES

Psychologic Techniques

The numerous available psychologic techniques can be divided into "natural childbirth," "psychoprophylaxis," and "medical hypnosis." Psychologic preparation for labor benefits most patients, but its unpredictability and the great amount of time necessary to implement it often makes it impractical for routine use. However, they, along with regional anesthesia, have the important advantage of preserving the mother's ability to respond to and with the baby immediately after birth and to receive the psychological benefits of participation in the birth process.

Sedative and Narcotic Management of Labor Pain

Use of excessive analgesics and sedatives may extend the latent and active phases of labor. However, when labor is well established, only certain general inhalational anesthetics will completely inhibit uterine contractions. (Spinal, peridural, and thiopental anesthesia uncomplicated by hypotension does not influence the force of uterine contractions but may reduce the effectiveness of conscious muscular expulsive efforts.) Doses of sedatives and narcotics sufficient to reduce labor pain significantly without blocks or other adjuncts almost universally cause depression of breathing, cardiovascular function, and alertness in the newborn baby. Recently, however, fentanyl (Sublimaze), in doses of 25 μg given intravenously by patient-controlled analgesia (PCA) pump with a 10-minute lockout, has been used by some to decrease the pain of labor.

Pudendal Block

Pudendal block is still a useful option to establish surgical anesthesia of the perineum with no effect on the course of labor and can be administered by the obstetrician. This block can provide adequate anesthesia for simple spontaneous delivery, even with episiotomy, and is sufficient to allow some motivated women to experience even indicated vacuum extraction or minor outlet forceps procedures. Approximately 10 mL of 1% lidocaine (Xylocaine) deposited on each pudendal nerve at the origin of the sacrosciatic ligament is usually sufficient and rarely causes complications.

Paracervical Block Anesthesia for Vaginal Delivery

This block has regrettably fallen from favor because of a fear of fetal bradycardia and possible cardiac depression. It provides excellent relief of labor pains in both the first and second stages of labor but should be combined with pudendal block for the delivery itself. It is established by infiltration of approximately 10 mL of 1% lidocaine (many centers forbid the use of bupivacaine [Marcaine] for this block) at positions corresponding to four and eight o'clock around the cervix during careful fetal heart monitoring. The anesthetist should wait between injections and observe the fetal heart rate while administering the drug. Bradycardia or fetal death can occur when paracervical block is administered in a high dosage, too rapidly, or without monitoring, but the incidence is low.

Continuous Lumbar Peridural Analgesia for Vaginal Delivery

Continuous lumbar peridural analgesia allows the use of smaller doses of local anesthetic drugs than does a caudal block. Complete anesthesia of the perineum is somewhat delayed with this method compared with a caudal block, but hypotension and toxic reactions are less frequent because of the smaller dose and the lesser vascularity at the site of injection. Minor slowing of total labor may occur because of the reduced reflex urge to push down vigorously in second stage labor and because of unnecessary degrees of muscle block. These inconveniences can be minimized by limiting the concentration of local anesthetic and the spread of block and by maintaining good coaching during the second stage to encourage pushing. Several large clinical studies show that *acceleration* of labor by minimizing the effects of pain and fear actually occurs as frequently as inhibition of labor by epidural anesthesia.

Epidural Technique for Vaginal Delivery

Establishment of the epidural block before the cervix is dilated 3 to 4 cm may slow the latent phase of labor. After the sterile preparation and drape, a special needle (a 17-gauge Weiss needle serves well) is placed in the epidural space, and a plastic catheter is inserted. A test dose given to detect intravascular or subarachnoid placement is very important. One common test protocol includes 3 mL of 1.5% lidocaine with 1:100,000 epinephrine given through the plastic catheter. If no excitement, convulsions, respiratory impairment, tachycardia, or other signs of intravascular or subarachnoid injection are apparent after 3 minutes, a therapeutic dose of 8 mL of 0.25% bupivacaine with 40 μg of fentanyl (Sublimaze) is given through the epidural catheter. Analgesia usually develops within 20 minutes with little loss of muscle tone. Analgesia for labor can be maintained with an infusion by pump of 10 to 14 mL per hour of a mixture of 0.125% bupivacaine with 5 μg per milliliter of fentanyl at a rate of 10 to 14 mL per hour into the same catheter. Bolus doses of 0 to 4 mL can be given if the analgesia level is inadequate. An additional dose just before delivery is sometimes needed to improve perineal anesthesia; some prefer 0.25% bupivacaine without fentanyl for this final dose.

Spinal Anesthesia ("Saddle Block") for Vaginal Delivery

Spinal anesthesia is usually administered in the primiparous patient when the head is at about plus two to three station late in second stage, but it may be established earlier in the multiparous patient. Hypotension occurs in approximately 18% of saddle block anesthetics, so blood pressure should be monitored carefully, especially immediately after the block and after delivery of the infant.

Spinal Block Technique for Vaginal Delivery

After arachnoid puncture with the smallest possible needle (many now prefer the Sprotte design to avoid "spinal headaches"), a dose of about 25 to 40 mg of lidocaine, or 0.5 mL of 0.75% bupivacaine in dextrose diluted to 1½ to 2 mL, should produce anesthesia to about T10 if the patient sits erect for about 30 seconds after the injection before lying down. Anesthesia will be complete during forceps manipulations and episiotomy.

Inhalation Analgesia

The intentional use of a potent inhalational anesthetic agent in exceedingly low concentrations (subanesthesia) is a safe and simple analgesic technique that has fallen from common use because of the expressed desire of many women to be entirely alert at the time of birth. However, this technique can allow the mother to remain conversant, cooperative, and self-controlled without danger to the baby. Constant inhalation of 40 to 50% nitrous oxide and oxygen, 0.5 to 0.8% enflurane (Ethrane), or 0.3 to 0.5% isoflurane (Forane) is effective in producing demonstrable analgesia and degrees of amnesia in approximately 90% of cases. All of these agents have essentially no effects on the fetus at these low concentrations.

General Anesthesia

When general anesthesia is necessary, the dose or depth and the duration of anesthesia prior to delivery must be minimized. Mixing of all intravenous and inhalational anesthetics with the fetal blood begins almost immediately after administration. The use of unconscious general anesthesia usually calls for endotracheal intubation owing to the possibility of aspiration of gastric contents or loss of patency of the airway. This technique usually requires two persons, one of whom presses the cricoid cartilage directly against the vertebrae, thereby "pinching" the esophagus closed (Sellick's maneuver).

Inhalation Anesthetic Agents

These anesthetics pass the placenta immediately, and in anesthetic concentrations all produce significant depression in the newborn. All but nitrous oxide can lead to postpartum uterine bleeding. Although they are of great help in certain obstetric complications (e.g., tetanic uterine contractions), their routine obstetric use is not recommended because their effects make the baby "sleepy." However, in low concentrations (i.e., 0.75% enflurane, or 0.6% isoflurane), they produce amnesia and some analgesia and reduce stress responses during light general endotracheal anesthesia along with nitrous oxide at 50%.

Thiopental

Thiopental (Pentothal) induction of maternal general anesthesia may cause some depression of breathing in the newborn. In full-term infants the danger is real but of small magnitude, and a dose of 3.5 mg per kg given intravenously is commonly used. It was mistakenly thought in the past that a long period between the injection and delivery allows "redistribution" of the drug in the baby, but it is clear now that the shortest interval practical between induction of anesthesia and delivery of the baby is safest. Greater caution should be used with thiopental when dealing with "high-risk" or premature babies.

Ketamine

Although slower in achieving induction, ketamine (Ketalar) in small doses (up to 0.75 mg per kg) is recognized as a safe alternative to thiopental as an induction agent in obstetrics. In small doses both immediate and delayed newborn alertness appear to be better than with thiopental, and the blood pressure of both mother and newborn are better supported. Neurologic complications and respiratory depression may be caused by larger ketamine doses. Rarely, hallucinations by mothers during emergence from ketamine anesthesia occur, but at these low doses they are very infrequent and are usually prevented by postpartum doses of diazepam (Valium).

CHOICE OF ANESTHESIA AND ANALGESIA IN COMPLICATED PREGNANCIES

Forceps

Forceps are rarely used in modern obstetrics but still have indications. During the use of forceps or vacuum extraction devices, a relaxed perineum and a quiet patient aid in preventing maternal vaginal lacerations and extension of the episiotomy and help to minimize trauma to the baby's head. These conditions are provided by spinal and peridural blocks, which also allow the mother to participate in the birth.

Breech Presentation

Vaginal delivery of babies presenting by breech became infrequent in recent years owing to evidence that both neonatal mortality and intellectual development appeared more favorable after cesarean birth of breech babies. However, the incidence of vaginal breech births is now increasing as the risk/benefit ratio is becoming better understood. Today many experts advocate epidural analgesia for breech births. An alternate choice for pain management in vaginal breech birth consists of good psychic support supplemented by minimal narcotics and tranquilizers, a paracervical block in the first stage, and a quick induction of general endotracheal anesthesia including succinylcholine (Anectine) when the infant's umbilicus becomes visible. This sequence, combined with the "following hand" pressure on the mother's abdomen just above the pubis, may obviate forceps and minimize the transfer of anesthetic to the baby.

Multiple Births

Useful methods of pain management for the vaginal delivery of the first baby of twins may include the use of limited doses of systemic analgesia (i.e., narcotics and tranquilizers) during the first and early second stage, occasionally supplemented by light inhalational or continuous epidural analgesia. Anesthesia for delivery of the first baby can also be provided by pudendal block and inhalational analgesia or by regional block. The second baby may be delivered under pudendal or local anesthesia in some cases. A significant increase in neonatal mortality is associated with multiple births if intrauterine manipulation (e.g., version and breech extraction) is attempted while the mother is under local or regional anesthesia. If the second infant is to be delivered by means of version and breech extraction, endotracheal halothane anesthesia may be used to relax the uterus, but preparations for needed active resuscitation of the baby should be made in advance.

Tetanic Contractions

The older standard method of rapid relaxation of the uterus during tetanic contractions used inhalation anesthesia. Endotracheal halothane at concentrations of only 1 to 2% is effective within 2 to 4 minutes, but hypotension is frequent, and endotracheal intubation using prophylactic cricoid pressure is recommended to guard against aspiration of vomitus. Intravenous "beta stimulator" catecholamines do not work as completely nor as rapidly. Regional anesthesia does not relax the uterus. Intravenous nitroglycerin (in 100- to 300-μg boluses) may relax the uterus but often causes dangerous maternal hypotension.

Fetal Distress

When fetal distress exists, further depression of the newborn by potent anesthetics given to the mother should be minimized. Although some doctors have advocated spinal anesthesia at this time, no time should be wasted, nor should hypotension be tolerated. If local anesthesia is not sufficient, general anesthesia may be produced rapidly and obstetric delivery expedited.

Antepartum Hemorrhage

Sudden antepartum bleeding leading to hypotensive maternal blood pressure is detrimental to the fetus. Hypovolemia is an added danger to the mother with anesthesia of any type. All forms of major regional anesthesia are frequently contraindicated in this emergency because the resulting sudden sympathetic blockade paralyzes the compensatory mechanisms ordinarily required to maintain the mother's blood pressure during hemorrhage. Management by local anesthesia, pudendal block, or subanesthetic inhalational analgesia is recommended when applicable, but maternal vascular volume should be restored as rapidly as possible with the appropriate fluid. Vasopressors should *not* be used in place of adequate volume replacement. Ketamine, 0.75 mg per kg, succinylcholine, oxygen, endotracheal intubation (by Sellick's technique), and 50% oxygen with 50% nitrous oxide is a popular method of obtaining general anesthesia in this emergency. Potent inhalation anesthetics may accentuate the hypotension caused by hypovolemia.

Pregnancy-Induced Hypertension (Toxemia of Pregnancy)

In a toxemic pregnancy, maternal liver and kidney function may be poor, convulsions are frequently encountered, severe maternal hypertension and increased sensitivity to vasopressors occur frequently, and the infant is often born prematurely and is undernourished. Most obstetric anesthesiologists favor continuous regional analgesia because of its antihypertensive quality and because of the minimal concomitant drug depression in the infant. However, some obstetricians still worry that hypotension develops more easily in response to regional block. Current worldwide experience does not validate this concern. Of course, care should be taken to evaluate and correct the hypovolemia frequently seen in toxemia before the regional blocks are placed. In managing general anesthesia, efforts to attenuate the hypertensive response to endotracheal intubation are important. Intravenous magnesium sulfate, which is frequently used by obstetricians, synergizes with anesthetic muscle relaxants and may contribute to newborn drug depression. Nitroglycerin, 100 to 300 μg by intravenous bolus, is sometimes used for this purpose.

Prematurity

Respiratory and cardiovascular depression is extremely common after the use of analgesic and anesthetic agents in premature infants. Continuous regional block is the analgesic method of choice during the first and second stages of labor. "Saddle block" is excellent for delivery but is not suitable for labor. Pudendal block is not dangerous but does not relax the birth canal sufficiently to minimize head trauma to the premature baby.

Diabetes

Anesthesia should be directed toward reducing stress. Although hypotension and other complications must be avoided, major regional analgesia is desirable when practical. Insulin and glucose control should be meticulous and should be frequently monitored during labor and the induction of anesthesia. Intravenous glucose intake must be carefully controlled because maternal hyperglycemia may stimulate excessive insulin release by the baby, leading to postpartum hypoglycemia.

Cardiac Disease

Fewer than 2% of pregnant patients suffer from severe heart disease, less than half the incidence noted 40 years ago. Although valvular sequelae of rheumatic fever still predominate, an increasing portion of pregnant cardiac patients today suffer from complicated congenital heart defects. Continuous regional analgesia is very popular for patients with a wide variety of acquired or congenital heart lesions. Great caution should be exercised in regard to the potential of regional anesthesia for precipitating heart failure by a sudden decrease in peripheral resistance. In addition, a potential for reversal of abnormal shunts because of changing vascular resistance should be borne in mind. Indications for invasive monitoring should be neither more nor less stringent than those used in patients with similar cardiac conditions about to undergo major surgical interventions. Certainly all pregnant cardiac patients should be continuously monitored with electrocardiography, and there shoud be continuing consultation with the physician caring for the cardiac condition.

Sickle Cell Disease

Sickle cell disease remains a grave threat to women with the SS configuration and their babies. Although some centers report excellent results with exchange transfusion in pregnant sickle cell patients, others disagree. Anesthesia for these patients also remains controversial. However, it should be noted that general anesthesia has not been followed by complications in a large reported series of surgical patients, and inhalation anesthetics have even been reported to be protective against sickling for several hours after anesthesia. Although stasis in the peripheral vascular bed and possible coagulation problems at the needle site have theoretically been objections to major regional analgesia in sickle cell disease, no objective evidence has ever been offered to support these objections.

Cesarean Section

Major regional analgesia is favored for cesarean section today in most large institutions because of its favorable effects on both mother and infant provided that the anesthesiologist is aware of and alert to the potential dangers. Prophylactic and therapeutic means of avoiding or treating common complications should be used. Such measures include preanesthetic intravenous volume expansion fluids, slight Trendelenburg position, prevention and correction of aortocaval compression by displacement of the uterus to the left, and preparation for administration of ephedrine, either prophylactically or therapeutically. Intravenous doses of 12.5 mg as needed are more controllable than intramuscular doses for either use.

ANESTHETIC TECHNIQUES FOR CESAREAN SECTION

Epidural Block Technique

When the patient is transferred to the operating table, she is placed in the left lateral position. An intravenous line is started with a 16- to 18-gauge plastic catheter, and 800 to 1500 mL of intravenous lactated Ringer's solution without dextrose is administered (to avoid rebound neonatal hypoglycemia). The epidural catheter is placed and tested for safety as outlined in the section on vaginal delivery. After the test dose, medication for cesarean section under epidural block could include 15 to 22 mL of bupivacaine 0.5% mixed with 100 μg of fentanyl or 4 mg morphine and administered in three divided doses.

Pain following extraction of the infant is treated by reinforcing the block routinely with 75% of the original dose of local anesthetic and fentanyl or morphine every hour, provided that a pinprick test verifies safe block level. During both epidural and spinal anesthesia, unpleasant sensations may be a problem for the mother even with high block levels. In such an event, intravenous analgesics and tranquilizers may be used in reduced doses. However, narcotics and benzodiazepines synergize their respiratory depressant effects when used together, particularly during high regional block analgesia. Extreme alertness for respiratory depression should always be exercised. Fentanyl, 25 μg per intravenous bolus, and midazolam (Versed), 0.5 mg per bolus, are common combinations. If analgesia remains inadequate, general endotracheal anesthesia with Sellick's technique can be instituted rather than continuing to reinforce intravenous sedation.

Spinal Anesthesia Technique

Bupivacaine, 0.75% in doses from 8 through 13 mg, with 20 μg of fentanyl or 0.2 mg of "spinal morphine" (Duramorph) mixed with 0.2 mL of 1:1000 fresh epinephrine, is adequate for subarachnoid block for cesarean section. After blocking, the patient is placed supine with a slight (10 degrees) Trendelenburg position, head on a pillow, and table tilted 15 degrees to the left. A pillow, balloon, or wedge is placed under the right hip to displace the uterus from the vena cava and aorta.

Arterial blood pressure is monitored at least every 60 seconds. If the systolic pressure falls 30% below the preanesthesia level or below 100 mmHg, the left uterine displacement is increased, the Trendelenburg position is steepened, the rate of intravenous infusion is increased, oxygen by face mask is administered, and ephedrine, 12.5 mg given intravenously in increments if necessary, can be given. Phenylephrine is not accepted by many anesthesiologists in this circumstance.

General Anesthesia

Premedication is usually omitted because of its effect on the baby. An intravenous infusion is started using a 16- or 18-gauge needle. Neutralization of acid stomach contents and suppression of further secretion of acid gastric content is desirable when possible by giving 30 mL of sodium bicitrate (Bicitra) orally. The patient is placed on the operating table in the left lateral recumbent position until the start of the skin preparation. The dangers of aortocaval compression are also present during general anesthesia, so the mother's right hip should be elevated on a pillow or the uterus deflected during cesarean section under general as well as regional anesthesia. During preparations, the patient is preoxygenated for 3 minutes. When the surgeon is ready, 0.6 mg of scopolamine and 0.3 mg of pancuronium are given about 3 minutes before induction.

Thiopental, 3.5 mg per kg intravenous, may depress even full-term infants slightly even in this small dose; however, the degree of "sleepiness" is not important in most full-term healthy babies. Ketamine in small doses (0.75 mg per kg intravenous) seems to be well tolerated but in higher doses may cause *profound* neurologic and respiratory problems in the baby. Many obstetric anesthesiologists still prefer muscle paralysis induced by succinylcholine, 2 mg per kg intravenous, followed by a variable intravenous infusion. However, others use 0.1 mg per kg of pancuronium (Pavulon) given intravenously and followed by smaller increments as needed.

Either thiopental, 3.5 mg per kg up to a maximum of 250 mg, or ketamine, 0.75 mg per kg up to 60 mg, is given as a bolus intravenously, followed by succinylcholine, 2 mg per kg, followed by a continuous drip of 0.2% succinylcholine. *Cricoid pressure should be instituted and maintained by someone other than the anesthetist as soon as consciousness is impaired.* Intubate the trachea and check ventilation in both lungs with a stethoscope before permitting the incision.

After tracheal intubation, many elect to administer only nitrous oxide, 4 liters per minute, and oxygen, 4 liters per minute, until the cord is clamped. In this case, the level of anesthesia can be deepened with thiopental, narcotics, or potent inhalation agents as soon as the cord is clamped. The continuing use of succinylcholine drip (or pancuronium) should be monitored with a nerve block stimulator. Some experts advocate adding a small dose of fentanyl, sufentanil (Sufenta), or alfentanil (Alfenta) or approximately one-half minimal alveolar concentration of a potent inhalation agent before the birth to reduce the maternal stress response and the possibility of memory. However, the possibility that respiratory depression in the baby exists after these drugs are administered should not be disregarded.

Pain After Vaginal Delivery

The intensity of pain in the period following vaginal delivery is rarely as severe as that in cesarean section. Therefore, a variety of oral analgesic agents are commonly employed for this purpose, and, rarely, a few doses of common parenteral opioid agents are used. In recent years a wide variety of antiprostaglandins has been employed with increasing success, sometimes without the need for other analgesics. In the occasional patient with a large episiotomy or perineal lacerations, it may be anticipated that the pain will be severe enough to warrant use of techniques described later in conjunction with cesarean section.

Pain After Cesarean Section

Again, a variety of methods of treatment of pain after cesarean section may be suitable. Oral and parenteral opioids or even milder oral analgesics represented by substances such as oxycodone, 5 mg, and acetaminophen, 325 mg orally (Percocet) every 6 hours, often in conjunction with antiprostaglandins (e.g., ibuprofen [Motrin], 400 mg orally every 6 hours), have become standard in treating this type of pain. Recent research shows that many deficiencies exist in this method including "peaks and valleys" in the intensity of pain due to the varying blood levels achieved by intermittent intramuscular injection. On the other hand, this method is by far the least costly of all those described in this section, and it may be expedient and sufficient in many patients.

Patient-Controlled Analgesia (PCA)

Although the concept of PCA is well over 25 years old, its popularity has surged in the past 4 years. This method has been shown to result in a less variable blood concentration of the analgesic agent. In addition, numerous studies verify that eliminating the peaks and valleys of analgesia, along with the undefinable psychologic comfort of the patient of knowing that she can instantly obtain relief from pain, clearly results in overall administration of a lesser total dose of analgesic agent during any given time period. Unexpected apnea from the respiratory depressant effects of the opioids has been reported but is not as frequent as that reported after intrathecal or epidural use of opioids as described later. However, because of the need for specialized electronic gear and the preparation by the pharmacy of large volumes of analgesic agent to be placed in the reservoir, this method of analgesia entails significant additional expense.

COMPLICATIONS OF GENERAL ANESTHESIA

Airway Obstruction

Eleven obstetric patients were reported to have died in New York City in one 2-year period owing to failure to achieve and maintain control of the patient's access to air (the "airway") and ventilation of the lungs during induction of general anesthesia for obstetric delivery. Therefore, it is essential that before induction of general anesthesia, the obstetrician and the anesthetist agree on the steps to be taken for the patient at hand should intubation of the trachea prove impossible. These will vary according to the condition of the mother and the baby. This "failed intubation" protocol should be instituted quickly and skillfully.

Aspiration of Gastric Contents

Aspiration of stomach contents is a major hazard during heavy sedation or general anesthesia and occurs even under major regional anesthesia. Gastric emptying may be slowed because of the pain of labor or by the administration of narcotic pain relievers. In addition, the patient frequently has recently eaten a meal just before the onset of labor. Emptying the stomach artificially by administering apomorphine or gastric lavage is very unpleasant, dangerous, and unreliable. Aspiration of gastric contents is now reported to be fatal in fewer than 10% of aspirations by obstetric patients in reporting university hospitals. Until very recently, though, careful reports from Great Britain demonstrated that 35% of all anesthetic-related obstetric deaths were directly caused by inhalation of stomach contents. Although the majority of these deaths occurred during attempted tracheal intubation under general anesthesia, only half of them occurred in patients with "difficult" intubation conditions. Forty percent of those who died received prophylactic antacids orally to prevent acid damage to the lungs, and half were receiving attempted prophylactic external cricoid pressure (Sellick's maneuver). Nonetheless, both measures are firmly indicated in obstetrics.

Treatment of aspiration pneumonia should be based on the principles of immediate establishment of unimpeded ventilation, suppression of transudation by positive end-expiratory intratracheal pressure, and careful monitoring for inadequate ventilation or the delayed development of bacterial pneumonia. Although steroid therapy after aspiration into the trachea has been advocated by many, evidence from animal research indicates that it is ineffective. So-called prophylactic antibiotics are almost universally avoided by experts because of the tendency to favor the growth of opportunistic organisms. The combination of ranitidine (Zantac), 150 mg PO, along with metoclopramide (Reglan), 10 mg PO given 90 minutes before surgery as prophylaxis against acid aspiration, has been reported to be effective in nearly eliminating these risk factors but has not yet been recommended by the United States Food and Drug Administration in obstetric patients.

COMPLICATIONS OF BLOCK ANESTHESIA

Hypotension and Circulatory Failure

Hypotension and circulatory failure may account for 34% of all maternal deaths due to anesthesia and are also a hazard to the fetus. The most frequent cause of maternal death is the aortocaval compression syndrome complicated by blockade of the sympathetic nervous system incidental to spinal or epidural anesthesia. This syndrome can be diagnosed by the presence of hypotension, dyspnea, and acute apprehension, often with tachycardia. It is treated by lifting the uterus to the left or placing the patient on her left side or tilting the patient to the left with a pillow. Further treatment of hypotension includes position change, vigorous fluid infusion, and, if necessary, intravenous ephedrine in 12.5-mg bolus doses. Large doses of alpha-agonist vasoconstrictors such as phenylephrine are NEVER used because they further depress uterine blood flow despite restoring maternal blood pressure.

Seizures Due to Local Anesthetics

Convulsions may constitute about 11% of all disastrous complications of regional anesthesia. Frequently incorrectly attributed to previously undiagnosed eclamptic seizure, unexpected neurologic events ranging from disorientation and bizarre behavior to tonic-clonic convulsions following the injection of a local anesthetic drug should be assumed to be due to the local anesthetic until proved otherwise even in pregnant patients. Local anesthetic-induced convulsions are rarely due to "allergy" but most often result from elevated blood concentrations of the local anesthetic. Subarachnoid ("spinal") anesthesia almost never results in convulsions owing to the very small dose of local anesthetic, which is usually injected to produce subarachnoid block. Although lidocaine-induced convulsions have relatively benign neurologic and cardiovascular sequela after prompt therapy, convulsions due to bupivacaine are much more serious and have been associated with conduction defects in the human myocardium that are very difficult to reverse once established. Emergency treatment of local anesthetic convulsions consists of skillful support of ventilation and monitoring and support when necessary of cardiovascular function. The injection of a small dose of rapid-acting barbiturate, such as 100 mg of thiopental sodium or a small dose of diazepam—for example, 5 mg given intravenously along with succinylcholine, 40 to 80 mg—followed by intermittent positive-pressure breathing, is very useful. Generally, the baby should not be delivered at this time because the fetal blood level of anesthetic will also be high until it has had time to be redistributed. Blood pressure should be monitored and supported with 12.5-mg boluses of ephedrine if necessary.

Massive Subarachnoid Instillation of Local Anesthetic ("Total Spinal")

Unintended total spinal anesthesia is still a frequent problem during attempted epidural anesthesia and may occur as often as one in every thousand attempted epidural blocks. The epidural catheter definitely can "migrate" into the subdural space from the epidural space some hours after original institution of the block, leading to a "total spinal" after a reinjection. The resulting duration of the respiratory and cardiovascular embarrassment can be expected to be relatively shorter than the planned duration of the intended subarachnoid block. But total spinal anesthesia resulting from unintended subarachnoid instillation of local anesthetic that was intended for the epidural space is a much more threatening emergency because the quantity of local anesthetic injected is frequently 4 to 10 times greater. Patients experiencing this unfortunate situation should be adequately sedated immediately until return of spontaneous vital functions is complete. Skillful application of intermittent positive-pressure breathing and monitoring and support of cardiovascular activity usually prevent the otherwise fatal outcome of this complication.

Unilateral or Uneven Peridural Block

Some desired segments are not blocked in as many as 10% of patients undergoing peridural blocks. The cause is frequently a laterally placed catheter, use of volumes that are too small, insufficiently strong concentrations of local anesthetic agent, or perhaps lateral positioning of the patient during injection. The remedy may lie in pulling back the catheter and injecting more anesthetic volume, placing the patient on the unblocked side, or injecting a larger volume of a more concentrated solution.

Inadvertent Dural Puncture During Attempted Peridural Block

Even a very skilled anesthetist may puncture the dura in 2% or less of attempts. A second attempt at an epidural in an adjacent interspace is routine in this event, but extreme care should then be taken to administer and observe test doses at every subsequent injection of the epidural catheter. Because postpartum headaches occur in from 25 to 75% of patients who have experienced inadvertent dural puncture by the epidural needle, immediate precautions against headache may be desirable. Immediate postpartum instillation of large volumes (up to 60 mL) of "normal" saline has been very successful. Bedrest, hydration, use of intravenous caffeine sodium benzoate or intravenous theophylline, or other conservative measures are often successful in treating these headaches once they are established. Persistent "spinal headaches" are usually eliminated by injections of autologous blood (10 mL) in the epidural space no sooner than the third postpartum day.

HAZARDS TO THE NEWBORN FROM OBSTETRIC ANESTHESIA

Three main factors may contribute to anesthesia-related morbidity in the newborn: (1) sedatives, analgesics, and anesthetics administered to the mother during labor; (2) trauma of labor and delivery; (3) asphyxia due to impaired exchange of respiratory gases during labor and delivery. Obstetric factors such as toxins from amnionitis, muscular depression due to magnesium sulfate, and other factors cannot be disregarded. The newborn is more susceptible to anesthetic overdose than the adult because the undeveloped brain is more susceptible to these drugs. Modern practice attempts to minimize the use of prepartum sedatives particularly by encouraging psychologic techniques such as prepared childbirth, regional analgesia techniques, and the concurrent use of synergistic but less depressant drugs. Phenothiazines, for example, add to the analgesia of narcotics, diminish nausea and vomiting, and cause little direct respiratory depression, although some may cause hypotension. Propiomazine (Largon) in incremental doses of 5 mg intravenously or promethazine (Phenergan) in increments of 12.5 mg given intravenously can often be used with good effect. Benzodiazepines such as midazolam (Versed) and diazepam (Valium) are sometimes used in laboring women but may be more dangerous to the newborn baby.

POSTPARTUM CARE

method of
ALEXANDER REITER, M.D.
Baylor College of Medicine
Houston, Texas

The postpartum period or puerperium, or the so-called fourth trimester of pregnancy, begins after the delivery of the newborn and the placenta and empirically ends 6 weeks afterwards. At that time, most of the anatomic and physiologic changes that occurred during the pregnancy have reversed. Some of the most dreadful obstetric complications, such as hemorrhage, eclamptic seizures, thromboembolic phenomena, and severe infections, may occur during the postpartum period. Immediate recognition and adequate management of these complications are essential for intact maternal survival.

PHYSIOLOGY AND MANAGEMENT

After the vaginal delivery of the newborn, the uterus becomes smaller and harder. The amount of vaginal bleeding is normally between 150 and 300 mL. The birth canal can be inspected while separation of the placenta is awaited. The examiner introduces two fingers into the vagina and applies gentle downward pressure on the perineum. To visualize the vaginal walls, the cervix is moved from side to side with a sponge stick. In order to inspect the cervix, the author applies a ring forceps on both the anterior and posterior cervical lip and gently pulls out until visualization is adequate. If lacerations of the birth canal are noted to bleed heavily, constant pressure over the bleeding area is applied with a sponge stick or a pad until the placenta separates and final repair can be achieved. On rare occasions, hemostatic sutures must be placed in order to control the bleeding before the placenta separates. As long as the uterus is firm and there is no abnormal bleeding, the examiner can wait for the spontaneous separation of the placenta. There is no consensus with regard to the length of time before intervening. The author considers 1 hour a reasonable period because chances of spontaneous separation afterward are minimal. The examiner manually removes the placenta, if necessary (under appropriate anesthesia), by placing a hand inside the uterus and dissecting the edge of the placenta from the uterine wall until it is completely loose. The separated placenta is then pulled out. The bladder needs to be empty because a full bladder may interfere with the delivery of the placenta.

The following are signs of spontaneous separation of placenta: the uterus becomes harder and globular in shape and rises higher in the abdomen as the placenta drops down into the lower uterine segment; there is a sudden increase in the amount of vaginal bleeding; and the umbilical cord protrudes farther out of the vagina. Once the separation occurs, the patient is asked to push down. The physician can facilitate the expulsion by expressing mild pressure on the fundus of the uterus. Twisting the placenta several times as it appears in the vagina and at the vulva causes the membranes to separate completely. If the membranes start to tear apart from the placenta, they should be grasped with a ring forceps and gently pulled out. Once delivered, the maternal surface of the placenta should be inspected for possible missing fragments, in which case the surface appears asymmetrical and rough. The presence of accessory vessels on the lateral margins of the fetal membranes may indicate a succenturiate lobe that might have been retained in the uterus. The placental fragments are removed either manually or by curettage.

After the delivery of the placenta, the episiotomy and other possible lacerations of the birth canal are repaired. At this time, the uterus is firm, and the fundus reaches the level of the umbilicus. Routine administration of oxytocin has been shown to reduce the overall blood loss. Oxytocin is usually administered intravenously at a concentration of 10 or 20 units in 1000 mL of a crystalloid solution. The rate of infusion is about 200 mL per hour. Intravenous bolus doses of oxytocin should be avoided because they may cause hypotension and arrhythmia.

Postpartum hemorrhage, defined as blood loss in excess of 500 mL in the first 12 hours after the delivery, is encountered in about 4% of cases. This is a significant complication in that hemorrhage accounts for about 10% of the non–abortion-related maternal mortality in the United States. Fifty percent of the cases of postpartum hemorrhage are caused by uterine atony; 20% are secondary to birth canal trauma; 20% are related to uterine rupture, placenta previa, or uterine inversion (after excessive traction of the umbilical cord); and 10% occur late in the postpartum period and are related to retained products of conception or to coagulopathies.

Aggressive management of postpartum hemorrhage is critical. Large-bore intravenous lines should be started immediately while blood products are made available. Clotting studies are obtained, and the patient's vital signs and urinary output are carefully monitored. The birth canal should be methodically inspected, and any source of bleeding should be repaired. If atony is suspected, the uterus is massaged through the abdominal wall. Ergot preparations such as ergonovine maleate (Ergotrate) or methylergonovine (Methergine), 0.2 mg, can be administered intramuscularly in patients who do not respond to oxytocin. Ergot drugs cause sustained uterine contractions that start shortly after administration and last for several hours. They may cause high blood pressure and should not be used in patients with a history of cardiac disease or hypertension. An alternative drug is intramuscular prostaglandin 15-methyl-F2-alpha (0.25 mg every 30 to 60 minutes).

A surgical approach is undertaken whenever the pharmacologic management fails to control the postpartum hemorrhage. The first step is the postpartum curettage, meant to remove possible products of conception. The author recommends that this procedure be done under continuous ultrasound guidance to minimize the risks of uterine perforation. Laparotomy with ligation of uterine or hypogastric arteries or hysterectomy is occasionally needed in the most difficult cases of postpartum hemorrhage.

During the first 1 or 2 hours after the delivery, the vital signs are monitored every 30 minutes, and the patient is observed carefully for signs of excessive blood loss (more than 500 mL). Pelvic and birth canal hematomas can enlarge rapidly, causing intense pain (never to be overlooked in this situation) and significant hemodynamic changes that are disproportional to the amount of external bleeding. Pelvic examination and inspection of the birth canal are performed, and hematomas, if present, are opened and drained. Sites of bleeding need to be controlled, but if they are not easily identified, hemostatic sutures are applied over the bleeding area. On occasion, a patient is unable to void spontaneously because of a combined effect of local edema and anesthetic drugs. The urethra can be catheterized in order to decompress an overdistended bladder that interferes with uterine contraction and causes pelvic pain and pressure.

During the first few days after the delivery, the patient might experience pain related to the episiotomy, and mild analgesics might be required. Normal healing is expected to be complete in 2 to 3 weeks. Extensive episiotomies or those complicated by lacerations of the sphincter or the wall of the rectum are usually more painful and necessitate stronger analgesic treatment. However, intense pain unresponsive to analgesics needs to be evaluated for the possibility of hematoma or perineal infection. Prolapsed hemorrhoids (especially if thrombotic) might be another cause of sustained perineal pain.

The pain associated with the physiologic uterine contractions usually decreases in intensity and becomes mild by the third or fourth postpartum day. Significant lower abdominal pain, especially if associated with fever, suggests the possibility of endometritis or urinary tract infection.

The most common sites of postpartum infection are the uterus (endometritis), the birth canal, the urinary tract, and the breasts (mastitis). The vaginal bleeding (lochia rubra) decreases over the first 3 to 4 postpartum days and becomes pale and thinner (lochia serosa between days 3 to 10). Then it becomes thicker and white-yellowish (lochia alba) and might persist for about 3 to 5 weeks. Foul-smelling lochia suggests endometritis. The author does not recommend the use of tampons during the postpartum period because of the risk of infection. They can, however, be used in patients who do not have lacerations of the birth canal and who change their tampons regularly every 3 to 4 hours.

The duration of the postpartum confinement varies between 12 hours and 3 days for patients with uncomplicated vaginal deliveries and is 4 to 5 days for patients with uncomplicated cesarean deliveries. This period is important not only for ascertaining the patient's hemodynamic stability but also for providing education and help in areas such as breast-feeding and care of the newborn.

Early discharge from the hospital, more and more encouraged by third-party payers, should be allowed only after the vaginal bleeding has been carefully evaluated and a stable hematocrit is available. Other laboratory tests to be assessed before the discharge are the blood type, the Rh factor (anti-Rh prophylaxis must be administered in the appropriate cases), and the rubella immune status. Prenatal vitamins and iron supplements are recommended for another 4 to 6 weeks. Upon the discharge from the hospital, the patient should receive specific instructions regarding her immediate lifestyle. Physical activity is not restricted, and the patient may return to normal activities and exercise whenever she desires. Persistent complaints of lethargy and fatigue must be evaluated for severe anemia and for hypothyroidism.

Postpartum psychological reactions (postpartum "blues") in the form of anxiety, restlessness, and extreme irritability occur in up to 70% of postpartum patients. These reactions usually resolve without therapy within 10 to 15 days. The more severe condition of postpartum depression is less common and has a strong association with previous psychological problems. This condition necessitates medical treatment.

Sexual activity may be resumed when the bleeding has subsided, the lacerations have healed, and the perineum is comfortable. The libido is, however, very much decreased in the postpartum period. Patients may return to work 6 weeks after delivery. This is regarded as the postpartum "disability" period.

Suppression of lactation, if desired, can be achieved by applying breast binders and ice packs, using mild analgesics, and avoiding nipple stimulaton. In cases of extreme breast engorgement, when the conservative methods have failed, oral bromocriptine (Parlodel), which is a dopamine receptor agonist, can be used in a dosage of 2.5 mg twice daily for 14 days. This is successful in about 90% of the cases. This drug should be avoided, however, in patients with hypertension or pregnancy-induced hypertension.

At the end of the postpartum period, the patient should have a gynecologic examination and a Papanicolaou smear. Contraceptive methods should be discussed on this occasion.

RESUSCITATION OF THE NEWBORN

method of
SCOTT A. JOHNSON, M.D., and
ALFRED L. GEST, M.D.
Baylor College of Medicine
Houston, Texas

At birth, the newborn must make rapid cardiopulmonary adaptations to make the transition from intrauterine to extrauterine life. An effective neonatal resuscitation protocol ensures the accomplishment of a successful transition to postnatal life.

In utero the placenta is the organ of respiration, and the lungs are filled with fluid. Because the lung does not function to oxygenate the blood in utero, oxygenated blood from the placenta through the umbilical vein traverses the ductus venosus, enters the inferior vena cava, and empties into the right atrium. This blood is then shunted through the foramen ovale into the left side of the heart, which in turn distributes oxygenated blood to the brain and peripheral circulation. The right side of the heart primarily receives blood with a lower oxygen content that is ejected into the pulmonary artery but is then diverted to the aorta rather than to the high-resistance lungs through the ductus arteriosus. This blood is then distributed to the placenta through the aorta and umbilical arteries to receive oxygen and nutrients and to release carbon dioxide and waste products.

As the newborn is delivered and takes the first few breaths, several changes occur that allow the lungs to become responsible for respiration: First, the lungs expand as they are filled with gas and fetal lung fluid gradually leaves the alveoli by moving into the extra-alveolar interstitium, which is eventually cleared by lung lymphatics. At the same time, the pulmonary vascular resistance decreases precipitously while pulmonary blood flow correspondingly increases. With occlusion of the umbilical cord, systemic vascular resistance increases. Even though the foramen ovale and ductus arteriosus remain anatomically open, the decrease in pulmonary vascular resistance and the increase in systemic vascular resistance effectively reverse the direction of blood flow through them. Elevated pulmonary vascular resistance caused by hypoxia, acidosis, and hypothemia leads to right-to-left shunting through the foramen ovale and ductus arteriosus, thus prolonging the fetal circulatory pathways and impairing oxygen delivery. It is apparent that minimization of hypoxia, acidosis, and hypothermia at birth helps to ensure a smooth transition to a normal postnatal circulation.

Fortunately, the first few breaths of most newborn infants are effective and allow the cardiopulmonary adaptations previously discussed to take place. However, some infants are asphyxiated in utero and are born with ineffective respirations or apnea, which leads to hypoxia and acidosis, making these adaptations difficult.

In animal studies total asphyxia initially causes a short period of increased respiratory effort, which is followed by apnea. This condition is known as primary apnea, and during this time spontaneous respirations can be restored by tactile stimulation. However, if asphyxia continues, the infant develops gasping respirations, the heart rate continues to decrease, and the blood pressure begins to fall. The infant then takes a last gasping breath (the "last gasp") and enters a period known as secondary apnea. Now the infant is unresponsive to stimulation, and only positive pressure ventilation restores spontaneous respiration. The longer the delay in resuscitation, the longer it takes for spontaneous respirations to occur. Because the fetus may experience asphyxia in utero, he or she may undergo primary and secondary apnea in utero. Therefore, when the infant is born apneic, one cannot differentiate between primary and secondary apnea, and one must assume that the infant is in secondary apnea and initiate positive pressure ventilation.

PREPARATION

Preparation is the essential first step in effective neonatal resuscitation. According to *The Textbook of Neonatal Resuscitation,* published by the American Heart Association and the American Academy of Pediatrics, 90% of hospitals where deliveries occur have only Level 1 nurseries. Therefore, it is essential to ensure that personnel who are adequately skilled in neonatal resuscitation are present at every delivery, whether or not perinatal problems are anticipated. In deliveries at which a normal, healthy infant is expected, one person (e.g., physician, nurse, respiratory therapist) who has the skills to perform a complete neonatal resuscitation must be present. If this person is also caring for the mother, another person who is capable of initiating and assisting with neonatal resuscitation must be present. It is inappropriate to have someone "on call" to provide neonatal resuscitation because this may cause unnecessary delay. During high-risk deliveries at which neonatal asphyxia is likely, two persons not involved in the care of the mother must be readily available, and one of these two must be skilled in endotracheal intubation and the administration of medications.

Equipment needed for a complete resuscitation is listed in Table 1. This equipment should be present in every delivery area and should be routinely checked to ensure that it is working properly. When the antepartum or intrapartum history suggests that an asphyxiated infant may be born, all equipment needed should be taken out of the packages and prepared for use. One should quickly check to ensure that the radiant warmer is heating, that oxygen is flowing through the tubing, that suction is functioning properly, that the resuscitation bag and mask can provide an adequate seal and generate pressure, and that the laryngoscope light source is functional. Several minutes into the resuscitation of a cyanotic infant is not the time to realize that the valve to the oxygen source was never opened. For multiple gestations, a full complement of equipment and personnel is needed for each infant.

TABLE 1. **Requirements for Resuscitation**

Environment
Radiant warmer
Blankets, towels (warm)
Wall clock with sweep second hand
Suction
Bulb syringe
Suction catheters (6, 8, 10 Fr)
Regulated wall suction
Meconium aspirators
Airway Management
Stethoscope
Oxygen
Flow meter
Oxygen tubing
Infant resuscitation bag with manometer and pressure relief valve
Masks (premature and infant sizes)
Laryngoscope
Size 0 and 1 laryngoscope blades
Endotracheal tubes (2.5-, 3.0-, 3.5-, 4.0-mm diameters)
Stylets
Vascular Access
Umbilical catheters (3.5 and 5.0 Fr)
Umbilical catheterization tray
Syringes (1-, 3-, 5-, 10-, 20-, and 60-mL)
Needles
Stopcocks
Suture
Sterile saline (10 mL)
IV catheters
IV tubing
Umbilical tape
Medications
Epinephrine (1:10,000)
Naloxone hydrochloride (Narcan) (1 mg/mL or 0.4 mg/mL)
IV solutions (normal saline, 10% dextrose)
Sodium bicarbonate (4.2%, 0.5 mEq/mL)
Albumin (5%)
Sterile water
Miscellaneous
Gloves
Masks, with eye shield
Quick reference card for ages and weights

INITIAL STEPS OF RESUSCITATION

Although there are certain aspects of neonatal resuscitation that make it unique, it should be noted that the basic ABCs of resuscitation in any age group still apply (*a*irway, *b*reathing, *c*irculation). Most infants respond to airway management and the initiation of positive pressure ventilation if needed. Chest compressions and, in particular, medications are rarely necessary. This also applies to infants with medical complications such as those in whom prenatal diagnosis has detected complex congenital heart disease or hydrops fetalis. The basic rules of neonatal resuscitation still apply, and one should not forget the ABCs in the excitement that sometimes accompanies delivery of an infant with a complex prenatally detected condition. As we begin to discuss the individual steps of neonatal resuscitation, the importance of continuous evaluation of the patient to assist in the necessary decision-making process involved in neonatal resuscitation cannot be overemphasized.

One very important and unique aspect of newborn resuscitation is temperature control. Simply keeping the newborn warm decreases morbidity more than any other component of resuscitation. In fact, paying attention to temperature should come before the "A" in the ABCs. Cold stress in the newborn leads to increased oxygen consumption and increased metabolic demand, which further complicates the resuscitation of the asphyxiated newborn. This is especially true in the very-low-birthweight infant (less than 1.0 kg). The large surface area of the newborn relative to body mass and the newborn's poor insulating ability (decreased body fat, particularly in preterm infants) accelerate heat loss. Heat can be lost by four different mechanisms: evaporation, convection, radiation, and conduction. Evaporative heat loss is increased by failure to dry off amniotic fluid. This evaporative heat loss is exacerbated in very-low-birthweight infants whose skin is thin and less keratinized. Convective heat loss occurs when ambient air temperature is less than the infant's skin temperature. Heat loss by radiation to cold objects in a delivery room is a major cause of thermal stress in newborns, and if the baby is placed on cool blankets or towels for resuscitation, heat loss by conduction can occur. It is easy to see how quickly a newborn can lose heat and how important it is for the first steps of resuscitation to include ways to minimize this heat loss. This is easily accomplished by placing the newborn under a prewarmed radiant heat source and quickly drying the infant with a prewarmed towel or blanket. Remember to remove the wet blanket or towel from the infant or evaporative heat loss will continue. Drying of the infant also has the added benefit of providing gentle stimulation, which may aid in the onset of spontaneous respirations.

Establishment of an open airway is accomplished by placing the neonate on his or her back with the neck in a neutral to slightly extended position on a flat radiant warmer bed. The neck should not be hyperextended or underextended, and the warmer bed should not be in the Trendelenburg position as was once recommended. If needed, a rolled blanket or towel may be placed under the shoulders, elevating them approximately 1 inch off the mattress. The newborn should now be in the best position to maintain an open airway.

When the infant has been correctly positioned, the mouth and nose should be quicky suctioned. The material in the mouth should be suctioned first to decrease the risk of aspiration should the infant gasp. A bulb syringe or mechanical suction device may be used. Deep suctioning of the esophagus and stomach or prolonged suctioning is contraindicated because it can produce a vagal response leading to apnea and bradycardia. According to the update to the *Interim Training Guidelines for Neonatal Resuscitation,* published by the American Heart Association and the American Academy of Pediatrics, suctioning should be limited to 3 to 5 seconds. This time limit in addition to avoidance of deep suctioning should lessen the risk of vagal-induced apnea or bradycardia.

The next step is to provide tactile stimulation. The infant has already been dried and suctioned, which in many cases will initiate respirations. If not, there are two (and only two) safe and appropriate ways of providing additional tactile stimulation: (1) slapping or flicking the soles of the feet and (2) rubbing the infant's back. Other actions such as slapping the baby's back or buttocks or blowing cool oxygen or air into the baby's face can result in unnecessary bruising and hyothermia, respectively. If there is no response to one or two flicks of the feet, it is not appropriate to then try to rub the infant's back. The time elapsed from placing the baby under the warmer to postioning, suctioning, and providing additional tactile stimulation should be 15 to 20 seconds. During this time period, the adequacy of respirations should be assessed. Because one must assume that apnea noted at birth may be secondary apnea, it is now time to proceed to positive pressure ventilation.

The initial steps of warming, positioning, suctioning, and applying tactile stimulation are applied in every newborn delivery. The remaining guidelines to resuscitation depend on the evaluation of the infant while those initial steps are being performed. Apgar scores are of little value to the pediatrician or neonatologist at the delivery. Continued need for resuscitation depends on three clinical signs: (1) respiratory effort, (2) heart rate, and (3) color. If the infant has a regular breathing pattern after tactile stimulation, proceed to check the heart rate. If the infant is gasping or apneic, positive pressure ventilation should be given. When respiratory effort has been evaluated and the appropriate action taken, the heart rate is monitored. If the heart rate is more than 100 beats per minute, proceed to evaluate the infant's color. If the heart rate is less than 100, even if the infant has spontaneous respirations, proceed to positive pressure ventilation. The heart rate can be monitored by auscultation or palpation of the pulse in the umbilical cord, although it is generally more prudent to auscultate, especially for the less experienced caregiver. Constant monitoring of the heart rate determines the extent of resuscitation, as will be discussed later. The infant's color should be evaluated next. Peripheral cyanosis (acrocyanosis) is common in the newborn, but central cyanosis is abnormal. Central cyanosis involves the entire body, including the mucous membranes. If central cyanosis is present in a newborn with adequate respirations and a heart rate of more than 100, free-flowing oxygen should be administered. In this instance, positive pressure ventilation is not indicated. Oxygen should be delivered at a flow rate of 5 liters per minute via an oxygen hose and held steadily (not waved back and forth) one-half inch from the infant's nares. This will deliver approximately 80% inspired oxygen to the infant. It is inappropriate to attempt to deliver free-flow oxygen with a bag and mask. It does not work! The infant should receive a high concentration of oxygen until he or she turns pink, then oxygen should be gradually withdrawn to the degree that the newborn can maintain a pink color.

MECONIUM-STAINED AMNIOTIC FLUID

Another situation unique to resuscitation of the newborn is that of meconium-stained amniotic fluid. Thin, watery meconium-stained fluid has not been proved to contribute to increased perinatal morbidity, and specific management of these infants is probably unnecessary. However, thick and particulate meconium-stained amniotic fluid can lead to meconium aspiration syndrome, with or without persistent pulmonary hypertension. To minimize this risk, the baby's mouth, pharynx, and nose should be suctioned with a No. 10 French catheter by the obstetrician as the baby's head is delivered but before the shoulders are delivered. After delivery, the baby should be placed under a radiant warmer and before drying, any remaining meconium should be suctioned from the hypopharynx. The trachea should then be suctioned under direct vision. This is best accomplished by intubating the infant with an endotracheal tube and applying suction (no more than 100 mmHg) as the endotracheal tube is withdrawn. Passing a suction catheter through the endotracheal tube is inappropriate because it may be too small to suction particulate meconium. Reintubation followed by repeat suctioning should be performed until all meconium is removed, provided the infant remains stable. Free-flow oxygen should be provided with all intubation attempts to minimize the risk of hypoxia. It is important to monitor the heart rate continuously because positive pressure ventilation may have to be initiated in the asphyxiated infant before all the meconium can be removed from the trachea. If positive pressure ventilation has to be initiated prior to removal of all meconium in the trachea, complete resuscitation (including chest compressions and medications if needed) should performed until the heart rate is over 100, at which time repeat tracheal suctioning can then be performed. Gastric contents should be suctioned for meconium to prevent the possibility of later regurgitation and aspiration. However, this should be done only after resuscitation is completed and the infant is stable.

POSITIVE PRESSURE VENTILATION

Positive pressure ventilation is sometimes needed during the course of neonatal resuscitation. This can be provided by bag-and-mask ventilation or by bag-and-endotracheal tube. Although an anesthesia bag may be used, it is a more difficult technique to master, and in our opinion it is not nearly as effective at delivering the higher pressures sometimes required to resuscitate a sick newborn. A self-inflating resuscitation bag is preferable and should be equipped with a face mask and an oxygen reservoir, which enables the bag to deliver a higher concentration of oxygen (90 to 100%). Without the oxygen reservoir, the self-inflating bag is unable to deliver a high concentration of oxygen. The flow of oxygen through the tubing should be increased to 8 to 10 liters per minute and should be connected to the oxygen inlet on the resuscitation bag. The self-inflating bags have a pressure-release valve, commonly called a pop-off valve, that usually releases at 25 to 35 cmH_2O pressure. It is often necessary to occlude this pop-off valve to generate a sufficient amount of pressure to ventilate a newborn's nonaerated lungs effectively, especially with the first few breaths. With the pop-off valve occluded, care should be taken not to overventilate the newborn because this may cause a pneumothorax. A pressure manometer should always be used in conjunction with the bag to prevent overdistention of the lung. Masks come in different shapes and sizes, with or without cushioned rims. The mask rim should be cushioned and should cover the chin, mouth, and nose but not the eyes. It is recommended that masks be available for full-term and premature infants. The bag-and-mask apparatus should already have been tested for adequacy by forming an airtight seal against the palm of one's hand and generating pressure. At the time of need for bag-and-mask ventilation, the baby should already be in the correct position for an open airway with the neck in a neutral to slightly extended position. The newborn has already been suctioned and tactilely stimulated not more than twice. If respirations remain inadequate, bag-and-mask ventilation should be initiated.

The ventilator should stand in a position that does not obstruct the view of the newborn's chest. The mask is placed over the baby's face, and light downward pressure is applied with one hand. Constant reevaluation is necessary to ensure that the seal is adequate and that chest expansion is occurring with each assisted ventilation. If chest expansion is inadequate, the most common problem is an inadequate seal. Second, the infant's airway could be blocked by improper positioning or occluded by secretions. It may be necessary to reposition the infant or suction the infant's mouth and nose. If a good seal is obtained and an airway is maintained, increasing the pressure may be necessary to move the chest. Pressures of 20 to 40 cmH_2O are often required in infants with respiratory conditions that decrease lung compliance. The infant should be ventilated at a rate of 40 to 60 times per minute. After 15 to 30 seconds of bag-and-mask ventilation, the heart rate determines the next step of resuscitation. If the heart rate is more than 100 and spontaneous respirations have begun, bag-and-mask ventilation is gradually decreased, free-flowing oxygen is provided, and one observes the infant for continuation of effective respirations. If the heart rate is 60 to 100 and increasing, bag-and-mask ventilation is continued. If the heart rate is 60 to 100 and not increasing, the adequacy of ventilation is reassessed, and if the heart rate remains less than 80, chest compressions are begun. If the heart rate is less than 60, the adequacy of ventilation is again assessed, and chest compressions are begun immediately. The adequacy of the seal between the mask and the baby's face cannot be overemphasized.

CHEST COMPRESSIONS

Chest compessions are performed on the lower third of the sternum, located between an imaginary line drawn between the nipples and the xyphoid process. Care must be taken to avoid applying pressure directly over the xyphoid. The thumb technique may be used by encircling the infant's body with both hands and placing the thumbs on the sternum and the fingers under the infant. The thumbs are used to compress the sternum. The two-finger method uses the tips of the first two fingers or the middle and ring finger placed in a perpendicular position over the lower sternum. Only the fingertips should rest on the chest and pressure should be applied directly downward to decrease the risk of fractured ribs or a pneumothorax. The amount of pressure used should be the amount sufficient to depress the sternum one-half to three-quarters of an inch. According to the new *Interim Training Guidelines for Neonatal Resuscitation,* published by the American Heart Association and the American Academy of Pediatrics in April, 1993, chest compressions should be interposed with ventilation in a ratio of 3:1. This amounts to 90 compressions and 30 breaths per minute. Therefore, the ventilation rate used during chest compressions is lower than the 40 to 60 range recommended when chest compressions are not being performed. The heart rate should be evaluated every 30 seconds and compressions continued until the heart rate is over 80.

ENDOTRACHEAL INTUBATION

Endotracheal intubation is indicated when prolonged positive pressure ventilation is required or bag-and-mask ventilation is deemed ineffective. It is also indicated in such special circumstances as infants born with thick or particulate meconium in the amniotic fluid or infants with congenital diaphragmatic hernia. Intubation is a skill that takes practice and that becomes better with experience. In preparation for intubation, the laryngoscope should be equipped with a No. 0 blade for premature infants and a No. 1 blade for full-term infants, although many skilled intubators find that a No. 0 blade is sufficient for full-term infants also. Double check to see that the light source is functional. Select the proper size of endotracheal tube based on the baby's weight. A 2.5-mm (internal diameter) tube is appropriate for an infant weighing less than 1.0 kg, 3.0 mm is best for infants weighing 1.0 to 2.0 kg, and 3.5 mm is appropriate for infants weighing more than 2.0 kg. Use of a stylet is optional but is usually unnecessary because the stiffness of the endotracheal tube is adequate for manipulation during intubation. Mechanical suctioning (not to exceed 100 mmHg) should be available as well as free-flow oxygen to provide a high concentration of oxygen during the procedure to minimize hypoxia. The resuscitation bag and mask remain at the bedside for use between intubation attempts; the bag will be connected to the endotracheal tube after intubation is completed.

When intubation is needed, the infant should already be in the proper position, that is, with the head in a midline position and the neck in a neutral to slightly extended position. The laryngoscope handle is held in the left hand and the blade is inserted between the tongue and the palate until the tip of the blade rests in the vallecula. Once inserted, the glottis is visualized by lifting the entire blade in an "up and outward" motion. With this motion, the intubator's entire arm should move in the desired direction. The laryngoscope should never be rotated in a "prying" or "can opener" type of maneuver. At least two people are required for endotracheal intubation. The second person prepares the tape for securing the tube in place, administers free-flow oxygen during the attempt, monitors the heart rate, limits the time of the attempt to no more than 20 seconds, assesses whether the attempt is successful, helps to determine the appropriateness of the position of the tube, and helps to secure the tube in place. The intubation attempt should not last more than 20 seconds. Bag-and-mask ventilation should be performed between attempts. Suctioning is sometimes necessary to provide adequate visualization of the glottis. Once the glottis is in view, the endotracheal tube is inserted with the right hand until the vocal cord guideline (the heavy black line near the tip of the tube) is at the level of the vocal cords. A guideline to confirm that the endotracheal tube is in a good location is to add 6 to the infant's weight in kilograms. This provides the centimeter mark at which the endotracheal should be taped at the lip. It is important for the intubator to hold the endotracheal tube securely until it is taped into position and always listen for equal breath sounds bilaterally in the axillae of the infant. One should be sure to record the position at which the tube is taped because this is useful for repositioning later and for determining whether the tube has inadvertently shifted in position.

Often one is so elated at passing the tube successfully that he or she fails to pay attention to the distance that it is inserted. Much harm can come from inserting an endotracheal tube too far. If it is inserted too far, it can rest in the right mainstem bronchus, causing poor oxygen and carbon dioxide exchange and overdistention of that lung segment, possibly leading to pulmonary interstitial emphysema and pneumothorax. In the premature infant, extra care should be taken to ensure good endotracheal tube placement because the "6 plus weight in kilograms" rule may be less reliable; the tube may need to be inserted less far. To ensure against esophageal intubation, listen for air entering the stomach and observe for gastric distention. This usually becomes apparent because secretions enter the endotracheal tube and the patient does not respond clinically. Always obtain a chest radiograph to confirm the position of the endotracheal tube.

MEDICATIONS

Resuscitation medications are rarely needed in the newborn. However, in the newborn whose heart rate remains less than 80 despite adequate ventilation with 100% oxygen and effective chest compressions for more than 30 seconds, or in the newborn with a heart rate of 0, medications should be administered. The initial medication in such a situation is epinephrine. Epinephrine increases cardiac output by increasing the heart rate and myocardial contractility and increases blood pressure by causing peripheral vasoconstriction. It should be given rapidly and can be given intravenously or via an endotracheal tube in a dose of 0.1 to 0.3 mL per kg of 1:10,000 solution. The intravenous route is preferable because plasma concentrations with the endotracheal route are sometimes low. However, intravenous access has usually not been established when the first dose of epinephrine is required, so it may be preferable to give the higher recommended dose when the drug is administered by the endotracheal route. Epinephrine may be repeated every 5 minutes if the heart rate remains less than 100. If there is no response to epinephrine, one should suspect metabolic acidosis in the asphyxiated infant. In this case, or in the case of documented metabolic acidosis, sodium bicarbonate is indicated in a dose of 2 mEq per kg. It can only be given intravenously. Intracranial hemorrhage has been associated with the use of bicarbonate in animal studies. To reduce that risk, sodium bicarbonate in the commercially available 4.2% solution (0.5 mEq per milliliter) should be given slowly over a minimum of 2 minutes, not to exceed a rate of 1 mEq per minute. Hypovolemia may be present in the newborn and is usually a known event (e.g., umbilical cord accidents) and is indicated by pallor, poor perfusion despite a normal pH and PO_2, and weak pulses despite a good heart rate. Hypovolemia must also be considered if there is no response to the administration of epinephrine and bicarbonate. A dose of 10 mL per kg of volume expander should be given slowly intravenously. In the premature infant, this volume should always be given over at least 30 minutes to decrease the risk of intraventricular hemorrhage. However, in the hypovolemic asphyxiated full-term infant it may be necessary to administer the volume over 5 to 10 minutes. It is essential to monitor the heart rate and discontinue medications once the heart rate is over 100.

In the special instance of a baby born with respiratory depression to a mother who received narcotics within 4 hours of delivery, naloxone hydrochloride (Narcan) in a dose of 0.1 mg per kg given rapidly is indicated. In our experience this is a rare occurrence, and we find that naloxone is often given when it is unwarranted. Remember that apnea can always be effectively controlled with bag-and-mask ventilation while the narcotic administration history is checked. When needed, naloxone may be given by endotracheal tube, intravenously, intramuscularly, or subcutaneously. The intravenous route is preferable. It should not be given if the mother had a narcotic addiction because this may precipitate withdrawal in the infant. The infant who receives naloxone should be observed because the narcotic causing the respiratory depression may have a longer duration of action than the naloxone, which has a duration of action of 1 to 4 hours. Therefore, the dose of naloxone may need to be repeated.

Successful neonatal resuscitation requires communication between the resuscitation team and the obstetric staff, advanced preparation, and skilled and knowledgeable personnel. This expertise should be available at all hospitals for every newborn delivery regardless of the presence of highly specialized perinatal services. We encourage all hospitals delivering babies to have skilled personnel available for all deliveries. Preferably, these personnel will have completed The Neonatal Resuscitation Program offered by the American Academy of Pediatrics and the American Heart Association.

CARE OF THE HIGH-RISK NEONATE

method of
C. W. GOWEN, JR., M.D.
Eastern Virginia Medical School
Norfolk, Virginia

THE NEONATE AT RISK: ANTICIPATING NEONATAL PROBLEMS

A high-risk neonate is one in whom the morbidity and mortality is expected to be greater than that in the general population. The high incidence of morbidity and mortality during the perinatal period makes it important to identify as early as possible those mothers and infants who are at greatest risk. Approximately 10% of all pregnancies are considered to be high risk. In addition, over 75% of poor pregnancy outcomes can be identified by maternal history, medical problems existing in the mother prior to pregnancy, complications of the pregnancy, and a history of previous neonatal disorders. It is noteworthy that the remaining 25% of cases of perinatal morbidity and mortality occur in patients without identifiable risks. There is increasing evidence that early identification of women with high-risk pregnancies and high-risk neonates followed by appropriate perinatal care will reduce the incidence of handicapping conditions and the incidence of infant mortality. Table 1 is a partial list of high-risk factors that should alert the physician to potential serious problems for the neonate.

Many neonatal problems may be susceptible to primary intervention through education and treatment of the mother. Improvements in the mother's general knowledge of reproduction and in her level of basic health care can prevent many subsequent problems. Likewise, because most teenage pregnancies are high risk, prevention of teenage pregnancy through education and contraception may avoid serious problems in the neonate. The percentage of infants weighing less than 1500 grams born to teenage mothers is more than 50% higher than the percentage born to mothers over 25 years of age. In addition, it is essen-

TABLE 1. **High-Risk Factors**

1. Birth before 37 weeks' or 42 weeks' gestation
2. Birthweight <2500 grams or >4000 grams
3. Deviations in expected size of neonate for gestational age
4. Maternal age <18 or >35 years
5. Poor, inadequate, or absent prenatal care
6. Family history of serious hereditary or familial abnormalities
7. Maternal history of
    - Low socioeconomic status, low level of education
    - Alcohol or substance abuse or addiction
    - Habit of smoking
    - Prolonged infertility
    - Poor nutritional status
    - Premature rupture of membranes
    - Pregnancy-induced hypertension
    - Chorioamnionitis
    - Polyhydramnios or oligohydramnios
    - Isoimmunization
    - Placental separation
8. Maternal medical complications
    - Diabetes mellitus
    - Thyroid and endocrine disorders
    - Cardiovascular disease
    - Hypertension or renal disease
    - Collagen vascular disease
    - Neoplastic disease
    - Hepatitis
    - Seizure disorder
9. Multiple gestation
10. Abnormal presentation at delivery
11. History of meconium staining
12. Several maternal emotional problems or stress
13. Serious accidents
14. General anesthesia during pregnancy or delivery

tial that good communication and cooperation exist between the obstetric and neonatal health care teams to ensure the best outcome for the neonate.

ASSESSMENT AND MANAGEMENT OF THE HIGH-RISK NEONATE

Transition at Birth

The normal process of labor is, to a mild degree, asphyxiating. With uterine contraction, the uterine blood flow decreases, and there is a resulting temporary decrease in placental perfusion and transplacental gas exchange. This is accompanied by a transient fetal hypoxia and hypercapnia. Although the intermittent nature of labor permits the fetus to "recover" between contractions, the overall effect is cumulative with progressive fetal hypoxia, hypercapnia, and metabolic acidosis. In most circumstances, this mild degree of asphyxia is not enough to interfere with the normal transition at birth. However, in severe conditions of asphyxia, the birth process can be interrupted.

With birth, the neonate must establish the lungs as the site of gas exchange. In addition, the circulatory system, which has shunted blood away from the lungs in utero, must now perfuse the lungs. In utero, the fetal lungs are filled with fluid. This active process of fluid secretion by the fetal lung is thought to be necessary for normal lung development. Near the time of birth, the secretion of fetal lung fluid slows (this is thought to be secondary to the hormonal changes that occur around the time of labor). Also, this fluid must be cleared from the lungs to allow for gas exchange. The first few breaths help clear this fluid from the lungs and help to establish normal lung function. In addition, passage through the vaginal canal may squeeze out lung fluid (thoracic squeeze); however, there is no passive entry of air into the lungs as a result of this squeeze. The thoracic squeeze along with the reduced volume of lung fluid that occurs near term gestation is associated with a more rapid development of normal lung function. Neonates born via cesarean section are more likely to be slower to develop normal lung function and may present with transient clinical signs of increased respiratory effort.

Expansion of the lungs is also a stimulus for surfactant release, which reduces alveolar surface tension, increases compliance, and helps to develop normal lung function. At the same time, ventilation lowers pulmonary vascular resistance through a rise in oxygenation, a fall in carbon dioxide, and a rise in pH. This fall in pulmonary vascular resistance, along with the catecholamine surge at birth, helps to accelerate the clearance of lung fluid and facilitates ventilation.

With the onset of ventilation, the fetal circulatory system assumes the function of an adult. Coincident with umbilical cord clamping and closure of the ductus venosus, there is a rise in systemic blood pressure. This rise in systemic pressure coupled with the fall in pulmonary vascular resistance and pressure decreases the right-to-left shunting of blood through the ductus arteriosus. With diminished ductal flow, pulmonary artery blood flow increases, resulting in increased pulmonary venous return to the left atrium and increased pressure in the left atrium. Once the left atrial pressure exceeds that of the right atrium, the foramen ovale closes. In the more mature neonate, the ductus arteriosus closes by 48 to 96 hours after delivery.

Following delivery, survival is dependent on the integration of cardiac and pulmonary functions. However, these functions can be influenced by a number of clinical conditions. The information provided in Table 2 is helpful as an approach to the differential diagnosis for neonates who do not establish effective adaptation at the time of birth.

The Apgar Score

The neonate's success in completing the transition to extrauterine life is evaluated by the Apgar score. The Apgar score, devised by Dr. Virginia Apgar, is a quick method of assessing the status of the newborn infant. The ease of scoring has led to its wide use. The Apgar score is composed of five components: heart rate, respiratory effort, muscle tone, reflex irritability, and skin color. Each component is given a score of 0, 1, or 2 (Table 3). Following delivery, each component is evaluated, and a total score can be calculated routinely at 1 minute and 5 minutes. The Apgar score is most helpful when used as a guide to selection of resuscitative measures specific to the needs of an individual neonate. When the Apgar score is less than 6 at 5 minutes, it is recommended that a 10-minute Apgar score be calculated.

The 1-minute Apgar score may be used to identify infants who require special attention. The 5-minute Apgar score, and especially the change in the score between 1 and 5 minutes, is a useful index of the effectiveness of the birth transition and any resuscitative efforts that have been made. The more immature the neonate, the less applicable the Apgar score. This reflects the immature neurologic and muscular status of the early gestational neonate. However, skin color, heart rate, and respiratory effort remain extremely valuable.

Neonatal Resuscitation

Resuscitation of the neonate is one of the major pediatric emergencies. There is no substitute for adequate training and periodic review of the techniques required. All health professionals who participate in newborn care should be certified in neonatal resuscitation by the American Heart Association/American Academy of Pediatrics program to ensure that personnel trained in neonatal resuscitation are available in the delivery room for all deliveries. Details about resuscitation are provided in the article on neonatal resuscitation.

TABLE 2. **Causes of Ineffective Adaptation at Birth**

Etiology	Major Effect	Clinical Examples
Immaturity	Respiratory distress Respiratory depression	Pulmonary/CNS immaturity
Hemorrhage	Hypovolemia/shock	Abruptio placentae, placenta previa, ruptured umbilical cord, fetomaternal transfusion
Postmaturity	Pulmonary hypertension	Meconium aspiration syndrome, persistent pulmonary hypertension
Infection	Pneumonia/sepsis	Congenital pneumonia, group B streptococcal sepsis
Developmental anomalies	Pulmonary insufficiency Oligohydramnios/polyhydramnios	Diaphragmatic hernia, choanal atresia, Potter's syndrome, pulmonary hypoplasia, gastrointestinal obstruction
Cyanotic heart disease	Persistent/progressive cyanosis	Transposition of the great arteries, tetralogy of Fallot, tricuspid atresia, truncus arteriosus, total anomalous pulmonary venous return
Drugs	Respiratory depression	Anesthetics, narcotics, tranquilizers, alcohol, magnesium sulfate
"Excessive" suctioning	Vagal stimulation	Bradycardia/apnea
Incorrect intubation	Persistent hypoxia	Intubation of esophagus or right mainstem bronchus

Adapted from Karotkin E, and Goldsmith J: Resuscitation. *In* Goldsmith J, and Karotkin E (eds): Assisted Ventilation of the Neonate, 2nd ed. Philadelphia, WB Saunders Co, 1988.

Physical Examination

The first 24 hours of life are particularly precarious as the neonate makes the transition from intrauterine to extrauterine life. During this critical period, careful observations are essential to identify problems and institute early interventions. In the delivery room, every neonate should have a brief physical examination to ensure that his or her status is stable and that no major anomalies exist. This physical examination can usually be performed in 1 to 2 minutes. The neonate's respiratory effort and air exchange should be observed closely. Symptoms of respiratory distress such as grunting, flaring, retractions, and cyanosis should be identified promptly. Particular attention should be given to the adequacy of the neonate's heart rate and clinical indicators of cardiovascular function. Pallor and poor perfusion need immediate further evaluation and possible intervention. The neonate should possess good muscle tone and be appropriately responsive. The extremities, facies, genitalia, abdomen, and back should be quickly inspected for any anomalies. Any abnormalities should be described and shown to the parents as soon as possible.

Once the neonate has been stabilized, vitamin K (1 mg) should be given intramuscularly to prevent hemorrhagic disease of the newborn, and an antibiotic solution or ointment or silver nitrate solution should be placed in both eyes for prevention of gonococcal ophthalmia.

The first comprehensive medical evaluation of the neonate should be performed as soon after birth as possible. The examination should begin with a thorough review of the mother's history of the pregnancy, labor, and delivery (Table 4). In addition, a medical history of the parents and their families should be documented, including genetic diseases.

As part of the initial physical examination, gestational maturation should be evaluated. The Dubowitz examination (neuromuscular and physical maturity) and more often the Ballard scoring system (Fig. 1) are the standards by which a neonate's gestational age is estimated following birth. Although physical maturity assessment is best performed in the first hours after birth, the neuromuscular examination may be affected by a variety of perinatal factors. Anesthetic agents, narcotics, and acute asphyxia can depress neuromuscular activity. Chronic stress in utero, as in maternal toxemia, hypertension, or prolonged rupture of the membranes, may result in neuromuscular maturity more advanced than gestational age. Such a disparity between neuromuscular and physical maturity should prompt a review of the maternal history of perinatal events. Continued depression of neuromuscular actvity should alert the physician to perform a close neurologic evaluation of the neonate.

Following determination of the gestational age, this information should be plotted on a birthweight versus gestational age graph. Using the information on these graphs, a neonate can be classified by ges-

TABLE 3. **Components of the Apgar Score**

Component	0	1	2
Heart rate	Absent	<100 beats per minute	>100 beats per minute
Respiratory effort	Apneic	Shallow, irregular, gasping	Vigorous cry
Reflex irritability	Absent	Grimace	Active avoidance
Muscle tone	Flaccid	Weak, passive	Active movement
Skin color	Pale, cyanotic	Pale, acrocyanotic	Pink

TABLE 4. **Components of the Maternal History**

Routine Prenatal Care
Ages of the mother and father
Marital status
Last menstrual period
Estimated date of confinement
Onset of prenatal care
Prepregnancy weight and weight gain during pregnancy
Previous Pregnancies
Number
Outcome of each
Previous prenatal, intrapartum, neonatal complications
Prenatal Maternal Laboratory Studies
Blood type and Rh
Antibody screen
HBsAg
HIV antibody
Underlying Maternal Systemic Illnesses
Pregnancy-Related Illnesses
Maternal Medications
Steroids
Tocolytics
Antibiotics
Sedatives, analgesics, anesthetics
Maternal Substance Use/Abuse
Tobacco
Alcohol
Marijuana, cocaine
Amphetamines, heroin, methadone
Phencyclidine (PCP)
Prenatal Fetal Laboratory Studies
Alpha-fetoprotein
Bacterial, viral cultures
Amniotic fluid lung maturity studies
Fetal chromosome studies
Fetal Status
Number
Ultrasound results
Time of rupture of membranes
Cord injuries/prolapse
Results of fetal heart rate monitoring
Maternal bleeding: placenta previa, abruption
History of oligohydramnios or polyhydramnios
Meconium staining
Delivery
Premature labor (use of tocolytics)
Method of delivery
Presentation
Use of instrumentation: forceps, vacuum
Preferred Method of Feeding
Desire for Circumcision

Adapted from D'Harlingue A, and Durand D: Recognition, stabilization, and transport of the high-risk newborn. *In* Klaus M, and Fanaroff A (eds): Care of the High-Risk Neonate, 4th ed. Philadelphia, WB Saunders Co, 1993.

tational age as preterm (less than 37 weeks), term (38 to 42 weeks), and post-term (greater than 42 weeks). In addition, neonates can be grouped by birthweight (small for gestational age [SGA], appropriate for gestational age [AGA], or large for gestational age [LGA]). Assignment of neonates to a specific gestational age group allows the physician to anticipate particular problems in the neonate and to develop a specific plan of medical care (Fig. 2).

Thermoregulation

Immediately after birth the neonate needs to be dried off to maintain body temperature. In the delivery room, evaporation is the most significant mechanism of heat loss. It is important to dry and immediately cover the head of the neonate. Because the surface area of the head is proportionally larger than the rest of the body, it contributes significantly to radiant heat loss. A radiant warmer is used to provide external heat to the neonate, who can then remain exposed so that other vital signs and skin color can be evaluated. Thermal (cold) stress can be detrimental because it places increasing metabolic demands on oxygen delivery and carbohydrate stores. Keeping neonates warm increases their chances of survival. Temperature maintenance is the keystone of effective stabilization.

The mortality rate for preterm neonates increases when they are exposed to a cold environment. The preterm neonate is at a disadvantage in maintaining body temperature because of a relatively large surface area and a lack of subcutaneous fat. The neonate must be maintained in a neutral thermal environment to ensure a normal core temperature and metabolic rate and to minimize oxygen requirements. As a rule, neonates are homeotherms who attempt to maintain their body temperature within a narrow range. They respond to heat loss by generating more heat, even at the risk of developing respiratory insufficiency, hypoglycemia, and metabolic acidosis. The risk of subsequent neurologic impairment has also been noted.

The optimal thermal environment for a given neonate depends on the neonate's maturity, size, and metabolic activity. If a neonate's internal (core) temperature is within the range of 36.5 to 37.5° C (97.6 to 99.5° F), the neonate's temperature can be considered normal. Measurement of axillary temperature provides a fairly good correlation with core temperature. A normal body temperature should not be confused with a "normal" metabolic rate.

The sick neonate who requires close observation, monitoring, and accessibility for procedures is best cared for under a radiant warmer. The neonate's skin temperature should be regulated automatically using a servocontrol skin probe (Thermistor) and maintained at around 37° C (98.6° F). The axillary temperature and the functioning of the radiant warmer, including temperature alarms, should be checked frequently, and temperature should be recorded at least every 2 to 3 hours. A neonate under a radiant warmer should not be covered because the cover will block the heat source. A hypothermic neonate (skin temperature less than 35.0° C [95.0° F]) can be warmed to a normal body temperature more rapidly with a radiant warmer than in an incubator. Fast rewarming under a radiant warmer has been suggested as a way of preventing asymptomatic hypoglycemia and prolonged metabolic acidosis. In contrast to similar studies in incubators, apnea during rewarming of infants under radiant warmers seems to be less frequent.

An alternative means of achieving a neutral thermal environment is to put the neonate in a double-walled incubator in which the controls have been pre-

MATURATIONAL ASSESSMENT OF GESTATIONAL AGE (New Ballard Score)

NAME ____ DATE/TIME OF BIRTH ____ SEX ____

HOSPITAL NO. ____ DATE/TIME OF EXAM ____ BIRTH WEIGHT ____

RACE ____ AGE WHEN EXAMINED ____ LENGTH ____

APGAR SCORE: 1 MINUTE ____ 5 MINUTES ____ 10 MINUTES ____ HEAD CIRC. ____

EXAMINER ____

NEUROMUSCULAR MATURITY

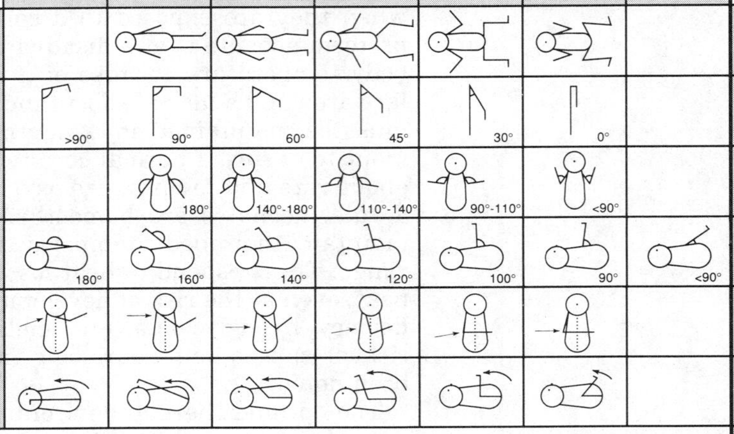

NEUROMUSCULAR MATURITY SIGN	SCORE -1	0	1	2	3	4	5	RECORD SCORE HERE
POSTURE								
SQUARE WINDOW (Wrist)	>90°	90°	60°	45°	30°	0°		
ARM RECOIL		180°	140°-180°	110°-140°	90°-110°	<90°		
POPLITEAL ANGLE	180°	160°	140°	120°	100°	90°	<90°	
SCARF SIGN								
HEEL TO EAR								

TOTAL NEUROMUSCULAR MATURITY SCORE

PHYSICAL MATURITY

PHYSICAL MATURITY SIGN	SCORE -1	0	1	2	3	4	5	RECORD SCORE HERE
SKIN	sticky friable transparent	gelatinous red translucent	smooth pink visible veins	superficial peeling &/or rash, few veins	cracking pale areas rare veins	parchment deep cracking no vessels	leathery cracked wrinkled	
LANUGO	none	sparse	abundant	thinning	bald areas	mostly bald		
PLANTAR SURFACE	heel-toe 40-50 mm:-1 <40 mm:-2	>50 mm no crease	faint red marks	anterior transverse crease only	creases ant. 2/3	creases over entire sole		
BREAST	imperceptible	barely perceptible	flat areola no bud	stippled areola 1-2 mm bud	raised areola 3-4 mm bud	full areola 5-10 mm bud		
EYE/EAR	lids fused loosely: -1 tightly: -2	lids open pinna flat stays folded	sl. curved pinna; soft; slow recoil	well-curved pinna; soft but ready recoil	formed & firm instant recoil	thick cartilage ear stiff		
GENITALS (Male)	scrotum flat, smooth	scrotum empty faint rugae	testes in upper canal rare rugae	testes descending few rugae	testes down good rugae	testes pendulous deep rugae		
GENITALS (Female)	clitoris prominent & labia flat	prominent clitoris & small labia minora	prominent clitoris & enlarging minora	majora & minora equally prominent	majora large minora small	majora cover clitoris & minora		

TOTAL PHYSICAL MATURITY SCORE

SCORE

Neuromuscular ____

Physical ____

Total ____

MATURITY RATING

score	weeks
-10	20
-5	22
0	24
5	26
10	28
15	30
20	32
25	34
30	36
35	38
40	40
45	42
50	44

GESTATIONAL AGE (weeks)

By dates ____

By ultrasound ____

By exam ____

Figure 1. Expanded new Ballard Score (NBS) includes extremely premature infants and has been refined to improve accuracy in more mature infants. (From Ballard JL, et al: New Ballard Score, expanded to include extremely premature infants. J Pediatr *119*[3]:417–423, 1991.)

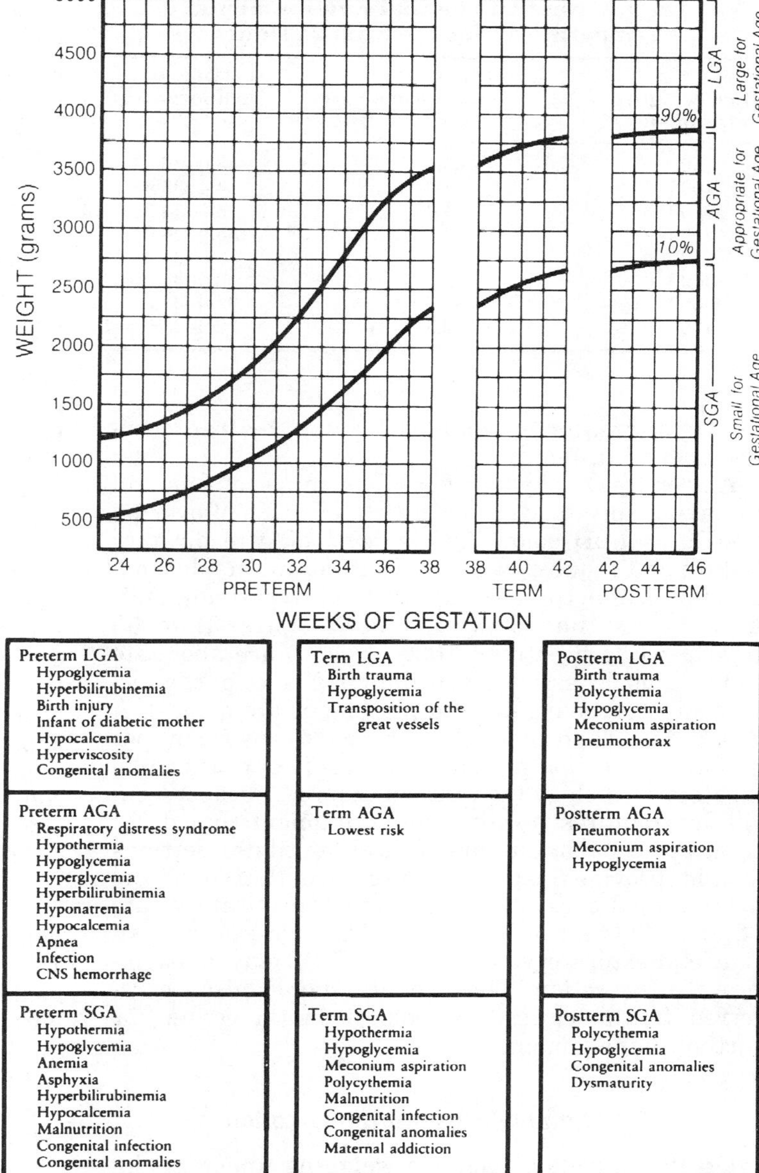

Figure 2. Neonatal morbidity risk. (Adapted from Lubchenco LO, et al: Neonatal mortality rate: Relationship to birthweight and gestational age. J Pediatr *81*:818, 1972; reprinted with permission from Coen RW, and Koffler H: Primary Care of the Newborn. Boston, Little, Brown and Company, 1987, p. 60.)

sent to provide specific air temperatures (Table 5). Humidity should be maintained in the neutral range of 40 to 60%, allowing no visible mist or moisture to form on the incubator walls. The neonate's temperature as well as the incubator settings and probe placement should be checked and recorded routinely. When single-walled incubators are used, neonates - 4ncan still lose heat by radiation to cold walls, windows, or environment. In addition, a normal axillary temperature does not necessarily mean that the neonate is in the correct ambient temperature because a cold-stressed neonate can maintain a normal temperature by increasing the metabolic rate.

Oxygenation and Ventilation

Proper oxygenation and ventilation of the high-risk neonate are very important to avoid hypoxic tissue damage and metabolic acidosis. Laboratory determinations of PaO_2, $PaCO_2$, pH, and hematocrit are necessary to ensure that body tissues are receiving proper amounts of oxygen.

Continuous transcutaneous oxygen measurements are beneficial and noninvasive. With adequate skin perfusion, the correlation between arterial oxygen tension and transcutaneous oxygen tension is very close. The transcutaneous method has been very useful in determining the concentration of oxygen needed to avoid hypoxia and to wean neonates from oxygen. In very sick hypotensive neonates, transcutaneous oxygen levels appear to reflect the shocked state rather than the level of oxygen in the arterial blood. Blood pressure, respiratory rate, and heart rate should be continuously monitored and recorded. Adjustments in inspired oxygen concentration should be made to maintain the PaO_2 at a level of 60 to 80

TABLE 5. **Neutral Thermal Environmental Temperatures for the First 24 Hours**

Birthweight (grams)	Starting Temperature (° C)	Range of Temperature (° C)
500	35.5	35.0–36.0
1000	34.9	34.4–35.4
1500	34.0	33.5–34.5
2000	33.5	33.0–34.0
2500	33.2	32.6–34.0
3000	33.0	32.0–34.0
3500	32.8	32.0–33.0
4000	32.5	32.0–33.0

mmHg or greater than 90% saturation by transcutaneous monitoring.

A neonate who by blood gas determination is found to have respiratory acidosis with a $PaCO_2$ of over 60 mmHg or a pH below 7.20 is developing respiratory failure and requires assisted ventilation. In addition, cardiovascular collapse, apnea, and hypoxemia (saturation less than 90% or a PaO_2 of less than 50 mmHg while breathing 100% oxygen) are adequate indications for assisted ventilation. Choice of the correct endotracheal tube and placement are critical. A chest radiograph should be obtained to ensure proper endotracheal tube placement and rule out other respiratory pathology (i.e., pneumothorax). Proper ventilation requires training and equipment that differ from those for adult care. Initial ventilator settings should provide inspiratory pressure that produces symmetrical chest movement and a respiratory rate of 30 to 60 breaths per minute. The addition of positive end-expiratory pressure (PEEP) may also improve oxygenation. The neonate should also be referred to the closest regional neonatal center for further management.

Fluid and Glucose Administration

On the first day, neonates weighing under 1.0 kg who are receiving intravenous fluids are given 5% dextrose in water at a rate of 100 to 120 mL of fluid per kg per day. Neonates between 1000 and 1500 grams are begun on 10% dextrose in water at a rate of 80 to 100 mL of fluid per kg per day, and neonates larger than 1500 grams are begun on 10% dextrose in water at a rate of 80 mL of fluid per kg per day. A neonate typically loses 1 to 2% of body weight per day for the first 3 to 4 days. Weight is the most accurate indicator of an infant's fluid status in the absence of third spacing. The intravenous fluid rate should be advanced by 20 to 30 mL of fluid per kg per day as long as the infant is following the expected weight curve, including the initial loss.

Factors that increase fluid requirements include extreme immaturity (due to increased evaporation and decreased ability to concentrate urine), environmental temperature, radiant warmers, skin breakdown, phototherapy, third spacing, tachypnea, hyperthermia, and excessive losses from the gastrointestinal tract through nasogastric tubes or stool output. Factors that decrease fluid requirements include plastic heat shield, high ambient or inspired humidity, and renal insufficiency. An acceptable urinary output is 1 to 4 mL of urine per kg per day. Fluid requirements need to be adjusted as determined by urine output, changes in daily weight, and serum electrolyte concentrations.

The blood glucose level should be monitored periodically using capillary whole blood reagent strips (Chemstrip, Dextrostix) to ensure normal gluose homeostasis with a level between 40 to 80 mg per dL. Whenever there is a borderline or low value, a true glucose level should be determined in the laboratory. Low blood glucose concentrations (less than 40 mg per dL) should be treated with a 10% glucose solution given at a rate of 2 to 3 mL of fluid per kg per dose. Sick premature neonates often develop hyperglycemia, which may result in an osmotic diuresis and dehydration.

Because a neonate's electrolyte status reflects the mother's, it is not necessary to obtain the neonate's serum electrolytes on admission unless there is a predisposing factor causing the mother to have an electrolyte imbalance. If intravenous fluids are required beyond the first 12 to 24 hours, serum electrolytes should be checked. If these levels are normal and if urine output is adequate, maintenance fluids should consist of a dextrose solution containing sodium chloride (3 mEq per kg per day) and potassium chloride (2 mEq per kg per day). Very-low-birthweight neonates (less than 1500 grams) may need more sodium because of increased renal losses. Hyponatremia is defined as a serum sodium concentration of less than 130 mEq per liter and can be associated with iatrogenic causes, syndrome of inappropriate antidiuretic hormone, renal disease, congestive heart failure, and fluid overload. Hypernatremia is defined as a serum sodium level of greater than 150 mEq per liter and is associated with extreme immaturity, dehydration, renal disease and iatrogenic causes.

Hypocalcemia

Hypocalcemia is a common occurrence in sick premature neonates, asphyxiated neonates, and neonates of diabetic or epileptic mothers. Other less common causes include maternal hyperparathyroidism, hypomagnesemia, and renal abnormalities. Normally, the serum calcium should be greater than 7 mg per 100 mL. Symptoms of hypocalcemia include seizures, irritability, listlessness, vomiting, and apnea. The treatment of neonatal hypocalcemia consists of calcium gluconate (10% solution) given at 200 mg per kg as a slow intravenous push. In high-risk situations, one may also give maintenance calcium in a dose of 200 to 400 mg per kg per day as a constant or intermittent infusion in the intravenous fluid while monitoring serum calcium levels. Whenever calcium is given as a "push," the heart rate should be closely monitored because too rapid an infusion can cause bradycardia or other arrhythmias. If these occur, the infusion should be stopped for a few minutes and then resumed at a slower rate.

Hematocrit

An initial hematocrit should be obtained in all neonates shortly after admission. Preferably, the hematocrit should be obtained by venipuncture because capillary hematocrits may be as much as 10 to 20% higher than central hematocrits. In a sick neonate, the hematocrit should be maintained at or above 45% to ensure optimal delivery of oxygen to the tissues. Usually, packed red cells are given at a dose of 10 mL per kg slowly over 1 to 2 hours to raise the hematocrit.

Polycythemia is defined as a central hematocrit greater than 65%. The most common causes include pregnancy-induced hypertension, maternal diabetes, maternal-to-fetal or fetal-to-fetal transfusion, delayed clamping of the umbilical cord, and "milking" the umbilical cord toward the neonate at birth. If the central hematocrit is greater than 65% and there are cardiopulmonary or neurologic signs consistent with hyperviscosity, or if the hematocrit is greater than 70% in an asymptomatic neonate, the hematocrit should be lowered. This can be accomplished by a partial exchange transfusion through an umbilical venous catheter. Aliquots of blood are removed and replaced with equal volumes of crystalloid or colloid solution to lower the hematocrit to a level of 50%. To calculate the partial exchange volume, the following formula is used:

Volume of exchange (mL) = Blood volume (0.8 × kg) × (observed hematocrit − desired hematocrit)/observed hematocrit

A simple phlebotomy should never be used to lower the hematocrit because it may result in acute hypovolemia.

Sepsis

Neonatal septicemia affects between 1 in 500 and 1 in 1600 newborns. This range in incidence depends on the prevalence of maternal and neonatal risk factors for sepsis (i.e., maternal fever, prematurity, prolonged rupture of membranes, chorioamnionitis, and birth asphyxia). The incidence of meningitis is a fraction of that of sepsis (approximately 25 to 30%) and is greatly dependent on the various etiologic agents because some (i.e., group B streptococci and *Escherichia coli)* are frequently associated with concomitant meningitis, whereas others (i.e., *Staphylococcus aureus)* rarely cause meningitis in the absence of anatomic defects of the central nervous system. During the last decade, the incidence of bacterial infections in the newborn has increased. This increase is due in part to the emergence of group B streptococci as frequently encountered agents and the improved outcome for high-risk neonates, who survive to develop one or more episodes of nosocomial infection.

An infection may be acquired during fetal life via the transplacental route or by rupture of the fetal membranes. Also, the neonate may be colonized by a pathogenic organism during the passage through the birth canal. The most common bacteria causing systemic infection include group B streptococci, *Escherichia coli, Klebsiella, Neisseria gonorrhoea,* Enterobacter, *Haemophilus influenzae,* and *Listeria monocytogenes. Chlamydia trachomatis* produces conjunctivitis and pneumonitis.

Any infection in the neonate may be devastating because a neonate's response to bacterial invasion is limited both by immature defense mechanisms and by the virulence of the infectious agent. Sepsis should be suspected when there has been rupture of the membranes for more than 24 hours or when the neonate is malodorous at birth. A neonate who is lethargic, intermittently mottled, and feeding poorly must be considered to be septic until proved otherwise. Overwhelming sepsis is characterized by temperature instability (hypothermia or hyperthermia), respiratory grunting, apnea, cyanosis, and shock.

The laboratory work-up for septicemia includes a complete blood count, platelet count, and appropriate cultures of the blood, urine, and cerebrospinal fluid. Urine or cerebrospinal fluid for countercurrent immunoelectrophoresis (CIE) may be useful as a rapid diagnostic test to provide presumptive diagnosis before the culture results are known. Chest and abdominal radiographs are needed if clinical symptoms or physical findings are abnormal. Blood gas analysis may be useful in early septicemia because it often reveals an insidious metabolic acidosis.

The neonate with suspected sepsis must be treated immediately after appropriate diagnostic studies are performed and before the exact etiologic agent is identified. Therapy consists of administration of antibiotics that protect against both gram-positive and gram-negative bacteria. Initial treatment is with a penicillin derivative (such as ampicillin) and an aminoglycoside (such as gentamicin) or a cephalosporin (such as cefotaxime). Antibiotic sensitivity patterns direct the choice of antibiotics once the infectious organism has been identified. Appropriate antibiotic doses are given in Table 6.

Intrauterine Growth Retardation

The growth of a fetus is influenced by hereditary and environmental factors that affect the supply of nutrients across the placenta. Intrauterine growth retardation (IUGR) and small for gestational age (SGA), although related, are not synonymous. IUGR is a deviation or reduced eventual fetal growth pattern that results from multiple adverse effects on the fetus. IUGR is due to processes that inhibit the normal growth pattern of the fetus. Deviations from the predicted weight at delivery may produce IUGR but may not produce an SGA neonate. SGA is a weight based on population norms and includes neonates weighing less than a predetermined weight (−2 SD, less than 5 percentiles) and represents pathologic

TABLE 6. **Common Antibiotic Therapy**

Ampicillin	Broad-spectrum antibiotic useful against group B streptococcus, *Listeria monocytogenes,* and susceptible *E. coli* species for sepsis and meningitis
Dosage	50 to 100 mg/kg per dose by IV or IM (for meningitis give higher dose)
Interval	For neonates <1 week of age, give every 12 hours For neonates >1 week of age, give every 8 hours
Cefotaxime	Useful for treatment of gram-negative neonatal sepsis and meningitis caused by susceptible gram-negative organisms such as *E. coli, H. influenzae, Klebsiella, Pseudomonas,* and disseminated gonococcal infections
Dosage	50 mg/kg per dose by IV or IM (for gonococcal infections, give 25 mg/kg per dose by IV or IM)
Interval	For neonates <1 week of age, give every 12 hours For neonates >1 week of age, give every 8 hours
Gentamicin	Useful for treatment of infections caused by aerobic gram-negative bacilli such as *Pseudomonas, Klebsiella,* and *E. coli.*
Dosage	2.5 mg/kg per dose IV
Interval	For neonates less than 30 weeks gestation, give every 24 hours For neonates less than 37 weeks gestation, give every 18 hours For all other neonates, give every 12 hours
Vancomycin	Drug of choice for serious infections caused by methicillin-resistant staphylococci (such as *Staphylococcus aureus* or *S. epidermidis*) and penicillin-resistant pneumococci
Dosage and Interval	For neonates less than 1200 grams, give 20 mg/kg per dose IV every 24 hours For neonates 1200–2000 grams, give 15 mg/kg per dose IV every 12 hours For neonates over 2000 grams, give 10 mg/kg per dose IV every 8 hours

(IUGR) and nonpathologic conditions. It is important to recognize growth retardation in utero so that the cause can be established and treated if possible. Potential problems presenting in the neonatal period include hypoglycemia, polycythemia, pulmonary hemorrhage, feeding disorders, and infections. Findings associated with IUGR include maternal, environmental, placental, and fetal factors; a partial list of these factors is presented in Table 7.

The long-term outcome for IUGR neonates depends on the cause of the growth retardation. Infants with chromosomal abnormalities or congenital infections subsequently have marked growth and developmental delays. Neonates whose intrauterine growth was affected by uteroplacental insufficiency from various placental lesions or maternal illness late in gestation will show normal growth patterns. Neurologic sequelae in this group are uncommon.

SPECIAL PROBLEMS IN THE DELIVERY ROOM

Meconium Aspiration

Meconium aspiration syndrome, a common cause of neonatal respiratory distress, is initiated by the aspiration of meconium-stained fluid. A distressed near-term fetus will pass meconium in utero in response to an asphyxiant insult. Gasping respirations that draw the meconium-stained amniotic fluid into the oropharynx and major airway passages may occur. If the meconium is not removed at delivery, the neonate may inhale it, or the meconium may be aspirated into the lower airways during bag-and-mask ventilation. The oropharynx and nasopharynx should be suctioned by the obstetrician with a catheter connected to wall suction as soon as the neonate's head is delivered. Bulb suction is probably inferior in removing meconium effectively. After suctioning, the neonate should be given to the neonatal resuscitation team without further stimulation, and immediate intubation of the trachea is then performed. The largest endotracheal tube that will not cause trauma to the vocal cords should be used for intubation. Once intubation has been achieved, the airway should be suctioned with a large catheter connected to wall suction. Special devices connected to wall suction that fit directly over the adapter of the endotracheal tube should be used. In effect, the endotracheal tube itself becomes a large suction catheter. Negative pressure is applied as the endotracheal tube is removed. If meconium is present in the lower airways, reintuba-

TABLE 7. **Findings Associated with Intrauterine Growth Retardation**

- Maternal factors
  - Congenital infections
  - Toxemia or chronic hypertension
  - Severe malnutrition
  - Smoking
  - Alcohol or narcotic usage
  - Young maternal age
- Placental factors
  - Infarcts
  - Thrombosis of fetal vessels
  - Premature partial separation
  - Single umbilical artery (associated with fetal renal anomalies)
- Environmental factors
  - Radiation exposure
  - Residence at high altitudes
  - Exposure to teratogens
- Fetal factors
  - Chromosomal abnormalities
  - Congenital malformations
  - Inborn errors of metabolism
  - Multiple gestation

tion and suctioning may need to be repeated several times. Unless clinically necessary, it is suggested that no positive pressure be applied to the airway until the first suctioning is completed.

These guidelines are applicable for the neonate who is depressed at birth. However, some neonates who pass meconium are pink, vigorous, and have active cough reflexes. They often resist intubation. It is suggested that these neonates not be intubated but closely observed clinically and allowed to clear their airways on their own.

Acute Hypovolemia

Not infrequently, neonates are born pale and "shocky" as a result of asphyxia or acute blood loss from a placental separation, a torn or cut umbilical cord, or in a cesarean section when the obstetrician must cut through an anterior placenta to deliver the neonate. Crossmatched blood may not be available for these neonates at the time of delivery. Expansion of the circulating volume by rapid administration of colloid may be necessary in an emergency. Vascular access is more rapidly obtained and maintained during resuscitation by passing an umbilical venous catheter. It is safest to pass the catheter only a few centimeters until blood return is obtained, so that fluid and drugs administered are less likely to enter directly into the liver and produce tissue damage. Albumin (5% salt-poor solution) can be administered at a dose of 10 to 15 mL per kg given over 5 to 10 minutes. The dose may be repeated if adequate perfusion or blood pressure is not obtained. Isotonic saline solution, plasma protein factor (Plasmanate), or fresh-frozen plasma may also be used in the same dose (10 to 15 mL per kg given over 10 to 15 minutes). When it is appreciated that a neonate has suffered massive acute blood loss, blood or packed red cells must be given rapidly at a dose of 10 to 15 mL per kg. The urgency of the situation makes it advisable to use uncrossmatched type O, Rh-negative blood or packed cells from the blood bank. Alternatively, blood drawn immediately from a placental vessel into a heparinized syringe (1000 units of heparin per milliliter) may be administered to the neonate after passage through a blood filter.

Congenital Diaphragmatic Hernia

Persistent cyanosis and respiratory distress, a scaphoid abdomen, and a barrel-shaped chest in a neonate should raise the suspicion of a congenital diaphragmatic hernia (CDH). Most commonly, CDH involves the left hemidiaphragm. Breath sounds over the left chest will be diminished or absent, and the cardiac sounds will be shifted to the right. The clinical signs are often not as obvious when the hernia is on the right side, making the diagnosis more difficult. One should pass a radiopaque feeding tube into the stomach and immediately obtain a chest roentgenogram. This defines the stomach and distinguishes a left diaphragmatic hernia from cystic adenomatous malformation of the lung. Once the diagnosis of CDH has been confirmed, the neonate must be treated promptly because this condition is a medical and surgical emergency. The trachea should be intubated with an endotracheal tube, and assisted ventilation should be implemented with a low inspiratory pressure and a rapid rate. Quick referral to a regional neonatal center for continuing care is recommended.

SPECIAL PROBLEMS OF THE TERM HIGH-RISK NEONATE

Hyperbilirubinemia

Hyperbilirubinemia is virtually universal in newborn infants during the first week of life. Mild to moderate jaundice may develop because (1) a large red blood cell mass is present at birth, (2) the hepatic glucuronide conjugation system is relatively immature, and (3) unconjugated bilirubin present in meconium may be reabsorbed. These factors result in clinically evident jaundice usually after the first 24 hours. Physiologic jaundice is defined as a bilirubin level that does not exceed 12 to 12.5 mg per dL and dissipates by the end of the first week. By definition, jaundice appearing during the first 24 hours after birth, rising above 12.5 mg per dL or persisting beyond the first week of life is pathologic and requires further evaluation.

Once significant jaundice is recognized, a diagnosis must be established. A careful review of the neonate's history, paying particular attention to traumatic delivery (bruises, cephalhematomas) and to a family history of jaundice (hemolytic conditions) is recommended. Specific information relating to possible sepsis should be evaluated. The mode of feeding should be established because breast-feeding has been associated with jaundice. Laboratory work-up should include determination of the serum bilirubin (total and direct components), mother's and neonate's blood type, and a direct Coombs' test. An indirect Coombs' test may be helpful if the direct Coombs' test is negative and there is evidence of hemolysis on the peripheral blood smear. The neonate's hematocrit should be determined and a peripheral blood smear should be examined to rule out abnormal red blood cell morphology. A white blood cell count with differential may be useful to rule out sepsis. The possibility of infection should lead the physician to obtain appropriate cultures and begin antibiotic therapy as necessary. Determination of the level of IgM in the cord blood may be useful to rule out congenital infection. Once formula or breast feedings have been established, the urine should be tested for reducing substances to rule out galactosemia. For persistent jaundice, thyroid function studies should be performed to rule out hypothyroidism.

Phototherapy is currently the method of choice for treating elevated bilirubin levels. In term neonates, phototherapy is initiated when serum bilirubin levels rise above 15 mg per dL. The neonate's eyes and genitalia should be shielded to prevent damage from the phototherapy light. Exchange transfusion is indicated when bilirubin levels exceed 20 mg per dL to minimize the risk of kernicterus.

Since the introduction of phototherapy, the number of exchange transfusions performed in the newborn intensive care nursery has decreased dramatically. However, most neonates with Rh incompatibility continue to require exchange transfusions because of rapidly rising bilirubin levels, profound anemia, heart failure, and generalized edema (hydrops).

Persistent Fetal Circulation

Persistent fetal circulation (PFC), or persistent pulmonary hypertension of the newborn, is a syndrome characterized primarily by right-to-left shunting of blood. This shunting occurs at the level of the foramen ovale or patent ductus arteriosus and is secondary to pulmonary artery hypertension. The pulmonary artery hypertension that occurs with this syndrome results from a variety of diseases that may cause reactive pulmonary arteriolar constriction, increased pulmonary arteriolar musculature, or hypoplasia of the pulmonary vascular bed. Some clinical conditions resulting in PFC include aspiration syndromes (i.e., meconium, amniotic fluid, blood), group B streptococcal pneumonia, diaphragmatic hernia, and cardiomyopathy. Common precipitating factors of PFC include asphyxia, hypoxia, hypothermia, hypoglycemia, and metabolic acidosis. Infants in respiratory distress or those who require oxygen should be evaluated for all of these conditions because if inappropriately treated, these neonates can deteriorate suddenly. Administration of oxygen is essential to obtain a stable PaO_2 of 90 to 100 mmHg and prevent hypoxia. Mechanical ventilation with hyperventilation is usually necessary. Efforts should be made to correct any acidosis, hypothermia, hypoglycemia, or hypotension immediately. Therapy is directed toward reducing the pulmonary artery pressure and increasing the systemic blood pressure to reduce right-to-left shunting. The modes of therapy presently available have major sequelae, and the mortality rate in the most severe cases is about 40 to 50%. Rapid recognition of the disease and referral to a regional neonatal center are essential.

Infants of Diabetic Mothers

The infant of a diabetic mother (IDM) may have a number of clinical problems including hypoglycemia, respiratory distress, polycythemia, hypocalcemia, hypomagnesemia, hyperbilirubinemia, congenital anomalies, and vascular thrombosis. There is also an increased risk of sepsis because of the higher frequency of urinary tract infections in pregnant diabetic patients. Fifty percent of IDM and 25% of infants of gestational diabetic mothers have blood glucose levels of less than 40 mg per dL during the first several hours after birth. Of these neonates, half are symptomatic. Therefore, it becomes necessary to monitor these neonates very carefully, usually on an hourly basis, for the first 6 hours. Blood glucose screening can be accomplished with capillary whole blood reagent strips (Dextrostix, Chemstrip). A screening blood glucose level of less than 40 mg per dL should prompt a blood glucose determination by the chemistry laboratory and an immediate glucose in water feeding as tolerated. For neonates who are unable to feed orally (e.g., due to prematurity or respiratory distress), a continuous intravenous infusion of glucose (10% dextrose in water solution at 90 to 120 mL per kg per day) is necessary to maintain glucose homeostasis. Frequent monitoring of glucose levels should be performed to maintain glucose levels at between 40 and 80 mg per dL. If the neonate becomes hypoglycemic, minibolus infusions of 200 mg of glucose per kg are preferred to the use of a large bolus of glucose or glucagon, which might result in acute hyperglycemia, thus potentiating wide swings in glucose levels and producing hyperinsulinemia and recurrent hypoglycemia. On occasion, it may become necessary to use glucagon or glucocorticosteroids to control hypoglycemia. Hypoglycemia may also accompany other conditions such as perinatal asphyxia, sepsis, hypothermia, cardiorespiratory failure, and conditions that affect gastrointestinal function and prevent enteral feedings.

The most common congenital malformations in the IDM involve the cardiovascular system and the skeletal system. Renal vascular thrombosis, which is peculiar to this group of neonates, has no immediate explanation. Treatment of hypocalcemia, polycythemia, and hyperbilirubinemia has been discussed previously.

SPECIAL PROBLEMS OF THE HIGH-RISK PRETERM NEONATE

Respiratory Distress Syndrome

Neonatal respiratory distress syndrome (RDS, surfactant deficiency syndrome, hyaline membrane disease) is the most common clinical problem affecting preterm neonates and remains a major cause of neonatal death. RDS is not a true disease per se but represents a phenomenon of developmental maturity. The syndrome affects approximately 90% of neonates who weigh less than 1500 grams at birth.

RDS presents clinically as progressive repiratory insufficiency with increasing requirement for supplemental oxygen. Clinical signs include tachypnea, inspiratory retractions (suprasternal, substernal, and intercostal), paradoxical seesaw respirations, nasal flaring, and audible respiratory grunting. Symptoms usually appear at birth or within the first hours of life. In the very small neonate, RDS usually is manifest at birth as respiratory failure.

The neonate with RDS has typical radiographic findings of overall hypoventilation, a nonspecific ground-glass appearance of the lungs, air bronchograms (alveolar atelectasis interspersed with dilated bronchioles), and increased pulmonary vascularity. A "white-out" on the chest radiograph should suggest pulmonary congestion and edema from a probable patent ductus arteriosus (PDA). Any of these radiographic findings may also represent pneumonia, but it is difficult to differentiate pulmonary infection from RDS. Antibiotics should be standard therapy until appropriate culture results are known.

The pathophysiology of RDS is incompletely understood and represents a combination of (1) anatomic immaturity of the lung parenchyma and chest wall, (2) a decrease in lung surfactant, (3) the presence of a PDA with left-to-right shunting resulting in pulmonary congestion, and (4) an increase in the interstitial and alveolar lung fluids. The major surfactants of the lung include phosphatidylcholine (lecithin), phosphatidylinositol (PI), and phosphatidylglycerol (PG). Lecithin and sphingomyelin form the basis of the L/S ratio, which is measured in the amniotic fluid. It is the presence of PG that ensures functional maturity of the lungs and stable alveoli at low lung volumes. Classic RDS does not occur in the presence of PG. Evaluation of surfactant from pulmonary effluent suctioned from the trachea or nasopharynx at birth has been shown to reflect the degree of pulmonary maturation closely and may be helpful in confirming the diagnosis of RDS.

The treatment of an infant with RDS should not be undertaken except at a facility where treatment is commonly established, where competent medical personnel (physicians, nurses, and respiratory therapists) are available, and where ventilatory and monitoring equipment are available. General management includes (1) surfactant replacement, (2) maintenance of body temperature within a neutral thermal environment, (3) maintenance of intravascular blood volume (perfusion) to prevent metabolic acidosis, (4) administration of intravenous fluids at a rate of 60 to 80 mg per kg per day, and (5) maintenance of the hematocrit above 45%. Oxygen should be administered to maintain the PaO_2 between 50 and 80 mmHg by monitoring oxygen levels in umbilical artery blood or using transcutaneous oxygen monitors. Respiratory support is initiated with oxygen administration. Ventilatory assistance should be considered when respiratory failure exists or when the oxygen concentration exceeds 60%. Continuous positive airway pressure (CPAP) may be useful in the larger preterm neonate when there is no apnea or respiratory failure. Mechanical ventilation is used to maintain the PaO_2 between 50 and 80 mmHg, $PaCO_2$ at 40 to 50 mmHg, and pH between 7.28 and 7.35. Serial arterial blood gases should be monitored closely, and the neonate should be weaned from mechanical ventilation rapidly to prevent complications of air leak (pneumothorax or pulmonary interstitial emphysema) or chronic lung disorders.

A left-to-right shunt through a PDA should be suspected in all neonates with bounding pulses, a systolic cardiac murmur, hyperdynamic precordium, hypercapnia, and systemic hypoperfusion. Its presence can be confirmed by Doppler echocardiography. Indomethacin (a prostaglandin synthetase inhibitor) is currently used to close a PDA medically. Surgical ligation is performed in infants in whom medical therapy has failed.

Bronchopulmonary Dysplasia

The incidence of bronchopulmonary dysplasia (BPD) is about 3 to 8% in neonates with RDS. Clinically, BPD is characterized by persistent inspiratory retractions and tachypnea. The physiologic abnormalities include decreased pulmonary compliance, increased airway resistance, intrapulmonary shunts, and a persistent oxygen requirement. Beginning shortly after the fifth day of life, radiographic alterations can be seen. These changes consist of progressive atelectasis alternating with areas of overinflation. Recovery to normal lung is possible; however, if continuous lung damage occurs, progressive interstitial fibrosis, emphysema, pulmonary hypertension, and cor pulmonale may result.

Treatment of neonates with BPD consists of removal of the source of lung injury. In the infant who is ventilator-dependent, higher $PaCO_2$ (50 to 60 mmHg) and lower pH (7.26 to 7.30) levels should be tolerated to wean the infant from mechanical ventilation and minimize barotrauma. Oxygen administered to the neonate should be reduced to the lowest concentration possible, but transcutaneous oxygen levels or earlobe oximetry of oxygen saturation should be monitored to avoid hypoxia. Pulmonary edema should be treated with diuretics and judicious fluid balance. Concerns about hypercalciuria and renal stones, hypochloremic acidosis, and chronic volume depletion must be kept in mind when using fluid restriction and diuretics. Serum electrolytes must be monitored and replacement of potassium, sodium, and chloride provided. Chest percussion is often helpful to prevent pulmonary superinfections. Proper nutrition, utilizing a 24-calorie formula, should be maximized to establish somatic growth. Limiting total fluid intake to 150 to 160 mL per kg per day is a common practice. Vitamin D and calcium supplementation are needed to prevent osteomalacia secondary to chronic diuretic therapy. After discharge, infants with BPD remain at high risk for poor growth, developmental delay, reactive airway disease, and sudden death. They are particularly prone to upper respiratory illnesses, which can rapidly progress to pulmonary insufficiency and failure.

Intraventricular Hemorrhage

Intraventricular hemorrhage (IVH) is the most common serious neurologic lesion of the neonatal period. With cranial computed tomography (CT) scan and ultrasound examinations, it has been established that significant hemorrhage occurs in a large percentage of premature neonates. The incidence is approximately 40 to 50% in neonates who weigh less than 1500 grams at birth. Neonates at greatest risk include those with asphyxia, hypoxia, acidosis, and pneumothorax.

Clinically, severe IVH may be suspected on the

basis of acute onset of shock, acidosis, seizures, hypoventilation, and a sudden drop in hematocrit in an otherwise stable neonate. Physical findings may include a full anterior fontanel, decreased muscle tone, and decreased spontaneous activity. Recent studies have shown that neonates with fluctuating arterial blood pressure are more likely to develop intraventricular hemorrhage. Neonates should be observed closely, and efforts to stabilize the fluctuating blood pressure should be attempted. Some specific factors associated with the development of these hemorrhages include rapid administration of volume expanders, rapid administration of hypertonic sodium bicarbonate solution, and excessively high ventilator settings; these activities should be avoided if possible.

Post-hemorrhagic hydrocephalus is found in approximately 20% of neonates with intraventricular hemorrhage. The process of dilatation evolves as a result of obstruction to the flow of cerebrospinal fluid by intraventricular blood clots or secondary to arachnoiditis, which inhibits cerebrospinal fluid reabsorption. Progressive ventricular enlargement is diagnosed earliest by cranial ultrasound. Clinically, increase in the head circumference may not develop until the second or third week. Treatment is directed at preventing further progression of the hydrocephalus. Serial lumbar punctures and ventricular taps through a ventriculostomy have had variable success. In neonates who do not respond, a ventriculoperitoneal shunt is placed. Prognosis is inversely related to the severity of the hemorrhage. The poorest neurologic outcome has been observed in infants with intraparenchymal hemorrhages or periventricular leukomalacia. Although many studies have looked at pharmacologic interventions (pancuronium, phenobarbital, indomethacin, ethamsylate,* vitamins E and K) for the prevention of hemorrhage, none has been shown unequivocally to be useful, and they cannot be recommended for routine administration until further support is obtained from carefully designed clinical trials.

Nutrition

The initial goals of management of the metabolic needs of the sick preterm neonate are to maintain a neutral thermal environment, to define fluid and electrolyte requirements, and to minimize problems that could produce a catabolic state. Optimal growth should parallel the known rate of intrauterine growth. However, this is rarely achieved.

Many factors interfere with normal gastrointestinal function in a preterm neonate. These include incompetent lower esophageal sphincter, delay in gastric emptying, poorly coordinated intestinal motility, and inefficient digestion and absorption of fat and proteins. Coordination of sucking and swallowing mechanisms do not usually occur until after 32 weeks' gestation. Sick preterm neonates may have significant delays in establishing normal sucking and swallowing mechanisms.

The goal of good nutrition is to provide the neonate with approximately 120 calories per kg per day to maintain optimal growth with a weight gain of 20 to 30 grams per day. Weight should be followed on a daily basis; length and head circumference should be plotted each week on a standard extrauterine growth curve.

During the first week, daily fluid and caloric requirements are not usually met by oral feedings, and supplementation with intravenous alimentation is necessary. During this period, serum electrolytes, total protein, calcium, phosphorus, and hematocrit should be followed at least two times per week. Enteral feedings should be started as soon as the neonate can tolerate them. Simultaneously, the quantity of intravenous calories is reduced as oral feedings are increased. Preterm neonates often require additional sodium and calcium. Breast milk or commercial formulas should be used, first at a slow rate and then gradually increased over several days as tolerated. Preterm neonates require special feeding techniques. Continuous nasogastric or transpyloric nasojejunal feedings in neonates weighing less than 1200 grams decrease the risk of gastroesophageal reflux. Tolerance for this method of feeding must be evaluated on an individual basis. Gavage feedings are generally used for neonates of around 32 weeks' gestation. Feedings are offered every 2 to 3 hours, a time consistent with expected gastric emptying. Oral nipple feedings should be initiated as soon as the neonate can coordinate suck and swallow mechanisms (usually around 33 to 34 weeks' gestation).

Chronic total parenteral nutrition may become necessary in neonates with interval feeding intolerance or congenital malformations of the gastrointestinal tract and intestinal resections. Suggested goals are a total caloric intake of 120 calories per kg per day; protein, 1 to 2.5 grams per kg per day; sodium, 3 to 4 mEq per kg per day; and calcium, 8 to 10 mEq per kg per day. Serum electrolytes, calcium, phosphorus, creatinine, and total bilirubin should be followed at least twice weekly. Problems of hyperglycemia and glycosuria require careful monitoring as dextrose concentrations in the feedings are increased. Fat emulsions should be used with great caution in preterm neonates, who are deficient in lipoprotein lipase. Infusions should be slow, given over 20 to 24 hours, and serum triglyceride levels should be monitored. The administration of emulsions is contraindicated in neonates with liver disease, thrombocytopenia, jaundice, or severe respiratory insufficiency. Complications of total parenteral nutrition include acidosis, infections, cholestasis (etiology unknown), and catheter-related problems.

Most neonatologists believe the colostrum and breast milk provide both immunologic and nutritional advantages. Breast milk is often better tolerated in the sick neonate. However, breast milk may present significant problems in the rapidly growing neonate owing to its low level of protein, sodium,

*Not available in the United States.

calcium, and phosphorus. It often is necessary to modify breast milk by adding a human milk fortifier (Similac Natural Care, Enfamil Human Milk Fortifier). Alternatives to breast milk are commercial formulas (24 calories per ounce) especially designed for premature neonates. These low–solute load preparations provide higher levels of protein, sodium, calcium, and phosphorus, resulting in approximate in utero rates of growth. A stage of rapid growth extends until the infant weights approximately 1800 grams, at which time the usual formulas for full-term infants can be used for continued growth.

Vitamin supplementation is an integral component of nutritional management. Infants on breast milk should receive supplements of vitamins C, D, and E. A multivitamin preparation such as Poly-Vi-Sol or Vi-Daylin, at a dose of 0.5 mL twice daily, provides adequate amounts of these vitamins. Use of a multivitamin preparation containing fluoride (based on local water supply) and iron should be considered prior to discharge. For the infant on commercial formula, the necessity and type of supplementation vary with the formula.

Necrotizing Enterocolitis

Necrotizing enterocolitis (NEC) is an acute inflammatory disease of the gastrointestinal tract. The incidence (10 to 30 per 1000 neonatal admissions) is highest in neonates who weigh less than 1500 grams at birth and are 32 weeks' gestation or less. At risk are neonates who have had asphyxia, acidosis, hypotension, umbilical vessel catheterization, and enteral feedings. Infection and overcrowding of the nursery appear to play roles in the genesis of this problem.

Typically, the neonate presents with feeding intolerance, temperature instability, apnea, and abdominal distention. There may be emesis, feeding residuals, and either occult or gross blood in the stool. If early signs are missed, overwhelming sepsis with shock and disseminated intravascular coagulation (DIC) may be manifest. Abdominal radiographs (including the left lateral decubitus view) should be obtained, and usually reveal a pattern of ileus with dilated loops of bowel, pneumatosis intestinalis (air in the bowel wall), or free air.

Treatment consists of stopping enteral feedings and placing the bowel at rest. A nasogastric tube should be placed and set to low intermittent suction. Intravenous fluids are started, and a sepsis work-up, including complete blood count and appropriate cultures (blood, urine, CSF, stool), are obtained. Antibiotic therapy (usually ampicillin and gentamicin) is initiated. Serial abdominal radiographs, platelet counts, and electrolyte determinations should be obtained every 4 to 6 hours. If hypotension occurs, fresh-frozen plasma, albumin, or whole blood (10 mL per kg) as well as dopamine (Intropin) (5 to 10 μg per kg per minute) should be administered to support the circulating volume. Surgical intervention is indicated for intestinal perforation, peritonitis, rapidly progressive pneumatosis intestinalis, and uncorrectable metabolic acidosis.

The neonate should be treated with antibiotics (adjusted for culture results) for 10 to 14 days to allow the bowel to heal adequately and should have no oral intake for at least 14 days. During this period, nutrition is provided with intravenous hyperalimentation. Enteral feedings are then reintroduced slowly and cautiously in small increments and diluted concentrations and increased as tolerated.

Prevention is the best approach to NEC. It is wise to introduce feedings cautiously to the preterm neonate. Feeding intolerance can be an early warning sign, and neonates with this sign require careful evaluation. Neonates with frequent apnea and bradycardia who have cyanoses, severe infections, asphyxia, and RDS should have their feedings withheld until clinically stable.

Hyperbilirubinemia

The development of jaundice in the preterm neonate is almost inevitable because of hepatic immaturity, increased enterohepatic circulation of bilirubin from delayed enteric feedings, and decreased red blood cell survival. The serum bilirubin level peaks at the end of the first week and may remain elevated for 3 to 4 weeks. Treatment is more critical in preterm neonates because of their increased propensity to develop kernicterus. Therapy is directed toward prevention with the early use of phototherapy. In our nursery, phototherapy is started immediately on nearly all neonates who weigh less than 1000 grams. Exchange transfusion is performed when the total serum indirect bilirubin level reaches 10 mg per dL in neonates weighing less than 1000 grams, or when it exceeds 1% of birthweight in neonates weighing more than 1000 grams (e.g., exchange transfusion is indicated when the indirect bilirubin level equals or exceeds 15 mg per dL in the 1500-gram neonate).

Apnea

Apnea is a common finding in preterm neonates, yet little is known about its physiologic mechanisms. It is probably one of the most troublesome respiratory problems in the premature infant. Apnea means the absence of respiratory gas flow. It may be central (no air flow and no respiratory effort), obstructive (no air flow but respiratory efforts are present), or mixed (central and obstructive) in origin. If apnea persists for 5 to 10 seconds and alternates with breathing, the condition is called periodic breathing. However, when apnea is prolonged, lasting longer than 20 seconds, the condition is referred to as simply apnea. Periodic breathing is thought to be a benign disorder, whereas apnea is a serious condition that may lead to severe hypoxia and brain damage. Apnea may be associated with bradycardia (heart rate below 80 beats per minute); however, some apneas may produce severe hypoxia without a major change in heart rate.

Approximately 40 to 50% of premature infants

breathe periodically during the neonatal period. The incidence is inversely related to gestational age (85% at 28 to 30 weeks of gestation). Additionally, up to 50% of infants with periodic breathing develop apnea during the neonatal period.

Neonates weighing less than 1800 grams and larger babies who are sick should have their heart rates and respirations continuously monitored. An attempt to determine the cause of apnea is important; however, none is usually found. Apnea is often associated with intraventricular hemorrhage, patent ductus arteriosus, RDS, pneumonia, sepsis (NEC), and, less commonly, hyperthermia, hypoglycemia, hypocalcemia, anemia, oversedation, and seizures. Precipitating causes of apnea such as cold stimulation of the face, rapid changes in oxygenation, and obstruction of the nasal airway by a feeding tube or secretions should be avoided.

The first consideration to be made is whether apnea is severe enough to be treated. If the episodes of apnea are infrequent, they can be managed by monitoring and tactile or auditory stimulation. If the episodes are severe and the cause unknown, theophylline can be used to abolish or reduce apnea by increasing alveolar ventilation through central stimulation. Theophylline is available in both intravenous and oral preparations. Theophylline should be given as a loading dose (4 to 6 mg per kg) followed by a maintenance dose (1.5 to 3.0 mg per kg per dose every 12 hours). Suggested therapeutic serum levels of theophylline vary from 5 to 15 mg per liter, aiming at a value near 10 mg per liter. Serum levels should be monitored once or twice per week. Side effects are dose-related and relatively few, usually an increase in heart rate, but hematemesis, jitteriness, seizures, and albuminuria are possible. Caffeine can also be used to treat apnea of prematurity (loading dose, 10 mg per kg; maintenance dose, 2.5 mg per kg per dose every 24 hours beginning 24 hours after loading dose; therapeutic level, 10 to 25 mg per liter).

Hypoxemia, caused by increasing frequency of apneic spells, is treated with 25 to 30% oxygen plus theophylline. More severe apnea may respond to the administration of continuous positive airway pressure, using nasal prongs or an endotracheal tube. Despite all other efforts, mechanical ventilation may be necessary in the most severe cases.

If apnea is simply a function of prematurity and immature respiratory control, it usually resolves by 34 to 36 weeks' gestational age. Theophylline can then be discontinued with continued observation and monitoring for an additional 7 days. If apnea or bradycardia persists, a detailed work-up of the nervous and cardiorespiratory systems should be performed. A 12- to 24-hour cardiorespiratory impedance pneumogram can be useful to determine the difference between true apneic or bradycardic spells and monitoring equipment alarms. However, skill and judgment are needed in the interpretation of pneumograms.

The decision about home monitoring should be made in consultation with a regional neonatal or apnea evaluation center. Parents must be made aware of the fact that home monitoring is expensive and has not been shown to prevent sudden infant death syndrome. If home monitoring is used, a well-organized system of technical, psychosocial, and medical support for the patient and family must be available.

SPECIAL CONSIDERATIONS

Congenital Malformations

Life-threatening congenital malformations require prompt recognition and medical attention. The neonate must be quickly stabilized and then transferred to a regional center where further evaluation and surgical correction can be performed. The role of the primary physician in efficient stabilization and support of the family is most important. When the physician is faced with the ethical dilemma of providing only supportive care, it is best to provide effective stabilization first and then obtain consultation from the closest regional neonatal center.

Gastrointestinal Obstruction

Obstruction of the gastrointestinal tract can occur anywhere along its length. A history of prematurity and polyhydramnios may be the first clue to a possible obstruction. Other clinical signs may include bilious vomiting, abdominal distention, a palpable abdominal mass, and failure to pass meconium. The presence of excess mucus or salivation within the first few hours after birth should suggest esophageal atresia with or without tracheoesophageal fistula. There may be associated respiratory distress with tachypnea, choking, and cyanosis. Early diagnosis is important to prevent possible aspiration and chemical pneumonitis. Resistance to passage of a nasogastric tube suggests the diagnosis. A radiograph of the chest and abdomen will show a radiopaque catheter curled in the blind esophageal pouch.

Associated abnormalities of the cardiovascular, genitourinary, and musculoskeletal systems are present in 50% of neonates. Air in the gastrointestinal tract indicates patency of a fistula. Management consists of placing a suction catheter in the blind upper esophageal pouch for continuous suction and positioning the infant in a prone position with the head elevated. The neonate should then be transferred to a local regional center for further evaluation and treatment.

Abdominal Wall Defects

Defects in the anterior abdominal wall are readily apparent at birth. An omphalocele represents a herniation of the intra-abdominal contents through a defect of the umbilical ring. It is usually covered by a sac composed of amnion and peritoneum. The size varies with the defect, ranging from a smal defect at the base of the umbilical cord to a large defect that includes not only the gastrointestinal tract but also the liver. Other congenital anomalies (Beckwith syndrome, trisomy 13 or 18, eutrophy of the bladder) are found in approximately 50% of neonates with an omphalocele. Gastroschisis is a defect of the abdominal wall just lateral to the umbilicus. Unlike the omphalocele, there is no peritoneal sac, and only 15% of neonates have associated anomalies (intestinal atresia).

Initial treatment should be directed at maintaining body temperature and fluid balance and preventing infection. A nasogastric catheter should be placed to prevent bowel distention. Exposed viscera should be covered with warm saline dressings. Appropriate culture should be obtained and antibiotics (ampicillin and gentamicin) administered. Intravenous fluids with glucose should be started, and blood pressure, heart rate, temperature, and perfusion should be monitored to permit early identification and treatment of hypovolemia or hypothermia.

Congenital Heart Defects

Heart defects are among the most common congenital abnormalities and usually present within the first hours after birth. Fortunately, there are only a limited number of ways that neonates with these defects present to the primary care physician. A cardiac disorder should be suspected in the presence of (1) congestive heart failure, (2) persistent cyanosis, (3) heart murmurs, and (4) dysrhythmias. Transposition of the great arteries, severe tetralogy of Fallot, and right heart lesions (pulmonary stenosis or atresia, tricuspid atresia) present early, within the first few hours of life, as the patent ductus arteriosus begins to close in response to extrauterine oxygenation. The neonate develops increasing cyanosis and hypoxemia or decreasing peripheral perfusion with congestive heart failure and metabolic acidosis. Aortic stenosis, coarctation, and hypoplastic left heart complex should be suspected in the neonate with increasing respiratory distress and poor perfusion; this condition is observable later within the first week of life. Often neonates with these lesions are thought to be septic and antibiotics are begun. Once the infant's condition has stabilized, diagnosis of the specific lesion is facilitated by echocardiography and cardiac catheterization performed by a skilled pediatric cardiologist.

The availability of prostaglandin E_1 (PGE_1, Prostin VR) has aided in the initial medical management of neonates with congenital heart lesions. PGE_1 relaxes the constricting ductus arteriosus and permits better perfusion of the pulmonary and systemic circulation across the patent ductus arteriosus. The medication is given by peripheral vein beginning at a dose of 0.025 to 0.05 μg per kg per minute. Side effects include flushing, hyperthermia, apnea, bradycardia, and seizures. Equipment for intubation and mechanical ventilation should be available prior to the administration of the medication. Consultation with a pediatric cardiologist or regional neonatal center should be sought prior to initiation of therapy.

Care of the Family of a High-Risk Neonate

The unique psychological process of parent-infant bonding is abruptly interrupted with the birth of a high-risk neonate. During the period following birth, the parents undergo a high degree of anxiety over the infant's clinical course and survival. This anxiety is further complicated by feelings of guilt as the parents look at possible personal reasons for the poor outcome of the pregnancy.

In all situations in which parents are suddenly presented with a sick neonate, it must be remembered that they are in a state of shock and may not be able to absorb information and explanations about the medical care of their infant. The clinical course needs to be reviewed with them on a daily basis, and they should be given the opportunity to ask questions and state their understanding of the situation. Parents often need help in adapting to the infant's situation, relieving associated feelings of guilt and anger, developing a mutual interaction with the infant, and learning to care for their baby. A supportive health care team (physicians, nurses, and social workers) and parent groups can provide families with an opportunity to express their feelings and level of stress. Before discharge home, the family should become involved in the nursery with routine daily care and begin taking over the responsibility of meeting the needs of their special infant.

When a neonate dies, it becomes especially important to recognize that parents will have unresolved feelings of shock, denial, guilt, anger, and depression. Opportunities to discuss their emotions as well as to ask questions about medical care should be provided around the time of death and in a follow-up visit 3 to 4 months later.

Discharge Planning

Discharge planning, like risk assessment, must be initiated early and reviewed regularly to meet the medical needs of the neonate and the psychosocial support requirements of the family. It is optimal if weekly meetings of the health care team can be held, so that information about the family unit can be reviewed and a comprehensive plan for each family developed. At discharge, this information, as well as medical problems, must be made available to the primary physician and health care providers.

NORMAL INFANT FEEDING

method of
LEWIS A. BARNESS, M.D.
University of South Florida
Tampa, Florida

The Committees on Nutrition of the American Academy of Pediatrics and the Canadian Pediatric Society strongly recommend breast-feeding for normal full-term infants. The most rapid growth and development of the entire life span occurs during the first few years of life, and nutrition during this time has not only immediate but also lasting effects.

PRENATAL CONSIDERATIONS

The physician who will be caring for the newborn should discuss with the parents their choice of feeding for the newborn. Mothers who wish to breast-feed should be encouraged to do so. They should be taught details of feeding procedures during prenatal visits. Breast care advice should include avoidance of soaps, alcohol, and ointments. Mothers with inverted or flat nipples should be instructed in the use of a shell inside the brassiere; in the last month of pregnancy this may facilitate eversion.

BREAST-FEEDING

Breast milk is the natural food for full-term human infants and suffices as the only food for the first few months of life. Breast-fed infants have an apparently lower incidence of allergies and respiratory infections in the first months compared with formula-fed infants. In societies and environments of high contamination by viruses or bacteria breast-feeding is essential to decrease morbidity.

Breast milk contains antibodies to those organisms to which the mother has been exposed. It contains lactoferrin, which improves iron absorption in the infant and also limits iron availability for *Escherichia coli* and other iron-requiring organisms. It contains secretory IgA, which consists of specific antibodies and also serves as a barrier in the intestine to prevent adherence of bacteria and other foreign substances to the intestinal mucosa.

Caloric density of breast milk is 67 to 70 kcal per dL. Electrolyte content is approximately 20 mEq per liter. Protein provides approximately 7 to 8% of the energy and consists of whey, 70 to 80%, which is highly soluble and easily absorbed, and casein, 20 to 30%. Fat provides approximately 50% of the energy and is unique in composition because it includes very-long-chain polyunsaturated fatty acids and a configuration that makes it easily absorbable. The balance of energy is supplied by carbohydrate, which consists almost entirely of lactose.

Breast-feeding should begin as soon after delivery as the condition of the mother and baby permits. Stimulus to secretion of human milk is best accomplished by completely emptying the breasts. The infant should be allowed to empty both breasts frequently, usually every 2 to 3 hours in the first few days. Early discharge practices militate against establishing a good milk supply in the first few days, when colostrum is the main secretion, and the mother will benefit from support by her family and physician. The infant's condition should be determined at 3 to 4 days of life to ascertain the adequacy of nursing.

The mother should use a sturdy, well-fitting nursing brassiere to support the breasts. The volume of milk produced usually increases about the third day. Breasts may become firm, swollen, and tender, resulting in engorgement. If the baby cannot latch on well to the full breast, hand expression of a small amount of milk allows the baby to suck, and complete emptying will relieve the engorgement.

After the milk supply is adequate, usually within 2 or 3 weeks, the infant may be satisfied with a 3- or 4-hour interval between feedings and should be fed when he or she indicates hunger. The baby should have four to eight wet diapers in 24 hours and may have no stools or as many as six soft stools daily.

Nipples should be kept dry, and ointments or lotions are not generally needed. If irritation develops, the nipples may be exposed to air or dry heat, and pure lanolin may be applied. Soap or alcohol should be avoided. Honey should not be placed on the nipples.

The mother's diet should include a vitamin supplement. Alcohol ingestion by the mother may make the baby lethargic. Most babies develop physiologic jaundice in the first week, and some develop breast milk jaundice, which may continue for 1 month. Neither cause of jaundice requires stopping nursing. Water should not be offered because it may interfere with nursing. Only the infant who is clinically dehydrated or is at risk for hypoglycemia should be offered glucose water.

Contraindications to breast-feeding include galactosemia in the infant; some maternal illnesses, such as breast cancer or systemic diseases; or maternal consumption of such medications as anticancer drugs, antithyroid or radioactive drugs, or antibiotics.

FORMULA FEEDING

Commercially prepared formulas are convenient to use, are designed to approach composition of human milk, and contain all known vitamins and minerals in quantities similar to that found in human milk. They are available as liquid ready-to-feed preparations (67 to 70 kcal per dL), as concentrate that requires dilution with equal quantities of boiled water, or as a powder, which requires mixing one scoop to two ounces of water. Each manufacturer makes the formula with small amounts or adequate amounts of iron. Because of the recognized deleterious effects of iron deficiency, the iron-supplemented formulas are recommended. Formulas are based on cow's milk protein, which is more commonly used, or soy protein. The latter is recommended for infants with cow's milk intolerance. Because some infants may be exquisitely sensitive to cow or soy protein, hydrolyzed protein formulas may be required.

Less expensive formulas can be made with 13 ounces of evaporated milk, 17 ounces of water, and 2 ounces of Karo syrup. These formulas are more likely than prepared formulas to cause gastrointestinal problems and in addition require supplementation with vitamins and iron.

VITAMINS AND MINERALS

The breast-fed baby requires no vitamin supplement except vitamin D, 10 μg per day. At about 4 to 6 months, iron supplements are given. The baby who is fed prepared infant formulas with iron requires no iron supplement. All babies are given vitamin K, 1 mg, at birth.

WEANING

Introduction of supplemental foods such as baby cereal or pureed fruits, vegetables, or meats should not be given until 4 to 6 months. Earlier introduction of supplements appears to be associated with a higher prevalence of allergy. At 4 to 6 months, each new food should be introduced at 5- to 7-day intervals to identify whether a food causes intolerance.

Whole cow's milk should not be given in the first year. Cow's milk has a high electrolyte and protein content, a high osmolality, and high calcium and phosphorus levels, which may cause constipation, poor iron absorption, and gastrointestinal bleeding.

DISEASES OF THE BREAST

method of
BLAKE CADY, M.D.
New England Deaconess Hospital
Boston, Massachusetts

The only disease of the female breast of major health consequence is carcinoma. Therefore, the entire role of physicians is to separate a large number of benign and relatively innocuous breast complaints and breast findings on physical examination from cancer. Although this separation is relatively easy in teenagers and patients in their twenties because of the rarity of breast cancer in these age groups and is also relatively easy in 60- and 70-year-old patients because of uncommon benign problems, it is a major problem for physicians with patients in their thirties, forties, and fifties. It can be seen from Table 1 that cancer of the breast is rare to extremely uncommon in women under the age of 35. By the age of 40 one woman in 200 has developed breast cancer. By the age of 50 two women in 100 have developed breast cancer. By the age of 60 4%, and by the age of 70, 6% of American women have developed breast cancer. It is not until over the age of 95 that the currently promulgated risk of one in eight women developing breast cancer actually becomes manifest. Although these figures are disturbing, they fail to explain that they are based on actuarial projections of women born in 1990 and are subject to the continuance of the recent increasing incidence of breast cancer into the future. In actual fact, there will be an estimated 182,000 female breast cancers in 1994 and approximately 46,000 deaths. Thus, about 25% of women who develop breast cancer actually die of the disease. Although breast cancers comprise 32% of all cancers in women, they account for 18% of deaths, well below the 22% of female cancer deaths caused by the rapidly increasing occurrence of lung cancer. These figures are certainly of concern, but they do not justify the near panic about breast cancer among the public and in the press. The increasing use of mammography and the resultant breast biopsies, particularly in younger women, have made many more women aware of breast cancer. The continued press coverage and the adoption of breast cancer as a feminist issue have considerably heightened awareness but also have increased anxiety and fright. Recent data actually indicate that the significant rise in incidence of breast cancer during the past 15 years has now peaked and is decreasing; the reason for this recent decline is multifaceted but may reflect the earlier detection of breast cancers discovered by mammographic screening during the past decades. A large number of cancers are detected by mammography many years before they ordinarily would have become manifest; in addition, many lesions are being discovered and labeled "cancer" that are "nondisease" in terms of their likelihood of progressive growth during a normal lifetime, such as lobular carcinoma in situ and tiny foci of noncomedo-type ductal carcinoma in situ. Actuarial projections of breast cancer risk for American women in the future will undoubtedly be revised downward in the coming years because of this declining incidence. Furthermore, substantial data indicate increasing curability of the breast cancers discovered by mammography because of the marked decline in the median size of the lesions under the impact of screening programs. This may well begin to have an impact on overall breast cancer survival and may help to reduce some of the fright and anxiety. Widespread assumptions by the media that not enough money has been spent on breast cancer research is belied by the fact that no human cancer has such a huge literature, copious research, or numbers of committed vigorous research laboratories as does breast cancer.

TABLE 1. **Chance of Developing Breast Cancer in Women Born in 1990**

Age	Risk	
25	One in 19,608	
30	One in 2,525	
35	One in 622	
40	One in 217	½%
45	One in 93	1%
50	One in 50	2%
55	One in 33	3%
60	One in 24	4%
65	One in 17	5%
70	One in 14	6%
75	One in 11	
80	One in 10	10%
85	One in 9	
Over 95	One in 8	

It is important for physicians dealing with women with breast complaints to realize that part of their professional obligation should be to put the breast cancer hysteria in perspective by encouraging screening and by recognizing that although breast cancer may be common, the actual death rate is low and becoming lower. It should be recognized at the same time that every woman that has breast pain or a perceived "mass" is terrified of breast cancer and needs careful empathetic attention, reassurance, and return visits to the practitioner's office to allay anxiety and minimize any chance that a breast cancer may be missed. Such cautionary notes are particularly true for women in their thirties in whom the uncommon breast cancer is masked by the very common benign breast complaints. The obscure presentation of the few aggressive cancers that present without a definitive mass and in association with pain and during pregnancy and lactation adds to the difficulty.

No discussion of the differential diagnosis of breast abnormalities is complete without understanding the basic biologic aspects of breast cancer. A significant proportion of breast cancer patients, perhaps 25%, present with a form of cancer that is aggressive, highly lethal, and frequently obscure in presentation. These lesions may be "inflammatory" or spread diffusely throughout the breast, or there may be a relatively small primary but multiple node metastases. These varieties not uncommonly defy early clinical recognition and escape mammographic detection. They occur at a younger median age and thus may comprise a significant proportion in young patients in whom diagnostic confusion is common and the emotional reaction to a poor prognosis and fatal outcome is even more disastrous and tragic. Whether this subset of breast cancers will ever be subject to early diagnosis that improves prognosis is problematic because, even if found at an early stage and at a small size, they still may carry their highly lethal implication. Although survival in this group of patients seems to have improved with modern multimodality therapy, these patients still contribute a high proportion of the deaths from breast cancer.

SCREENING

Mammographic screening, which discovers breast cancer at a preclinical or prepalpable stage, has increased dramatically in the past 2 decades. There is clear evidence from randomized prospective trials that mortality rates from patients in mammographic screening programs are as much as 33% lower, presumably owing to earlier discovery of disease. Although this reduction in mortality may be a reflection of "lead time bias," it is hoped that the extreme earliness of detection common today may actually move the diagnosis to the premetastatic state and thus truly increase the cure rate over time. The impact of the mammographic screening program is clearly dramatic, showing statistically significant declines in the mean diameter of breast cancers. Figure 1 and Table 2 display this declining mean maximum diameter of breast cancer at the New England Deaconess Hospital during the past 60 years; note the accelerating trend to small size beginning in 1968 and continuing unabated through 1988. There is no current sign of plateauing of this curve. Thirteen percent of all cancers encountered between 1984 and 1988 were less than 1 cm in diameter (Table 2). The Surveillance Epidemiology and End Results (SEER) study of 10% of American cancers also shows this marked increase in small cancers and a modest decline in larger cancers, the median diameter of all breast cancers being only 2 cm by 1989. It is important to realize that the hypothesis of all randomized trials of mammography is that if patients are *offered* mammographic screening, mortality will decrease. In actual fact, a significant proportion of the experimental groups declined mammography, and a significant proportion of the control groups had mammography anyway; thus, the already significant decrease in mortality may actually under-represent the achievement of mammography in patients who actually follow screening guidelines.

Considerable controversy exists about the best age to begin mammographic screening. Prospective trials have failed to show a significant decrease in death rate in patients under the age of 50, whereas the decline in death rate in women between the ages of 50 and 70 is highly significant. The original guidelines for mammographic screening suggested a single baseline film at age 35, yearly or bi-annual films after the age of 40, and annual mammograms after age 50. Economic projections indicated that the cost of mammography between the ages of 40 and 49 may be too high to justify screening as a public health policy. Nevertheless, in terms of mammographic usage, more than 50% of women between 40 and 49 have regular mammograms, but less than 50% of women in their fifties do, and only a third of women in their sixties undergo routine screening. Thus, the age group that may have the least benefit is the group most concerned about breast cancer in terms of actually following mammographic screening guidelines. With continued promotion and education of both physicians and patients, the great majority of American women between the ages of 50 and 70 will be encouraged to follow

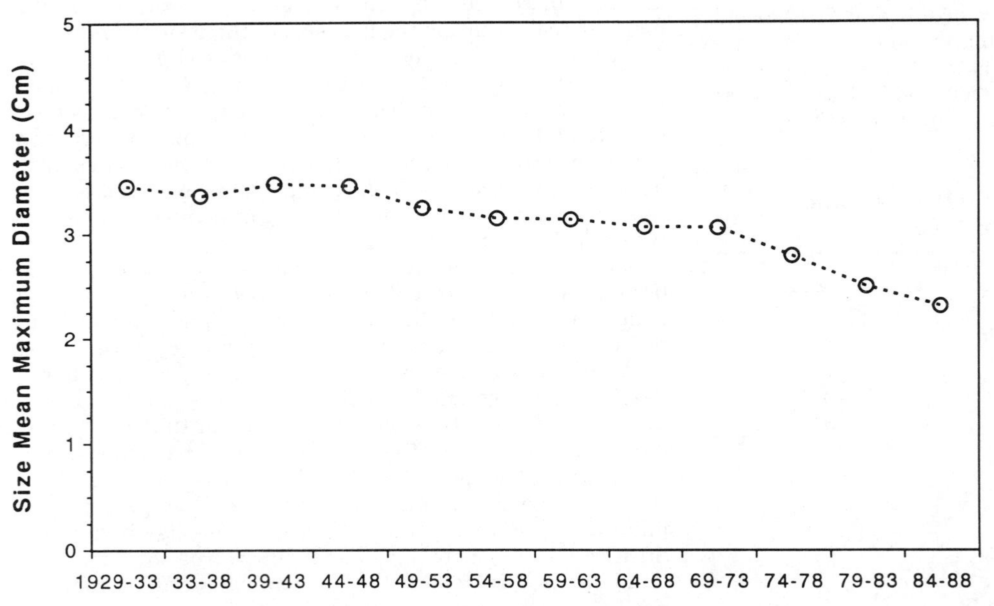

Figure 1. Size of invasive breast cancer.

TABLE 2. **Size of Invasive Breast Cancer, New England Deaconess Hospital**

Years	Cases (No.)	Mean Maximum Diameter (cm)	Medium Median Diameter (cm)	Less Than 1 cm	
				No.	*%*
1929–1938	665	3.40			
1939–1948	890	3.47			
1949–1958	910	3.20			
1959–1968	889	3.11			
	3354				
1969–1973	315	3.06	2.5	8	3
1974–1978	337	2.79	2.4	14	5
1979–1983	382	2.50	2.0	26	8
1984–1988	499	2.31	2.0	58	13
	1533				

Adapted from Cady B, Stone MD, Wayne J, et al: New therapeutic possibilities in primary invasive breast cancer. Ann Surg *218*:338–349, 1993.

regular mammographic screening guidelines. Whether mammography will continue to be encouraged between the ages of 40 and 50 is not yet clear, but with the realization of the biases of the prospective studies, at present the established guidelines should be followed.

One problem with current mammographic screening guidelines is that no upper age limit has been accepted. Women voluntarily stopped participating above the age of 75 in prospective trials, and with the increasing competing risks of death over the age of 75, the value of mammography is considerably less. Whether an upper age limit should be formally adopted is debated, but clearly practitioners should realize the declining value of routine mammographic screening in older women and rationalize its utilization in women over the age of 70 or 75.

Self-examination as a screening technique has not proved to be effective. In addition, most women find it difficult, uncomfortable, and anxiety-provoking to practice regularly. It is the unusual woman who can consciously and without anxiety perform a careful monthly breast self-examination. Emphasis on self-examination as a technique should be curtailed because of poor acceptability and compliance. Focus on mammography screening with its proven benefits should be encouraged.

Other techniques of screening for breast cancer in asymptomatic women have not been effective. Thermography has long been abandoned, and ultrasonography should be used only for specific diagnostic purposes associated with prior mammography. In the future, magnetic resonance imaging may play a role, but its costs are prohibitive as a screening technology.

DIFFERENTIAL DIAGNOSIS OF BREAST SIGNS AND SYMPTOMS

The principal breast signs and symptoms that require a differential diagnosis include pain, actual masses, patient-perceived "masses," breast swelling, nipple discharge, and axillary nodal enlargement. Lesions seen only by screening mammography that are frequently benign require some differential diagnostic course of action and risk assessment also.

Pain

Painful breasts are extremely common in menstruating women but particularly so in women in the late thirties and forties. Pain usually is cyclic in association with menstrual periods but may be more or less continuous for periods of months. Pain is almost always a manifestation of physiologic changes in the breast and not cancer. As a general rule, it is safe to say that painful areas in the breast indicate a benign process; however, in a very small subset of patients, particularly young women, breast cancers may present with pain and discomfort either with or without a mass. Because of the presentation with pain, these patients are dismissed as having functional changes, and the result is a disproportionate number of malpractice suits for failure to make the correct diagnosis, unfortunately. Many women have a prolonged period of discomfort or pain in the breast at some time during their menstrual life that causes concern and anxiety. The patient's immediate interpretation of a painful breast is that cancer must be the cause, following misconceptions that all cancers are associated with pain. Thus, large numbers of women seen in practitioners' offices require careful assessment of pain and reassurance if indeed the problems are functional and not carcinoma. Rarely is a breast operation warranted to diagnose the cause of breast pain, but on occasion a patient's complaints may be so forceful, localized, and persistent that the most appropriate form of reassurance is an open biopsy or needle aspiration cytology of the painful area. In general, complaints of pain in the breast should be placed in perspective and managed with minor medication and reassurance after careful and detailed examination; particular emphasis should be placed on the use of routine mammography and return visits. Hormonal treatments of breast pain are rarely justified. Painful breasts in women in their late thirties or forties may be a manifestation of gross cystic disease. Some of these lesions may be palpable and others can be seen by mammography. Complaints of breast pain justify screening mammography both for reassurance and because patients over 35 are in the screening age group. Despite evidence that the breast cancer death rate is not reduced in patients under the age of 50 with screening mammography, with breast complaints the mammogram is no longer a "screening" technique but is used for diagnosis. Mammography has wide usefulness in reassurance of symptomatic patients.

Patients taking post-menopausal estrogens may have painful breasts much like premenstrual women; this sign should be evaluated and assessed particularly in terms of continuing the post-menopausal estrogens. Even without post-menopausal estrogens, occasional post-menopausal patients have painful breasts, presumably because of low levels of physiologic estrogens; after menopause, mammography should be part of the diagnostic work-up if a recent screening mammogram has not been obtained.

Masses

Masses that are perceived by the patient and those that are felt by the physician may be quite different. Patients who sense a difference in an area of the breast but are not able to explain its detailed anatomy may describe such an area as a "mass," whereas physicians examining that breast area for cancer would not label the perceived change as a mass without noting the usual unilateral palpable mass of greater or lesser distinctiveness and texture difference. Defined palpable masses in a woman's breast detected by a physical examination always need resolution by needle aspiration or excision regardless of the mammographic findings. At least 15% of mammograms are interpreted as normal in the presence of known palpable cancer. Mammography, both in concept and in practice, is of no value in evaluating palpable lesions but is designed for and is best used as a screening tool in the absence of palpable findings. Mammograms obtained to help evaluate a palpable lesion are *not* used to make a differential diagnosis of the palpable lesion but for evaluating the remainder of the ipsilateral and contralateral breast for the presence of nonpalpable abnormalities. A common misconception is that mammography is used to define a palpable mass, but no concept could be more dangerous to the patient or the physician because there is a high rate of false-negative mammograms in the presence of known carcinoma. Thus, every palpable mass must be resolved by tissue sampling either by fine-needle aspiration or by open excisional biopsy. This is as true in a teenager with a fibroadenoma as it is in 65-year-old woman with a clinically apparent cancer. There is no justification for following a palpable fibroadenoma or mass in any patient without pathologic confirmation. Although the physician may be convinced that the palpable discrete nodule is benign, the patient's family may be frightened and anxious, and the patient undoubtedly palpates it anxiously every day. Anxiety and concern are relieved promptly by simple excision of palpable abnormalities under local anesthesia.

The "masses" perceived by patients but not felt as distinctive or discrete masses by physicians frequently cause difficulty. A certain proportion of breast cancers appear with very subtle early findings that are perceived by patients as changes described as masses but are not felt as discrete well-defined lesions by even experienced examining physicians. Thus, women who persist in describing perceived masses not palpable by the physician are candidates for "blind" needle aspiration cytology or open biopsy as the best way of managing risk by the physician and relieving the concern of the patient. Such patients should have frequent re-examinations or referral if they persist in their complaints of abnormality if unconfirmed by the physician.

Nipple Discharge

Nipple discharge is not an uncommon presentation in the late premenopausal age groups, and needs careful characterization in terms of quantity, color, type, spontaneousness, and bilaterality. The most common discharge is a unilateral and serous fluid that stains clothing but is unaccompanied by other symptoms or signs. Discharge is usually the result of ductal abnormalities that are largely benign, such as intraductal papilloma. If the discharge is copious, spontaneous, and persistent it should be resolved by excision of the major lactiferous ducts. Bloody nipple discharge implies a higher risk of duct epithelial abnormalities, usually intraductal papilloma but possibly ductal carcinoma in situ, and should be an indication for biopsy preceded by mammography.

Bilateral discharges of greenish, whitish, or blackish color in small quantities are physiologic and are not important as long as they are not copious enough to cause significant symptoms. Galactorrhea describes a copious bilateral thin breast discharge and may be a manifestation of a pituitary microadenoma. Patients with a small quantity of occasional normal breast discharge of the colors described do not warrant a work-up for pituitary adenoma. Only patients with true galactorrhea justify hormonal diagnostic studies.

There is no role for cytology examination for nipple discharge because these are not reliable and should not be used to resolve therapeutic or diagnostic problems. Radiologic ductograms are unreliable, difficult, and may miss an early manifestation of breast cancer; ductograms should be used only with great caution.

Skin Changes

Complaints of edema, swelling, or erythema carry a high index of suspicion for carcinoma. Except in lactating women, breast infections seldom occur and it is a mistake to assume that any breast swelling, redness, or tenderness is the result of infection warranting antibiotics. All such breast changes should be assumed to be inflammatory carcinoma of the breast until proved otherwise; antibiotics should never be used initially in these situations. Only in lactating women are breast abscesses and breast infections common. Aspiration cytology, dermal punch biopsy, and open biopsy should be the first steps in evaluation rather than treatment with antibiotics.

Pregnancy and Lactation Changes

Breast engorgement in pregnancy and lactation sometimes causes differential diagnostic problems. Any perceived changes such as masses, erythema, or edema need careful assessment; the use of aspiration cytology should be considered to help resolve the underlying anxiety about the presence of carcinoma after mammography has been performed. Breast carcinoma occurs approximately once in every 3000 pregnancies, and thus, although rare, it is hardly unknown and should constantly be considered in examining women who are having breast complaints out of the ordinary during pregnancy or lactation. In recent years the age of initial pregnancy has increased, and many women are having children at an age when breast cancer is more common, i.e., in the late thirties and early forties. The risk of breast cancer is increased with delayed childbirth, and the risk for women who first become pregnant after the age of 40 is considerably higher than the risk in nulliparous women.

Periductal Mastitis

Rarely, patients may have abscesses in the periareolar area that persist and recur despite repeated incision and drainage. Such patients occasionally require central breast excision to prevent repetition of recurrent abscesses.

RISK ASSESSMENT

In addition to the woman's complaints and physical findings, it is necessary to make an estimate of the general risk category for breast cancer. All American women are at risk (see Table 1), but some well-defined groups have a considerably increased risk. This estimate is most important in terms of family history, but age of first full-term pregnancy, country of origin, a previous breast biopsy, the particular histology of previous benign breast biopsies, and a previous breast cancer are all critical aspects of risk assessment. The aphorism, "the most common antecedent of a breast cancer is a previous breast cancer," needs reaffirmation as smaller, earlier carcinomas are treated with breast preservation. In such women a large volume of high-risk breast tissue remains, and the number of such patients with two, three, four or more breast cancers will increase in the future. Any woman who has had a cancer treated by excision and breast preservation is at some risk for recurrence as well as new cancer development, and any significant breast changes or complaints need to be evaluated fully.

A family history of breast cancer is an extremely important aspect of history taking and risk assessment and should be obtained specifically. In particular, the characterization of the age and relationship of the relative and the number of generations of breast cancer occurrence need to be documented. The highest-risk patient has a premenopausal first-degree (mother, sister, or daughter) relative with breast cancer; further incremental increases in risk occur if bilateral disease, successive generations, or multiple affected siblings at each generation have occurred. With a single premenopausal first-degree relative with a single breast cancer, the relative risk ratio of cancer developing compared to the normal population is on the order of 3, whereas with multiple relatives spanning two or three generations of premenopausal women the relative risk ratio may be as high as 8. Because of the frequency of breast carcinoma in post-menopausal women, a single first-degree post-menopausal relative with breast cancer communicates relatively little risk to the patient, probably a risk ratio on the order of 1.3. However, multiple affected family members in successive generations, even though post-menopausal, convey a higher risk ratio but never the level of risk of premenopausal cancers. In the future, genetic screening of women of such high-risk breast cancer families may allow prediction of which family members are at risk of genetically predisposed breast cancers. Even in these families, however, the high incidence of sporadic diet-related post-menopausal breast cancer may affect members over and above their risk of genetic cancer. Thus, there is still a need to screen for sporadic breast cancer with mammography in such high genetic-risk families.

In recent years it has become clear that biopsies of "benign" breast tissues may have ductal epithelial abnormalities that imply significant risk of the later development of carcinoma. Thus, atypical ductal and atypical lobular hyperplasia constitute roughly 4% of benign breast biopsies but confer a risk of future breast cancer development that may reach 0.5% per year in the 10 to 15 years after biopsy (Fig. 2). Breast biopsies that reveal nonproliferative or no atypical hyperplasia in the duct epithelium do not indicate any increased risk of breast cancer, however. Breast biopsies with lobular carcinoma in situ indicate a risk of later invasive breast cancer in either the ipsilateral or contralateral breast of about 1% per year. This cumulative risk of 20% by 20 years may be doubled by a family history of breast cancer.

Although patients with a biopsy diagnosis of atypical ductal or atypical lobular hyperplasia or lobular carcinoma in situ may be at appreciable risk of eventual development of invasive breast cancer, the meaningful risk in these patients is not that of developing breast cancer but the risk of ever dying of the cancer that does appear. In patients who undergo yearly screening by mammography, the risk of death from cancers discovered probably does not exceed 10% and may be more on the order of 5% of the cancers that develop. Long-term survival studies of the Breast Cancer Detection Demonstration Project (BCDDP) show about a 95% survival of patients with mammographically discovered cancers. Thus, the meaningful risk is not the 15%, 20%, or 25% risk of developing cancer but the 1 or 2% risk of dying of the cancer that may arise in a retained breast after the biopsy that revealed the abnormal pathology (Table 3). Such patients should be followed by yearly high-quality mammography and careful physical examination assessment, perhaps by a specialist. Some patients in very-high-risk groups as described may be suitable candidates for "prophylactic" mastectomy if the risk in a breast cancer family is extremely high or the patient is unwilling to suffer the continued fear of cancer development. However, these risks, although high, are spread out over many years and, with continued progress in cancer control, may never become manifest.

Despite delineation of these particular high-risk groups, only 5 to 10% of American women with breast cancer can be so characterized, and thus in some respects all women should be considered at high risk.

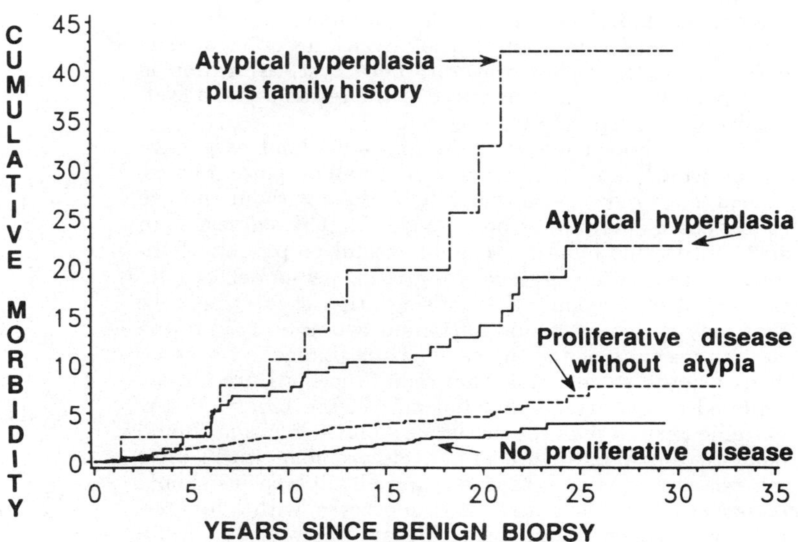

Figure 2. Proportion of patients who have developed invasive breast cancer as a function of time since their benign breast biopsy. (Adapted from Dupont WD, Page DL: Hum Pathol *20*:723–725, 1989.)

TABLE 3. **Risk of Ipsilateral Invasive Breast Cancer and Death as Price of Breast Preservation with Yearly Mammograms and PE After Adequate Local Excision (Author's Estimation)**

	Family History	Yearly Risk	Cumulative 10-year	10-year Risk of Death	Cumulative 20-year	20-year Risk of Death
Normal women, no biopsy						
Age 40	no	.25%	2.5%	.1%	5%	.25%
	yes	.5%	5.0%	.25%	10%	.5%
Age 55	no	.5%	5.0%	.25%	10%	.5%
	yes	1.0%	10.0%	.5%	20%	1.0%
Women with biopsy						
No proliferative disease, all ages	no	.1%	1.0%	.05%	2%	.1%
	yes	.1%	1.0%	.05%	2%	.1%
Proliferative disease without atypia (PDWA)	no	.25%	2.5%	.1%	5%	.25%
	yes	.5%	5.0%	.25%	10%	.5%
ADH or ALH	no	0.5%	5.0%	.25%	10%	.5%
	yes	1.0%	10.0%	.5%	20%	1.0%
LCIS	no	1.0%	10.0%	.5%	20%	1.0%
DCIS	yes	2.0%	20.0%	1.0%	40%	2.0%
Noncomedo	no	1.0%	10.0%	.5%	20%	1.0%
	yes	2.0%	20.0%	1.0%	40%	2.0%
Comedo	no	2.0%	20.0%	1.0%	40%	2.0%
	yes	4.0%	40.0%	2.0%	>50%	>2.5%

Abbreviations: PE = physical examination; PDWA = proliferative disease without atypia; ADH = atypical ductal hyperplasia; ALH = atypical lobular hyperplasia; LCIS = lobular carcinoma in situ; DCIS = ductal carcinoma in situ.

DIAGNOSTIC WORK-UP

There are two tracks of diagnostic studies to be appreciated. One is the diagnostic sequence following discovery of a mammographic abnormality, whereas the other follows the discovery of a palpable breast abnormality. A palpable breast abnormality or mass that warrants biopsy should, with few exceptions, be preceded by mammography. However, women in their teens, twenties, and early thirties who have a palpable abnormality that is to be biopsied do not need preliminary mammography because the great majority of these lesions are benign, and mammography is of relatively little use in the dense young menstruating woman's breast. However, in any woman in her late thirties or older who has a palpable abnormality, mammography should precede biopsy. It must be constantly reiterated that a negative mammogram in the presence of a palpable mass means nothing as far as the mass is concerned and should be ignored because mammography is intended for screening normal breast tissue.

As a standard practice, every palpable mass should undergo needle aspiration in the physician's office at first detection. If the lesion proves to be a cyst, aspiration is therapeutic as well as diagnostic. If the lesion is not a cyst, aspiration cytology can be obtained.

Biopsy of breast masses can, almost without exception, be performed under local anesthesia on an outpatient basis; indeed, such biopsies can usually be done without the use of diazepam (Valium) or heavy sedation. Critical issues in such outpatient biopsies include careful empathetic handling of the patient by operating room personnel, careful placement of incisions with consideration of later surgery that may be required, and particular attention paid to the cosmetic results of the incisions. Thus, Langer's line incisions are the preferred option; radial incisions are largely confined to the extreme medial part of the breast. In the extreme periphery of the breast, the biopsy incision should be more central in the breast to avoid problems with a later mastectomy incision if that is required. All biopsies should be performed as part of a two-step process, with a lumpectomy performed at the initial biopsy, followed by careful analysis of the final pathology and discussions with the patient and family about therapeutic choices. Breast biopsy resulting from mammographic findings adheres to similar principles. In the absence of a palpable lesion, the biopsy must be preceded by a localization mammogram.

The biopsy specimen, whether previously palpable or not, must be excised as a coherent intact piece. It should be sent for radiologic examination to ensure that the calcification or mass precipitating the biopsy is included in the excised tissue if it was detected mammographically.

The principles of breast biopsy include performance of a lumpectomy on all palpable masses except those that are obviously fibroadenomas with a 1-cm margin around the mass. Careful inking and orientation of the excised specimen is required for contemporary management of breast cancer. The most satisfactory inking technique currently available is the five-colored Davidson Marking System,* which defines the margin and reliably orients the specimen.

Accurate analysis of breast pathology can be extremely difficult and taxing even for experienced pathologists. Concordance among pathologists is difficult to achieve in diagnoses of atypical ductal or lobular hyperplasia, lobular carcinoma in situ, or ductal carcinoma in situ because these lesions occupy borderline gray areas in a diagnostic spectrum and are heavily dependent on experience. Thus, it is frequently useful in such borderline cases to have pathologic consultation. Critical decisions about risk assessment and therapy exist with atypical hyperplasia and in situ carcinoma; controversy regarding microinvasion or minimal invasion may be encountered as well as a diagnosis of lymph vessel or blood vessel invasion. Therapeutic plans may depend on sophisticated pathologic description of the amount of surrounding ductal carcinoma in situ with invasive breast cancers and the level of abnormal ductal epithelium in benign breast biopsies. Classification of the form of ductal carcinoma in situ is also critical. Comedo ductal carcinoma in situ carries vastly different implications for the

*R. Davidson Marking System, Bradley Products, Bloomington, MN.

likelihood of recurrence, the possibility of microinvasion, and the progressive nature of the disease than noncomedo, cribriform, or micropapillary varieties of ductal carcinoma in situ (DCIS).

Invasive carcinoma of the breast also needs sophisticated interpretation because there are some varieties of low-grade histology that may be safely handled by more conservative treatment than the usual breast cancer. Tubular carcinoma, which makes up roughly 10% of all mammographically discovered invasive carcinomas, papillary carcinoma, and medullary carcinoma with lymphoid stroma are all low-grade varieties that have an extremely favorable outcome. Invasive ductal carcinoma of the breast also requires description of nuclear grade, lymph vessel invasion, perineural invasion, differentiation, and careful assessment of size. Perineural invasion, lymphatic invasion, extremely poor differentiation, poor nuclear grade, diffuse involvement of the breast, subdermal lymphatic invasion, and large size are all indicators of poor prognosis. In addition, selective prognostic indicators from the primary tissue such as S phase by flow cytometry, estrogen and progesterone receptor studies, and a host of other biochemical determinations may offer significant prognostic information, but at present exact relationships are not carefully documented, and these tests are not reproducible or reliable enough to justify their routine use. Commercial laboratories marketing panels of such prognostically related tests should be viewed with great skepticism and caution because the reliability, quality control, and implications for decision making for therapy are not well established.

Sophisticated analysis of axillary nodal pathology also is required, and the mere designation of positive nodes is not sufficient. The extent of nodal involvement, definition of microscopic (≤2 mm) or macroscopic size (Table 4), the exact number of lymph nodes involved, and evidence of extranodal disease are all important factors. Patients with a small cancer and only one or two nodes with micrometastases have an excellent prognosis. However, even small cancers with features such as perineural or lymph vessel involvement with poor nuclear grade, even with negative lymph nodes, may have a poor prognosis.

STAGING WORK-UP

Once a cancer has been diagnosed, it may be important to perform staging studies. Chest radiographs, bone scans, or liver function tests are not required for noninvasive carcinomas or for mammographically discovered or palpable small invasive cancers (T1a or T1b) (Table 4). They are also probably not useful for T1c carcinomas with negative nodes. False-positive bone scans occur in 3% of cases, whereas true positive bone scans in early cancers occur in less than 1%. However, for patients with a T2 primary cancer, axillary metastases, or evidence of an extremely poor prognosis based on primary features, staging studies should be performed to confirm that the disease is still localized. Liver scans should *not* be performed except in the presence of abnormal liver biochemical tests.

TABLE 4. **Stage of Breast Cancer**

TNM		
T_1	Tumor	2 cm or less
	T_{1a}	0.5 cm or less
	T_{1b}	>0.5 cm up to 1 cm
	T_{1c}	>1.0 cm up to 2 cm
T_2	Tumor	>2 cm up to 5 cm
T_3	Tumor	>5 cm
N_1	Metastases to movable ipsilateral axillary lymph nodes	
	N_{1a}	Only micrometastases (0.2 cm or less)
	N_{1b}	Metastases larger than 0.2 cm
	Na_{1b1}	1 to 3 less than 2 cm
	N_{1b1}	4 or more less than 2 cm
	N_{1b3}	Extranodal extension < 2 cm
	N_{1b4}	Extranodal extension > 2 cm
Stage I		$T_1N_0M_0$
Stage IIa		$T_0N_1M_0$
		$T_1N_1M_0$
		$T_2N_0M_0$
Stage IIb		$T_2N_1M_0$
		$T_3N_0M_0$

Note: The prognosis of patients with N_{1a} is similar to that of N_0.

TREATMENT

The contemporary treatment of primary breast cancer and benign but high-risk pathology is extraordinary complex and confusing, and there are a variety of options available in the fields of surgery, radiotherapy, and chemotherapy. The combinations and permutations of the various components of multimodality therapy are such that 20 or more separate treatment options, all of them reasonable for individual patient presentations, are available. The complexities of analyzing these options for physicians and explaining them to patients tax everyone's ingenuity and patience. However, patient input in decision making is critical. Even when a clear therapeutic plan is apparent from the cancer presentation, considerable effort must still be expended in patient discussion and presentation of options. All this careful therapeutic decision process requires comprehensive information from the pathologic analysis of the biopsy and the diagnostic and staging work-up as well as careful assessment of patient characteristics for explanation of treatment selection to the patient and family. There is no more confusing area of contemporary oncology than the comprehensive and sophisticated treatment of primary breast cancer and its explanation to patients. This next section attempts to summarize the major aspects of therapeutic selection in these patients.

High-Risk Benign Pathology (Atypical Ductal Hyperplasia and Atypical Lobular Hyperplasia)

Patients with atypical hyperplasia on biopsy have a risk of later invasive breast cancer that may total 5% or 10% at the rate of approximately 0.5% per year (see Fig. 2). If in addition a family history of breast cancer is present, the risk is probably doubled. Although most such patients should continue careful screening because the risk of death is extremely low, bilateral mastectomy for prevention may at least be considered in highly selected patients. Use of tamoxifen for prevention of breast cancer has not been proved and should not be used on an ad hoc basis outside the context of a clinical trial. Obviously, such patients are at increased risk during subsequent years for the development of breast cancer, and they need careful monitoring with yearly mammograms and physical examination and reporting of changes in the breast for sophisticated follow-up.

Lobular Carcinoma In-Situ

Lobular carcinoma in situ (LCIS) has clearly been established as a risk indicator and is not a true in situ cancer. Thus, later invasive cancers that develop after a diagnosis of LCIS are as liable to occur in the opposite breast as the same breast. This risk amounts to roughly 1% per year for at least 15 to 20 years following diagnosis. If there is a family history, that risk is apparently doubled. These patients also require close follow-up; if a family history is present, bilateral prophylactic mastectomy for prevention of invasive breast cancer may be perceived by the patient or the physician as a logical procedure. Without a family history, patients should be followed carefully. There is no role for unilateral mastectomy. Although the risk of developing cancer may be significant over a prolonged time (±20%), the risk of ever dying of the cancer that develops as the price of retaining the breast is very small (1 to 2%; see Table 3); decisions about breast conservation in such situations depend on the patient's risk acceptance, fear of cancer, and desires about breast preservation.

Most women with LCIS without a family history elect to be observed carefully, particularly when careful definition of risks and future problems are explained. The 20% risk of developing breast cancer is spread over a 20-year period at an apparently constant low yearly rate. This provides the patients with a good deal of security, especially when they understand that continual developments in cancer management may occur during the years ahead.

Ductal Carcinoma In Situ

Ductal carcinoma in situ (DCIS) is separated into comedo and noncomedo forms. The comedo variety has multiple markers of progressive growth in terms of nuclear grade, neu-oncogene overexpression, size, incidence of microinvasion, and growth patterns that indicate that it is a true in situ cancer with later recurrences appearing in the same area of the same breast. In contrast, noncomedo varieties are found frequently as incidental findings in autopsy studies and in breasts removed for other reasons; if of small size, they have a minimal risk of recurrence and later development of invasive disease, particularly when found by mammographic screening. DCIS is found with markedly increased frequency in mammographic screening programs. Before mammography, DCIS constituted roughly 1% of cases but now comprises 10 to 15% of all cancers and 25 to 50% of all mammographically discovered cancers.

Noncomedo Ductal Carcinoma In Situ

A significant proportion of small, mammographically discovered, ductal carcinoma in situ in the current screening programs are of the noncomedo variety. Local excision only with careful follow-up has a 5 to 10% recurrence rate over 10 years, with half the recurrences appearing as small invasive cancers and the other half as noninvasive cancers. With proper follow-up these recurrences are usually detected at an early enough stage as to be almost totally curable. A recent report of the National Surgical Adjuvant Breast Program (NSABP) that suggests that all patients with DCIS should receive radiation therapy after local excision is a flawed study; most of these patients can be handled by local excision only as long as the extent of the lesion is less than 2 or $2\frac{1}{2}$ cm in diameter, the guidelines of Schnitt (Table 5) are followed, and the patients are carefully informed. The median diameter of mammographically discovered noncomedo DCIS tends to be very small (5 to 6 mm). Such small lesions are relatively innocuous and can be handled readily by local excision only, with appropriate precautions and patient education. Obviously, selection of mastectomy for treatment of ductal carcinoma in situ is one standard therapeutic option and may be selected in certain situations by patient choice or consideration of other high-risk factors such as a strong family history. However, it seems illogical to propose wide use of mastectomy for noninvasive breast cancer when breast conservation is widely applied for fully invasive breast cancer.

Comedo Ductal Carcinoma In Situ

Most mammographically discovered DCIS is of the comedo variety because of its association with mammographic microcalcifications owing to the intraluminal ductal necrosis. The comedo variety of ductal carcinoma in situ is associated with a high incidence of local recurrence even when the lesions are small in size and detected by mammographic screening if

TABLE 5. **Guidelines for the Evaluation of Patients with Mammographically Detected Ductal Carcinoma in Situ with Microcalcifications Being Considered for Breast-Conserving Treatment**

1. Careful mammographic evaluation of the breast before biopsy, including magnification views, to determine the extent of the microcalcifications
2. Needle localization for the biopsy
3. Specimen radiography, preferably with magnification views as well as contact views, to confirm that the lesion has been excised and to direct pathologic sampling
4. Careful gross description of the excised specimen by the pathologist.
5. Inking of the specimen margins by the surgeon or pathologist before sectioning, to facilitate evaluation of margins on permanent sections
6. On microscopic examination, description of the relation between the calcifications and the lesion and the distance from the tumor to the inked margins of resection
7. Post-biopsy mammography with magnification views to confirm that all suspicious microcalcifications have been removed. (NB: Since the pathologic extent of the lesion is commonly greater than its mammographic extent, the absence of microcalcifications on a post-biopsy mammogram does not ensure the absence of residual DCIS in the breast.)
8. Repeat excision of the primary site if residual microcalcifications are seen on post-biopsy mammography, or if tumor extends close to the margins of resection microscopically, or if margins were not assessed on the original resection

Adapted from Schnitt SJ, et al. Current concepts: Ductal carcinoma in situ (intraductal carcinoma) of the breast. N Engl J Med *31*:898–903, 1988.

treated merely by local excision and breast preservation. This local recurrence rate, even in lesions less than $2\frac{1}{2}$ cm in diameter, may be 30%, and thus careful discussion of management options with the patient before selecting therapy is essential. Again, the risk of death may be only a small fraction of the recurrence rate with careful screening (see Table 3). Treatment options are local excision only, local excision plus radiation, which seems to reduce the local recurrence rate by one-half, or mastectomy; treatment is selected depending on lesion size, family history, patient preference, adequacy of excision, appearance of the mammogram, and a variety of other factors. For comedo DCIS greater than $2\frac{1}{2}$ but less than 5 cm in diameter, total excision with negative margins may be appropriate, particularly if accompanied by radiation therapy. For comedo DCIS greater than 5 cm in diameter, mastectomy is the preferred option because the incidence of microinvasion and multifocal disease is greater than 50% and recurrence is almost certain. The presence of scattered microcalcifications on mammography in patients with DCIS suggests that the disease is more widespread than measured and may warrant biopsy, more extensive removal of breast tissue, or mastectomy. No patient with ductal carcinoma in situ, whether treated with local excision or mastectomy, needs axillary nodal dissection because the incidence of axillary metastases is at most 2%.

Nonpalpable, Small, Mammographically Discovered Invasive Cancer

T1a invasive breast cancers are 5 mm or less in diameter. T1b cancers are greater than 5 mm but 1 cm or less in diameter. T1c lesions are greater than 1 cm but 2 cm or less in diameter (see Table 4). A high proportion of current mammographically discovered invasive breast cancers are T1a or T1b. Such patients with small nonpalpable mammographically discovered invasive breast cancers have an extremely low risk of axillary lymph node involvement ($\pm 5\%$). Such breast cancers are highly suitable for local excision and breast preservation. Whether to perform axillary node dissection also in such cases is under investigation at present. Local recurrence rates in these small cancers may be so low that radiation therapy may produce only small therapeutic gains. Standard therapeutic options now include mastectomy or lumpectomy, axillary lymph node dissection, and adjuvant radiation therapy. Even these small invasive breast cancers may have pathologic features suggesting poor prognosis, such as lymph vessel invasion or poor nuclear grade, that indicate that despite the small size the cancer may have a poor biologic behavior pattern. Such patients may be appropriate candidates for adjuvant therapy. In general, such patients have an excellent prognosis, with a long-term survival approaching 95%.

Small Palpable Invasive Breast Cancer

Palpable breast cancers are generally 1 cm or greater in diameter. Palpable T1c invasive breast cancers have a positive lymph node incidence of 20% or more. If axillary nodes are negative, such patients may have an exceptionally good prognosis, but if there are axillary node metastases larger than micrometastases (see Table 4), patients are candidates for systemic adjuvant therapy. Therefore, for patients with palpable T1 tumors, axillary dissection may provide prognostic information that determines selection for adjuvant therapy. These patients should also have analysis of the primary cancer for prognostic features. Adjuvant breast radiation therapy should be used because the high risk of local in-breast recurrence can be markedly reduced by such treatment.

T2 Invasive Breast Cancer

T2 cancers are greater than 2 cm but 5 cm or less in diameter. Such cancers comprise less than 50% of invasive breast cancers today, have a high risk of systemic metastases, a high risk of axillary lymph node metastases, and a modest prognosis. Therefore, these patients are almost all candidates for systemic adjuvant therapy.

Local treatment options for such patients include breast conservation and radiation therapy or mastectomy. Various factors enter into the decision about breast conservation such as the relationship between the size of the cancer and the size of the breast, the extent of the surrounding intraductal disease (extensive intraductal component or EIC), the location of the cancer within the breast, and individual prognostic factors within the primary cancer. However, most of these patients are candidates for breast conservation, and the choice between breast preservation or mastectomy depends heavily on the patient's desire to keep the breast as well as on technical factors such as the ability to achieve negative margins if extensive ductal carcinoma in situ surrounds the invasive cancer (EIC+) and whether the breast will have a suitable cosmetic appearance following adequate local excision.

Histologically negative surgical margins following adequate gross tumor excision are not critical if the patient does not have extensive intraductal carcinoma surrounding the invasive disease (EIC−) but are highly important if such ductal carcinoma in situ is present (EIC+) because recurrence rates may approach 40 or 50% if negative margins cannot be achieved in the latter patients despite the use of adjuvant radiotherapy.

Advanced Primary Breast Cancer

Advanced primary presentations still occur in about 5% of breast cancer patients. These include inflammatory breast cancer, T3 primary breast cancer (lesions greater than 5 cm in diameter), and those with extensive nodal metastases. Such patients have an extremely high risk of distant metastases. Although some of these patients may have an initial mastectomy followed by adjuvant therapy, it is more common today to begin treatent with adjuvant systemic multidrug chemotherapy for several cycles and then use either mastectomy or radiation therapy or radiation therapy followed by planned mastectomy. Although such patients in the past have been considered categorically incurable, the long-term survival rate in such patients with contemporary multimodality and multidrug chemotherapy seems to be significantly improved, with perhaps 40% achieving a disease-free 5-year survival. What the survival of such patients at 10 and 15 years will be is not clearly defined at the present time. These patients all require careful individual therapeutic decisions. Clearly, patient input is essential in these situations, but multimodality usage and the resort to mastectomy are more commonly accepted. These cancers are not usually suitable for local excision of the primary tumor, even with radiation therapy, but individualization of therapy is critical and allows some options.

In all invasive breast cancers the details of local tumor management do not govern survival. Thus, in all prospective trials comparing local excision with or without radiation therapy versus mastectomy, survival rates at 5, 10, and 15 years are exactly equivalent. These results demonstrate the basic principle in breast cancer management that the details of local tumor treatment do not govern survival but of course do have an impact on the ability to preserve the breast. Local recurrence is associated with distant metastatic disease but does not cause it. Local recurrence does not reduce the potential for survival but is associated with a more aggressive disease, with metastases occurring either at the time of the local recurrence or thereafter. Local recurrences in a preserved breast generally require mastectomy for treatment, but approximately 25 to 33% may be adequately treated by another local excision.

Virtually every patient except the aged woman is a candidate for breast reconstruction if mastectomy is performed. Reconstruction can be performed simultaneously with mastectomy or after a delay. Immediate reconstruction is to be preferred because it is perfectly safe and eliminates the need for later surgery. Whether to use silicone breast implants or tissue transfer techniques is a decision to be made by the patient in consultation with a plastic surgeon. There is no scientific evidence whatsoever that silicone implants have any health risk despite the media hysteria created in 1992.

Radiation Therapy

Radiation therapy is an adjunct to the local excision of primary breast cancer with breast preservation and is a critical part of modern breast cancer management. However, there are different styles of breast radiation therapy, including that advocated by the NSABP, which consists of 5000 cGy to the whole breast without a local boost dose, and that promulgated at the Joint Center for Radiation Therapy at Harvard Medical School, which limits whole breast radiation therapy to 4500 cGy and adds a boost of roughly 1500 cGy to bring the radiation dose to the local excision site to 6000 cGy. It is unclear at present which technique is to be preferred, but local failure rates overall range from 3 to 10%.

Post-mastectomy radiation therapy to the chest wall is seldom necessary. However, if direct involvement of the pectoral muscles or chest wall occurs or if there are features of the cancer indicating an extremely high risk of chest wall recurrence, post-mastectomy radiation therapy may be justified. There are no data suggesting that routine chest wall radiation therapy following mastectomy is associated with improved survival, however.

Radiation therapy of regional lymph nodes in the apex of the axilla, supraclavicular space, or internal mammary lymph node chain should no longer be performed routinely. Numerous studies have indicated that regional lymph node radiation therapy, although it reduces recurrence in those lymph nodes, does not alter survival in any way. When the majority of patients enter treatment facilities with a relatively low risk of internal mammary, supraclavicular, or axillary apex nodal metastases, it seems unjustified to radiate routinely these areas during radiation of the breast. Almost without exception if these lymph nodes are the site of recurrent disease, they can be treated at that time by systemic therapy or by localized radiation therapy.

Systemic Adjuvant Therapy

Systemic adjuvant therapy consists of either chemotherapy or hormonal therapy. Multidrug chemotherapy reduces recurrence rates in premenopausal women, and hormonal therapy reduces recurrences in post-menopausal women. Table 6 illustrates the proportional and absolute reductions in recurrence achieved by the use of adjuvant systemic therapy as determined by a large meta-analysis of the many prospective trials conducted throughout the world. For cancers with a very good prognosis marked by small size and negative nodes, the proportional gain is the same, but the absolute gain may be quite small. As an example, if a patient has a 10% risk of systemic

TABLE 6. **Analysis of Adjuvant Systemic Therapy**

Adjuvant Therapy	Proportional Reduction in Annual Odds of Death (%)	Absolute Reduction in 10-Year Mortality per 100 Women Treated
Age <50		
Chemotherapy*	25 ± 5	10 ± 3
Ovarian ablation	28 ± 9	11 ± 4
Age ≥50		
Tamoxifen†	20 ± 2	8 ± 1
Chemotherapy*	12 ± 4	5 ± 2

*Results include trials comparing chemotherapy alone vs. no treatment and chemotherapy plus tamoxifen vs. the same tamoxifen alone.

†Results include trials comparing tamoxifen alone vs. no treatment and tamoxifen plus chemotherapy vs. the same chemotherapy alone.

Modified from Early Breast Cancer Trialists' Collaborative Group: Lancet *1*:1–15, 71–85, 1992. © by The Lancet Ltd, 1992.

metastases and a proportional reduction of 25% by systemic therapy, the patient would then have a 92.5% rather than a 90% survival rate. However, this also indicates that 97.5% of patients would not benefit. Thus, the absolute gains that can be achieved from proportional reduction in recurrence depends entirely on the degree of risk of failure.

In general, premenopausal patients who might benefit from adjuvant systemic therapy should receive the usual multidrug chemotherapy with cyclophosphamide (Cytoxan), methotrexate (Folex), and fluorouracil (Adrucil), whereas post-menopausal patients should receive hormonal therapy with tamoxifen. Whether the use of tamoxifen therapy in premenopausal patients after systemic chemotherapy or systemic chemotherapy in addition to tamoxifen in post-menopausal patients will significantly improve outcome is a question that has yet to be answered.

An attempt to improve the effectiveness of adjuvant systemic chemotherapy by increasing the dose intensity of chemotherapy is also under active study. Bone marrow autotransplantation with superlethal doses of chemotherapy is currently undergoing an experimental trial in highly selected patients. Such programs are extraordinarily expensive, highly toxic, and of no proven benefit at the present time. They should be avoided except in the context of a clinical trial. Other programs of dose intensification are under study. In general, the use of adjuvant chemotherapy has moved toward shorter, more intense periods of chemotherapy. It is to be expected that the routine duration of adjuvant chemotherapy in the future will be less than 6 months. In contrast, programs of adjuvant anti-estrogens (tamoxifen) have proved more effective with a longer duration because the basic mechanism of action of these drugs is of cancer micrometastasis suppression rather than the cancericidal action characteristic of chemotherapy.

CONCLUSION

Modern breast cancer management is complex and varied. Large numbers of therapeutic options exist for almost all patients. Careful balancing of the risks and benefits of the various therapeutic alternatives needs to be recognized. Clearly, the most important decision the patient must make is whether to attempt breast conservation or not. This decision depends heavily on personal attitudes but also on the perceptions of the community, the biases of the physicians and surgeons in the local area, the accessibility of radiation therapy resources, and a host of pathologic and technical features. However, patients should not consider mastectomy a less satisfactory treatment option, because it remains the gold standard of therapy. Although no better than local excision and radiation therapy in terms of survival and cure, mastectomy is fully equivalent, less complicated, and less expensive and it is well tolerated by the great majority of patients. Indeed, controlled trials of psychological, emotional, and psychosexual function of patients randomly assigned to mastectomy or breast conservation fail to reveal any significant differences in basic psychosocial functioning or psychiatric measurements. Only in the realm of improved body image and sexual functioning is there some advantage for breast conservation versus mastectomy. With this balance, patient preference obviously is paramount in selecting surgical therapy. Selection of other aspects of therapy depends heavily on the perceived risk of recurrence as well as the potential proportional and absolute reductions in recurrence.

ENDOMETRIOSIS

method of
DEBORAH A. METZGER, PH.D., M.D.
University of Connecticut Health Center
Farmington, Connecticut

Endometriosis is a progressive, often debilitating disease that affects 10 to 15% of women during their reproductive years. Although not usually life-threatening, endometriosis may significantly impair health and fertility potential. Timely diagnosis and selection of optimal therapy is therefore of the utmost clinical significance because new and improved methods of treatment continue to be sought in the hope of finding a cure for this pervasive disease.

ETIOLOGY AND PATHOGENESIS

Although reference to endometriosis was made in the medical literature throughout the nineteenth century, it was not until 1925 that Sampson introduced the first accurate description of a disease that he defined as "the presence of ectopic tissue which possesses the histological structure and function of the uterine mucosa."

Many theories have been proposed to explain the development of endometriosis, but the most popular and widely accepted theory is that of Sampson, who proposed that during menstruation viable endometrial cells reflux through the fallopian tubes and become implanted on the surrounding pelvic structures. By a similar mechanism, viable endometrial cells may be implanted in open wounds or be transported to distant sites within vascular or lymphatic channels. Other theories include (1) coelomic metaplasia, whereby the mesothelium covering the abdominal and pelvic organs undergoes metaplastic transformation in response to inflammation or hormonal stimuli and (2) activation of embryonic rests of müllerian tissue.

Although these theories may explain how viable endometrial cells reach ectopic sites, none offers insight into why some women are predisposed to the disease whereas others are protected. Practically all menstruating women have menstrual reflux and the appropriate hormonal milieu, yet the disease develops in only a few. Clinical and epidemiologic studies have suggested a familial predisposition. Another association has been postulated between the amount of retrograde menstruation and the functional status of the immune system. Several studies have demonstrated that women with a greater amount of retrograde menstruation such as those with short cycle lengths, menorrhagia, or outflow obstruction, have a much higher chance of developing endometriosis. In addition, there may be subtle alterations in the immune system that modify a woman's risk of developing endometriosis. Thus, a woman with a poor immune system may develop endometriosis even though the amount of retrograde menstruation is small. Likewise, a woman with a well-functioning immune system may not develop endometriosis even though she has a large volume of retrograde menstruation.

Regardless of the origins of ectopic endometrium, it is apparent that hormonal factors are of central importance in the pathogenesis of endometriosis. Like endometrium found in the uterine cavity, endometriosis implants respond to the fluctuating blood levels of ovarian hormones during the menstrual cycle. At the end of each menstrual cycle, endometriosis implants break down and bleed, causing pain or elicting an inflammatory reaction with subsequent scarring, fibrosis, and adhesions of the affected tissues.

SYMPTOMS AND SIGNS

Endometriosis should be suspected in any patient with the triad of dysmenorrhea, dyspareunia, and infertility. However, it should be kept in mind that the symptoms of endometriosis may be quite variable and are for the most part determined by the areas of involvement. Although it occurs most frequently in the pelvis, endometriosis has been found in most areas of the body. After the pelvic organs, the next most commonly affected locations include the appendix, terminal ileum, cervix, perineum, abdominal scars, umbilicus, inguinal region, and ureter. Only rarely is endometriosis encountered on the diaphragm, extremities, pleura, lungs, gallbaldder, spleen, stomach, or kidney.

Symptoms of pain tend to be most severe at the time of menstruation, although some women experience the most intense pain around the time of ovulation. Severity of symptoms does not always correlate with the extent of the disease, and not infrequently, patients with extensive disease exhibit minimal symptoms, whereas some with minimal disease may have marked symptoms. Patients with infertility may not exhibit any pain or significant dysmenorrhea.

The most common physical findings of pelvic endometriosis are generalized pelvic tenderness, nodular induration of the uterosacral ligaments, ovarian enlargement and a fixed, retroverted uterus. Just as the symptoms of endometriosis can be quite variable depending on the tissues and organs involved, the pelvic findings may also be confused with other gynecologic disorders such as pelvic inflammatory disease, pelvic masses, and ectopic pregnancy.

DIAGNOSIS

Because endometriosis is a progressive and potentially crippling disease, it is of the utmost importance that a definitive diagnosis be established as early as possible so that therapy aimed at arresting the disease and preventing its complications can be instituted.

A definitive diagnosis of endometriosis can be made only by direct visualization of the pelvis. Laparoscopy is the procedure of choice because it provides a panoramic view of the entire abdomen. Thorough intraoperative examination of the pelvis is essential with particular attention directed to the ovaries, the anterior cul-de-sac, the broad ligament under the ovaries, uterosacral ligaments, and the posterior cul-de-sac. Typical endometriosis implants appear as stellate-scarred lesions surrounded by reddish-blue, "powder burn" implants on the peritoneal surfaces of the pelvis. Atypical endometriosis is considerably more difficult to recognize and may appear as clear vesicles, pinkish implants, red petichiae, nodules, or white-erythematous plaques. Because some implants may not be readily visible because they are nonpigmented, their presence may be detected only as irregularities of light reflection from the peritoneal surface. The rate of diagnosis of endometriosis increases when these atypical implants are biopsied.

TREATMENT

The goals of treatment of endometriosis are to decrease pain, limit the recurrence of disease, and maintain or enhance fertility. In planning therapy, many variables must be considered, such as age of the patient, extent of disease, degree of symptoms, and desire for immediate or deferred fertility. Hormonal therapy, surgery, and expectant management have been used alone or in combination to treat endometriosis. The indications for treatment consist of pain (50% of patients with endometriosis), infertility (25%), or both (25%). Although the rationale in treating endometriosis has been no different whether the major indication was pain or infertility, it is becoming increasingly apparent that the approach to managing a patient with pelvic pain differs from that of the patient with infertility, and these situations will be considered separately in this discussion.

Treatment Modalities

Surgical Management. Not surprisingly, many gynecologists have approached endometriosis as a surgical disease under the assumption that if all disease can be excised and proper anatomic relationships restored, the patient could be cured. Traditionally conservative resection of endometriosis was performed by laparotomy, but laparoscopic surgery is being used increasingly for all stages of disease. In addition to establishing a diagnosis of endometriosis, laparoscopy permits various therapeutic surgical procedures including ablation or excision of implants, salpingolysis, ovariolysis, transection of the uterosacral ligaments, presacral neurectomy, and extirpation of the adnexae. Laparoscopic surgery is being used increasingly to treat more advanced stages of endometriosis that require ablation or excision of large endometriomas, management of deep-seated cul-de-sac implants, and extensive adhesiolysis.

Successful conservative surgery for endometriosis is dependent on several factors: (1) proper identification of both typical and atypical endometriosis implants; (2) complete ablation or excision of all implants; (3) treatment of cul-de-sac disease; (4) excision of ovarian endometrioma capsules to decrease risk of recurrence; (5) prevention of adhesion formation; and (6) adjunctive pain-relieving measures such as uterosacral nerve transection, presacral neurectomy, or uterine suspension in selected patients.

Medical Management. The whole spectrum of sex steroids, including estrogens, progestins, and androgens, singly or in combination, has been used to treat endometriosis. Early therapy, which utilized high doses of sex steroids, has been replaced with medications specifically developed for the treatment of endometriosis that are associated with significantly fewer side effects.

The three commonly used classes of hormonal suppressive agents for endometriosis are progestins, danazol, and gonadotropin-releasing hormone (GnRH) agonists. Only the latter two are approved by the U.S. Food and Drug Administration for the treatment of endometriosis. Danazol (Danocrine), a synthetic isoxazol derivative of ethisterone, was the first medication specifically marketed for endometriosis. It is unclear how danazol acts, but four possibilities exist: (1) it inhibits GnRH release, (2) it inhibits follicle-stimulating hormone (FSH) and LH synthesis or release, (3) it inhibits steroidogenic enzymes, or (4) it interacts with steroid hormone receptors in target tissues. Doses of 400 to 800 mg per day are administered for 6 to 9 months. The adverse effects of danazol reflect its mild androgenic and anti-estrogenic properties, almosts all of which are readily reversible once the medication is stopped. Perhaps the major drawback to danazol is its cost, which amounts to $1.25 for a 200-mg tablet.

Oral medroxyprogesterone acetate (MPA) (Provera), at a dose of 30 to 50 mg per day, has also been successful in the management of minimal to moderate endometriosis. MPA acts by suppressing LH release and estradiol production. Side effects consist of breast tenderness, bloating, weight gain, and depression, all of which are generally mild and well tolerated. It is by far the least expensive of the endometriosis medications.

Observations that oophorectomy is the most effective treatment for endometriosis led to the development of GnRH agonists, which produce a readily reversible "medical oophorectomy" by suppressing LH and FSH release. This results in decreased ovarian activity and hypoestrogenemia similar to that observed in menopausal or castrated women. Currently, GnRH agonists are available as monthly injections or nasal spray preparations that must be self-administered several times daily. The adverse effects of GnRH analogues are similar to postmenopausal symptoms—hot flashes and bone loss. This bone loss is completely regained within a year of discontinuation of treatment. A 6-month course of treatment costs approximately $2000.

Results of multiple studies indicate that relief of pain occurs in the majority of patients during suppressive therapy; the chance of recurrence of pain increases with the severity of disease and time elapsed after cessation of treatment. It is not clear which of the currently available hormonal therapies is the most effective. Therefore, until more data become available, cost and patient tolerance of side effects may be the most important determinants in the selection of a specific agent.

Pain

The management of the patient with pain associated with endometriosis continues to be a challenge despite the availability of a variety of both medical and surgical treatments for this condition. Part of the difficulty in managing these patients lies in our limited understanding of the pathophysiology of pain associated with this disease, the subjective nature of pain, and the many anatomic factors that may contribute to pain.

The basic principles of pain management with endometriosis require an integrated therapeutic approach. Often there is a sense of failure and disappointment on the part of both physician and patient when symptoms recur, and for this reason it is important to acknowledge that endometriosis is a chronic condition requiring long-term solutions and a multidisciplinary approach. Patients who have experienced pain for 6 months or longer may develop chronic pain syndrome characterized by (1) incomplete relief by most previous treatments, (2) significantly impaired physical function at home or work, (3) signs of depression, (4) pain out of proportion to pathology, and (5) altered family roles. These patients often benefit from intensive psychological support during treatment.

When taking a pain history, it is important to inquire about (1) the pain characteristics: site, duration, change with activity, relation to position, association with bowel or bladder function, (2) chronology of the pain, (3) patient perception of cause of the pain, and (4) degree of interference with activities.

Localization of tenderness on physical examination generally corresponds to the location of the anatomic sources of the pain, and for this reason it is important to perform a careful pelvic examination to map the areas of maximal tenderness. However, the level of reported pain is not related to the extent of disease. To make evaluation even more complicated, pain in these patients may result from sources other than endometriosis or adhesions such as pelvic floor muscle spasm, interstitial cystitis, irritable bowel syndrome, or ilioinguinal nerve entrapment. Following many surgical procedures, the pain due to endometriosis implants may be replaced by pain from adhesions.

For patients with dysmenorrhea or mild pelvic pain as their presenting symptom, initial treatment may consist of a 2- to 3-month trial of oral contraceptives and nonsteroidal anti-inflammatory agents. Patients who fail to obtain adequate relief, develop recurrence of symptoms while being treated conservatively, or have more severe pain require definitive diagnosis and aggressive treatment.

The approach that has been successful in providing long-term relief includes an initial diagnostic or operative laparoscopy during which all visible disease is ablated or excised. Patients with severe dysmenorrhea that has failed to respond to medical therapy are offered a presacral neurectomy. Postoperatively, a 6-month course of hormonal therapy is administered such as GnRH agonists (with or without norethindrone to control hot flashes and limit bone loss), high-dose progestins, or danazol. At the end of the course of hormonal therapy, the patient is given continuous oral contraceptives (low progestin pills are better tolerated and as effective as high progestin pills) until fertility is desired.

Controlled studies show that hormonal therapy has a high degree of efficacy when relief of pain and dysmenorrhea are used as end points. However, although the majority of women continue to experience significant relief of general pelvic pain and dyspareunia after the medications are stopped, dysmenorrhea invariably returns with the resumption of cyclic menses.

Although hormonal therapy has had a prominent role in the treatment of symptomatic endometriosis, several factors limit its effectiveness. Apparently successful treatment may be only a temporary remission, with approximately 25 to 30% of patients reporting recurrence of symptoms within 6 months of treatment. It is not clear whether recurrence is due to reactivation of residual disease or the acquisition of new implants. Women who are more likely to have recurrences include those with severe disease or large endometriomas.

For patients with recurrent or intractable pain associated with endometriosis, hysterectomy remains the definitive treatment. In young women remote from menopause, removal of one or both ovaries is controversial despite the fact that the ovaries are the most common site of endometrial implants and the growth of endometrial implants is driven by cyclic ovarian activity. If a woman's symptoms are severe enough to warrant a hysterectomy, all remaining ovarian tissue should be removed at the same time. Reoperation for an ovarian remnant or residual ovary is one of the most challenging surgical procedures and is associated with a high risk of additional surgical procedures.

Postoperative hormonal replacement can be commenced immediately following surgery and should include both estrogen and a progestin. The progestin attenuates the growth-promoting effects of estrogen and decreases the possibility of recurrent pain due to endometriosis. Alternatively, the patient can be treated with progestins alone for 3 to 6 months to suppress residual endometriosis and hot flashes; this is followed by either estrogen alone or combined continuous estrogen and progestin. In women who have recurrence of pain following total abdominal hysterectomy and bilateral salpingo-oophorectomy, the differential diagnosis includes recurrent endometriosis, ovarian remnant, adhesions or other sources of pain unrelated to endometriosis, or the surgical procedure itself.

Infertility

Despite the apparent association between infertility and endometriosis, there is a paucity of evidence identifying the specific mechanisms of infertility resulting from this enigmatic disease. Three separate factors may play a role in infertility associated with endometriosis: implants, ovarian endometriomas, and adhesions. Each may contribute separately to a reduction in fertility by different mechanisms, which include alterations in immune system function, peritoneal fluid composition, anatomic relationships, and ovarian function. To confuse the issue even further, a high rate of additional infertility factors has been noted in these couples, including male factor, cervical factor, luteal phase defect, and tubal factor. Despite this confusion, controlled studies suggest that the presence of endometriosis implants significantly compromises fertility potential.

The type of endometriosis encountered in women presenting with infertility is generally asymptomatic, and the indication for performing laparoscopy is part of an infertility evaluation. For patients with endometriosis and infertility, it is important to stress the importance of a complete and thorough work-up of infertility factors. In many couples, endometriosis is not the only problem affecting their ability to conceive.

Surgical Treatment. Theoretically, pregnancy rates following conservative surgery should be equivalent for each stage of disease because the surgery is intended to excise all visible disease as well as correct anatomic distortion and lyse adhesions. When conservative resection of endometriosis is performed by laparotomy, pregnancy rates decline with disease severity. In contrast, compared with expectant management of minimal and mild disease, laser laparoscopic treatment of endometriosis appears to have a fertility-enhancing effect significantly above that reported for other types of treatment, i.e., expectant management, hormonal therapy, or laparotomy. Indeed, for severe endometriosis, pregnancy rates following laser laparoscopy appear to be much better than those reported after laparotomy (65% vs. 40%). This discrepancy in pregnancy rates may be due to the greater risk of reformation of adhesions with laparotomy, particularly in more severe disease.

Other Fertility-Enhancing Treatments. For patients who fail to conceive following laparoscopic surgery, there are several fertility-enhancing regimens that have demonstrated value. Repeat surgery may be of benefit by diminishing the amount of endometriosis that has recurred. Although the numbers are small and the surgical procedures were performed by laparotomy, the reported pregnancy rates of 25 to 40% are promising and may offer a treatment option to women who cannot or do not want to undergo advanced reproductive technologies.

Recently, the combined therapy of superovulation and intrauterine insemination was introduced as a method of treating infertile couples with patent fallopian tubes when more traditional therapy has failed. Treatment with clomiphene citrate (Clomid), and intrauterine insemination improves fecundity compared wtih periovulatory intercourse in couples with either unexplained infertility or surgically corrected endometriosis. Cycle fecundity rates as high as 9.5% have been reported. The efficacy of human menopausal gonadotropins and intrauterine insemination appears to be stage-specific, with cycle fecundity remaining fairly constant for Stages I to III but dropping precipitously for Stage IV (8.3%, 11%, 14.3%, and 0%, respectively). This may reflect the fact that superovulation with intrauterine insemination is dependent on an intact ovum pickup mechanism, which may be altered by adhesions in severe disease.

Gamete intra-fallopian transfer (GIFT) allows direct insertion of gametes into the fallopian tube, thus ensuring that the gametes make it to the proper location. Pregnancy rates are comparable to those reported in women with other infertility diagnoses. Moreover, the laparoscopic retrieval of oocytes provides an opportunity to treat endometriosis under the same anesthesia without adversely affecting the probability of conception. Likewise, in vitro fertilization (IVF) offers an opportunity for conception, particularly in women with tubal damage, when assessment of fertilizing capacity of the gametes is indicated and other treatments have failed.

Treatments That Have No Efficacy in Enhancing Fertility. Recent studies suggest that hormonal treatment of mild and moderate endometriosis may not offer any advantage over expectant management for enhancing fertility. Moreover, the period of time during actual treatment delays conception because all of these hormonal agents are effective contraceptives. In addition, women are exposed to the risks and side effects of these hormonal agents without receiving any benefit. Thus, medical therapy has no place in enhancing conception in the treatment of endometriosis-associated infertility.

Very few studies have reported pregnancy rates using preoperative or postoperative hormonal therapy, and fewer still have compared results with a control group. Despite the paucity of published studies, some trends can be gleaned from these data. It appears that neither preoperative nor postoperative hormonal therapy is effective for the treatment of infertility associated with endometriosis.

DYSFUNCTIONAL UTERINE BLEEDING

method of
MICHAEL M. MILLER, M.D.
University of Arkansas for Medical Sciences
Little Rock, Arkansas

Normal menstruation occurs every 29 days with a range of 23 to 39 days. Abnormal uterine bleeding (AUB) is defined as unexpected, irregular, prolonged, or heavy (more than 80 mL) bleeding. It affects virtually all women at some point in their lives but is most common during the pubertal and perimenopausal periods. Dysfunctional uterine bleeding (DUB) due to anovulation or other ovulatory dysfunction accounts for approximately 85% of AUB. DUB is a diagnosis of exclusion that requires a thorough evaluation to rule out other causes of AUB including uterine, cervical, vaginal or vulvar pathology, pregnancy, neoplasia, infection, blood dyscrasia, cirrhosis, kidney failure, or medication (Table 1).

TABLE 1. **Differential Diagnosis of Abnormal Vaginal Bleeding**

Dysfunctional uterine bleeding: 85% of cases
Disorders of pregnancy: Ectopic, abortion, abnormal placentation
Infection: Pelvic inflammatory disease, chronic endometritis
Cervical pathology: Erosions, polyps, cervicitis, carcinoma
Uterine problems: Submucous myomas, endometrial polyps, carcinoma
Ovarian pathology: Inadequate luteal phase, polycystic ovarian disease, granulosa-theca cell tumors, ovarian abscess
Vaginal pathology: Trauma, foreign bodies, infection, carcinoma
Blood dyscrasias: Thrombocytopenia, leukemia, coagulation disorders
Endocrine disorders: Hypothyroidism or hyperthyroidism, adrenal disease, hyperprolactinemia
Systemic disease: Cirrhosis, renal failure
Iatrogenic: Various medications, hormones, intrauterine devices

Modified from Jewelewicz R: Dysfunctional uterine bleeding. *In* Rakel RR (ed): Conn's Current Therapy 1993. Philadelphia, WB Saunders Co, 1993.

ETIOLOGY

Anovulation accounts for 90% of cases of DUB. Bleeding results from two mechanisms. Estrogen withdrawal bleeding commonly occurs in adolescence, perimenopause, and in patients with levonorgestrel implants (Norplant). Estradiol produced during folliculogenesis stimulates endometrial growth but fails to induce a luteinizing hormone (LH) surge. Subsequent follicular atresia results in declining estradiol levels and concomitant endometrial sloughing. Estrogen breakthrough bleeding occurs in chronic anovulatory disorders such as polycystic ovarian disease, adrenal disease, hyperprolactinemia, and hypothyroidism. Chronic estrogen exposure unopposed by progesterone stimulates growth of an unstable thickened endometrium that breaks down and bleeds when the blood supply is outgrown. Anovulatory patients can present with bleeding that is profuse or light and irregular, prolonged or cyclic.

Dysfunctional ovulation occurs in 10% of patients with DUB. Mechanisms include a persistent corpus luteal cyst or a prolonged follicular phase or luteal phase defect. Patients can present with oligomenorrhea, prolonged periods (menorrhagia), or intermenstrual bleeding.

DIFFERENTIAL DIAGNOSIS AND EVLUATION

The diagnosis of DUB requires a thorough evaluation to rule out other causes of AUB. In addition, the occurrence or lack of ovulation should be established by charting basal body temperature or serial weekly serum progesterone levels. A rise of 0.5° F in temperature from the follicular to the luteal phase or a progesterone level of more than 3 ng per mL are diagnostic of ovulation. A medical history should include questions about the method of contraception, unprotected intercourse, bleeding or bruising tendencies, chronic illness, and drug use including nonsteroidal anti-inflammatory drugs, anticoagulants, or sex steroids. An examination of the skin and gums for petechiae, bleeding, and bruising is necessary. If a lower abdominal mass is palpated, a pregnancy test should be obtained. The perineum, vulva, and vagina should be evaluated for trauma or other lesions. The cervix should be evaluated for softness, a bluish hue, or dilatation suggesting pregnancy, the presence of copious mucus that is consistent with chronic anovulation, and any other lesion. A bimanual examination is required to evaluate uterine size, consistency, shape, and adnexal pathology. A vaginal probe ultrasound examination is extremely useful to evaluate the adnexa, the uterus for fibroids or pregnancy, and the endometrium for irregularity or excessive thickness (more than 10 to 12 mm), suggesting polyps or hyperplasia.

Initial laboratory evaluation includes a pregnancy test and a complete blood count to assess the amount of bleeding and an erythrocyte sedimentation test to screen for pelvic infection. A platelet count, coagulation profile, and bleeding times are required in ovulatory patients with unexplained DUB and in any adolescent with severe hemorrhage. Before hormonal therapy is initiated an endometrial biopsy should be obtained in any patient over 35 years of age with DUB and in all patients with prolonged chronic anovulation regardless of age. A hysterosalpingogram or, preferably, a hysteroscopy should be done in any patient with DUB that is unexplained or unresponsive to hormonal therapy to thoroughly evaluate the endometrium.

THERAPY

Treatment is based on the severity of symptoms, the desires of the patient, and the cause of the problem. Ovulatory patients with a normal hemoglobin and mild irregular bleeding need reassurance. If desired, oral contraceptives will provide cycle regularity. Infertile patients require a thorough evaluation beyond the scope of this text.

Anovulatory patients require treatment with cyclical progestins such as medroxyprogesterone acetate (Provera) 10 mg for 12 days every 4 weeks to prevent endometrial hyperplasia. Adolescents should be treated every 6 weeks to allow discontinuation if regular ovulatory cycles develop. When contraception is needed oral contraceptives should be used as a progestin source. Infertility patients require ovulation induction, generally with clomiphene citrate (Clomid or Serophene) if serum prolactin and thyroid-stimulating hormone levels are normal.

Acute hemorrhage must be treated promptly. Estrogen-induced bleeding responds to progestogens unless prolonged bleeding has resulted in a denuded endometrium that requires estrogen for regrowth. Hemodynamically stable patients will stop bleeding within 2 days after initiation of treatment with three oral contraceptive tablets per day for 1 week, 2 per day for 1 week and 1 per day for 1 week. This will be followed by a moderately heavy withdrawal bleed. Patients should then be cycled with progestins or oral contraceptives. Antiemetic therapy is usually required with this regimen.

Patients with significant anemia will respond within 6 to 12 hours to 25 mg of intravenous conjugated estrogen (Premarin) every 4 hours for three doses. Oral contraceptives or medroxyprogesterone acetate (Provera), 20 mg per day, should be started when bleeding slows and continued for 2 to 3 weeks. A heavy withdrawal bleed will occur. Alternatively, when the duration of acute bleeding is less than 1 week patients usually respond to oral megestrol acetate (Megace), 40 mg every 6 hours for 3 days and then daily for a total of 14 days. The withdrawal bleed will be lighter than that in the intravenous estrogen protocol. A dilation and curettage is rarely required to control hemorrhage, but when necessary it should be done with a hysteroscopy to prevent missing pathology. If uncontrolled hemorrhage persists, the need for transfusion can be reduced by inserting a Foley catheter through the cervix and inflating the balloon to 30 mL. This can be followed by hypogastric artery embolization when preservation of childbearing potential if desired. It this is not a concern, a hysterectomy can be performed.

AMENORRHEA

method of
TONY ZREIK, M.D., and
DAVID L. OLIVE, M.D.
Yale University School of Medicine
New Haven, Connecticut

Amenorrhea is the end result of a number of different pathologic states, some congenital, others benign, and occasionally, one of several that are life-threatening. For this reason, correct diagnosis is critically important. This article outlines a diagnostic approach to this symptom that is both comprehensive and cost effective.

PRIMARY AMENORRHEA

The incidence of primary amenorrhea is less than 1:1000, and it is defined as no spontaneous menses by the age of 16; however, a diagnostic work-up should be initiated by age 14 in the girl who has had no menstruation and failure of development of secondary sexual characteristics. Similarly, evaluation should be performed in the girl who has failed to menstruate within 4 years following the onset of thelarche and adrenarche. Patients with primary amenorrhea and normal external genitalia can be placed in one of four diagnostic categories, depending on the presence or absence of breast development and whether or not a uterus is present. Patients with ambiguous genitalia or cryptomenorrhea will not be considered here.

No Breast Development; Uterus Present

In this category, the abnormality may be due to a hypothalamic failure to release gonadotropin-releasing hormone (GnRH), or to a failure of pituitary or gonadal function.

When the defect is at the hypothalamic level, the inability to secrete GnRH may be due to disorders of neurotransmitter action (norepinephrine, dopamine) necessary to induce adequate GnRH synthesis or release, or both (Fig. 1). Pituitary failure, on the other hand, may be due to isolated gonadotropin deficiency, pituitary adenomas, mumps, encephalitis, or prepubertal hypothyroidism.

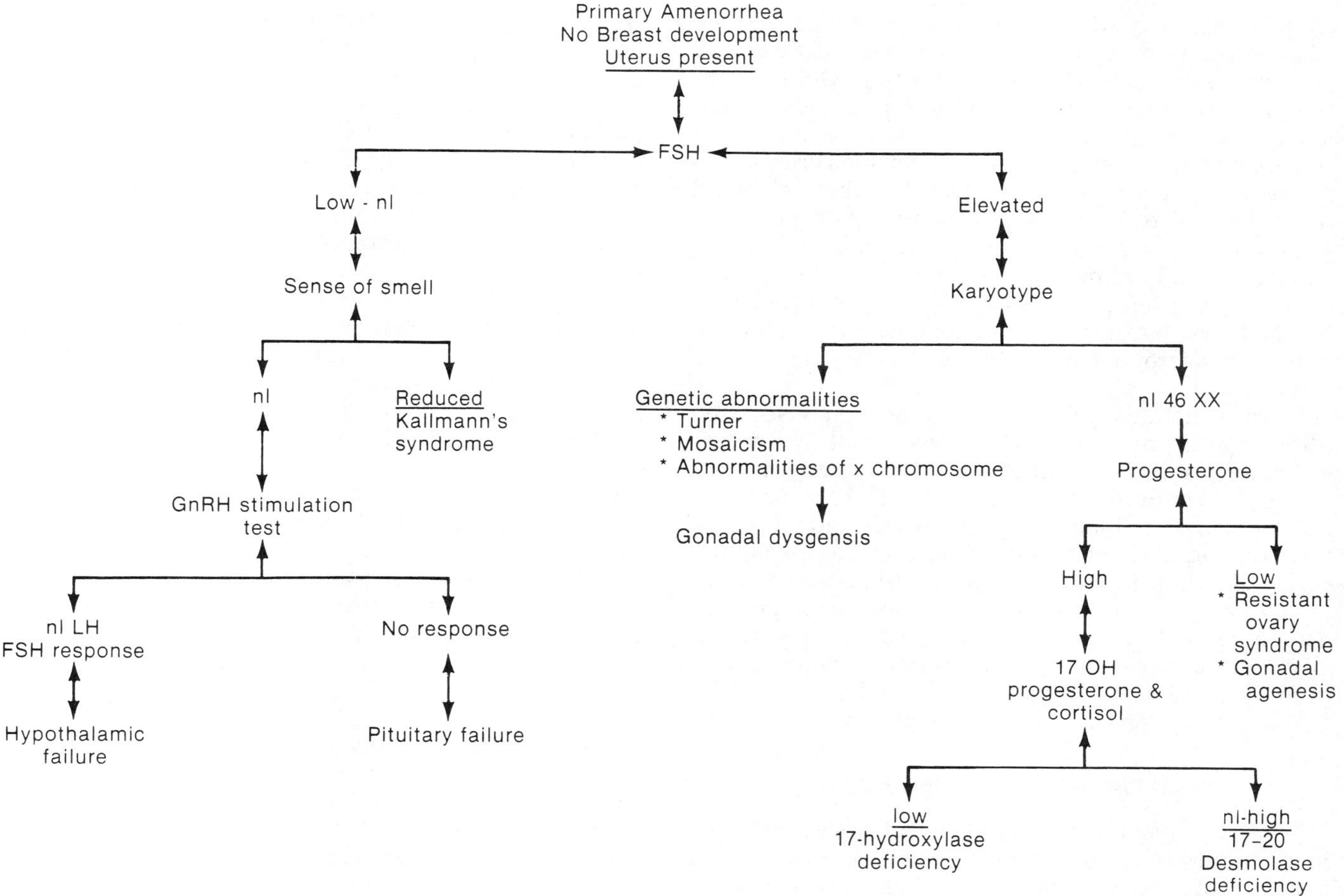

Figure 1.

Gonadal failure is generally due to chromosomal abnormalities or to enzyme deficiency states. Chromosomal abnormalities are the most common cause of primary amenorrhea, and they consist of Turner's syndrome, Turner's mosaicism, and structural abnormalities of the X chromosome. Patients with these conditions have streak gonads that lack primary follicles and are incapable of ovarian steroid synthesis; thus, the negative feedback on the hypothalamic-pituitary axis is missing, leading to elevated gonadotropins in the postmenopausal range. Enzyme deficiency states such as 17-hydroxylase deficiency and 17-20 desmolase deficiency also produce gonadal failure. These patients with 17-hydroxylase deficiency and a 46XX karyotype present with primary amenorrhea, no breast development, a prepubertal uterus, and slightly eunuchoid habitus. The enzyme deficiency results in reduction in cortisol production, which, in turn, causes an increase in adrenocorticotropic hormone (ACTH) release necessary to maintain cortisol production. This may lead to excessive production of mineralocorticoids (DOC, corticosterone), which, in turn, can result in sodium retention, hypertension, and loss of potassium. The diagnosis of 17-hydroxylase deficiency should be suspected when an elevated serum progesterone level, a low 17-α hydroxyprogesterone level, and an elevated serum DOC level are obtained. The diagnosis can then be confirmed by performing an ACTH stimulation test, which induces markedly elevated progesterone levels with little change in the serum 17-α hydroxyprogesterone levels.

Individuals with any of these disorders cannot synthesize ovarian steroids; thus, these patients have elevated gonadotropins because they lack the negative feedback of sex steroids on the hypothalamic-pituitary axis. The work-up of these patients with primary amenorrhea, no breast development, and uterus present begins with measurement of serum follicle-stimulating hormone (FSH). This value distinguishes central (hypothalamic and pituitary) abnormalities from primary gonadal failure; an elevated FSH level points to an ovarian etiology, whereas a low or normal FSH level indicates a hypothalamic or pituitary disorder. When primary gonadal failure is suspected following the discovery of an elevated FSH serum level, a karyotype is necessary to rule out genetic abnormalities, most commonly Turner's syndrome.

The central nervous system abnormalities can be differentiated as hypothalamic or pituitary in origin by performing a GnRH stimulation test (100 to 150 μg intravenously over 30 seconds) following a week of priming with estradiol. An elevation of FSH and luteinizing hormone (LH) in response to GnRH stimulation indicates a hypothalamic failure. These patients should be evaluated for the presence of a central nervous system neoplasm (such as craniopharyngiomas), and a qualitative test for olfaction should be performed to rule out Kallmann's syndrome (hypothalamic hypogonadotropic hypogonadism with anosmia and other abnormalities, including cleft palate, deafness, and renal anomalies). Treatment consists of hormonal replacement therapy or ovulation induction with gonadotropins if the patient is trying to conceive.

In rare instances, GnRH elicits no response, even after proper pretreatment with estradiol, indicating a pituitary failure. Evaluation of these patients consists of a computed tomography (CT) scan or magnetic resonance imaging (MRI) to rule out pituitary tumors, and treatment consists of cyclic estrogen and progestin therapy to develop the breast and other secondary sexual characteristics as well as to prevent osteoporosis. If pregnancy is desired, the treatment of choice is exogenous gonadotropin therapy. Clomiphene citrate (Clomid) has been found to be ineffective in inducing ovulation in such patients.

Breast Development, Uterus Absent

There are two disorders in this category; androgen insensitivity (testicular feminization), and congenital absence of the uterus (Mayer-Rokitansky-Küster-Hauser syndrome, or müllerian agenesis).

The former is an X-linked inherited disorder; patients have a 46XX karyotype, testes and female phenotype, with the clinical features of lack of axillary and pubic hair, abnormal but developed breasts, and a blind vaginal pouch.

Management consists of removing the gonads postpubertally and placing the patient on hormonal replacement therapy once full development is attained. This is the only exception to the rule that gonads, in the presence of a Y chromosome, should be removed prior to puberty. The reasoning behind this approach is that pubertal development is better achieved with endogenous hormones, and that gonadal tumors in these patients have not been encountered prior to puberty.

Congenital absence of the uterus is due to a failure of development of the müllerian system and is the second most common cause of primary amenorrhea. This disorder is characterized by the presence of ovaries and normal secondary sex characteristics, along with absence of the uterus and the absence of a vagina or one that is hypoplastic. Patients with müllerian agenesis should be evaluated for associated extragenital anomalies. Approximately 40% of patients have associated renal anomalies necessitating intravenous pyelogram (IVP) as part of the work-up. Moreover, 12% of patients have skeletal abnormalities, mostly involving the spine: examples include spina bifida, scoliosis, and congenital fusion of the cervical spine (Klippel-Feil anomaly). Additional extragenital anomalies include rib and limb abnormalities, congenital heart disease, and inguinal hernias.

Treatment of the genital anomalies of patients with müllerian agenesis consists of development of an artificial or pseudovaginal pouch. This procedure is occasionally performed via surgical reconstruction. Surgery, however, should be reserved for those patients in whom the progressive vaginal dilatation has failed.

Differences between müllerian agenesis and testicular feminization include a 46XX karyotype and normal female sexual hair in the müllerian agenesis, as opposed to a 46XY karyotype and absent to sparse sexual hair seen with testicular feminization.

The simplest, least expensive test used to differentiate the two conditions is measurement of the serum testosterone level. A normal male testosterone concentration is consistent with androgen insensitivity; however, a testosterone level in the normal female range indicates congenital absence of the uterus. For more definitive evaluation, a karyotype may be used to distinguish these two conditions.

No Breast Development, No Uterus

This condition is extremely rare; all reported cases have a male karyotype, elevated gonadotropins and female levels of serum testosterone. Two enzyme defects in the male have been reported to cause this condition: 17-hydroxylase deficiency, and 17-20 desmolase deficiency, both leading to failure of androgen and estrogen synthesis. These patients have abdominal testes that require removal followed by estrogen replacement therapy.

In addition to these enzyme defects in the male, a case of agonadism presenting with primary amenorrhea, no breast development, and uterine agenesis has been reported. The absence of the uterus in this patient was thought to be secondary to vanishing testicular tissue, which is possibly present early in embryonic life; thus, the syndrome of agonadism is also referred to as the vanishing testes syndrome.

Breast Development, Uterus Present

This group comprises one third of patients with primary amenorrhea. Approximately 20% of patients in this group have elevated prolactin levels and should be evaluated for hyperprolactinemia. The remaining 80% have the same disorders seen with secondary amenorrhea, and they should be evaluated accordingly.

SECONDARY AMENORRHEA

Secondary amenorrhea is defined as the absence of menses for 6 months in a woman previously having regular menses, or 12 months if the woman was previously oligomenorrheic.

Initial investigation should rule out pregnancy and thyroid disease. Amenorrhea secondary to excess prolactin, cortisol, or androgen excess states is not discussed in this section. Included here are conditions involving abnormalities of the hypothalamic-pituitary ovarian axis as well as intrauterine synechiae (Fig. 2).

Hypothalamic Dysfunction

In most instances of hypothalamic dysfunction, there are abnormalities of GnRH pulsatile release, as determined by abnormalities in LH pulses. This dysfunction appears to be related to either a central nervous system neurotransmitter alteration or a hypothalamic derangement, which is most commonly idiopathic in nature. Other causes include medications such as phenothiazines and other psychotropic drugs.

Stress, exercise, weight loss, and anorexia nervosa have all been associated with secondary amenorrhea, as have hypothalamic lesions such as craniopharyngiomas, tuberculous granulomas, sarcoidosis, and meningoencephalitis.

Pituitary Dysfunction

Amenorrhea may be the first symptom of a pituitary tumor; the most common pituitary lesion resulting in secondary amenorrhea is a prolactin-secreting tumor. However, chromophobe adenomas and nonneoplastic lesions including Sheehan's syndrome (acute pituitary infarction in association with severe postpartum hemorrhage) have also been shown to cause secondary amenorrhea.

Ovarian Dysfunction

The etiology of premature ovarian failure, which is defined as menopause prior to the age of 40, is unknown in most cases but may be due to specific sex chromosome anomalies (45X, 47XXY, and mosaicism), or to autoimmune antibodies directed against steroid-producing cells of the ovary.

In fact, the association between premature ovarian failure and autoimmune disease entities is well established; these entities include Hashimoto's thyroiditis, Graves' disease, hypoparathyroidism, juvenile

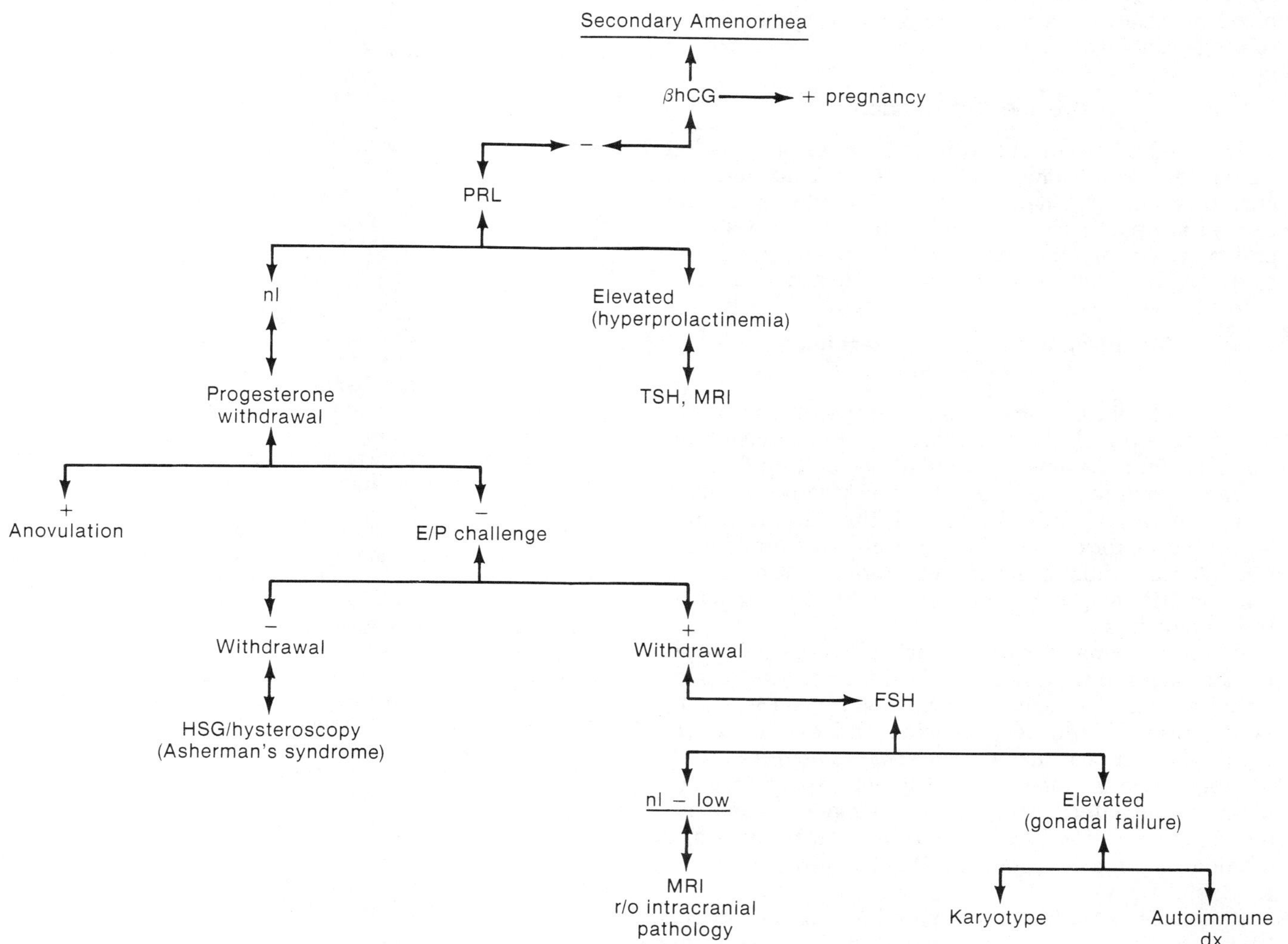

Figure 2.

onset diabetes mellitus, myasthenia gravis, pernicious anemia, and idiopathic thrombocytopenic purpura. The diagnosis of autoimmune oophoritis requires the demonstration of circulating tissue-specific antiovarian antibodies.

Loss of ovarian function may also be secondary to castration, hemorrhage, infection, or perhaps to destruction of follicles by physical insult such as irradiation (with as little as 50 cGy to the ovaries), or chemotherapy (especially alkylating agents such as cyclophosphamide).

Multicomponent Dysfunction

Patients with this abnormality are commonly referred to as having polycystic ovarian disease. Patients with this condition have normal or elevated serum estrogen levels but are chronically anovulatory. All components of the hypothalamic-pituitary-ovarian axis may be functional but dyssynchronous; thus, the polycystic ovary is the result of a functional derangement rather than a specific deficiency state.

Most patients present with oligomenorrhea, but some may have secondary or even primary amenorrhea. Estrogen levels are generally greater than 40 picograms per mL; thus, bleeding occurs in response to progestin withdrawal.

Uterine Dysfunction

The formation of intrauterine adhesions, called Asherman's syndrome, is often due to dilatation and curettage performed either in pregnancy or in the immediate postpartum period; it may also be due to endometritis, myomectomy, or metroplasty. Such patients ovulate normally, but menses do not occur.

Diagnosing the Cause of Secondary Amenorrhea

After adequate history and physical examination are obtained, including nutritional and exercise habits, a serum pregnancy test should be obtained.

Once pregnancy is excluded, a serum prolactin level is obtained. If it is elevated, the patient should be evaluated for causes of hyperprolactinemia including hypothyroidism, drugs, and renal failure. A CT scan or MRI may also be necessary to rule out pituitary adenomas.

When a normal serum prolactin level is obtained, menses are induced by administration of a progestational agent. If a positive withdrawal bleed is noted, anovulation should be suspected and evaluated accordingly. If no withdrawal bleeding is achieved with a progestational agent, an estrogen/progestin challenge is initiated (conjugated estrogen [Premarin] 0.625 mg orally per day for 25 days, with 10 mg orally of medroxyprogesterone acetate [Provera] daily for the last 10 days).

If menses again fail to occur, end-organ dysfunction (Asherman's syndrome) is suspected and can be diagnosed by hysterosalpingogram or hysteroscopy.

However, if withdrawal bleeding occurs following an estrogen/progestin challenge, a serum FSH level should be obtained. A low to normal FSH level indicates a central (hypothalamic or pituitary) origin of the amenorrhea and necessitates a CT scan or an MRI to rule out intracranial pathology. When elevated levels of FSH are obtained in a patient younger than 40 years of age, the diagnosis is premature ovarian failure. This warrants further evaluation using the following methods: a karyotype to rule out sex chromosome anomalies, and thyroid function tests with thyroid antibodies, cortisol, rheumatoid factor and antinuclear antibodies to rule out a possible autoimmune origin of the ovarian failure.

DYSMENORRHEA

method of
KURT T. BARNHART, M.D., and
STEVEN J. SONDHEIMER, M.D.
Hospital of the University of Pennsylvania
Philadelphia, Pennsylvania

Primary dysmenorrhea is defined as menstrual pain without pelvic pathology. The pelvic examination of a women with primary dysmenorrhea is, by definition, normal. Primary dysmenorrhea is primarily a problem of younger women, occurring more frequently during the teenage years and early twenties. The initial onset of primary dysmenorrhea is 6 months to 1 year after menarche, coincident with the onset of ovulatory cycles. Ovulation is a prerequisite for primary dysmenorrhea. The onset of dysmenorrhea is usually hours prior to the onset of menses and lasts up to 72 hours. The pain is characterized by intermittent crampy lower abdominal or pelvic pain, concentrated in the midline (suprapubic) region but possibly radiating to the lower back or inner thighs. It may also be associated with diarrhea or nausea and vomiting. The incidence of dysmenorrhea declines after vaginal delivery, but pregnancy does not cure this disorder. Dysmenorrhea is not relieved by exercise, but may improve with orgasm. Dysmenorrhea does not have prodromal affective symptoms prior to the menses and should be distinguished from premenstrual syndrome.

Secondary dysmenorrhea is defined as painful menstruation secondary to an underlying pelvic pathology. The onset of secondary dysmenorrhea typically occurs at a later age and the symptoms may be associated with anovulatory cycle, may persist after the menses, and can usually be related to a causative pelvic pathology. Common causes of secondary dysmenorrhea are endometriosis, adenomyosis, uterine fibroids, uterine polyps, ovarian neoplasms (benign or malignant), pelvic inflammatory disease, müllerian congenital anomalies (such as a partially communicating or noncommunicating uterine horn, transverse vaginal septum, or imperforate hymen), intrauterine adhesions, acquired cervical stenosis, or use of an intrauterine device.

DISTINGUISHING PRIMARY FROM SECONDARY DYSMENORRHEA

Often when a women presents reporting dysmenorrhea, the distinction between primary and secondary dysmenorrhea can be made by carefully obtaining the patient's history and performing a physical examination. Primary dysmenorrhea is rarely found in a woman who has had years of relatively painless menses. Dysmenorrhea with heavy vaginal bleeding may suggest the possibility of uterine fibroids. Irregular vaginal bleeding or spotting may suggest a uterine polyp, a submucosal uterine fibroid, or possibly a chlamydial infection. A history of progressive dysmenorrhea and infertility is suggestive of endometriosis. Dysmenorrhea in a parous woman with a mildly enlarged globularly shaped uterus is consistent with adenomyosis. Increased dysmenorrhea accompanied by decreased menstrual flow, or spotting, after a dilatation and curettage may suggest an Asherman's syndrome. Primary amenorrhea accompanied with dysmenorrhea is suggestive of a imperforate hymen or possible vaginal or cervical agenesis. Dysmenorrhea in a woman just after menarche accompanied by a foul-smelling or currant jelly–like discharge is suggestive of a partially communicating uterine horn or duplicated vagina.

Physical examination also helps in the diagnosis of many causes of secondary dysmenorrhea. A speculum examination may confirm the diagnosis of an imperforate hymen or a partially occluded vaginal septum. A polyp, or pedunculated myoma may be visualized at the external cervical os or in the cervical canal. A bimanual examination, complete with a rectovaginal examination, may detect an irregularly enlarged uterus consistent with uterine myomas; a bulky uterus consistent with adenomyosis; cervical motion tenderness, consistent with pelvic inflammatory disease; adnexal enlargement suggesting an ovarian neoplasm; a fixed uterus or adnexa consistent with pelvic adhesions or endometriosis, or tender uterosacral nodularity also consistent with endometriosis. If the diagnosis is still in doubt, a vaginal ultrasound examination may be help in identifying a small submucosal fibroid or an ovarian neoplasm, and may suggest adenomyosis or a congenital müllerian anomaly. A hysteroscopy may be helpful in diagnosing a uterine polyp, an submucosal fibroid, or Asherman's syndrome. The use of magnetic resonance imaging (MRI) may be helpful in the diagnosis of congenital müllerian anomalies or adenomyosis.

Secondary dysmenorrhea should be distinguished from chronic pain syndrome. Although chronic pelvic pain, by definition, is not associated with pelvic pathology and may be amplified at menstruation, it does not have any true cyclic relation to menstruation. In patients recalcitrant to therapy for presumed primary dysmenorrhea, a laparoscopy may be useful to rule out conditions difficult to diagnose clinically, such as pelvic adhesions, pelvic inflammatory disease, and endometriosis.

ETIOLOGY OF PRIMARY DYSMENORRHEA

The pain of primary dysmenorrhea is thought to be secondary to excessive uterine contractions from an excess of uterine prostaglandins (PG). An abnormally high release of PG E_2 and $F_2\alpha$ from the endometrium can increase uterine myometrial contractility, which can cause uterine ischemia and pain. PGs may also be responsible for the systemic side effects of dysmenorrhea, such as nausea, vomiting, and diarrhea. PGs are synthesized from the phospholipids found in the cell membranes, which are converted to arachidonic acid by the enzyme phospholipase A_2. PGs are produced in the cyclooxygenase pathway, where arachidonic acid is converted to PG E_2 and $F_2\alpha$ by cyclic endoperoxidase and prostaglandin synthetase. PG production is dependent on cyclic and sequential production of estrogen and progesterone in an ovulatory cycle. In the luteal phase, as luteolysis occurs, progesterone levels fall, destabilizing lysosomal membranes, thereby releasing phospholipase A_2 and starting the cascade of PG production. Direct evidence supporting this hypothesis is that patients with dysmenorrhea have significantly higher levels of PG in endometrial biopsies and washings than women without dysmenorrhea. Multiple clinical trials have also demonstrated that nonsterodial anti-inflammatory drugs are effective in the treatment of dysmenorrhea presumably by blocking PG synthesis at the level of the cyclooxgenase pathway. Other theories possibly explaining the etiology of dysmenorrhea include the hypersensitization of uterine pain receptors by PGs, which reduces the threshold for painful stimuli; an increase in the leukotrienes, (a potent vasoconstrictor also produced from arachidonic acid), which induce stronger uterine muscle contractions; and an increase in vasopressin levels, which can cause dysfunctional and strong uterine contractions.

TREATMENT OF PRIMARY DYSMENORRHEA

In the treatment of dysmenorrhea, two important considerations are (1) to rule out and diagnose the

TABLE 1. **Prostaglandin Synthetase Inhibitors**

Drug	Brand Name	Dosage
Phenylpropionic acid derivatives		
Ibuprofen	Motrin, Advil, Nuprin, Rufen	400–600 mg q 6 hr
Naproxen	Naprosyn	250–500 mg q 6 hr
Naproxen sodium	Anaprox	275–550 mg q 6 hr
Ketoprofen	Orudis	50 mg q 8 hr
Flurbiprofen*	Ansaid	50 mg q 6 hr
Acetic acid derivatives		
Indomethacin	Indocin	25–50 mg q 6 hr
Ketorolac tromethamine	Toradol	10 mg q 6 hr
Fenamates		
Mefenamic acid	Ponstel	250–500 mg q 6 hr
Meclofenamate sodium*	Meclomen	50–100 mg q 6 hr
Oxicams		
Piroxicam*	Feldene	20–40 mg daily

*Commonly used, but not specifically labeled by the FDA for treatment of dysmenorrhea.
Modified from MacKay TH, and Chang JR: Dysmenorrhea. *In* Rakel RE (ed): Conn's Current Therapy 1993. Philadelphia, WB Saunders Co, 1993.

cause of secondary amenorrhea and (2) to address the psychosocial situations that may surround the patient with dysmenorrhea. Empiric treatment for primary dysmenorrhea can be started in a patient with a history consistent with primary dysmenorrhea and a pelvic examination that did not reveal an obvious abnormality. It is important, however, to understand any social situation that may be aggravating the dysmenorrhea and take the time to explain the condition and alleviate any concerns the patient may have about this condition.

The most common medical treatments for dysmenorrhea are oral contraceptive pills and nonsteroidal anti-inflammatory drugs. Oral contraceptive pills relieve primary dysmenorrhea in 90% of women with this condition. Oral contraceptive pills decrease dysmenorrhea by inhibiting ovulation, decreasing uterine motility, decreasing the concentration of prostaglandins in the endometrium, decreasing endometrial growth, and therefore, decreasing menstrual bleeding. Monophasic combined estrogen and progesterone pills are more effective than triphasic combination pills in suppressing ovulation and have also been shown to be more effective in relieving dysmenorrhea. Relief from dysmenorrhea also seems to be gestagen related. Relief can be obtained by progestin-only contraceptive pills (Micronor, Ovrette), medroxy progesterone acetate (Depo Provera) injections and progestin implants like levonorgestrel (Norplant). Progesterone-medicated intrauterine devices also decrease dysmenorrhea. Hormonal contraception should be considered in the treatment of dysmenorrhea in any woman, not just those in need of contraception, since it not only effectively treats dysmenorrhea but offers other health benefits including reliable contraception, a reduction of iron-deficient anemia, protection against endometrial cancer, and possibly, preventing or slowing the progression of endometriosis.

Nonsteriodal anti-inflammatory medications are also effective in the treatment of dysmenorrhea in 75% to 90% of cases and may be used alone or in combination with oral contraceptive pills. Prostaglandin sythetase inhibitors are divided into separate classes, including derivatives of phenylpropionic acid (naproxen [Naprosyn], ketoprofen [Orudis], flurbiprofen [Ansaid]), acetic acid (ketorolac [Toradol], indomethacin [Indocin]) and the fenamates (Ponstel). The commonly used agents are listed in Table 1. To be effective, these agents should not be taken on an as-needed basis but continuously, starting before the onset of menses and continuing for 2 to 3 days. The loading dose and the maintenance dose may be increased as needed. These agents are only recommended for short-term treatment (5 days or less). Clinically, there are no clear guidelines in selecting the most appropriate agent; therefore, selection is based on clinical experience, patient convenience, and cost. As a given patient's relief from a particular agent can be idiosyncratic, if adequate relief is not obtained, it may be useful to try a second or even a third agent, particularly from a different class.

New and less proven treatments that are usually reserved for patients with severe dysmenorrhea that is resistant to standard treatments include the use of beta agonists and calcium channel blockers such as Nicardipine hydrochloride (Cardene)* and nifedipine* to decrease uterine contractility. These agents have also been shown to inhibit PG $F_2\alpha$ and vasopressin. A presacral neurectomy, or laparoscopic uterosacral ablation, should not be used to treat primary dysmenorrhea unless all other therapies have failed in a patient with incapacitating pain.

*Not FDA approved for this indication.

PREMENSTRUAL SYNDROME (PMS)

method of
C. JAMES CHUONG, M.D., M.P.H.
Baylor College of Medicine
Houston, Texas

Premenstrual syndrome (PMS) is defined as the cyclic psychological and somatic changes that occur for 10 to 14 days during the luteal phase of the ovulatory cycle. All the changes disappear dramatically within 2 days following the onset of menstrual flow or the onset of the following cycle in the case of hysterectomy, and the patients are free of symptoms for at least 2 weeks afterward. Psychological changes include irritability, tension, anxiety, mood swings, emotional lability, restlessness, decreased concentration, depression, aggression, lethargy, poor coordination, craving for sweet or salty food, crying easily, and increased or decreased sexual desire. Somatic changes include generalized swelling; breast tenderness; abdominal bloating; swelling of face, hands, and feet; weight gain; change in bowel habits; headache; dizziness; hot flushes; and acne.

For many years, both physicians and patients were ignorant of this syndrome; however, recent reports have drawn great interest from patients, media persons, and health care professionals. The social and economic concerns are further enhanced by the high prevalence of premenstrual symptom and the increased number and role of women in the work force. There is now a definite demand for professional attention to the condition.

ETIOLOGY

Numerous hypotheses regarding etiology have been proposed in the past 50 years. Although many investigators believe that PMS, like all physical diseases, arises from disordered physiology, others attempt to explain premenstrual symptoms on a psychogenic basis, and the pathophysiology remains elusive. Central nervous system (CNS) hormone dysregulation has been linked to PMS by the similarity of symptoms or by association with other emotional syndromes. These hormones include small peptides with opiate receptor activity (endogenous opioid peptides) such as serotonin, norepinephrine, dopamine, α-melanocyte–stimulating hormone, melatonin, and acetylcholine. Other theories include hypothalamic-pituitary-adrenal dysregulation, progesterone deficiency or withdrawal, fluid retention, hyperprolactinemia, abnormal prostaglandin metabolism, hypoglycemia, and thyroid dysfunction. However, no definite etiology has been identified, and PMS is still considered as a multifactorial psychosocial-neuroendocrinologic disorder.

DIAGNOSIS

The most important factor at the first visit is to devote considerable time listening to the patient relate her history. One should assess the patient's psychiatric history and explore her relationship with her family members and coworkers, if any. External stress associated with these relationships can make the premenstrual symptoms worse. Premenstrual changes may be confused with other gynecologic or psychiatric problems. The evaluation should include not only a detailed history but the formulation of a differential diagnosis of each complaint and a thorough physical and psychological examination, with laboratory and radiologic examinations, if indicated, and referral to other specialists when appropriate. It has been shown that PMS is associated with the number of deliveries, postpartum depression, past birth control pill use, alcohol and drug use, and history of PMS in first-degree relatives. It is also important to differentiate PMS from psychiatric disorders with premenstrual aggravation. As an aid to understanding the psychological status of patients presenting with premenstrual symptoms, the Minnesota Multiphasic Personality Inventory (MMPI) may be administered whenever necessary.

It is critical in establishing the diagnosis of PMS that symptoms occur specifically during the luteal phase of the cycle and that there is a symptom-free period of at least 1 week following the cessation of menstruation. Symptoms continuing after the fifth day of the menstrual cycle are not generally considered as PMS. There are still no uniformly accepted objective criteria for the diagnosis of PMS, and we have to depend on the patient's subjective report. Prospective recording of symptoms for at least 1 to 2 months using a daily diary, specific mood assessment charts, or specific visual linear analogue scales is much more predictive of premenstrual changes than are retrospective reports, which tend to overdiagnose PMS. Keeping careful records is also helpful in increasing the patient's awareness of the problems.

Laboratory Evaluation

Thyroid dysfunction, hyperandrogenism, diabetes mellitus, hypoglycemia, and hyperprolactinemia can cause somatic and affective symptoms that are occasionally mistaken for PMS. Therefore, thyroid work-up and measurement of serum afternoon cortisol, testosterone, glucose, and prolactin levels may be performed to rule out the underlying medical problems. However, the routine use of peripheral hormonal tests for patients with premenstrual complaints is not only costly but also not indicated at this time. This conclusion is based on the findings that no differences in hormone concentrations were observed in the serum levels or patterns of secretion of progesterone, estradiol, follicle-stimulating hormone, luteinizing hormone, sex hormone–binding globulin, dehydroepiandrosterone sulfate, dihydrotestosterone, prolactin, cortisol, growth hormone, or aldosterone during the follicular and luteal phases between PMS patients and controls.

MANAGEMENT

Treatment of PMS requires a multidisciplinary team that integrates the efforts of a gynecologist, an endocrinologist, a psychiatrist or psychologist, a social worker, and a nutritionist.

Patient Education

The patient should be reassured that this is a problem common to many women and that "she is not going crazy." It is most important that the woman be allowed to express herself and to describe her problems. The physician must attempt to familiarize the patient with the nature of the syndrome. With this knowledge and awareness, the patient may recognize the changes in herself and find a way to cope. The articulate patient can be encouraged to write a diary of her moods, feelings, activities, and functions during this premenstrual period. The diary can serve as another mode of ventilation and describe the pattern of the patient's premenstrual tension as well. She can then become more conscious of the changes that seem to occur in that week. Particularly important is the physician's sensitivity in helping the patient repair her emotional environment. The patient should be encouraged to join a local PMS support group, if one is available.

Diet and Exercise

The PMS Prevention Diet emphasizes whole fresh foods. Eating regular frequent small meals; decreasing the intake of salts, fats, sugar, and caffeine; and increasing exercise are helpful. Foods that are high in refined sugars and fats and that are highly processed are to be avoided. Intake of foods made from whole grains, legumes, seeds, nuts, vegetables, fruits, and vegetable oils should be encouraged.

Previous studies revealed that women who participated in sports experienced less premenstrual anxiety than nonathletic women. How exercise helps PMS is not clear, but exercise was noted to increase beta-endorphin levels, which may explain the sense of well-being reported by some patients. If beta-endorphin withdrawal contributes to PMS, it might be corrected, at least partially, by exercise.

Pharmacologic Therapy

If no improvement is reported within 1 to 2 months using the approach of education, diet, and exercise, pharmacologic therapy is added.

Treatment of Specific Symptoms

In a double-blind, placebo-controlled study, it was noted that 250 mg of prostaglandin synthetase inhibitor mefenamic acid (Ponstel), administered daily during the luteal phase, significantly improved many symptoms, particularly fatigue, headache, general aches and pains, and mood swings. Nonsteroidal anti-inflammatory agents such as acetylsalicylic acid (aspirin) or acetaminophen (Tylenol) with or without codeine are also used to relieve headaches, muscle, and joint pain.

Sumatriptan (Imitrex), a 5-hydroxytryptamine receptor agonist, has been shown to be effective and well tolerated by patients for menstruation-associated migraine as it is for nonmenstrual migraine. In a double-blind, placebo-controlled study, women were treated for a menstruation-associated migraine (1 day before and 4 days after the onset of menstrual flow) with 6 mg of sumatriptan in a 0.5-mL subcutaneous injection. A second injection was available to those who did not have significant improvement of headache 1 hour after the first injection. At 1 hour, 80% of the sumatriptan-treated patients had significant headache relief, compared with 19% of the placebo group. Other associated symptoms, such as nausea and photophobia were also improved. The most common adverse side effects were injection-site reactions, dizziness, tingling, nausea and vomiting, warm sensation, and chest tightness. Most adverse side effects lasted less than 1 hour. Clinical trials using other forms of the medication, such as rectal suppositories and oral pills, are currently under way.

Studies have shown significant improvement in reduction in weight and psychological symptoms using spironolactone (Aldactone), a potassium-sparing diuretic. If the patient gains weight, experiences bloatedness and edema premenstrually, and weight loss occurs dramatically after the onset of menstruation, spironolactone, 25 mg four times a day, or 100 mg once daily during the luteal phase, is recommended.

The dopaminergic agonist bromocriptine (Parlodel), 5 mg at night daily from days 10 to 26 of the cycle, was noted to produce a significant reduction in breast tenderness and swelling but was ineffective in controlling other symptoms of PMS. Danazol (Danocrine), 200 mg once or twice daily, could effectively suppress breast and other generalized symptoms.

Treatment of Generalized Symptoms

Naltrexone (Trexan).* The beta-endorphin withdrawal and deficiency hypothesis suggests treatment of PMS with exogenous beta-endorphin, but it is not practical because of addiction and the route of administration (intramuscular or intravenous). An opiate antagonist, given before the periovulatory beta-endorphin peak and withdrawal, might offer a rational treatment for PMS by keeping a rather constant level of beta-endorphin. Naltrexone is an oral pure narcotic antagonist that has been used in the treatment of withdrawal symptoms for patients with heroin addiction. Unlike drugs that have mixed agonist and antagonist effects, it does not cause addiction or withdrawal.

Recent studies suggest that naltrexone alleviates PMS symptoms and may be an effective treatment for this syndrome. The acceptability of this medication in the study was good, with only low incidence of nausea, decreased appetite, dizziness, and fainting, which may be minimized by further dividing or decreasing the dosage. Previously, we demonstrated a decrease of plasma beta-endorphin in PMS patients periovulatorily and near menses, and proposed that the premenstrual decrease of beta-endorphin may be responsible for the PMS symptoms. It is possible that naltrexone inhibited beta-endorphin withdrawal prevented the decrease of beta-endorphin levels, and thus, reduced the severity of symptoms significantly.

Vitamins and Minerals. It has been suggested that deficiencies of vitamins and minerals are related to PMS. However, recent studies did not demonstrate serum vitamin A, B_6, or E or magnesium deficiency in PMS patients compared with the controls in peripheral blood obtained at 2- or 3-day intervals throughout three menstrual cycles. However, serum zinc deficiency and copper excess were found during the luteal phase in PMS patients. Because copper competes with zinc for intestinal absorption and serum protein binding sites, the availability of zinc in patients premenstrually was reduced further by the elevated copper. PMS patients were also found to have lower serum calcium levels in the peripheral blood than controls. Whether these peripheral concentrations reflect central changes requires further studies.

Although deficiencies of vitamins and minerals in patients with PMS could not be demonstrated, a number of these supplements have appeared widely on the market over the past few years. It was reported that a combination tablet of vitamin B_6 and other essential micronutrients reduced the severity of many PMS symptoms at daily doses of 2 to 12 tablets that contained 100 to 600 mg of vitamin B_6. In contrast, another study showed that 150 mg of vitamin B_6 could improve only those premenstrual symptoms related to automatic reactions and behavioral changes but not the physical or affective symptoms. The efficacy of vitamin E in the treatment of PMS was studied in a double-blind, placebo-controlled trial. A significant improvement in certain affective and physical symptoms was noted in subjects treated with daily 400 IU of vitamin E.

The effects of vitamins and minerals in these studies could be due to a pharmacologic response rather than correction of a deficiency state. The roles of these supplements in beta-endorphin and other central neurohormone activities need to be clarified. Until these issues are addressed, the supplementation of vitamins and minerals can be considered only as empirical therapy for PMS.

Serotonin Uptake Inhibitor. Enhancement of serotonin synthesis and neurotransmission by administration of tryptophan or of serotonin-specific drugs has been used to treat some types of depressive illness. Administration of large doses of pyridoxine (vitamin B_6), a cofactor in serotonin synthesis, has been observed to alleviate depression, anxiety, irritability, and a number of other PMS symptoms. A recent study showed that carbohydrate consumption was effective in alleviating many of the luteal mood changes of the subjects with PMS and, in that capacity, thus exerted a therapeutic, not a nutritional, effect. The authors suggested that the absence of a complete remission may reflect the severity of the subjects' symptoms or the use of a nutrient instead of

*Not FDA approved for this indication.

a drug to relieve those patients' symptoms. Subsequently, a double-blind, placebo-controlled study was conducted using one of the serotonin uptake inhibitors, D-fenfluramine (Pondimin),* at 30 mg daily during the luteal phase. It significantly improved depressed mood and reduced calorie and carbohydrate intake. These results support the hypothesis that serotonin is involved in both the affective and appetitive symptoms of PMS. Studies using other serotonin uptake inhibitors in PMS, such as sertraline (Zoloft)* and fluvoxamine (Luvox)† are currently under investigation.

Progesterone.* Several studies have shown that a progesterone vaginal suppository is not superior to placebo in double-blind, placebo-controlled clinical trials despite higher circulating progesterone levels. An early study reported complete relief of symptoms in more than 83% of a group of 86 women with PMS. Although others question its efficacy, progesterone has remained one of the popular medications. Estrogen and progesterone have been noted to increase beta-endorphin levels in hypophyseal portal blood samples collected from ovariectomized monkeys. It is possible that the beneficial effect of progesterone is mediated by beta-endorphin; however, such data on human subjects are still lacking.

Psychotropic Agents. Several psychotropic agents have been used in the treatment of PMS, such as diazepam (Valium),* alprazolam (Xanax),* buspirone hydrocholoride (BuSpar),* clorazepate dipotassium (Tranxene),* clonazepam (Klonopin),* amitriptyline hydrochloloride (Elavil),* and tricyclic agents. Because of the required long-term therapy for PMS patients, these agents may produce undesirable side effects over time. It is recommended that these agents be given only to patients with severe symptoms as a short-term adjuvant to other therapies.

Medical Oophorectomy. In a cross-over study, it was demonstrated that elimination of ovarian cyclicity through down-regulation of pituitary gonadotropin secretion with a daily subcutaneous injection of gonadotropin-releasing hormone agonist resulted in marked attenuation of premenstrual symptoms. The therapy was rapidly reversible with no influence on subsequent cycles. Medical oophorectomy is supposed to prevent the fluctuation and deficiency of beta-endorphin levels by causing temporary cessation of cyclic ovarian activity. Studies using monthly leuprolide acetate (Lupron Depot),* daily nafarelin acetate (Synarel),* and other gonadotropin-releasing hormone agonists showed similar results. Danazol (Danocrine), at a dosage of 600 to 800 mg daily, can also achieve reversible medical oophorectomy. One study showed PMS symptoms were improved with danazol, 200 mg daily for 90 days, during the anovulatory cycles but not during the ovulatory cycles.

The safety and side effects of long-term medical oophorectomy remain to be determined. Studies using "add-back" synthetic sex steroid therapy to prevent bone loss in patients given gonadotropin-releasing hormone agonists are currently under investigation. The use of gonadotropin-releasing hormone antagonists, which can achieve medical oophorectomy in a much more rapid fashion with rapid reversal, is anticipated in the near future, assuming its side effects, such as effects caused by histamine release, can be minimized.

Bilateral Oophorectomy With or Without Hysterectomy. Two studies showed that total abdominal hysterectomy and salpingo-oophorectomy with low-dose estrogen replacement was effective in relieving the symptoms in women with severe, debilitating PMS who did not respond to conventional interventions. Most patients in the studies were placed on danazol, 400 mg daily or higher dosages, for 3 to 9 months, to suppress menstrual cyclicity. A lasting benefit from ovarian suppression was ensured prior to the surgery. The surgical solution to PMS should be considered only as the last resort after careful screening of patients and after all forms of medical therapies have failed. Only those who have completed childbearing should be considered for this option. Because PMS is related to ovarian function, bilateral oophorectomy alone by laparoscopy should be sufficient.

Continuous estrogen and progestin replacement after surgery can avoid monthly withdrawal bleeding and PMS-like symptoms. Concurrent hysterectomy is also indicated if the patient has other gynecologic conditions, such as fibroid uterus, severe dysmenorrhea, and severe menorrhagia. Patients who underwent hysterectomy alone with intact ovaries were noted to have persistent cyclic luteal phase symptoms in the absence of menstrual flow, as shown on the symptom calendar and basal body temperature chart. Endometrial ablation is not expected to improve the symptoms because ovarian function is still preserved.

MENOPAUSE

method of
DANIEL R. MISHELL, Jr., M.D.
University of Southern California School of Medicine and Women's Hospital
Los Angeles, California

The mean age of menopause is about 51 years, with a normal distribution curve and 95% confidence limits between ages 45 and 55. The average life expectancy for a woman in the United States is about 78 years, and about one-third of a woman's life will be spent after menopause. This time of life should be considered an estrogen-deficiency state, and improvement in both the quality and the quantity of life can be obtained with the use of estrogen replacement during the postmenopausal years.

*Not FDA approved for this indication.
†Investigational drug in the United States.

GENITOURINARY EFFECTS

Atrophy of the genitourinary tract can produce symptoms of atrophic vaginitis, with itching, burning, dyspareunia, and possible vaginal bleeding. Local estrogen therapy rapidly relieves these symptoms, but because vaginal administration of estrogen results in irregular systemic absorption, estrogen is best administered systemically for long-term prevention of vaginal atrophy as well as osteoporosis. Estrogen deficiency may also cause uterine prolapse because the supporting ligaments lose their tonicity. In addition, cystocele and rectocele may develop as a result of estrogen deficiency. These changes can be prevented or alleviated by administering estrogen. The trigone of the bladder and the urethra are embryologically derived from estrogen-dependent tissue, and postmenopausal estrogen deficiency causes atrophy of these structures, producing symptoms of urinary urgency, incontinence, dysuria, and urinary frequency. Because of atrophy of collagen in the periurethral fascia, urinary stress incontinence can also occur. If these symptoms develop after menopause, estrogen replacement alleviates the problem in a high percentage of women.

CENTRAL NERVOUS SYSTEM CHANGES

The pathognomonic symptom of the menopause is the hot flush or flash, which is caused by a decrease in circulating estrogen levels. The best treatment for the hot flush is estrogen, which has been shown to alleviate symptoms better than placebo. It is best to administer estrogen at bedtime to prevent the hot flushes that can interfere with sleep. The usual initial dosage is 0.625 mg of conjugated estrogen (Premarin), or 1 mg of estradiol (Estrace), although higher doses may be necessary, especially when the ovaries are removed in a premenopausal individual. For women with contraindications to estrogen therapy (e.g., cancer of the breast or endometrium), other medications that are effective in treating hot flushes include oral medroxyprogesterone acetate (Provera) in a dosage of 10 mg per day. Hot flushes can also be relieved by a single injection of Depo-Provera,* 150 mg given once every 3 months. In addition, clonidine (Catapres) in a dosage of 150 μg per day can also reduce the incidence of hot flushes.

Symptoms such as anxiety, depression, irritability, and fatigue increase after the menopause, and it has been shown that estrogen replacement significantly relieves these symptoms even in women who do not have hot flushes that interfere with sleep. In addition to decreasing the incidence of depression, recent studies show that estrogen users are less likely to develop Alzheimer's disease. Because urinary incontinence and dementia are the two major reasons why women are admitted to chronic care facilities, estrogen replacement can enable them to stay in a self-care environment.

*This use is not listed by the manufacturer.

Studies have shown that postmenopausal estrogen users have a significantly thicker skin and a greater amount of collagen in the dermis than do postmenopausal women who do not use estrogen. Thus, systemic estrogen use can retard the wrinkling and thinning of the skin that occurs postmenopausally.

OSTEOPOROSIS

Postmenopausal osteoporosis affects about 25% of women but is uncommon in black persons and in obese women. In thin white and Asian women, about 1% to 1.5% of bone mass is lost each year after the menopause. Bone loss is more rapid in trabecular bone, which is found mainly in the thoracic spine, than in cortical bone, which is present in the axial skeleton. Beginning about age 60, fractures occur in the vertebral spine as well as the distal portion of the radius, which is also composed of trabecular bone. The incidence of fractures of the neck of the femur, which is made up mainly of cortical bone, usually start to increase at about age 70 and increase at a logarithmic rate thereafter. Estrogen therapy reduces the bone loss associated with postmenopausal osteoporosis and thus reduces the fracture rate in women, prolonging their productive life span as well as providing great savings in health care costs. Supplemental calcium therapy and weight-bearing exercise are ancillary measures that, by themselves, will retard but not prevent postmenopausal bone loss. The following factors are known to increase the risk of osteoporosis: (1) white or Asian race; (2) reduced weight for height; (3) early spontaneous menopause or early surgical menopause; (4) family history of osteoporosis, (5) a diet low in calcium intake, high in caffeine intake, or high in alcohol intake; (6) cigarette smoking; and (7) sedentary lifestyle. Routine screening by densitometry or computed tomography scanning is not cost effective and is not recommended to determine whether osteoporosis is developing postmenopausally.

Osteoporosis is associated with an increased rate of bone resorption, and the administration of estrogen will return the resorption rate to normal. Numerous prospective and retrospective epidemiologic studies have shown that estrogen therapy reduces the amount of postmenopausal bone loss: When estrogen is discontinued, the rate of bone loss rapidly increases to the same rate as that occurring immediately postmenopausally. Therefore, estrogen replacement therapy should be maintained as long as a woman is ambulatory. The minimum dosage of estrogen needed to prevent osteoporosis is 0.625 mg of conjugated equine estrogen (Premarin), 0.625 of piperazine estrone sulfate (Ogen), or 0.5 mg of micronized estradiol (Estrace). It is recommended that in addition to estrogen, about 700 mg of calcium should be ingested daily, and weight-bearing exercise such as walking should be encouraged. Supplemental use of vitamin D is of no benefit. There is no need for additional calcium supplementation beyond the 700 mg of daily dietary calcium in women receiving adequate estrogen replacement.

CARDIOVASCULAR EFFECTS

Because estrogen replacement regimens have a minimal effect on liver globulins, postmenopausal estrogen users do not have an increase in mean blood pressure compared with women not ingesting estrogen. It is safe to provide estrogen replacement for postmenopausal women with or without pre-existing hypertension. Because natural estrogens do not produce a hypercoagulable state, available data indicate that postmenopausal women with or without a past history of thrombophlebitis do not have an increased incidence of thrombophlebitis with estrogen replacement therapy. Use of estrogen replacement has been shown in numerous retrospective as well as prospective epidemiologic studies to reduce the risk of myocardial infarction by about 50%. Estrogen replacement also reduces the risk of stroke by about 50%. Oral estrogen increases levels of the cardioproductive high-density lipoprotein cholesterol as well as directly increasing coronary artery blood flow. The substantial reduction of rate of myocardial infarction, which is the major cause of mortality in women, is a major beneficial effect of estrogen. Age-adjusted data from several studies indicate that the mortality rate from all causes is significantly lower in estrogen users than in nonusers (Table 1).

NEOPLASTIC EFFECTS

Six meta-analyses, each combining the data of several epidemiologic studies, have shown there is no significantly increased risk of breast cancer in women using estrogen replacement therapy compared with nonusers. Only a few of any epidemiologic studies investigating the relation of estrogen use and breast cancer have shown an increased risk of breast cancer in some subsets of postmenopausal estrogen users, specifically long-term users of high doses of estradiol but not conjugated equine estrogen. Several studies show no effect of conjugated equine estrogen on this cancer. Because estrogen can stimulate the growth of a nonpalpable breast cancer, it is advisable that all women have mammograms performed before the initiation of estrogen therapy. If no tumor is found, patients can be told that oral estrogen use will not increase the risk of developing breast cancer. There is a significantly increased risk of developing endometrial cancer in postmenopausal women who are ingesting estrogen without progestins. This risk increases with increased duration of estrogen use as well as with increased dosage. The endometrial cancer that develops in estrogen users is usually well differentiated and is usually cured by performing a simple hysterectomy. The increased risk of developing this endometrial carcinoma in women receiving estrogen replacement can be eliminated by also administering progestins. The duration of progestin therapy is more important than the dosage, and it is now recommended that the progestin be administered for at least 12 days per month. The addition of progestin to the estrogen therapy acts synergistically to cause a slight increase in bone density. However, progestins reverse some of the beneficial effects of estrogen on serum lipids and, thus, should not be given to women who do not have a uterus. Several epidemiologic studies investigating the use of progestins with estrogen and the risk of breast cancer have yielded conflicting results. Therefore, a beneficial effect of progestin on breast cancer risk has not been substantiated.

TABLE 1. **Relative Risk Estimates from Cohort Studies of Use of Estrogen Replacement Therapy and Mortality from Cardiovascular Disease, Cerebrovascular Diseases, and All Causes**

Study	Relative Risk		
	CHD	*CVD*	*AC*
Burch et al	0.4*	0.9	0.4*
Stamper et al	0.6	—	0.51*
Wilson et al	1.9	—	0.97
Henderson and Paganini-Hill et al	0.6*	0.5*	0.8*
Petitti et al	0.5*	—	0.7*
Bush et al	0.4*	0.4	0.5*
Hunt et al	0.5*	0.6	0.6*
Criqui et al	0.7	—	0.7*

Abbreviations: AC = all causes; CHD = cardiovascular disease; CVD = cerebrovascular disease.

*$p < 0.05$

From Henderson BE, Paganini-Hill A, and Ross RK: Decreased mortality in users of estrogen replacement therapy. Arch Int Med *151*:74–78, 1991.

TREATMENT REGIMENS

The treatment regimen most commonly used in the United States is the sequential regimen of 0.625 mg of conjugated estrogen or 1 mg of estradiol orally for the first 25 days each month. Beginning on day 12 to 15 of estrogen treatment, 5 to 10 mg of medroxyprogesterone acetate is added daily for 10 to 13 days. With this regimen, more than half the women have regular withdrawal bleeding, an annoying problem that decreases patient compliance to continued use. It is not necessary to have withdrawal bleeding to slough the endometrium to reduce the risk of endometrial cancer. A continuous regimen in which the estrogen is given daily together with a small dose of oral progestin, such as 2.5 or 5 mg of medroxyprogesterone acetate, reduces the chance of developing uterine bleeding as well as avoiding a week off treatment, in which symptoms may appear. Data from several recent studies indicate that most women do not bleed on this regimen, and the endometrium usually remains atrophic. A routine pretreatment endometrial biopsy is unnecessary, because it is not cost effective, and routine annual endometrial biopsies are not necessary unless breakthrough bleeding occurs. For women who do bleed, if a sonogram of the uterus reveals the endometrial thickness to be less than 5 mm, a biopsy is probably unnecessary because the endometrium is nearly always atrophic.

Estrogen replacement therapy is indicated for nearly all postmenopausal women because of its numerous beneficial effects. Contraindications to estrogen replacement are uncommon. These include a history of breast cancer, recent history of endometrial cancer, active liver disease, or the presence of thrombophlebitis. A past history of thrombophlebitis hypertension or diabetes mellitus is not an absolute contraindication for estrogen replacement therapy.

VULVOVAGINITIS

method of
MAURIZIO MACCATO, M.D.
Baylor College of Medicine
Houston, Texas

Vulvovaginitis is one of the most common gynecologic disorders. It has both infectious and noninfectious causes. The most common infectious causes include several different species of yeasts, *Trichomonas vaginalis,* and *Gardnerella vaginalis* with its associated proliferation of anaerobic bacteria. In the postmenopausal woman, atrophic vaginitis is the most common noninfectious cause of vaginitis. In prepubertal girls, *Neisseria gonorrhoeae,* Group A beta-hemolytic streptococcus *(Streptococcus pyogenes),* other bacteria, pinworms, and foreign bodies in the vagina are also possible causes of vaginitis.

DIAGNOSIS

Proper therapy of this condition is based on the careful determination of the etiologic agent. The history and physical examination provide clues as to the cause of the vaginitis. Confirmation of such suspicion is generally obtained by straightforward laboratory tests that can be performed, in the majority of cases, directly in the office of the practitioner. The evaluation of the patient should include a menstrual history, especially in postmenopausal women, when the development of symptoms may be associated with a significant decrease in estrogen level. The sexual history and the history of use of medications such as antibiotics, oral contraceptives, or immunosuppressive agents should be obtained. The pelvic examination is vital to determine the correct type of vaginitis.

It is important to point out that in the majority of cases, the history and physical examination alone should not be relied on to make the definitive diagnosis because there is a significant degree of overlap between the signs and symptoms associated with the various types of vaginitis. Therefore, the etiologic agent should be confirmed by laboratory testing, as will be discussed in the following section.

MONILIAL VULVOVAGINITIS

One of the most common causes of infectious vulvovaginitis is a yeast, usually *Candida albicans.* Other organisms are *Candida glabarata* and *Candida tropicalis.* A handful of case reports of less common yeasts have appeared in the literature. *Candida albicans* is responsible for more than 90% of all cases of yeast vaginitis. Itching is the most common symptom associated with vulvovaginal candidiasis. An unusual odor is not a prominent feature of this vaginitis. The physical examination reveals a discharge that is usually white and clumpy. Plaques of secretions may be adherent to the mucous membrane of the vagina, and on their removal, a reddened and irritated base is noted.

The confirmatory test for vulvovaginal candidiasis is the examination of the discharge by wet mount or KOH preparation. A drop of vaginal secretion is suspended in a drop of saline, and it is examined under the microscope. The identifications of yeast in the wet mount confirms the diagnosis suspected on clinical grounds. The examination of a drop of vaginal fluid suspended in a solution of 10% KOH may help in identification of the yeast by lysing epithelial cells. The pH of the vaginal discharge is usually normal (i.e., less than 4.5). The so-called whiff test is negative. In this test, the application of 10% KOH to a sample of the vaginal discharge will not release the amine odor characteristic of bacterial vaginosis. It should be noticed that in approximately 30% of patients with vulvovaginal candidiasis, the examination of the discharge for yeast forms by wet mount will not reveal the presence of either cellular or hyphal forms. Therefore, in the presence of the appropriate signs and symptoms (i.e., a normal pH and a negative whiff test), it is reasonable to assume that the symptoms are caused by yeast, and an adequate antifungal therapy may be prescribed. Culture of the vaginal secretion for yeast is another method to confirm the diagnosis.

Recurrent monilial vulvovaginitis is a vexing problem for both patients and physicians alike. The etiology of such recurrent infections is frequently unclear. Therapy of the sexual partner is rarely associated with a decrease in the rate of recurrence. It is possible that the source of the patient's continued colonization of the vagina may be the lower gastrointestinal tract. Unfortunately, therapy of the gastrointestinal tract with oral antifungal agents does not reliably decrease the incidence of recurrent infection. Therapy of such infection is frequently based on long-term suppression of the causative agents of the vaginitis as is discussed in the following section.

Treatment

First-line therapy for vulvovaginal candidiasis are vaginal creams containing an antifungal agent, most frequently of the imidazole class. Common topical drugs are summarized in Table 1. The two alternative agents (boric acid gelatin capsules 600 mg, intravaginally, twice daily for 2 weeks, and gentian violet used as a 1% aqueous solution) have been used with success, especially in the therapy of species of *Candida* other than *Candida albicans.* Gentian violet is

TABLE 1. **Topical Agents Used in the Initial Therapy of Fungal Vulvovaginitis**

Generic Name	Trade Name
Miconazole	Monistat
Clotrimazole	Lotrimin, Mycelex
Butoconazole	Femstat
Terconazole	Terazol
Tioconazole	Vagistat
Nystatin	Mycostatin
Alternatives	
Gentian violet (1% aqueous solution)	
Boric acid (gelatin capsules)	

an aniline dye that is mutagenic and has been associated with possible teratogenic effects, and it is therefore seldom used.

Oral antifungal agents include ketoconazole (Nizoral), fluconazole (Diflucan), and itraconazole (Sporanox). All three have demonstrated activity against vulvovaginal candidiasis. They have not, at this point, been considered as first-line therapy because of their systemic effects. In particular, ketoconazole has been associated with liver dysfunction in some patients. The role of the oral antifungal agents may be found in long-term suppression of recurrent candidal vaginitis in specific patients. They may also have a role in the prevention of infection in patients with immunodeficiencies.

BACTERIAL VAGINOSIS

On physical examination, bacterial vaginosis is characterized by a grayish discharge, which is at times profuse and associated with an amine odor. Itching is generally not a significant problem. The examination of the discharge on a wet mount reveals epithelial cells that have bacteria adherent to them, which are the so-called clue cells. The performance of a whiff test on the discharge will reveal the characteristic fishy odor of amines. The pH of the vaginal discharge is usually greater than 4.7. Although the microbiology of bacterial vaginosis is exceedingly complex, the presence of *Gardnerella vaginalis* and an increased number of anaerobic bacteria and a decrease in the number of *Lactobacillus* appears to be the dominant characteristic of the microbiology of the vagina affected by bacterial vaginosis.

Treatment

With the above-noted changes in microbiology, the therapy of bacterial vaginosis hinges on the use of antibiotics that decrease the number of anaerobic organisms and are effective against *Gardnerella vaginalis.* The use of metronidazole (Flagyl) has been advocated. Metronidazole can be administered either as an oral agent at a dose of 500 mg twice daily for 1 week or as an intravaginal cream (MetroGel). Other agents that have demonstrated efficacy in the conditions are clindamycin (Cleocin), either orally or intravaginally (as a 2% cream), and amoxicillin-clavulanic acid (Augmentin). Amoxicillin-clavulanic acid also is effective against *Gardnerella vaginalis,* an organism that is only partially susceptible to Flagyl. The advantage of intravaginal versus systemic therapy with metronidazole or clindamycin is the reduction in the risk of possible side effects from these agents, especially diarrhea with clindamycin and an Antabuse effect with metronidazole. With the use of amoxicillin-clavulanic acid, it is wise to anticipate the possible development of yeast overgrowth in the vagina.

The problem of chronic recurrent bacterial vaginosis again is the subject of much current research. It appears that the treatment of the sexual partner in recurrent bacterial vaginitis may decrease the risk of recurrence.

TRICHOMONIASIS

Trichomonas vaginalis is the flagellate protozoan responsible for the development of trichomonas vaginitis. The organism is both species specific and site specific. It causes a vaginitis with a profuse, greenish, malodorous discharge. Irritation of the cervix often leads to punctate lesions in the cervix, giving it the characteristic appearance of a so-called strawberry cervix, often best appreciated on colposcopy.

The pH of the vaginal discharge is above 4.5, and because of a proliferation of anaerobic organisms, the whiff test is again positive. Motile *Trichomonas vaginalis* are usually easily identified on wet mount of the discharge. The organism may be cultured as well in Diamond's media. Trichomoniasis is almost invariably a sexually transmitted condition. Treatment of the partner, therefore, is indispensable in order to prevent re-infection. However, in rare occasions, the transmission of trichomonas by nonsexual methods has been demonstrated. It has also been noted that trichomonas may remain asymptomatic for long periods of time. Recurrent trichomoniasis is usually related to failure of adequate therapy of all sexual partners involved. In rare occasions, it may be secondary to the presence of true resistance to metronidazole of the organism. Table 2 summarizes the characteristics of the most common vaginal infections.

TABLE 2. **Characteristics of Vaginal Infections**

	Vaginal Discharge	Symptoms	Wet Mount	pH
Fungal	White, sometimes curdy	Itching	Budding yeast, pseudohyphae	<4.5
Bacterial vaginosis	Gray, homogeneous	Malodorous discharge	Clue cells	>4.5
Trichomoniasis	Greenish, sometimes frothy	Malodorous discharge, itching	Trichomonads, white blood cells	>4.5

Treatment

The current recommended treatment for trichomoniasis is oral metronidazole (Flagyl). The dose of metronidazole varies from 250 mg orally three times a day for a week to 500 mg twice a day for 1 week or a single oral dose of 2 grams. It appears that 250 mg orally three times a day may have a slightly higher cure rate than the single dose of 2 grams. The decision of which regimen to use should be based on the requirements of the specific patient and the likelihood of adequate compliance of the patient to the various regimens. Again, it is important to ensure treatment of all sexual partners.

Strains of *Trichomonas vaginalis* resistant to metronidazole have been identified. In these cases, the use of combined oral and intravaginal metronidazole or intravenous metronidazole has been advocated. It has been observed that clotrimazole (Mycelex) used intravaginally provides some relief of the symptoms. The therapy is however, not curative. The use of a vaginal douche with 20% sodium chloride has been used with some success as well. It is important to remember that metronidazole has an Antabuse-like effect and, therefore while the patient is on therapy with metronidazole, she should avoid alcohol. Metronidazole also is not recommended during the first trimester of pregnancy because of concerns about mutagenicity. No teratogenetic effect, however, has ever been described in humans, even when it is used in the first trimester.

POSTMENOPAUSAL PATIENTS

Atrophic vaginitis has to be included in the differential diagnosis of vaginitis in postmenopausal women. The diagnosis is suspected because of the absence of identifiable infectious disease etiologies for the vaginitis in the presence of a hypoestrogenic state. On wet mount, a large number of white blood cells are noted.

The therapy involves the supplementation of estrogen either orally or intravaginally. It is important to remember that the hypoestrogenic vagina has a pH of greater than 5.0. Vaginal and vulval pruritus also are commonly associated with malignancies of the vulva, and therefore, evaluation of the patients for such a possibility is imperative.

PREMENARCHEAL GIRLS

In premenarcheal women the etiology of vaginitis may not be confined to the same organisms discussed earlier. *Neisseria gonorrhoeae, Streptococcus pyogenes,* and shigella and other bacteria may all be associated with the development of vaginitis. In this population, it is, therefore, useful to routinely obtain cultures of the vaginal discharge. The presence of a foreign body in the vagina is also a frequent finding in young girls presenting with vaginitis. Therefore, careful inspection of the vagina for such an occurrence is important. Therapy of this type of vaginitis is based on the etiologic agents.

TOXIC SHOCK SYNDROME

method of
GARY R. SCHWARTZ, M.D., and
SETH W. WRIGHT, M.D.
Vanderbilt University Medical Center
Nashville, Tennessee

Toxic shock syndrome (TSS) is a toxin-mediated illness characterized by fever, hypotension, erythroderma, delayed desquamation, and multisystem organ dysfunction. The syndrome was first described by Todd and coworkers in 1978 in seven children, and an association with *Staphylococcus aureus* was postulated at that time. Shortly thereafter, numerous cases of this newly recognized syndrome were reported, primarily in menstruating young women. In 1980, there were 890 reported cases, 91% of which were associated with menstruation. Epidemiologic investigation revealed an association with the use of superabsorbent tampons, and in September 1980, the popular tampon Rely was voluntarily withdrawn from the market following massive lay media coverage.

The incidence of TSS has fallen dramatically in recent years, with only 44 definitive cases reported to the Centers for Disease Control and Prevention (CDC) in 1992. Presumably, the decline in cases is a result of changes in the composition of tampons and education of consumers, although there probably is underdiagnosis and underreporting of cases. The case-fatality rate was originally reported at 13% in 1980, but the rate has fallen dramatically since then. There was one reported death from TSS in 1992. The number of nonmenstrual cases of TSS, accounting for 45% of all cases of TSS in 1992, has not significantly decreased. Table 1 lists some of the nonmenstrual causes of toxic shock syndrome.

PATHOGENESIS

Toxic shock syndrome is caused by one or more exotoxins produced by *S. aureus.* An exotoxin, toxic shock syndrome toxin 1 (TSST-1), was identified in 1984 and is believed to play a central role in the pathogenesis of the disease. TSST-1–producing strains of *S. aureus* are found in the majority of patients with TSS. TSST-1 has both a direct effect and the ability to stimulate production of interleukin-1 and tumor necrosis factor. In addition to TSST-1, there must be additional toxins that mediate TSS because TSST-1 cannot be isolated from all patients with the syndrome.

Because exotoxin–producing strains of *S. aureus* are very common but the disease is rare, there must be other factors that make a host susceptible. Increased susceptibility may be related to the ability of the immune system to produce antibodies against TSST-1. It has been found that most

TABLE 1. **Nonmenstrual Causes of Toxic Shock Syndrome**

Surgical infections
Abscesses
Infected burns and skin wounds
Nasal packing
Childbirth
Septic abortion
Barrier contraceptives
Postinfluenzal complications
Osteomyelitis
Endocarditis

patients with TSS have very low levels of antibodies against TSST-1, whereas most controls have high levels of antibodies. Convalescent titers of anti-TSST-1 also remain low in the majority of patients recovering from TSS. Why some individuals do not mount an adequate antibody response is not known.

CLINICAL PRESENTATION

The diagnosis of TSS is made clinically because there are no laboratory tests specific for the disease. The disease classically presents with the abrupt onset of fever, shock, and multisystem organ dysfunction. A hallmark of TSS is the rapidity of the onset of symptoms, which often occurs within 48 hours. Table 2 lists the current CDC case definition.

Cutaneous findings are always present in patients with the disease. The characteristic rash is a nonpruritic, blanching, erythroderma that resembles a sunburn. It occurs on the trunk but spreads to the extremities with accentuation in the flexural areas. The rash can be subtle, particularly in dark-skinned individuals. Prominent nonpitting edema of the face, eyelids, hands, and soles may also be seen. Conjunctival injection and a strawberry tongue are frequently noted. Desquamation of the skin is always noted during convalescence in survivors. By definition, hypotension or an orthostatic change in blood pressure usually is present. The mechanism is probably multifactorial, involving decreased vascular tone, capillary leakage, depressed myocardial function, and volume loss from fever, vomiting and diarrhea. Patients may develop adult respiratory distress syndrome with hypoxia and pulmonary edema. The pulmonary edema primarily results from capillary leakage, but myocardial depression may cause cardiogenic shock in some patients. Exudative pleural effusions due to capillary leakage are almost universally seen.

TABLE 2. **Centers for Disease Control and Prevention Case Definition for Toxic Shock Syndrome**

Fever:
  Temperature ≥38.9° C (102° F)
Rash:
  Diffuse macular erythroderma
Desquamation:
  1 to 2 weeks after onset of illness, particularly of palms and soles
Hypotension:
  Systolic BP ≤90 mm Hg for adults or below fifth percentile by age for children below 16 years old, or orthostatic drop in diastolic BP ≥15 mm Hg from lying to sitting, orthostatic syncope, or orthostatic dizziness.
Multisystem involvement—three or more of the following:
  GI: Vomiting or diarrhea at onset of illness
  Musculoskeletal: Severe myalgia or creatine kinase level at least twice the upper level of normal
  Mucous membrane: Vaginal, oropharyngeal, or conjunctival hyperemia
  Renal: BUN or creatinine at least twice the upper limit of normal or urinary sediment with pyuria (≥5 leukocytes per high power field) in the absence of urinary tract infection
  Hepatic: Total bilirubin, SGOT, or SGPT at least twice the upper limit of normal
  Hematologic: Platelets ≤100,000/mm^3
  CNS: Disorientation or alterations in consciousness without focal neurologic signs when fever and hypotension are absent
Negative results on the following test, if obtained:
  Blood, throat, or CSF fluid cultures (blood cultures may be positive for *S. aureus*)
  Rise in titer to Rocky Mountain spotted fever, leptospirosis, or rubeola

Abbreviations: BUN = blood urea nitrogen; CSF = cerebrospinal fluid; SGOT = serum glutamic-oxaloacetic transaminase; SGPT = serum glutamate pyruvate transaminase.

Gastrointestinal involvement is almost always present. Usually, the first symptom is vomiting, followed by abdominal pain and watery diarrhea. The stools may contain blood and have leukocytes on microscopic examination. Liver enzymes are elevated in over half the patients. Hepatomegaly is common. Myalgias and arthralgias are common early symptoms, and they may be severe. Lumbar, cervical, and abdominal muscles are most commonly involved and may be tender to the touch. The creatinine kinase is elevated in over half the patients. The pelvic examination may reveal a tampon still in place if the disease is menstrually related. Examination may also reveal hyperemia of the thighs and external genitalia and a malodorous vaginal discharge. A Gram's stain of the discharge may reveal gram-positive cocci. Evidence of acute renal insufficiency is common in TSS and is exhibited by increased urea nitrogen and creatinine. The renal dysfunction may be oliguric or nonoliguric and is usually reversible. Dialysis may be required when severe azotemia is present.

There is a wide spectrum of neurologic manifestations of TSS. Most patients report having a headache, and meningismus may be present. Hallucinations, disorientation, confusion, and agitation are all common. Examination of the cerebrospinal fluid shows normal glucose and protein levels and, occasionally, an elevated white cell count. Cerebral edema has been reported in fatal cases. Neuropsychiatric sequelae such as difficulty with memory and concentration may be found in up to 50% of patients.

Laboratory abnormalities are frequently present and reflect the multisystem effect of TSST-1. There are no specific laboratory diagnostic tests for TSS; however, many nonspecific abnormalities are discovered on laboratory evaluation. The complete blood cell count usually shows a normal or low normochromic normocytic red cell pattern, leukocytosis with many immature white cell forms, and mild thrombocytopenia. Also present may be electrolyte abnormalities, including hyponatremia, hypokalemia, hypomagnesemia, hypocalcemia, hypoalbuminemia, and hypophosphatemia. An elevated lactate is commonly due to hypotension.

The differential diagnosis of toxic shock syndrome is lengthy, primarily consisting of diseases characterized by fever and rash. Table 3 lists some of the disorders that should be considered when evaluating patients with signs and symptoms suggestive of TSS. One recently described illness, caused by a virulent strain of *Streptococcus pyogenes,* merits mentioning. This toxin-mediated illness is characterized by fever, hypotension, rash, and multisystem organ dysfunction and may be clinically indistinguishable from TSS.

MANAGEMENT

The key to management of TSS is early diagnosis followed by rapid and aggressive treatment. Treatment is directed at removing the source of the infection, general stabilization of the patient, management of complications, and prevention of recurrent disease. Most patients are critically ill and require admission to the intensive care unit. Less severely ill patients can be admitted to a general medical ward, but close supervision by medical and nursing personnel is mandatory.

In all cases, the underlying source of the toxin

TABLE 3. **Differential Diagnosis of Toxic Shock Syndrome**

Kawasaki disease
Staphylococcal scalded skin syndrome
Scarlet fever
Streptococcal toxic shock–like syndrome
Rocky Mountain spotted fever
Leptospirosis
Stevens-Johnson syndrome
Septic shock
Meningococcemia
Measles

must be removed to eliminate any preformed toxin and to prevent the formation of additional toxin. In menstruating women, this involves the removal of the tampon, followed by irrigation of the vagina. If the patient has recently had an operation, the operative site must be closely examined for signs of infection. Any skin abscess or operative site should be explored and drained. Any operative packing material should be removed.

Aggressive fluid resuscitation is the mainstay of therapy for most patients, and large volumes may be required. Normal saline and lactated Ringer's solution are the preferred fluids because there is some evidence that the use of colloid solutions may be associated with a higher incidence of noncardiogenic pulmonary edema. Fluids are best administered through a large-bore peripheral catheter or through a central venous line. Patients with persistent shock after an adequate fluid challenge may require invasive monitoring with a Swan-Ganz catheter and arterial line to determine hemodynamic parameters. Additional fluid challenges should be administered to obtain a pulmonary capillary wedge pressure of 15 to 20 mm Hg. Patients with persistent hypotension that is not responsive to fluids require a pressor, such as dopamine or norepinephrine. Patients with evidence of myocardial dysfunction (manifested by low cardiac index and high wedge pressure) require inotropic support with dobutamine or amrinone. Urine output should be monitored with a indwelling catheter.

The respiratory status of critically ill patients should be monitored with continuous pulse oximetry, and blood gas analysis should be performed as indicated. The combination of hypoxemia, pulmonary infiltrates, and a low or normal pulmonary capillary wedge pressure is suggestive of adult respiratory distress syndrome. Positive pressure ventilation via endotracheal intubation is indicated in patients with adult respiratory distress syndrome. High-peak end-expiratory pressure and a high F_IO_2 may be required to provide adequate oxygenation.

Antibiotics with antistaphylococcal coverage should be started in all patients with TSS. A beta-lactamase–resistant penicillin such as nafcillin (Nafcil), 1 to 2 grams every 4 hours, is recommended for most patients. An alternative agent is cefazolin (Ancef), 1 to 2 grams every 6 hours, or vancomycin (Vancocin), 1 gram twice daily. Toxic shock syndrome and gram-negative sepsis may appear very similar clinically, and antibiotic treatment with a aminoglycoside such as gentamicin (Garamycin) should be added if the diagnosis is in doubt. Parenteral antibiotic coverage can be switched to the oral form when tolerated by the patient. Antibiotics should be continued for a 14-day course. It should be noted that the administration of antibiotics has not been shown to alter the course of the disease but is instrumental in the prevention of recurrent illness.

One retrospective study has suggested that corticosteroid therapy may decrease the severity of the illness and the duration of fever, although this has not been confirmed in a prospective study. We would recommend that corticosteroids be given only to severely ill patients with persistent hypotension and those with known or suspected adrenal insufficiency. When they are given, corticosteroids should be used early in the course of the disease. The suggested agent is methylprednisolone (Solu-Medrol), 10-30 mg per kg per day in divided doses.

Pooled immunoglobulin contains high levels of antibodies to TSST-1 and may be useful in neutralizing the circulating toxin in severely ill patients. The efficacy of immunoglobulin has not been proved in clinical trials, but animal studies suggest that this therapy would improve outcome. Immunoglobulin therapy might be most beneficial when the source of infection cannot be easily removed, such as endocarditis or tracheitis. This therapy is very expensive and we suggest that its use be reserved only for the sickest patients.

SEQUELAE

Most patients fully recover from TSS. All surviving patients have desquamation, usually of the palms and soles. Sequelae from prolonged shock may include delayed hair and nail growth as well as renal failure requiring long-term dialysis. Neuropsychological complications such as memory loss, depression, and difficulty concentrating have been reported.

TSS is known to recur in patients with menstrual-related cases. Usually, the recurrence is within several months of the initial presentation, and the recurrent episode is generally milder than the initial episode. The incidence of recurrent disease is decreased with administration of antistaphylococcal antibiotics and changes in the pattern of tampon use.

CHLAMYDIA TRACHOMATIS INFECTION

method of
KIMBERLY A. WORKOWSKI, M.D.
Emory University
Atlanta, Georgia

Chlamydia trachomatis is the most common bacterial sexually transmitted pathogen in the United States, accounting for an estimated four million infections annually. In most instances, the initial lower genital tract infection is asymptomatic and hence difficult to recognize clinically. Undetected infections can cause serious sequelae, including pelvic inflammatory disease, infertility, and ectopic pregnancy. Thus, as a leading cause of pelvic inflammatory disease and infertility, chlamydial infections are an important threat to women's reproductive health.

EPIDEMIOLOGY

Although the prevalence of genital chlamydial infection has ranged from 2% to 20% in various settings, precise epidemiologic data are not currently available due to the lack of uniform reporting nationwide. Demographic factors associated with an increased risk of chlamydial infection include young age, nonwhite race, multiple sexual partners, single marital status, concurrent gonorrhea, and nonbarrier contraceptive methods (Table 1). Transmission rates vary depending on the presence of symptoms in the index case and whether the sexual encounter is casual or continuous. Recent studies using DNA amplification techniques indicate that approximately 50% to 75% of male partners and 55% to 60% of female partners are infected.

BIOLOGY

Chlamydia are distinguished from all other microorganisms on the basis of their unique life cycle involving an alteration between two highly specialized morphologic forms adapted to either intracellular or extracellular environments. *C. trachomatis* is one of the three species within the genus *Chlamydia. C. trachomatis* can be differentiated into 18 serovars or strains based on monoclonal antibody-based typing assays. Serovars A, B, Ba, and C are associated with endemic trachoma, serovars D to L with genital tract disease, and L1 to L3 with lymphogranuloma venereum. Chlamydia are obligate intracellular parasites that infect squamocolumnar epithelial cells, causing damage from replication of the organism as well as from the resultant inflammatory response.

CLINICAL MANIFESTATIONS

Cervicitis

Clinical recognition of chlamydial cervicitis depends on a high index of suspicion and careful examination because the majority of women are asymptomatic (Table 2). Findings suggestive of chlamydial infection include easily induced endocervical bleeding, mucopurulent endocervical discharge, and hypertrophic ectopy. Gram's stain of endocervical secretions from women with chlamydial cervicitis usually shows more than 30 polymorphonuclear leukocytes per 1000× field.

Urethritis

Although urethral symptoms may develop in women with chlamydial infection, the majority of women with urethral infection do not have dysuria or frequency. However, chlamydial urethritis should be suspected in young women with dysuria lasting more than 7 to 10 days, lack of hematuria and suprapubic tenderness, use of birth control pills, and sterile pyuria.

TABLE 1. **Demographic Risk Factors**

Age <19	Single marital status
Nonwhite race	Nonbarrier contraceptives
Multiple sexual partners	

Endometritis and Salpingitis

Histologic evidence of endometritis is present in approximately 50% of women with mucopurulent cervicitis and almost all of those with salpingitis. The presence of endometritis in women with chlamydial cervicitis correlates with a history of intermenstrual bleeding. The proportion of women with cervical chlamydial infection who develop upper genital tract infection (endometritis, salpingitis, pelvic peritonitis) is thought to be significant. One study has shown that 30% of women with both gonococcal and chlamydial infections treated only for gonorrhea subsequently developed salpingitis. Studies of the long-term complications of salpingitis underscore the impact of *so-called* silent infection. Infertility due to obstructed fallopian tubes and ectopic pregnancy have been correlated with serologic evidence of chlamydial infection.

Perihepatitis

Recent studies have suggested that chlamydia is more commonly associated with perihepatitis than gonococcal infection. Perihepatitis should be suspected in women with right upper quadrant pain, fever, nausea and vomiting, and salpingitis.

Neonatal Infection

The attack rate of chlamydial conjunctivitis in infants varies from 18% to 50% and that of chlamydial pneumonitis, 3% to 18%. Chlamydial pneumonitis is clinically indistinguishable from pneumonitis caused by other pathogens. Other infant infections implicated to be caused by *C. trachomatis* include otitis media, bronchiolitis, and vulvovaginitis.

Diagnostic Testing

Isolation of *Chlamydia trachomatis* by cell culture is the most sensitive and specific test available for detection. However, isolation rates depend on strict sample handling and culture procedures. As such, specimens should be immediately placed in specific transport media and frozen at −70° C if specimens cannot be inoculated into tissue culture within 24 hours of acquisition. Additionally, the use of cell culture is beyond the capability of most laboratories due to its technical demands, labor intensity, and high cost. As a result, nonculture methods to detect chlamydia in genital specimens primarily based on antigen detection or nucleic acid hybridization methods offer reasonable alternatives. At present, there are three nonculture based assays used for the detection of *C. trachomatis* antigens: a fluorescent monoclonal antibody for direct visualization of the organism, enzyme immunoassays for antigen detection, and a nucleic acid hybridization test. Compared with cell culture, these tests have a reported sensitivity of 70% to 90% in populations in which the prevalence of chlamydial infection exceeds 8%. However, in populations in which the prevalence of chlamydial infection is below 5%, the positive predictive value of a nonculture test may be less than 50%. Confirmatory testing can be performed using blocking antibodies, competitive probes, or a different nonculture test to confirm the initial result. The recent commercial development of nucleic acid amplification methods using the polymerase chain reaction offers more sensitive assays and

TABLE 2. **Spectrum of *C. trachomatis* Infections in Women**

Diagnosis	Clinical Criteria	Laboratory Criteria	
		Presumptive	*Confirmation*
Mucopurulent cervicitis	Mucopurulent cervical discharge, cervical ectopy and edema, easily induced endocervical bleeding	Cervical Gram's stain ≥30 polymorphonuclear leukocytes/1000X (nonmenstruating women)	Culture, direct antigen test (cervix), polymerase chain reaction (PCR)
Acute urethral syndrome	Dysuria—frequency >7 days; new sexual partner	Pyuria, no bacteriuria	Culture or direct antigen test (cervix, urethra)
Pelvic inflammatory disease	Lower abdominal pain, adnexal tenderness, mucopurulent cervical discharge	Cervical mucopus	Culture or direct antigen test (cervix, endometrium, tube)
Perihepatitis	Right upper quadrant pain, nausea, vomiting, fever, salpingitis	Cervical mucopus	*C. trachomatis* serology

may soon provide extremely accurate noninvasive methods (urine testing) for screening asymptomatic patients.

TREATMENT

The recommended treatment regimens for uncomplicated chlamydial urethral, cervical, and rectal infections are doxycycline (Vibramycin), 100 mg twice daily for seven days, or azithromycin (Zithromax) in a single 1-gram dose (Table 3). Azithromycin offers the advantage of single-dose therapy with proven efficacy in recent comparative trials with doxycycline in the treatment of uncomplicated chlamydial infections. Alternative regimens include a 7-day regimen of either ofloxacin (Floxin), 300 mg twice daily; erythromycin base, 500 mg four times daily; erythromycin ethylsuccinate, 800 mg four times daily; or a 10-day regimen of sulfisoxazole (Gantrisin), 500 mg four times daily.

Pregnant women with chlamydial infection should not be treated with doxycycline, ofloxacin, or erythromycin estolate. Azithromycin has not yet been evaluated in pregnancy. Recommendations for treatment in pregnancy include a 7-day regimen of either erythromycin base, 500 mg four times daily, or erythromycin ethylsuccinate, 800 mg four times daily. An alternative regimen for pregnant patients intolerant to erythromycin is amoxicillin, 500 mg three times daily for 10 days.

TABLE 3. **Treatment Regimens for Uncomplicated Urethral, Endocervical, or Rectal Chlamydial Infections**

Recommended Regimens
- Doxycycline (Vibramycin) 100 mg orally twice daily for 7 days
  or
- Azithromycin (Zithromax) 1 gm orally in single dose

Alternative Regimens
- Ofloxacin (Floxin) 300 mg orally twice daily for 7 days
- Erythromycin base 500 mg orally four times daily for 7 days
- Erythromycin ethylsuccinate (EES) 800 mg orally four times daily for 7 days
- Sulfisoxazole (Gantrisin) 500 mg orally four times daily for 10 days

In Pregnancy
- Erythromycin 500 mg orally four times daily for 7 days
- Amoxicillin 500 mg orally three times daily for 10 days

Although routine test of cure during the immediate post-treatment period is not recommended for the standard treatment regimens, re-testing should be considered after using the alternative regimens of either amoxicillin or sulfisoxazole. However, use of a nonculture test for confirming organism eradication should be performed at least 3 to 4 weeks after antimicrobial therapy due to the possibility of prolonged antigen shedding resulting in a false-positive test.

Additionally, screening for other sexually transmitted diseases should be considered, along with referral of the sexual partner for evaluation and treatment.

PELVIC INFLAMMATORY DISEASE

method of
W. P. FLEMING, M.D.
Las Cruces, New Mexico

Pelvic inflammatory disease (PID) is an imprecise medical term used to describe infection of the female upper genital tract, which commonly involves the uterine cervix, the endometrium, the fallopian tubes, the ovaries, and the pelvic peritoneum. Salpingitis and salpingo-oophoritis are synonymous terms.

PID is a worldwide problem that affects 1 to 2% of women of reproductive age annualy. PID is the most common serious infection in young women aged 16 to 25. The initial presentation of PID varies widely from mild asymptomatic infection to the ruptured tubo-ovarian abscess, which is a surgical emergency. Delayed morbidity may not be apparent for years after the initial infection. The late manifestations are a result of tubal damage and pelvic adhesion formation, which predispose the patient to ectopic pregnancy, chronic pelvic pain, and infertility. Women with acute PID can expect a 6- to 10-fold increased risk of ectopic pregnancy and a 4-fold increased risk of developing chronic pelvic pain. The incidence of infertility due to tubal occlusion following one episode of PID ranges from 6% to 30% depending on the severity of the infection and rises to 50% to 60% in women who experience three or more episodes.

ETIOLOGY

In more than 99% of cases, PID occurs as a result of ascending infection that begins with disruption of the barriers of the endocervical canal, which normally prevent entry of microorganisms into the uterus and beyond via the fallopian tubes. A small number of cases occur as a result of intraperitoneal spread of an infection from an acute intra-abdominal process, such as appendicitis. Most cases of ascending infection occur spontaneously in sexually active females, but in approximately 15% of patients, the onset of acute PID is a direct result of an antecedent iatrogenic procedure that disturbs the normal endocervical barrier. Such procedures include uterine dilatation and curettage, hysteroscopy, hysterosalpingography, insertion of an intrauterine device, cervical biopsies, and cervical destruction procedures such as cryotherapy and laser ablation.

Acute PID is a polymicrobial infection caused by a number of aerobic and anaerobic bacteria. The sexually transmitted microorganisms *Chlamydia trachomatis* and *Neisseria gonorrhoeae* are the implicated pathogens in the majority of cases. Both of these organisms incite an inflammatory process that leads to mucopurulent endocervicitis. *Chlamydia* has surpassed *N. gonorrhoeae* as the most common cause of PID. Coinfection with *N. gonorrhoeae* and *C. trachomatis* is common, but in 25 to 50% of cases, neither organism is detectable. The nonsexually transmitted bacteria found in proven cases of PID are usually representative of the normal vaginal flora. Such bacteria include the aerobes *Escherichia coli, Haemophilus influenzae, Gardnerella vaginalis, Streptococcus,* and the anaerobes *Peptococcus, Peptostreptococcus,* and *Bacteroides* spp. *Ureaplasma urealyticum and Mycoplasma hominis* have been cultured from infected fallopian tubes, but their role as primary etiologic agents of PID remains unclear. Although uncommon in the United States, tuberculosis of the upper genital tract is a widespread cause of chronic pelvic inflammatory disease and infertility in many countries especially Asia, Latin America, and the Middle East. *Actinomyces israelii* is a rare cause of PID that is almost exclusively associated with use of the intrauterine device.

RISK FACTORS

Acute PID is a disease of young, sexually active menstruating women. The rate of PID is highest among 15- to 19-year-old adolescents, and the rate decreases with advancing age. Three fourths of cases occur in women under the age of 25. Multiple studies, including recent reports, have shown that PID occurs more frequently in users of the intrauterine device. PID occurs only rarely in women who are amenorrheic or pregnant, or those who have had a previous tubal ligation. Intestinal disease, diabetes mellitus, or genital malignancy is usually found in postmenopausal women who are discovered to have salpingitis.

DIAGNOSIS

The clinical diagnosis of acute PID is difficult. In the absence of diagnostic laparoscopy, which is the gold standard for confirmation of PID, misdiagnosis is very common. Reliance on strict clinical and laboratory criteria alone leads to a high percentage of both false-positive and false-negative diagnoses. Unfortunately, laparoscopy is invasive, expensive, and impractical for diagnosis in the majority of cases. Laparoscopy has limitations in that it will not detect endometritis, and mild inflammation of the fallopian tubes may go undetected on direct visualization. Moreover, observer bias in the absence of an inflammatory exudate may lead to a false-positive diagnosis. In the absence of laparoscopic evaluation, consideration of risk factors along with the constellation of signs and symptoms of the disease improves diagnostic accuracy.

The chief complaint in women who present with PID is abdominal pain. The pain may be mild or even absent in a small number of women with laparoscopically proven PID. The lower abdominal pain usually occurs during or within a few days of the menses. The fact that many cases of PID go unrecognized is underscored by the fact that one half of women who are found to have infertility secondary to tubal occlusion recall no history of previous pelvic infection. Other symptoms that occur commonly include abnormal uterine, bleeding, dyspareunia, and vaginal discharge. Fever (>38° C [100.4° F]) is present in one third of patients, and a small number report urinary symptoms, nausea, and emesis. The physical examination in women with PID is most remarkable for lower abdominal and cervical motion tenderness. Cervical and vaginal leukocytosis is common. Laboratory tests are of limited use in the diagnosis. The most helpful diagnostic test is Gram's stain of cervical secretions, which when indicative of *N. gonorrhoeae* in symptomatic women, yields strong presumptive evidence of salpingitis. The presence of plasma cells on an endometrial biopsy is useful in the diagnosis of PID. Purulent fluid obtained by culdocentesis supports the diagnosis, but other causes of peritonitis, such as acute appendicitis, must be excluded. The importance of performing a sensitive pregnancy test in all patients thought to have PID in order to exclude the diagnosis of ectopic gestation cannot be overemphasized. Ultrasonography has little use in the diagnosis of uncomplicated PID, but it may be useful in patients who are so tender on examination that a pelvic mass cannot be confirmed or excluded.

Diagnostic laparoscopy should be performed for women in whom the diagnosis is uncertain and in those who do not respond to therapy.

TREATMENT

The treatment of PID is based on the consensus that PID is a polymicrobial infection. Antibiotic choices should include agents effective in the elimination of *C. trachomatis* and pencillin-resistant *N. gonorrhoeae* while maintaining satisfactory empiric coverage of other likely pathogens. In many European countries, hospitalization for parenteral antibiotics is standard practice, but in the United States, 75% of women with acute PID are treated as outpatients. Table 1 lists indications for inpatient management. Ambulatory patients who do not respond to treatment within 72 hours should be hospitalized.

Unfortunately, no single antibiotic regimen has been established as a satisfactory form of treatment for women with acute PID. Table 2 outlines the antibiotic regimens recommended by the Centers for Dis-

TABLE 1. **Indications for Hospital Management of PID**

Uncertain diagnosis
Nulliparity
Adolescence
Pregnancy
Failed outpatient therapy
Presence of an intrauterine device
Presence of a tubo-ovarian abscess or complex
Nausea and emesis
Severe peritonitis
Human immunodeficiency virus infection

TABLE 2. **Recommendations of the Centers for Disease Control and Prevention for Treatment of Pelvic Inflammatory Disease**

Outpatient

Cefoxitin (Mefoxin), 2 gm IM plus probenecid (Benemid), 1 gm orally, in a single dose concurrently, or ceftriaxone (Rocephin), 250 mg IM or other parenteral third-generation cephalosporin (e.g., ceftizoxime [Cefizox] or cefotaxime [Claforan]), PLUS doxycycline (Vibramycin), 100 mg orally bid for 14 days

OR

Ofloxacin (Floxin), 400 mg orally bid for 14 days, PLUS either clindamycin (Cleocin), 450 mg orally qid, or metronidazole (Flagyl), 500 mg orally bid for 14 days

Inpatient*

Cefoxitin 2 gm IV q 6 h or cefotetan (Cefotan), 2 gm IV q 12 h, PLUS doxycycline 100 mg IV or orally q 12 h

OR

Clindamycin 900 mg IV q 8 h, PLUS gentamicin loading dose IV or IM (2 mg/kg of body weight), followed by a maintenance dose (1.5 mg per kg) q 8 h

*Parenteral treatment should be continued for at least 48 hours after the patient demonstrates improvement followed by an oral antibiotic regimen of doxycycline 100 mg orally bid or clindamycin 450 mg orally qid to complete a total of 14 days coverage.

ease Control and Prevention (CDC). Two alternative inpatient regimens that appear to be effective include ampicillin/sulbactam (Unasyn), plus doxycycline (Vibramycin), and ofloxacin (Floxin), plus either clindamycin (Cleocin), or metronidazole (Flagyl).

Surgical intervention in the management of PID decreased markedly in the last decade. Operative intervention is usually restricted to ruptured tubo-ovarian abscesses, persistent tubo-ovarian complexes, and drainage of pelvic abscesses through a colpotomy incision or percutaneous aspiration under ultrasonographic guidance. Conservative surgery is usually preferred.

The complete treatment of pelvic inflammatory disease extends beyond antibiotic therapy to include patient education with emphasis on safe sexual practices, follow-up clinical evaluation, and treatment of sexual partners to eliminate persistent reservoirs of reinfection.

UTERINE LEIOMYOMA

method of
LEILA R. HAJJAR, M.D., and
GEORGE H. NOLAN, M.D., M.P.H.
Henry Ford Medical Center
Detroit, Michigan

Uterine leiomyomas (fibroids, myomas), benign uterine smooth muscle tumors that likely arise as a result of somatic mutation, are the most common pelvic tumor in the women. Their clinical prevalence is estimated to be 20 to 30%, whereas extensive pathologic examination of hysterectomy specimens shows their presence in 77% of all specimens. Although a higher prevalence is often stated for blacks, the often-cited data supporting this belief are less than convincing. It is clear that blacks face a two to three times greater frequency of hysterectomy for this condition than do whites. The presence of myoma becomes more apparent with advancing age, and their prevalence is increased in obese women. Age at the time of last childbirth, parity, and menopausal status are each negatively associated with clinically detectable myoma and are factors reducing the prevalence of hysterectomy for this diagnosis. Women with two or more live births have 50% less risk of hysterectomy for myoma than do women who have not given birth. The age-specific incidence of hysterectomy for myoma peaks between 45 and 50 years. Case reports suggest that growth of myoma is stimulated by estrogens, clomiphene, tamoxifen, and obesity, but data relating to oral contraceptives do not tend to incriminate the pills as consistent stimuli.

CLINICAL ASPECTS

Approximately 33% of women with uterine leiomyoma are clinically symptomatic. The clinical symptoms range from pelvic discomfort to the most common and consistent problem of menorrhagia. Other problems attributed to myoma include infertility, pregnancy wastage, pregnancy problems, and neoplastic degeneration. The problems attributed to myoma are related to their size, number, and location. We prefer classifying them by location: **intracavitary** (pedunculated), **intramural** (submucosal, intramyometrial and subserous) and **subserosal** (pedunculated).

A definitive explanation for myoma-associated menorrhagia is not established, but obstruction of the venous plexi of the adjacent myometrium and endometrium is a plausible theory. This theory has been expanded to explain alleged myoma-associated infertility and abortion.

Pregnancy complications related to myoma are uncommon, as is rapid growth of these tumors during pregnancy. Pain that occurs as a result of intramyometrial hemorrhage and distention of the pseudocapsule may be severe. Preterm labor, albeit uncommon, may be associated with intramyometrial hemorrhage. Labor in patients with leiomyoma is similar to that of patients without leiomyoma unless malpresentation, an uncommon complication, occurs. When malpresentation complicates pregnancies associated with myoma, more than one myoma usually is present.

Leiomyosarcoma are rare, having an incidence less than 0.5% and a range of 0.13 to 0.5%. The incidence of this problem in women undergoing hysterectomy who are younger than 40 years of age is 0.2%. The etiology of leiomyosarcoma is unknown and many question whether they actually arise from leiomyoma.

DIAGNOSIS

The diagnosis of leiomyoma is arrived at clinically through the pelvic examination. The use of the ultrasound and computerized tomography should be reserved for defining the status of the ovaries and monitoring the growth of myoma. These diagnostic tools may also be useful adjuncts in confirming the diagnosis of acute hemorrhage into a myoma in women with an acute onset of severe pelvic pain that is otherwise unexplained.

MANAGEMENT

The primary approach to the management of the patient with uterine leiomyoma is observation and is based on the fact that these tumors are usually incidental findings and are benign. When there are associated problems, the approaches to management may involve medical or surgical therapy, or both.

The need for intervention because of uterine size has been lessened by the availability of ultrasound and computerized tomography. Thus, the routine removal of myoma because the uterus approaches 12 weeks' gestational size is not recommended. Medical therapy, with a gonadotrophin-releasing hormone (GnRH) agonist* may be used to reduce uterine size. They exert an effect by the eventual suppression of estrogen. The effect of these agents is temporary. Thus, medical therapy is used to temporarily reduce the size, symptoms and findings associated with myoma during preparation for surgery.

Gonadotropin-releasing hormone agonist therapy reduces menorrhagia and causes amenorrhea, thus allowing erythrocyte production to overcome anemia. There are direct benefits from agonist therapy preceding the surgical approaches because the size of the myoma is reduced and the vascularity of the uterus is lessened. In borderline situations, reduction in the size of myoma may allow vaginal hysterectomy rather than abdominal procedures. In other instances, myomectomy becomes an alternative to hysterectomy. Myomectomy is technically simpler and is associated with less blood loss. It must be emphasized that there are significant side effects associated with the use of GnRH agonists. Approximately 30% of patients undergoing treatment experience irregular vaginal bleeding, hair loss, vaginal dryness and irritation, depression, and musculoskeletal stiffness. Hot flushes complicate therapy in 80 to 100% of patients within 3 to 4 weeks of the onset of therapy. When the medication is withdrawn, menses can be expected to return within 3 to 4 weeks and uterine myoma size approaches pretreatment size within 3 to 4 months. Leuprolide acetate (Lupron), 3.75 mg intramuscularly every 28 days, is one schedule we have followed. Finally, medical therapy with a GnRH agonist for leiomyoma must be short-term at this time because of the cost of therapy, the side effects, and the risk of missing a leiomyosarcoma.

Progestins have been used to shrink myoma, but their effect is variable and remains controversial for this purpose. They inhibit endometrial growth, cause endometrial atrophy, and eventually reduce uterine bleeding.

The primary approach to managing symptomatic leiomyoma is surgical. Most patients are currently managed by hysterectomy. Myomectomy is indicated when fertility issues must be resolved. At present, the advances in endoscopic surgery allow laparoscopic myomectomy using lasers in cases in which there are few myoma of small size. Similarly, hysteroscopic removal of submucous myoma is now regularly performed. Hysteroscopic removal is a reasonable consideration when there are up to four myomas, when they are from 5 to 9 cm in size, and when at least 50% of the myomas are within the uterine cavity. Patients should understand that when myomectomy is contemplated, usually for multiple small myomas, there is a substantial probability that new myomas will become prominent. This is not as likely when there is a single large myoma.

*Not FDA approved for this indication.

CANCER OF THE ENDOMETRIUM

method of
AL ELBENDARY, M.D., and
ANDREW BERCHUCK, M.D.
Duke University
Durham, North Carolina

Endometrial cancer is the most common gynecologic malignancy, and approximately 40,000 women develop this disease in the United States each year. The median age of patients with this disease is 60 years. The vast majority of endometrial cancers are adenocarcinomas, whereas the next most common type of uterine malignancy, sarcomas, comprise only 3% to 5% of cases. Most endometrial adenocarcinomas resemble normal endometrium and are called endometrioid adenocarcinomas. Frequently, benign squamous metaplasia is found, in which case the cancer is called an adenoacanthoma. The prognosis of an adenoacanthoma is similar to that of a pure endometrioid cancer. In contrast, there are three histologic variants that appear to have a worse prognosis—adenosquamous, clear cell, and papillary serous adenocarcinomas. These variants, which are similar to sarcomas, occur infrequently and are associated with advanced-stage disease, aggressive biologic behavior, and poor survival.

ETIOLOGY AND DIAGNOSIS

Endometrial adenocarcinoma often develops in a hormonal milieu characterized by unopposed stimulation of the endometrium by estrogen. The source of estrogen may be either endogenous or exogenous. The most common cause of unopposed endogenous estrogen during the reproductive years is chronic anovulation. After menopause, endogenous estrogenic stimulation most often occurs in obese women, who convert androstenedione of adrenal origin to estrone in adipose tissue. In addition, in the past, continuously administered exogenous estrogen also was a significant cause of unopposed estrogenic stimulation of the endometrium leading to endometrial cancer. Because this problem has been appreciated, iatrogenic overstimulation of the endometrium has become less common. More recently, however, tamoxifen (Nolvadex) use has been associated with the development of endometrial cancer because this hormone also acts as a weak estrogen.

Endometrial cancers often are preceded by or accompanied by hyperplasia of the endometrium. Most patients who develop endometrial hyperplasia or cancer present because of abnormal uterine bleeding. In premenopausal patients, this frequently is exhibited as irregular, noncyclic bleeding, whereas in postmenopausal patients reappearance of bleeding after spontaneous menopause is noted. All patients older than 35 years of age with abnormal uterine bleeding should undergo endometrial biopsy for diagnostic purposes. Biopsy may be performed in the operating room under anesthesia, but in most instances, it is performed in the office using a narrow plastic sampling device (Pipelle).

Following endometrial biopsy, endocervical curettage also often is performed, and the specimen submitted separately. Fractional curettage allows one to determine whether or not an endometrial cancer has spread to the endocervix. In addition, endocervical curettage enables one to diagnose a primary endocervical cancer, which also can cause abnormal bleeding. Finally, the Papanicolaou smear has poor sensitivity for detecting endometrial cancer (50%), and a normal smear should not be considered reassuring in a patient with abnormal uterine bleeding.

TREATMENT

Preoperative Evaluation

If endometrial biopsy reveals hyperplasia, in most cases, regression can be induced with progestins. On the other hand, hysterectomy is considered an acceptable form of treatment in women who have completed childbearing, because hyperplasia is a premalignant lesion. If a uterine cancer is found on biopsy, the patient should be prepared to undergo surgical therapy. Because the median age of these patients is approximately 60 years, however, a careful medical evaluation must be performed prior to surgery. Many women with endometrial cancer are obese and have accompanying medical conditions such as diabetes mellitus and hypertension. These medical problems should be adequately controlled prior to bringing the patient to the operating room, in order to avoid perioperative complications.

In addition to a complete history and physical examination and routine preoperative blood tests, a chest radiograph should be performed to exclude the presence of lung metastases. In general, imaging studies of the pelvis such as ultrasound, computed tomography, and magnetic resonance imaging scans are not useful for patients with early stage disease, because surgical exploration is indicated regardless of the findings. These scans and other diagnostic procedures such as sigmoidoscopy, barium enema, cystoscopy, and intravenous pyelography should be employed selectively in the minority of patients in whom the cancer appears to have spread outside the uterus.

Surgical Therapy

Following the initial evaluation, almost all patients are found to be suitable for primary surgical therapy. Occasionally, however, in patients with severe cardiovascular or other medical diseases, surgery may be considered unacceptably risky. In these cases, curative treatment often can be accomplished with a combination of external pelvic radiation and intracavitary radiation. For patients with cancer confined to the uterus, the cure rate with radiation therapy alone is approximately 50%, which is 25% less than that for surgery alone. Patients in whom neither surgery nor radiation therapy can be accomplished are best treated with progestins such as megestrol acetate (Megace), 40 mg four times daily. Well to moderately differentiated endometrial cancers often respond well to progestin therapy, which in some cases may be curative.

Most patients who undergo surgery for endometrial cancer have an increased risk of developing deep venous thrombophlebitis and pulmonary emboli owing to their advanced age and obesity. Therefore, these patients should receive thromboembolism prophylaxis. Either minidose heparin or an intermittent pneumatic compression device is acceptable. In addition, because the vagina normally is heavily colonized by bacteria, prophylactic antibiotics usually are administered perioperatively to decrease the risk of pelvic infection. Finally, on the evening prior to surgery, the patient's bowel is cleansed with oral magnesium citrate and enemas.

The cornerstone of therapy for the vast majority of patients with endometrial cancer is surgical exploration, with removal of the uterus, fallopian tubes, and ovaries. Exploration is performed through a midline lower abdominal incision to allow access to the upper abdomen. Approximately 100 mL of saline is instilled into the pelvis, which is aspirated and submitted for cytology, and then hysterectomy and bilateral salpingo-oophorectomy are performed. After the specimen has been extirpated, the uterus is opened and the cavity is inspected. The location of the cancer and gross depth of invasion into the uterine wall are noted. In addition, a sample of tumor is submitted for determination of estrogen and progesterone receptor levels.

Most endometrial adenocarcinomas are either well or moderately differentiated, and these cancers usually are confined to the inner part of the uterine wall. Because these cancers have a low incidence of occult metastases, further surgical staging beyond gross inspection and palpation usually is not performed (Table 1). If the cancer is poorly differentiated or invades into the outer half of the uterine wall, however, we sample the regional lymph nodes. Because the lymphatic drainage of the uterus is both to the pelvic sidewall via the cardinal ligaments and to the aortic area via the infundibulopelvic ligaments, lymph nodes in both of these areas are sampled. Because lymph node sampling increases the duration and potential morbidity of the operation, however, it is not

TABLE 1. **FIGO Staging of Endometrial Carcinoma**

Stage I—Confined to the Uterus	
IA	No invasion
IB	Inner 1/2 uterine invasion
IC	Outer 1/2 uterine invasion
Stage II—Cervical Involvement	
IIA	Endocervical gland involvement
IIB	Cervical stromal invasion
Stage III	
IIIA	Positive peritoneal cytology, adnexal metastases, uterine serosal involvement
IIIB	Vaginal metastases
IIIC	Pelvic or aortic lymph node metastases
Stage IV	
IVA	Bladder or rectal involvement
IVB	Distant metastases

Note: Within each stage, the histologic grade also is recorded (e.g., G1 = well differentiated, G2 = moderately differentiated, G3 = poorly differentiated).

performed in patients who are considered to be at high risk for perioperative complications.

Approximately 5% to 10% of patients with endometrial cancer are found to have grossly visible extrauterine disease at surgical exploration. The most common sites of metastases are the ovaries, peritoneal surfaces, and lymph nodes. In these cases, attempts usually are made to remove the extrauterine metastases. Following surgery, either chemotherapy or external radiation is administered, but only a small proportion of these patients are long-term survivors. In addition, although uterine papillary serous cancer frequently is only superficially invasive, it has a propensity to spread throughout the peritoneal cavity, similar to epithelial ovarian cancer. Even when these cancers appear to be confined to the uterus, intraperitoneal recurrence is common. In these patients, we routinely biopsy the omentum and peritoneal surfaces. If microscopic metastatic disease is found, whole abdominal radiation, intraperitoneal ^{32}P, or chemotherapy is employed. However, survival continues to be poor.

Adjuvant Radiation Therapy

Most patients with endometrial cancer have disease that appears to be confined to the uterus, and survival rates for this group are excellent with surgery alone. Because 10% to 20% of patients develop recurrent cancer, however, there has been interest in adjuvant therapy for selected subsets of high-risk patients. In this regard, it has been shown that there are several prognostic factors predictive of a higher risk of recurrence (e.g., cervical involvement, poor histologic grade, deep myometrial invasion). Historically, external pelvic irradiation has been employed most frequently as adjuvant therapy for patients with high-risk endometrial cancer. Because these cancers usually are at least moderately radiosensitive, it is hoped that irradiation will eradicate microscopic residual disease in the pelvis. In the past, as many as 30% to 40% of patients with early stage disease have been considered candidates for adjuvant pelvic radiation therapy on the basis of clinicopathologic prognostic factors. Although many patients have received adjuvant pelvic radiation therapy over the years, an unequivocal survival benefit has not been demonstrated. More recently, because occult spread of early stage endometrial cancer usually is via lymphatics, selective lymph node sampling has been used to identify more accurately the 10% to 20% of patients who are most likely to benefit from adjuvant radiation therapy. In addition, if aortic lymph nodes are involved, the radiation field can be tailored to include this area, which is not part of the standard pelvic field. Finally, surgical staging allows patients who do not appear to have occult metastatic disease to be spared the potential morbidity of irradiation.

Approximately 10% to 15% of patients with early-stage endometrial cancer are found to have malignant cells in pelvic peritoneal washings obtained at laparotomy. Most, but not all, series have shown that positive cytology is associated with an increased risk of recurrence even when there is no other evidence of metastatic disease. When positive cytology is the only evidence of extrauterine spread, we have used radioactive ^{32}P intraperitoneally as adjuvant therapy. Survival of these patients has been better than that of a historical control group. When positive cytology and lymph node metastases are found, we do not combine ^{32}P instillation and external irradiation, however, because an unacceptably high proportion of patients treated in this fashion subsequently have developed small bowel obstruction due to radiation enteritis.

Following surgery, the patient is seen every 3 months for the first year, every 4 months for the second year, and every 6 months the third through fifth years. A chest radiograph is ordered on a yearly basis to search for recurrent disease in the lungs. Seventy-five percent of patients who develop recurrence do so within 3 years of primary therapy, and by 5 years, 90% of recurrences will have occurred. After 5 years of follow-up, the patient is seen on a yearly basis. In the past, endometrial cancer has been considered an absolute contraindication to estrogen replacement therapy because many of these cancers express estrogen receptors. In practice, however, estrogen replacement has not been proved to be detrimental in these patients. We are most comfortable in recommending estrogen replacement for women with cancers that have a low risk of recurrence or in whom 2 years have elapsed since surgery.

RECURRENT DISEASE

Endometrial cancer initially recurs locally in the pelvis in 50% of patients, at distant sites in 25%, and both locally and at distant sites in 25%. A significant proportion of pelvic recurrences are confined to the vagina and can be cured with radiation therapy. Pelvic sidewall recurrences also usually are treated with radiation, but salvage rates are much poorer. Treatment of distant metastases is with either progestin therapy or cytotoxic chemotherapy. Approximately 25% of patients with metastatic disease will have a significant response to progestins, and some of these responses are prolonged. A favorable response to progestins usually occurs in well-differentiated cancers that express steroid receptors. Unfortunately, most cancers that recur are poorly differentiated and do not express steroid receptors. We use the receptor status of the tumor to determine whether or not progestin therapy is appropriate.

If the cancer is steroid receptor negative, patients with metastatic disease are treated using cytotoxic chemotherapy. Most frequently we have used a combination of doxorubicin (Adriamycin)* and cisplatin (Platinol),* administered every 3 weeks for six cycles. Although a substantial proportion of patients have objective responses, few are cured. Thus, although survival rates are excellent following surgery in patients with early-stage disease, further improvement

*Not FDA approved for this indication.

in survival for patients with endometrial cancer awaits the development of effective treatment of metastatic disease.

CANCER OF THE UTERINE CERVIX

method of
F. J. MONTZ, M.D.
*University of California,
Los Angeles School of Medicine
Los Angeles, California*

Despite the availability of an efficient screening tool and inexpensive and effective therapies for the nonmalignant progenitor processes, cervical cancer has maintained its position as the most common malignant disease process of the female reproductive tract in the world. In industrialized countries such as the United States, cervical cancer trails both ovarian and endometrial malignancies in incidence and as a cause of cancer death. Unfortunately, available screening and therapy for premalignant diseases of the uterine cervix is not universally applied and this disease remains as a significant, if not the most significant, cause of cancer morbidity in many nonindustrialized and theoretically less wealthy societies.

RISK FACTORS

In many instances, cervical cancer is a sexually transmitted disease, a reality that has been appreciated for decades, though only recently understood. It is now accepted that age at first intercourse, interval from menarche to coitarche, number of sexual partners at a young age (younger than 20 years), exposure to the human papillomavirus, and intercourse with the so-called "high risk male" (history of sexually transmitted diseases, penile cancer, numerous sexual partners, prior mate with cervical cancer) all significantly increase a woman's risk of developing cervical cancer of the squamous variety. Interestingly, parity does not appear to be an independent risk factor. Other proposed risk factors include cigarette smoking, herpes simplex virus infection, and sex steroid–containing medications (e.g., oral contraceptive pills). However, monogamy or celibacy, use of barrier contraceptive devices, and vitamin A and folic acid supplementation may offer some protective effect. It has been well documented that chronically immunosuppressed patients (e.g., renal transplant recipients, patients with human immunodeficiency virus infection) are predisposed to developing premalignant cervical dysplasias and, therefore, cervical cancer.

The incidence of adenocarcinoma of the cervix is rising, a rise that is purportedly due to an increased use of oral contraceptive steroids. This theory, however, is unproved and controversial, as are similar theories that attempt to relate increasing human papillomavirus rates to increasing cervical adenocarcinoma rates. However, it is recognized that patients with Peutz-Jeghers syndrome have an increased frequency of a rare subtype of adenocarcinoma of the cervix.

SCREENING

Cervical cancer screening relies almost exclusively on the collection and evaluation of exfoliative cytology. The Pap smear, named after George Papanicolaou, who pioneered its use in the early 1940s, has almost single-handedly been responsible for the remarkable decrease in the frequency of squamous cervical cancer. Screening should begin at time of first intercourse or age 18 (whichever comes first) and continue on a yearly basis thereafter. There may be a subgroup of low-risk women who have had serial normal Pap smears in whom the screening frequency can be spaced to once every 3 years, although this latter point is controversial.

HISTOLOGY

The vast majority of cervical malignancies are squamous in cell type. Large cell nonkeratinizing cancer comprises approximately 70% to 75% of all cervical cancer primaries with large cell keratinizing making up another 15%. Adenocarcinoma is responsible for 10% of cervical malignancies, with this proportion allegedly increasing. Fortunately, the highly aggressive small cell variant occurs in only 3% to 5% of cases. There appears to be a direct relationship between cell type and 5-year survival. After adjusting for disease stage, it appears that those patients with a nonkeratinizing type have the best prognosis (60 ± %), those with the small cell carcinoma have the worst prognosis (± 13%), and those with the keratinizing and adeno cell types have an intermediate prognosis (40 ± % and 50 ± %, respectively).

DIAGNOSIS

The goal of cervical screening is to diagnose non-invasive precursors of the disease process and, subsequently, to treat such precursors adequately so as to prevent the development of a cervical malignancy. Unfortunately, the system for screening that exists (i.e., Pap smears) is not a perfect one, with innumerable opportunities for failure. Patient non-compliance, unsatisfactory sample collection, and inadequate pathologic interpretation are the most common causes for failure. Suboptimal health care professional follow-up and therapy does occur but is much less common.

So as to ensure adequate sensitivity of the test, it is important that the health care provider remember that any significantly abnormal Pap smear is presumed to represent an underlying premalignant disease process until proved otherwise (e.g., after colposcopy with directed biopsy, as indicated). It is not uncommon that patients with grossly evident cervical malignancies have Pap smears that fail to demonstrate malignant cells and have only inflammatory or infectious changes or excessive blood. These later changes should instill the health care professional with a healthy degree of suspicion because they may be masking malignant cells. Unfortunately, only 20% of patients with cervical cancer are asymptomatic at the time of diagnosis of the malignancy. The most common presenting symptom (80% to 90% of symptomatic patients) is some form of abnormal vaginal bleeding, which is often alleged by the subject to be an abnormality of menstruation. Post-coital bleeding, though widely recognized as a symptom of cervical cancer, is relatively uncommon. The two other common symptoms, comprising about 10% each, are vaginal discharge and pelvic pain.

The evaluation of the patient who has findings that are suspicious for cervical cancer must include a thorough pelvic examination, with emphasis on the rectovaginal portion, a Pap smear, and a biopsy of any suspicious change of the ectocervix or endocervix. Such changes may be as subtle as a heaping white lesion or as virulent appearing as a briskly bleeding ulcer.

Cervical cancer is initially a locally invasive process, starting in most cases at the squamo-columnar junction and spreading outward to the vagina and parametria. Bladder, rectal, and distal (lymphatic) spread is usually a later finding in the disease course, but it can occur early. As is discussed later, it is the extent of the disease (i.e., its "Stage") that most accurately predicts chance of cure.

STAGING

Staging of cervical cancer under the International Federation of Gynecology and Obstetrics (FIGO) rules is clinical (Table 1). Physical examination findings and directed biopsies are paramount, and information obtained from simple radiographic investigations (intravenous pyelogram and chest x-ray study) are permissible. Findings from more invasive radiographic investigations (computed tomography [CT] and magnetic resonance imaging) may be clinically valuable, but they cannot be used to change the patient's stage. Cystoscopy and proctoscopy appear to have merit only in those instances when the disease is locally advanced. The value of surgical staging whether via laparoscopy or laparotomy, is controversial and surgical staging should be performed only on investigational study protocols.

THERAPY

Stage Ia

Stage Ia includes a broad spectrum of diseases that must be viewed as a continuum. It is imperative that the treating physician remember, however, that this diagnosis can only be made following a cone biopsy with pathologically clear surgical margins or a hysterectomy. A simple biopsy is not adequate to ensure that there is not a more deeply invasive disease process. Those lesions in which invasion is only microscopic and minimal (Stage Ia1) can be treated with a cone biopsy only, although traditional therapy would be surgical extirpation via hysterectomy. Management of Stage Ia2 disease must be individualized. In those patients with lesions that have less than 3 millimeters of invasion and do not have high-risk histology (e.g., lymph vascular space invasion), a simple extrafascial hysterectomy should be performed. Patients either with lymph vascular space invasion or with a depth of invasion that is greater than 3 mm should be treated with a radical hysterectomy and

TABLE 1. **FIGO Staging of Carcinoma of the Cervix Uteri**

Preinvasive Carcinoma

Stage 0 *Carcinoma in situ,* intraepithelial carcinoma (Cases of Stage 0 should not be included in any therapeutic statistics).

Invasive Carcinoma

Stage I* Carcinoma strictly confined to the cervix (extension to the corpus should be disregarded).

Stage Ia Preclinical carcinomas of the cervix, that is, those diagnosed only by microscopy.

Stage Ia1 Minimal microscopically evident stromal invasion.

Stage Ia2 Lesions detected microscopically that can be measured. The upper limit of the measurement should not show a depth of invasion of more than 5 mm taken from the base of the epithelium, either surface or glandular, from which it originates, and a second dimension, the horizontal spread, must not exceed 7 mm. Larger lesions should be staged as Ib.

Stage Ib Lesions of greater dimensions than Stage 1a2, whether seen clinically or not. Preformed space involvement should not alter the staging but should be specifically recorded so as to determine whether it should affect treatment decisions in the future.

Stage II† The carcinoma extends beyond the cervix but has not extended onto the wall. The carcinoma involves the vagina, but not the lower third.

Stage IIa No obvious parametrial involvement.

Stage IIb Obvious parametrial involvement.

Stage III† The carcinoma has extended into the pelvic wall. On rectal examination, there is no cancer-free space between the tumor and the pelvic wall. The tumor involves the lower third of the vagina. All cases with hydronephrosis or nonfunctioning kidney.

Stage IIIa No extension to the pelvic wall.

Stage IIIb Extension into the pelvic wall and/or hydronephrosis or non-functioning kidney.

Stage IV‡ The carcinoma has extended beyond the true pelvis or has clinically involved the mucosa of the bladder or rectum. A bullous edema as such does not permit a case to be allotted to Stage IV.

Stage IVa Spread of the growth to adjacent organs.

Stage IVb Spread to distant organs.

*Stage Ia carcinoma should include minimal microscopically evident stromal invasion as well as small cancerous tumors of measurable size. Stage Ia should be subdivided into those lesions with minute foci of invasion visible only microscopically as Stage Ia1, and the macroscopically measurable microcarcinomas as Stage Ia2, in order to gain further knowledge of the clinical behavior of these lesions. The term Ib occult should be omitted.

The diagnosis of both Stages Ia1 and Ia2 should be based on microscopic examination of removed tissue, preferably a cone, which must include the entire lesion. As noted earlier, the lower limit of Stage Ia2 should be that it can be measured macroscopically (even if dots need to be placed on the slide before measurement) and the upper limit of Ia2 is given by measurement of the two largest dimensions in any given section. The depth of invasion should not be more than 5 mm taken from the base of the epithelium, either surface or glandular, from which it originates. The second dimension, the horizontal spread, must not exceed 7 mm. Vascular space involvement, either venous or lymphatic, should not alter the staging but should be specifically recorded because it may affect treatment decisions in the future. Lesions of greater size should be staged as Ib. As a rule, it is impossible to estimate clinically whether a cancer of the cervix has extended to the corpus. Extension to the corpus should therefore be disregarded.

†A patient with a growth fixed to the pelvic wall by a short and indurated, but not nodular, parametrium should be allotted to Stage IIb. At clinical examination, it is impossible to decide whether a smooth, indurated parametrium is truly cancerous or only inflammatory. Therefore the case should be placed in Stage III only if the parametrium is nodular to the pelvic wall or the growth itself extends to the pelvic wall. The presence of hydronephrosis or nonfunctioning kidney due to stenosis of the ureter by cancer permits a case to be allotted to Stage III even if, according to other findings, the case should be allotted to Stage I or II.

‡The presence of bullous edema as such should not permit a case to be allotted to Stage IV. Ridges and furrows into the bladder wall should be interpreted as signs of submucous involvement of the bladder if they remain fixed to the growth at palpation (i.e., examination from the vagina or the rectum during cystoscopy). A cytologic finding of malignant cells in washings from the urinary bladder requires further examination and a biopsy from the wall of the bladder. From Berek J: Practical Gynecologic Oncology. Baltimore, MD, Williams & Wilkins, 1988, p. 326.

bilateral pelvic lymphadenectomy. I prefer to perform a Type II radical hysterectomy in these cases because there is a lower rate of morbidity associated with them. Oophorectomy is not mandatory and should be performed only if indicated for independent reasons.

Stages Ib and IIa

In those instances in which the lesion is less than 4 cm in maximal diameter and the patient is medically a candidate for radical pelvic surgery, my preference is to perform a Type III radical hysterectomy with bilateral pelvic lymphadenectomy and para-aortic lymph node sampling. Again, oophorectomy should be completed only as needed for specific indications. Should the patient be found to have two or more positive pelvic nodes, parametrial or margin involvement, or a clinically enlarged lymph node at the time of surgery, I recommend that she receive postoperative pelvic radiotherapy. Unfortunately, such a regimen of radiotherapy after radical hysterectomy has a significant risk of long-term bowel or bladder dysfunction. Therefore, in patients with large lesions (≥4 cm) who are more likely to have either microscopic parametrial disease or pelvic lymph node involvement, I prefer to treat the patient preoperatively with chemoradiation in an attempt to maximize chance of cure while minimizing associated toxicities (see Stages IIb to IVa later) using whole pelvis radiation and a single intracavitary implant. This is followed by an extrafascial hysterectomy and para-aortic node sampling. Any patient who is not a surgical candidate should be treated similarly, but with two intracavitary implants so as to optimize the probability of central disease control.

Stages IIb to IVa

We encourage all of our patients to participate in extant Gyncologic Oncology Group cooperative protocols, which evaluate various chemotherapy and radiation regimens. Entry into these studies requires that the patient have undergone surgical staging with para-aortic lymph node sampling. For those patients who are not candidates or who refuse to participate, I would perform a CT scan of the abdomen. In patients in whom there is no suspicious para-aortic adenopathy on CT, I would perform an extraperitoneal or laparoscopic para-aortic lymph node sampling. In the setting in which these same nodes are radiographically suspicious for spread of disease, I would perform a CT scan of the chest. If this study is positive, I would obtain confirmation of disease spread through fine-needle aspiration and treat the patient as described for Stage IVb. In cases in which the scan is negative, I would proceed to a scalene node sampling in an outpatient setting. If the scalene nodes were positive, I would treat the patient as listed for Stage IVb disease; should such nodes be negative, I would attempt to surgically resect the enlarged para-aortic lymph nodes. Patients with negative para-aortic nodes should be treated with whole pelvis radiation and two intracavitary applications of cesium while receiving a radiation sensitizer, such as hydroxyurea (Hydrea),* cisplatin (Platinol),* or 5-fluorouracil (Efudex).* Cisplatin has a theoretic advantage because it is not only a known radiosensitizer but the most effective chemotherapeutic agent against metastatic squamous carcinoma of the cervix. Unfortunately, this advantage is counterbalanced by significant associated toxicity. Which of the numerous recommended regimens has the best therapeutic index is presently unknown but is actively being investigated in cooperative group trials. For patients who have disease extending to the para-aortic nodes but not beyond, I would recommend that the radiation field be extended via a so-called chimney port to the level of the diaphragm. In those patients with massive locally invasive disease fistula formation during the course of radiotherapy, if such has not occurred prior to the institution of therapy, is common. In an attempt to limit fistula-related morbidity while maximizing the patient's quality of life, I prefer to immediately divert the fecal stream via an end colostomy, while using percutaneous nephrostomes as a temporizing measure in patients with urinary fistulas, delaying the definitive and often complex procedure for a later time when local disease control has been confirmed.

Stage IVb

The goal in patients with distant metastases is to limit suffering to as great an extent as possible, because the disease is universally fatal. Rapid-course pelvic teletherapy, with or without systemic chemotherapy depending upon the patient's desire, is my preference. Urinary or fecal diversion should be performed in the least invasive manner possible and only in an attempt to alleviate specific symptoms.

Recurrent Disease

Almost 50% of all patients with cervical cancer have a recurrence of their disease, with the vast majority of these women dying from these recurrences. Where and when the disease recurs depends on the extent of the disease at time of institution of therapy and what initial treatment modalities were employed. A general caveat is that whatever modalities were not used in the initial therapy should be used for treatment of the recurrence. Unfortunately, by using multimodality primary therapy, we are improving cure rates but do limit subsequent therapeutic options if a recurrence occurs. Prior to beginning any further therapy, thorough evaluation of the extent of the recurrence (examination under anesthesia, CT scan) must be undertaken. In patients who have local recurrence following a radical hysterectomy, I prefer to employ chemoradiation with an appropriate port initially, followed by an exenteration only in those patients who fail to respond completely and fulfill the

*Not FDA approved for this indication.

criteria listed later. In those patients who have local failure following chemotherapy and radiation, exenterative therapy should be offered immediately. However, this option can be offered to the patients only after ensuring that the disease is truly localized in the pelvis because up to 60% of these patients will have a component of distant failure and therefore will not be candidates for exenteration. The development of advanced reconstructive techniques now allows us to perform neovagina construction, continent urinary diversion, and primary anastomosis of the rectosigmoid. All of these accessory procedures make exenteration much less of a disfiguring and disabling operation. One must remember that this procedure is of unquestionably high risk, with a 3% to 5% mortality rate and a morbidity rate that is greater than 60%. Therefore, there must be remarkable commitment on behalf of both the surgeon and patient before undertaking such a radical procedure.

SPECIAL TREATMENT PROBLEMS

There are numerous special treatment problems (active pelvic infections, either gynecologic or colorectal; anatomic distortions such as of the pelvis or kidney, or those resulting from prior surgery; disease diagnosis following simple hysterectomy) that make the treatment of cervical cancer uniquely challenging. Of all of these problems, the one that is probably the most difficult to deal with is cervical cancer complicating an intrauterine pregnancy, particularly if the pregnancy is one that is desired. A discussion of this topic is beyond the scope of this text, but it must be noted that many of the traditional recommendations were based on scanty data. In our institution, treatment decisions are highly individualized, with significant emphasis being given to the patients' desires regarding maintenance of the pregnancy.

PROGNOSIS

Interested readers are encouraged to review the Annual Report on Gynecologic Cancer published by the International Federation of Gynecology and Obstetrics to obtain specific information on 5-year survival rates for any given disease stage treated in a select geographic location. In general, 5-year survival rates are approximately 75% for Stage I, 55% for State II, 35% for Stage III, and less than 5% for Stage IV. Results are remarkably heterogeneous because any given stage can have a wide variation in size, cell type, and grade, with certain institutions being more likely to see more advanced disease within a given stage.

TUMORS OF THE VULVA

method of
RAYMOND H. KAUFMAN, M.D.
Baylor College of Medicine
Houston, Texas

Both benign and malignant neoplasms are found on the vulva. Careful inspection of the vulva and vagina is still the best means of accessing the disease processes involving this area. The colposcope can be of some help in carefully examining the vulvar tissues; however, the use of a hand magnifying glass (2–4×) usually suffices. Vulvar biopsies should be liberally performed in the office because, in many instances, a specific diagnosis is based on the findings of the biopsy. Small discrete lesions are best handled by an excisional biopsy. For biopsy of larger or widespread lesions, the Keyes cutaneous dermal punch biopsy instrument should be used. A 4-mm punch is usually adequate for providing a tissue specimen.

After obtaining the biopsy, the tissue specimen should be oriented on a small piece of filter paper or paper towel before it is dropped into the fixative. This approach allows for proper sectioning of the specimen, avoiding tangential cuts and occasionally erroneous diagnosis. Washing the vulva with 4% to 5% acetic acid frequently highlights mucosal lesions such as intraepithelial neoplasia, which often turns acetowhite after the application of the solution. This change is also often seen in the presence of human papillomavirus (HPV) infection involving the vulvar tissues. Staining of the vulva with 1% toluidine blue is sometimes of help in selecting a biopsy site. The vulva is washed with 1% toluidine blue. After allowing the stain to dry, the tissues are then washed with 1% acetic acid, which should remove the toluidine blue. Lesions such as invasive and intraepithelial carcinoma retain the blue color after being washed with acetic acid.

BENIGN TUMORS OF THE VULVA

A wide spectrum of benign, solid, and cystic tumors involve the vulva. These tumors can easily be classified based on the tissue of origin, embryologic derivation, morphologic findings, or gross appearance. We divide the benign tumors of the vulva into solid and cystic tumors. They are classified as in Table 1.

If a benign tumor is not causing the patient discomfort and the diagnosis is apparent on the basis of gross inspection, it can be left alone. However, if the clinician is not absolutely sure of the exact nature of the tumor, a biopsy should be obtained.

Benign Solid Tumors

The most common of the benign solid tumors affecting the vulva are the acrochordon (often called fibroepithelial polyp), fibroma, lipoma, neurofibroma, and solid tumors arising in the Bartholin and vestibular glands. When the diagnosis is in doubt or the tumor is causing discomfort, the tumor should be widely excised either in the office using local anesthesia or in the hospital while the patient is under general anesthesia. Wide local excision with primary closure of the defect is all that is required.

Benign Cystic Tumors

The most common cystic tumors involving the vulva are the epidermal inclusion cyst and develop-

TABLE 1. **Classification of Benign Vulvar Tumors**

Benign Solid Tumors
- Epidermal origin
  - Condyloma acuminatum
  - Molluscum contagiosum
  - Acrochordon
  - Seborrheic keratosis
  - Nevus
- Epidermal appendage origin
  - Hidradenoma
  - Sebaceous adenoma
  - Basal cell carcinoma
- Mesodermal origin
  - Fibroma
  - Lipoma
  - Neurofibroma
  - Leiomyoma
  - Granular cell myoblastoma
  - Hemangioma
  - Pyogenic granuloma
  - Lymphangioma
- Bartholin's and vestibular gland origin
  - Adenofibroma
  - Mucous adenoma
- Urethral origin
  - Caruncle
  - Prolapse of the urethral mucosa

Benign Cystic Tumors
- Epidermal origin
  - Epidermal inclusion cysts
  - Pilonidal cysts
- Epidermal appendage origin
  - Sebaceous cysts
  - Hidradenoma
  - Fox-Fordyce disease
  - Syringoma
- Embryonic remnant origin
  - Mesonephric (Gartner's) cysts
  - Paromesonephic (müllerian) cysts
  - Urogenital sinus cysts
  - Cysts of canal of Nuck (hydrocele)
  - Adenosis
  - Cysts of supernumerary mammary glands
  - Dermoid cysts
- Bartholin's gland origin
  - Duct cysts
  - Abscess
- Urethral and paraurethral origin
  - Paraurethral (Skene's duct) cysts
  - Urethral diverticula
- Miscellaneous oigin
  - Endometriosis
  - Cystic lymphangioma
  - Liquified hematoma

mental cysts of urogenital sinus, paramesonephric duct, mesonephric duct, and ectopic mammary gland origin. Once again, if the clinician is confident of the diagnosis and the patient is asymptomatic, these tumors can be left untreated. If the diagnosis is in doubt or if the patient has symptoms related to the mass, a local excision is usually adequate therapy.

The hidradenoma is often a confusing tumor for clinicians as well as pathologists. Hidradenomas are not uncommonly confused with a primary or metastatic adenocarcinoma of the vulva. The distinction is made on the basis of the characteristic pattern of the tumor, as well as the absence of nuclear atypia and multilayering of cells. This tumor is easily removed in the office by local excision using local anesthesia.

Bartholin's duct cyst and abscess are seen in approximately 2% of new gynecologic patients. The cysts arise within the duct system of the Bartholin gland. Occlusion of the duct usually occurs near the opening of the main duct into the vestibule. Most cysts involve only the main duct and thus are unilocular, although occasionally one or more loculi lie deep in the main cyst. The majority of patients with small Bartholin's duct cysts are asymptomatic. If the cyst becomes enlarged, discomfort and pressure may be experienced by the patient, as may discomfort during coitus and walking. Treatment under these circumstances is best managed by marsupialization. The incision for marsupialization should be made medially enough that the new orifice of the duct is located close to the original opening of the Bartholin duct into the vestibule. An incision 4 to 6 cm in length is made extending through the wall of the cyst. After evacuation of the contents, the lining of the cyst is sewn to the mucosal and skin surfaces with interrupted fine, absorbable sutures.

An acute Bartholin abscess may arise primarily or may occur in the presence of a previous Bartholin duct cyst. Culture of the contents of an abscess reveals a wide spectrum of organisms. The chief symptoms of a Bartholin abscess consist of pain and tenderness over the affected gland. The rapidity of development and the extent of involvement depend on the size of an infected cyst and the virulence of the infectious agent. Objective signs include unilateral swelling over the site of the affected gland, redness of the overlying skin, and frequently, edema of the surrounding labia. An acute Bartholin abscess usually requires surgical therapy, but local application of heat in the form of hot, wet dressings or sitz baths may promote spontaneous drainage within 72 hours. If treatment is begun early enough with a broad-spectrum antibiotic, occasionally formation of an abscess can be prevented. Incision and drainage of the abscess can be accomplished in the physician's office. Marsupialization of the abscess through the use of a Word catheter, an inflatable bulb-tipped closed catheter, is effective treatment. The catheter is inserted into the abscess cavity after a small stab incision is made into the abscess close to the hymenal ring, and the contents of the abscess are evacuated. After the catheter is inserted, the balloon is inflated with 2 mL of saline. The distal end of the catheter is then tucked into the vagina. The catheter should be left in place for at least 4 to 6 weeks, after which time the balloon is deflated and the catheter is removed. The patient rarely notes the presence of the catheter and may engage in sexual activity without disturbing it.

MALIGNANT NEOPLASMS OF THE VULVA

Both intraepithelial and invasive neoplasms are found on the vulva. The International Society for the Study of Vulvar Diseases has classified intraepithelial neoplastic disorders of the vulvar skin and mucosa as follows:

I. Squamous (may include changes resulting from HPV infection)
   A. Vulvar intraepithelial neoplasia (VIN)-1 (mild dysplasia)
   B. VIN-2 (moderate dysplasia)
   C. VIN-3 (severe dysplasia; carcinoma in situ)
II. Other
   A. Paget's disease
   B. Melanoma, level one

The incidence of VIN-3 has nearly doubled between 1973 to 1976 and 1985 to 1987 (Sturgeon et al).* During this same period of time, however, the incidence rate of invasive carcinoma remained stable. Sturgeon and colleagues reported that the incidence of VIN-3 increased from 1.1 to 2.1 cases per 100,000 women years. The largest increase occurred in white women under the age of 35. The peak incidence of in situ carcinoma decreased over time from women over the age of 54 to women between the ages of 35 and 54. Several possible factors may explain the increased incidence of this disease and its occurrence at a younger age. Heightened awareness of neoplasia on the part of the physician plays some role in its more frequent diagnosis. Associated with this factor is an increasing tendency to perform biopsies on questionable lesions. A third factor is the increased occurrence of viral infections involving the lower genital tract. The association of HPV with the development of lower genital tract neoplasia is now well accepted. Whereas most cases of condylomata acuminata of the lower genital tract are associated with infection by HPV Type 6 and HPV Type 11, vulvar squamous cell carcinomas of the vulva are most often associated with HPV Types 16 and 18. However, it has been postulated that possibly two forms of invasive squamous cell carcinoma of the vulva are seen. One is observed most often in younger women who smoke and whose lesions morphologically resemble the changes seen with intraepithelial neoplasia and whose tumors have a high association with HPV infection. The other type of cancer is seen more often in older women with a more well-differentiated type of squamous cell carcinoma who do not smoke and whose lesions are infrequently associated with HPV infection.

The diagnosis of vulvar intraepithelial neoplasia must be established by biopsy before treatment is undertaken. Very often, the lesions are multifocal. If this is the case, often several biopsies should be taken from different sites to establish that the lesion is, in fact, intraepithelial and not invasive.

Treatment of VIN-3

Opinion regarding management of intraepithelial squamous cell carcinoma of the vulva has changed radically since the early 1970s. The treatment should be individualized on the basis of the location and extent of the lesion. Both wide local excision and laser surgery are appropriate under proper circumstances. If wide local excision is chosen as a method of treatment, the entire lesion should be surgically removed, taking with it at least 0.5 to 1 centimeter of normal tissue. Frozen sections should be taken from the distal margins of the excised tissue to be certain that there is no residual disease. If disease is noted along the margins of the excised tissue, more skin and mucosa should be removed until the margins are free of disease. Recurrence of disease is related to the presence or absence of free margins. When extensive VIN-3 is present, wide local excision may consist of performance of a wide superficial skinning vulvectomy. The skin and a small amount of subcutaneous tissue are removed, leaving the bulk of the vulvar structures intact. Often, the defect can be closed primarily, but occasionally, it will be necessary to use a skin graft to adequately cover the denuded vulvar surfaces. If the disease extends into the anal canal, it is necessary to remove the anal mucosa up to the level of the pectinate line. The rectal mucosa can then be undermined and pulled down to cover the defect.

The use of the carbon dioxide laser in treating VIN is becoming increasing popular. It is an excellent tool for the treatment of this disease, especially disease that is localized. Prior to using this approach, however, an occult invasive carcinoma must be excluded through adequate biopsies. Lesions demonstrating thickening of the tissues or those that appear ulcerated are best treated by excision rather than by laser. When the laser is used, the lesion and a surrounding 0.5 to 1 centimeter of normal tissue should be ablated down to a depth of 1 to 3 millimeters, depending on the location of the lesion. On skin surfaces, the ablation should be carried down to a depth of 3 millimeters to remove any possible disease that has extended down into the superficial skin appendages. A depth of destruction to 1 millimeter is adequate on mucosal surfaces.

We prefer not to use the carbon dioxide laser in treating extensive vulvar intraepithelial neoplasia. Attempts to remove the entire lesion in one session prove to be time consuming, uncomfortable for the patient, and associated with significant postoperative discomfort.

The primary complications observed following laser therapy to the vulva are pain, bleeding, and discharge. Usually, the degree of pain is related to the area of the vulva treated and to the depth of treatment. The pain usually becomes most severe 4 to 5 days after therapy and may persist for another 5 to 10 days. The use of analgesics and warm sitz baths is of value in alleviating the symptoms.

Paget's disease of the vulva requires more aggressive treatment than does squamous cell carcinoma in situ. Underlying adnexal carcinoma occurs in a small number of patients. Added to this possibility is that of concomitant invasive disease. In addition, the intraepidermal migration of Paget's cells can occur, and

---

*Sturgeon SR, Brinton LA, Devesa SS, et al. In situ and invasive vulvar cancer incidence trends (1973–1987). Am J Obstet Gynecol 1992; *166*:1482.

an adequate margin of normal-appearing tissue must be removed. Our approach to therapy is that of wide local excision of the lesion. When the disease involves large areas of the vulva, a wide superficial vulvectomy can be performed. This is carried out in the form of a so-called skinning vulvectomy with removal of the skin and underlying adnexal structures, leaving the subcutaneous fat in place. If an underlying adnexal or invasive carcinoma is found, a second procedure consisting of a more extensive vulvectomy and inguinal-femoral lymphadenectomy should be performed.

Invasive Neoplasms of the Vulva

Malignant vulvar tumors have been classified as in Table 2. The most common of the malignant tumors is squamous cell carcinoma. This lesion most commonly presents as a raised granular tumor on the vulva, but it also may appear as a thickened white plaque or granular ulceration. Often, invasive squamous cell carcinoma is seen in association with lichen sclerosus, which in the past led to the concept that lichen sclerosus was a precursor of invasive carcinoma. However, the likelihood that an individual with lichen sclerosus will ultimately develop invasive carcinoma of the vulva is less than 5%. In addition to the presence of a mass, the patient often complains of pruritus, bleeding from the vulva, discharge, and occasionally, pain. The diagnosis is established on the basis of a biopsy.

Treatment

Treatment to a large extent depends upon the stage of disease. Also of importance is an understanding of the method of spread of vulvar carcinoma. This is by direct extension and via the lymphatics to the ipsilateral inguinal and femoral lymph nodes. From here, the cancer may spread to the contralateral groin nodes or to the deep pelvic lymph nodes, or both.

TABLE 2. **Malignant Tumors of the Vulva**

- Epithelial tumors of the skin and mucosa
  - Squamous cell origin
    - Squamous cell carcinoma
    - Verrucous carcinoma
  - Basal cell carcinoma
  - Melanoma
  - Adenocarcinoma
    - Paget's disease
    - Skin appendage
- Malignant tumors of the urethra
- Bartholin gland carcinoma
  - Squamous cell carcinoma
  - Adenocarcinoma
  - Adenoid cystic carcinoma
  - Adenosquamous carcinoma
  - Transitional cell carcinoma
- Carcinoma and sarcoma of ectopic breast tissue
- Soft tissue sarcomas
  - Embryonal rhabdomyosarcoma
  - Leiomyosarcoma
  - Malignant fibrous histiocytoma
  - Epithelial sarcoma

Surgical staging also plays a role in the decision as to appropriate therapy. The International Federation of Gynecology and Obstetrics (FIGO) staging system for carcinoma of the vulva is surgically determined, as indicated in Table 3.

Prior to formulation of a treatment plan, the patient should be carefully evaluated to search for the presence of distant metastasis, although this is highly unlikely in a Stage I or II lesion. Certainly, a preoperative chest x-ray study, bone scan, and CT scan of the pelvis should be used in the search for enlarged lymph nodes, especially in those individuals with Stage III or IV disease.

Whereas in the past, radical vulvectomy with bilateral femoral-inguinal lymph node dissection was considered the standard of care for all cases of invasive carcinoma of the vulva, this is no longer true today. Treatment is individualized and based on the knowledge of the natural spread of vulvar carcinoma.

Treatment of Stage I Carcinoma. With a tumor localized to one side of the vulva, a partial deep vulvectomy with ipsilateral groin node dissection is considered adequate treatment. This allows for preservation of much of the normal vulvar anatomy and is also associated with less postoperative morbidity than occurs with radical vulvectomy. In excising the tumor, at least a 2- to 3-centimeter margin of normal skin should be removed surrounding the tumor, and the subcutaneous fat should be excised down to the fascia. A groin dissection should be performed through a separate incision. If there is no evidence of spread to the groin lymph nodes, no further therapy is required. If, however, positive nodes are found, then the contralateral lymph nodes should be removed or the contralateral groin should be treated with external beam radiotherapy. The deep pelvic nodes should also receive external beam therapy. In the presence of a mid-line lesion, a bilateral inguinal-femoral lymph node dissection should be performed. Following surgical excision of the lesion and groin lymph nodes, suction drainage should be left in place until the drainage has decreased to a negligible amount.

Treatment of Stage II Disease. Depending on the size of the tumor, an operative procedure similar to that recommended for Stage I disease can be carried out for Stage II disease. Occasionally, however, when the lesion is of sufficient size, it is necessary to perform a complete deep vulvectomy in order to remove the entire tumor along with an adequate margin of normal tissue. When this procedure is performed, the inguinal and femoral lymph nodes are removed through separate groin incisions. Often, in order to close a large defect, it is necessary to produce skin flaps with attached subcutaneous fat to cover the defect.

Treatment of Stage III Disease. A Stage III tumor that has spread to the lower urethra and vagina is also treated by vulvectomy with removal of the lower portion of the urethra or vagina, or both, to allow for at least a 2-centimeter margin of normal tissue. When the anus is involved with the tumor, it

TABLE 3. **FIGO Staging System for Carcinoma of the Vulva**

Stage 0	Carcinoma in situ; intraepithelial carcinoma.
Stage I	Tumors confined to the vulva and/or perineum; 2 cm or less in greatest dimension; nodes are not palpable
Stage II	Tumor confined to the vulva and/or perineum; more than 2 cm in greatest dimension; nodes are not palpable.
Stage III	Tumor of any size with: Adjacent spread to the lower urethra and/or the vagina, or the anus, and/or — Unilateral regional lymph node metastasis
Stage IVA	Tumor invades any of the following: Upper urethra, bladder mucosa, rectal mucosa, or pelvic bone, as well as/or bilateral regional node metastasis
Stage IVB	Any distant metastasis, including pelvic lymph nodes

may be necessary to perform a vulvectomy with abdominoperineal resection while removing the anus. Bilateral inguinal and femoral lymph nodes should be removed through separate groin incisions. Occasionally, it is necessary to use a full-thickness skin flap using the gracilis muscle to cover a large vulvar defect that cannot be covered by a rhomboid flap.

In the presence of a large, bulky lesion, the use of radiotherapy may decrease its size to the point where a less radical excision is required.

Treatment of Stage IV Disease. Therapy of Stage IV vulvar carcinoma must be individualized. Depending on whether or not there is evidence of distant metastasis, local palliative excision or radiation therapy, or both, is utilized. In the absence of distant metastasis, the patients are managed as described for Stage III disease.

Verrucous Carcinoma

Verrucous carcinoma, often called condyloma of Buschke-Löwenstein, appears as a large, irregular cauliflower lesion. It locally invades the vulvar tissue without the development of metastasis. Like condyloma acuminata, it has been found to be associated with HPV Type 6. A biopsy usually confirms the diagnosis. The lesion can usually be easily distinguished from invasive squamous cell carcinoma in that large, broad areas of relatively well-differentiated squamous cells are noted to be pushing down into the dermis rather than invading it.

Treatment

The treatment of verrucous carcinoma consists of wide local excision. Rarely is it necessary to consider performing a groin lymph node dissection. Only if enlarged, suspicious lymph nodes are palpated should a groin dissection be performed. Radiation therapy is contraindicated in the management of this tumor because radiation frequently transforms it into an aggressive neoplasm that may metastasize.

Basal Cell Carcinoma

Basal cell carcinoma usually arises as a solitary, ulcerated lesion with raised, round, pearly edges. If it is left untreated, this lesion will continue to invade the vulvar tissues destructively. Only rarely does basal cell carcinoma metastasize.

Treatment

Treatment consists of wide local excision of the neoplasm. It is not necessary to perform a regional lymph node dissection because spread to the lymph nodes is extremely rare.

Melanoma

Very uncommonly, melanoma occurs as a primary vulvar lesion. When it does occur, however, early diagnosis is mandatory if cure is to be achieved. Prognosis is directly related to the depth of invasion of the tumor. Several methods for microstaging melanoma have been proposed. The staging systems of Clark and Breslow are most commonly used by the pathologist. They are listed in Table 4.

The diagnosis is established on the basis of biopsy. The microstaging is finally determined following excision of the neoplasm.

Treatment

Level one and two melanomas have an extremely good prognosis. Melanoma that extends into the subcutaneous fat carries with it an almost hopeless outlook.

Tumors invading less than 1 millimeter can be treated by wide local excision, removing the underlying subcutaneous fat. When the level of extension is deeper than 1 millimeter, a wide radical excision of the neoplasm is recommended, along with ipsilateral inguinofemoral lymph node removal. The lymph node dissection is more prognostic than therapeutic because once spread to the regional lymph nodes has occurred, the prognosis is extremely poor regardless of additional adjunctive therapy that is attempted.

Bartholin's Gland Carcinoma

The diagnosis of Bartholin's gland carcinoma is established when the neoplasm is localized to the re-

TABLE 4. **Levels of Melanoma**

Clark's Levels	Breslow's Levels (modified)
1. Intraepithelial	<0.76 mm
2. Extends into papillary dermis	0.76–1.49 mm
3. Fills papillary dermis	1.50–2.49 mm
4. Extends into reticular dermis	2.50–3.99 mm
5. Extends into subcutaneous fat	≥ 4 mm

gion of Bartholin's gland and histologic evidence of Bartholin's gland structures is contiguous to the tumor. In addition, the skin overlying the neoplasm should be intact. Suspicion of a malignancy of the Bartholin gland should be aroused when the postmenopausal woman suddenly develops what is thought to be a Bartholin duct abscess or cyst. Another finding that should arouse suspicion is the presence of a solid mass developing in this region.

Treatment

Bartholin's gland carcinomas are managed in a manner similar to that for invasive squamous cell carcinoma of the vulva.

Soft Tissue Sarcoma

Soft tissue sarcomas are extremely rare. They usually appear as rapidly growing solid tumors. The diagnosis is made on the basis of biopsy or histologic examination of the surgical specimen. Therapy consists primarily of wide local excision. Radiotherapy is of little use in the management of most vulvar sarcomas.

THROMBOPHLEBITIS IN OBSTETRICS AND GYNECOLOGY

method of
ANTHONY J. COMEROTA, M.D., and
RUSSELL N. HARADA, M.D.
Temple University Hospital
Philadelphia, Pennsylvania

DEEP VENOUS THROMBOSIS

Thrombophlebitis is a poor term because it carries the connotation of an inflammatory etiology or response. This is not often the case, and "venous thrombosis" is more descriptive of the underlying problem. In absolute numbers, deep venous thrombosis (DVT) represents a relatively uncommon complication of pregnancy, with an incidence of only 0.02% to 0.3%. Despite this low incidence, the pregnant woman faces a sixfold risk of venous thromboembolism compared with the nonpregnant woman, and venous thromboembolism is a leading cause of maternal mortality, representing 14.3% of all deaths. Additionally, the incidence of deep venous thrombosis following gynecologic procedures ranges from 10% to 30%.

Factors that identify the high-risk patient include a history of previous deep venous thrombosis or pulmonary embolism, age greater than 30 years, obesity, prolonged bed rest, malignancy, pelvic operation, prolonged operative procedure (over 2 hours in duration), shortened prothrombin time or partial thromboplastin time, birth control pills, complications during delivery, and cesarean section. Hypercoagulable states also predispose obstetric patients to venous thromboembolism. The period of greatest risk is the immediate postpartum period, especially following cesarean section. The risk of DVT may be 20 times higher in the puerperium following cesarean section than in the nonpregnant population.

Two basic pathophysiologic processes account for the occurrence of venous thromboembolism during pregnancy. The first is by compression of the pelvic veins and vena cava by the gravid uterus. The second is the hypercoagulability that occurs as a result of pregnancy. Pregnant patients have an increase in clotting factors, especially factors II, VII, VIII, and X, as well as an increase in fibrin split products and a decrease in clotting inhibitors. Plasma fibrinolytic activity and antithrombin III levels are also decreased. There is evidence that platelet counts increase following labor. Exogenous estrogen increase certain clotting factors, decrease the level of antithrombin III, and decrease vascular tone, which may promote venous stasis.

Diagnosis

The clinical diagnosis of deep venous thrombosis is elusive, and the initial diagnosis is erroneous at least 50% of the time. The symptoms and signs of DVT include swelling, edema, pain, and a change in limb color. The level of thrombosis determines the site of swelling. Swelling in the thigh usually signifies iliofemoral DVT, whereas femoral-popliteal DVT usually causes swelling in the calf and foot. A palpable cord may be present, and Homan's sign is positive when pain is elicited with passive dorsiflexion of the foot; however, these findings (or their absence) are frequently misleading. With extensive thrombosis of the iliofemoral system, a clinical picture of massive lower extremity edema and blanching, referred to as phlegmasia alba dolens (milk leg), may occur. In the most severe form of iliofemoral DVT, the arterial supply to the leg is compromised, and the threatened limb becomes blue; this condition is referred to as phlegmasia cerulea dolens (painful blue leg). Although the left leg is more frequently involved with DVT in general, the predilection for left-sided DVT is more pronounced in the pregnant patient. The diagnosis should be suspected when swelling occurs, especially when it is associated with atypical pelvic and lower abdominal complaints. Because the medical and nonmedical implications of the diagnosis of DVT are serious and the complications associated with therapy are real, patients should not be treated on the basis of clinical impression alone and the diagnosis should be proved by some objective means.

Objective diagnostic studies for DVT can be divided into invasive and noninvasive methods. Ascending phlebography is traditionally accepted as the diagnostic gold standard for DVT. It involves the injection of contrast into the venous system, usually via a foot vein. Radiographs of the limb will show either partially occluding venous thrombi or nonfilling, which indicates occlusion. Although ascending phlebography is highly accurate in diagnosing DVT, it is invasive and uncomfortable, exposes the fetus to the potential harmful effects of radiation, may actually cause DVT, and subjects the patient to an intravenous contrast agent. Because of these disadvantages, several noninvasive diagnostic methods have been developed.

Indirect methods of noninvasive testing measure some aspect of physiology that is expected to be abnormal owing to luminal obstruction. This is in contrast to the direct methods of noninvasive testing, which image the venous system, detailing areas of thrombosis. The indirect methods include impedance plethysmography and phleborrheography. Both of these tests suffer from inaccuracies in detecting nonoccluding and calf vein thrombosis, and are completely unreliable for evaluating the asymptomatic high-risk patient. In our vascular laboratory, these tests have been largely replaced by direct methods owing to the improved accuracy with venous duplex imaging and therefore are not discussed further.

Direct noninvasive methods include continuous wave Doppler and venous duplex imaging. Continuous wave Doppler examines the velocity patterns of venous flow with ultrasound, whereas duplex imaging combines B-mode ultrasound, which allows examination of the morphology of the venous system, with continuous wave Doppler. Continuous wave Doppler is performed by placing the probe over different segments of the extremity and listening to the change in the velocity signal with respiratory excursion and Valsalva augmentation maneuvers. Although this technique is reported to be fairly accurate in detecting occluding thrombus, thrombus that partially occludes the vessel lumen is often missed. Venous duplex imaging is the noninvasive diagnostic method of choice for acute DVT. Venous duplex imaging provides an anatomic and functional evaluation of the deep limb veins. Because ultrasound rather than ionizing radiation is used, there is no risk to the fetus. A recent literature review of over 3500 patients by comparing venous duplex imaging and phlebography found that the sensitivity, specificity, and positive and negative predictive values for venous duplex imaging in symptomatic patients were 95%.* For the surveillance of high-risk asymptomatic patients, the overall sensitivity was only 54%. Of these high-risk asymptomatic patients, the sensitivity of detecting proximal DVT was much better than that of detecting calf DVT (93% verses 54%, respectively). Duplex imaging is highly accurate in detecting proximal DVT but will miss calf DVT in about 20% to 40% of cases. We believe that venous duplex imaging is the best noninvasive test for diagnosing acute DVT.

Treatment

The treatment of DVT in pregnant patients is different from that in nonpregnant patients, in that the use of warfarin compounds may have detrimental effects on the fetus. Thrombolytic agents have a generic added risk compared with standard anticoagulation, and there is little experience with their use in the pregnant patient.

The major sequela of DVT is pulmonary embolism in the acute stage and the post-thrombotic syndrome chronically. Ideal treatment eliminates the clot, thereby removing the risk of pulmonary embolism. The post-thrombotic syndrome, manifested by swelling, brawny induration, hyperpigmentation, and ulceration, may occur several years after DVT, and is a potential source of great morbidity and expense. Eliminating the thrombus prior to anatomic or functional damage of the venous valves and restoring venous patency minimize the development of the post-thrombotic syndrome. Streptokinase, urokinase, and tissue plasminogen activator are the currently available thrombolytic agents that can potentially achieve these goals pharmacologically, and venous thrombectomy can achieve them mechanically.

Thrombolytic Therapy

The thrombolytic agents are produced from different sources and possess different mechanisms of action. Streptokinase (SK) is a filtrate of beta-hemolytic streptococci, which activates plasminogen indirectly through the formation of activator complexes. Urokinase (UK) is produced by cultured fetal kidney cells and acts on plasminogen directly by breaking the arginyl-valyl bond. Recombinant tissue plasminogen activator, a naturally occurring enzyme present in all tissues, is manufactured by recombinant DNA technology. Recombinant tissue plasminogen activator binds to fibrin present on the surface of thrombus and activates plasminogen by breaking the arginyl-valyl bond. Plasmin production is the net result of the use of all thrombolytic agents, and is the active enzyme that dissolves thrombus. All three agents are most effective when given within 7 days of the onset of thrombosis, and they are more effective if given earlier. Contraindications to thrombolytic therapy are listed in Table 1.

TABLE 1. **Contraindications to Thrombolytic Therapy**

Absolute contraindications
Current active bleeding
Intracranial disease
Recent eye operation (3 months)
Relative contraindications
Within 10 days of major surgery
Postpartum—10 days
Recent external cardiac massage
Active peptic ulcer or other gastrointestinal pathology
Biopsy of a noncompressible site
Hemorrhagic coagulopathy
Pregnancy
Diabetic hemorrhagic retinopathy
Recent serious trauma
Uncontrolled hypertension
Severe hepatic or renal disease
Atrial fibrillation or cardiac thrombus
Arterial aneurysmal disease

*Comerata AJ, Katz ML, and Hashemi H: Venous duplex imaging for the diagnosis of acute DVT. Haemostasis *23*(Suppl 1):62–72, 1993.

When administered systemically, a loading dose of each agent must be given. This is especially important when administering SK to overcome circulating antistreptococcal antibodies. Patients who had streptococcal infections or were treated with SK within the past 6 months frequently do not respond, owing to the high circulating titers of antistreptococcal antibodies. UK and tissue plasminogen activator are the lytic agents of choice in this setting. Prior to administering streptokinase, 100 mg of hydrocortisone (Solu-Cortef) is given intravenously. Steroids minimize the pyretic response to streptokinase and may be repeated during the course of therapy if necessary. Acetaminophen, 650 mg every 4 hours, is used to treat the mild pyretic response as well as arthralgias and myalgias that may be associated with SK infusion. UK is given systemically as a loading dose of 4400 units per kg and a subsequent infusion of 4400 units per kg per hour. Patients frequently develop a pyretic response to UK. Therefore, pretreatment with antihistamines, steroids, and acetaminophen is routine in our practice.

There is much less experience treating acute DVT with recombinant plasminogen factor; therefore dosing schedules have not been well established. A reasonable treatment scheme would be a loading dose of 10 mg and a continuous infusion of 0.05 mg per kg per hour, with a maximal dose of 100 mg. An alternative treatment would be 50 mg infused over 2 hours with a repeat dose of 30 to 50 mg given intravenously over 6 hours. Table 2 summarizes the dosaging, advantages, and disadvantages of each thrombolytic agent. UK and tissue plasminogen activator have fewer side effects than SK; however, these agents are more costly. Factoring in the treatment of complications and lengths of treatment, the overall cost of UK therapy may be similar to that of SK. Fibrinogen levels should be monitored to modify infusion rates because levels of 50 to 100 mg have been associated with an increased incidence of bleeding complications.

Anticoagulation Therapy

Standard anticoagulation is used to stop thrombus propagation, thereby allowing the patient's endogenous fibrinolysis to reduce thrombus burden and recanalize occluded veins. Intravenous or high-dose subcutaneous porcine sodium heparin is the anticoagulant of choice. Low-dose subcutaneous heparin is inadequate therapy for established deep venous thrombosis. Continuous intravenous heparin infusion is the method chosen for most patients, because it allows constant anticoagulation with fewer bleeding complications than the intermittent intravenous bolus technique. Use of intramuscular heparin should be avoided owing variable blood levels and the high risk of hematoma formation. Evidence exists that anticoagulation with heparin stimulates endogenous fibrinolytic activity.

Patients are given a loading dose of 100 units per kg as an intravenous bolus, followed by 12 to 15 units per kg per hour as a continuous infusion. After 8 to 12 hours, the partial thromboplastin time (PTT) is monitored and should be prolonged to 70 to 90 seconds. In patients who are not in the postoperative period and who have no other risk factors for bleeding complications, we prefer to maintain the PTT higher than 100 seconds. This ensures consistent anticoagulation, and if it is maintained for only 2 to 4 days, there is no increased hemorrhagic complication rate compared with that in patients with PTT values titrated to 70 to 90 seconds. If the patient is not therapeutically anticoagulated, a repeat bolus injection of 3000 to 5000 units of heparin is administered, and the continuous infusion is increased by 100 to 200 units per hour. The PTT is then rechecked in 6 to 8 hours. Heparin requirements frequently decrease as the thrombotic process is controlled, because fewer procoagulants are produced.

All patients receiving heparin must be carefully monitored for the rare heparin-induced platelet aggregation reaction (including patients receiving low-dose subcutaneous heparin); therefore, platelet

TABLE 2. **Comparison of Thrombolytic Agents**

	Streptokinase (Streptase, Kabikinase)	**Urokinase (Abbokinase)**	**Tissue Plasminogen Activator (Activase)**
Half-life	Bimodal: 16 and 83 min	15 min	4–7 min
Advantages	Relatively inexpensive	Nonantigenic; predictable dose-response relationship; decreased bleeding complications (5%–10%)	Nonantigenic; high affinity for thrombus-bound fibrin; may be faster acting and more potent
Disadvantages	Dose-reponse relationship variable; allergic reactions; increased bleeding complications (15% to 20%); not effective in patients with previous therapy or streptococcal infection within last 6 months	Expensive	Expensive
Systemic Dosing	Loading dose: 250,000 U IV over 30 min; 100,000 U IV/h	Loading dose: 4400 U/kg IV over 10 min; 4400 U/kg IV/h	50 mg infused over 2 h; repeat 30–50 mg IV over 4–6 h, as necessary
Regional Dosing	5,000–10,000 U/h	30,000–50,000 U/h	0.1 U/kg/h
Wholesale Cost	$50 (250,000 U)	$137.50 (250,000 U)	$1,350 (50 mg)

counts should be checked at least three times a week. A drop in the platelet count heralds this reaction, and heparin must be discontinued and the patient anticoagulated with warfarin. Failure of heparin therapy is most commonly associated with an inadequate dose. In rare instances, patients are encountered who have a congenital deficiency of antithrombin III. They will not respond to heparin and require anticoagulation with warfarin.

On the first day of treatment, after the heparin bolus, patients are started on warfarin, which inhibits the hepatic synthesis of the vitamin K–dependent clotting factors. Because existing clotting factors are variably degraded, warfarin compounds do not rapidly achieve anticoagulation, and require a minimum of 3 to 5 days before a true anticoagulant effect can be obtained. Most patients are given warfarin, 10 mg for 3 days, and the prothrombin time (PT) is monitored daily. Elderly patients and those with hepatic dysfunction or minimal hepatic reserve are begun on smaller doses. Subsequent doses of warfarin are based on the daily PT. The goal is to prolong the international normalized ratio to 2.0. When the PT approaches the therapeutic level, the continuous heparin infusion is converted to a bolus heparin infusion of 5000 units every 6 hours. Subsequent PT specimens are drawn immediately prior to a bolus heparin dose, since heparin infusions have an effect on the PT in the presence of warfarin. Having achieved a therapeutic level of anticoagulation with warfarin, heparin is discontinued and the patient's daily dose of warfarin is stabilized. The PT is monitored at biweekly intervals. The effect of the warfarin drugs can be reversed by administering 10 to 25 mg of vitamin K (AquaMEPHYTON) intravenously. The clotting factors can be rapidly restored, if necessary, by fresh frozen plasma. Patients remain anticoagulated for 6 months. If the initial episode of DVT was extensive, if the patient tolerates oral anticoagulation well and has a low risk of bleeding complications, oral anticoagulation is frequently extended to 12 months. Patients who are treated for recurrent venous thromboembolism or who are found to have an inherited or acquired hypercoagulable state are treated indefinitely.

An attractive alternative to oral anticoagulation is long-term self-administered subcutaneous heparin. The heparin dose required is that necessary to keep the midinterval PTT at 1.5 times the control. Following the 5 to 7 days of full anticoagulation for the acute process, the heparin is administered subcutaneously every 12 hours. The PTT is checked 6 hours following heparin injection (midinterval PTT). Once the appropriate heparin dose has been determined, further PTTs need not be obtained, and the patient self-administers this dose every 12 hours following discharge. This has been shown to be as effective as oral anticoagulation and is associated with minimal bleeding complications.

Once a diagnosis is established, treatment should be stratified based on the level of the thrombus and the patient's associated risk factors for the various treatment options. In general, patients who are not at high risk for bleeding complications should have calf DVT treated to avoid the 20% to 30% risk of extension into the proximal venous system, as well as the associated risk of pulmonary embolism when asymptomatic extension occurs. Anticoagulation therapy is generally sufficient treatment to prevent extension into the proximal venous system. In the absence of contraindications, we believe acute femoral popliteal venous thrombosis should be treated with systemic thrombolytic therapy in an effort to regain patency of the deep venous system and preserve the long-term valvular function. There are data suggesting that valvular function can be maintained and the risk of the post-thrombotic syndrome reduced. Standard anticoagulation is initiated following systemic thrombolysis.

Catheter-Directed Thrombolysis and Venous Thrombectomy

The morbidity of iliofemoral DVT may be considerable and can be avoided. Extensive iliofemoral DVT should be treated aggressively, with the goal of removing the thrombus from the iliofemoral venous system and restoring unobstructed venous outflow to the involved lower extremity. Prior to treatment, an iliofemoral phlebogram on the involved leg and contralateral iliocavagram is performed to establish the full extent of the thrombus. If a patient has no contraindication to thrombolytic therapy, direct intrathrombus infusion of a fibrinolytic agent via a catheter with multiple side holes has been shown to be very effective. A heparin infusion is started concurrently with catheter-directed thrombolysis and is continued following the completion of thrombolysis. If a catheter cannot be appropriately positioned or if the patient has a contraindication to thrombolytic therapy, a venous thrombectomy with an arteriovenous fistula and/or venous bypass is indicated. Surgical thrombectomy is especially appropriate in patients with extensive DVT causing phlegmasia cerulea dolens or phlegmasia alba dolens. Contemporary results with venous thrombectomy are substantially better than those reported two decades or more earlier, owing to improved technique, completion phlebography, the application of an arteriovenous fistula, continuing perioperative anticoagulation, and the application of external pneumatic compression garments.

Historically, patients with DVT were kept at bed rest with their legs elevated for about 7 days. This was thought to be important to minimize the potential for dislodgement of the thrombus. At present, we allow ambulation of the patient as soon as anticoagulation is instituted to help prevent further propagation of the thrombus. When they are immobile, we routinely apply pneumatic compression devices to patients with DVT. Prolonged sitting or standing is discouraged, and the thrombus is monitored by venous duplex imaging for possible propagation or dislodgement. We have seen no detrimental effects since instituting this protocol.

Vena Cava Interruption

Vena caval interruption techniques are indicated when pulmonary emboli occur despite anticoagulation therapy, if there is a contraindication to anticoagulation therapy, or if discontinuation of anticoagulation therapy is required following a complication. Vena caval interruption should also follow pulmonary embolectomy. Vena caval filters are effective in preventing recurrent pulmonary embolism, with an incidence following insertion of 2% to 4%. These are the preferred techniques, and most can be inserted percutaneously.

Caval ligation is indicated in patients with septic emboli that do not respond to antibiotic and anticoagulant therapy, multiple small pulmonary emboli in patients with minimal pulmonary functional reserve, paradoxical embolism to the arterial tree, and recurrent pulmonary emboli following vena caval plication.

DEEP VENOUS THROMBOSIS OF PREGNANCY

Treatment of DVT in the pregnant patient warrants special consideration, because coumarin derivatives (warfarin [Coumadin]) must be avoided and pregnancy is at least a relative contraindication to the use of thrombolytic agents. There is little experience with SK being used for the treatment of DVT during pregnancy. The therapeutic regimen used in one study did not differ significantly from that routinely recommended. Using radiolabeled SK, it was determined that the drug did not cross the placenta. In two patients so treated, no radioactivity was detected in the cord blood, nor was there any evidence of activation of the fibrinolytic system in the neonate when SK was given to the mother immediately before delivery. However, the neonates were found to have elevated levels of antistreptococcal antibodies. Until more data are available from carefully performed studies, thrombolytic agents should be withheld.

Drugs with a molecular weight of less than 1000 daltons pass through the placental membrane. Because of their low molecular weight, coumarin anticoagulants readily cross the placental barrier. Administration of coumarin derivatives to women during the first trimester causes a specific constellation of malformations in at least 25% of the offspring. This is known as the warfarin embryopathy or fetal warfarin syndrome, the most consistent features of which are nasal hypoplasia and stippled epiphyses. The use of coumarin derivatives at any other time during pregnancy may increase the risk of central nervous system anomalies in the fetus. Although the warfarin embryopathy syndrome is considered the most characteristic teratogenic consequence of oral anticoagulants, the sequelae of central nervous system abnormalities are more significant and debilitating than the warfarin embryopathy itself. In addition to the teratogenic effects of warfarin, the coagulation system of the fetus can be affected. The fetus has low levels of vitamin K–dependent clotting factors throughout gestation, and the coumarin drugs further deplete these already low levels. Hence, the coagulopathy present in the fetus is not necessarily related to that of the mother, and may persist long after the mother's coagulation parameters have returned to normal following discontinuation of the drug. This, therefore, places the fetus at an increased risk of hemorrhage, especially during delivery.

Patients with DVT during pregnancy should be treated acutely with continuous intravenous heparin. Anticoagulation for the duration of pregnancy should be maintained, with intermittent subcutaneous heparin given every 12 hours, maintaining the mid-interval PTT at 1.5 times control. Subcutaneous heparin should be discontinued just prior to delivery, and intravenous heparin is restarted in the immediate postpartum period. Following delivery, the patient can be converted to warfarin and maintained on adequate anticoagulation for a total of at least 6 months. During all subsequent pregnancies, the patient should be prophylactically treated with subcutaneous heparin, 5000 units every 12 hours. We emphasize that any female of childbearing potential should be thoroughly counseled on the need for effective contraception while taking oral anticoagulants.

Calf vein thrombosis during pregnancy is usually treated with external elastic compression stockings with a 20 to 30 mmHg ankle gradient and continued ambulation, with ongoing surveillance with venous duplex imaging. Acute iliofemoral venous thrombosis during pregnancy represents a particularly severe problem. It has been shown that these patients have a greater risk of post-thrombotic sequelae, which is especially morbid because these patients are so young. Our current recommendation would be venous thrombectomy with arteriovenous fistula. When this procedure is followed by heparin anticoagulation, this appears to be safe and effective therapy. There is no need to interrupt pregnancy except for a specific obstetric reason. Because this is a particularly young group of patients, and because the long-term results appear good without an adverse effect on the fetus, venous thrombectomy with an arteriovenous fistula should be seriously considered for severe iliofemoral DVT in these patients.

It remains to be seen whether the low-molecular weight heparins (LMWH) (e.g., enoxaparin sodium [Lovenox]) are effective for treating DVT during pregnancy. With average molecular weights of 3,200 to 6,500 daltons, these drugs do not cross the placenta. LMWH compounds are more completely absorbed from the subcutaneous tissues than is unfractionated heparin, and may further improve efficiency of prophylaxis. Although there is evidence that the incidence of heparin-induced thrombocytopenia may be reduced with LMWH, it does occur, and platelet counts need to be monitored. Two recent randomized, prospective trials comparing subcutaneous LMWH to intravenous unfractionated heparin in the treatment of proximal DVT revealed no difference in the incidence of thromboembolic events but a reduction in bleeding complications with LMWH. Because of these beneficial properties, LMWH hold promise for the treatment of DVT during pregnancy.

SUPERFICIAL THROMBOPHLEBITIS

Thrombophlebitis located in the superficial veins of the leg may be related to an acute inflammatory response or to true intraluminal thrombosis similar to DVT. These are clearly two separate pathologic entities. The associated thrombosis of these superficial veins frequently extends 8 to 10 centimeters higher than appreciated clinically; therefore, all patients should be evaluated with venous duplex imaging.

Superficial thrombophlebitis is associated with acute inflammation of the tissues surrounding the vein and the skin overlying the superficial veins, and the condition should be treated with the local application of moist heat, nonsteroidal anti-inflammatory medications, and external support stockings. If this condition recurs in multiple areas, thrombophlebitis migrans should be suspected and an underlying cause for this problem should be investigated. Collagen vascular disease and malignancy are common etiologies, and the underlying disease should be treated primarily. Recurrent superficial phlebitis warrants excision of the involved veins after the acute process has subsided.

Superficial vein thrombosis limited to the calf is similarly treated with external compression, nonsteroidal anti-inflammatory medications, and continued ambulation. If the process continues to extend to the major superficial veins above the knee, especially the greater saphenous vein, surgical therapy is recommended. Prior to ligation and excision of the involved veins, a venous duplex scan should be performed to exclude involvement of the deep venous system. If the deep veins are normal, then the involved superficial and greater saphenous veins are removed. Long-term anticoagulation is not required. If the deep venous system is involved, then the routine approach with anticoagulant therapy should be instituted.

OVARIAN VEIN THROMBOSIS

Ovarian vein thrombosis is a rare disorder that usually occurs within the first week of delivery or abortion. The disease can be clinically silent; however, more commonly patients present with fever, lower abdominal pain, and tenderness. Unlike DVT, over 90% of cases occur on the right side. Therefore, patients are often operated on for a presumed acute appendicitis, and the diagnosis is often made at the time of exploratory laparotomy. It is important to inspect the ovarian veins at the time of laparotomy for presumed acute appendicitis in the postpartum female. The best techniques for preoperative and postoperative diagnosis are computed tomography and magnetic resonance imaging. Ovarian vein thrombosis is most often treated with a standard anticoagulation regimen, including heparin for 5 to 7 days, followed by at least 6 months of warfarin therapy.

SEPTIC THROMBOPHLEBITIS

Septic thrombophlebitis is usually related to prolonged use of indwelling catheters in superficial veins. If the involved vein has a localized process that is adequately drained, the application of moist heat and administration of appropriate systemic antibiotics are sufficient to treat the problem. If there is loculated pus within the thrombosed vein, then the involved vein should be excised. Septic thrombophlebitis involving the pelvic veins requires treatment with both heparin and parenteral antibiotics.

CONTRACEPTION

method of

AMY E. POLLACK, M.D., M.P.H.
Columbia University
New York, New York

and

CASSANDRA MOORE, M.A., M.P.H.
Columbia University
New York, New York

Many contraceptive methods are currently available in the U.S. market, each with distinct advantages and disadvantages. Factors including cost, availability, ease of use, and personal health issues affect individual choice of a contraceptive method. As the risk of being infected with human immunodeficiency virus (HIV) and other sexually transmitted diseases (STD) continues, contraceptors and their family planning or health care providers must consider the risks and benefits of each method in the context of the unique needs of the user, in terms of both contraception and disease protection. Women at risk for STDs and acquired immune deficiency syndrome (AIDS) should be encouraged to use condoms in addition to other highly effective contraceptive methods. Although spermicidal preparations provide some protection against the most common STDs, the latex condom is the only contraceptive that provides proven protection against the transmission of HIV.

HORMONAL CONTRACEPTIVES

Oral Contraceptives

Oral contraceptives are highly effective and easily reversible and provide a method of birth control unrelated to the coital act. Combined oral contraceptives (COCs) prevent pregnancy primarily by suppressing ovulation through complementary estrogenic and progestogenic effects. Estrogenic effects include suppression of luteinizing hormone and follicle-stimulating hormone, and a direct effect on uterine secretions that leads to an inhibition of ovum implantation. Progestogenic effects include thickening of cervical mucus, which obstructs sperm transport, and inhibition of implantation through suppression of the endometrium.

Studies of modern low-dose COCs have shown reduced cardiovascular risk and significant protective effects against menorrhagia and anemia, benign breast disease, and ovarian and uterine cancer. The effect of COCs on plasma lipoprotein levels varies with the androgenicity of the progestin in the formulation. In general, estrogens increase triglyceride and high-density lipoprotein components, while progestins with androgenic effects (e.g., norgestrel and norethindrone) increase low-density lipoprotein levels. However, low-dose COCs containing norethindrone (0.5 mg per dose or less) decrease low-density lipoprotein levels and increase high-density lipoprotein levels, indicating that the effects of the estrogen component may overcome the androgenic effects of the progestin component to produce a positive impact on cardiovascular health. Recently, three new progestins—desogestrel, norgestimate, and gestodene—were developed with the intent of reducing androgenic effects while retaining the beneficial progestogenic effects. Studies on COC formulations containing the new progestins indicate they may reduce both nuisance side effects and the minimal lipoprotein changes associated with androgenic effects of progestins. Nuisance side effects such as nausea and breast tenderness often diminish with time with all low-dose COCs. Persistent problems can usually be remedied by pill changes, once it is determined whether the complaint is estrogen or progestin related.

Several prescription drugs (e.g., ampicillin, tetracycline, rifampin, anticonvulsants) can have an impact on the metabolism of oral contraceptives, either reducing the contraceptive effect, or reducing or increasing the effect of the other drug. An additional contraceptive method may be used if short-term drug treatment is prescribed, but an alternative contraceptive method should be considered if a long course of medication is prescribed.

Oral contraceptives are optimally suited to healthy, nonsmoking women. Women over 35 who smoke are not good candidates for oral contraceptives. If a woman has no cardiovascular risk factors and takes a low-dose pill, she may continue taking oral contraceptives through menopause, and at that time can switch directly to estrogen/progestin replacement therapy. In addition, oral contraceptive use in perimenopause may have a bone-sparing effect, which aids in the prevention of osteoporosis.

The progestin-only pill (POP), which contains no estrogen and a low-dose of progestin, is an alternative for women who experience estrogen-related side effects or complications. Although POPs are slightly less effective than COCs, they are appropriate for lactating women because they do not affect milk supply. Disadvantages of progestin-only pills include a higher incidence of irregular bleeding, and fewer noncontraceptive benefits than with COCs.

Implants and Injectables

The levonorgestrel implant (Norplant) and the injectable progestin medroxyprogesterone acetate (Depo-Provera, or DMPA) are long-acting progestin-only contraceptives (Table 1). Implants and injectables are highly effective contraceptive methods that afford a high degree of privacy and are not temporally related to sexual activity. Neither method requires remembering to take a pill each day. Norplant consists of six progestin-containing capsules that are implanted under the skin of the upper arm. The progestin slowly diffuses through the nonbiodegradable polydimethylsiloxane (Silastic) of the slender flexible capsules, creating a constant efflux of progestin. Norplant is effective within 24 hours of insertion and provides reliable contraception for up to 5 years. Baseline fertility is restored soon after removal. Relatively few systemic side effects of Norplant have been documented; irregular bleeding for the first 6 months is the most common complaint. Approximately 10% of all users develop amenorrhea within the first year of use.

Depo-Provera (150 mg intramuscularly every 3 months) is effective within 8 hours. Although the client should be punctual about receiving injections every 3 months, the progestogenic effects of the last injection may persist for an additional 2 to 4 weeks, giving the woman a grace period during which she may still be protected against pregnancy. The return of fertility after cessation of DMPA use is delayed an average of 10 months. No serious side effects have been associated with DMPA, but amenorrhea occurs in 50% of users within the first year of use.

No hormonal contraceptive method provides protection against the transmission of STDs or HIV. Cervical ectopy, a common estrogenic effect found in oral contraceptive users, may increase the risk of contracting some STDs. Women at risk for STDs or HIV should be cautioned to use condoms in addition to any hormonal contraceptive.

BARRIER METHODS

Male and Female Condoms

The latex male condom fits tightly over the erect penis, collecting the ejaculate and providing a barrier between the penis and vagina that is impermeable to sperm, viruses, and bacteria. Natural membrane condoms made of processed collagenous tissue are permeable to some viruses and bacteria, including HIV. No data exist indicating that spermicidally treated condoms are more protective, against either pregnancy or disease, than untreated latex condoms. To be effective, condoms must be used properly and consistently.

Correct male condom use requires (1) never reusing a condom; (2) avoiding damage by teeth, fingernails, or other sharp objects; (3) putting the condom on after the penis is fully erect, but before any genital contact with the partner; (4) ensuring that no air is trapped in the tip of the condom; (5) ensuring adequate lubrication during intercourse, possibly requiring use of lubricants; (6) using only water-based lubricants with latex condoms (any kind of oil and most lotions can weaken the latex); (7) holding the condom firmly against the base of the penis during withdrawal and withdrawing while the penis is still erect to prevent condom slippage.

TABLE 1. **Efficacy of Contraceptive Methods**

Method	**Percentage of Women Experiencing Accidental Pregnancy within First Year of Use** — *Typical Use**	*Perfect Use†*	**Percentage of Women Continuing Use at 1 Year‡**
Chance§	85	85	
Spermicides‖	21	6	43
Periodic abstinence	20		67
Calendar		9	
Ovulation method		3	
Sympto-thermal¶		2	
Postovulation		1	
Withdrawal	19	4	
Cap**			
Parous women	36	26	45
Nulliparous women	18	9	58
Sponge			
Parous women	36	20	45
Nulliparous women	18	9	58
Diaphragm**	18	6	58
Condom††			
Female (Reality)	21	5	56
Male	12	3	63
Pill	3		72
Progestin only		0.5	
Combined		0.1	
Intrauterine device			
Progesterone T	2.0	1.5	81
Copper T 380A	0.8	0.6	78
LNg 20	0.1	0.1	81
Depo-Provera	0.3	0.3	70
Norplant (6 capsules)	0.09	0.09	85
Sterilization			
Female	0.4	0.4	100
Male	0.15	0.10	100

Emergency contraceptive pills: Treatment initiated within 72 hours after unprotected intercourse reduces the risk of pregnancy by at least 75%.‡‡

Lactational amenorrhea method: The lactational amenorrhea method is a highly effective, *temporary* method of contraception.§§

*Among typical couples who initiate use of a method (not necessarily for the first time), the percentage who experience an accidental pregnancy during the first year if they do not stop use for any other reason.

†Among couples who initiate use of a method (not necessarily for the first time) and who use it perfectly (both consistently and correctly), the percentage who experience an accidental pregnancy during the first year if they do not stop use for any other reason.

‡Among couples attempting to avoid pregnancy, the percentage who continue to use a method for 1 year.

§The percents failing in columns 2 and 3 are based on data from populations in which contraception is not used and from women who cease using contraception in order to become pregnant. Among such populations, about 89% become pregnant within 1 year. The estimate was lowered slightly (to 85%) to represent the percent who would become pregnant within 1 year among women now relying on reversible methods of contraception if they abandoned contraception altogether.

‖Foams, creams, gels, vaginal suppositories, and vaginal film.

¶Cervical mucus (ovulation) method supplemented by calendar in the pre-ovulatory phase and by basal body temperature in the post-ovulatory phase.

**With spermicidal cream or jelly.

††Without spermicides.

‡‡The treatment schedule is one dose as soon as possible (but no later than 72 hours) after unprotected intercourse, and a second dose 12 hours after the first dose. The hormones that have been studied in the clinical trials of postcoital hormonal contraception are found in Nordette, Levlen, Lo/Ovral (one dose is equal to four pills), Triphasil, Tri-Levlen (one dose is equal to four pills), and Ovral (one dose is equal to two pills).

§§However, to maintain effective protection against pregnancy, another method of contraception must be used as soon as menstruation resumes, the frequency or duration of breast-feeding is reduced, bottle feeding is introduced, or the baby reaches 6 months of age.

Adapted from Hatcher RA, Trussell J, Stewart F, et al: Contraceptive Technology, 16th ed. New York, Irvington, 1994.

The female condom (Reality) consists of a polyurethane pouch with a large ring at either end. One ring fits into the vagina and is secured behind the pubic bone, the other remains outside the vagina anchoring the open end of the pouch. Like the male condom, the female condom is impermeable to sperm, viruses, and bacteria. Additionally, the female condom creates a barrier between the base of the penis and the vulva and perineum. The female condom is currently available in the United States and several other countries; the cost is approximately four times the cost of a male condom.

Diaphragms and Cervical Caps

The diaphragm and cervical cap have few side effects, allow women to control their contraceptive method, and provide some protection against several sexually transmitted diseases. The diaphragm and cap can be inserted before sexual activity, and must remain in place for at least 6 hours after the last act of intercourse. The diaphragm has been recommended for continuous use up to 24 hours, and the cervical cap has been recommended for use up to 72 hours. Diaphragm users should insert additional spermicide into the vagina prior to each act of intercourse, but additional spermicide is unnecessary with the cervical cap. Both the diaphragm and cervical cap prevent entrance of sperm into the cervical os and provide a repository for spermicide.

The diaphragm is a rubber dome-shaped device with a flexible rim that covers the cervix. The posterior rim rests in the posterior fornix of the vagina and the anterior rim fits behind the pubic bone. Four types of diaphragms are available in the United States. The flat spring is thin-rimmed for women with firm vaginal tone (e.g., the nullipara), or women with a shallow pubic notch. The coil spring has a sturdier rim, making it appropriate for women with average vaginal tone. The arcing spring has the sturdiest rim and an arc shape when folded; it is suitable for women with lax vaginal tone, rectocele, or cystocele. The wide-seal diaphragm has a flexible flange 1.5 cm wide inside the rim and is available in various spring types.

Only the Prentif Cavity Rim Cervical Cap is approved for use in the United States. The cervical cap is shaped like a large thimble; the deep, soft rubber cap has a firm rounded rim with a groove along the inner circumference of the rim, which forms a seal by suction between the rim and the surface of the cervix. The cap is available in four sizes. Women with extensive scarring of the cervix, an anteverted or short cervix, or a cervix that is flush with the vaginal vault are not good candidates for a cervical cap.

Neither the diaphragm nor the cervical cap has user effectiveness rates equivalent to those for hormonal contraceptive methods, but effectiveness can be increased by coupling diaphragm or cap use with condom use during the fertile period. After pregnancy or late abortion, cervical or vaginal anatomy may change, requiring refitting of the diaphragm or cap.

Contraceptive Sponge

The contraceptive sponge (Today Sponge) is a small polyurethane pillow permeated with 1 gram of nonoxynol-9 spermicide. A concave dimple on one side of the sponge is designed to cover the cervix. The sponge functions as a barrier between sperm and the cervical os, as a trap for sperm, and as a constant-release mechanism for spermicide. The spermicide contained in the sponge is activated when it is moistened with water. The sponge is inserted deep into the vagina covering the cervix, where it provides protection up to 24 hours, after which it must be removed and discarded. The sponge is manufactured in one size only, and is available without prescription.

Sponge user effectiveness rates are highest for nulliparous women who have received instruction on proper insertion; reported failure rates with parous users have been as high as twice those of nulliparous women. Recent data from several studies have indicated that very frequent or continuous use of the sponge may cause vaginal or vulvar ulceration, which could increase the risk of contracting STDs or HIV if exposed.

Toxic shock syndrome, although very rare, is a risk for diaphragm, cervical cap, and sponge users. Women should be cautioned to remove the device immediately after the recommended use period, and they should be aware of the signs of toxic shock syndrome.

VAGINAL SPERMICIDES

Vaginal spermicides are available without prescription in the form of creams, foams, gels, film, and suppositories. Most spermicidal preparations contain 100 to 150 mg nonoxynol-9 or octoxynol per application. Creams, foams, and gels are effective immediately on insertion, but film and suppositories require a delay to allow for melting or effervescence. The effective period for all five products is 1 hour after insertion. Although vaginal spermicides have been shown to kill almost all viruses and bacteria associated with STDs and HIV in vitro, their effectiveness for HIV protection in vivo has not been proved.

INTRAUTERINE DEVICES

The intrauterine device (IUD) is a highly effective method of contraception that can be used privately and does not require daily attention. Two types of IUD are available in the United States. The Copper T380A (ParaGard), made of polyethylene wrapped with copper, has the highest rate of effectiveness and is effective for 10 years after insertion. The Progestasert, a flexible plastic device with progestin in the stem, is effective for 1 year. The IUD provides contraception by immobilizing sperm, inhibiting fertilization, and inhibiting implantation.

The primary concern regarding IUD use is pelvic inflammatory disease. Pelvic inflammatory disease may develop following insertion owing to the introduction of vaginal bacteria or an undiagnosed pathogen into the uterine cavity. Prophylactic antibiotics administered prior to insertion may decrease the risk of infection, but this protection is unproved in the scientific literature. IUDs provide no protection against STDs or HIV; the risk of subsequent pelvic inflammatory disease, STD, or HIV infection among IUD users is reduced by limiting IUD use to monogamous couples. Side effects associated with IUD use include heavier menstrual bleeding and cramping. If the IUD user becomes pregnant, there is an increased risk of ectopic pregnancy. Intrauterine pregnancy with an IUD in place results in a high rate of spontaneous abortion and an increased risk of septic abortion in the second trimester. Therefore, the IUD should be removed as soon as possible.

STERILIZATION

Female Sterilization

Tubal sterilization provides a safe, highly effective, permanent method of contraception for women who are certain they wish to end their fertility. Sterilization does not affect hormone production or sexual function. Women continue to ovulate, but ova entering the fallopian tubes are blocked at the site of occlusion, where they disintegrate and are reabsorbed by the body.

Two methods of accessing the fallopian tubes are currently popular. Minilaparotomy requires a 2- to 3-centimeter suprapubic or subumbilical incision (for postpartum procedures). Using a uterine manipulator, the clinician maneuvers each tube into the incision; lifts it with a special hook, forceps, or a finger; occludes the tube; and replaces it into the abdomen. Laparoscopy is the most popular method of assessing the tubes for tubal occlusion in the United States. It is most frequently performed on an outpatient basis and produces only a tiny scar. A hollow needle is introduced into the abdomen just below the navel, and the abdomen is inflated with nitrous oxide or carbon dioxide. The needle is withdrawn and a sharp trocar is used to make a puncture through which a laparoscope is inserted. The operating instruments are introduced into the abdomen through an operating channel in the laparoscope or a second puncture site in the lower abdomen. After the tubes are accessed using either procedure, tubal occlusion is accomplished by either ligation (via minilaparotomy), cauterization, or application of special clips or bands.

The long-term health effects of tubal occlusion appear to include a reduced risk of ovarian cancer. Investigation into the existence and extent of so-called post–tubal ligation syndrome, a collection of psychological symptoms and physical signs related to changes in the menstrual cycle, continues, but a physical basis for the condition has yet to be convincingly demonstrated.

Sterilization reversal involves expensive, complicated microsurgery. Patency rates following reconstructive surgery range from 50 to 70%. Because of the permanent nature of sterilization, proper patient counseling is imperative. The strongest indicator of future regret of the decision to end fertility is age less than 30 years at the time of sterilization. Young women are more likely to experience life changes such as remarriage, the death of a child, or changes in emotional or economic situations that could create the desire for a pregnancy.

Male Sterilization

Any couple considering sterilization should receive information about vasectomy as well as tubal sterilization, because vasectomy is generally simpler, safer, and less expensive than female sterilization. Vasectomy terminates fertility but does not alter testicular volume, spermatogenesis, or testicular hormonal function. Occlusion is accomplished by ligation, cautery, or clipping of the vasa deferentia, thus preventing delivery of sperm but not semen to the penis. Two surgical methods of accessing the vasa deferentia for sterilization are currently in use.

Traditional vasectomy employs one or two small incisions in the scrotum through which the vasa are lifted and then occluded by ligation, clips, or cauterization. No-scalpel vasectomy (NSV) uses a sharp instrument to pierce the scrotal skin. The single opening is stretched to allow retraction of the vas for occlusion and does not require a suture closure. No-scalpel vasectomy is quick and less invasive than traditional vasectomy and entails less pain, bleeding, and edema. Both procedures are performed on an outpatient basis, using local anesthesia.

Recent reviews of the scientific literature have led both the World Health Organization and the National Institutes of Health to conclude that it is unlikely that there is an association between vasectomy and prostate or testicular cancer. Cardiovascular disease also appears to be unrelated to vasectomy.

Restoration of fertility after vasectomy involves reconnection of the severed ends of the vasa deferentia by means of complex microsurgery. Patency rates can be as high as 85% to 95%, but are lower if vasectomy was performed over 10 years previously. Even with patency rates of 85%, pregnancy rates are only 50% to 70% and fall to 20% to 30% if the epididymis is obstructed. If a long segment of the vas was excised successful reversal is unlikely.

POSTCOITAL CONTRACEPTION

The most common method of postcoital contraception in the United States is a regimen of 100 mcg of ethinyl estradiol and 1.0 mg norgestrel (two Ovral), taken within 72 hours of unprotected intercourse, and repeated 12 hours later. Although this method is highly effective, it frequently causes nausea and vomiting, and may be prescribed with an antiemetic.

FERTILITY AWARENESS

The term natural family planning refers to several fertility awareness methods that prescribe abstinence during the ovulatory period. Although these methods have no physical side effects, planned periodic abstinence has a low rate of effectiveness, may inhibit sexual spontaneity, and requires detailed record keeping. Natural family planning methods have the greatest chance of success with couples who clearly understand the method and are highly motivated to use it correctly.

The basal body temperature method requires accurate daily recording of first morning temperature; postovulation is indicated by a 0.4° to 0.8° temperature rise. The cervical mucus method requires daily recording of changes in cervical mucus; ovulation occurs around the time spinnbarkeit mucus (a profuse, clear, egg white–like substance) is observed. Symptothermal charting combines both methods. These methods are most effective if the couple abstains from intercourse from the cessation of menses until 3 days after the rise in basal body temperature or 4 days after peak mucus production.

Section 16

Psychiatric Disorders

ALCOHOL-RELATED PROBLEMS

method of
STEPHEN JURD, M.B., B.S.
Sydney University
Sydney, New South Wales, Australia

In a substantial proportion of all patients presenting for medical treatment alcohol is a causal factor or a coexisting health risk. In family practice, one in every six patients is at risk, and in hospital practice one in five. Community statistics indicate that lifelong prevalence of alcohol abuse among men is in the range of 19 to 30%. Usual estimates of point prevalence of serious drinking problems (alcohol dependence) range from 3 to 5% of the adult male population. Women have approximately half the risk of males.

THE DOCTOR'S ROLE

There is no doubt that much alcohol-related illness goes undiagnosed. Therefore, the doctor's principal role is that of case identification and provision of information to the patient. The usual situation is that neither doctor nor patient has considered behavioral change as a health strategy. The next stage depends on the severity of the presenting problem and the patient's willingness to accept treatment.

LEVELS OF SEVERITY

Essentially there are three levels of severity that require clinical attention: hazardous, harmful, and dependent drinking. The first two levels have been defined from epidemiologic studies that have indicated an increased risk of a variety of disorders once these limits are exceeded. A standard drink is a 1-fluid ounce (30-mL) "shot" of whiskey, a 2-fluid ounce (60-mL) glass of fortified wine, a 4-ounce (120-mL) glass of table wine, and a 10-fluid ounce (300-mL) glass of beer.

Hazardous Drinking. Drinking more than four standard drinks (40 grams of alcohol) daily in males or more than two standard drinks (20 grams of alcohol) a day in females confers a significant risk of alcohol-related problems. To maintain low-risk drinking, there should be two or three alcohol-free days each week and no episodes of drinking more than six drinks on one occasion.

Harmful Drinking. This exists when known alcohol-related harm, such as any of the problems listed in Table 1, occurs in the presence of hazardous drinking.

Alcohol Dependence Syndrome. This syndrome is a complex biopsychosocial disorder that has internationally accepted major features:

1. Subjective awareness of compulsion to drink, usually manifest by multiple attempts to control, cut down, or abstain.
2. Stereotyped, narrowed pattern of drinking—i.e., the drinking predicts the social life rather than vice versa.
3. Increased importance of drinking over other activities, eroding work, family, and personal responsibilities.
4. Pharmacologic tolerance, resulting in an increased capacity to drink without showing signs of intoxication.
5. Repeated withdrawal symptoms (e.g., nausea, tremor, irritability, and anxiety, especially in the morning).
6. Relieving or preventing withdrawal by drinking.
7. Reinstatement of pathologic drinking after a period of abstinence.

These features, as in any syndrome, tend to predict each other's presence, but not always. Generally, the presence of three features is required for a diagnosis of alcohol-dependence syndrome, though the presence of any feature is relevant. Dependence ranges from the most mild degree to the most severe. Severe dependence is usually complicated by multiple problems. The presence of dependence does not mean that affected individuals will experience serious withdrawal, but the more severe the dependence, the more likely it is that clinically significant withdrawal will occur.

ALCOHOL-RELATED PROBLEMS

An attempt to summarize the many complications of excessive drinking is made in Table 1. The ubiquity of excessive drinking means that many of these problems present in relative isolation, leading alcohol to be considered the modern "great imitator" of other diseases.

FAMILY PROBLEMS

Every problem drinker seriously affects the lives of at least four other people. The family disruption may result in the development of psychiatric symptoms in family members. Domestic violence commonly coexists with alcohol problems and cannot be managed without dealing with the alcohol problem. Some family members are assisted by Al-Anon, a self-help group for relatives of problem drinkers. This group is available to families regardless of whether the drinker accepts treatment.

DIAGNOSIS

The high incidence of alcohol problems in clinical practice and the low diagnosis rate indicate a need for a much higher index of suspicion. Meticulous assessment is required wherever one of the problems listed in Table 1 presents.

History of Alcohol Use. An attitude of nonjudgmental acceptance of heavy drinking as a common human behavior should pervade all history-taking efforts. One technique that emerges from this attitude is the "top-high" technique, in which one deliberately overestimates the amount consumed and places the onus of denial on the patient: for example, "I bet you could drink two bottles of whiskey in a day." A variant of this technique can be used when taking

TABLE 1. **Alcohol-Related Problems**

Trauma	**Psychiatric Problems**	**Neurologic Problems**
Motor vehicle accidents	Suicide	Peripheral neuropathy
Falls	Parasuicide	Subdural hematoma
Fractures	Depression	Wernicke-Korsakoff psychosis
Head injuries	Paranoia	**Muscular Problems**
Industrial injuries	Dementia	Myopathy
Drownings	Alcohol withdrawal delirium	Rhabdomyolysis
Domestic fires	Anxiety	**Hematologic Disorders**
Social Problems	Phobias	Macrocytosis
Financial problems	Panic attacks	Anemia
Marital conflict	**Gastrointestinal Disorders**	Thrombocytopenia
Absenteeism	Gastritis	Leukopenia
Unemployment	Ulcers	**Metabolic Disorders**
Drunk driving	Reflux esophagitis	Obesity
Convictions	Esophageal varices	Gout
Assault	Diarrhea	Hyperlipidemia
Homicide	Vomiting	Diabetes
Domestic violence	Fatty liver	Impotence
Indirect Presentations*	Mallory-Weiss syndrome	Gynecomastia
Spouse	Cirrhosis	**Obstetric Problems**
Injury	Pancreatitis	Low birthweight
Depression	**Cardiovascular Problems**	Fetal alcohol syndrome
Psychosomatic illness	Hypertension	Second-trimester abortion
Children	Arrhythmias	**Oncologic Problems**
Abuse	**Respiratory Problems**	Oropharyngeal cancers
Depression	Lung abscess	Esophogeal cancers
Anxiety	Sleep apnea	
School refusal	Tuberculosis	

*Indirect presentations occur when family members display problems consequent on the drinking of their relative.

a daily drinking estimate by asking whether a patient has his first drink of the day before or after breakfast! This having been ascertained, the clinician builds up a picture of the typical drinking that occurs in a day. This eventually allows the clinician to estimate how many standard drinks (10 grams of alcohol) are consumed during an average day. The perceived benefits and the social setting of the drinking should also be elicited.

Physical Examination. During the physical examination the physician looks for the following signs.

1. Signs of trauma.
2. Signs of liver disease—tender hepatomegaly, spider nevi, secondary lunules, palmar erythema, bruising, parotid enlargement, ascites.
3. Conjunctival injection, facial telangiectasia, tongue and hand tremors.
4. Hypertension, obesity.
5. Withdrawal features, commonly anxiety, sweating, and tachycardia.
6. Evidence of intoxication—alcohol on the breath, ataxia, disinhibition.

Clinical Investigations. These are used to confirm the suspected diagnosis. Because all tests have a low sensitivity, negative test results cannot exclude alcohol problems.

1. Liver function tests will show some abnormality in about 50% of cases; the gamma-glutamyl transpeptidase measurement is the most sensitive.
2. The mean corpuscular volume is elevated.
3. Blood alcohol levels may be detected, especially in emergencies. Apparent sobriety with a substantial blood alcohol level may clarify the situation.
4. Screening devices such as the Alcohol Use Disorders Identification Test (AUDIT) (Fig. 1) can assist in identifying individuals who need more detailed assessment.

TREATMENT

Brief Intervention

Following a thorough assessment as outlined previously, patients whose alcohol use is hazardous or harmful but not dependent should receive a brief (10- to 15-minute) intervention along these lines:

Feedback. Explain why alcohol is relevant to the patient, providing details about any abnormal test results and never explaining away minor abnormalities if they fit the clinical situation. Indicate to patients who have no clinically apparent harm how their drinking behavior puts them at risk.

Listen. Pay careful attention to the way the patient responds to the information provided. Defensiveness may interfere with communication and requires clarification.

Outline Benefits. Provide an account of the future prospects, outlining the benefits to the patient if drinking behavior is altered.

Set Goals. Inform the patient of the limits of low-risk drinking. If harm is manifest, a brief (1- to 3-month) period of abstinence may be indicated.

Set Strategies. Provide suggestions about altering behaviors—e.g., start with a nonalcoholic drink, avoid heavy drinking parties, resurrect an old hobby, engage in physical fitness activities, alternate alcoholic and nonalcoholic drinks, avoid buying rounds of drinks..

Evaluate. Encourage each patient to return for a review of his or her progress with attempts at behavioral change. Exceeding the drinking goals set should

WORLD HEALTH ORGANIZATION

A U D I T

Please place a mark in the box next to your answer

1 How often do you have a drink containing alcohol?

☐ never ☐ monthly or less ☐ 2 to 4 times a month ☐ 2 to 3 times a week ☐ 4 or more times a week

2 How many 'standard' drinks (see below) containing alcohol do you have on a typical day when you are drinking?

☐ 1 or 2 ☐ 3 or 4 ☐ 5 or 6 ☐ 7 to 9 ☐ 10 or more

3 How often do you have six or more drinks on one occasion?

☐ never ☐ less than monthly ☐ monthly ☐ weekly ☐ daily or almost daily

4 How often during the last year have you found that you were not able to stop drinking once you had started?

☐ never ☐ less than monthly ☐ monthly ☐ weekly ☐ daily or almost daily

5 How often during the last year have you failed to do what was normally expected from you because of drinking?

☐ never ☐ less than monthly ☐ monthly ☐ weekly ☐ daily or almost daily

6 How often during the last year have you needed a drink in the morning to get yourself going after a heavy drinking session?

☐ never ☐ less than monthly ☐ monthly ☐ weekly ☐ daily or almost daily

7 How often during the last year have you had a feeling of guilt or remorse after drinking?

☐ never ☐ less than monthly ☐ monthly ☐ weekly ☐ daily or almost daily

8 How often during the last year have you been unable to remember what happened the night before because you had been drinking?

☐ never ☐ less than monthly ☐ monthly ☐ weekly ☐ daily or almost daily

9 Have you or someone else been injured as a result of your drinking?

☐ no ☐ yes, but not in the last year ☐ yes, during the last year

10 Has a relative, a friend, a doctor or other health worker been concerned about your drinking or suggested you cut down?

☐ no ☐ yes, but not in the last year ☐ yes, during the last year

ONE STANDARD DRINK APPROXIMATELY = Middy of Beer = Small Glass of Wine = Small Glass of Sherry or Port = 1 Nip of Spirits

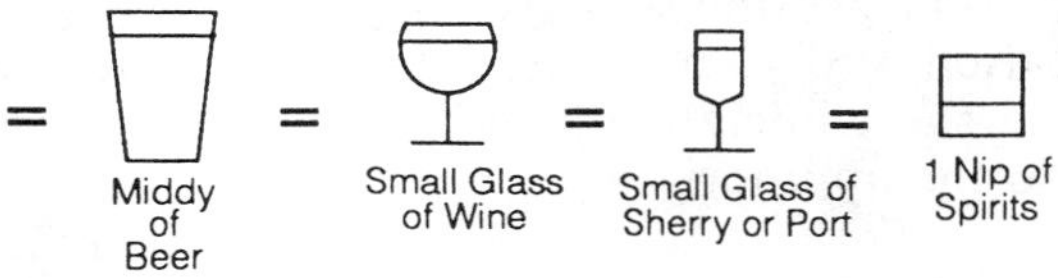

NOTE: A schooner of normal strength beer contains about 1 1/2 standard drinks; a bottle about 3. The average light beer is about half the strength of normal beer.

Figure 1. One standard drink equals approximately one 10-oz glass of beer; one 4-oz glass of wine; one 2-oz glass of sherry or port; or one shot of spirits. *Note:* The average light beer is about half the strength of normal beer.

(From Saunders JB, Aasland OG, Amundsen A, & Grant M (1993). Alcohol consumption and related problems among primary health care patients: WHO Collaborative Project on Early Detection of Persons with Harmful Alcohol Consumption-I. **Addiction,** 88: 349–362; and Saunders JB, Aasland OG, Babor TF, de la Fuente JR, & Grant M (1993). Development of the Alcohol Use Disorders Identification Test (AUDIT); WHO Collaborative Project on Early Detection of Persons with Harmful Alcohol Consumption-II. **Addiction,** 88: 791–804.) For further information contact the Drug and Alcohol Department, Royal Prince Alfred Hospital, Sydney.

not be seen as a failure but as part of a learning process.

If clinically significant medical problems are present, closer follow-up is indicated, with regular monitoring of any abnormal test results. Despite all efforts by clinicians, some people who are dependent will not disclose their symptoms, so prolonged inability to change drinking behavior should indicate a need to consider a diagnosis of alcohol dependence.

ALCOHOL DEPENDENCE

The seventh feature of alcohol dependence is a return to pathologic use after a period of abstinence. The more severe the dependence, the more inevitable the return to damaging drinking habits. Under these circumstances, the only solution is lifelong total abstinence. This is a tall order for those who value alcohol highly and is why members of Alcoholics Anonymous (AA) say they do it "one day at a time." AA is a worldwide self-help organization founded in 1935 in Akron, Ohio, that has over 1,500,000 members. It is based on spiritual principles and encourages altruistic endeavor but makes no demands of its members apart from a desire to stay sober. AA can be an invaluable source of support for patients who espouse abstinence as a goal.

If patients are physically dependent, they will experience some withdrawal symptoms. These can be a potent stimulant to return to drinking. Often an inpatient detoxification program is necessary to allow the patient to withdraw safely from alcohol. Occasionally sedatives such as chlordiazepoxide (Librium) or diazepam (Valium) may ease withdrawal, but great care should be taken to taper the dose to ensure that the sedative is stopped prior to discharge. At least relative malnutrition is the rule in alcohol dependence, so multivitamins, particularly vitamin B (thiamine), should be prescribed. Regular contact with the clinician, particularly early in the abstinence period, can be helpful, as can referral to a counselor skilled in drug and alcohol problems. Commonly difficulties with personal relationships and family situations require attention. Patients with more severe or complicated problems or continual relapses may benefit from an inpatient rehabilitation program. These exist in a variety of forms, and the clinician should attempt to match the patient to the appropriate program.

LONG-TERM FOLLOW-UP

It is rare for patients to change ingrained habits without a struggle. Maintenance of a nonjudgmental stance and positive expectations despite a relapse are useful. Often patients learn from a relapse and are better able to pursue complete recovery. Experience indicates that even the most profoundly damaged patients can attain long-term sobriety.

DRUG ABUSE

method of
DAVID J. ROBERTS, M.D.
North Memorial Medical Center
Robbinsdale, Minnesota

Despite its legality, alcohol abuse overshadows all other forms of drug abuse in the United States. The cost of alcohol-associated absenteeism, loss of productivity, and alcohol-related accidents at home and work is enormous, and the associated human suffering is incalculable. Alcoholism is discussed elsewhere. This chapter focuses on the complications of recreational abuse of other legal and illegal drugs.

DIAGNOSIS OF DRUG ABUSE

The most common and easily recognized presentation of drug abuse is acute intoxication, with signs and symptoms such as obtundation, slurred speech (e.g., depressant drugs); agitation, tachycardia (e.g., stimulant drugs); and auditory or visual hallucinations (e.g., hallucinogenic drugs). The youth or adult who presents with obtundation and an obvious alcohol odor demands no diagnostic acumen. The patient who presents with a first seizure, however, may easily undergo a traditional work-up, and the diagnosis of cocaine abuse may be overlooked because no one thought to obtain a urine drug screen within the 4-day detection period for this drug. Table 1 lists the less common presentations of drug abuse.

Accidents are another common presentation of drug abuse. The physical examination is often limited to the injured extremity, and signs of drug abuse—easily detected by a more complete examination—are overlooked. Now that the legality of drug testing has been established, even mandated in some cases, more and more employers are requiring routine urine drug screening after workplace accidents. A study of Georgia Power Company employees between 1983 and 1987 showed that drug users had a significantly higher annual rate of lost time (0.008 days per individual vs. 0.000) and vehicular accidents (0.23 days vs. 0.109). In addition, drug users had significantly higher annual medical benefits usage ($1377 vs. $163 for matched controls) and higher annual absenteeism (165 hours vs. 47 hours). In 1987, the National Institute on Drug Abuse (NIDA) estimated that occupational drug abuse cost the United States $100 billion in lost productivity alone. Many trauma centers include a blood alcohol test in their routine screening for major trauma cases, but it is clear that any drug of abuse can affect judgment and the ability to operate a motor vehicle or any machinery.

URINE DRUG SCREENING

Urine is preferred to blood for routine qualitative screening for abused drugs. Most common drugs of abuse, with the exception of solvents, can be readily and inexpensively detected by immunoassay screening. Because of the enormous impact of a positive test, especially for employment, a positive test should always be confirmed by a second, unrelated technique, usually gas chromatography or mass spectrometry. Table 2 lists the average detection periods for drugs. In addition to a thorough physical examination, several readily obtainable studies can detect most complications of drug abuse: rhythm strip, complete blood count, electrolytes, glucose, blood urea nitrogen, and urinalysis.

TABLE 1. **Less Common Presentations of Drug Abuse**

Presentation	Drug
Seizure	Cocaine, amphetamines, "designer drug," PCP, propoxyphene, solvent; withdrawal
Subcutaneous abscess, especially antecubital	Parenteral drugs, especially cocaine
Stains on face or hands	Solvents
Cyanosis	Nitrites (methemoglobinemia)
Accidents	All drugs of abuse
Unusual odors	Solvents, alcohol, chloral hydrate, ethchlorvynol, marijuana
Nystagmus	Alcohol, PCP, solvents, mescaline, sedative hypnotics
Miosis	Narcotics, PCP
Mydriasis	Amphetamines, cocaine, LSD, glutethimide, meperidine, hypoxia secondary to respiratory depression
Ischemic chest pain at unusually young age	Cocaine, amphetamines
Acute psychiatric disorders (e.g., hyperventilation, panic, dysphoria, psychosis)	Alcohol, amphetamines, cocaine, PCP, hallucinogens, marijuana
Neuropathy	Nitrous oxide, toluene
Myoglobinuria	Cocaine, amphetamines, PCP
Salivation, drooling	PCP (cholinergic effects)
Hyperthermia	Cocaine, amphetamines, PCP, withdrawal
Hypothermia	Alcohol, barbiturates, ethchlorvynol
Pulmonary edema	Narcotics, barbiturates, ethchlorvynol, meprobamate
Confusional state in elderly	Alcohol, sedative hypnotics, narcotics, withdrawal
Tachydysrhythmias	Stimulants, hallucinogens, propoxyphene
Neonatal withdrawal	Maternal abuse of alcohol, narcotics, cocaine, amphetamines

STIMULANT DRUGS

Table 3 lists the commonly abused stimulant drugs. Most people using stimulant drugs achieve the desired effects of increased alertness and energy, decreased fatigue, euphoria, and anorexia, and they never present to an emergency department. What makes a user a patient is some undesired or frightening effect, either psychological (e.g., panic attack, dysphoric reaction) or physiologic (e.g., tachycardia, chest pain). Cocaine and amphetamines are the dominant drugs of abuse in this class, and their effects and toxicity are similar. Cocaine is rapidly metabolized by the liver, and its effects usually dissipate in minutes, but the effects of amphetamines can persist for hours. Either drug, depending on the dose and individual susceptibility, can precipitate acute anxiety states, paranoia, hallucinations, acute psychosis, and violent behavior.

TABLE 2. **Detection Periods for Drugs of Abuse in Blood and Urine**

Drug	Detection Period
Alcohol, ethyl	3–10 h
Amphetamine	1–2 days
Barbiturates	
Secobarbital	24 h
Phenobarbital	2–6 weeks
Benzodiazepines, heavy	3–5 days
abuse	3–6 weeks
Cocaine	5 h
Benzoylecgonine (cocaine metabolite)	2–4 days
Codeine	1–2 days
Heroin	1–2 days
Hydromorphone (Dilaudid)	1–2 days
LSD	8 h
Methaqualone (Quaalude)	2 weeks
Methadone (Dolophine)	2–3 days
Morphine	1–2 days
PCP (phencyclidine)	2–8 days
Propoxyphene (Darvon)	6 h
Propoxyphene metabolites	6–48 h
THC metabolite (marijuana)	
1 joint, urine	2 days
3 times weekly, urine	2 weeks
Daily, urine	3–6 weeks
Blood	8 h

With permission of Harry G. McCoy, Pharm.D., Clinical Director, Med Tox Laboratories, St. Paul, MN.

In addition to undesired behavioral effects, patients may present with various unpleasant physiologic effects. A first seizure in an adolescent or young adult demands that cocaine and other stimulants be ruled out. The patient, fearing parental or legal consequences, often denies drug abuse. If initial history and testing are negative for common causes of seizure, such as previous or acute head injury, family history of seizure, metabolic derangement, or central nervous system (CNS) infection and disease, drug abuse should be pursued more aggressively. Other common causes for seizure, such as carbon monoxide and acute overdose of other medications, should not be overlooked. The attending physician should also consider withdrawal from a drug of abuse and look for supporting signs, such as tachycardia, diaphoresis, tremor, or agitation.

An especially dangerous presentation of cocaine abuse is ischemic chest pain in the young, healthy-appearing patient. If the history of cocaine use is not

TABLE 3. **Commonly Abused Stimulant Drugs**

Amphetamines	Phencyclidine
Cocaine	Phenylpropanolamine
Caffeine	Ephedrine
Nicotine	Pseudoephedrine

volunteered or elicited, the patient is likely to be sent home with reassurance and an analgesic. Myocardial infarction is a recognized complication of cocaine abuse, even in the absence of traditional risk factors. Some risk management protocols suggest obtaining an electrocardiogram (ECG) in all cases of chest pain in patients older than 25, but if cocaine use is suspected, an ECG should be obtained at any age. Cardiac monitoring may reveal various dysrhythmias, such as sinus tachycardia, paroxysmal supraventricular tachycardia, premature ventricular contraction, ventricular tachycardia, and ventricular fibrillation.

Phencyclidine (PCP, "angel dust") is abused for its stimulant and mood-altering effects, but it is pharmacologically more complex than most other drugs of abuse. Because it affects multiple neurotransmitters in the brain, it can produce CNS stimulation and depression, hallucinations, analgesia, and cholinergic effects. Its behavioral effects include dysphoria, violence, psychosis, and catatonia. Because of a combination of hyperactivity and delusion of strength, PCP abusers may suffer serious injuries and rhabdomyolysis. Because of its analgesic effects, patients on PCP may not complain of pain, and a complete physical examination is indicated. Using a purely psychiatric approach in cases of drug abuse (i.e., interviewing the patient fully clothed) invites overlooking serious injuries and complications. A combined psychiatric and medical approach is well rewarded.

Treatment

Milder panic or dysphoric reactions may respond to reassurance and the continuous presence of a friend, nurse, or counselor until the drug effect subsides. Other patients may benefit from a short-acting benzodiazepine, such as 0.25 mg of triazolam (Halcion), which may be given sublingually. Making the patient comfortable with a "downer" could be construed as enabling the drug abuse, so referral for chemical dependency evaluation and treatment should also be made.

Violent patients present an immediate threat to themselves and others. Initial restraint is most safely achieved by five staff members, one for each limb and one for the head. Physical restraints can then be applied. Many patients, however, continue to thrash dangerously after being restrained, and some form of chemical restraint is often needed. Chemical restraints bring their own risks of toxicity, such as respiratory depression, but their benefits usually outweigh their risks. The most popular drugs for chemical restraint have been short-acting benzodiazepines and haloperidol (Haldol), a butyrophenone. These drugs have a better safety profile than barbiturates and phenothiazines, and their use, dosage, and effectiveness have been well documented in the emergency medicine literature. A common protocol is 5 mg of haloperidol plus 2 mg of lorazepam (Ativan) intravenously or intramuscularly. Most other benzodiazepines are not well absorbed intramuscularly. The combined use of the two drugs obviates the need for an excessive dose of either drug alone. If necessary, the dose can be repeated in 30 minutes. Dystonic reactions occasionally complicate haloperidol use and are controlled by diphenhydramine (Benadryl), 50 mg four times daily, or benztropine (Cogentin), 1 to 2 mg twice daily. Use of chemical restraint obligates the physician to even closer physiologic monitoring.

Dysrhythmias range from mild sinus tachycardia to life-threatening ventricular arrhythmias. Sinus tachycardia is usually well tolerated and self-limited, and the associated anxiety may be treated with reassurance or a small dose of a short-acting benzodiazepine. Hemodynamically significant PSVT should be treated with an intravenous beta blocker, such as 5 mg of metoprolol (Lopressor), or a calcium channel blocker, such as 5 mg of verapamil (Isoptin). Each drug can be safely repeated in a few minutes if necessary. Drug-driven tachycardias are less likely to respond to vagal maneuvers, and the likelihood of recurrence of PSVT after adenosine is high. If the supraventricular tachycardia is associated with hypertension, labetalol (Normodyne, Trandate), which blocks both alpha and beta receptors, or verapamil makes the most sense. Initially, labetalol can be administered intravenously in a dose of 20 mg over 2 minutes. There have been some reports of hypertension worsening after the administration of other beta blockers, especially propranolol (Inderal), because of unopposed alpha effect. Hypertension may be accompanied by reflex bradycardia, especially in younger patients. The bradycardia resolves spontaneously with normalization of the blood pressure and does not require treatment. Hypertensive emergencies can also be controlled with nitroprusside (Nipride) infusions. Ventricular arrhythmias should be treated with lidocaine (Xylocaine), beta blockers, or cardioversion.

The toxicity of stimulant drugs is not limited to behavioral and cardiovascular effects. Other serious effects include seizures, cerebrovascular accidents, hyperthermia, rhabdomyolysis, and acute tubular necrosis. Seizures usually complicate *overdoses* of stimulant drugs, but they may also occur with recreational use. Seizures are best controlled with intravenous diazepam (Valium). If more seizures are expected, the patient should be loaded intravenously with phenytoin (Dilantin) at a rate of 25 to 50 mg per minute for a total dose of 15 to 18 mg per kg. Alternatively, phenobarbital (Luminal) can be loaded at 18 mg per kg. Seizures and hyperactivity can result in hyperthermia. Failing to measure body temperature is a common oversight in the setting of drug abuse or overdose. Rhabdomyolysis is suggested by a urine dipstick positive for blood when the microscopic examination shows no erythrocytes. If rhabdomyolysis is suspected, intravenous hydration should begin immediately. Alkalinization of the urine with intravenous sodium bicarbonate may offer additional benefit because myoglobin is more likely to precipitate and damage renal tubules in the normally acidic urine.

If the patient presents shortly after ingestion of a stimulant drug, gastric emptying (e.g., induced emesis, lavage) is worthwhile. If presentation is delayed beyond 1 hour, charcoal administration is more appropriate (initial dose, 50 grams). Repeat oral charcoal, 25 grams every 2 to 4 hours, is indicated in the asymptomatic cocaine body packer. Induced emesis or endoscopic attempts at removal may result in packet rupture and immediate lethal toxicity. Whole-bowel irrigation may also be helpful. Plain abdominal radiographs or contrast studies may help detect and quantitate the packets, although not all are radiopaque. Drugs other than cocaine, such as heroin, may also be smuggled by body packing, and clinical presentation may vary. Extracorporeal methods to remove stimulant drugs (e.g., hemodialysis, hemoperfusion, plasmapheresis, exchange transfusion) are ineffective.

Withdrawal

In contrast to withdrawal from alcohol and sedative hypnotic drugs, physiologic withdrawal from stimulant drugs is seldom severe or life-threatening, and events such as seizures are rare. Serious depression and suicidal ideation, however, may occur and require treatment with antidepressant medication.

HALLUCINOGENS

Table 4 lists the common hallucinogenic drugs. Hallucinations may be the desired effect sought by the user of these drugs, but occasionally the hallucinations are frightening, especially to the inexperienced user. A "bad trip" may bring a young user to the emergency department or crisis intervention center for treatment. The hallucinations may also be accompanied by a panic reaction or psychosis. The most commonly abused drug in this class is lysergic acid diethylamide (LSD). Known for its induction of vivid visual hallucinations, LSD may also demonstrate sympathomimetic effects, such as mydriasis, hypertension, and tachycardia, but these effects are usually mild and seldom require treatment. Mescaline is a less potent hallucinogen that is related chemically to epinephrine and exhibits sympathomimetic effects. Designer drugs, such as MDA, MDMA ("ecstasy"), MDEA, and others, have been synthesized in an effort to escape criminal designation. They are more potent stimulants and hallucinogens. Their adrenergic effects may be more pronounced, and seizures and death have been associated with their use, as well as persistent extrapyramidal and choreiform movements resembling parkinsonism.

TABLE 4. **Commonly Abused Hallucinogens**

Lysergic acid diethylamide (LSD)
Mescaline
Designer drugs (e.g., MDA, MDMA, MDEA)
Marijuana and hashish (tetrahydrocannabinol)
Peyote (cactus)
Mushrooms (psilocybin, psilocin)
Morning glory seeds

TABLE 5. **Commonly Abused Narcotics**

Heroin	Hydrocodone
Opium	Codeine
Morphine	Propoxyphene
Hydromorphone	Pentazocine
Methadone	Diphenoxylate
Oxycodone	Fentanyl

Of all the illegal drugs of abuse, marijuana is the most popular. NIDA estimated in 1986 that there were about 18,000,000 users of this drug, outnumbered only by the users of alcohol, nicotine, and caffeine. Its widespread use among young people guarantees that it will remain a problem. According to the 1990 National School-Based Youth Risk Behavior Survey, almost one-third (31.4%) of all students in grades 9 through 12 had used marijuana at least once. In a 1987 to 1989 study of accidents by the Federal Railroad Administration, cannabinoids were the most commonly encountered single drug finding for years 1 (61%) and 2 (47%). Although grouped here with the hallucinogens, marijuana does not usually cause hallucinations at the doses smoked or ingested. It is used for its mood-altering effects, and patients usually present as a result of accidents or dysphoric reactions.

Treatment

Those suffering "bad trips" and dysphoric reactions may be "talked down," as in the case of stimulant drugs. Those experiencing more severe reactions or psychosis may require sedation with benzodiazepines or haloperidol. Even if haloperidol is used only briefly, the doses required raise the risk of extrapyramidal reactions, and the author prescribes 50 mg of diphenhydramine every 6 hours or 2 mg of benztropine every day for 2 days after the last dose.

NARCOTICS

Table 5 lists the commonly abused narcotics. Although stimulants and hallucinogens generally cause CNS excitation, narcotics, sedative hypnotics, and solvents cause various degrees of CNS depression.

Narcotic abuse classically presents as miosis, respiratory depression, and CNS depression (i.e., narcotic toxidrome). Exceptions are meperidine (Demerol) and diphenoxylate (Lomotil), which produce mydriasis or no pupillary change because of their anticholinergic effect. Propoxyphene (Darvon), meperidine, and codeine can cause seizures. Nausea, vomiting, and hypotension also occur. Cardiac arrhythmias occur with propoxyphene, but they can follow any narcotic dose large enough to cause hypoxia or pulmonary edema, which is more likely after intravenous administration. Parenteral drug abuse is associated with a variety of infectious complications, such as subcutaneous abscesses, septic emboli, pneumonia, endocarditis, hepatitis, and acquired immune deficiency syndrome (AIDS).

Treatment

As with any drug abuse emergency, attention should be directed first to the basics of airway, breathing, and circulation because most drugs lack a specific antidote or antagonist. For the respiratory depression induced by narcotics, however, naloxone (Narcan) is a rapid, safe, and effective antidote. Narcosis is reversed within seconds. The initial dose should be 2 mg. Synthetic narcotics, such as codeine, methadone, pentazocine (Talwin), and propoxyphene, may require higher doses, and narcotic overdose is not ruled out until 10 mg have been given. Suddenly aroused narcotic abusers may become agitated and violent, and the staff should be prepared to restrain them. Because the duration of many narcotics exceeds that of naloxone, these patients require prolonged observation or admission. An intravenous naloxone infusion at an hourly rate equal to two-thirds of the arousal dose maintains normal respirations.

Withdrawal

Narcotic withdrawal is not as serious as that from alcohol and sedative hypnotic drugs, and many patients can withdraw without medication. Withdrawal symptoms begin soon after the first missed dose of narcotic, peak at about 48 hours, and subside in 7 to 10 days, depending on the half-life of the abused opioid. Early symptoms include lacrimation, rhinorrhea, and diaphoresis. Soon the patient becomes restless and irritable, and examination often shows sinus tachycardia, mydriasis, and tremor. Appetite and sleep are disturbed, and the patient often complains of abdominal cramps and general achiness. Nausea, vomiting, and diarrhea can be troublesome. Treatment is symptomatic: non-narcotic antidiarrheal agents, non-narcotic analgesics, and antiemetics. Clonidine (Catapres) has also been shown to mitigate the withdrawal syndrome. Narcotics, other than methadone for maintenance therapy in strictly supervised programs, should not be used for managing narcotic withdrawal.

SEDATIVE HYPNOTIC DRUGS

Table 6 lists the commonly abused sedative hypnotic drugs. This diverse class of drugs includes barbiturates, benzodiazepines, and non-barbiturate non-benzodiazepines. They are all CNS depressants, and acute intoxication resembles that of alcohol and narcotics. Patients may present with slurred speech, ataxia, slowed mentation, impaired memory, and somnolence. Overdose can result in coma, respiratory depression, and hypotension. Lesser doses, as with alcohol, may cause emotional lability and acute dysphoric reactions. Their disinhibitory effect may also result in aggressiveness and violent behavior. The clinical presentation may also be confused by the concomitant abuse of other drugs, as when a sedative hypnotic is used to counteract the unpleasant excitation of stimulant or hallucinogenic drugs. Sedative hypnotic drugs are abused by the old and young. Drug abuse should be considered in any elderly patient who presents with confusion or acute or chronic dementia.

TABLE 6. **Commonly Abused Sedative Hypnotic Drugs**

Benzodiazepines	**Propanediol Carbamate**
Alprazolam	Meprobamate
Chlorazepate	Ethinamate*
Chlordiazepoxide	**Piperidinediones**
Clonazepam	Glutethimide
Diazepam	Methyprylon
Flurazepam	**Quinazolines**
Halazepam	Methaqualone
Lorazepam	**Barbiturates**
Midazolam	Amobarbital
Oxazepam	Barbital
Prazepam	Butabarbital
Temazepam	Pentobarbital
Triazolam	Phenobarbital
Alcohols	Secobarbital
Chloral hydrate	
Ethchlorvynol	

*Not available in the United States.

Some sedative hypnotic drugs have important effects other than CNS depression. For example, barbiturates, especially in overdose, can cause hypotension, hypothermia, skin blisters, and pulmonary edema. Chloral hydrate can cause cardiac disturbances, such as atrial fibrillation, aberrant conduction, PVCs, and ventricular tachycardia. Glutethimide (Doriden) has anticholinergic activity and can cause mydriasis, urinary retention, tachycardia, and hypertension.

Treatment

Treatment of sedative hypnotic intoxication is usually supportive, with special attention to preserving the airway and ventilation. Traditionally, unconscious patients are treated empirically with naloxone and glucose to rule out narcotics and hypoglycemia. No other specific antagonist is available except flumazenil (Mazicon), which rapidly and effectively reverses the CNS depression of benzodiazepines. For the treatment of overdose, the recommended initial dose is 0.2 mg intravenously over 30 seconds. If no arousal occurs, a second dose of 0.3 mg is given over 30 seconds. If necessary, further doses of 0.5 mg can be administered over 30 seconds, up to a total dose of 3.0 mg.

If a patient presents in an acute state of sedation, gastric decontamination is indicated. Activated charcoal should also be administered, and repeat doses may remove additional drug by "intestinal dialysis," shortening the half-life of the drug and its associated coma. Alkaline diuresis enhances excretion of phenobarbital but not the shorter acting barbiturates. Hemodialysis and hemoperfusion can also remove long-acting barbiturates, but expense and complications of these therapies should be considered because most patients recover with good supportive care. A re-

TABLE 7. **Commonly Abused Solvents and Inhalants**

Product	Solvent or Inhalant
Gasoline	Various hydrocarbons, tetraethyl lead
Typewriter correction fluid	Trichloroethane, trichloroethylene, perchloroethylene
Lighter fluid	Butane
Model glue or cement	Toluene, xylene
Adhesives	Toluene
Nail polish remover	Acetone, amyl acetate
Aerosol cans (paints, fabric protector)	Fluorocarbons
Paints, varnishes, lacquers	Trichloroethylene, toluene, methylene chloride
Spot remover, dry cleaning chemicals	Trichloroethane, trichloroethylene, tetrachloroethylene
Hair styling mousse	Propane, butane, isobutane
Anesthetic, whipped cream propellant	Nitrous oxide
"Aphrodisiac" inhalants	Amyl, butyl, and isobutyl nitrites

gional poison center should be consulted for advice on specific drugs and problems.

Withdrawal

Withdrawal from these drugs is probably more dangerous than from other drugs of abuse. In contrast to withdrawal from alcohol and narcotics, which usually begins within hours to days after the last dose, withdrawal from long-acting sedative hypnotic drugs may be delayed for many days. Detoxification from alcohol is usually accomplished within a few days, but withdrawal from sedative hypnotics may require 2 to 3 weeks.

Signs and symptoms are similar to alcohol withdrawal. Patients are restless, tremulous, and diaphoretic. They frequently complain of nausea, vomiting, and abdominal pain. Hyperreflexia and myoclonic jerks may precede generalized seizures, which may be severe and prolonged. Hallucinations and delirium complicate severe cases. Withdrawal should be managed by toxicologists or experienced physicians in a hospital or other institutional setting. Withdrawal is usually ameliorated by slowly tapering doses of intermediate-acting to long-acting barbiturates or benzodiazepines.

SOLVENTS

No discussion of drug abuse would be complete without including solvents and other inhalants. No dealer or pusher is needed to obtain these chemicals, which are in many household products. Table 7 lists the commonly abused solvents. They are generally abused by the most inexperienced drug seekers: adolescents and preadolescents.

Solvents are volatile, lipid-soluble substances that have CNS depressant effects. Abusers may sniff the open containers, "huff" rags soaked with the solvent, or "bag" the vapors from a plastic bag. Bagging is probably the most dangerous because the vapors are more concentrated and the abuser can lose consciousness and suffocate. Solvent vapors can also induce hypoxia both by respiratory depression and by displacement of oxygen. Asphyxiation was commonly assumed to be the cause of death until it was appreciated that solvents, especially halogenated hydrocarbons, could sensitize the heart to catecholamines and cause ventricular tachycardia and fibrillation. All too often the presentation is sudden death; few successful resuscitations have been reported. More commonly, however, the patient presents with slurred speech, ataxia, and somnolence. A solvent, rather than alcohol, odor is usually conspicuous. Chronic abuse can result in toxicity to the bone marrow, liver, and peripheral nerves. Toluene is especially noxious, causing electrolyte imbalance, renal tubular acidosis, and neurotoxicity. Urine drug screens generally do not detect solvents. Physicians should alert the toxicology laboratory about what chemical is suspected.

Treatment

Treatment of solvent abuse is mainly supportive, assuring a stable airway and ventilation. Supplemental oxygen may be helpful. There is no other way to enhance excretion as with ingested drugs of abuse. The heart should be monitored initially for arrhythmias. Antiarrhythmic drugs, such as lidocaine and beta blockers, should be administered for life-threatening ventricular arrhythmias. A complete blood count, electrolytes, liver enzymes, and urinalysis should be obtained to rule out toxicity of solvents such as toluene. Toluene intoxication may require intravenous fluids, electrolyte replacement, and administration of sodium bicarbonate if acidosis is significant. Methemoglobinemia may complicate abuse of nitrites and require treatment with methylene blue. Peripheral neuropathy secondary to chronic nitrous oxide abuse may respond to vitamin B_{12} and thiamine.

Knowledge and therapies are continuously expanding in toxicology. When an unfamiliar drug is encountered, it is always wise to consult a toxicologist, regional poison center, or a standard reference such as *Clinical Management of Poisoning and Drug Overdose,* edited by Lester Haddad and James Winchester. As with all drugs of abuse, medical treatment of complications should be followed by psychiatric or chemical dependency evaluation and treatment.

ANXIETY DISORDERS

method of
C. KNIGHT ALDRICH, M.D.
University of Virginia
Charlottesville, Virginia

DIAGNOSIS AND CLASSIFICATION

There are two major groups of anxiety disorders in addition to anxiety that is a symptom of either a disease like hyperthyroidism or overuse of a substance like caffeine. In the first group, anxiety is manifest *directly* by its symptoms, which are the same as the symptoms of fear (most anxiety is essentially fear of the unknown). This group includes three disorders: (1) adjustment disorder with anxious mood, perhaps the most common type, in which the anxiety occurs in response to an evident acute or long-term situational stress; (2) the persistent generalized anxiety disorder, in which the precipitating stresses are usually more obscure; and (3) intermittent panic attacks and panic disorder, in which the anxiety is episodic.

In the second group, anxiety is manifest *indirectly*. This group includes, among other disorders: (1) phobias, in which the anxiety occurs in response to social situations or to specific stimuli such as heights or air travel; (2) obsessive-compulsive disorders, characterized by persistent interfering thoughts or ritualized behaviors; (3) post-traumatic stress disorders, in which severe anxiety is associated with the re-experience of a past overwhelming stressor; and (4) somatoform disorders, in which the patient concentrates on the physical manifestations of anxiety (somatoform disorders are discussed in more detail later).

The various anxiety disorders are not discrete entities; they tend to overlap, not only with each other but also with depression. Although classification is useful in planning the symptomatic treatment of anxiety, most treatment requires individualized diagnosis as well. For individualized diagnosis it is very important to obtain a history of the condition's *duration* and, if possible, of its *precipitant*. The diagnosis of any of the anxiety disorders stems from (1) symptoms that are characteristic of anxiety, and (2) a history of psychosocial stresses that can be correlated with the symptoms. Without both of these elements, the patient should be considered undiagnosed.

SYMPTOMATIC TREATMENT

Because symptomatic treatment is simpler and less time-consuming to carry out than treatment aimed at causes, it is tempting to rely on it too much. It is usually indicated in *self-limited* conditions ("I get symptoms every time I visit my in-laws, but when the visit is over I am all right") or in *chronic* conditions ("As long as I can remember I have been nervous and tense"). Symptomatic treatment includes supportive psychotherapy, relaxation techniques, behavior modification, which is most useful in patients with phobias and obsessive-compulsive conditions, and drugs. Drugs are the most widely used symptomatic treatment; unfortunately, however, they have side effects, and many of them encourage drug dependency.

The most commonly used drug treatments for anxiety disorders are the *benzodiazepines,* which should be used only in combination with psychosocial measures and preferably for short periods of up to a month. Several of the benzodiazepines appear to be effective in generalized anxiety disorders and phobias; alprazolam seems to have advantages in panic states. The *tricyclic antidepressants* also may be effective in these disorders and are usually better choices for chronic conditions. One of the tricyclics, clomipramine (Anafranil), is the drug treatment of choice in obsessive-compulsive disorders.

PSYCHOTHERAPY

If psychotherapy aimed at causes is indicated and feasible, the sooner it is initiated the better, preferably by the primary care physician. The indications for psychotherapy provided by primary care physicians include a definable onset of the symptoms, often a loss of some kind. In such patients the goal of therapy is to help the patient return to a previous level of reasonably satisfactory adaptation, not to try to reconstruct the personality. The focus of treatment is therefore on the precipitants of the condition, not on the childhood predisposing factors; thus a physician would try to help a patient express and cope with unresolved grief resulting from the death of a relative rather than to change the personality characteristics that have kept him or her from dealing with the grief.

The kind of psychotherapy that primary care physicians can adapt to their practices ordinarily takes no more than 15 to 20 minutes a week and in the long run saves time for both physician and patient. Castelnuovo-Tedesco's book, *The Twenty-Minute Hour,* and Stuart and Lieberman's *The Fifteen-Minute Hour: Applied Psychotherapy for the Primary Care Physician,* describe the details of techniques that can make working with patients with anxiety disorders successful and enjoyable. Even brief restorative psychotherapy, however, requires two major shifts from the primary care physicians' usual modus operandi:

1. An emphasis on *empathic listening* rather than on advice-giving is needed. Because most physicians' day-to-day activities are active—manipulating, prescribing, advising—they may view relatively passive listening as somehow not giving the patient his money's worth. Actually, empathic listening is the most effective psychotherapeutic technique.
2. Setting the *duration* of each session by time rather than by task is another change for most physicians. Not having a "wrap-up" at the end of the session usually stimulates the patient to continue to work on the problem between sessions. A statement such as "We're about at the end of this week's session, so perhaps we can look at this problem again next week" encourages the patient to think about the situation during the intervening time.

SOMATOFORM DISORDERS

Of all anxiety disorders seen by the primary care physician, somatoform disorders are, if not the most frequent, surely the most time-consuming and frustrating to treat. Somatoform disorders include several related conditions; the two most frequent are called *somatization disorders,* in which the signs of anxiety are perceived by the patient as evidence of organic disease, and *hypochondriasis,* characterized by a fear of organic disease. Conversion disorders, somatoform pain disorders, and body dysmorphic disorders are other types of somatoform disorders.

Whether the treatment of somatoform disorders gets off to a good start depends on how and when the tentative diagnosis is made and communicated to the patient. When the tentative diagnosis is made in positive rather than negative terms and when it is communicated to the patient early in the process, it is much easier for the physician to overcome the patient's resistance to recognizing and dealing with the psychosocial aspects of the condition.

The Positive Diagnosis. Primary care physicians usually can tell within the first few minutes of history-taking whether anxiety plays a significant role in the cause of a patient's symptoms. When the anxiety occurs in response to an organic illness, physicians usually deal with it along with the underlying condition, but when there is no evidence of significant organic illness in the history, physicians often delay mentioning the possibility of a psychosocial factor until they have accumulated enough negative examination or laboratory evidence to "prove" their case to their patients. Reliance on negative evidence, however, not only can lead to an inaccurate diagnosis but also can reduce the physician's therapeutic effectiveness. A diagnosis made on the basis of an absence of physical examination and laboratory findings is much less convincing to either the doctor or the patient than a positive diagnosis made by the doctor and then confirmed by laboratory findings. To be convincing to patients physicians need to make it evident that they are not simply falling back on a diagnosis of somatization because they cannot find anything else.

The exploration of psychosocial causative factors in patients with somatoform disorders does not have to be approached head on. The physician can start with a question like, "Can you tell me how your symptoms are affected by tension?" rather than, "Does tension cause your symptoms?" Most patients acknowledge that tension has an impact on their symptoms; if so, the physician's next question can be, "What kinds of tension cause the problems?", which leads naturally to an exploration of the current stresses in the patient's life. In this exploration it is important not to ask leading questions; thus, the physician should ask, "Could you tell me about your family?" rather than, "Things are all right at home, aren't they?"

Taking the psychosocial history along with the rest of the medical history rather than at the end helps the patient to perceive that the physician is as interested in the psychosocial component of the history as in the biologic component and thus to become more accepting of its relevance.

Early Discussion of the Tentative Diagnosis. Because a positive diagnosis of anxiety does not exclude the possibility of coexisting conditions, it is not necessary or even desirable to rule out everything else before conveying the positive diagnosis to the patient. The optimal time for making this statement is at the completion of the history, at which time the physician can say something like, "From the nature of your symptoms and from what you have told me about the tensions in your life and how they affect your symptoms, I suspect that tension has a lot to do with your condition. Later on we are going to have to look at these tensions more closely; perhaps together we can find ways of dealing with them that can help to reduce your symptoms."

Does this approach put the physician out on a limb if there are coexisting organic conditions? Not at all, because he or she goes on to say, "I want to make sure, however, that there is nothing else that might be contributing to your symptoms, so I may order some tests after we finish the physical examination. I don't see any reason right now to expect that anything else will turn up, but I am sure you will agree that we ought to be thorough. In any case, we will have to do some more exploring of your tensions." With this approach, each negative laboratory report strengthens the tentative diagnosis and increases the patient's confidence in it; if "anything else" turns up, it is *in addition to, not instead of,* the anxiety. On the other hand, if patients believe that the physician expects each test to reveal an organic cause for the symptoms and test after test does not, they are less likely to accept an eventual diagnosis of anxiety.

Reassurance. Doctors tend to use negative test results to reassure somatizing patients and are often surprised, and annoyed, to find that patients are only reassured temporarily if at all (anxiety resulting from somatic disease, however, usually responds well to understanding and warranted reassurance about its nature and prognosis). The reason for the disappointing results of reassurance for patients with somatizing disorders is that they are, at least initially, more frightened of their hidden conflicts than they are of organic disease. For them, somatization acts as a protection against facing the unknown underlying causes of their anxiety; they therefore desperately hang on to the somatic disguise. They are not aware of this process—if they were it wouldn't work—so although they may be momentarily reassured by evidence that they have no organic disease, they soon fall back on their old defenses.

The kind of reassurance that results from the doctor's interest in exploring and working with the patient's problems and the doctor's optimism that together they may find better solutions helps the patient begin to give up the defensive somatization and to accept appropriate treatment for the underlying anxiety.

BULIMIA NERVOSA

method of
ARNOLD E. ANDERSEN, M.D.
University of Iowa
Iowa City, Iowa

Bulimia nervosa is a fascinating disorder of abnormal eating behavior with significant medical aspects that occurs primarily in adolescents and young adults. It has been recognized as a distinct diagnostic disorder only since 1979 but quickly came to be seen as an important disease entity in which previous cases were probably undiagnosed rather than nonexistent. Although much remains unknown about the disorder in terms of its fundamental mechanism, enough data have been tested on a firm empirical basis to give guidance to practitioners.

The term bulimia comes from the words for ox plus hunger. The central feature is the experience of compulsive binge-eating during which the patient feels out of control, usually ingesting large quantities of food rapidly, especially fats and sweets. The binge is followed by remorse and, in 80% of cases, by purging, food restriction, or strenuous exercise. A disorder of adolescence and young adults primarily, it can occur at virtually any age from 7 to 70.

Table 1 summarizes the basic facts of bulimia nervosa as a syndrome. This disorder, which occurs in 90% of cases in females, is often preceded by a full or partial syndrome of anorexia nervosa. In many ways bulimia represents an unsuccessful attempt at substantial weight loss by an individual whose mind and body are not cooperating. Appetite breaks through the food restriction attempt like an express train, provoking binge-eating. The essential feature of bulimia nervosa as a syndrome is the progression of binge-eating from being initially a response to hunger to an all-purpose, nonspecific method of dealing with a wide variety of emotional distress, especially depression, anxiety, anger, feeling stuck, or boredom. Once this happens, the disorder is no longer driven physiologically by hunger but primarily psychologically by relief of emotional distress plus variable amounts of hunger.

Table 2 shows a comparison of bulimia nervosa and anorexia nervosa, the opposite side of the same coin of an attempt to lose weight. The essential shared feature is the morbid fear of fatness, which is out of proportion to reality, and the associated relentless pursuit of thinness. In males (who account for 10% of cases of bulimia) the goal of shape change usually predominates over weight change. Studies document the distressing finding that by sixth grade half of girls feel fat and by age 21 more than 70% have felt fat enough to have dieted. Young people are subjected to systematic indoctrination that body weight, especially in women, should be below average to ensure attractiveness and social acceptance. Moderate personal distress about feeling overweight, even for women in a healthy weight range, is essentially culturally normal now but cannot be defended on that basis.

Bulimia nervosa is the third most common source of chronic morbidity in female adolescents. It has a potential association with death, either acute or long-term (follow-up studies of anorexia nervosa, for example, have found a 19% earlier than expected death rate). Finally, it imposes a major psychological, social, and financial burden involving themes of shame, secrecy, hidden medical symptomatology, and the loss of meaningful quality of life, especially during the pre-adult developmental years.

TABLE 1. **Basic Facts About Bulimia Nervosa**

A. Natural History
1. Bulimia represents a failed attempt at anorexia nervosa in which appetite has broken through the dieting pattern
2. Ninety percent of patients are female
3. Up to half of patients have experienced a preceding full or partial anorexia nervosa syndrome
4. Most common ages: mid-teens to mid-twenties
5. Three to 5% of teenage girls meet full criteria; up to 15% meet partial criteria

B. Stages of Illness
1. Pre-illness
   a. Socioculturally "normative" dissatisfaction with body with sporadic dieting plans or attempts
   b. Hunger-induced overeating episodes
2. Bulimia nervosa syndrome
   a. Trigger for binge episodes switches to primarily distressed mood (depression, anxiety, anger, "trapped" feeling, boredom) plus variable contribution from hunger
   b. Morbid fear of fatness or pursuit of thinness is present
3. Chronic "professional" stages of bulimia nervosa
   a. Patient develops an identity based on the illness
   b. Medical symptoms are severe, often stable, and are resistant to change

C. Predisposing Features (none absolutely required)
1. Lives in society that values or promotes thinness
2. Develops overvalued beliefs about benefits of thinness and phobic fears of fatness
3. Adolescent or young adult (no age excluded)
4. Dieting behavior
5. Family history of
   a. Mood disorder
   b. Obesity
6. More impulsive, dramatic, emotionally reactive personality
7. Personal history of early maturation or weight above that of peers
8. Membership in interest group that promotes thinness—ballet, modeling, cheerleading, wrestling, etc.
9. History of sexual abuse or physical abuse?

DIAGNOSIS

As with appendicitis, the beginning of accurate diagnosis is the need to think of the condition as an ever-present possibility. Second, diagnosis is aided by understanding this disorder as the response of a vulnerable individual to the interaction of sociocultural norms promoting weight loss with the physiologic regulation of the limbic system promoting weight stability. The disorder begins with self-induced attempts at weight loss, followed by unwanted binge-eating and then by a variety of means of getting rid of the unwanted caloric intake. Chronic bulimia becomes sustained by a combination of biomedical factors as well as its capacity to provide a personal, almost professional, identity to the developing individual. The most common bulimic disorder is bulimia nervosa at a normal weight, followed by binge-eating disorder, a relatively recently defined syndrome of binge-eating without purging that may occur in up to 25% of medically obese individuals, and last by the bulimic subtype of anorexia nervosa.

Table 3 lists the diagnostic features of bulimia nervosa binge-eating disorder and the bulimic subtype of anorexia nervosa. Milder versions of each of these conditions that do not meet full criteria are called atypical eating disorders, or, more formally, Eating Disorders Not Otherwise Specified (EDNOS).

The essential feature of the diagnosis of bulimia nervosa is the experience of compulsive binge episodes in an individual who feels out of control during the binge and afterward attempts to avoid weight gain from the extra calories

TABLE 2. **Comparison of Bulimia Nervosa and Anorexia Nervosa**

	Bulimia Nervosa	Anorexia Nervosa
Gender	10:1 female-male	10:1 female-male
Typical age of onset	15–25	12–22 (slightly younger)
Possible age of onset	10–70	7–75
Family history of depression	+ + +	+ +
Family history of obesity	+ +	+
Personality features	More dramatic, impulsive, emotionally reactive	More perfectionistic, anxious, self critical
Amenorrhea (females)	None or intermittent	Present
Binge-eating	Defining feature	No—restricting subtype; yes—bulimic subtype
Weight	Normal or overweight	<85% of normal
Fear of fatness, pursuit of thinness	Essential feature	Essential feature
Causes of death	Suicide—50%; medical complications—50%	Starvation—65%; suicide—35%
Alcohol or other drug abuse	+ +	+
Depressive syndrome in patient	+ + +	+
Response to antidepressants	+ +	+
Common co-morbid psychological disorders	Mood disorders, especially bipolar II alcohol or drug abuse	Mood disorders, especially major depression; OCD
Need for hospitalization	Seldom	Usually
Prevalence of full syndrome	2–5% female adolescents	0.5–1% female adolescents
Partial syndrome	5–15%	5%
Sexual experiences	Reticent or impulsive, more experienced, sometimes promiscuous	Usually reticent, inexperienced
Compulsive exercise	+/−	+ +
Food content	High fat, lower protein; typically 4000 kcal/day	Lower fat; higher protein; typically 600–700 kcal/day
Gastrointestinal symptoms due to illness	+ + +	+
Gastrointestinal symptoms due to nutritional rehabilitation	+ +	+ + +
Brain shrinkage	+/−	+ +
Social class	Population spectrum	Upper socioeconomic status

+ = mild; + + = moderate; + + + = strong relationship; +/− = may or may not be present (equivocal relationship).

by purging, exercise, or fasting. This is quite different from culturally normative episodes of feasting or gorging in groups (e.g., in dorms before examinations), no matter how excessive they may seem. To exclude cases of experimental binge-eating or the occurrence of a short-term self-correcting condition, there is a diagnostic requirement for the presence of binges twice a week for at least 3 months and for an association with an irrational fear of fatness or a relentless pursuit of thinness. The most common diagnostic error is to call self-induced vomiting by itself, without binges, bulimia nervosa. An accurate diagnosis first excludes the weight loss syndrome of anorexia nervosa.

About 20% of bulimic individuals meet the criteria for binge-eating disorder, a subtype of binge-eating that lacks any post-binge purge. These patients are more often actually overweight, tend to be older, are predominantly female, and often have a more passive nurturing personality with a low sense of self-esteem and low assertiveness. The bulimic subtype of anorexia nervosa requires the presence of both substantial weight loss, more than 15%, or failure to gain weight normally, a morbid fear of fatness, and binge-purge behavior. These individuals bear the burdens of both starvation from anorexia and the medical complications of binge-purge episodes.

Table 4 lists some of the occult signs and symptoms of bulimia nervosa. In contrast to anorexia nervosa, which in many ways is a public disorder through the visibility of the starved body, bulimia nervosa remains a very private disorder for many persons. Bulimic patients may test the physician for trust and understanding by bringing to them other concerns before the bulimic symptomatology is introduced, if it is introduced at all. Signs of binge-eating in the home or elsewhere, signs of vomiting not related to short-term illness such as the flu, substantial weight fluctuations for no clear reason, and unexplained low potassium levels in a young person are some of the most common occult signs and symptoms. Even more rare are calluses on the knuckles where they hit the teeth when inducing vomiting. Chronic laxative abuse in this age group tends to occur more because of bulimia nervosa than because of constipation.

Finally, eating disorders seldom travel alone. They almost always have companions in their posse. The most common co-morbid conditions are mood disorders, which occur in 40 to 70% of patients with bulimia nervosa, personality disorders or vulnerable personality traits, especially impulsivity and mood lability, alcohol and other drug abuse, and anxiety states. The outcome of treatment may have as much to do with the management and treatment of the co-morbid mood disorder and personality traits as with the binge-eating itself.

Physical Examination

A thorough examination reveals the general body condition including any degree of starvation and the appearance of health or illness. Overall, the vital signs should be carefully assessed, and pulse irregularity or hypotension should be sought diligently. At times signs of dehydration such as tenting of the skin are present; these usually indicate de-

TABLE 3. **Diagnostic Criteria for Bulimia Nervosa and Binge-Eating Disorder, Bulimic Subtype of Anorexia Nervosa**

A. Bulimia Nervosa at Normal Weight
1. Anorexia nervosa criteria not fulfilled
2. Presence of binge episodes—large amounts of food, often high in fats and sweets, usually eaten quickly and privately while feeling out of control, to the point of physical discomfort. Ceases with social interruption or running out of food; followed by guilt and self-blame; two episodes per week for 3 months
3. Preoccupation with desire to be thinner or different in shape, or irrational fear of becoming fat
4. Generally, distortion of body image, rejection of body, excess dissatisfaction with body size or shape
5. Usually (in 80% of cases) followed by efforts to compensate for binge episodes by
   a. Self-induced vomiting
   b. Periods of food restriction or abstention
   c. Laxative, diuretic, emetic, or diet pill abuse

B. Binge-Eating Disorder
1. Affects a smaller number of typically overweight, older (thirties to forties) patients with more passive and nurturing personalities. They binge but do not purge or restrict food afterward (about 20% of normal-weight bulimia nervosa patients and about 25% of overweight patients are binge-disordered eaters)

C. Anorexia Nervosa, Bulimic Subtype
1. Self-induced weight loss or failure to gain weight normally with resulting weight more than 15% below normal
2. Inappropriate, excessive, fear of fatness or pursuit of thinness
3. Reproductive hormone abnormality: for females, 3 months of secondary amenorrhea or primary amenorrhea; for males, decreased sexual drive and function with lowered testosterone
4. Binge episodes (as in bulimia nervosa), followed by efforts to compensate for binge food ingested (vomiting, food restriction, medication abuse, compulsive exercise)

D. Eating Disorders Not Otherwise Specified (EDNOS)
Milder versions that do not meet full criteria—for example, one binge episode per week, or bingeing lasting for less than 3 months

hydration secondary to sustained diuretic or laxative abuse because of the patient's confusion between water weight and true body weight. The parotid glands are assessed for visible swelling and tenderness, a side effect of self-induced vomiting. The teeth may have obvious loss of enamel on the lingual surface and multiple caries. Palpation may elicit discomfort in the subxiphoid area caused by esophagitis. The abdomen in general may be variably distended or tender to palpation. Examination of the periphery occasionally shows scars on the knuckles caused by abrasions where the teeth scraped the knuckles during induction of vomiting. Many superficial cuts may indicate self-harm associated with a borderline personality.

A simple recording of height and weight is essential, and, if possible, a determination of body fat is performed as a baseline index. The simple act of weighing may result in anxiety, however, and some patients prefer being weighed backward with no mention of weight.

TABLE 4. **Occult Signs and Symptoms of Bulimia Nervosa**

1. Unexplained weight cycles or weight fluctuations, especially in adolescent or young adults
2. Signs of vomiting or purging
   a. External: laxative packages, vomitus materials found, ipecac purchase
   b. Internal: erosion of lingual surface of dental enamel, unexplained hypokalemia
3. Signs of binge-eating
   a. Unusual eating patterns
   b. Exit after or during meals to bathroom
   c. Unexplained disappearance of large amounts of food
4. Parotid gland enlargement
5. Scars on knuckles of hand from self-induced vomiting (Russell's sign)
6. Unexplained amenorrhea
7. Preoccupation with weight, size, shape
8. New onset of vegetarianism

Laboratory Studies

A few basic laboratory studies are essential, including measurement of electrolytes, a complete blood count, a chemistry panel (including kidney function tests, liver chemistries, calcium, phosphate, serum albumin, total protein, uric acid, and lipids). A low serum albumin is one of the few indications of potentially increased mortality due to eating disorders. Cholesterol may be paradoxically high. Renal damage may be secondary to diuretic or laxative abuse. The electrocardiogram is vital to assess rhythm, composition of QRS complexes and other indications of possible arrhythmias due to hypokalemia, and myocardial damage. Cardiac damage caused by the emetine component of Ipecac may masquerade as symptoms similar to those produced by viral myocarditis.

The key to the use of laboratory tests is to develop a systematic method of assessment of the bulimic patient to quantitate the severity of medical symptomatology and to detect any potentially serious, possibly life-threatening, abnormalities such as hypokalemia. A potassium level below 2 occurs with sustained diuretic abuse, but the patient may look completely normal. The tests are not used to look for an alternative cause of either the binge-eating or the self-induced vomiting. When the central psychopathologic abnormality is present along with the characteristic behavior of binge episodes, medical tests are used for medical management, not diagnosis.

Tests To Be Considered

1. Occasionally, specialized gastrointestinal studies are necessary, especially when there is persistent distress despite clinical improvement in binge-purge behavior. These include swallowing studies, gastric emptying, assessment of reflux, and either gastroscopy or indwelling PH probes if persistent symptoms exist.
2. Bone mineral density determination, by dual photon absorptiometry or other means, makes sense if patients have had a previous anorexic episode or amenorrhea for more than 6 months. Forty percent of anorexic patients with the bulimic subtype are below the critical fracture threshold of 0.965 gram per cm^2 compared with the normal level of 1.2 grams per cm^2. This is another medical sign that cannot be determined by visual inspection.
3. Thyroid function tests are usually not necessary but may be helpful if depressive symptoms persist after weight and eating behavior have become normal. A slight increase in thyroid-stimulating hormone (TSH) level suggests borderline thyroid hypofunction, which will diminish response to antidepressants. A persisting low triiodothyronine (T_3) level suggests that weight is not truly normal.
4. If weight has been restored to a seemingly adequate point but menstrual disturbance continues, determination of luteinizing hormone, follicle-stimulating hor-

mone, and estrogen (blood or urine) levels are helpful in finding the occasional patient with premature menopause versus the more probable situation of continued hypothalamic hypogonadism due to too low a weight for that patient. An ovarian sonogram may be used to document the degree to which ovarian function has returned to normal, a single dominant cyst being present just before ovulation resumes. In males, a return to normal testosterone level is a necessary but not sufficient criterion of treatment success in patients with any degree of underweight.

5. Other tests that are occasionally indicated include magnetic resonance imaging (MRI) to detect atypical features to rule out pituitary microademonas or other CNS lesions. In the presence of seizures, usually secondary to electrolyte abnormalities, an electroencephalogram (EEG) is useful to rule out a seizure focus. Medical information may also be used psychotherapeutically. Although it is not helpful to frighten patients with the finding of a severe medical abnormality, by sharing test results of, for example, a shrunken brain or an abnormal electrocardiogram, the physician may encourage the patient to become a therapeutic partner by recognizing the seriousness of the disorder.

TREATMENT

Before treatment is begun, a basic decision should be made about whether to refer the patient to a specialist in eating disorders. This is not a disorder of willful adolescents or self-indulgent patients who are simply lacking in determination to stop a bad habit. Adjunctive treatment with a local support group of an eating disorders association adds efficacy. If treatment is undertaken, two simple preliminary steps help in the subsequent formal treatment. The first is to ask the patient to keep a record for 1 or 2 weeks of the eating behavior. Records of the time of day, location, food eaten, type of eating (normal versus binge), and a few words about context including mood state, thoughts, or events going on around the patient enable the clinician to notice typical behavioral patterns that are helpful in directing treatment goals. For example, patients often skip breakfast and have a light lunch, followed by a late afternoon binge. Binges often occur in a somewhat predicable fashion around the times of emotional distress at work, in personal relationships, or with mood fluctuations.

The second pre-treatment foundation is patient psychoeducation. Although accurate information by itself rarely cures a serious medical or psychiatric illness, it often allows the patient to make sense of the rationale and the sequence of treatment steps. For example, it may help to share with the patient information from recent studies showing that early food restriction during the day promotes bingeing later in the afternoon; severe abuse of laxatives leading to a diarrheal output of more than 6 liters per day cuts down calorie absorption by only 20%; yo-yo dieting produces more heart disease than mild sustained obesity; storage of calcium in the "retirement bank" must be done by age 35 because after that there is an inevitable decrease in bone mineral density; the sooner treatment is started, the better the outcome; and, conversely, the duration of symptomatology is no barrier to improvement.

Because the binge behavior and the subsequent purging (which are present in 80% of cases) are a source of shame and guilt to the patient, a trusting relationship is necessary. Occasionally, especially if the patient has experienced previous sexual abuse, the gender of the therapist may make a difference, but on the whole, competence and nonpossessive warmth are more important than gender.

After baseline diary documentation of eating behavior patterns and the triggers of binge episodes and after adequate time has been allowed for patient education in psychologic mechanisms, treatment begins with a prescription for normal nutritional intake (Table 5). Patients may object that they will gain

TABLE 5. **Basis of Treatment of Bulimia Nervosa**

A. Make the diagnosis of type of bulimic syndrome
B. Form trusting relationship with patient
C. Decide on treatment yourself vs. referral
D. Undertake psychoeducation
E. Prospective patient keeps record of food intake on 3 by 5 cards for 1 to 2 weeks to assess baseline pattern of energy intake and to identify triggers of binge episodes: time, location, food eaten (meal or snack, normal or binge meal), mood, events
F. Institute prescribed normal nutrition
    1. At least 25% of energy intake eaten at breakfast
    2. No skipped meals
    3. Low to moderate fat and protein, with no conscious dieting; total energy intake is proportional to age, weight and activity
    4. Follow pattern of food "exchanges" or portions for each meal, not calories
G. No weight loss for overweight patients considered until eating pattern is normal, then, if appropriate, very slow, long-term, nondieting weight reduction is undertaken, emphasizing moderate regular physical activity and low-fat foods
H. Persuade the patient to rethink the excessive value placed on weight and shape; cognitive-behavioral therapy (group or individual) produces best results
I. Antidepressants can be used, especially serotonin re-uptake inhibitors: fluoxetine (Prozac),* sertraline (Zoloft),* paroxetine (Paxil)* at standard doses with gradual introduction *if* depressive symptoms persist after binges are interrupted, weight is stable, psychotherapy has been tried, especially if patient has strong family history of mood disorder preceding the bulimia mood disorder. Consider use of lights for strong seasonal component to binges or depression
J. Gradual elimination of binge episodes is accomplished by accurate identification of cognitive and emotional triggers of mood distress or hunger, and substitution of healthy behaviors
K. Consider hospitalization if:
    1. Significant medical symptoms or signs are present
    2. Suicidal ideation or behavior
    3. Intractable binge-eating and or purging does not respond to outpatient treatment
    4. Significant co-morbid symptoms exist: alcoholism, other drug abuse
    5. Toxic or barren environment
L. Most bulimia nervosa patients do best at upper-normal or slightly above "normal" weight range. Factors determining healthy weight goals (range, 4–5 pounds) include normal periods, absence of chronic hunger, no excess coldness or other signs of unphysiologic low weight
M. Be prepared to treat probable cluster of co-morbid psychiatric conditions: mood disorders, personality disorders, alcohol and other drug abuse, anxiety states

*Not FDA approved for this indication.

weight, but they actually do much better in maintaining a stable weight with regular balanced meals. At least 25% of the daily energy intake should be taken at breakfast. No meals may be skipped. Each meal ideally includes a 3- to 4-ounce portion of low-fat protein, carbohydrate equivalent to a minimum of two slices of bread, and fruits and vegetables. A program of "exchange groups," as used for diabetes, or other forms of portion management is much more helpful than an emphasis on calories. A dietitian may or may not be consulted depending on the experience of the clinician.

No attempts to change weight should be considered initially. Normalization of the pattern of food intake takes precedence over weight change. Weight may change during the early stages of treatment in either direction owing to physiologic equilibration. An early challenge in the treatment of bulimia patients with normal weight is to persuade them to accept on faith that their weight will become normal for them if they eat regular meals containing low to moderate amounts of fat, exercise moderately, and deal directly with the stresses that produce binge-eating.

Usually, bulimia patients fare better if their weight approximates the upper part of the weight range for age and height in a normal population rather than the lower part. If weight reduction is undertaken, a loss of 1 or 2 pounds a month, at most, for however long it takes to achieve a target goal range is much healthier and more likely to stay off than a rapid weight loss. For underweight patients with the bulimic subtype of anorexia nervosa, weight restoration of 2 to 3 pounds per week may be undertaken, beginning with about 1500 kcal of energy intake and increasing to approximately 3500 kcal by 500-kcal increments each week. Excess weight in patients with binge-eating disorders often decreases moderately on a regimen of fluoxetine (Prozac).*

After nutritional normalization and agreement by the patient on avoidance of voluntary rapid weight change, the treatment emphasis shifts to gradually extinguishing the binge episodes through identification of the immediate triggers of binges (depressed mood, feeling stuck or bored, hunger, etc.) and the substitution of healthy alternatives. This is an area where personal record-keeping is essential because the specific issues differ from individual to individual. Rather than stopping an unhealthy behavior (bingeing), a more successful alternative is to start a healthy behavior that is incompatible with bingeing. If, for example, a patient is very anxious after a work assignment, trying to "not binge" is about as successful as trying to obey a command to stand in the corner and "not think" about a pink polar bear. Instead, the patient may go directly on a brisk half-hour walk, call up a buddy, practice relaxation, or go to a meeting of a self-help group.

The second aspect of the psychological component of treatment consists of a more general, usually cognitive-behavioral approach to correcting the underlying issues—revising the overvaluation of thinness, refuting the irrational fear of normal weight, counteracting feelings of low self-esteem or lack of effectiveness, and dealing with the consequences of past traumatic experiences. A combination of individual and group treatment, or either alone, may be helpful. The data indicate a better and longer lasting outcome with cognitive-behavioral therapy than with any kind of medication, even though medication may be useful in specific cases. A cost-effective approach is to begin with group cognitive-behavioral therapy and then consider additional individual forms of treatment, either psychotherapy or psychopharmacology, for patients who have not decreased symptoms by at least 50% at the end of six group treatment sessions. The essence of cognitive-behavioral therapy is to persuade the patient that he or she has, in the context of our sociocultural endorsement, placed an excessively high value on the benefits of changing body weight or shape. The healthy alternative to weight loss is to discover the goals behind the search for thinness or shape change, to endorse them (they are rarely abnormal), and to find healthy means of achieving them.

The last word on the role of antidepressants for bulimia has not been said, but these drugs appear to be helpful for some bulimic patients. There are three general guidelines for the use of antidepressants. First, they are best given, when possible, after a trial of standard treatment including the achievement of normal eating behavior and a trial of cognitive-behavioral psychotherapy if depression persists. Second, in binge-eating disorders (bingeing without purging), I recommend initial treatment with selective serotonin re-uptake inhibitors (SSRIs), starting with fluoxetine (Prozac) or one of the alternative serotonin re-uptake inhibitors such as sertraline (Zoloft)* or paroxetine (Paxil)* along with, rather than after, a trial of psychotherapy. The SSRIs have the advantage of not increasing carbohydrate craving and sometimes produce a mild decrease in weight as well as a decrease in depressive and sometimes in obsessional symptoms. Third, when a pharmacologic trial is undertaken, it confuses any future treatment unless it is done right; drug treatment should be continued long enough (6 to 8 weeks) and maintained at adequate doses (blood level monitoring for tricyclic antidepressants should be performed if they are used) to assess the results before concluding that the medication is not effective.

Hospitalization should be considered if significant medical signs and symptoms are initially serious and urgent, if suicidal ideation or behaviors exist, if intractable binge-eating or purging does not respond to a trial of outpatient treatment, if there is significant co-morbid symptomatology (especially alcohol and other drug abuse), or if the environment is "toxic" or barren, especially in the presence of ongoing sexual abuse or lack of outpatient treatment facilities. The

*This drug has not been approved by the Food and Drug Administration (FDA) for this indication.

*This drug has not been approved by the FDA for this indication.

general rule is that most anorexia nervosa patients require hospitalization whereas most bulimia nervosa patients may be treated as outpatients.

One advantage of having the primary physician treat patients with mild to moderate bulimia nervosa or binge-eating disorder is that the patient's mood and behavioral pattern throughout the year may come to be anticipated. A surprisingly high percentage of bulimia patients have a form of either seasonal depressive disorder or seasonal bipolar II mood disorder (hypomania alternating with depression). In seasonal depressive disorders the patient tends to have a lower mood in the fall and winter, with increased sleep needs and increased carbohydrate craving, often with weight gain, in contrast to the decreased appetite, decreased sleep, and weight loss seen in classic major depressive illness. Addition of therapeutic full-spectrum lights (now easily available) of between 2500 and 10,000 lux for 2 to ½ hours respectively per day, according to the strength of the lights, may be all that is necessary to interrupt a seasonal depressive disorder associated with and sustaining binge-eating or to achieve more complete results from partially successful antidepressant treatment of the seasonal mood disorder.

DELIRIUM

method of
PETER V. RABINS, M.D., M.P.H.
Johns Hopkins Medical Institutions
Baltimore, Maryland

Delirium is among the most common psychiatric disorders in the medically ill. Among the elderly, 10 to 30% of acutely hospitalized patients are admitted with or develop delirium. Prompt identification and evaluation are important because delirium is often caused by a treatable disorder, and the associated impairment is usually reversible.

RECOGNITION AND DIAGNOSIS

The two clinical hallmarks of delirium are (1) impaired cognitive function and (2) altered level of alertness or consciousness. Diminished cognitive performance can be subtle in mild delirium, but it is usually easy to identify with a standard mental status examination of cognitive performance, such as the Mini-Mental State Exam (MMSE) or the Short Portable Mental Status Examination. The MMSE is particularly useful because it measures nonmemory functions. Like all screening instruments, however, it can miss mild delirium. Altered level of consciousness and impaired attention have proved more difficult to operationalize. Generally, delirious patients appear drowsy or inaccessible, and their ability to attend or participate in a conversation fluctuates. On occasion they are hyperalert or hypervigilant. Whether the patient is drowsy or alert, examiners find themselves repeating questions, explaining things several times, or repeatedly needing to awaken or alert the patient when assessing or talking with a delirious patient.

A number of associated symptoms should raise the suspicion of delirium. These include (1) disorders of perception, e.g., hallucinations, illusions, or misinterpretations; (2) wide fluctuations in behavior; (3) disturbances in the sleep-wake cycle; and (4) activity level changes, either increased or decreased from usual level. Delirium usually develops acutely and is short-lived, lasting several days to several weeks. On occasion it becomes chronic. Pre-existing cognitive disorder (dementia), older age, and more severe medical illness are risk factors.

CLINICAL MANAGEMENT

Prompt early recognition is an important part of the management of delirium because correction of the underlying cause is the primary focus of management. Although delirium often has a treatable cause, it is frequently superimposed on a chronic condition.

Evaluation

As can be seen in Table 1, the differential diagnosis of delirium covers a wide variety of causes; disorders in almost every organ system can be etiologic. After delirium has been identified, the first step in the evaluation is to review the physical examination, history, and recent medications. These often suggest one or several causes. These high-likelihood causes should be assessed with the appropriate studies and clinical responses. For example, if drug withdrawal is suspected, a test dose of the agent thought to be involved would be a first step. If a toxic drug reaction is suspected, a blood specimen should be drawn to determine the blood level and the potentially offending agent withdrawn if possible. Because metabolic and infectious causes commonly result in delirium, it is usually prudent to order a complete blood count, metabolic panel, urinalysis, and chest radiograph in all patients in whom delirium is suspected. When no specific cause is identified by the history, physical examination, or review of the medical record, the

TABLE 1. **Common Causes of Delirium**

Metabolic
Electrolyte disturbances are most common. Hypoxia, calcium imbalance, liver failure, renal failure. Most endocrine disorders can present with delirium often due to excess or deficient actions of the hormone
Infectious
Any systemic infection can cause delirium, even upper respiratory and urinary tract infections. Fever is not always present, especially in the debilitated elderly
Vascular
Any condition leading to decreased brain perfusion (e.g., congestive heart failure, circulatory failure); anemia; stroke; hypertensive encephalopathy; autoimmune vasculitis
Toxic
Medications and psychoactive substances are most common. Drugs from many classes can cause delirium. Heavy metals. Drug withdrawal
Intrinsic Brain Disorders
Mass lesions (tumor, subdural hematoma), postictal state, sequelae of concussion and brain injury
Psychiatric
Severe depression and mania can mimic delirium. Hysterical fugue states can also mimic

search for a cause should begin by focusing on the common infectious, metabolic, and toxic causes.

If hypoxia is in the differential diagnosis, arterial blood gases should be obtained. Unsuspected alcohol and drug withdrawal are common causes of delirium, and a high level of suspicion is warranted; signs of vasomotor instability (orthostatic hypotension, tachycardia) are common indicators of withdrawal. Improvement in cognition, behavior, and vital signs after a single dose of a short-acting benzodiazepine (e.g., lorazepam [Ativan], 0.5 to 1 mg) suggests alcohol or benzodiazepine withdrawal. If central nervous system pathology is possible or has not been ruled out, computed tomography head scan or magnetic resonance imaging can identify subdural hematomas, acute stroke, or intracranial masses. A lumbar puncture should be done when there is no papilledema or evidence of intracranial mass.

Medications are among the most common causes of delirium because the majority of pharmacologically active substances can cause cognitive impairment. A high level of suspicion is warranted. Any change in a medication during the 30 days preceding the development of delirium should be closely reviewed as a potential cause. Anticholinergic toxicity is a common cause of delirium because a wide variety of pharmacologic compounds have anticholinergic activity. Table 2 reproduces an index of anticholinergic activity developed by Tune. Plasma blood levels (e.g., digoxin, quinidine, antidepressant, anticonvulsant) should be obtained whenever possible.

The electroencephalogram (EEG) can be helpful at several stages of assessment and management. The characteristic EEG change in delirium is generalized slowing. In mild delirium, the EEG is helpful in confirming the diagnosis. Improvement from baseline of the EEG to normal is a helpful objective finding when the clinician is unsure whether there has been progress. A diffusely slow EEG is also seen in moderate and severe dementia, so the EEG is not useful in distinguishing between delirium and dementia.

TABLE 2. **Anticholinergic Properties of the 13 Most Commonly Prescribed Medications***

Medication†	Anticholinergic Drug Level (ng/mL of Atropine Equivalents)
Cimetidine	0.86
Prednisolone	0.55
Theophylline anhydrous	0.44
Digoxin	0.25
Furosemide	0.22
Nifedipine	0.22
Ranitidine	0.22
Isosorbide dinitrate	0.15
Warfarin	0.12
Dipyridamole	0.11
Codeine	0.11
Dyazide	0.08
Captopril	0.02

*All others have no anticholinergic properties.

†At a 10^{-8} Molar concentration.

From Tune L, Carr S, Hoag E, Cooper T: Anticholinergic effects of drugs commonly prescribed for the elderly: Potential means for assessing risk of delirium. Am J Psychiatry *149*:1393–1394, 1992.

SYMPTOM MANAGEMENT

The associated symptoms—hallucinations, delusions, agitation—require treatment if they lead to dangerous behavior or are of significant distress to the patient. Although no well-designed trials of psychopharmacologic management have been published, most experts recommend haloperidol (Haldol) at beginning doses of 0.5 mg twice a day when pharmacotherapy is indicated. Some clinicians use low-dose benzodiazepines in this circumstance, but because they are more likely to cause sedation and respiratory depression, they are usually not recommended.

Environmental adjustments are also widely recommended but little studied. Lighting that is adequate but not too bright is thought to decrease misperceptions and illusions. Frequent orientation and reassurance, as often as every 15 minutes, appear to be helpful to many patients.

It is important to explain, in common language, to patients, their families, and attendants that delirium is the cause of the cognitive and behavioral disorder. Delirium is often frightening to the patient and caregiver. Identifying and explaining it can relieve some of this concern.

MOOD DISORDERS

method of
DAVID A. SOLOMON, M.D., and
MARTIN B. KELLER, M.D.
Brown University
Providence, Rhode Island

Although psychiatrists as well as primary care physicians have become increasingly aware that mood disorders are chronic and recurrent illnesses, posing a public health problem and affecting lifetime productivity, they remain underdiagnosed and undertreated. It is important for the medical field to adjust to the conceptual shift that mood disorders are medical disorders analogous to diabetes or hypertension. The consequences of these disorders can be very serious, ranging from social and physical disability to suicide. The physical, social, and role functioning of patients with a depressive disorder, for example, is often significantly worse than that associated with hypertension, angina, diabetes, advanced coronary artery disease, arthritis, back problems, lung problems, and gastrointestinal disorders. Patients with depression tend to have significantly more days in bed, worse perceived current health, and more bodily pain than do patients with major chronic medical conditions.

PREVALENCE

Mood disorders have a high lifetime prevalence: 5% for major depression; 3% for dysthymia; 1% for bipolar disorder; and 8% for affective disorders. Each year depression alone affects 10 to 14 million people in the United States.

The median age at onset for major depression is 25 years; the corresponding age for a bipolar disorder is 19 years. Half of all patients who recover from an episode of major depression at a tertiary care center will have a recurrence within 2 years. The natural history of bipolar disorders is marked by even higher rates of recurrence.

Co-morbidity is frequently seen in mood disorders. Although anxiety and depression are two separate disorders, research shows that approximately 60% of patients with depression have some anxiety symptoms, and 25% of those patients have panic attacks. Other co-morbid conditions include substance abuse and chronic medical conditions.

LOW LEVEL OF TREATMENT

Many patients suffering from depression for at least 2 years still receive minimal, insufficient, or no treatment at all. Research demonstrates that half of the patients who recover from a major depression receive no preventive treatment prior to their next episode. There are several explanations for low levels of somatic treatment. Patients may not seek evaluation, or clinicians may miss the initial diagnosis. Patients may refuse treatment or not comply with it. Some physicians prefer psychosocial treatment, and others may be concerned with medical contraindications or the issue of overdose attempts by patients with suicidal ideation. When medication is prescribed, the dose may be inadequate or side effects may arise and necessitate discontinuation.

Based on treatment research gathered for over a decade, it is clear that low levels of treatment alone do not cause the high rate of chronicity, relapse, and recurrence found in patients suffering from mood disorders. It is, however, clinically important to note that most of the available data reflect that the majority of patients do not receive adequate treatment for their mood disorders.

Further, there is a tendency for patients receiving the lowest levels of somatotherapy to remain ill for the longest period of time. This suggests that some severely ill patients who previously may have been thought to be resistant to treatment may in fact have received inadequate levels of treatment and for too short a period of time. Some researchers have concentrated on whether early intervention shortens the length of an episode, whereas others have focused on assessing the prospective pattern of recurrence following short-term treatment and recovery. Both areas of research are still being investigated. There is concurrence, however, among most researchers that prophylactic drug treatment can reduce the risk of recurrence.

COSTS

The low levels of treatment given for mood disorders lead to disruption of patients' social and physical functioning and create a heavy economic burden on patients and society. The direct costs of these illnesses include hospitalization and medication. Some of the more subtle but equally precarious economic strains come from repeated hospital stays, nursing home care, and the support costs of outpatient care including medical doctors, psychologists, and social workers.

Also troublesome are the indirect costs that influence the economic burden of mood disorders. The high morbidity of these illnesses reduces the productivity and therefore the income of both the patient and the employer. Other productivity losses are incurred by absenteeism, decreased quality of life, increased strain on relationships, and overall value of time spent by caregivers. Mortality is the ultimate loss in productivity.

Additional expenses are incurred by the social welfare administration and criminal justice system, which assist in treating, maintaining, and tracking those patients who make their way into those systems. Although current figures estimate that depressive disorders alone pose a $50 billion burden nationally, it is hard to quantify the effect of welfare dependence, disability, human loss and suffering, lost income and homelessness, and unreported or unrecognized illness, especially in primary care. It is crucial to recognize the significance of the costs of untreated mood disorders. Besides absenteeism, low productivity, safety risks, and high employee turnover are also factors.

CLINICAL DESCRIPTIONS

Mood disorders are diagnosed by the clinical history and mental status examination. Criteria for each diagnosis are specified in the *Diagnostic and Statistical Manual of Mental Disorders,* 4th edition* (DSM-IV). The primary disorders described subsequently are major depression, dysthymia, and bipolar disorder. Criteria are included here because, as of mid-1994, the 1987 criteria found in DSM-IIIR will have been revised. Descriptions of other mood syndromes such as hypomania and cyclothymia as well as modifiers of mood disorders, such as psychotic, catatonic, melancholic, atypical, postpartum, single episode, recurrent, rapid cycling, and seasonal pattern, can be found in DSM-IV.

Major Depression

According to the DSM-IV criteria, to diagnose an episode of major depression, at least five of the following symptoms must be present during the same 2-week period, and they must represent a change from the patient's previous level of functioning. Further, at least one of the symptoms must be either (1) depressed mood or (2) loss of interest or pleasure.

1. Depressed mood most of the day, nearly every day, as indicated by either subjective report (i.e., feels sad or empty) or observation made by others (i.e., appears tearful) Note: In children and adolescents, this can be an irritable mood.

*From American Psychiatric Association: *Diagnostic and Statistical Manual of Mental Disorders,* 4th ed., Washington, D.C., American Psychiatric Association, 1994.

2. Markedly diminished interest or pleasure in all, or almost all, activities most of the day, nearly every day (as indicated either by subjective account or observation made by others).

3. Significant weight loss when not dieting or weight gain (i.e., more than 5% of body weight in a month), or a decrease or increase in appetite nearly every day. Note: In children, consider failure to make expected weight gains.

4. Insomnia or hypersomnia nearly every day.

5. Psychomotor agitation or retardation nearly every day (observable by others, not merely subjective feelings of restlessness or being slowed down).

6. Fatigue or loss of energy nearly every day.

7. Feelings of worthlessness or excessive or inappropriate guilt (which may be delusional) nearly every day (not merely self-reproach or guilt about being sick).

8. Diminished ability to think or concentrate, or indecisiveness, nearly every day (either by subjective account or as observed by others).

9. Recurrent thoughts of death (not just fear of dying), recurrent suicidal ideation without a specific plan, or a suicide attempt or a specific plan for committing suicide.

The definition, or criteria, also states that these symptoms cause clinically significant distress or impairment in social, occupational, or other important areas of functioning and are not due to the direct effects of a substance (i.e., drugs of abuse, medication) or a general medical condition (e.g., hypothyroidism). Major depression should not be diagnosed in the context of bereavement (i.e., after the loss of a loved one) unless the symptoms persist for longer than 2 months or are characterized by marked functional impairment, morbid preoccupation with worthlessness, suicidal ideation, psychotic symptoms, or psychomotor retardation.

Dysthymia

Dysthymic disorder is defined by

A. Depressed mood for most of the day, for more days than not, as indicated by subjective account or observation made by others, for at least 2 years. In children and adolescents, mood can be irritable, and duration must be at least 1 year.

B. In addition, criteria include the presence, while depressed, of at least two of the following:
   1. poor appetite or overeating
   2. insomnia or hypersomnia
   3. low energy or fatigue
   4. low self-esteem
   5. poor concentration or difficulty in making decisions
   6. feelings of hopelessness.

C. During the 2-year period (1 year for children and adolescents) of the disturbance, the person has never been without the symptoms in A and B for more than 2 months at a time.

D. No major depressive episode has existed during the first 2 years of the disturbance (1 year for children and adolescents)—i.e., the episode is not better accounted for by chronic major depressive disorder, or major depressive disorder in partial remission.
Note: There may have been a previous major depressive episode provided there was a full remission (no significant signs or symptoms for 2 months) before the dysthymic disorder developed. In addition, after these 2 years (1 year for children and adolescents) of dysthymic disorder, there may be superimposed episodes of major depressive disorder, in which case both diagnoses may be given.

E. Patient has never had a manic episode or an unequivocal hypomanic episode.

F. The disorder does not occur exclusively during the course of a chronic psychotic disorder such as schizophrenia or delusional disorder.

G. The disorder is not due to the direct effects of a substance (e.g., drugs of abuse, medication) or a general medical condition (e.g., hypothyroidism).

Bipolar Disorder

Bipolar disorder is characterized by recurrent episodes of mania and major depression. Between episodes, patients may experience full remission but are just as likely to suffer significant morbidity that falls short of meeting the full criteria for a mood episode. Such subsyndromal symptoms increase the risk of relapse. Within the DSM-IV diagnosis of bipolar disorder there are many categories of distinction including hypomanic, single episode, depressed, cyclothymic, and due to a medical condition, and there are even examples of bipolar disorder not otherwise specified. For the purposes of common use and brevity, this article outlines the criteria for manic episode as follows:

A. A distinct period of abnormally and persistently elevated, expansive, or irritable mood lasting at least 1 week (or any duration if hospitalization is necessary).

B. During the period of mood disturbance, at least three of the following symptoms persist (four if the mood is irritable) and are present to a significant degree:
   1. inflated self-esteem or grandiosity
   2. decreased need for sleep (e.g., feels rested after only 3 hours of sleep)
   3. more talkative than usual or feels pressure to keep talking
   4. flight of ideas or subjective experience that thoughts are racing
   5. distractibility (i.e., attention too easily drawn to unimportant or irrelevant external stimuli)
   6. increase in goal-directed activity (either socially, at work or school, or sexually) or psychomotor agitation
   7. excessive involvement in pleasurable activities that have a high potential for painful consequences (e.g., unrestrained buying sprees, sexual indiscretions, or foolish business investments).

C. Mood disturbance is sufficiently severe to cause marked impairment in occupational functioning or in the usual social activities or relationships with others or necessitates hospitalization to prevent harm to self or others.
D. The disorder is not due to direct effects of substance (e.g., drugs of abuse or medication) or a general medical condition (e.g., hyperthyroidism).

Note: Manic episodes that are clearly precipitated by somatic antidepressant treatment (e.g., medication, electroconvulsive therapy, light therapy) should not count toward a diagnosis of bipolar disorder.

GENETICS

Evidence of the heritability of mood disorders comes from genetic-epidemiologic studies, using three different methods. Twin, family, and adoption studies indicate that major depression and bipolar disorder are at least partially caused by genetic transmission. In family studies, for example, relatives of patients are two to three times more likely to incur a mood disorder than are relatives of case controls. Twin studies, conducted over a span of 50 years, reveal an average concordance rate of 65% for monozygotic twins and 14% for dizygotic twins. There appears to be at least a partial overlap in the genetic transmission of major depression and bipolar disorder. Furthermore, the heritability of these disorders, as shown by twin studies, is comparable to that of illnesses such as diabetes and hypertension.

More recent findings have made use of the techniques of molecular genetics. These genetic mapping studies have reported a linkage of bipolar disorder to markers on the X chromosome (color blindness, glucose-6-phosphate dehydrogenase deficiency, factor IX, and the Xg blood group), and a linkage of bipolar illness and major depression to markers on chromosome 11 (insulin-*ras* oncogene) and chromosome 6 (human leukocyte antigen). None of these findings has been consistently replicated, meaning either that these specific linkages do not exist or that genetic heterogeneity is present in the population.

When counseling patients and their families about childbearing and the risk of a child's incurring the illness, the following figures may be useful. If one parent has a mood disorder and the other is not ill, there is roughly a 30% risk of having a child with a mood disorder. If one parent has bipolar disorder and the other parent has a mood disorder, the risk is 50 to 75%. Finally, first-degree relatives of patients with a bipolar disorder have at least a 25% chance of developing a mood disorder.

COURSE AND OUTCOME

Clinical research has consistently provided evidence that mood disorders are chronic and recurrent conditions. Despite the previously widely held clinical belief that depressed patients tend to make complete recoveries from acute depressive episodes, a significant percentage of patients suffering from mood disorders remain chronically ill. More than 20% of patients remain ill with major depression for 2 years, and 12% fail to recover after 5 years. Patients spend as much as 20% of their lifetime in depressive episodes. Up to 20% may commit suicide.

Factors found to predict a slower time to recovery are longer duration and increased severity of the initial episode, prior history of a nonaffective psychiatric disorder (suggesting that the depression in these subjects was secondary), lower family income, and being married. Research data confirm that a significant percentage of depressed patients experience multiple episodes or lengthy episodes without returning to the "pre-depression" state of well-being. This differs from earlier theories that depression consisted of discrete episodes of illness alternating with clearly defined well periods.

Probabilities of recovery calculated for intervals ranging from 1 week to 5 years show that the chances of recovery from major depression are highest within the first 6 months following accurate diagnosis and treatment. The longer patients remain ill, the less likely recovery becomes, as suggested by the fact that only 18% of patients observed are still depressed after 1 year, whereas 54% recovered during the first 6 months after enrollment in the study. The majority of patients who do not recover during the 5 years experience subsyndromal symptoms of depression most of the time. Their illness resembles chronic minor depression or dysthymia with episodes of major depression rather than major depression alone.

Among patients who do recover from acute episodes of major depression, relapse is frequent, although the risk of relapse tends to decrease the longer the patients remain well. Among patients who relapse, the probability of remaining ill for 1 year or more is 22%.

DIFFERENTIAL DIAGNOSIS

Clinicians, particularly in the primary care setting, may encounter patients with mixed anxiety and depressive symptoms that do not meet the full criteria for either an anxiety or mood disorder. It appears that a significant number of patients in the community, as many as 10% of patients with depressive symptoms, fall into this subclinical population. This is an area that is receiving extensive attention; in DSM-IV, this problem is discussed in an appendix on the mixed anxiety-depression syndrome.

The differential diagnosis of major depression includes organic mood syndrome with depression, primary degenerative dementia of the Alzheimer type, multi-infarct dementia, schizoaffective disorder of the depressive type, and uncomplicated bereavement. The differential diagnosis of mania includes organic mood syndrome with mania, schizoaffective disorder of the bipolar type, attention-deficit hyperactivity disorder, and borderline personality disorder.

TREATMENT

Three types of treatment are currently used for severe depression: pharmacotherapy, psychotherapy, and electroconvulsive therapy. Antidepressant medications are usually the first approach in treatment because of their demonstrated efficacy and rapid effect. Three classes of antidepressants are generally used for treating major depression: tricyclic antidepressants (TCAs) such as imipramine, monoamine oxidase inhibitors (MAOIs) such as phenelzine, and selective serotonin re-uptake inhibitors (SSRIs) such as fluoxetine. In addition, there are several atypical compounds. Prescriptions for antidepressant medications require close monitoring of the patient because of the risk of overdose or suicide.

TCAs are effective and widely used and have historically been the first-line antidepressant. They are rapidly absorbed and metabolized in the liver. Their mechanism of action is a function of their ability to block re-uptake of the neurotransmitters norepinephrine and serotonin. These medications interact with many other pharmacologic agents including MAOIs, alcohol, oral contraceptives, antihistamines, beta-adrenergic blockers, clonidine, diuretics, class II antiarrhythmics, and anticholinergic drugs. Even when used within the therapeutic range, they cause significant and sometimes unacceptable side effects: sedation, increased heart rate, cardiac rhythm disturbances, postural hypotension, dry mouth, blurred vision, constipation, urinary retention, sexual dysfunction, and weight gain. The elimination half-life is such that the TCAs can be given once a day and, because of their hypnotic effect, are usually administered at bedtime (Table 1).

The MAOIs inhibit the enzyme that degrades biogenic amines, including catecholamines. The MAOIs are effective antidepressants but are less widely used than TCAs because they produce severe adverse interactions with sympathomimetic drugs and food products containing amines such as tyramine. They are, however, more effective than TCAs in treating depression characterized by symptoms of anxiety, phobic features, panic attacks, hysterical features, or reversed vegetative symptoms (e.g., increased sleep, increased appetite). Patients taking MAOIs must be educated about the importance of avoiding medications, foods, and beverages that contain vasoactive amines and the hypertensive crisis that can ensue. MAOIs are prescribed on a twice-a-day or three-times-a-day basis (Table 2).

The recent introduction of a new class of antidepressant medications, the SSRIs, has had a profound impact on depression pharmacotherapy. As denoted by their name, the SSRIs are highly selective in blocking the re-uptake of serotonin and have little direct effect on norepinephrine. The SSRIs have a relatively mild side effect profile and are usually better tolerated than TCAs and MAOIs. The elimination half-life is such that the SSRIs can be given once a day and, because of their stimulating effect, are usually administered in the morning (Table 3).

TABLE 1. **Tricyclic Antidepressants: Preparations and Doses**

Generic Name	Brand Name	Dosage Forms	Usual Dosage Range (mg/day)*
Amitriptyline	Elavil, Endep	10, 25, 50, 75, 100, 150 mg	100–300
Clomipramine	Anafranil	25, 50, 75 mg	100–250
Desipramine	Norpramin	10, 25, 50, 75, 100, 150 mg	100–300
	Pertofrane	25, 50 mg	
Doxepin	Sinequan Adapin	10, 25, 50, 75, 100, 150 mg	100–300
Imipramine	Tofranil Janimine Sk-Pramine	10, 25, 50, 75, 100, 125, 150 mg	100–300
Imipramine pamoate	Tofranil PM (sustained release)	5, 100, 125, 150 mg	150–300
Maprotiline	Ludiomil	25, 50, 75 mg	100–150
Nortriptyline	Pamelor Aventyl	10, 25, 50, 75 mg	50–150
Protriptyline	Vivactil	5, 10 mg	15–60
Trimipramine	Surmontil	25, 50, 100 mg	150–300

Common or Troublesome Side Effects of Tricyclic Drugs

Anticholinergic	Dry mouth and nasal passages, constipation, urinary hesitance, esophageal reflux
Autonomic	Orthostatic hypotension, palpitations, intracardiac conduction slowing, increased sweating, increased blood pressure, tremors
Allergic	Skin rashes
Central nervous system	Stimulation, sedation, delirium, myoclonic twitches (generally at high dosages), nausea, speech blockage, seizures, and extrapyramidal symptoms
Other	Weight gain and impotence

*Dosage ranges are approximate.

The atypical compounds are a heterogeneous group of drugs with novel structures and mechanisms of action. Venlafaxine was approved quite recently and is given in three divided doses. Bupropion is also prescribed on a three-times-a-day basis. Both amox-

TABLE 2. **Monoamine Oxidase Inhibitors: Preparations and Doses**

Generic Name	Brand Name	Dosage Forms	Usual Dosage Range (mg/day)*
Isocarboxazid	Marplan	10 mg	20–50
Phenelzine	Nardil	15 mg	45–90
Selegiline†	Eldepryl	5 mg	20–50
Tranylcypromine	Parnate	10 mg	30–50

Common or Troublesome Side Effects of MAOIs

Anticholinergic	Dry mouth, constipation, urinary hesitance
Autonomic	Orthostatic hypotension, hypertensive crisis (interactions with food or medications), hyperpyrexic reactions, myoclonic twitches, muscle cramps and myositis-like reactions
Central nervous system	Stimulation during the day, sedation (particularly daytime and due to insomnia during the night), insomnia during the night
Other	Weight gain, anorgasmia, sexual impotence

*Dosage ranges are approximate.
†Not FDA approved for this indication.

TABLE 3. **Selective Serotonin Re-Uptake Inhibitors: Preparations and Doses**

Generic Name	Brand Name	Dosage Forms	Usual Dosage Range (mg/day)*
Fluoxetine	Prozac	10, 20 mg	20–40
Fluvoxamine†	Luvox	50, 100 mg	50–300
Paroxetine	Paxil	20, 30 mg	20–50
Sertraline	Zoloft	50, 100 mg	50–200

Common or Troublesome Side Effects of SSRIs

Anticholinergic	Nausea, diarrhea, vomiting
Autonomic	Restlessness, nervousness, tremulousness
Central nervous system	Insomnia and daytime drowsiness
Other	Sexual dysfunction and headaches

*Dosage ranges are approximate.
†Investigational drug in the United States.

apine, which has some properties of a neuroleptic, and trazodone should be considered second-line drugs. Amoxapine is given once a day, usually at bedtime, whereas trazodone is prescribed in two or three divided doses. As of this writing, a new drug application has been submitted to the Food and Drug Administration (FDA) for nefazodone,* a compound structurally related to trazodone. Nefazodone is also administered in two or three divided doses (Table 4).

Somatic treatments are the most effective for severe depression, but psychotherapy has been proved to be effective either as an alternative or in combination with medication. Candidates for psychotherapy as an alternative to medication include those who refuse medication, those for whom antidepressant pharmacotherapy is contraindicated, those who cannot tolerate the side effects, and those whose depressive symptoms are refractory to pharmacotherapy. Psychotherapy is most useful as an adjunct to pharmacotherapy.

Three psychotherapeutic approaches have been modified or developed specifically for the treatment of depression: cognitive therapy, behavioral therapy, and interpersonal therapy. Cognitive therapy is based on the premise that depression results from faulty cognition, which leads to an unrealistic outlook and set of expectations. Therapy aims to identify the specific distorted cognitions and replace them with corrected patterns of thinking. Behavioral psychotherapy views depression as a result of the loss of positive reinforcement. Therapy seeks to create specific systems of self-reinforcement that will improve the balance of positive versus negative interactions. Interpersonal psychotherapy (IPT) is based on the premise that difficulties in interpersonal relationships are the cause or result of depression, and it focuses on the resolution of current conflicts. IPT was developed especially for the treatment of depression. Each of these are short-term interventions, usually involving 12 to 20 sessions over 12 to 16 weeks.

It had been thought that because psychotherapeutic techniques help patients develop more effective coping strategies, these techniques would produce more lasting benefits in the long-term treatment of depression. In the few studies available, IPT and a combination of cognitive and behavioral therapies have been effective in preventing relapse. Nevertheless, somatic therapy appears to provide even better results.

*Nefazodone is an investigational drug in the United States.

The treatment of bipolar disorder and acute mania requires attention to both specific and nonspecific antimanic medications. Nonspecific medication includes antipsychotic drugs such as haloperidol and chlorpromazine. It should be noted that there are some medications that can induce mania, including tricyclic antidepressants, amphetamines, and steroids. Over-the-counter stimulants and the caffeine found in coffee, tea, and sodas may also have the same result (Table 5).

Electroconvulsive therapy (ECT) is usually reserved for severely depressed or manic patients who have not responded to pharmacotherapy, for whom medication is contraindicated, or for whom immediate effective intervention is essential (e.g., suicidal patients). It has been debated whether ECT is more rapidly effective than medication. ECT is not considered to have lasting effects, and maintenance medication must be administered following a course of ECT.

The results of most studies point to a combination of pharmacologic and psychotherapeutic treatments as being most effective in the management of mood disorders. A three-phase plan for pharmacologic treatment of depression has been proposed that includes acute, continuation, and maintenance stages as the best means of preventing recurrence.

CONTINUATION AND MAINTENANCE

A number of investigators have recently explored the role played by maintenance treatment in the outcome of major depressive disorder. They uniformly note that surprisingly few studies have attempted to address the questions of whether and how early intervention influences the subsequent course of patients' illness, whether somatotherapy shortens episodes and decreases their likelihood, and how the discontinuation of medication impacts the course of the illness.

Research shows that it takes a median of 25 weeks for patients to achieve stabilization from an initial episode of major depression. Continuation therapy is the uninterrupted extension of pharmacotherapy after the acute episode has resolved. Medication is thus continued to consolidate the remission and forestall relapse of the acute episode. When therapy is extended for longer periods for the purpose of preventing recurrence of a new episode, this prophylaxis is referred to as maintenance therapy. Maintenance treatment is particularly important for patients at high risk of repeated episodes. Risk factors for recurrent episodes include history of frequent or multiple episodes, double depression (major depression plus pre-existing dysthymia), onset after age 60, long du-

TABLE 4. **Atypical Compounds: Preparations and Doses**

Generic Name	Brand Name	Dosage Forms	Usual Dosage Range (mg/day)*
Amoxapine	Asendin	25, 50, 100, 150 mg	200–300
Bupropion	Wellbutrin	75, 100 mg	200–450
Nefazodone†	New drug application		100–400
Trazodone	Desyrel	50, 100, 150, 300 mg	150–400
Venlafaxine	Effexor	37.5, 50, 75, 100 mg	75–375

Common or Troublesome Side Effects of Atypical Compounds

Amoxapine	Sedation, dry mouth, constipation, nausea, blurred vision, anxiety, restlessness. In addition, neuroleptic side effects may occur, including akathisia, tremor, tardive dyskinesia, and neuroleptic malignant syndrome
Bupropion	Agitation, restlessness, insomnia. Risk of seizures may be higher than for other antidepressants, and the total daily dose should not exceed 450 mg
Nefazodone†	Dizziness, headache, nausea, drowsiness, asthenia
Trazodone	Sedation (trazodone is often used as a hypnotic), orthostatic hypotension, nausea, vomiting, priapism
Venlafaxine	Anorexia, nausea, sedation, dizziness. Less commonly, palpitations, fatigue, headache, constipation, anxiety, dry mouth, sexual dysfunction, diaphoresis, increased blood pressure and increased heart rate

*Dosage ranges are approximate.
†Investigational drug in the United States.

ration of individual episodes, family history of affective disorder, co-morbid anxiety disorder, or substance abuse.

Studies of maintenance pharmacotherapy suggest that such treatment results in a 30 to 40% reduction in relapses (i.e., a 50% relapse rate in patients on maintenance treatment as opposed to an 80% relapse rate in patients not receiving maintenance therapy). However, the costs and benefits of such treatment must be carefully weighed on a case-by-case basis because long-term somatotherapy entails both economic expense and the risk of side effects. For patients with short illness cycles, severe symptoms, or inter-episode dysthymia, the benefits of treatment frequently outweigh the costs.

TABLE 5. **Specific Antimanic Medications**

Generic Name	Brand Name	Dosage Forms	Therapeutic Plasma Levels
Lithium carbonate	Eskalith	300 mg	0.8–1.0 mM/L
	Lithane	300 mg	
	Lithonate	300 mg	
	Lithotabs	300 mg	
	Eskalith CR (sustained release)	450 mg	
Lithium citrate syrup	Cibalith-S	8 mEq/5 mL (480-mL bottle)	0.8–1.0 mM/L
Carbamazepine	Tegretol	200 mg (chewable: 100 mg)	4–12 μg/mL
Valproic acid	Depakote Depakene	125, 250, 500 mg	50–125 μg/mL

Common or Troublesome Side Effects of Antimanic Compounds

Lithium	Gastrointestinal distress (nausea, vomiting, diarrhea), impaired renal function (polyuria), tremor, hypothyroidism, electrocardiographic changes, acne, psoriasis
Carbamazepine	Sedation, gastrointestinal distress, tremor, leukopenia, hepatotoxicity
Valproic acid	Sedation, gastrointestinal distress, tremor, hepatotoxicity, alopecia

Contrary to long-held clinical wisdom, patients with mood disorders experience a significant risk of chronicity, relapse, and recurrence. For example, patients with "double depression" may never return to a pre-illness healthy personality because the underlying dysthymia frequently persists even after acute episodes of major depression have ended.

Given these facts, and given the high levels of morbidity and mortality associated with mood disorders, it is especially disturbing that these illnesses are underdiagnosed and undertreated. It is imperative that clinicians who treat major depression remain aware of its pernicious nature and of the many effective options available for its treatment. Primary care physicians should seek psychiatric consultation or referral for patients who fail to respond to acute therapy, deteriorate during maintenance treatment, develop new co-morbidity, or desire to discontinue prophylactic treatment.

Given the complexity of treatment decisions, no single report to date fully describes or explains the reason for the gap between the availability of treatments demonstrated by controlled clinical trials to be effective for depression, and the treatment actually received by individual patients in clinical practice. However, the accumulation of concordant findings from different investigators with complementary strengths and weaknesses provides strong evidence that such a gap exists.

Research has demonstrated that there is a need for a conceptual shift in the understanding of major depression. It is a chronic medical disorder, analogous to diabetes or hypertension, and requires long-term maintenance treatment. The approach to treatment should include early recognition, treatment of the acute episode, stabilization to avoid relapse, and maintenance to prevent recurrence. The need for continuation and maintenance treatment is an issue that now deserves increased attention, especially with the availability of new classes of antidepressant drugs that have excellent efficacy and more favorable side effect profiles.

SCHIZOPHRENIC DISORDERS

method of
CARMEN M. McINTYRE, M.D., and
GEORGE M. SIMPSON, M.D.
Medical College of Pennsylvania
Philadelphia, Pennsylvania

Schizophrenia is a serious mental disorder affecting millions of people worldwide and resulting in major impairments in social and occupational functioning in those afflicted. It is a psychotic disorder, meaning that one's ability to perceive reality correctly is impaired. Recognition of the disorder has increased during the past decade, yet it remains poorly understood. This is probably because it is a heterogeneous group of disorders that varies among individuals as well as within an individual over time. In 1896, Emil Kraepelin described dementia praecox as an illness occurring before age 40 that had a chronic deteriorating course. Patients had delusions and hallucinations, exhibited severe functional deterioration, and were cognitively impaired. In 1911, Eugen Bleuler used the term schizophrenia and de-emphasized the chronic deterioration. He instead stressed the importance of disturbances in four primary areas: associations, affect, autism, and ambivalence. Secondary symptoms included delusions and hallucinations. In 1959, Kurt Schneider organized the clinical signs and symptoms into first-rank and second-rank symptoms according to how pathognomonic they are.

Currently in the United States, the diagnosis of schizophrenia is based on the criteria listed in the revised third edition of the *Diagnostic and Statistical Manual* (DSM-IIIR). A 6-month duration of illness that includes deterioration in work, social, or self-care functioning is required for diagnosis. The active phase of the illness includes symptoms such as delusions, hallucinations, thought disturbances such as incoherence or loosening of associations, catatonia, and flat or inappropriate affect. The prodromal and residual phases include odd beliefs and unusual perceptual experiences, bizarre behavior, social isolation or withdrawal, poor self-care, speech and affect abnormalities, and lack of initiative or interest.

Despite the narrowly defined criteria, there are no pathognomonic signs and symptoms for schizophrenia, and the syndrome varies widely. Nevertheless, at least two symptom clusters are distinguishable. Positive symptoms (so-called Type I schizophrenia) are the more florid psychotic symptoms such as delusions, hallucinations, and thought disorder. Negative symptoms, the so-called Type II syndrome, are characterized by emotional withdrawal, apathy, flat or blunted affect, and loss of volition. It has been hypothesized that Type I and Type II are independent disease processes that may or may not coexist in a given individual and have different treatment and prognostic implications.

EPIDEMIOLOGY

The lifetime prevalence rate for schizophrenia is about 1% worldwide, with a U.S. incidence rate of 200,000 new cases yearly. Peak age of onset for males is between 15 and 25, and for women between 25 and 35. Onset before age 10 or after age 50 is rare. Mortality rates from natural causes are higher in patients with schizophrenia. About half of patients with this illness attempt suicide, and 10% succeed.

The course of illness and prognosis are variable. Classically, schizophrenia has been described as chronically deteriorating, with exacerbations and relative remissions, yet never returning to the previous baseline level of functioning. Others have reported a more optimistic early course, but for the majority of those afflicted, deterioration progresses for 5 to 10 years and then plateaus. Other practitioners suggest that recovery rates of 10 to 60% occur, and 20 to 30% of patients are able to lead relatively normal lives. Another 20 to 30% have moderate symptoms, and 40 to 60% have significant impairment for the rest of their lives. These discrepancies are at least in part related to methodologic inconsistencies underlying diagnostic practices.

Although schizophrenia is observed in all cultural and socioeconomic groups, there is a disproportionate representation of the lower socioeconomic classes in urban areas. This may result from a decline in status or a failure to rise in status in afflicted persons, who may also tend to congregate in these areas. It is estimated that at least a third of the homeless population suffers from schizophrenia.

Seasonality of birth is correlated with incidence of schizophrenia. More patients are born during the late spring and early winter months—in the northern hemisphere, January to April, and in the southern hemisphere, July to September.

ETIOLOGY

The cause of schizophrenia is not known. The predominant opinion is that there is a biologic diathesis, or vulnerability, to a spectrum of schizophreniform disorders that can be affected by biologic or environmental stressors. Typically, the initial onset of illness, known as the first break, may be precipitated by stressors common to young adults, such as college, work, or marriage. Exacerbations also frequently follow stressors as well as noncompliance with treatment.

There is evidence that schizophrenia is, at least in part, a heritable disorder. Familial studies, including adoption studies, show that first-degree relatives of patients with schizophrenia have an incidence of illness that is five to 10 times higher than that of the general population. The incidence in second-degree relatives is two to three times higher. Twin studies strongly support a genetic hypothesis. Concordance rates for illness in monozygotic twins are about 58% and for dizygotic twins about 13%. Such studies have resulted in an estimate of a likelihood of heritability of schizophrenia of between 60 and 90%. Genetic studies indicate a complex model of transmission that is probably multifactorial and polygenic. There is unconfirmed evidence from linkage studies that a susceptibility locus exists on human chromosome 5.

The Helsinki study demonstrated a high incidence of schizophrenia among those exposed in utero to the influenza A2 virus during the second trimester. Seasonality of birth also raises the possibility of a viral cause, and recent United Kingdom studies confirm this finding. Perinatal insults have also been considered predisposing factors, as has drug abuse including cannabis use.

Further evidence of a biologic cause of schizophrenia exists in brain imaging studies. Patients have a greater rate of abnormal brain morphology than normals, although none of the abnormalities are specific to, nor found globally in, schizophrenia. Computed tomography studies demonstrate that a majority of patients show lateral and third ventricle enlargement, and a significant proportion show cortical atrophy. Magnetic resonance imaging studies have found that patients have smaller brain volumes, as well as changes in the temporal lobe in some. Functional brain imaging studies such as position emission tomography (PET) and single-photon emission computed tomography (SPECT) have demonstrated an increased density of D2 receptors in the striatum. This lends support to the dopamine hypothesis of schizophrenia; that is, the concept that hyperdopaminergia is central to the illness. Some postmortem studies have shown that patients have increased presynaptic dopamine or its metabolites in mesolimbic and mesocortical areas of the brain.

Type I schizophrenia is more responsive to typical antipsychotics, which are primarily dopamine receptor blockers, whereas Type II schizophrenia is more refractory to treatment. It is hypothesized that the former group of patients has an excess of dopamine, whereas the latter group has a deficit of dopamine. Other neurotransmitters are implicated in the illness, including serotonin (5-HT), norepinephrine, and gamma-aminobutyric acid.

TREATMENT

Acute Care

Correct diagnosis of schizophrenia requires first a thorough medical evaluation to ensure that organic causes of the symptoms are ruled out, including drugs such as amphetamines, cocaine, marijuana, and corticosteroids, as well as epilepsy, delirium, and dementia. Brain imaging studies are indicated in patients with neurologic findings or in older patients with a first presentation of psychosis. The history is important in making a diagnosis, and collateral sources, such as family, friends, and past hospitalization records, are usually required for adequate information. Hospitalization may be indicated for diagnostic purposes or for stabilization of medication. When the patient is dangerous to self or others (e.g., is suicidal, homicidal, or unable to care for himself), then compulsory hospitalization may be necessary. Identification of target symptoms helps to organize treatment planning.

Although hospitalization, by providing a safe, structured, and therapeutic environment, may be helpful in itself, the mainstay of acute treatment is antipsychotic medication. These medications, also known as major tranquilizers or neuroleptics, have been shown repeatedly to be more effective than placebo. Introduced in the early 1950s, the older, or typical, antipsychotics are postsynaptic dopamine receptor blockers. They may be categorized according to potency. Low-potency agents include chlorpromazine (Thorazine) and thioridazine (Mellaril). Dosage comparisons are frequently reported as chlorpromazine equivalents, thus assigning a rating of 1.00 to chlorpromazine. Mid-potency agents include perphenazine (Trilafon), which has an equivalence of about 11, and loxapine (Loxitane), which has an equivalence of about 7. High-potency agents include trifluoperazine (Stelazine) and fluphenazine (Prolixin), which have equivalences of 35 and 50, respectively.

The choice of antipsychotic depends first on the history. An agent that has worked and has been tolerated in the past should be used again. In the absence of such a history, the choice of agent depends mainly on the side effect profile of the medication that seems most suitable for the patient. Although all typical neuroleptics have the potential to cause similar side effects, agents with a lower potency typically cause more anticholinergic side effects such as dry mouth, constipation, and orthostatic hypotension. They also tend to cause more sedation and weight gain. Higher potency agents tend to cause more extrapyramidal side effects (EPS) such as dystonia, pseudoparkinsonism, and akathisia. Acute dystonic reactions are reportedly more likely to result in men than in women, in black males than in white males, and in younger people than in older people. Thus, chlorpromazine may be more appropriate for an agitated young man, and haloperidol (Haldol), a high-potency neuroleptic, may be better tolerated by an elderly female.

Potential risks as well as benefits should be discussed at the appropriate time with the patient, especially because some side effects may be permanent or severe. All antipsychotics reduce the seizure threshold, increase blood prolactin levels, and may cause, although rarely, leukopenias. Neuroleptic malignant syndrome (NMS), or extrapyramidal symptoms with fever, is a rare but serious and sometimes fatal complication. It is manifested by hyperpyrexia and muscle rigidity as the key features, with elevated blood levels of creatinine phosphokinase, an elevated white blood cell count, increased heart rate with diaphoresis, and a decreased level of consciousness as other features. Although it may occur at any time during antipsychotic treatment, it more commonly occurs shortly after initiating or increasing the dosage of neuroleptics and is more common if high doses are used. Treatment is symptomatic and supportive and consists of withdrawal of the antipsychotic agents, cooling the body, and hydration. Treating the muscle rigidity rigorously is important, and anticholinergics such as benztropine (Cogentin) may be used if the temperature is below 103°F (39.4°C). In patients with a higher temperature or who show lack of response to anticholinergics, dantrolene (Dantrium), 200 mg a day, or bromocriptine (Parlodel), 5 mg every 4 hours to 60 mg a day, may be beneficial.

Tardive dyskinesia (TD) may occur with chronic use of antipsychotics but may develop after only a few months of use. In a small proportion of cases it can be physically disabling and may be permanent. TD consists of abnormal, involuntary, irregular body movements and frequently begins with tongue, lip, mouth, and face movements. Other muscle groups may also be affected, including muscles of the neck, arm and shoulder, trunk and diaphragm, and leg and foot. Movements may range from tongue darting to gross, incapacitating disfigurement. The rate of development is about 3 to 4% per year of exposure to antipsychotics, and elderly women and patients with affective disorders (e.g., depression) are at greatest risk. The onset and severity of TD are in part dose related. There is no completely effective treatment, but at least 40% of patients improve if antipsychotics are discontinued. Thus, decreasing the dose of neuroleptic is often recommended at the initial onset of

TD. Agents such as clonazepam (Klonopin),* reserpine (Serpasil),* clozapine (Clozaril),* and vitamin E* have been used for treatment with some positive results. Patients with a subtype of disease with dystonia may respond to anticholinergic agents.

Starting dosage of antipsychotics is variable. There is a tendency to use high doses with rapid titration in caring for patients with acute disease. There is strong evidence, however, that this so-called rapid neuroleptization offers no benefit over low or moderate doses and is, in fact, undesirable. One study demonstrated that 20 mg of haloperidol produced greater improvements during the first 2 weeks, but then the ratings showed significant deterioration in progress during subsequent weeks compared to patients receiving doses of 5 and 10 mg. The initial superior results are probably due to sedation. Deterioration is due to side effects such as blunted affect, emotional withdrawal, akinesia and akathisia, which are more likely to occur at these higher doses. The onset of uncomfortable side effects frequently results in treatment noncompliance as well.

Thus, a more conservative approach is to start with low doses, such as 2 mg of haloperidol or fluphenazine, 25 mg of loxapine, or even 50 mg of chlorpromazine given twice daily. Dosage can be started at twice this level for agitated patients; if sedation is desirable early in the course of treatment, temporary use of benzodiazepines is useful and produces fewer adverse effects. The initial dose can be increased every 2 to 3 days until side effects appear or until the equivalent of 15 mg of haloperidol is reached. Another approach is to regulate the dose according to the plasma level of the neuroleptic. Antipsychotic dosages resulting in plasma levels higher than 10 mg/dL of haloperidol, or 300 to 600 mg/dL of chlorpromazine show no advantage over lower doses (e.g., 3 to 4 mg/dL of haloperidol) and result in more adverse effects. Patients with more chronic disease with histories of high-dose treatment may require higher doses of neuroleptics, but even here it is not clear that high doses were required initially. A history of response is most useful in these patients.

The time course of clinical improvement may be slow. The most rapid improvement occurs during the first 2 weeks, with continued improvement possible through 12 weeks or longer. Most responders to typical antipsychotics show improvement by the second week. Therefore, there is no reason to titrate medications more frequently than weekly once an adequate dose has been achieved. An adequate trial of a neuroleptic is at least 6 weeks of treatment.

Side effects are managed either by lowering the dose of neuroleptic or by using adjunctive medications. Acute dystonia usually occurs very early in the treatment course and consists of muscle spasms and abnormal postures. It frequently becomes manifest as protrusion or twisting of the tongue, or torticollis. In severe cases, intramuscular anticholinergic agents such as benztropine are effective. Oral anticholinergics are sufficient for milder forms. Anticholinergics result in a dramatic response, which usually takes place before 96 hours of treatment; thus, there is little need to continue anticholinergics.

Parkinsonism is a frequent adverse effect and results in akinesia, rigidity, tremor, and postural abnormalities. The akinesia and masked facies may be mistaken for negative symptoms. An incidence of parkinsonism as high as 90% following 3 months of treatment has been reported. Micrographia may be detected before more obvious signs and symptoms appear. Antiparkinson agents such as benztropine, trihexyphenidyl (Artane), and amantadine (Symmetrel) are beneficial in alleviating this effect.

Akathisia, a state of motor restlessness, is a particularly troubling and treatment-resistant side effect. If present, the patient complains of "inner anxiety" and of a drive to remain in motion. Ankle and leg movements while sitting and shifting of weight and rocking while standing as well as intrusive behavior are likely presentations of akathisia that may be mistaken for agitation or decompensation. Beta blockers, such as propranolol (Inderal), in doses of up to 80 mg, are partially helpful. Other, less effective, treatments include benzodiazepines and antiparkinson agents.

It should be remembered that all treatments for side effects have their own array of adverse effects and so are not generally recommended for prophylactic use but for symptomatic use only.

MAINTENANCE CARE

Following recovery from an acute episode of schizophrenia, the dosage of antipsychotic medication can usually be decreased slowly after 3 to 6 months of stability. Relapse rates as high as 30% during the first year of maintenance therapy with conventional medications have been reported. It is therefore important to remain flexible in dosing, increasing the dose to previous therapeutic levels as soon as any decompensation is detected. Following discontinuation of neuroleptic treatment in patients who had been in remission for 3 to 5 years, at least two-thirds suffered a relapse within 18 months, most within 3 to 7 months. Thus, in a patient with a history of more than one prior active phase, continuous rather than intermittent treatment is preferable.

Depot neuroleptics are useful in maintenance therapy. This type of drug formulation is given intramuscularly and provides a tissue concentration of at least 1 week's duration in a single dose. A more reliable steady-state blood level is achieved, compliance is improved, and the risk of EPS is no higher with depot neuroleptics. Conversion from oral haloperidol to haloperidol decanoate is 20 times the oral dose for the initial month but not exceeding 100 mg. The balance may be given 3 to 7 days later. The maintenance dose is 10 to 15 times the daily oral dose monthly, not to exceed 450 mg a month. Because of a larger first-pass metabolic effect, conversion from oral to depot fluphenazine decanoate is more complicated. Low do-

*This drug has not been approved by the Food and Drug Administration (FDA) for this indication.

sages (e.g., 6.25 mg) to start coupled with oral supplementation is recommended, the goal being 6.25 to 37.5 mg every 2 weeks. Roughly 25 mg of fluphenazine decanoate every 2 weeks corresponds to a daily oral dose of 20 mg. As little as 5 mg every 2 weeks may be effective in preventing relapse.

It is essential to provide patient and family education as well as medication therapy. It is important to remove the myths and stigma about the illness. Education of the family also provides collateral observers who can report adverse effects and exacerbations of the illness as well as collaborate in other treatment activities. Family environments with high expressed emotion—that is, families that are critical or overinvolved, are associated with poor outcomes. Family therapy is a useful intervention that can help change these behaviors, and support groups for families are helpful. In general, involvement of the family improves compliance and treatment overall.

Supportive and behaviorally oriented group therapies are helpful. Social skill training in patients is an important part of rehabilitation. A total program of care ideally incorporates the aforementioned treatment modalities with day treatment programs and vocational training as available in the community.

ATYPICAL ANTIPSYCHOTICS

Despite the treatment modalities just mentioned, a poor outcome frequently occurs in schizophrenia. Many patients do not respond to conventional medications, and the adverse effects of these drugs limit their usefulness. There is much research in the areas of early identification of nonresponders and development of better antipsychotics.

The discovery of clozapine in the early 1960s and clinical claims of its efficacy in the 1970s resulted in the knowledge that antipsychotic activity could be obtained in the absence of EPS. This led to the description of clozapine as an atypical neuroleptic. After reports of agranulocytosis produced by this drug appeared in the 1970s, it disappeared but was later introduced when adequate substitutes were not found. Studies demonstrated its efficacy in treatment-resistant schizophrenia, showing that patients who had previously failed multiple trials of typical neuroleptics responded significantly in both positive and, most important, negative symptoms. These studies also confirmed that this drug has little or no effect in producing EPS and in fact is helpful in the treatment of tardive dyskinesia.

Clozapine is used widely throughout the world now, mainly for patients who have failed to respond adequately to typical antipsychotics or who are exquisitely sensitive to extrapyramidal side effects. Extension of the use of this agent to dual diagnostic categories is now taking place. Clozapine affects multiple neurotransmitter systems, its serotonin receptor action being an important one. Its effect on the D2 receptor is less potent than that of typical neuroleptics, and it also has effects on the D1 and D4 receptors. It is believed that the combination of the effect on the D2 receptor with that on serotonin transmission is what makes this agent different from typical antipsychotics. Concern about agranulocytosis as well as an increased incidence of seizures at higher doses have limited the use of clozapine.

A variety of such agents are currently undergoing investigation. Risperidone (Risperdal) is one such agent that has been designed to affect these two neurotransmitter systems. This drug is available in Europe as well as in North America, and its antipsychotic activity has been shown to be efficacious. Its therapeutic effects occur at dosages of 4 to 8 mg, which appear to produce little in the way of extrapyramidal side effects. Higher dosages, 12 mg and above, have been associated with EPS. In several studies, low doses (4 to 6 mg) of risperidone were shown to be more effective on both positive and negative symptoms than comparable single doses of haloperidol (10 to 20 mg). Unlike clozapine, this agent may be used earlier in the treatment course of schizophrenia and for a wider array of disorders because it has not been shown to have any effects on white cell production.

PANIC DISORDER AND AGORAPHOBIA

method of
OLGA BRAWMAN-MINTZER, M.D., and
R. BRUCE LYDIARD, PH.D., M.D.
Medical University of South Carolina
Charleston, South Carolina

Panic disorder (PD) is classified as an anxiety disorder in the revised third edition of the *Diagnostic and Statistical Manual* (DSM-IIIR) of the American Psychiatric Association. Each of the anxiety disorders is defined by distinctive cognitive, behavioral, and physiologic signs and symptoms. The essential feature for a diagnosis of panic disorder is the recurrence of unexpected panic attacks, described as sudden and intensely distressing feelings of apprehension, impending doom, or loss of mental or physical self-control that are often spontaneous and unexpected, generally lasting 20 to 30 minutes, and associated with at least four of the following somatic symptoms suggestive of autonomic arousal: shortness of breath or dyspnea, dizziness, unsteady feeling or faintness, palpitations or tachycardia, trembling or shaking, sweating, choking, nausea or abdominal distress, depersonalization or derealization, numbness or tingling sensation, flushes or chills, chest pain or discomfort, fear of dying, fear of going crazy, and fear of doing something uncontrollable. Many patients also develop agoraphobia—an irrational fear of being alone or in public places, frequently leading to an increasingly restricted lifestyle marked by avoiding those situations that might trigger an attack.

Patients with unrecognized and untreated PD are likely to make repeated office visits, presenting with multiple unexplained or atypical somatic complaints, and are often subjected to unnecessary laboratory testing. Data from population surveys showed that of individuals meeting diagnostic criteria for PD, 42% had visited an emergency room for emotional problems in the year before the survey.

The cause of PD is uncertain and involves an interaction between several biologic and psychological determinants. As many as 10% of the U.S. population have had a single panic attack at some time in their lives. One to 2% suffer from PD, and an additional 2 to 3% suffer from agoraphobia with or without panic attacks. Panic disorder tends to be familial; up to 18% of first-degree relatives of a patient diagnosed with PD also have panic disorder. About two-thirds of patients with PD are female. The peak age of onset is the middle twenties. Co-morbid conditions frequently occur and can result in failure to make the proper diagnosis and in treatment resistance. Depression and self-medication with alcohol are frequent psychiatric complications of PD; co-morbid medical conditions such as irritable bowel syndrome (IBS) are also frequently seen.

TREATMENT

Tricyclic Antidepressants. The tricyclic antidepressants (TCAs) have been traditionally regarded as the mainstay of antipanic treatment. Imipramine (Tofranil)* and clomipramine (Anafranil)* have the most extensively documented effectiveness. However, many other TCAs are probably effective in the treatment of PD, including desipramine* and nortriptyline.* It is preferable to initiate TCA treatment at 10 mg per day because of the sensitivity of PD patients to the anticholinergic and adrenergic properties of these drugs. Higher initial doses may lead to jitteriness, insomnia, tremulousness, and increased anxiety. TCA dosage should be increased every 1 to 3 days by 10 mg daily to 50 mg, and then by 25 mg each week until a therapeutic response or unacceptable side effects appear. Oral doses of 100 to 150 mg per day or a steady-state total plasma concentration of approximately 125 to 150 ng per milliliter have been shown to be associated with optimal response; however, higher doses (150 to 300 mg) may be needed. After initial stabilization, maintenance treatment (for up to a year) with lower effective doses (half the stabilization dose) is usually indicated.

Monoamine Oxidase Inhibitors. The monoamine oxidase inhibitors (MAOIs) have been found to be as effective as (or possibly more effective than) TCAs in the treatment of PD. The usual therapeutic dose is 30 to 90 mg per day of phenelzine (Nardil)* or 30 to 60 mg of tranylcypromine (Parnate).* The starting dose is usually 1 tablet per day (15 mg of phenelzine or 10 mg of tranylcypromine), increasing the dose by 1 tablet every 3 to 4 days as needed. After a dose of 3 tablets per day is reached, we recommend keeping the dose constant for approximately 3 weeks and then increasing it if necessary. The main side effects of MAOIs are orthostatic hypotension, weight gain, and sexual dysfunction. Certain drug-drug and drug-food interactions (pressor amines, narcotics, and food containing tyramine) may produce hypertensive crisis or delirium. Patients receiving MAOIs should therefore receive a list of foods and medications to avoid and should check with their physician prior to starting any new drug. Maintenance of the dietary and drug restrictions is recommended for at least 14 days after stopping the medication or before switching to a different agent and for 5 weeks before prescribing any selective serotonin re-uptake inhibitor (SSRI).

Benzodiazepines. Benzodiazepines have been found to be very effective in the treatment of PD. The most extensively studied benzodiazepine in the treatment of PD is alprazolam (Xanax), although clonazepam (Klonopin),* lorazepam (Ativan),* and diazepam (Valium)* are also effective. The starting dose of alprazolam is generally 0.5 mg two to three times per day. The usual dosage range is 2 to 6 mg per day. Recent research suggests that many patients may obtain substantial clinical improvement while receiving a relatively low dose of alprazolam (e.g., 2 mg per day). The main side effects include sedation and fatigue and, at higher doses, ataxia, slurred speech, and some memory impairment. Therefore, patients should be advised, at least initially, not to use benzodiazepines while driving or operating machinery. Another problem has been the occurrence of "breakthrough" anxiety prior to receiving the next scheduled dose, a phenomenon believed to be related to alprazolam's relatively short elimination half-life (10 to 14 hours). Switching to a longer-acting benzodiazepine such as clonazepam (elimination half-life 20 to 50 hours) may be beneficial. Clonazepam is started at a dosage of 0.5 mg or less once daily, with a goal of 1 to 3 mg per day in two divided doses. It appears at present that maintenance treatment with benzodiazepines (e.g., for 6 months) is effective in preventing relapse of panic symptoms, and there is no evidence to support the concern that long-term treatment of PD with benzodiazepines is associated with a pattern of progressive dosage increases. Nevertheless, all benzodiazepines produce transient withdrawal symptoms if they are stopped abruptly. To minimize the occurrence of withdrawal symptoms, we recommend a gradual tapering schedule at a rate of no more than a 25% dose reduction per week or an even slower taper (lasting up to 4 to 6 months) if necessary. The last 50% of the taper should be even more gradual, with the daily dose decreasing by the lowest possible amount. We also recommend continuing to use divided doses of short half-life benzodiazepines (e.g., alprazolam) or using longer half-life benzodiazepines (e.g., clonazepam) that can be used at once-a-day dosing schedules.

Selective Serotonin Re-uptake Inhibitors (SSRIs). Fluoxetine (Prozac)* and other newer SSRIs such as sertraline (Zoloft)* and paroxetine

*This drug has not been approved by the FDA for this indication.

*This drug has not been approved by the FDA for this indication.

(Paxil)* have been widely used and are believed to be effective in the treatment of PD. Frequently observed side effects of SSRIs in patients with PD include restlessness and arousal; therefore, the starting doses may need to be lower than the usual antidepressant doses (5 to 10 mg per day of fluoxetine, and 25 mg per day of sertraline). The usual maintenance dose range for fluoxetine is 20 to 40 mg per day; for sertraline, 50 to 200 mg per day; and for paroxetine, 20 to 60 mg per day.

Anticonvulsants. The anticonvulsant valproate* in doses of 1000 to 1500 mg per day has been found useful in patients with PD, especially those with coexisting alcohol abuse or dependence.

Other Agents. The beta blocker propranolol (Inderal)* may provide symptomatic relief in some patients with residual somatic symptoms (e.g., palpitations and tachycardia) when combined with the ongoing treatment regimen, but it is not indicated as a first-line treatment in PD. Other agents such as buspirone (BuSpar),* an azapirone with partial serotonergic agonist properties, and verapamil,* a calcium channel blocker, may have limited antipanic effects in a small number of patients but are probably of limited value. Cognitive behavioral therapy, including education, cognitive restructuring, training in breathing, and desensitization to interoceptive cues, is beneficial for many patients.

In practice, effective treatment of PD frequently requires the combined use of different agents. We favor the use of agents with antidepressant properties, given the high risk of depression in the PD population over the long term. Despite the lack of definitive research supporting their effectiveness, the SSRIs are probably the initial treatment choice for many clinicians who work extensively with these patients because patient acceptability is high owing to the relatively few side effects, and this has advantages for long-term management. The addition of cognitive-behavioral treatment may improve treatment outcome in many patients. It should be noted that this illness often has a chronic or intermittent course, and drug therapy may be required for many years.

*This drug has not been approved by the FDA for this indication.

Section 17

Physical and Chemical Injuries

BURNS

method of
KAREN FRYE, M.D., and
DAVID HEIMBACH, M.D.
University of Washington
Seattle, Washington

Each year in the United States approximately 2 million individuals are burned seriously enough to cause them to see a physician; about 70,000 of these require hospitalization, and about 5000 die. It has been estimated that more than 90% of burns are completely preventable and are caused by carelessness or ignorance, and nearly half are smoking or alcohol related. Although prevention of burns is the obvious long-term solution to burn care, advances in the care of burned patients during the past 20 years have been among the most dramatic in all of medicine. The development of specialized treatment centers staffed by highly trained individuals from many disciplines has improved the medical, physical, and psychosocial outlook of the burned patient and has served as a model for care in other complex diseases. As with other forms of trauma, burns frequently affect children and young adults. The hospital expenses and the social costs related to time away from work or school are staggering. Although most burns are limited in extent, a significant burn of the hand or foot may keep manual workers away from work for a year or more and in some cases may permanently prevent them from returning to their former activity. The eventual outcome for the burned patient is related to the severity of the injury, the individual physical characteristics and the motivation of the patient, and, very importantly, the quality of the treatment of the acute burn. Because of space limitations, this chapter can deal only with the initial assessment and treatment of burns, the proper triage of the severely burned patient, and the principles of care of burns on an outpatient basis.

The primary rule for the emergency physician is, "Forget about the burn." As with any form of trauma, the ABCs—airway, breathing, circulation—must be followed. Although a burn is usually readily apparent and is a dramatic injury, a careful search for other life-threatening injuries must take priority. Only after an overall assessment of the patient's general condition has been made should attention be directed to the specific problem of the burns.

TREATMENT

Smoke Inhalation

In the fire-burned patient, the airway and breathing may be compromised by smoke inhalation. Any patient with flame burns that occurred in a closed space who has carbonaceous sputum and a carboxyhemoglobin level in the fire (see following discussion) of greater than 9% is at risk and should be closely watched for progressive airway obstruction or compromise of oxygenation. Anyone suspected of having smoke poisoning should have blood drawn for determination of arterial blood gases. One of the earliest indicators is an improper P/F ratio (i.e., the arterial oxygen content [PaO_2] to the inspired oxygen concentration [F_IO_2]). A ratio of 400:500 is normal, whereas patients with impending pulmonary problems have a ratio of less than 300 (e.g., a PaO_2 of less than 120 with an F_IO_2 of 0.40). A ratio of less than 250 is an indication for vigorous pulmonary therapy. All surgeons agree that in the presence of increasing laryngeal edema, nasotracheal or orotracheal intubation is indicated. A tracheostomy is never an emergency procedure.

Patients with mild symptoms of smoke poisoning are treated with highly humidified air, vigorous pulmonary toilet, and bronchodilators as needed. Blood for blood gas determination is drawn at least every 4 hours, and the P/F ratio is calculated. Increasing symptoms, difficulty in handling secretions, and a falling P/F ratio are all indications for intubation and respiratory assistance with a volume ventilator. The decision for hospital admission and the need for specialized care rest on the severity of symptoms due to the smoke and the presence and magnitude of associated burns. Any patient who is symptomatic following smoke inhalation and has more than trivial burns should be admitted. If the burns cover more than 15% of the total body surface area (TBSA; see following discussion), the patient should be referred to a special care unit.

Carbon Monoxide Poisoning

Carbon monoxide (CO) poisoning is the most common cause of death in fires and may be a source of long-term morbidity in survivors. Carbon monoxide has an affinity for hemoglobin 200 times that of oxygen, and reversibly displaces oxygen on the hemoglobin molecule. Carboxyhemoglobin levels are reported as the percentage of hemoglobin bound to CO and are easily measured in the emergency room. Levels of less than 10% do not cause symptoms and may be found in heavy smokers or in people living in polluted cities. At levels of 20%, healthy persons complain of headache, nausea, vomiting, and loss of manual dexterity. At 30%, they become confused and lethargic and may show depressed ST segments on electrocardiography. In a fire, this level may lead to death because the victim loses both the interest and the ability to flee the smoke. At levels between 40 and 60% the patient lapses into coma, and levels much above 60% are usually fatal. In very smoky fires, carboxyhemoglobin levels of 40 to 50% may be reached after only 2 to 3 minutes of exposure.

Carbon monoxide is reversibly bound to the heme pigments (hemoglobin and myoglobin) and enzymes (cytochromes) and, despite its intense affinity, readily dissociates according to the laws of mass action. The half-life of carboxyhemoglobin in room air is between 4 and 5 hours. In an individual breathing 100% oxygen, the half-life is reduced to 45 to 60 minutes. Thus, a patient seen in the emergency room after 1 hour of breathing 100% oxygen who has a carboxyhemoglobin level of 10% can be assumed to have had levels of greater than 20% in the fire. There is clear agreement that all patients who have been burned in an enclosed space or who have any suggestion of neurologic symptoms should be administered 100% oxygen while measurement of carboxyhemoglobin levels is awaited. Oxygen should be instituted in the field by the paramedics using a tight-fitting mask or, when necessary, endotracheal intubation if the personnel are adequately trained in tube insertion. Although often recommended, hyperbaric oxygen treatment is not of proven benefit.

BURN SEVERITY

Prognosis and all treatment plans, including initial resuscitation efforts, are directly tied to the size of the burn. A general idea of burn size is provided by the "rule of nines." Each upper extremity accounts for 9% of the TBSA; each lower extremity accounts for 18%; the anterior and posterior trunk each account for 18%; the head and neck account for 9%; and the perineum accounts for 1%. Although the rule of nines provides a reasonably accurate estimate of burn size, a number of more precise charts have been developed and are available in nearly every emergency room. For smaller burns an accurate assessment can be made of burn size by using the hand of the patient. The palmar surface, including the fingers, amounts to 1% of the TBSA.

BURN HEALING

Burns that do not extend all the way through the dermis leave behind epithelial lined skin appendages—sweat glands and hair follicles with attached sebaceous glands. Once the dead dermal tissue has been removed, epithelial cells swarm from the surface of each appendage to meet swarming cells from the neighboring appendages, thus forming a new, fragile epidermis on top of a thinned or scarred dermal bed. Because skin appendages vary in depth, the deeper the burn, the fewer the appendages that contribute to healing, and the longer the burn takes to heal. The longer it takes to heal, the less the dermis remaining and the greater the inflammatory response, so the scarring is much greater.

CLASSIFICATION OF BURNS

Burns are classified by increasing depth as first-degree, superficial dermal, deep dermal, full-thickness, and fourth-degree.

First-Degree Burns

First-degree burns involve only the epidermis. First-degree burns do not blister. They become erythematous because of dermal vasodilation, and they are very painful, both spontaneously and when touched. Over a period of 2 to 3 days both the erythema and the pain subside. By about day 4 the injured epithelium desquamates in the phenomenon of "peeling," which is known to everyone following a sunburn.

Superficial Dermal Burns

Superficial dermal burns include the upper layers of the dermis and characteristically form blisters in which fluid collects at the interface of the epidermis and dermis. Blistering may not occur for some hours following injury, and burns originally appearing to be first degree may in fact be diagnosed as superficial dermal burns after 12 to 24 hours. Once blisters are removed, the wound is pink and wet and is painful as currents of air pass over it. The wound is hypersensitive, and the burns blanch with pressure. If infection is prevented, superficial dermal burns heal spontaneously in less than 3 weeks and will do so with no functional impairment. They rarely cause hypertrophic scarring, but in pigmented individuals the healed burn may never completely match the color of the surrounding normal skin.

Deep Dermal Burns

Deep dermal burns also blister, but the wound surface is usually a mottled pink and white color immediately following the injury. The patient complains of discomfort rather than pain. When pressure is applied to the burn, capillary refill occurs slowly or may be absent. The wound is often less sensitive to pinprick than the surrounding normal skin. By the second day the wound may be white and is usually fairly dry. If infection is prevented, such burns heal in 3 to 9 weeks but invariably do so with considerable scar formation. Unless active physical therapy is continued throughout the healing process, joint function may be impaired, and hypertrophic scarring, particularly in pigmented individuals and children, is common.

Full-Thickness Burns

Full-thickness burns involve all layers of the dermis and can heal only by wound contracture, by epithelialization from the wound margin, or by skin grafting. Full-thickness burns are classically described as being leathery, firm, depressed compared to the adjoining normal skin, and insensitive to light touch or pinprick. Unfortunately, the difference in depth between a deep dermal burn and a full-thickness burn may be less than a millimeter. Full-thickness burns can masquerade with many of the clinical findings of a deep dermal burn. Like deep dermal burns they may be mottled in appearance. They rarely blanch on pressure, and they may have a dry, white appearance. In some cases the burn may be translucent with clotted vessels visible in the depths. Some full-thickness burns, particularly immersion scalds, may have a red appearance and can be confused by the uninitiated with a superficial dermal burn. They can be distinguished, however, because these red, full-thickness burns do not blanch with pressure. Full-thickness burns develop a classic burn *eschar*. An eschar represents the structurally intact but dead and denatured dermis that, over days and weeks, separates from the underlying viable tissue.

Fourth-Degree Burns

Fourth-degree burns involve not only all layers of the skin but also subcutaneous fat and deeper structures. These burns almost always have a charred appearance, and frequently only the cause of the burn gives a clue to the amount of underlying tissue destruction. Electrical burns, contact burns, some immersion burns, and burns sustained by patients who are unconscious at the time of burning may all be fourth degree.

Although these descriptions appear to separate burns nicely into categories, many burns have a mixture of characteristics, giving the observer very imprecise diagnostic clues. Considerable research is currently under way to devise instruments that can diagnose the depth of injury more precisely. Much of the current methods of burn treatment depends on a knowledge of the depth of the burn.

ELECTRICAL BURNS

Electrical burns are really thermal burns from very high-intensity heat. Electricity as it meets the resistance of body tissues is converted to heat in direct proportion to the amperage of the current and the electrical resistance of the body parts through which it passes. The smaller the size of the body part through which the electricity passes, the more intense the heat and the less the heat is dissipated. Therefore, fingers, hands, forearms, feet, and lower legs are frequently totally destroyed by high-voltage current (greater than 1000 volts), whereas larger volume areas, like the trunk, usually dissipate the current enough to prevent extensive damage to the viscera, although organ damage underlying contact points on the abdomen or chest may result. Although cutaneous manifestations may appear to be limited, the skin injury is only the tip of an iceberg because massive underlying tissue destruction may take place. This underlying tissue destruction may result in myoglobinuria, coloring the urine a burgundy or claret wine color. If myoglobinuria is visible grossly, it should be treated by maintaining the urine output at 100 mL per hour during resuscitation. An increase in the amount of fluids alone may accomplish this, but if it does not, mannitol is given (12.5 grams followed by another 12.5 grams in 30 to 45 minutes). Extremities should be assessed for compartment syndrome. When indicated, fasciotomies must be performed.

Electrical burns cause a particular set of other injuries and complications that must be considered during the initial evaluation. Injuries related to a fall are common. The intense associated muscle contractions may cause fractures of the thoracolumbar vertebrae, humerus, or femur and may dislocate shoulders or hips. Electrical cardiac damage may present in a similar manner or as a myocardial contusion or infarction. Alternatively, the conduction system may be deranged; in some cases, actual rupture of the heart wall or rupture of papillary muscle, leading to sudden valvular incompetence and refractory cardiac failure, can occur. Household current at 110 volts generally either does no damage or induces ventricular fibrillation. If no cardiac abnormalities are detected in the emergency room following shocks of 110 to 220 volts, the likelihood that they will appear later is small; if the initial electrocardiogram is normal, the patient can usually go home. It is likely that cardiac dysrhythmias induced by high-voltage electrical shocks will be present on admission. However, common practice is to admit all patients with high-voltage electrical injury for cardiac monitoring for 24 hours.

CHEMICAL BURNS

Chemical burns, usually caused by strong acids or alkalies, are most often the result of industrial accidents, drain cleaners, assaults, or the improper use of harsh solvents. In contrast to a thermal burn, chemical burns cause progressive damage until the chemicals are inactivated by reaction with the tissue or dilution by flushing with water. Although individual circumstances vary, acid burns may be more self-limiting than alkali burns. Acid tends to "tan" the skin, creating an impermeable barrier that limits further penetration of the acid. Alkalies, on the other hand, combine with cutaneous lipids to create soap and thereby continue "dissolving" the skin until they are neutralized. A full-thickness chemical burn may appear deceptively superficial, causing clinically only a mild brownish discoloration of the skin. The skin may appear to remain intact during the first few days after the burn and only then begins to slough spontaneously. Unless the observer can be absolutely sure, chemical burns should be considered deep dermal or full-thickness until proved otherwise. Initial treatment consists of copious rinsing with tap water for as long as 30 minutes; this should be encouraged at the site of the accident before transport to the emergency room. Patients with chemical burns of the eye should have copious saline lavage until the pH of the eye returns to normal.

BURN RESUSCITATION

All patients with dermal or full-thickness burns greater than 15% TBSA should be considered candidates for intravenous fluid replacement to prevent the decreased plasma volume that is a universal accompaniment of the capillary permeability resulting from the burn. Because of its simplicity, its ease of administration, and its minimal need for blood chemistry monitoring, the formula developed by Baxter, known as the Baxter or Parkland formula, has been adopted by most hospitals and the American College of Surgeons. The Baxter formula recommends the administration of crystalloid as lactated Ringer's solution (or equivalent) during the first 24 hours while the capillaries are still permeable to albumin. The formula calls for the administration of 4 mL of lactated Ringer's solution per kg of body weight for each 1% of body surface burned during the first 24 hours post-injury. Half of this fluid should be given during the first 8 hours and the second half during the next 16 hours. If after 12 to 15 hours the patient requires substantially more fluid than that indicated by the Baxter formula (more than 1.5 times the calculated amount), colloid, given as albumin, may be needed. Fluid therapy during the second 24 hours consists of maintenance fluids. Colloid in the form of albumin is administered if needed to maintain normal vital signs and urine output.

Children weighing up to about 45 kg will be under-resuscitated if only burn fluid is given, so they should be given their usual daily maintenance fluids in addition to the burn formula. Maintenance treatment should be given uniformly over 24 hours (Table 1).

The Baxter formula is merely a guideline, and adjustments in fluid rate are made based on the clinical response of the patient. The adequacy of resuscitation can be judged by frequent measurements of vital signs, hourly urine output, and observation of general mental and physical response. Despite the myriad of new monitoring devices, urine output remains one of the most sensitive and reliable methods of assessment of fluid resuscitation efforts. A urine output of 30 to 50 mL per hour in adults and 1.5 mL per kg per hour in children ensures that renal perfusion is adequate. The patient should be alert and cooperative; confusion and combativeness are signs of inadequate resuscitation or warn of other causes of hypoxia.

OTHER CONSIDERATIONS

The need for tetanus prophylaxis is determined by the patient's current immunization status. The treating physician should follow the recommendation of the American College of Surgeons, which includes routine immunization at 10 years and reimmunization at 5 years for any tetanus-prone wound. All medications administered during the "shock phase" of burn care should be given intravenously. Subcutaneous and intramuscular injections are undependably absorbed and should be avoided. Pain control is best managed with small intravenous doses of morphine, usually in the range of 2 to 3 mg, given every 5 to 10 minutes until pain control is adequate without affecting blood pressure or respiration.

All patients undergoing intravenous resuscitation should have a Foley catheter placed for hourly monitoring of urine output. Arterial lines may be useful in patients who need frequent blood gas determinations or repeated blood sampling; however, necessary laboratory work during the resuscitation phase is relatively minimal. Blood for baseline chemistry measurements and a complete blood count should be drawn. Only if major operative procedures such as fasciotomy or multiple escharotomies are contemplated is it necessary to type and crossmatch blood. Blood gas determinations are mandatory in any patient with a suspected inhalation injury, and arterial pH measurement is useful in the assessment of the overall treatment of shock. If the Baxter formula is used for resuscitation, frequent electrolyte determinations are not necessary because they will remain in the normal range.

TABLE 1. **Fluid Replacement in Burn Patients**

Examples	Hours 1–8	Hours 8–16	Hours 16–24	Day 2
70-kg adult with 50% burn	(4 × 70 × 50 × 0.5) RL = 7000 mL ~ 875 mL/hour	(4 × 70 × 50 × 0.25) RL = 3500 mL ~ 450 mL/hour	(4 × 70 × 50 × 0.25) RL = 3500 mL ~ 450 mL/hour	RL maintenance only + albumin to keep urine and vital signs stable
15-kg child with 50% burn (~ 1300 mL maintenance)	(4 × 15 × 0.5) RL = 1500 mL ~ 200 mL/hour + 50 mL/hour maintenance	(4 × 15 × 0.25) RL = 750 mL ~ 100 mL/hour + 50 mL/hour maintenance	(4 × 15 × 0.25) RL = 750 mL ~ 100 mL/hour + 50 mL/hour maintenance	Maintenance only + albumin to keep urine and vital signs stable

RL = Lactated Ringer's solution.

The blood glucose level is commonly elevated because of the glycogenolytic effect of elevated catecholamines, the gluconeogenic effect of elevated glucocorticoids, elevated glucagon levels, and relative insulin resistance. This well-described form of "stress diabetes" can become a problem in normal patients if glucose-containing solutions are given during resuscitation, and it frequently becomes a serious problem in patients with pre-existing diabetes. All diabetic patients require careful monitoring of blood and urine glucose levels, and most will need supplemental insulin during resuscitation.

Patients with a greater than 20% TBSA burn have an increased metabolism. If the burn is greater than 30% TBSA, tube feedings will probably be necessary. Immediately on admission the patient is started on a regular diet or tube feedings or both. If oral feedings are not tolerated, sucralfate (Carafate)* or antacids (30 to 50 mL per hour) are started as prophylaxis against stress ulcers.

An extremity with a circumferential full-thickness burn must have its distal circulation assessed. Pulses should be monitored by Doppler echocardiography; if absent, an escharotomy is indicated.

Patients with periorbital burns of the face should be assessed for a corneal abrasion.

Psychosocial care should begin immediately. The patient and family must be comforted, and a realistic outlook regarding the prognosis of the burns should be given, at least to the patient's family. In house fires, loved ones, pets, and many or all possessions may have been destroyed. If the family is not available, some member of the team, usually the social worker, should find out the extent of the damage with the hope of being able to comfort the patient. If the patient is a child and if the circumstances of the burn are suspicious, physicians are required by law to report any suspected case of child abuse or neglect to local authorities.

BURN SEVERITY—TRANSFER PROTOCOLS

Severity of injury is determined by the size of the total burn, the depth of the burn, the age of the patient, and associated medical problems or injuries. Burns have been classified by the American Burn Association and the American College of Surgeons Committee on Trauma into categories of minor, moderate, and severe. Moderate burns are defined as partial-thickness burns of 15 to 25% TBSA in adults (10 to 20% in children); full-thickness burns of less than 10% TBSA; and burns that *do not* involve the face, hands, feet, or perineum. Because of the significant cosmetic and functional risk, all but very superficial burns of the face, hands, feet, and perineum should be treated by a physician with a special interest in burn care in a facility that is accustomed to dealing with such problems. Major burns and most full-thickness burns in infants, the elderly, or patients with associated disease or injuries should also be cared for in a specialized facility. Patients with moderate burns can be cared for in a community hospital by a knowledgeable physician as long as the *other* members of the health care team have the resources and knowledge to ensure a good result. Newer techniques of early wound closure have made burn care more complex, and an increasing number of patients with small but significant burns are being referred to specialized care facilities to take advantage of these concepts.

The criteria for admission of patients with minor and moderate burns to the hospital vary according to physician preference, the patient's social circumstances, and the ability to provide close follow-up care. Even tiny superficial burns may require admission because of the patient's inability or unwillingness to care for the wound (alcoholics, homeless people, drug abusers, mentally impaired patients). In general, the physician should have a low threshold for admission of elderly patients and small children. Any patient (child or adult) in whom abuse is suspected *must* be admitted.

Once an airway has been established and resuscitation is under way, burned patients are eminently suitable for transport. Resuscitation can continue en route, and, for the most part, the patient will remain stable for several days. This was well proved during the Viet Nam war; military burn victims were first transported from Viet Nam to Japan, and then from Japan to the military Burn Center in San Antonio, Texas. The transport was generally accomplished during the first 2 weeks after the burn, and very few complications occurred in more than 3000 patients transferred during the war.

Hospitals without specialized burn care facilities should decide where they will refer patients, and work out transfer agreements and treatment protocols with the chosen burn center well in advance of need. If this is done, definitive care can begin at the initial hospital and continue without interruption during transport and at the burn center. In general, transfer should be made from physician to physician, and contact should be established between them as soon as the patient arrives in the emergency room of the initial hospital. The mode of transport and the arrangements for procuring it should be well known to all involved.

TREATMENT OF BURNS IN OUTPATIENTS

Using the guidelines described earlier, the condition of the severely burned patient should be stabilized, and the patient should be well on his or her way to receive optimal care. However, the great majority of patients who sustain burns do not require hospitalization at all. In many cases, the burn, if merely kept clean, heals spontaneously in less than 3 weeks with acceptable cosmetic results and no functional impairment. Unfortunately, good results in treating superficial minor burns may entice the unwary physician to treat more complex burns by the same methods. For the patient, the consequences of

*This drug has not been approved by the FDA for this indication.

such a mistake can be unnecessary hospitalization, joint dysfunction, hypertrophic scarring that may be difficult to correct, and excessive loss of time from work or school.

First-Degree Burns

Although first-degree burns are very painful, victims rarely seek medical attention unless the area burned is extensive. These patients do not require hospitalization, but control of the pain is extremely important. Aspirin or codeine may be adequate for small injuries, but for large burns, liberal use of a more potent narcotic for 2 to 3 days is indicated. For topical medication we recommend one of the many proprietary compounds containing extracts of the aloe vera plant in concentrations of at least 60%. Aloe vera has some antimicrobial properties and is an effective temporary analgesic. Anecdotal evidence suggests that it may decrease subsequent pruritus and peeling.

Burns from ultraviolet rays (sunlight, sun lamp) may initially appear to be only epidermal, but the injury may in fact be a superficial dermal burn with blistering becoming apparent only after 12 to 24 hours. Therefore, the patient with such a burn should be cautioned about blisters and should be asked to return if they form because wound management then becomes more important owing to the potential for infection and subsequent scarring.

Superficial Dermal Burns

Treatment of superficial dermal burns presents little problem. If the wound is kept clean, the patient is kept comfortable, and the joints are kept active, these wounds heal in less than 3 weeks with minimal scarring and no joint impairment.

Initially, the wound should be cleansed and gently débrided, and loose skin should be removed. Small blisters may be left intact. Larger blisters are difficult to protect, and blister fluid is a reasonable culture medium for bacteria that live in the skin appendages. Therefore, blisters should usually be totally removed with forceps and scissors. In some instances, the blister fluid can be aspirated with a large-bore needle, allowing the blistered epidermis to remain on the wound as a biologic dressing. This dead epidermis, however, is fragile, tends to contract, and rarely stays in place except over small areas. After débridement, these wounds are ideally managed with a biologic dressing such as porcine xenograft (pig skin). Pig skin is available frozen or treated with glutaraldehyde, permitting a long shelf life. Once it has been applied, burn pain is markedly diminished, and if the xenograft "sticks," no further treatment is necessary except for a periodic wound check. When the burn reepithelializes, the xenograft desiccates and peels away from the new epidermis. Other synthetic dressings, such as those made from plastic film (Op-Site, Tegaderm, or Epigard), or those made with composite materials (Biobrane), have achieved some popularity, but the authors have little experience with them.

The most common treatment is application of silver sulfadiazine (Silvadene) and a light dressing with daily dressing changes. Some very small burns do not require topical agents. For small facial burns, antibiotic ointment may be a better choice than silver sulfadiazine cream because it is less drying. We prescribe a home treatment regimen in which the patient cleanses the wound daily with tap water and reapplies the topical agent and a light dressing. During dressing changes and as often as possible, all involved joints should be put through a full range of motion. The dressing may be unnecessary while the patient is at home, but we recommend that the patient dress the wound before leaving the house. This method is highly successful, but it is inconvenient, and the dressing changes may be fairly painful, requiring good patient cooperation and prescription of adequate pain medication. Acetaminophen with codeine, or oxycodone tablets are usually sufficient to manage pain during dressing changes and exercise. The patient usually should return every 5 to 7 days until the wound heals or the patient has demonstrated an ability to manage the wound without supervision.

Deep Dermal and Full-Thickness Burns

Treatment of these burns is a matter of much graver concern than treatment of superficial burns. Full-thickness burns heal only by contraction and epithelialization from the periphery. Epithelium does not begin to migrate until the eschar is removed; the growth rate then is only about 1 mm per day. Thus, healing of even a small full-thickness burn may involve many weeks of discomfort and disability. Deep dermal burns may take 4 to 8 weeks to heal and then may leave an unacceptable scar. If a joint is involved, some loss of joint function is the rule rather than the exception. Thus, we have adopted a policy of early excision and grafting for such wounds.

Initial outpatient treatment can be followed by elective surgery as soon as it can be scheduled. Small wounds can be treated with outpatient surgery; larger wounds over dynamically important areas can be closed with only a day or two of hospitalization. The excision and grafting procedures should be done by a surgeon experienced in burn wound excision. We believe that the advantages of this aggressive approach—a pain-free patient with normal joint function, a better cosmetic result, and a rapid return to work or school—more than compensate for the brief hospitalization and the very small risk associated with a minor operation.

Should the excision and grafting plan not be acceptable to the patient or the treating physician, the standard method of daily cleansing and application of silver sulfadiazine cream is used. Full-thickness burns eventually need grafting after about 3 to 4 weeks. Deep dermal burns should be seen by the physician frequently during the healing process; active physical therapy is crucial to ensure a successful outcome.

DISTURBANCES DUE TO COLD

method of
SCOTT OSLUND, M.D.,
REBECCA SMITH-COGGINS, M.D., and
PAUL AUERBACH, M.D., M.S.
Stanford University Hospital
Stanford, California

ACCIDENTAL HYPOTHERMIA

Accidental hypothermia occurs when the core temperature of a human accidentally drops below 35° C (95° F). Mild hypothermia is defined as a core temperature of 35° to 33° C (95° to 91.4° F). Moderate hypothermia is 32° to 28° C (89.6° to 82.4° F), and severe hypothermia is 27° C (80.6° F) or less. The causes of accidental hypothermia are decreased heat production, increased heat loss, and impaired thermoregulation. Hypothermia can be associated with several clinical entities (Table 1).

Pathophysiology

Cardiovascular effects are often encountered. In the initial excitatory state of mild hypothermia, heart rate, cardiac output, and blood pressure rise. However, at 28° C the heart rate may drop to half its normal rate owing to decreased spontaneous depolarization of pacemaker cells that are refractory to atropine. Mean arterial pressure, cardiac index, and threshold for ventricular fibrillation (VF) are also decreased. Systemic vascular resistance is increased. Rough handling of a hypothermic patient can induce VF owing to ventricular irritability. Prolongation of the cardiac cycle may be noted, as evidenced by prolonged PR, QRS, and QTC intervals. A J, or Osborn, wave may appear on the electrocardiogram (ECG) at the junction of the QRS complex and ST segment and is seen best in leads II and V_6. The cause of the J wave deflection is not precisely known but may be due to late depolarization or early repolarization of the left ventricle secondary to ion shifts in cold myocardium. The J wave is not pathognomonic for hypothermia and is seen in lesions of the central nervous system, in patients with cardiac ischemia, or sepsis, and in young healthy patients. When pronounced, J waves may simulate the ECG findings of a myocardial infarction.

The typical sequence of dysrhythmias is a progression from sinus bradycardia to atrial fibrillation with a slow ventricular response, to VF, and eventually to asystole. Causes of VF and asystole may include tissue hypoxia, acid-base disturbances, hypovolemia, coronary vasoconstriction, and increased blood viscosity. Pre-existing ventricular dysrhythmias initially suppressed by hypothermia may reappear as patients are rewarmed. Atrial dysrhythmias, including atrial fibrillation, are usually innocent and convert to sinus rhythm on rewarming. Other ECG changes, such as T wave inversion, muscle tremor artifact, atrioventricular block, and premature ventricular contractions, may be seen. Even after rewarming, cardiovascular function may remain temporarily depressed.

With rewarming, a patient's core temperature may paradoxically decline. This phenomenon is called afterdrop. Simple equilibration between a warm core and cooler extremities is one explanation. Another possibility is a reversal of peripheral vasoconstriction and arteriovenous shunting, which allows warm arterial blood to perfuse cold tissue. Cooler venous blood returning to the core may potentiate dysrhythmias. This is especially true if frozen extremities are thawed prior to attaining thermal stabilization of the core temperature.

Hypothermia has numerous effects on the central nervous system. In mild hypothermia, amnesia, dysarthria, ataxia, and apathy appear. If the core temperature drops below 32° C (89.6° F), the patient can become stuporous. Below 26° C (78.8° F), deep tendon reflexes disappear, and the patient ceases to respond to pain. At 23° C (73.4° F), corneal and oculocephalic reflexes are lost, and at 19° C (66.2° F), a flat electroencephalogram (EEG) will appear. The lowest core temperatures in adult and infant survivors of accidental hypothermia were 16° C (60.8° F) and 15° C (59.2° F), respectively. The lowest core temperature in a survivor of intentional hypothermia was 9° C.

Initial tachypnea is followed by a progressive decrease in respiratory rate and tidal volume. Cold-induced bronchorrhea and depression of cough and gag reflexes predispose to aspiration pneumonia. Shallow respirations may be secondary to decreased pulmonary and chest wall compliance and contraction of intercostal muscles and diaphragm. Ventilation-perfusion mismatches may result in decreased oxygenation. Noncardiogenic pulmonary edema may occur.

Despite a decrease in renal blood flow, hypothermia induces a diuresis of dilute urine that is ineffective in clearing nitrogenous wastes. Inhibition of antidiuretic hormone release and decreased renal tubular function have been suggested as possible causes of this "cold diuresis." However, it may simply be due to relative hypervolemia associated with diffuse vasoconstriction. Ensuing hemoconcentration may in turn lead to intravascular thrombosis. Immobilization predisposes a hypothermic patient to rhabdomyolysis. With muscle breakdown, myoglobin is released and broken down into globin and ferrihemate. Studies suggest that ferrihemate has a direct toxic effect on the kidney. Increased renal vascular resistance and a subsequent dim-

TABLE 1. **Factors Predisposing to Hypothermia**

Decreased Heat Production	**Impaired Thermoregulation**
Hypopituitarism	Neuropathies
Hypoadrenalism	Diabetes mellitus
Hypothyroidism	Acute spinal cord transection
Hypoglycemia	CNS trauma
Malnutrition	Stroke
Dehydration	Subarachnoid hemorrhage
Age extremes	Toxicologic
Impaired shivering	Pharmacologic
Overexertion	Metabolic
Hypoxia	**Miscellaneous Clinical States**
Immobility	
Increased Heat Loss	Trauma
Immersion in a body of water	Sepsis
Exposure (cold, wind, rain)	Pneumonia
Toxicologic	Endocarditis
Burns	Pancreatitis
Exfoliative dermatitis	Peritonitis
Shock	Meningitis
Altitude	Encephalitis
	Tuberculosis
	Myocardial infarction
	Bradycardia
	Vascular diseases
	Psychiatric disorders

inution of glomerular filtration rate and renal blood flow can result in acute tubular necrosis.

Coagulopathies are common in hypothermic patients. Clotting factors are enzymatically less active when cold. When cold blood samples from a hypothermic patient are warmed to 37° C in the laboratory, the enzymes become normoactive, and prothrombin (PT) and partial thromboplastin times (PTT) are reported by the laboratory to be normal. This results in the paradox of normal clotting times reported in an oozing patient. The required treatment is rewarming, not administration of clotting factors. Thrombocytopenia also accounts for bleeding in the hypothermic patient. In a study of intentional hypothermia, the average platelet count dropped from 184,000 to 37,000 per cubic milliliter. Bone marrow suppression and hepatic and splenic sequestration are thought to be the mechanisms of thrombocytopenia. Disseminated intravascular coagulation (DIC) may be seen in patients with hypothermia secondary to release of thromboplastin from cold tissue. Hyperviscosity due to hemoconcentration and "stiff" erythrocytes may contribute to circulatory collapse.

Acid-base disturbances are common but do not follow a uniform pattern. Patients may become acidotic from respiratory depression and carbon dioxide (CO_2) retention or from lactic acid production secondary to shivering and poor tissue perfusion. Alkalosis may result from diminished CO_2 production secondary to low metabolic rate, or from iatrogenic hyperventilation and exogenous sodium bicarbonate administration. Arterial blood gas (ABG) specimens should be interpreted without corrections made for temperature. Prior to analysis, the sample should be warmed in the usual fashion. An uncorrected pH of 7.4 and PCO_2 of 40 mmHg generally indicate adequate alveolar ventilation and acid-base balance at any patient temperature.

Hyperkalemia may be due to underlying disease or may be associated with metabolic acidosis, rhabdomyolysis, or renal failure. Severe potassium elevation lowers the threshold for ventricular fibrillation. However, hypokalemia is seen more commonly. In acute hypothermia, hyperglycemia may occur secondary to increased glycogenolysis and decreased glucose utilization and insulin release. Exogenous insulin is rarely effective below 30° C and should not be administered to avoid the iatrogenic hypoglycemia seen with rewarming. If hyperglycemia persists during rewarming, hemorrhagic pancreatitis or diabetic ketoacidosis should be suspected. In that case, insulin is used with extreme caution. If hypothermia is chronic, hypoglycemia is usually due to depleted glycogen stores.

Clinical Presentation

Historical factors do not always suggest hypothermia. Patients may present with nonspecific symptoms of hunger, nausea, dizziness, or fatigue. Persons may be uncooperative, uncoordinated, moody, or apathetic. The elderly may demonstrate signs and symptoms that mimic senility or a cerebrovascular accident. Psychosis, neurosis, anxiety, and perseveration have also been reported. Inappropriate and maladaptive behavior have been observed, most notably "paradoxical undressing"—a phenomenon in which hypothermic persons undress in cold weather.

MANAGEMENT

It has been stated that "no one is dead until warm and dead." In general, resuscitation measures should not be discontinued unless there is no improvement with hospital rewarming to 35° C. However, every clinical situation is unique, so it may be appropriate to discontinue resuscitation efforts at a lower core temperature, particularly if there are major co-morbid conditions, obvious lethal injuries, or significant dangers to rescuers. However, cold, stiff, and cyanotic patients with fixed and dilated pupils have been resuscitated. The core temperature should be checked rectally to confirm hypothermia. Placement of the rectal thermometer into cold stool may yield an artificially low core temperature.

Initial management of the hypothermic patient includes removing all wet clothing, insulating with blankets, and preventing further heat loss. Attention to the airway, breathing, and circulation (ABCs) is critical. If the patient is in respiratory arrest, rescue breathing should be initiated. Adequate oxygenation is the key to the electrical stability of the myocardium, but overzealous ventilation can induce hypocapnea and ventricular irritability. Intubation of the hypothermic patient is indicated for the same reasons that exist in normothermic patients. Blind nasotracheal or fiberoptic intubation may be necessary if cold-induced trismus is present. If rapid-sequence induction is used, hypothermia will prolong the duration of neuromuscular blockade. Peripheral pulses are very difficult to palpate in patients with vasoconstriction and bradycardia. If there is no evidence of perfusion after careful assessment of blood pressure and pulses (which may require use of a Doppler echocardiogram), cardiopulmonary resuscitation (CPR) should be initiated. Closed chest compressions maintain neurologic viability in hypothermic patients far longer than in normothermic patients. There have been many neurologically intact survivors after prolonged periods of chest compression (one patient recovered after 6½ hours of chest compressions). If appropriate, a single attempt at defibrillation at 2 watt-seconds per kg up to 200 watt-seconds should be attempted. Defibrillation is rarely successful at temperatures below 28° to 30° C (82.4° to 86° F). Transient ventricular dysrhythmias can generally be ignored. However, if treatment is necessary, bretylium (Bretylol) has been found to be effective. It possesses direct antifibrillatory properties and increases the VF threshold, action potential duration, and effective refractory period. Of note, in one study of nonaccidental hypothermia, 100 mg per kg of magnesium sulfate* given intravenously resulted in spontaneous defibrillation within minutes.

All medication should be given intravenously because oral and intramuscular absorption is erratic. In general, pharmacologic manipulation of the pulse and blood pressure should be avoided. Vasopressors are dysrhythmogenic and useless if the vasculature is maximally constricted. Exogenous administration of catecholamines may further jeopardize a frozen extremity. If a patient is severely hypotensive and is not responding to crystalloid infusion and rewarming, low-dose dopamine (Intropin) (1 to 5 μg per kg

*Exceeds dosage recommended by the manufacturer.

per minute) may be started. If myxedema coma is suspected as the cause of hypothermia, 250 to 500 μg of levothyroxine (T_4) should be administered immediately; daily injections of 100 μg should be continued for 5 to 7 days. Steroids are not routinely indicated in the hypothermic patient unless adrenal failure or prior steroid dependence is present.

An initial 250- to 500-mL fluid bolus of 5% dextrose in normal saline heated to 40° to 42° C (104° to 107.6° F) should be given. Lactated Ringer's solution should be avoided because of the theoretical problem of poor lactate metabolism by a cold liver. Intravenous fluids should be warmed to 40° to 42° C prior to administration. Fluid warming may be accomplished using a microwave oven; at high power, 1 liter of crystalloid should take approximately 2 minutes to reach 40° to 42° C. However, because ovens vary, each unit should be individually calibrated. Heating blood in a microwave oven will result in hemolysis.

A nasogastric tube is indicated in patients with moderate to severe hypothermia for the treatment of ileus. An indwelling bladder catheter with a temperature probe is helpful in monitoring core temperature. An arterial line is useful for monitoring blood pressure, following acid-base status, and checking serial laboratory values. Pulmonary arterial catheters should be avoided because they have a tendency to induce dysrhythmias in hypothermic myocardium. Likewise, central venous catheters should not be inserted past the junction of the superior vena cava and the right atrium.

Immediate laboratory tests should include measurements of glucose, ABG (uncorrected for temperature), complete blood count (CBC), electrolytes, blood urea nitrogen (BUN), creatinine, calcium, magnesium, amylase, lipase, PT, PTT, platelet count, and fibrinogen level. Potassium levels of less than 3 mEq per liter should be corrected by administering potassium intravenously at a rate no greater than 10 to 20 mEq per hour. Potassium replacement must be undertaken carefully because supplementation in hypothermic patients may result in normothermic toxicity. A urine or blood toxicologic screen should be considered if a toxic agent for which there is therapy is suspected as a contributing cause of the hypothermia. A chest radiograph should be obtained. Radiographs of the cervical spine may be indicated in the unconscious patient.

Whether to rewarm a patient passively or actively is the next critical decision. In mild hypothermia, patients can be rewarmed *passively.* This technique involves covering the patient with insulating material. Ambulances and emergency departments frequently stock aluminized body covers that significantly reduce heat loss. Recommended rewarming rates vary from 0.5° C to 2.0° C per hour.

In moderate to severe cases (core temperature less than 32° C), *active rewarming*—the transfer of exogenous heat—is usually required. Active external rewarming is indicated in patients with *mild* hypothermia if the patient is very young or old or has cardiovascular instability, spinal shock, central nervous system (CNS) dysfunction, pharmacologically induced peripheral vasodilation, or an underlying endocrine insufficiency. Both active external rewarming (AER) and active core rewarming (ACR) are possible.

Immersion in a water bath of 40° C (104.4° F) is one form of AER. Cardiac monitoring of an immersed patient is difficult. *Hot water bottles* or *heating blankets* applied to the trunk allow easier monitoring, but care should be taken to avoid skin burns. Forced air warming systems are also efficient in transferring heat. In AER, the extremities should be left unheated to avoid sudden peripheral vasodilatation, which may lead to decreased shivering and cardiovascular collapse.

Airway rewarming is an easy, safe, and effective method of ACR. Humidified inhalation improves oxygenation and bronchorrhea but does not wash out surfactant. The oxygen should be humidified and warmed to 45° C (113° F). Spontaneously breathing patients can be treated with heated nebulization. Intubated patients require a ventilator with a heating humidifier. Airway rewarming rates range from 1.0° to 2.5° C per hour.

Rewarming with *peritoneal lavage* is accomplished by inserting two catheters through a standard peritoneal incision to hasten rewarming. The crystalloid (10 to 20 mL per kg) should be heated to 40° to 45° C (104° to 113° F), infused, left in place for 20 minutes, and then drained. At 6 liters per hour, rewarming rates average 1° to 3° C per hour. Abdominal adhesions increase the complication rate and minimize heat exchange. However, peritoneal lavage offers the additional advantage of detoxification from rhabdomyolysis or drug overdose if hemodialysis is unavailable. Drugs removed by peritoneal dialysis include aspirin, cimetidine, isoniazid, phenobarbital, and many others. A nephrologist, toxicologist, or poison control specialist should be consulted for specific detoxification guidelines.

Using a Foley catheter, *bladder irrigation* may be done with 200- to 300-mL aliquots of warmed crystalloid. The small surface area available for heat exchange is a disadvantage of this technique.

Gastrointestinal irrigation has been used to rewarm patients. Using a commercially available kit designed for gastric decontamination (or a nasogastric tube), 200- to 300-mL aliquots of crystalloid warmed to 40° to 42° C (104° to 107.6° F) are instilled into the stomach and drained using a Y connector and clamp. Regurgitation with possible aspiration is a complication of this procedure. Rewarming rates range from 1.0° to 2.0° C per hour.

Instilling heated irrigant into the thorax through a tube thoracostomy is another option. With this technique, 200- to 300-mL aliquots of warmed crystalloid should be infused through a Y connector, left in place for several minutes, and then drained. Because clinical experience with this technique is extremely limited, it should be reserved for cardiac arrest resuscitations.

Extracorporeal rewarming, such as cardiopulmonary bypass (CPB) and hemodialysis, has been used successfully in severely hypothermic patients. These techniques should be considered in patients with severe hypothermia that does not respond to less invasive rewarming measures or in patients with a completely frozen extremity or rhabdomyolysis associated with severe electrolyte disturbances. The advantage of CPB is preservation of blood flow if cardiac activity is absent. In CPB, blood is generally shunted in a femoral-femoral circuit. Complications of CPB include air embolism, hemolysis, DIC, vessel damage, and pulmonary edema. Hemodialysis is likely to be a more widely available and practical rewarming technique with the advent of two-way flow catheters that allow cannulation of a single vessel. If CPB and hemodialysis are not available and the patient is severely hypothermic, all other rewarming techniques should be used in combination.

Diathermy involves the transmission of heat by conversion of energy, e.g., ultrasound or low-frequency microwave radiation. Using these two modalities, potentially large quantities of heat are transferable. Presently, these techniques are experimental.

PERIPHERAL COLD INJURIES

Frostbite occurs when tissue temperature drops below 0° C (32° F). Trench foot and immersion foot are nonfreezing injuries resulting from exposure to wet cold. A nonfreezing injury after exposure to dry cold is called chilblain (pernio).

The "pre-freeze" phase of frostbite consists of tissue cooling, increased blood viscosity, and microvascular constriction. As tissue freezes, extracellular ice crystals form. Intracellular water migrates extracellularly, resulting in intracellular dehydration and hyperosmolality. Cell membranes subsequently become denatured, leading to cellular shrinkage and collapse. With cell death, vasoactive compounds are activated and released. Thromboxane A_2 and prostaglandin F_2 account for much of the injury associated with frostbite. In vivo, they contribute to platelet and erythrocyte aggregation, which leads to vascular occlusion and arteriovenous shunting. This "freezing cascade" is unique to peripheral cold injuries.

Clinical Presentation

Unlike with burns, classification of frostbite by degrees is often inaccurate. "Frostnip" is a superficial insult producing transient numbness or tingling that resolves with rewarming. This does not represent true frostbite because there is no tissue destruction. A history of complete and acute anesthesia in a painful cold digit suggests a severe frostbite injury. All patients with frostbite have a sensory deficit in pain, temperature, or light touch. The ears, nose, penis, and distal extremities are locations at greatest risk. On examination, frozen tissues can appear mottled, violaceous, pale yellow, or waxy.

Chilblain is a form of dry cold injury that often develops after repetitive exposure. It typically occurs in young females, especially those with Raynaud's phenomenon. Patients present with "cold sores," usually involving the face and dorsa of the hands and feet. Plaques, blue nodules, and ulcerations may eventually develop.

Trench foot is produced by prolonged exposure to cold moisture at above-freezing temperatures. Initially, the feet appear erythematous, edematous, and cyanotic. There is often numbness and leg cramping. After warming, the skin remains erythematous, dry, and very painful to touch. Bullae may form that are indistinguishable from those associated with frostbite. This vesiculation may proceed to ulceration and liquefaction gangrene. In milder cases, hyperhidrosis, cold sensitivity, and painful ambulation persist for years.

TABLE 2. **Treatment of Frostbite**

Before Thawing	After Thawing
Stabilize core temperature	Clear vesicles: aspirate if intact; débride if broken
Do not massage frozen part	Hemorrhagic vesicles: aspirate, do not débride
Avoid partial thawing and refreezing	Topical aloe vera every 6 hours (inhibits mediators)
Thawing	Nonsteroidal anti-inflammatory agents (for pain and mediator inhibition); these may increase propensity to infection
Parenteral analgesia and hydration	Tetanus prophylaxis
Rapid rewarming of entire part in 38° to 40° C circulating water	Elevate part in cradle
Requires 10 to 30 minutes with gentle motion of the part by the patient without friction massage	Whirlpool hydrotherapy two to three times daily for 20 to 30 minutes
	Avoid vasoconstrictors, including nicotine

Treatment

Before thawing, frozen parts should not be massaged or exposed to excessive or extreme focal dry heat (Table 2). A circulating tank of warm water, 38° to 40° C (100.4° to 104° F), is ideal for thawing frozen tissue. Temperatures greater than 42° C (107.6° F) should be avoided. Premature termination of rewarming secondary to pain is a common error. Therefore, parenteral analgesics should be given.

Rapid rewarming produces initial hyperemia. With rewarming, favorable signs include warmth, normal color, varying degrees of sensation, and early formation of clear vesicles or bullae. A residual violaceous hue or development of small hemorrhagic blebs is more ominous. In patients with severe frostbite, a dry black eschar may form and eventually mummifies. The final demarcation between viable and dead tissue may take several months, hence the surgical maxim, "frostbite in January, amputate in July."

There is no conclusive evidence that enhanced tissue salvage results in patients with frostbite with administration of dextran (Rheomacrodex), heparin, steroids, dimethylsulfoxide (Rimso-50), dipyridamole (Persantine), calcium channel blockers, or hyperbaric oxygen. A long-acting alpha blocker, phenoxybenzamine (Dibenzyline), 10 mg per day (up to a maximum of 60 mg per day), may decrease refractory vasospasm during the clinical course. A "medical" sympathectomy has the theoretical benefit of producing vasodilatation, decreased edema, and tissue salvage. It is achieved by injecting reserpine (Serpasil)* 0.5 mg intra-arterially. The injection produces local depletion of arterial wall norepinephrine for 2 to 4 weeks; no undesirable side effects have been observed at this dose. Treatment of chilblains may respond to nifedipine (Procardia) at a dose of 20 to 60 mg daily.

DISTURBANCES DUE TO HEAT

method of
PETER HANSON, M.D.
University of Wisconsin Clinical Science Center
Madison, Wisconsin

Heat illness represents a continuum of morbid responses to heat exposure in which fluid and electrolyte balance, cardiovascular regulation, and central nervous system function are progressively impaired. Heat illnesses occur most frequently in athletes, military recruits, and outdoor workers who perform sustained activity in warm, humid environments. Episodic heat illness is also associated with seasonal heat waves and commonly affects the elderly, homeless, and patients taking medications with anticholinergic activity.

HEAT SYNCOPE

Heat syncope usually occurs in the setting of heat exposure and orthostatic stress such as standing in military formation. Another cause is inappropriate use of whirlpool and sauna baths, especially after exercise or alcohol ingestion. Cutaneous vasodilation, the absence of muscle venous pump activity, and moderate fluid loss due to sweating all contribute to reduced central venous return and low ventricular filling volumes. Syncope is probably mediated by activation of ventricular stretch receptors due to inadequate filling, causing vagal reflex bradycardia and loss of sympathetic vasomotor tone (Bezold-Jarisch reflex). Treatment is supportive; vital signs should be monitored closely and the airway protected from tongue obstruction or emesis. Venous return is initially enhanced by raising the lower extremities and cooling the skin. Volume repletion may be required if orthostatic intolerance persists (see later discussion). Victims of heat syncope should be questioned about the possible role of drugs or alcohol or a history of recurrent orthostatic intolerance.

*Not available in the United States.

HEAT EXHAUSTION

Heat exhaustion is a syndrome of progressive volume depletion due to sustained sweat loss with inadequate fluid replacement; it typically occurs in athletes (football players, runners) who are inadequately acclimatized. Symptoms include progressive fatigue, weakness, nausea, and dizziness. Rectal temperature is moderately increased (38° to 39.5° C), the skin is cool and vasoconstricted, and active sweating is present. Supine heart rate is mildly elevated, and blood pressure is in the low normal or hypotensive range (Table 1). With orthostatic stress there is a marked decrease in blood pressure with systolic values falling to below 90 mmHg. Laboratory studies reveal hemoconcentration, variable electrolyte patterns (due to the combined effects of sweat losses and hemoconcentration), and increased urine specific gravity. Initial treatment is similar to that given for heat syncope but with added emphasis on active cooling and intravascular volume repletion using oral (e.g., 2.5 grams of NaCl per liter) or intravenous electrolyte fluids (Table 2). If intravenous fluids are required, one-half or one-quarter normal saline may be more appropriate because these approximate the sodium concentration of unacclimatized sweat. Glucose and water

TABLE 1. **Clinical Findings in Heat Illness**

	Heat Exhaustion	Heat Stroke
Level of consciousness	Mild confusion Presyncope on standing	Marked alteration Delirium, coma
Skin	Vasoconstricted Active sweating	Vasodilated Dry or sweating
Rectal temperature	38° to 40° C	>42° C
Cardiovascular signs	Heart rate 90 to 120 bpm Systolic blood pressure usually <110 mmHg with marked orthostatic drop of >20 mmHg	Heart rate >120 bpm Systolic blood pressure varies—low if in shock Low vascular resistance
Laboratory studies	Hemoconcentration Variable electrolyte levels Mild increase in muscle enzymes	Multisystem abnormalities: ↑ muscle, hepatic enzymes ↑ uric acid, lactate, K^+ ↓ coagulation factors ↓ platelets + myoglobinuria + hemoglobinuria

↑ = increased, ↓ = decreased, + = present (abnormal finding).

TABLE 2. **Treatment of Heat Illnesses**

	Evaluation and Therapy	Additional Considerations
Heat syncope	Elevate legs, restore venous return and vasomotor tone Fluid replacement and cooling of skin as needed	Possible drug effects Baroreflex disorders (if recurrent)
Heat exhaustion	Monitor VS, rectal temperature Fluid replacement PO or IV to restore orthostatic BP and urine output	Laboratory studies (CBC, electrolytes, BUN, creatinine, U/A) for severe hypotension or suspected prior hyperthermia
Heat stroke	Treat as multisystem injury with continuous VS monitoring Immediate cooling to <39° C (avoid body immersion) Comprehensive baseline laboratory tests (see text) Initiate diuresis with mannitol or loop diuretic Fluid replacement as needed to maintain BP and urine output Judicious use of vasopressors, inotropic agents if needed	Watch for: Rhabdomyolysis Renal failure (ATN) Hepatic failure Disseminated intravascular coagulation Hypoglycemia

Abbreviations: BP = blood pressure; VS = vital signs; ATN = acute tubular necrosis; U/A = urinalysis; CBC = complete blood count; BUN = blood urea nitrogen.

should be used with caution because hyponatremia may occur if hypotonic fluid replacement is excessive. Intravenous fluid therapy should be guided by stabilization of vital signs and normalization of orthostatic hypotension, serum electrolyte values, and urine output. Extensive laboratory work is usually unnecessary unless there is evidence of concomitant hyperthermia as discussed subsequently.

HEAT STROKE

Heat stroke is a critical extension of the heat exhaustion syndrome that may present in a classic or exertional form. *Classic heat stroke* occurs with prolonged heat exposure, progressive hyperthermia, and eventual cessation of sweating. *Exertional heat stroke* occurs over a shorter time and is associated with the combined effects of heat exposure and high-intensity exercise. Sweating is usually present but is inadequate to provide effective cooling.

In both forms of heat stroke there is marked central nervous system impairment ranging from delirium to coma and convulsions. The rectal temperature exceeds 42° C but may be lower after transport to a medical facility. The skin is warm and flushed unless circulatory collapse has occurred. There is moderate to severe tachycardia and variable blood pressure values depending on cardiac function and vasomotor tone.

Emergency treatment requires a multisystem management approach. Immediate cooling of body temperature is essential. Immersion in an ice bath is now discouraged because intense cutaneous vasoconstriction may inhibit heat loss. Alternative methods that are highly effective include application of ice packs to the neck, axillae, and groin (areas of vascular countercurrent exchange) and spraying of the skin with tepid water while fanning vigorously to promote evaporative cooling. Rectal temperature must be monitored continuously. Active cooling should be discontinued when body temperature falls to 39° C. Consciousness usually returns at this point. Insertion of large-bore intravenous catheter lines and a Foley catheter is also essential.

The hemodynamic state resembles that characteristic of a low vascular resistance circulatory failure. Cardiovascular support may require the judicious use of vasopressors (dopamine or norepinephrine) along with inotropic agents (dobutamine) and intravenous fluids (saline). However, fluid should be administered in small boluses of 250 to 500 mL to avoid cerebral or pulmonary edema. Urine output should be monitored carefully, and mannitol (0.5 grams per kg) or furosemide (Lasix) (1 mg per kg) should be administered to initiate diuresis. Comprehensive laboratory studies include a complete blood count (CBC) with platelet count, liver function panel, creatinine kinase, coagulation panel, glucose, lactate, electrolytes, calcium, uric acid, blood urea nitrogen (BUN), creatinine, and arterial blood gases. The urine should be tested for the presence of hemoglobin or myoglobin (Table 2).

Major complications include hypoglycemia, metabolic acidosis, renal failure due to acute tubular necrosis, rhabdomyolysis, disseminated intravascular coagulation syndrome, and hepatic failure. Some recent studies suggest that endotoxemia originating from increased gastrointestinal permeability may also play a role in the clinical manifestations of heat stroke syndrome. Patients with documented or suspected heat stroke should always be admitted for observation because these complications may not develop for 24 to 48 hours. Some studies have indicated that victims of exertional heat stroke may exhibit abnormal thermoregulatory responses to exercise and remain at risk for repeated episodes of heat illness during heat exposure and exercise.

SPIDER BITES AND SCORPION STINGS

method of
PHILIP C. ANDERSON, M.D.
University of Missouri-Columbia
Columbia, Missouri

NORTH AMERICAN BROWN RECLUSE SPIDER (*Loxosceles reclusa*)

Many bites of the North American brown recluse spider (*Loxosceles reclusa*) are so trivial that they may not even be noticed, and most do not require medical care. Cutaneous loxoscelism consists of a quickly developing painful local necrosis of the skin at the site of the bite. Look for the sinking blue macule on the skin that signifies the underlying distinctive infarct caused by this venom. Rarely, severe hemolysis ensues after a bite. This hemolytic type of systemic loxoscelism is encountered mostly in small children. Finally, a wide variety of toxic erythemas, edemas, and other systemic allergic reactions to the bite may occur. Brown recluse spider bites are seen mostly from April through July in the Ohio–lower Mississippi–Missouri River region, which is the natural habitat of this spider.

The most important consideration in initial diagnosis is to avoid confusing an early necrotizing infection of the skin, such as streptococcal necrotizing fasciitis, with a recluse spider bite. Clinically significant recluse spider bites are almost invariably single necrotic lesions, usually measuring 0.5 to 2 cm in size, self-limited in spread, and lacking adenopathy or sustained general toxicity. If the patient is exceptionally toxic, hypotensive, or mentally confused, or if tender local lymph nodes are found, or if the necrosis is present in multiple sites or is progressive, exudative, or otherwise unusual, prompt evaluation for infection is crucial. A deep disk of skin should be obtained for histologic evaluation, Gram's stain, and culture.

A thoroughly credible diagnosis of loxoscelism depends on prompt recovery of the spider or fragments of the spider near the bite with expert independent identification by an entomologist. At the very least, the presence of numerous recluse spiders should be readily confirmed in the household or in the neighborhood. The clinical literature on loxoscelism overall is unreliable because these logical precautions about diagnosis have been ignored; in turn, the reader should ignore such unproven case reports. Remember, there are many other causes of focal cutaneous necrosis, including various infections, local thromboses, punctures, trauma, drug reactions, other bites, Arthus reactions, emboli to the skin, artifacts, and more. Even if one recovers a brownish spider next to the bite, all experts agree that several other common spiders, including *Lycosa* and *Chiracanthium,* can cause painful necrotic ulcers of the skin.

In the important cases of severe systemic North American loxoscelism that have been reported, the painful necrosis of the skin begins within a few hours of the bite, and hemolysis with hematuria usually is seen within 8 to 12 hours. An abrupt drop in the hemoglobin value from 14 grams to 4 grams is often seen in this severe syndrome, the child becoming suddenly very ill, pale, restless, and even comatose. Most reliably, the Coombs' test remains negative, and lactate dehydrogenase (LDH) values soar, sometimes to over 5000 units per liter. The free hemoglobin in the plasma damages the kidney, causing episodes of black hematuria followed by anuria. (Our own sparse experience with blood transfusion for these severely anemic children indicates that hemolysis usually becomes worse with this treatment, and so simple hydration is the primary treatment. Peritoneal dialysis may be necessary.) The simplest method of ruling out hemolytic loxoscelism is to test for blood in the urine. The hematocrit shows the hemolysis even when hemoglobin tests do not. The laboratory can perform an accurate serum free–hemoglobin test only if it has been properly warned and instructed.

Patients with milder hemolysis may appear a bit jaundiced, the plasma free–hemoglobin and LDH may increase briefly, and transient hematuria may occur. No laboratory tests can yet confirm distinctively an early diagnosis of cutaneous loxoscelism, nor are there any immunologic tests that can confirm the diagnosis retrospectively. Progress in developing such tests seems imminent.

Formerly a "cave" spider, the recluse spider now has become a house spider but still is found around wooded river banks. Billions of recluse spiders share homes with millions of American citizens with very little conflict. Also called the violin spider, Missouri brown spider, or fiddle-back spider, the recluse spider is small, long-legged, and smooth and may be tan to black. The distinctive violin marking may not always be visible. Cleanliness in the home or good "bug control" will not prevent spider bites, nor can recluse spiders be eliminated even by using illegal excess amounts of pesticides. Spiders are insensitive to many insecticides. However, eating in bed or leaving crumbs that are subsequently attractive to the spider may not be smart. I recommend shaking out one's bathrobe after a long absence. On entering an attic or storeroom to open boxes, give these shy spiders a chance to vacate the space because recluse spiders nest in and under cardboard boxes; they will avoid you if they can. Patients recovered from proven loxoscelism usually do not react noticeably to subsequent bites.

TREATMENT

No therapy at all is needed for simple cutaneous loxoscelism beyond a tetanus booster if one is due. Unnecessary treatments include the use of commercial antivenoms, antibiotics, antihistamines, steroids, hyperbaric oxygen, vasodilators, and dapsone. No proper studies have proved any benefit from any such therapies. More important, nearly all untreated patients have no problems whatever and heal very well. Don't accept marginal treatments that have not been randomly well tested against placebo. The manufacturer's directions cite a relative contraindication to the use of dapsone in any patient with an illness that involves hemolysis. Pain can be controlled by splinting, resting, and elevating the injured body part as well as by medication.

Treatment of hemolysis in patients with systemic loxoscelism depends on achieving prompt hydration and restoring homeostasis in the hospital. Expert nephrologists, usually pediatricians, may give assistance. However terrible the first laboratory results seem, the crisis is short because the venom is quickly destroyed and the hemolytic episode is brief. Therapists become concerned about the many bizarre laboratory findings, especially the alarmingly low hemoglobin and the sudden anuria. Reliably we find a consumption of fibrinogen and an early rise in fibrin degradation products. This disorder is like a disseminated intravascular coagulopathy (DIC) that most closely resembles the hemolysis-uremia syndrome. Some medical centers employ steroids, heparin, or other means, and the local peer-reviewed approach to the treatment of DIC is probably the best plan. We use low-dose heparin. No one plan for the treatment of systemic loxoscelism has been thoroughly studied; proven cases are too few. Seek advice from experienced physicians as problems arise.

The various toxic erythemas, urticarias, and angioedemas caused by loxoscelism (without hemolysis or DIC) are self-limited, but the patient may be very uncomfortable. Prednisone* therapy seems to relieve most of these problems promptly, but no proper study entirely supports such a claim.

Plainly, cutaneous loxoscelism has been much overtreated. The impulse to excise the lesion widely, as was once vigorously promoted, is especially ill advised in view of the excellent progress made without it and because such excisions seem to delay healing. Wide excision is not practiced today by experts.

BLACK WIDOW SPIDER BITES

Latrodectus venom is a neurotoxin that exerts all its damage by dumping acetylcholine and vasopressors from the nervous system. No reaction in the skin may be seen at all. After a proven bite, symptoms may be negligible, or the victim may experience hypertension, headache, muscular rigidity and spasm, hyperreflexia, vomiting, abdominal pain, agitation, or psychosis. Such a state is easily distinguished from an infection in that patients display flaccidity, hypotension, and depression, as for example, with appendicitis.

These spiders are known for a bright red hourglass mark on the abdomen, although this feature is variable. They are found outdoors, especially in barns, woodpiles, electrical boxes, around livestock, and, notoriously, under the seat in old-fashioned outhouses.

Treatment consists of providing relief of symptoms with generous doses of muscle relaxants such as diazepam (Valium) and with a 10% solution of calcium gluconate intravenously, in 10-mL increments, with rehydration. Recent experience with the antivenom (antivenin [Latrodectus mactans]) is obscure. Severe relapses and odd late vasomotor reactions are common, so the patient should be followed for a few days after apparent recovery has occurred.

SCORPIONS

In most of the United States, stings of native scorpions such as *Centruroides vittatus* cause about the same harm as stings by hornets. The exception is the sting of the small Mexican scorpion, *Centruroides sculpturatus.* This scorpion may be encountered in Arizona or a few other border sites. The venom has actions similar to the venom of the black widow spider, and similar modes of treatment with relaxants, calcium gluconate, and antivenom may be useful. Most stings in healthy adults are not dire, but deaths and severe illnesses do occur, mostly in children in whom damage to the neurologic system may be severe. Because scorpion stings are unusually variable, local experts should be consulted. For stings by the lesser U.S. scorpions, cool packs, splinting, rest, and relaxants should suffice.

*This drug has not been approved by the FDA for this indication.

VENOMOUS SNAKEBITE

method of
RICHARD F. CLARK, M.D.
San Diego Regional Poison Center
San Diego, California

The great majority of poisonous snakebites in the United States are inflicted by members of the Crotalidae family. Genera of crotalid (also called pit vipers) found in this country include *Crotalus* (rattlesnakes), *Sistrurus* (massasaugas), and *Akistrodon* (copperheads and cottonmouths). *Crotalus* envenomations tend to be most severe and frequently result from intentional handling or mishandling of captured or "pet" snakes. Crotalids are not aggressive and strike only when threatened.

Pit vipers can be identified by several characteristic features. Their heads are triangular, and they have elliptical pupils and a facial "pit" located below each nostril. The pit is actually an organ sensitive to temperature change that allows the snake to locate warm-blooded prey. Crotalids have evolved an efficient venom delivery apparatus consisting of curved, hinged, hollow front fangs connected to a muscular gland. The fangs may be up to 2 cm in length and can penetrate muscular compartments. *Crotalus* species also have terminal horny scales that have evolved into a "rattle" (except *Crotalus catalinensis,* found only on Santa Catalina Island in California). Although most defensive strikes are preceded by a rattling sound, a frightened snake may strike without this warning.

The clinical spectrum produced by crotalid envenomation depends on the site of envenomation, the type and geographic location of snake, the patient's overall state of health, and perhaps even the time of year. Although bites may produce significant morbidity, fatalities are rare. A review of over 2200 crotalid envenomations reported during the past 2 years noted only two fatalities. One of these resulted from airway loss in a patient envenomated on the lip, and the other resulted from a severe anaphylactic reaction following the administration of antivenom. More than 25% of all snakebites are "dry bites," in which no venom is actually injected. Clinical findings in these patients consist only of one or more puncture wounds.

Crotalid venom contains a complex of enzymes that are cytotoxic, hemotoxic, and neurotoxic and can damage vascular endothelium. A variety of heavy metals and amino acids are also present within the venom, but their significance is unclear. The first clinical evidence of crotalid envenomation is pain and swelling in proximity to the puncture wounds, usually within 6 to 8 hours of the bite. Many victims complain of a metallic taste in the mouth soon after being envenomated. Systemic effects such as fasciculations, weakness, dizziness, and gastroenteritis are frequent. Hypotension may occur but is less common. Edema may progress rapidly and may involve the entire extremity. Hemorrhagic blisters resembling the thermal injuries seen in burns or frostbite frequently form around the punctures, enlarging over several days. When the blisters are unroofed, third-degree tissue destruction is often noted and can result in significant soft tissue defects or even autoamputation of the digit. Although swelling of the affected extremity can be massive, circulatory compromise is rare. Compartment syndrome (compartment pressures of more than 30 mmHg) may occasionally develop as a result of direct intramuscular envenomation.

The other significant clinical effect of crotalid envenomation is hematologic toxicity. Venom components may have "thrombin-like" effects on fibrinogen molecules within the circulation, resulting in falling fibrinogen levels. A lack of significant cross-linking of fibrin monomers usually does not lead to intravascular coagulation, but elevations in prothrombin (PT) and partial thromboplastin (PTT) times are frequently documented. Thrombocytopenia is also common in victims of significant envenomation and may be seen in the absence of dropping fibrinogen levels. Massive envenomations, especially those into vascular structures, may produce laboratory and physical findings consistent with disseminated intravascular coagulation, and these patients are at high risk for bleeding.

Two other poisonous snakes within the family of Elapidae are found in the United States—the Eastern (*Micrurus fulvius fulvius*) and Texas (*Micrurus fulvius tenere*) coral snakes. The Sonoran coral snake (*Micruroides euryxanthus euryxanthus*) is limited to parts of Arizona and rarely produces severe toxicity. Coral snakes are brightly colored with black, red, and yellow ringed stripes and can be separated from similarly colored nonpoisonous snakes in North America by the contiguity of the red and yellow rings (remembered by the mnemonic "red on yellow, kill a fellow; red on black, venom lack"). Coral snakes have small oval heads and small mouths with short, fixed, posterior fangs and must chew to inject venom. Envenomations from these snakes are infrequent but can be life-threatening. Coral snake venom contains mostly neurotoxic components that can cause weakness, lethargy, respiratory insufficiency, and paralysis but do not usually cause tissue injury. Regional poison centers can aid in the identification and management of both exotic and native snakebites.

TREATMENT

Numerous misconceptions exist about efficacious therapies for crotalid envenomation. First, although many varieties of suction devices have been used to remove snake venom, none has proved effective in influencing patient outcome. It has long been recommended to use these devices or even one's own mouth to remove venom after incising the puncture site. In reality, because crotalid fangs are curved and may be up to several millimeters long, it is impossible to estimate accurately the site or depth of the actual venom injection. Bacterial inoculation of the wound may also occur during these procedures. No attempt therefore should be made to remove the venom.

Second, there is no evidence that placing a tourniquet proximal to the envenomation site on an extremity affects the outcome. Animal studies have confirmed that a "constricting band" retards the lymphatic flow of venom in a swine model. It is far more likely that an overzealous victim or pre-hospital care provider will create an obstruction to either venous or arterial blood flow in this situation. Therefore, a tourniquet is not recommended.

Third, ice should be used sparingly on a snakebitten extremity. Although ice can be an effective prehospital analgesic, extended exposure in these patients can cause thermal injury and further compromise the circulation. Limiting movement of the extremity with a splint or sling may provide some pain relief during transport to a hospital.

Finally, *prophylactic* fasciotomy has been initiated on arrival of patients with crotalid envenomations in some institutions whenever an extremity demonstrates massive edema, even when signs and symptoms of compartment syndrome are not yet present. Compartment syndrome is uncommon in aggressively treated envenomations, and fasciotomy is indicated only in patients with a severe envenomation when intracompartmental pressures are measured as elevated and signs and symptoms of impaired circulation are documented.

The proper definitive management of crotalid envenomation should focus on rapid transportation to a health care facility, aggressive use of antivenom as indicated later, and good supportive care. As stated earlier, fatalities from crotalid envenomation are rare in this country. All patients should be observed for 6 to 12 hours after the bite for signs of toxicity. If no signs or symptoms have been documented by that time, the victim can be sent home as long as follow-up care is available. If envenomation appears to be evident, with swelling, pain, or early systemic effects such as nausea, vomiting, or dizziness, the patient should be placed in a monitored setting, intravenous access should be established, and the patient should be closely followed. Blood should be drawn and evaluated, and special attention should be paid to hematology results including a complete blood count, fibrinogen level, fibrin split products, platelet count, and coagulation studies. These tests should be repeated as the patient's condition indicates. Intravenous rehydration should be initiated because large amounts of fluid can be third-spaced into the affected extremity and rhabdomyolysis often occurs in which there are massive elevations in creatine phosphokinase (CPK) resulting from severe swelling of muscular compartments and direct venom effects on myocytes.

A grading scale has been devised for crotalid envenomation and may aid in determining the need for antivenom. Minimal envenomation consists of localized pain and edema, but laboratory tests are normal, and there is an absence of systemic symptoms. Moderate envenomation shows spreading pain and edema, mild to moderately abnormal coagulation studies (fibrinogen level less than 100 mg/dL) or thrombocytopenia (platelet count less than 100,000), and mild systemic effects such as dizziness, nausea, and vomiting. Severe envenomations are evident by rapidly spreading and extensive pain and edema, hypotension, pulmonary edema, severe gastroenteritis, marked coagulopathy or thrombocytopenia, disseminated intravascular coagulation, or altered neurologic function such as depressed mentation.

Polyvalent antivenin (Crotalidae) should be used for patients with moderate to severe envenomations. Crotalidae antivenin is horse serum derived from the venoms of four crotalids found in North and South America: *Crotalus atrox, Crotalus adamanteus, Crotalus durissus terrificus,* and *Bothrops atrox.* The antivenom can reverse hemotoxicity and slow the progression of edema, but the equine origin of this product can promote both immediate and delayed hypersensitivity reactions. Patients likely to develop hypersensitivity reactions include those with allergies to horses or horse serum, and severe asthmatics. These patients should not receive antivenom unless they are severely envenomated. Blood products are not usually needed if antivenom is used aggressively and should be reserved for the actively bleeding or hemolyzing individual.

Crotalidae antivenin is reconstituted and infused intravenously in normal saline solution. We administer antivenom in 10-vial increments, infusing the contents of 10 vials over 30 to 60 minutes. Skin testing is performed with horse serum test solution (included with antivenom) prior to the infusion. Approximately 0.1 mL of the solution is injected subcutaneously, and the patient is observed for 10 to 15 minutes. Although a reaction to the horse serum skin test may identify some allergic individuals, it is not 100% sensitive. A negative test does not rule out the possibility that the patient may have an anaphylactic reaction to the antivenom. Hypersensitivity or allergic reactions should be managed as in any other situation with epinephrine and histamine receptor blockers such as diphenhydramine. Epinephrine can be administered subcutaneously or as a continuous infusion in severe cases. If antivenom is infusing when the reaction is observed, it should be stopped.

After each infusion of crotalid antivenom, the patient should be re-evaluated for ongoing toxicity. A bitten extremity can be splinted and elevated for comfort. Analgesics such as morphine should be administered liberally. Hematology tests should be repeated an hour or so after the end of the infusion. If signs of bleeding or toxicity continue, more antivenom is required. An "average" moderate or severe envenomation may require 20 to 30 vials before resolution of signs and symptoms is noted. Mild swelling may not respond immediately to antivenom and may progress over several days. Elevation of the affected extremity can distribute edema to more proximal structures, relieving pain and possibly avoiding severe elevations in compartmental pressure. Distal blood flow and neurologic function of the bitten extremity should be monitored. Because crotalid venom has some antibacterial properties, empirical antibiotic coverage is not usually required unless secondary wound infection occurs. Patients can be discharged once hematologic toxicity has been reversed and swelling is decreasing. Tetanus toxoid boosters should be provided as indicated. Physical therapy may be required in some of these patients to improve range of motion of the extremity.

Clinically significant bites from coral snakes require more aggressive administration of antivenom because these effects are not easily reversed. Coral snake antivenom (antivenin [*Micrurus fulvius*]) should be administered in 5- to 10-vial increments. Loss of neurologic function may begin soon after envenomation and can progress to paralysis and respiratory arrest. Coral snake antivenom should be administered to all patients who have definitely been bitten by one of these snakes or have developed signs or symptoms of toxicity.

Delayed hypersensitivity reactions are seen in the majority of patients receiving crotalid antivenom. Symptoms usually begin 5 to 10 days after administration of antivenom and resemble the symptoms of a viral syndrome with myalgias, arthralgias, urticarial rashes, and occasionally low-grade fever. Once recognized, these manifestations can be reduced with antihistamines and corticosteroids but rarely pose any life-threatening danger. All patients receiving antivenom should be warned after they recover of the possibility of more severe immediate hypersensitivity on readministration of horse serum products.

Most patients survive snakebites if standard advanced life-support techniques are applied. Supplemental information on the treatment of severe envenomations or infrequently encountered toxicities can be obtained from medical toxicologists or regional poison centers.

HAZARDOUS MARINE ANIMALS

method of
BRUCE FLAREAU, M.D., and
DAVID O. PARRISH, M.D.
Bayfront Family Practice Center
St. Petersburg, Florida

The uniqueness of the marine environment carries with it a number of inherent dangers. The many hazardous marine animals include sharks, stingrays, barracudas, and sea snakes as well as less notorious animals such as stinging jellyfish and sea urchins. There are even hazards from the ingestion of sea animals. Although many of these injuries have specific treatment caveats, the approach to marine injury starts with the basics of first aid and general medical care. In the following discussion we provide an overview of the general approach to a variety of the more common marine injuries.

FIRST AID

In the approach to a marine injury, one must consider specific difficulties that relate to the environment in which the accident occurs. Thus, before administering initial or definitive treatment, one must remove the patient from the water to avoid drowning or further insult while simultaneously ensuring one's own safety. Basic life-support procedures should follow if necessary. Once the airway has been cleared, breathing is established, and circulation is ensured, other problems may be addressed. Wounds should be covered and bleeding controlled with direct pressure. Next, attention may be directed toward removing any remnants of marine life from the patient and neutralizing any toxins. If one is unable to remove or neutralize the toxin or venom, one must prepare to deal with the effects of these toxins. This situation applies in patients with injuries containing sea snake venom, stingray toxins, or poisonous octopus or scorpion fish venom, among others. Once the toxins have been addressed, attention should be directed toward the need for therapeutic or prophylactic antibiotics. Other areas of concern for which the physician should be prepared include anaphylaxis, near-drowning, alcohol or illicit drug use, and barotrauma relating to diving injuries. As with any accident victim, a careful history is important, including previous medical problems and medications.

MARINE TRAUMA

Open Wounds and General Wound Management

Bites. Open wounds and general wound management are certainly no different for marine trauma. Sharks may produce crush and laceration injuries depending on the size of the shark. Such crush injuries can devitalize tissue and require considerable débridement before closure is undertaken. The great barracuda and moray eels can also produce puncture wounds and lacerations that require attention. Large bite wounds should be managed initially by ensuring hemostasis. Apply direct pressure for immediate control while placing the patient in a supine position and monitoring for signs of shock. If there is considerable bleeding, placement of a tourniquet may be necessary until the bleeding can be controlled. As in similar cases, to avoid tissue hypoxia the tourniquet should not be placed so that it prevents all blood flow for a prolonged period of time. Once the patient is stable or if the wound is less severe, the next step is to clean the wound thoroughly. If there is doubt about tissue viability, the wound should probably not be closed primarily. Apply topical antiseptic and consider prophylactic antibiotics to cover the most common organisms. Administer systemic antibiotics if the wound shows signs of infection (see later section on infectious disease).

Coral Wounds. True corals inflict open cuts or abrasions when the victim brushes against them. These lacerations tend to heal slowly, with the patient experiencing discomfort for as long as several weeks to months. This slow resolution may be the result of infection or retained particles of the coral itself and may be accompanied by granuloma or keloid formation. For this reason, vigorous cleansing, irrigation with saline, and débridement of the wound are recommended. In addition, hydrogen peroxide should be used to remove small coral particles from within the wound. Systemic antibiotics are usually unnecessary but if used should cover *Vibrio* species (see later section on infectious disease). Following initial therapy, daily scrubbing or wet to dry dressings with subsequent topical antibiotic dressing may be needed. These measures will minimize granuloma and keloid formation. Topical steroids may be necessary for pruritus or if keloid tissue begins to form. Once established, keloids may be better addressed with intra-lesional steroids.

Puncture Wounds

Puncture wounds can be produced by various marine animals such as sea urchins, starfish, bristleworms, and certain types of fish.

Sea Urchins. Depending on the type of sea urchin, the spines may or may not contain toxins. Contact with those that do may cause intense pain and burning. Other symptoms typically include erythema and swelling but may also include hemorrhage, paresthesia, paralysis, respiratory failure, and, in rare cases, death. These symptoms may occur when the victim handles, steps on, or brushes against the spines. Treatment includes débridement of the wound as well as surgical removal of spines that have lodged at or near a joint. Immersing the lesion in nonscalding hot water may help with pain control, neutralize the toxins, and sometimes dissolve spines. This may also work on other types of spiny corals as well as certain types of fish spines. Purple dye leached from sea urchin spines may be mistaken for retained spines. Even so, attempts should be made to remove all fragments because any retained pieces may form the nidus for a granuloma. It should be realized that although the spines should usually be removed, more tissue destruction may occur in attempting an unsuccessful removal than in allowing the spine to dissolve on its own. Antibiotic therapy is usually unnecessary. Starfish and bristleworms are treated similarly.

Catfish and Scorpion Fish. Like sea urchins, catfish and scorpion fish pose a special concern of possible retained fragments from the embedded spine of the fish. The fragment is radiopaque, and wounds of this type should routinely be radiographed. Treatment is the same as that given for stingray envenomations. Antivenom is available for scorpion fish envenomations.

Infectious Disease

Patients with marine-acquired wounds should receive tetanus prophylaxis as with any tetanus-prone wound.

Microbiology and Antibiotic Selection. Marine infections may involve a host of organisms. Commonly, streptococci and staphylococci are the infecting agents. Of equal concern, however, are the marine-specific bacteria such as the *Vibrio* species, *Mycobacterium marinum, Erysipelothrix,* and *Pseudomonas* species. Of these, *Vibrio* appears to be the most prevalent. Because they are resistant to penicillins and cephalosporins, *Vibrio* species require a quinolone, sulfa agent, or tetracycline for adequate treatment. Owing to the side effect of photosensitivity, tetracycline is poorly tolerated in the Sunbelt, and for this reason a quinolone such as ciprofloxacin (Cipro) or ofloxacin (Floxin) or trimethoprim-sulfamethoxazole (Bactrim or Septra) is often the selected agent. Any marine infection not responding to a penicillin or cephalosporin should be given a trial with one of these agents. It should be remembered that because the quinolones are not the best coverage for a likely streptococcal infection, they may not be the best first-line treatment.

Fish Handler's Disease. Fish handler's disease is a condition manifested by a blister-like rash on the hands of marine-exposed individuals. Actually a cutaneous infection caused by *Erysipelothrix,* it should be treated with penicillin, erythromycin, or a cephalosporin.

COMMON MARINE ENVENOMATIONS

General Approach

Always remove the patient from the water, administer first aid, and prepare for shock, anaphylaxis, hypothermia, or other environmental hazards.

Animal-Specific Approach

Stingrays. One of the most common marine injuries is envenomation by a stingray. As the unwary beachgoer wades into the water and disturbs the fish, it reflexly strikes with its barbed "tail." Actually a caudal appendage, the tail contains a heat-labile poison that accounts for most of the morbidity. The venom reaches maximal effect within 30 to 60 minutes. Treatment involves getting the victim safely out of the water and immersing the involved extremity in the hottest water the individual can tolerate (approximately 40° C). This denatures the protein venom and minimizes any destruction. After immersing the extremity for 20 to 40 minutes, the wound can be cleaned out and treated like any other puncture wound. In the interim, local anesthesia either into the wound or as a field block may help the patient who is in excruciating pain. Less common are systemic symptoms that include seizures, limb paralysis, hypotension, and bradycardia. Tetanus prophylaxis should be given as for all tetanus-prone wounds. Antimicrobial prophylaxis is optional, but if given it should cover *Vibrio* species (see later section on infectious disease). Avoidance is the best treatment. In areas where stingray attacks are common, the "stingray shuffle" becomes a way of life. This involves shuffling the feet to scare the fish away, thus avoiding coming into contact with its wing and suffering the consequences of its tail.

Jellyfish. Another common marine envenomation is that caused by the jellyfish. Unlike the stingray injury, however, these lesions are superficial and involve microscopic injection cells called nematocysts. These cells carry spearlike lances that can inject venom into the victim even after the jellyfish has been long dead. Thus, people may be exposed on the beach if they touch dead jellyfish that have washed ashore. These nematocysts are sensitive to changes in osmolarity and therefore fire to stimuli such as fresh water. For this reason, first aid involves soaking the area in vinegar to stop the cysts from firing. Careful removal of any remaining tentacles should be done by scraping the wound and then irrigating it with an isotonic solution such as seawater or saline. Reactions range from minor to severe depending on the organism. The Portuguese man-of-war and the deadly box jellyfish are perhaps the most notorious examples of jellyfish envenomations. Common signs and symptoms are pain, erythema, lacrimation, arrhythmia, mental confusion, spasms, and shock. Treatment is supportive by alleviating the pain, inhibiting further discharge, removing nematocysts that remain, and avoiding shock. Intravenous calcium gluconate given slowly at a dose of 0.1 to 0.2 mL per kg can sometimes relieve muscle spasms and may be lifesaving if severe spasms involve the diaphragm. Antivenom is available for box jellyfish stings from the National Zoo, Washington, D.C.

Corals. Of the corals, fire coral is by far the most feared by scuba divers. Many an unsuspecting diver has unexpectedly brushed against this coral, which takes many shapes and forms. Symptoms include intense pain, burning, erythema, and reactive adenopathy. Treatment includes denaturing the poison with vinegar or meat tenderizer. Most dive vessels carry this on board for the unfortunate diver. Other organisms in this category include sea anemones and hydroids, exposures to which are treated in a similar fashion.

Sponges. Sponges are capable of producing both irritant and contact dermatitis. The local dermatitis is characterized by erythema and pruritus, but it may form vesicles and cause desquamation. Small spicules may cause a burning or weeping lesion. Adhesive tape may be used acutely to débride the wound of any retained spicules. Dilute vinegar soaks and topical steroids may facilitate healing.

Mollusks. Cone shells are known to inflict envenomations that can be deadly, and care should be taken to avoid the venomous sting. If the victim is stung, the venom may produce perioral and peripheral paresthesia that can be followed by respiratory failure and death. The blue octopus bite can produce similar neurologic symptoms and paralysis. Treatment is supportive.

Sea Snakes. Sea snakes inhabit the warm temperate Pacific and Indian Oceans. There are no sea snakes in the Atlantic or Caribbean. Sea snakes have two to four hollow maxillary fangs with associated venom glands. Most fangs are too short to penetrate a diver's wet suit. Bites may resemble a pinprick and often number one to eight bites per victim but may go as high as 20. Little to no local reaction occurs, but neurologic symptoms occur 2 to 3 hours later and may include ascending paralysis, dysarthria, dysphagia, ptosis, ophthalmoplegia, and myopathy and myonecrosis with secondary myoglobinurea; death is rare. Supportive treatment is given in addition to antivenom obtained in regional poison centers.

AQUATIC DERMATOLOGY

Otitis Externa

The very common otitis externa, or "swimmer's ear," is precipitated by maceration of a wet ear canal.

This may be controlled by using ear solutions such as those containing boric acid, peroxide, or vinegar and alcohol. These solutions produce a slight antibacterial action with a drying effect, which prevents prolonged moisture and decreases the risk of maceration. Swimmers with long hair or other situations that cause the ears to remain wet for extended periods of time should consider use of a prophylactic ear solution. Typical signs include tenderness with pressure at the tragus or pain with traction on the earlobe. Debris can be suctioned out of the ear canal and a polymyxin B–neomycin-hydrocortisone (Cortisporin) solution or suspension applied. It is used four times a day for 5 to 10 days based on the patient's clinical response. If the canal is swollen enough to impede passage of the topical drops, a wick may have to be placed to ensure that the medication reaches its destination. A suspension is usually used if there is any concern about a perforated tympanic membrane, thus avoiding the irritating middle ear reaction. Occasionally, owing to the cortisone in the Cortisporin, there is a slight flare of the condition, but it usually resolves. If not, or if Cortisporin is not effective, gentamicin drops* can be used. If there is concern that otitis media is complicating the patient's condition, systemic antibiotics may be added. Extended spectrum agents such as amoxicillin-clavulinic acid (Augmentin) may be used if there is concern about *Haemophilus influenzae* resistance.

Dermatitis

There are numerous types of contact dermatitis. Treatment usually consists of removing any irritants or toxins and then applying topical or occasionally systemic steroids. This may be necessary because of the intense pruritic nature of some of these dermatoses. Antibiotics are usually not necessary.

Sea Lice. Seabather's eruption is caused by various newly determined larvae. The lesions are normally under the swimsuit where, owing to the pressure of the suit, the trapped larvae sting the individual. The treatment is topical steroids, although oral steroids are occasionally necessary.

Swimmer's Itch. Swimmer's itch may be a more serious problem. The marine swimmer's itch, or cercarial dermatitis, is typified by pruritic papules that occur on the exposed body areas by the boring action of the schistosome larvae. This condition may be treated by local or oral steroids. However, in fresh water these papules may be caused by schistosomes that are human parasites (*mansoni, haematobium, japonicum,* and *mekongi*) and may create the liver, lung, and bladder problems of schistosomiasis (bilharziasis). Insect repellents containing dimethyl phthalate may provide some protection, although avoidance is the preferred method. Treatment is the same as for sea lice.

Other Dermatitides. There is also a seawater-induced pruritus that can present with wheals or a blotchy rash. Various possible causes have been suggested for this aquagenic pruritus. Antihistamines may be used prophylactically or as treatment. Steroids can be used if necessary.

*This drug has not been approved by the FDA for this indication.

Bends

Decompression sickness Type I may manifest in the skin as a condition termed cutis marmorata. This involves nitrogen bubble obstruction of the cutaneous lymphatics with a secondary reticular-appearing rash. It may herald a more serious condition that may require recompression or oxygen therapy to relieve the symptoms.

MARINE INGESTION

Scombroid

Scombroid poisoning is the result of ingestion of decaying fish. The amino acid histidine is converted to histamine by bacteria, and the individual has a massive histamine exposure that presents much like anaphylaxis. Treatment is geared toward gastric lavage, cardiovascular support, and antihistamine therapy.

Ciguatera

Ciguatera is acquired by ingesting fish that themselves have ingested the offending dinoflagellate. Thought to be a type of flora found on the reef, it becomes concentrated during its progress up the food chain until a critical mass is ingested by the patient. The majority of fish implicated are grouper, snapper, jack, and barracuda, although almost any fish can be involved. The offending agent, known as ciguatoxin, is tasteless and is unaffected by refrigeration or cooking. The illness usually begins within 6 hours of ingestion and is characterized by gastrointestinal and neurologic symptoms. Initially the gastrointestinal symptoms predominate with abdominal cramps, nausea, vomiting, and diarrhea. These usually resolve within 24 to 48 hours and may be followed by neurologic symptoms, typically by the third to fifth day. In severe cases, bradycardia, shock, respiratory failure, and rarely death may occur. One unifying feature of this ingestion is the sensation of hot-cold reversal that may occur 3 to 5 days after the ingestion and may last for months in some individuals. Recurrent episodes tend to have increased severity, and thus victims should eliminate fish and fish derivatives from their diet. Other foods such as nuts and alcohol may precipitate recurrence and should be avoided for at least 6 months. Treatment is supportive for patients seeking care but may also involve diphenhydramine (Benadryl) for concomitant pruritus and mannitol for neurologic symptoms. Doses of mannitol of up to 1 gram per kg at a rate of 500 mL per hour have been used with success in small studies. Fortunately, the disease is usually self-limited;

however, preventive measures are certainly recommended.

Paralytic Shellfish Poisoning

The dinoflagellate again may cause this disease, manifested by tingling of the mouth and face that may spread to generalized paresthesia. Paralysis may ensue, with death being a very rare possibility. Gastric lavage to remove any remaining toxins is indicated, followed by supportive care.

Fugu (Tetrodotoxin)

Fugu is a Japanese delicacy from the puffer fish. The meat can be toxic if prepared improperly owing to the poisonous organs and skin of the fish. An old Biblical adage admonishing one not to eat fish without scales applies to the puffer fish, porcupine fish, and ocean sunfish, all of which contain the deadly tetrodotoxin. If the fish is improperly prepared and eaten, perioral paresthesia may progress to total paralysis and death. Gastric lavage with respiratory and cardiovascular support are the only known treatments.

ACUTE POISONINGS

method of
HOWARD C. MOFENSON, M.D.,
THOMAS R. CARACCIO, PHARM.D., and
JOSEPH GREENSHER, M.D.
Long Island Regional Poison Control Center
East Meadow, New York

BASIC MANAGEMENT OF POISONINGS

The severity of the manifestations of acute poisoning exposures varies greatly with the age and intent of the victim. Accidental poisoning exposures make up 80 to 85% of all poisoning episodes and are most frequent in children under 5 years of age. Many of these episodes are actually ingestions of relatively nontoxic substances that require minimal medical care. Intentional poisonings constitute 10 to 15% of poisonings, and often these patients require the highest standards of medical and nursing care and the occasional use of sophisticated equipment for recovery. Suicide attempts represent a significant number of these poisonings, and the use of toxic substances is often involved. The majority of the drug-related suicide attempts involve a central nervous system (CNS) depressant, and "coma management" is vital to the treatment.

Sixty percent of patients who take a drug overdose do so with their own prescribed medication and 15% with drugs prescribed for relatives. The top poisoning categories for all ages are over-the-counter analgesics, sedative-hypnotics, benzodiazepines, cleaning agents and petroleum products, alcohol and substance abuse, pesticides, tricyclic antidepressants, plants, carbon monoxide, and opioids.

ASSESSMENT AND MAINTENANCE OF VITAL FUNCTIONS

Upper airway obstruction is the most common cause of death in intoxicated patients outside the hospital. Any patient who is comatose and has absent protective airway reflexes is able to tolerate an endotracheal tube (cuffed for those over the age of 7 to 9 years) and should have it inserted as soon as possible.

Ventilation is required if the respiratory rate and depth are inadequate.

The circulatory status is best assessed by the blood pressure and heart rate and rhythm. The circulatory clinical status and tissue perfusion may be inferred from the skin temperature, the return of color after pressure blanching (capillary filling), and the urine output. Intra-arterial blood pressure measurements are essential for adequate monitoring.

If the circulation fails to improve after adequate ventilation and oxygenation, a 15- to 20-cm elevation of the foot of the bed may aid by increasing the venous return to the heart. A fluid challenge also may improve the circulatory status if hypovolemia is the cause. If these measures fail, plasma expanders and similar products may be required. As a last resort, vasopressors may be needed. If these measures fail to produce a response, a central venous pressure or pulmonary artery wedge pressure (PAWP) line should be inserted to monitor for heart failure and fluid overload.

The level of consciousness of all intoxicated patients should be assessed and the time of assessment recorded. The Glasgow Coma Score used in head trauma is not useful in intoxications because alcohol, depressant drugs, and hypotension may give falsely lowered scores. The Reed Coma Scale is preferred (Table 1).

PREVENTION OF ABSORPTION AND REDUCTION OF LOCAL DAMAGE

Ocular exposure should be immediately treated with water or saline irrigation for 20 minutes with eyelids fully retracted. Do not use neutralizing chemicals. All caustic and corrosive injuries should be evaluated by an ophthalmologist.

Dermal exposure is treated immediately with rinsing, not a forceful flushing in a shower, which might result in deeper penetration of the toxic substance. The skin should be rinsed with copious amounts of water for at least 30 minutes. Hair shampoo, cleansing of fingernails and navel, and irrigation of the eyes are necessary in an extensive exposure. The clothes may have to be discarded. Leather goods are irreversibly contaminated and must be abandoned. Caustic (alkali) exposures often require hours of irrigation until the "soapy" feeling of the burn is gone. Dermal absorption may occur with pesticides, hydrocarbons, and cyanide.

Injected exposures to drugs and toxins or those introduced by envenomation may require a proximal tourniquet and early suction. (See Antidotes 4 through 6 in Table 4.)

Inhalation exposure to toxic substances is treated by immediately removing the victim from the contaminated environment.

Gastrointestinal exposure is the most common

TABLE 1. **Level of Consciousness (Reed Coma Scale)**

Stage	Conscious Level	Pain Response	Reflexes	Respiration	Circulation
0	Asleep	Normal	Normal	Normal	Normal
1	Coma	Decreased	Normal	Normal	Normal
2	Coma	None	Normal	Normal	Normal
3*	Coma	None	None	Normal	Normal
4†	Coma	None	None	Abnormal	Abnormal

*Patients in Stages 3 and 4 require intubation and placement in an intensive care unit.
†Patients in Stage 4 need intervention to sustain life.

route of poisoning, and an estimate of what, when, and how much of the toxic substance was ingested must be made. If there is a possibility of potential intoxication, gastrointestinal decontamination is performed rather than waiting for symptoms to develop.

Gastrointestinal Decontamination

To decrease gastrointestinal absorption, emesis should be induced or gastric aspiration and lavage performed. Neither of these methods is completely effective; each removes only 30 to 50% of the ingested substance. They are recommended up to 3 to 4 hours postingestion; however, there are few indications for induced emesis in the emergency department in an adult because it delays the administration of activated charcoal, which is more effective.

Emesis

Relative contraindications to the induction of emesis are (1) petroleum distillate ingestion of high-viscosity agents; (2) ingestions of agents that are likely to rapidly produce coma (short-acting barbiturates) or convulsions (propoxyphene, camphor, isoniazid, strychnine, tricyclic antidepressants) in less than 30 minutes and therefore may predispose to aspiration during emesis; and (3) prior significant vomiting.

Absolute contraindications to the induction of emesis are (1) caustic (alkali) or corrosive (acid) ingestions; (2) convulsions because of the danger of aspiration and possible induction of laryngospasm; (3) coma because of the possibility of aspiration with the loss of protective airway reflexes; (4) absence of a cough reflex—absence of the gag reflex is not a reliable indication of lack of airway protection because a number of healthy people lack gag reflexes; (5) hematemesis, in which vomiting may produce additional damage; (6) age under 6 months, because of immature protective airway reflexes; (7) foreign bodies—emesis is ineffective and risks obstruction or aspiration; and (8) absence of bowel sounds (when no bowel sounds are present, gastric lavage is preferred).

Inducing Emesis

Syrup of ipecac is the preferred agent but never fluid extract of ipecac, which is too potent, or salt water, which has produced fatal hypernatremia. Emesis is not recommended to be induced at home in children younger than 1 year of age but can be performed in a medical facility under supervision when indicated. The dose of syrup of ipecac in the 6- to 9-month-old infant is 5 mL; in the 9- to 12-month-old, 10 mL; and in the 1- to 12-year-old, 15 mL. In children over 12 years and in adults, the dose is 30 mL. The dose may be repeated *once* if the child does not vomit in 15 to 20 minutes. The vomitus should be inspected for remnants of pills or toxic substances, and the appearance and odor should be noted.

Apomorphine is a parenteral emetic that must be freshly prepared. Its use is fraught with complications, although it produces more rapid onset of emesis than syrup of ipecac. We do not recommend its use in the cooperative patient. Naloxone (Narcan) should be available to reverse CNS depression.

Gastric aspiration and lavage may be preferable to the induction of emesis in cooperative adolescents or adults because a large tube can be introduced through the oral cavity. Contraindications to gastric aspiration and lavage in intoxicated patients are (1) caustic (alkali) and corrosive (acid) ingestions because of the risk of esophageal perforation; (2) uncontrolled convulsions because of the danger of aspiration and injury during the procedure; (3) ingestions of petroleum distillate products; (4) coma or absent protective airway reflexes, which require the insertion of an endotracheal tube to protect against aspiration; (5) significant cardiac dysrhythmias, which should be controlled first; and (6) hematemesis, which may be a relative contraindication.

The best results with gastric aspiration and lavage are obtained with the largest possible orogastric tube that can be reasonably passed (nasogastric tubes are not large enough for this purpose). In adults, use a large-bore orogastric Lavacuator hose or a No. 42 French Ewald tube; in children, use a No. 22–28 French orogastric-type tube.

The amount of fluid used varies with the patient's age and size, but in general, aliquots of 150 to 200 mL per lavage are used in adolescents or adults and 5 mL per kg or 50 to 100 mL per lavage in children younger than 5 years of age.

Continuous gastric suction has been used for substances that have an enterohepatic recirculation or are actively secreted into the gastrointestinal tract, such as tricyclic antidepressants (imipramine [Tofranil]) and local anesthetics such as mepivacaine (Carbocaine) (Table 2).

TABLE 2. **Substances with Enterohepatic Recirculation**

Chloral hydrate
Colchicine
Digitalis preparations (digoxin, digitoxin)
Glutethimide
Halogenated hydrocarbons (DDT derivatives)
Isoniazid
Methaqualone
Nonsteroidal anti-inflammatory agents
Phencyclidine
Phenothiazines
Phenytoin
Salicylates
Tricyclic antidepressants

Activated charcoal is produced by combustion of organic material in the absence of air until the carbon particle is formed. There are few relative contraindications to the use of activated charcoal: (1) It should not be administered before, concomitantly with, or shortly after syrup of ipecac because it may adsorb the ipecac and interfere with its emetic properties; (2) it should not be given before, concomitantly with, or shortly after oral antidotes unless it has been proved not to interfere significantly with their absorption; (3) it does not effectively adsorb caustics and corrosives and may produce vomiting or cling to the esophageal or gastric mucosa and falsely appear as a burn on endoscopy; and (4) it should not be given if there are no bowel sounds. Activated charcoal has no absolute contraindications, but it does not effectively adsorb alcohols, boric acid, caustics, corrosives, cyanide, metals, and drugs insoluble in aqueous acid solution (Table 3). Activated charcoal is a stool marker, indicating that the toxin has passed through the gastrointestinal tract and that no further significant absorption from the original ingestion will occur.

The dose of activated charcoal is 1 gram per kg per dose orally, with a minimum of 15 grams. The usual adolescent and adult dose is 60 to 100 grams. It is administered as a slurry mixed with water or by orogastric tube. A continuous nasogastric drip of activated charcoal, 0.25 gram per kg per hour, is an alternative in children. It should not be mixed with milk, marmalade, or starch because these interfere with charcoal's adsorptive action. Charcoal is administered with a cathartic initially. Subsequently, cathartics should be given every 24 hours.

Activated charcoal may be administered orally every 4 hours as long as bowel sounds are present, and it may be especially beneficial in intoxications that have an enterohepatic recirculation (see Table 2). Repeated dosing with oral activated charcoal has been shown to increase the clearance of many drugs without allowing enterohepatic recirculation (see later discussion of individual poisonings).

TABLE 3. **Substances Poorly Adsorbed by Activated Charcoal**

C—caustics and corrosives
H—heavy metals (arsenic, iron, lead, lithium, mercury)
A—alcohols (ethanol, methanol) and glycols (ethylene glycols)
C—chlorine and iodine
O—other substances insoluble in water
A—aliphatic and poorly absorbed hydrocarbons
L—laxatives (sodium, magnesium, sorbitol)

Catharsis is used to hasten the elimination of any remaining toxin in the gastrointestinal tract. Cathartics are relatively contraindicated (1) when ileus is indicated by absence of bowel sounds, (2) in intestinal obstruction or evidence of intestinal perforation, and (3) in cases with a pre-existing electrolyte disturbance. Magnesium sulfate (Epsom salts) is contraindicated in renal failure; sodium sulfate (Glauber's salts), in heart failure or diseases requiring sodium restriction. Magnesium sulfate or sodium sulfate is administered in doses of 250 mg per kg per dose as 20% solutions. The adolescent and adult dose is 30 grams. Sorbitol is given at 2.8 mL per kg to a maximum of 214 mL of a 70% solution, in adults. The cathartic should be given with the initial dose of activated charcoal. Sorbitol should be used with caution in children younger than age 3 years and is not recommended in children under 1 year of age.

Dilutional treatment is indicated for the immediate management of caustic and corrosive poisonings but is otherwise not useful. Contraindications to dilution are (1) inability of the patient to swallow, resulting in aspiration of the diluting fluid, and (2) signs of upper airway obstruction, esophageal perforation, and shock. The administration of large quantities of diluting fluid—above 30 mL in children and 250 mL in adults—may produce vomiting, re-exposing the vital tissues to the effects of local damage and possible aspiration.

Neutralization has not been proved to be scientifically effective.

In whole-bowel irrigation bowel-cleansing solutions of polyethylene glycol with electrolytes are used. It may be indicated with ingestions of substances that are poorly absorbed by activated charcoal, such as iron, lithium, or sustained-release preparations. The procedure has been used successfully with iron overdose when abdominal radiographs reveal incomplete emptying of excess ingested iron. There are additional implications in other ingestions, e.g., body packing of illicit drugs, such as cocaine and heroin. The procedure is to administer, orally or by nasogastric tube, the solution (GoLytely or Colyte), 0.5 liter per hour in children younger than 5 years of age and 2 liters per hour in adolescents and adults. The end point is reached when the rectal effluent is clear. This takes approximately 2 to 4 hours. These measures should not be used if there is extensive hematemesis, ileus, or signs of bowel obstruction, perforation, or peritonitis.

USE OF ANTIDOTES

Antidotes are available for only a relatively small number of poisons. An available antidote should be administered only after the vital functions have been established. Table 4 summarizes the commonly used antidotes and their indications and methods of administration. Most informational, so-called first aid measures and antidotes on commercial product labels are notorious for their inaccuracy; it is preferable to contact the Regional Poison Control Center rather than follow the recommendations on these labels.

ENHANCEMENT OF ELIMINATION

The medical methods for elimination of absorbed toxic substances are diuresis, dialysis, hemoperfusion, exchange transfusion, plasmapheresis, enzyme induction, and inhibition. Methods of increasing urinary excretion of toxic chemicals and drugs are being studied extensively, but the other modalities have not been well evaluated.

In general, these methods are needed in only a minority of instances and should be reserved for life-threatening circumstances or when a definite benefit is anticipated.

Diuresis

Diuresis increases the renal clearance of compounds that are partially reabsorbed in the renal tubules. Forced-fluid diuresis is based on the principle that it will shorten exposure to reabsorption at the distal renal tubules. The risks of diuresis are fluid overload, with cerebral and pulmonary edema, and disturbances in acid-base and electrolyte balance. Failure to produce a diuresis may imply prerenal or renal failure. If renal failure is present, dialysis should be considered.

Osmotic diuresis is meant to increase the osmotic gradient and prevent reabsorption from the proximal loop and distal tubules. Mannitol is used to initiate this type of diuresis, and then fluids are added in sufficient amounts to produce a diuresis similar to forced-fluid diuresis.

Acid and alkaline diuresis is based on the principle that inhibition of reabsorption of certain toxic agents can be encouraged by adjusting the urinary pH so the substance is maintained in its ionized form, which interferes with its passage back into the blood. Electrolyte and acid-base monitoring are necessary. Hypokalemia and hypocalcemia are frequent complications. Acid diuresis is accomplished by using ammonium chloride (Antidote 2, Table 4). Although it may enhance the elimination of weak bases, such as amphetamines and fenfluramine (Pondimin), it is not recommended. Ammonium chloride is contraindicated if rhabdomyolysis is present. Alkaline diuresis with sodium bicarbonate can be used in the therapy of weak acids, such as salicylates, and long-acting barbiturates, such as phenobarbital (Antidote 39, Table 4).

Dialysis

Dialysis is the extrarenal means of removing certain toxins from the body and can substitute for the kidney when renal failure occurs. Dialysis is never the first measure instituted; however, it may be lifesaving later in the course of a severe intoxication. It is needed in only a small minority of intoxicated patients (Table 5). Peritoneal dialysis is only one-twentieth as effective as hemodialysis. It is easier to use and less hazardous to the patient but also less reliable in removing the toxin; thus it is seldom used. Hemodialysis is the most effective means of dialysis but requires experience with sophisticated equipment. The patient-related criteria for dialysis are anticipated prolonged coma and the likelihood of complications, renal impairment, and deterioration despite careful medical management. Most dialyzable substances have a volume of distribution (Vd) of less than 1 liter per kg and protein binding of less than 50%.

Hemoperfusion

Hemoperfusion is the extracorporeal exposure of the patient's blood to an adsorbing surface (charcoal or resin). This procedure has extended extracorporeal removal to a large range of substances that were formerly either poorly dialyzable or nondialyzable. Hemoperfusion may be used for agents that have high protein binding, low aqueous solubility, and poor distribution in the plasma water. In these cases, hemodialysis is relatively ineffective. Hemoperfusion has proved useful in glutethimide intoxication, barbiturate overdose even with short-acting barbiturates, and intoxication with theophylline, cyclic antidepressants, or chlorophenothane (DDT). Activated charcoal cartridges are the primary type of hemoperfusion that is currently available. In general, supportive care is all that is required. Analysis of studies with hemodialysis and hemoperfusion does not indicate that they reduce morbidity or mortality substantially except in certain cases (Table 6).

SUPPORTIVE CARE, OBSERVATION, AND THERAPY OF COMPLICATIONS

The comatose patient is on the threshold of death and must be stabilized initially by establishing an airway. Intubation should be accomplished in any comatose patient.

An intravenous line should be inserted in all comatose patients, and blood should be collected for appropriate tests, including toxicologic analysis (10 mL of clotted blood, initial gastric aspirate, 100 mL of urine). The initial management of the comatose patient should include the administration of 100% oxygen, 100 mg of thiamine intravenously, 50% glucose as an intravenous bolus, and 2 to 10 mg of naloxone (Narcan) intravenously. Other causes associated with coma and mimicking intoxications should be eliminated by examination and laboratory tests (trauma, infection, cerebrovascular accident, hypoxia, and endocrine-metabolic causes).

Pulmonary edema complicating poisoning may be cardiac or noncardiac in origin. Fluid overload during

Text continued on page 1098

TABLE 4. **Antidotes***

Medication	Indications	Comments
1. ***N*-Acetylcysteine** (NAC, Mucomyst, Mead Johnson). Glutathione precursor that prevents accumulation and helps detoxify acetaminophen metabolites. **Dose:** *Adult,* 140 mg/kg PO of 5% solution as loading dose, then 70 mg/kg PO q 4 h for 17 doses as maintenance dose. *Child,* same as for adult. **Packaged:** 10 and 20% solution in 4-, 10-, and 30-mL vials.	Acetaminophen toxicity. Most effective within first 8 h (to make more palatable, administer through a straw inserted into closed container of citrus juice). **AR:** Stomatitis, nausea, vomiting. See Acetaminophen in text. The full course of therapy is required in any patient whose level falls in the toxic range.	IV preparation experimental.‡ The dose of NAC should be repeated if the patient vomits within 1 h after administration. Methods to stop vomiting of the NAC are: (a) placement of a tube in the duodenum, (b) slow administration over 1 h, (c) ½ h before NAC dose use metoclopramide (Reglan), 1 mg/kg intravenously over 15 min (max dose 10 mg) q 6 h; infants 0.1 mg/kg/dose IM, IV. Droperidol (Inapsine), 1.25 mg IV; for extrapyramidal reactions, use diphenhydramine (see 18).
2. **Ammonium chloride.**	Not recommended.	
3. **Amyl nitrate.**	See 14, Cyanide antidote kit.	
4. **Antivenin,** black widow spider (*Latrodectum mactans*). **Dose:** 1–2 vials infused over 1 h. **Packaged:** 6000 U/vial with 2.5 mL sterile water and 1 mL horse serum 1:10 dilution.	Envenomation by black widow spider or of all *Latrodectus* species producing severe symptoms. Most healthy adults survive with supportive care. Antivenin is used in elderly or infants or if there is underlying medical condition causing hemodynamic instability. **AR:** Same as for 5, Antivenin Polyvalent because derived from horse serum.	Preliminary sensitivity test. Supportive care alone is standard management.
5. **Antivenin Polyvalent** for Crotalidae (pit vipers), Wyeth, IV only. **Dose:** Depends on degree of envenomation: minimal: 5–8 vials; moderate: 8–12 vials; severe: 13–30 vials. Dilute in 500–2000 mL of crystalloid solution and start IV at a slow rate, increasing after the first 20 min, if no reaction occurs. **Packaged:** 1 vial (10 mL) lyophilized serum, 1 vial (10 mL) bacteriostatic water for injection, 1 vial (1 mL) normal horse serum.	Venoms of crotalids (pit vipers) of North and South America. **AR:** Anaphylactic shock reaction occurs within 30 min. Serum sickness usually occurs 5–44 days after administration. It may occur in less than 5 days, especially in those who have received horse serum products in the past. Signs and symptoms include fever, edema, arthralgia, nausea, and vomiting, as well as pain and muscle weakness.	Consider consulting with regional poison control center and herpetologist. Administer IV. Preliminary sensitivity test. Never inject in fingers, toes, or bite site.
6. **Antivenin,** North American coral snake, Wyeth, IV only. **Dose:** 3–5 vials (30–50 mL) by slow IV injection. First 1–2 mL should be injected over 3–5 min. **Packaged:** 1 vial antivenin, 10 mL. 1 vial bacteriostatic water 10 mL for injection.	*Micrurus fulvius* (Eastern coral snake); *Micrurus tenere* (Texas coral snake). **AR:** Anaphylaxis (sensitivity reaction). Usually 30 min after administration. Signs/symptoms: Flushing, itching, edema of face, cough, dyspnea, cyanosis. Neurologic manifestations—usually involve the shoulders and arms. Pain and muscle weakness are frequently present, and permanent atrophy may develop.	Same as for Antivenin polyvalent: for Crotalidae. Will not neutralize the venom of *Micrurus euryxanthus* (Arizona or Sonoran coral snake).

Abbreviations: AR = adverse reaction to antidotes; MP = monitoring parameters; FDA = US Food and Drug Administration; Conc. = concentration; ECG = electrocardiogram; TIBC = total iron-binding capacity; G6PD = glucose-6-phosphate dehydrogenase; CNS = central nervous system; GI = gastrointestinal; AV = atrioventricular; EEG = electroencephalogram; RBC = red blood count; CBC = complete blood count.

*This is for information purposes and is not intended to substitute for independent judgment. It is always advisable to review the package insert for the most up-to-date information. Contact Regional Poison Control Center for additional details on use.

†This dose may exceed the manufacturer's recommended dose.

‡Investigational drug in the United States.

¶Not FDA approved for this indication.

TABLE 4. **Antidotes*** *Continued*

Medication	Indications	Comments
7. **Atropine** (various manufacturers). Antagonizes cholinergic stimuli at muscarinic recptors. **Dose:** *Adult,* initial dose 2–4 mg IV. Dose every 10–15 min as necessary until cessation of secretions. Severe poisoning may require doses up to 2000 mg. *Child,* initial dose of 0.02 mg/kg to a max of 2 mg every 10–15 min as necessary until cessation of secretions. Use preservative-free atropine if infusion. **Packaged:** 0.3 mg/mL; 0.4 mg/mL in 0.5-, 1-, 20-, and 30-ml vials; 1 mg/mL in 1- and 10-mL vials.	Carbamate and organophosphate insecticide poisonings. Rarely needed in cholinergic mushroom intoxication (*Amanita muscaria, Clitocybe, Inocybe* spp.). Lack of signs of atropinization confirms diagnosis of cholinesterase inhibition. **AR:** Flushing and dryness of skin, blurred vision, rapid and irregular pulse, fever, and loss of neuromuscular coordination. **Diagnostic Test:** *Child:* 0.01 mg/kg IV. *Adult:* 1 mg total.	If cyanosis, establish respiration first because atropine in cyanotic patients may cause ventricular fibrillation. If severe signs of atropinization, may correct with physostigmine in doses equal to one-half dose of atropine. If symptomatic, administer until the end point of drying secretions and clearing of lungs. Hallucinations, flushing of the skin, dilated pupils, tachycardia, and elevation of body temperature are not end points and do not preclude atropine administration. Atropinization should be maintained for 12–24 h, then taper dose and observe for relapse. Atropine has been administered successfully by IV infusion, although this method has not received FDA approval. **Dose:** Place 8 mg of atropine in 100 mL D5W or saline. Conc. = 0.08 mg/mL. Dose range = 0.02–0.08 mg/kg/h or 0.25–1 mL/kg/h. Severe poisoning may require supplemental doses of intravenous atropine intermittently in doses of 2–4 mg until drying of secretions occurs.
8. **BAL**	See 17, Dimercaprol.	
9. **Bicarbonate**	See 39, Sodium bicarbonate.	
10. **Botulism antitoxin,** Connaught Medical Research Labs. **Dose:** *Adult,* 1 vial IV stat, then 1 vial IM, repeat in 2–4 h if symptoms appear in 12–24 h. *Child,* check with state health department.	Prevention or treatment of botulism.	Contact local or state health department for full management guidelines.
11. **Calcium disodium edetate** (EDTA, Disodium Versenate, Riker). **Dose:** *Adult,* max 4 gm. *Child,* max 1 gm. Moderate toxicity: IM or IV, 50 mg/kg/day for 3–5 days. Severe toxicity: IV or IM, 75 mg/kg/day for 4–5 days. Dose divided into 3–6 doses daily. Dilute 1 gm in 250–500 mL saline or D5W, infuse over 4 h bid for 5–7 days. For lead levels over 69 μg/dL or if symptoms of lead poisoning or encephalopathy: Add BAL alone initially, 4 mg/kg, then combination BAL and EDTA at different sites. EDTA dose: 12.5 mg/kg IM. (See Lead in text for latest recommendations.) Modify dose in renal failure. **Packaged:** 200 mg/mL ampules.	For chelation of cadmium, chromium, cobalt, copper, lead, magnesium, nickel, selenium, tellurium, tungsten, uranium, vanadium, and zinc poisoning. **AR:** 1. Thrombophlebitis. 2. Nausea, vomiting. 3. Hypotension. 4. Transient bone marrow suppression. 5. Nephrotoxicity, reversible tubular necrosis, (particularly in acid urine). 6. Fever 4–8 h after infusion. 7. Increased prothrombin time.	Hydrate first and establish renal flow. Avoid plain sodium EDTA because hypocalcemia may result. Procaine 0.25–1 mL of 0.5% for each mL of IM EDTA to reduce pain. Do not use EDTA orally. Limit use to 7 days (otherwise loss of other ions and cardiac dysrhythmias may occur). **MP:** Calcium levels, urinalysis, renal profile, erythrocyte protoporphyrin, blood lead, and liver profile. Contraindicated in iron intoxication, hepatic impairment, and renal failure.

Abbreviations: AR = adverse reaction to antidotes; MP = monitoring parameters; FDA = US Food and Drug Administration; Conc. = concentration; ECG = electrocardiogram; TIBC = total iron-binding capacity; G6PD = glucose-6-phosphate dehydrogenase; CNS = central nervous system; GI = gastrointestinal; AV = atrioventricular; EEG = electroencephalogram; RBC = red blood count; CBC = complete blood count.

*This is for information purposes and is not intended to substitute for independent judgment. It is always advisable to review the package insert for the most up-to-date information. Contact Regional Poison Control Center for additional details on use.

†This dose may exceed the manufacturer's recommended dose.

‡Investigational drug in the United States.

¶Not FDA approved for this indication.

Table continued on following page

TABLE 4. **Antidotes*** *Continued*

Medication	Indications	Comments
12. (A) **Calcium gluconate** 10%. **Dose:** IV 0.2–0.5 mL/kg of elemental calcium up to max 10 mL (1 gm) over 5–10 min with continuous ECG monitoring. Titrate to adequate response. **Packaged:** 10% solution in 10-mL vial.	Calcium channel blocker poisoning, e.g., nifedipine (Procardia), verapamil (Calan), diltiazem (Cardizem). It improves the blood pressure but does not affect the dysrhythmias. Hypocalcemia as result of poisonings. Black widow spider envenomation.	Repeat dose as needed. Monitor calcium levels. Contraindicated with digitalis poisoning.
(B) **Calcium chloride.** **Dose:** IV 0.2 mL/kg up to max 10 mL (1 gm) with continuous IV monitoring. Titrate to adequate response. Rate should not exceed 2 mL/min.	Hydrofluoric acid (HF) exposure (if irrigation with cool water fails to control the pain). **AR:** IV bradycardia, asystole, necrosis with extravasation.	Infiltration with calcium gluconate should be considered if HF exposure results in immediate tissue damage and erythema and pain persist following adequate irrigation.
(C) **Infiltration of calcium gluconate.** **Dose:** Infiltrate each square cm of the affected dermis and subcutaneous tissue with about 0.5 mL of 10% calcium gluconate using a 30-gauge needle. Repeat as needed to control pain. **Packaged:** 10% solution in 10-mL vial.		
(D) **Calcium gel:** 3.5 gm USP calcium gluconate powder added to 5 oz of water-soluble lubricating jelly.	Dermal exposure of hydrofluoric acid less than 20%.	Gel must have direct access to burn area; if pain persists, calcium gluconate injection may be needed. Placing a loose-fitting surgical glove over the gel when the fingers are involved helps to keep preparation in contact with burn area.
13. **Chemet.**	See 42, Succimer.	
14. **Cyanide antidote kit,** Lilly. Nitrite-induced methemoglobin attracts cyanide off cytochrome oxidase, and thiosulfate forms nontoxic thiocyanate. **Doses:** *Adult,* amyl nitrite. Inhale for 30 sec of every min. Use a new ampule every 3 min. Reapply until sodium nitrite can be given. Then inject IV 300 mg (10 ml of 3% solution of sodium nitrite) over 20 min. Alternative: IV infusion, 300 mg in 50–100 mL of 0.9% saline over 20 min. Then inject 12.5 gm (50 mL of 25% solution) of sodium thiosulfate over 20 min. *Child,* use the following chart for children's dosage. **Packaged:** 2- to 10-mL ampules sodium nitrite injection; 2- to 50-mL ampules sodium thiosulfate injection; 0.3-mL amyl nitrite inhalant.	Cyanide poisoning. **AR:** Hypotension, methemoglobinemia.	*Note:* If a child is given the adult dose of sodium nitrite, a fatal methemoglobinemia may result. Do not use methylene blue for methemoglobinemia in cyanide therapy. Observe for hypotension and have epinephrine available. Cyanide kits should have amyl nitrite changed annually. Administer oxygen 100% between inhalations of amyl nitrite. Monitor hemoglobin, arterial blood gases, methemoglobin concentration (nitrite given to obtain a methemoglobin of 25%). Some add nitrite ampule to resuscitation bag.

Chart should be used to determine dose of sodium nitrite and sodium thiosulfate in children on the basis of hemoglobin concentration on left. The average child with a normal hemoglobin requires 0.33–0.39 mL/kg of sodium nitrite up to 10 mL over 20 min.

Hemoglobin	*Initial Child Dose of Sodium Nitrite 3% (do not exceed 10 mL)*	*Initial Child Dose of Sodium Thiosulfate (do not exceed 12.5 gm)*
8 gm	0.22 mL/kg (6.6 mg/kg)	1.10 mL/kg
10 gm	0.27 mL/kg (8.7 mg/kg)	1.35 mL/kg
12 gm	0.33 mL/kg (10 mg/kg)	1.65 mL/kg
14 gm	0.39 mL/kg (11.6 mg/kg)	1.95 mL/kg

If signs of poisoning reappear, repeat above procedure at one-half the above doses. Each agent should be given at a rate of over 20 min.

Abbreviations: AR = adverse reaction to antidotes; MP = monitoring parameters; FDA = US Food and Drug Administration; Conc. = concentration; ECG = electrocardiogram; TIBC = total iron-binding capacity; G6PD = glucose-6-phosphate dehydrogenase; CNS = central nervous system; GI = gastrointestinal; AV = atrioventricular; EEG = electroencephalogram; RBC = red blood count; CBC = complete blood count.

*This is for information purposes and is not intended to substitute for independent judgment. It is always advisable to review the package insert for the most up-to-date information. Contact Regional Poison Control Center for additional details on use.

†This dose may exceed the manufacturer's recommended dose.

‡Investigational drug in the United States.

¶Not FDA approved for this indication.

TABLE 4. **Antidotes*** *Continued*

Medication	Indications	Comments
15. **Deferoxamine mesylate** (DFOM, Desferal, Ciba). Has a remarkable affinity for ferric iron and chelates it. **Therapeutic Dose:** *Adult,* 90 mg/kg† IM or IV q 8 h to maximum of 1 gm per injection; may repeat to maximum of 6 gm in 24 h. *Child,* same as adult. IV administration can be given by slow infusion at rate not exceeding 15 mg/kg/h. **Packaged:** 500 mg/ampule (powder).	DFOM is useful in the treatment of symptomatic iron poisoning or cases where the serum iron is greater than 500 μg/dL. If the DFOM challenge test is positive, it is not a definite indication that therapy is necessary in the asymptomatic patient. Oral DFOM is not recommended. Iron intoxication. Therapeutic—see dose in left column. *Diagnostic trial:* Give deferoxamine, 50 mg/kg IM (up to 1 gm). If serum iron exceeds TIBC, unbound iron is excreted in urine, producing a "vin rosé" color of chelated iron complex in the urine (pink-orange). However, may be negative with high serum iron exceeding TIBC. **AR:** Flushing of the skin, generalized erythema, urticaria, hypotension, and shock may occur. Blindness has occurred rarely in patients receiving long-term, high-dose DFOM therapy. Continuous infusions of DFOM over 24 h has produced severe pulmonary manifestations such as adult respiratory distress syndrome. Contraindicated in patients with renal disease or anuria.	Therapy is usually continued until serum iron < 100 μg/dL, or when positive "vin rosé" urine turns clear, or when patient is asymptomatic. Therapy is rarely required over 24 h. Establish a good renal flow. To be effective, DFOM should be administered in first 12–16 h. In mild to moderate iron intoxication or shock, IV route only. Monitor serum iron levels, urine output, and urine color.
16. **Diazepam** (Valium, Roche). **Dose:** *Adult,* 5–10 mg IV (max 20 mg) at a rate of 5 mg/min until seizure is controlled. May be repeated 2 or 3 times. *Child,* 0.1–0.3 mg/kg up to 10 mg IV slowly over 2 min. **Packaged:** 5 mg/mL; 2-, 10-mL vials.	Any intoxication that provokes seizures when specific therapy is not available, e.g., amphetamines, PCP, barbiturate and alcohol withdrawal. Chloroquine poisoning. **AR:** Confusion, somnolence, coma, hypotension.	Intramuscular absorption is erratic. Establish airway and administer 100% oxygen and glucose.
17. **Dimercaprol** (BAL, Hynson, Westcott, and Dunning). **Dose:** Recommendations vary; contact regional poison control center. Prevents inhibition of sulfhydryl enzymes. Given deep IM only. *For severe lead poisoning*—see 11, Calcium disodium edetate. *For mild arsenic or gold poisoning*—2.5 mg/kg q 6 h for 2 days, then q 12 h on the third day, and once daily thereafter for 10 days. *For severe arsenic or gold poisoning*—3–5 mg/kg q 6 h for 3 days, then q 12 h thereafter for 10 days.† *For mercury poisoning*—5 mg/kg initially, followed by 2.5 mg/kg 1 or 2 times daily for 10 days. **Packaged:** 100 mg/mL 10% in oil in 3-mL ampules.	For chelation of antimony, arsenic, bismuth, chromates, copper, gold, lead, mercury, and nickel. **AR:** 30% of patients have reactions: fever (30% of children), hypertension, tachycardia, may cause hemolysis in G6PD deficiency patients. Doses greater than recommended may cause various adverse effects: nausea, vomiting, headache, chest pain, tachycardia, and hypertension.	Contraindicated in instances of hepatic insufficiency, with the exception of postarsenic jaundice. Should be discontinued or used only with extreme caution if acute renal insufficiency is present. Monitor blood pressure and heart rate (both may increase), urinalysis, qualitative urine excretion of heavy metal. Contraindicated in iron, silver, uranium, selenium, and cadmium poisoning.
18. **Dimercaptosuccinic acid** (DMSA).	See 42, Succimer.	
19. **Diphenhydramine** (Benadryl, Parke-Davis). Antiparkinsonian action. **Dose:** *Adult,* 10–50 mg IV over 2 min. *Child,* 1–2 mg/kg IV up to 50 mg over 2 min. Max in 24 h: 400 mg. **Packaged:** 10 mg/mL in 10- and 30-mL vials. 50 mg/mL in 1-, 5-, 10-, and 30-mL vials. Capsules, tablets 25 and 50 mg. Elixir, syrup 12.5 mg/5mL.	Used to treat extrapyramidal symptoms and dystonia induced by phenothiazines and related drugs. **AR:** Fatal dose, 20–40 mg/kg. Dry mouth, drowsiness.	Continue with oral diphenhydramine, 5 mg/kg/day to 25 mg 3 times a day for 72 h, to avoid recurrence.

Abbreviations: AR = adverse reaction to antidotes; MP = monitoring parameters; FDA = US Food and Drug Administration; Conc. = concentration; ECG = electrocardiogram; TIBC = total iron-binding capacity; G6PD = glucose-6-phosphate dehydrogenase; CNS = central nervous system; GI = gastrointestinal; AV = atrioventricular; EEG = electroencephalogram; RBC = red blood count; CBC = complete blood count.

*This is for information purposes and is not intended to substitute for independent judgment. It is always advisable to review the package insert for the most up-to-date information. Contact Regional Poison Control Center for additional details on use.

†This dose may exceed the manufacturer's recommended dose.

‡Investigational drug in the United States.

¶Not FDA approved for this indication.

Table continued on following page

TABLE 4. **Antidotes*** *Continued*

Medication	Indications	Comments
20. **EDTA.**	See 11, Calcium disodium edetate.	
21. **Ethanol** (ETOH). Competitively inhibits alcohol dehydrogenase. **Dose:** *Loading*—administer 7.6–10.0 mL/kg of 10% ETOH in D5W over 30 min IV or 0.8–1.0 mL/kg 95% ETOH PO in 6 oz of orange juice over 30 min. While administering loading dose, start maintenance. *Maintenance:* Volume of 10% ETOH needed IV or 95% oral solution (not in dialysis). See chart on maintenance dose, below. If patient is on dialysis, add 91 mL/h in addition to regular maintenance dose. See comments to prepare 10% solution if not commercially available. **Packaged:** 10% ethanol in D5W 1000 mL; 95% ethanol. May be given as 50% solution orally.	Methanol, ethylene glycol poisoning. Ethanol infusion therapy may be started in cases of suspected methanol and ethylene glycol poisoning presenting with increased anion gap and osmolal gap, or if the urine shows the crystalluria of ethylene glycol poisoning or the hyperemia of the optic disk of methanol intoxication. **AR:** CNS depression, hypoglycemia.	Monitor blood ethanol 1 h after starting infusion and q 4–6 h. Maintain a blood ethanol concentration of 100–200 mg/dL. Monitor blood glucose, electrolytes, blood gases, urinalysis, and renal profile at least daily. Continue infusion until safe concentration of ethylene glycol or methanol is reached. Ethanol-induced hypoglycemia may occur. Dialysis, preferably hemodialysis, should be considered in severe intoxication not controlled by ethanol alone. To prepare 10% ethanol for infusion therapy: Remove 100 mL from 1 L D5W and replace with 100 mL of tax-free bulk absolute alcohol after passing through 0.22-μ filter; 50-mL vials of pyrogen-free absolute ethanol for injection are available from Pharm-Serv, 218–20 96th Avenue, Queen's Village, NY 11429. Telephone 718–475–1601.

Maintenance Dose:

Patient Category	mL/kg/h using 10% IV	mL/kg/h using 50% oral
Nondrinker	0.83	0.17
Occasional drinker	1.40	0.28
Alcoholic	1.96	0.39

Medication	Indications	Comments
22. **Fab** (antibody fragment, Digibind). **Dose:** The average dose used during clinical testing was 10 vials. Dosage details are specified by the manufacturer. It should be administered by the IV route over 30 min. Calculate on basis of body burden either by known amount ingested or by serum digoxin concentration. *Calculation of dose of Fab*: 1. Known amount ingested multiplied by bioavailability (0.8) = body burden. Body burden divided by 0.6 = number of vials. 2. Known serum digoxin (obtained 6 h postingestion) multiplied by volume distribution (5.6 L/kg) and weight in kg divided by 1000 = body burden. Body burden divided by 0.6 = number of vials.	Toxicity due to digoxin, digitoxin, oleander tea, with the following: 1. Imminent cardiac arrest or shock. 2. Hyperkalemia > 5.5 mEq/L. 3. Serum digoxin > 10 ng/mL at 6–12 h postingestion in adults. 4. Life-threatening dysrhythmias. 5. Ingestion over 10 mg in adults or 4 mg in child (0.3 mg/kg). 6. Bradycardia or second- or third-degree heart block unresponsive to atropine.	Contact regional poison control center. Preliminary sensitivity test. Administer through a 0.22-μ filter. Fab causes a rise in measured bound digoxin but a fall in free digoxin. 40 mg binds 0.6 mg digoxin.
23. **Flumazenil** (Mazicon, Roche Labs), Benzodiazepine (BZP) receptor antagonist. **Dose:** 1. *Management of BZP overdose:* (Caution) 0.2 mg (2 mL) IV over 30 sec; may repeat after 30 sec with 0.3 mg (3 mL). Further doses of 0.5 mg over 30 sec. If no response in 5 min and max of 5 mg, cause of sedation is unlikely to be BZP. 2. *Reversal of conscious sedation or in general anesthesia:* 0.2 mg (2 mL) IV over 15 sec; may repeat in 45 sec. Doses may be repeated at 60-sec intervals to max dose of 1 mg (10 mL). If resedation, repeated doses may be administered at 20-min intervals to max 1 mg (0.2 mg/min). Max 3 mg should be given in any 1 h. **Packaged:** 0.1 mg/mL in 5- and 10-mL multiple-use vials.	1. Reversal of the sedative effects of BZP general anesthesia. 2. Sedation with BZP for procedures. 3. Caution in management of overdose. **AR:** Convulsions, dizziness, injection site pain, increased sweating, headache and abnormal or blurred vision (3–9%).	Not treatment for hypoventilation. Caution with overdoses. Flumazenil is not recommended for cyclic antidepressant poisoning, if patient has seizures or increased intracranial pressure. Flumazenil has been associated with seizures in long-term benzodiazepine use or dependency.

Abbreviations: AR = adverse reaction to antidotes; MP = monitoring parameters; FDA = US Food and Drug Administration; Conc. = concentration; ECG = electrocardiogram; TIBC = total iron-binding capacity; G6PD = glucose-6-phosphate dehydrogenase; CNS = central nervous system; GI = gastrointestinal; AV = atrioventricular; EEG = electroencephalogram; RBC = red blood count; CBC = complete blood count.

*This is for information purposes and is not intended to substitute for independent judgment. It is always advisable to review the package insert for the most up-to-date information. Contact Regional Poison Control Center for additional details on use.

†This dose may exceed the manufacturer's recommended dose.

‡Investigational drug in the United States.

¶Not FDA approved for this indication.

TABLE 4. **Antidotes*** *Continued*

Medication	Indications	Comments
24. **Folic acid.**	See 28, Leucovorin.	
25. **Folinic acid.**	See 28, Leucovorin.	
26. **Glucagon.** Works by stimulating production of cyclic adenyl monophosphate. **Dose:** 50–150 μg/kg over 1 min IV followed by a continuous infusion of 1–5 mg/h in dextrose and then taper over 5–12 h. 2 mg of phenol per 1 mg glucagon. 50 mg is the maximum amount of phenol recommended; therefore, toxicity may result when high doses of glucagon are used. **Packaged:** 1-mg (1-unit) vial with 1-mL diluent with glycerin and phenol; also in 10-mL size.	Beta blocker, quinidine, and calcium channel blocker intoxication. **AR:** Glucagon is generally well tolerated—most frequent reactions are nausea, vomiting.	Do not dissolve the lyophilized glucagon in the solvent packaged with it when administering IV infusion because of possible phenol toxicity. Use D5W, not 0.9% saline. Effects of single dose observed in 5–10 min and last for 15–30 min. A constant infusion may be necessary to sustain desired effects.
27. **Labetalol hydrochloride** (Normodyne, Schering; Trandate, Glaxo). Nonselective beta and mild alpha blocker. **Dose:** IV 20 mg over 2 min. Additional injections of 40 or 80 mg can be given at 10-min intervals until desired supine blood pressure achieved. Max dose 300 mg. Alternative: Slow IV infusion: 200 mg (40 mL) is added to 160 or 250 mL of D5W and given at 2 mg/min. Titrate infusion according to response. **Packaged:** Solution 5 mg/mL in 20 mL.	Hypertensive crises secondary to cocaine. **AR:** GI disturbances, orthostatic hypotension, bronchospasm, congestive heart failure, AV conduction disturbances, and peripheral vascular reactions.	Concomitant diuretic enhances therapeutic response. Patient should be kept in a supine position during infusion. **MP:** Monitor blood pressure during and after administration.
28. **Leucovorin.** **Dose:** For methanol poisoning: 1 mg/kg up to 50 mg IV q 4 h for 6 doses. For methotrexate overdose: See Comments. **Packaged:** 3 mg/mL (1 mL), 5 mg/mL (1 and 5 mL), 50 mg/vial.	1. **Methanol poisoning¶:** Active form of folic acid used to enhance metabolism of formic acid in animals to carbon dioxide and water. 2. **Methotrexate (MTX) overdose:** Supplies tetrahydrofolate cofactor, which is blocked by methotrexate. **AR:** Allergic sensitization.	For MTX overdose, initial dose can give IV or IM in MTX equivalent dose up to 75 mg. If a MTX blood level is measured 6 h postingestion, and is above 10^{-8} molar or is unavailable, give 12 mg q 6 h after the MTX level is below 10^{-8} molar. Alternatively, if GI function is adequate, may give orally 10 mg/M^2 q 6 h until MTX levels are lowered to less than 10^{-8} molar. Leucovorin in doses of 5–15 mg PO per day has also been recommended to counteract hematologic toxicity from folic acid antagonists such as trimethoprim and pyrimethamine.
29. **Methylene blue,** Harvey and others. Methylene blue reduces the ferric ion of methemoglobin to the ferrous ion of hemoglobin. **Dose:** *Adult,* 0.1–0.2 mL/kg of 1% solution (1–2 mg/kg) over 5 min IV. Max adults 7 mg/kg. *Child,* same as adults. Max infants 4 mg/kg. May repeat in 1 h if necessary. Repeat only once. **Packaged:** 1% 10-mL ampules.	Methemoglobinemia. **AR:** GI (nausea, vomiting), headache, hypertension, dizziness, mental confusion, restlessness, dyspnea, hemolysis, blue skin, blue urine, burning sensation in vein when IV dose exceeds 7 mg/kg. Treatment is unnecessary unless methemoglobin is over 30% or respiratory distress is present.	Saliva, urine, and other body fluids may turn blue. Contraindications: Renal insufficiency, cyanide poisonings when sodium nitrite is used to induce methemoglobinemia; in G6PD deficiency patients. Monitor hemolysis, methemoglobin level, and arterial blood gases. Avoid extravasation because of local necrosis.

Abbreviations: AR = adverse reaction to antidotes; MP = monitoring parameters; FDA = US Food and Drug Administration; Conc. = concentration; ECG = electrocardiogram; TIBC = total iron-binding capacity; G6PD = glucose-6-phosphate dehydrogenase; CNS = central nervous system; GI = gastrointestinal; AV = atrioventricular; EEG = electroencephalogram; RBC = red blood count; CBC = complete blood count.

*This is for information purposes and is not intended to substitute for independent judgment. It is always advisable to review the package insert for the most up-to-date information. Contact Regional Poison Control Center for additional details on use.

†This dose may exceed the manufacturer's recommended dose.

‡Investigational drug in the United States.

¶Not FDA approved for this indication.

Table continued on following page

TABLE 4. **Antidotes*** *Continued*

Medication	Indications	Comments
30. **Naloxone** (Narcan). Pure opioid antagonist. **Dose:** *Adult,* 0.4–2.0 mg IV and repeat at 3-min intervals until respiratory function is stable. Before excluding opioid intoxication on the basis of a lack of naloxone response, a minimum of 2 mg in a child or 10 mg in an adult should be administered. *Child,* initial dose is 0.1 mg/kg IV. **Packaged:** 0.02 mg/mL, 0.4 mg/mL ampule, 10-mL multidose vial.	1. Comatose patient (not just a lethargic patient). 2. Ineffective ventilation or an adult respiratory rate <12. 3. Pinpoint pupils. 4. Circumstantial evidence of opioid intoxication, e.g., known drug abuser, track marks, opioid paraphernalia. **AR:** Relatively free of adverse reactions. Rare reports of pulmonary edema. Should be administered with caution in pregnancy.	Naloxone infusion therapy should be used if a large initial dose was required, repeated boluses are necessary, or a long-acting opiate is involved. In infusion therapy the initial response dose is administered every hour and may need to be boostered in a half-hour after starting. The infusion may be tapered after 12 h of therapy. Naloxone infusion: calculate daily fluid requirements, add initial response dose of naloxone multiplied by 24 to the solution. Divide fluid by 24 h for naloxone infusion rate per hour. Does not cause CNS depression. Routes: IV and endotracheal are preferred routes. Pentazocine (Talwin), dextramethorphan, propoxyphene (Darvon), and codeine may require larger doses.
31. **Nicotinamide,** various manufacturers. **Dose:** *Adult,* 500 mg IM or IV slowly, then 200–400 mg q 4 h. If symptoms develop, the frequency of injections should be increased to every 2 h (max 3 gm/day). *Child,* One-half suggested adult dose. **Packaged:** 100 mg/mL: 2-, 5-, 10-, 30-mL vials; 25- and 50-mg tablets.	Vacor poisoning: phenylurea pesticide intoxication. *Note:* Vacor 2% is now available only to professional exterminators. 0.5% Vacor is available to the general public and can be toxic to children if swallowed. **AR:** Large doses—flushing, pruritus, sensation of burning, nausea, vomiting, anaphylactic shock.	Nicotinamide is most effective when given within 1 h of ingestion. Do not use niacin or nicotinic acid in place of nicotinamide. Monitor liver profile.
32. **Oxygen** 100%. **Dose:** *Adult,* 100% oxygen by inhalation or 100% oxygen in hyperbaric chamber at 2–3 atm. *Child,* Same as adult.	Carbon monoxide or cyanide exposure, methemoglobinemia. Any inhalation intoxication.	Half-life of carboxyhemoglobin is 240 min in room air 21% oxygen; if a patient is hyperventilated with 100% oxygen, half-life of carboxyhemoglobin is 90 min; in chamber at 2 atm, half-life is 25–30 min.
33. **Pancuronium bromide** (Pavulon, organon). Nondepolarizing (competitive) blocking agent. **Dose:** *Adults and children,* initially, 0.1 mg/kg IV; for intubation, 0.1 mg/kg IV, repeated as required (generally every 40–60 min).† **Packaged:** Solution 1 mg/mL in 10 mL. 2 mg/mL in 2- and 5-ml containers.	Neuromuscular blocking agent. Used for intubation and seizure control, acts in 2 min, lasts 40–60 min. **AR:** Main hazard is inadequate postoperative ventilation. Tachycardia and slight increase in arterial pressure may occur due to vagolytic action.	The required dose varies greatly, and a peripheral nerve stimulator aids in determining appropriate amount. Should monitor EEG, because motor effect may be abolished without decreasing electrical discharge from brain.
34. **D-Penicillamine** (Cuprimine, Merck; Depen, Wallace). Effective chelator and promotes excretion in urine. **Dose:** 250 mg 4 times daily PO for up to 5 days for long-term (20–40 days) therapy; 30–40 mg/kg/day in children. Max 1 gm/day. For chronic therapy, 25 mg/kg/day in 4 doses. **Packaged:** 125- and 250-mg capsules.	For chelation of heavy metals: arsenic, cadmium, chromates, cobalt, copper, lead, mercury, nickel, and zinc. **MP:** Routine urinalysis, white blood count differential, hemoglobin determination, direct platelet count, renal and hepatic profiles. Collect 24-h urine, quantify for heavy metal. **AR:** Leukopenia (2%); thrombocytopenia (4%); GI–nausea, vomiting, anaphylactic shock, diarrhea (17%); fever, rash, lupus syndrome, renal and hepatic injury.	This is not considered standard therapy for lead poisoning after chelation therapy. May produce ampicillin-like rash, allergic reactions, neutropenia, and nephropathy. Contraindication: hypersensitivity to penicillin.

Abbreviations: AR = adverse reaction to antidotes; MP = monitoring parameters; FDA = US Food and Drug Administration; Conc. = concentration; ECG = electrocardiogram; TIBC = total iron-binding capacity; G6PD = glucose-6-phosphate dehydrogenase; CNS = central nervous system; GI = gastrointestinal; AV = atrioventricular; EEG = electroencephalogram; RBC = red blood count; CBC = complete blood count.

*This is for information purposes and is not intended to substitute for independent judgment. It is always advisable to review the package insert for the most up-to-date information. Contact Regional Poison Control Center for additional details on use.

†This dose may exceed the manufacturer's recommended dose.

‡Investigational drug in the United States.

¶Not FDA approved for this indication.

TABLE 4. **Antidotes*** *Continued*

Medication	Indications	Comments
35. **Physostigmine salicylate** (Antilirium, O'Neil). Cholinesterase inhibitor; a diagnostic trial is not recommended. **Dose:** *Adult,* 1–2 mg IV over 2 min; may repeat every 5 min to max dose of 6 mg. *Child,* IV, 0.5 mg (0.02 mg/kg) over paralysis, 2 min to a max dose of 2 mg q 30–60 min if symptoms recur.† Once effect accomplished, give lowest effective dose. **Packaged:** 1 mg/mL in 2 mL/ampule.	Not advised for use in diagnostic testing or for routine use in treating anticholinergic effects. Reserve for life-threatening complications. **AR:** Death may result from respiratory paralysis, hypertension/ hypotension, bradycardia/ tachycardia/asystole, hypersalivation, respiratory difficulties/convulsions (cholinergic crisis).	Do not consider for toxicities due to the following: antidepressants, amoxapine, maprotiline, nomifensine, bupropion, trazodone, imipramine. IV administration should be at a slow controlled rate, not more than 1 mg/ min. Rapid administration can cause adverse reactions.
36. **Pralidoxime chloride** (2-PAM, Protopam, Ayerst). Cholinesterase reactivator; acts by removing phosphate. **Dose:** *Adults,* 1–2 gm IV infused in 100–250 mL saline IV over 15–30 min. Repeat in 1 h if needed. Repeat q 8–12 h when needed; if toxicity is severe, can give 0.5 gm/h infusion. *Child,* 25–50 mg/kg IV over 30 min. No faster than 10 mg/kg/min. Max 12 gm/24 h. **Packaged:** 1 gm/20-mL vials.	Organophosphate insecticide (OPI) poisoning. Not usually needed in carbamate insecticide poisoning. Most effective if started in first 24 h before bonding of phosphate. **AR:** Rapid IV injection has produced tachycardia, muscle rigidity, transient neuromuscular blockade. IM: conjunctival hyperemia, subconjunctival hemorrhage, especially if concentrations exceed 5%. Oral: nausea, vomiting, diarrhea, malaise.	Should be used only after initial treatment with atropine. Draw blood for RBC cholinesterase level before giving 2-PAM. The use of 2-PAM may require a reduction in the dose of atropine. The end point is absence of fasciculations and return of muscle strength. **MP:** Monitor renal profile and reduce dose accordingly. Half-life: 1–2 h. Reversal of OPI effects at 4 μg/mL of 2-PAM. Start early because "aging" of PO_4 on acetylcholinesterase makes it more difficult to reverse.
37. **Protamine sulfate.** **Dose:** 1 mg neutralizes 90–115 U of heparin, max dose 50 mg IV over 5 min at 10 mg/mL. **Packaged:** 5 mL (50 mg); 25 mL (250 mg).	Heparin overdose. **AR:** Rapid administration causes anaphylactoid reactions.	**MP:** Monitor thromboplastin times. Doses of up to 200 mg have been tolerated over 2 h in an adult.
38. **Pyridoxine** (vitamin B_6). Gamma amino acid agonist. **Dose:** *Unknown amount ingested*: 5 gm over 5 min IV. *Known amount:* Add 1 gm of pyridoxine for each gram of INH ingested IV over 5 min. **Packaged:** 50 and 100 mg/mL; 10, 30 mL.	Isoniazid (INH), monomethyl hydrazine mushrooms. **AR:** Unlikely owing to the fact that vitamin B_6 is water-soluble. However, nausea, vomiting, somnolence, and paresthesia have been reported from chronic high doses; up to 52 gm IV and up to 357 mg/kg have been tolerated.	Pyridoxine is given as 5–10% solution IV mixed with water. It may be repeated every 5–20 min until seizures cease. Some administer pyridoxine over 30–60 min. **MP:** Correct acidosis, monitor liver profile, acid-base parameters. Lethal dose of pyridoxine in animals is 1 gm/kg.
39. **Sodium bicarbonate.** **Dose:** IV 1–3 mEq/kg as needed to keep pH 7.5 (generally 2 mEq/kg q 6 h). When alkalinization is desired to correct acidosis to a pH of 7.3, use 2 mEq/kg to raise pH 0.1 unit. **Packaged:** 50 mL, 50-mEq ampule.	To promote urinary alkalinization for salicylates, phenobarbital (weak acids with low volume of distribution and excreted in urine unchanged). To correct severe acidosis. To promote protein binding and supply sodium ions into Purkinje cells in cyclic antidepressant intoxication. **AR:** Large doses in patients with renal insufficiency may cause metabolic alkalosis. In patients with ketoacidosis, rapid alkalinization with sodium bicarbonate may result in clouding of consciousness, cerebral dysfunction, seizures, hypoxia, and lactic acidosis.	Alkaline diuresis. The assessment of the need for bicarbonate should be based on both the blood and urine pH. Maintain the blood pH at 7.5. Keep the urinary output at 3–6 mL/ kg/h. May use a diuretic to enhance diuresis. Potassium is necessary to produce alkaline diuresis. Monitor electrolytes, calcium, pH of both urine and blood, arterial blood gases.

Abbreviations: AR = adverse reaction to antidotes; MP = monitoring parameters; FDA = US Food and Drug Administration; Conc. = concentration; ECG = electrocardiogram; TIBC = total iron-binding capacity; G6PD = glucose-6-phosphate dehydrogenase; CNS = central nervous system; GI = gastrointestinal; AV = atrioventricular; EEG = electroencephalogram; RBC = red blood count; CBC = complete blood count.

*This is for information purposes and is not intended to substitute for independent judgment. It is always advisable to review the package insert for the most up-to-date information. Contact Regional Poison Control Center for additional details on use.

†This dose may exceed the manufacturer's recommended dose.

‡Investigational drug in the United States.

¶Not FDA approved for this indication.

Table continued on following page

TABLE 4. **Antidotes*** *Continued*

Medication	Indications	Comments
40. **Sodium nitrite.**	See 14, Cyanide antidote kit.	
41. **Sodium thiosulfate.**	See 14, Cyanide antidote kit.	
42. **Succimer** (DMSA, Chemet, McNeil Consumer Products). **Dose:** 10 mg/kg or 350 mg/M^2 q 8 h for 5 days, then 10 mg/kg or 350 mg/M^2 q 12 h for 14 more days (see following chart). Therapy course lasts 19 days. **Packaged:** 100-mg capsule.	For chelation in children only whose blood lead is >45 μg/dL. **AR:** Rashes, nausea, vomiting, an elevation of serum transaminases occur in 6–10% of patients.	A minimum of 2 weeks between courses is recommended unless the venous lead indicates a need for more prompt therapy. Patients who have received CaEDTA or BAL may use succimer after an interval of 4 weeks. In young children the capsule can be opened and sprinkled on soft food. Monitor venous lead before therapy, on day 7, and weekly for rebound. Monitor the following tests: CBC, platelets, ferritin, liver.
43. **Vitamin K** (Aqua MEPHYTON, Merck). Promotes hepatic biosynthesis of prothrombin and other coagulation factors. Competitive antagonist of warfarin. It may be administered orally in the absence of vomiting. **Dose:** *Adult,* 2.5–10 mg IV, depending on potential for hemorrhage. Oral dose is 15–25 mg/day. Severe bleeding, 5–25 mg slow IV push. Rate 1 mg/min. Repeat q 4–8 h depending on prothrombin time. *Child,* 1–5 mg IV may be given orally when vomiting ceases at a dose of 5–10 mg/day. **Packaged:** 2 mg/mL in 0.5-mL ampules. 2.5- or 5-mL vials. Child oral dose 5–10 mg.	Overdose of warfarin (Coumadin) or superwarfarins, salicylate intoxication.	Fatalities from anaphylactic reaction have been reported following IV route. It takes 24 h for vitamin K to be effective. The need for further vitamin K is determined by the prothrombin time. If bleeding is severe, fresh blood or plasma transfusion may be needed.

Pediatric Dosing Chart (Succimer)

lbs	kg	Dose (mg)	No. of Capsules
18–35	8–15	100	1
36–55	16–23	200	2
56–75	24–34	300	3
76–100	35–44	400	4
>100	>45	500	5

Abbreviations: AR = adverse reaction to antidotes; MP = monitoring parameters; FDA = US Food and Drug Administration; Conc. = concentration; ECG = electrocardiogram; TIBC = total iron-binding capacity; G6PD = glucose-6-phosphate dehydrogenase; CNS = central nervous system; GI = gastrointestinal; AV = atrioventricular; EEG = electroencephalogram; RBC = red blood count; CBC = complete blood count.

*This is for information purposes and is not intended to substitute for independent judgment. It is always advisable to review the package insert for the most up-to-date information. Contact Regional Poison Control Center for additional details on use.

†This dose may exceed the manufacturer's recommended dose.

‡Investigational drug in the United States.

¶Not FDA approved for this indication.

forced diuresis may cause the cardiac variety, particularly if the drugs used have an antidiuretic effect (opioids, barbiturates, and salicylates). Some toxic agents produce increased pulmonary capillary permeability, and other agents may cause a massive sympathetic discharge resulting in neurogenic pulmonary edema (opioids and salicylates). Management consists of minimizing fluid administration and administering diuretics and oxygen. If renal failure is present, dialysis may be necessary. The noncardiac type of pulmonary edema occurs with inhaled toxins, such as ammonia, chlorine, and oxides of nitrogen, or with drugs, such as salicylates, opioids, paraquat, and intravenous ethchlorvynol (Placidyl). This type does not respond to cardiac measures, and oxygen with intensive respiratory management using mechanical ventilation with positive end-expiratory pressure (PEEP) is necessary.

Hypotension and circulatory shock may be caused by heart failure due to myocardial depression, hypovolemia (fluid loss or venous pooling), decrease in peripheral vasculature resistance (adrenergic blockage), or loss of vasomotor tone caused by central nervous system depression.

Renal failure may be due to tubular necrosis as a result of hypotension, hypoxia, or a direct effect of the poison (e.g., salicylate, paraquat, acetaminophen, carbon tetrachloride) on the tubular cells. With hemoglobinuria or myoglobinuria, hemoglobin or myoglobin may precipitate in the renal tubules and produce renal failure.

Cerebral edema in intoxicated patients is produced by hypoxia, hypercapnia, hypotension, hypoglycemia, and drug-impaired capillary integrity. Computed tomography may aid in diagnosis. Therapy consists of correction of the arterial blood gas and metabolic abnormalities and the hypotension. Reduction of the increased intracranial pressure may be accomplished by giving 20% mannitol, 0.5 gram per kg, infused over a 30-minute period, and hyperventilation to reduce the $PaCO_2$ to 25 mmHg. The head should be elevated, and intracranial pressure monitoring should be considered. Fluid administration should be minimized.

Seizures are caused by many substances, such as amphetamines, camphor, chlorinated hydrocarbon insecticides, cocaine, isoniazid, lithium, phencyclidine, phenothiazines, propoxyphene, strychnine, tricyclic antidepressants, and drug withdrawal from ethanol and sedative hypnotics. Recurring or protracted seizures require intravenous diazepam (Valium) and phenytoin and, if seizure persists, a neuromuscular blocking agent and assisted ventilation.

Cardiac dysrhythmias occur with poisoning. A wide QT interval occurs with phenothiazines, and a wide QRS complex occurs with tricyclic antidepressants, quinine, or quinidine overdose. Digitalis, cocaine, cyanide, propranolol, theophylline, and amphetamines are among the more frequent toxic causes of dysrhythmias. Correction of metabolic disturbances and adequate oxygenation correct some of the dysrhythmias; others may require antidysrhythmic drugs or a cardiac pacemaker or cardioversion.

TABLE 5. **Dialysis: Indications and Contraindications**

Immediate Consideration of Dialysis: Life-Threatening Toxicities

Etyhlene glycol with refractory acidosis
Methanol with refractory acidosis and levels consistently over 50 mg/dL
Lithium levels consistently elevated over 4 mEq/L
Amanita phalloides

Severe Toxicities Due to Dialyzable Drugs (Stage 3 or higher on Reed Coma Scale)

Alcohol*	Iodides
Ammonia	Isoniazid*
Amphetamines	Meprobamate
Anilines	Paraldehyde
Antibiotics	Potassium*
Barbiturates* (long-acting)	Quinidine
Boric acid	Quinine
Bromides*	Salicylates*
Calcium	Strychnine
Chloral hydrate*	Thiocyanates
Fluorides	(Certain other drugs also dialyzable)

Conditions Requiring Dialysis for General Supportive Therapy

Uncontrollable metabolic acidosis or alkalosis
Uncontrollable electrolyte disturbance, particularly sodium or potassium
Overhydration
Renal failure
Hyperosmolality not responding to conservative therapy
Marked hypothermia
Stage 3 or higher on Reed Coma Scale

Dialysis Contraindicated on Pharmacologic Basis Except for Supportive Care: Nondialyzable Drug Toxicities

Antidepressants (tricyclic and monoamine oxidase inhibitors)
Antihistamines
Barbiturates (short-acting)
Belladonna alkaloids
Benzodiazepines (Valium, Librium)
Digitalis and derivatives
Hallucinogens
Meprobamate (Equanil, Miltown)
Methyprylon (Noludar)
Opioids (heroin, Lomotil)
Phenothiazines (Thorazine, Compazine)
Phenytoin (Dilantin)

*Most useful.

TABLE 6. **Plasma Concentrations Above Which Removal by Extracorporeal Means May Be Indicated**

Drug	Plasma Concentration (mg/dL)*	Method of Choice
Phenobarbital	10	HP>HD
Other barbiturates	5	HP
Glutethimide	4	HP
Methaqualone	4	HP
Salicylates	80	HD>HP
Ethchlorvynol	15	HP
Meprobamate	10	HP
Trichloroethanol	5	HP
Paraquat	0.1	HP>HD
Theophylline	6 (chronic) 10 (acute)	HP
Methanol	50	HD
Ethylene glycol	Unknown	HD
Lithium	4 mEq/L	HD
Ethanol	500	HD

Abbreviations: HP = hemoperfusion; HD = hemodialysis.
*1 mg/dL = 10 μg/mL.
Modified from Haddad L, and Winchester JF (eds): Clinical Management of Poisoning and Drug Overdose. Philadelphia, W. B. Saunders, 1983, p 162.

Metabolic acidosis with an increased anion gap is seen with many agents in overdose. There is a mnemonic by which to remember these agents: MUD PILES (*m*ethanol, *u*remia, *d*iabetic ketoacidosis, *p*araldehyde and *p*henformin, *i*ron and *i*soniazid, *l*actic acidosis, *e*thylene glycol and *e*thanol, and *s*alicylate, *s*tarvation, and *s*olvents such as toluene). Assessment of the arterial blood gases, serum electrolytes, and plasma osmolality may be a clue to the etiologic agent. Intravenous sodium bicarbonate may be needed when the pH is below 7.1 if there is adequate ventilation.

Hematemesis can be produced by caustics and corrosives, iron, lithium, mercury, phosphorus, arsenic, mushrooms, plant poisons, fluoride, and organophosphates. Therapy consists of fluid and blood replacement and iced saline lavage if there is no esophageal damage. Although controversial, antacids, H_2 blockers, sucralfate, or misoprostol may be used.

TOXICOKINETICS FOR THE PRACTICING PHYSICIAN

Toxicokinetics is clinical pharmacokinetics from the viewpoint of the toxicologist. Pharmacokinetics is a mathematic description of what the body does to a drug. Knowledge of the toxicokinetics of a specific toxic agent allows the physician to plan a rational approach to the definitive management of the intoxicated patient after the vital functions have been stabilized.

The LD_{50} (the lethal dose for 50% of experimental animals) and the MLD (the minimum lethal dose) are seldom relevant in human intoxications but indicate potential toxicity of the substance. Protein binding of toxic agents influences the volume distribution, elimination, and action of the drug. Diuresis and dialysis are usually reserved for drugs with less than 50% protein binding. The therapeutic blood range for a drug is the range of drug concentrations at which the majority of the treated population can be expected to receive therapeutic benefit. The toxic blood range is the range of drug concentrations at which this majority would be expected to have toxic manifestations. The drug range values are not absolute. Blood concentrations are a quantitative aid in determining whether more specific measures need to be instituted in correlation with the clinical manifestations. The apparent volume of distribution (Vd) is the percentage of body mass in which the drug is distributed. It is determined by dividing the amount absorbed by the blood concentration. When a substance has a large volume of distribution, as do most lipid-soluble chemicals (above 1 liter per kg), and is concentrated in the body fat, it is not available for diuresis, dialysis, or exchange transfusion. Elimination routes of detoxification allow the physician to make therapeutic decisions, such as using ethanol to interfere with the metabolism of methanol and ethylene glycol into more toxic metabolites. Urine identification is usually qualitative and allows only the identification of an agent.

Never manage a poisoned patient solely by laboratory tests, and always treat according to the manifestations of poisoning, not the laboratory test results. The laboratory toxicology analyst should be given whatever historical information is available so that the agent can be sought and identified as rapidly as possible. Toxicologic analysis is like a mini research project, unlike most other laboratory tests. Specimens for toxicologic analysis require the patient's name, date, time of exposure, time specimen was drawn, therapeutic drugs administered, patient's manifestations, and other relevant data. The toxicologic specimens that should be obtained for analysis are (1) vomitus or initial gastric aspiration; (2) blood, 10 mL (ask the analyst about the type of container and anticoagulant); and (3) urine, 100 mL. Acetaminophen plasma concentrations should be assessed in all suicide attempts.

COMMON POISONS AND THERAPY

Abbreviations Used in the Following List of Common Poisons

t½	= half-life (time required for blood level to drop by 50% of the original value)
Vd	= volume of distribution (liter per kg)
TLV	= threshold limit value in air
TWA	= time-weighted average
PPM	= parts per million in air and water

Conversion Factors

1 gram	= 1000 milligrams (mg)
1 milligram (mg)	= 1000 micrograms (μg)
1 microgram (μg)	= 1000 nanograms (ng)
Standard International Units:	
1 mole	= mol wt in grams per liter (L)
1 millimole	= mol wt in milligrams per L
1 micromole	= mol wt in micrograms per L
Blood levels:	
1 microgram per mL	= 100 micrograms per dL
	= 1 milligram per L
	= 1000 nanograms per mL
100 mg per dL	= 0.1 gram per dL
	= 1000 mg (1 gram) per L
	= 1 mg per mL

Acetaminophen, APAP (Tylenol). *Toxic dose:* Child, 3 grams or more; adult, 7.5 grams or more. Liver toxicity, 140 mg per kg. *Toxicokinetics:* Absorption time, 0.5 to 1 hour. Vd, 0.9 L per kg. Route of elimination by liver. Draw peak blood level after 4 hours in overdose. *Manifestations:* First 24 hours: malaise, nausea, vomiting, and drowsiness, followed by a latent period of 24 hours to 5 days; then hepatic symptoms, disturbances in clotting mechanism, and renal damage. *Management:* (1) Activated charcoal may be given when *N*-acetylcysteine (NAC) is contemplated. In these circumstances, separate activated charcoal from NAC by 1 to 2 hours. (2) *N*-Acetylcysteine for toxic overdose (Antidote 1, Table 4). Start and give a full course if a toxic dose has been ingested or if blood concentrations are above the toxic line on the nomogram shown in Figure 1. (3) In this instance, a saline sulfate cathartic is preferred to sorbitol. Treat at lower APAP plasma levels if patient has history of alcoholism or is taking enzyme inducer medication, i.e., anticonvulsants. *Laboratory aids:* APAP level, optimally at 4 to 6 hours. Plot levels on nomogram in Figure 1 as a guide for treatment. Monitor liver and renal profiles daily.

Acids. See Caustics and Corrosives.

Alcohols

1. Ethanol (grain alcohol). *Manifestations:* Blood ethanol levels over 30 mg per dL produce euphoria; over 50, incoordination and intoxication; over 100, ataxia; over 300, stupor; and over 500, coma. Levels of 500 to 700 mg per dL may be fatal. Chronic alcoholic patients tolerate higher levels, and the correlation may not be valid. *Management:* (1) Gastrointestinal decontamination. Caution: The rapid onset of CNS depression may preclude the induction of emesis. Activated charcoal and cathartics are not indicated. (2) Give 0.25 gram per kg of dextrose, 50%, intravenously if the blood glucose level is less than 60 mg per dL. (3) Thiamine, 100 mg intravenously, if chronic alcoholism is suspected, to prevent Wernicke-Korsakoff syndrome. (4) Hemodialysis is indicated in severe cases when conventional therapy is ineffective (rarely needed). (5) Treat seizures with diazepam (Valium) followed by phenytoin (Dilantin) if patient is unresponsive. (6) Treat withdrawal with hydration and chlordiazepoxide (Librium) or diazepam. Large doses of sedatives may be required for delirium tremens. *Laboratory aids:* Arterial blood gases, electrolytes, blood ethanol levels, glucose; determine anion and osmolar gap and check for ketosis. Chest radiograph to determine whether aspiration pneumonia is present. Liver function tests and bilirubin levels.

2. Isopropanol (rubbing alcohol). Normal propyl alcohol is related to isopropanol but is more toxic. *Manifestations:* Ethanol-like intoxication with ace-

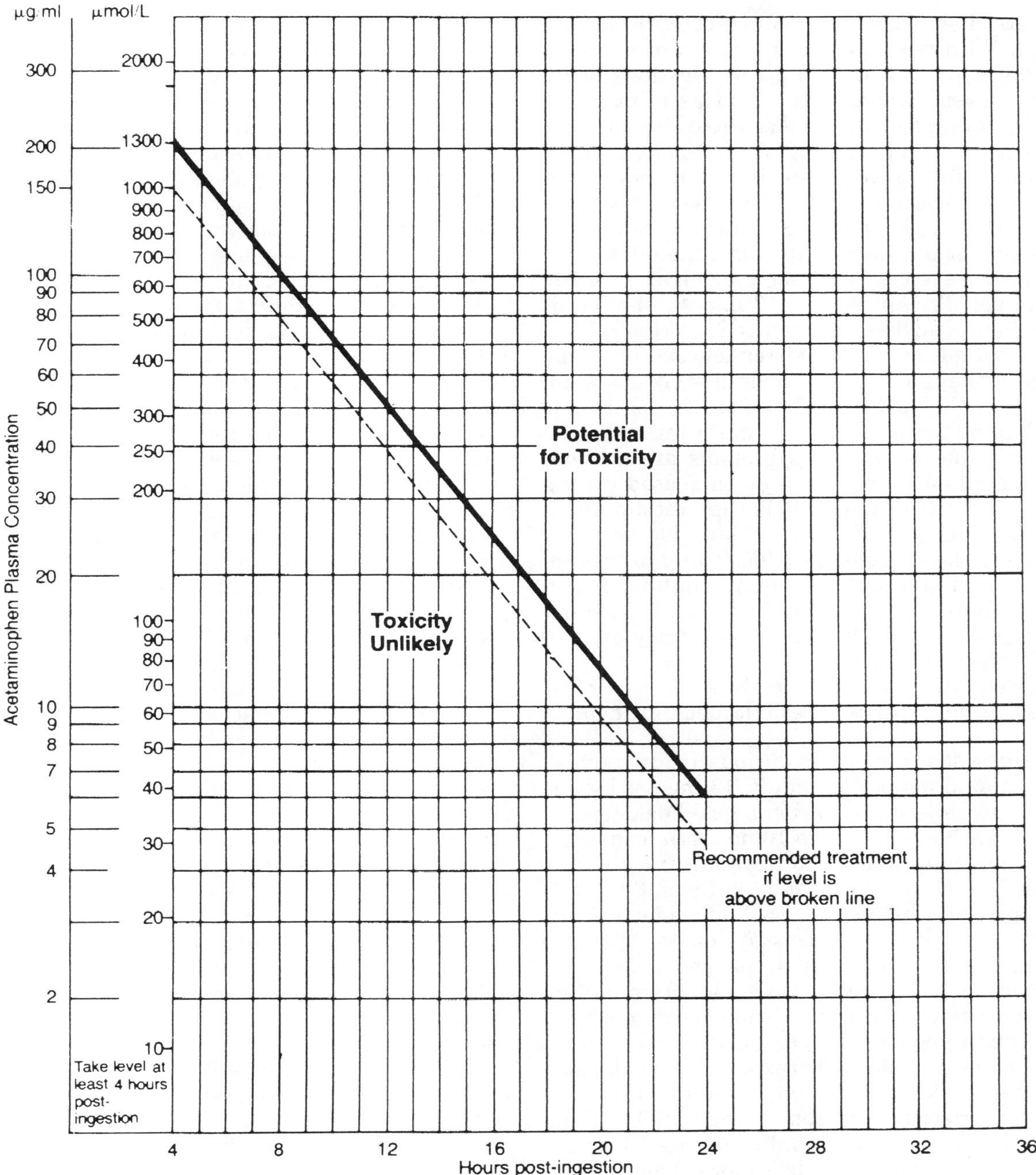

Figure 1. Nomogram for acetaminophen intoxication. Start *N*-acetylcysteine therapy if levels and time coordinates are above the lower line on the nomogram. Continue and complete therapy even if subsequent values fall below the toxic zone. The nomogram is useful only in acute, single ingestions. Serum levels drawn before 4 hours may not represent peak levels. (From Rumack BH, and Matthew H: Acetaminophen poisoning and toxicity. Pediatrics *55*:871, 1975. Reproduced by permission of Pediatrics.)

tone odor to breath, acetonuria, acetonemia without systemic acidosis, gastritis. With worsening acidosis, there is multiorgan failure, with death from complications of intractable acidosis. *Management:* (1) Gastrointestinal decontamination. Activated charcoal and cathartics not indicated. (2) Hemodialysis in life-threatening overdose (rarely needed). *Laboratory aids:* Isopropyl alcohol levels, acetone, glucose, and arterial blood gases. The lack of excess acetone in the blood (normal 0.3 to 2 mg per dL) within 30 to 60 minutes or acetone in the urine within 3 hours excludes the possibility of significant isopropanol exposure.

3. METHANOL (wood alcohol). *Toxic dose:* One teaspoonful is potentially lethal for a 2-year-old child and can cause blindness in an adult. The toxic blood level of methanol is above 20 mg per dL, the potentially fatal level over 50 mg per dL. *Manifestations:* Metabolism may delay onset for 12 to 18 hours or longer if ethanol is ingested concomitantly. Hyper-

emia of optic disk, violent abdominal colic, blindness, and shock. With worsening acidosis, there is multiorgan failure, with death from complications of intractable acidosis. *Management:* (1) Gastrointestinal decontamination up to 1 hour. Activated charcoal and cathartics are not indicated. (2) Treat acidosis vigorously with sodium bicarbonate intravenously. (3) If methanol is clinically suspected because of metabolic acidosis, with an anion gap if methanol concentration above 20 mg per dL, immediately initiate ethanol IV or PO to produce a blood ethanol concentration of 100 to 150 mg per dL (Antidote 21, Table 4). (4) Folinic acid and folic acid have been used successfully in animal investigations. Administer leucovorin, 1 mg per kg up to 50 mg IV every 4 hours for six doses. (5) Consider hemodialysis if the blood methanol level is greater than 50 mg per dL or if significant metabolic acidosis or visual or mental symptoms are present. *Note:* The ethanol dose has to be increased during dialysis therapy. (6) Continue therapy (ethanol and hemodialysis) until blood methanol level is preferably undetectable, and there is no acidosis and no mental or visual disturbances. This often requires 2 to 5 days. (7) Ophthalmology consultation. *Laboratory aids:* Methanol and ethanol levels, electrolytes, glucose, and arterial blood gases.

Alkali. See Caustics and Corrosives.

Amitriptyline (Elavil). See Tricyclic Antidepressants.

Amphetamines (diet pills, various trade names). *Toxicity:* Child, 5 mg per kg; adult, 12 mg per kg has been reported as lethal. *Toxicokinetics:* Peak time of action is 2 to 4 hours. t½, 8 to 10 hours in acid urine (pH less than 6.0) and 16 to 31 hours in alkaline urine (pH, 7.5). *Route of elimination:* Liver, 60%; kidney, 30 to 40% at alkaline urine pH; at acid urine pH, 50 to 70%. *Manifestations:* Dysrhythmias, hyperpyrexia, convulsions, hypertension, paranoia, violence. *Management:* (1) Gastrointestinal decontamination. Avoid induced emesis because of rapid onset of action. (2) Control extreme agitation or convulsions with diazepam. Chlorpromazine (Thorazine) may be dangerous if ingestion is not pure amphetamine. (3) Treat hypertensive crisis with nitroprusside at 0.3 to 2 mg per kg per minute; maximum infusion rate 10 μg per kg per minute; should never last more than 10 minutes. (4) Acidification diuresis is not recommended. (5) Treat hyperpyrexia symptomatically. (6) If focal neurologic symptoms are present, consider cerebrovascular accident. Obtain computed tomography scan. (7) Observe for suicidal depression that may follow intoxication. (8) In life-threatening agitation, use haloperidol (Haldol). (9) Significant life-threatening tachydysrhythmia may respond to the alpha and beta blocker labetalol (Normodyne; Antidote 27, Table 4) or other appropriate antidysrhythmic agents. In a severely hemodynamically compromised patient, use immediate synchronized cardioversion. *Laboratory aids:* Monitor for rhabdomyolysis (creatine phosphokinase [CPK]), myoglobinuria, hyperkalemia, and disseminated intravascular coagulation. Toxic blood level, 10 μg per dL.

Aniline. See Nitrites and Nitrates.

Anticholinergic Agents. Examples are antihistamines—hydroxyzine (Atarax), diphenhydramine (Benadryl); antipsychotics (neuroleptics)—phenothiazines (Thorazine); antidepressant drugs (tricyclic antidepressants)—imipramine (Tofranil); antiparkinsonian drugs—trihexyphenidyl (Artane), benztropine (Cogentin); over-the-counter sleep, cold, and hay fever medicines (methapyrilene); ophthalmic products (atropine); plants—jimsonweed (*Datura stramonium*), deadly nightshade (*Atropa belladonna*), henbane (*Hyoscyamus niger*); and antispasmodic agents for the bowel (atropine). *Toxicokinetics:* See Table 7. *Manifestations:* Anticholinergic signs—hyperpyrexia, dilated pupils, flushing of skin, dry mucosa, tachycardia, delirium, hallucinations, coma, and convulsions. *Management:* (1) Gastrointestinal decontamination up to 12 hours postingestion. *Note:* Caution with emesis if diphenhydramine overdose because of rapid onset of action and seizures. (2) Control seizures with diazepam. (3) Control ventricular dysrhythmias with lidocaine. (4) Physostigmine (Antidote 35, Table 4) for life-threatening anticholinergic effects refractory to conventional treatments. (5) Relieve urinary retention by catheterization to avoid reabsorption. (6) Treat cardiac dysrhythmias only if tissue perfusion is not adequate or if the patient is hypotensive. (7) Control hyperpexia by external cooling. No antipyretics.

Anticonvulsants. See Table 8. *Toxic dose:* Specific anticonvulsant blood levels and the clinical manifestations indicate toxicity. In general, the ingestion of five times the therapeutic dose is expected to have the potential for toxicity. *Management:* (1) Gastrointestinal decontamination up to 12 hours postingestion. Repeated doses of activated charcoal shorten t½ of carbamazepine, phenobarbital, primidone, phenytoin, and possibly others. Naloxone (Antidote 30, Table 4) may improve valproic acid–induced coma. (2) Monitor specific anticonvulsant blood levels. (3) The effectiveness of hemoperfusion and dialysis has not been established.

Antidepressants. See Tricyclic Antidepressants.

Antifreeze. See Alcohols (Methanol) and Ethylene Glycol.

Antihistamines (H_1 Receptor Antagonists). See Anticholinergic Agents. Newer nonsedating long-acting preparations—terfenadine and astemizole—may produce prolonged QT intervals and torsades de pointes. In patients who have impaired hepatic function or are receiving cimetidine, ketoconazole, or macrolide antibiotics the metabolism of terfenadine and astemizole may be inhibited. All children who ingest these newer nonsedating antihistamines or adults who ingest more than the therapeutic dose require close cardiac monitoring for 24 hours. Gastrointestinal decontamination is advised.

Arsenic and Arsine Gas. *Toxic dose:* In humans, the inorganic arsenic trioxide toxic dose is 5 to 50 mg; the potential fatal dose is 120 mg or 1 to 2 mg per kg. Sodium arsenite is nine times more toxic than arsenic trioxide. Organic arsenic is less toxic. The maximum allowable concentration for prolonged exposure

TABLE 7. **Toxicokinetics of Anticholinergic Agents**

Drug	Potential Fatal Dose	Time to Peak Effect	Volume of Distribution (L/kg)	Half-life (h)	Excretion Route
Atropine	Child: 10–20 mg; adult: 100 mg	1–2 h, may be prolonged in overdose	2.3	2–3	Renal (30–50%); hepatic (50–70%)
Diphenhydramine	Child: 25 mg/kg; adult: 2–8 gm	2 h, may be prolonged in overdose	3.3–6.8	3–10	98% hepatic

is 0.05 PPM. See Table 9. Humans are more sensitive than rodents to arsenic. Acute poisoning results from accidental ingestion of arsenic-containing pesticides. (Ant traps sold in some states contain arsenic.) *Toxicokinetics:* Arsenates are water soluble and arsenite is lipid soluble. The soluble forms of arsenic are rapidly absorbed by inhalation and ingestion. Crosses placenta and can cause fetal damage. Distributes into spleen, liver, kidneys. *Excretion:* In urine, 90%. Following acute ingestion, it takes 10 days to clear a single dose; chronic ingestion takes up to 70 days. *Arsine gas:* Forms when active hydrogen comes in contact with arsenic. This may occur when zinc, antimony, lead, or iron is contaminated with arsenic and comes in contact with acid. This causes arsine inhalation intoxication characterized by a latent period of 2 to 48 hours and a triad of abdominal pain, jaundice (due to hemolysis), and hematuria. *Manifestations:* Gastroenteritis, neurologic and cardiac abnormalities, subsequent renal involvement. A garlic odor to the breath may be a clue. Smaller doses and prolonged low-level exposure produce subacute (stomatitis) and chronic (peripheral neuropathy) symptoms. *Management:* (1) Gastrointestinal decontamination. Activated charcoal is ineffective. Cathartics are not advised because of potential for diarrhea. Follow with abdominal radiographs because arsenic is radiopaque. Consider whole-bowel washout if usual methods fail to remove arsenic. (2) Intravenous fluids to correct dehydration and electrolyte deficiencies. (3) Treat shock with oxygen, blood, and fluids as needed. (4) In severe cases, administer BAL (dimercaprol) (Antidote 17, Table 4). (5) In chronic poisoning, D-penicillamine (Antidote 34, Table 4) may be used to chelate arsenic. Therapy should be continued in 5-day cycles until the urine arsenic is less than 50 μg per liter. (6) Treat liver and renal impairment. (7) Hemodialysis is effective in acute poisoning and can be used concurrently with chelation therapy in severe cases, especially if renal failure develops. (8) Arsine

TABLE 8. **Anticonvulsants**

Drug	Peak Time of Action: Steady State (h)	Volume of Distribution (L/kg)	Half-life (h)	Route of Elimination (%)	Protein Binding (%)	Blood Level (μg/mL)	Comment*
Carbamazepine (Tegretol)	8–24 (2–4 days)	1.0	18–54	Liver (98)	70	Therapeutic, 4–10	Related to tricyclic antidepressants, can cause dysrhythmias
Ethosuximide (Zarontin)	24–48 (5–8 days)	0.8	36–55	Liver (80–90)	0	Therapeutic, 40–100	
Phenytoin (Dilantin)	PO 6–12 IV, 1 (5–10 days)	1.0	24; varies in toxic doses: zero-order kinetics	Liver (95)	90	Therapeutic, 10–20; toxic, 20–30; nystagmus only, 30–40; ataxia, 40+; coma, convulsions	Dysrhythmias with parenteral use only
Primidone (Mysoline)	?3–4 days	0.6	Parent, 3–12; metabolites, 30–36	Liver	60	Therapeutic, 6–12 primidone and 15–40 phenobarbital (PB); toxic, over 50 primidone and over 40 PB (see Barbiturates)	Metabolized to active metabolites phenylethylmalonamide and PB; overdose gives white crystals in urine†
Valproic acid (Depakene)	? 1–2 days	0.4	5–15	Liver (80–100)	84–96	Therapeutic, 50–100	Produces nausea and vomiting, changes in liver function
Clonazepam (Clonopin)	?		20–60	Liver (98)	90	Therapeutic, 20–70 ng/mL	
Phenobarbital (Luminal)	3–6 h	0.75	50–120	Liver	30	Therapeutic, 15–40	

*Manifestations: The major manifestations of these agents are depression of consciousness and respiratory depression. Other significant manifestations are mentioned in this column.

†Primidone produces whorls of shimmering white crystals in the urine from precipitation of intact primidone in massive overdose.

TABLE 9. **Comparative Acute Toxicities of Some Common Arsenicals**

Arsenic Compound	Lethal Dose
Arsenate	5–50 mg/kg
Arsenites	<5 mg/kg
Arsenic trioxide (insoluble)	120 mg total
Arsenic trioxide (soluble)*	13 mg total

*Nine times as toxic as insoluble form.

intoxication is treated by exchange transfusion and hemodialysis if renal failure occurs. BAL is ineffective. *Laboratory aids:* Blood arsenic and 24-hour urine arsenic levels. Excessive exposure is indicated by a level of 50 μg per liter of arsenic in urine, but persons whose diets are rich in seafood may excrete larger amounts. View values over 50 μg per day with suspicion. Monitor electrocardiogram (ECG) and renal function. A blood arsenic level above 1.0 mg per liter is toxic, and one of 9 to 15 mg per liter is potentially fatal (false values occur in inexperienced laboratories).

Aspirin. See Salicylates.

Atropine. See Anticholinergic Agents.

Barbiturates. See Table 10. *Management:* (1) Gastrointestinal decontamination up to 8 to 12 hours postingestion. Avoid emesis in short-acting barbiturate intoxications. Activated charcoal and a cathartic in repeated doses have been shown to reduce the serum half-life of phenobarbital and increased the nonrenal clearance by over 50%. Give every 4 hours while the patient is comatose. (2) Supportive and symptomatic care is all that is necessary in the majority of cases. (3) Alkalinization with sodium bicarbonate, 2 mEq per kg IV during the first hour, followed by sufficient sodium bicarbonate (Antidote 39, Table 4) to keep the urinary pH at 7.5 to 8.0, enhances excretion of long-acting barbiturates. Alkalinization is not useful for short-acting barbiturate intoxication. Forced diuresis should be used with caution because of fluid overload. At present, alkalinization without diuresis is advocated. (4) In severe cases that do not respond to conservative measures, consider hemodialysis and hemoperfusion. (5) Treat any bullae as a local second-degree skin burn. (6) Give intensive care monitoring to the comatose patient. *Treatment of withdrawal: In an emergency,* use pentothal or diazepam intravenously. If the patient is stable, a pentobarbital is given orally and the patient examined after 1 hour for signs of intoxication (nystagmus, slurred speech, and ataxia). If none is present, the dose is repeated every 3 hours until these signs develop. This is the stabilizing dose; the patient is maintained on this dose for 72 hours and then changed to phenobarbital, 30 mg substituted for each 100 mg of pentobarbital. The phenobarbital is tapered, decreasing by 10% or 30 mg every 3 to 5 days. *Laboratory aids:* Emergency plasma barbiturate concentrations rarely alter management.

Benzene. See Hydrocarbons.

Benzodiazepines (BZP). See Table 11. *Toxicity:* Low toxic potential. More than 500 mg has been ingested without respiratory depression. Benzodiazepines have an additive effect with sedatives, such as alcohol and barbiturates. Most patients intoxicated with benzodiazepines alone recover within 24 hours. Many of these agents have active metabolites with a long plasma t½, so performance in skilled tasks, such as driving, may be impaired. Withdrawal may be delayed. *Manifestations:* CNS depression. Deep coma leading to respiratory depression suggests presence of other drugs. *Management:* (1) Gastrointestinal decontamination. (2) Supportive and symptomatic care. (3) Flumazenil (Romazicon) is a recently approved specific benzodiazepine antagonist. It is not a treatment for hypoventilation and should be used with caution in overdose cases because of dependency and seizures (Antidote 23, Table 4). (4) Withdrawal, if it occurs, is treated with a long-acting benzodiazepine on a tapering schedule. *Laboratory aids:* Document benzodiazepines in urine. Quantitative blood levels are not useful.

Bleach. Household bleaches are 4 to 6% sodium hypochlorite. Commercial types are 10 to 20%. *Manifestations:* Difficulty in swallowing; pain in mouth, throat, chest, or abdomen. General household strength bleach does not produce burns; commercial strength bleach may. Inhalation of gases produced by mixing chlorine bleach with acids (toilet bowl cleaner and rust removers—chlorine gas) or with household ammonia (chloramine gas) causes irritation of mucous membranes, eyes, and upper respiratory tract. *Management:* (1) Ingestion—avoid gastrointestinal decontamination procedures. Dilute with small amounts of water or milk. Avoid acids. (2) Esophagoscopy only if unusually large amounts have been ingested, the patient is symptomatic, or the product was stronger than the average household bleach. (3) Inhalation—Remove from contaminated area. Observe for pulmonary edema. (4) Ocular exposure requires immediate gentle irrigation with water for at least 15 minutes, followed by fluorescein dye stain to detect any damage.

Botulism. See article Food-Borne Illness in Section 2.

Brake Fluid. See Ethylene Glycol.

Calcium Channel Blockers. Used in treatment of effort angina, supraventricular tachycardia, and hypertension. See Table 12. *Manifestations:* Hypotension, bradycardia within 1 to 5 hours, CNS depression, and gastric distress. Manifestations are delayed after ingestion of slow-release preparations. *Management:* (1) Gastrointestinal decontamination. If long-acting preparation, consider whole-bowel washout. If patient is symptomatic, obtain cardiac consult. May need pacemaker. (2) Treat hypotension and bradycardia with positioning, fluids, and calcium gluconate or chloride (Antidote 12B, Table 4). Dopamine or norepinephrine may be used if necessary. If calcium fails, use sodium bicarbonate, glucagon, or both (Antidote 26, Table 4). (3) Heart block—may respond to intravenous calcium (Antidote 12B, Table 4) or atropine sulfate, 0.5 to 1 mg, if no response. (4) Ventricular

TABLE 10. **Features of Barbiturates***

Feature	Long-Acting (LAB)	Intermediate-Acting (IAB) Acting (SAB)	Short-Acting (SAB)
Duration	>8 h	3–8 h	<3 h
Medical use	Anticonvulsants	Sedative hypnotics	
Half-life	>50 h	<50 h	<50 h
DEA	Schedule IV	Schedule II	Schedule II

Feature	Barbital	Phenobarbital†	Amobarbital	Pentobarbital	Secobarbital
Trade name	Veronal	Luminal	Amytal	Nembutal	Seconal
Slang name	—	Purple hearts	Blues	Yellows	Red devils
pKa	7.8	7.24	7.9	7.96	7.9
Elimination route	Renal 20% Hepatic 80%	Renal 30% Hepatic 70%	Hepatic 98%	Hepatic >90%	Hepatic >90%
Onset IV	22 min	12 min	—	0.1 min	0.1 min
Onset oral	1 h	20–60 min	13–30 min	15–30 min	10–30 min
Peak conc oral	12–18 h	6–18 h	3–4 h	2–4 h	1–2 h
Protein-bound	6%	20–40%	40–60%	40–65%	40–60%
Oral doses					
Fatal dose	10 gm 75 mg/kg	8 gm 65 mg/kg	5 gm 40 mg/kg	3 gm 50 mg/kg	3 gm 30 mg/kg
Toxic dose	>8 mg/kg	15–35 mg/kg	>6 mg/kg	>6 mg/kg	>6 mg/kg
Adult nontolerant		300 mg	200–300 mg	200–300 mg	200 mg
Therapeutic dose	2–6 mg/kg	2–6 mg/kg	2–6 mg/kg	2–6 mg/kg	6 mg/kg
Adult dose	300–500 mg	100–200 mg	100–200 mg	100–200 mg	100–200 mg
Blood concentrations					
Therapeutic	5–8 μg/mL	15–40 μg/mL	5–6 μg/mL	1–5 μg/mL	1–5 μg/mL
Toxic	>30 μg/mL	>40 μg/mL	10–30 μg/mL	>10 μg/mL	>10 μg/mL
Lethal‡	>100 μg/mL	>100 μg/mL	>50 μg/mL	>35 μg/mL	>35 μg/mL
Duration	16 h	6–8 h	6 h	6 h	6 h
Elimination t½	56–96 h	50–120 h	15–40 h	15–30 h	22–29 h
Volume of distribution	—	0.75 L/kg	0.5 L/kg	0.65 L/kg	1.5 L/kg
Available					
Capsule (mg)	—	16	65, 200	50, 100	50, 100
Tablet (mg)	—	16, 32, 65, 100	15, 30, 50, 100	—	100
Elixir (mg/5 mL)	—	15, 20	—	20	—
Suppository (mg)	—			30, 60, 120, 200	—
Manifestations					
Low dose: Euphoria, ataxia, incoordination, nystagmus on lateral gaze					
High dose: Flaccid coma, hypotension, respiratory depression, pulmonary edema (particularly with the short-acting barbiturates), subcutaneous bullae (6%), dermatographia					

Abbreviations: DEA = Drug Enforcement Agency; conc = concentration; nontol = nontolerant; therap = therapeutic; t½ = half-life; elimin = elimination.
*Classification into long acting, intermediate, and short acting has no relationship to the duration of coma.
†The half-life (t½) in children is approximately 50% of adult.
‡These levels are not absolute, and tolerance occurs.

pacing may be required in the severely intoxicated patient. (5) Patients receiving digitalis run the risk of toxicity and should be carefully monitored. (6) Extracorporeal washout measures are generally not considered to be useful. *Laboratory aids:* Specific drug levels, blood sugar and calcium, ECG.

Camphor (External analgesic rubs, Vicks Vaporub 4.8%, Campho-Phenique 11%). Many camphorated oil products were removed from the marketplace in September, 1982. Five milliliters of camphorated oil (20% camphor) equals 1 gram of camphor. *Toxicity:* More than 10 mg per kg may cause seizures. Adult, 5 grams has been fatal; child, 1 gram. *Toxicokinetics:* Time to onset of manifestations, 5 to 90 minutes. Readily and rapidly absorbed through the skin, mucous membranes, and gastrointestinal tract, and crosses the placenta. *Route of elimination:* Rapidly metabolized in liver to the glucuronide form, which is excreted in urine. Pulmonary excretion causes a distinctive odor on the breath. *Manifestations:* Nausea, vomiting, and burning epigastric pain. Seizures may occur suddenly and without warning within 5 minutes of ingestion. Apnea and vision disturbances may occur. *Management:* (1) Induction of emesis is contraindicated because of early seizures. (2) Remove residual drug by gastric lavage. (3) Administer activated charcoal and a saline cathartic. Avoid giving oils or alcohol. (4) Treat seizures with intravenous diazepam. (5) Treat apnea with respiratory support.

Carbon Monoxide (CO). This is an odorless gas produced from incomplete combustion; it is found also as an in vivo metabolic breakdown product of methylene chloride (paint removers). Observe for the symptoms described in Table 13. Contrary to popular belief, the skin rarely shows a cherry-red color in the living patient. *Toxicokinetics:* CO is rapidly absorbed

TABLE 11. **Benzodiazepines (BZPs)**

Drug	Oral Dosage Range	Time to Peak Oral Plasma Levels (h)	Half-life: t1/2 (h)	Major Active Metabolites (Half-life in h)	Elimination Rate
Anxiolytics					
Diazepam (Valium)	6–40 mg/day	1–2	20–50	Desmethyldiazepam ($t\frac{1}{2}$ = 30–60 h)	Slow
Chlordiazepoxide (Librium, Libritabs, various others)	15–100 mg/day	2–4	5–30	Desmethylchlordiazepoxide, demoxepam, desmethyldiazepam	Slow
Clorazepate (Tranxene)	15–60 mg/day	1–2.5	30–60	Desmethyldiazepam	Slow
Prazepam (Centrax)	20–60 mg/day	6	78	3-Hydroxyprazepam, desmethyldiazepam	Slow
Halazepam (Paxipam)	60–160 mg/day	1–3	7	*N*-3-Hydroxyhalazepam, desmethyldiazepam	Slow
Oxazepam (Serax)	30–120 mg/day	1–2	3–10	None	Rapid to intermediate
Lorazepam (Ativan)	2–6 mg/day	2	10–20	None	Intermediate
Alprazolam (Xanax)	0.75–4 mg/day	0.7–1.6	12–19	α-Hydroxyalprazolam	Intermediate
Hypnotics					
Flurazepam (Dalmane)	15–60 mg	3–6	50–100	Desalkylflurazepam ($t\frac{1}{2}$ = 50–100 h)	Slow
Midazolam (Versed)	5–30 mg/day IV	0.3–0.8	3–5	None	—
Flunitrazepam (Rohypnol—investigational, Roche)	1–2 mg	<1	—	7-Aminoflunitrazepam ($t\frac{1}{2}$ = 23 h), *N*-desmethylflunitrazepam ($t\frac{1}{2}$ = 31 h)	—
Temazepam (Restoril)	15–30 mg	2–3	9–12	None	Intermediate
Triazolam (Halcion)	0.125–0.5 mg	0.5–1.5	2–3	α-Hydroxytriazolam	Rapid
Quazepam (Doral)	7.5–15 mg	1–2	>24	2-Oxoquazepam *N*-desalkylflurazepam	Intermediate
Estazolam (ProSom)	1–2 mg	1–2	12–15	1-Oxo estazolam	Intermediate
Anticonvulsants					
Clonazepam (Klonopin)	1.5–20 mg/day	1–4	24–48	None	—
Zolpidem* (Ambien)	5–20 mg/day	2	1.5–2.5	None	Rapid

*Not a benzodiazepine chemically but an imidazopyridine that is a selective benzodiazepine-1 receptor agonist.

through the lungs. The rate of absorption is directly related to alveolar ventilation. Elimination occurs through the lungs. The $t\frac{1}{2}$ in room air equals 5 to 6 hours; in 100% oxygen, 90 minutes; in hyperbaric oxygen, 20 minutes. The nomogram pictured in Figure 2 can be used to decide quickly whether serious CO intoxication is likely to have occurred and to select patients at high risk or who need early management in the intensive care unit or hyperbaric oxygen. *Management:* (1) Remove the patient from contaminated area and expose to fresh air. Establish vital functions. (2) Give 100% oxygen to all patients until the carboxyhemoglobin level falls to 5% or less. Assisted ventilation may be necessary. The exposed pregnant woman should be kept in 100% oxygen for several hours after the carboxyhemoglobin level is zero because carboxyhemoglobin concentrates in the fetus and oxygen is needed five times longer to ensure elimination of CO from fetal circulation. CO or hypoxia may be teratogenic. (3) Monitor arterial blood gases and carboxyhemoglobin levels. Determine carboxyhemoglobin level at time of exposure by using nomogram. *Note:* A near-normal carboxyhemoglobin level does not rule out significant CO poisoning. (4) Only if pH is below 7.1 after correction of hypoxia and adequate ventilation, give sodium bicarbonate to correct acidosis. (5) Indications for 100% oxygen and, if possible, therapy with hyperbaric oxygen: (a) carboxyhemoglobin level higher than 25%; (b) carboxyhemoglobin level higher than 15% in a child or in a patient with cardiovascular disease; (c) carboxyhemoglobin level higher than 10% in a pregnant woman (and monitor fetus); (d) abnormal or ischemic chest pain or ECG abnormality; (e) abnormal chest radiograph; (f) presence of hypoxia, myoglobinuria, or abnormal renal function; (g) history of unconsciousness, syncope, or neuropsychiatric symptoms. Most important indication for hyperbaric chamber is history of unconsciousness. A list of hyperbaric oxygen chambers can be obtained by contacting a Regional Poison Control Center. (6) Treat seizures with intravenous diazepam. (7) Monitor ECG, chest radiograph, and serum CPK and lactate dehydrogenase levels. (8) Treat cerebral edema with elevation of the patient's head, minimizing intravenous fluid and hyperventilation; if needed, mannitol and intracranial pressure monitor. (9) Reevaluate after recovery for neuropsychiatric sequelae. *Laboratory aids:* Arterial blood gases show metabolic acidosis and normal oxygen tension but reduced oxygen saturation, as measured by a co-oximeter.

Carbon Tetrachloride. See Hydrocarbons.

Caustics and Corrosives. Common acid substances are hydrochloric acid, sulfuric acid (battery acid), carbolic acid (phenol), nitric acid, oxalic acid, hydrofluoric acid, and aqua regia (mixture of hydrochloric and nitric acids). These are used as cleaning agents. Common alkali substances are sodium or po-

TABLE 12. **Kinetics of the Calcium Channel Blockers**

Parameter	Nifedipine	Verapamil	Diltiazem	Nicardipine	Nimodipine	Felodipine*	Amlodipine	Bepridil	Isradipine
Class	Dihydropyridine	Phenylalkylamine	Benzothiazepine	Dihydropyridine	Dihydropyridine	Dihydropyridine	Dihydropyridine	Dihydropyridine	Dihydropyridine
Trade name	Procardia	Calan, Isoptin	Cardizem	Cardene	Nimotop	Plendil	Norvasc	Vascor	DynaCirc
Preparations	10-, 20-mg cap	40-, 80-, 120-mg tab	30-, 60-, 90-, 120-mg tab	20-, 30-mg cap	30 mg	None	2.5-, 5-, 10-mg tab	200-, 300-, 400-mg tab	2.5-, 5-mg cap
Slow-release preparation	30-, 60-, 90-mg cap	120-, 180-, 240-mg tab	60-, 90-, 120-, 180-, 240-, 300-mg tab	30-, 40-, 60-mg	None	5, 10 mg	See above	None	None
Bioavailability	65–70%	20–30%	40%	35%	3–30%	20%	60–65%	60%	17%
Mean toxic dose	340 mg	3.2 gm	? rare toxicity	NA	NA	NA	—	—	—
Serious toxic amount	Lowest 200 mg	40 mg/kg child 2–3 gm adult	Up to 300 mg well tolerated by adults	NA	NA	NA	—	—	—
Dose range	—	—	—	—	—	—	2.5–10 mg/d	200–400 mg/d	2.5–15 mg/d
Max daily dose	—	—	—	—	—	—	10 mg/d	400 mg/d	20 mg/d
Onset of action	—	—	—	—	—	—	—	—	—
Oral	<20 min	30–120 min	<15 min	<20 min	<20 min	—			
IV	<1 min	<3 min	<1 min	—	—	—			
SL	3–5 min	—	—	—	—	—			
Peak action									
Oral	30–90 min	60–90 min	30–60 min	60 min	60 min	2.5–6 h	6–9	2–3	2–3
SL	20 min	—	—	—	—	—			
Sustained	—	4–8 h	3–4 h	—	—	—			
Peak blood conc	30–60 min	90–120 min	120–180 min	60 min	NA	NA	—	—	—
Half-life	3–6 h	6–12 h	4–9 h	8 h	1–8 h	24 h	35–50 h	33–42 h	5–10.7 h
Duration	4–12 h	6–12 h	—	4–6 h	NA	—	24 h	24 h	12 h
Protein binding	92–98%	90–99%	70–85%	>95%	>95%	NA	98%	99%	97%
Volume of distribution	1–5 L/kg	4.5–7 L/kg	3–5 L/kg	NA	—	—	21 L/kg	8 L/kg	3 L/kg
Elimination	Renal 50–70%	Hepatic 60–65%	Renal 70–80%	Hepatic	—	—	Hepatic	Hepatic	Hepatic
Metabolite	Inactive	Active mild norverapamil	Active 50% parent diacetyldiltiazem	NA	NA	NA	Pyridine deriv. (not active)	17 metabolites (one active)	None active

Abbreviations: cap = capsules; tab = tablets; NA = no available information; SL = sublingual; conc = concentration.
*Anonymous: Felodipine—another calcium channel blocker for hypertension. Med Lett *33:*115–116, 1991.

tassium hydroxide (lye), sodium hypochlorite (Clorox [bleach]), sodium carbonate (nonphosphate detergents), potassium permanganate, ammonia, electric dishwashing agents, cement, and flat disk batteries. *Toxicity:* Acids produce mucosal coagulation necrosis. They usually do not penetrate deeply (exception: hydrofluoric acid). The gastric mucosa is the primary site of injury. Alkalis produce liquefaction necrosis and saponification and penetrate deeply. Oropharyngeal and esophageal damage by solids is more frequent than by liquids. Liquids are more likely to produce gastric damage. *Toxic dose:* Adult potential fatal dose of concentrated acid or alkali is 5 mL. The absence of oral burns does not exclude the possibility of esophageal burns (seen in 10 to 15% of patients). *Management:* (1) Dilute with milk or water immediately up to 30 mL in children or 250 mL in adults. Neutralization with acidic or alkalinic agents is contraindicated. Dilute only if patient can swallow. Contraindications to dilution are an inability to swallow and signs of respiratory distress, shock, or esophageal perforation. (2) Gastrointestinal decontamination is contraindicated. In acid ingestions, however, some authorities advocate nasogastric intubation and aspiration in the early postingestion phase. Patient should receive only intravenous fluids following dilution until surgical consultation is obtained. Dermal and ocular decontamination should be carried out. (3) Endoscopy at 12 to 48 hours postingestion may be indicated to assess severity of burn. (4) Steroids are controversial. (5) Antibiotics are not useful prophylactically. (6) Barium swallow may be necessary at 10 days to 3 weeks to assess severity of damage. (7) Esophageal dilation may need to be performed at 2- to 4-week intervals if evidence of stricture is found. (8) Interposition of the colon may be necessary if dilation fails to provide an adequate-sized esophagus. (9) Inhalation management requires immediate removal from the environment, and clinical, radiographic, and arterial blood gas evaluation when ap-

TABLE 13. **Progression of Signs and Symptoms with Carbon Monoxide (CO) Exposure**

CO in Atmosphere (PPM)	Duration of Exposure	Saturation of Blood (%)	Signs/Symptoms
Up to 0.01	Indefinite	1–10	None
0.01–0.02	Indefinite	10–20	Tightness across forehead, slight headache, dilation of cutaneous vessels
0.02–0.03	5–6 h	20–30	Headache, throbbing temples
0.04–0.06	4–5 h	30–40	Severe headache, weakness and dizziness, nausea and vomiting, collapse, leukocytosis
0.07–0.10	3–4 h	40–50	Above, plus increased tendency to collapse and syncope, increased pulse and respiratory rate
0.11–0.15	1.5–3 h	50–60	Increased pulse and respiratory rate, syncope, Cheyne-Stokes respirations, coma with intermittent convulsions
0.16–0.30	1–1.5 h	60–70	Coma with intermittent convulsions, depressed heart action and respirations, death possible
0.50–1.00	1–2 h	70–80	Weak pulse, depressed respirations, respiratory failure, and death

propriate. Oxygen and respiratory support may be required.

Chloral Hydrate. See Sedative Hypnotics.

Chlordane. See Organochlorine Insecticides.

Chlordiazepoxide (Librium). See Benzodiazepines.

Chlorine Gas. Chlorine gas is a yellow greenish gas with an irritating odor used in bleach, in manufacture of plastics, and for water purification. Exposure usually results from transportation mishaps, industrial accidents, chemistry experiments, the mixing of household cleaners with bleach containing hypochlorite, and accidental release around swimming pools. Its density is greater than that of air, and an odor is detected at concentrations of less than 0.04 to 0.2 PPM. Chlorine acts as an oxidizing agent and also reacts with tissue water to form hypochlorous and hydrochloric acids and generate free oxygen radicals. *Toxic dose:* The threshold limit value is less than 1 PPM, but mild mucous irritation occurs in some patients; 30 PPM produces choking and chest pain; 60 PPM produces pulmonary edema; 400 PPM for 30 minutes is lethal; and 1000 PPM is fatal in a few minutes. *Management:* (1) Remove the patient from contaminated environment and stabilize vital functions. Decontamination procedures for dermal and ocular contamination as indicated. Protect rescue personnel with breathing apparatus. There are patients who have responded to nebulized 3.75% sodium bicarbonate (4 mL) (prepared by diluting 2 mL of 7.5% IV sodium bicarbonate with 2 mL saline). Classification—If patient is symptomless or presents with a cough that clears up in less than 1 hour, advise rest for 12 hours and report if symptoms occur; no vigorous exercise for 24 hours. If symptoms persist beyond period of exposure, admit to hospital and treat with bronchodilators (use aerosol beta agonists and theophylline, not epinephrine) and humidified oxygen. Noncardiac pulmonary edema is treated with positive end-expiratory pressure (PEEP); corticosteroids are controversial; furosemide (Lasix) may be used. For conjunctival irritation, copious water irrigation and fluorescein stain for corneal damage. For dermal burns, copious water irrigation and conventional treatment of burns. *Laboratory aids:* Chest radiograph (may not reflect damage for 24 hours), arterial blood gases, cardiac monitor for dysrhythmias.

Chlorpromazine (Thorazine). See Phenothiazines and Other Major Neuroleptics.

Clinitest Tablets. See Caustics and Corrosives.

Cocaine (Benzoylmethylecgonine). *Toxic dose:* The potential fatal dose is 1200 mg, but death has occurred with 20 mg parenterally. *Toxicokinetics:* See Table 14. *Manifestations:* Hypertension, convulsions, hyperthermia, and cardiac dysrhythmias. *Management:* (1) Supportive care. Avoid induction of emesis or gastric lavage because of rapid onset of action of cocaine. Blood pressure and thermal monitoring. Phenytoin may be effective for ventricular dysrhythmias, whereas lidocaine may be ineffective and enhance toxicity. Nitroprusside infusion, 0.5 to 10 μg per kg per minute, may be used for severe hypertension. Avoid propranolol. Control anxiety and convulsions with diazepam. Labetalol intravenously (Antidote 27, Table 4) has been used to control life-

TABLE 14. **Pharmacotoxicokinetics of Cocaine**

Type	Route	Time to Onset of Action	Peak	Duration Half-life	Possible Fatal Dose (Adult)
Hydrochloride	Insufflation	1–5 min	15–60 min	60–75 min	750–800 mg
	Ingested	Delayed	50–90 min	Sustained	1.4 gm
	IV	30–120 s	5–11 min	60–90 min	20–800 mg
Coca paste	Smoked			Not known	
Crack and free base	Smoked	(Fastest) 5–10 s	5–11 s	Up to 20 min	Not known

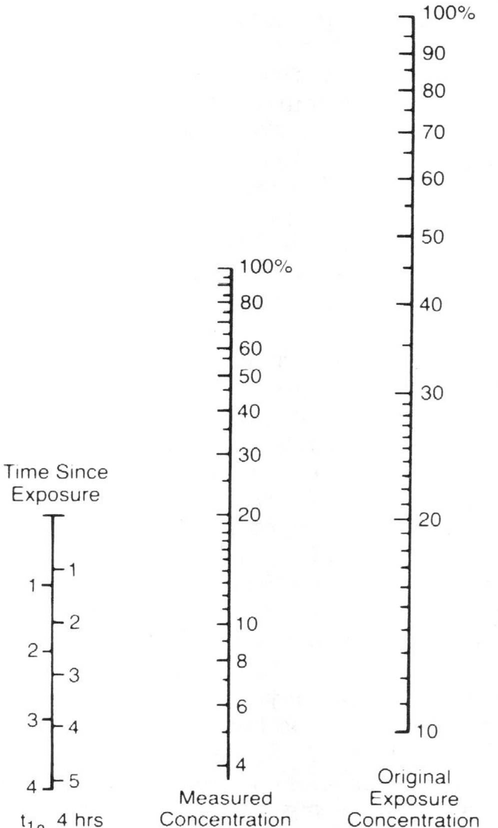

Figure 2. Nomogram for calculating carboxyhemoglobin concentration at time of exposure. The time since exposure is given on two scales to allow for the effects of previous oxygen administration on the half-life of carboxyhemoglobin (left-hand scale assumes a half-life of 3 hours). *Note*: The nomogram assumes a half-life of carboxyhemoglobin of 4 hours in a subject breathing room air. Most patients will not have received supplementary oxygen before admission, and at best this will have been administered via a face mask, giving a maximum fractional inspired oxygen concentration of 50 to 60% with little effect on carboxyhemoglobin elimination. The scale on the left side of the time column makes allowances for prior oxygen supplements by assuming a short half-life of 3 hours. The nomogram may help decide quickly whether serious carbon monoxide intoxication is likely to have occurred and may help select patients at high risk for early management in the intensive care unit. The nomogram may be an oversimplification because patients usually are not resuscitated with constant concentrations of oxygen, and many patients may hyperventilate, thus changing elimination characteristics. (Redrawn from Clark CJ, et al: Blood carboxyhaemoglobin and cyanide levels in fire survivors. Lancet *1*:1332, 1981.)

threatening hypertension and tachycardia but has been shown to increase the mortality in mice given cocaine. Most cases of hypertension and tachycardia are transient and can be managed without drugs or careful titration of benzodiazepines. A nonthreatening environment to reduce all sensory stimuli and protect patient from injury is required. Apply precautions against suicide attempts and monitor the fetus if patient is a pregnant woman. The management of the "body packer" and "body stuffer" is to administer repeated doses of activated charcoal (except plastic vials), secure venous access, and have drugs readily available for treating life-threatening manifestations until contraband is passed in the stool. Surgical removal may be indicated if material does not pass the pylorus. Endoscopy may be used to remove hard plastic vials, but not the bags, containing crack. Whole-body irrigation may be useful if plastic vials or bags were ingested.

Codeine. See Opioids.

Corrosives. See Caustics and Corrosives.

Cyanide. See Table 15. Hydrocyanic acid and sodium and potassium salts act rapidly and are extremely poisonous. The acid is extremely volatile, producing cyanide, which has a distinctive odor of bitter almonds and can produce death within minutes after inhalation. Cyanide interferes with the cytochrome oxidase system. *Classes of cyanides and derivatives:* (1) Hydrogen cyanide and simple salts in large doses act to produce death in 15 minutes. (2) Halogenated cyanides, such as cyanogen chloride, produce irritant and vesicant gases that may cause pulmonary edema. (3) Nitriles, such as acrylonitrile and acetonitrile (artificial nail removers). (4) Residential fires. Cyanides are used as fumigants (hydrogen cyanide), in synthetic rubber (acrylonitrile), in fertilizers (cyanamide), in metal refining (salts), and in the home in some silver and furniture polishes. Cyanide in the seeds of fruit stones is harmful only if the capsule is broken. *Manifestations:* Seizures, stupor, cardiac dysrhythmias, pulmonary edema, lactic acidemia, decreased arterial venous oxygen difference. Bright red venous blood. *Management:* Attendants should not administer mouth-to-mouth resuscitation. (1) Immediately, 100% oxygen. If inhaled, remove patient from contaminated atmosphere. (2) Cyanide antidote kit (Antidote 14, Table 4). Use antidote only if certain of diagnosis or residential fires involving plastics, urethane, or upholstery plus: (a) significant toxicity (impairment of consciousness); (b) manifestations not corrected by oxygen and out of proportion to carboxyhemoglobin level; and (c) lactic acidosis and bright red venous blood with high or normal PaO_2. (3) Gastrointestinal decontamination by gastric lavage. *No* syrup of ipecac. Activated charcoal is used but is not very effective (1 gram binds only 35 mg of cyanide). (4) Treat seizures with intravenous diazepam. (5) Correct acidosis. (6) Other antidotes: In Europe, dicobalt edetate, 600 mg, is used intravenously, followed by 300 mg if the response is not satisfactory. Hydroxycobalamin (vitamin B_{12}) is a useful antidote but must be given immediately after exposure in large doses. Dose: 1800 mg of vitamin B_{12} per dL of potassium cyanide (KCN) is usually required (forms cyanocobalamin).

DDT and Derivatives. See Organochlorine Insecticides.

Desipramine (Norpramin, Pertofrane). See Tricyclic Antidepressants.

Diazepam (Valium). See Benzodiazepines.

Digitalis Preparations. See Table 16. *Manifestations:* Manifestations may be delayed 9 to 18 hours. Abdominal pain, nausea, vomiting, diarrhea, dysrhythmias, heart block, CNS depression, colored-halo vision. No dysrhythmia on ECG is characteristic of

TABLE 15. **Sources of Cyanide and Their Toxicity**

Plants Containing Cyanide Glycosides

Common Name	*Part of Plant**	*Botanical Name*
Apple	Seeds	*Malus* spp
Apricot	Seeds	*Prunus armeniaca*
Arrow grass		*Triglochin* spp
Bamboo	Sprouts, stems	Tribe Bambuseae
Bermuda grass		*Cynodon dactylon*
Bird's-foot trefoil		*Lotus corniculatus*
Bitter almond	Seeds	*Prunus amygdalus amara*
Blackthorn, sloe		*Prunus spinosa*
Calabash tree		*Crescentia cujete*
Cassava	Beans and roots	*Manihot esculenta*
Catclaw		*Acacia greggi*
Cherry laurel		*Prunus laurocerasus*
Chokecherry		*Prunus virginiana*
Cotoneaster		*Cotoneaster* spp
Cycad nut		*Zamia pumila*
Elderberry	Leaves and shoots	*Sambucus* spp
Eucalyptus		*Eucalyptus cladocalyx*
False sago palm		*Cycas circinalis*
Flax		*Linum usitatissimum*
Hyacinth bean	Bean	*Dolichos lablab*
Hydrangea	Leaves and bulb	*Hydrangea* spp
Jetbead		*Rhodotypos tetrapetala*
Johnson grass		*Sorghum halepense*
Lima bean		*Phaseolus lunatus* (not in United States)
Mountain mahogany		*Cercocarpus montanus*
Passionflower (African)		*Adenia volkensii*
Peach	Seed	*Prunus persica*
Pear	Seeds	*Pyrus communis*
Plains bahia		*Bahia oppositifolia*
Plum	Seed	*Prunus domestica*
Poison suckleya		*Suckleya suckleyana*
Queen's delight		*Stillingia sylvatica*
Sudan grass		*Sorghum* spp
Velvet grass		*Holcus lanatus*
Vetch	Seed	*Vicia sativa*

*In most cases, cyanide is distributed throughout the plant.

Hydrogen Cyanide Liberated from Samples of Carcinogenic Glycosides

Sample	*HCN (mg/gm or mL)*
Laetrile (amygdalin)	
Sigma	55.9
Tablet yellow	400
Kemdalin	14.1
Apricot seeds	2.92
Peach seeds	2.60
Apple seeds	0.61
Laetrile is 500-mg tablet for oral use, which is 6% cyanide by weight	

Forms of Cyanide and Their Toxicity

Product	*Toxicity (Potential Lethal Dose)*
Hydrocyanic acid	50 mg (1.0 mg/kg)
Potassium/sodium cyanide	150–300 mg (2 mg/kg)
Ferriferrocyanide (Prussian blue)	50 gm
Sodium nitroprusside	5 mg/kg causes toxicity
Bitter almonds	
Oil	2 oz
Almonds	50–60 (each contains 0.001 gm of cyanide)
Pulp	240 gm
Apricot	
Wild	100 gm of moist seed = 217 mg of cyanide
Cultivated	100 gm = 8.7 mg of cyanide

digitalis toxicity. *Management:* (1) Gastrointestinal decontamination. Avoid ipecac syrup; it may increase the vagal effect if patient is symptomatic. Repeated doses of activated charcoal may interrupt enterohepatic recirculation. (2) Treat hemodynamically unstable ventricular dysrhythmias with Fab (antibody fragment [Digibind], Antidote 22, Table 4). Antidysrhythmic agents and pacemaker should be used only when Fab therapy fails. Phenytoin and lidocaine also may be administered for ventricular dysrhythmias. Magnesium sulfate, 20 mL 20% IV given slowly over 20 minutes, has been useful for malignant ventricular dysrhythmias, such as torsades de pointes. (3) Treat bradycardia and second-degree and third-degree atrioventricular block with atropine or low-dose phenytoin, 25 mg per dose IV in adults. If patient is unresponsive, use Fab (Digibind, Antidote 22, Table 4). Insertion of a pacemaker should be seriously considered. Avoid isoproterenol, which causes dysrhythmias. External pacing may be needed. (4) Treat hyperkalemia (above 5.5 mEq per liter) with Fab (antibody fragment [Digibind], Antidote 22, Table 4). Avoid calcium. Hemodialysis is treatment of choice for severe or refractory hyperkalemia. (5) Direct current countershock may cause life-threatening dysrhythmias. (6) Specific Fab antibody fragments (Digibind, Antidote 22, Table 4) have been used if cardiac arrest or shock is imminent; the dose is 10 mg in an adult, 4 mg (or over 0.3 mg per kg) in a child, or lower (0.2 mg per kg) in an adolescent. Fab is also given for hyperkalemia (serum potassium >5.5 mEq per liter), or serum digoxin toxicity (>10 ng per mL in adults or >5 ng per mL in children) at 6 to 8 hours postingestion, or life-threatening dysrhythmias. Contact Poison Control Center for calculation of Fab or use package insert. *Laboratory aids:* Monitor ECG and potassium and digitalis levels. Draw digoxin levels 6 to 8 hours postingestion, as well as when it is given by the IV route. An endogenous digoxin-like substance that cross-reacts with most common immunoassay antibodies, with values as high as 4.1 ng per mL, has been reported in newborns, patients with chronic renal failure, and patients with abnormal immunoglobulin levels. The bound digoxin blood concentrations rise after use of Fab, but the free (usually unmeasured) digoxin level falls.

Diphenhydramine (Benadryl). See Anticholinergic Agents.

Doxepin (Sinequan, Adapin). See Tricyclic Antidepressants.

Ethchlorvynol (Placidyl). See Sedative Hypnotics.

Ethyl Alcohol. See Alcohols.

Ethylene Glycol (solvent, antifreeze). *Toxic dose:* Death has occurred after a 60 mL ingestion of 95% ethylene glycol; fatal dose = 1.4 mL per kg of 100% solution. The TLV is 50 PPM. *Toxicokinetics:* Time of onset, 30 minutes to 12 hours for CNS and metabolic abnormalities to occur (Phase I). Twelve to 36 hours postingestion, cardiopulmonary depression (Phase II). In Phase III (2 to 3 days postingestion), renal failure occurs. The t½ is 3 hours (during ethanol

TABLE 16. **Toxicity and Kinetics of Common Digitalis Preparations**

Characteristic	Digoxin	Digitoxin
Trade name	Lanoxin	Crystodigin
Loading dose (LD) over 18–24 h	Varies with age	Varies with age
Premature infant	0.005 mg/kg	
Child <10 years	0.020–0.060 mg/kg	<2 years 0.025–0.040 mg/kg
Child >10 years	0.010–0.015 mg/kg	>2 years 0.020–0.040 mg/kg
Total adult	0.5–7.5 mg	0.8–1.4 mg
Maintenance dose (MD)	25–35% of LD	10% of LD
Total adult	0.125–0.50 mg	0.05–0.20 mg
Toxic dose		
Child	0.3 mg/kg	NA
Normal adult	2 mg	3–5 mg
Adult fatal dose	10–20 mg	3–10 mg
Gastrointestinal absorption	50–80%	90–100%
Tablet bioavailable	60–75%	
Capsule bioavailable	95%	
Elixir bioavailable	85%	
Onset oral	15–30 min	25–120 min
Peak IV	1.5–6 h	4–12 h
Peak oral	3–6 h	4–12 h
Duration of action	3–6 days	2–3 weeks
Protein bound	25%	>90%
Volume of distribution		
In neonate	7.5–10 L/kg	
In infants and children	16 L/kg	
In adults	5–8 L/kg	0.6 L/kg
Fetal plasma concentrations equal maternal concentrations		
Half-life		
In premature infants	37–170 h	
In neonates	35–69 h	
In infants	19–35 h	
In adults	26–45 h (1½ days)	6–8 days or longer
Shorter in overdose	6–22 h	
Elimination	Renal 75%	Liver 80%
Active metabolite	None	8% converted digoxin
Plasma concentration should be measured 6–8 h after last dose		
Therap plasma concentration	0.5–2 ng/mL	15–30 ng/mL
Toxic plasma concentration	>4 ng/mL; varies	>35 ng/mμg/mL
There is considerable overlap between therapeutic and toxic ranges		
Normal blood concentrations do not exclude toxicity		
Serious toxic concentration	>10 ng/mL	
Healthy children tolerate high concentrations better than adults		
Enterohepatic recirculation	Up to 14%	30%
Availability		
Capsules	0.05, 0.1, 0.2 mg	
Tablets	0.125, 0.25, 0.50 mg	0.05, 0.1, 0.15, 0.2 mg
Elixir	0.05 mg/mL	0.05 mg/mL

Sources: Clinical Data Handbook 1988, pp 472–474; AMA Drug Evaluations 1986, pp 425–427.
SI conversion factor: ng/ml × 1.281 = mmol/L; NA = not available.

therapy this is prolonged to 17 hours). Urine oxalate or monohydrate crystals may be seen 4 to 8 hours postingestion but are not always present. *Management:* (1) Gastrointestinal decontamination up to 30 minutes postingestion. Activated charcoal and cathartics are not indicated. (2) Treat seizures with intravenous diazepam. Exclude hypocalcemia and treat if necessary. (3) Correct acidosis with intravenous sodium bicarbonate. (4) Initiate ethanol therapy to block metabolism (Antidote 21, Table 4) if the blood ethylene glycol level is higher than 20 mg per dL, or if the patient is symptomatic or acidotic with increased anion gap or osmolar gap. Ethanol should be administered intravenously or orally to produce a blood ethanol concentration of 100 to 150 mg per dL. (5) Early hemodialysis is indicated if the ingestion was large; if the blood ethylene glycol level is greater than 50 mg per dL; if severe acid-base or electrolyte abnormalities occur despite conventional therapy; or if renal failure occurs. (6) Thiamine (100 mg per day) and pyridoxine (50 mg four times daily) have been recommended for 48 hours but have not been extensively studied. (7) Continue therapy (ethanol and hemodialysis) until the plasma ethylene glycol level is below 10 mg per dL, the acidosis has cleared, the creatinine level is normal, and urinary output is adequate. *Laboratory aids:* Complete blood count, electrolytes, urinalysis (look for oxalate ["envelope"] and monohydrate ["hemp seed"] crystals), and arterial blood gases. The oral mucosa and urine fluoresce if ethylene glycol is present. Obtain ethylene glycol and ethanol levels, plasma osmolarity (use freezing point depression method). Calcium, creatinine, and blood urea nitrogen studies. An ethylene glycol level of 20 mg per dL is usually toxic (levels are very difficult to obtain). The oral mucosa and urine will appear fluorescent under Wood's light if ethylene glycol is present. Propylene glycol, a vehicle in many liquid and IV medications (phenytoin, diazepam), may produce spurious ethylene glycol levels.

Flurazepam (Dalmane). See Benzodiazepines.

Fluoxetine (Prozac). *Toxic dose:* >3.5 mg per kg in children. Adult fatal dose, 6 grams. Over 1800 mg has produced seizures. *Manifestations:* Minimal risk of cardiovascular or neurologic complications. *Toxicokinetics:* See Table 30. *Management:* See Tricyclic Antidepressants.

Glutethimide (Doriden). See Sedative Hypnotics.

Hallucinogens

1. LSD (lysergic acid diethylamide). *Toxic dose:* ≥35 μg. Street doses are typically 50 to 300 μg. *Toxicokinetics:* Peak effect, 1 to 2 hours. Duration, 12 to 24 hours. t½, 3 hours. Route of elimination, hepatic.

2. MORNING GLORY SEEDS (*Rivea corymbosa* or *Ipomoea*). These have one-tenth the potency of LSD.

3. MESCALINE/PEYOTE (trimethoxyphenylethylamine, or the toxic principle of *Lophophora williamsii*). *Toxic dose:* ≥5 mg per kg. Each button of mescaline contains 45 mg (4 to 12 produce symptoms). *Toxicokinetics:* Peak effect, 4 to 6 hours. Duration, 14 hours.

4. PSILOCYBIN. Similar in effect to LSD but short acting. Peak effect, 90 minutes. Duration, 5 to 6 hours.

5. NUTMEG (*Myristica*). *Toxic dose:* 5 to 15 grams (1 to 3 nutmegs). Peak effect, 3 to 6 hours. Duration, up to 60 hours.

6. MARIJUANA (*Cannabis sativa*) (Δ^9-tetrahydrocannabinol, THC). One joint equals 500 mg of marijuana; when the plant is smoked, 50% is destroyed. *Toxicokinetics:* Time of onset, 2 to 3 minutes (smoked). Duration, 2 to 3 hours. t½, 28 to 47 hours (shorter for chronic user). *Note:* 1% of the metabolite can be detected in urine up to 2 weeks after use. *Manifestations:* Visual illusions, sensory perceptual distortions, depersonalization, and derealization. *Management:* "Talk-down" technique.

7. INHALANTS. Nitrites (amyl and isobutyl nitrite)—act immediately; aromatic hydrocarbon in airplane model glues, plastic cements (benzene, toluene, xylene)—see Hydrocarbons; *nitrous oxide* and *halogenated hydrocarbons.*

8. TRYPTAMINE DERIVATIVES (DMT, *N*-dimethyltryptamine; DET, diethyltryptamine; DPT, dipropyltryptamine). Rapid onset of action, but duration is only 1 to 2 hours.

9. STP OR DOM (2,5-dimethoxy-4-methylamphetamine). Acts like LSD but lasts 72 hours or longer.

10. MDA (3-methoxy-4,5-ethylenedioxyamphetamine). Related to amphetamine, produces a mild LSD-like reaction lasting 6 to 10 hours ("love pill").

See also Alcohols, Amphetamines, Anticholinergic Agents, Barbiturates, Cocaine, Opioids, Phencyclidine, Phenothiazines and Other Major Neuroleptics, and Tricyclic Antidepressants.

Haloperidol (Haldol). See Phenothiazines and Other Major Neuroleptics.

Heroin. See Opioids.

Hydrocarbons

1. PETROLEUM DISTILLATES. Gasoline (petroleum spirit), 2 to 5% benzene; kerosene (coal oil, kerosene, jet aviation fuel No. 1, charcoal lighter fluid); petroleum naphtha (cigarette lighter fluid, ligroin, racing fuel); petroleum ether (benzine); turpentine (pine oil, oil of turpentine); and mineral spirits (Stoddard solvent, white spirits, varsol, mineral turpentine, petroleum spirit). *Manifestations:* Materials aspirated during the process of ingestion may produce pneumonitis. Hypoxia associated with aspiration is the cause of CNS depression, not absorption. It is *unlikely* that a child accidentally or an adult during siphoning of gasoline would ingest a sufficient quantity to warrant the induction of emesis.

2. AROMATIC HYDROCARBONS. *Benzene,* a solvent used in manufacturing dyes, phenol, and nitrobenzene, has a TLV of 10 PPM by inhalation according to the Occupational Safety and Health Administration (OSHA). The National Institute for Occupational Safety and Health (NIOSH) value is 1 PPM. The adult ingested toxic dose is 15 mL. Chronic exposure may cause leukemia. A level of 200 PPM is fatal in 5 minutes. *Toluene,* used in manufacturing TNT, has an OSHA TLV of 200 PPM by inhalation; the NIOSH figure is 100. The adult ingested toxic dose is 50 mL. *Styrene* has an OSHA TLV of 100 PPM by inhalation. *Xylene,* used in the manufacture of perfumes, has an OSHA TLV of 100 PPM by inhalation. The adult ingested toxic dose is 50 mL. *Manifestations:* Asphyxiation, CNS depression, defatting dermatitis, and aspiration pneumonitis. A bite into a tube of household plastic cement by a young child does not warrant the induction of emesis. Ingestion of hydrocarbon with a benzene fraction over 5% may warrant induction of emesis.

3. ALIPHATIC HALOGENATED HYDROCARBONS. See Table 17 for common examples. *Manifestations:* Myocardial sensitization and irritability, hepatorenal toxicity, and CNS depression. Dichloromethane may be converted into carbon monoxide in the body. Trichloroethylene concentrates in the fetus (pregnant women should not be exposed) and causes a disulfiram (Antabuse) reaction ("degreaser's flush") when associated with ingestion of ethanol. The decision to induce emesis must be based on the toxicity of the agent.

4. DANGEROUS ADDITIVES. Dangerous additives to the hydrocarbons, such as heavy metals, nitrobenzene, aniline dyes, insecticides, and demothing agents, may warrant the induction of emesis.

5. HEAVY HYDROCARBONS. These have high viscosity, low volatility, and minimal absorption, so emesis

TABLE 17. **Common Examples of Aliphatic Halogenated Hydrocarbons**

	Estimated Toxic Dose (Ingested 100%)†	TLV-TWA (PPM ACGIH)	Synonyms
1,2-Dichloromethane*	0.3 ml/kg,* one swallow adult, lethal >0.5 mL/kg	1	Methylene chloride
1,2-Dichloroethylene	150–200 mL toxic in adults or large intentional ingestion	200	Acetylene dichloride
1,2-Dichloropropane	0.3 mL/kg toxic, one swallow	75	Propylene dichloride
Tetrabromoethane	1 mL/kg toxic, several swallows	—	Acetylene tetrabromide
Tetrachloroethane	0.3 mL/kg toxic, one swallow	1	Acetylene tetrachloride
Tetrachloroethylene	1 mL/kg toxic, several swallows	50	Perchloroethylene
Tetrachloromethane	0.3 mL/kg toxic, one swallow	5	
1,1,1-Trichloroethane	5.0 mL/kg fatal, 150–200 mL toxic in adults or large intentional ingestion	350	Methyl chloroform, Triethane, Glamorene Spot Remover, Scotchgard Typewriter fluid
Trichlorethylene	0.3 mL/kg toxic, >one swallow	50	Vapor degreaser, typewriter correction fluid, fire retardant
Trichloromethane	0.3 mL/kg toxic, one swallow	10	Cleaning agent, fumigant, insecticide
1,1,2-Trichloro-1,2,2-fluoroethane	>200 mL? toxic adult		
1,1,2-Trichloroethane	0.5 mL/kg toxic, >2.0 mL/kg lethal	10	Vinyl trichloride
Carbon tetrachloride	3–5 mL total amount Lethal 4 mL total	2	

Abbreviations: ACGIH = American Conference of Government Industrial Hygienists; PPM = parts per million; TLV = threshold limit value for 8-hour workday; TWA = time-weighted average concentration for normal workday and 40-hour workweek to which nearly all workers may be repeatedly exposed.

*Amount of methylene chloride in a single Christmas tree bubbling fluid light (0.5 mL) is nontoxic if ingested by small children.

†Estimated fatal dose assumes pure 100% of the halogenated hydrocarbon in the ingested product. At this dose it is recommended that medical evaluation is needed. *A swallow* in 2-year-old is approximately 5 mL (0.3 mL/kg), in adult, 15–20 mL. *Large intentional amount* is 120–150 mL in adults. The decision for medical evaluation should be based on the most toxic substance present at concentrations exceeding 10 to 20%.

is unwarranted. Examples are asphalt (tar), machine oil, motor oil (lubricating oil, engine oil), diesel oil (engine fuel, home heating oil), petrolatum liquid (mineral oil, suntan oils), petrolatum jelly (Vaseline), paraffin wax, transmission oil, cutting oil, and greases and glues.

6. PRODUCTS TREATED AS PETROLEUM DISTILLATES. Essential oils (e.g., turpentine, pine oil) are treated as petroleum distillates. Mineral seal oil (signal oil), found in some furniture polishes, is a heavy, viscous oil that *never* warrants emesis; it can produce severe pneumonia if aspirated. It has minimal absorption. *Management:* Dermal decontamination. Removal from the environment in inhalation.

FIRST AID TREATMENT. See Table 18. *The use of activated charcoal, oils, and cathartics is not advised in petroleum distillate ingestions. General management:* (1) In the asymptomatic patient: observe several hours for development of respiratory distress. (2) In the symptomatic patient: supportive respiratory care for respiratory distress. Bronchospasm may be treated with intravenous aminophylline. Avoid epinephrine. Monitor ECG; arterial blood gases; liver, pulmonary, and renal function; serum electrolytes; serial radiographs. Observe for signs of intravascular hemolysis and disseminated intravascular coagulation. If cyanosis is present that does not respond to oxygen or the arterial PaO_2 is normal, suspect methemoglobinemia that may require therapy with methylene blue. Steroids have not been shown to be beneficial. Antimicrobial agents are not useful in prophylaxis. (Fever or leukocytosis may be produced by the chemical pneumonitis itself.) It is not necessary to treat pneumatoceles. Most infiltrations resolve spontaneously in 1 week except for lipoid pneumonia, which may last up to 6 weeks.

Imipramine (Tofranil). See Tricyclic Antidepressants.

Iron. The iron content of some preparations appears in Table 19. *Toxic dose:* Range, 20 to 60 mg per kg or greater of elemental iron. Dose to induce emesis, ≥20 mg per kg. The potential fatal dose is 180 mg per kg (600 mg of elemental iron). *Toxicokinetics:* Absorption occurs chiefly in the small intestine. For excretion there is no normal route except blood loss or gastrointestinal desquamation. *Manifestations:* Phase I—mucosal injury possibly with hematemesis (1 to 6 hours postingestion). Phase II—patient ap-

TABLE 18. **Initial Management of Hydrocarbon Ingestions**

Symptoms	Contents	Amount	Initial Management
None	Petroleum distillate only	<5 mL/kg	None
None	Heavy hydrocarbon	Any amount	None*
	Mineral seal oil		None
None	Petroleum distillate with dangerous additive (heavy metals, pesticide)	Depends on toxicity of additive	Gastric lavage with small-bore tube
	>15 mL/kg or 150–200 mL		
	Aromatic	>1 mL/kg	
	Halogenated hydrocarbons†		
	A. Very toxic compounds	>0.3 mL/kg	Gastric lavage
	B. Moderate toxic compounds	>0.5 mL/kg	Gastric lavage
	C. Low toxic compounds	>1.0 mL/kg	Gastric lavage
	D. Christmas bubbling light		
Loss of protective airway reflexes, coma, seizures	Petroleum distillate with dangerous additive, aromatic or halogenated hydrocarbons	Gastric lavage‡	Endotracheal tube prior to gastric lavage

*Emesis may be necessary if machine oil contains triorthocresyl phosphate (TOCP), which causes weakness, sensory impairment, and "partially reversible damage to the spinal cord."

†Amounts of halogenated hydrocarbons ingested assume 100% of product.

A. More than one swallow in adult or 0.3 mL/kg in a child of 100% of 1,2-dichloromethane (methylene chloride), 1,2-dichloropropane (propylene dichloride), tetrachloroethane (acetylene tetrachloride), tetrachloromethane, trichloroethylene, tetrachloroethylene, trichloromethane, tetrabromoethane (acetylene tetrabromide).

B. Several swallows in an adult or 0.5 mL/kg in a child of 100% 1,2-dichloroethane (ethylene dichloride), 1,2-dichloroethylene (acetylene dichloride), 1,1,2-trichloroethane (vinyl trichloride), tetrabromoethane and tetrachloroethylene (perchloroethylene), 1,1,2,2-tetrachloroethylene.

C. A large intentional ingestion in an adult (150–200 mL) or over 1 mL/kg in a child of 100% 1,2-dichloroethylene or tetrachloromethane, 1,1,1-trichloroethane methyl chloroform), 1,1,2-trichloro-1,2,2-fluoroethane.

D. The amount of dichloromethane (methylene chloride) in a single Christmas tree bubbling fluid light (0.5 mL) is nontoxic if ingested by small children.

‡See footnotes A to D and hydrocarbon amounts above.

pears improved (2 to 24 hours). Phase III—cardiovascular collapse and severe metabolic acidosis (12 to 48 hours). Phase IV—hepatic injury associated with jaundice (2 to 4 days). Phase V—sequelae of intestinal stricture and obstruction or anemia (2 to 6 weeks). Patients asymptomatic for 6 hours rarely develop serious intoxication manifestations. *Management:* (1) Gastrointestinal decontamination. Emesis should be induced in ingestions of elemental iron of over 20 mg per kg. Emesis should be followed by gastric lavage in an adult or in a child who has ingested a chewable or liquid preparation. The solution to be used for lavage is saline 0.9% or 1 to 1.5% sodium bicarbonate to form ferrous carbonate salts, which are poorly absorbed. One hundred milliliters of this solution should be left in the stomach (prepared by dilution of a sodium bicarbonate ampule with saline). The use of deferoxamine (Desferal) in the gastrointestinal tract is not recommended. The use of diluted Fleet's enema solution risks severe hypertonic phosphate poisoning. Activated charcoal is not recommended. (2) Postlavage abdominal radiograph—if significant amounts of residual radiopaque material are present, consider whole-bowel irrigation with polyethylene glycol solution first. Removal by endoscopy or surgery may also be required because coalesced tablets have produced hemorrhagic infarction and perforation peritonitis. (3) Diagnostic chelation test—deferoxamine not reliable. (4) Indications for chelation therapy with deferoxamine are serum iron levels over 500 mg per dL or systemic signs of intoxication independent of serum iron level. Chelation should be performed within 12 to 18 hours to be effective (Antidote 15, Table 4). *Laboratory aids:* Serum iron levels correlate with the clinical course. Iron levels taken at 2 to 6 hours that are below 350 mg per dL predict an asymptomatic course; levels of 350 to 500 are associated with mild gastrointestinal symptoms (rarely serious); and levels greater than 500 suggest the possibility of serious Phase III manifes-

TABLE 19. **Iron Content of Some Preparations**

Iron Salt	Elemental Iron Content (%)	Average Tablet Strength (mg)	Elemental Iron/ Tablet (mg)	Average $FeSO_4$ Strength (mg)
Ferrous sulfate (hydrous)	20	300	60	Drp 75/0.6 mL
	20	SR 160	32	Syp 90/5 mL
	20	195	39	Solu 125/mL
	20	325	65	Elxr 220/5 mL
Ferrous sulfate (dried)	30	200	60	
	30	SR 160	48	
Ferrous gluconate	12	320	36	Elxr 320/5 mL
Ferrous fumarate	33	200	67	
	33	SR 324	107	Drp 45/0.6 mL
	33	Chewable 100	33	Susp 100/5 mL

Abbreviations: SR = slow release; Drp = dropper; Syp = syrup; Solu = solution; Elxr = elixir; Susp = suspension.

tations. Draw serum iron (SI) before administering deferoxamine because it interferes with analysis. Total iron-binding capacity is not necessary. An SI at 8 to 12 hours is useful to exclude delayed absorption from a bezoar or sustained-release preparation. White blood cell counts greater than 15,000 per μL, blood glucose levels over 150 mg per dL, radiopaque material present on abdominal radiograph, vomiting, and diarrhea predict iron levels greater than 300 mg per dL. Monitor complete blood counts, blood glucose, serum iron, stools, and vomitus for occult blood; electrolytes; acid-base balance; urinalysis and urinary output; liver function tests; blood urea nitrogen; and creatinine. Obtain type and match of blood in severe cases. Abdominal radiographs. Follow-up is necessary for sequelae in significant intoxications—gastrointestinal series for intestinal strictures and anemia secondary to blood loss. Patients who develop fever or toxic symptoms following iron overdose should have blood and stool cultures checked for *Yersinia enterocolitica.*

Isoniazid (INH, Nydrazid). This is an antituberculosis drug frequently used in suicide attempts by Native Americans and Eskimos. *Mechanism of toxicity:* It produces pyridoxine deficiency (doubles excretion of pyridoxine). *Toxic dose:* 1.5 grams, 35 to 40 mg per kg, produces convulsions; severe toxicity is seen at 6 to 10 grams; 200 mg per kg is an obligatory convulsant. *Toxicokinetics:* Absorption is rapid, with a peak in 1 to 2 hours (clinical symptoms may start in 30 minutes). Volume of distribution is 0.6 liter per kg. It passes the placenta and into breast milk at 50% of the maternal serum level. Not protein bound. Elimination is by the liver, which produces a hepatotoxic metabolite, acetylisoniazid. The t½: Slow acetylators (2 to 4 hours) may develop peripheral neuropathy (50% of blacks and whites). Fast acetylators (0.7 to 2 hours) may develop hepatitis (90% of Asians and a majority of patients with diabetes). Excreted unchanged, 10 to 40%. *Major toxic manifestations:* Visual disturbances, convulsions (≥90% with one or more seizures), coma, resistant severe acidosis (due to lactate secondary to hypoxia, convulsions, and metabolic blocks). *Management:* (1) Control seizures with large doses of pyridoxine, 1 gram for each gram of isoniazid ingested (Antidote 38, Table 4). If the dose ingested is unknown, give at least 5 grams of pyridoxine intravenously. Diazepam is given and works synergistically to control seizures. (2) Correct acidosis with fluids and sodium bicarbonate (pyridoxine may spontaneously correct the acidosis). (3) After patient is stabilized, or if asymptomatic, gastrointestinal decontamination procedures may be carried out, keeping in mind the rapid onset of convulsions. Asymptomatic patients should be observed for 4 hours. (4) Hemodialysis is rarely needed but may be used as an adjunct for uncontrollable acidosis and seizures. Hemoperfusion has not been adequately evaluated. Diuresis is ineffective. *Laboratory aids:* Isoniazid toxic levels are above 10 to 20 μg per mL. Monitor the blood glucose (often hyperglycemia), electrolytes (often hyperkalemia), bicarbonate, arterial blood gases, liver function tests, blood urea nitrogen (BUN), and creatinine. If convulsions persist obtain an electroencephalogram (EEG). Monitor the temperature closely (often hyperpyrexia).

Isopropyl Alcohol. See Alcohols.

Kerosene. See Hydrocarbons.

Lead. *Acute* lead poisoning is rare. *Acute toxic dose:* 0.5 gram. *Management:* (1) Gastrointestinal decontamination. (2) Supportive care, including measures to deal with the hepatic and renal failure and intravascular hemolysis. (3) Ethylenediaminetetraacetic acid (EDTA) in all severe cases if lead levels confirm absorption. *Chronic* lead poisoning occurs most often in children 6 months to 6 years of age who are exposed in their environment and in adults in certain occupations. *Chronic toxic dose:* Determined by blood lead level and clinical findings. A level of 10 μg per dL or over is the threshold of concern in children; 40 μg per dL or over in adult workers; 30 μg per dL or over for those planning pregnancy. Medical removal from work at 60 μg per dL. *Toxicokinetics:* Absorption—10 to 15% of the ingested dose is absorbed in adults; in children up to 40% is absorbed with iron deficiency anemia. Inhalation absorption is rapid and complete. Vd—95% present in bone. In blood, 95% is in red blood cells. t½, 35 days; in bone, 10 years. The major elimination route for inorganic lead is renal. Organic lead is metabolized in the liver to inorganic lead; 9% is excreted in the urine per day. *Manifestations of acute symptoms of chronic lead poisoning* (ABCDE): Anorexia, apathy, anemia; behavior disturbances; clumsiness; developmental deterioration; and emesis. Manifestations of encephalopathy are remembered by the mnemonic PAINT: *P,* persistent forceful vomiting; *A,* ataxia; *I,* intermittent stupor and lucidity; *N,* neurologic coma and convulsions; *T,* tired and lethargic. In adults, one may see peripheral neuropathies and "lead gum lines." *Management:* (1) Gastrointestinal decontamination with enemas if radiopaque foreign bodies are noted. Do not delay therapy until clear. (2) Remove from exposure. For children, see Table 20. Dimercaptosuccinic acid, a derivative of BAL, is an oral agent approved by the FDA for chelation in children only with venous blood lead levels of over 45 μg per dL. The recommended dose is 10 mg per kg every 8 hours for 5 days, then every 12 hours for 14 days (Antidote 42, Table 4). *Laboratory aids:* (1) Provocation mobilization test—500 mg of EDTA per M^2 of body surface area for one dose given deeply intramuscularly with 0.5% procaine diluted 1:1; collect the urine for 8 hours. A ratio of micrograms excreted in the urine to milligrams of Ca-EDTA administered greater than 0.6 represents an increased lead body burden, and chelation should be carried out. (2) Evaluate complete blood count, levels of serum iron, or ferritin; repeat blood lead levels and erythrocyte protoporphyrin. (3) Flat plate of the abdomen and long bone radiographs (knees usually). (4) Renal function tests. (5) Monitor electrolytes, serum calcium, phosphorus, blood glucose.

Lindane. See Organochlorine Insecticides.

Lithium (Eskalith, Lithane). Most cases of intoxi-

TABLE 20. **Choice of Chelation Therapy Based on Symptoms and Blood Lead Concentration**

Clinical Presentation	Treatment	Comments
Symptomatic Children		
Acute encephalopathy	BAL, 450 mg/M^2/24 h $CaNa_2$-EDTA, 1500 mg/M^2/24 h	BAL, 75/M^2 q 4 h After 4 h, start infusion of EDTA or use IM* q 4 h† Duration, 5 days Interrupt therapy for 2 days If blood Pb >70 µg/dL, BAL and EDTA for 5 more days; EDTA alone if blood Pb = 45–69 µg/dL Other cycles depend on blood Pb rebound
Blood Pb >70 µg/dL	BAL, 300 mg/M^2/24 h $CaNa_2$-EDTA, 1000 mg/M^2/24 h Do not use $CaNa_2$-EDTA alone if symptomatic	BAL, 50 mg/M^2 q 4 h After 4 h, start infusion of EDTA or use IM q 4 h† Duration, 5 days Interrupt therapy for 2 days Discontinue BAL in 3 days if blood Pb <50 µg/dL; BAL and EDTA for 5 more days if blood Pb >50 µg/dL Other cycles depend on blood Pb rebound
Asymptomatic Children		
BEFORE TREATMENT, MEASURE VENOUS BLOOD LEAD		
Blood Pb > 70 µg/dL	BAL, 300 mg/M^2/24 h $CaNa_2$-EDTA, 100 mg/M^2/24 h	BAL, 50 mg/M^2 IM q 4 h After 4 h, start infusion of EDTA or use IM q 4 h Duration, 5 days Discontinue BAL in 3 days if blood PB <50 µg/dL Give second course of EDTA if blood PB >45 µg/dL within 5 days Other cycles depend on blood Pb rebound
Blood Pb = 45–69 µg/dL‡	$CaNa_2$-EDTA, 1000 mg/M^2/24 h	EDTA, IM q 4 h or IV Duration, 5 days Give second course of EDTA if blood Pb >45 µg/dL within 7–14 days; wait 5–7 days before giving second course If lead exposure controlled, give single IV/IM dose on outpatient basis Other cycles depend on blood Pb rebound
Blood Pb = 25–44 µg/dL		Provocation, EDTA test
Ratio >0.6	$CaNa_2$-EDTA, 1000 mg/M^2/24 h	Duration, 5 days IM or IV
Ratio <0.6		Provocation test periodically
Guidelines for Chelation of Excess Lead in Adults		
Inorganic Lead§		
SYMPTOMATIC CASES		
Acute encepalopathy	BAL-EDTA	Same as for children
Abdominal pain, weakness, and colic	BAL-EDTA	Course for 3–5 days followed by oral penicillamine until urine lead is <500 µg/24 h or 2 months, whichever less
Painless peripheral neuropathy	D-Penicillamine	For 1–2 months If blood lead >100 µg/dL, BAL-EDTA first course 3–5 days, followed by oral penicillamine
ASYMPTOMATIC CASES		
Blood Lead Concentrations		
100 µg/dL	BAL-EDTA	
80–100 µg/dL	Penicillamine alone	
40–79 and EP >60 µg/dL	Provocative test	
Organic Lead	No chelation therapy	

Note: OSHA requires that workers be removed from the work environment when lead levels exceed 50 µg/dL and until they are below 40 µg/dL.

*Dimercaprol.
†Some physicians prefer to give EDTA IM to avoid large fluid volumes in high intracranial pressure.
‡DSMA may be used.
§Data from Rempel D: The lead exposed worker: JAMA *262*:532–534, 1989. Copyright 1989, American Medical Association.
Abbreviations: BAL = British antilewisite; Blood Pb = venous blood lead concentration; $CaNa_2$ = calcium disodium; DSMA = 2,3 dimercaptosuccinic acid; EDTA = ethylene diaminotetraacetic acid; EP = erythrocyte protoporphyrin; IM = intramuscularly; IV = intravenously.
Modified from Piomelli S, et al: Management of childhood lead poisoning. J Pediatr *103*:527, 1984, and CDC Prevention of Childhood Lead Poisoning 1991.

cation have occurred as therapeutic overdoses. The toxic dose is determined by serum levels, although intoxication has occurred with levels in the therapeutic range. *Toxicokinetics:* Absorption is rapid, with complete peaking in 1 to 4 hours. Vd is 0.5 to 0.9 liter per kg. It is not protein bound. The t½ therapeutically is 18 to 24 hours. Eighty-nine to 98% is excreted by the kidney unchanged, one-third to two-thirds in 6 to 12 hours. Excretion is decreased in the presence of hyponatremia and dehydration. The cerebrospinal fluid concentration is one-half the plasma concentration. The breast milk level is 50% of the maternal serum level—toxic to the nursling. *Manifestations:* The first sign of toxicity may be diarrhea. Fine tremor of hands, lethargy, weakness, polyuria and polydipsia, goiter and hypothyroidism, and fasciculations are side effects. Severe toxicity is manifested by ataxia, impaired mental state, coma, and seizures (limbs held in hyperextension with eyes open in "coma vigil"). Cardiovascular manifestations are dysrhythmias, hypotension, flat T waves, and increased QT interval. *Management:* (1) Gastrointestinal decontamination may not be useful after 2 hours because of rapid absorption. In slow-release preparations, decontamination may be useful up to 24 hours postingestion. Activated charcoal is not indicated. Sodium polystyrene sulfonate (Kayexalate), 60 mL orally four times a day, is useful in preventing absorption. Determine serum sodium level before administration because this agent may aggravate existing hypernatremia. (2) Hospitalize if intoxication is suspected because seizures may occur unexpectedly. (3) Restore normothermia and fluid and electrolyte balance, particularly sodium. If diabetes insipidus is present, an infusion of sodium may cause hypernatremia. Current evidence supports saline infusion as enhancing excretion of lithium. (4) Hemodialysis is the treatment of choice for severe intoxication. Lithium is the most dialyzable toxin known. Long runs should be used until the lithium level is less than 1 mEq per liter because of extensive re-equilibration rebound. Monitor levels every 4 hours after dialysis. Dialysis may have to be repeated. Expect a time lag in neurologic recovery. If hemodialysis is not available or delayed, peritoneal dialysis can be used but is less effective. (5) Monitor ECG. Refractory dysrhythmias may be treated with magnesium sulfate and sodium bicarbonate. (6) Avoid thiazides and spironolactone diuretics, which increase lithium levels. *Laboratory aids:* Lithium level determinations should be performed every 4 hours. Although they do not always correlate with the manifestations at low levels, they are predictive in severe intoxications. Levels of 0.6 to 1.2 mEq per liter are usually therapeutic. Levels over 4.0 mEq per liter are usually severely toxic. Other tests to be monitored are complete blood count (lithium causes leukocytosis), renal function, thyroid, ECG, and electrolytes. Factors that predispose to lithium toxicity are febrile illness, sodium depletion, concomitant drugs (thiazide and spironolactone diuretics), impaired renal function, advanced age, and fluid loss in vomiting and diarrheal illness.

Lomotil (Diphenoxylate and Atropine). See Opioids and Anticholinergic Agents.

LSD (Lysergic Acid Diethylamide). See Hallucinogens.

Marijuana. See Hallucinogens.

Meperidine (Demerol). See Opioids.

Meprobamate (Equanil, Miltown). See Sedative Hypnotics.

Mercury. *Management:* (1) Inhalation of elemental mercury—remove from exposure. (2) Ingestion of mercuric salt—gastrointestinal decontamination. Do not induce emesis. A protein solution such as egg white or 5% salt-poor albumin can be given to reduce salt to mercurous ion (less toxic). Activated charcoal does adsorb mercuric chloride. (3) Chelating agents (do not use Ca-EDTA because of nephrotoxicity): Dimercaprol (BAL) enhances mercury excretion through the bile as well as the urine and is the first choice if renal impairment from the mercury exists (Antidote 17, Table 4). Alternatives are penicillamine (Antidote 34, Table 4) and *N*-acetyl-DL-penicillamine (investigational use). Use of BAL in methyl mercury intoxication increases the brain mercury and appears to be contraindicated; penicillamine and its analogue should be used (decreases mercury in brain). Another chelator, 2,3-dimercaptosuccinic acid, holds promise of less toxicity and more specific therapy.* (4) Monitor fluid and electrolyte levels, renal function, hemoglobin levels. Obtain blood and urine mercury levels (consult the laboratory for proper collection technique and containers). (5) Hemodialysis early in the symptomatic patient is useful. (6) Newer but not established approaches are use of polythiol resin to bind the methyl mercury excreted in the bile; heat and sauna treatment to increase mercury excretion through perspiration; and a regional dialyzer system using L-cysteine. (7) Surgical excision of *local injection sites. Laboratory aids:* (1) Blood levels are below 2 to 4 μg per dL and urine levels below 10 to 20 μg per liter in 90% of the adult population. Levels above 4 μg per dL in blood and 20 μg per liter in urine probably should be considered abnormal. Blood levels are not always reliable. Exposed industrial workers' urine levels are 150 to 200 μg per liter. (2) In asymptomatic patients with urine levels under 300 μg per liter, a chelating challenge with BAL or penicillamine may bring a significant increase that may aid in establishing the diagnosis. (3) Approximately 150 μg per liter of mercury in urine is equivalent to 3.5 μg per dL in blood. (4) Methyl mercury is excreted mainly through the feces, so urine mercury would not be a reliable measurement. (5) Mercury is also excreted in the sweat and saliva. The parotid fluid level is approximately two-thirds that of the blood. Because the hair is porous, it may absorb mercury from the atmosphere; however, hair concentrations of 400 to 500 μg per gram are likely to be associated with neurologic symptoms. Radiographs of the abdomen for ingestion and chest radiographs for injections may be helpful in showing radiopaque material.

*Not approved by the FDA for this purpose.

Methadone. See Opioids.

Methanol. See Alcohols.

Methaqualone. See Sedative Hypnotics.

Methyprylon (Noludar). See Sedative Hypnotics.

Narcotic Analgesics. See Opioids.

Neuroleptics. See Phenothiazines and Other Major Neuroleptics.

Nitrites (NO_2) and Nitrates (NO_3). These are readily available in both inorganic and organic forms. Organic nitrates used for angina pectoris are listed in Table 21. Inorganic nitrates have more toxicologic importance in natural foods and contaminated well water. *Potential fatal doses:* Nitrite, 1 gram; nitrate, 10 grams; nitrobenzene, 2 mL; nitroglycerin, 0.2 gram; and aniline dye (pure), 5 to 30 grams. *Toxicokinetics:* Time to onset of action of nitroglycerin sublingually is 1 to 3 minutes, with a time to peak action of 3 to 15 minutes and a duration of 20 to 30 minutes. Other routes have a slower onset (2 to 5 minutes) and longer duration of action (1.5 to 6 hours). Nitrites are potent oxidizing agents converting ferrous to ferric iron, which cannot carry oxygen. Normally humans have 0.7% of methemoglobin, which is converted by methemoglobin reductase into oxygen-carrying hemoglobin. Liver detoxification by dinitration is the route of elimination. *Toxic manifestations* depend on the level of methemoglobinemia. At 10%, "chocolate cyanosis" occurs; at 10 to 20%, headache, dizziness, and tachypnea occur; and at 50%, mental alterations are present and coma and convulsions may occur. Headache, flushing, and sweating are due to the vasodilatory effect; hypotension, tachycardia, and syncope may also occur. Severe hypoxia may produce pulmonary edema and encephalopathy. Levels above 50% produce metabolic acidosis and ECG changes; cardiovascular collapse occurs at levels of 70%. *Management:* (1) Dermal decontamination, if indicated. Aniline dyes may be removed with 5% acetic acid (vinegar). (2) Gastrointestinal decontamination if ingested. (3) Hypotension can be treated by the Trendelenburg position and fluid challenge. Vasoconstrictors (dopamine or norepinephrine) are rarely needed. (4) Methylene blue (Antidote 29, Table 4) is indicated for methemoglobin levels above 30%, dyspnea, metabolic acidosis (lactic acidosis), or an altered mental state. (5) Oxygen, 100%, or a hyperbaric chamber should be used in symptomatic patients if methylene blue fails or is not effective, e.g., as in chlorate intoxication or glucose-6-phosphate dehydrogenase deficiency. *Laboratory aids:* Methemoglobin levels, arterial blood gases. Blood has a chocolate-brown appearance and fails to turn red on exposure to oxygen. Methemoglobulin levels and oxygen saturation should be measured by co-oximeter, not by pulse oximetry.

TABLE 21. **Organic Nitrates for Angina Pectoris**

Drug and Route	Trade Name	Time to Onset of Action (min)	Duration (h)
Nitroglycerin			
Oral	Many	Varies	4–6
Sublingual	Many	1–3	¼–½
2% ointment	Nitro-Bid Nitrol	15	3–6
Transdermal	Nitrodur	30	2–4
Isosorbide dinitrate	Isordil		
Sublingual		1–3	1.3–3
Oral		2–5	4–6
Chewable		2–5	2–3
Timed release		Varies	—
Isosorbide mononitrate	Ismo	1–2	6–12
Pentaerythritol tetranitrate, oral	Peritrate	2–5	3–5
Erythrityl tetranitrate, oral	Cardilate	2–5	4–6

Nortriptyline (Aventyl, Pamelor). See Tricyclic Antidepressants.

Opioids (Narcotic Opiates). See Table 22. The major metabolic pathway differs for each opioid but they are 90% metabolized in the liver. Patients should be observed for CNS and respiratory depression and hypotension. Pulmonary edema is a potentially lethal complication of mainlining (intravenous use). *Manifestations:* All opiate agonists produce miotic pupils (except meperidine and Lomotil early), respiratory and CNS depression, physical dependence, and withdrawal symptoms. *Management:* (1) Supportive care, particularly an endotracheal tube and assisted ventilation. (2) Gastrointestinal decontamination up to 12 hours postingestion, because opiates delay gastric emptying time, but this is of no benefit if overdose is by injection. Convulsions occur rapidly with propoxyphene (Darvon) and codeine overdose, and this may be an indication not to use an emetic for gastrointestinal decontamination in this drug overdose. (3) Naloxone (Narcan) (Antidote 30, Table 4) may be given in bolus intravenous doses and by continuous drip. Naloxone must be titrated against the clinical response and precipitation of withdrawal in narcotic addicts. It should be repeated as often as necessary, because the effects of many opioids in overdose can last 24 to 48 hours, whereas the action of naloxone lasts only 2 to 3 hours. *Larger doses are needed for buprenorphine, codeine, designer drugs, dextromethorphan, diphenoxylate, methadone, pentazocine, and propoxyphene.* (4) Pulmonary edema does not respond to naloxone, and patient needs respiratory supportive care. Fluids should be given cautiously in opioid overdose because these agents stimulate antidiuretic hormone effect and pulmonary edema is frequent. (5) *If the patient is comatose, give 50% glucose* (3 to 4% of comatose narcotic overdose patients have hypoglycemia). (6) *If the patient is agitated,* consider hypoxia rather than withdrawal and treat as such. (7) *Observe for withdrawal* signs and symptoms (nausea, vomiting, cramps, diarrhea, dilated pupils, rhinorrhea, piloerection). If these occur, stop naloxone.

OPIOID ADDICT WITHDRAWAL SCORE. Signs and symptoms of withdrawal are diarrhea, dilated pupils, gooseflesh, hyperactive bowel sounds, hypertension, insomnia, lacrimation, muscle cramps, restlessness, tachycardia, and yawning. Each sign or symptom is

TABLE 22. **Opioids (Narcotic Opiates)***

Drugs		Equivalent IM		Time to Peak Action (h)	Half-life (h)	Duration of Action (h)	Potential Toxic Dose (mg)
Generic	*Trade*	*Dose† (mg)*	*Oral† (mg)*				
Alphaprodine‡	Nisentil	40–60	—	—	2	1–2	—
Butorphanol	Stadol	2	—	0.5–1.0	3	2.5–3.5	—
Camphorated tincture of opium	Paregoric	—	25 mL	—	—	4–5	—
Codeine	Various	120	200	—	3	4–6	800
Diacetylmorphine	Heroin	5	60	—	0.5	3–4	100
Diphenoxylate	Lomotil	—	10	Delayed by atropine	2.5	14	300
Fentanyl	Sublimaze	0.1–0.2	—	0.5	4–6	0.5–2	—
Hydrocodone	Hycodan	5–10	5–10	—	3.8	3–4	100
Hydromorphone	Dilaudid	1.5	6.0	0.5–1.5	2–3	2–4	100
Meperidine	Demerol	50–100	75–100	0.5–1	2–5	3–4	1000
Methadone	Dolophine	10.0	20	2–4	22–97	4–12	120
Morphine	Various	10.0	60	0.3–1.5	2–3	3–4	200
Nalbuphine	Nubain	10.0	—	0.5–1.0	3–4	3–4	—
Oxycodone	Percodan	—	15	—	—	3–4	—
Oxymorphone	Numorphan	1.0	—	1	2–3	4–5	—
Pentazocine	Talwin	—	30–60	1	2–6	3–4	—
Propoxyphene	Darvon	—	65–100	2–4	8–24	2–4	500

*"Ts and blues" are a combination of pentazocine (Talwin) and tripelennamine (Pyribenzamine) used intravenously. Pentazocine now has naloxone added to it to counter this abuse. Innovar is fentanyl plus droperidol, used as an IV anesthetic.
†Dose equivalent to 10 mg of morphine.
‡Not available in the United States.

given 0, 1, or 2 points, depending on the severity. A score of 1 to 5 is mild; 6 to 10, moderate; and 11 to 15, severe. Seizures are unusual with withdrawal. They indicate severity regardless of the rest of the score. *Management:* Mild withdrawal is treated with diazepam orally, 10 mg every 6 hours; moderate withdrawal, with intramuscular diazepam; and severe withdrawal, with diazepam and diphenoxylate (Lomotil) for the diarrhea. Methadone orally may be used, 20 to 40 mg every 12 hours, decreased by 5 mg every 12 hours. When 10 mg is reached, add Lomotil. Clonidine (Catapres), 6 μg per kg every 6 hours, can be used with informed consent. (This is an unlisted use of clonidine; the manufacturer states that relief from withdrawal symptoms has been reported with 0.8 mg per day.) *Laboratory aids:* For acute overdose obtain levels of blood gases, blood glucose, and electrolytes; chest radiographs; and ECG. Blood opioid levels confirm diagnosis but are not useful for making a therapeutic decision. For drug abusers, consider testing for hepatitis B, syphilis, and human immunodeficiency virus (HIV) antibody (HIV testing usually requires consent).

PROPOXYPHENE (Darvon). *Manifestations:* Onset may be as early as 30 minutes after ingestion. Convulsions occur early. Patients may develop diabetes insipidus, pulmonary edema, and hypoglycemia. *Elimination:* Metabolism is 90% by demethylation in the liver. Peak plasma level of 1 to 2 hours after oral dose. Half-life is 1 to 5 hours. As little as 10 mg per kg has caused symptoms, and 35 mg per kg has caused cardiopulmonary arrest. Therapeutic blood level is less than 200 μg per mL. *Treatment* (in addition to the general management): (1) Emesis can be dangerous because of the rapid onset of seizures. (2) Indications for naloxone are respiratory depression, seizure activity, coma, and miotic pupils. Signs of naloxone effect are dilation of pupils, increased rate and depth of respirations, reversal of hypotension, and improvement of obtunded or comatose state. Larger doses of naloxone are often required and can be continued as an infusion of the initial response dose every hour. (3) Naloxone and intravenous glucose should be tried first to control seizures. If these fail, diazepam may be tried.

Organochlorine Insecticides (DDT derivatives). See Table 23 for a listing of these agents. The *toxic dose* varies greatly. For chlorophenothane (DDT), 200 to 250 mg per kg is fatal; 16 mg per kg causes seizures. For methoxychlor, 500 to 600 mg per kg is fatal. For chlordane, 200 mg per kg is fatal (chlordane house air guidelines are below 5 μg per M^3; the occupational TLV is 500 μg per M^3). These insecticides interfere with axon transmission of nerve impulses. Metabolism varies; they resist degradation in human tissue and the environment. They accumulate in adipose tissue; the elimination route is via the liver. *Manifestations:* CNS stimulation, convulsions, late respiratory depression, increased myocardial irritability usually develop within 1 to 2 hours and may last for 1 week or more. Endrin produces liver toxicity with guarded prognosis. Chronic exposure causes liver and kidney damage. *Management:* (1) Dermal decontamination, discard contaminated leather goods. Protect personnel. Gastrointestinal decontamination, no oils. Emesis can be dangerous, owing to rapid seizures. Many of these agents are dissolved in petroleum distillates, presenting an aspiration hazard. (2) No adrenergic stimulants (epinephrine) should be used because of myocardial irritability. (3)

TABLE 23. **Organochlorine Pesticides (DDT Derivatives)**

Chemical Name	Trade Name	Toxicity Rating	Fatal Dose (Adult)	Elimination Time	Comment
Endrin	Hexadrin	Highest	NA	Hours–days	Banned
Lindane	1% in Kwell; Benesan; Isotox; Gamene	Moderate to high	10 gm	Hours–days	Scabicide; general garden insecticide
Endosulfan	Thiodan	Moderate	NA	Hours–days	
Benzene hexachloride	BHC, HCH	Moderate	NA	Weeks–months	Banned, produces porphyria (cutanea tarda)
Dieldrin	Dieldrite	High	3 gm	Weeks–months	Banned in 1974
Aldrin	Aldrite	High	3 gm	Weeks–months	Banned in 1974
Chlordane (10% is heptachlor)	Chlordan	High	3 gm	Weeks–months	Restricted in 1979; termiticide
Toxophene	Toxakil Strobane-T	High	2 gm	Hours–days	
Heptachlor	—	Moderate	NA	Weeks–months	Malignancy in rats; banned in 1976
Chlorophenothane	DDT	Moderate	NA	Months–years	Banned in 1972
Mirex	—	Moderate	NA	Months–years	Banned; red anticide
Chlordecone	Kepone	Moderate	NA	Months–years	Tidewater, Virginia, contamination
Methoxychlor	Marlate	Low	600 mg/kg	Hours–days	
Ethylan	Perthane	Low	NA	Hours–days	
Dicofol	Kelthane	Low	NA	Hours–days	
Chlorobenzilate	Acaraben	Low	NA	Hours–days	Banned

Abbreviation: NA = not available.

Cholestyramine, 4 grams every 8 hours, has been reported to increase the fecal excretion. (4) Anticonvulsants, if needed.

Organophosphate and Carbamate Insecticides (OPIs). These may cause (1) irreversible inhibition of cholinesterase, either direct (TEPP) or delayed (parathion or malathion), or (2) reversible inhibition of cholinesterase (carbamates). Examples of OPIs are listed in Table 24. Absorption is by all routes. The onset of acute toxicity is usually before 12 hours and always before 24 hours, unless the agents are absorbed by the dermal route or are liquid soluble (fenthion), which may delay onset for 24 hours. Inhalation produces intoxication within minutes. *Toxic manifestations:* Garlic odor of the breath, gastric contents, or container; miosis and muscle twitching are helpful clues to acute OPI poisoning. Early, cholinergic crisis—cramps, diarrhea, excess secretion, bronchospasms, bradycardia. Later, sympathetic and nicotine effects occur—twitching, fasciculations, weakness, tachycardia and hypertension, and convulsions. CNS effects are anxiety, confusion, emotional lability, and coma. Delayed respiratory paralysis and neurologic disorders have been described. *Management:* (1) Basic life support and decontamination with careful protection of personnel. (2) Atropine (Antidote 7, Table 4), if patient is symptomatic, every 10 to 30 minutes until drying of secretions and clearing of lungs occur. Maintain for 12 to 24 hours, then taper the dose and observe for relapse. (3) Intravenous pralidoxime (2-PAM) is required after atropinization (Antidote 36, Table 4). It should be given early. Its use may require reduction in the dose of atropine. (4) Careful dermal and gastrointestinal decontamination when patient is stable. (5) Suction secretions until atropinization drying is achieved. Intubation and assisted ventilation may be needed. (6) *Do not* use morphine, aminophylline, phenothiazine, or reserpine-like drugs or succinylcholine. *Laboratory aids:* Draw blood for red blood cell cholinesterase determination before giving pralidoxime. Levels are usually more than 90% depressed for severe symptoms. A postexposure rise of 10 to 15% determined at least 10 to 14 days without exposure is important in the diagnosis. Monitor chest radiograph, blood glucose, arterial blood gases, ECG, blood coagulation status, liver function, and the urine for the metabolite alkyl phosphate *p*-nitrophenol. *Note:* If the diagnosis is probable, do not delay therapy until it is confirmed by laboratory tests. Atropine is both a diagnostic and a therapeutic agent. A test dose of 1 mg in adults and 0.01 mg per kg in children may be administered parenterally. In the presence of severe cholinesterase inhibition, the patient fails to develop signs of atropinization.

PROPHYLAXIS. It is not medically advisable to administer atropine or pralidoxime prophylactically to workers exposed to organophosphate pesticides.

CARBAMATES (esters of carbonic acid). Carbamates cause reversible carbamylation of acetylcholinesterase. Pralidoxime is usually not indicated in the management, but atropine may be required. The major differences from OPI are (1) toxicity is less and of shorter duration, (2) they rarely produce overt CNS effects because of poor penetration, and (3) cholinesterase returns to normal rapidly, so blood values are not useful in confirming the diagnosis. Some common examples of carbamates are Ziram, Temik (alkicarb) (taken up by plants and fruit), Matacil (aminocarb, carazol), Vydate (oxamyl), Isolan, furadan (Carbo-

TABLE 24. **Examples of Common Organophosphate Insecticides (OPIs)**

Common Name	Trade Name(s)	EFD (gm/70 kg)	LD_{50} (mg/kg)
Agricultural Products (25–50% formulations, highly toxic; LD_{50} is 1–40 mg/kg)			
Azinphosmethyl	Guthion	0.2	10.0
Chlortriphos	Calathion		
Demeton[1]	Systox		1.5
Disulfoton[1]	Di-Syston	0.2	12.0
Ethyl-nitrophenyl thiobenzene PO_4	EPN		
Fonofon	Dyfonate		
Mevinphos	Phosdrin	0.15	
Methamidophos[2]	Monitor		
Monocrotophos	Azodrin		21.0
Octamethyldiphosphoramide	OMPA, Schradan		
Parathion	Thiophos	0.10	2.5
Ethyl parathion	Parathion		
Methyl parathion	Dalf		
Phorate	Thimet		
Terbufos	Counter		
Tetraethyl pyrophosphate	TEPP, Tetron	0.05	1.5
Animal Insecticides (moderately toxic; LD_{50} is 40–200 mg/kg)			
Chlorfenvinophos (tick dip)	Supona, Dermaton		
Coumaphos	Co-ral		
DEF	DeGreen		
Dichlorvos[3]	DDVP, Vapona		46
Dimethoate[4]	Cygon, De-fend		>500
Fenthione[5]	Baytex		40
Leptophos	Phosvel		
Phosmet	Imidon		
Ronnel	Korlan	10.0	
Trichlorfon	Dylox		
Household and Garden Pest Control (1–2% formulations, low toxicity; LD_{50} is 200–1400 mg/kg)			
Acephate[6]	Oerthene		>1000
Bromophos			>1000
Chlorpyrifos[7] (toxic dose is 300 mg/kg)	Lorsban, Dursban, Pyrinex		>500
Diazinon[1,8]	Spectracide, Dimpylate	25.0	>400
Dichlorvos[9]	DDVP, Vapona (plastic strip)		
Malathion (>92%, <24 h)	Cythion	60.0	1375
Merphos	Folex		>1000
Temephos	Abate		<2000

[1]Most OPIs degrade in the environment in a few days to nontoxic radicals. These may be taken up by the plants and fruits.
[2]Delayed neuropathy.
[3]Found in flea collars and No-Pest Strips.
[4]Half-life is <24 h.
[5]Long-acting.
[6]Half-life is 1–6 days.
[7]Some authors classify this as moderately toxic; half-life is 27 h.
[8]In rats, half-life is 12 h.
[9]Some authors classify this as moderately toxic.
Abbreviations: EFD = estimated fatal dose, common lawn chemical has 14.3%; LD_{50} = dose that is fatal in 50% of animals.

furan), Lannate (methomyl, Nudrin), Zectran (mexacarbate), and Mesural (methiocarb). These agents are all highly toxic. Moderately toxic are Baygon (propoxur) and Sevin (carbaryl). Some of these agents may be formulated in wood alcohol and have the added toxicity of methyl alcohol.

Paradichlorobenzene. See Hydrocarbons.

Paraquat and Diquat. Paraquat is a quaternary ammonia herbicide rapidly inactivated in the soil by clay particles. Nonindustrial preparations of 0.2% are unlikely to cause serious intoxications. *Toxic dose:* Commercial preparations such as Gramoxone 20% are very toxic; one mouthful has produced death. Systemic absorption in the course of occupational use is apparently minimal. Paraquat on marijuana leaves is pyrolyzed to nontoxic dipyridyl. *Toxicokinetics:* "Hit and run" toxin. Less than 20% is absorbed. The peak is 1 hour postingestion. The route of elimination is the kidney. Most of the dose is eliminated in the first 40 hours; it is detected in urine for 15 days. Volume of distribution is over 500 liters per kg. *Manifestations:* Local corrosive effect on skin and mucous membranes. Acute renal failure in 48 hours (often reversible). Pulmonary effects in 72 hours are progressive, and oxygen aggravates the pulmonary fibrosis. Diquat does not produce effects on the lungs but produces convulsions and gastrointestinal distention. Long-term exposure may cause cataracts. Chlormequat's target organ is the kidney. *Management:* (1) Gastrointestinal decontamination despite corrosive effects should be done cautiously with a nasogastric tube. Repeated doses of activated charcoal are recommended. Dermal and ocular decontamination as needed. (2) Hemodialysis and hemoperfusion may be carried out in tandem. Hemoperfusion with charcoal alone, if started within 2 hours after ingestion, may be effective; if started after 2 hours, however, the results are poor. Continue hemoperfusion until blood paraquat levels cannot be detected. (3) Diuresis may be of value but consider the risk of fluid overload. (4) Niacin and vitamin E have not been effective. (5) Avoid oxygen unless absolutely necessary (PaO_2 below 60 mmHg) because this aggravates fibrosis. Some use hypoxic air, F_IO_2 10 to 20%. (6) Corticosteroids may help prevent adrenocortical necrosis. (7) Sepsis often develops within 7 to 10 days and should be treated appropriately. *Laboratory aids:* Blood levels above 2 μg per mL at 4 hours or above 0.10 μg per mL at 24 hours are usually fatal. Blood level testing and advice may be obtained from ICI America, 800–327–8633. Monitor renal, liver, and pulmonary functions and chest radiographs. Urine test for paraquat exposure—alkalinization and sodium dithionite give an intense blue-green color in exposure.

Parathion. See Organophosphate Insecticides.

Pentazocine (Talwin). See Opioids.

Perphenazine. See Phenothiazines and Other Major Neuroleptics.

Petroleum Products. See Hydrocarbons.

Phencyclidine (angel dust, PCP, peace pill, hog). This is the "drug of deceit" because it is substituted for many other drugs, such as THC and mescaline. There are now at least 38 analogues. Smoking may give cyanide poisoning. Improper mixing has caused explosions. *Toxic dose:* Two to 5 mg smoked or "snorted" produces drunken behavior, agitation, and excitement. Five to 10 mg produces stupor, coma, and myoclonus convulsions. Ten to 25 mg smoked, snorted, or taken orally results in prolonged coma and respiratory failure. It is usually fatal over 25 mg (250 ng per mL blood concentration). *Toxicokinetics:* Weak base. Rapidly absorbed when smoked, snorted, or ingested and secreted into stomach gastric juice. Absorbed in alkaline intestine, but ion trapping takes place in acid gastric media. Half-life is 30 to 60 minutes. Lipophilic drug with extensive Vd. The onset of action if smoked is 2 to 5 minutes (peak in 15 to 30 minutes); orally, 30 to 60 minutes. The duration at low doses is 4 to 6 hours and normality returns in 24 hours. At large overdoses, coma may last 6 to 10 days (waxes and wanes). An adverse reaction in overdose occurs in 1 to 2 hours. *Route of elimination:* By liver metabolism (50%). Urinary excretion of conjugates and free PCP. *Manifestations:* Sympathomimetic, cholinergic, cerebellar. Observe for violent behavior, paranoid schizophrenia, self-destructive behavior. Clues to diagnosis are bursts of horizontal, vertical, and rotary nystagmus, coma with eyes open. *Management* (avoid overtreatment of mild intoxications): (1) Gastrointestinal decontamination up to 4 hours postingestion, but this may not be effective because PCP is rapidly absorbed. Insert nasogastric tube into stomach for administration of activated charcoal every 6 hours because PCP is secreted into the stomach even if it is smoked or snorted. (2) Protect patient and others from harm. "Talk down" is usually ineffective. Low sensory environment. Diazepam (Valium) may be used orally or intramuscularly in the uncooperative patient. (3) For behavioral disorders and toxic psychosis—diazepam. (4) Seizures and muscle spasm—control with diazepam, 2.5 mg, up to 10 mg (Antidote 16, Table 4). (5) Dystonia reaction—diphenhydramine (Benadryl) intravenously (Antidote 19, Table 4). (6) Hyperthermia—external cooling. (7) Hypertensive crisis (dopaminergic)—use nitroprusside, 0.3 to 2 μg per kg per minute. Maximum infusion rate—10 μg per kg per minute; should never last more than 10 minutes. (8) Acid diuresis ion trapping (controversial). Ammonium chloride use is not recommended because of rhabdomyolysis and the danger of myoglobin precipitation in the renal tubules (Antidote 2, Table 4). (9) Avoid phenothiazines in the acute phase of intoxication because they lower the convulsive threshold. May be needed later for psychosis. *Laboratory aids:* (1) Elevation of CPK level is a clue to the amount of rhabdomyolysis occurring and the chance of myoglobinuria developing. Values up to 20,000 units have been reported. (2) Test urine for myoglobin and pigmented casts. Test urine with orthotoluidine; a positive test without red blood cells on microscopic examination suggests myoglobinuria. (3) Monitor urine and blood pH and urinary output if acidifying patient. (4) Measure PCP level. (5) Evaluate blood urea nitrogen, ammonia, electrolytes, blood glucose levels (20% of patients have hypoglycemia). (6) Test for PCP in gastric juice; levels are 40 to 50 times higher than in blood. *Complications:* Rhabdomyolysis, myoglobinuria, and renal failure. Dopaminogenic hypertensive crisis, cerebrovascular accident, encephalopathy, and malignant hyperthermia. Schizophrenic paranoid psychosis (induced in chronic users or precipitated in acute users). Loss of memory for months. Delayed toxicity and "flashbacks" occur. Teratogenic cases have been reported. Children have been intoxicated from inhalation in a room where adults were smoking PCP. PCP-induced depression and suicide have been reported.

Phenobarbital. See Barbiturates.

Phenothiazines and Other Major Neuroleptics. Phenothiazines are represented by aliphatic compounds: chlorpromazine (Thorazine), promethazine (Phenergan), promazine (Sparine), triflupromazine (Vesprin), methoxypromazine (Tentone);* piperazine compounds (dimethylamine series); acetophenazine (Tindal), fluphenazine (Prolixin), prochlorperazine (Compazine), perphenazine (Trilafon), trifluoperazine (Stelazine); and piperidine compounds: mesoridazine (Serentil), thioridazine (Mellaril), pipamazine (Mornidine).* Nonphenothiazines are the thioxanthines: chlorprothixene (Taractan), thiothixene (Navane); butyrophenones: haloperidol (Haldol), droperidol (Inapsine); dibenzoxazepines: loxapine (Loxitane, Daxolin); and dihydroindolones: molindone (Moban, Lidone). These have pharmacologic properties similar to those of the phenothiazines. See Table 25. *Manifestations:* If patient is asymptomatic, monitor vital signs and ECG for at least 6 to 12 hours. Clues to phenothiazine overdose

*Not available in the United States.

TABLE 25. **Pharmacokinetics of Phenothiazines and Related Compounds**

Medication	Metabolism	Dose Equivalent	Absorption	Volume of Distribution (L/kg)	Half-life (h)	Therapy
Aliphatic Type						
Moderate cardiotoxic and hypotensive effects; low sedation; moderate extrapyramidal effects; moderate anticholinergic effects						
Chlorpromazine (Thorazine) (high sedation)	Hepatic	100 mg	Rapid	10–20	16–30	PO: child, 2 mg/kg/24 h; max <12 years old, 75 mg/24 h; adult, 200–2000 mg/24 h
Promethazine (Phenergan)	Hepatic	25 mg	Rapid	—	12	PO: child, 0.1–0.5 mg/kg/dose; adult; 12.5–25 mg/dose (25–200 mg/24 h)
Piperazine						
Least cardiotoxic and hypotensive effects; very high extrapyramidal effects; moderate anticholinergic effects						
Prochlorperazine (Compazine)	Hepatic	15 mg	Slow	10–35	8–12	PO: child, 0.1 mg/kg/dose (not <2 years old); adult, 10 mg/dose
Fluphenazine HCl (Prolixin) (injectible deconate salt)	Hepatic	2 mg	Rapid	—	2–12 (6.8–9.6 days)	PO: adult, 2.5–10 mg/24h
Piperidine						
Highest cardiotoxic and hypotensive effects; low extrapyramidal effects; high anticholinergic effects						
Thioridazine (Mellaril) (high sedation)	Hepatic	100 mg	Slow	3.5	26–36	PO: child, 1 mg/kg/24 h (not <3 years old); adult, 150–300 mg/24 h
Butyrophenone						
Low cardiotoxic and hypotensive effects; low sedation; very high extrapyramidal effects; very low anticholinergic effects						
Haloperidol (Haldol)	Hepatic	2–15 mg	Rapid	20–30	12–22	PO: child, 0.1 mg/kg/24 h; adult, 20–100 mg/24 h
Droperidol (Inapsine)	Hepatic	2.5–10 mg	N/A	Large	2.2	IM/IV: child, 0.1–1.5 mg/kg/dose; adult, 2.5–10 mg/dose
Thioxanthene						
Low cardiotoxic and hypotensive effects: low sedation; high extrapyramidal effects; low anticholinergic effects						
Thiothixene (Navane)	Hepatic	2 mg	N/A	Large	34	PO: child, 0.25 mg/kg/24 h; adult, 16–60 mg/24 h (max, 60 mg)
Dibenzorazepine						
Low cardiotoxic and hypotensive effects; low sedation; high extrapyramidal effects; low anticholinergic effects						
Loxapine (Loxitane)	Hepatic	15 mg	N/A	Large	3–4	PO: adult, initially 10 mg bid to max of 50 mg
Dihydroindolones						
Molindone (Moban)	Hepatic	10 mg	Rapid	Large	1.5	PO: adult, initially 50–75 mg/24 h increased up to 225 mg

Peak levels occur mainly 1–4 h postingestion, and these drugs have enterohepatic recirculation. The pharmacokinetics of most phenothiazines resemble those of chlorpromazine. See kinetics for details.

Abbreviations: PO = per os (orally); IM = intramuscularly; IV = intravenously; N/A = not available.

are miosis, tremor, hypotension, hypothermia, respiratory depression, radiopaque pills on radiograph of abdomen, and increased QT waves on the ECG. Anticholinergic actions are also present. Major problems are respiratory depression, myocardial toxicity (quinidine-like), neurogenic hypotension (antidopaminogenic), and idiosyncratic reaction, which may occur at therapeutic levels. Idiosyncratic reaction consists of opisthotonos, torticollis, orolingual dyskinesia, and oculogyric crisis (painful upward gaze) and can be mistaken for a psychotic episode. Extrapyramidal crisis is frequent in children and women. Malignant neuroleptic syndrome may occur. It is characterized by hyperthermia, muscle rigidity, and autonomic dysfunction. Death is usually due to cardiac effects. Phenothiazines are metabolized by the liver into many metabolites. Some remain in the body longer than 6 months. *Management:* (1) Gastrointestinal decontamination. Emesis induction may be useful within 30 minutes after ingestion if symptoms have not occurred. If symptoms are already present, many of these agents have antiemetic action, so lavage may be required. Always provide gastric lavage to comatose patients after the airway is protected regardless of the time of ingestion because of inhibition of gastric motility. (2) Extrapyramidal signs (idiosyncratic reaction) can be treated with diphenhydramine (Benadryl) (Antidote 19, Table 4), or benztropine (Cogentin), 1 to 2 mg intravenously slowly. Symptoms recur, and these drugs should be continued orally for

TABLE 26. **Pharmacokinetic Properties of Beta Blockers**

Drug Name	Solubility and Absorption (%)	Plasma Half-life (h)	Elimination Route	Time to Peak Concentration (h)	Protein Binding (%)	Volume of Distribution (L/kg)	Beta$_1$ Cardiac Selective
Acebutolol* (Sectral) Dose: 400–800 mg MDD: 800 mg TPC: 200–2000 ng/mL	Moderate, lipid (90)	3–4, metabolite diacetolol	Hepatic, active metabolite	—	26	1.2	+
Alprenolol* (Aptin,§ Betapin; Betacard) Dose: 200–800 mg MDD: 800 mg TPC: 50–200 ng/mL	Lipid (10)	3.1	Hepatic	1–3	85	3.4	–
Atenolol (Tenormin) Dose: 50–100 mg MDD: 100 mg TPC: 200–500 ng/mL	Water (46–62)	6–9	Renal, 95%	2–4	3–10	0.7	+
Betaxolol (Betoptic) (Kerlone) Dose: 1 drop in eye twice daily MDD: Not available	Water (70–90)	12–22	Hepatic, 3–12%	—	50–60	4.9–13	+
Bisoprolol (Zebeta) Dose: 5–20 mg	Water (82–94)	9–12	Renal, 50%	3–4	30	2.9	+
Carteolol (Cartrul) Dose: 2.5–10 mg MDD: 40 mg	Lipid (84)	6–11	Renal, 60%	—	15	NA	–
Esmolol (Brevibloc) Dose: IV 50–500 μg/kg/min (loading dose) MDD: 300 μg/kg/min	Water	9 min	Hepatic, plasma esterases	—	55	3.4	+
Labetalol (Normodyne, Trandate) Dose: 400–800 mg MDD: 1–2 gm	Water (50)	6–8	Hepatic, 95% Blocks alpha (weakly) and beta activity	—	50	11	–
Levobunolol (Betagan) Dose: Ophthalmologic: 1 drop twice daily, 0.5%, 1%	Water (100)	6.1	Hepatic	—	—	—	–
Metoprolol (Lopressor) Dose: 50–100 mg MDD: 450 mg TPC: 50–100 ng/mL	Lipid (>95)	3–4	Hepatic	1–2	10	5.6	+
Nadolol (Corgard) Dose: 40–320 mg MDD: 320 mg TPC: 20–400 ng/mL	Water (15–25)	14–23	Renal, 70%	3–4	25	2.1	–
Oxprenolol (Trasicor)¶ Dose: 80–320 mg MDD: 480 mg TPC: 80–100 ng/mL	Lipid (70–95)	1.5–3	Hepatic	1–2	80	1.5	–
Penbutolol (Levatol) Dose: 20–80 mg MDD: 80 mg	Lipid (100)	4–8	Hepatic	1–1.5	80–90	0.5	–
Pindolol* (Visken) Dose: 20–60 mg MDD: 60 mg TPC: 50–150 ng/mL	Lipid (>90)	3–4	Hepatic, 60%; renal, 40%	1.25	57	2.0	–
Practolol* (Eraldin)¶ Dose: 25–600 mg MDD: 800 mg TPC: 1500–5000 ng/mL	No longer available in United States because of adverse reactions Water (100)	6–8	Renal	3	40	—	+
Propranolol (Inderal) Dose: 40–160 mg MDD: 480 mg TPC: 50–100 ng/mL	Lipid (100) (70% first pass)	2–3	Hepatic; renal (<1%), active hydroxy metabolite	1.5	90–95	3.6	–

TABLE 26. **Pharmacokinetic Properties of Beta Blockers** *Continued*

Drug Name	Solubility and Absorption (%)	Plasma Half-life (h)	Elimination Route	Time to Peak Concentration (h)	Protein Binding (%)	Volume of Distribution (L/kg)	$Beta_1$ Cardiac Selective
Sotalol (Betapace)	Prolongs QT and may produce torsades de pointes						
Dose: 80–320 mg MDD: 480 mg TPC: 500–4000 ng/mL	Water (70)	5–13	Renal	2–3	54	0.7	–
Timolol†‡ Dose: 20 mg (Blocadren); ophthalmologic (Timoptic, 0.25%, 0.5%), 1 drop twice daily MDD: 60 mg TPC: 5–10 ng/mL	Lipid (>90)	3–5	Hepatic, 80%; renal, 20%	4–5	<10	5.5	–

Abbreviations: MDD = maximum daily dose; TPC = therapeutic plasma concentration.
*Partial agonists.
†Substantial first pass.
‡Mitochondrial calcium protection during ischemia.
§Investigational drug in the United States.
¶Not available in the United States.

2 to 3 days. *This is not the treatment of overdose,* only of the idiosyncratic reaction. (3) Monitor ECG for dysrhythmias and treat with antidysrhythmic agents. Avoid quinidine, procainamide, or disopyramide. Treat the membrane depressant effects with IV sodium bicarbonate. (4) Hypotension is treated with the Trendelenburg position or fluid challenge or both. Vasopressors are used only if these fail. Dopamine (Intropin) should *not* be used to treat the hypotension because these drugs are antidopaminogenic. If a pressor agent is needed, use norepinephrine (Levarterenol, Levophed). (5) Treat neuroleptic malignant syndrome by discontinuing the offending agent, reducing temperature with external cooling, and correcting any metabolic imbalance. Dantrolene, bromocriptine, and amantadine are agents that have been shown to be useful pharmacologic adjuncts for the management of this syndrome. (6) Treat hypothermia or hyperthermia with external physical measures (not drugs). (7) Physostigmine should be avoided because it can produce seizures and cardiac toxicity. *Laboratory aids:* A ferric chloride test of urine can confirm exposure to phenothiazines if there is a sufficient blood level. Blood levels are *not* useful in management. A radiograph of the abdomen is useful to detect undissolved tablets, which may be radiopaque. Monitor arterial blood gases, renal and hepatic function, and levels of electrolytes and blood glucose for creatinine kinase and myoglobinemia in neuroleptic malignant syndrome.

Phenylpropanolamine (PPA). See Amphetamines.

Primidone. See Anticonvulsants.

Propoxyphene. See Opioids.

Propranolol and Beta Blockers. Some of these agents available in the United States at this time are listed in Table 25. Beta blockers generally act as negative cardiac ionotropes and chronotropes, although some have partial agonist activity with the opposite effect. *Toxic dose:* Varies considerably. *Toxicokinetics:* Time to peak action is 1 to 2 hours orally; the effects last 24 to 48 hours. In drugs with long half-lives, e.g., nadolol, it may take many days to recover from overdose toxicity (Table 26). *Manifestations:* Observe for bradycardia and hypotension. Fat-soluble drugs have more CNS effects. Partial agonists may initially produce tachycardia and hypertension (oxprenolol, pindolol). ECG changes include varying degrees of atrioventricular conduction delay or frank asystole. May cause hypoglycemia. *Management:* (1) Gastrointestinal decontamination with gastric lavage and activated charcoal/cathartic. Before gastric lavage, treatment with atropine, 0.01 mg per kg for a child and 0.5 mg for an adult, has been suggested to decrease the vagal effect in patients with bradycardia or significant intoxications. Avoid induced emesis because of early onset of seizures and vagal stimulation. Asymptomatic patients may be discharged after 12 to 24 hours of observation. (2) Treat hypoglycemia (frequent in children) and hyperkalemia. (3) Control convulsions. (4) Cardiovascular manifestations: Bradycardia—if patient is hemodynamically stable and asymptomatic, no therapy. If patient is unstable (hypotension or atriovenous block), use atropine, glucagon, isoproterenol, and pacemaker. Ventricular tachycardia or premature beats—use lidocaine, phenytoin, or overdrive pacing. Myocardial depression and hypotension—correct dysrhythmias, institute Trendelenburg positioning and fluids. Monitor with pulmonary arterial wedge pressure (PAWP) catheter. If low cardiac output with low PAWP, give more fluids. If low cardiac output with normal PAWP, use glucagon (Antidote 26, Table 4). Avoid quinidine, procainamide, and disopyramide (Norpace). Glucagon is probably the drug of choice because it works through an adenyl cyclase mechanism not affected by the beta blockers. It is given as a bolus and may be continued as an infusion (Antidote 26, Table 4). If bronchospasm is present, give aminophylline. Hemodialysis or hemoperfusion for low-volume distribution drugs that are low–protein binding and water soluble (nadolol, atenolol, and sotalol) particularly with evidence of renal failure. If hypoglycemia is present, give intravenous glucose. *Laboratory aids:* Monitor blood glucose, potassium, ECG, PAWP. Toxic blood level of propranolol is over 2 μg per mL.

Quinidine and Quinine (antidysrhythmic and antimalarial agents). *Toxic dose:* Quinidine in child is 60 mg per kg; in adult, 2 to 8 grams. Quinine is 15 mg per kg, child; 1 gram, adult. *Toxicokinetics:* There is 95 to 100% absorption, with peak action in 2 to 6 hours. Half-life is 3 to 4 hours (quinidine gluconate, 8 to 12 hours). Large Vd. Metabolized predominantly by the liver. *Manifestations:* Cinchonism (headache, nausea, vomiting, tinnitus, deafness, diplopia, dilated pupils). Myocardial depression, dysrhythmias, ECG changes—widening of PR and QT intervals and QRS complexes. Rashes and flushing. Hemolysis in glucose-6-phosphate dehydrogenase deficiency. Dementia reported. Quinidine produces more cardiovascular damage and quinine produces more ocular damage. *Management:* (1) Obtain an immediate cardiac consultation. Electrophysiologic support of the heart should be readily available. (2) Gastrointestinal decontamination. Avoid emesis because of rapid onset of seizures and coma. (3) Monitor ECG and liver function. (4) May need antidysrhythmic drugs (but avoid Class IA antidysrhythmics), and pacemaker and alkalinization. Treat torsades de pointes in adults with magnesium sulfate, 2 grams IV over 2 to 3 minutes. *Laboratory aids:* Quinidine: Therapeutic level 2 to 6 μg per mL. Toxic greater than 8 μg per mL. Fatal greater than 16 μg per mL. Quinine: Therapeutic level 7 μg per mL. Toxic greater than 10 μg per mL.

Salicylates. *Toxic dose:* See Table 27. Methyl salicylate (oil of wintergreen): 1 mL equals 1.4 grams of salicylate. One teaspoonful equals 21 adult aspirins. *Toxicokinetics:* Plasma concentration is significant in 30 minutes and peaks in 1 to 2 hours but may be delayed 6 hours or more in overdose with enteric-coated, sustained-release preparations or concretions. Half-life is 3 to 6 hours (therapeutic) to 12 to 36 hours (toxic). Urine pH influences urine salicylate elimination. *Manifestations of acute ingestion* (see Table 27): The metabolic disturbance in adults and older children is usually respiratory alkalosis; in children younger than 5 years of age, the initial respiratory alkalosis usually changes to metabolic or mixed metabolic acidosis and respiratory alkalosis, with acidosis predominating within a few hours. *Management:* Do not wait for 6-hour salicylate level to start treatment of symptomatic patients. If hemodialysis may be required, suggest immediate consult with nephrologist. (1) Gastrointestinal decontamination is useful up to 12 hours postingestion because some factors delay absorption (food, enteric-coated tablets, other drugs); pylorospasm may delay emptying; and concretions may form. Activated charcoal should be administered every 4 hours until stools are black. Concretions may be removed by lavage, whole-body irrigation, endoscopy, or gastrostomy. (2) Intravenous fluid should be given as recommended in Table 28. Alkalinization enhances salicylate excretion. Potassium is essential to produce adequate alkalinization. Monitor both the urine and blood pH. Do not use the urine pH alone to assess the need for alkalinization (Antidote 39, Table 4). (3) Fluid retention can be treated with mannitol (20%), 0.5 gram per kg over 30 minutes, or furosemide, 1 mg per kg intravenously. (4) Hyperpyrexia should be treated with external cooling. (5) Patients with abnormal bleeding or hypoprothrombinemia will need vitamin K, 10 to 50 mg intravenously, and, if bleeding continues, fresh blood or platelet transfusion (Antidote 43, Table 4). (6) Hemodialysis is indicated if there is persistent acidosis (pH $<$7.0) and lack of response to fluid or alkali in 6 hours; if serum salicylate levels are initially greater than 160 mg per dL or greater than 120 mg per dL at 6 hours postingestion (do *not* use the salicylate level as the sole criterion for dialysis); or if there are coma and uncontrollable seizures, congestive heart failure, acute renal failure, and progressive deterioration despite good management. Lower levels such as 30 to 60 μg per mL may be an indication for hemodialysis in chronic salicylism with altered mental status. (7) Chronic toxicity is usually a more severe intoxication because of the cumulative pharmacokinetics of salicylates. Management needs are outlined in Table 29. *Laboratory aids:* The metabolic acidosis of salicylism has a moderately elevated anion gap. Hyperglycemia or hypoglycemia may exist. Serum salicylate levels used in conjunction with the Done nomogram (Fig. 3) are useful predictors of expected severity following *acute single ingestions.* The Done nomogram is *not* useful in chronic intoxications or in methyl salicylate,

TABLE 27. **Quantities of Aspirin Ingested: Deposition and Manifestations***

Category	Amount Ingested (mg/kg)	Toxicity Expected	Gastrointestinal Decontamination	Manifestations Anticipated
Nontoxic	$<$150	No	No	None
Mild intoxication	150–200	Yes	Yes (ECF)	Vomiting, tinnitus, mild hyperventilation
Moderate intoxication	200–300	Yes	Yes (ECF)	Hyperpnea, lethargy or excitability
Severe intoxication	300–500	Yes	Yes (ECF)	Coma, convulsions, severe hyperpnea
Very severe intoxication	$>$500	Yes	Yes (ECF)	Potentially fatal

Abbreviation: ECF = emergency care facility.
*See toxic dose indications for gastrointestinal decontamination.

TABLE 28. **Recommendations for Fluid Management for Moderate or Severe Salicylism***

Purpose	Rate (mL/kg/h)	Duration (h)	Electrolyte Concentration (mEq/L) *Na*	*K*	*Cl*	*HCO_3*	Glucose (%)
Volume expansion	20	0.5–1.0	100	0	77	23	5–10
Administered as 0.45% saline with 23 mEq/L $NaHCO_3$							
Hydration Ongoing losses Alkalinization	4–8	Until therapeutic blood serum concentration 30 mg/dL	56	40	56	1–2 mEq/kg child; 50–100 mEq adult	5–10
Administered as 0.33% saline and $NaHCO_3$ to obtain urine pH 7.5–8.0, blood pH 7.5							
			mEq/kg/day				
Maintenance	2–6	—	3	2	4		

*For severe acidosis (pH <7.15), may require 1–2 mEq/kg of sodium bicarbonate every 1–2 h. Usual fluid loss is 200–300 mL/kg, but carefully monitor for fluid overload. Potassium may be needed in excess of 40 mEq/L when alkalinizing.

phenyl salicylate, or homomethyl salicylate ingestions. The salicylate level for use in the Done nomogram should be obtained 6 hours postingestion. Before 6 hours, levels in the toxic range should be treated, and patients with levels below the toxic range should be retested if a potentially toxic dose is ingested. Monitor urine output, urine pH, electrolytes, arterial blood gases, blood glucose, prothrombin time, renal function, serum salicylate level, and urine salicylate with the ferric chloride test. Arterial blood pH should be kept at 7.5. *Prognosis:* Persistent vigorous treatment of salicylate ingestion is essential because recovery has occurred despite decerebrate rigidity.

Sedative Hypnotics, Nonbarbiturate. See Table 30. *Management:* Primarily supportive (especially intubation and ventilator therapy with continuous positive airway pressure for adult respiratory distress syndrome) and with the use of hemoperfusion or hemodialysis in patients who are severely intoxicated and fail to respond to good supportive care and whose intoxication is life-threatening. Avoid emesis because of rapid onset of convulsions, apnea, and coma. (1) *Chloral hydrate* management includes cautious gastrointestinal decontamination. Avoid the use of epinephrine and catecholamines that may produce dysrhythmias. Propranolol, 0.1 mg per kg in 1-mg increments, appears to be more effective than lidocaine for ventricular dysrhythmias. Charcoal hemoperfusion may effectively remove chloral hydrate and its metabolite in patients who fail to respond and have potentially fatal plasma levels (20 μg per mL or higher). Hemodialysis may be ineffective because of lipid solubility. (2) *Ethchlorvynol* management includes gastrointestinal decontamination up to several hours postingestion. Charcoal hemoperfusion is the best method of extracorporeal removal when other measures fail in a life-threatening situation (ingestion of over 10 grams or 100 mg per kg, with serum levels of over 100 μg per mL in the first 12 hours or 70 μg per mL after 12 hours in patients with prolonged life-threatening coma). External rewarming if temperature is below 32° C. (3) *Glutethimide* management includes gastrointestinal decontamination up to 24 hours postingestion. Concretions may form. Charcoal hemoperfusion appears to be the best method of extracorporeal removal in life-threatening protracted coma when the patient has ingested over 10 grams and has a serum level of over 30 μg per mL. Treat hyperthermia with external cooling. (4) *Meprobamate* management includes gastrointestinal decontamination up to several hours postingestion, with charcoal hemoperfusion in prolonged coma with life-threatening complications. Concretions may form in the stomach and may require whole-bowel irrigation, endoscopy, or surgical removal. (5) *Methaqualone* management includes gastrointestinal decontamination up to 12 hours postingestion. Forced diuresis, dialysis, and hemoperfusion are not indicated. Fatalities are rare. (6) *Methyprylon* manage-

TABLE 29. **Management of Chronic Salicylate Intoxication**

Classification	Urine pH	Blood pH	Hydration	$NaHCO_3$ (mEq/L)	Potassium (mEq/L)
Mild	Alkaline	Alkaline	Yes	Yes†	20
Moderate	Acid*	Alkaline	Yes	pH 7.5†	40
Severe	Acid	Acid	Yes	pH 7.5	40‡ 80§

*Paradoxical acid urine and alkaline blood indicate potassium depletion.
†Bicarbonate administered to keep blood pH at 7.5 and urine pH at 7.5–8.0.
‡Normal serum potassium and electrocardiogram (ECG).
§Low serum potassium and/or abnormal ECG indicating potassium deficiency.

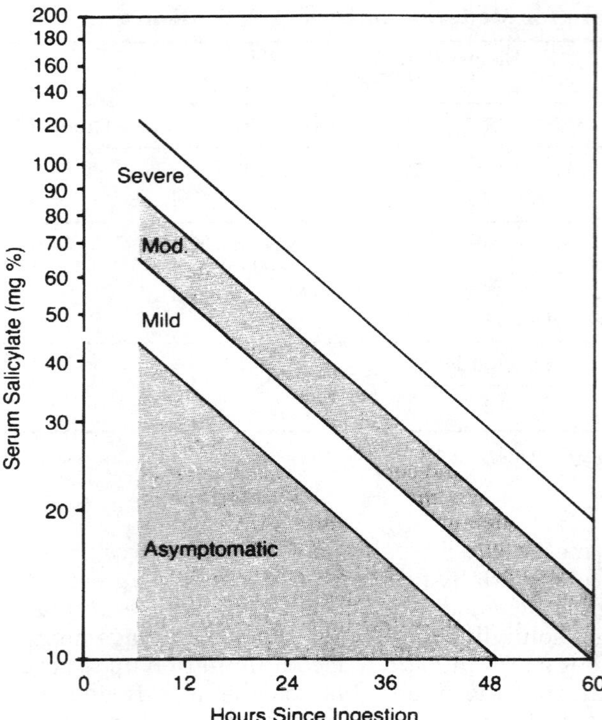

Figure 3. The Done nomogram for salicylate intoxication. For limitations of use, see *Laboratory aids*. (Redrawn from Done A: Salicylate intoxication: Significance of measurements of salicylate in blood in cases of acute ingestion. Pediatrics *26*:800, 1960. Reproduced by permission of Pediatrics.)

ment includes gastrointestinal decontamination and may require treatment of the hypotension with vasopressors of the alpha-adrenergic variety—e.g., levarterenol (Levophed). The hypotension usually does not respond to position or fluids alone. This is a dialyzable drug, but dialysis usually is not necessary. Fatalities are rare.

Strychnine. Primarily available as a rodenticide and component of cathartics and "tonics." Adulterant of "street drugs," particularly marijuana and cocaine. *Toxic dose:* 5 to 10 mg; fatal in doses of 15 to 30 mg. *Toxicokinetics:* Rapid absorption. Manifestations may occur within 15 to 30 minutes. Low protein binding. Hepatic metabolism, which appears to be saturable. Twenty percent is excreted in urine. Has been found in the urine up to 48 hours after a 700-mg dose. *Manifestations:* Interferes with postsynaptic neurotransmitter inhibition by glycine. Hyperacusis is often the first sign. Mild cases—face stiffness (trismus and risus sardonicus). Moderate cases—extensor muscle thrusts. Severe cases—tetanic convulsions with opisthotonos. Death occurs within 1 to 3 hours after ingestion. The prognosis for recovery improves if the patient survives beyond 5 hours. The complications of intoxication are lactic acidosis, hyperthermia, rhabdomyolysis and renal damage from precipitation of myoglobin in the renal tubules, and death from hypoxia. *Management:* (1) Emesis is contraindicated because of rapid absorption and the early onset of seizures. Gastric aspiration and lavage may be used after the seizures are controlled. Activated charcoal should be given and repeated. (2) Control convulsions with diazepam or phenobarbital. (3) Supportive care for respiratory depression. (4) Acid diuresis and dialysis do not appear to be justified on the basis of available studies. (5) Paralysis with assisted ventilation is useful.

Tear Gas (lacrimators). CS (chlorobenzylidine), "riot control"; CN powder (chloroacetophenone, 1%); Mace (chloroacetophenone). *Management:* Dermal and ocular decontamination. Protect attendants from contamination. Ophthalmologic evaluation. Oxygen therapy may be needed for dyspnea and respiratory distress.

Theophylline. *Toxic dose:* Acute, single dose greater than 10 mg per kg yields mild toxicity. Greater than 20 mg per kg, moderate manifestations. *Toxicokinetics:* Absorption is complete. Peak levels occur within 60 minutes after ingestion of liquid preparations; 1 to 3 hours after regular tablets; and 3 to 10 hours after slow-release preparations. Vd, 0.3 to 0.7 liter per kg. Protein binding, 15 to 40%. Half-life varies: 3.5 hours average in a child and 4.5 hours in an adult (range from 3 to 9 hours). In neonates and young infants the drug's half-life is much longer. Overdose increases the half-life. *Elimination:* Hepatic metabolism, 90% (demethylation and oxidation); 8 to 10% is excreted unchanged in the urine. *Manifestations:* Acute toxicity generally correlates with blood levels; chronic toxicity does not. Ten to 20 μg per mL is the therapeutic range, but mild gastrointestinal toxicity may occur in some. Twenty to 40 μg per mL is moderate toxicity, with gastrointestinal and CNS stimulation. Over 50 μg per mL—seizures and dysrhythmias may occur, but they may also occur at lower levels and without gastrointestinal symptoms. Children tolerate higher serum levels. Chronic intoxication is more serious and difficult to treat. Many factors increase theophylline concentration. *Management:* (1) Gastrointestinal decontamination in acute overdose, up to 4 hours with regular preparations and up to 8 to 12 hours with slow-release preparations. Test aspirate or vomitus for blood. Give activated charcoal every 4 hours until serum theophylline levels are less than 20 μg per mL. Do not induce emesis if hematemesis exists. If there is intractable vomiting, administer the antiemetic metoclopramide, 0.4 mg per kg per dose intravenously (maximum, 0.5 mg per kg per 24 hours) in infants and children, and 10 mg slowly over 15 minutes every 6 to 8 hours in adults. Alternative: droperidol, 2.5 mg intravenously or 0.05 to 0.1 mg per kg per dose every 6 to 8 hours if needed. Both drugs may cause extrapyramidal symptoms. Ondansetron is not recommended because it inhibits metabolism of theophylline. (2) Monitor ECG, obtain theophylline levels every 4 hours they remain until in the therapeutic range of 10 to 20 μg per mL. (3) Control seizures with diazepam. If coma, convulsions, or vomiting exists, intubate immediately. (4) Hypotension is treated with fluid challenge and, if this fails, vasopressors. (5) Hematemesis is managed with saline lavage and blood

TABLE 30. **Nonbarbiturate Sedative Hypnotic Drugs**

Drug	Absorption and Toxic Dose	Time to Peak Effect (h)	Volume of Distribution (L/kg)	Protein Binding (%)	Elimination Route	Serum Half-life (h)	Toxic Level (μg/mL)	Manifestations and Comment*
Chloral hydrate (Noctec)	Rapid TD, 2 gm FD, 4–10 gm	1–2	0.75–0.9	40	Hepatic 90% to active metabolite trichloroethanol (TCE)	4–8 min TCE: 8–12 h	100 (80 TCE—very toxic)	Pear-like odor; dysrhythmias (especially ventricular), hepatotoxicity, irritant to mucosa of GI tract; ARDS; radiopaque capsules
Ethchlorvynol (Placidyl)	Rapid TD, 2.5 gm FD, 10–25 gm	1–2	3–4	35–50	Hepatic 90%	10–25 in OD over 100	20–80	Prolonged coma up to 200 h, apnea, hypothermia, pulmonary edema, pink gastric aspirate, pungent odor
Glutethimide (Doriden) (highest mortality of all sedative hypnotics, 14%)	Slow, erratic TD, 5 gm FD, 10 gm	6	Large, 2–2.7	50	Hepatic 98% to toxic metabolite 4-hydroxyglutarimide	10–40 in OD over 100	20–80	Prolonged, cyclic comas up to 120 h, anticholinergic signs, convulsions, recurrent apnea, hyperthermia
Meprobamate (Equanil, Miltown)	Rapid TD, 10–20 gm FD, 10–20 gm	4–8	10	20	Hepatic 90%	6–16	30–100	Coma, convulsions, pulmonary edema, apnea, concretions in stomach
Methaqualone (Quaaludes, "love drugs")	Rapid TD, 800 mg FD 3–8 gm	1–3	2–6	80	Hepatic 90%	10–40	8–10	Hypertonia, hyperreflexia, convulsions, apnea, acts "drunk," bleeding tendencies
Methyprylon (Noludar)	Rapid TD, 3 gm FD, 8–20 gm	2–4	1–2	—	Hepatic 97%	3–6 in OD over 50	30	Hyperactive, coma lasts 30 h, miosis, persistent hypotension, pulmonary edema; mortality rare

Abbreviations: TD = toxic dose; FD = fatal dose; OD = overdose; ARDS = adult respiratory distress syndrome; GI = gastrointestinal.
*Comment includes other features besides the typical manifestations of all these agents—coma, respiratory depression, psychological and physiologic withdrawal, hypotension, hypothermia (except glutethimide hyperthermia).

replacement if needed. (6) Charcoal hemoperfusion is the management of choice in life-threatening convulsions, dysrhythmias, hematemesis, or intractable vomiting refractory to conventional measures. It is recommended for acute intoxications with serum theophylline concentrations of 70 to 100 μg per mL, or with chronic overdoses with drug levels of 40 to 60 μg per mL, especially if the patient has risk factors that increase serum levels, e.g., age younger than 6 months or older than 60 years, liver disease, heart failure, viral infections, pneumonia, fever greater than 102° F; medications: macrolide antibiotics, oral contraceptives, cimetidine, beta blockers, carbamazepine, and caffeine. Differences in slow-release preparations from regular preparations: few or no gastrointestinal symptoms with high levels; peak concentration times may be 10 to 24 hours postingestion; and onset of seizures may occur 10 to 12 hours postingestion. *Laboratory aids:* Monitor theophylline levels, check for occult blood in vomitus and stools, monitor vital signs and hemoglobin and hematocrit (for hemorrhage). Monitor cardiac, renal, and hepatic function, electrolytes, blood glucose, arterial blood gases, and acid-base balance.

Toluene. See Hydrocarbons.

Tranquilizers. See Sedative Hypnotics.

Trichloroethylene. See Hydrocarbons.

Tricyclic Antidepressants (TCADs). See Table 31. These agents are generally rapidly absorbed from the gastrointestinal tract, but absorption may be prolonged in overdose owing to anticholinergic action. Their bioavailability has considerable variation among patients, and they are highly bound to plasma and tissue proteins. Protein binding decreases with decreasing pH. The Vd is large, usually 10 to 20 liters per kg. The TCADs are metabolized primarily in the liver. *N*-Demethylation of the tertiary amines yields the active secondary amine metabolites; hydroxylation gives rise to inactive metabolites. Forty percent is excreted in the feces and only 3% in the urine unchanged. The t½ varies from 9 to 198 hours. In an overdose, the half-life may be much longer. Tricyclic tertiary amines (metabolized to active metabolites) are amitriptyline (Elavil), imipramine (Tofranil), and doxepin (Sinequan). Tricyclic secondary amines (metabolized to nonactive metabolites) are desipramine (Norpramin, Pertofrane), protriptyline (Vivactil), and nortriptyline (Pamelor). Tricyclic dibenzoxazepine (metabolized to a major metabolite) is amoxapine (Asendin). *Manifestations:* The onset of action varies from less than 1 hour to 12 hours after ingestion. The phases of intoxication are (1) consciousness with dry mouth, mydriasis, ataxia, increased deep tendon reflexes, and changes in the ST segment; (2) Stages I

TABLE 31. **Kinetics of Cyclic Antidepressants**

Antidepressant (Trade Name)	Absorption	Time to Peak Effect (h)	Volume of Distribution (L/kg)	Half-life (h)	Protein Binding (%)	Elimination	Toxic Level (ng/mL)	Availability	Therapeutic Plasma Level (Range)	Usual Dose: *Adult (mg)*	Usual Dose: *Child (mg/kg/24 h)*
Tricyclic Tertiary Amines (metabolized to active metabolites)											
Amitriptyline (Elavil)	Slow	2–12	8–10	15–19	82–96	Hepatic	>500	Tab 10, 25, 75, 100, 150, mg	50–250	75–300	1.5–2.0
Imipramine (Tofranil)	Rapid (29–77%)	1–2	5–20	8–16	76–96	Hepatic	>500	Tab 10, 25, 50, mg; Cap 75, 100, 125, 150 mg	150–250	75–300	3–7
Doxepin (Sinequan, Adapin)	Rapid complete	2–4	20	15–19	95	Hepatic	>150	Cap 25, 50, 75, 100, 150 mg	150–250	75–300	
Trimipramine (Surmontil)	Rapid	2	NA	NA	Large	Renal		Cap 25, 50, 100 mg	100–200	75–300	
Tricyclic Secondary Amines (metabolized to nonactive metabolites)											
Desipramine (Norpramin, Pertofrane)	Rapid incomplete	4–6	28–60	18–28	73–92	Hepatic	>500	Tab 10, 25, 50, 100, 150 mg; Cap 10, 50 mg	125–300	75–300	
Protriptyline (Vivactil)						Hepatic	NA	Tab 5, 10 mg	70–260	20–60	
Nortriptyline (Aventyl)	Slow (46–77%)	7–8	21–57	50–150	93–65	Hepatic	>500	Cap 10, 25, 75 mg	50–150	75–200	1.5–2.0
Tetracyclic Dibenzoxapines (metabolized to major metabolites)											
Amoxapine (Asendin)	Rapid	1.5	Large	8–30	90	Renal and hepatic	NA	Tab 25, 50, 100, 150 mg	200–600	150–600	
Maprotiline (Ludiomil)		8–24	22.6	27–58	88	Hepatic	Over 300	Tab 25, 50, 75 mg	200–600	75–300	
Triazolopyridines											
Trazodone (Desyrel)	Rapid	0.5–2	NA	4–13	89–95	Hepatic	NA	Tab 50, 100, 150 mg	800–1600	50–600	
Unclassified or Bicyclics (metabolized to active metabolite)											
Fluoxetine (Prozac)	Rapid	4–6	14–102	24–96	94	Hepatic	>400	Cap 20 mg; syrup 20 mg/5 mL, 4-oz bottles	NA	20–80	
Norfluoxetine (active metabolite) peak 76 h, half-life 5–7 days											
Dibenzazepines											
Clomipramine* (Anafranil)	Rapid	3–5	12	21	98	Hepatic	500	Cap 25, 50, 75 mg		25 increasing up to 100, max 200	
Dimethylclomipramine (DM) (primary active metabolite) half-life 54–77 h											
Aminoketones											
Bupropion (Wellbutrin)	Rapid 5–20% bioavailability	2	NA	8–24	80%	Hepatic	NA	Tab 75, 100 mg		100 bid increasing up to 150 tid	
Several active metabolites relate to toxicity											

Abbreviations: Toxic level = toxic serum concentration; NA = not available; Tab = tablets; Cap = capsules.
*Available to psychiatrists free of charge to treat patients 1–800–842–2422 (Med Lett *30:*102–104, 1988).

and II coma with hypertension, tachycardia above 160, mydriasis, and supraventricular tachycardia; and (3) Stages III and IV coma with hypotension, heart rate under 120, respiratory depression, tonic-clonic seizures, and ventricular dysrhythmias. The CNS effects occur early, and seizures are common. *Cardiovascular toxicity* is frequent in the serious poisonings and results from anticholinergic effects, sympathomimetic activity (by blocking reuptake of catecholamines), quinidine activity, catecholamine depletion, and alpha-adrenergic blockade. Cardiotoxic effects include cardiac dysrhythmias, hypertension, hypotension, and pulmonary edema.

Toxic dose: The TCADs have a narrow margin of safety. In a child, a 375-mg dose and in adults, as little as 500 to 750 mg has been fatal. The following dosages may serve as a guide to the degree of imipramine toxicity: Less than 10 mg per kg produces light coma, mydriasis, and tachycardia and has a good prognosis. At 20 mg per kg, Stage III manifestations are produced. At 30 mg per kg, fatalities may result. At 50 mg per kg, the mortality rate is increased. Over 70 mg per kg is rarely survived. Relative adult dosage equivalents may serve as a guide: amitriptyline, 100 mg; amoxapine, 125 mg; desipramine, 75 mg; doxepin, 100 mg; imipramine, 75 mg; maprotiline, 75 mg; nortriptyline, 50 mg; and trazodone, 200 mg (see Table 30). Therapeutic blood levels are in the range of 50 to 170 ng per mL. If the QRS interval is less than 0.10 second for 6 hours, the prognosis is good. If it is greater than 0.10 second, seizures may occur, and if it is over 0.16 second, serious dysrhythmia may occur. In general, most antidepressants possess anticholinergic activity. The tricyclics produce dysrhythmias, hypotension, and seizures. The tetracyclics (amoxaprine, maprotiline) produce convulsions that may result in rhabdomyolysis and renal dysfunction. The new agents trazodone and fluoxetine appear to have mild sedative effects and cardiotoxicity, although orthostatic hypotension, vertigo, and priapism have been reported. Bupropion (Wellbutrin) is a phenylaminoketone antidepressant that produces dose-related seizures. Nomifensine (Merital) was withdrawn in 1986 because of reports of hemolytic anemia associated with it. *Management:* (1) Maintenance of vital functions. If the patient is asymptomatic, there should be vascular access, and cardiac monitoring should continue for at least 6 hours from admission or 8 to 12 hours postingestion. All children should be observed closely for 24 hours in an intensive care unit. If patient is symptomatic, obtain cardiac consultation and monitor in an intensive care unit until the patient is asymptomatic and shows no ECG abnormalities for at least 72 hours. (2) Gastrointestinal decontamination (omit emesis) if the patient is alert. Intact pills have been recovered by lavage up to 18 hours after ingestion. Suspected cases should have ECG monitoring. (3) Activated charcoal initially with a cathartic. No more than two doses of activated charcoal is advised. (4) Control seizures with intravenous diazepam. Intravenous phenytoin (Dilantin) may be added in patients with seizures not responding to diazepam alone. If not immediately successful, consider an aggressive approach to airway management and rapid-sequence intubation with paralysis by short nonpolarizing neuromuscular blockers such as vecuronium. (5) Cardiovascular complications of TCAD intoxication, including a QRS complex of over 0.16 second, ventricular tachycardia, severe conduction blocks, hypotension, or seizures, should *first* be treated by alkalinization of blood with sodium bicarbonate to a pH of 7.5 to 7.55 (Antidote 39, Table 4). Administer 1 mEq per kg of sodium bicarbonate undiluted as a bolus and repeated twice a few minutes apart. If it does not affect cardiotoxicity, an infusion of $NaHCO_3$ may follow to keep blood pH at 7.5 to 7.55 but not higher. Monitor serum sodium, potassium, and blood pH because fatal alkalemia and hypernatremia have been reported. Continuous infusion of bicarbonate by itself is of limited usefulness in TCAD intoxication because of its delayed onset. The combination of hyperventilation and sodium bicarbonate has produced fatal alkalemia. Alkalinization increases the protein binding of the TCAD. Serum potassium levels should be monitored because a sudden increase in blood pH can aggravate or precipitate hypokalemia. Specific cardiovascular complications should be treated as follows: *Hypotension*—norepinephrine (Levophed), a predominantly alpha-adrenergic drug, is preferred over dopamine. (Hypertension that occurs early rarely requires treatment.) *Serious conduction defects* are best managed with phenytoin, and patients may need a temporary transvenous pacemaker. *Sinus tachycardia* usually does not require treatment except for alkalinization. *Supraventricular tachycardia* with hemodynamic instability requires synchronized cardioversion, 0.25 to 1.0 watt-second per kg, after sedation. *Ventricular tachycardia*—after alkalinization and phenytoin, intravenous lidocaine (for one dose only) may be required for persistent ventricular tachycardia. Synchronized cardioversion may be needed if lidocaine fails. *Ventricular fibrillation* should be treated with direct current countershock. *Torsades de pointes* is treated with magnesium sulfate IV 20%, 2 grams over 2 to 3 minutes, followed by a continuous infusion of 5 to 10 mg per minute of isoproterenol, lidocaine, phenytoin, and bretylium and atrial or ventricular overdrive pacing to shorten the QT interval. *Laboratory aids:* Arterial blood gases with blood pH, ECG, serum electrolytes, blood urea nitrogen and creatinine, serum phenytoin level, urine output, and, in severe cases, central venous pressure, PAWP, or both should be monitored.

Turpentine. See Hydrocarbons.

Xylene. See Hydrocarbons.

Section 18

Appendices and Index

REFERENCE INTERVALS FOR THE INTERPRETATION OF LABORATORY TESTS

method of
WILLIAM Z. BORER, M.D.
Thomas Jefferson University Hospital
Philadelphia, Pennsylvania

Most of the tests performed in a clinical laboratory are quantitative in nature. That is, the amount of a substance present in blood or serum is measured and reported in terms of concentration, activity (e.g., enzyme activity), or counts (e.g., blood cell counts). The laboratory must provide reference values to assist the clinician in the interpretation of laboratory results. These reference ranges comprise the physiologic quantities of substance (concentrations, activities, or counts) that are to be expected in healthy individuals. Deviation above or below the reference range may be associated with a disease process, and the severity of the disease process may be associated with the magnitude of the deviation. Unfortunately, there is rarely a sharp demarcation between physiologic and pathologic values, and the transition between these two is often gradual as the disease process progresses.

The terms normal and abnormal have been used to describe the laboratory values that fall inside or outside of the reference range, respectively. Use of these terms is now discouraged because it is virtually impossible to define normality and because "normal" may be confused with the statistical term Gaussian. Reference ranges are established from statistical studies in groups of healthy volunteers. Although these study subjects must be free of disease, they may have lifestyles or habits that result in subtle variations in their laboratory values. Examples of these variables include diet, body mass, exercise, and geographic location. Age and gender may also affect reference values. When the data from a large cohort of healthy subjects fit a Gaussian distribution, the usual statistical approach is to define the reference limits as two standard deviations above and below the mean. By definition, the reference range excludes the highest and the lowest 2.5% of the population. Non-Gaussian distributions are handled by different statistical methods, but the result is similar in that the reference range is defined by the central 95% of the population. In other words, the odds are 1 in 20 that a healthy individual will have a laboratory result that falls outside the reference range. If 12 laboratory tests are performed, the odds increase to about 1 in 2 that at least one of the results will be outside the reference range. This means that all healthy individuals are likely to have a few laboratory results that are unexpected. The clinician must then integrate these data with other clinical information such as the history and physical examination to arrive at the appropriate clinical decision. The reference range for many tests (especially enzyme and immunochemical measurements) varies with the method used. It is important that each laboratory establish reference ranges appropriate for the methods that it employs.

SI UNITS

During the past decade a concerted effort has been made to introduce SI units (le Système International d'Unités). The rationale for conversion to SI units is sound. Laboratory data are scientifically more informative when the units are based on molar concentration rather than mass concentration. For example, the conversion of glucose to lactate and pyruvate or the binding of a drug to albumin is more easily understood in units of molar concentration. Another example is illustrated as follows:

Conventional Units
1.0 gram of hemoglobin
Combines with 1.37 mL of oxygen
Contains 3.4 mg of iron
Forms 34.9 mg of bilirubin

SI Units
4.0 mmol of hemoglobin
Combines with 4.0 mmol of oxygen
Contains 4.0 mmol of iron
Forms 4.0 mmol of bilirubin

Another advantage of SI units involves the standardization of nomenclature to facilitate global com-

TABLE 1. **Base SI Units**

Property	Base Unit	Symbol
Length	meter	m
Mass	kilogram	kg
Amount of substance	mole	mol
Time	second	s
Thermodynamic temperature	kelvin	K
Electric current	ampere	A
Luminous intensity	candela	cd
Catalytic amount	katal	kat

TABLE 2. **Derived SI Units and Non-SI Units Retained for Use with the SI**

Property	Unit	Symbol
Area	square meter	m^2
Volume	cubic meter	m^3
	liter	L
Mass concentration	kilogram/cubic meter	kg/m^3
	gram/liter	gL
Substance concentration	mole/cubic meter	mol/m^3
	mole/liter	mol/L
Temperature	degree Celsius	°C = K − 273.15

munication of medical and scientific information. The units, symbols, and prefixes employed in the International System are shown in Tables 1, 2, and 3.

Unfortunately, problems have arisen with the implementation of SI units in the United States. Their introduction in 1987 prompted many medical journals to report laboratory values in both SI and conventional units in anticipation of complete conversion to SI units in the early 1990s. The lack of a coordinated effort toward this goal has forced a retrenchment on the issue. Physicians continue to think and practice using laboratory results expressed in conventional units, and few if any American hospitals or clinical laboratories use SI units exclusively. It is not likely that complete conversion to SI units will occur in the foreseeable future, yet most medical journals will probably continue to publish both set of units. For this reason, the tables of reference ranges in this appendix are given in both conventional units and SI units.

TABLE 3. **Standard Prefixes**

Prefix	Multiplication Factor	Symbol
yocto	10^{-24}	y
zepto	10^{-21}	z
atto	10^{-18}	a
femto	10^{-15}	f
pico	10^{-12}	p
nano	10^{-9}	n
micro	10^{-6}	μ
milli	10^{-3}	m
centi	10^{-2}	c
deci	10^{-1}	d
deca	10^{1}	da
hecto	10^{2}	h
kilo	10^{3}	k
mega	10^{6}	M
giga	10^{9}	G
tera	10^{12}	T

REFERENCES

AMA Drug Evaluations, Annual. Chicago, American Medical Association, 1994.

Bick RL (ed): Hematology—Clinical and Laboratory Practice. St. Louis, Mosby–Year Book, 1993.

Borer WZ: Selection and use of laboratory tests. *In* Tietz NW, Conn RB, and Pruden EL (eds): Applied Laboratory Medicine. Philadelphia, WB Saunders Co, 1992, pp 1–5.

Campion EW: A retreat from SI units. N Engl J Med *327*:49, 1992.

Friedman RB, and Young DS: Effects of Disease on Clinical Laboratory Tests, 2nd ed. Washington, DC, AACC Press, 1989.

Henry JB: Clinical Diagnosis and Management by Laboratory Methods, 18th ed. Philadelphia, WB Saunders Co, 1991.

Hicks JM, and Young DS: DORA '92–'93: Directory of Rare Analysis. Washington, DC, AACC Press, 1992.

Jacobs DS, Kasten BL, Demott WR, and Wolfson DC: Laboratory Test Handbook, 2nd ed. Baltimore, Williams & Wilkins Co, 1990.

Kaplan LA, and Pesce AJ: Clinical Chemistry—Theory, Analysis, and Correlation, 2nd ed. St. Louis, CV Mosby, 1989.

Kjeldsberg CR, and Knight JA: Body Fluids–Laboratory Examination of Amniotic, Cerebrospinal, Seminal, Serous and Synovial Fluids, 3rd ed. Chicago, ASCP Press, 1993.

Laposata M: SI Unit Conversion Guide. Boston, New England Journal of Medicine Books, 1992.

Scully RE, McNeely WF, Mark EJ, and McNeely BU: Normal reference laboratory values. N Engl J Med *327*:718–724, 1992.

Speicher CE: The Right Test—A Physician's Guide to Laboratory Medicine, 2nd ed. Philadelphia, WB Saunders Co, 1993.

Tietz NW (ed): Clinical Guide to Laboratory Tests, 2nd ed. Philadelphia, WB Saunders Co, 1990.

Wallach J: Interpretation of Diagnostic Tests—A Synopsis of Laboratory Medicine, 5th ed. Boston, Little, Brown and Co, 1992.

Young DS: Implementation of SI units for clinical laboratory data. Ann Intern Med *106*:114–129, 1987.

Young DS: Determination and validation of reference intervals. Arch Pathol Lab Med *116*:704–709, 1992.

Young DS: Effects of Drugs on Clinical Laboratory Tests, 3rd ed. Washington, DC, AACC Press, 1990.

TABLES OF REFERENCE VALUES

Some of the values included in the tables have been established by the Clinical Laboratories at Thomas Jefferson University Hospital, Philadelphia, PA, and have not been published elsewhere. Other values have been compiled from the sources just cited. These tables are provided for information and educational purposes only. They are intended to complement data derived from other sources including the medical history and physical examination. Users must exercise individual judgment in using the information provided in this appendix.

Reference Values for Hematology

	Conventional Units	SI Units
Acid hemolysis (Ham test)	No hemolysis	No hemolysis
Alkaline phosphatase, leukocyte	Total score 14–100	Total score 14–100
Cell counts		
Erythrocytes		
Males	4.6–6.2 million/mm^3	4.6–6.2 × 10^{12}/L
Females	4.2–5.4 million/mm^3	4.2–5.4 × 10^{12}/L
Children (varies with age)	4.5–5.1 million/mm^3	4.5–5.1 × 10^{12}/L
Leukocytes, total	4500–11,000/mm^3	4.5–11.0 × 10^9/L
Leukocytes, differential*		
Myelocytes	0%	O/L
Band neutrophils	3–5%	150–400 × 10^6/L
Segmented neutrophils	54–62%	3000–5800 × 10^6/L
Lymphocytes	25–33%	1500–3000 × 10^6/L
Monocytes	3–7%	300–500 × 10^6/L
Eosinophils	1–3%	50–250 × 10^6/L
Basophils	0–1%	15–50 × 10^6/L
Platelets	150,000–350,000/mm^3	150–350 × 10^9/L
Reticulocytes	25,000–75,000/mm^3 (0.5–1.5% of erythrocytes)	25–75 × 10^9/L
Coagulation tests		
Bleeding time (template)	2.75–8.0 min	2.75–8.0 min
Coagulation time (glass tube)	5–15 min	5–15 min
D-dimer	<0.5 μg/mL	<0.5 mg/L
Factor VIII and other coagulation factors	50–150% of normal	0.5–1.5 of normal
Fibrin split products (Thrombo-Welco test)	<10 μg/mL	<10 mg/L
Fibrinogen	200–400 mg/dL	2.0–4.0 g/L
Partial thromboplastin time (PTT)	20–35 s	20–35 s
Prothrombin time (PT)	12.0–14.0 s	12.0–14.0 s
Coombs' test		
Direct	Negative	Negative
Indirect	Negative	Negative
Corpuscular values of erythrocytes		
Mean corpuscular hemoglobin (MCH)	26–34 pg/cell	26–34 pg/cell
Mean corpuscular volume (MCV)	80–96 μm^3	80–96 fL
Mean corpuscular hemoglobin concentration (MCHC)	32–36 g/dL	320–360 g/L
Haptoglobin	20–165 mg/dL	0.20–1.65 g/L
Hematocrit		
Males	40–54 ml/dL	0.40–0.54
Females	37–47 ml/dL	0.37–0.47
Newborn	49–54 ml/dL	0.49–0.54
Children (varies with age)	35–49 ml/dL	0.35–0.49
Hemoglobin		
Males	13.0–18.0 g/dL	8.1–11.2 mmol/L
Females	12.0–16.0 g/dL	7.4–9.9 mmol/L
Newborn	16.5–19.5 g/dL	10.2–12.1 mmol/L
Children (varies with age)	11.2–16.5 g/dL	7.0–10.2 mmol/L
Hemoglobin, fetal	<1.0% of total	<0.01 of total
Hemoglobin A_{1C}	3–5% of total	0.03–0.05 of total
Hemoglobin A_2	1.5–3.0% of total	0.015–0.03 of total
Hemoglobin, plasma	0.0–5.0 mg/dL	0–3.2 μmol/L
Methemoglobin	30–130 mg/dL	19–80 μmol/L
Sedimentation rate (ESR)		
Wintrobe		
Males	0–5 mm/h	0–5 mm/h
Females	0–15 mm/h	0–15 mm/h
Westergren		
Males	0–15 mm/h	0–15 mm/h
Females	0–20 mm/h	0–20 mm/h

*Conventional units are percentages; SI units are absolute counts.

Reference Values* for Clinical Chemistry (Blood, Serum, and Plasma)

	Conventional Units	SI Units
Acetoacetate plus acetone		
Qualitative	Negative	Negative
Quantitative	0.3–2.0 mg/dL	30–200 μmol/L
Acid phosphatase, serum (thymolphthalein monophosphate substrate)	0.1–0.6 U/L	0.1–0.6 U/L
ACTH (see Corticotropin)		
Alanine aminotransferase (ALT, SGPT), serum	1–45 U/L	1–45 U/L
Albumin, serum	3.3–5.2 g/dL	33–52 g/L
Aldolase, serum	0.0–7.0 U/L	0.0–7.0 U/L
Aldosterone, plasma		
Standing	5–30 ng/dL	140–830 pmol/L
Recumbent	3–10 ng/dL	80–275 pmol/L
Alkaline phosphatase (ALP), serum		
Adult	35–150 U/L	35–150 U/L
Adolescent	100–500 U/L	100–500 U/L
Child	100–350 U/L	100–350 U/L
Ammonia nitrogen, plasma	10–50 μmol/L	10–50 μmol/L
Amylase, serum	25–125 U/L	25–125 U/L
Anion gap, serum, calculated	8–16 mEq/L	8–16 mmol/L
Ascorbic acid, blood	0.4–1.5 mg/dL	23–85 μmol/L
Aspartate aminotransferase (AST, SGOT) serum	1–36 U/L	1–36 U/L
Base excess, arterial blood, calculated	0 ± 2 mEq/L	0 ± 2 mmol/L
Bicarbonate		
Venous plasma	23–29 mEq/L	23–29 mmol/L
Arterial blood	21–27 mEq/L	21–27 mmol/L
Bile acids, serum	0.3–3.0 mg/dL	0.8–7.6 μmol/L
Bilirubin, serum		
Conjugated	0.1–0.4 mg/dL	1.7–6.8 μmol/L
Total	0.3–1.1 mg/dL	5.1–19 μmol/L
Calcium, serum	8.4–10.6 mg/dL	2.10–2.65 mmol/L
Calcium, ionized, serum	4.25–5.25 mg/dL	1.05–1.30 mmol/L
Carbon dioxide, total, serum or plasma	24–31 mEq/L	24–31 mmol/L
Carbon dioxide tension (PCO_2), blood	35–45 mmHg	35–45 mmHg
Beta-carotene, serum	60–260 μg/dL	1.1–8.6 μmol/L
Ceruloplasmin, serum	23–44 mg/dL	230–440 mg/L
Chloride, serum or plasma	96–106 mEq/L	96–106 mmol/L
Cholesterol, serum or EDTA plasma		
Desirable range	<200 mg/dL	<5.20 mmol/L
Low-density lipoprotein cholesterol	60–180 mg/dL	1.55–4.65 mmol/L
High-density lipoprotein cholesterol	30–80 mg/dL	0.80–2.05 mmol/L
Copper	70–140 μg/dL	11–22 μmol/L
Corticotropin (ACTH), plasma, 8 A.M.	10–80 pg/mL	2–18 pmol/L
Cortisol, plasma		
8:00 A.M.	6–23 μg/dL	170–630 nmol/L
4:00 P.M.	3–15 μg/dL	80–410 nmol/L
10:00 P.M.	<50% of 8:00 A.M. value	<50% of 8:00 A.M. value
Creatine, serum		
Males	0.2–0.5 mg/dL	15–40 μmol/L
Females	0.3–0.9 mg/dL	25–70 μmol/L
Creatine kinase (CK, CPK), serum		
Males	55–170 U/L	55–170 U/L
Females	30–135 U/L	30–135 U/L
Creatine kinase MB isoenzyme, serum	<5% of total CK activity <5.0 ng/mL by immunoassay	
Creatinine, serum	0.6–1.2 mg/dL	50–110 μmol/L
Ferritin, serum	20–200 ng/mL	20–200 μg/L
Fibrinogen, plasma	200–400 mg/dL	2.0–4.0 g/L
Folate		
Serum	2.0–9.0 ng/mL	4.5–20.4 nmol/L
Erythrocytes	170–700 ng/mL	385–1590 nmol/L
Follicle-stimulating hormone (FSH), plasma		
Males	4–25 mU/mL	4–25 U/L
Females, premenopausal	4–30 mU/mL	4–30 U/L
Females, postmenopausal	40–250 mU/mL	40–250 U/L
Gamma-glutamyltransferase (GGT), serum	5–40 U/L	5–40 U/L
Gastrin, fasting, serum	0–110 pg/mL	0–110 mg/L
Glucose, fasting, plasma or serum	70–115 mg/dL	3.9–6.4 nmol/L
Growth hormone (hGH), plasma, adult, fasting	0–6 ng/mL	0–6 μg/L
Haptoglobin, serum	20–165 mg/dL	0.20–1.65 g/L
Immunoglobulins, serum (see Immunologic Procedures)		
Insulin, fasting, plasma	5–25 μU/mL	36–179 pmol/L
Iron, serum	75–175 μg/dL	13–31 μmol/L

Reference Values* for Clinical Chemistry (Blood, Serum, and Plasma) *Continued*

	Conventional Units	SI Units
Iron-binding capacity, serum		
Total	250–410 μg/dL	45–73 μmol/L
Saturation	20–55%	0.20–0.55
Lactate		
Venous blood	5.0–20.0 mg/dL	0.6–2.2 mmol/L
Arterial blood	5.0–15.0 mg/dL	0.6–1.7 mmol/L
Lactate dehydrogenase (LD, LDH), serum	110–220 U/L	110–220 U/L
Lipase, serum	10–140 U/L	10–140 U/L
Lutropin (LH), serum		
Males	1–9 IU/L	1–9 U/L
Females		
Follicular phase	2–10 IU/L	2–10 U/L
Midcycle	15–65 U/L	15–65 U/L
Luteal phase	1–12 U/L	1–12 U/L
Postmenopausal	12–65 U/L	12–65 U/L
Magnesium, serum	1.3–2.1 mg/dL	0.65–1.05 mmol/L
Osmolality	275–295 mOsm/kg water	275–295 mOsm/kg water
Oxygen, blood, arterial, room air		
Partial pressure (PaO_2)	80–100 mmHg	80–100 mmHg
Saturation (SaO_2)	95–98%	95–98%
pH, arterial blood	7.35–7.45	7.35–7.45
Phosphate, inorganic, serum		
Adult	3.0–4.5 mg/dL	1.0–1.5 mmol/L
Child	4.0–7.0 mg/dL	1.3–2.3 mmol/L
Potassium		
Serum	3.5–5.0 mEq/L	3.5–5.0 mmol/L
Plasma	3.5–4.5 mEq/L	3.5–4.5 mmol/L
Progesterone, serum, adult		
Males	0.0–0.4 ng/mL	0.0–1.3 mmol/L
Females		
Follicular phase	0.1–1.5 ng/mL	0.3–4.8 mmol/L
Luteal phase	2.5–28.0 ng/mL	8.0–89.0 mmol/L
Prolactin, serum		
Males	1.0–15.0 ng/mL	1.0–15.0 μg/L
Females	1.0–20.0 ng/mL	1.0–20.0 μg/L
Protein, serum, electrophoresis		
Total	6.0–8.0 g/dL	60–80 g/L
Albumin	3.5–5.5 g/dL	35–55 g/L
Globulins		
$Alpha_1$	0.2–0.4 g/dL	2–4 g/L
$Alpha_2$	0.5–0.9 g/dL	5–9 g/L
Beta	0.6–1.1 g/dL	6–11 g/L
Gamma	0.7–1.7 g/dL	7–17 g/L
Pyruvate, blood	0.3–0.9 mg/dL	0.03–0.10 mmol/L
Rheumatoid factor	0.0–30 IU/mL	0.0–30 kIU/L
Sodium, serum or plasma	135–145 mEq/L	135–145 mmol/L
Testosterone, plasma		
Males, adult	300–1200 ng/dL	10.4–41.6 nmol/L
Females, adult	20–75 ng/dL	0.7–2.6 nmol/L
Pregnant females	40–200 ng/dL	1.4–6.9 nmol/L
Thyroglobulin	3–42 ng/mL	3–42 μg/L
Thyrotropin (hTSH), serum	0.4–4.8 μIU/mL	0.4–4.8 mIU/L
Thyrotropin-releasing hormone (TRH)	5–60 pg/mL	5–60 ng/L
Thyroxine (FT_4), free, serum	0.9–2.1 ng/dL	12–27 pmol/L
Thyroxine (T_4), serum	4.5–12.0 μg/dL	58–154 nmol/L
Thyroxine-binding globulin (TBG)	15.0–34.0 μg/mL	15.0–34.0 mg/L
Transferrin	250–430 mg/dL	250–430 g/L
Triglycerides, serum, 12-h fast	40–150 mg/dL	0.4–15.0 g/L
Triiodothyronine (T_3), serum	70–190 ng/dL	1.1–2.9 nmol/L
Triiodothyronine uptake, resin (T_3RU)	25–38%	0.25–0.38
Urate		
Males	2.5–8.0 mg/dL	150–480 μmol/L
Females	2.2–7.0 mg/dL	130–420 μmol/L
Urea, serum or plasma	24–49 mg/dL	4.0–8.2 nmol/L
Urea nitrogen, serum or plasma	11–23 mg/dL	8.0–16.4 nmol/L
Viscosity, serum	1.4–1.8 × water	1.4–1.8 × water
Vitamin A, serum	20–80 μg/dL	0.70–2.80 μmol/L
Vitamin B_{12}, serum	180–900 pg/mL	133–664 pmol/L

*Reference values may vary depending upon the method and sample source used.

Reference Values for Therapeutic Drug Monitoring (Serum)

	Therapeutic Range	Toxic Concentrations	Proprietary Names
Analgesics			
Acetaminophen	10–20 μg/mL	>250 μg/mL	Tylenol Datril
Salicylate	100–250 μg/mL	>300 μg/mL	Aspirin Ascriptin Bufferin
Antibiotics			
Amikacin	25–30 μg/mL	Peak >35 μg/mL Trough >10 μg/mL	Amikin
Chloramphenicol	10–20 μg/L	>25 μg/mL	Chloromycetin
Gentamicin	5–10 μg/mL	Peak >10 μg/mL Trough >2 μg/mL	Garamycin
Tobramycin	5–10 μg/mL	Peak >10 μg/mL Trough >2 μg/mL	Nebcin
Vancomycin	5–10 μg/mL	Peak >40 μg/mL Trough >10 μg/mL	Vancocin
Anticonvulsants			
Carbamazepine	5–12 μg/mL	>15 μg/mL	Tegretol
Ethosuxamide	40–100 μg/mL	>150 μg/mL	Zarontin
Phenobarbital	15–40 μg/mL	40–100 ng/mL (varies widely)	
Phenytoin	10–20 μg/mL	>20 μg/mL	Dilantin
Primidone	5–12 μg/mL	>15 μg/mL	Mysoline
Valproic acid	50–100 μg/mL	>100 μg/mL	Depakene
Antineoplastics and Immunosuppressives			
Cyclosporine	50–400 mg/mL	>400 ng/mL	Sandimmune
Methotrexate (high dose, 48 h)	Variable	>1 μmol/L 48 h after dose	Mexate Folex
Bronchodilators and Respiratory Stimulants			
Caffeine	3–15 ng/mL	>30 ng/mL	
Theophylline (Aminophylline)	10–20 μg/mL	>20 μg/mL	Accurbron Elixophyllin Quibron Theobid
Cardiovascular Drugs			
Amiodarone*	1.0–2.0 μg/mL	>2.0 μg/mL	Cordarone
Digitoxin†	15–25 ng/mL	>35 ng/mL	Crystodigin
Digoxin‡	0.8–2.0 ng/mL	>2.4 ng/mL	Lanoxin
Disopyramide	2–5 μg/mL	>7 μg/mL	Norpace
Flecainide	0.2–1.0 ng/mL	>1 ng/mL	Tambocor
Lidocaine	1.5–5.0 μg/mL	>6 μg/mL	Xylocaine
Mexiletine	0.7–2.0 ng/mL	>2 ng/mL	Mexitil
Procainamide	4–10 μg/mL	>12 μg/mL	Pronestyl
Procainamide plus NAPA	8–30 μg/mL	>30 μg/mL	
Propranolol	50–100 ng/mL	Variable	Inderal
Quinidine	2–5 μg/mL	>6 μg/mL	Cardioquin Quinaglute
Tocainide	4–10 ng/mL	>10 ng/mL	Tonocard
Psychopharmacologic Drugs			
Amitriptyline	120–150 ng/mL	>500 ng/mL	Amitril Elavil Triavil
Bupropion	25–100 ng/mL	Not applicable	Wellbutrin
Desipramine	150–300 ng/mL	>500 ng/mL	Norpramin Pertofrane
Imipramine	125–250 ng/mL	>400 ng/mL	Tofranil
Lithium§	0.6–1.5 mEq/L	>1.5 mEq/L	Lithobid
Nortriptyline	50–150 mg/mL	>500 ng/mL	Aventyl Pamelor

*Specimen must be obtained more than 8 hours after last dose.
†Specimen must be obtained 12–24 hours after last dose.
‡Specimen must be obtained more than 6 hours after last dose.
§Specimen must be obtained 12 hours after last dose.

Reference Values for Clinical Chemistry (Urine)*

	Conventional Units	SI Units
Acetone and acetoacetate, qualitative	Negative	Negative
Albumin		
Qualitative	Negative	Negative
Quantitative	10–100 mg/24 h	0.15–1.5 μmol/d
Aldosterone	3–20 μg/24 h	8.3–55 nmol/d
δ-Aminolevulinic acid (δ-ALA)	1.3–7.0 mg/24 h	10–53 μmol/d
Amylase	<17 U/h	<17 U/h
Amylase/creatinine clearance ratio	0.01–0.04	0.01–0.04
Bilirubin, qualitative	Negative	Negative
Calcium (regular diet)	<250 mg/24 h	<6.3 nmol/d
Catecholamines		
Epinephrine	<10 μg/24 h	<55 nmol/d
Norepinephrine	<100 μg/24 h	<590 nmol/d
Total free catecholamines	4–126 μg/24 h	24–745 nmol/d
Total metanephrines	0.1–1.6 mg/24 h	0.5–8.1 μmol/d
Chloride (varies with intake)	110–250 mEq/24 h	110–250 mmol/d
Copper	0–50 μg/24 h	0–0.80 μmol/d
Cortisol, free	10–100 μg/24 h	27.6–276 nmol/d
Creatine		
Males	0–40 mg/24 h	0–0.30 mmol/d
Females	0–80 mg/24 h	0–0.60 mmol/d
Creatinine	15–25 mg/kg/24 h	0.13–0.22 mmol/kg/d
Creatinine clearance (endogenous)		
Males	110–150 mL/min/1.73 m^2	110–150 mL/min/1.73 m^2
Females	105–132 mL/min/1.73 m^2	105–132 mL/min/1.73 m^2
Cystine or cysteine	Negative	Negative
Dehydroepiandrosterone		
Males	0.2–2.0 mg/24 h	0.7–6.9 μmol/d
Females	0.2–1.8 mg/24 h	0.7–6.2 μmol/d
Estrogens, total		
Males	4–25 μg/24 h	14–90 nmol/d
Females	5–100 μg/24 h	18–360 nmol/d
Glucose (as reducing substance)	<250 mg/24 h	<250 mg/d
Hemoglobin and myoglobin, qualitative	Negative	Negative
Homogentisic acid, qualitative	Negative	Negative
17-Ketogenic steroids		
Males	5–23 mg/24 h	17–80 μmol/d
Females	3–15 mg/24 h	10–52 μmol/d
17-Hydroxycorticosteroids		
Males	3–9 mg/24 h	8.3–25 μmol/d
Females	2–8 mg/24 h	5.5–22 μmol/d
5-Hydroxyindoleacetic acid		
Qualitative	Negative	Negative
Quantitative	2–6 mg/24 h	10–31 μmol/d
17-Ketosteroids		
Males	8–22 mg/24 h	28–76 μmol/d
Females	6–15 mg/24 h	21–52 μmol/d
Magnesium	6–10 mEq/24 h	3–5 mmol/d
Metanephrines	0.05–1.2 ng/mg creatinine	0.03–0.70 mmol/mmol creatinine
Osmolality	38–1400 mOsm/kg water	38–1400 mOsm/kg water
pH	4.6–8.0	4.6–8.0
Phenylpyruvic acid, qualitative	Negative	Negative
Phosphate	0.4–1.3 g/24 h	13–42 mmol/d
Porphobilinogen		
Qualitative	Negative	Negative
Quantitative	<2 mg/24 h	<9 μmol/d
Porphyrins		
Coproporphyrin	50–250 μg/24 h	77–380 nmol/d
Uroporphyrin	10–30 μg/24 h	12–36 nmol/d
Potassium	25–125 mEq/24 h	25–125 mmol/d
Pregnanediol		
Males	0–1.9 mg/24 h	0–6.0 μmol/d
Females		
Proliferative phase	0–2.6 mg/24 h	0–8.0 μmol/d
Luteal phase	2.6–10.6 mg/24 h	8–33 μmol/d
Postmenopausal	0.2–1.0 mg/24 h	0.6–3.1 μmol/d
Pregnenetriol	0–2.5 mg/24 h	0–7.4 μmol/d
Protein, total		
Qualitative	Negative	Negative
Quantitative	10–150 mg/24 h	10–150 mg/d
Protein/creatinine ratio	<0.2	<0.2
Sodium (regular diet)	60–260 mEq/24 h	60–260 mmol/d
Specific gravity		
Random specimen	1.003–1.030	1.003–1.030
24-Hour collection	1.015–1.025	1.015–1.025
Urate (regular diet)	250–750 mg/24 h	1.5–4.4 mmol/d
Urobilinogen	0.5–4.0 mg/24 h	0.6–6.8 μmol/d
Vanillylmandelic acid (VMA)	1–8 mg/24 h	5–40 μmol/d

*May vary depending on the method used.

Reference Values for Toxic Substances

	Conventional Units	SI Units
Arsenic, urine	<130 μg/24 h	<1.7 μmol/d
Bromides, serum, inorganic	<100 mg/dL	<10 mmol/L
Toxic symptoms	140–1000 mg/dL	14–100 mmol/L
Carboxyhemoglobin, blood		
Urban environment	<5% (% saturation)	<0.05 (saturation)
Smokers	<12% (% saturation)	<0.12 (saturation)
Symptoms		
Headache	>15% (% saturation)	>0.15 (saturation)
Nausea and vomiting	>25% (% saturation)	>0.25 (saturation)
Potentially lethal	>50% (% saturation)	>0.50 (saturation)
Ethanol, blood	<0.05 mg/dL	<1.0 mmol/L
	<0.005%	
Intoxication	>100 mg/dL	>22 mmol/L
	>0.1%	
Marked intoxication	300–400 mg/dL	65–87 mmol/L
	0.3–0.4%	
Alcoholic stupor	400–500 mg/dL	87–109 mmol/L
	0.4–0.5%	
Coma	>500 mg/dL	>109 mmol/L
	>0.5%	
Lead, blood		
Adults	<25 μg/dL	<1.2 μmol/L
Children	<15 μg/dL	<0.7 μmol/L
Lead, urine	<80 μg/24 h	<0.4 μmol/L
Mercury, urine	<30 μg/24 h	<150 nmol/d

Reference Values for Cerebrospinal Fluid

	Conventional Units	SI Units
Cells	<5 mm^3; all mononuclear	<5 × 10^6/L, all mononuclear
Electrophoresis	Albumin predominant	Albumin predominant
Glucose	50–75 mg/dL (20 mg/dL less than in serum)	2.8–4.2 mmol/L (1.1 mmol less than in serum)
IgG		
Children under 14	<8% of total protein	<0.08 of total protein
Adults	<14% of total protein	<0.14% of total protein
IgG index $\left(\frac{\text{CSF/serum IgG ratio}}{\text{CSF/serum albumin ratio}}\right)$	0.3–0.6	0.3–0.6
Oligoclonal banding on electrophoresis	Absent	Absent
Pressure	70–180 mmH_2O	70–180 mmH_2O
Protein, total	15–45 mg/dL	150–450 mg/L

Reference Values for Immunologic Procedures

		Conventional Units	SI Units
Complement, serum			
C3		85–175 mg/dL	0.85–1.75 g/L
C4		15–45 mg/dL	150–450 mg/L
Total hemolytic (CH_{50})		150–250 U/mL	150–250 U/mL
Immunoglobulins, serum, adult			
IgG		640–1350 mg/dL	6.4–13.5 g/L
IgA		70–310 mg/dL	0.70–3.1 g/L
IgM		90–350 mg/dL	0.90–3.5 g/L
IgD		0–6.0 mg/dL	0–60 mg/L
IgE		0–430 ng/dL	0–430 μg/L
Lymphocyte subsets, whole blood, heparinized			
Antigen	*Cell Type*	*Percentage*	*Absolute*
CD3	Total T cells	56–77%	860–1880
CD19	Total B cells	7–17%	140–370
Cd3 and CD4	Helper-inducer cells	32–54%	550–1190
CD3 and CD8	Suppressor-cytotoxic cells	24–37%	430–1060
CD3 and DR	Activated T cells	5–14%	70–310
CD2	E rosette T cells	73–87%	1040–2160
CD16 and CD56	Natural killer (NK) cells	8–22%	130–500

Helper/suppressor ratio: 0.8–1.8

Reference Values for Tests of Gastrointestinal Function

	Conventional Units
Bentiromide test	6-h urinary arylamine excretion greater than 57% excludes pancreatic insufficiency
Carotene, serum	60–250 ng/dL
D-Xylose absorption test	5-h urinary excretion >20% of ingested dose
Fecal fat estimation	
Qualitative	No fat globules seen by high-power microscope
Quantitative	<6 g/24 h (>95% coefficient of fat absorption)
Gastric acid output	
Basal	
Males	0–10.5 mmol/h
Females	0–5.6 mmol/h
Maximum (after histamine or pentagastrin)	
Males	9–48 mmol/h
Females	6–31 mmol/h
Ratio: basal-maximum	
Males	0–0.31
Females	0–0.29
Secretin test, pancreatic fluid	
Volume	>1.8 mL/kg/h
Bicarbonate	>80 mEq/L

Reference Values for Semen Analysis

	Conventional Units	SI Units
Volume	2–5 mL	2–5 mL
Liquefaction	Complete in 15 min	Complete in 15 min
pH	7.2–8.0	7.2–8.0
Leukocytes	Occasional or absent	Occasional or absent
Spermatozoa		
Count	60–150 × 10^6/mL	60–150 × 10^6/mL
Motility	>80% motile	>0.80 motile
Morphology	80–90% normal forms	0.80–0.90 normal forms
Fructose	>150 mg/dL	>8.33 mmol/L

DRUGS APPROVED IN 1993

prepared by
MARGARET A. NOYES
University of Houston
Houston, Texas

Generic Name	Trade Name and (Manufacturer)	Dosage Form	FDA Rating	Approved Use
Aprotinin	Trasylol (Miles)	1.4 mg/mL injection 100- and 200-mL vials	1, P, V	Prevents blood loss during heart surgery
Calcipotriene	Dovonex (Westwood-Squibb)	0.005% ointment	1, S	Psoriasis
Cisapride	Propulsid (Janssen)	10-mg tablets	1, S	Nighttime heartburn
Cladribine	Leustatin (Ortho Biotech)	1-mg/mL injection, 10 mL vials	1, P, V	Hairy cell leukemia
Dornase alfa (DNase)	Pulmozyme (Genentech)	1 mg/mL inhalation solution 2.5-mL ampules	Biological	Cystic fibrosis
Enoxaparin	Lovenox (Rhone-Poulenc Rorer)	30-mg/0.3-mL injection, prefilled syringes	1, P	Anticoagulant
Felbamate	Felbatol (Wallace Labs)	400- and 600-mg tablets, 600 mg/5 mL suspension	1, P, V	Epilepsy
Fenofibrate	Lipidil (Fournier Research)	100-mg capsules	1, S	Lowering serum triglycerides
Fluvastatin sodium	Lescol (Sandoz)	20- and 40-mg capsules	1, S	Lowering serum cholesterol
Gabapentin	Neurontin (Parke-Davis)	100-, 300-, 400-mg capsules	1, P	Epilepsy
Gadodiamide	Omniscan injection (Sanofi Winthrop)	287 mg/mL injection 10 and 20 mL vials	1, S	Diagnostic imaging agent
Granisetron HCl	Kytril (SmithKline Beecham)	1 mg/mL injection, 1-mL vials	1, S	Prevents nausea and vomiting during cancer chemotherapy
Interferon beta-1b	Betaseron (Berlex)	0.3-mg/vial powder for injection reconstitutes to 0.25 mg/mL	Biological	Multiple sclerosis
Levocabastine HCl	Livostin (Iolab)	0.05% oph. suspension 2.5-, 5-, and 10-ml dropper bottles	1, P	Allergic conjunctivitis
Levomethadyl acetate	ORLAAM (BioDevelopment)	10 mg/mL solution 474 mL containers	1, P, V	Opiate addiction
Lodoxamide tromethamine	Alomide (Alcon Labs)	0.1% oph. solution 10-mL Drop-Tainers	1, S, V	Eye disorders
Loratadine	Claritin (Schering)	10-mg tablets	1, S	Allergic rhinitis
Perflubron	Imagent GI (Alliance)	Oral liquid, 200-mL containers	1, P	Diagnostic bowel imaging agent
Perindopril erbumine	Aceon (Ortho Pharm.)	2-, 4-, and 8-mg tablets	1, S	Hypertension
Piperacillin/Tazobactam	Zosyn (Lederle)	Injection, 2, 3, and 4-gm piperacillin/vial	1, 4, S	Antibiotic
Rimantadine HCl	Flumadine (Forest Labs)	100-mg tablets 50 mg/5 mL syrup	1, P	Preventing influenza
Risperidone	Risperdal (Janssen)	1-, 2-, 3-, and 4-mg tablets	1, P	Psychotic disorders
Strontium-89 chloride	Metastron (Medi-Physics/Amersham)	10.9 to 22.6 mg/mL injection, 10-mL vials	1, P	Analgesic (skeletal metastases)
Tacrine HCl	Cognex (Parke-Davis)	10-, 20-, 30-, and 40-mg capsules	1, P	Alzheimer's disease
Torsemide	Demadex (Boehringer Mannheim)	5-, 10-, 20-, and 100-mg tablets 10 mg/mL injection	1, S	Edema
Trimetrexate glucuronate	NeuTrexin (US Bioscience)	Powder for injection, 25-mg/5-mL vial	1, P, AA, V, E	PCP in AIDS patients
Venlafaxine HCl	Effexor (Wyeth-Ayerst)	25-, 37.5-, 50-, 75-, and 100-mg tablets	1, S	Depression

Abbreviations: AIDS = acquired immune deficiency syndrome; HIV = human immunodeficiency virus; PCP = pneumocystis carinii pneumonia.
Ratings: 1 New molecular entity.
4 New combination of ingredients.
P Therapeutic advance (no other effective agent or more effective than standard therapy).
S Therapeutic qualities are similar to drugs on the market.
V Orphan drug.
E Treatment for a severely disabling or life-threatening illness.
AA Indicated for AIDS or HIV-related disease.

NOMOGRAM FOR THE DETERMINATION OF BODY SURFACE AREA OF CHILDREN AND ADULTS

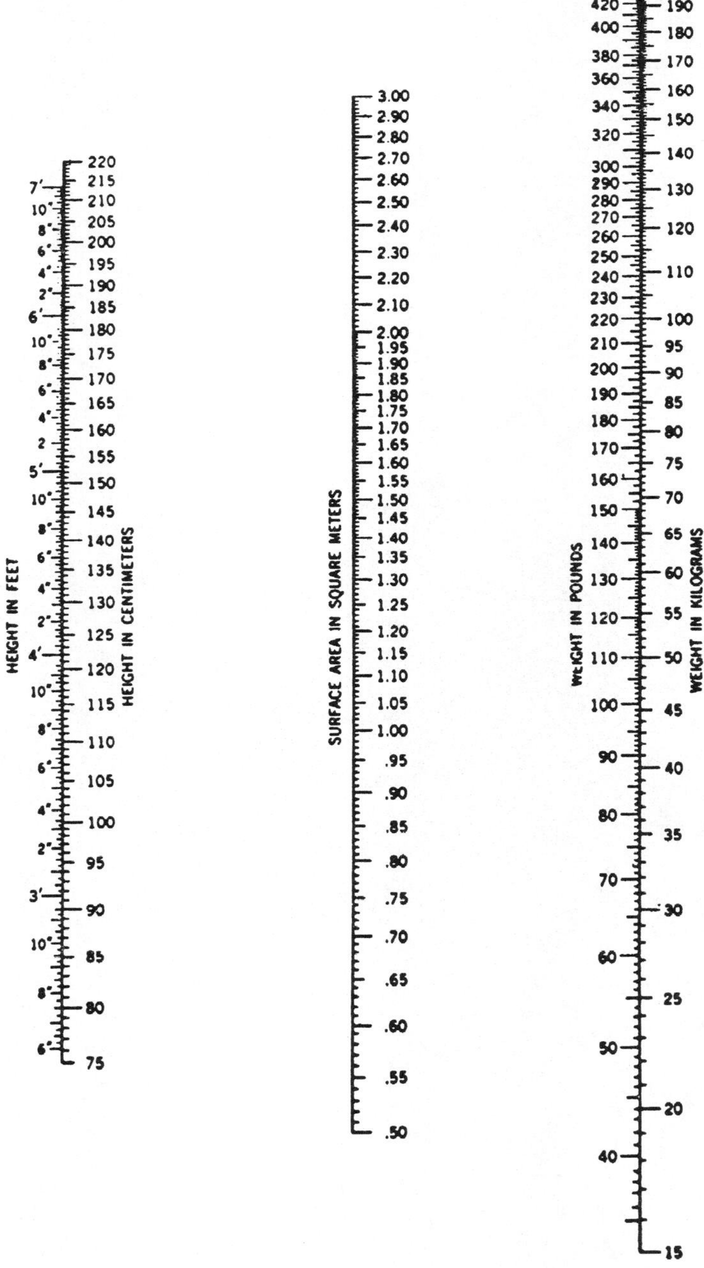

From Boothby WM, Sandiford RB: Boston Med Surg J *185*:337, 1921.

Index

Note: Page numbers followed by (t) refer to tables; page numbers in *italics* refer to illustrations.

ABCD mnemonic, in recognition of malignant skin lesions, 732, 735
Abdomen, defects in wall of, in preterm infant, 976–977
pain in. See *Abdominal pain.*
sensation of distention of, 8
Abdominal aorta, aneurysm of, 213, 295
occlusive disease of, 216–217
Abdominal irradiation, for Hodgkin's disease, 356, *356*
Abdominal pain, cholecystitis and, 403, 404
diabetic ketoacidosis and, 500
irritable bowel syndrome and, 436(t), 437(t)
pancreatitis and, 459, 465
pelvic inflammatory disease and, 1013
sickle cell disease and, 323
Abdominal wall, defects of, in preterm infant, 976–977
Abetalipoproteinemia, 456
Abruptio placentae, 942, 943
Abscess, amebic, 55
treatment of, 15(t), 54(t), 54–55
anorectal, 439–440
fistulizing Crohn's disease and, 434
Bartholin's gland, 1022
brain, 788–790, 789(t), 790(t)
breast, 982
liver, amebic, 55
treatment of, 15(t), 54(t), 54–55
lung, 171–172
orbital, 204
pancreatic, 461, 463
subperiosteal, 204
Absence seizures, 823
treatment of, 808, 810, 810(t), 811(t), 816–818, 823
Absorption, disorders of. See *Malabsorption.*
Abstinence method, of contraception, 1035
Abstinence syndrome. See *Withdrawal (abstinence syndrome).*
ABVD chemotherapy regimen, for Hodgkin's disease, 351, 351(t), 352, 352(t)
Acalculous cholecystitis, 404
Accelerated phase, of chronic myelogenous leukemia, 371
Accidental hypothermia, 1073–1074
Acebutolol, 219(t), 1124(t)
for angina pectoris, 219(t)
for hypertension, 270(t)
Acetaminophen, for fever, 20–21
for headache, 834
for influenza, 189
for laryngitis, 28(t), 29
for migraine, 834
for pain, in relapsing fever, 116
for painful renal calculi, 662
for postpartum pain, 953
for sore throat, due to common cold, 188
Acetaminophen *(Continued)*
poisoning by, 1100
nomogram for, *1101*
therapeutic vs. toxic levels of, 1138(t)
use of, in patient receiving amphotericin B, 165, 169
in patient receiving streptokinase, 1028
Acetazolamide, for glaucoma, 867(t)
Acetic acid–hydrocortisone, for otitis externa, 106(t)
Acetohexamide, for diabetes mellitus, 491(t)
Acetylcysteine, as antidote, 1090(t)
for cough, 25
Acetylsalicylic acid. See *Aspirin.*
Achalasia, 419–420
Acid injury, 1069, 1107
Acidosis, diabetic, 499–502, 500(t)
hypothermia and, 1074
neonatal, bicarbonate for, 961–962
poisoning and, 1099
renal dysfunction and, 638, 647, 663
sepsis and, 60
Acne, 703–705
industrial agents causing, 783, 784
Acne keloidalis, 738
Acquired aortic diseases, 213–217
Acquired hemochromatosis, 346, 346(t), 347, 1113–1115
chelation therapy for, 316, 347, 1093(t)
toxic iron ingestion and, 1113–1115
transfusion and, 316, 401
Acquired immunodeficiency syndrome (AIDS), 42–52
antibodies to Epstein-Barr virus in, 52
aspergillosis in, 49
AZT (azidothymidine, zidovudine) for, 43–44, 45(t)
bacterial infections in, 45–47, 46(t)
barriers to transmission of, condoms as, 1031
blastomycosis in, 170
brain lesions in, 50, 52, 132–133, 790, 790(t)
candidiasis in, 48
CDC criteria for, 43(t)
chancroid in, 666
coccidioidomycosis in, 49
cryptococcosis in, 48
cryptosporidiosis in, 51, 483
cytomegalovirus infection in, 51–52
diarrhea in, 12
dideoxycytidine for, 44, 44(t), 45(t)
dideoxyinosine for, 44, 44(t), 45(t)
encephalopathy in, 52
enteropathy in, 458
esophagitis in, 48, 52
fungal infections in, 46(t), 48–50, 168, 170
herpes simplex virus infection in, 52
histoplasmosis in, 49, 168
Acquired immunodeficiency syndrome (AIDS) *(Continued)*
isosporiasis in, 51, 483
Kaposi's sarcoma in, 656–657
malabsorption in, 458
microsporidiosis in, 51, 483
molluscum contagiosum in, 52
mycobacterial infections in, 45–47, 207, 208, 211, 291
neuropathy in, 886–887
opportunistic infections in, 45–52, 46(t)
and bacteremia, 58(t)
oral lesions in, 52, 756, 757
papovavirus infections in, 52
pericarditis in, 291
Pneumocystis carinii pneumonia in, 49–50, 50(t)
pneumonia in, 47, 48, 49, 50(t), 52, 184
pox virus infections in, 52
progressive multifocal leukoencephalopathy in, 52
protozoan infections in, 46(t), 50–51, 483
risk factors for transmission of, 42(t)
salmonellosis in, 47
sulfonamide use in, and allergic drug reaction, 698
syphilis in, 47, 674
thrombocytopenia in, 341
toxoplasmosis in, 50–51, 132–133, 790
transfusion-transmitted, 334, 401
tuberculosis in, 45–46, 46(t), 207, 208
vaccination in, 128
varicella-zoster virus infection in, 52
viral infections (non-HIV) in, 46(t), 51–52
zidovudine (azidothymidine, AZT) for, 43–44, 45(t)
Acquired myasthenia gravis, 856–862
treatment of, 857(t)–860(t), 857–862
Acquired nevi, 729–731
Acquired polyneuropathies, in children, 888
Acral lentiginous melanoma, 732
Acromegaly, 548–550
Acromioclavicular separation, 930
Actinic lesions. See *Sun exposure.*
Activated charcoal, for poisoning, 1043, 1044, 1088
Activated factor VII, 338
Activated prothrombin complex concentrates, 397, 397(t)
for hemophiliac patient with factor VIII inhibitors, 338
Active hepatitis, chronic, 444
Active rewarming, of hypothermic patient, 1075
Acupuncture, for pain, 4
Acyanotic congenital heart disease, 243
Acyclovir, for herpes simplex virus infection, 741, 751, 844
in immunocompromised patient, 52
in patient with erythema multiforme, 765

Acyclovir *(Continued)*
for Kaposi's varicelliform eruption, 764
for sporadic encephalitis, 844, 845(t)
for varicella-zoster virus infection, 67, 68, 69, 742
in immunocompromised patient, 52, 69, 190, 369, 386
Addiction, fear of, 1
types of. See under *Drug abuse.*
vs. drug tolerance, 1
Addison's disease, 550
Adenocarcinoma. See also *Carcinoma.*
of endometrium, 1015–1018
of esophagus, 421
of kidney, 649–651
of uterus, 1015–1018
Adenoidectomy, in management of otitis media, 174
Adenoma(s), of adrenal gland. See *Adrenal tumors.*
of colon, 476
of pituitary gland, and acromegaly, 548–550
and amenorrhea, 997
and Cushing's disease, 554, 555, 556, 557
and hyperprolactinemia, 575–577
of salivary gland, 754
Adenosine, for supraventricular tachycardia, 238, 239(t)
in children, 244, 244(t)
Adolescent(s), asthma in, 678–682
diabetes mellitus in, 493–499
epilepsy in, 806–819
Adrenal cancer, 648–649
Adrenal crisis, 553
Adrenalectomy, for aldosteronism, 571
for cancer, 649
for Cushing's disease or syndrome, 555, 556
for pheochromocytoma, 591
Adrenal insufficiency, 550(t), 550–554, *552*
hypopituitarism and, 572, 573
Adrenalitis, due to cytomegalovirus infection, in AIDS, 51
Adrenal resection. See *Adrenalectomy.*
Adrenal tumors, 648–649
and aldosteronism, 570, 571, 571(t), 572
and Cushing's syndrome, 554, 556
and excess catecholamine production, 588–592, 649
Adrenergic agonists, for glaucoma, 867(t), 867–868
Adrenocortical insufficiency, 550(t), 550–554, *552*
hypopituitarism and, 572, 573
Adrenocorticotropic hormone (ACTH), for gout, 504
for infantile spasms, 822
for postinfectious encephalitis, 845, 845(t)
for ulcerative colitis, 429(t), 431
Adrenocorticotropic hormone–secreting tumors, 554, 555, 556, 557
Adrenocorticotropic hormone stimulation test, for adrenal insufficiency, 551
Adrenoleukodystrophy, 888
Adult respiratory distress syndrome, 147, 148, 149
Advanced life support, in management of cardiac arrest, 224–226
Aerobic gram-negative bacillary pneumonia, 179(t), 183
Aerophagia, 8–9
Aerophobia, 111
Affective display, lability of, in multiple sclerosis, 855
African-Americans, sickle cell syndromes affecting, 318(t). See also *Sickle cell disease.*
African trypanosomiasis, 747
Age, gestational, 964–965
morbidity in relation to, *967*
Agenesis, müllerian, 996
Aging, of skin, due to sun exposure, 785
Agitated rabies, 111
Agitation, in Alzheimer's disease, 793
Agoraphobia, 1064
Agranulocytosis, clozapine therapy and, 1064
AIDS. See *Acquired immunodeficiency syndrome (AIDS).*
Air swallowing, 8–9
Airway(s), establishment of, in neonatal resuscitation, 959
foreign body impaction in, 182
obstruction of, and hoarseness, 25
as complication of obstetric anesthesia, 953
due to lymphoid tissue swelling, in mononucleosis, 104
due to poisoning, 1086
opening of, in management of cardiac arrest, 224(t)
warming of, to raise temperature of hypothermic patient, 1075
Airway device, for patient with status epilepticus, 818
Akathisia, levodopa usage and, 874–875
use of neuroleptics and, 1063
ALA-dehydratase deficiency, 389, 390(t)
Albendazole, for enterobiasis, 484
for helminthiasis, 481(t), 482(t), 483, 484, 485, 486
for larva migrans, 748
for microsporidiosis, 15(t), 483
for trichinosis, 134
Albumin, 396–397
for hemolytic disease of newborn, 333
Albuterol, for asthma, 681(t)
in pediatric patient, 685(t)
for chronic obstructive pulmonary disease, 154
Alcohol, as antidote, 1094(t)
poisoning by, 1100–1102
Alcohol consumption, 1037
and gastritis, 442
and hepatitis, 406
and hypertension, 267
and neuropathy, 884
and pancreatitis, 460, 461, 464
and sleep disturbances, 33
and thrombocytopenia, 341
excessive, 1037–1040
Alcohol dependence syndrome, 1037, 1040
Alcoholic patient, 1037–1040
Alcoholics Anonymous, 1040
Alcohol-related problems, 1037–1040, 1038(t)
screening test for, *1039*
Alcohol Use Disorders Identification Test (AUDIT), *1039*
Alcohol withdrawal, management of, 1040
Aldosteronism, 569–572, 570(t), 571(t)
Alimentary tract. See *Gastrointestinal tract.*
Aliphatic halogenated hydrocarbons, poisoning by, 1112, 1113(t)
Alkali injury, 1069, 1107
Alkalosis, hypothermia and, 1074
Allergen(s), avoidance of, by asthmatic patient, 684
by patient with hypersensitivity pneumonitis, 202
by patient with rhinitis, 692–693
food, and atopic dermatitis, 763
and pruritus ani, 776
inhaled, alveolitis in reaction to, 201–202, 202(t)
asthma in reaction to. See *Asthma.*
hoarseness caused by, 29
rhinitis in reaction to, 203, 691–695
occupational, 679(t)
photosensitizing, 786(t)
effects of exposure to, 786
Allergic alveolitis (hypersensitivity pneumonitis), 201–202, 202(t)
Allergic conjunctivitis, 65, 66(t)
Allergic contact dermatitis, 772, 773
Allergic fungal sinusitis, 203
Allergic reaction(s), 675–702. See also *Asthma.*
to crotalid antivenin, 1082
to drugs, 695(t), 695–700, 696(t), 698(t)
to inhaled antigens, 29, 201, 202, 202(t), 203, 691–695. See also *Asthma.*
to insect stings, 700–702
to penicillin, 676, 697–698
and management of patient at risk for endocarditis, 119(t), 263(t)
and management of patient with endocarditis, 261
and management of patient with syphilis, 673(t)
to photosensitizing agents, 786
to radiocontrast media, 700
prevention of, 677(t), 700
to transfusion, 399–400
Allergic rhinitis, 203, 691–695
cough management in, 24
treatment of, 692–695, 693(t), 694(t)
Alloimmunization, in transfusion recipient, 400
Allopurinol, for hyperuricemia or hyperuricosuria, 505, 664
in polycythemia, 389
for leishmaniasis, 86
for tumor lysis syndrome, 368
Allylamines, for dermatophytosis, 722–723, 749, 750
Aloe vera, for burns, 1072
Alopecia, 706–709, 706(t)–709(t)
Alopecia areata, 708
nail lesions associated with, 723–724
Alpha-adrenergic blocking agents, for hypertension, 272(t), 273–274, 278
in patient with pheochromocytoma, 588–589, 591(t)
for prostatic hyperplasia, 632
Alpha$_1$-antitrypsin deficiency, and chronic obstructive pulmonary disease, 153
Alpha-fetoprotein, measurement of serum levels of, 935
Alpha granule deficiency, 339
Alpha heavy chain disease, 456
Alpha-methyl-L-tyrosine, for hypertension due to pheochromocytoma, 590, 591(t)
Alphaprodine, 1119(t)
Alpha-thalassemia, 315, 315(t), 316, 317
Alprazolam, 1106(t)
for anxiety, in Alzheimer's disease, 793
for panic disorder, 1065
for tinnitus, 39
Alprenolol, 1124(t)
Alveolar process, lesions of, 757

Alveolar ventilation, ineffective, 148
Alveolitis, allergic (hypersensitivity pneumonitis), 201–202, 202(t)
Alzheimer's disease, 790–794, 792(t), 793(t)
Amalgam tattoo, 757
Amantadine, for influenza, 81–82, 174, 189, 190
in patient with COPD, 153
in patient with renal disease, 82(t)
for Parkinson's disease, 877
Ambulances, defibrillators in, 224
Amebiasis, 15(t), 53–55, 54(t), 480(t), 482–483
cutaneous, 748
Amenorrhea, 994–998, *995*, *997*
American College of Rheumatology criteria, for rheumatoid arthritis, 902(t)
Amikacin, for atypical mycobacterial infection, 211
for meningitis, 102(t)
for neutropenia and infection, 328
therapeutic vs. toxic levels of, 1138(t)
Amiloride, for diabetes insipidus, 561(t), 562
for hypertension, 270(t)
for hypokalemia, in aldosteronism, 571
Amino acids, in parenteral nutrition, 533–534, 534(t), 537
Aminocaproic acid, use of, in bleeding hemophiliac patient, 337
in patient with disseminated intravascular coagulation, 344
Aminoglutethimide, for Cushing's syndrome, 557(t), 558
Aminophylline. See *Theophylline*.
Aminosalicylates, for Crohn's disease, 433, 435
for ulcerative colitis, 428–430, 429(t)
Amiodarone, for arrhythmias, 238(t)
in mitral valve prolapse syndrome, 252
for atrial fibrillation, 228(t)
therapeutic vs. toxic levels of, 1138(t)
Amitriptyline, 1130(t)
for ankylosing spondylitis, 913
for cutaneous dysesthesia, 776
for depression, 1058(t)
in insomnia, 34
in multiple sclerosis, 855
for headache, 832, 835
for lability of affective display, in multiple sclerosis, 855
for migraine, 835
for muscle-contraction headache, 832
for neuropathic pain, 888
for post-herpetic neuralgia, 743
for sleep disturbance, in depression, 34
in muscle pain syndromes, 920
for tinnitus, 39
for urticaria, 778
therapeutic vs. toxic levels of, 1130(t), 1138(t)
Amlodipine, 1107(t)
for angina pectoris, 221(t)
for hypertension, 277(t)
Ammonia, elevated serum levels of, in Reye's syndrome, 847
Amniotic fluid, analysis of, 936, 936(t)
in evaluation of fetal hemolytic disease, 331, *331*
meconium staining of, 959, 970
Amobarbital, poisoning by, 1105(t)
Amorolfine, for onychomycosis, 722
Amoxapine, 1130(t)
adverse effects of, 1060(t)
for depression, 1060(t)
Amoxicillin, for acute exacerbations of chronic obstructive pulmonary disease, 23
for arthritis, in Lyme disease, 120(t)
for bacterial vaginosis, 1007
for bronchitis, 175(t)
in COPD, 23
for carditis, in Lyme disease, 120(t)
for chancroid, 666(t)
for chlamydial infection, in pregnant patient, 1012, 1012(t)
for endocarditis, 260(t)
for enteric fever, 139
for enterocolitis (gastroenteritis), in salmonellosis, 14(t), 138
for *Gardnerella vaginalis* infection, 1007
for *Helicobacter pylori* infection, 442, 471
for Lyme disease, 120(t), 121
for otitis externa, 106(t)
for otitis media, 173(t)
for pharyngitis, 206(t)
for salmonellosis, 14(t), 138, 139, 141(t)
for streptococcal pharyngitis, 206(t)
for typhoid fever, 141(t)
in carrier patient, 142
rash in reaction to, 697
Amoxicillin prophylaxis, for endocarditis, 119(t), 263(t)
Amphetamines, abuse of or poisoning by, 1041, 1102
Amphotericin B, adverse effects of, 165, 167, 169
for blastomycosis, 169–170
for candidiasis, 595(t)
in AIDS, 48
for coccidioidomycosis, 165
in AIDS, 49
for cryptococcosis, in AIDS, 48
for endocarditis, 260(t), 261
for histoplasmosis, 167, 168
in AIDS, 49, 168
for infection in neutropenic patient, 328, 362, 369
for leishmaniasis, 86, 747
for necrotizing infections, 80
medications for adverse effects of, 165, 167, 169
Ampicillin, for bacteremia or sepsis, 57(t)
in newborn, 970(t)
in patient with salmonellosis, 138
for cellulitis, 740
for endocarditis, 259, 260(t)
for enteric fever, 139
for enterocolitis (gastroenteritis), in patient with salmonellosis, 14(t), 138
for meningitis, 99, 100(t), 101, 101(t), 102(t)
for necrotizing infections, 79
for osteomyelitis, 928(t)
for pyelonephritis, in female patient, 622
for salmonellosis, 14(t), 138, 139, 141(t), 928(t)
in carrier patient, 140, 142
for sepsis or bacteremia, 57(t)
in newborn, 970(t)
in salmonellosis, 138
for shigellosis, 14(t)
for typhoid fever, 141(t)
in carrier patient, 142
for urinary tract infection, in female patient, 622
in male patient, 595(t)
rash in reaction to, 697
Ampicillin prophylaxis, for endocarditis, 119(t), 263(t)
Amrinone, for heart failure, 254
in children, 245, 245(t)
Amylase, elevated serum levels of, causes of, 459, 459(t)
Amyl nitrite, for cyanide poisoning, 1092(t)
Amyloid angiopathy, cerebral, 797
Amyotrophy, neuralgic, 880
Anaerobic osteomyelitis, treatment of, 928, 928(t)
Anagen effluvium, 708, 708(t)
Anagrelide, for polycythemia, 389
Anal canal, 438
hemorrhoids lining, 440–441
Anal fissure, 439
Anal fistula, 440
Analgesics, 1–3
adjuvant, 3
for back pain, 40
for breakthrough pain, 2
in sickle cell disease, 321
for burns, 1072
for labor pain, 948, 949
for low back pain, 40
for pancreatitis, 460, 467
for post-herpetic neuralgia, 743
for postpartum pain, 953
for renal calculi, 662
for sore throat, due to common cold, 188
narcotic. See *Narcotics*.
negative effect of, in patient with muscle-contraction headache, 831
non-narcotic, 1, 3. See also particular types, e.g., *Nonsteroidal anti-inflammatory drugs*.
vs. narcotic analgesics, 322(t)
postoperative use of, as aid to prevention of atelectasis, 152
problems with use of, in ulcerative colitis, 428
therapeutic vs. toxic levels of, 1138(t)
Anal pruritus, 775–776
Anaphylactic reaction, 675–678, 676(t), 677(t)
to drugs, 695, 696(t)
to insect stings, 701–702
to transfusion, 400
Anaphylactoid reaction, 675
to radiocontrast media, 700
prevention of, 677(t), 700
Anaplastic thyroid cancer, 586, 587
Ancrod, for thrombosis due to heparin-induced thrombocytopenia, 193, 340
Ancylostoma duodenale infestation, 481(t)
Androgen deprivation therapy, for prostatic cancer, 655–656
for prostatic hyperplasia, 632
Androgenetic alopecia, 706(t), 706–707
Anemia, aplastic, 299–302
bleeding associated with, 300
bone marrow transplantation for, 301, 311
cobalamin (vitamin B_{12}) deficiency and, 311, 312
colony-stimulating factors for, 301–302
Fanconi's, 299
folate deficiency and, 313
hemolytic, 305–311
autoimmune, 305(t), 305–308
fetal/neonatal, 329–334, 330(t)
gallstones associated with, 317
microangiopathic, *Escherichia coli* infection and, 11, 344
nonimmune, 308–311, 309(t)
sickle cell disease and, 324. See also *Sickle cell disease*.
thalassemia and, 316, 317

Anemia *(Continued)*
hyperhemolytic, sickle cell disease and, 324, 324(t). See also *Sickle cell disease.*
immunosuppressives for, 301, 308
iron deficiency, 302–305, 303(t)
lupus erythematosus and, 717
megaloblastic, 311(t), 311–314
multiple myeloma and, 386
neutropenia and infection in, 300, 301
pernicious, 311–314
renal failure and, 639, 647–648
sickle cell, 324(t), 324–325. See also *Sickle cell disease.*
splenectomy for, 307–308, 310
steroids for, 301, 307, 311
systemic lupus erythematosus and, 717
thalassemia and, 316, 317
transfusion for, 300–301, 307, 308, 310, 312
viral infection and, 299
vitamin B_{12} (cobalamin) deficiency and, 311, 312
Anesthesia, in surgery for pheochromocytoma, 591
in treatment of pain, 4
local, agents inducing, 700(t)
allergic reaction to, 699
seizures due to, 954
in surgical drainage of carbuncle, 738
obstetric, 948–955
Aneurysm, aortic, 213–215, 294–295
rupture of, 213, 295
aortic arch, 214
cerebral, hemorrhage due to, 797
femoral artery, 295
iliac artery, 295
left ventricular, myocardial infarction and, 283
popliteal artery, 295
Angel dust (phencyclidine), 1042
poisoning by, 1122
Angina pectoris, 217–222
drugs for, 218(t), 219(t), 219–221, 221(t), 1118(t)
surgery for, 222
Angioedema, 753, 778
drug reaction and, 276, 695–696, 700
Angiomyolipoma, of kidney, 652
Angiopathy, amyloid, cerebral, 797
Angioplasty, for occlusive disease of lower extremity arteries, 293
Angiostrongyliasis, 481(t), 484
Angiotensin-converting enzyme inhibitors, adverse effects of, 275–276
angioedema in reaction to, 276, 700
cough due to, 25, 275, 700
for heart failure, 255–256
in children, 245(t)
for hypertension, 274–276, 275(t), 278, 278(t)
in aldosteronism, 572
in renal failure, 646
in scleroderma-related renal failure, 718–719
for myocardial infarction, 281(t), 282, 284
Animal bites. See *Bite(s).*
Anisakiasis, 481(t), 484–485
Anisoylated plasminogen-streptokinase activator complex, for myocardial infarction, 281, 281(t)
Ankle sprains, 930
Ankylosing spondylitis, 911–914, 912(t), 913(t)
Ann Arbor staging, of Hodgkin's disease, 350(t), 355(t)
Anorectal lesions, 438–441
fistulizing Crohn's disease and, 434
Anorexia nervosa, 1048, 1049(t)
bulimic subtype of, 1049, 1050(t)
Antacids, for gastritis, 442(t)
for peptic ulcer, 470
use of, in burned patient, 1071
Antepartum care, 933–940. See also *Prenatal care.*
Antepartum hemorrhage, 941–944, 951
Anterior myocardial infarction, and heart block, 236. See also *Myocardial infarction.*
Anterior urethra, trauma to, 625, 626
Anthelmintics, 481(t)–482(t), 483–486
for trichinosis, 134
Anthralin, for psoriasis, 713
Anthralin-induced contact dermatitis, as stimulus to hair growth, 708
Antiandrogen therapy, for prostatic cancer, 655–656
for prostatic hyperplasia, 632
Antianxiety drugs, 1046, 1106(t)
poisoning by, 1104
Antiarrhythmics, 238(t)
for atrial fibrillation, 228, 228(t), 229, 240
for premature atrial complexes, 231
for supraventricular tachycardia, 238, 239(t)
in pediatric patient, 244(t)
for tachycardia, in patient with tetanus, 131
for ventricular dysrhythmias associated with mitral valve prolapse syndrome, 252
for ventricular fibrillation, 224(t), 225
for ventricular tachycardia, 241, 241(t)
in pediatric patient, 244(t)
pediatric dosages of, 244(t)
risks and benefits of use of, after surgery for congenital heart disease, 247
in heart failure, 256
therapeutic vs. toxic levels of, 1138(t)
Antibiotics. See *Antimicrobial(s)*; *Antimicrobial prophylaxis*; and specific agents, e.g., *Penicillin.*
Antibody (antibodies), cold- or warm-reactive, and hemolytic anemia, 305(t), 305–308
to Epstein-Barr virus, in AIDS patients, 52
to Rh antigens, 329–334
Anticholinergics, adverse effects of, 1054
delirium due to, 1054
drugs acting as, 1054(t)
for allergic rhinitis, 694
for asthma, in pediatric patient, 686
for chronic obstructive pulmonary disease, 153
for glaucoma, 868
for nausea and vomiting, 6, 6(t), 8
for side effects of neuroleptics, 826, 1062, 1063
for urinary incontinence, 606
in children, 604
poisoning by, 1102, 1103(t)
risks and benefits of use of, in ulcerative colitis, 428
Anticipatory emesis, 7–8
Anticoagulants. See also *Heparin* and *Warfarin.*
for stroke, 229, 800(t)
Anticoagulants *(Continued)*
for thromboembolism, 192, 193, 194, 195, 296, 1028–1029
in pregnant patient, 1030
hemorrhage risk with, factors potentiating, 194(t)
intracerebral, 796, 801
use of, prior to cardioversion for atrial fibrillation, 229
Anticonvulsants, 811(t), 1103(t)
poisoning by, 1102, 1103(t)
teratogenic effects of, 809
therapeutic vs. toxic levels of, 1103(t), 1138(t)
use of, in epilepsy, 807–823, 810(t), 811(t), 818(t), 1103(t)
in head trauma, 890, 894
in lupus erythematosus, 716
in mania, 1060(t)
in metastatic brain disease, 157, 158(t)
in pain, 3
in painful neuropathies, 888
in porphyria, 391
in post-herpetic neuralgia, 743
in preeclampsia, 946(t), 947
in Reye's syndrome, 847
in status epilepticus, 818(t), 819, 820
in stimulant abuse, 1042
in trigeminal neuralgia, 863
Antidepressants, 1058(t), 1058–1059, 1059(t), 1060(t), 1130(t)
adverse effects of, 1058, 1058(t), 1059(t), 1060(t)
atypical, 1058–1059, 1060(t). See also specific agents, e.g., *Trazodone.*
adverse effects of, 1060(t)
low-dose, for patient with possible cutaneous dysesthesia, 776
pediatric dosages of, 1130(t)
poisoning by, 1129–1131
therapeutic vs. toxic levels of, 1130(t), 1138(t)
use of, 1058–1059
in Alzheimer's disease, 793
in anxiety, 1046
in attention deficit hyperactivity disorder, 827
in bulimia nervosa, 1052
in insomnia, 34
in mood disorders, 1058–1059
in multiple sclerosis, 855
in pain, 3
in painful neuropathies, 888
in panic disorder, 1065
in post-herpetic neuralgia, 743
Antidiarrheals, 16
for AIDS enteropathy, 458
for food poisoning, 78
for salmonellosis, 137
for ulcerative colitis, 427–428
Antidiuretic hormone (vasopressin), for colonic diverticular bleeding, 425
for diabetes insipidus, 560, 561(t), 562, 574–575
for esophageal variceal bleeding, 414
for hemorrhagic portal hypertensive gastropathy, 443
Antidotes, for poisoning, 1088–1089, 1090(t)–1098(t)
Antiemetics/antinauseants, 5–8, 6(t), 7(t), 78, 116, 137, 289, 842, 874
Antifibrinolytic drugs, use of, in bleeding hemophiliac patient, 337
in patient with disseminated intravascular coagulation, 344

Antifreeze (ethylene glycol), poisoning by, 1110–1112
Antifungals. See specific agents, e.g., *Ketoconazole.*
Antigen(s), allergenic. See *Allergen(s).*
carcinoembryonic, 477
Rh, development of antibodies to, 329–334
Antihemophilic factor. See *Coagulation factor VIII concentrates* and *Cryoprecipitate.*
Antihistamines. See also specific agents, e.g., *Diphenhydramine.*
for allergic drug reaction, 696, 696(t), 697
for allergic rhinitis, 693, 693(t)
for anaphylactic reaction, 677, 677(t)
for cough associated with allergic rhinitis, 24
for nausea and vomiting, 6, 6(t), 8
for pain, in sickle cell disease, 321
for pemphigoid gestationis, 774
for pruritus, 37, 37(t)
in atopic dermatitis, 763
in contact dermatitis, 773, 782
in erythema multiforme, 764
for urticaria, 37, 696, 696(t), 777, 778
for vertigo, 838(t)
in Meniere's disease, 842
use of, in asthmatic patient, 686
Antimalarials, 93–98, 94(t), 97(t)
Antimicrobial(s). See also *Antimicrobial prophylaxis* and specific agents, e.g., *Penicillin.*
for acne, 704, 705, 784
for acute exacerbations of chronic obstructive pulmonary disease, 23, 154–155
for amebiasis, 15(t), 54, 54(t), 55, 480(t), 482–483
for arthritis, following venereal infection, 914
in Lyme disease, 120(t), 123
for aspiration pneumonia, 179(t), 183
for atypical mycobacterial infections, 211, 212
in AIDS, 47, 211
for atypical pneumonia, 179(t), 181, 182
for bacteremia or sepsis, 56–59, 57(t)
in newborn, 969, 970(t)
in patient with salmonellosis, 138
for bacterial endocarditis. See *Antimicrobial(s), for endocarditis.*
for bacterial meningitis, 99–101, 100(t), 101(t), 102(t), 120(t)
for bacterial overgrowth, in small intestine, 457
for bacterial pericarditis, 291
for bacterial peritonitis, in cirrhosis, 411
for bacterial pneumonia, 179(t), 180, 181, 182, 183, 186, 186(t), 187
in AIDS, 184
for bacterial prostatitis, 633
for bacterial sinusitis, 203
for bacterial vaginosis, 1007
for *Blastocystis hominis* infection, 483
for blastomycosis, 169, 170
for brain abscess, 789, 789(t)
for bronchitis, 174, 175, 175(t), 176, 176(t)
in patient with COPD, 23
for brucellosis, 62, 63
for bullous impetigo, 737
for bullous pemphigoid, 769
for *Campylobacter jejuni* infection, 14, 14(t)
for candidiasis, 595(t), 750, 751, 1007, 1007(t)
in AIDS, 48
Antimicrobial(s) *(Continued)*
for carbuncles, 738–739
for carditis, in Lyme disease, 120(t), 122
for cellulitis, 740
for chancroid, 666, 666(t)
for chlamydial infection, 66, 66(t), 109, 182, 668(t), 669, 669(t), 670, 671, 1012, 1012(t)
in pregnant patient, 1012, 1012(t)
for cholera, 13, 14(t), 71–72, 75
for *Clostridium difficile*–associated diarrhea, 14(t)
for coccidioidomycosis, 165
in AIDS, 49
for colonic diverticulitis, 425
for community-acquired pneumonia, 179(t), 180, 181, 182, 183
in AIDS, 184
for conjunctivitis, 66, 66(t)
in newborn, 64, 64(t)
for Crohn's disease, 433, 434
for cryptococcosis, in AIDS, 48
for cryptosporidiosis, 483
for cystitis, in female patient, 597, 600
in male patient, 595
for diarrhea, 13–16, 14(t), 15(t), 78
for *Dientamoeba fragilis* infection, 480(t), 483
for diphtheria, 73
for diverticulitis, 425
for endocarditis, 259, 260(t), 261
in brucellosis, 63
in Q fever, 110
in rat-bite fever, 114
for *Entamoeba histolytica* infection, 15(t), 54, 54(t), 55, 480(t), 482–483
for enteric fever, 139
for enterocolitis (gastroenteritis), in salmonellosis, 14(t), 16, 138
for epididymitis, 608–609
for fistulizing Crohn's disease, 434
for food poisoning, 78
for *Gardnerella vaginalis* infection, 1007
for gastroenteritis (enterocolitis), in salmonellosis, 14(t), 16, 138
for giardiasis, 15(t), 455, 480, 480(t), 482
for gingivitis, 757
for gonorrhea, 66, 66(t), 667(t), 667–669
in pediatric patient, 64, 64(t), 669
for gram-negative bacillary pneumonia, 179(t), 183
for granuloma inguinale, 671
for guttate psoriasis, 713
for *Haemophilus influenzae* infection, 180
for *Helicobacter pylori* infection, 442, 471
for histoplasmosis, 167, 168
in AIDS, 49
for hospital-acquired pneumonia, 186, 186(t), 187
for impetigo, 737
for intestinal infection, 13–16, 14(t), 15(t), 455, 480(t), 480–483
for isosporiasis, 455, 483
in AIDS, 51
for legionnaires' disease, 191
for leishmaniasis, 86
for leprosy, 87, 88, 89
for lung abscess, 172
for Lyme disease, 120(t), 121, 122, 123, 887
for lymphogranuloma venereum, 671
for malaria, 94(t), 95, 97(t), 98
for meningitis, 99–101, 100(t), 101(t), 102(t), 165
in Lyme disease, 120(t)
Antimicrobial(s) *(Continued)*
for *Moraxella catarrhalis* infection, 180
for mycobacterial infections, 87, 88, 89, 207, 208, 208(t), 211, 212
in AIDS, 46, 47, 208, 211
for mycoplasmal pneumonia, 181, 190
for necrotizing enterocolitis, 975
for necrotizing infections, 79
for neonatal sepsis, 969, 970(t)
for neurobrucellosis, 63
for neurosyphilis, 672, 673(t)
for neutropenia and infection, 328
in patient with leukemia, 362, 368–369
for nonbullous impetigo, 737
for nongonococcal urethritis, 608, 669(t), 669–670
for nosocomial pneumonia, 186, 186(t), 187
for oil-induced acne, 784
for ophthalmia neonatorum, 64, 64(t)
for osteomyelitis, 927–929, 928(t)
for otitis externa, 105, 106(t), 107, 1085
for otitis media, 173, 173(t)
for pelvic inflammatory disease, 668(t), 1013, 1014, 1014(t)
for pericarditis, 291
for peritonitis, in cirrhosis, 411
for pertussis, 144–145
for pharyngitis, 205, 206, 206(t)
for plague, 107–108
for pneumococcal pneumonia, 180
for *Pneumocystis carinii* pneumonia, in AIDS, 49–50, 50(t)
for pneumonia, 179(t), 180, 181, 182, 183, 186, 186(t), 187, 190
in AIDS, 49–50, 50(t), 184
for pressure ulcer, 761
for prostatitis, 633
for protozoan infection, in AIDS, 50, 51
of intestine, 15(t), 455, 480(t), 480–483
for psittacosis, 109
for psoriasis, 713
for pyelonephritis, 622
in female patient, 598, 599, 600, 622
in male patient, 595, 621, 621(t)
for Q fever, 110
for rat-bite fever, 114
for reactive arthritis, 914
for relapsing fever, 116, 116(t)
Jarisch-Herxheimer reaction to, 116
for rheumatic fever, 118
for rickettsioses, 110, 124, 143, 143(t)
for Rocky Mountain spotted fever, 124
for salmonellosis, 14(t), 16, 137–141, 141(t), 928(t)
in carrier patient, 140, 142
for sepsis or bacteremia, 56–59, 57(t)
in newborn, 969, 970(t)
in patient with salmonellosis, 138
for shigellosis, 13, 14(t)
for sinusitis, 203
for spontaneous bacterial peritonitis, 411
for syphilis, 672, 673, 673(t)
Jarisch-Herxheimer reaction to, 672
for tetanus, 129
for toxic shock syndrome, 1010
for toxoplasmosis, 131, 132, 132(t), 133
in AIDS, 50, 133
for traveler's diarrhea, 13, 14(t), 78
for trichomoniasis, 1008
for tropical sprue, 454
for tuberculosis, 207, 208, 208(t)
in AIDS, 46, 208
for tularemia, 136
for typhoid fever, 140–141, 141(t)

Antimicrobial(s) *(Continued)*
in carrier patient, 142
for typhus fevers, 143, 143(t)
for urethritis, 608, 669(t), 669–670
for urinary tract infection, in female patient, 597, 598, 599, 600, 622
in male patient, 595, 595(t), 621, 621(t)
for vaginitis, 1007, 1007(t), 1008
for vibrio infections, 13, 14(t), 71–72, 75, 1083
for Whipple's disease, 455
for whooping cough, 144–145
for *Yersinia enterocolitica* infection, 16
Jarisch-Herxheimer reaction to, 116, 672
nephrotoxicity of, 644
pediatric dosages of, for bacterial meningitis, 102(t)
for intestinal protozoal infection, 480(t)
for neonatal sepsis, 970(t)
for osteomyelitis, 928(t)
for relapsing fever, 116(t)
for typhoid fever, 141(t)
for urinary tract infection, 595(t)
pros and cons of use of, in ulcerative colitis, 430
reaction to, allergic, 697–699. See also *Penicillin allergy.*
role of, in *Clostridium difficile*–associated diarrhea, 12, 13
therapeutic vs. toxic levels of, 1138(t)
Antimicrobial prophylaxis, for bronchitis, 176
for cystitis, 597, 621
for endocarditis, 263, 263(t)
in child with heart disease, 247
in patient with mitral valve prolapse, 251
in patient with rheumatic heart disease, 119, 119(t)
indications for, 262(t)
for *Pneumocystis carinii* pneumonia, in AIDS patient, 50(t)
for recurrent rheumatic fever, 118(t), 118–119
for streptococcal infection, 118(t), 118–119
for toxoplasmosis, 133
for urinary tract infection, 597
in leukemic patient, 362
in neutropenic patient, 362
Antimonials, for leishmaniasis, 84–86, 747
Antinauseants/antiemetics, 5–8, 6(t), 7(t), 78, 116, 137, 289, 842, 874
Anti-oxidants, in management of diabetes mellitus, 498
Antiplatelet drugs, as cause of bleeding, 340
Antipsychotic drugs. See *Neuroleptic(s).*
Antipyretics, 20–21
Antiretroviral medications, adverse effects of, 44
for acquired immunodeficiency syndrome, 43–45, 44(t), 45(t)
Antithrombin III concentrates, 397, 397(t)
Antithymocyte globulin, for aplastic anemia, 301
Antithyroid drugs, 581, 582, 583
Antitoxin, botulism, 1091(t)
diphtheria, 72, 73, 73(t)
desensitization to, 72–73, 73(t)
tetanus, 129
Antitussives, 23(t)
for common cold, 188
Antivenin, black widow spider, 1090(t)
coral snake, 1082, 1090(t)
pit viper, 1081, 1082, 1090(t)
Anxiety, 1046–1047, 1064
Anxiety *(Continued)*
Alzheimer's disease and, 792–793
drugs for, 1046, 1106(t)
poisoning by, 1104
Aorta, acquired diseases of, 213–217
aneurysm of, 213–215, 294–295
rupture of, 213, 295
Aortic arch, aneurysm of, 214
Aortitis, 217
Aortobifemoral graft, 216, 217, 293
Aortoiliac occlusive disease, 216–217, 292, 293
APAP. See *Acetaminophen.*
Apgar score, 963, 964(t)
Aphthous ulcers, 752–753
Aplastic anemia, 299–302
Aplastic crisis, due to parvovirus B19 infection, 401
in thalassemia, 317
Apnea, during sleep, 34
in preterm infant, 975–976
Apomorphine, for poisoning, 78, 1087
Apoplexy, pituitary, 549
Apraclonidine, for glaucoma, 867(t), 868
Areflexic bladder, 605–606
Arginine vasopressin. See *Antidiuretic hormone (vasopressin).*
Aromatic hydrocarbons, poisoning by, 1112
Arrhythmia(s), 237
development of, after heart surgery, 247
during cardiac rehabilitation, 287, 288
drugs for. See *Antiarrhythmics.*
electrical shock and, 1069
hypothermia and, 1073
iron overload and, 346
myocardial infarction and, 283
narcotic abuse and, 1043
pheochromocytoma and, 589, 591
poisoning and, 1099
renal failure and, 639
solvent abuse and, 1045
stimulant abuse and, 1042
ventricular, 237, 240(t), 240–241. See also *Ventricular tachycardia.*
evaluation of, in cardiac rehabilitation patient, 287, 288
heart failure and, 256
neonatal, 244
mitral valve prolapse and, 252
nonsustained, 232, 240–241
sustained, 241
Arsenic, cancers and keratoses caused by, 734
poisoning by, 882, 1102–1104, 1104(t)
Arsine gas, poisoning by, 1103
Artemisinin derivatives, for malaria, 96
Arterial disease, peripheral, 292–295
reduced claudication in, due to exercise, 288
Arteriovenous hemodialysis, continuous, for renal failure, 640, 640(t)
Arteriovenous malformation, cerebral, and hemorrhage, 797
Arteritis, giant cell (temporal), 830, 922–923
Takayasu's, 217
Arthralgia. See also *Arthritis.*
rubella and, 125
sodium stibogluconate–induced, 86
Arthritis, degenerative, 922, 922(t)
gouty, 503, 504
lupus erythematosus and, 715–716
Lyme disease and, 120(t), 123
rat-bite fever and, 114
reactive, 914
rheumatic fever and, 117, 118, 118(t)
Arthritis *(Continued)*
rheumatoid, 901–907, 902(t)
juvenile, 907–911, 908(t), 909(t)
treatment of, 901–911, 902(t), 904(t), 908(t), 909(t)
sites of, in ankylosing spondylitis, 912
Streptobacillus moniliformis infection and, 114
TMJ involvement in, 911, 918–919
Arthropathy. See also *Arthritis.*
hereditary hemochromatosis and, 346
5-ASA (mesalamine), for Crohn's disease, 433, 435
for ulcerative colitis, 428–429, 429(t)
Ascariasis, 481(t), 483, 484, 486
Ascending aorta, aneurysm of, 214
dissection of, 215, 216
Ascending urinary tract infection, and pyelonephritis, 621
Ascites, cirrhotic, 409–411, 410(t)
pancreatitis and, 463
Ascorbic acid. See *Vitamin C (ascorbic acid).*
Aseptic meningitis, 99, 843
Asparaginase, for leukemia, 366, 367
Aspergillosis, in AIDS, 49
Aspiration, 182
gastric acid, 182
as complication of obstetric anesthesia, 953, 954
meconium, reduction of risk of, 959–960, 970–971
pneumonia due to, 179(t), 182–183
as complication of obstetric anesthesia, 953–954
prevention of, in management of dysphagia, 418, 419
Aspiration syndrome, 182
Aspirin, adverse effects of, 21, 340, 442, 699
for arthritis, 901–903, 902(t)
in rheumatic fever, 118(t)
for carditis, in rheumatic fever, 118, 118(t)
for fever, in pericarditis, 289
for membranous glomerulopathy, 615
for myocardial infarction, 281, 281(t), 284
for pain, 1
for rheumatic carditis, 118, 118(t)
for rheumatoid arthritis, 901–903, 902(t)
for sore throat, due to common cold, 188
for stroke, 229, 799, 800(t)
for thrombotic thrombocytopenic purpura, 345
gastric inflammation or ulceration due to, 442
poisoning by, 1126(t)
thrombocytopenia induced by, 340
use of, in patient with mitral valve prolapse, 251
in patient with polycythemia, 389
to improve outcome of pregnancy, 934
Assist-control mode, of mechanical ventilation, 150
Astemizole, adverse effects of, 1102
for allergic rhinitis, 693(t)
for pruritus, 37, 37(t)
for urticaria, 696(t), 778
Asthma, 148, 678–691, 680(t), 684(t)
classification of, 680, 680(t), 683, 684(t)
cough management in, 24
drug effects and, 679
exercise-induced, 679, 691
in adults and adolescents, 678–682
in children, 682–691
occupational, allergens causing, 679(t)
treatment of, 149, 680–691, 681(t), 684(t), 685(t), 686(t), *687*, *689*, *690*

Asthma *(Continued)*
viral respiratory tract infections and, 679
Astrocytoma, 830, 897
Asymptomatic bacteriuria, in female patient, 598–599, 601, 621
in male patient, 596
Asystole, cardiac arrest due to, 222, 223, 225
treatment of, 224(t), 225
Ataxia, cerebellar, varicella and, 68
Atelectasis, 151(t), 151–152
Atenolol, 219(t), 1124(t)
for angina pectoris, 219(t)
for arrhythmias, in children, 244(t)
for hypertension, 270(t), 278(t)
in pregnant patient, 938(t)
for migraine, 835
for myocardial infarction, 282(t)
Atheroembolism, lower extremity arterial occlusion due to, 294
Atherosclerosis, 213
coronary artery. See *Coronary artery disease.*
lower extremity arterial occlusion due to, 292, 293
renal artery, 644–645
Atony, uterine, 956
Atopic dermatitis (eczema), 762–764
Atovaquone, adverse effects of, 132(t)
for *Pneumocystis carinii* pneumonia, in AIDS, 50(t)
for toxoplasmosis, 131, 132(t)
Atracurium, use of, in management of tetanus, 129, 130
Atrial complexes, premature, 230–231
Atrial fibrillation, 227(t), 227–230, 228(t), 238(t), 240
myocardial infarction and, 283
stroke risk associated with, 229, 801, 801(t)
Atrial flutter, 238(t), 239–240
Atrial septal defect, timing of surgery for, 247, 248
Atrioventricular block (heart block), 233–236, 234(t)
cardiac arrest due to, 227
infectious endocarditis and, 261
Lyme disease and, 122
myocardial infarction and, 236, 284
Atrioventricular junction, radiofrequency ablation of, 229
Atrioventricular nodal re-entrant tachycardia, 239(t)
Atrioventricular reciprocating tachycardia, 239(t)
Atrophic gastritis, 443
Atrophic vaginitis, 1004, 1008
Atropine, as antidote, 1091(t)
for asthma, in pediatric patient, 686
for cardiac arrest, 224(t)
for heart block, 234, 235
in patient with myocardial infarction, 284
for mushroom poisoning, 77
poisoning by, 1103(t)
pretreatment with, for patient receiving edrophonium or neostigmine, 858
Attapulgite, for diarrhea, 16
Attention deficit hyperactivity disorder, in Tourette syndrome, 824, 827
Attention-focusing, problems with, in multiple sclerosis, 855
Atypical antidepressants, 1058–1059, 1060(t). See also specific agents, e.g., *Trazodone.*
adverse effects of, 1060(t)
Atypical antipsychotic drugs, 1064
Atypical hyperplasia, of breast tissue, 985
Atypical mycobacterial infections, 209–212, 211(t)
and pericarditis, 291
in AIDS, 45, 46, 47, 211, 291
Atypical nevus, 730, 735
Atypical pneumonia, 179(t), 181–182
AUDIT (Alcohol Use Disorders Identification Test), *1039*
Aura, migraine with, 833, *833*
Auranofin, for rheumatoid arthritis, 904(t)
Aurothioglucose, for rheumatoid arthritis, 904(t)
Autogenic training, in therapy for muscle-contraction headache, 832
Autogenous vein grafts, in surgery for occlusive disease of lower extremity arteries, 293–294
Autoimmune disease, vertigo in, 840(t)
Autoimmune hemolytic anemia, 305(t), 305–308
Autoimmune myasthenia gravis, 856–862
treatment of, 857(t)–860(t), 857–862
Autoimmune thyroiditis, 592(t), 592–593
Automated external defibrillators, 224
Autotransplantation, of pancreatic tissue, for pancreatitis, 469
Avascular necrosis, in sickle cell disease, 324
Axillary-subclavian venous thrombosis, 297
Axillofemoral graft, 217, 293
Axonal neuropathy, distal, 880
in children, 888
Azathioprine, adverse effects of, 859, 904(t)
for autoimmune hemolytic anemia, 308
for bullous pemphigoid, 769
for chronic actinic dermatitis, 786
for chronic demyelinating inflammatory polyneuropathy, 885
for cicatricial pemphigoid, 770
for Crohn's disease, 434, 435
for inflammatory myopathies, 718
for multiple sclerosis, 851
for myasthenia gravis, 859
for pemphigus vulgaris, 767
for rheumatoid arthritis, 904(t), 906
for ulcerative colitis, 431
Azatidine, for cough associated with allergic rhinitis, 24
Azidothymidine (AZT, zidovudine), adverse effects of, 44
for acquired immunodeficiency syndrome, 43–44, 45(t)
Azithromycin, adverse effects of, 132(t)
for atypical mycobacterial infection, 211
for bronchitis, 176(t)
for chancroid, 666(t)
for chlamydial infection, 668(t), 669(t), 669–670, 1012, 1012(t)
for cryptosporidiosis, 483
for Lyme disease, 120(t), 121
for mycoplasmal pneumonia, 181
for pharyngitis, 206(t)
for pneumonia, 181
for streptococcal pharyngitis, 206(t)
for toxoplasmosis, 131, 132(t)
for urethritis, 669(t), 669–670
Azlocillin, for neutropenia and infection, 328
Azole antifungals. See specific agents, e.g., *Ketoconazole.*
AZT (azidothymidine, zidovudine), adverse effects of, 44
for acquired immunodeficiency syndrome, 43–44, 45(t)
Aztreonam, for endocarditis, 260(t)
for meningitis, 102(t)
for osteomyelitis, 928(t)
for typhoid fever, 141

Bacille Calmette-Guerin, for bladder cancer, 653
Bacillus cereus toxins, food-borne, 74, 75(t)
Bacitracin, for *Clostridium difficile*–associated diarrhea, 14(t)
for conjunctivitis, 66, 66(t)
in newborn, 64, 64(t)
Bacitracin-polymyxin, for sunburn, 785
Back pain, 39–41
atypical clinical features associated with, 39(t)
fracture of osteopenic vertebra and, 522, 523
metastatic lung cancer and, 158
Baclofen, for spasticity, in multiple sclerosis, 852
for trigeminal neuralgia, 863
Bacteremia, 55–62, 57(t), 58(t), *61*. See also *Sepsis.*
salmonellosis and, 138
Bacterial conjunctivitis, 66, 66(t)
in newborn, 64, 64(t)
Bacterial contamination, of blood for transfusion, 401
Bacterial endocarditis. See *Infectious endocarditis.*
Bacterial infection, of bone, 63, 138, 204, 923–929, 928(t)
in patient with sickle cell disease, 325, 924
of lungs, 172, 176–187, 179(t), 186(t), 191
in AIDS patient, 47
in patient with influenza, 80
of skin, 736–740
and necrosis, 79, 740
in patient with varicella, 67
secondary to contact dermatitis, 782–783
of urinary tract, 595–601
and acute-on-chronic renal failure, 644
and bacteremia, 57(t)
in female patient, 596(t), 596–601
in male patient, 595(t), 595–596, 669–670
opportunistic, in AIDS patient, 45–47, 46(t)
Bacterial labyrinthitis, 839(t)
Bacterial meningitis, 98–103, 100(t), 101(t), 102(t)
Bacterial overgrowth, in small intestine, 456–457
Bacterial pericarditis, 291
Bacterial peritonitis, spontaneous, 411
Bacterial pneumonia, 176–187, 179(t), 186(t), 191
AIDS and, 47
influenza and, 80
Bacterial prostatitis, 633–634
Bacterial sinusitis, 203
common cold and, 188
Bacterial toxins, food sources of, 75(t)
Bacterial vaginosis, 1007, 1007(t)
Bacteriuria, 596
asymptomatic, in female patient, 598–599, 601, 621
in male patient, 596
BAL (dimercaprol), as antidote, 1093(t)
for arsenic poisoning, 882

BAL (dimercaprol) *(Continued)*
for lead poisoning, 1116(t)
Baldness, 706–709, 706(t)–709(t)
nail lesions associated with, 723–724
Ballard score, in assessment of newborn, *966*
Balloon angioplasty, for occlusive disease of lower extremity arteries, 293
Balloon compression, of trigeminal nerve, 863
Balloon dilatation, of esophagus, for achalasia, 419–420
Balloon tamponade, for bleeding esophageal varices, 414–415
Barber's itch, 738
Barbital, poisoning by, 1105(t)
Barbiturate(s), 1105(t)
for intracranial hypertension, in Reye's syndrome, 847
poisoning by, 1044, 1104, 1105(t)
withdrawal from, 1104
Barrett's esophagus, 421
Barrier contraceptives, 1032–1034
Bartholin's gland, abscess of, 1022
cancer of, 1025–1026
cysts of, 1022
Basal cell carcinoma, of skin, 709–711
of vulva, 1025
Basic life suppport, in management of cardiac arrest, 223
Bathing instructions, for patient with atopic dermatitis, 763
for patient with impetigo, 737
for patient with pruritus, 36
for patient with varicella, 67
Baxter formula, for fluid replacement therapy, in burned patient, 1070
BCNU (carmustine), for brain cancer, 897
for multiple myeloma, 384(t)
Beats, premature, 230–233
ventricular, 231–233, 240, 241
Beclomethasone, for allergic rhinitis, 694, 694(t)
for asthma, 681(t)
in pediatric patient, 688
possible adverse effects of, 685
Bed(s), for patients with pressure ulcers, 760
Bed rest, in management of low back pain, 40
in management of ulcerative colitis, 426
Bedsores, 759–762
Behavioral therapy, for Alzheimer's disease, 793
for bulimia nervosa, 1052
for depression, 1059
for insomnia, 35, 35(t)
for nocturnal enuresis, 603–604
for obesity, 515
for panic disorder, 1066
for temporomandibular disorders, 917
Belching, 8
Bell's palsy (facial paralysis), 869–871, *870*
Lyme disease and, 120(t), 123
Benazepril, for hypertension, 275(t)
Bendroflumethiazide, for hypertension, 270(t)
Benign migratory glossitis, 755
Benign positional vertigo, 837
treatment of, 837, *839*
Benign prostatic hyperplasia, 627–633, 628(t)–630(t)
Benign rolandic epilepsy, 822–823
Benzamides (substituted benzamides). See *Metoclopramide.*
Benzene, poisoning by, 1112
Benznidazole, for trypanosomiasis, 747
Benzodiazepines, 1106(t). See also specific agents, e.g., *Diazepam.*
for anxiety, 1046, 1106(t)
in Alzheimer's disease, 793
for insomnia, 35
for nausea and vomiting, 7
for nocturnal myoclonus, 34
for panic disorder, 1065
for schizophrenic disorders, 1063
for stimulant overdose, 1042
poisoning by, 1104
flumazenil for, 1044, 1094(t)
Benzonatate, for cough, 22, 25
Benzoylmethylecgonine (cocaine), abuse of or poisoning by, 1041, 1042, 1043, 1108(t), 1108–1109
Benzoyl peroxide, for acne, 704, 784
for oil acne, 784
for pruritic folliculitis of pregnancy, 775
for stasis ulcer, 759
Benztropine, for effects of haloperidol, 1042, 1043
for neuroleptic malignant syndrome, 1062
Bepridil, 1107(t)
Bernard-Soulier syndrome, 339
Beta-adrenergic agonists, for asthma, 680, 681, 681(t)
in pediatric patient, 685(t), 686, *687*, 688, 689, *689*, *690*, 691
for chronic obstructive pulmonary disease, 153, 154, *155*
in prophylaxis against exercise-induced asthma, 679
Beta-adrenergic blocking agents, 219(t), 1124(t)–1125(t)
for angina pectoris, 219, 219(t), 220, 221
for arrhythmias, 238(t)
in children, 244(t)
in patient with pheochromocytoma, 589
in stimulant-abusing patient, 1042
for atrial fibrillation, 228, 228(t)
for glaucoma, 867, 867(t)
for headache, 835
for heart failure, 256
for hypertension, 269–270, 270(t), 278, 278(t)
in patient with porphyria, 391
for hyperthyroidism, 583, 584
for migraine, 835
for myocardial infarction, 281(t), 282, 282(t), 284
for supraventricular tachycardia, 238, 239(t)
for tachycardia, in patient with pheochromocytoma, 589
in stimulant-abusing patient, 1042
for thyroid storm, 584
for ventricular tachycardia, 241(t)
poisoning by, 1125–1126
side effects of, adverse, 220(t)
altered glucose metabolism due to, 266
changes in lipid levels due to, 266
use of, by patient in cardiac rehabilitation, 288
Beta-carotene, for erythropoietic protoporphyria, 392
Beta-hemolytic streptococcal infection. See also *Streptococcal infection.*
necrosis due to, 78, 79
pharyngitis due to, 117, 204–207, 206(t)
Betamethasone, for aphthous ulcers, 753
for atopic dermatitis, 763
for cicatricial pemphigoid, 770
Betamethasone *(Continued)*
for contact dermatitis, 782
for lichen simplex chronicus, 776
for pemphigoid gestationis, 774
for polymorphic eruption of pregnancy, 775
for scabies, 745
Beta-thalassemia, 315, 315(t), 316, 317
Betaxolol, 219(t), 1124(t)
for angina pectoris, 219(t)
for glaucoma, 867, 867(t)
for hypertension, 270(t)
Bicarbonate, as antidote, 1097(t)
for acidosis, in cyanotic infant, 244(t)
in newborn, 961–962
in patient with renal failure, 638, 639(t), 647
for cardiac arrest, 226
for diabetic ketoacidosis, 502
use of, to alkalinize urine, in child with tumor lysis syndrome, 368
in patient with cystine stones, 664
Bifascicular block, 235, 236
Bifonazole, for onychomycosis, 722
Bile acid sequestrants. See also *Cholestyramine.*
for hyperlipoproteinemia, 508
Bile reflux gastritis, 443
Bilharziasis (schistosomiasis), 481(t), 485
cutaneous, 748, 1085
Biliary colic, 403
Biliary tract disease, malabsorption due to, 456
signs of, 450, 452(t)
Bilirubinemia, neonatal, 971–972, 975
hemolytic disease and, 330, 331, 333
Billowing mitral leaflets. See *Mitral valve prolapse.*
Binge eating, 1048, 1049, 1050(t)
occurrence of, in bulimia nervosa, 1048, 1049
therapeutic approach to, 1052
Biofeedback, in management of tinnitus, 39
in therapy for muscle-contraction headache, 832
Biopsy, of breast masses, 984
of liver, in hereditary hemochromatosis, 346–347
of skin, in malignant or premalignant disease, 732, 733
of small intestine, in malabsorption, 453(t). See also *Malabsorption.*
Biotin, 518(t), 519
deficiency of, 518(t), 519
for brittle nails, 721
Bipolar disorder, 1056–1057
mania in, 1056–1057
treatment of, 1059, 1060(t)
multiple sclerosis and, 854–855
Bird fancier's disease, antigens in, 202(t)
Bisacodyl, for bowel dysfunction, in multiple sclerosis, 853
Bismuth, for diarrhea, 16, 78
in salmonellosis, 137
for *Helicobacter pylori* infection, 442, 471
Bisoprolol, 1124(t)
for hypertension, 270(t), 278(t)
Bisphosphonates, for osteoporosis, 525
for Paget's disease of bone, 528–529
Bite(s), and need for rabies prophylaxis, 112
fly, and tularemia, 134
kissing bug, and trypanosomiasis, 747
marine animal, 1083, 1084
mite, and typhus fever, 143

Bite(s) *(Continued)*
mosquito, and malaria, 91
pathogens transmitted by, and bacteremia, 58(t)
rat, 113, 114
sandfly, and leishmaniasis, 83, 747
snake, 1080–1082
antivenin for, 1081, 1082, 1090(t)
spider, 1078–1080
antivenin for, 1090(t)
tick, and Lyme disease, 120
and paralysis, 887
and relapsing fever, 115, 115(t), 116, 117
and tularemia, 134
and typhus fever, 143
tsetse fly, and trypanosomiasis, 747
Black pigment gallstones, 402
Black widow spider bites, 1080
antivenin for, 1090(t)
Bladder. See *Urinary bladder*; *Urinary incontinence.*
Blastocystis hominis infection, 480(t), 483
Blastomycosis, 168–170
in AIDS patient, 170
in renal transplant recipient, 170
Blast phase, of chronic myelogenous leukemia, 371–372
Bleach, poisoning by, 1104
Bleeding. See *Hemorrhage*; *Hemorrhagic* entries.
Bleomycin, for cutaneous T-cell lymphoma, 381
for Hodgkin's disease, 351(t)
for non-Hodgkin's lymphoma, 376(t)
for penile cancer, 656
for testicular cancer, 658
for urethral cancer, 653
for warts, 724, 728–729
Blepharitis, seborrheic, 713
Blisters, burn, 1072
fever, 741, 751
hemorrhagic, due to snake bite, 1080
Bloating, 8
Block (conduction block), along peripheral nerves, 885
in heart, 233–236, 234(t)
cardiac arrest due to, 227
infectious endocarditis and, 261
Lyme disease and, 122
myocardial infarction and, 236, 284
Block anesthesia, for delivery, 948, 949
complications of, 954–955
Blood, laboratory reference values for, 1135(t)–1137(t)
Blood loss. See *Hemorrhage*; *Hemorrhagic* entries.
Blood pressure measurement, 264
abnormal findings on. See *Hypertension*; *Hypotension.*
Blood transfusion. See *Transfusion.*
"Bloody show," 942
Blowfly larvae, in skin, 748–749
Blue nevus, 731
Body clock, and insomnia, 34
Body lice, 746
Body surface area, nomogram for, *1143*
"rule of nines" for, 1068
Body weight reduction, by hypertensive patient, 267
by obese patient, 512–515
Body weight standards, 511, 512(t)
Bone(s), defective mineralization of, liver disease and, 409
fractures of. See *Fracture(s).*
Bone(s) *(Continued)*
infections of, 63, 138, 204, 923–929, 928(t)
sickle cell disease and, 325, 924
mass of, loss of, 521–526, 522(t)
liver disease and, 409
menopause and, 525, 1004–1005
necrosis of, sickle cell disease and, 324
Paget's disease of, 527–530
pain in, metastatic lung cancer and, 157
Paget's disease and, 527
sarcoidosis involving, 198
solitary plasmacytoma of, 386
Bone marrow infarction, in sickle cell disease, 319
Bone marrow relapse, in leukemia, 364, 367
Bone marrow transplantation, for aplastic anemia, 301
for hemolytic anemia, 311
for leukemia, 363, 364, 367, 371
for multiple myeloma, 383, 384, 385
for thalassemia, 317
Boot, Unna, for stasis ulcer, 759
Borderline isolated systolic hypertension, 263, 264(t). See also *Hypertension.*
Borderline leprosy, 87
Bordetella pertussis infection, 144(t), 144–146, 145(t)
Boric acid, for candidal vulvovaginitis, 1006
Boric acid dressings, for venous stasis ulcer, 759
Borrelia burgdorferi infection, and Lyme disease, 119–124, 120(t), 887
Borrelia species, infection by, and relapsing fever, 114–117, 115(t)
Botfly larvae, in skin, 748–749
Botulinum toxin injections, for spasmodic dysphonia, 32
Botulism, 75–76
Botulism antitoxin, 1091(t)
Bougienage, of esophagus, 421
Boutonneuse fever, 143(t)
Bowenoid papulosis, 735–736
Bowen's disease, 734
Brace, for low back pain, 40
Brain. See also *Central nervous system.*
abscess of, 788–790, 789(t), 790(t)
amyloid angiopathy of, 797
aneurysmal or arteriovenous hemorrhage in, 797
astrocytoma of, 830, 897
cancer metastatic to, 157, 158(t), 829–830, 895–896
cancer of, 830, 895–900
edema of. See also *Intracranial hypertension.*
poisoning and, 1098
glioma of, 830, 896–898
hemorrhage in, 794–798, 795(t), 801
intraventricular, in preterm infant, 973–974
infarction of, sickle cell disease and, 325
infection of, abscess due to, 788–790, 789(t), 790(t)
AIDS and, 50, 132–133, 790, 790(t)
Plasmodium schizonts in, 93, 96
tapeworm larvae in, 485
toxoplasmal, in AIDS, 50, 132–133, 790
viral, 68, 111, 127, 844(t), 844–845, 845(t)
inflammation of. See *Encephalitis.*
ischemia of. See *Stroke syndrome.*
lymphoma of, 899
Brain *(Continued)*
malaria (*Plasmodium* schizonts) involving, 93, 96
meninges of, infection/inflammation of. See *Meningitis.*
tumors of, 830, 898
headache associated with, 830
oligodendroglioma of, 830, 896, 898
perfusion pressure in, maintenance of, 891, 894, 894(t)
surgery of, for abscess, 789–790
for tumors, 896, 897, 898
tapeworm larvae in, 485
toxic damage to. See *Encephalopathy.*
toxoplasmosis of, AIDS and, 50, 132–133, 790
trauma to. See *Head, trauma to.*
tumors of, 829–830, 895–900
headache associated with, 829, 830
vascular disease of, ischemic. See *Stroke syndrome.*
leading to hemorrhage, 797
sickle cell syndromes and, 325
viral infection of, 68, 111, 127, 844(t), 844–845, 845(t)
white matter lesions in, 888
AIDS and, 52
Breakthrough pain, drugs for, 2
in sickle cell disease, 321
Breast(s), abscesses in, 982
biopsy of, 984
cancer of, 979–989
evaluation of, 986(t)
mortality risk associated with, 983, 984(t)
risk of, 979, 979(t), 983, *983*
size of, 980, *980*, 981(t)
staging of, 985(t)
treatment of, 985–989, 988(t)
engorgement of, bromocriptine for, 957
hyperplastic tissue changes in, atypical, 985
infection of, 982
"masses" in, 982
milk production in, 978
pain in, 981
resection of, for cancer, 987, 988
tumors of. See *Breast(s), cancer of.*
Breast-feeding, 978
Breech presentation, anesthesia for, 950
Breslow levels, in assessment of melanoma, 732, 1025(t)
Bretylium, for arrhythmias, 238(t)
for ventricular fibrillation, 224(t), 225
in hypothermic patient, 1074
Brill-Zinsser disease, 142
Brittle nails, 721
Bromocriptine, for acromegaly, 549–550
for breast engorgement, 957
for Cushing's syndrome, 556–557, 557(t)
for hyperprolactinemia, 575, 576, 577
for neuroleptic malignant syndrome, 1062
for Parkinson's disease, 877
for premenstrual syndrome, 1002
Brompheniramine, for rhinitis, 693(t)
Bronchitis, 174–176
acute, 174
treatment of, in patient with COPD, 23
antimicrobials for, 174–176, 175(t), 176(t)
chronic, exacerbations of, 175–176
obstructive, 152
Bronchodilators, for asthma, 24, 680, 681, 681(t)

Bronchodilators *(Continued)*
in pediatric patient, 685(t), 686, *687*, 688
for chronic obstructive pulmonary disease, 153–154, *155*
for cough due to asthma, 24
Bronchogenic carcinoma, 156–163, *157*
chemotherapy for, 161, 162, 162(t), 163
metastases of, effects of, 157–158, 158(t)
pleural effusion associated with, 158, 158(t)
radiation therapy for, 161, 162, 163
signs and symptoms of, 156, 156(t)
staging of, 160(t)
surgery for, 159, 161, 161(t)
conditions contraindicating, 159–160, 160(t)
Bronchopleural fistula, 171
Bronchopulmonary dysplasia, 973
Bronchospasm, anaphylaxis and, 677, 677(t)
asthma and. See *Asthma*.
Brown pigment gallstones, 402
Brown recluse spider bites, 1078–1080
Brucellosis, 62–63
Bubonic plague, 107, 108
Buccal mucosa, lesions of, 753–754
Bulimia nervosa, 1048(t)–1051(t), 1048–1053
Bulk-forming agents, for constipation, 18
Bullous diseases, of skin, 737, 766–772
Bullous impetigo, 737
Bullous pemphigoid, 768–769
Bumetanide, for heart failure, 255
for hypertension, 270(t)
Bundle branch block, 235, 236
Bupivacaine, for delivery, 949, 952
Buprenorphine, for pain, 2(t)
Bupropion, 1130(t)
adverse effects of, 1060(t)
for depression, 1060(t)
Burkitt's lymphoma (small non–cleaved cell lymphoma), 377
Burn(s), 1067–1073
chemical, 1069–1070, 1106–1108
electrical, 1069
infection risk with, and bacteremia, 58(t)
Burn care facilities, specialized, transfer to, 1071
Burning tongue syndrome, 755–756
Burow's solution, for contact dermatitis, 782
for decubitus dermatitis, 761
irrigation of ear canal with, in treatment of otitis externa, 106(t)
Bursitis, 920–921
Buschke-Lowenstein giant condyloma, 1025
Buspirone, for panic disorder, 1065
Busulfan, for leukemia, 370
for multiple myeloma, 384(t)
Butorphanol, 1119(t)
for headache, 829
for pain, 2, 2(t)
Butyrophenones, for nausea and vomiting, 6, 6(t)
Bypass, cardiopulmonary, and thrombocytopenia, 340
in hypothermic patient, 1075–1076
coronary artery, for heart failure, 256
gastric, as therapy for obesity, 516
veins for, in surgery for occlusive disease of lower extremity arteries, 293–294

"Cafe coronary," 182
Caffeine, for apnea of prematurity, 976
for pain, 3
therapeutic vs. toxic levels of, 1138(t)
Calcipotriene, for psoriasis, 713
Calcitonin, for osteoporosis, 523–524
for Paget's disease of bone, 528, 529
Calcium, abnormal serum levels of. See *Hypercalcemia*; *Hypocalcemia*.
elevated urinary levels of, 663(t)
need for, in female patient with secondary hypogonadism, 573
in patient receiving prednisone, 903
in patient with parathyroid disorders, 568, 569
rationale for use of, in prevention of osteoporosis, 525
Calcium acetate, for hyperphosphatemia, 567–568, 647
Calcium carbonate, for hyperphosphatemia, 567–568, 647
for hypoparathyroidism, 568
for osteoporosis, 525
Calcium channel blockers, 221(t), 1107(t)
adverse effects of, 277
for angina pectoris, 220–221, 221(t)
for atrial fibrillation, 228, 228(t)
for hypertension, 276–277, 277(t)
in aldosteronism, 572
in renal failure, 646
for myocardial infarction, 283, 284
for Raynaud's phenomenon, 718
for supraventricular tachycardia, 239(t)
poisoning by, 1104–1105, 1107(t)
Calcium chloride, for hydrofluoric acid exposure, 1092(t)
for hyperkalemia, in renal failure, 639(t)
Calcium disodium edetate, as antidote, 1091(t)
for lead poisoning, 1116(t)
Calcium gel, for hydrofluoric acid exposure, 1092(t)
Calcium gluconate, as antidote, 1092(t)
for hyperkalemia, in renal failure, 638
for hypocalcemia, 569
for muscle spasms due to jellyfish sting, 1084
for neonatal hypocalcemia, 968
for symptoms of spider bite, 1080
Calcium stones, 662–663, 663(t)
Calculi, cholecystic, 9, 402–405
hemolytic anemia and, 317
pancreatitis due to, 461
salmonellosis and, 140, 142
renal, 661–665, 662(t), 663(t)
sarcoidosis and, 199
salivary gland, 756–757
ureteral. See *Calculi, renal*.
Calf vein thrombosis, 297–298, 1030
Calorie requirements, determination of, 514(t), 532, 532(t)
in pediatric patient, 539, 539(t)
Calorie-restricted diet, for obesity, 513, 513(t), 514, 515
Calymmatobacterium granulomatis infection, 670–671
CAMP chemotherapy regimen, for lung cancer, 162(t)
Camphor, poisoning by, 1105
Campylobacter jejuni infection, 14, 14(t)
Cancer, arsenic ingestion and, 734
chemotherapy for. See *Chemotherapy*.
germ cell, of testis, 657–658
in patient treated for Hodgkin's disease, 354, 359
in patient treated for polycythemia, 388
Cancer *(Continued)*
metastasis of, from lung, 157–158, 158(t)
sites of, in patient with pheochromocytoma, 592
to brain, 157, 158(t), 829–830, 895–896
nonseminomatous germ cell, of testis, 657–658
of adrenal gland, 556, 648–649
and aldosteronism, 570, 571, 572
of Bartholin's gland, 1025–1026
of bladder, 652–653
of blood-forming organs. See *Leukemia*.
of brain, 830, 895–900
of breast, 979–989
evaluation of, 986(t)
mortality risk associated with, 983, 984(t)
risk of, 979, 979(t), 983, *983*
size of, 980, *980*, 981(t)
staging of, 985(t)
treatment of, 985–989, 988(t)
of buccal mucosa, 753–754
of cervix, 1018–1021, 1019(t)
of colon, 476–479
risk factors for, 432, 476
of endometrium, 1015–1018, 1016(t)
risk of, in relation to postmenopausal estrogen use, 1005
of esophagus, 421
of floor of mouth, 757
of genitourinary tract, 648–658
of kidney, 649–652
of larynx, 32–33
of lip, 752
of liver, cirrhosis and, 412–413
porphyria and, 393
viral hepatitis and, 412, 445
of lung, 156–163, *157*
chemotherapy for, 161, 162, 162(t), 163
metastases of, effects of, 157–158, 158(t)
pleural effusion associated with, 158, 158(t)
radiation therapy for, 161, 162, 163
signs and symptoms of, 156, 156(t)
staging of, 160(t)
surgery for, 159, 161, 161(t)
conditions contraindicating, 159–160, 160(t)
of lymphoid tissue. See *Lymphoma*.
of mouth, 752, 753, 754, 756, 757
of pancreas, 465
of penis, 656–657
of prostate, 653–656
of rectum, 476–479
of salivary glands, 754
of scrotum, 658
of skin, 377–382, 709–711, 731–733
lesions predisposing to, 733–736
recognition of, mnemonic for, 732, 735
sun exposure and, 786
of stomach, 473–475
of testis, 657–658
of thyroid, 584(t), 584–587
of tongue, 756
of upper urinary tract, 652
of urethra, 653
of urinary bladder, 652–653
of urogenital tract, 648–658
of uterine cervix, 1018–1021, 1019(t)
of uterus, 1015–1018, 1016(t)
leiomyoma and, 1014
of vulva, 1022–1026, 1024(t), 1025(t)
papillomavirus infection and, 727, 1023
pemphigus associated with, 768

Cancer *(Continued)*
radiation exposure and, 736
radiation therapy for. See *Radiation therapy.*
surgery for. See *Surgery, for cancer.*
Candidiasis, 750
AIDS and, 48
cheilitis due to, 751
cystitis due to, 596
treatment of, 595(t), 596
endocarditis treatment in, 260(t)
esophageal, AIDS and, 48
susceptibility to, multiple myeloma and, 386
vulvovaginal, 1006
treatment of, 776, 1006–1007, 1007(t)
Canker sore, 752
Cannabinoids, for nausea and vomiting, 6, 6(t)
Cantharidin, for molluscum contagiosum, 744
Cap, cervical, 1033, 1034
CAP-BOP chemotherapy regimen, for non-Hodgkin's lymphoma, 376, 376(t)
CAP chemotherapy regimen, for lung cancer, 162(t)
Capillariasis, 481(t), 484
Capsaicin, for neuropathic pain, 888
for post-herpetic neuralgia, 743
Captopril, anticholinergic properties of, 1054(t)
for heart failure, 256
in children, 245(t)
for hypertension, 273(t), 275(t), 278(t)
for myocardial infarction, 282
Carbachol, for glaucoma, 867(t)
Carbamate insecticides, poisoning by, 1120–1121
Carbamazepine, 811(t), 1103(t)
adverse effects of, 1060(t)
for agitation, in Alzheimer's disease, 793
for epilepsy, 808, 809, 810(t), 810–812, 811(t), 818
in pediatric patient, 823
for mania, 1060(t)
in multiple sclerosis, 854–855
for neuropathic pain, 888
for post-herpetic neuralgia, 743
for trigeminal neuralgia, 863
therapeutic vs. toxic levels of, 1138(t)
Carbidopa-levodopa, for Parkinson's disease, 873–876, 878
Carbohydrate(s), for porphyria, 391
in parenteral nutrition, 533
Carbonic anhydrase inhibitors, adverse effects of, 868
for glaucoma, 867(t), 868
Carbon monoxide, poisoning by, 1105–1106, 1108(t)
nomogram for, *1109*
Carbon monoxide poisoning, 1067–1068
Carbuncles, 738–739
surgical drainage of, 738, *739*
Carcinoembryonic antigen, 477
Carcinoma, anaplastic, of thyroid, 586, 587
basal cell, of skin, 709–711
of vulva, 1025
bronchogenic, 156–163, *157*
chemotherapy for, 161, 162, 162(t), 163
metastases of, effects of, 157–158, 158(t)
pleural effusion associated with, 158, 158(t)
radiation therapy for, 161, 162, 163
signs and symptoms of, 156, 156(t)
Carcinoma *(Continued)*
staging of, 160(t)
surgery for, 159, 161, 161(t)
conditions contraindicating, 159–160, 160(t)
ductal (in situ), 986(t), 986–987
follicular, of thyroid, 585, 587
hepatocellular, cirrhosis and, 412–413
porphyria and, 393
viral hepatitis and, 412, 445
Hürthle cell, 585, 587
lobular (in situ), 986
medullary, of thyroid, 585, 586, 587
non-small cell, of lung, *157*, 160–162
of adrenal gland, 556, 648–649
and aldosteronism, 570, 571, 572
of Bartholin's gland, 1025–1026
of bladder, 652–653
of breast, 979–989
evaluation of, 986(t)
mortality risk associated with, 983, 984(t)
risk of, 979, 979(t), 983, *983*
size of, 980, *980*, 981(t)
staging of, 985(t)
treatment of, 985–989, 988(t)
of buccal mucosa, 753–754
of cervix, 1018–1021, 1019(t)
of colon, 476–479
risk factors for, 432, 476
of endometrium, 1015–1018, 1016(t)
of esophagus, 421
of floor of mouth, 757
of genitourinary tract, 648–656
of kidney, 649–651
of larynx, 32–33
of lip, 752
of liver, cirrhosis and, 412–413
porphyria and, 393
viral hepatitis and, 412, 445
of lung, 156–163, *157*
chemotherapy for, 161, 162, 162(t), 163
metastases of, effects of, 157–158, 158(t)
pleural effusion associated with, 158, 158(t)
radiation therapy for, 161, 162, 163
signs and symptoms of, 156, 156(t)
staging of, 160(t)
surgery for, 159, 161, 161(t)
conditions contraindicating, 159–160, 160(t)
of mouth, 752, 753, 754, 756, 757
of penis, 656
of prostate, 653–656
of rectum, 476–479
of salivary glands, 754
of scrotum, 658
of skin, 709–711
of stomach, 473–475
of thyroid, 584–585
of tongue, 756
of upper urinary tract, 652
of urethra, 653
of urogenital tract, 648–656
of uterine cervix, 1018–1021, 1019(t)
of uterus, 1015–1018, 1016(t)
of vulva, 1022–1025, 1025(t)
papillary, of thyroid, 584–585, 587
papillomavirus infection and, 727, 1023
radiation exposure and, 736
renal cell, 649–651
small cell, of lung, 162–163
squamous cell, of esophagus, 421
of larynx, 32
Carcinoma *(Continued)*
of mouth, 752, 756, 757
of skin, 709–711
of vulva, 1023, 1024
transitional cell, of urinary collecting system, 652–653
verrucous, of oral cavity, 753–754
of vulva, 1025
Cardiac. See also *Heart* entries.
Cardiac arrest, 222–227
asystole and, 222, 223, 225
coronary artery disease and, 222. See also *Coronary artery disease.*
electromechanical dissociation and, 222
heart block and, 227
management of, *223*, 223–226
advanced life support in, 224–226
basic life support in, 223
cardiopulmonary resuscitation in, 223, 224(t), 226
"chain of survival" in, *223*
defibrillation in, 223, 224, 224(t), 225
drugs in, 224, 224(t), 225, 226
early access in, 223
treatment protocols in, 224(t), 225
prevention of, 226–227
pulseless electrical activity and, 222, 223, 225
risk factors for, 222. See also sub-entries under *Cardiac death, risk of.*
ventricular fibrillation and, 222, 223, 225
ventricular tachycardia and, 222, 223, 225
Cardiac arrhythmias. See *Arrhythmia(s).*
Cardiac catheterization, in patient with myocardial infarction, 283
Cardiac death, 222. See also *Cardiac arrest.*
risk of, coronary artery disease and, 222. See also *Coronary artery disease.*
ischemic heart disease and, 222
mitral valve prolapse syndrome and, 252
myocardial infarction and, 222, 226
ventricular dysfunction and, 222, 240
ventricular ectopy and, 222, 227, 232, 252
Cardiac emboli, and occlusion of lower extremity arteries, 294
and stroke, 801
Cardiac output, low, in heart failure, 254–255
Cardiac rehabilitation, 285–289
Cardiac tamponade, 289–290
Cardiac trauma, and pericarditis, 291
Cardioembolic stroke, 801
Cardiogenic shock, 255
as complication of myocardial infarction, 284(t)
Cardiomyoplasty, for heart failure, 256–257
Cardiopulmonary bypass, and thrombocytopenia, 340
in hypothermic patient, 1075–1076
Cardiopulmonary resuscitation (CPR), 223, 224(t), 226
in hypothermic patient, 1074
Cardiovascular syphilis, 673(t)
Cardiovascular system, disease of, in diabetes mellitus, 493
effects of estrogen on, 1005, 1005(t)
effects of renal failure on, 639
Cardioversion, for arrhythmias associated with myocardial infarction, 283
for atrial fibrillation, 228, 229

Cardioversion *(Continued)*
for cardiac arrest, 223, 224, 224(t), 225
for ventricular fibrillation, 224(t), 225
in hypothermic patient, 1074
in pediatric patient, 244(t)
Cardioverter-defibrillator, implantable, for ventricular tachycardia, 241, 241(t)
Carditis. See also *Infectious endocarditis; Pericarditis.*
Lyme disease and, 120(t), 122
radiation-induced, 359
rheumatic, 117, 118, 118(t), 119, 250
Caries, dental, radiation-induced xerostomia and, 359
Carmustine (BCNU), for brain cancer, 897
for leukemia, 384(t)
Carotenoderma, 780
Carotid endarterectomy, 800
Carpal tunnel syndrome, 880
Carriers, of salmonellosis, 139–140, 142
of typhoid fever, 142
Carteolol, 219(t), 1124(t)
for angina pectoris, 219(t)
for glaucoma, 867(t)
Catarrhal stage, of pertussis, 144, 144(t)
Catecholamine-secreting tumors, 588–592, 649
Catfish, effects of contact with, 1083
Cathartics, 18–19
abuse of, 18
in bulimia nervosa, 1049
for constipation, 18–19
for poisoning, 78, 1088
Catheter-directed thrombolysis, 1029
Catheter infection, 57(t), 537, 596, 599
Catheterization, cardiac, after myocardial infarction, 283
intermittent, for bladder dysfunction, 605
subclavian vein, in parenteral nutrition, 535–536, 537
Caustic/corrosive injury, 1069–1070, 1106–1108
to esophagus, 422
CDC criteria, for acquired immunodeficiency syndrome, 43(t)
for Reye's syndrome, 846(t)
for toxic shock syndrome, 1009(t)
Cefaclor, allergic reaction to, 698
for bronchitis, 175(t)
for otitis media, 173(t)
Cefadroxil, for streptococcal pharyngitis, 206(t)
Cefazolin, for cellulitis, 740
for endocarditis, 260(t)
for osteomyelitis, 928(t)
for pneumococcal pneumonia, 180
for pneumonia, 179(t), 180
for pyelonephritis, in female patient, 622
for toxic shock syndrome, 1010
Cefixime, for bronchitis, 175(t)
for gonorrhea, 667, 667(t), 668
for otitis externa, 106(t)
for otitis media, 173(t)
Cefoperazone, for neutropenia and infection, 328
for salmonellosis, 14(t)
Cefotaxime, for bacteremia or sepsis, 57(t)
in newborn, 970(t)
in patient with Reye's syndrome, 847
in patient with salmonellosis, 138
for brain abscess, 789(t)
for endocarditis, 260(t)
for enteric fever, 139
for Lyme disease, 123
for meningitis, 102(t)
Cefotaxime *(Continued)*
for osteomyelitis, 928(t)
for peritonitis, in cirrhosis, 411
for pneumonia, 179(t)
for pyelonephritis, in female patient, 622
in male patient, 621(t)
for salmonellosis, 138, 139
for sepsis. See *Cefotaxime, for bacteremia or sepsis.*
for spontaneous bacterial peritonitis, 411
Cefotetan, for pelvic inflammatory disease, 668(t), 1014(t)
for pyelonephritis, in male patient, 621(t)
Cefoxitin, for bacteremia, 57(t)
for pelvic inflammatory disease, 668(t), 1014(t)
Cefpodoxime, for bronchitis, 176(t)
for otitis media, 173(t)
for streptococcal pharyngitis, 206(t)
Cefprozil, for bronchitis, 176(t)
for streptococcal pharyngitis, 206(t)
Ceftazidime, for bacteremia, 57(t)
for brain abscess, 789(t)
for endocarditis, 260(t)
for meningitis, 102(t)
for neutropenia and infection, 328
for osteomyelitis, 928(t)
for otitis externa, 106(t), 107
for pneumonia, 179(t)
for pressure ulcer, 761
Ceftizoxime, for meningitis, 102(t)
for pyelonephritis, in male patient, 621(t)
Ceftriaxone, for arthritis, in Lyme disease, 120(t)
for bacteremia, in salmonellosis, 138
for carditis, in Lyme disease, 120(t), 122
for chancroid, 666(t)
for conjunctivitis, 66, 66(t)
in newborn with gonococcal infection, 64, 64(t), 669
for endocarditis, in brucellosis, 63
for enteric fever, 139
for enterocolitis (gastroenteritis), in salmonellosis, 14(t)
for gonorrhea, 64, 64(t), 66, 66(t), 667, 667(t), 668, 669
for Lyme disease, 120(t), 122, 887
for meningitis, 102(t)
in gonococcal disease, 669
in Lyme disease, 120(t)
for ophthalmia neonatorum, 64, 64(t)
for pelvic inflammatory disease, 1014(t)
for pyelonephritis, in female patient, 598
in male patient, 621(t)
for relapsing fever, 116(t)
for salmonellosis, 14(t), 138, 139, 141, 141(t)
for syphilis, 672
for typhoid fever, 141, 141(t)
Cefuroxime, for bronchitis, 175(t)
for Lyme disease, 120(t), 121
for otitis externa, 106(t)
for pharyngitis, 206(t)
for pneumococcal pneumonia, 180
for pneumonia, 179(t), 180, 186(t)
for streptococcal pharyngitis, 206(t)
Celiac sprue, 453
Cellular blue nevus, 731
Cellulitis, 739–740
bacteremia as complication of, 57(t)
periorbital, 204, 739–740
Centers for Disease Control and Prevention criteria, for AIDS, 43(t)
for Reye's syndrome, 846(t)
for toxic shock syndrome, 1009(t)
Central diabetes insipidus, 559, 562
Centrally acting sympatholytics, for hypertension, 272, 272(t)
in renal failure, 646
Central nervous system. See also *Brain.*
as "sanctuary" site, in leukemia, 367–368
brucellosis involving, 63
effects of hypothermia on, 1073
lesions of, and diabetes insipidus, 559, 562
in sickle cell disease, 325–326
lupus erythematosus involving, 716–717
lymphoma of, 899
sarcoidosis involving, 198
syphilis involving, 672, 673, 673(t)
AIDS and, 47
Trichinella larval migration through, 133
Central (total) parenteral nutrition, 535, 536. See also *Parenteral nutrition.*
complications of, 536–538
Central sleep apnea, 34
Central venous catheter, in parenteral nutrition, 535, 536, 537
Centruroides species, stings by, 1080
Cephalexin, for carbuncles, 739
Cephalosporin(s). See specific agents, e.g., *Cefotaxime; Ceftriaxone.*
Cephalosporin allergy, 698
Cephalothin, for endocarditis, 260(t)
Cephradine, for carbuncles, 739
for urinary tract infection, in male patient, 595(t)
CEPP chemotherapy regimen, for non-Hodgkin's lymphoma, 376(t)
Cercarial dermatitis, 748, 1085
Cerebellar ataxia, varicella and, 68
Cerebral lesions. See *Brain; Central nervous system.*
Cerebrospinal fluid, laboratory reference values for, 1140(t)
Cerebrospinal fluid drainage, in reduction of intracranial pressure, 891, 893, 894(t)
via shunt, and meningitis, 99–100
Cerebrovascular disease, ischemic. See *Stroke syndrome.*
leading to hemorrhage, 797
sickle cell disease and, 325
Cervical cap, 1033, 1034
Cervicitis, 1011, 1012(t)
Cervix, cancer of, 1018–1021, 1019(t)
inflammation/infection of, 1011, 1012(t)
Papanicolaou smear of, in screening for cancer, 1018
tumors of, 1018–1021
Cesarean section, anesthesia for, 952–953
pain following, 953
third-trimester bleeding as indication for, 943
Cestode infestation, 481(t), 482(t), 485, 486
Chagas' disease, 747–748
"Chain of survival," in management of cardiac arrest, *223*. See also *Cardiac arrest, management of.*
Chancroid, 666, 666(t)
Charcoal, activated, for poisoning, 1043, 1044, 1088
Charcot-Marie-Tooth disease, 886
Chédiak-Higashi syndrome, 339
Cheek-chewing, 753
Cheilitis, 736, 751, 752
Chelation therapy, for iron overload, 316, 347, 1093(t)
for lead poisoning, 1116(t)
Chemical conjunctivitis, 64

Chemical injury, 1069–1070, 1106–1108
  to esophagus, 422
Chemical pneumonitis, due to aspiration, 182
Chemical restraint, of stimulant-abusing patient, 1042
Chemotherapy, for cancer, of bladder, 653
    of brain, 896, 897, 898, 899
    of breast, 988(t), 988–989
    of cervix, 1020
    of colon, 479
    of endometrium, 1017
    of lung, 161, 162, 162(t), 163
    of penis, 656
    of rectum, 479
    of skin, 380, 381, 733
    of stomach, 475
    of testis, 658
    of urethra, 653
    of uterine cervix, 1020
    of uterus, 1017
    problems with, 353(t), 354, 363
    vomiting and nausea due to, 7(t), 7–8
  for cutaneous T-cell lymphoma, 380, 381
  for Hodgkin's disease, 349–354, 351(t), 352(t)
    radiation therapy combined with, 349, 350, 352, 357, 357(t), 358
  for leukemia, 362, 363, 364, 366–368, 367(t), 370, 371, 374
  for lymphoma, 349–354, 351(t), 352(t), 375–377, 376(t), *377*, 380, 381
    radiation therapy combined with, 349, 350, 352, 357, 357(t), 358
  for melanoma, 733
  for multiple myeloma, 383, 384, 384(t)
  for non-Hodgkin's lymphoma, 375–377, 376(t), *377*
  for pheochromocytoma, 592
Chest compressions, in cardiopulmonary resuscitation, 224(t)
    and survival of hypothermic patient, 1074
  in neonatal resuscitation, 960–961
Chest pain. See also *Angina pectoris.*
  aortic dissection and, 215
  cocaine abuse and, 1041–1042
  sickle cell disease and, 322
Chest physical therapy, for acute exacerbations of COPD, 155
  in prevention of atelectasis, 152
Chest syndrome, acute, in sickle cell disease, 322–323
Chickenpox. See *Varicella-zoster virus infection.*
Chilblain (pernio), 1076, 1077
Child(ren). See also *Newborn.*
  acute leukemia in, 365–369
  amebicidal dosages for, 54(t), 480(t)
  anthelmintic dosages for, 481(t)–482(t)
  antiarrhythmics for, 244(t), 247
  antidepressant dosages for, 1130(t)
  antimalarial dosages for, 94(t), 97(t)
  antimicrobial dosages for. See *Antimicrobial(s), pediatric dosages of.*
  arthritis in, rheumatoid, 907–911, 908(t), 909(t)
  asthma in, 682–691
  bacterial urinary tract infection in, 595, 599–601
  congenital conditions in. See *Congenital* entries.
  dehydration in, 540–547, 541(t), 542(t), *546*
  diabetes mellitus in, 493–499
Child(ren) *(Continued)*
  digitalis dosages for, 1111(t)
  enuresis in, 601–604
  epilepsy in, 819–823
  exanthema subitum in, 744
  feeding of, 977–979
  fluid replacement therapy for, 538–547
    in cases of burn injury, 1070, 1070(t)
  gonorrhea in, 669
  head trauma in, 892–895
  heart disease in, 241–249
  hoarseness in, 26
  hyperlipoproteinemia in, 509
  immunization of, 74, 81(t), 105, 127, 128, 145–146
    in cases of AIDS, 128
    in cases of hemophilia, 336
  laryngeal papilloma in, 32
  leukemia in, 365–369
  myasthenia gravis in, 860–861
  polyneuropathies in, 887–888
  rheumatoid arthritis in, 907–911, 908(t), 909(t)
  seizures in, 819–823
  urinary tract infection in, 595, 599–601
  vaginitis in, 1006, 1008
Chinese restaurant syndrome, 77
Chlamydial infection, 108–109, 1010–1012
  cervicitis due to, 1011, 1012(t)
  conjunctivitis due to, 66, 66(t)
    neonatal, 64, 64(t), 1011
  cough due to, 23
  endometritis due to, 1011
  gonococcal infection concurrent with, 667, 668(t)
  lymphogranuloma venereum due to, 671
  neonatal, 1011
    conjunctivitis due to, 64, 64(t), 1011
    pneumonitis due to, 1011
  pelvic inflammatory disease due to, 1012(t), 1013
  perihepatitis due to, 1011, 1012(t)
  pneumonia or pneumonitis due to, 181–182
    neonatal, 1011
  risk factors for, 1011(t)
  salpingitis due to, 1011
  urethritis due to, 669–670, 1011, 1012(t)
Chloasma, 780
Chloracne, 784
Chloral hydrate, 1129(t)
  for insomnia, in Alzheimer's disease, 793
  poisoning by, 1044, 1127, 1129(t)
Chlorambucil, for cicatricial pemphigoid, 770
  for cutaneous T-cell lymphoma, 381
  for glomerulopathy, 613, 614, 615, 619, 620
  for leukemia, 374
  for non-Hodgkin's lymphoma, 375
  for pemphigus vulgaris, 767
  for polycythemia, 388
Chloramphenicol, for brain abscess, 789
  for enteric fever, 139
  for granuloma inguinale, 671
  for Lyme disease, 120(t)
  for meningitis, 101(t), 102(t)
    in Lyme disease, 120(t)
    in plague, 108
  for plague, 108
  for relapsing fever, 116(t)
  for rickettsioses, 124, 143, 143(t)
  for Rocky Mountain spotted fever, 124
  for salmonellosis, 139, 140, 141(t)
  for typhoid fever, 140, 141(t)
Chloramphenicol *(Continued)*
  for typhus fevers, 143, 143(t)
  therapeutic vs. toxic levels of, 1138(t)
Chlordiazepoxide, 1106(t)
Chlorhexidine, in oral hygiene, for AIDS patient with gingivitis, 757
Chlorine gas, poisoning by, 1108
2-Chlorodeoxyadenosine, for leukemia, 372
Chloroquine, adverse effects of, 93
  for amebiasis, 15(t)
  for lupus erythematosus, 715
  for malaria, 93, 94(t), 97(t), 98
Chlorothiazide, for renal failure, 638
Chlorpheniramine, for allergic rhinitis, 693(t)
  for pemphigoid gestationis, 774
  for pruritus, 37(t)
Chlorpromazine, 1123(t)
  for headache, 829
  for nausea and vomiting, 6, 6(t)
  for schizophrenic disorders, 1063
  potency of, as neuroleptic, 1062
Chlorpropamide, for diabetes insipidus, 561, 561(t)
  for diabetes mellitus, 491(t)
Chlorthalidone, for hypertension, 270(t)
Cholecystectomy, for calculi or inflammation, 403, 404
Cholecystitis, 9, 402–405. See also *Cholelithiasis.*
Cholelithiasis, 9, 402–405
  hemolytic anemia and, 317
  pancreatitis due to, 461
  salmonellosis and, 140, 142
Cholera, 13, 69–72, 75
  antimicrobials for, 13, 14(t), 71–72, 75
  rehydration in management of, 70, 70(t), 71
  stool in, 71(t)
Cholestasis, sickle cell disease and, 323
Cholesterol, 506
  serum levels of, abnormal elevation in. See *Hyperlipoproteinemia.*
    effects of diuretics on, 265, 266(t)
Cholesterol gallstones, 402
Cholesterol pericarditis, 292
Cholestyramine, for diarrhea, in short bowel syndrome, 458
  for hepatic dysfunction, in porphyria, 392
  for hyperlipoproteinemia, 508
  for pruritus, 37
    in liver disease, 408
  for thyroid storm, 584
Choline magnesium trisalicylate, for rheumatoid arthritis, 902(t)
Cholinergic agents, for glaucoma, 867(t), 868
Cholinergic crisis, 861–862
Cholinergic urticaria, 778
Choline salicylate, for pain, 1
  for rheumatoid arthritis, 902(t)
Cholinesterase inhibitors, for glaucoma, 867(t), 868
  for myasthenia gravis, 857(t), 857–858
CHOP-bleo chemotherapy regimen, for non-Hodgkin's lymphoma, 376, 376(t)
CHOP chemotherapy regimen, for cutaneous T-cell lymphoma, 381
  for gastric lymphoma, 475
  for non-Hodgkin's lymphoma, 376, 376(t)
Chorea, levodopa usage and, 874
  rheumatic fever and, 117, 118, 118(t)
Chorionic villus sampling, 936
Christmas disease, 335
Chylomicrons, 506, 506(t)

Chylomicrons *(Continued)*
elevated serum levels of, 507
Cicatricial alopecia, 708–709, 709(t)
Cicatricial pemphigoid, 769–770
Ciguatera, 75(t), 76, 78, 1085–1086
Cimetidine, anticholinergic properties of, 1054(t)
for anaphylactic reaction to insect sting, 701
for effects of esophageal dysmotility, in scleroderma, 718
for erythema multiforme, 765
for gastritis, 442(t)
for peptic ulcer, 9, 470
for pruritus, 37
Cinchonism, 95, 1126
Cinnamon flavoring, oral mucosal reaction to, 754
Ciprofloxacin, for atypical mycobacterial infection, 211
for bronchitis, 176(t)
for *Campylobacter jejuni* infection, 14(t)
for chancroid, 666(t)
for cystitis, in female patient, 597
for enteric fever, 139
for enterocolitis (gastroenteritis), in salmonellosis, 14(t), 138
for epididymitis, 609
for gonorrhea, 667(t), 668
for legionnaires' disease, 191
for meningitis, 102(t)
for osteomyelitis, 928(t)
in salmonellosis, 138
for otitis externa, 106(t), 107
for pressure ulcer, 761
for prostatitis, 633, 634
for pyelonephritis, in male patient, 621(t)
for salmonellosis, 14(t), 138, 139, 141(t), 928(t)
in carrier patient, 140, 142
for shigellosis, 14(t)
for traveler's diarrhea, 14(t), 78
for typhoid fever, 141(t)
in carrier patient, 142
for urinary tract infection, in female patient, 597
in male patient, 595(t), 621(t)
Ciprofloxacin prophylaxis, for cystitis, in female patient, 597
Cirrhosis, 405(t), 405–413
complications of, 340, 406–413, 407(t), 408(t), 410(t)
portal hypertension and bleeding esophageal varices as, 406–407, 413–417
hepatitis and, 406, 445
hereditary hemochromatosis and, 346, 406
thrombocytopenia in, 340, 412
Cirrhotic ascites, 409–411, 410(t)
Cisapride, for constipation, 19
for indigestion (dyspepsia), 9
Cisplatin, for bladder cancer, 653
for cervical cancer, 1020
for cutaneous T-cell lymphoma, 381
for lung cancer, 162, 162(t)
for lymphoma, 376(t), 381
for multiple myeloma, 384, 384(t)
for non-Hodgkin's lymphoma, 376(t)
for penile cancer, 656
for testicular cancer, 658
for urethral cancer, 653
Citrate solutions, alkalinization of urine with, in treatment of renal calculi, 664
Clarithromycin, adverse effects of, 132(t)
Clarithromycin *(Continued)*
for atypical mycobacterial infection, 211
for bronchitis, 176(t)
for *Helicobacter pylori* infection, 471
for legionnaires' disease, 191
for mycoplasmal pneumonia, 181
for pharyngitis, 206(t)
for pneumonia, 181
for streptococcal pharyngitis, 206(t)
for toxoplasmosis, 131, 132(t)
Clark levels, in assessment of melanoma, 732, 732(t), 1025(t)
Classic heat stroke, 1078
Claudication, 216, 292, 293
effect of exercise on, 288
Clean intermittent catheterization, for bladder dysfunction, 605
Clemastine, for allergic rhinitis, 693(t)
for pruritus, 37, 37(t)
Clindamycin, adverse effects of, 132(t)
for aspiration pneumonia, 179(t), 183
for bacteremia, 57(t)
for bacterial pneumonia, 179(t), 183
for bacterial vaginosis, 1007
for cellulitis, 740
for lung abscess, 172
for necrotizing infections, 79
for osteomyelitis, 928(t)
for pelvic inflammatory disease, 668(t), 1014(t)
for pneumonia, 179(t), 183
for toxoplasmosis, 131, 132(t)
in AIDS, 50, 133
Clindamycin prophylaxis, for endocarditis, 119(t), 263(t)
Clioquinol, for pemphigoid gestationis, 774
Clobetasol, for lupus erythematosus, 715
for paronychia, 722
for pemphigoid gestationis, 774
for scabies, 745
for vitiligo, 781
Clofazimine, adverse effects of, 88
for atypical mycobacterial infection, 211
for erythema nodosum leprosum, 90
for leprosy, 88, 89
Clofibrate, for hyperlipoproteinemia, 509
Clomipramine, 1130(t)
for depression, 1058(t)
for obsessive-compulsive disorder, 1046
in Tourette syndrome, 827, 828
for panic disorder, 1065
for post-herpetic neuralgia, 743
Clonazepam, 811(t), 1103(t)
for panic disorder, 1065
for seizures, 1106(t)
in epileptic patient, 808, 810, 810(t), 811(t), 817–818
in patient with porphyria, 391
for tics, in Tourette syndrome, 826
Clonidine, for hot flushes, 1004
for hypertension, 272(t), 273, 273(t)
for manifestations of Tourette syndrome, 826, 827
Clorazepate, 1106(t)
Clostridium botulinum toxin, effects of, 75–76
food sources of, 75(t), 76
injections of, for spasmodic dysphonia, 32
Clostridium difficile–associated diarrhea, 12, 13, 14, 14(t)
Clostridium perfringens toxin, food sources of, 75(t)
Clostridium tetani infection, 128–131
Clotrimazole, for candidiasis, 751
for seborrheic dermatitis, 713
Cloxacillin, for carbuncles, 738–739
Clozapine, agranulocytosis due to, 1064
for levodopa-induced psychosis, 876
for schizophrenic disorders, 1064
Cluster headache, 835–836
CNOP chemotherapy regimen, for non-Hodgkin's lymphoma, 376(t)
Coagulation factor deficiencies, 334–338
bleeding due to, 335, 336, 336(t), 337
replacement therapy for, 336(t), 337, 397
Coagulation factor VII, activated, 338
Coagulation factor VIII concentrates, 337, 397, 397(t)
for hemophiliac patient, 336(t), 337, 397
porcine, 338
Coagulation factor VIII inhibitors, 338
Coagulation factor IX concentrates, 337, 397, 397(t)
for hemophiliac patient, 336(t), 337, 397
Coagulopathy, 334–338
cirrhosis and, 412
disseminated intravascular, 342–344
relapsing fever and, 116–117
hypothermia and, 1074
snake bite and, 1081
Coated tongue, 755
Cobalamin. See *Vitamin B_{12}* (cobalamin).
Cocaine, abuse of or poisoning by, 1041, 1042, 1043, 1108(t), 1108–1109
Coccidioidomycosis, 163–165
in AIDS, 49
Codeine, 1119(t)
anticholinergic properties of, 1054(t)
for cough, 22, 23(t), 25
due to common cold, 188
in pericarditis, 289
for migraine, 834
for pain, 2(t)
for painful renal calculi, 662
Cognitive impairment, Alzheimer's disease and, 791
delirium and, 1053
dementia and, 790
multiple sclerosis and, 854
Cognitive therapy, for bulimia nervosa, 1052
for depression, 1059
for obesity, 515
for panic disorder, 1066
Colchicine, adverse effects of, 503–504
for cirrhosis, 406
for gout, 503, 504
for keloids, 726
for pulmonary scleroderma, 719
for urticarial vasculitis, 778
for vasculitis, 720
Cold (common cold), 187–189
Cold agglutinin disease, 305–306, 307, 308
Cold exposure, effects of, 1073–1077
Cold hemoglobinuria, paroxysmal, 306, 307, 308
Cold sores, 741, 751
Cold stress, prevention of, in newborn, 958–959, 965
Cold urticaria, 778
Colectomy, for cancer, 478
for diverticular disease, 425
for ulcerative colitis, 431
Colestipol, for hyperlipoproteinemia, 508
Colic, biliary, 403
Colitis, amebic, 53, 54, 54(t), 55
antibiotic-associated (*Clostridium difficile*–mediated), and diarrhea, 12, 13, 14, 14(t)
cytomegaloviral, in AIDS, 52

Colitis *(Continued)*
hemorrhagic, 11, 13
infectious, 11
pseudomembranous, 12
ulcerative, 426–433, 429(t)
Collagen injections, for intrinsic urethral sphincter deficiency, 607
Colon, adenomas of, 476
amebiasis of, 53, 54, 54(t), 55
cancer of, 476–479
risk factors for, 432, 476
dilatation of, ulcerative colitis and, 431–432
diverticular disease of, 424–426
hemorrhage from, diverticular disease and, 424, 425
inflammation of. See *Colitis.*
perforation of, diverticulitis and, 425
polyps of, 476
resection of. See *Colectomy.*
strictures of, ulcerative colitis and, 432
toxic dilatation of, ulcerative colitis and, 431–432
tumors of, 476–479
risk factors for, 432, 476
ulcerative disease of, 426–433, 429(t)
Colony-stimulating factors, adverse effects of, 329
for aplastic anemia, 301–302
for neutropenia, 328
use of, in patient treated for multiple myeloma, 383, 385
Coma, Glasgow scale for, 890(t)
induction of, in patient with head trauma, 891(t), 892, 894, 894(t)
myxedema, 579
hypothermia due to, 1075
poisoning and, 1089
Reed scale for, 1087(t)
Reye's syndrome and, 847(t)
Combined oral contraceptives. See *Oral contraceptives.*
Comedo ductal carcinoma in situ, 986–987
Comedonal acne, 703–704
COMLA chemotherapy regimen, for non-Hodgkin's lymphoma, 376, 376(t)
Common cold, 187–189
Community-acquired infection, bacteremia as complication of, 57(t)
pneumonia due to, 179(t), 179–184, 191
Compartment syndrome, snake bite and, 1081
Complete heart block (third-degree atrioventricular block), 227, 234–235
myocardial infarction and, 236
Complex(es), premature, 230–233
ventricular, 231–233, 240, 241
Complex partial seizures, treatment of, 808, 809, 810(t), 810–816, 811(t)
Complicated silicosis, 199, 200(t)
Compound nevi, 729
Compresses, for contact dermatitis, 773, 782
Compression(s), chest, in cardiopulmonary resuscitation, 224(t)
and survival of hypothermic patient, 1074
in neonatal resuscitation, 960–961
intermittent pneumatic, in prevention of deep venous thrombosis, 195
Compression dressing, wet-to-dry, for stasis ulcer, 759
Compression neuropathies, 880
Conditioned insomnia, 34–35
Condom(s), for females, 1033
Condom(s) *(Continued)*
for males, 1031, 1032
Conduction block, along peripheral nerves, 885
in heart, 233–236, 234(t)
cardiac arrest due to, 227
infectious endocarditis and, 261
Lyme disease and, 122
myocardial infarction and, 236, 284
Condyloma, giant, 1025
Condyloma acuminatum, 727, 728, 729, 735, 1023
Cone shells, effects of contact with, 1084
Congenital diaphragmatic hernia, 971
Congenital erythropoietic porphyria, 390(t), 392
Congenital heart disease, 241–249, 977
Congenital malformations, as indication for patient transfer to specialty care center, 976
Congenital nevi, 731, 735
Congenital rubella, 125, 126
Congenital syphilis, 673, 673(t)
Congenital toxoplasmosis, 132
Congenital varicella, 68
Congestive heart failure. See *Heart failure.*
Conjunctivitis, 63–66, 64(t), 66(t)
chlamydial, 66, 66(t)
in newborn, 64, 64(t), 1011
cicatricial pemphigoid and, 769
gonococcal, 66, 66(t)
in newborn, 64, 64(t), 668–669
herpes simplex virus infection and, 65, 66, 741
neonatal, 63–65, 64(t)
due to chlamydial infection, 64, 64(t), 1011
due to gonococcal infection, 64, 64(t), 668–669
Connective tissue diseases, 715–719
esophageal motility disorders in, 420, 718
pericarditis associated with, 291
Consolidation therapy, for leukemia. See *Chemotherapy, for leukemia.*
Constipation, 16–19
causes of, 17(t)
treatment of, 17–19
in irritable bowel syndrome, 437(t)
in multiple sclerosis, 853
in typhoid fever, 141
Constrictive pericarditis, 290
Contact dermatitis, 772–773, 782–783
allergic, 772, 773
anthralin-induced, as stimulus to hair growth, 708
irritant, 772, 773
treatment of, 773, 773(t)
Contact urticaria, 779
Contamination, of blood for transfusion, 401
Continuous arteriovenous hemodialysis, for renal failure, 640, 640(t)
Continuous lumbar peridural analgesia, for delivery, 949
Continuous positive airway pressure, for relief of symptoms of pulmonary edema, in heart failure, 254
Continuous venovenous hemodialysis, for renal failure, 640, 640(t)
Contraceptives, 1031–1035, 1033(t)
oral. See *Oral contraceptives.*
use of, by patient with systemic lupus erythematosus, 717
Contractions, tetanic, of uterus, 950
Contrast media, anaphylactoid reaction to, 700
prevention of, 677(t), 700
nephrotoxicity of, 644
Convalescent stage, of pertussis, 144, 144(t)
Convulsions. See *Anticonvulsants* and *Seizure(s).*
Cooling, of patient with heat stroke, 1078
COP-BLAM chemotherapy regimen, for non-Hodgkin's lymphoma, 376, 376(t)
COP-bleo chemotherapy regimen, for cutaneous T-cell lymphoma, 381
COPD (chronic obstructive pulmonary disease), 148, 152–156
management of acute exacerbations of, 23, 154–155
therapy for, 149, 152–156, *155*
Copolymer-1, for multiple sclerosis, 851
Coproporphyria, 390(t), 393
Coral, effects of contact with, 1083, 1084
Coral snake envenomation, 1081, 1082
antivenin for, 1082, 1090(t)
Core rewarming, of hypothermic patient, 1075
Cornea, herpes simplex virus infection of, 741
Coronary artery bypass, for heart failure, 256
Coronary artery disease, 217, 218, 222
cardiac arrest due to, 222
reduction of risk of, by lowering blood pressure, 265, 265(t)
by lowering serum cholesterol levels, 285, 507, 508, 508(t)
by providing estrogen replacement, 1005(t)
risk factors for, 222, 507, 507(t)
treatment of, in patient with hypothyroidism, 579
Corrosive/caustic injury, 1069–1070, 1106–1108
to esophagus, 422
Corset(s), for low back pain, 40
Corticosteroids. See *Steroids* and see also specific drugs, e.g., *Prednisone.*
Cortisone, 553(t)
for adrenocortical insufficiency, 552
in patient with hypopituitarism, 573
perioperative administration of, 903
use of, in patient treated for Cushing's syndrome, 558–559
Corynebacterium diphtheriae infection, 72–74, 73(t)
Cosmetics, use of, to camouflage vitiligo, 781
Cough, 21–25, 22(t)
causes of, 22(t)
pertussis and, 144
secretion-mobilizing effect of, in prevention of atelectasis, 151
treatment of, 21–25, 23(t), 28(t), 29
in patient with common cold, 188
in patient with pericarditis, 289
use of angiotensin-converting enzyme inhibitors and, 25, 275, 700
Cough suppressants, 22, 23(t)
for common cold, 188
Counseling, genetic, about mood disorders, 1057
pre-conception, 933–934
psychological, for obese patient, 516
Cow's milk, 979
Coxiella burnetii infection, 109–110
Coxsackievirus infection, 744

CP chemotherapy regimen, for cutaneous T-cell lymphoma, 381
CPR (cardiopulmonary resuscitation), 223, 224(t), 226
in hypothermic patient, 1074
Crab lice, 746
Crack (cocaine), poisoning by, 1108(t)
Creeping eruption, 748
Crescentic glomerulonephritis, idiopathic, 616–617
Cricopharyngeal dysfunction, 417–418
Critical illness polyneuropathy, 883
Crohn's disease, 433–435, 455
Cromolyn, for allergic rhinitis, 694
for asthma, 680, 681(t)
in pediatric patient, 684–685, 685(t)
in prophylaxis against exercise-induced asthma, 679
Crotalid envenomation, 1080–1082
antivenin for, 1081, 1082, 1090(t)
Crotamiton, for scabies, 746
Croup, viral, 190
Cryopathic hemolytic syndromes, 305(t), 305–308
Cryoprecipitate, 334, 395
for disseminated intravascular coagulopathy, 343
in relapsing fever, 116, 117
for hemophilia, 337
Cryotherapy, for actinic keratosis, 733–734
for keloids, 725–726
for molluscum contagiosum, 744
for myxoid cysts, 725
for prostate cancer, 655
for prostatic hyperplasia, 631
for skin cancer, 711
for warts, 727
Cryptococcosis, in AIDS, 48
Cryptosporidiosis, 15(t), 483, 485
in AIDS, 51, 483
Cubital tunnel syndrome, 880
"Culture-negative" endocarditis, 258, 261
Curettage, for molluscum contagiosum, 744
for skin cancer, 710
Cushing's disease, 554, 555, 556, 557
Cushing's syndrome, 554–559, 558(t)
Cutaneous lesions. See *Skin* and *Dermatitis*.
CVP chemotherapy regimen, for non-Hodgkin's lymphoma, 375
Cyanide, poisoning by, 1109, 1110(t)
antidote for, 1092(t)
Cyanosis, in newborn, 959
in newborn or infant with heart disease, 242–243, 246
treatment of, 243, 244(t)
Cyclobenzaprine, for sleep disturbance, in muscle pain syndromes, 920
Cyclodestructive surgery, for glaucoma, 869
Cyclophosphamide, adverse effects of, 904(t)
for autoimmune hemolytic anemia, 308
for breast cancer, 989
for bullous pemphigoid, 769
for cicatricial pemphigoid, 770
for cutaneous T-cell lymphoma, 381
for glomerulopathy, 613, 614, 619, 620
in lupus erythematosus, 716
for inflammatory myopathies, 718
for leukemia, 367, 374
for lung cancer, 162(t)
for lymphoma, 375, 376(t), 381
for multiple myeloma, 383, 384(t)
for multiple sclerosis, 851–852
for myasthenia gravis, 859
Cyclophosphamide *(Continued)*
for nephritis, in lupus erythematosus, 716
for neuropathy, in vasculitis, 886
for non-Hodgkin's lymphoma, 375, 376(t)
for pemphigus vulgaris, 767
for renal disease, 613, 614, 619, 620
in lupus erythematosus, 716
for rheumatoid arthritis, 904(t), 906
for testicular cancer, 658
for vasculitis, 886
Cyclospora species, infection by, 15(t), 480(t), 483
Cyclosporine, for aplastic anemia, 301
for chronic actinic dermatitis, 786
for epidermolysis bullosa acquisita, 771
for glomerulopathy, 614
for myasthenia gravis, 859
for pemphigus vulgaris, 767
for psoriasis involving nails, 723
therapeutic vs. toxic levels of, 1138(t)
Cyproheptadine, for Cushing's syndrome, 556, 557(t)
for pruritus, 37(t)
in polycythemia, 389
for urticaria, 777, 778
Cyst(s), Bartholin's gland, 1022
echinococcal, in liver, 485
mucous, of lip, 752
myxoid, 725
Cystic duct, obstruction of, 404
Cysticercosis, 482(t), 485
Cystic fibrosis, pancreatitis in, 464
Cystine stones, 664
Cystitis, in female patient, 596–598, 600, 621
in male patient, 595, 596
Cytarabine, for leukemia, 362, 367, 367(t), 368
for multiple myeloma, 384, 384(t)
for non-Hodgkin's lymphoma, 376(t)
Cytomegalic inclusion disease, 743
Cytomegalovirus infection, 743
and adrenalitis, in AIDS, 51
and colitis, in AIDS, 52
and esophagitis, in AIDS, 52
and pneumonia or pneumonitis, 190
in AIDS, 52
and retinitis, in AIDS, 51, 52
in AIDS, 51–52
transfusion-transmitted, 401
prevention of, 396
Cytomegalovirus-negative blood products, 396

Dacarbazine, for Hodgkin's disease, 351(t)
for melanoma, 733
Danazol, for angioedema, 778
for endometriosis, 991
for idiopathic thrombocytopenic purpura, 341
for premenstrual syndrome, 1002, 1003
for thrombocytopenia, in patient with lupus erythematosus, 717
Dandruff, 712
Dantrolene, for neuroleptic malignant syndrome, 1062
for spasticity, 760
in multiple sclerosis, 852
for tetanus, 130
Dapsone, adverse effects of, 87
for bullous pemphigoid, 769
for cicatricial pemphigoid, 770
Dapsone *(Continued)*
for dermatitis herpetiformis, 771
for epidermolysis bullosa acquisita, 770
for erythema multiforme, 765
for leishmaniasis, 86
for leprosy, 87, 88, 89
for linear IgA dermatitis, 772
for *Pneumocystis carinii* pneumonia, in AIDS, 50(t)
for toxoplasmosis, in AIDS, 50, 133
for urticarial vasculitis, 778
for vasculitis, 720
Daunorubicin, for leukemia, 362, 367, 368
DDAVP. See *Desmopressin (DDAVP)*.
DDC (dideoxycytidine), adverse effects of, 44
for acquired immunodeficiency syndrome, 44, 44(t), 45(t)
DDI (dideoxyinosine), adverse effects of, 44
for acquired immunodeficiency syndrome, 44, 44(t), 45(t)
DDT derivatives, poisoning by, 1119–1120, 1120(t)
Death, cardiac, 222. See also *Cardiac arrest*.
risk of, coronary artery disease and, 222
ischemic heart disease and, 222
mitral valve prolapse syndrome and, 252
myocardial infarction and, 222, 226
ventricular dysfunction and, 222, 240
ventricular ectopy and, 222, 227, 232, 252
Debridement, for necrotizing gingivitis, 757
for necrotizing infections, 79
for pressure ulcer, 761
Decompressive microvascular surgery, for trigeminal neuralgia, 864
Decongestant(s), for allergic rhinitis, 693
for common cold, 188
for cough, 21
for respiratory tract infection, 28(t), 29, 188
Decongestant–cough suppressant combinations, 22, 23(t)
Decontamination, gastrointestinal, for poisoning, 1087–1088
Decubitus dermatitis, 760, 761
Decubitus ulcers, 759–762
Deep dermal burns, 1068–1069, 1072
Deep inspiration(s), in prevention of atelectasis, 151
Deep penetrating nevus, 731
Deep venous thrombosis, 192, 296–298
in female patient, 1026–1031
prophylaxis for, 195, 297(t)
risk factors for, 192(t), 195(t), 296(t)
treatment of, 297, 1027–1029, 1028(t)
in pregnant patient, 1030
Deferoxamine, for iron overload, 316, 347, 1093(t)
use of vitamin C with, 316, 347
Defibrillation. See *Cardioversion*.
Degenerative dementia, 790
Degenerative joint disease, 922, 922(t)
Degenerative mitral valve prolapse, 250, 250(t)
Deglycerolized red blood cells, frozen, 394
Dehydration, 71, 540–547, 541(t), 542(t), *546*
cholera and, 70, 71
food poisoning and, 78
pancreatitis and, 459

Dehydration *(Continued)*
pediatric cases of, 540–547, 541(t), 542(t), *546*
Dehydroemetine, for amebiasis, 15(t), 54(t), 55, 480(t), 748
Delayed emesis, 7
Delayed transfusion reactions, 399
Delirium, 1053(t), 1053–1054
anticholinergic medications and, 1054
Delivery, anesthesia for, 948–955
cesarean, anesthesia for, 952–953
pain following, 953
third-trimester bleeding as indication for, 943
estimated date of, 934
labor pain and, 948, 949
premature labor and, 938–939, 939(t)
vaginal, anesthesia for, 949
pain following, 953
Delta hepatitis, 446
Demecarium bromide, for glaucoma, 867(t)
Dementia, 790, 791, 791(t)
Demyelinating polyneuropathy, chronic inflammatory, 884–885
in children, 887–888
Denervation, for pain, in pancreatitis, 468–469
Dental caries, radiation-induced xerostomia and, 359
Dental procedures, prophylaxis against endocarditis in, 119(t), 262(t), 263(t)
Dental sinus tract, 757
Dentures, irritation from, effects of, 754, 757–758
Deoxycoformycin, for leukemia, 372
Dependency, addictive/habituating drug. See *Drug abuse*.
steroid, in patients with pericarditis, 291
vs. drug addiction, 1
Depolarizations, early (premature beats), 230–233, 240, 241
Depression, 1054–1060. See also *Antidepressants*.
Alzheimer's disease and, 792–793
hemiplegia and, 803
multiple sclerosis and, 853, 854, 855
postpartum, 957
sleep disturbance and, 33–34, 34(t)
treatment of, 1058(t), 1058–1060, 1059(t), 1060(t)
de Quervain's thyroiditis, 593–594
Dermal burns, 1068–1069, 1072
Dermatitis, actinic, chronic, 786
atopic (eczema), 762–764
cercarial, 748, 1085
contact, 772–773, 782–783
allergic, 772, 773
anthralin-induced, as stimulus to hair growth, 708
irritant, 772, 773
treatment of, 773, 773(t)
decubitus, 760, 761
fiberglass, 783
immunoglobulin A deposition and, 771–772
linear IgA, 771–772
marine, 748, 1085
seborrheic, 712–713
Dermatitis herpetiformis, 453–454, 771
Dermatomyositis/polymyositis, 717–718
and dysphagia, 420
Dermatophytosis, 722–723, 749–750
Dermatosis (dermatoses), linear IgA, 771–772
occupational, 781–784
Dermatosis (dermatoses) *(Continued)*
pregnancy-related, 773–775, 774(t)
sun exposure and. See *Sun exposure*.
Descending thoracic aorta, aneurysm of, 214
dissection of, 215, 216
Desensitization, to diphtheria antitoxin, 72–73, 73(t)
to penicillin, 698(t)
to sulfasalazine, 428
Desipramine, 1130(t)
for attention deficit hyperactivity disorder, in Tourette syndrome, 827
for depression, 1058(t)
in Alzheimer's disease, 793
for panic disorder, 1065
therapeutic vs. toxic levels of, 1130(t), 1138(t)
Desmopressin (DDAVP), for coagulopathy, in cirrrhosis, 412
for diabetes insipidus, 560–561, 561(t), 562, 563, 575
for hemophilia, 337
for platelet disorders, 339, 340
in renal failure, 639
for urinary incontinence, 603, 604
for von Willebrand's disease, 336(t)
Desquamation, toxic shock syndrome and, 1009, 1010
Desquamative gingivitis, 758
Detrusor dysfunction, and incontinence, 605, 606
Dexamethasone, 553(t)
for adrenocortical insufficiency, 553
in patient with hypopituitarism, 573
for alopecia, 707
for brucellosis, 63
for effects of brain tumors, 899
for effects of metastatic disease, in patient with lung cancer, 157, 158(t)
for enteric fever, 139
for intracranial hypertension, 796, 845
for laryngitis, 30
for lymphoma, 376(t)
for meningitis, 103
for multiple myeloma, 383, 384, 384(t)
for nausea and vomiting, 6, 6(t), 7, 7(t)
for neurobrucellosis, 63
for non-Hodgkin's lymphoma, 376(t)
for salmonellosis, 139, 141
for typhoid fever, 141
for vomiting and nausea, 6, 6(t), 7, 7(t)
use of, in patient being treated for Cushing's syndrome, 556
Dextroamphetamine, use of, in patient receiving opiates for pain, 2
Dextromethorphan, for cough, 22, 23(t), 28(t), 29, 188
Dextrose, calories provided by, in parenteral nutrition, 533
use of, in newborn, 968
in patient receiving insulin for diabetic ketoacidosis, 501, 502
DHAP chemotherapy regimen, for non-Hodgkin's lymphoma, 376, 376(t)
Diabetes Control and Complications Trial, 487, 488(t)
Diabetes insipidus, 559–563, 561(t)
hypopituitarism and, 574–575
Diabetes mellitus, 487–499
acidosis in, 499–502, 500(t)
cardiovascular disease in, 493
classification of, 487, 488(t)
complications of, 492–493, 493(t), 497, 498, 499–502
Diabetes mellitus *(Continued)*
diagnosis of, 487–488, 488(t), 494
gastroparesis in, 884
goiter in, 498
hereditary hemochromatosis and, 346
hypercholesterolemia in, 498
hyperglycemia in, 493, 496, 499
hypertension in, 498
hypoglycemia in, 497
in adults, 487–493
in children and adolescents, 493–499
in pregnant patients, 937–938, 951
effects of, on offspring, 972
insulin-dependent, 487, 489–490, 493–499
hereditary hemochromatosis and, 346
ketoacidosis in, 499–502, 500(t)
management of, 488–492, 493(t), 494–497
anti-oxidants in, 498
diet in, 490, 494
exercise in, 490–491
glucose monitoring in, 488, 495–496, 498
goals of, 489
insulin in, 489, 490, 491, 492, 494–496, 938, 938(t)
intercurrent illness and, 496–497, 1071
oral hypoglycemic agents in, 491, 491(t), 492
pancreas transplantation in, 490
pancreatitis and, 467
patient education in, 488, 494
standards of care in, 492, 492(t)
nephropathy in, 493, 498, 645
neuropathy in, 493, 498, 499, 883–884
non–insulin-dependent, 487, 490–492
pancreatitis and, 467
psychosocial impact of, 497
retinopathy in, 493, 498, 499
Type I, 487, 489–490, 493–499
hereditary hemochromatosis and, 346
Type II, 487, 490–492
Diabetic acidosis, 499–502, 500(t)
Diabetic gastroparesis, 884
Diabetic ketoacidosis, 499–502, 500(t)
Diabetic nephropathy, 493, 498, 645
Diabetic neuropathy, 493, 498, 499, 883–884
Diabetic retinopathy, 493, 498, 499
Diacetylmorphine, 1119(t)
Dialysis, for hyperkalemia, in renal failure, 639(t)
for poisoning, 1089, 1099(t)
for renal failure, 640(t), 640–641, 648
pericarditis associated with, 291
Diaphragmatic hernia, congenital, 971
Diaphragm contraceptive, 1033–1034
Diarrhea, 9–16, *10*, 11(t), 14(t), 15(t)
acute, infectious, 9–16, *10*, 14(t), 15(t)
noninfectious causes of, 11(t)
AIDS and, 12
antibiotic-associated (*Clostridium difficile*–mediated), 12, 13, 14, 14(t)
bloody, *Escherichia coli* infection and, 11, 13
bowel resection and, 458
dehydrating, cholera and, 70, 71
fluid required by child in, *546*
food poisoning and, 12, 75, 78
infectious, acute, 9–16, *10*, 14(t), 15(t)
inflammatory, 9, 11
malabsorption and, 451(t). See also *Malabsorption*.
noninfectious causes of, 11(t)

Diarrhea *(Continued)*
noninflammatory, 11–12
traveler's, 12, 13, 14(t), 78
treatment of, 12–16, 14(t), 15(t)
in cholera, 13, 14(t), 70, 71
in food poisoning, 78
in irritable bowel syndrome, 437(t)
in salmonellosis, 14(t), 16, 137
in ulcerative colitis, 427–428
Diastolic heart failure, 257
Diastolic hypertension. See *Hypertension.*
Diazepam, 1106(t)
as antidote, 1093(t)
for epilepsy, 818(t), 819
in pediatric patient, 820, 821
for febrile seizures, 821
for headache due to trauma, 889
for panic disorder, 1065
for seizures, in epileptic patient, 818(t), 819, 820, 821
in patient with head trauma, 890
for spasticity, 760
in patient with multiple sclerosis, 852
for status epilepticus, 818(t), 819
in pediatric patient, 820
for symptoms of spider bite, 1080
for tetanus, 130
for vertigo, 838(t), 842
use of, as antidote, 1093(t)
in patient with sickle cell disease, 322
Diazoxide, for hypertension, 273(t)
in pregnant patient, 946(t)
Dichlorphenamide, for glaucoma, 867(t)
Diclofenac, for gout, 503(t)
for rheumatoid arthritis, 902(t)
Dicloxacillin, for carbuncles, 739
for otitis externa, 106(t)
Dicyclomine, for irritable bowel syndrome, 9, 437(t)
Dideoxycytidine (DDC), adverse effects of, 44
for acquired immunodeficiency syndrome, 44, 44(t), 45(t)
Dideoxyinosine (DDI), adverse effects of, 44
for acquired immunodeficiency syndrome, 44, 44(t), 45(t)
Dientamoeba fragilis infection, 480(t), 483
Diet. See also *Dietary recommendations*; *Nutritional support.*
after cholera treatment, 72
after rehydration therapy for diarrhea, 12–13
after small bowel resection, 458
after surgery for obesity, 517
and prevention of colorectal cancer, 476
for bulimic patient, 1051(t), 1051–1052
for diabetic patient, 490, 494
for infant, 977–979
for obese patient, 512–515, 513(t)
for preterm infant, 974–975
gluten-free, 453
for dermatitis herpetiformis, 771
high-fiber, for constipation, 18
for irritable bowel syndrome, 437
liquid, for diabetic patient with intercurrent illness, 496
low-calorie, for obesity, 513, 513(t), 514, 515
low-fat, for hyperlipoproteinemia, 507–508
for obesity, 513
low-phosphate, for renal disease or renal failure, 567
low-potassium, for hyperkalemia, in renal failure, 647
Diet *(Continued)*
low-protein, for portosystemic encephalopathy, 407
for renal disease or renal failure, 612, 645, 648
low-sodium, for cirrhotic ascites, 410
for hypertension, 267
in aldosteronism, 572
for Meniere's disease, 842
for renal disease or renal failure, 611, 646, 648
very-low-calorie, for obesity, 514–515
Dietary recommendations, in aldosteronism, 572
in bulimia nervosa, 1051(t), 1051–1052
in celiac sprue, 453
in cirrhotic ascites, 410
in constipation, 18
in coronary artery disease, 507–508
in dermatitis herpetiformis, 771
in diabetes mellitus, 490, 494
in gluten-sensitive enteropathy, 453, 771
in hyperkalemia, 647
in hyperlipoproteinemia, 507–508
in hypertension, 267, 267(t)
in hypertension due to aldosteronism, 572
in irritable bowel syndrome, 437
in Meniere's disease, 842
in obesity, 512–515
in pancreatitis, 460, 467
in peptic ulcer disease, 470
in portosystemic encephalopathy, 407
in premenstrual syndrome, 1001
in renal disease or renal failure, 567, 611, 612, 645, 646, 648
in short bowel syndrome, 458
in sprue, 453
in ulcerative colitis, 427
Diffuse alopecia, 707(t), 707–708
Diffuse cutaneous leishmaniasis, 83
Diffuse otitis externa, 105, 106(t)
Diffuse ulcerative nongranulomatous enteritis, idiopathic, 456
Diflorasone, for vitiligo, 781
Diflunisal, for pain, 1
for rheumatoid arthritis, 902(t)
Digestion, disorders of, 8, 9. See also *Malabsorption.*
Digitalis preparations, 1111(t)
anticholinergic properties of, 1054(t)
for atrial fibrillation, 228(t)
for heart failure, 256
in children, 245(t)
for supraventricular tachycardia, 239(t)
pediatric dosages of, 1111(t)
poisoning by, 1109–1110, 1111(t)
therapeutic vs. toxic levels of, 1111(t), 1138(t)
Digitolingual paresthesias, migraine and, 833, *833*
Dihydroergotamine, for headache, 829
Diiodohydroxyquin (iodoquinol), adverse effects of, 482
for *Blastocystis hominis* infection, 483
for *Dientamoeba fragilis* infection, 480(t)
for *Entamoeba histolytica* infection, 15(t), 54, 54(t), 480(t), 482
Dilatation, esophageal, 419, 420, 421
urethral, for prostatic hyperplasia, 631
for strictures, 659–661
Diloxanide, for amebiasis, 15(t), 53, 54(t), 480(t), 482
Diltiazem, 1107(t)
for angina pectoris, 221(t)
Diltiazem *(Continued)*
for atrial fibrillation, 228(t)
for hypertension, 277(t)
for myocardial infarction, 283, 284
for Raynaud's phenomenon, 718
poisoning by, 1107(t)
Dimenhydrinate, for nausea and vomiting, 6(t)
for vertigo, 838(t)
in Meniere's disease, 842
Dimercaprol (BAL), as antidote, 1093(t)
for arsenic poisoning, 882
for lead poisoning, 1116(t)
Dinitrochlorobenzene, for warts, 729
Diphencyprone, for warts, 724
Diphenhydramine, as antidote, 1093(t)
for allergic drug reaction, 696(t), 697
for allergic rhinitis, 693(t)
for anaphylactic reaction, 677, 677(t), 696(t), 701
for effects of dopamine antagonists, 5–6
for effects of haloperidol, 1042, 1043
for nausea and vomiting, 6(t), 7(t)
for oral erythema multiforme, 764
for pain, in sickle cell disease, 321
for pruritus, 37, 37(t)
in erythema multiforme, 764
for urticaria, 696(t), 777
poisoning by, 1103(t)
use of, in patient receiving amphotericin B, 165, 169
in patient receiving vancomycin, 699
in patient undergoing radiocontrast studies, 677(t), 700
Diphenoxylate, 1119(t)
for diarrhea, in ulcerative colitis, 427, 428
Diphtheria, 72–74, 73(t)
Diphtheria antitoxin, 72, 73, 73(t)
desensitization to, 72–73, 73(t)
Diphtheria toxoid, 74
Diphtheritic pseudomembrane, 72
Diphyllobothrium latum infestation, 481(t), 485
Dipivefrin, for glaucoma, 867(t), 868
Dipylidium caninum infestation, 481(t), 485
Dipyridamole, anticholinergic properties of, 1054(t)
for thrombotic thrombocytopenic purpura, 345
use of, in patient with mitral valve prolapse, 251
Diquat, poisoning by, 1121
Disabled patient, cardiac rehabilitation in, 288
Discharge, of newborn, from special care nursery, 977
Disease-modifying antirheumatic agents, 903–906, 904(t)
use of, in pediatric patient, 909–910
Dislocation, of shoulder, 929–930
Disopyramide, for arrhythmias, 238(t)
for atrial fibrillation, 228(t)
therapeutic vs. toxic levels of, 1138(t)
Dissection, aortic, 215–216
Disseminated coccidioidomycosis, 164, 165
Disseminated gonococcal infection, 668, 669
Disseminated histoplasmosis, 166, 168
Disseminated intravascular coagulopathy, 342–344
relapsing fever and, 116–117
Disseminated Lyme disease, 122–124
Dissociation, electromechanical, 225
cardiac arrest due to, 222

Distal axonopathy, 880
Diuresis, induction of, in poisoning victim, 1089
Diuretics, for cirrhotic ascites, 410
for diabetes insipidus, 561, 561(t)
for heart failure, 254, 255
in children, 245(t)
for hyperkalemia, in renal failure, 638, 639(t)
for hypertension, 268–269, 270(t), 277–278
for hypokalemia, in aldosteronism, 571
for Meniere's disease, 842
for renal disease or renal failure, 611, 638, 646
high dosages of, and changes in serum cholesterol levels, 265, 266(t)
and changes in serum glucose levels, 266, 267(t)
Diverticula, of gastrointestinal tract, 418, 422–426
Dobutamine, for heart failure, 254
in children, 245(t)
Docusate sodium, use of, in multiple sclerosis, 853
Domperidone, for levodopa-induced nausea and vomiting, 874
Donath-Landsteiner hemolytic anemia, 306, 307, 308
Donovanosis, 670–671
Dopamine, for heart failure, 254
in children, 245(t)
for hypotension, in anaphylaxis, 677, 677(t)
in hypothermia, 1074
in sepsis, 60
for renal failure, 638
Dopamine receptor agonists, for Parkinson's disease, 877, 878
Doxazosin, for hypertension, 272(t), 274
in patient with pheochromocytoma, 588–589, 591(t)
Doxepin, 1130(t)
for depression, 1058(t)
for headache, 832
for muscle-contraction headache, 832
for neuropathic pain, 888
for pruritus, 37
for urticaria, 696(t), 778
Doxorubicin, for bladder cancer, 653
for cutaneous T-cell lymphoma, 381
for Hodgkin's disease, 351(t)
for lung cancer, 162(t)
for lymphoma, 351(t), 376(t), 381
for multiple myeloma, 383, 384(t)
for non-Hodgkin's lymphoma, 376(t)
for testicular cancer, 658
for urethral cancer, 653
Doxycycline, adverse effects of, 98
for acne, 704
for acute exacerbations of chronic obstructive pulmonary disease, 23
for arthritis, in Lyme disease, 120(t)
for bronchitis, 175(t)
in COPD, 23
for brucellosis, 62
for carditis, in Lyme disease, 120(t)
for chlamydial infection, 23, 109, 668(t), 669, 669(t), 671, 1012, 1012(t)
for cholera, 14(t), 71, 75
for legionnaires' disease, 191
for Lyme disease, 120(t), 121
for lymphogranuloma venereum, 671
for malaria, 97(t), 98
for meningitis, in Lyme disease, 120(t)
Doxycycline *(Continued)*
for mycoplasmal pneumonia, 181, 190
for nongonococcal urethritis, 608, 669, 669(t)
for pelvic inflammatory disease, 668(t), 1014(t)
for pneumonia, 179(t), 181, 190
for prostatitis, 634
for psittacosis, 109
for Q fever, 110
for relapsing fever, 116, 116(t)
for rickettsioses, 110, 124, 143(t)
for Rocky Mountain spotted fever, 124
for syphilis, 672, 673(t)
for typhus fevers, 143(t)
for urethritis, 608, 669, 669(t)
Drainage, of anorectal abscess, 440
of blood, from brain, 795, 797
of buboes, in chancroid, 666
of carbuncles, 738, *739*
of cerebrospinal fluid, in reduction of intracranial pressure, 891, 893, 894(t)
via shunt, and meningitis, 99–100
of lung abscess, 172
of lymph nodes, in tularemia, 136
of pancreatic duct, for pain of pancreatitis, 467–468
of pericardial effusion, 289
of pleural fluid, 171
of sinuses, 203
Dressing changes, in burned patient, 1072
Dressings, for pressure ulcer, 761
for stasis ulcer, 759
Dronabinol, for nausea and vomiting, 6, 6(t)
Droperidol, 1123(t)
for nausea and vomiting, 6, 6(t)
for vertigo, 838(t)
Drug abuse, 1040–1045, 1041(t)
alcoholic. See *Alcohol* entries.
barbiturate, 1044, 1104, 1105(t)
benzodiazepine, 1104
flumazenil for, 1044, 1094(t)
hallucinogenic, 1043, 1043(t), 1112
inhalant, 1045, 1045(t)
intravenous, endocarditis associated with, 57(t), 257, 258(t), 259
narcotic, 1043(t), 1043–1044, 1118–1119
naloxone for, 1044, 1096(t), 1118, 1119
sedative hypnotic, 1044(t), 1044–1045, 1127–1128, 1129(t)
solvent, 1045, 1045(t), 1110–1112
stimulant, 1041(t), 1041–1043, 1102, 1108(t), 1108–1109
withdrawal in. See *Withdrawal (abstinence syndrome).*
Drug addiction, fear of, 1
types of. See under *Drug abuse.*
vs. drug tolerance, 1
Drug approvals (1993), 1142(t)
Drug effects, and addiction. See *Drug abuse.*
and alopecia, 708
and asthma, 679
and delirium, 1054
and dyskinesia, 874–875, 1062
and erythema multiforme, 765
and hemolytic anemia, 305(t), 306, 306(t), 307, 308
in patient with G6PD deficiency, 310, 310(t)
and insomnia, 33
and intoxication. See *Poisoning.*
and intracerebral hemorrhage, 796–797
and malabsorption, 456
Drug effects *(Continued)*
and neuropathies, 884, 888
and pancreatitis, 462, 462(t)
and pericarditis, 291
and pruritus, 36
and renal failure, 644
and respiratory depression, naloxone for, 962, 1044
and thrombocytopenia, 340, 341(t)
Drug monitoring, therapeutic, laboratory reference values for, 1138(t)
Drug precautions, for patient with G6PD deficiency, 310, 310(t)
for patient with porphyria, 391(t), 392
for patient with renal failure, 641(t), 644, 648
Drug reactions, 695(t), 695–700
treatment of, 695–700, 696(t), 698(t)
Drug tolerance, vs. addiction, 1. See also *Drug abuse.*
Drug withdrawal, and abstinence syndrome. See *Withdrawal (abstinence syndrome).*
Dry mouth, 751
due to radiation therapy, 359
Ductal carcinoma in situ, 986(t), 986–987
Ductal hyperplasia, atypical, 985
Dumb rabies, 112
Duncan's syndrome, 104
Duodenum, diverticula of, 423
ulcer of, 469–472
Helicobacter pylori infection and, 469, 471–472
NSAID-induced, 469, 472
Dural puncture, during attempted peridural block, 954–955
Dyazide, anticholinergic properties of, 1054(t)
Dyclonine, for herpetic gingivostomatitis, 757
for oral erythema multiforme, 764
Dye exposure, and urticaria, 778
Dysesthesia, cutaneous, low-dose antidepressants for, 776
painful, multiple sclerosis and, 854
Dysfunctional uterine bleeding, 993–994
Dysfunctional voiding. See also *Incontinence.*
in girls, 601, 604
Dyskinesia, levodopa usage and, 874–875
tardive, use of neuroleptics and, 1062
Dysmenorrhea, 998–1000
treatment of, 999(t), 999–1000
Dyspepsia, 9, 441, 470
Dysphagia, 417(t), 417–422, 418(t), 419(t)
hemiplegia and, 806
myasthenia gravis and, 856
Dysphonia, muscle tension, 31
spasmodic, 32
Dysplasia, bronchopulmonary, 973
Dysplastic nevus, 730, 735
Dyspnea, transfusion-induced, 400
Dysreflexia, sympathetic, as complication of tetanus, 130
Dysthymia, 1056
Dystonia, drug-induced, 874, 1062, 1063
medications for, 1042
Dystrophy, twenty-nail, 723–724

Ear(s), infection/inflammation of, 105–107, 106(t), 172–174, 175(t)
common cold and, 188
exposure to moisture and, 1084–1085

Ear(s) *(Continued)*
pain in, otitis externa and, 105, 106
tinnitus and, 38
wetting of, otitis externa due to, 1084–1085
Early access, in management of cardiac arrest, 223
Early depolarizations (premature beats), 230–233, 240, 241
Early Lyme disease, 120(t), 120–121
Early syphilis, 671, 672, 673, 673(t)
Eating, binge, 1048, 1050(t)
occurrence of, in bulimia nervosa, 1048, 1049
therapeutic approach to, 1052
swallowing difficulties in, 417(t), 417–422, 418(t), 419(t)
Eating behavior, disturbances of, 1048(t)–1051(t), 1048–1053
Echinococcal cysts, in liver, 485
Echothiophate, for glaucoma, 867(t)
Eclamptic convulsions, 946(t), 947
Ectopic ACTH syndrome, 556
Ectopic beats, premature, 230–233
ventricular, 231–233, 240, 241
ventricular, cardiac death due to, 222, 227, 232, 252
development of, during cardiac rehabilitation, 287, 288
mitral valve prolapse and, 252
premature, 231–233, 240, 241
Ectopic pregnancy, 940–941
Eczema (atopic dermatitis), 762–764
EDAP chemotherapy regimen, for multiple myeloma, 384, 384(t)
Edema, angioneurotic, 753, 778
drug reaction and, 276, 695–696, 700
cerebral, poisoning and, 1098
nephrotic syndrome and, 611
pulmonary, congestive heart failure and. See *Heart failure*.
malaria and, 96
poisoning and, 1089, 1098
renal failure and, 639
transfusion and, 400
snake bite and, 1081
Edrophonium, bradycardia as side effect of, 858
use of, in myasthenia gravis, 856–857
in supraventricular tachycardia, 239(t)
EDTA (ethylenediamine tetra-acetic acid), as antidote, 1091(t)
for lead poisoning, 1116(t)
Effluvium, anagen, 708, 708(t)
telogen, 707(t), 707–708
Effusion, pericardial, 289, 290
pleural, 170(t), 170–171
lung cancer and, 158, 158(t)
Eflornithine, for trypanosomiasis, 747
Elbow pain, overuse injury and, 921, 931
Elderly patient, cardiac rehabilitation in, 288
gallstone disease in, 404–405
hypertension treatment in, 265, 265(t), 279
laryngeal degeneration in, 33
meningitis in, 99, 100(t)
Electrical activity, pulseless, 225
cardiac arrest due to, 222, 223, 225
treatment of, 224(t), 225, 225(t)
Electrical burns, 1069
Electrical stimulation, in amelioration of neuropathic pain, 888
in management of tinnitus, 39
Electroconvulsive therapy, for depression, 1059
Electrodesiccation, for molluscum contagiosum, 744
for skin cancer, 710
Electrolyte(s). See also *Fluid replacement therapy*.
in rehydration solutions, 71(t)
in stool of cholera patient, 71(t)
Electrolyte losses, gastrointestinal, 540(t)
Electromechanical dissociation, 225
cardiac arrest due to, 222
Electron beam radiation therapy, for cutaneous T-cell lymphoma, 381
Embolism. See also *Thromboembolism*.
atrial fibrillation and, 229, 801
lower extremity arterial occlusion due to, 294
mitral valve prolapse and, 251–252
pulmonary, 192–195, 296
diagnosis of, 192, *193*
differential diagnosis of, 192(t)
prevention of, 195
treatment of, 192–194, 195(t), 297, 1030
sources of, 294(t)
Emergency management, of asthma, 688–689, *690*
of cardiac arrest, *223*, 223–226
advanced life support in, 224–226
basic life support in, 223
cardiopulmonary resuscitation in, 223, 224(t), 226
"chain of survival" in, *223*
defibrillation in, 223, 224, 224(t), 225
drugs in, 224, 224(t), 225, 226
early access in, 223
treatment protocols in, 224(t), 225
of dehydration, in pediatric patient, 543
of hypertension, 273(t)
of suspected myocardial infarction, 280, 280(t)
Emesis. See *Vomiting*.
Emollients, for atopic dermatitis, 763
for contact dermatitis, 773
Emphysematous cholecystitis, 405
Empyema, of chest, 171
of gallbladder, 405
Enalapril, for heart failure, 255
in children, 245(t)
for hypertension, 275(t), 278(t)
Encephalitis, epidemic, 844(t), 845, 845(t)
postinfectious, 844(t), 845, 845(t)
rabies and, 111
sporadic, 844(t), 844–845, 845(t)
toxoplasmal, in AIDS, 50, 132–133, 790
varicella and, 68
viral, 68, 111, 127, 844(t), 844–845, 845(t)
Encephalomyelitis, measles and, 127
Encephalopathy, AIDS and, 52
lead-induced, 1115
treatment of, in children, 1116(t)
portosystemic, 407(t), 407–408
Endarterectomy, carotid, 800
Endocarditis, infectious. See *Infectious endocarditis*.
Endolymphatic hydrops, 841
Endolymphatic sac-enhancement surgery, for Meniere's disease, 842–843
Endometriosis, 989–993
Endometritis, bacteremia as complication of, 57(t)
chlamydial, 1011
Endometrium, cancer of, 1015–1018, 1016(t)
risk of, in relation to postmenopausal estrogen use, 1005
Endoscopic retrieval, of esophageal foreign body, 422
Endoscopic sclerotherapy, for bleeding esophageal varices, 414, 415, 415(t), 416
Endotracheal intubation, of newborn, 961
of patient with Guillain-Barré syndrome, 882
End-stage renal disease, 642, 642(t), 648
Enoxaprin, approved use of, 298
Entamoeba histolytica infection, 15(t), 53–55, 54(t), 480(t), 482–483
of skin, 748
Entamoeba polecki infection, treatment of, 480(t)
Enteral nutrition, conditions contraindicating, 530–531, 531(t)
delivery of, to preterm infant, 974
Enteric fever, 138–139
Enteritis, radiation injury and, 455
ulcerative nongranulomatous, idiopathic, 456
Enterobacteriaceae, bone infection by, treatment of, 927–928, 928(t)
Enterobius vermicularis infestation, 481(t), 484, 486, 748
Enterococcal endocarditis, treatment of, 259, 260(t)
Enterocolitis, necrotizing, 975
salmonellosis and, 14(t), 16, 137–138
Enterocytozoon bieneusi infection, 15(t), 483
in AIDS, 51
Enterohepatically recirculated drugs, 1088(t)
Enteropathy, AIDS and, 458
gluten-sensitive, 453
and dermatitis herpetiformis, 771
Entrapment, of popliteal artery, 293
Entrapment neuropathies, 880
Enuresis, 604–608
in children, 601–604
Eosinophilic gastroenteritis, 456
EP chemotherapy regimen, for lung cancer, 162(t)
Ephedrine, use of, before administration of radiocontrast media, 677(t)
Epidemic encephalitis, 844(t), 845, 845(t)
Epidemic influenza. See *Influenza*.
Epidemic typhus (louse-borne typhus), 142, 143(t)
Epidermal necrolysis, toxic, 765
Epidermolysis bullosa acquisita, 770–771
Epididymitis, 608–609
Epidural anesthetic injection, for delivery, 949, 952
complications of, 954
for low back pain, 41
Epigastric pain, causes of, 441
peptic ulcer and, 470
Epilepsy, 806–823, 807(t)
in adolescents and adults, 806–819
in infants and children, 819–823
in newborn, 821
in pregnant patients, 809
treatment of, 807–823, 810(t), 811(t), 818(t), 1103(t)
poisoning by drugs used in, 1102, 1103(t)
therapeutic vs. toxic levels of drugs used in, 1138(t)
Epinephrine, adverse effects of, 867–868

Epinephrine *(Continued)*
for anaphylaxis, 677, 677(t), 678, 695, 696(t), 701, 702
for angioedema, 696
for asthma, 681
for cardiac arrest, 224(t), 225, 226
for glaucoma, 867(t)
for urticaria, 777
in neonatal resuscitation, 961
in prevention of allergic reaction to contrast media, 700
Epinephryl borate, for glaucoma, 867(t)
Epiphrenic diverticula, 423
Episiotomy, pain due to, 956
Episodic vertigo, 837–841
treatment of, 837–841, 838(t)–840(t), *839*
Epstein-Barr virus, antibodies to, in AIDS patients, 52
infection by, 103–104
Epulis fissuratum, 757–758
Erection, abnormal, in sickle cell disease, 323
Ergonovine, for postpartum hemorrhage, 956
Ergotamine, for cluster headache, 836
for headache due to trauma, 889
for migraine, 834
Erosive lichen planus, 753
Eructation, 8
Eruption(s), creeping, 748
drug reaction and, 696–697
light, polymorphous, 786
papulosquamous, 711–715
polymorphic, in pregnancy, 775
seabather's, 748, 1085
varicelliform, Kaposi's, 741, 764
Erysipelas, 739
Erythema chronicum migrans, Lyme disease and, 120–121
Erythema infectiosum, 744
Erythema marginatum, in rheumatic fever, 117
Erythema migrans, 755
Erythema multiforme, 764(t), 764–766, 765(t)
Erythema nodosum, sarcoidosis and, 198
Erythema nodosum leprosum, 90
Erythrityl tetranitrate, for angina pectoris, 218(t), 1118(t)
Erythroblastosis fetalis, 329–334, 330(t)
Erythrocytes. See *Red blood cells.*
Erythroderma, psoriatic, 714
toxic shock syndrome and, 1009
Erythromycin, for acne, 704
for bronchitis, 175(t)
for bullous pemphigoid, 769
for *Campylobacter jejuni* infection, 14(t)
for chancroid, 666(t)
for chlamydial infection, 66, 66(t), 109, 668(t), 669, 669(t), 671, 1012, 1012(t)
in newborn, 64, 64(t)
in pregnant patients, 1012, 1012(t)
for cholera, 72
for conjunctivitis, 66, 66(t)
in newborn, 64, 64(t)
for diphtheria, 73
for granuloma inguinale, 671
for guttate psoriasis, 713
for legionnaires' disease, 191
for lymphogranuloma venereum, 671
for mycoplasmal pneumonia, 181, 190
for pertussis, 144
for pneumonia, 179(t), 181, 190
for psittacosis, 109
for psoriasis, 713
Erythromycin *(Continued)*
for rat-bite fever, 114
for relapsing fever, 116(t)
for rheumatic fever, 118
for secondary bacterial infection, in contact dermatitis, 783
for urethritis, 669, 669(t)
for whooping cough, 144
Erythromycin prophylaxis, for endocarditis, 119(t), 263(t)
for recurrent rheumatic fever, 118(t)
for streptococcal infection, 118(t)
Erythromycin-sulfisoxazole, for otitis media, 173(t)
Erythroplakia, 736, 757
Erythroplasia of Queyrat, 734
Erythropoietic porphyria, congenital, 390(t), 392
Erythropoietic protoporphyria, 390(t), 392
Erythropoietin, for anemia, in patient with multiple myeloma, 386
in patient with renal failure, 647–648
for AZT (zidovudine) toxicity, 44
ESAP chemotherapy regimen, for non-Hodgkin's lymphoma, 376, 376(t)
Eschar, separation of, from pressure ulcer, 761
Escherichia coli infection, 11, 13
hemolytic uremic syndrome following, 11, 344
Escherichia coli toxins, food sources of, 75(t)
Esmolol, 219(t), 1124(t)
for angina pectoris, 219(t)
for arrhythmias, 238(t)
in patient with pheochromocytoma, 591
for atrial fibrillation, 228(t)
for myocardial infarction, 282(t)
for thyroid storm, 584
Esophageal dysphagia, 419, 419(t)
Esophagitis, in AIDS, 48, 52
Esophagus, achalasia of, 419–420
adenocarcinoma of, 421
balloon dilatation of, 419–420
Barrett's, 421
bleeding from varices of, 413–417, *414*, 415(t)
bougienage of, 421
cancer of, 421
candidal infection of, in AIDS, 48
carcinoma of, 421
caustic injury to, 422
cytomegalovirus infection of, in AIDS, 52
dilatation of, 419, 420, 421
diverticula of, 418, 422–423
effect of dermatomyositis/polymyositis on, 420
foreign body in, 422
hemorrhage from varices of, 413–417, *414*, 415(t)
infection/inflammation of, in AIDS, 48, 52
motility disorders of, 419–420
dermatomyositis/polymyositis and, 420
scleroderma and, 420, 718
obstruction of, 417(t), 417–422, 418(t), 419(t)
peptic stricture of, 420–421
pill-induced injury to, 421
pneumatic dilatation of, 419–420
radiation injury to, 422
reflux of gastric contents into, 24, 30, 420–421
in scleroderma, 420, 718
Esophagus *(Continued)*
rings of, 421
scleroderma involving, 420, 718
spasm of, 420
squamous cell carcinoma of, 421
strictures of, 420, 421, 422
tumors of, 421
varices of, bleeding from, 413–417, *414*, 415(t)
webs in, 421
Estazolam, 1106(t)
Estimated date of delivery, 934
Estradiol, for gonadotropin deficiency, 573
for osteoporosis, 1004
postmenopausal use of, to reduce recurrence of cystitis, 598
Estrogen(s). See also *Oral contraceptives.*
for acne, 705
for atrophic vaginitis, 1004
for dysfunctional uterine bleeding, 994
for gonadotropin deficiency, 573
for hot flushes, 1004
for hyperlipoproteinemia, 509
for osteoporosis, 525, 1004
for platelet disorders, in renal failure, 639
postmenopausal use of, 567, 1004–1006
and reduced risk of cardiovascular or cerebrovascular disease, 1005, 1005(t)
to lower rate of recurrent cystitis, 598
to prevent osteoporosis, 525, 1004
Ethacrynic acid, for hypertension, 270(t)
Ethambutol, for atypical mycobacterial infection, 211
for tuberculosis, 207, 208, 208(t)
in AIDS, 46
Ethanol. See *Alcohol* entries.
Ethchlorvynol, 1129(t)
poisoning by, 1127, 1129(t)
Ethinyl estradiol, for gonadotropin deficiency, 573
Ethinyl estradiol contraceptive, 1035
Ethionamide, adverse effects of, 88
for leprosy, 88, 89
Ethosuximide, 811(t), 1103(t)
for epilepsy, 808, 810, 810(t), 811(t), 816
in pediatric patient, 823
therapeutic vs. toxic levels of, 1138(t)
Ethotoin, for epilepsy, 816
Ethylenediamine tetra-acetic acid (EDTA), as antidote, 1091(t)
for lead poisoning, 1116(t)
Ethylene glycol, poisoning by, 1110–1112
Etidronate, for osteoporosis, 525
for Paget's disease of bone, 529
Etodolac, for arthritis, in lupus erythematosus, 715
for rheumatoid arthritis, 902(t)
Etomidate-induced coma, in management of head trauma, 891(t), 892, 894, 894(t)
Etoposide. See *VP16 (etoposide).*
Exanthema subitum, 744
Exenteration, pelvic, for cervical cancer, 1021
Exercise. See also *Physical therapy.*
after sports injury, 930, 931, 932
by diabetic patient, 490–491
by hypertensive patient, 268
by obese patient, 515–516
by patient with COPD, 153
by patient with multiple myeloma, 387
in cardiac rehabilitation, 286, 287, 288
in relief of pain, 4, 920
in lower back, 40

Exercise *(Continued)*
in relief of premenstrual syndrome, 1001
in vestibular rehabilitation, 840
range-of-motion, for patient with bursitis or tendinitis, 921
Exercise-induced asthma, 679, 691
Exercise testing, in cardiac rehabilitation, 287
Exertional heat stroke, 1078
Exhaustion, heat exposure and, 1077(t), 1077–1078, 1078(t)
Exostoses, mandibular, 757
Expectorants, for cough, 23(t)
External ear, infection/inflammation of, 105–107, 106(t)
exposure to moisture and, 1084–1085
External hemorrhoids, 440, 441
External rewarming, of hypothermic patient, 1075
Extracorporeal photophoresis, for cutaneous T-cell lymphoma, 382
Extracorporeal rewarming, of hypothermic patient, 1075–1076
Extramedullary plasmacytoma, 386
Extrapyramidal effects, of neuroleptics, 1062
Extremity, lower. See *Lower extremity*.
upper, deep venous thrombosis in, 296, 297
Exudative pleural effusion, 170, 170(t)
Eye(s), care of, in facial paralysis (Bell's palsy), 871
elevated pressure in, 866
treatment of, 866–869, 867(t)
examination of, in child with rheumatoid arthritis, 911
in diabetic patient, 498–499
inflammation of. See also such inflammations as *Conjunctivitis*.
due to cytomegalovirus infection, in AIDS, 51, 52
due to herpes simplex virus infection, 65, 66, 741
due to varicella-zoster virus infection, 742
in Graves' disease, 583
in juvenile rheumatoid arthritis, 911
in leprosy, 91
in sarcoidosis, 198
in toxoplasmosis, 132
irrigation of, after chemical exposure, 1070, 1086
neovascularization in, and retinopathy, in sickle cell disease, 326
orbit of, as site of infection, 204, 739–740
painful congestion of, in tularemia, 135
painful movement of, in optic neuritis, 864
weakened muscles of, in myasthenia gravis, 856, 860
Eyelashes, louse infestation of, 746

Fab, as antidote, 1094(t)
FAB (French-American-British) classification, of acute lymphoblastic (lymphocytic) leukemia, 364(t), 365(t)
of acute myelogenous leukemia, 361(t)
Facial pain, due to temporomandibular disorders, 914
in region of trigeminal nerve, 862–864
in multiple sclerosis, 854
Facial paralysis (Bell's palsy), 869–871, *870*
in Lyme disease, 120(t), 123
Factor deficiencies, 334–338
bleeding due to, 335, 336, 336(t), 337
replacement therapy for, 336(t), 337, 397
Factor VII, activated, 338
Factor VIII concentrates, 337, 397, 397(t)
for hemophiliac patient, 336(t), 337, 397
porcine, 338
Factor VIII inhibitors, 338
Factor IX concentrates, 337, 397, 397(t)
for hemophiliac patient, 336(t), 337, 397
Fallopian tube, implantation of fertilized ovum in, 940
infection of. See also *Pelvic inflammatory disease*.
chlamydial, 1011
occlusion of, to effect sterilization, 1035
resection of, in surgery for ectopic pregnancy, 941
in surgery for endometrial cancer, 1016
FAM chemotherapy regimen, for metastatic gastric cancer, 475
Familial adenomatous polyposis, 476
Familial medullary thyroid cancer, 585
Family planning, natural, 1035
Famotidine, for gastritis, 442(t)
for peptic ulcer, 9, 470
Fanconi's anemia, 299
Farmer's lung disease, antigens in, 202(t)
Fascicular block, 235, 236
Fasciitis, necrotizing, 78, 740
plantar, 921, 932
Fasciolopsis buski infestation, 481(t), 485
Fasciotomy, for snake bite, 1081
Fat emulsions, in parenteral nutrition, 533, 538
Fatigue, in multiple sclerosis, 853–854
Fat malabsorption, 450
due to pancreatic insufficiency, 466–467
Fat-restricted diet, for hyperlipoproteinemia, 507–508
for obesity, 513
Febrile seizures, 820–821
Feces, examination of, for fat, 450
in cholera, 71(t)
in food poisoning, 77
Feeding, of infants, 977–979
of preterm infants, 974–975
Feet. See *Foot (feet)*.
Felbamate, for epilepsy, 810, 810(t), 811(t), 812
in pediatric patient, 822
Felodipine, 1107(t)
for hypertension, 277(t)
Female patient. See also sex-specific entries (*Menstruation*; *Pregnancy*) and particular organs (e.g., *Uterus*).
androgenetic alopecia in, 706, 707
bacteremia in, 57(t)
bacterial urinary tract infection in, 596(t), 596–601, 621–622
bulimia nervosa in, 1048
chlamydial infection in, 1011, 1012(t)
contraceptives for, 1031–1035
gonadotropin deficiency in, 573–574
pelvic inflammatory disease in, 57(t), 668, 668(t), 1012(t), 1012–1014, 1013(t), 1014(t)
sterilization of, 1034–1035
thrombophlebitis in, 1026–1031
Feminization, testicular, 996
Femoral artery, aneurysm of, 295
Femorofemoral graft, 293
Femoropopliteal arterial occlusion, 292–293
Femorotibial arterial occlusion, 292–293
Fenfluramine, for obesity, 516, 516(t)
for premenstrual syndrome, 1003
Fenoprofen, for rheumatoid arthritis, 902(t)
Fentanyl, 1119(t)
for cesarean section, 952
for pain, 2
in labor, 948, 949
transdermal, 2
Ferrous sulfate, for iron deficiency, 303
iron content of preparations of, 1114(t)
Fertility awareness, and contraception, 1035
Fertility-enhancing therapy, for patient with endometriosis, 992–993
Fertilized ovum, ectopic implantation of, 940
Fetal circulation, persistent, 972
Fetal distress, 950–951
Fetal epilepsy syndrome, 809
Fetal surveillance, 939–940, 940(t)
Fetal warfarin syndrome, 1030
Fetus. See also *Fetal* entries.
diagnosis of genetic disorders in, 315–316, 935–936
heart disease in, 242
hemolytic disease of, 329–334, 330(t)
impaired development of, rubella and, 125
nonstress testing of, 939, 940
retarded growth of, 969–970, 970(t)
ultrasonographic assessment of, 331, 936–937, 937(t)
Fever, 19–21
boutonneuse, 143(t)
development of, after surgery for congenital heart disease, 247
drug reaction and, 697
enteric, 138–139
Haverhill, 113, 114
neutropenia and. See *Neutropenia, and infection*.
pancreatitis and, 459
pericarditis and, 289
Pontiac, 191
Q, 109–110
rat-bite, 113–114, 114(t)
relapsing, 114–117, 115(t), 116(t)
rheumatic, 117(t), 117–119, 118(t)
and carditis, 117, 118, 118(t), 119, 250
seizures associated with, 820–821
spotted, 143, 143(t)
Rocky Mountain, 124–125, 143(t)
transfusion and, 399
typhoid, 140–142, 141(t)
typhus, 142–143, 143(t)
Fever blisters, 741, 751
Fiberglass dermatitis, 783
Fiber-rich diet, for constipation, 18
for irritable bowel syndrome, 437
Fibric acid derivatives, for hyperlipoproteinemia, 509
Fibrillation, atrial, 227(t), 227–230, 228(t), 238(t), 240
myocardial infarction and, 283
stroke risk associated with, 229, 801, 801(t)
ventricular, 241
cardiac arrest due to, 222, 223, 225
myocardial infarction and, 283
treatment of, 224(t), 225
in hypothermic patient, 1074
Fibroid, of uterus, 1014–1015
Fibroma, in oral cavity, 753, 758
due to ill-fitting dentures, 757–758
Fibrosis, cystic, pancreatitis in, 464

Fibrosis *(Continued)*
hepatic, hemochromatosis and, 346
myocardial, scleroderma and, 719
pulmonary, lupus erythematosus and, 716
silicosis and, 199
Fibrostenotic Crohn's disease, 435
Fibrous hyperplasia, focal, of buccal mucosa, 753
inflammatory, 757–758
Fifth disease, 744
Filter, inferior vena caval, for thromboembolism, 194, 297, 1030
Finasteride, for benign prostatic hyperplasia, 632
Finger injuries, sports-related, 931
Fire coral, effects of contact with, 1084
First aid, for person wounded or poisoned by contact with marine animals, 1082–1083
First-degree atrioventricular block, 233–234
First-degree burns, 1068, 1072
Fish, contact with, bite wounds or envenomation due to, 1083
ingestion of, toxins consumed in, 75(t), 76, 1085, 1086
Fish-handler's disease, 1084
Fissured tongue, 755
Fistula, anal, 440
bronchopleural, 171
Fistulizing Crohn's disease, 434–435
Flatus, excessive, 8
Flat warts, 727
Flatworm infestation, 481(t), 482(t), 485, 486
Flea-borne typhus, 142
Flecainide, for arrhythmias, 238(t)
for atrial fibrillation, 228(t)
therapeutic vs. toxic levels of, 1138(t)
Fleroxacin, for cystitis, in female patient, 597
Floor of mouth, lesions of, 756–757
Fluclorolone, for polymorphic eruption of pregnancy, 775
Fluconazole, for candidiasis, 595(t), 751, 1007
in AIDS patient, 48
in patient with multiple myeloma, 386
for coccidioidomycosis, 165
for cryptococcosis, in AIDS patient, 48
for onychomycosis, 722
for vulvovaginitis, 1007
Flucytosine, for cryptococcosis, in AIDS patient, 48
for endocarditis, 260(t)
Fludarabine, for leukemia, 374
Fludrocortisone, 553(t)
for adrenocortical insufficiency, 552
for orthostatic hypotension, in diabetes mellitus, 884
use of, in patient receiving mitotane, 558
Fluid management, in patient with acute renal failure, 637–638
Fluid overload, in chronic renal failure, 646
Fluid replacement solutions, 70, 70(t), 71
electrolyte content of, 71(t)
Fluid replacement therapy, for burned patient, 1070, 1070(t)
for child or infant, 538–547, 539(t), 540(t)
for child with burn injury, 1070, 1070(t)
for child with complications of leukemia, 368
for diabetic patient with intercurrent illness, 496
Fluid replacement therapy *(Continued)*
for newborn, 968
for patient bitten by pit viper, 1081
for patient with head trauma, 890, 891
in acute infectious diarrhea, 12
in adrenal crisis, 553
in cholera, 70, 70(t), 71
in dehydration, 78
in diabetes insipidus, 560
in diabetic ketoacidosis, 501
in enterocolitis due to salmonellosis, 137
in food poisoning, 78
in heat illnesses, 1077, 1078
in hypotension accompanying anaphylaxis, 677, 677(t), 696(t)
in hypothermia, 1075
in pancreatitis, 459
in plague, 108
in Reye's syndrome, 846
in salicylate poisoning, 1127(t)
in salmonellosis, 137
in sepsis, 60
in toxic shock syndrome, 1010
Fluke infestation, 481(t), 485
Flumazenil, for benzodiazepine overdose, 1044, 1094(t)
Flunisolide, for allergic rhinitis, 694, 694(t)
for asthma, 681(t)
Flunitrazepam, 1106(t)
Fluocinolone, for contact dermatitis, 782
Fluocinonide, for alopecia, 708
Fluoride, for osteoporosis, 525–526
Fluoride gel, applied to prevent tooth decay, in xerostomia, 751
Fluoroquinolones. See specific agents, e.g., *Ciprofloxacin.*
5-Fluorouracil, for actinic keratosis, 734, 785
for breast cancer, 989
for colorectal cancer, 479
for gastric cancer, 475
for warts, 729
Fluoxetine, 1130(t)
for bulimia nervosa, 1052
for depression, 1059(t)
in Alzheimer's disease, 793
in multiple sclerosis, 855
for obsessive-compulsive disorder, in Tourette syndrome, 828
for panic disorder, 1066
poisoning by, 1112
Fluoxymesterone, for paroxysmal nocturnal hemoglobinuria, 311
Fluphenazine, 1123(t)
for post-herpetic neuralgia, 743
for schizophrenic disorders, 1063–1064
potency of, as neuroleptic, 1062
Flurazepam, 1106(t)
Flurbiprofen, for dysmenorrhea, 999(t)
for gout, 503(t)
for rheumatoid arthritis, 902(t)
Flutamide, for benign prostatic hyperplasia, 632
Flutter, atrial, 238(t), 239–240
Fluvastatin, for hyperlipoproteinemia, 508
Fluvoxamine, for depression, 1059(t)
Fly bites, and tularemia, 134
Flying squirrel–borne typhus, 143(t)
Focal fibrous hyperplasia, of buccal mucosa, 753
Focal glomerulosclerosis, 614
Folate, deficiency of, 311, 313
for anemic patient, 313
for female patient with epilepsy, 809
for patient using sulfasalazine, 427
Folate *(Continued)*
for patient with thalassemia, 317
for patient with tropical sprue, 454
repigmentation with, in vitiligo, 781
Folinic acid (leucovorin), as antidote, 1095(t)
use of, with pyrimethamine, 50, 131
Follicle-stimulating hormone, for effects of hypopituitarism, 574
Follicular carcinoma, of thyroid, 585, 587
Folliculitis, 737–739
pruritic, in pregnancy, 775
Folliculitis decalvans, 709
Food allergens, and atopic dermatitis, 763
and pruritus ani, 776
Food-borne illnesses, 12, 74–78, 75(t), 137, 1085–1086
Foot (feet), effects of cold immersion on, 1076
fungal infection of, 749
overuse injury to, 921, 932
pain in, sickle cell disease and, 323
warts on, 727
Forceps delivery, 950
Fordyce granules, 751
Foreign body impaction, in airway, 182
in esophagus, 422
Formula feedings, for infants, 978
for preterm infants, 975
Foscarnet, for cytomegalovirus infection, in AIDS, 52
for herpes simplex virus infection, 742
Fosinopril, for hypertension, 275(t)
Fosphenytoin, for epilepsy, 815, 819
for status epilepticus, 819
Fourth-degree burns, 1069
Fracture(s), hip, in osteoporosis, 526
pelvic, and bladder trauma, 624
vertebral, in ankylosing spondylitis, 913
in osteoporosis, 522, 523, 524
Francisella tularensis infection, 134–136
Free-base cocaine, poisoning by, 1108(t)
Freezing injury, 1076–1079
French-American-British (FAB) classification, of acute lymphoblastic (lymphocytic) leukemia, 364(t), 365(t)
of acute myelogenous leukemia, 361(t)
Fresh frozen plasma, 395
for disseminated intravascular coagulopathy, 343
in relapsing fever, 117
for hemophilia, 337
for thrombotic thrombocytopenic purpura, 345
Frontal bone, infection of, 204
Frostbite, 1076–1077
treatment of, 1076(t), 1076–1077
Frostnip, 1076
Frozen deglycerolized red blood cells, 394
Fugu, poisoning by, 1086
Full-spectrum lights, in interruption of seasonal mood disorder, 1053
Full-thickness burns, 1069, 1072
Fulminant hepatic failure, due to hepatitis, 444
Fungal infection, and endocarditis, 260(t), 261
in AIDS patient, 46(t), 48–50, 168, 170
in neutropenic patient, 328
in patient with multiple myeloma, 386
of lungs, 163–170
in AIDS patient, 48, 49
of nails, 723–724, 750
of scalp, 709, 749
of sinuses, 203

Fungal infection *(Continued)*
of skin, 749–750
and necrosis, 80
vs. bacterial or protozoal pathogens, in colonization of vagina, 1007(t)
Furazolidone, adverse effects of, 482
for cholera, 14(t), 71
for giardiasis, 15(t), 480(t), 482
for isosporiasis, 455
for salmonellosis, 141(t)
for traveler's diarrhea, 14(t)
for typhoid fever, 141(t)
Furious rabies, 111
Furosemide, anticholinergic properties of, 1054(t)
for cirrhotic ascites, 410
for heart failure, 254, 255
in children, 245(t)
for hyperkalemia, in renal failure, 639(t)
for hypertension, 270(t)
for intracranial hypertension, 795(t), 796
for renal disease or renal failure, 611, 638
Furuncles, 738

Gabapentin, for epilepsy, 810, 810(t), 811(t), 812–813
GABHS infection (group A beta-hemolytic streptococcal infection). See also *Streptococcal infection.*
necrosis due to, 78, 79
pharyngitis due to, 117, 204–207, 206(t)
Gallbladder, inflammation of, 9, 402–405. See also *Gallstones.*
resection of, for calculi or inflammation, 403, 404
Gallstones, 9, 402–405
hemolytic anemia and, 317
pancreatitis due to, 461
salmonellosis and, 140, 142
Gamma globulin. See *Immune globulin.*
Gammopathy, monoclonal, 383, 885
Ganciclovir, for cytomegalovirus infection, 190
in AIDS, 51, 52
Gangrene, 740
and eschar in pressure ulcer, 761
Gardnerella vaginalis infection, 1007
Gaseousness, 8–9
Gastric acid, aspiration of, 182
as complication of obstetric anesthesia, 953, 954
excessive secretion of, 457
reflux of. See *Gastroesophageal reflux.*
Gastric atony and dilation, in patient with migraine, 833, *834*
Gastric diverticula, 423
Gastric emptying, disordered, in diabetes mellitus, 884
Gastric inflammation. See *Gastritis.*
Gastric lavage, for poisoning, 1087
in warming of hypothermic patient, 1075
Gastric surgery, for cancer, 474, 475
for obesity, 516–517
for polyps, 472
for ulcer, 472
Gastric tumors, 472–475
Gastric ulcer, 469–472
Helicobacter pylori infection and, 469, 472
malignant, 474
NSAID-induced, 469, 472
Gastrinoma, 457
Gastritis, 441–443, 442(t)
Gastroenteritis, 442
eosinophilic, 456
salmonellosis and, 14(t), 16, 137–138
Gastroesophageal reflux, and cough, 24
and dysphagia, 420, 421
and laryngitis, 30
and stricture formation, 420–421
in scleroderma, 420, 718
Gastrointestinal electrolyte losses, 540(t)
Gastrointestinal tract, decontamination of, for poisoning, 1087–1088
diverticula of, 418, 422–426
dysfunction of, in patient with migraine, 833, *834*
effects of iron therapy on, 303
exposure of, to toxins, 1086–1087. See also *Poisoning.*
hemorrhage from, due to portal hypertension, 407, 413–417, 443
infection of, causing bacteremia, 57(t)
obstruction of, in preterm infant, 976
scleroderma involving, 420, 718
surgery of, prophylaxis against endocarditis in, 119(t), 263(t)
tests of function of, laboratory reference values for, 1141(t)
Gastrointestinal tularemia, 135
Gastroparesis, diabetic, 884
Gastropathy, portal hypertensive, 407, 443
Gastroplasty, for obesity, 516
Gemfibrozil, for hyperlipoproteinemia, 509
General anesthesia, for delivery, 949–950, 952–953
complications of, 953–954
Generalized gingival hyperplasia, 758
Generalized myasthenia gravis, 860–861
Generalized pustular psoriasis, 713
Gene therapy, for thalassemia, 317
Genetic counseling, about mood disorders, 1057
Genital lesions. See also sex-specific organ entries.
Haemophilus ducreyi infection and, 666
herpes simplex virus infection and, 741
human papillomavirus infection and, 727, 728, 729, 735, 1023
trauma and, 626
Genitourinary tract. See *Genital lesions* (and sex-specific organ entries); *Urinary* entries; *Urogenital tract.*
Gentamicin, for bacteremia or sepsis, 57(t)
in newborn, 970(t)
for conjunctivitis, in newborn with gonococcal infection, 64
for endocarditis, 259, 260(t)
for granuloma inguinale, 671
for meningitis, 102(t)
for neutropenia and infection, 328
for pelvic inflammatory disease, 668(t), 1014(t)
for pericarditis, 291
for prostatitis, 633
for sepsis or bacteremia, 57(t)
in newborn, 970(t)
for toxic shock syndrome, 1010
for tularemia, 136
for urinary tract infection, in male patient, 595(t)
therapeutic vs. toxic levels of, 1138(t)
Gentamicin prophylaxis, for endocarditis, 119(t), 263(t)
Gentian violet, for candidal vulvovaginitis, 1006
Geographic tongue, 755
German measles, 125–127
Germ cell tumor, of testis, 657–658
Gestational age, 964–965
morbidity in relation to, *967*
Giant cell arteritis (temporal arteritis), 830, 922–923
Giant cell granuloma, peripheral, 758
Giant condyloma of Buschke-Lowenstein, 1025
Giant nevus, 731, 735
Giardiasis, 455, 479–480
treatment of, 15(t), 455, 480, 480(t), 482
Gilles de la Tourette syndrome, 823–828
Gingival lesions, 757, 758
cicatricial pemphigoid and, 769, 770
herpes simplex virus infection and, 740, 757
Glandular tularemia, 135
Glanzmann's thrombasthenia, 339
Glasgow coma scale, 890(t)
Glass fibers, exposure to, and dermatitis, 783
Glaucoma, 866–869, 867(t)
Glioma, 830, 896–898
Glipizide, for diabetes mellitus, 491, 491(t), 492
Global hypoventilation, 148, 149
Glomerular diseases, 609–620. See also *Glomerulonephritis.*
vs. tubulointerstitial or vascular diseases, 642, 643(t)
Glomerulonephritis, 615–617
lupus erythematosus and, 716
poststreptococcal, 617–618, 737
Glomerulosclerosis, focal, 614
Glossitis, 755
Glossopyrosis, idiopathic, 755–756
Glucagon, as antidote, 1095(t)
for anaphylaxis, 677, 677(t), 695, 696(t)
for hypoglycemia, in diabetes mellitus, 497
use of, in management of foreign body in esophagus, 422
Glucocorticoid-suppressible hyperaldosteronism, 570, 571, 572
Glucocorticoid therapy. See *Steroids* and see also specific drugs, e.g., *Prednisone.*
Glucose, abnormal serum levels of. See *Hyperglycemia*; *Hypoglycemia.*
metabolism of, effects of antihypertensive drugs on, 266, 267(t)
monitoring of serum levels of, in diabetic patient, 488, 495–496, 498. See also *Diabetes mellitus.*
in infant of diabetic mother, 972
in newborn, 968, 972
use of, in coma due to poisoning, 1089
in diabetic hypoglycemia, 497
in hyperkalemia due to renal failure, 638, 639(t)
in neonatal hypoglycemia, 968, 972
in porphyria, 883
in Reye's syndrome, 846, 847, 847(t)
in status epilepticus, 818(t)
Glucose-6-phospate dehydrogenase deficiency, 309, 310, 310(t)
Gluten-free diet, 453
for dermatitis herpetiformis, 771
Gluten-sensitive enteropathy, 453
and dermatitis herpetiformis, 771
Glutethimide, 1129(t)
poisoning by, 1044, 1127, 1129(t)
Glyburide, for diabetes mellitus, 491, 491(t), 492
Glycerin, for glaucoma, 867(t), 868

Glycerol, for intracranial hypertension, 795(t), 796
Glycerol rhizolysis, percutaneous, for trigeminal neuralgia, 863
Glycolic acid, for melasma, 780
Goiter, 563–565, 592, 593
  diabetes mellitus and, 498
Gold therapy, adverse effects of, 340, 904–905
  for pemphigus vulgaris, 767
  for rheumatoid arthritis, 904, 904(t)
    in pediatric patient, 910
Gonadotropin(s), deficiency of, 573–574
  for effects of hypopituitarism, 574
Gonadotropin-releasing hormone, for effects of hypopituitarism, 574
Gonadotropin-releasing hormone agonists, for endometriosis, 991
  for premenstrual syndrome, 1003
  for prostatic cancer, 656
  for prostatic hyperplasia, 632
  for uterine leiomyoma, 1015
Gonorrhea, 666–669, 667(t), 1013
  conjunctivitis due to, 64, 64(t), 66, 66(t)
  neonatal, 64, 64(t), 668–669
Goserelin, in postpartum management of pemphigoid gestationis, 774–775
Gout, 502–505
  treatment of, 503(t), 503–505
    in patient with polycythemia, 389
G6PD deficiency, 309, 310, 310(t)
Graft(s), aortobifemoral, 216, 217, 293
  autogenous vein, in surgery for occlusive disease of lower extremity arteries, 293–294
  axillofemoral, 217, 293
  femorofemoral, 293
  prosthetic, in repair of aortic lesions, 213, 214, 216, 217
    in surgery for aortoiliac occlusive disease, 216, 217, 293
    in surgery for occlusive disease of lower extremity arteries, 293, 294
  skin, for stasis ulcer, 759
  xenogeneic, in management of burns, 1072
Graft-versus-host disease, transfusion-associated, 400
    prevention of, 396
Grain alcohol. See *Alcohol* entries.
Gram-negative organisms, endocarditis due to, 259
    treatment of, 259, 260(t), 261
  pneumonia due to, 179(t), 183, 186
Granisetron, for nausea and vomiting, 5, 6(t)
Granule(s), Fordyce, 751
Granulocyte colony-stimulating factor. See *Growth factors, hematopoietic.*
Granulocyte-macrophage colony-stimulating factor. See *Growth factors, hematopoietic.*
Granulocyte transfusion, 395
Granuloma, giant cell, peripheral, 758
  pulmonary, coccidioidomycosis and, 164
  pyogenic, oral, 758
  sarcoid, 196
Granuloma inguinale, 670–671
Graves' disease, 580–584
Gray platelet syndrome, 339
Great arteries, transposition of, repair of, 246
Greater trochanteric bursitis, 921
Griseofulvin, for dermatophytosis, 722, 749, 750
Griseofulvin *(Continued)*
  for molluscum contagiosum, 744
  for onychomycosis, 722, 750
  for tinea, 749, 750
Group A beta-hemolytic streptococcal infection (GABHS infection). See also *Streptococcal infection.*
  necrosis due to, 78, 79
  pharyngitis due to, 117, 204–207, 206(t)
Growth factors, hematopoietic, adverse effects of, 329
    for aplastic anemia, 301–302
    for neutropenia, 328
    use of, in patient treated for multiple myeloma, 383, 385
Growth hormone, deficiency of, 574
  hypersecretion of, 548–550
Growth retardation, intrauterine, 969–970, 970(t)
  ulcerative colitis and, 432
Guaifenesin, for cough, 23(t)
  for upper respiratory tract infection, 28(t)
Guanabenz, for hypertension, 272(t), 273
Guanadrel, for hypertension, 271, 272(t)
Guanethidine, for hypertension, 271, 272(t)
Guanfacine, for hypertension, 272(t), 273
Guillain-Barre syndrome, 881–882, 887
  vs. chronic demyelinating inflammatory polyneuropathy, 885
Gummatous syphilis, 673(t)
Guttate hypomelanosis, idiopathic, 781
Guttate psoriasis, 713

HACEK pathogens, endocarditis due to, 259
    treatment of, 259, 260(t), 261
Haemophilus ducreyi infection, 666, 666(t)
Haemophilus influenzae infection, cellulitis due to, 740
  conjunctivitis due to, neonatal, 64, 64(t)
  meningitis due to, 99, 100, 101, 101(t)
  pneumonia due to, 180
    AIDS and, 47
Haemophilus species, bone infection by, treatment of, 927, 928(t)
Hair follicle infections, 737–739
Hair loss, 706–709, 706(t)–709(t)
  nail lesions associated with, 723–724
Hairy cell leukemia, 372–373
Hairy leukoplakia, in AIDS, 52, 756
Hairy tongue, 755
Halazepam, 1106(t)
Hallucinogens, 1043(t)
  abuse of or poisoning by, 1043, 1112
Halobetasol, for scabies, 745
Halofantrine, adverse effects of, 96
  for malaria, 94(t), 95
Halogenated hydrocarbons, poisoning by, 1112, 1113(t)
Haloperidol, 1123(t)
  adverse effects of, drugs for, 1042, 1043
  for agitation, in Alzheimer's disease, 793
  for chorea, in rheumatic fever, 118
  for delirium, 1054
  for nausea and vomiting, 6, 6(t)
  for schizophrenic disorders, 1063
  for stimulant overdose, 1042
  for tics, in Tourette syndrome, 825–826
Hand(s), fungal infection of, 750
  pain in, sickle cell disease and, 323
  trauma to, sports-related, 931
Hand-foot-mouth disease, 744
Hand-foot syndrome, in sickle cell disease, 323
Hansen's disease, 87–91
Hard palate, lesions of, 754
Harmful drinking, 1037
Hashimoto's disease, 592–593
Haverhill fever, 113, 114
Hazardous drinking, 1037
Hazardous marine animals, effects of contact with, 1082–1084
Head, pain in. See *Headache.*
  positioning of, in management of dysphagia, 418
    in treatment of vertigo, 837, *839*
    to lower intracranial pressure, 795, 891
  trauma to, 889(t), 889–895
    and formation of subdural hematoma, 830–831, 889
    and vertigo, 839(t)
    in adults, 889–892
    in children, 892–895
Headache, 828–836, *832*, 916
  dural puncture and, 955
  head trauma and, 889
  migraine, 832–835
    aura and paresthesias associated with, 833, *833*
    gastric atony and dilation accompanying, 833, *834*
    vertigo associated with, 840(t)
Head lice, 709, 746
Healing, of burns, 1068
Hearing loss, Meniere's disease and, 841
Heart. See also *Cardiac* entries.
  catheterization of, in patient with myocardial infarction, 283
  emboli originating in, and occlusion of lower extremity arteries, 294
    and stroke, 801
  functional assessment of, in patient with diphtheria, 73
  hypoplastic, surgery for, 246
  inflammation of. See *Carditis*; *Infectious endocarditis*; *Pericarditis.*
  iron deposition in, effects of, 346
  lupus erythematosus involving, 716
  scleroderma involving, 719
  tamponade of, 289–290
  transplantation of, 246, 257
  trauma to, and pericarditis, 291
Heart attack. See *Cardiac arrest* and *Myocardial infarction.*
Heart block, 233–236, 234(t)
  cardiac arrest due to, 227
  infectious endocarditis and, 261
  Lyme disease and, 122
  myocardial infarction and, 236, 284
Heart disease, congenital, 241–249, 977
  coronary. See *Coronary artery disease.*
  endocarditis risk in, 257, 262(t)
  fetal, 242
  in pregnant patient, 248–249, 951
  ischemic, 217–218
    angina as symptom of, 217, 218
    cardiac arrest due to, 222
    coronary atherosclerosis and, 218. See also *Coronary artery disease.*
  lupus erythematosus and, 716
  rheumatic, 117, 118, 250, 250(t)
    prophylaxis against endocarditis in, 119, 119(t)
  scleroderma and, 719
  sickle cell syndromes and, 326

Heart disease *(Continued)*
uncorrected congenital cases of, effects of, 248
valvular. See *Mitral* entries and *Infectious endocarditis.*
Heart failure, 252–257
congenital heart disease and, 242, 243–245, 977
hereditary hemochromatosis and, 346
infectious endocarditis and, 261
mitral regurgitation and, 250, 261
rheumatic carditis and, 250
sickle cell disease and, 326
treatment of, 253–257
in cardiac rehabilitation, 288
in patient with chronic renal failure, 643–644
in pediatric patient, 245, 245(t)
Heart sounds/heart murmurs, mitral valve prolapse and, 251
Heart transplantation, for congestive heart failure, 257
for hypoplastic left heart syndrome, 246
Heated irrigating solutions, in rewarming of hypothermic patient, 1075
Heat illnesses, 1077(t), 1077–1078, 1078(t)
Heavy hydrocarbons, 1112–1113
Hebra's disease, 764–765
Heel pain, overuse injury and, 921, 932
Helicobacter pylori infection, and gastritis, 442
and peptic ulcer disease, 469, 471–472
Helminthiasis, 479, 481(t)–482(t), 483–486
cutaneous, 748
Hemangioma, in oral cavity, 756
Hemarthrosis, hemophilia and, 335, 336(t), 337
Hematemesis, gastritis and, 441, 442
poisoning and, 1099
Hematogenous osteomyelitis, 924, 925
Hematogenous pyelonephritis, 620–621
Hematologic laboratory reference values, 1135(t)–1137(t)
Hematoma. See also *Hemorrhage.*
formation of, in hemophilia, 335
intracerebral. See *Hemorrhage, intracerebral.*
subdural, 830–831
headache associated with, 830
head trauma and, 830–831, 889
Hematopoietic growth factors, adverse effects of, 329
for aplastic anemia, 301–302
for neutropenia, 328
use of, in patient treated for multiple myeloma, 383, 385
Hematuria, hemophilia and, 337
Heme, defects in synthesis of, and porphyria, 389, 390(t). See also *Porphyria.*
Hemiacidrin, for struvite stones, 664
Hemicrania, paroxysmal, 836
Hemin, for porphyria, 391, 883
Hemiplegic patient, incapacitated by stroke. See *Stroke syndrome.*
rehabilitation for, 801–806, *802*, 802(t)–804(t)
Hemochromatosis, 345–348, 346(t)
acquired, 346, 346(t), 347, 1113–1115
chelation therapy for, 316, 347, 1093(t)
toxic iron ingestion and, 1113–1115
transfusion and, 316, 401
hereditary, 346, 347, 406
phlebotomy for, 347
screening for, 347, *348*
Hemochromatosis *(Continued)*
toxic iron ingestion and, 1113–1115
transfusion and, 316, 401
Hemodialysis, for poisoning, 1089
for renal failure, 640, 640(t), 648
Hemofiltration, for renal failure, 640
Hemoglobin H disease, 315, 315(t), 317
Hemoglobinopathies, 314–327
Hemoglobin SC disease. See *Sickle cell disease.*
Hemoglobinuria, march, 310
paroxysmal cold, 306, 307, 308
paroxysmal nocturnal, 299, 309, 310, 311
Hemolytic anemia, 305–311
autoimmune, 305(t), 305–308
fetal/neonatal, 329–334, 330(t)
gallstones associated with, 317
microangiopathic, *Escherichia coli* infection and, 11, 344
nonimmune, 308–311, 309(t)
sickle cell disease and, 324. See also *Sickle cell disease.*
thalassemia and, 316, 317
Hemolytic disease of fetus and newborn, 329–334, 330(t)
Hemolytic loxoscelism, 1079
Hemolytic transfusion reactions, 398–399
Hemolytic uremic syndrome, 11, 344
Hemoperfusion, for poisoning, 1089, 1099(t)
Hemophilia, 334–338
bleeding due to, 335, 336, 336(t), 337
replacement therapy for, 336(t), 337, 397
Hemorrhage. See also *Hemorrhagic* entries.
antepartum, 941–944, 951
aplastic anemia and, 300
cerebral, 794–798, 795(t), 801
neonatal, 973–974
cirrhosis and, 412
colonic, diverticular disease and, 424, 425
disseminated intravascular coagulopathy and, 342–343
diverticular, 424, 425
drug-induced, 796–797
esophageal variceal, 413–417, *414*, 415(t)
gastrointestinal, portal hypertension and, 407, 413–417, 443
hemophilia and, 335, 336, 336(t), 337
heparin use and, 193
hypertensive, intracerebral, 794
prevention of recurrence of, 795(t), 796
intestinal, typhoid fever and, 142
intracerebral, 794–798, 795(t)
anticoagulant use and, 796, 801
neonatal, 973–974
intracranial, 794–798
headache associated with, 829, 830
head trauma and, 830–831, 889
hemophilia and, 335
neonatal, 973–974
risk of, with anticoagulant use, 796, 801
surgery for, 795, 797, 891
intramuscular, hemophilia and, 335, 336, 337
intraventricular, neonatal, 973–974
joint, hemophilia and, 335, 336(t), 337
malaria and, 96
mucocutaneous, hemophilia and, 335, 336(t), 337
muscle, hemophilia and, 335, 336, 337
oral, hemophilia and, 335, 337
platelet disorders and, 339–342
postpartum, 956
Hemorrhage *(Continued)*
risk factors for, during anticoagulant therapy, 194(t)
subarachnoid, 829
headache associated with, 829
transplacental, Rh isoimmunization due to, 329–334
uterine, dysfunctional, 993–994
vaginal, late in pregnancy, 941–944
pathologic causes of, 993(t)
variceal, esophageal, 413–417, *414*, 415(t)
vitamin K deficiency and, 520, 521
Hemorrhagic blisters, due to snake bite, 1080
Hemorrhagic colitis (hemorrhagic diarrhea), 11, 13
Hemorrhoids, 440–441
Hemosiderosis. See *Iron overload.*
Heparin, for disseminated intravascular coagulopathy, 343–344
in relapsing fever, 116
for myocardial infarction, 282
for stroke, 797, 800(t)
for thromboembolism, 192, 193, 194, 195, 296, 1028, 1029
in pregnancy, 297, 1030
hemorrhage associated with use of, 193
risk factors for, 194(t)
low molecular weight, 298, 1030
for deep venous thrombosis, 195, 298, 1030–1031
modifying dosage of, based on activated partial thromboplastin time, 192, 193(t)
resistance to, 194
thrombocytopenia induced by, 193, 340
Hepatic abscess, amebic, 55
treatment of, 15(t), 54(t), 54–55
Hepatic crisis, in sickle cell disease, 323
Hepatic encephalopathy, 407(t), 407–408
Hepatic failure, in porphyria, 392
in viral hepatitis, 444
Hepatic fibrosis, in hereditary hemochromatosis, 346
Hepatic iron deposition, 346, 347
Hepatic transplantation, 413, 416
Hepatitis, 443–450
alcoholic, 406
cirrhosis due to, 406, 445
hepatocellular carcinoma risk in, 412, 445
immunization against, 447–448, 448(t)
interferon for, 406, 448–449, 449(t)
Q fever and, 109–110
transfusion-transmitted, 401, 446
Hepatoerythropoietic porphyria, 390(t), 392
Hepatoma, cirrhosis and, 412–413
porphyria and, 393
viral hepatitis and, 412, 445
Hepatomegaly, in sickle cell disease, 323
Hepatorenal syndrome, 411–412
Hereditary angioedema, 778
Hereditary hemochromatosis, 346, 347, 406
phlebotomy for, 347
screening for, 347, *348*
Hereditary metabolic disorders, and Reye's syndrome, 846, 846(t)
Hereditary myasthenic syndromes, 862
Hereditary neuropathies, 886
Hereditary nonpolyposis colorectal cancer syndromes, 476
Hereditary pancreatitis, 465
Hermansky-Pudlak syndrome, 339
Hernia, diaphragmatic, congenital, 971

Herpes labialis, 751
Herpes simplex virus infection, 740–742
acyclovir for, 741, 751, 844
in immunocompromised patient, 52
in patient with erythema multiforme, 765
AIDS and, 52
cerebral, 844
cutaneous, 740–742
erythema multiforme associated with, 764
foscarnet for, 742
genital, 740–741
immunodeficiency and, 52, 756
ocular, 65, 66, 741
oral, 740, 741, 751, 754, 756, 757
Herpes virus 6 infection, 744
Herpes zoster (shingles). See *Varicella-zoster virus infection.*
Herpetic gingivostomatitis, 740, 757
Herpetiform aphthous ulcers, 753
Heterophyes heterophyes infestation, 481(t), 485
Hidradenitis suppurativa, 739
Hidradenoma, vulvar, 1022
High-density lipoprotein, 506, 506(t)
diminished serum levels of, treatment of, 510
High-fiber diet, for constipation, 18
for irritable bowel syndrome, 437
High-grade lymphoma, 375(t), 376–377
High-risk newborn, 962, 962(t)
care of, 962–977
Hip fracture, osteoporosis and, 526
Hip replacement, complications of, in ankylosing spondylitis, 913
His bundle branch block, 235, 236
Histoplasmosis, 166–168
in AIDS, 49, 168
HIV (human immunodeficiency virus) infection. See *Acquired immunodeficiency syndrome (AIDS).*
HLA typing, in hereditary hemochromatosis, 347
Hoarseness, 25–33, 31(t)
treatment of, 26(t)–28(t), 27–33
Hodgkin's disease, 348(t)–350(t), 348–359, *358*
staging of, 350(t), 355(t)
treatment of, 349–359, 351(t), *356*
complications of, 353(t), 354, 359
results of, 352(t), 357(t)
Hog (phencyclidine), 1042
poisoning by, 1122
Home parenteral nutrition, 535. See also *Parenteral nutrition.*
Homosexual patient, AIDS in, 42
diarrhea in, 11
Hookworm infestation, 481(t), 483, 484, 486
and creeping eruption, 748
HOP chemotherapy regimen, for cutaneous T-cell lymphoma, 381
Hormonal contraception, 1031–1032
Horse serum hypersensitivity, 72
Hospital-acquired infection, bacteremia as complication of, 57(t)
pneumonia due to, 184–187, 186(t)
Hospitalization, for bulimia or anorexia nervosa, 1051(t), 1052–1053
for pelvic inflammatory disease, 668(t), 1013(t)
for pneumonia, 184
for schizophrenic disorders, 1062
Hot flushes, 1004
Hot water immersion, for lesions due to contact with hazardous marine animals, 1083, 1084
H_1 receptor antagonists. See *Antihistamines* and specific agents, e.g., *Diphenhydramine.*
H_2 receptor antagonists, for anaphylactic reaction to insect sting, 701
for effects of esophageal dysmotility, in scleroderma, 718
for gastritis, 442(t)
for peptic ulcer, 9, 470, 471, 472
Human chorionic gonadotropin, for effects of hypopituitarism, 574
Human colony-stimulating factors, adverse effects of, 329
for aplastic anemia, 301–302
for neutropenia, 328
use of, in patient treated for multiple myeloma, 383, 385
Human diploid cell vaccine, 112
Human immunodeficiency virus (HIV) infection. See *Acquired immunodeficiency syndrome (AIDS).*
Human milk, 978
Human papillomavirus infection. See *Papillomavirus infection.*
Human tetanus immune globulin, 129
Humidification, in relief of nasal or laryngeal irritation, 28(t), 29
"Humidifier lung," antigens in, 202(t)
Hürthle cell carcinoma, 585, 587
Hydergine, for Alzheimer's disease, 792
Hydralazine, for hypertension, 274
in patient with intracerebral hemorrhage, 795(t), 796
in pregnant patient, 938(t), 946(t), 947
Hydrocarbons, poisoning by, 1112–1113, 1113(t), 1114(t)
Hydrochlorothiazide, for calcium stone disease, 663(t)
for diabetes insipidus, 561(t)
for hypertension, 270(t)
for Meniere's disease, 842
Hydrocodone, 1119(t)
for cough, 23(t)
for pain, 2(t)
Hydrocolloid dressing, for pressure ulcer, 761
Hydrocortisone, 553(t)
for adrenal crisis, 553
for adrenocortical insufficiency, 552
in patient with hypopituitarism, 573
for anaphylactic reaction, 677, 677(t)
for atopic dermatitis, 763
for leukemia, 367(t)
for lichen simplex chronicus, 776
for pruritic folliculitis of pregnancy, 775
for pruritus, 37, 776
for seborrheic dermatitis, 713
for ulcerative colitis, 429(t), 430, 431
perioperative administration of, 903
potency of preparations of, 773(t)
"replacement" with, in discontinuation of steroid therapy, 553
use of, in patient receiving amphotericin B, 169
in patient receiving streptokinase, 1028
in patient treated for Cushing's syndrome, 558–559
Hydrocortisone–acetic acid, for otitis externa, 106(t)
Hydrocortisone-polymyxin-neomycin, for otitis externa, 106(t), 1085
Hydrofluoric acid exposure, calcium preparations for, 1092(t)
Hydromorphone, 1119(t)
for pain, 2(t)
in sickle cell disease, 321
oral doses of, equivalent to parenteral doses, 2(t), 323(t)
Hydrophilic solutions, for brittle nails, 721
Hydrophobia, 111
Hydrops, endolymphatic, 841
Hydrops fetalis, 330
Hydroquinone, for melasma, 780
Hydroxocobalamin. See *Vitamin B_{12} (cobalamin).*
Hydroxychloroquine, for chronic actinic dermatitis, 786
for inflammatory myopathies, 718
for juvenile rheumatoid arthritis, 909–910
for lupus erythematosus, 715, 787
for malaria, 95
for pemphigus foliaceus, 768
for polymorphous light eruption, 786
for porphyria, 787
for rheumatoid arthritis, 904(t), 905
in pediatric patient, 909–910
for urticarial vasculitis, 778
17-Hydroxylase deficiency, 995
3-Hydroxy-3-methylglutaryl coenzyme A reductase inhibitors, for hyperlipoproteinemia, 508
Hydroxyurea, for leukemia, 370
for polycythemia, 388
for thalassemia, 317
Hydroxyzine, for allergic drug reaction, 697
for headache, 829
for nausea and vomiting, 6(t)
for pain, in sickle cell disease, 321
for pruritus, 37, 37(t)
in atopic dermatitis, 763
in contact dermatitis, 773
in erythema multiforme, 764
in scabies, 745
for urticaria, 777, 778
use of, in patient receiving vancomycin, 699
Hymenolepis nana infestation, 481(t), 485
Hymenoptera stings, allergic reactions to, 700–702
Hyoscyamine, for urinary incontinence, 606
Hyperactivity disorder, with attention deficit, in Tourette syndrome, 824, 827
Hyperacute headache, subarachnoid hemorrhage and, 829
Hyperadrenocorticism, 554–559
Hyperaldosteronism, 569–572, 570(t), 571(t)
Hyperammonemia, in Reye's syndrome, 847
Hyperamylasemia, causes of, 459, 459(t)
Hyperbaric oxygen facilities, as source of treatment, for patient with necrotizing skin infection, 80
Hyperbilirubinemia, neonatal, 971–972, 975
hemolytic disease and, 330, 331, 333
Hypercalcemia, 565
hyperparathyroidism and, 565
multiple myeloma and, 385
sarcoidosis and, 199
Hypercalciuria, 663(t)
Hypercapnic respiratory failure (ventilatory pump failure), 147, 148, 149

Hypercholesterolemia. See *Hyperlipoproteinemia.*
Hypercyanotic spells, in congenital heart disease, 246
Hyperemesis gravidarum, 8
Hypergastrinemia, 457
Hyperglycemia, diabetes mellitus and, 493, 496, 499. See also *Diabetes mellitus.*
  neonatal, 968
  risk of, in patient receiving parenteral nutrition, 537
Hyperkalemia, renal failure and, 638, 639(t), 646–647
Hyperleukocytosis, 362
Hyperlipoproteinemia, 505–510, 506(t)
  diabetes mellitus and, 498
  nephrotic syndrome and, 611, 612
  pancreatitis due to, 462
  treatment of, 507–510, 508(t)
Hypermobility, urethral, and incontinence, 607
Hypernatremia, 545, 545(t)
  dehydration due to, 542, 542(t), 545–547
  neonatal, 968
Hyperosmotic laxative agents, 18
  in management of poisoning, 1088
Hyperoxaluria, 663
Hyperparathyroidism, 565–568
  pancreatitis due to, 462
  renal failure and, 567, 647
  risk of calcium stone disease in, 662
Hyperphosphatemia, renal failure and, 567, 638, 647
Hyperpigmentation, 779–780
  agents causing, 780(t), 784
Hyperplasia, atypical, of breast tissue, 985
  fibrous, of oral mucosa, 753, 757–758
  gingival, 758
  papillary, inflammatory, 754
  prostatic, benign, 627–633, 628(t)–630(t)
Hyperprolactinemia, 575–577, 576(t)
Hyperreflexic bladder, 606
Hypersensitivity, horse serum, 72
Hypersensitivity pneumonitis, 201–202, 202(t)
Hypertension, 263–280, 264(t)
  alcohol consumption and, 267
  aldosteronism and, 569, 570, 571, 572
  aortic dissection associated with, 215
  cerebral hemorrhage due to, 794
    prevention of recurrence of, 795(t), 796
  diabetes mellitus and, 498
  emergency management of, 273(t)
  induction of, in maintenance of cerebral perfusion pressure, 891, 894, 894(t)
  intracranial. See *Intracranial hypertension.*
  mineralocorticoid, 569–570, 570(t)
  pharmacotherapy for, 268–280, 270(t), 272(t), 273(t), 275(t), 277(t)–279(t)
    effects of, on elderly patient, 265, 265(t), 279
    on glucose metabolism, 266, 267(t)
    on lipid levels, 265, 266, 266(t)
    on risk or severity of coronary artery disease and stroke, 265, 265(t)
  pheochromocytoma and, 588–591, 591(t)
  porphyria and, 391
  portal, 406–407
    gastrointestinal bleeding associated with, 407, 413–417, 443
  pregnancy and, 937, 938(t), 944–948, 945(t)–947(t), 951
  pulmonary, in newborn, 972
  renal, 280, 612, 639, 644, 645, 646
Hypertension *(Continued)*
  scleroderma and, 718–719
  scleroderma and, 718–719
  systolic, borderline isolated, 263, 264(t)
  tetanus and, 131
  treatment of, 267–280. See also *Hypertension, pharmacotherapy for.*
    emergency drug therapy in, 273(t)
    J curve of response to, 264
    lifestyle modifications in, 267(t), 267–268
    perioperative, 279–280
  white coat, 264
Hypertensive crisis, treatment of, 273(t)
Hyperthermia, microwave, for prostatic hyperplasia, 631
Hyperthyroidism, 580–584, 581(t), 593, 594
Hypertriglyceridemia, 507
  treatment of, 509–510
Hypertrophic scars, 725
Hyperuricemia, 503, 504, 505
  renal failure and, 639
Hyperventilation, as means of reducing intracranial pressure, 795, 892, 893, 894(t)
Hyperviscosity syndrome, 386
Hypnotic(s), 1106(t), 1129(t)
  abuse of or poisoning by, 1044(t), 1044–1045, 1104, 1127–1128, 1129(t)
  induction of coma with, in management of head trauma, 894, 894(t)
  short-term use of, in insomnia, 35
  withdrawal from, 1045
Hypoadrenalism, 550(t), 550–554, *552*
Hypocalcemia, hypoparathyrodism and, 569
  renal failure and, 638
Hypochondriasis, 1047
Hypoglycemia, diabetes mellitus and, 497. See also *Diabetes mellitus.*
  malaria and, 96
  neonatal, 968
    maternal diabetes mellitus and, 972
  prevention of, in patient receiving parenteral nutrition, 537
  Reye's syndrome and, 847
Hypoglycemic agents, for diabetes mellitus, 491, 491(t), 492
Hypogonadism, 573–574
Hypokalemia, aldosteronism and, 569, 570, 571
Hypomagnesemia, and hypoparathyroidism, 566, 569
Hypomelanosis, guttate, idiopathic, 781
Hyponatremia, 544, *545*
  dehydration due to, 542, 542(t), 544–545
  neonatal, 968
Hypoparathyroidism, 566, 568–569
Hypopharyngeal (pharyngoesophageal) diverticulum (Zenker's diverticulum), 418, 422
Hypopigmentation, 780–781
  agents causing, 784
Hypopituitarism, 572–575
Hypoplastic left heart syndrome, surgery for, 246
Hyporeflexic bladder, 605–606
Hypotension, anaphylaxis and, 677, 677(t), 696(t)
  dopamine for, in anaphylaxis, 677, 677(t)
    in hypothermia, 1074
    in sepsis, 60
  norepinephrine for, in anaphylaxis, 677, 677(t)
    in heart failure, 254
Hypotension *(Continued)*
  obstetric anesthesia and, 954
  orthostatic, in diabetes mellitus, 884
    resulting from use of levodopa, 874
  poisoning and, 1098
  sepsis and, 60
  toxic shock syndrome and, 1009, 1009(t)
Hypothalamic dysfunction, and amenorrhea, 997
Hypothermia, 1073–1076
  factors predisposing to, 1073(t)
  induction of, in lowering of intracranial pressure, 894
Hypothyroidism, 577–580, 592, 593, 594
  in hypopituitarism, 573
  secondary to therapy for Hodgkin's disease, 354, 359
  treatment of, 578–580
    in hypopituitarism, 573
    in thyroiditis, 592, 593, 594
Hypoventilation, global, 148, 149
Hypovolemic shock, in newborn, 971
Hypoxemic respiratory failure, 147, 148, 149
Hysterectomy, for cervical cancer, 1019, 1020
  for endometrial cancer, 1016
  for endometriosis, 992
  for leiomyoma, 1015
  for premenstrual syndrome, 1003

Ibuprofen, adverse effects of, 21
  for arthritis, in lupus erythematosus, 715
  for dysmenorrhea, 999(t)
  for fever, 21
  for gout, 503(t)
  for juvenile rheumatoid arthritis, 908
  for pain, 1
    in passage of kidney stone, 662
    in pericarditis, 289
    in sickle cell disease, 321
  for postpartum pain, 953
  for rheumatoid arthritis, 902(t)
    in pediatric patient, 908
Idiopathic chronic ulcerative jejunoileitis, 456
Idiopathic facial paralysis (Bell's palsy), 869–871, *870*
  Lyme disease and, 120(t), 123
Idiopathic glomerulopathies, 614–617
Idiopathic glossopyrosis, 755–756
Idiopathic guttate hypomelanosis, 781
Idiopathic hyperaldosteronism, 570, 571, 571(t), 572
Idiopathic hyperprolactinemia, 577
Idiopathic hypoparathyroidism, 566
Idiopathic pericarditis, 290–291
Idiopathic thrombocytopenic purpura, 341, 344
Ifosfamide, for non-Hodgkin's lymphoma, 376(t)
IgA deposition, linear, and dermatitis, 771–772
  renal, and nephritis, 617
Ileitis (Crohn's disease), 433–435, 455
Ileostomy, for ulcerative colitis, 431
Ileum, diverticula of, 423–424
  lymphoma of, 457
  resection of, malabsorption following, 458
Ileus, gallstone, 405
Iliac artery, aneurysm of, 295
  stenosis of, 216, 293

Iliofemoral venous thrombosis, 1026, 1029, 1030
Imaging costs, 925(t)
Imidazole antifungals. See specific agents, e.g., *Ketoconazole*.
Imipenem, for endocarditis, 260(t)
Imipramine, 1130(t)
for attention deficit hyperactivity disorder, in Tourette syndrome, 827
for depression, 1058(t)
in multiple sclerosis, 855
for lability of affective display, in multiple sclerosis, 855
for panic disorder, 1065
for urinary incontinence, 606, 607
in children, 603
therapeutic vs. toxic levels of, 1130(t), 1138(t)
Immune complex reaction, to drugs, 697
Immune globulin, 397–398
for fetal hemolytic disease, 333–334
for Guillain-Barré syndrome, 882, 887
for hepatitis, 448
for measles, 128
for myasthenia gravis, 860, 860(t)
for neutropenia, 328
for thrombocytopenia, 340, 341, 342(t)
in patient with leukemia, 374
in patient with lupus erythematosus, 717
for toxic shock syndrome, 1010
Immune hemolytic anemia, drug-induced, 305(t), 306, 306(t), 307, 308
Immune-mediated polyneuropathies, 884–886
Immune-mediated transfusion reactions, 398(t), 398–400
Immunization, against diphtheria, 74
against German measles, 126–127
against hepatitis, 447–448, 448(t)
against influenza, 81, 81(t), 189
in patient with chronic airway disease, 153, 176
against measles, 128
in AIDS patient, 128
against mumps, 105
against pertussis, 145–146
reactions to vaccine in, 145(t)
against plague, 108
against pneumococcal pneumonia, in patient with chronic airway disease, 153, 176
against Q fever, 110
against rabies, 112, 113
against rubella, 126–127
against rubeola, 128
in AIDS patient, 128
against tetanus, 129
in burned patient, 1070
against tularemia, 136
against typhoid fever, 142
against varicella-zoster virus infection, 69
against whooping cough, 145–146
reactions to vaccine in, 145(t)
before splenectomy, 308, 316
of AIDS patient, 128
of child, 74, 81(t), 105, 127, 128, 145–146
in cases of AIDS, 128
in cases of hemophilia, 336
of hemophiliac patient, 336
Immunodeficiency, acquired. See *Acquired immunodeficiency syndrome (AIDS)*.
acyclovir treatment of viral infection in, 52, 69, 369
Immunodeficiency *(Continued)*
brain abscess in, 790
herpes simplex virus infection in, 52, 756
infection risk in, and bacteremia, 58(t)
malignant skin lesions in, 736
pneumonia in, 47, 48, 49, 50(t), 52, 179(t), 183–184
varicella-zoster virus infection in, 52, 69, 190, 386
X-linked, Epstein-Barr virus infection in, 104
Immunogens, for warts, 724, 729
Immunoglobulin deposition, linear, and dermatitis, 771–772
renal, and nephritis, 617
Immunology, laboratory reference values in, 1141(t)
Immunosuppressive effects, of transfusion, 400
Immunosuppressives, for anemia, 301, 308
for aplastic anemia, 301
for autoimmune hemolytic anemia, 308
for bullous pemphigoid, 769
for chronic demyelinating inflammatory polyneuropathy, 885
for cicatricial pemphigoid, 770
for Crohn's disease, 434, 435
for glomerulopathy, 613, 614, 615, 619–620
for hemolytic anemia, 308
for inflammatory bowel disease, 431, 434, 435
for inflammatory myopathies, 718
for juvenile rheumatoid arthritis, 910
for multiple sclerosis, 851–852
for myasthenia gravis, 859
for neuropathy, 885
in vasculitis, 886
for pemphigus vulgaris, 767
for renal disease, 613, 614, 615, 619–620
for rheumatoid arthritis, 904(t), 905, 906
in pediatric patient, 910
for ulcerative colitis, 431
for vasculitis, 886
for warm antibody autoimmune hemolytic anemia, 308
Immunotherapy, for allergic rhinitis, 694–695
for insect sting allergy, 702
Impacted foreign body, in airway, 182
in esophagus, 422
Impetigo, 736–737
Implantable cardioverter-defibrillator, for ventricular tachycardia, 241, 241(t)
Implantable contraceptive, 1032
IMVP-16 chemotherapy regimen, for non-Hodgkin's lymphoma, 376, 376(t)
Inborn errors of metabolism, and Reye's syndrome, 846, 846(t)
Incontinence, urinary, 604–608
in children, 601–604
in patients with multiple sclerosis, 852–853
Indapamide, for hypertension, 270(t)
Indeterminate leprosy, 87
Indigestion, 9
Indomethacin, for diabetes insipidus, 561(t)
for dysmenorrhea, 999(t)
for gout, 503, 503(t)
for juvenile rheumatoid arthritis, 909, 909(t)
for migraine, 834
for pain, 1
for paroxysmal hemicrania, 836
for rheumatoid arthritis, 902(t)
Indomethacin *(Continued)*
in pediatric patient, 909, 909(t)
for urticarial vasculitis, 778
Induction therapy, for leukemia. See *Leukemia, chemotherapy for*.
Indwelling urinary catheter, infection associated with, 596, 599
Infant(s). See *Child(ren)*; *Congenital* entries; *Newborn*.
Infantile spasms, 821–822
Infarction, bone marrow, in sickle cell disease, 319
cerebral, in sickle cell disease, 325
myocardial. See *Myocardial infarction*.
pulmonary, in sickle cell disease, 322, 323
renal, in sickle cell disease, 326
right ventricular, 284(t)
sites of, in sickle cell disease, 319, 322, 323, 325, 326
Infection(s), catheter, 57(t), 537, 596, 599
community-acquired, bacteremia as complication of, 57(t)
pneumonia due to, 179(t), 179–184, 191
disseminated intravascular coagulopathy associated with, 342
hospital-acquired, bacteremia as complication of, 57(t)
pneumonia due to, 184–187, 186(t)
leukemia and, 362, 368–369, 372
multiple myeloma and, 58(t), 386
mycosis fungoides and, 379
necrotizing, 78–80, 740
neonatal, sepsis due to, 969, 970(t)
neutropenia and. See *Neutropenia, and infection*.
nosocomial, bacteremia as complication of, 57(t)
pneumonia due to, 184–187, 186(t)
opportunistic, AIDS and, 45–52, 46(t), 58(t). See also specific infections under *Acquired immunodeficiency syndrome (AIDS)*.
postpartum, 956
postsplenectomy, 310
bacteremia as complication of, 58(t)
prophylaxis against, 308, 316
renal disease and, 610, 639
sickle cell disease and, 325
transfusion-transmitted, 334, 401, 446
types of, in patient with hereditary hemochromatosis, 346
Infectious bronchitis, 174–176
acute, 174
antimicrobials for, 174, 175, 175(t), 176, 176(t)
chronic, exacerbations of, 175–176
Infectious colitis, 11
Infectious diarrhea, acute, 9–16, *10*, 14(t), 15(t)
Infectious endocarditis, 257–263
antimicrobials for, 63, 110, 114, 259, 260(t), 261
bacteremia as complication of, 57(t)
brucellosis and, 63
causes of, 257, 258(t), 259, 261
diagnosis of, 257–258
prophylaxis against, 262(t), 262–263, 263(t)
in child with heart disease, 247
in patient with mitral valve prolapse, 251
in patient with rheumatic heart disease, 119, 119(t)

Infectious endocarditis *(Continued)*
Q fever and, 110
rat-bite fever and, 114
surgery for, 261, 262
treatment of, 258–262, 260(t)
Infectious laryngitis, 30
Infectious mononucleosis, 103–104
Infectious neuropathies, 886–887
Infectious pericarditis, 291
Inferior myocardial infarction, and heart block, 236. See also *Myocardial infarction.*
Inferior vena caval filter, for thromboembolism, 194, 297, 1030
Infertility, endometriosis and, 992
treatment of Hodgkin's disease and, 354, 359
Inflammatory acne, 703, 704
Inflammatory bowel disease, 426–435
ankylosing spondylitis and, 913
Inflammatory diarrhea, 9, 11
Inflammatory fibrous hyperplasia, 757–758
Inflammatory myopathies, idiopathic, 717, 718
Inflammatory papillary hyperplasia, 754
Inflammatory polyneuropathy, demyelinating, chronic, 884–885
Influenza, 80–82, 189, 190
acetaminophen for, 189
amantadine for, 81–82, 174, 189, 190
in patient with COPD, 153
in patient with renal disease, 82(t)
immunization against, 81, 81(t), 189
in patient with chronic airway disease, 153, 176
rimantadine for, 81–82, 189, 190
Infrarenal aorta, aneurysm of, 213, 295
chronic occlusion of, 216
stenosis of, 216
Ingested toxins. See *Poisoning.*
Ingrown nails, 724
INH. See *Isoniazid.*
Inhalant abuse, 1045, 1045(t)
Inhalation analgesia/anesthesia, for delivery, 949, 950
Inhalation exposure, to toxins, 1086
oxygen for, 1096(t)
Inhalation injury, 1067
Inhaled antigens, alveolitis in reaction to, 201–202, 202(t)
asthma in reaction to. See *Asthma.*
hoarseness caused by, 29
rhinitis in reaction to, 203
Inhalers, metered-dose, 153
Inhibitors, coagulation factor VIII, 338
Injectable contraceptive, 1032
Injection exposure, to toxins, 1086
Injury. See *Trauma.*
Insecticides, poisoning by, 1119–1121, 1120(t), 1121(t)
Insect stings, allergic reactions to, 700–702
Insomnia, 33(t), 33–35
Alzheimer's disease and, 793
behavioral therapy for, 35, 35(t)
depression and, 33–34, 34(t)
muscle pain syndromes and, 920
sleep hygiene for, 35, 35(t)
Inspiration(s), deep, in prevention of atelectasis, 151
Insulin, 489(t)
for diabetes complicating pancreatitis, 467
for diabetes mellitus, 489, 490, 491, 492, 494–496
in pregnancy, 938, 938(t)
Insulin *(Continued)*
for diabetic ketoacidosis, 501–502
for hyperkalemia, in renal failure, 638, 639(t)
relative or absolute deficiency of, and diabetic ketoacidosis, 499
Insulin-dependent diabetes mellitus, 487, 489–490, 493–499
hereditary hemochromatosis and, 346
Insurability, after surgery for congenital heart disease, 248
Interferon(s), adverse effects of, 449, 449(t), 850
for cutaneous T-cell lymphoma, 381
for hepatitis, 406, 448–449, 449(t)
for kidney cancer, 651
for laryngeal papilloma, 32
for leukemia, 371, 372
for multiple myeloma, 384(t), 385
for multiple sclerosis, 850–851, 865
for polycythemia, 389
for varicella-zoster virus infection, 743
for warts, 729
Interleukin-2, for kidney cancer, 651
Intermediate-grade lymphoma, 375(t), 375–376, *377*
Intermittent acute porphyria, 389, 390(t)
Intermittent catheterization, for bladder dysfunction, 605
Intermittent pneumatic compression, in prevention of deep venous thrombosis, 195
Internal hemorrhoids, 440, 441
International system of units (S.I. units), 1133(t), 1133–1134, 1134(t)
International Working Formulation, for classification of lymphoma, 375, 375(t)
Interocclusal splints, for temporomandibular disorders, 918
Interpersonal psychotherapy, for depression, 1059
Intervention strategies, for alcohol-related problems, 1038
Intestine, amebiasis of, 15(t), 53–55, 54(t), 482–483
bleeding in, typhoid fever and, 142
cleansing of, hyperosmotic solutions for, 18
in management of poisoning, 1088
dysmotility of, multiple sclerosis and, 853
functional disorders of, 436(t)
helminthic infestation of, 479, 481(t)–482(t), 483–486
infections of, 455–456, 479–486, 480(t)–482(t)
bacteremia as complication of, 57(t)
diarrhea due to, 9–16, *10*, 14(t), 15(t)
helminthic, 479, 481(t)–482(t), 483–486
parasitic, 15(t), 16, 455–456, 479–486, 480(t)–482(t)
protozoan, 15(t), 53–55, 54(t), 455, 479–483, 480(t), 485
AIDS and, 51, 483
inflammatory disease of, 426–435
ankylosing spondylitis and, 913
large. See *Colon.*
obstruction of, Crohn's disease and, 435
parasitic infestation of, 15(t), 16, 455–456, 479–486, 480(t)–482(t)
perforation of, diverticulitis and, 425
typhoid fever and, 142
protozoan infections of, 15(t), 53–55, 54(t), 455, 479–483, 480(t), 485
AIDS and, 51, 483
Intestine *(Continued)*
small. See *Small intestine.*
syndrome of irritability of, 8, 9, 435–438, 436(t), 437(t)
vascular disease of, portal hypertension and, 407
Intoxication. See *Poisoning.*
Intra-atrial re-entry, 239(t)
Intracranial hemorrhage, 794–798
anticoagulant use and, 796, 801
hemophilia and, 335
neonatal, 973–974
subarachnoid, 829
headache associated with, 829
subdural, 830–831
headache associated with, 830
head trauma and, 830–831, 889
surgery for, 795, 797, 891
Intracranial hypertension, cerebral hemorrhage and, 795–796, 797
encephalitis and, 68, 845
meningitis and, 99
poisoning and, 1098
reduction of, in adult with head trauma, 889, 890, 891, 891(t), 892
in child with head trauma, 893–894, 894(t)
Reye's syndrome and, 847
Intradermal nevi, 729
Intraepithelial neoplasia, vulvar, 1023
Intrahepatic cholestasis, sickle cell disease and, 323
Intrahepatic portosystemic shunt, for bleeding esophageal varices, 415, 415(t), 416
Intramural esophageal diverticulosis, 423
Intramuscular hemorrhage, hemophilia and, 335, 336, 337
Intraocular pressure, elevated, 866
treatment of, 866–869, 867(t)
Intrauterine device, 1034
Intrauterine growth retardation, 969–970, 970(t)
Intravascular coagulopathy, disseminated, 342–344
relapsing fever and, 116–117
Intravenous drug abuse. See also *Drug abuse.*
and endocarditis, 257, 258(t), 259
leading to bacteremia, 57(t)
Intraventricular hemorrhage, neonatal, 973–974
Intrinsic factor, deficiency of, 311
Intrinsic surgical infections, and pyelonephritis, 620
Intrinsic urethral sphincter deficiency, and incontinence, 607–608
Intubation, of hypothermic patient, 1074
of newborn, 961
of patient with Guillain-Barré syndrome, 882
of patient with head trauma, 890
of patient with tetanus, 129
Invasive otitis externa, 105–107, 106(t)
Iodine, for thyroid storm, 584
radioactive, for hyperthyroidism, 582–583
Iodoquinol (diiodohydroxyquin), adverse effects of, 482
for *Blastocystis hominis* infection, 483
for *Dientamoeba fragilis* infection, 480(t)
for *Entamoeba histolytica* infection, 15(t), 54, 54(t), 480(t), 482
Iopanoic acid, for thyroid storm, 584

Ipecac, for patient exhibiting allergic drug reaction, 695
  for poisoning victim, 78, 1087
Ipodate sodium, for thyroid storm, 584
Ipratropium, for allergic rhinitis, 694
  for asthma, in pediatric patient, 685(t), 686
  for chronic obstructive pulmonary disease, 153, *155*
Iridectomy, laser, for glaucoma, 869
Iridocyclitis, juvenile rheumatoid arthritis and, 911
  leprosy and, 91
Iritis, ankylosing spondylitis and, 912, 913
Iron absorption, 345
  defective, 304
Iron chelation therapy, 316, 347, 1093(t)
Iron deficiency, 302–305, 303(t)
  in patient with pernicious anemia, 314
Iron dextran, 304–305
  for patient receiving parenteral nutrition, 534–535
Iron index, hepatic, 347
Iron malabsorption, 304
Iron overload, 345–348, 346(t)
  primary, 346, 347, 406
    phlebotomy for, 347
    screening for, 347, *348*
  secondary, 346, 346(t), 347, 1113–1115
    chelation therapy for, 316, 347, 1093(t)
    toxic iron ingestion and, 1113–1115
    transfusion and, 316, 401
Iron therapy, 302–305
  for cyanotic infant, 244(t)
  gastrointestinal side effects of, 303
  iron content of preparations used in, 1114(t)
Irradiated blood products, 396, 396(t)
Irritable bowel syndrome, 8, 9, 435–438, 436(t), 437(t)
Irritant contact dermatitis, 772, 773
Irritation fibroma, of buccal mucosa, 753
Ischemia, cerebrovascular. See *Stroke syndrome.*
  lower limb, arterial occlusion and, 292, 293, 294
  myocardial. See *Ischemic heart disease.*
  nephropathic, 644–645
  sickle cell disease and, 319, *319*, *320*
Ischemic heart disease, 217–218
  angina pectoris as symptom of, 217, 218
  cardiac arrest due to, 222
  coronary artery disease and, 218. See also *Coronary artery disease.*
Ischemic nephropathy, 644–645
Islet cell autotransplantation, for pancreatitis, 469
Isocarboxazid, for depression, 1058(t)
Isoimmunization, Rh, 329–334, 939
Isolated borderline systolic hypertension, 263, 264(t). See also *Hypertension.*
Isolation, for diphtheria, 73
  for pertussis, 145
  for plague, 108
  for varicella, 69
  for whooping cough, 145
Isometheptene, for migraine, 834
Isonatremic dehydration, 542, 542(t), 543–544
Isoniazid, adverse effects of, 1115
    pyridoxine (vitamin B_6) for, 884
  for atypical mycobacterial infection, 211
  for tuberculosis, 207, 208, 208(t)
    in AIDS, 46, 208
    in silicosis, 201
Isoniazid *(Continued)*
  poisoning by, 1115
  use of, with antimicrobials effective against brucellosis, 63
Isoniazid prophylaxis, for tuberculosis, 209, *210*
Isopropanol, poisoning by, 1100–1101
Isoproterenol, for heart block, 235
Isosorbide, for glaucoma, 867(t), 868
Isosorbide dinitrate, anticholinergic properties of, 1054(t)
  for achalasia, 419
  for angina pectoris, 218(t), 1118(t)
  for esophageal motor disorders, 419
Isosorbide mononitrate, for angina pectoris, 218(t), 1118(t)
Isosporiasis, 15(t), 455, 480(t), 483
  in AIDS, 51, 483
Isotretinoin. See *Tretinoin.*
Isradipine, 1107(t)
  for angina pectoris, 221(t)
  for hypertension, 277(t)
Itching. See *Pruritus.*
Itraconazole, adverse effects of, 167
  drug interactions with, 167
  for blastomycosis, 169, 170
  for candidiasis, 1007
  for coccidioidomycosis, 165
  for histoplasmosis, 167, 168
  for onychomycosis, 722
  for vulvovaginitis, 1007
Ivermectin, for strongyloidiasis, 15(t), 481(t), 484, 486
Ixodid tick bite, and Lyme disease, 120

Jarisch-Herxheimer reaction, to antimicrobial therapy, 116, 672
Jaundice, neonatal, 971, 975
    hemolytic disease and, 330
Jejunoileitis, chronic ulcerative, idiopathic, 456
Jejunum, diverticulum of, 423–424
Jellyfish stings, 1084
Job recommendations, for patient with low back pain, 41
Job-related asthma, allergens causing, 679(t)
Job-related dermatoses, 781–784
Job-related pulmonary disease, 199(t), 199–201
Joint(s), bleeding into, hemophilia and, 335, 336(t), 337
  deformation of, sarcoidosis and, 198
  disease of. See also *Arthritis.*
    hereditary hemochromatosis and, 346
  pain in. See also *Arthritis.*
    rubella and, 125
    sodium stibogluconate–induced, 86
Jones criteria (revised), for diagnosis of rheumatic fever, 117, 117(t)
Junctional complexes, premature, 231
Junctional nevi, 729
Juvenile laryngeal papillomatosis, 32
Juvenile rheumatoid arthritis, 907–911, 908(t), 909(t)

Kala-azar (visceral leishmaniasis), 83–86, 747
Kaposi's sarcoma, in AIDS, 656–657
Kaposi's varicelliform eruption, 741, 764
Keloids, 725–726
Keratitis, herpes simplex virus infection and, 741
Keratoacanthoma, 734–735
Keratolytics, for warts, 728
Keratosis, actinic, 733–734, 736, 751–752, 785–786
Kerion, 709, 749
Kernicterus, erythroblastosis fetalis and, 330
Ketamine, in obstetric anesthesia, 950, 952
Ketoacidosis, diabetic, 499–502, 500(t)
Ketoconazole, adverse effects of, 167
  drug interactions with, 167
  for candidiasis, 750, 1007
    in AIDS, 48
  for Cushing's syndrome, 557, 557(t)
  for dermatophytosis, 749
  for histoplasmosis, 167, 168
  for leishmaniasis, 86, 747
  for seborrheic dermatitis, 712, 713
  for tinea, 749, 750, 781
  for vulvovaginitis, 1007
Ketoprofen, for dysmenorrhea, 999(t)
  for gout, 503(t)
  for pain, 1
  for rheumatoid arthritis, 902(t)
Ketorolac, for dysmenorrhea, 999(t)
  for headache, 1, 829
  for migraine, 1
  for pain, 1
    in sickle cell disease, 321
Ketotifen, for atopic dermatitis, 764
Kidneys. See *Renal* entries.
Kissing bug bite, and trypanosomiasis, 747
Knee injuries, sports-related, 930, 931, 932
Krabbe's disease, 888

Labetalol, 219(t), 1124(t)
  as antidote, 1095(t)
  for angina pectoris, 219(t)
  for hypertension, 270(t), 270–271, 273(t)
    in patient with intracerebral hemorrhage, 793, 795(t), 796
    in patient with pheochromocytoma, 589–590, 591(t)
    in pregnant patient, 938(t)
  for tachycardia, in stimulant-abusing patient, 1042
Labial mucosa, lesions of, 752–753
Lability of affective display, in multiple sclerosis, 855
Labor. See also *Delivery.*
  pain in, management of, 948, 949
  preterm, 938–939, 939(t)
  psychological preparation for, 948
Laboratory reference values, 1133–1134, 1135(t)–1141(t)
Labyrinthitis, bacterial, 839(t)
Lactated Ringer's solution, use of, in burned patient, 1070, 1070(t)
    in diabetic patient with intercurrent illness, 496
Lactation, 978
Lactulose, for constipation, 18
    in typhoid fever, 141
  for portosystemic encephalopathy, 408
Lamotrigine, for epilepsy, 810, 810(t), 811(t), 813
Laparoscopic surgery, for ectopic pregnancy, 941
  for gallbladder disease, 403, 404
Large intestine. See *Colon.*
Larva migrans, 748

Laryngeal tumors, 32–33
Laryngitis, 25–33, 31(t)
  treatment of, 26(t)–28(t), 27–33
Laser therapy, for glaucoma, 868–869
  for keloids, 726
  for laryngeal papilloma, 32
  for prostatic hyperplasia, 631
  for vulvar intraepithelial neoplasia, 1023
  for warts, 728
Lassitude, in multiple sclerosis, 854
Late latent syphilis, 673(t)
Late syphilis, 671, 672, 673, 673(t)
Latex, anaphylactic reaction to, 676
Latex condom, 1031, 1032
Latrodectism, 1080
  antivenin for, 1090(t)
Laughing and weeping, in multiple sclerosis, 855
Lavage, gastric, for poisoning, 1087
    in warming of hypothermic patient, 1075
  peritoneal, in warming of hypothermic patient, 1075
Laxatives, 18–19
  abuse of, 18
    in bulimia nervosa, 1049
  for constipation, 18–19
    in multiple sclerosis, 853
  for poisoning, 78, 1088
Lead, poisoning by, 1115
    chelation therapy for, 1116(t)
Left anterior fascicular block, 235, 236
Left bundle branch block, 235, 236
Left posterior fascicular block, 235, 236
Left ventricular aneurysm, myocardial infarction and, 283
Left ventricular dysfunction, asymptomatic, management of, 255
  heart failure due to, 253
Leg. See *Lower extremity*; *Foot (feet)*.
Legionnaires' disease, 190–192
Leiomyoma, uterine, 1014–1015
Leiomyosarcoma, uterine, 1014
Leishmaniasis, *83*, 83–87, 747
Lennox-Gastaut syndrome, 822
Lentiginous melanoma, acral, 732
Lentigo (lentigines), 780
Lentigo maligna, 732, 735
Lepromatous leprosy, 87
Leprosy, 87–91
Leriche's syndrome, 216, 292
Leucovorin (folinic acid), as antidote, 1095(t)
  use of, with pyrimethamine, 50, 131
Leukemia, 359–374
  acute, 359–369
    in adults, 359–364
    in children, 365–369
  bone marrow transplantation for, 363, 364, 367, 371
  chemotherapy for, 362, 363, 364, 366–368, 367(t), 370, 371, 374
  chronic, 369–374
  complications of, management of, 362, 368, 369, 372
  FAB classification of, 361(t), 364(t), 365(t)
  hairy cell, 372–373
  in adults, 359–364
  in children, 365–369
  in patients treated for Hodgkin's disease, 354, 359
  in patients treated for polycythemia, 388
  interferon for, 371, 372
Leukemia *(Continued)*
  lymphoblastic (lymphocytic), acute, 363–368, 364(t), 365(t)
    chronic, 373(t), 373–374
    in adults, 363–364
    in children, 365–368
  MOPP chemotherapy regimen and, 354
  myelogenous, acute, 360–363, 361(t)
    chronic, 369–372
  nonlymphocytic, acute, 368–369
  plasma cell, 386–387
  secondary, 354, 359, 362–363, 388
Leukocyte-depleted blood products, 396
Leukodystrophy, metachromatic, 888
Leukoedema, 753
Leukoencephalopathy, in AIDS, 52
Leukopenia. See also *Neutropenia*.
  systemic lupus erythematosus and, 717
Leukoplakia, oral, 736, 756
    in AIDS, 52, 756
Leuprolide, for premenstrual syndrome, 1003
  for uterine leiomyoma, 1015
Levamisole, for colon cancer, 479
Levobunolol, 1124(t)
  for glaucoma, 867(t)
Levocarnitine, for Reye's syndrome, 846
Levodopa, adverse effects of, 873–877, 874(t), 876(t)
  for Parkinson's disease, 873–876, 878
Levonorgestrel implant, 1032
Levorphanol, for pain, 2(t)
Lhermitte's sign, following radiation therapy, 359
Libido, loss of, in hereditary hemochromatosis, 346
Lichen planus, 714, 723, 753
Lichen simplex chronicus, 776
Lidocaine, for arrhythmias, 238(t)
    in children, 244(t)
    in patient with pheochromocytoma, 591
  for delivery, 949
  for tinnitus, 39
  for vaginal delivery, 949
  for ventricular fibrillation, 224(t), 225
    in patient with myocardial infarction, 283
  for ventricular tachycardia, 241
    in patient with myocardial infarction, 283
  injection of, in skin around carbuncle, 738
  therapeutic vs. toxic levels of, 1138(t)
  viscous, for herpetic gingivostomatitis, 757
    for oral erythema multiforme, 764
Life support, basic and advanced, in management of cardiac arrest, 223–226
Light(s), full-spectrum, in interruption of seasonal mood disorder, 1053
Light eruption, polymorphous, 786
Lindane, for pediculosis, 746
  for scabies, 745, 746
Linea alba, oral, 753
Linear IgA dermatoses, 771–772
Lip(s), lesions of, 736, 751–752
Lipase, for pancreatic insufficiency, 457, 467
Lipids, in parenteral nutrition, 533, 538
Lipoid nephrosis, 612–614
Lipoproteins, 506, 506(t)
  serum levels of, abnormal elevation in. See *Hyperlipoproteinemia*.
Lipoproteins *(Continued)*
    effects of antihypertensive drugs on, 265–266, 266(t)
Liposomal amphotericin B, for leishmaniasis, 86
Liquid diet, for diabetic patient with intercurrent illness, 496
Liquor carbonis detergens, for atopic dermatitis, 763
Lisinopril, for heart failure, 255
  for hypertension, 275(t), 278(t)
Listeria monocytogenes infection, meningitis due to, 100(t), 101
Listeriosis, food-borne, 76
Lithium, adverse effects of, 1060(t)
  for cluster headache, 836
  for mania, 1060(t)
  poisoning by, 1117
  therapeutic vs. toxic levels of, 1138(t)
Liver, amebic abscess of, 55
    treatment of, 15(t), 54(t), 54–55
  biopsy of, results of, in hereditary hemochromatosis, 346–347
  cancer of, cirrhosis and, 412–413
    porphyria and, 393
    viral hepatitis and, 412, 445
  cirrhosis of, 405(t), 405–413
    complications of, 340, 406–413, 407(t), 408(t), 410(t)
      portal hypertension and bleeding esophageal varices as, 406–407, 413–417
    hepatitis and, 406, 445
    hereditary hemochromatosis and, 346, 406
    thrombocytopenia in, 340, 412
  cysts in, echinococcal, 485
  disease of, 405–413. See also *Liver, cirrhosis of*.
    infectious, viral. See *Viral hepatitis*.
    malabsorption due to, 456
    malignant, cirrhosis and, 412–413
      porphyria and, 393
      viral hepatitis and, 412, 445
  dysfunction of, total parenteral nutrition and, 538
  echinococcal cysts in, 485
  enlargement of, sickle cell disease and, 323
  failure of, porphyria and, 392
    viral hepatitis and, 444
  fibrosis of, hereditary hemochromatosis and, 346
  infection of, viral. See *Viral hepatitis*.
  iron deposition in, 346, 347
  malignant disease of, cirrhosis and, 412–413
    porphyria and, 393
    viral hepatitis and, 412, 445
  peritoneal capsule of, inflammation of, due to chlamydial infection, 1011, 1012(t)
  sarcoidosis involving, 198–199
  transplantation of, indications for, 413, 416
  tumors of, cirrhosis and, 412–413
    porphyria and, 393
    viral hepatitis and, 412, 445
  viral infection of. See *Viral hepatitis*.
Lobectomy, pulmonary, for cancer, 161, 161(t)
Lobular carcinoma in situ, 986
Lobular hyperplasia, atypical, 985
Local anesthesia, agents inducing, 700(t)
  allergic reaction to, 699

Local anesthesia *(Continued)*
seizures due to, 954
in surgical drainage of carbuncle, 738
Localized otitis externa, 105, 106(t)
Locomotor system, disorders of, 901–932
Lodoxamide, for allergic conjunctivitis, 65
Lomefloxacin, for bronchitis, 176(t)
for cystitis, in female patient, 597
Lomustine, for brain cancer, 898
Long-term vascular access devices, in parenteral nutrition, 535, 536, 537
Loop diuretics. See also *Diuretics*; *Furosemide*.
for hypertension, 269, 270(t)
Loperamide, for diarrhea, 16
in food poisoning, 78
in irritable bowel syndrome, 437(t)
in ulcerative colitis, 427, 428
Loracarbef, for bronchitis, 176(t)
for otitis media, 173(t)
Loratadine, for allergic rhinitis, 693(t)
for pruritus, 37, 37(t)
for urticaria, 696(t), 778
Lorazepam, 1106(t)
for epilepsy, in pediatric patient, 820, 821
for nausea and vomiting, 6(t), 7, 7(t)
for panic disorder, 1065
for seizures, in epileptic patient, 820, 821
in patient with Reye's syndrome, 847
for status epilepticus, in pediatric patient, 820
for stimulant overdose, 1042
response to, significance of, in delirium, 1054
Lordosis, activities or positions minimizing, 40
Louse-borne relapsing fever, 115, 115(t), 116, 117
Louse-borne typhus (epidemic typhus), 142, 143(t)
Louse infestation, 709, 746
Lovastatin, for hyperlipoproteinemia, 508
Low back pain, 39–41
atypical clinical features associated with, 39(t)
Low-calorie diet, for obesity, 513, 513(t), 514, 515
Low-density lipoprotein, 506, 506(t)
elevated serum levels of. See *Hyperlipoproteinemia*.
Low-density lipoprotein cholesterol, elevated serum levels of, in diabetes mellitus, 498
Lower extremity, arterial aneurysms in, 295
arterial occlusion in, 292(t), 292–294
claudication in, 216, 292, 293
effect of exercise on, 288
deep venous thrombosis in, 296–298, 1026, 1029, 1030, 1031
ischemia of, due to arterial occlusion, 292, 293, 294
periodic movements of, and insomnia, 34
superficial venous thrombosis in, 1031
ulcers of, 758(t), 758–759
in sickle cell disease, 324
Low-fat diet, for hyperlipoproteinemia, 507–508
for obesity, 513
Low-grade lymphoma, 375, 375(t)
Low molecular weight heparins, 298, 1030
for deep venous thrombosis, 195, 298, 1030–1031
Low-phosphate diet, for renal disease or renal failure, 567
Low-potassium diet, for hyperkalemia, in renal failure, 647
Low-protein diet, for portosystemic encephalopathy, 407
for renal disease or renal failure, 612, 645, 648
Low-sodium diet, for cirrhotic ascites, 410
for hypertension, 267
in aldosteronism, 572
for Meniere's disease, 842
for renal disease or renal failure, 611, 646, 648
Loxapine, 1123(t)
for agitation, in Alzheimer's disease, 793
for schizophrenic disorders, 1063
potency of, as neuroleptic, 1062
Loxoscelism, 1078–1080
LSD (lysergic acid diethylamide), abuse of or poisoning by, 1043, 1112
Lubricant laxatives, 18
Lucio phenomenon, 90
Lumbar peridural analgesia, for delivery, 949
Lumbosacral spine, limiting stress on, 40
Lung(s), abscess of, 171–172
atelectasis of, 151(t), 151–152
bacterial infections of, 172, 176–187, 179(t), 186(t), 191
AIDS and, 47
influenza and, 80
blastomycosis of, 168, 169
cancer of, 156–163, *157*
chemotherapy for, 161, 162, 162(t), 163
metastases of, effects of, 157–158, 158(t)
pleural effusion associated with, 158, 158(t)
radiation therapy for, 161, 162, 163
signs and symptoms of, 156, 156(t)
staging of, 160(t)
surgery for, 159, 161, 161(t)
conditions contraindicating, 159–160, 160(t)
chronic obstructive disease of, 148, 152–156
management of acute exacerbations of, 23, 154–155
therapy for, 149, 152–156, *155*
coccidioidomycosis of, 163, 164
disease of, chronic obstructive, 148, 152–156
management of acute exacerbations of, 23, 154–155
therapy for, 149, 152–156, *155*
infectious. See *Lung(s), infections of*; *Pneumonia*.
inflammatory. See *Pneumonitis*.
lupus erythematosus and, 716
malignant, 156–163
occupational, 199(t), 199–201
pericarditis accompanying, 291
scleroderma and, 719
sickle cell syndromes and, 322–323
edema of, congestive heart failure and. See *Heart failure*.
malaria and, 96
poisoning and, 1089, 1098
renal failure and, 639
transfusion and, 400
embolism in, 192–195, 296
diagnosis of, 192, *193*
differential diagnosis of, 192(t)
prevention of, 195
Lung(s) *(Continued)*
treatment of, 192–194, 195(t), 297, 1030
fibrosis of, lupus erythematosus and, 716
silicosis and, 199
function of, adaptive, in newborn, 963
fungal infections of, 163–170
AIDS and, 48, 49
granuloma of, coccidioidomycosis and, 164
histoplasmosis of, 166
treatment of, 167–168
infarction of, sickle cell disease and, 322, 323
infections of. See also *Pneumonia*.
abscess due to, 171–172
AIDS and, 45, 47, 48, 49, 52, 184
bacterial, 176–187, 179(t), 186(t), 191
AIDS and, 47
influenza and, 80
fungal, 163–170
AIDS and, 48, 49
mycobacterial, 207–208, 210, 211, 212
AIDS and, 45
silicosis and, 201
mycoplasmal, 190
routes of, in tularemia, 135
viral, 68, 80, 189–190
inflammation of. See *Pneumonitis*.
lupus erythematosus involving, 716
malignant disease of, 156–163
mycobacterial infections of, 207–208, 210, 211, 212
AIDS and, 45
silicosis and, 201
mycoplasmal infections of, 190
nodule(s) of, silicosis and, 199
solitary, 159
non–small cell carcinoma of, *157*, 160–162
obstructive disease of, chronic, 148, 152–156
management of acute exacerbations of, 23, 154–155
therapy for, 149, 152–156, *155*
occupational disease of, 199(t), 199–201
resection of, for cancer, 161, 161(t)
sarcoidosis involving, 198
scleroderma involving, 719
silicosis of, 199(t), 199–201, 200(t)
small cell carcinoma of, 162–163
solitary nodule of, 159
stretching of, promotion of, in prevention of atelectasis, 151
transplantation of, for chronic obstructive pulmonary disease, 155(t), 156
tuberculosis of, 207–208, 208(t)
AIDS and, 45
silicosis and, 201
tumors of, 156–163
viral infections of, 68, 80, 189–190
Lupoid sycosis, 738
Lupus erythematosus, 715–717
photosensitivity in, 715, 787
Lupus nephritis, 716
Luteinizing hormone–releasing hormone analogues. See *Gonadotropin-releasing hormone agonists*.
Lyme disease, 119–124, 120(t), 887
Lymphangiectasia, intestinal, 457
Lymphangioma, in oral cavity, 756
Lymph nodes, drainage of, in tularemia, 136
enlargement of, in sarcoidosis, 198

Lymphoblastic (lymphocytic) leukemia, acute, 363–368, 364(t), 365(t)
chronic, 373(t), 373–374
in adults, 363–364
in children, 365–368
Lymphoblastic lymphoma, 376–377
Lymphocytic leukemia. See *Lymphoblastic (lymphocytic) leukemia.*
Lymphogranuloma venereum, 671
Lymphoid tissue, airway obstruction by, in infectious mononucleosis, 104
Lymphokine-activated killer cells, for kidney cancer, 651
Lymphoma, 374–377, 375(t)
Burkitt's (small non–cleaved cell lymphoma), 377
central nervous system, 899
chemotherapy for, 349–354, 351(t), 352(t), 375–377, 376(t), *377*, 380, 381
radiation therapy combined with, 349, 350, 352, 357, 357(t), 358
gastric, 475
high-grade, 375(t), 376–377
Hodgkin's, 348(t)–350(t), 348–359, *358*
staging of, 350(t), 355(t)
treatment of, 349–359, 351(t), *356*
complications of, 353(t), 354, 359
results of, 352(t), 357(t)
intermediate-grade, 375(t), 375–376, *377*
International Working Formulation for classification of, 375, 375(t)
intestinal, 457
risk of, in patient with dermatitis herpetiformis, 771
low-grade, 375, 375(t)
lymphoblastic, 376–377
mediastinal, 357
non-Hodgkin's, 364, 374–377, 375(t)
treatment of, 375–377, 376(t), *377*
radiation therapy for, 349, 354–359, *356*, 357(t), 381
chemotherapy combined with, 349, 350, 352, 357, 357(t), 358
small non–cleaved cell (Burkitt's lymphoma), 377
subdiaphragmatic, treatment of, 355–356, *356*, 358
supradiaphragmatic, treatment of, 355, *356*, 357
T-cell, cutaneous, 377–382, 378(t), 379(t), 380(t)
thyroid, 586, 587
Lysergic acid diethylamide (LSD), abuse of or poisoning by, 1043, 1112

MACOP-B chemotherapy regimen, for non-Hodgkin's lymphoma, 376, 376(t)
Macroadenoma, pituitary. See *Pituitary, adenoma of.*
Macroglossia, 756
Macronutrients, in parenteral solutions, 533–534
imbalance of, 537–538
Macule, melanotic, 751
Magnesium citrate, for poisoning, 78
use of, in sickle cell disease, 322
Magnesium deficiency, and hypoparathyroidism, 566, 569
Magnesium gluconate, for calcium stone disease, 663(t)
Magnesium oxide, for calcium stone disease, 663(t)
Magnesium salicylate, for pain, 1
Magnesium sulfate, for hypoparathyroidism, 569
for poisoning, 1088
for seizures, in patient with porphyria, 391
in pregnant patient, 946(t), 947
for ventricular fibrillation, 225
in hypothermic patient, 1074
Magnesium sulfate paste, for pressure ulcer, 761
Major aphthous ulcers, 752–753
Major depression, 1055–1056. See also *Depression*; *Antidepressants.*
Malabsorption, 450–458
biliary tract disease and, 450, 452(t), 456
diagnosis of, 450–453, 451(t)–453(t), *454*
fat, 450
pancreatic insufficiency and, 466–467
iron, 304
pancreatic disease and, 450, 452(t), 457, 466–467
signs of, 450, 451(t), 452(t)
systemic diseases causing, 458, 458(t)
vitamin, signs of, 451(t)
vitamin B_{12} (cobalamin), 311
tropical sprue and, 454–455
Malaria, 91–98, *92*, 94(t), 97(t)
Maldigestion, 8, 9. See also *Malabsorption.*
Male patient. See also sex-specific organ entries.
androgenetic alopecia in, 706, 706(t), 707
condoms for, 1032
gonadotropin deficiency in, 574
osteoporosis in, 526
sterilization of, 1035
urinary tract infection in, 595(t), 595–596, 621, 669–670
Malignant external otitis, 105–107, 106(t)
Malignant tumors. See *Cancer*; specific types.
Malnutrition, 530, 531
renal disease and, 610, 639
Mandibular exostoses, 757
Mandibular tori, 757
Mania, 1056–1057
management of, 1059, 1060(t)
multiple sclerosis and, 854–855
Manning criteria, for irritable bowel syndrome, 436(t)
Mannitol, for ciguatera, 1085
for glaucoma, 867(t), 868
for heat stroke, 1078
for increased intracranial pressure, 795(t), 796, 847(t), 1098
in adult with head trauma, 889, 890, 891, 891(t), 892
in child with head trauma, 893, 894(t)
for myoglobinuria, in burned patient, 1069
Mantle field irradiation, for Hodgkin's disease, 355, *356*, 357
Maprotiline, 1130(t)
for depression, 1058(t)
March hemoglobinuria, 310
Marijuana, abuse of or poisoning by, 1043, 1112
Marine animals, contact with, bite wounds or envenomation due to, 1082–1084
ingestion of, toxins consumed in, 75(t), 76, 1085, 1086
Marine dermatitis, 748, 1085
Marine microbiota, infection by, 1083–1084
Marrow infarction, in sickle cell disease, 319
Marrow transplantation. See *Bone marrow transplantation.*
Masking, in management of tinnitus, 39
Masoprocol, for actinic keratosis, 734
Mastectomy, for cancer, 987, 988
Mastitis, 982
Mattresses, for patients with pressure ulcers, 760
Maturational assessment, of newborn, 964, *966*
Maturity-onset diabetes of youth (MODY), 487
M-BACOD chemotherapy regimen, for non-Hodgkin's lymphoma, 376, 376(t)
Meal replacement products, for obese patient, 514
Measles, 127–128
immunization against, 128
in AIDS patient, 128
Mebendazole, for enterobiasis, 484, 748
for helminthiasis, 481(t), 482(t), 483, 484, 486
for trichinosis, 134, 482(t), 484
Mechanical ventilation, 149–151
as etiologic factor in pneumonia, 185
as means of preventing atelectasis, 151
in newborn, 960, 968
for respiratory distress syndrome, 973
in patient with myasthenia gravis, 861
in patient with septic syndrome, 60
Mechlorethamine (nitrogen mustard), for cutaneous T-cell lymphoma, 380, 381
for Hodgkin's disease, 351(t)
for non-Hodgkin's lymphoma, 376(t)
Meckel's diverticulum, 424
Meclizine, for nausea and vomiting, 6(t)
for vertigo, 838, 838(t)
in Meniere's disease, 842
Meclofenamate, for dysmenorrhea, 999(t)
for gout, 503(t)
for rheumatoid arthritis, 902(t)
Meconium, suctioning of, 959–960, 970–971
Median nerve, compression of, in carpal tunnel, 880
Mediastinal lymphoma, 357
Medroxyprogesterone, for dysfunctional uterine bleeding, 994
for endometriosis, 991
for gonadotropin deficiency, 573
for hot flushes, 1004
postmenopausal use of, 567, 1005
Medroxyprogesterone contraceptive, 1032
Medullary carcinoma, of thyroid, 585, 586, 587
Mefenamic acid, for dysmenorrhea, 999(t)
for premenstrual syndrome, 1001
Mefloquine, adverse effects of, 95, 98
for malaria, 94(t), 95, 97, 97(t)
Megacolon, toxic, ulcerative colitis and, 431–432
Megaloblastic anemia, 311(t), 311–314
Megestrol, for dysfunctional uterine bleeding, 994
for endometrial cancer, 1016
Meglumine antimoniate, for leishmaniasis, 84, 747
Melanocytic nevi, 729–731, 735
melanoma associated with, 729, 730, 731, 735
Melanoma, 731–733, 732(t)
acral lentiginous, 732
lentigo maligna, 732, 735
nevi and, 729, 730, 731, 735
nodular, 732

Melanoma *(Continued)*
superficial spreading, 732
vulvar, 1025, 1025(t)
Melanonychia, 724
Melanotic macule, 751
Melarsoprol, for trypanosomiasis, 747
Melasma, 780
Melphalan, for multiple myeloma, 383, 384(t)
Membranoproliferative glomerulonephritis, 615–616
Membranous glomerulopathy, 615
Mendelsohn's maneuver, to improve pharyngeal emptying, 418
Mendelson's syndrome, 182
Meniere's disease, 838(t), 841–843
differential diagnosis of, 842, 842(t)
Meningeal plague, 107, 108
Meningeal plasma cell disease, 387
Meningioma, 830, 898
headache associated with, 830
Meningitis, 828–829
aseptic, 99, 843
bacteremia as complication of, 57(t)
bacterial, 98–103, 100(t), 101(t), 102(t)
coccidioidal, treatment of, 165
cryptococcal, in AIDS, 48
gonococcal, 669
headache associated with, 828
Lyme disease and, 120(t), 122–123
plague and, 107, 108
relapsing fever and, 116
viral, 843–844
differential diagnosis of, 843(t)
Meniscal tears, due to twisting motion of knee, 930
Menopause, 1003–1006
hot flushes associated with, 1004
osteoporosis following, 525, 1004–1005
use of estrogens following, 567, 1004–1006
and reduced risk of cardiovascular or cerebrovascular disease, 1005, 1005(t)
to lower rate of recurrent cystitis, 598
to prevent osteoporosis, 525, 1004
use of progestins following, 567, 1005
vaginitis following, 1008
Menstruation, absence of, 994–998, *995*, *997*
cessation of. See *Menopause.*
painful, 998–1000
treatment of, 999(t), 999–1000
symptoms preceding, 1000–1003
toxic shock syndrome associated with, 1008
Meperidine, 1119(t)
adverse effects of, 2
for headache, 829
for pain, 2(t)
in sickle cell disease, 321
oral doses of, equivalent to parenteral doses, 2(t), 323(t)
use of, in child receiving intra-articular steroid injection, 909
in patient receiving amphotericin B, 165, 169
Meprobamate, 1129(t)
poisoning by, 1127, 1129(t)
Meralgia paresthetica, 880
6-Mercaptopurine, for Crohn's disease, 434, 435
for leukemia, 366–367
for ulcerative colitis, 431
Mercury, poisoning by, 1117
Mesalamine (5-ASA), for Crohn's disease, 433, 435
for ulcerative colitis, 428–429, 429(t)
Mesangial nephropathy (IgA mesangial nephropathy), 617
Mescaline, abuse of or poisoning by, 1043, 1112
Metabolic acidosis, diabetic, 499–502, 500(t)
neonatal, 961–962
poisoning and, 1099
renal failure and, 638, 647
sepsis and, 60
Metabolic disorders, inherited, and Reye's syndrome, 846, 846(t)
Metabolic pericarditis, 291
Metachromatic leukodystrophy, 888
Metagonimus yokogawai infestation, 481(t), 485
Metaproterenol, for asthma, 681(t)
in pediatric patient, 685(t)
for chronic obstructive pulmonary disease, 154
Metered-dose inhalers, 153
Methadone, 1119(t)
for pain, 2, 2(t)
Methanol, poisoning by, 1101–1102
Methaqualone, 1129(t)
poisoning by, 1127, 1129(t)
Methazolamide, for glaucoma, 867(t)
Methimazole, for hyperthyroidism, 582, 583
Methotrexate, adverse effects of, 904(t), 910
for ankylosing spondylitis, 913
for bladder cancer, 653
for breast cancer, 989
for bullous pemphigoid, 769
for cutaneous T-cell lymphoma, 381
for ectopic pregnancy, 941
for inflammatory myopathies, 718
for juvenile rheumatoid arthritis, 910
for leukemia, 366, 367, 367(t)
for lung cancer, 162(t)
for lymphoma, 376(t), 381
for multiple sclerosis, 852
for non-Hodgkin's lymphoma, 376(t)
for pemphigus vulgaris, 767
for penile cancer, 656
for rheumatoid arthritis, 904(t), 905
in pediatric patient, 910
for urethral cancer, 653
therapeutic vs. toxic levels of, 1138(t)
8-Methoxypsoralen. See *Psoralen–ultraviolet A therapy.*
Methyclothiazide, for hypertension, 270(t)
Methyldopa, for hypertension, 272, 272(t)
in pregnant patient, 938(t), 947(t), 948
hemolysis induced by, 307, 308
Methylene blue, as antidote, 1095(t)
Methylergonovine, for postpartum hemorrhage, 956
Methylphenidate, for attention deficit hyperactivity disorder, in Tourette syndrome, 827
Methylprednisolone, for anaphylaxis, 696(t), 701
for anemia, 301, 307
for ankylosing spondylitis, 913
for aplastic anemia, 301
for asthma, 681
in pediatric patient, 685(t)
for autoimmune hemolytic anemia, 307
for bullous pemphigoid, 769
for chronic obstructive pulmonary disease, 154
Methylprednisolone *(Continued)*
for hemolytic anemia, 307
for juvenile rheumatoid arthritis, 909, 909(t)
for multiple sclerosis, 849, 851
for nausea and vomiting, 6, 6(t)
for neuropathy, in patient with vasculitis, 886
for optic neuritis, 865
for oropharyngeal lymphoid swelling, in patient with mononucleosis, 104
for postinfectious encephalitis, 845, 845(t)
for renal disease, 614, 615
in patient with lupus erythematosus, 716
for rheumatoid arthritis, 903
in pediatric patient, 909, 909(t)
for sarcoidosis, 198
for toxic shock syndrome, 1010
for ulcerative colitis, 431
for vasculitis, 720, 886
for vomiting and nausea, 6, 6(t)
for warm antibody autoimmune hemolytic anemia, 307
perioperative administration of, 553
in patient being treated for Cushing's syndrome, 558
Methyprylon, 1129(t)
poisoning by, 1127–1128, 1129(t)
Methysergide, for cluster headache, 836
for migraine, 835
Metipranolol, for glaucoma, 867(t)
Metoclopramide, for bile reflux gastritis, 443
for diabetic gastroparesis, 884
for effects of esophageal dysmotility, in scleroderma, 718
for gastrointestinal dysfunction, in migraine, 833–834
for headache, 829
for nausea and vomiting, 5, 6(t), 7, 7(t)
Metolazone, for hypertension, 270(t)
for renal disease or renal failure, 611, 638
Metoprolol, 219(t), 1124(t)
for angina pectoris, 219(t)
for arrhythmias, 238(t)
for atrial fibrillation, 228(t)
for hypertension, 270(t)
for migraine, 835
for myocardial infarction, 282(t)
for tachycardia, in stimulant-abusing patient, 1042
Metronidazole, adverse effects of, 54, 480
for amebiasis, 15(t), 54, 54(t), 480(t), 483, 748
for bacteremia, 57(t)
for bacterial overgrowth in small intestine, 457
for bacterial vaginosis, 1007
for *Blastocystis hominis* infection, 483
for brain abscess, 789, 789(t)
for *Clostridium difficile*–associated diarrhea, 14(t)
for Crohn's disease, 433, 434, 455
for *Entamoeba histolytica* infection, 15(t), 54, 54(t), 480(t), 483
for *Entamoeba polecki* infection, 480(t)
for fistulizing Crohn's disease, 434
for giardiasis, 15(t), 455, 480, 480(t)
for *Helicobacter pylori* infection, 442, 471
for osteomyelitis, 928(t)
for pelvic inflammatory disease, 1014(t)
for pressure ulcer, 761

Metronidazole *(Continued)*
for tetanus, 129
for trichomoniasis, 1008
for vaginal infections, 1007, 1008
Metyrapone, for Cushing's syndrome, 557, 557(t)
Metyrosine, for hypertension due to pheochromocytoma, 590, 591(t)
Mexiletine, for arrhythmias, 238(t)
therapeutic vs. toxic levels of, 1138(t)
Mezlocillin, for meningitis, 102(t)
for neutropenia and infection, 328
Miconazole, for seborrheic dermatitis, 713
Microadenoma, pituitary. See *Pituitary, adenoma of.*
Microangiopathic hemolytic anemia, *Escherichia coli* infection and, 11, 344
Micrographic surgery, for skin cancer, 711
Micronutrients, in parenteral solutions, 534, 535(t)
imbalance of, 538
Microsporidiosis, 15(t), 483
in AIDS, 51, 483
Microvascular decompressive surgery, for trigeminal neuralgia, 864
Microwave hyperthermia, for prostatic hyperplasia, 631
Midazolam, 1106(t)
for child receiving intra-articular steroid injection, 909
Mid-borderline leprosy, 87
Middle ear, infection/inflammation of, 172–174, 175(t)
common cold and, 188
Midesophageal diverticula, 423
Mifepristone, for Cushing's syndrome, 557(t), 558
Migraine, 832–835
aura and paresthesias associated with, 833, *833*
gastric atony and dilation accompanying, 833, *834*
vertigo associated with, 840(t)
Migraine status, 834
Migratory glossitis, benign, 755
Milk, cow, 979
human, 978
Milker's nodules, 744–745
MINE chemotherapy regimen, for non-Hodgkin's lymphoma, 376, 376(t)
Mineral(s), in parenteral nutrition, 534, 535(t)
Mineralocorticoid hypertension, 569–570, 570(t)
Mineralocorticoid therapy. See *Steroids.*
Minimal change nephrotic syndrome, 612–614
Minocycline, for acne, 704, 784
for nongonococcal urethritis, 608
for oil-induced acne, 784
for reactive arthritis, 914
Minoxidil, for alopecia, 707, 708
for hypertension, 274
Misoprostol, for NSAID-induced gastroduodenal mucosal damage, 442, 471, 472
Mite-borne typhus, 143, 143(t)
Mitomycin, for bladder cancer, 653
for lung cancer, 162, 162(t)
Mitotane, for adrenal cancer, 649
for Cushing's syndrome, 557, 557(t), 558
Mitoxantrone, for non-Hodgkin's lymphoma, 376(t)
Mitral regurgitation, heart failure due to, 250, 261
Mitral regurgitation *(Continued)*
mitral valve prolapse and, 250, 251
myocardial infarction and, 284(t)
rheumatic carditis and, 250
Mitral valve prolapse, 249–252, 250(t)
sickle cell disease and, 326
Mitral valve prolapse syndrome, 250–252
Mivacurium, use of, in management of tetanus, 129
Mixed gallstones, 402
Mobitz Type I heart block, 234
Mobitz Type II heart block, 227, 234
MODY (maturity-onset diabetes of youth), 487
Mohs' micrographic surgery, for skin cancer, 711
Moisturizers, for nasal or laryngeal irritation, 28(t), 29
for pruritus, 37
Molindone, 1123(t)
Molluscum contagiosum, 744
in AIDS, 52
Mollusks, envenomation by, 1084
Mometasone, for scabies, 745
Moniliasis. See *Candidiasis.*
Monoamine oxidase inhibitors, adverse effects of, 1058(t)
for depression, 1058, 1058(t)
for panic disorder, 1065
Monobenzone, for vitiligo, 781
Monoclonal gammopathy, 383, 885
Mononeuropathies, 879(t), 879–880, 886
in children, 888
Mononucleosis, 103–104
Monosodium glutamate, effects of, manifested as Chinese restaurant syndrome, 77
Mood disorders, 1054–1060
seasonal, and bulimia nervosa, 1053
treatment of, 1058(t), 1058–1060, 1059(t), 1060(t). See also *Antidepressants.*
MOPP-ABV chemotherapy regimen, for Hodgkin's disease, 351(t)
MOPP-ABVD chemotherapy regimen, for Hodgkin's disease, 351(t), 352, 352(t)
MOPP chemotherapy regimen, complications associated with, 354
for Hodgkin's disease, 351, 351(t), 352, 352(t), 357, 357(t), 358
Moraxella catarrhalis infection, 180
Morphine, 1119(t)
for cesarean section, 952
for pain, 2(t)
in burns, 1070
in myocardial infarction, 289
in pericarditis, 289
in sickle cell disease, 321, 322
oral doses of, equivalent to parenteral doses, 2(t), 323(t)
sedation with, in management of head trauma, 890, 891, 891(t), 893, 894(t)
use of, in cyanotic infant, 244(t)
in patient with heart failure, 254
Mosquito bites, and malaria, 91
Motility disorders, of esophagus, 419–420
in dermatomyositis/polymyositis, 420
in scleroderma, 420, 718
Motion sickness, 8, 837
Motor fluctuations, levodopa usage and, 875, 876
Motor tics, in Tourette syndrome, 824
treatment of, 825–827
Mouth, actinic lesions of, 736, 751–752
bleeding from, in hemophilia, 335, 337
Mouth *(Continued)*
cicatricial pemphigoid involving, 769, 770
coxsackievirus infection of, 744
diseases of, 750–758
premalignant, 736
dry, 751
due to radiation therapy, 359
erythema multiforme involving, 764
erythroplakia of, 736, 757
herpes simplex virus infection of, 740, 741, 751, 754, 756, 757
leukoplakia of, 736, 756
in AIDS, 52, 756
pemphigus involving, 768
premalignant diseases of, 736
preoperative prophylaxis against infection from, in prevention of endocarditis, 119(t), 262(t), 263(t)
suctioning of, in neonatal resuscitation, 959
ulcers of, 752–753, 755, 756, 757
in tularemia, 135
Mouth rinse, for AIDS patient with gingivitis, 757
for patient with oral erythema multiforme, 764–765
MP chemotherapy regimen, for multiple myeloma, 383, 384(t)
Mucocele, of lip, 752
Mucocutaneous bleeding, in hemophilia, 335, 336(t), 337
Mucocutaneous leishmaniasis, 83–86
Mucolytics, for cough, 25
Mucopurulent cervicitis, 1011, 1012(t)
Müllerian agenesis, 996
Multibacillary leprosy, 87, 89
Multifocal atrial tachycardia, 238(t), 239
Multifocal leukoencephalopathy, in AIDS, 52
Multiple endocrine neoplasia, 585, 586, 587, 588
Multiple gestation, delivery in, anesthesia for, 950
Multiple myeloma, 382–387, 384(t)
and bacteremia, 58(t)
Multiple sclerosis, 848–855, 849(t), *850*
disorders misdiagnosed as, 849(t)
optic neuritis as harbinger of, 865
Mumps, 104–105
Mupirocin, for carbuncles, 739
for impetigo, 737
Murine typhus, 143(t)
Muscle(s), hemorrhage in, hemophilia and, 335, 336, 337
idiopathic inflammatory diseases of, 717, 718
Muscle-contraction headache, 831–832, *832*
Muscle-contraction vascular headache, 831
Muscle pain, 919, 920
multiple sclerosis and, 854
stiffness with, in polymyalgia rheumatica, 922
syndromes of, 919–920
differential diagnosis of, 919(t)
trichinosis and, 133
Muscle relaxants, allergic reaction to, 699–700
Muscle spasms, infantile seizure syndrome and, 821–822
jellyfish sting and, 1084
tetanus and, 129
Muscle spasticity, treatment of, 760
in multiple sclerosis, 852
Muscle tension dysphonia, 31

Muscle weakness, sites of, in myasthenia gravis, 856, 860
Mushroom poisoning, 75(t), 76–77
M-VAC chemotherapy regimen, for bladder cancer, 653
for urethral cancer, 653
MVP chemotherapy regimen, for lung cancer, 162(t)
Myasthenia gravis, 856–862
treatment of, 857(t)–860(t), 857–862
Myasthenic crisis, 861–862
Myasthenic syndromes, 862
Mycobacterial infections, 207–212
and leprosy, 87–91
and pericarditis, 291
and tuberculosis, 207–209, 208(t), 209(t), *210*
in AIDS, 45–46, 46(t), 207, 208
in silicosis, 201
atypical, 209–212, 211(t)
and pericarditis, 291
in AIDS, 45, 46, 47, 211, 291
in AIDS, 45–47, 207, 208, 211, 291
in silicosis, 201
nontuberculous. See *Mycobacterial infections, atypical.*
Mycoplasmal pneumonia, 181, 190
Mycoses. See *Fungal infection.*
Mycosis fungoides, 378–382, 379(t), 380(t)
Myelogenous leukemia, acute, 360–363, 361(t)
chronic, 369–372
Myeloma, 382–387, 384(t)
and bacteremia, 58(t)
Myelosuppressives. See specific agents, e.g., *Hydroxyurea.*
Myiasis, cutaneous, 748–749
Myocardial fibrosis, scleroderma and, 719
Myocardial infarction, 280–285
complications of, 236, 253, 283–284, 284(t)
heart block associated with, 236, 284
heart failure following, 253
initial work-up in, 280(t)
premature ventricular complexes occurring during, 232
recurrent, prevention of, 284–285
risk of sudden cardiac death following, 222, 226
risk stratification following, 284
treatment of, 281(t), 281–283, 282(t)
Myocardial ischemia, 217–218
angina pectoris as symptom of, 217, 218
cardiac arrest due to, 222
coronary artery disease and, 218. See also *Coronary artery disease.*
Myocardial sarcoidosis, 198
Myoclonus, levodopa-induced, 874
nocturnal, 34
Myofascial pain, 919–920
Myoglobinuria, in burned patient, 1069
Myomas (fibroids), of uterus, 1014–1015
Myomectomy, for leiomyoma, 1015
Myopathy, inflammatory, idiopathic, 717, 718
Myringotomy, in management of otitis media, 174
Myxedema coma, 579
hypothermia due to, 1075
Myxoid cysts, 725

Nabumetone, for arthritis, in lupus erythematosus, 715
Nabumetone *(Continued)*
for juvenile rheumatoid arthritis, 908–909
for pain, 1
for rheumatoid arthritis, 902(t), 908–909
Nadolol, 219(t), 1124(t)
for angina pectoris, 219(t)
for hypertension, 270(t), 278(t)
Nafarelin, for premenstrual syndrome, 1003
Nafcillin, for bacteremia, 57(t)
for brain abscess, 789(t)
for endocarditis, 259, 260(t)
for meningitis, 102(t)
for osteomyelitis, 928(t)
for toxic shock syndrome, 1010
Nail(s), diseases of, 721–725, 750
pigmentation of, significance of, 724, 780
Nalbuphine, 1119(t)
for pain, 2(t)
Nalidixic acid, for shigellosis, 14(t)
Naloxone, for drug-induced respiratory depression, 1044
in newborn, 962
for narcotic overdose, 1044, 1096(t), 1118, 1119
for pruritus, in liver disease, 409
in resuscitation of comatose poisoning victim, 1089
Naltrexone, for premenstrual syndrome, 1002
Nandrolone decanoate, for aplastic anemia, 302
Nanophyetus salmincola infestation, 481(t), 485
Naproxen, for arthritis, in lupus erythematosus, 715
for dysmenorrhea, 999(t)
for gout, 503(t)
for rheumatoid arthritis, 902(t)
in pediatric patient, 908
Narcotics, 1119(t)
abuse of or poisoning by, 1043(t), 1043–1044, 1118–1119
naloxone for, 1044, 1096(t), 1118, 1119
for headache, 829
for pain, 1–3, 2(t)
in renal calculous disease, 662
in sickle cell disease, 321, 322, 322(t)
subsequent to varicella-zoster virus infection, 743
oral doses of, equivalent to parenteral doses, 2(t), 323(t)
tolerance to, 1
vs. non-narcotic analgesics, 322(t)
withdrawal from, 1044, 1118–1119
Nasal decongestants, for allergic rhinitis, 693
for common cold, 188
for upper respiratory tract infection, 28(t), 29
Nasal infection, viral, 203
Nasal mucosa, inflammation of, 203, 691(t)
inhaled allergens and. See *Rhinitis, allergic.*
Nasal saline spray, 28(t), 29
Natural family planning, 1035
Nausea, 4–8
causes of, 5(t)
drugs for, 5–8, 6(t), 7(t), 78, 116, 137, 289, 842, 874
pancreatitis and, 459
Necator americanus infestation, 481(t)
Neck, pain in, due to thyroiditis, 593
Necrolysis, toxic epidermal, 765
Necrosis, avascular, in sickle cell disease, 324
cutaneous, due to infection, 78–80, 740
due to recluse spider bite, 1079
pancreatic, 461, 463
soft tissue, due to infection, 78–80, 740
Necrotizing enterocolitis, 975
Necrotizing fasciitis, 78, 740
Necrotizing infections, 78–80, 740
Necrotizing ulcerative gingivitis, acute, 757
Nedocromil sodium, for asthma, 680, 681(t)
in pediatric patient, 685, 685(t)
in prophylaxis against exercise-induced asthma, 679
Nefazodone, adverse effects of, 1060(t)
for depression, 1060(t)
Neisseria gonorrhoeae infection, 666–669, 667(t), 1013
conjunctivitis due to, 64, 64(t), 66, 66(t)
neonatal, 64, 64(t), 668–669
Neisseria meningitidis infection, 99, 100, 100(t), 101
Nematode infestation, 481(t), 482(t), 483–484, 486
cutaneous, 748
Neomycin, for portosystemic encephalopathy, 408
for Reye's syndrome, 846, 847(t)
Neomycin-polymyxin-hydrocortisone, for otitis externa, 106(t), 1085
Neonate. See *Newborn* and *Congenital* entries, and see also *Child(ren).*
Neostigmine, for myasthenia gravis, 857, 857(t), 858
Nephrectomy, for cancer, 650, 651, 652
Nephritis. See *Glomerulonephritis*; *Pyelonephritis.*
Nephrogenic diabetes insipidus, 559, 562–563
Nephrolithiasis, 661–665, 662(t), 663(t)
sarcoidosis and, 199
Nephropathy. See *Renal disease.*
Nephrosis, lipoid, 612–614
Nephrotic syndrome, 609–612
minimal change, 612–614
sickle cell disease and, 327
Nerve blocks, for pain, 4
Nerve fiber fatigue, in multiple sclerosis, 854
Nervous system, central. See *Central nervous system* and see also *Brain.*
peripheral, disorders of, 879(t), 879–888, 881(t). See also *Neuropathy (neuropathies).*
Neuralgia, amyotrophy and, 880
post-herpetic, 742, 743
trigeminal, 862–864
in multiple sclerosis, 854
Neuritis, leprosy and, 90
optic, 864–866
Neurobrucellosis, 63
Neurocysticercosis, 485
Neurogenic hoarseness, 31–32
Neurolabyrinthitis, viral, 839(t)
Neuroleptic(s), 1062–1064, 1123(t)
adverse effects of, 826, 1062, 1063
atypical, 1064
for agitation, in Alzheimer's disease, 793
for schizophrenic disorders, 1062–1064
for tics, in Tourette syndrome, 825–826
poisoning by, 1122–1123, 1125
Neuroleptic malignant syndrome, 1062
Neuromuscular disease, and dysphagia, 417–418

Neuromuscular maturity, in newborn, 964, *965*
Neuropathic conduction blocks, 885
Neuropathic pain, 888
  diabetes mellitus and, 883
Neuropathy (neuropathies), 879(t), 879–888, 881(t)
  diabetes mellitus and, 493, 498, 499, 883–884
  dideoxyinosine-induced, 44
  Lyme disease and, 122–123, 887
  peripheral, 879(t), 879–888, 881(t)
  porphyria and, 389, 882–883
Neurosurgery, for pain, 4
Neurosyphilis, 672, 673, 673(t)
  in AIDS, 47
Neurotoxic shellfish poisoning, 75(t), 76
Neutropenia, 327(t), 327–329
  and infection, 327, 328, 362, 368–369
    as cause of bacteremia, 57(t), 58(t), 59
    in aplastic anemia, 300, 301
    in leukemia, 362, 368–369
Nevus (nevi), 729–731, 735
  melanoma associated with, 729, 730, 731, 735
Newborn. See also *Child(ren)* and *Congenital* entries.
  adaptive capacity of, factors compromising, 964(t)
  anesthesia-related morbidity in, 955
  antimicrobial dosages for, in treatment of bacterial meningitis, 102(t)
    in treatment of sepsis, 970(t)
  care of, 962–977
  chlamydial infection in, 64, 64(t), 1011
  conjunctivitis in, 63–65, 64(t), 668–669, 1011
  epilepsy in, 821
  feeding of, 977–979
  gonorrhea in, 668–669
    conjunctivitis due to, 64, 64(t), 668–669
  heart failure in, 242, 243–245, 977
    treatment of, 245, 245(t)
  hemolytic disease of, 329–334, 330(t)
  high-risk, 962, 962(t)
    care of, 962–977
  myasthenia gravis in, 862
  ophthalmia in, 63–65, 64(t), 668–669, 1011
  pneumonitis in, chlamydial infection and, 1011
  resuscitation of, 957–962, 958(t)
    certification for, 963
  seizures in, 821
  varicella-zoster virus infection in, 68–69
Niacin, 518(t), 519
  adverse effects of, 508–509
  deficiency of, 518(t), 519
  for hyperlipoproteinemia, 508
Niacinamide (nicotinamide), for bullous pemphigoid, 769
  use of, as antidote, 1096(t)
Nicardipine, 1107(t)
  for angina pectoris, 221(t)
  for hypertension, 277(t)
Niclosamide, for helminthiasis, 481(t), 482(t), 485, 486
Nicotinamide (niacinamide), for bullous pemphigoid, 769
  use of, as antidote, 1096(t)
Nicotine patch, for smoker with COPD, 152–153
Nicotine stomatitis, 754
Nicotinic acid. See *Niacin.*
Nifedipine, 1107(t)
  anticholinergic properties of, 1054(t)
  for achalasia, 419
  for angina pectoris, 221(t)
  for chilblains, 1077
  for esophageal motor disorders, 419
  for hypertension, 273(t), 277(t)
    in aldosteronism, 572
    in pregnant patient, 938(t)
  for Raynaud's phenomenon, 718
  for urticaria, 778
  poisoning by, 1107(t)
Nifurtimox, for trypanosomiasis, 747
Nil disease, 612–614
Nimodipine, 1107(t)
Nipple discharge, 982
Nipple irritation, from breast-feeding, 978
Nitrates. See also specific agents, e.g., *Nitroglycerin.*
  for angina pectoris, 218(t), 219, 221, 1118(t)
  poisoning by, 1118
Nitrites, for cyanide poisoning, 1092(t)
  poisoning by, 1118
Nitrofurantoin, for prostatitis, 634
Nitrofurantoin prophylaxis, for cystitis, in female patient, 621
  for pyelonephritis, in female patient, 599
Nitrogen mustard (mechlorethamine), for cutaneous T-cell lymphoma, 380, 381
  for Hodgkin's disease, 351(t)
  for non-Hodgkin's lymphoma, 376(t)
Nitroglycerin, for angina pectoris, 218(t), 219, 221, 1118(t)
  for bleeding esophageal varices, 414
  for heart failure, 254
  for hypertension, 273(t)
  for myocardial infarction, 282
Nitroglycerin ointment, for pressure ulcer, 761
Nitroprusside, for hypertension, 273(t)
    in patient with intracerebral hemorrhage, 793, 795(t), 796
    in patient with pheochromocytoma, 591
Nizatidine, for peptic ulcer, 9, 470
Nocturnal enuresis, 602–604
Nocturnal hemoglobinuria, paroxysmal, 299, 309, 310, 311
Nocturnal myoclonus, 34
Nodular melanoma, 732
Nodule(s), milker's, 744–745
  pulmonary, silicosis and, 199
    solitary, 159
  subcutaneous, in rheumatic fever, 117
  thyroid, 563, 564, 565, 586
  vocal fold, 30
Non-A, non-B hepatitis, 446
  transfusion-transmitted, 401, 446
Nonbarbiturate sedative hypnotic drugs, 1129(t)
  poisoning by, 1127–1128, 1129(t)
Nonbullous impetigo, 736–737
Noncomedo ductal carcinoma in situ, 986
Nongonococcal urethritis, 608, 669(t), 669–670
Nongranulomatous enteritis, ulcerative, idiopathic diffuse, 456
Non-Hodgkin's lymphoma, 364, 374–377, 375(t)
  treatment of, 375–377, 376(t), *377*
Nonimmune hemolytic anemia, 308–311, 309(t)
Nonimmune transfusion reactions, 398(t), 400–401
Noninflammatory diarrhea, 11–12
Non-insulin-dependent diabetes mellitus, 487, 490–492
Nonlymphocytic leukemia, acute, 368–369
Non-narcotic analgesics, 1, 3. See also particular types, e.g., *Nonsteroidal anti-inflammatory drugs.*
  vs. narcotic analgesics, 322(t)
Nonpolyposis colorectal cancer syndromes, hereditary, 476
Nonseminomatous germ cell cancer, of testis, 657–658
Non-small cell carcinoma, of lung, *157*, 160–162
Nonsteroidal anti-inflammatory drugs, adverse effects of, 340, 442, 469, 472, 644, 699, 901
  for ankylosing spondylitis, 913(t)
  for arthritis, 901–903, 902(t), 908(t), 908–909
    in lupus erythematosus, 715
  for back pain, 40
  for diabetes insipidus, 561(t), 562
  for dysmenorrhea, 999(t), 1000
  for fever, 21
  for gout, 503, 503(t), 504
  for juvenile rheumatoid arthritis, 908(t), 908–909
  for pain, 1, 40
    in pericarditis, 289
    in sickle cell disease, 321
  for painful menstruation, 999(t), 1000
  for premenstrual syndrome, 1001
  for rheumatoid arthritis, 901–903, 902(t)
    in pediatric patient, 908(t), 908–909
  gastric inflammation due to, 442
  peptic ulcer due to, 469, 472
  renal failure due to, 644
  thrombocytopenia induced by, 340
Nonstress testing, of fetus, 939, 940
Nonsustained ventricular arrhythmias, 232, 240–241
Nontuberculous mycobacteria. See *Mycobacterial infections, atypical.*
Nonvital tooth, sinus tract from, 757
Norepinephrine, for hypotension, in anaphylaxis, 677, 677(t)
    in heart failure, 254
Norfloxacin, for cystitis, in female patient, 597
  for salmonellosis, 138
  for shigellosis, 14(t)
  for traveler's diarrhea, 14(t)
  for typhoid fever, in carrier patient, 142
  for urinary tract infection, in female patient, 597
Norfloxacin prophylaxis, for bacterial peritonitis, in cirrhosis, 411
  for cystitis, 597
Norgestrel contraceptive, 1035
North American brown recluse spider bites, 1078–1148
North Asian tick typhus, 143(t)
Nortriptyline, 1130(t)
  for attention deficit hyperactivity disorder, in Tourette syndrome, 827
  for cutaneous dysesthesia, 776
  for depression, 1058(t)
    in Alzheimer's disease, 793
  for panic disorder, 1065
  for post-herpetic neuralgia, 743
  therapeutic vs. toxic levels of, 1130(t), 1138(t)
Norwegian scabies, 745
Nose. See *Nasal* entries; *Rhinitis.*

Nosocomial infection, bacteremia as complication of, 57(t)
  pneumonia due to, 184–187, 186(t)
NSAIDs. See *Nonsteroidal anti-inflammatory drugs.*
Nursing care, of patient with head trauma, 892
Nutrition. See *Diet*; *Dietary recommendations*; *Nutritional support*; *Parenteral nutrition.*
Nutritional assessment, 531
Nutritional support, 530–538, 531(t)
  for burned patient, 1071
  for child with leukemia, 369
  for preterm infant, 974
  in pancreatitis, 461
  in renal failure, 640
  in ulcerative colitis, 427
Nystatin, for candidiasis, 751

Obesity, 510–517, 511(t)
  physical assessment in, 513(t)
  treatment of, 512–517, 513(t), 516(t)
Objective tinnitus, 38
Obsessive-compulsive disorder, 1046
  in Tourette syndrome, 824, 827–828
Obstetric anesthesia, 948–955
Obstetric history, information included in, 934, 965(t)
Obstructive pulmonary disease, chronic, 148, 152–156
    management of acute exacerbations of, 23, 154–155
    therapy for, 149, 152–156, *155*
Obstructive sleep apnea, 34
Occlusal therapy, for temporomandibular disorders, 918
Occupational asthma, allergens causing, 679(t)
Occupational dermatoses, 781–784
Occupational pulmonary disease, 199(t), 199–201
Occupational recommendations, for patient with low back pain, 41
Occupational therapy, in management of rheumatoid arthritis, 907, 911
  in rehabilitation of hemiplegic patient, 805
Octopus bites, 1084
Octreotide, for acromegaly, 550
  for AIDS enteropathy, 458
  for Cushing's syndrome, 557, 557(t)
Ocular lesions. See *Eye(s).*
Oculoglandular tularemia, 135
Odontalgia, causes and effects of, 916
Odynophagia, 419
Oesophagostomum species, infestation by, 484
Ofloxacin, for bronchitis, 176(t)
  for chlamydial infection, 668(t), 669(t), 670, 1012, 1012(t)
  for cystitis, in female patient, 597
  for enteric fever, 139
  for gonorrhea, 667(t), 668
  for pelvic inflammatory disease, 668(t), 1014(t)
  for prostatitis, 633, 634
  for pyelonephritis, in male patient, 621(t)
  for salmonellosis, 139
  for traveler's diarrhea, 14(t)
  for urethritis, 669(t), 670
  for urinary tract infection, in female patient, 597
Ofloxacin *(Continued)*
    in male patient, 621(t)
Ofloxacin prophylaxis, for cystitis, in female patient, 597
Oil, occupational exposure to, and acne, 783–784
Oligodendroglioma, 830, 896, 898
Olsalazine, for Crohn's disease, 433
  for ulcerative colitis, 429, 429(t)
Omeprazole, for gastroesophageal reflux, 9, 30
  for peptic ulcer, 9, 471, 472
  for Zollinger-Ellison syndrome, 457
Oncocytoma, 651–652
Ondansetron, for nausea and vomiting, 5, 6(t), 7, 7(t), 8
One-rescuer cardiopulmonary resuscitation, 224(t)
On/off phenomenon, with levodopa usage, 875
Onycholysis, 722
Onychomycosis, 722–723, 750
Oophorectomy, for endometrial cancer, 1016
  for endometriosis, 992
  for premenstrual syndrome, 1003
Ophthalmia neonatorum, 63–65, 64(t), 668–669, 1011
Opiates/opioids. See *Narcotics.*
Opium tincture, 1119(t)
Opportunistic infections, in AIDS, 45–52, 46(t). See also specific infections under *Acquired immunodeficiency syndrome (AIDS).*
    and bacteremia, 58(t)
Optic neuritis, 864–866
Oral cavity. See *Mouth.*
Oral contraceptives, 1031–1032
  for dysfunctional uterine bleeding, 994
  for dysmenorrhea, 1000
  hormones in. See *Estrogen(s)*; *Progestin(s).*
  postcoital use of, 1035
Oral decongestants, for allergic rhinitis, 693
  for cough, 21
  for upper respiratory tract infection, 28(t), 29
Oral hypoglycemic agents, for diabetes mellitus, 491, 491(t), 492
Oral/pharyngeal dysphagia, 417(t), 417–419, 418(t)
Oral rehydration solutions, 70, 70(t), 71, 546(t)
  for patient with diarrhea, 12
  in cholera, 70, 70(t), 71
  in salmonellosis, 137
  in management of food poisoning, 78
Oral surgery, prophylaxis against endocarditis in, 119(t), 263(t)
Orbit, of eye, as site of infection, 204, 739–740
Orchiectomy, for cancer, 656, 657
Orf, 744
Organ failure, in sickle cell disease, 325–327, 326(t)
Organochlorine insecticides, poisoning by, 1119–1120, 1120(t)
Organophosphate insecticides, poisoning by, 1120, 1121(t)
Ornithosis, 108–109
Oropharyngeal lymphoid tissues, swelling of, in infectious mononucleosis, 104
Oropharyngeal tularemia, 135
Orthostatic hypotension, in diabetic patient, 884
  in patient using levodopa, 874
Osmotic agents. See also specific agents, e.g., *Mannitol.*
  for glaucoma, 867(t), 868
  laxative, 18, 1088
Ossifying fibroma, peripheral, 758
Osteoarthritis, 922, 922(t)
Osteodystrophy, renal, 647
Osteomalacia, liver disease and, 409
Osteomyelitis, 63, 138, 923–929, 928(t)
  frontal bone involvement in, 204
  sickle cell disease and, 325, 924
Osteonecrosis, sickle cell disease and, 324
Osteoporosis, 521–526, 522(t)
  liver disease and, 409
  postmenopausal, 525, 1004–1005
Otalgia, external otitis and, 105, 106
Otitis externa, 105–107, 106(t)
  exposure to moisture and, 1084–1085
Otitis media, 172–174, 175(t)
  common cold and, 188
Ovarian vein thrombosis, 1031
Ovary (ovaries), dysfunction of, 997–998
  resection of, for endometrial cancer, 1016
    for endometriosis, 992
    for premenstrual syndrome, 1003
Overdose. See *Poisoning.*
Overflow incontinence, 605
Overgrowth, bacterial, in small intestine, 456–457
Overuse injuries, 920, 921
  sports-related, 931(t), 931–932
Ovum, fertilized, ectopic implantation of, 940
Oxacillin, for endocarditis, 259, 260(t)
  for meningitis, 102(t)
  for osteomyelitis, 928(t)
  for pericarditis, 291
Oxamniquine, for schistosomiasis, 481(t), 485
Oxaprozin, for rheumatoid arthritis, 902(t)
Oxazepam, 1106(t)
  for anxiety, in Alzheimer's disease, 793
Oxprenolol, 1124(t)
Oxybutynin, for urinary incontinence, 606
  in multiple sclerosis, 853
Oxycodone, 1119(t)
  for pain, 2(t)
  for painful renal calculi, 662
  for postpartum pain, 953
Oxygen, warmed and humidified, for hypothermic patient, 1075
Oxygen therapy, for anaphylactic reaction, 677(t)
  for asthma, 149
    in pediatric patient, 689
  for carbon monoxide poisoning, 1068
  for chronic obstructive pulmonary disease, 149, 155–156
  for cluster headache, 836
  for inhalation intoxication, 1096(t)
  in comatose poisoning victim, 1089
  in newborn, 959
Oxymetazoline, for common cold, 188
  for upper respiratory tract infection, 28(t), 29
Oxymorphone, 1119(t)
  for pain, 2(t)
Oxytocin, for postpartum hemorrhage, 956

Pacemaker, for atrial fibrillation, 229

Pacemaker *(Continued)*
for heart block, 236
Paclitaxel, for lung cancer, 162(t)
Paget's disease, of bone, 527–530
of vulva, 1023–1024
Pain, 1–4
abdominal, diabetic ketoacidosis and, 500
gallstones and, 403, 404
irritable bowel syndrome and, 436(t), 437(t)
pancreatitis and, 459, 465
pelvic inflammatory disease and, 1013
sickle cell disease and, 323
amyotrophy and, 880
anorectal, causes of, 439, 441
back, 39–41
atypical clinical features associated with, 39(t)
fracture of osteopenic vertebra and, 522, 523
metastatic lung cancer and, 158
bone, metastatic lung cancer and, 157
Paget's disease and, 527
bone marrow infarction and, in sickle cell disease, 319
breakthrough, drugs for, 2
in sickle cell disease, 321
breast, 981
burns and, 1070, 1072
bursitis and, 921
chest. See also *Angina pectoris.*
aortic dissection and, 215
cocaine abuse and, 1041–1042
sickle cell disease and, 322
drugs for. See *Analgesics*; *Narcotics, for pain.*
ear, external otitis and, 105, 106
tinnitus and, 38
elbow, overuse injury and, 921, 931
epigastric, causes of, 441
peptic ulcer and, 470
episiotomy and, 956
facial, due to temporomandibular disorders, 914
in region of trigeminal nerve, 862–864
in multiple sclerosis, 854
hand and foot, in sickle cell disease, 323
head. See *Headache.*
heel, overuse injury and, 921, 932
joint. See also *Arthritis.*
rubella and, 125
sodium stibogluconate–induced, 86
knee, sports injuries and, 930, 931, 932
labor, management of, 948, 949
lower extremity, deep venous thrombosis and, 1026
menstrual, 998–1000
treatment of, 999(t), 999–1000
metastatic lung cancer and, 157–158
multiple myeloma and, 386
multiple sclerosis and, 854
muscular, 919, 920
multiple sclerosis and, 854
stiffness with, in polymyalgia rheumatica, 922
syndromes of, 919–920
differential diagnosis of, 919(t)
trichinosis and, 133
myofascial, 919–920
neck, thyroiditis and, 593
neuropathic, 888
diabetes mellitus and, 883
ocular, optic neuritis and, 864
tularemia and, 135
opiates for. See *Narcotics, for pain.*
Pain *(Continued)*
oral, herpetic gingivostomatitis and, 757
overuse injuries and, 921, 931, 931(t), 932
pancreatitis and, 459, 460, 465, 466(t), 467–469
patellofemoral, overuse injury and, 931–932
pelvic, endometriosis and, 990, 991, 992
pericarditis and, 289
porphyria and, 391
postpartum, 953, 956
prostate, 634
relapsing fever and, 116
rest, 292
right upper quadrant, sickle cell disease and, 323
shoulder, 921, 921(t)
sports injuries and, 929, 930, 931
sickle cell disease and, 319(t), 319–324, *320*, *321*, 321(t), 322(t)
snake bite and, 1081
somatoform, TMJ disorders with, 915
spider bite and, 1079
swallowing and, 419
tendinitis and, 921
throat, common cold and, 188
treatment of, 28(t)
tooth, causes and effects of, 916
varicella-zoster virus infection and, 742, 743
vulvar, following laser therapy for intraepithelial neoplasia, 1023
Painless thyroiditis, 594
Palate, lesions of, 754–755
Palsy, Bell's (facial paralysis), 869–871, *870*
Lyme disease and, 120(t), 123
Pamidronate, for Paget's disease of bone, 529
Pancreas, abscess of, 461, 463
autotransplantation of, for pancreatitis, 469
cancer of, 465
disease of, malabsorption due to, 457, 466–467
signs of, 450, 452(t)
fluid collections proximal to, 461, 463
inflammation of, 458–469, 464(t)
dideoxyinosine-induced, 44
insulin secretion by, impaired. See *Diabetes mellitus.*
iron deposition in, effects of, 346
necrosis of, 461, 463
pseudocysts of, 461, 463
resection of, for pancreatitis, 463, 468
tests of function of, 451
transplantation of, for diabetes mellitus, 490
for pancreatitis, 469
tumors of, 465
Pancreas divisum, 464–465
Pancreatic duct, drainage of, for pain of pancreatitis, 467–468
Pancreatic enzymes, for malabsorption, 457, 467
Pancreatic insufficiency, 457, 466–467
Pancreatitis, 458–469, 464(t)
acute, 458–463, 464(t)
chronic, 463–469, 464(t), 466(t)
dideoxyinosine-induced, 44
drugs causing, 462, 462(t)
prognosis in, Ranson's criteria for, 460, 460(t)
Pancuronium bromide, as antidote, 1096(t)
in management of head trauma, 890
Pancuronium bromide *(Continued)*
in treatment of tetanus, 130
Panic disorder, 1064–1066
Pantothenic acid, 518(t), 519
deficiency of, 518(t), 519
Papanicolaou smear, in screening for cervical cancer, 1018
Papillary carcinoma, of thyroid, 584–585, 587
Papillary hyperplasia, inflammatory, 754
Papilloma, laryngeal, 32
oral mucosal, 755
Papillomatosis, irritation from dentures and, 754
Papillomavirus infection, 727–729
and cancer, 727, 1023
of genitalia, 727, 728, 729, 735, 1023
and cancer, 727, 1023
of nails, 724
of skin, 727–729, 735
Papovavirus infections, in AIDS, 52
Papulosis, bowenoid, 735–736
Papulosquamous eruptions, 711–715
Paracentesis, for cirrhotic ascites, 410
Paracervical block anesthesia, for vaginal delivery, 949
Paraganglioma, 588
Paralysis, facial (Bell's palsy), 869–871, *870*
Lyme disease and, 120(t), 123
rabies and, 112
shellfish ingestion and, 1086
shellfish poisoning and, 76
therapeutic induction of, in patient with head trauma, 890, 893, 894(t)
tick, 887
vocal fold, 31–32
Paraneoplastic pemphigus, 768
Paraplegia, risk of, in surgery for aortic lesions, 214, 216
Parapsoriasis, 714–715
Paraquat, poisoning by, 1121–1122
Parasitosis, cutaneous, 745–749, 1085
intestinal, 15(t), 16, 455–456, 479–486, 480(t)–482(t)
Parasympatholytic agents. See *Anticholinergics.*
Parasympathomimetic agents, for glaucoma, 867(t), 868
Parathyroid disorders, 565–569
pancreatitis due to, 462
renal failure and, 567, 647
risk of calcium stone disease in, 662
Parathyroidectomy, for hyperparathyroidism, 568
Paravaccinia virus infection, 744–745
Parenteral fluid and electrolyte therapy. See *Fluid replacement therapy.*
Parenteral nutrition, 530–538, 531(t), 534(t), 535(t)
for preterm infant, 974
in pancreatitis, 461
in renal failure, 640
in ulcerative colitis, 427
Paresthesias, migraine and, 833, *833*
Parkinsonism, 871, 872(t)
use of neuroleptics and, 1063
Parkinson's disease, 871–879
Parkland formula, for fluid replacement therapy, in burned patient, 1070
Paromomycin, for amebiasis, 15(t), 54, 54(t), 480(t)
for cryptosporidiosis, 15(t), 483
for *Dientamoeba fragilis* infection, 480(t)

Paromomycin *(Continued)*
for *Entamoeba histolytica* infection, 15(t), 54, 54(t), 480(t)
for giardiasis, 15(t), 480(t), 482
for leishmaniasis, 86
Paronychia, 721–722
Parotitis, 104
Paroxetine, for depression, 1059(t)
in Alzheimer's disease, 793
for panic disorder, 1066
Paroxysmal cold hemoglobinuria, 306, 307, 308
Paroxysmal hemicrania, 836
Paroxysmal nocturnal hemoglobinuria, 299, 309, 310, 311
Paroxysmal stage, of pertussis, 144, 144(t)
Paroxysmal supraventricular tachycardia, 237–239, 238(t), 239(t)
Partial seizures, treatment of, 808, 809, 810(t), 810–816, 811(t)
Parulis, 757
Parvovirus B19 infection, 744
and aplastic crisis, 401
in thalassemia, 317
transfusion-transmitted, 401
Passive rewarming, of hypothermic patient, 1075
Patch testing, in dermatitis, 783
Patellofemoral pain syndrome, 931–932
Patient-controlled anesthesia, for delivery, 953
Patient education, as aid to management,
in asthma, 681, 682, 683
in bulimia nervosa, 1051
in contact dermatitis, 772–773
in diabetes mellitus, 488, 494
in multiple sclerosis, 848
in muscle pain syndromes, 920
in porphyria, 391–392
in premenstrual syndrome, 1001
in pruritus, 36–37
in temporomandibular disorders, 917
in Tourette syndrome, 825
in cardiac rehabilitation, 285
in prevention of low back pain, 40, 41
Paucibacillary leprosy, 87, 89
PCP (phencyclidine), 1042
poisoning by, 1122
PCV chemotherapy regimen, for brain cancer, 898
Peace pill (phencyclidine), 1042
poisoning by, 1122
Pediculosis, 709, 746
PEEP (positive end-expiratory pressure), 150–151
Pelvic exenteration, for cervical cancer, 1021
Pelvic fracture, and bladder trauma, 624
Pelvic inflammatory disease, 668, 668(t), 1012(t), 1012–1014, 1013(t), 1014(t)
bacteremia as complication of, 57(t)
Pelvic irradiation, for Hodgkin's disease, 356, *356*
Pelvic pain, due to endometriosis, 990, 991, 992
Pemphigoid, 768–770
bullous, 768–769
cicatricial, 769–770
Pemphigoid gestationis, 773–775
Pemphigus, 766–768
paraneoplastic, 768
Pemphigus foliaceus, 767–768
Pemphigus vulgaris, 755, 766–767
Penbutolol, 219(t), 1124(t)
for angina pectoris, 219(t)
Penetrating nevus, 731
Penicillamine, adverse effects of, 862, 905
as antidote, 1096(t)
for arsenic poisoning, 882
for cystine stones, 664
for lead poisoning, 1116(t)
for rheumatoid arthritis, 904(t), 905
for scleroderma, 718, 719
myasthenic syndrome induced by, 862
Penicillin, allergy to. See *Penicillin allergy*.
desensitization to, 698(t)
for arthritis, in Lyme disease, 120(t)
for aspiration pneumonia, 179(t)
for bacteremia, 57(t)
for brain abscess, 789, 789(t)
for carditis, in Lyme disease, 120(t), 122
for cellulitis, 740
for conjunctivitis, in newborn with gonococcal infection, 64, 64(t)
for diphtheria, 73
for endocarditis, 259, 260(t), 261
in patient with rat-bite fever, 114
for gingivitis, 757
for gonorrhea, 64, 64(t)
for guttate psoriasis, 713
for lung abscess, 172
for Lyme disease, 120(t), 122, 887
for meningitis, 100, 101(t), 102(t)
in Lyme disease, 120(t)
for neurosyphilis, 672, 673(t)
in AIDS patient, 47
for ophthalmia neonatorum, 64, 64(t)
for osteomyelitis, 928(t)
for pharyngitis, 205
for pneumonia, 179(t)
for psoriasis, 713
for rat-bite fever, 114
for relapsing fever, 116, 116(t)
for rheumatic fever, 117
for streptococcal pharyngitis, 205
for syphilis, 672, 673, 673(t)
in AIDS patient, 47
for tetanus, 129
for Whipple's disease, 455
Penicillin allergy, 676, 697–698
and management of patient at risk for endocarditis, 119(t), 263(t)
and management of patient with endocarditis, 261
and management of patient with syphilis, 673(t)
Penicillin prophylaxis, after rat bite, 114
after splenectomy, 308, 316
for diphtheria, 74
for recurrent rheumatic fever, 118, 118(t)
for streptococcal infection, 118, 118(t)
Penis, abnormal erection of, in sickle cell disease, 323
cancer of, 656–657
carcinoma of, 656
Kaposi's sarcoma of, 656–657
plaque on, in erythroplasia of Queyrat, 734
resection of, for cancer, 656
sarcoma of, 656–657
trauma to, 626
tumors of, 656–657
Pentaerythritol tetranitrate, for angina pectoris, 218(t), 1118(t)
Pentamidine, for leishmaniasis, 86, 747
for *Pneumocystis carinii* pneumonia, in AIDS, 50(t)
for trypanosomiasis, 747
Pentavalent antimonials, for leishmaniasis, 84–86
Pentazocine, 1119(t)
for pain, 2(t)
in pericarditis, 289
Pentobarbital, for intracranial hypertension, 847(t)
poisoning by, 1105(t)
Pentoxifylline, for leg or heel ulcers, 759, 761
Peptic stricture, of esophagus, 420–421
Peptic ulcer disease, 9, 469–472
Helicobacter pylori infection and, 469, 471–472
medications for, 9, 470–472
NSAID-induced, 469, 472
surgery for, 472
bile reflux gastritis following, 443
Percutaneous balloon compression, of trigeminal nerve, 863
Percutaneous rhizolysis, for trigeminal neuralgia, 863
Percutaneous transluminal angioplasty, for occlusive disease of lower extremity arteries, 293
Perforation, of colon, in diverticulitis, 425
of gallbladder, 405
of intestine, in typhoid fever, 142
Pergolide, for Parkinson's disease, 877
Pericardial effusion, 289, 290
Pericardiectomy, 290
Pericardiocentesis, 289
Pericardiotomy, complications of, in pediatric patient, 247
Pericarditis, 289–292, 290(t)
infectious endocarditis and, 261–262
lupus erythematosus and, 716
myocardial infarction and, 283
radiation-induced, 291, 359
Periductal mastitis, 982
Peridural block anesthesia, for delivery, 949
complications of, 954–955
Perihepatitis, chlamydial infection and, 1011, 1012(t)
Perindopril, for hypertension, 275(t)
Perineoplastic thyroiditis, 594
Periodic leg movement disorder, 34
Periorbital cellulitis, 204, 739–740
Periorbital hyperpigmentation, 779
Peripheral adrenergic inhibitors, for hypertension, 271–272, 272(t)
Peripheral arterial disease, 292–295
reduced claudication in, due to exercise, 288
Peripheral blood stem cells, collection of, in management of myeloma, 383, 385
Peripheral cold injuries, 1076–1077
Peripheral facial paralysis (Bell's palsy), 869–871, *870*
Lyme disease and, 120(t), 123
Peripheral giant cell granuloma, 758
Peripheral iridectomy, for glaucoma, 869
Peripheral neuropathies, 879(t), 879–888, 881(t). See also *Neuropathy (neuropathies)*.
Peripheral ossifying fibroma, 758
Peripheral parenteral nutrition, 535. See also *Parenteral nutrition*.
Peripheral vascular disease, 292–295
reduced claudication in, due to exercise, 288
Peripheral vestibulopathy, 837, 839(t)
Peritoneal dialysis, for poisoning, 1089
for renal failure, 640(t), 641, 648
Peritoneal lavage, in warming of hypothermic patient, 1075

Peritoneovenous shunt, for cirrhotic ascites, 410
Peritonitis, bacteremia as complication of, 57(t)
bacterial, spontaneous, 411
Permethrin, for pediculosis, 746
for scabies, 746
Pernicious anemia, 311–314
Pernio (chilblain), 1076, 1077
Peroneal nerve, compression of, 880
Perphenazine, for nausea and vomiting, 6, 6(t)
for post-herpetic neuralgia, 743
potency of, as neuroleptic, 1062
Persistent fetal circulation, 972
Persistent hepatitis, chronic, 444
Pertussis, 144(t), 144–146, 145(t)
Pesticides, poisoning by, 1119–1121, 1120(t), 1121(t)
Petroleum distillates, poisoning by, 1112, 1113, 1114(t)
Petroleum jelly, for brittle nails, 721
for nasal irritation, 28(t)
for pediculosis, 746
Peyote, poisoning by, 1112
Pharyngeal (oral/pharyngeal) dysphagia, 417(t), 417–419, 418(t)
Pharyngitis, gonococcal, 667
streptococcal, 204–207, 206(t)
rheumatic fever associated with, 117, 118, 119
tularemia and, 135
Pharyngoesophageal (hypopharyngeal) diverticulum (Zenker's diverticulum), 418, 422
Phase lag syndrome, and insomnia, 34
Phencyclidine, 1042
poisoning by, 1122
Phenelzine, for depression, 1058(t)
for panic disorder, 1065
Phenobarbital, 811(t), 1103(t)
for chorea, in rheumatic fever, 118
for headache due to trauma, 889
for hemolytic disease of newborn, 333
for seizures, in epilepsy, 809, 810, 810(t), 811(t), 813–814, 818(t), 819
in pediatric patient, 820, 821
in stimulant abuse, 1042
for status epilepticus, 818(t), 819
in pediatric patient, 820
poisoning by, 1105(t)
therapeutic vs. toxic levels of, 1138(t)
Phenobarbital-induced coma, in management of head trauma, 894, 894(t)
Phenothiazines, 1123(t)
for delivery, 955
for nausea and vomiting, 6, 6(t)
for post-herpetic neuralgia, 743
for schizophrenic disorders, 1063
poisoning by, 1122–1123, 1125
Phenoxybenzamine, for hypertension due to pheochromocytoma, 588, 589, 591(t)
in management of frostbite, 1077
Phentermine, for obesity, 516, 516(t)
Phentolamine, for hypertension due to pheochromocytoma, 590, 591
Phenylephrine, for cough, 23(t)
for cyanotic congenital heart disease, 244(t)
induction of hypertension with, in maintenance of cerebral perfusion pressure, 891, 894, 894(t)
Phenylpropanolamine, for cough, 23(t)
Phenytoin, 811(t), 1103(t)
Phenytoin *(Continued)*
for arrhythmias, in children, 244(t)
for neuropathic pain, 888
for post-herpetic neuralgia, 743
for seizures, in epilepsy, 808, 809, 810, 810(t), 811(t), 814–815, 818, 818(t), 819
in children, 820, 821
in head trauma, 894
in metastatic brain disease, 157
in Reye's syndrome, 847
in stimulant abuse, 1042
for status epilepticus, 818(t), 819
in pediatric patient, 820
for trigeminal neuralgia, 863
therapeutic vs. toxic levels of, 1103(t), 1138(t)
Pheochromoblastoma, 591–592
Pheochromocytoma, 588–592, *589*, 590(t), 591(t), 649
Phlebotomy (venesection), for iron overload, 347
for polycythemia, 388
for porphyria cutanea tarda, 393
Phlegmasia alba dolens, 1026
Phlegmasia cerulea dolens, 1026
Phobias, 1046
Phosphate binders, for renal failure, 567–568, 647
Phosphate-restricted diet, for renal insufficiency, 567
Phosphate therapy, for calcium stone disease, 663(t)
for hyperparathyroidism, 567
rationale for, in diabetic ketoacidosis, 502
Phosphorus, excess of, in renal insufficiency, 567, 638, 647
radioactive, for polycythemia, 388, 389
Photoaging, 785
Photoallergens, 786(t)
effects of exposure to, 786
Photochemotherapy, for cutaneous T-cell lymphoma, 380, 381, 382
for pruritus, 37
for psoriasis, 713, 723
for vitiligo, 781
Photophoresis, extracorporeal, for cutaneous T-cell lymphoma, 382
Photosensitivity. See also *Sun exposure*.
agents inducing, 786(t)
effects of, 786
lupus erythematosus and, 715, 787
porphyria and, 392, 786–787
Phototherapy, for neonatal hyperbilirubinemia, 333, 971, 975
Phototoxins, 786(t)
effects of exposure to, 786
Physical manipulation, in management of low back pain, 40
Physical maturity, in newborn, 964, *965*
Physical restraint, of stimulant-abusing patient, 1042
Physical therapy. See also *Exercise*.
for ankylosing spondylitis, 913(t)
for hemiplegia, 803–805
for muscle-contraction headache, 832
for muscle pain syndromes, 920
for pain, 4
for rheumatoid arthritis, 907, 911
for spasticity, in multiple sclerosis, 852
for temporomandibular disorders, 917
Physical urticaria, 778–779
Physostigmine, as antidote, 1097(t)
for glaucoma, 867(t)
Physostigmine *(Continued)*
for pediculosis, 746
Pigmentary disorders, 779–781
agents causing, 780(t), 784
hereditary hemochromatosis and, 346
Pigmentation, of nails, significance of, 724, 780
Pigmented nevi, 729–731, 735
melanoma associated with, 729, 730, 731, 735
Pigment gallstones, 402
Pill contraceptives. See *Oral contraceptives*.
Pill-induced esophageal injury, 421
Pilocarpine, for glaucoma, 867(t)
Pimozide, for tics, in Tourette syndrome, 826
Pindolol, 219(t), 1124(t)
for angina pectoris, 219(t)
for hypertension, 270(t)
Pinworm, 481(t), 484, 486, 748
Piperacillin, for endocarditis, 260(t)
for meningitis, 102(t)
for neutropenia and infection, 328
for osteomyelitis, 928(t)
Pirbuterol, for asthma, 681(t)
Piroxicam, for dysmenorrhea, 999(t)
for pain, 1
for rheumatoid arthritis, 902(t)
Pituitary, adenoma of, and acromegaly, 548–550
and amenorrhea, 997
and Cushing's disease, 554, 555, 556, 557
and hyperprolactinemia, 575–577
effects of iron overload on, 346
hypofunctioning of, 572–575
Pituitary apoplexy, 549
Pit viper envenomation, 1080–1082
antivenin for, 1081, 1082, 1090(t)
Pityriasis rosea, 714
Pityriasis rubra pilaris, 714
Placenta, blood passage through, and Rh isoimmunization, 329–334
delivery of, 955
Placenta accreta, 943
Placental abruption, 942, 943
Placental mosaicism, 936
Placenta previa, 942, 943
Plague, 107–108
Plantar fasciitis, 921, 932
Plantar warts, 727
Plaque, penile, in erythroplasia of Queyrat, 734
Plasma, blood, laboratory reference values for, 1136(t)–1137(t)
fresh frozen, 395
for disseminated intravascular coagulopathy, 343
in relapsing fever, 117
for hemophilia, 337
for thrombotic thrombocytopenic purpura, 345
Plasma cell leukemia, 386–387
Plasmacytoma, solitary, 386
Plasma exchange, for chronic demyelinating inflammatory polyneuropathy, 885
for glomerulopathy, 617
for Guillain-Barré syndrome, 882
for myasthenia gravis, 859–860
for neuropathy, 882, 885
for pemphigus vulgaris, 767
for thrombotic thrombocytopenic purpura, 345
Plasma protein fraction, 396–397

Plasma volume expanders, 396–397
Plasmodium species, infection by, 91–98, *92*, 94(t), 97(t)
Platelet(s), 338
  disorders of, 338–342. See also *Thrombocytopenia.*
    and bleeding, 339–342
    in renal failure, 340, 639
  transfusion of, 394–395
    in anemic patient, 300–301
    in patient with disseminated intravascular coagulopathy, 343
    in thrombocytopenic patient, 342(t)
    in thrombocytopenic patient with leukemia, 369
Platyhelminth infestation, 481(t), 482(t), 485, 486
Pleomorphic adenoma, 754
Pleural disease, pericarditis accompanying, 291
Pleural space, effusion in, 170(t), 170–171
    lung cancer and, 158, 158(t)
  leak of air in, complicating central venous catheter placement, 536–537
  pus in, 171
Pleuritis, lupus erythematosus and, 716
Pleurodesis, for malignant pleural effusion, 158, 158(t)
Plicamycin, for Paget's disease of bone, 529
PMS (premenstrual syndrome), 1000–1003
Pneumatic compression, intermittent, in prevention of deep venous thrombosis, 195
Pneumatic esophageal dilatation, for achalasia, 419–420
Pneumococcal meningitis, 99, 100, 100(t), 101, 101(t)
Pneumococcal pneumonia, 179–180
  AIDS and, 47
  immunization against, in patient with chronic airway disease, 153, 176
Pneumocystis carinii pneumonia, in AIDS, 49–50, 50(t)
Pneumonectomy, for cancer, 161, 161(t)
Pneumonia, 176–187, 189–190
  AIDS and, 47, 48, 49, 50(t), 52, 184
  aspiration, 179(t), 182–183
    obstetric anesthesia and, 953–954
  atypical, 179(t), 181–182
  bacteremia as complication of, 57(t)
  bacterial, 176–187, 179(t), 186(t), 191
    AIDS and, 47
    influenza and, 80
  Bordetella pertussis infection and, 144
  chlamydial, 181–182
  community-acquired, 179(t), 179–184, 191
    bacteremia as complication of, 57(t)
  cryptococcal, in AIDS, 48
  cytomegaloviral, 190
    AIDS and, 52
  diagnosis of, 177(t), 177–179, 187
  gram-negative bacillary, 179(t), 183
  Haemophilus influenzae infection and, 180
    in AIDS, 47
  hospital-acquired, 184–187, 186(t)
    bacteremia as complication of, 57(t)
  hospitalization for, 184
  influenza and, 80
  Legionella pneumophila infection and, 191
  mechanical ventilation and, 185
  Moraxella catarrhalis infection and, 180
  mycoplasmal, 181, 190
Pneumonia *(Continued)*
  nosocomial, 184–187, 186(t)
    bacteremia as complication of, 57(t)
  pertussis and, 144
  plague and, 107
  pneumococcal, 179–180
    AIDS and, 47
    immunization against, in patient with chronic airway disease, 153, 176
  Pneumocystis carinii, in AIDS, 49–50, 50(t)
  Q fever and, 109
  staphylococcal, 180–181, 187
  streptococcal. See *Pneumonia, pneumococcal.*
  varicella-zoster virus infection and, 68
    in immunocompromised patient, 190
  viral, 68, 80, 189–190
  whooping cough and, 144
Pneumonic plague, 107
Pneumonitis, chemical, due to aspiration, 182
  chlamydial, in newborn, 1011
  cytomegaloviral, in AIDS patient, 52
  hypersensitivity, 201–202, 202(t)
  lupus erythematosus and, 716
  radiation-induced, 359
  varicella and, 68
Pneumothorax, as complication of central venous catheter placement, 536–537
Podophyllin, for bowenoid papulosis, 736
  for condyloma acuminatum, 728
Podophyllotoxin, for condyloma acuminatum, 728
Poisoning, 1086–1131
  activated charcoal for, 1043, 1044, 1088
  alcohol. See *Alcohol* entries.
  antidotes for, 1088–1089, 1090(t)–1098(t)
  arsenic, 882, 1102–1104, 1104(t)
  barbiturate, 1044, 1104, 1105(t)
  benzodiazepine, 1104
    flumazenil for, 1044, 1094(t)
  carbon monoxide, 1067–1068, 1105–1106, 1108(t)
    nomogram for, *1109*
  cathartics for, 78, 1088
  contact with marine animals and, 1082–1084
  dialysis for, 1089, 1099(t)
  diuresis in management of, 1089
  food-borne, 12, 74–78, 75(t), 137, 1085–1086
  gastrointestinal decontamination for, 1087–1088
  hallucinogenic, 1043, 1043(t), 1112
  hemoperfusion for, 1089, 1099(t)
  induction of emesis for, 78, 1088
  iron. See *Iron overload.*
  laboratory determination of, reference values for, 1140(t)
  lithium, 1117
  management of, 1086–1089, 1090(t)–1099(t), 1098–1131
  narcotic, 1043(t), 1043–1044, 1118–1119
    naloxone for, 1044, 1096(t), 1118, 1119
  neuropathies due to, 884, 888
  sedative hypnotic, 1044(t), 1044–1045, 1127–1128, 1129(t)
  snake venom, 1080–1082
    antivenin for, 1081, 1082, 1090(t)
  solvent, 1045, 1045(t), 1110–1112
  spider venom, 1079–1080
    antivenin for, 1090(t)
  stabilization measures in, 1089
Poisoning *(Continued)*
  stimulant, 1041(t), 1041–1043, 1102, 1108(t), 1108–1109
  vs. therapeutic drug levels, 1138(t)
Polycythemia, 387–389, 388(t)
  in newborn, 969
Polyethylene glycol solutions, bowel-cleansing, 18
    in management of poisoning, 1088
Polymorphic eruption of pregnancy, 775
Polymorphous light eruption, 786
Polymyalgia rheumatica, 922, 923
Polymyositis, 420, 717
Polymyxin, for conjunctivitis, 66, 66(t)
  in newborn, 64, 64(t)
Polymyxin-bacitracin, for sunburn, 785
Polymyxin-neomycin-hydrocortisone, for otitis externa, 106(t), 1085
Polyneuropathies, 879(t), 880–888, 881(t). See also *Neuropathy (neuropathies).*
Polyp(s), colonic, 476
  gastric, 472–473
Pontiac fever, 191
Popliteal artery, aneurysm of, 295
  entrapment of, 293
Porcine factor VIII, 338
Porcine xenograft, for burns, 1072
Porphyria, 389–393, 390(t), 882–883, 887
  drug precautions in, 391(t), 392
  photosensitivity in, 392, 786–787
Porphyria cutanea tarda, 390(t), 393, 786–787
Portal hypertension, 406–407
  and bleeding esophageal varices, 413–417
  and gastropathy, 407, 443
  and intestinal vasculopathy, 407
Portosystemic encephalopathy, 407(t), 407–408
Portosystemic shunt, for bleeding esophageal varices, 415, 415(t), 416
Positional vertigo, 837
  treatment of, 837, *839*
Positioning, of head, in management of dysphagia, 418
    in treatment of vertigo, 837, *839*
    to lower intracranial pressure, 795, 891
Positive end-expiratory pressure (PEEP), 150–151
Positive pressure ventilation, for newborn, 960
Postcoital contraception, 1035
Posterior urethra, trauma to, 625, 626
Post-herpetic neuralgia, 742, 743
Postinfectious encephalitis, 844(t), 845, 845(t)
Postinfectious glomerulonephritis, 617–618, 737
Postmenopausal patient. See *Menopause.*
Postpartum care, 955–957
Postpartum pain, 953, 956
Postpartum thyroiditis, 593
Postpericardiotomy syndrome, in pediatric patient, 247
Poststreptococcal glomerulonephritis, 617–618, 737
Post-thrombotic syndrome, 1027
Post-transfusion purpura, 400
Post-traumatic stress disorder, 1046
Postural hypotension, in diabetic patients, 884
Potassium, concentration of, factors affecting, 646(t)

Potassium *(Continued)*
shifts in, in diabetic ketoacidosis, 500, 502
deficiency of, in aldosteronism, 569, 570, 571
excess of, in renal failure, 638, 639(t), 646–647
Potassium chloride, for diabetic ketoacidosis, 502
Potassium citrate, alkalinization of urine with, in treatment of renal calculi, 664
Potassium iodide, for hyperthyroidism, 583, 584
Potassium-restricted diet, for hyperkalemia, in renal failure, 647
Potassium-sparing diuretics. See also *Diuretics*; *Spironolactone*.
for hypertension, 270(t)
"Pouchitis," 431
Poxvirus infection, 744
in AIDS, 52
PPD (purified protein derivative) reaction, positive, definition of, 209, 209(t)
Practolol, 1124(t)
Pralidoxime, as antidote, 1097(t)
Pravastatin, for hyperlipoproteinemia, 508
Prazepam, 1106(t)
Praziquantel, for helminthiasis, 481(t), 482(t), 485, 486
Prazosin, for hypertension, 272(t)
in patient with pheochromocytoma, 588–589, 591(t)
Precipitated sulfur in petrolatum, for scabies, 746
Pre-conception counseling, 933–934
Prednisolone, anticholinergic properties of, 1054(t)
for gout, 504
Prednisone, 553(t)
for acne, 705
for adrenocortical insufficiency, in patient with hypopituitarism, 573
for allergic drug reaction, 696, 696(t), 697, 698
for allergic rhinitis, 694
for anaphylactic reaction, 701
for anemia, 307, 311
for ankylosing spondylitis, 913
for arthritis, 903, 909, 909(t)
in patient with lupus erythematosus, 716
for asthma, 680, 682
in pediatric patient, 685(t)
for atopic dermatitis, 764
for autoimmune hemolytic anemia, 307
in patient with leukemia, 374
for Bell's palsy, 871
for brucellosis, 63
for bullous pemphigoid, 769
for carditis, in patient with rheumatic fever, 118, 118(t)
for celiac sprue, 453
for chronic demyelinating inflammatory polyneuropathy, 885
for chronic obstructive pulmonary disease, 154
for cluster headache, 836
for complications of diphtheria, 73
for contact dermatitis, 773, 782
for Crohn's disease, 433
for cutaneous T-cell lymphoma, 381
for eosinophilic gastroenteritis, 456
for epidermolysis bullosa acquisita, 770
for erythema nodosum leprosum, 90
for facial paralysis, 871
Prednisone *(Continued)*
for giant cell arteritis, 923
for glomerulopathy, 613, 614, 615, 618(t), 618–619
in patient with lupus erythematosus, 716
for headache, 832
for hemolytic anemia, 307, 311
for Hodgkin's disease, 351(t)
for hypersensitivity pneumonitis, 202
for idiopathic thrombocytopenic purpura, 341
for juvenile rheumatoid arthritis, 909, 909(t)
for leukemia, 366, 367, 374
for lichen planus, 723
for linear IgA dermatitis, 772
for lupus erythematosus, 715, 716, 717
for lymphoma, 351(t), 375, 376(t), 381
for membranous glomerulopathy, 615
for minimal change nephrotic syndrome, 613
for multiple myeloma, 383, 384(t)
for multiple sclerosis, 849
for myasthenia gravis, 858(t), 858–859, 859(t)
for nephritis, in patient with lupus erythematosus, 716
for neurobrucellosis, 63
for neuropathy, 885
in patient with vasculitis, 886
for neutropenia, 328
for non-Hodgkin's lymphoma, 375, 376(t)
for optic neuritis, 865
for paronychia, 722
for paroxysmal nocturnal hemoglobinuria, 311
for pemphigoid gestationis, 774
for pemphigus vulgaris, 766, 767
for pericarditis, in patient with lupus erythematosus, 716
for pleuritis, in patient with lupus erythematosus, 716
for *Pneumocystis carinii* pneumonia, in AIDS patient, 50(t)
for pneumonitis accompanying lupus erythematosus, 716
for pneumonitis or alveolitis due to allergen inhalation, 202
for polymorphic eruption of pregnancy, 775
for polymyalgia rheumatica, 923
for post-herpetic neuralgia, 743
for pulmonary fibrosis, in patient with lupus erythematosus, 716
for renal disease, 613, 614, 615, 618(t), 618–619
in patient with lupus erythematosus, 716
for reversal reaction in leprosy, 90
for rheumatic carditis, 118, 118(t)
for rheumatoid arthritis, 903
in pediatric patient, 909, 909(t)
for sarcoidosis, 197
for serum sickness, 678
for skin lesions induced by sun exposure, in patient with lupus erythematosus, 715, 787
for sunburn, 785
for systemic lupus erythematosus, 715, 716, 717
for temporal arteritis, 923
for thrombocytopenia, in patient with lupus erythematosus, 717
for thyroiditis, 593
Prednisone *(Continued)*
for toxoplasmosis, in newborn, 132
for ulcerative colitis, 429(t), 430
for urticaria, 696(t), 777
for vasculitis, 720, 886
for warm antibody autoimmune hemolytic anemia, 307
risk of dependency on, in patient with pericarditis, 289
use of, in patient treated for acromegaly, 549
in patient treated for Cushing's syndrome, 559
in patient undergoing radiocontrast studies, 677(t), 700
in polytherapy for seizures complicating lupus erythematosus, 716
Preeclampsia, 937, 945(t), 945–947
Pregnancy, abruptio placentae in, 942, 943
"bloody show" in, 942
breast cancer in, 982
breast-feeding following, 978
brucellosis treatment in, 62–63
care during, 933–940. See also *Prenatal care*.
care following, 955–957
cervical cancer treatment in, 1021
chickenpox in, 68
chlamydiosis treatment in, 1012, 1012(t)
deep venous thrombosis in, 297, 1026, 1030
delivery in. See *Delivery*.
depression following, 957
diabetes mellitus in, 937–938, 951
effect of, on offspring, 972
ectopic, 940–941
epilepsy treatment in, 809
folliculitis in, pruritic, 775
German measles in, 125, 126
granuloma inguinale treatment in, 671
hemorrhage following, 956
hemorrhage late in, 941–944, 951
hyperemesis in, 8
hypertension in, 937, 938(t), 944–948, 945(t)–947(t), 951
hyperthyroidism in, 583
hypoparathyroidism in, 569
hypothyroidism in, 579
infection following, 956
in patient with heart disease, 248–249, 951
in patient with myasthenia gravis, 862
in patient with rheumatoid arthritis, 906
in patient with systemic lupus erythematosus, 717
in patient with ulcerative colitis, 433
laboratory tests in, 934(t), 934–935
Lyme disease in, treatment of, 120(t)
malaria treatment and prophylaxis in, 96, 97, 98
nausea and vomiting in, 8
pain following, 953, 956
pemphigoid in, 773–775
pheochromocytoma treatment in, 592
placenta in, and late second-trimester or third-trimester bleeding, 941–944
polymorphic eruption in, 775
preeclampsia in, 937, 945(t), 945–947
prurigo in, 775
pruritic folliculitis in, 775
pyelonephritis in, 598, 599, 622
Rh isoimmunization in, 329–334
Rh prophylaxis during, 334, 939, 939(t), 943
rubella in, 125, 126

Pregnancy *(Continued)*
skin diseases in, 773–775, 774(t)
syphilis in, 673, 673(t)
tampon use following, 956
thrombosis in, 297, 1026, 1030
thrombotic thrombocytopenic purpura in, 345
thyroiditis following, 593
toxoplasmosis in, 132
tubal, 940
tuberculosis treatment in, 209
uterine cervical cancer treatment in, 1021
uterine rupture in, 944
vaginal bleeding late in, 941–944
varicella in, 68
vasa praevia in, 942, 944
venous thrombosis in, 297, 1026, 1030
visits to physician during, 934–935
vomiting and nausea in, 8
Premalignant skin lesions, 733–736
Premature beats, 230–233
ventricular, 231–233, 240, 241
Premenstrual syndrome (PMS), 1000–1003
Prenatal care, 935–936
amniocentesis in, 331, 936, 936(t)
chorionic villus sampling in, 936
diagnosis of genetic disorders in, 315–316, 935–936
fetal ultrasonography in, 331, 936–937, 937(t)
measurement of alpha-fetoprotein levels in, 935
nonstress testing of fetus in, 939, 940
Prepackaged foods, for obese patient, 514
Presbylaryngis, 33
Preseptal cellulitis, 204
Pressure application, for keloids, 726
Pressure-assist mode, of mechanical ventilation, 150
Pressure ulcers, 759–762
Preterm infants, cardiac disease in, 242
delivery of, 951
problems requiring special care in, 972–976
Preterm labor, 938–939, 939(t)
Priapism, in sickle cell disease, 323
Primaquine, for malaria, 94(t), 94–95, 97(t)
Primary aldosteronism, 569–572, 570(t), 571(t)
Primary amenorrhea, 994–996, *995*
Primary dysmenorrhea, 998–1000
treatment of, 999(t), 999–1000
Primary glomerulopathies, 609–620
Primary herpetic gingivostomatitis, 740, 757
Primary hyperparathyroidism, 565
treatment of, 566–567, 567(t)
Primary iron overload, 346, 347, 406
phlebotomy for, 347
screening for, 347, *348*
Primidone, 811(t), 1103(t)
for epilepsy, 809, 810, 810(t), 811(t), 815–816
therapeutic vs. toxic levels of, 1103(t), 1138(t)
Prinzmetal's angina pectoris, 219
Probenecid, for arthritis, in Lyme disease, 120(t)
for endocarditis, 260(t)
for hyperuricemia, 505
for neurosyphilis, 672
for pelvic inflammatory disease, 668(t), 1014(t)
for salmonellosis carriers, 140, 142
Probenecid *(Continued)*
for syphilis, 672
for typhoid fever carriers, 142
Probucol, for hyperlipoproteinemia, 509
Procainamide, for arrhythmias, 238(t)
in children, 244(t)
for atrial fibrillation, 228(t), 229
for ventricular fibrillation, 225
for ventricular tachycardia, 241
therapeutic vs. toxic levels of, 1138(t)
Procarbazine, for brain cancer, 898
for Hodgkin's disease, 351(t)
for lung cancer, 162(t)
for non-Hodgkin's lymphoma, 376(t)
Prochlorperazine, 1123(t)
for headache, 829
for nausea and vomiting, 6, 6(t), 7(t)
in patient with food poisoning, 78
in patient with pericarditis, 289
in patient with salmonellosis, 137
for vertigo, 838(t)
use of, in patient with sickle cell disease, 322
Proctitis, 11, 667
Progestin(s), for dysfunctional uterine bleeding, 994
for dysmenorrhea, 1000
for endometrial cancer, 1016, 1017
for endometriosis, 991
for gonadotropin deficiency, 573
possible beneficial effect of, in premenstrual syndrome, 1003
postmenopausal use of, 567, 1005
Progestin-only contraceptives, 1032
Progressive glomerulonephritis, 616–617
Progressive multifocal leukoencephalopathy, in AIDS, 52
Proguanil, for malaria, 97(t), 98
Prolactin, hypersecretion of, 575–577, 576(t)
Prolapse, mitral valve, 249–252, 250(t)
sickle cell disease and, 326
ProMACE-CytaBOM chemotherapy regimen, for non-Hodgkin's lymphoma, 376, 376(t)
ProMACE-MOPP chemotherapy regimen, for non-Hodgkin's lymphoma, 376, 376(t)
Promethazine, 1123(t)
for delivery, 955
for nausea and vomiting, 6, 6(t)
in relapsing fever, 116
in salmonellosis, 137
for pemphigoid gestationis, 774
for vertigo, 838(t)
Propafenone, for atrial fibrillation, 228(t)
Propantheline, for urinary incontinence, 606
Propiomazine, for delivery, 955
Propofol, use of, in management of tetanus, 130
Propoxyphene, 1119(t)
poisoning by, 1119
Propranolol, 1124(t)
for akathisia due to neuroleptic medication, 1063
for arrhythmias, in child, 244(t)
in patient with pheochromocytoma, 589
for atrial fibrillation, 228(t)
for cyanotic congenital heart disease, 244(t)
for esophageal variceal bleeding, 415, 415(t)
for headache, 835
Propranolol *(Continued)*
for hemorrhagic portal hypertensive gastropathy, 407, 443
for hypertension, 270(t), 278(t)
in patient with porphyria, 391
for hyperthyroidism, 583, 584, 594
for migraine, 835
for panic disorder, 1066
for tachycardia, in patient with pheochromocytoma, 589
in patient with postpartum thyroiditis, 593
for thyroid storm, 584
poisoning by, 1125–1126
therapeutic vs. toxic levels of, 1138(t)
Propylthiouracil, for hyperthyroidism, 582, 583
Prostaglandin E_1, for congenital heart disease, 243, 244(t), 977
Prostaglandin $F_{2\alpha}$, for postpartum hemorrhage, 956
Prostaglandin synthetase inhibitors. See *Nonsteroidal anti-inflammatory drugs.*
Prostate, cancer of, 653–656
hyperplasia of, benign, 627–633, 628(t)–630(t)
inflammation of, 633(t), 633–635
resection of, for benign hyperplasia, 630
for cancer, 655
tumors of, 653–656
Prostatectomy, for benign hyperplasia, 630
for cancer, 655
Prostatic stent, for benign hyperplasia, 631
Prostatitis, 633(t), 633–635
Prostatodynia, 634
Prosthetic graft(s), in repair of aortic lesions, 213, 214, 216, 217
in surgery for aortoiliac occlusive disease, 216, 217, 293
in surgery for occlusive disease of lower extremity arteries, 293, 294
Prosthetic valve(s), infection of. See *Prosthetic valve endocarditis.*
mechanical destruction of red blood cells by, 310
metal, in pediatric patient, 248
Prosthetic valve endocarditis, 258(t), 259, 260(t), 261
bacteremia as complication of, 57(t)
Protamine, allergic reaction to, 699
as antidote, 1097(t)
Protein, determination of requirements for, 532, 532(t)
intake of, estimated from urinary urea nitrogen excretion, 612(t)
provision of, in parenteral nutrition, 533–534, 534(t)
Protein malnutrition, in nephrotic syndrome, 610
Protein-restricted diet, for portosystemic encephalopathy, 407
for renal disease or renal failure, 612, 645, 648
Prothionamide, for leprosy, 87
Prothrombin complex concentrates, 397, 397(t)
for bleeding hemophiliac patient, 336(t)
for hemophiliac patient with factor VIII inhibitors, 338
Proton beam therapy, for acromegaly, 549
Proton pump inhibitors. See *Omeprazole.*
Protoporphyria, erythropoietic, 390(t), 392
Protozoa, food sources of, 75(t)
Protozoan infection. See also specific infections.

Protozoan infection *(Continued)*
AIDS and, 46(t), 50–51, 483
intestinal, 15(t), 53–55, 54(t), 455, 479–483, 480(t), 485
AIDS and, 51, 483
transfusion-transmitted, 401
Protriptyline, 1130(t)
for depression, 1058(t), 1119
Proximal subungual onychomycosis, 750
Prurigo of pregnancy, 775
Pruritic folliculitis of pregnancy, 775
Pruritus, 35–37, 36(t), 775–776
anal, 775–776
atopic dermatitis and, 762, 763
cirrhosis and, 408(t), 408–409
dermatitis herpetiformis and, 771
marine dermatitis and, 748, 1085
scabies and, 745
treatment of, 36–37, 37(t)
in atopic dermatitis, 763
in contact dermatitis, 773, 782
in erythema multiforme, 764
in liver disease, 408(t), 408–409
in management of keloids, 726
in pediculosis, 746
in pityriasis rosea, 714
in polycythemia, 389
in scabies, 745
in varicella, 67
vulvar, 775–776
Pruritus ani, 775–776
Pruritus vulvae, 775–776
Pseudocysts, pancreatic, 461, 463
Pseudoephedrine, for cough, 21, 23(t), 24
for upper respiratory tract infection, 28(t)
for urinary incontinence, 607
Pseudohypoparathyroidism, 566
Pseudomembrane, diphtheritic, 72
Pseudomembranous colitis, 12
Pseudomonas aeruginosa infection, AIDS and, 47
endocarditis due to, 259
treatment of, 259, 260(t)
meningitis due to, 101
otitis externa due to, 106(t), 106–107
Pseudomonas species, bone infection by, treatment of, 928, 928(t)
Psittacosis, 108–109
Psoralen–ultraviolet A therapy, for cutaneous T-cell lymphoma, 380, 381, 382
for pruritus, 37
for psoriasis, 713, 723
for vitiligo, 781
Psoriasis, 713–714
ankylosing spondylitis and, 914
nail involvement in, 723
Psychiatric disorders, 1037–1066
and insomnia, 33
Psychogenic cough, 25
Psychological counseling, for obese patient, 516
Psychological preparation, for labor, 948
Psychologist, in treatment of pain, 3
Psychopharmacologic preparations, therapeutic vs. toxic levels of, 1130(t), 1138(t)
Psychophysiologic insomnia, 34–35
Psychosis, 1061–1064
drugs for. See *Neuroleptic(s).*
levodopa-induced, 876
Psychosocial impact, of diabetes mellitus, 497
Psychosocial support, of burned patient, 1071
Psychosocial support *(Continued)*
of child with leukemia, 369
of family of high-risk newborn, 977
of family of young leukemia patient, 369
of obese patient, 515
Psychotherapy, for anxiety, 1046
for depression, 1059
Pubic lice, 746
Pudendal block anesthesia, for delivery, 948
Puffer fish, poisoning by, 1086
Pulmonary abscess, 171–172
Pulmonary disease, chronic obstructive, 148, 152–156
management of acute exacerbations of, 23, 154–155
therapy for, 149, 152–156, *155*
infectious. See *Lung(s), infections of*; *Pneumonia.*
inflammatory. See *Pneumonitis.*
lupus erythematosus and, 716
malignant, 156–163
occupational, 199(t), 199–201
pericarditis accompanying, 291
scleroderma and, 719
sickle cell syndromes and, 322–323
Pulmonary edema, congestive heart failure and. See *Heart failure.*
malaria and, 96
poisoning and, 1089, 1098
renal failure and, 639
transfusion and, 400
Pulmonary embolism, 192–195, 296
diagnosis of, 192, *193*
differential diagnosis of, 192(t)
prevention of, 195
treatment of, 192–194, 195(t), 297, 1030
Pulmonary fibrosis, lupus erythematosus and, 716
silicosis and, 199
Pulmonary function, adaptive, in newborn, 963
Pulmonary granuloma, coccidioidomycosis and, 164
Pulmonary hypertension, causes of, in newborn, 972
Pulmonary infarction, sickle cell disease and, 322, 323
Pulmonary infections. See *Lung(s), infections of*; *Pneumonia.*
Pulmonary nodule(s), silicosis and, 199
solitary, 159
Pulmonary sarcoidosis, 198
Pulmonary scleroderma, 719
Pulmonary silicosis, 199(t), 199–201, 200(t)
Pulmonary tularemia, 135
Pulseless electrical activity, 225
cardiac arrest due to, 222, 223, 225
treatment of, 224(t), 225, 225(t)
Pulseless ventricular tachycardia, treatment of, 224(t), 225
Purified protein derivative (PPD) reaction, positive, definition of, 209, 209(t)
Purpura, post-transfusion, 341, 400
thrombocytopenic, idiopathic, 341, 344
thrombotic, 344–345
Pus, in gallbladder, 405
in pleural space, 171
Pustular psoriasis, generalized, 713
PUVA therapy, for cutaneous T-cell lymphoma, 380, 381, 382
for pruritus, 37
for psoriasis, 713, 723
for vitiligo, 781
Pyelonephritis, 620–622
Pyelonephritis *(Continued)*
in female patient, 598, 599, 600, 621–622
in male patient, 595, 621
Pyogenic granuloma, oral, 758
Pyrantel pamoate, for enterobiasis, 484, 748
for helminthiasis, 481(t), 482(t), 484, 486
for trichinosis, 134
Pyrazinamide, for tuberculosis, 207, 208, 208(t)
in AIDS, 46
Pyrethrin, for pediculosis, 746
Pyridostigmine, for myasthenia gravis, 857, 857(t), 858
Pyridoxine. See *Vitamin B_6 (pyridoxine).*
Pyrimethamine, adverse effects of, 132(t)
for isosporiasis, 15(t), 483
for *Pneumocystis carinii* pneumonia, in AIDS patient, 50(t)
for toxoplasmosis, 131, 132, 132(t), 133
in AIDS patient, 50, 51, 132
use of leucovorin (folinic acid) with, 50, 131
Pyrimethamine-sulfadoxine, for malaria, 94(t), 95, 97(t), 98
for *Pneumocystis carinii* pneumonia, in AIDS patient, 50(t)

Q fever, 109–110
Qinghaosu derivatives, for malaria, 96
Quazepam, 1106(t)
Queensland tick typhus, 143(t)
Quinacrine, adverse effects of, 482
for giardiasis, 15(t), 455, 480, 480(t)
Quinapril, for hypertension, 275(t)
Quinidine, adverse effects of, 340, 1126
for arrhythmias, 238(t)
for atrial fibrillation, 228(t)
for malaria, 94(t), 95
therapeutic vs. toxic levels of, 1138(t)
Quinine, adverse effects of, 95, 340, 1126
for malaria, 94(t), 95
Quinolone(s). See specific agents, e.g., *Ciprofloxacin.*
Quinolone reaction, 699

Rabies, 110–113
Rabies immune globulin, 112
Rabies vaccine (adsorbed), 112
Radial nerve, compression of, 880
Radiation therapy, electron beam, for cutaneous T-cell lymphoma, 381
for acromegaly, 549
for cancer, complications of, 422, 455, 736
of brain, 896, 897, 898
of breast, 987, 988
of cervix, 1020
of endometrium, 1016, 1017
of lung, 161, 162, 163
of prostate, 655
of rectum, 479
of skin, 711
of stomach, 475
of testis, 657
of uterine cervix, 1020
of uterus, 1016, 1017
of vulva, 1024, 1025
problems with, 359
for Cushing's disease, 556
for cutaneous T-cell lymphoma, 381

Radiation therapy *(Continued)*
for Hodgkin's disease, 349, 354–359, *356*, 357(t)
chemotherapy combined with, 349, 350, 352, 357, 357(t), 358
for hyperprolactinemia, 575
for keloids, 726
for lymphoma, 349, 354–359, *356*, 357(t), 381
chemotherapy combined with, 349, 350, 352, 357, 357(t), 358
for multiple myeloma, 383, 386
for mycosis fungoides, 381
for pheochromocytoma, 592
for prolactinoma, 575
proton beam, for acromegaly, 549
Radiation-treated blood products, 396, 396(t)
Radioactive iodine, for hyperthyroidism, 582–583
Radioactive phosphorus, for polycythemia, 388, 389
Radiocontrast media, anaphylactoid reaction to, 700
prevention of, 677(t), 700
nephrotoxicity of, 644
Radiofrequency ablation therapy, for atrial fibrillation, 229
Radiofrequency rhizolysis, percutaneous, for trigeminal neuralgia, 863
Ramipril, for heart failure, 255
for hypertension, 275(t)
Ranitidine, anticholinergic properties of, 1054(t)
for effects of esophageal dysmotility, in scleroderma, 718
for gastritis, 442(t)
for gastroesophageal reflux, 24, 30
for hypotension, in anaphylaxis, 677, 677(t), 701
for peptic ulcer, 9, 470
use of, in patient receiving methylprednisolone, 849
Ranson's criteria, for prognosis in pancreatitis, 460, 460(t)
Rapidly progressive glomerulonephritis, 616–617
Rash. See *Eruption(s)*.
Rat-bite fever, 113–114, 114(t)
Rauwolfia alkaloids, for hypertension, 271–272, 272(t), 278(t)
Raynaud's phenomenon, scleroderma and, 718
Reactivated toxoplasmosis, 132–133
Reactive arthritis, 914
Reactive cheilitis, 752
Reassurance, of patient with muscle pain syndrome, 920
of patient with somatoform disorder, 1047
of patient with tinnitus, 39
Reciprocating tachycardia, 239(t)
Recluse spider bites, 1078–1080
Rectum, cancer of, 476–479
infection of, 11, 667
tumors of, 476–479
Recurrence sites, in patients with endometrial cancer, 1017
Recurrent acute pericarditis, 290
Recurrent cervical cancer, 1020–1021
Recurrent herpes simplex virus infection, 741
oral, 741, 754
Recurrent myocardial infarction, prevention of, 284–285
Recurrent streptococcal pharyngitis, 206–207
Recurrent variceal hemorrhage, 415
prevention of, 415(t), 415–416
Red blood cells, increase in mass of, 387–389, 388(t)
in newborn, 969
membrane of, destruction of. See *Hemolytic* entries.
transfusion of, 394, 396
in child with leukemia, 369
in patient with aplastic anemia, 301
in patient with hemolytic anemia, 307, 308, 310
in pregnant patient with vaginal bleeding, 942, 943
Reed coma scale, 1087(t)
Re-entrant tachycardia, 239(t)
Reflux, gastroesophageal, and cough, 24
and dysphagia, 420, 421
and laryngitis, 30
and stricture formation, 420–421
in patients with scleroderma, 420, 718
vesicoureteral, in girls with urinary tract infection, 601
Reflux gastritis, 443
Regurgitation, mitral, heart failure due to, 250, 261
mitral valve prolapse and, 250, 251
myocardial infarction and, 284(t)
rheumatic carditis and, 250
Rehabilitation, after stroke, 801–806, *802*, 802(t)–804(t)
cardiac, 285–289
in management of hemiplegia, 801–806, *802*, 802(t)–804(t)
in management of polyneuropathies, 888
vestibular, 840–841
Rehydration solutions. See *Fluid replacement therapy*; *Oral rehydration solutions*.
Relapsing fever, 114–117, 115(t), 116(t)
Relapsing vestibulopathy, 838, 840(t)
Relaxation therapy, for muscle-contraction headache, 832
Remission induction therapy, for leukemia. See *Leukemia, chemotherapy for*.
Renal artery, atherosclerosis of, 644–645
Renal calculi, 661–665, 662(t), 663(t)
sarcoidosis and, 199
Renal cancer, 649–652
Renal cell carcinoma, 649–651
Renal disease, 609–620
amantadine dosage adjustments necessary in, 82(t)
calculous, 661–665, 662(t), 663(t)
sarcoidosis and, 199
diabetes insipidus due to, 559, 562–563
diabetes mellitus and, 493, 498, 645
drug dosage adjustments necessary in, 641(t), 648
end-stage, 642, 642(t), 648
hypertension in, 612, 639, 644, 645, 718–719
treatment of, 280, 646
infectious, 595, 598, 599, 600, 617–618, 620–622, 737
inflammatory, 615–617
infection and, 595, 598, 599, 600, 617–618, 620–622, 737
lupus erythematosus and, 716
malignant, 649–652
malnutrition in, 610, 639
neoplastic, 649–652
risk of infection in, 610, 639
Renal disease *(Continued)*
sarcoidosis and, 199
scleroderma and, 718
sickle cell syndromes and, 327
systemic lupus erythematosus and, 716
Renal failure, 635–648
acute, 635(t), 635–642, 637(t)
anemia associated with, 639, 647–648
chronic, 642(t), 642–648, 643(t), 646(t)
cirrhosis and, 411–412
dialysis for, 640(t), 640–641, 648
drug dosage adjustments necessary in, 641(t), 648
hyperkalemia in, 638, 646–647
treatment of, 638, 639(t)
hyperparathyroidism associated with, 567, 647
hyperphosphatemia in, 567, 638, 647
hypertension in. See *Renal disease, hypertension in.*
indices of, 543(t), 637, 637(t)
malaria and, 96
metabolic acidosis in, 638, 647
multiple myeloma and, 385–386
neuropathy associated with, 884
platelet disorders associated with, 340, 639
poisoning and, 1098
scleroderma and, 718
sickle cell disease and, 327
Renal function, in dehydrated child, 543
in hypothermic patient, 1073–1074
Renal infarction, sickle cell disease and, 326
Renal osteodystrophy, 647
Renal transplantation, 648
blastomycosis following, 170
Renal trauma, 623–624
Renal tubular dysfunction, and acidosis, 663
in nephrotic syndrome, 611
Renal tumors, 649–652
Renal vein thrombosis, 610, 612
Reserpine, for Cushing's syndrome, 557, 557(t)
for hypertension, 271–272, 272(t)
medical sympathectomy with, in management of frostbite, 1076
Respiratory depression, drug-induced, naloxone for, 962, 1044
Respiratory distress syndrome, adult, 147, 148, 149
malaria and, 96
neonatal, 972–973
Respiratory failure, 147–151
acute, 147–151
hypercapnic, 147, 148, 149
hypoxemic, 147, 148, 149
myasthenia gravis and, 861–862
Respiratory function, effects of hypothermia on, 1073
Respiratory syncytial virus infection, 190
Respiratory tract infections. See also *Lung(s), infections of*; *Pneumonia*.
bacterial. See *Lung(s), bacterial infections of.*
bronchitis due to, 174
cough due to, 23, 24
exacerbations of COPD due to, 154
fungal, 163–170
in AIDS, 48, 49
pneumonia due to. See *Pneumonia*.
symptomatic treatment of, 28(t), 29–30
viral, 68, 80, 187–190
effect of, in asthma, 679

Respiratory tract surgery, prophylaxis against endocarditis in, 119(t), 263(t)
Rest, in management of low back pain, 40
 in management of ulcerative colitis, 426
Restless legs syndrome, 34
Rest pain, 292
Restraint, of stimulant-abusing patient, 1042
Resuscitation, of burned patient, 1070
 of hypothermic patient, 1074
 of newborn, 957–962, 958(t)
  certification for, 963
 of patient in cardiac arrest, 223, 224(t), 226
 of patient with pancreatitis, 459–460
 of pregnant patient with vaginal bleeding, 943
Retardation, growth, intrauterine, 969–970, 970(t)
  ulcerative colitis and, 432
Reticular lichen planus, 753
Retinitis, cytomegaloviral, in AIDS, 51, 52
Retinochoroiditis, toxoplasmosis and, 132
Retinopathy, diabetic, 493, 498, 499
 sickle cell disease and, 326
Reversal reactions, in leprosy, 90
Rewarming. See *Warming.*
Reye's syndrome, 68, 845–848, 846(t), 847(t)
Rhabdomyolysis, stimulant abuse and, 1042
Rheumatic fever, 117(t), 117–119, 118(t)
Rheumatic heart disease, 117, 118, 250, 250(t)
 prophylaxis against endocarditis in, 119, 119(t)
Rheumatoid arthritis, 901–907, 902(t)
 juvenile, 907–911, 908(t), 909(t)
 treatment of, 901–911, 902(t), 904(t), 908(t), 909(t)
Rhinitis, 203, 691(t)
 allergic, 203, 691–695
  cough management in, 24
  treatment of, 692–695, 693(t), 694(t)
Rhinophyma, 705
Rhinosinusitis, viral, 203
Rh isoimmunization, 329–334, 939
Rhizolysis, percutaneous, for trigeminal neuralgia, 863
Rho(D) immune globulin, for pregnant patient, 334, 939, 939(t), 943
 for thrombocytopenic HIV-positive patient, 341
Rho(d) immune globulin, for transfusion recipient, 398
Ribavirin, for respiratory syncytial virus infection, 190
Riboflavin (vitamin B_2), 518(t), 519
 deficiency of, 518(t), 519
Rickettsialpox, 143(t)
Rickettsioses, 109–110, 124–125, 142–143, 143(t)
Riedel's thyroiditis, 594
Rifabutin, for atypical mycobacterial infection, in AIDS, 47, 211
Rifampin, adverse effects of, 88
 for atypical mycobacterial infection, 211
 for brucellosis, 62, 63
 for chlamydial infection, 109
 for endocarditis, 260(t)
 for legionnaires' disease, 191
 for leprosy, 87, 88, 89
 for meningitis, 102(t)
 for mycobacterial infections, 87, 88, 89, 207, 208, 208(t), 211
Rifampin *(Continued)*
  in AIDS, 46, 208
 for psittacosis, 109
 for Q fever, 110
 for salmonellosis carriers, 140
 for tuberculosis, 207, 208, 208(t)
  in AIDS, 46, 208
Rifampin prophylaxis, for tuberculosis, 209
Right bundle branch block, 235, 236
Right upper quadrant pain, sickle cell disease and, 323
Right ventricular failure, 254
Right ventricular infarction, 284(t)
Rimantadine, for influenza, 81–82, 189, 190
Ring(s), esophageal, 421
Ringer's lactate solution, use of, in burned patient, 1070, 1070(t)
  in diabetic patient with intercurrent illness, 496
Ringworm, 749
Risperidone, for schizophrenic disorders, 1064
Rocky Mountain spotted fever, 124–125, 143(t)
Rolandic epilepsy, benign, 822–823
Rome criteria, for irritable bowel syndrome, 436(t)
Rosacea, 705
Roseola infantum, 744
Roundworm infestation, 481(t), 482(t), 483–484, 486
 cutaneous, 748
Rubbing alcohol, poisoning by, 1100–1101
Rubella, 125–127
Rubeola, 127–128
 immunization against, 128
  in AIDS patient, 128
"Rule of nines," for body surface area, 1068
Rupture, of aortic aneurysm, 213, 295
 of spleen, in infectious mononucleosis, 104
 of uterus, in pregnancy, 944

Salicylates. See also *Aspirin.*
 for fever, 21
 for rheumatoid arthritis, 901–903, 902(t)
 poisoning by, 1126(t), 1126–1127, 1127(t)
  nomogram for, *1128*
 therapeutic vs. toxic levels of, 1138(t)
Salicylic acid, for seborrheic dermatitis, 712
 for warts, 728
Salicylsalicylic acid, for rheumatoid arthritis, 902(t)
Saline dressings, for venous stasis ulcer, 759
Saline irrigation, at site of surgically drained carbuncle, 738
Saline laxatives, for constipation, 18
Saline nasal spray, 28(t), 29
Salivary gland(s), swelling of, due to calculus, 756
  in mumps, 104
  in sarcoidosis, 198
 tumors of, 754
Salmeterol, for asthma, 680, 681(t)
 for chronic obstructive pulmonary disease, 154
Salmonellosis, 136–142
 and bacteremia, 138
 and enteric fever, 138–139
Salmonellosis *(Continued)*
 and enterocolitis (gastroenteritis), 14(t), 16, 137–138
 and typhoid fever, 140–142, 141(t)
 food-borne, 75(t)
 in AIDS patients, 47
 osteomyelitis treatment in, 928(t)
Salmonellosis carriers, 139–140, 142
Salpingectomy, for ectopic pregnancy, 941
Salpingitis. See also *Pelvic inflammatory disease.*
 chlamydial, 1011
Salpingo-oophorectomy, for endometrial cancer, 1016
"Sanctuary" sites, in leukemia, 364, 367–368
Sandfly, leishmaniasis transmission by, 83, 747
Sarcoidosis, 195–199
Sarcoma, Kaposi's, in AIDS, 656–657
 penile, 656–657
 vulvar, 1026
Sarcoptes scabiei infestation, 745–746
Scabies, 745–746
Scalp, fungal infections of, 709, 749
 hair loss from, 706–709, 706(t)–709(t)
  nail lesions associated with, 723–724
 louse infestation of, 709, 746
 seborrheic dermatitis of, 712
 trauma to, 709, 889
Scarring, hypertrophic, 725
Scarring acne, 704–705
Schatzki's ring, 421
Schilling test (vitamin B_{12} absorption test), 452, 452(t)
Schistosomiasis (bilharziasis), 481(t), 485
 cutaneous, 748, 1085
Schizophrenia, drugs for. See *Neuroleptic(s).*
Schizophrenic disorders, 1061–1064
School environment, of child with asthma, 691
Scintillating scotoma, migraine and, 833, *833*
Scleroderma, 718–719
 esophageal involvement in, 420, 718
Sclerosis, multiple, 848–855, 849(t), *850*
  disorders misdiagnosed as, 849(t)
  optic neuritis as harbinger of, 865
 systemic (scleroderma), 718–719
  esophageal involvement in, 420, 718
Sclerotherapy, for bleeding esophageal varices, 414, 415, 415(t), 416
 for myxoid cysts, 725
Scombroid poisoning, 75(t), 76, 78, 1085
Scopolamine, for nausea and vomiting, 6, 6(t), 8
 for vertigo, 838(t)
Scorpion fish, envenomation by, 1083
Scorpion stings, 1080
Scotoma, scintillating, migraine and, 833, *833*
Screening, for breast cancer, 980–981
 for cervical cancer, 1018
 for colorectal cancer, 477
 for hereditary hemochromatosis, 347, *348*
 for iron deficiency, 302
 for malabsorption, 450
 for prostate cancer, 654
 for thalassemia, 315
Scrotum, cancer of, 658
 swelling of, in epididymitis, 608
 trauma to, 626
 tumors of, 658
Scrub typhus, 143, 143(t)

Scurvy, 517, 518(t)
Seabather's eruption, 748, 1085
Seafood toxins, effects of ingestion of, 76, 1085, 1086
Sea snake bites, 1084
Seasonal mood disorders, and bulimia nervosa, 1053
Sea urchins, effects of contact with, 1083
Seborrheic dermatitis, 712–713
Secobarbital, poisoning by, 1105(t)
Secondary amenorrhea, 996–998, *997*
Secondary dysmenorrhea, 998, 999
Secondary glomerulopathies, 609
Secondary hyperparathyroidism, 565–566
  treatment of, 567–568
Secondary iron overload, 346, 346(t), 347, 1113–1115
  chelation therapy for, 316, 347, 1093(t)
  toxic iron ingestion and, 1113–1115
  transfusion and, 316, 401
Secondary leukemia, 354, 359, 362–363, 388
Second-degree atrioventricular block, 234
  Mobitz Type I, 234
  Mobitz Type II, 227, 234
Sedation, and therapeutic paralysis, in patient with head trauma, 890, 891, 891(t), 893, 894(t)
Sedatives, 1129(t)
  abuse of or poisoning by, 1044(t), 1044–1045, 1127–1128, 1129(t)
  use of, for chorea, in rheumatic fever, 118
    in alcohol withdrawal, 1040
    in ulcerative colitis, 428
  withdrawal from, 1045
Seizure(s), cerebral metastatic disease and, 157, 158(t)
  drugs for. See *Anticonvulsants.*
  eclamptic, 946(t), 947
  epileptic, 806–823, 807(t)
    in adolescents and adults, 806–819
    in infants and children, 819–823
    in newborn, 821
    in pregnant patients, 809
    treatment of, 807–823, 810(t), 811(t), 818(t), 1103(t)
      poisoning by drugs used in, 1102, 1103(t)
      therapeutic vs. toxic levels of drugs used in, 1138(t)
  febrile, 820–821
  head trauma and, 890, 894
  hypoglycemic, 497
  local anesthetics causing, 954
  lupus erythematosus and, 716
  neonatal, 821
  poisoning and, 1099
  porphyria and, 391
  Reye's syndrome and, 847
  sickle cell disease and, 326
  stimulant abuse and, 1041, 1042
Selective serotonin re-uptake inhibitors, adverse effects of, 1059(t)
  for bulimia nervosa, 1052
  for depression, 1058, 1059(t)
  for obsessive-compulsive disorder, in Tourette syndrome, 827–828
  for panic disorder, 1065–1066
  for premenstrual syndrome, 1002–1003
Selegiline, for depression, 1058(t)
  for Parkinson's disease, 877, 878
Selenium sulfide, for seborrheic dermatitis, 712
  for tinea, 750, 781
Semen, laboratory reference values for, 1141(t)
Seminoma, 657
Sepsis, 60, *61*, 62
  catheter, 57(t)
  neonatal, 969
    antimicrobial therapy for, 969, 970(t)
  Reye's syndrome and, 847
Septata intestinalis infection, 15(t), 483
Septicemic plague, 107
Septic shock, 60
Sequestration, and hepatomegaly, in sickle cell disease, 323
  and splenomegaly, in sickle cell disease, 323
    in thrombocytopenia, 342
Seronegative myasthenia gravis, 861
Serotonin antagonists, for nausea and vomiting, 5, 6(t)
Serotonin re-uptake inhibitors. See *Selective serotonin re-uptake inhibitors.*
Sertraline, for depression, 1059(t)
    in Alzheimer's disease, 793
  for panic disorder, 1066
Serum, laboratory reference values for, 1136(t)–1137(t)
Serum sickness, 73, 675, 678, 678(t)
Sexual dysfunction, in hereditary hemochromatosis, 346
Sexually transmitted diseases, 666–674, 1010–1014
Sezary's syndrome, 378, 379(t), 380(t), 381
Shampoos, for seborrheic dermatitis, 712
  for tinea, 749
Shark bites, 1083
Shellfish poisoning, 75(t), 76, 1086
Shigellosis, 13, 14(t)
Shingles (herpes zoster). See *Varicella-zoster virus infection.*
Shock, cardiogenic, 255
    as complication of myocardial infarction, 284(t)
  hypovolemic, in newborn, 971
  poisoning and, 1098
  septic, 60
  toxic, 1008–1010, 1008(t)–1010(t)
    patients at risk for, 1008, 1034
Short bowel syndrome, 457–458
Shoulder pain, 921, 921(t)
  sports injuries and, 929, 930, 931
Shoulder subluxation, in hemiplegia, 805
Shunt surgery, for bleeding esophageal varices, 415, 415(t), 416
  for cirrhotic ascites, 410
  for congenital heart disease, 246
  to drain CSF, meningitis following, 99–100
S.I. units (international system of units), 1133(t), 1133–1134, 1134(t)
Sialolithiasis, 756–757
Sickle cell disease, 318(t), 318–327, 319(t), 326(t)
  anemia in, 324(t), 324–325
  infection risk in, and bacteremia, 58(t)
  ischemia in, 319, *319*, *320*
  obstetric anesthetic implications of, 951
  organ failure in, 325–327, 326(t)
  osteomyelitis in, 325, 924
  pain in, 319(t), 319–324, *320*, *321*, 321(t), 322(t)
  transfusion for, 323, 325, 325(t)
Silastic gel sheeting, for keloids, 726
Silicosis, 199(t), 199–201, 200(t)
Silver nitrate, conjunctivitis secondary to use of, 64
Silver sulfadiazine, for burns, 1072
  for sunburn, 785
Simple partial seizures, treatment of, 808, 809, 810(t), 810–816, 811(t)
Simple silicosis, 199, 200(t)
Simvastatin, for hyperlipoproteinemia, 508
Single ventricle, surgery for, 246
Sinoatrial block, 233
Sinoatrial node re-entry, 239(t)
Sinusitis, 23, 24, 202(t), 202–204
  common cold and, 188
Sinus pause, 233
Sinus tachycardia, 237, 238(t)
Sinus tract, dental, 757
Skin. See also *Dermatitis*; *Dermatosis (dermatoses).*
  acne of, 703–705
    industrial agents causing, 783, 784
  aging of, sun exposure and, 785
  bacterial infections of, 736–740
    contact dermatits and, 782–783
    necrotizing, 79, 740
    varicella and, 67
  basal cell carcinoma of, 709–711
  biopsy of, in malignant or premalignant disease, 732, 733
  blowfly/botfly larvae infesting, 748–749
  bullous diseases of, 737, 766–772
  burns of, 1067–1073
  cancer of, 377–382, 709–711, 731–733
    lesions predisposing to, 733–736
    recognition of, mnemonic for, 732, 735
    sun exposure and, 786
  carcinoma of, 709–711
  cleaning of, in diphtheria, 73
  cold injuries to, 1076
  coxsackievirus infection of, 744
  cytomegalovirus infection of, 743
  desquamation of, toxic shock syndrome and, 1009, 1010
  Entamoeba histolytica infection of, 748
  eruptions of. See *Eruption(s).*
  erythema of. See *Erythema* entries.
  fungal infections of, 749–750
    necrotizing, 80
  grafting of, for stasis ulcer, 759
  helminth infestation of, 748
  hemorrhagic blisters of, snake bite and, 1080
  herpes simplex virus infection of, 740–742
  herpes virus 6 infection of, 744
  hookworm larvae penetrating, 748
  infections of, 736–750
    bacteremia as complication of, 57(t)
    bacterial, 736–740
      contact dermatits and, 782–783
      necrotizing, 79, 740
      varicella and, 67
    fungal, 80, 749–750
    necrotizing, 78–80, 740
    parasitic, 745–749, 1085
    viral, 66–69, 727–729, 735, 740–745. See also specific infections, e.g., *Varicella-zoster virus infection.*
  inflammation of. See *Dermatitis.*
  itching of. See *Pruritus.*
  keloids of, 725–726
  leishmaniasis involving, 83–86, 747
  louse infestation of, 746
  lupus erythematosus involving, 715, 787
  melanoma of, 731–733, 732(t)
    lentigo maligna and, 735
    nevi and, 729, 730, 731, 735

Skin *(Continued)*
necrosis of, brown recluse spider bite and, 1079
necrotizing infections of, 78–80, 740
nevi of, 729–731, 735
melanoma associated with, 729, 730, 731, 735
papillomavirus infection of, 727–729, 735
papulosquamous diseases of, 711–715
parasitic infestation of, 745–749, 1085
paravaccinia virus infection of, 744–745
parvovirus B19 infection of, 744
photoaging of, 785
photosensitivity of. See also *Sun exposure*.
agents inducing, 786(t)
effects of, 786
lupus erythematosus and, 715, 787
porphyria and, 392, 786–787
pigmentary disorders of, 779–781
agents causing, 780(t), 784
hereditary hemochromatosis and, 346
poxvirus infection of, 744
AIDS and, 52
pregnancy-related diseases of, 773–775, 774(t)
premalignant lesions of, 733–736
rinsing of, after chemical exposure, 1070, 1086
roundworm infestation of, 748
sarcoidosis involving, 198
Sarcoptes scabiei infestation of, 745–746
schistosome larvae penetrating, 748, 1085
scrapings of, in classification of leprosy, 87
squamous cell carcinoma of, 709–711
T-cell lymphoma involving, 377–382, 378(t), 379(t), 380(t)
thickening of, scleroderma and, 718
toxic necrolysis of epidermis of, 765
traumatic effects of cold exposure on, 1076
Trypansoma species infecting, 747
tumors of, 377–382, 709–711, 731–733
premalignant, 733–736
recognition of malignant transformation of, mnemonic for, 732, 735
sun exposure and, 786
ulcers of, 758(t), 758–762
leishmaniasis and, 86
sickle cell disease and, 324
tularemia and, 135
urticaria of. See *Urticaria*.
varicella-zoster virus infection of. See *Varicella-zoster virus infection*.
vasculitic lesions of, 719–721
viral infections of, 66–69, 727–729, 735, 740–745. See also specific infections, e.g., *Varicella-zoster virus infection*.
warts on, 727–729, 735
water-exposed, lesions of, 748, 1076, 1085
Skull, trauma to. See *Trauma, to head*.
Sleep apnea, 34
Sleep disturbances, 33(t), 33–35
Alzheimer's disease and, 793
depression and, 33–34, 34(t)
treatment of, 35, 35(t)
in muscle pain syndromes, 920
Sleep hygiene, 35, 35(t)
Sling, for shoulder subluxation in hemiplegia, 805
Small cell carcinoma, of lung, 162–163
Small intestine, bacterial overgrowth in, 456–457
biopsy of, in malabsorption, 453(t). See also *Malabsorption*.
diverticula of, 423–424
effects of gluten sensitivity on, 453
eosinophilic infiltration of, 456
inflammation of terminal portion of (Crohn's disease), 433–435, 455
lymphangiectasia of, 457
lymphoma of, 457
risk of, in patient with dermatitis herpetiformis, 771
malabsorption in. See *Malabsorption*.
obstruction of, by gallstone, 405
radiation injury to, 455
resection of, malabsorption following, 458
Trichinella larvae in, 133
Small non-cleaved cell lymphoma (Burkitt's lymphoma), 377
Smoke inhalation, 1067
Smoking, and stomatitis, 754
Smoking cessation, 152(t)
as aid to management, in COPD, 152–153
in peptic ulcer disease, 470
sources of information on, 152(t)
Snake bite, 1080–1082
antivenin for, 1081, 1082, 1090(t)
Sodium bicarbonate. See *Bicarbonate*.
Sodium etidronate, for osteoporosis, 525
for Paget's disease of bone, 529
Sodium fluoride, for osteoporosis, 525–526
Sodium imbalance, dehydration due to, 542, 542(t), 544–547
neonatal, 968
Sodium iodide, for thyroid storm, 584
Sodium nitrite, for cyanide poisoning, 1092(t)
Sodium nitroprusside, for hypertension, 273(t)
in patient with intracerebral hemorrhage, 793, 795(t), 796
in patient with pheochromocytoma, 591
Sodium polystyrene sulfonate, for hyperkalemia, in renal failure, 638, 639(t)
Sodium-restricted diet, for cirrhotic ascites, 410
for hypertension, 267
in aldosteronism, 572
for Meniere's disease, 842
for renal disease or renal failure, 611, 646, 648
Sodium stibogluconate, adverse effects of, 85(t), 85–86
for leishmaniasis, 84, 85, 86, 747
Sodium sulfate, for poisoning, 1088
Sodium tetradecyl sulfate, for myxoid cysts, 725
Sodium thiosulfate, for cyanide poisoning, 1092(t)
Sodoku, 113
Soft palate, lesions of, 755
Soft tissue, destruction of, due to snake bite, 1080
infections of, bacteremia as complication of, 57(t)
necrotizing, 78–80, 740
solitary plasmacytoma of, 386
Soft tissue sarcoma, vulvar, 1026
Solitary plasmacytoma, 386
Solitary pulmonary nodule, 159
Solvents, abuse of or poisoning by, 1045, 1045(t), 1110–1112
Somatoform disorders, 915, 1046–1047
Sorbitol, for constipation, 18
for poisoning, 1088
Sore, canker, 752
cold, 741, 751
pressure, 759–762
Sore throat, common cold and, 188
treatment of, 28(t)
Sotalol, 219(t), 1125(t)
for angina pectoris, 219(t)
for arrhythmias, 238(t)
in mitral valve prolapse syndrome, 252
for atrial fibrillation, 228(t)
South American trypanosomiasis, 747–748
Spasm(s), esophageal, 420
muscular, infantile seizure syndrome and, 821–822
jellyfish sting and, 1084
tetanus and, 129
Spasmodic dysphonia, 32
Spasticity, treatment of, 760
in multiple sclerosis, 852
in stroke syndrome, 806
Specialized burn care facilities, transfer to, 1071
Spectinomycin, for gonorrhea, 667(t), 668, 669
Speech therapy, in rehabilitation of hemiplegic patient, 805
Spent-phase polycythemia, treatment of, 389
Spermicides, 1034
Sphincter, urethral, intrinsic deficiency of, 607–608
Spider bites, 1078–1080
antivenin for, 1090(t)
Spinal anesthesia, for delivery, 949, 952
total, as unintended effect of epidural block, 954
Spinal cord compression, lung cancer metastases and, 158(t)
Spindle cell nevus, 731
Spine. See *Vertebra(e)*.
Spiramycin, adverse effects of, 132(t)
for toxoplasmosis, 131, 132, 132(t)
Spirillum minus infection, 113, 114, 114(t)
Spironolactone, for acne, 705
for alopecia, 707
for cirrhotic ascites, 410
for Cushing's syndrome, 557(t), 558
for heart failure, 255
in children, 245(t)
for hypertension, 270(t)
for hypokalemia, in aldosteronism, 571
for nephrotic syndrome, 611
for premenstrual syndrome, 1002
Spitz nevus, 731
Spleen, effects of sickle cell disease on, 323–324
enlargement of. See *Splenomegaly*.
resection of. See *Splenectomy*.
rupture of, in infectious mononucleosis, 104
Splenectomy, for hemolytic anemia, 307–308, 310
for idiopathic thrombocytopenic purpura, 341
for leukemia, 372
for thalassemia, 316
infection following, 310
bacteremia as complication of, 58(t)
prophylaxis against, 308, 316

Splenic vein thrombosis, in pancreatitis, 463
Splenomegaly, sickle cell disease and, 323
thrombocytopenia associated with, 342
Splint(s), interocclusal, for temporomandibular disorders, 918
Spondylitis, ankylosing, 911–914, 912(t), 913(t)
brucellosis and, 63
Spondyloarthropathies, 911–912, 912(t)
Sponge contraceptive (vaginal sponge), 1034
Sponge spicules, effects of contact with, 1084
Spontaneous bacterial peritonitis, 411
Sporadic encephalitis, 844(t), 844–845, 845(t)
Sports injuries, 929(t), 929–932, 930(t), 931(t)
Sports participation, after surgery for congenital heart disease, 248
Spotted fever, 143, 143(t)
Rocky Mountain, 124–125, 143(t)
Sprains, 929, 929(t)
sports-related, 930, 931
Spreading melanoma, superficial, 732
Sprue, 453–455
Squamous cell carcinoma, of esophagus, 421
of larynx, 32
of mouth, 752, 756, 757
of skin, 709–711
of vulva, 1023, 1024
Squamous cell papilloma, of larynx, 32
Squaric acid dibutyl ester, for warts, 724
Stable angina pectoris, 217–218, 221
Staging, of breast cancer, 985(t)
of chronic lymphocytic leukemia, 373(t)
of cutaneous T-cell lymphoma, 379(t)
of gynecologic cancer, 1016(t), 1019(t), 1025(t)
of Hodgkin's disease, 350(t), 355(t)
of kidney cancer, 650
of lung cancer, 160(t)
of melanoma, 732(t), 1025(t)
of mycosis fungoides, 379(t)
of non-Hodgkin's lymphoma, 375
of prostate cancer, 653
of Sezary's syndrome, 379(t)
Standards of care, in management of diabetes mellitus, 492, 492(t)
Stanozolol, for angioedema, 778
Staphylococcal infection, brain abscess due to, 789, 789(t)
carbuncles due to, 739
endocarditis due to, 259, 260(t)
treatment of, 259, 260(t)
folliculitis due to, 737
furuncles due to, 738
impetigo due to, 737
meningitis due to, 101, 101(t)
osteomyelitis due to, treatment of, 927, 928(t)
otitis externa due to, 106(t)
pneumonia due to, 180–181, 187
secondary to AIDS, 47
toxic shock syndrome due to, 1008–1010
Staphylococcal toxins, food-borne, 74, 75(t)
Stasis ulcers, 758–759
Status asthmaticus, 148, 149
Status epilepticus, 818
treatment of, 818, 818(t), 819, 820
Steatorrhea, 450
Stenosis, carotid artery, 800
Stenosis *(Continued)*
coronary artery. See *Coronary artery disease*.
iliac artery, 216, 293
infrarenal aortic, 216
intestinal, Crohn's disease and, 435
Sterilization, 1034–1035
Steroids, 553(t). See also specific drugs, e.g., *Prednisone*.
for acne, 705
for adrenocortical insufficiency, 552, 553
in patient with hypopituitarism, 573
for aldosteronism, 572
for allergic drug reaction, 696, 697, 698
for allergic rhinitis, 694, 694(t)
for alopecia, 708
for anaphylactic reaction, 677, 677(t), 701
for anemia, 301, 307, 311
for ankylosing spondylitis, 913
for aphthous ulcers, 752, 753
for aplastic anemia, 301
for arthritis, 909, 909(t)
for asthma, 24, 680, 681, 681(t)
in pediatric patient, 685, 685(t), *687*, 688, 689
for atopic dermatitis, 763, 764
for autoimmune hemolytic anemia, 307
for Bell's palsy, 871
for brucellosis, 63
for bullous pemphigoid, 769
for carditis, in patient with rheumatic fever, 118, 118(t)
for central nervous system lymphoma, 899
for chronic inflammatory demyelinating polyradiculoneuropathy, 885
for chronic obstructive pulmonary disease, 153, 154, *155*
for contact dermatitis, 773, 773(t), 782
for cough, in asthmatic patient, 24
for Crohn's disease, 433
for effects of brain tumors, 899
for effects of metastatic disease, in patient with lung cancer, 157, 158(t)
for enteric fever, 139
for eosinophilic gastroenteritis, 456
for epidermolysis bullosa acquisita, 770
for erythema nodosum leprosum, 90
for facial paralysis, 871
for giant cell arteritis, 923
for glaucoma, 868
for glomerulopathy, 613, 614, 615, 618(t), 618–619
in patient with lupus erythematosus, 716
for gout, 504
for headache, 832
for hemolytic anemia, 307, 311
for hypersensitivity pneumonitis, 202
for hyperthyroidism, 584
for idiopathic guttate hypomelanosis, 781
for idiopathic thrombocytopenic purpura, 341
for increased intracranial pressure, 796
for inflammatory myopathies, 718
for juvenile rheumatoid arthritis, 909, 909(t)
for keloids, 725
for laryngitis, 30
for lichen planus, 714, 723, 753
for lichen simplex chronicus, 776
for linear IgA dermatitis, 772
for lupus erythematosus, 715, 716, 717
for meningitis, 103
for multiple sclerosis, 849, 851
Steroids *(Continued)*
for myasthenia gravis, 858(t), 858–859, 859(t)
for nausea and vomiting, 6, 6(t)
for neurobrucellosis, 63
for neuropathy, 885
in patient with vasculitis, 886
for neutropenia, 328
for optic neuritis, 865
for oropharyngeal lymphoid swelling, in patient with mononucleosis, 104
for pain, 3, 4
for papulosquamous eruptions, 712(t)
for paraneoplastic pemphigus, 768
for paronychia, 722
for paroxysmal nocturnal hemoglobinuria, 311
for pemphigoid gestationis, 774
for pemphigus foliaceus, 768
for pemphigus vulgaris, 766–767
for photosensitivity and skin lesions, in patient with lupus erythematosus, 787
for *Pneumocystis carinii* pneumonia, in AIDS patient, 49, 50(t)
for polymorphic eruption of pregnancy, 775
for polymyalgia rheumatica, 923
for post-herpetic neuralgia, 743
for postinfectious encephalitis, 845, 845(t)
for pruritus, 37
for psoriasis, 713
for psoriasis involving nails, 723
for pulmonary scleroderma, 719
for renal disease, 613, 614, 615, 618(t), 618–619
in patient with lupus erythematosus, 716
for reversal reaction in leprosy, 90
for rheumatic carditis, 118, 118(t)
for rheumatoid arthritis, 903
in pediatric patient, 909, 909(t)
for salmonellosis, 139, 141
for sarcoidosis, 197, 198
for scabies, 745
for scleroderma, 718, 719
for seborrheic dermatitis, 712, 713
for serum sickness, 678
for sunburn, 785
for systemic lupus erythematosus, 715, 716, 717
for temporal arteritis, 923
for thyroid storm, 584
for toxic shock syndrome, 1010
for toxoplasmosis, 132
for trichinosis, 484
for typhoid fever, 141
for ulcerative colitis, 429(t), 430–431
for urticaria, 696, 696(t), 777
for vasculitis, 720, 886
for vitiligo, 781
for vomiting and nausea, 6, 6(t)
for warm antibody autoimmune hemolytic anemia, 307
perioperative administration of, 553, 903
in patient being treated for Cushing's syndrome, 558
potency of topical formulations of, 712(t), 773(t)
risk of dependency on, in patients with pericarditis, 290
topical, 711–712, 712(t), 773(t)
ocular, for glaucoma, 868
potency of, 712(t), 773(t)

Steroids *(Continued)*
use of, in patient receiving amphotericin B, 169
in patient receiving streptokinase, 1028
in patient treated for acromegaly, 549
in patient treated for Cushing's syndrome, 558–559
withdrawal from (discontinuation of), and adrenal insufficiency, 553
Stevens-Johnson syndrome, 765–766
Stibogluconate, adverse effects of, 85(t), 85–86
for leishmaniasis, 84, 85, 86, 747
Stimulant(s), abuse of or poisoning by, 1041(t), 1041–1043, 1102, 1108(t), 1108–1109
for attention deficit hyperactivity disorder, in Tourette syndrome, 827
withdrawal from, 1043
Stimulant laxatives, 18–19
Sting(s), allergic reactions to, 700–702
jellyfish, 1084
scorpion, 1080
Stingrays, envenomation by, 1084
Stomach. See *Gastric* entries; *Gastritis.*
Stomatitis, 754, 757
Stool, examination of, for fat, 450
in cholera, 71(t)
in food poisoning, 77
Stool softeners, 18
use of, in multiple sclerosis, 853
Storage pool deficiencies, 339
Strains, 929, 929(t)
Streak pigmentation, 780
Streptobacillus moniliformis infection, 113, 114, 114(t)
Streptococcal infection, brain abscess due to, 789, 789(t)
cellulitis due to, 740
endocarditis due to, 258, 260(t)
treatment of, 259, 260(t)
glomerulonephritis due to, 617–618, 737
impetigo due to, 737
meningitis due to, 99, 100, 100(t), 101, 101(t)
necrotizing, 78, 79
osteomyelitis due to, treatment of, 927, 928(t)
pharyngitis due to, 204–207, 206(t)
rheumatic fever associated with, 117, 118, 119
pneumonia due to, 179–180
AIDS and, 47
prophylaxis against, 118(t), 118–119
rheumatic carditis due to, 117, 118, 119, 250
rheumatic fever due to, 117, 118, 119
toxic shock due to, 1009
Streptokinase, for deep venous thrombosis, 297, 1027, 1027(t), 1028
for myocardial infarction, 281, 281(t)
for pulmonary embolism, 195(t)
Streptomycin, for atypical mycobacterial infection, 211, 212
for brucellosis, 62, 63
for endocarditis, 259, 260(t)
in patient with rat-bite fever, 114
for granuloma inguinale, 671
for plague, 107–108
for rat-bite fever, 114
for tuberculosis, 207, 208, 208(t)
for tularemia, 136
for Whipple's disease, 455
Stress, illness and, 532(t)
Stress *(Continued)*
thermal, in newborn, 958, 965
"Stress diabetes," in burned patient, 1071
Stress disorder, post-traumatic, 1046
Stress gastritis, 443
Stress incontinence, 607
Stricture(s), colonic, in ulcerative colitis, 432
esophageal, 420, 421, 422
urethral, 658–661, *660*
Stroke, heat, 1077(t), 1078, 1078(t)
Stroke syndrome, 798–801, 798(t)–801(t)
atrial fibrillation and, 229, 800(t), 801, 801(t)
reduction of risk of, 799–800, 800(t)
by lowering blood pressure, 265, 265(t)
by providing estrogen replacement, 1005, 1005(t)
rehabilitation for, 801–806, *802*, 802(t)–804(t)
vertigo in, 839(t)
Strongyloidiasis, 15(t), 455–456, 481(t), 483, 484, 486
Struvite stones, 663–664
Strychnine, poisoning by, 1128
Stuttering priapism, in sickle cell disease, 323
Styrene, poisoning by, 1112
Subacute headache, 829
Subacute thyroiditis, 593–594
Subarachnoid space, bacteria in, effects of, 102–103
selection of drug therapy for, based on species causing meningitis, 99, 100(t)
hemorrhage into, 829
headache associated with, 829
Subclavian vein, catheterization of, in parenteral nutrition, 535–536, 537
Subclinical hypothyroidism, 580
Subcutaneous nodules, in rheumatic fever, 117
Subdiaphragmatic irradiation, for Hodgkin's disease, 355–356, *356*, 358
Subdural hematoma, 830–831
headache associated with, 830
head trauma and, 830–831, 889
Subjective tinnitus, 38
Subperiosteal abscess, 204
Substituted benzamides. See *Metoclopramide.*
Subungual onychomycosis, 750
Suby's solution G, for struvite stones, 664
Succimer, as antidote, 1098(t)
Sucralfate, for bile reflux gastritis, 443
for gastritis, 442(t)
for peptic ulcer, 471
use of, in burned patient, 1071
Suctioning, of mouth of newborn, 959
of trachea of newborn, to remove meconium, 959, 960, 970–971
Sudden cardiac death, 222. See also *Cardiac arrest.*
risk of, coronary artery disease and, 222
ischemic heart disease and, 222
mitral valve prolapse syndrome and, 252
myocardial infarction and, 222, 226
ventricular dysfunction and, 222, 240
ventricular ectopy and, 222, 227, 232, 252
Sulfadiazine, adverse effects of, 132(t)
for toxoplasmosis, 131, 132, 132(t)
in AIDS patient, 50, 51, 133
Sulfadiazine prophylaxis, for recurrent rheumatic fever, 118(t)
for streptococcal infection, 118(t)
Sulfadoxine-pyrimethamine, for malaria, 94(t), 95, 97(t), 98
for *Pneumocystis carinii* pneumonia, in AIDS, 50(t)
Sulfamethoxazole, for lymphogranuloma venereum, 671
use of, with trimethoprim. See *Trimethoprim-sulfamethoxazole.*
Sulfapyridine, for bullous pemphigoid, 769
for dermatitis herpetiformis, 771
for linear IgA dermatitis, 772
Sulfasalazine, adverse effects of, 428
for ankylosing spondylitis, 913
for Crohn's disease, 433
for rheumatoid arthritis, 904(t), 906
for ulcerative colitis, 428, 429(t)
Sulfinpyrazone, for hyperuricemia, 505
Sulfisoxazole, for chlamydial infection, 1012, 1012(t)
Sulfonamide(s), 699(t)
allergic reaction to, 698–699
therapeutic applications of. See under specific sulfa drugs, e.g., *Sulfadiazine.*
Sulfonylureas, for diabetes mellitus, 491, 491(t), 492
Sulindac, for rheumatoid arthritis, 902(t)
Sumatriptan, for acute headache, 829
for cluster headache, 836
for menstrual migraine, 1002
for migraine, 835
Sun avoidance, 785
need for, in porphyria, 392, 787
in systemic lupus erythematosus, 715, 787
timing of, 785
for patient with dysplastic nevi, 735
for patient with erythema multiforme, 765
Sunburn, 784–785
Sun exposure, 784–787
and acute to chronic to neoplastic dermatoses, 785(t)
and aging of skin, 785
and allergic or toxic reactions to sensitizing agents, 786
and chronic dermatitis, 786
and exacerbation of existing lesions or diseases. See under *Sun avoidance.*
and hyperpigmentation, 779
and irradiation, 784, 785(t)
and keratosis or cheilitis, 733–734, 736, 751–752, 785–786
and polymorphous eruption, 786
and skin cancer, 786
and urticaria, 786
avoidance of. See *Sun avoidance.*
protection from, 779, 785
Sunscreens, 779, 785
Superficial dermal burns, 1068, 1072
Superficial fungal infections, of skin, 749–750
Superficial spreading melanoma, 732
Superficial thrombophlebitis, 1031
Superficial venous thrombosis, 1031
Superficial white onychomycosis, 750
Suppurative thyroiditis, 594
Supradiaphragmatic irradiation, for Hodgkin's disease, 355, *356*, 357
Supraglottic swallow, in management of dysphagia, 418

Supraventricular tachycardia, 237–240, 238(t), 239(t)
diagnosis of, in newborn with heart failure, 244
treatment of, 238–240, 239(t), 240(t)
in pediatric patient, 244, 244(t)
Suramin, for prostate cancer, 656
for trypanosomiasis, 747
Surface area of body, nomogram for, *1143*
"rule of nines" for, 1068
Surgery. See also specific procedures, e.g., *Splenectomy*.
atelectasis following, 151
bile reflux gastritis following, 443
cardiopulmonary bypass during, and thrombocytopenia, 340
diabetes insipidus following, 562
for achalasia, 420
for acromegaly, 548, 549, 550
for actinic keratosis, 752
for adrenal tumors, 556, 571, 591, 649
for aldosteronism, 571
for alopecia, 707, 709
for amebic liver abscess, 55
for anal fissure, 439
for anal fistula, 440
for angina pectoris, 222
for anorectal abscess, 440
for aortic aneurysm, 213, 214, 295
for aortic dissection, 215–216
for aortitis, 217
for aortoiliac occlusion, 216–217, 293
for ascites, 410
for atrial fibrillation, 229
for back pain, 41
for Bartholin's gland cysts, 1022
for bladder cancer, 652, 653
for bladder dysfunction, 606
for bladder trauma, 625
for Bowen's disease, 734
for brain abscess, 789–790
for brain hemorrhage, 795, 797
for brain tumors, 896, 897, 898
for breast cancer, 986, 987, 988
for bronchopleural fistula, 171
for burns, 1072
for cancer, of adrenal gland, 556, 649
of bladder, 652, 653
of brain, 896, 897, 898
of breast, 986, 987, 988
of cervix, 1019, 1020, 1021
of colon, 478
of endometrium, 1016
of kidney, 650–651
of liver, 413
of lung, 159, 161, 161(t)
conditions contraindicating, 159–160, 160(t)
of penis, 656
of prostate, 655, 656
of rectum, 478–479
of scrotum, 658
of skin, 711, 732–733
of stomach, 474–475
of testis, 657, 658
of thyroid, 586, 587
of upper urinary tract, 652
of urethra, 653
of urinary bladder, 652, 653
of uterine cervix, 1019, 1020, 1021
of uterus, 1016
of vulva, 1023, 1024, 1025
for carbuncles, 738, 739, *739*
for carotid artery stenosis, 800
for cervical cancer, 1019, 1020, 1021

Surgery *(Continued)*
for cholecystic disease, 403, 404
for chronic obstructive pulmonary disease, 156
for cirrhotic ascites, 410
for colonic cancer, 478
for colonic dilatation, in ulcerative colitis, 432
for colonic diverticula, 425–426
for colonic tumors, 478
for congenital heart disease, 245, 246, 247
complications of, 247–248
recent developments in, 249
for Crohn's disease, 434, 435
for Cushing's disease or syndrome, 555, 556
for deep venous thrombosis, 297, 1029
for diverticula, of gastrointestinal tract, 418, 422, 423, 424, 425
for duodenal ulcer, 472
for ectopic pregnancy, 941
for embolism, 294, 297
for empyema, 171
for endocarditis, 261, 262
for endometrial cancer, 1016
for endometriosis, 990, 992
for epilepsy, 818
for esophageal diverticula, 418, 422, 423
for esophageal motility disorders, 420
for esophageal variceal bleeding, 415, 415(t), 416
for fibroids, 1015
for gallbladder disease, 403, 404
for gastrointestinal diverticula, 418, 422, 423, 424, 425
for glaucoma, 868–869
for goiter, 565
for head trauma and intracranial hemorrhage, 891
for heart block treatable by pacing, 236
for heart failure, 256–257
in pediatric patient, 245
for hemorrhoids, 441
for hyperparathyroidism, 567, 568
for hyperprolactinemia, 575, 577
for hyperthyroidism, 583
for intracranial hemorrhage, 795, 797, 891
for keloids, 726
for kidney cancer, 650–651
for kidney stones, 662
for kidney trauma, 624
for leiomyoma, 1015
for liver abscess, 55
for liver cancer, 413
for low back pain, 41
for lung cancer, 159, 161, 161(t)
conditions contraindicating, 159–160, 160(t)
for melanoma, 732–733, 1025
for Meniere's disease, 842–843
for mitral valve prolapse, 250, 252
for myasthenia gravis, 858, 860, 861
for myoma, 1015
for necrotizing infections, 79
for nevi, 730, 731, 735
for obesity, 516–517
for occlusive disease of lower extremity arteries, 293–294
for osteomyelitis, 926–927
for otitis media, 174
for Paget's disease of vulva, 1024
for pain, 4
in pancreatitis, 467–469

Surgery *(Continued)*
of lower back, 41
for pancreatic anomalies, 462
for pancreatitis, 463, 467–469
for pelvic inflammatory disease, 1014
for penile cancer, 656
for penile trauma, 626
for peptic ulcer, 472
bile reflux gastritis following, 443
for pericarditis or pericardial effusion, 290, 291
for pheochromocytoma, 591
for pituitary tumors, 548, 549, 550, 575, 577
for postpartum hemorrhage, 956
for premenstrual syndrome, 1003
for pressure ulcer, 761
for prolactinoma, 575, 577
for prostatic cancer, 655, 656
for prostatic hyperplasia, 630–631
for rectal cancer, 478–479
for rheumatoid arthritis, 906–907
for salmonellosis complications, 142
for scrotal cancer, 658
for scrotal trauma, 626
for seizures, 818
for skin cancer, 711, 732–733
for small intestinal diverticula, 423, 424
for stasis ulcer, 759
for stomach tumors, 472, 474–475
for stomach ulcer, 472
for temporomandibular disorders, 918
for testicular cancer, 657, 658
for testicular trauma, 626
for thromboembolism, 194, 297, 1029, 1030
for thymoma, 861
for thyroid cancer, 586, 587
for toxic colonic dilatation, in ulcerative colitis, 432
for trigeminal neuralgia, 863–864
for tumors, of adrenal gland, 556, 571, 591, 649
of bladder, 652, 653
of brain, 896, 897, 898
of breast, 986, 987, 988
of cervix, 1019, 1020, 1021
of colon, 478
of endometrium, 1016
of kidney, 650–651
of liver, 413
of lung, 159, 161, 161(t)
conditions contraindicating, 159–160, 160(t)
of penis, 656
of pituitary, 548, 549, 550, 575, 577
of prostate, 655, 656
of rectum, 478–479
of scrotum, 658
of skin, 711, 732–733
of stomach, 472, 474–475
of testis, 657, 658
of thymus, 861
of thyroid, 586, 587
of upper urinary tract, 652
of urethra, 653
of urinary bladder, 652, 653
of uterine cervix, 1019, 1020, 1021
of uterus, 1015, 1016
of vulva, 1021, 1023, 1024, 1025
for typhoid fever complications, 142
for ulcerative colitis, 431
for upper urinary tract tumors, 652
for ureteral trauma, 624
for urethral cancer, 653

Surgery *(Continued)*
for urethral sphincter deficiency, 607
for urethral stricture, 661
for urethral trauma, 626
for urinary bladder cancer, 652, 653
for urinary bladder dysfunction, 606
for urinary bladder trauma, 625
for uterine cancer, 1016
for uterine cervical cancer, 1019, 1020, 1021
for uterine rupture, in pregnant patient, 944
for uterine tumors, 1015, 1016
for variceal bleeding, from esophagus, 415, 415(t), 416
for venous thrombosis, 297, 1029
for venous ulcer, 759
for ventricular tachycardia, 241, 241(t)
for vocal fold paralysis, 32
for vulvar tumors, 1021, 1023, 1024, 1025
for warts, 727–728
hypoparathyroidism following, 566
in hemophiliac patient, 337–338
in hypertensive patient, 279–280
in patient with hypothyroidism, 579
in patient with porphyria, 392
malabsorption following, 458
meningitis following, 99–100
nausea and vomiting following, 8
prophylaxis against endocarditis in, 119(t), 262(t), 263(t)
pyelonephritis following, 620
sterilization via, 1035
Sustained ventricular arrhythmias, 241
Swallowing, 417
difficulty in, 417(t), 417–422, 418(t), 419(t)
hemiplegia and, 806
myasthenia gravis and, 856
of air, 8–9
Swimmer's itch, 748, 1085
Sycosis barbae, 738
Sympathetic dysreflexia, as complication of tetanus, 130
Syncope, heat exposure and, 1077, 1078(t)
mitral valve prolapse syndrome and, 252
Syphilis, 671–674, 673(t)
and vestibulopathy, 840(t)
in AIDS, 47, 674
Syrup of ipecac, for patient exhibiting allergic drug reaction, 695
for poisoning victim, 78, 1087
Systemic disease, and malabsorption, 458, 458(t)
and pruritus, 36, 36(t)
Systemic hyperpigmentation, 779–780, 780(t)
Systemic lupus erythematosus, 715–717
photosensitivity in, 715, 787
Systemic sclerosis (scleroderma), 718–719
esophageal involvement in, 420, 718
Systolic hypertension. See *Hypertension*.

Tachycardia, 236–241, 238(t), 239(t)
cardiac arrest due to, 222, 223, 225
cardiac death due to, 232
diagnosis of, in newborn with heart failure, 244
myocardial infarction and, 283
pheochromocytoma and, 589
stimulant abuse and, 1042
treatment of, 224(t), 225, 238–241, 239(t), 240(t), 241(t)

Tachycardia *(Continued)*
in patient with tetanus, 131
in pediatric patient, 244, 244(t)
Tacrine, for Alzheimer's disease, 791
Tactile stimulation, in neonatal resuscitation, 959
Taeniasis, 481(t), 485, 486
Takayasu's arteritis, 217
Tamoxifen, for breast cancer, 989
Tamponade, cardiac, 289–290
Tamponade treatment, of bleeding esophageal varices, 414–415
Tampon use, and toxic shock syndrome, 1008
in postpartum period, 956
Tapeworm infestation, 481(t), 482(t), 485, 486
Tardive dyskinesia, use of neuroleptics and, 1062
Tar preparations, for psoriasis, 713
Tattoo, amalgam, 757
T-cell lymphoma, cutaneous, 377–382, 378(t), 379(t), 380(t)
Tear gas exposure, management of, 1128
Teeth, nonvital, sinus tract from, 757
pain in, causes and effects of, 916
prevention of decay of, in xerostomia, 751
Telangiectasia, oral, 752
Telogen effluvium, 707(t), 707–708
Temazepam, 1106(t)
Temporal arteritis (giant cell arteritis), 830, 922–923
Temporary catheter, in parenteral nutrition, 535–536, 537
Temporomandibular disorders, 914–919
arthritic, 911, 918–919
Tendinitis, 920–921
Tennis elbow, 921, 931
Terazosin, for hypertension, 272(t)
in patient with pheochromocytoma, 588–589, 591(t)
for prostatic hyperplasia, 632
for spastic external urinary sphincter, 634
Terbinafine, for onychomycosis, 722–723
Terbutaline, for asthma, 681(t)
for chronic obstructive pulmonary disease, 154
Terfenadine, adverse effects of, 1102
for allergic rhinitis, 693(t)
for pruritus, 37, 37(t)
for urticaria, 696(t), 778
Tertiary hyperparathyroidism, 566
treatment of, 568
Testicular feminization, 996
Testis (testes), as "sanctuary" site, in leukemia, 364, 368
cancer of, 657–658
resection of, for cancer, 656, 657
trauma to, 626
tumors of, 657–658
Testosterone, for gonadotropin deficiency, 574
Tetanic contractions, of uterus, 950
Tetanus, 128–131
Tetanus immunization, 129
in burned patient, 1070
Tetracyclic antidepressants, 1130(t). See also *Antidepressants*.
Tetracycline, adverse effects of, 483
for acne, 704, 784
for bacterial overgrowth in small intestine, 457
for brucellosis, 62
for bullous pemphigoid, 769

Tetracycline *(Continued)*
for *Campylobacter jejuni* infection, 14(t)
for chlamydial infection, 66, 66(t), 109, 671
for cholera, 13, 14(t), 71, 75
for conjunctivitis, 66, 66(t)
for *Dientamoeba fragilis* infection, 480(t)
for gingivitis, 757
for granuloma inguinale, 671
for *Helicobacter pylori* infection, 442, 471
for lymphogranuloma venereum, 671
for malaria, 94(t), 95
for mycoplasmal pneumonia, 181, 190
for oil-induced acne, 784
for plague, 108
for pneumonia, 179(t), 181, 190
for psittacosis, 109
for Q fever, 110
for rat-bite fever, 114
for reactive arthritis, 914
for rickettsioses, 110, 124, 143, 143(t)
for Rocky Mountain spotted fever, 124
for syphilis, 672
for tropical sprue, 454
for typhus fevers, 143, 143(t)
Tetralogy of Fallot, repair of, 246
Tetrodotoxin, effects of ingestion of, 1086
Thalassemia, 314–317, 315(t)
pericarditis in, 292
Thalidomide, for erythema nodosum leprosum, 90
Thawing, of frostbitten tissue, 1076
Theophylline, anticholinergic properties of, 1054(t)
factors affecting clearance of, 154(t)
for apnea of prematurity, 976
for asthma, 680, 681
in pediatric patient, 686, 686(t)
for bronchospasm accompanying anaphylaxis, 677(t)
for chronic obstructive pulmonary disease, 153
poisoning by, 1128–1129
precautions in use of, 154
therapeutic vs. toxic levels of, 1138(t)
Therapeutic drug monitoring, laboratory reference values for, 1138(t)
Thermoregulation, neonatal, 958–959, 965, 967
neutral environmental temperatures in, 968(t)
Thiabendazole, for helminthiasis, 15(t), 456, 481(t), 484, 486
for larva migrans, 748
for trichinosis, 134
Thiamine. See *Vitamin B_1 (thiamine)*.
Thiazide diuretics. See also *Diuretics*.
for diabetes insipidus, 561, 561(t)
for hypertension, 269, 270(t)
Thiethylperazine, for nausea and vomiting, 6, 6(t)
Thiopental, in obstetric anesthesia, 950, 952
Thioridazine, 1123(t)
for agitation, in Alzheimer's disease, 793
for post-herpetic neuralgia, 743
potency of, as neuroleptic, 1062
Thiothixene, 1123(t)
Third-degree atrioventricular block (complete heart block), 227, 234–235
myocardial infarction and, 236
Thoracic aorta, aneurysm of, 213–214
Thoracoabdominal aorta, aneurysm of, 214–215, 295
Throat soreness, common cold and, 188

Throat soreness *(Continued)*
treatment of, 28(t)
Thrombasthenia, Glanzmann's, 339
Thrombocytopenia, 338–342, 341(t), 342(t)
aspirin use and, 340
cirrhosis and, 340, 412
heparin use and, 193, 340
hypothermia and, 1074
lupus erythematosus and, 717
malaria and, 96
snake bite and, 1081
transfusion for, 342(t)
in leukemia, 369
Thrombocytopenic purpura, idiopathic, 341, 344
thrombotic, 344–345
Thromboembolism. See also *Thrombosis.*
heparin for, 192, 193, 194, 195, 296, 1028, 1029
in pregnancy, 297, 1030
pregnancy and, 1026
pulmonary. See *Pulmonary embolism.*
risk factors for, 192(t), 195(t), 296(t), 1026
vena caval filter for, 194, 297, 1030
warfarin for, 195, 296, 1029
Thrombolytic therapy, conditions contraindicating, 282(t), 1027(t)
for deep venous thrombosis, 297, 1027–1028, 1028(t)
for myocardial infarction, 281, 281(t)
for pulmonary embolism, 194, 195(t)
intracerebral hemorrhage due to, 796
Thrombophlebitis, in female patient, 1026–1031
septic, 1031
superficial, 1031
Thrombosis. See also *Thromboembolism.*
axillary-subclavian, 297
calf vein, 297–298, 1030
hemorrhoidal, 441
iliofemoral, 1026, 1029, 1030
ovarian vein, 1031
renal vein, 610, 612
splenic vein, pancreatitis and, 463
venous, deep, 192, 296–298
in female patient, 1026–1031
prophylaxis for, 195, 297(t)
risk factors for, 192(t), 195(t), 296(t)
treatment of, 297, 1027–1029, 1028(t)
in pregnant patient, 1030
disseminated intravascular coagulopathy and, 343
heparin-induced thrombocytopenia and, 193, 340
nephrotic syndrome and, 610, 612
pancreatitis and, 463
polycythemia and, 388
subclinical, central venous catheter placement and, 537
superficial, 1031
Thrombotic thrombocytopenic purpura, 344–345
Thymectomy, for myasthenia gravis, 858, 860, 861
Thymoma, 856, 861
Thyroid, cancer of, 584(t), 584–587
enlarged (goiter), 563–565, 592, 593
diabetes mellitus and, 498
inflammation of, 592(t), 592–594
lymphoma of, 586, 587
nodules of, 563, 564, 565, 586
resection of, for cancer, 586, 587
for hyperthyroidism, 583
Thyroid *(Continued)*
tumors of, 584–587
thyroiditis in area of, 594
Thyroid deficiency, 577–580, 592, 593, 594
in hypopituitarism, 573
secondary to therapy for Hodgkin's disease, 354, 359
treatment of, 578–580
in hypopituitarism, 573
in thyroiditis, 592, 593, 594
Thyroidectomy, for cancer, 586, 587
for hyperthyroidism, 583
Thyroid excess, 580–584, 581(t), 593, 594
Thyroid hormone. See *Thyroxine.*
Thyroiditis, 592(t), 592–594
Thyroid-stimulating hormone, deficiency of, in hypopituitarism, 573
Thyroid storm, 583–584
Thyroxine, 578
adverse effects of, 578
for autoimmune thyroiditis, 592, 593
for goiter, 564
for hypothyroidism, 578–580
in hypopituitarism, 573
in thyroiditis, 592, 593, 594
for myxedema coma, 579, 1075
for postpartum thyroiditis, 593
for subacute thyroiditis, 594
Tic(s), in Tourette syndrome, 824, 827
treatment of, 825–827
Ticarcillin, for meningitis, 102(t)
for neutropenia and infection, 328
for otitis externa, 106(t), 107
Tic douloureux (trigeminal neuralgia), 862–864
in multiple sclerosis, 854
Tick bites, and Lyme disease, 120
and relapsing fever, 115, 115(t), 116, 117
and tularemia, 134
and typhus fever, 143
Tick-borne relapsing fever, 115, 115(t), 116, 117
Tick paralysis, 887
Ticlodipine, stroke prophylaxis with, 799–800, 800(t)
thrombocytopenia induced by, 340
Timolol, 219(t), 1125(t)
for angina pectoris, 219(t)
for glaucoma, 867(t)
Tinea, 709, 749, 750, 781
Tinidazole, for amebiasis, 15(t), 54(t), 54–55, 480(t), 483
for giardiasis, 15(t), 480(t), 482
Tinnitus, 38(t), 38–39
Tiopronin, for cystine stones, 664
Tissue plasminogen activator, for deep venous thrombosis, 297, 1027, 1027(t), 1028
for myocardial infarction, 281, 281(t)
for pulmonary embolism, 195(t)
TMP-SMX. See *Trimethoprim-sulfamethoxazole.*
Tobramycin, for conjunctivitis, in newborn, 64, 64(t)
for endocarditis, 260(t)
for meningitis, 102(t)
for neutropenia and infection, 328
for ophthalmia neonatorum, 64, 64(t)
for otitis externa, 106(t), 107
therapeutic vs. toxic levels of, 1138(t)
Tocainide, for arrhythmias, 238(t)
for tinnitus, 39
therapeutic vs. toxic levels of, 1138(t)
Tocopherol (vitamin E), for premenstrual syndrome, 1002
Tocopherol (vitamin E) *(Continued)*
for yellow nail syndrome, 724
Tolazamide, for diabetes mellitus, 491(t)
Tolbutamide, for diabetes mellitus, 491(t)
Tolerance, drug, vs. addiction, 1. See also *Drug abuse.*
Tolmetin, for gout, 503(t)
for rheumatoid arthritis, 902(t)
in pediatric patient, 908
Toluene, poisoning by, 1045, 1112
Tongue, lesions of, 755–756
Tonic-clonic seizures, treatment of, 808, 809, 810(t), 810–816, 811(t)
Tonic-clonic status epilepticus, 818
treatment of, 818(t), 818–819
Tonsillopharyngitis. See *Pharyngitis.*
Tonsils, lesions of, 755
Tooth (teeth), nonvital, sinus tract from, 757
pain in, causes and effects of, 916
prevention of decay of, in xerostomia, 751
Topical antifungal agents, for tinea, 749, 781
for vulvovaginitis, 1006, 1007(t)
Topical fluoride gel, applied to prevent tooth decay, in xerostomia, 751
Topical steroids, 711–712, 712(t), 773(t)
ocular, for glaucoma, 868
potency of, 712(t), 773(t)
Torsades de pointes, 241
Torsemide, for hypertension, 270(t)
Torus (tori), mandibular, 757
palatal, 754
Total parenteral nutrition, 535, 536. See also *Parenteral nutrition.*
complications of, 536–538
Total skin electron beam radiotherapy, for cutaneous T-cell lymphoma, 381
Tourette syndrome, 823–828
Tourniquet, for wound from marine animal bite, 1083
use of, in anaphylaxis, 677, 677(t)
Toxemia, typhoid fever and, 141
Toxic colonic dilatation, in ulcerative colitis, 431–432
Toxic conjunctivitis, 65, 66(t)
Toxic epidermal necrolysis, 765
Toxic neuropathies, 884, 888
Toxicokinetics, 1099–1100
Toxic shock syndrome, 1008–1010, 1008(t)–1010(t)
patients at risk for, 1008, 1034
Toxin ingestion. See *Poisoning.*
Toxoid, diphtheria, 74
Toxoplasmosis, 131(t), 131–133
AIDS and, 50–51, 132–133, 790
drugs for, 131, 132, 132(t), 133
Trabeculoplasty, for glaucoma, 868–869
Trachea, suctioning of, to remove meconium, 959, 960, 970–971
Traction alopecia, 709
Tranexamic acid, use of, in bleeding hemophiliac patient, 337
Transcutaneous electrical nerve stimulation, for neuropathic pain, 888
Transdermal fentanyl, 2
Transection, aortic, 216
Transfer, to specialized burn care facilities, 1071
Transfusion, 393–397
adverse reactions to, 398(t), 398–401
AIDS transmitted by, 334, 401
cytomegalovirus infection transmitted by, 401
prevention of, 396

Transfusion *(Continued)*
for anemia, 300–301, 307, 308, 310, 312
for aplastic anemia, 300–301
for autoimmune hemolytic anemia, 307, 308
for cerebral infarction, in sickle cell disease, 325
for cold agglutinin disease, 308
for disseminated intravascular coagulopathy, 343
in relapsing fever, 116–117
for erythroblastosis fetalis, 333
for hemolytic anemia, 307, 308, 310
in fetus or newborn, 333
for hemophilia, 336(t), 337
in patient with factor VIII inhibitors, 338
for hepatic crisis, in sickle cell disease, 323
for hyperbilirubinemia, in newborn, 333, 972, 975
for hypovolemic shock, in newborn, 971
for leukemia-related blood dyscrasias, 362, 369
for malaria, 95
for megaloblastic anemia, 312
for sickle cell disease, 323, 325, 325(t)
for thalassemia, 316
for thrombocytopenia, 342(t)
for thrombotic thrombocytopenic purpura, 345
for vaginal bleeding, in pregnant patient, 942, 943
for warm antibody autoimmune hemolytic anemia, 307
graft-versus-host disease due to, 400
prevention of, 396
hepatitis transmitted by, 401, 446
HIV infection transmitted by, 334, 401
infections transmitted by, 334, 401, 446
iron overload due to, 316, 401
massive, complications of, 400–401
purpura following, 341, 400
thrombocytopenia due to, 341
viral infections transmitted by, 334, 401, 446
Transfusion reactions, 398(t), 398–401
Transient hypertension, in pregnancy, 945
Transient hypothyroidism, 579–580
Transient ischemic attack, and vestibulopathy, 840(t)
management of, 800(t). See also *Stroke syndrome.*
Transient neonatal myasthenia gravis, 862
Transitional cell carcinoma, of urinary collecting system, 652–653
Transjugular intrahepatic portosystemic shunt, for bleeding esophageal varices, 415, 415(t), 416
Transluminal angioplasty, for occlusive disease of lower extremity arteries, 293
Transplacental hemorrhage, and Rh isoimmunization, 329–334
Transplantation, autologous pancreatic tissue, for pancreatitis, 469
bone marrow, for aplastic anemia, 301
for hemolytic anemia, 311
for leukemia, 363, 364, 367, 371
for multiple myeloma, 383, 384, 385
for thalassemia, 317
heart, for congestive heart failure, 257
for hypoplastic left heart syndrome, 246
islet cell (autologous), for pancreatitis, 469

Transplantation *(Continued)*
kidney, 648
blastomycosis following, 170
liver, indications for, 413, 416
lung, for chronic obstructive pulmonary disease, 155(t), 156
pancreas, for diabetes mellitus, 490
for pancreatitis, 469
Transposition of great arteries, repair of, 246
Transudative pleural effusion, 170, 170(t)
Transurethral prostate surgery, 630–631
Tranylcypromine, for depression, 1058(t)
for panic disorder, 1065
Trauma, burn, 1067–1073
caustic/corrosive, 422, 1069–1070, 1106–1108
contact with marine animals and, 1082–1084
diabetes insipidus following, 562
sports-related, 929(t), 929–932, 930(t), 931(t)
stress disorder following, 1046
to ankle, sports-related, 930
to aorta, 216
to bladder, 624–625
to brain. See *Trauma, to head.*
to elbow, overuse and, 921, 931
to fingers, sports-related, 931
to foot, overuse and, 921, 932
to genitalia, 626
to genitourinary tract, 623–626
to hand, sports-related, 931
to head, 889(t), 889–895
and formation of subdural hematoma, 830–831, 889
and vertigo, 839(t)
in adults, 889–892
in children, 892–895
to heart, and pericarditis, 291
to heel, overuse and, 921, 932
to kidney, 623–624
to knee, sports-related, 930, 931, 932
to oral cavity, 755
to penis, 626
to pericardium, 291
to scalp, 709, 889
to scrotum, 626
to shoulder, sports-related, 929, 930, 931
to skin exposed to cold, 1076
to skull. See *Trauma, to head.*
to testis, 626
to ureter, 624
to urethra, 625–626
to urinary bladder, 624–625
to urogenital tract, 623–626
to wrist, sports-related, 931
Travelers, diarrhea in, 12, 13, 14(t), 78
malaria prevention in, 97, 98
Trazodone, 1130(t)
adverse effects of, 1060(t)
for agitation, in Alzheimer's disease, 793
for depression, 1060(t)
in Alzheimer's disease, 793
for insomnia, 33
in Alzheimer's disease, 793
for pain, in neuropathic disorders, 888
Trematode infestation, 481(t), 485, 486
Trench foot, 1076
Trench mouth, 757
Treponema pallidum infection, 671–674, 673(t)
and vestibulopathy, 840(t)
in AIDS, 47, 674
Tretinoin, adverse effects of, 705

Tretinoin *(Continued)*
for acne, 704, 705, 784
for actinic keratosis, 734
for chloracne, 784
for keloids, 726–727
for lichen planus, 714
for oil acne, 784
for periorbital hyperpigmentation, 779
for photoaging, 785
for rosacea, 705
Triamcinolone, for allergic rhinitis, 694, 694(t)
for alopecia, 708
for asthma, 24, 681(t)
for bullous pemphigoid, 769
for cicatricial pemphigoid, 770
for contact dermatitis, 782
for cough, in asthmatic patient, 24
for fluorouracil-induced inflammation, 786
for idiopathic guttate hypomelanosis, 781
for keloids, 725
for lichen planus, 723
for lichen simplex chronicus, 776
for myxoid cysts, 725
for post-herpetic neuralgia, 743
for psoriasis involving nails, 723
for scabies, 745
for seborrheic dermatitis, 713
Triamterene, for hypertension, 270(t)
for hypokalemia, in aldosteronism, 571
for Meniere's disease, 842
Triazolam, 1106(t)
for stimulant overdose, 1042
Trichinosis, 133–134, 482(t), 484
Trichloroacetic acid, for lentigines, 780
for warts, 728
Trichomoniasis, vaginal, 1007(t), 1007–1008
Trichostrongyliasis, 481(t), 484
Trichotillomania, 709
Trichuriasis, 482(t), 483, 486
Tricyclic antidepressants. See *Antidepressants.*
Trifascicular block, 235, 236
Trifluoperazine, potency of, as neuroleptic, 1062
Trifluorothymidine, for viral conjunctivitis, in newborn, 64(t), 65
Trigeminal neuralgia (tic douloureux), 862–864
in multiple sclerosis, 854
Triglycerides, 506
elevated serum levels of, 507
treatment of, 509–510
Trimeprazine, for pruritus, 37, 37(t)
Trimethaphan, for hypertension, 273(t)
in patient with intracerebral hemorrhage, 795(t), 796
Trimethobenzamide, for nausea and vomiting, in Meniere's disease, 842
Trimethoprim. See also *Trimethoprim-sulfamethoxazole.*
for *Pneumocystis carinii* pneumonia, in AIDS, 50(t)
for prostatitis, 634
Trimethoprim-sulfamethoxazole, for acute exacerbations of chronic obstructive pulmonary disease, 23
for bacteremia, in salmonellosis, 138
for bronchitis, 175(t)
in patient with COPD, 23
for brucellosis, 62, 63
for cholera, 14(t), 72
for *Cyclospora* infection, 15(t), 480(t), 483

Trimethoprim-sulfamethoxazole *(Continued)*
for cystitis, in female patient, 597
for enteric fever, 139
for enterocolitis (gastroenteritis), in salmonellosis, 14(t), 138
for epididymitis, 609
for granuloma inguinale, 671
for isosporiasis, 15(t), 455, 480(t)
in AIDS, 51
for legionnaires' disease, 191
for meningitis, 101(t), 102(t)
for neutropenia and infection, in leukemia, 369
for osteomyelitis, 928(t)
for otitis media, 173(t)
for pertussis, 144–145
for *Pneumocystis carinii* pneumonia, in AIDS, 50(t)
for prostatitis, 634
for pyelonephritis, in female patient, 598
for salmonellosis, 14(t), 138, 139, 141(t), 928(t)
in carrier patient, 140
for shigellosis, 14(t)
for traveler's diarrhea, 14(t)
for typhoid fever, 141(t)
for urinary tract infection, in female patient, 597
in male patient, 595(t)
for Whipple's disease, 455
for whooping cough, 144–145
Trimethoprim-sulfamethoxazole prophylaxis, for cystitis, in female patient, 597, 621
for *Pneumocystis carinii* pneumonia, in AIDS, 50(t)
for toxoplasmosis, 133
Trimipramine, 1130(t)
for depression, 1058(t)
for depression with insomnia, 34
for insomnia, in depression, 34
Tripelennamine, for allergic rhinitis, 693(t)
Trisulfapyrimidine, for toxoplasmosis, 131
Trochanteric bursitis, 921
Tropical sprue, 454–455
Trypanosomiasis, 747–748
Tsetse fly bite, and trypanosomiasis, 747
Tubal pregnancy, 940
Tubal sterilization, 1034–1035
Tuberculoid leprosy, 87
Tuberculosis, 207–209, 208(t), 209(t), *210*
acquired immunodeficiency syndrome and, 45–46, 46(t), 207, 208
silicosis and, 201
Tuberculous pericarditis, 291
Tube thoracostomy, delivery of heated solution via, in warming of hypothermic patient, 1075
Tularemia, 134–136
Tumor(s), ACTH-secreting, 554, 555, 556, 557
aldosterone-secreting, 570, 571, 571(t), 572
arsenic ingestion and, 734
catecholamine-secreting, 588–592, 649
chemotherapy for. See *Chemotherapy*.
gastrin-secreting, 457
germ cell, of testis, 657–658
growth hormone–secreting, 548–550
Hodgkin's disease treatment and, 354, 359
malignant. See *Cancer*; specific types.
of adrenal gland, 648–649
and aldosteronism, 570, 571, 571(t), 572
Tumor(s) *(Continued)*
and Cushing's syndrome, 554, 556
and excess catecholamine production, 588–592, 649
of Bartholin's gland, 1025–1026
of bladder, 652–653
of brain, 829–830, 895–900
headache associated with, 829, 830
of breast, 979–989
of buccal mucosa, 753–754
of cervix, 1018–1021
of colon, 476–479
risk factors for, 432, 476
of endometrium, 1015–1018
of esophagus, 421
of floor of mouth, 757
of genitourinary tract, 648–658
of kidney, 649–652
of larynx, 32–33
of lip, 752
of liver, cirrhosis and, 412–413
porphyria and, 393
viral hepatitis and, 412, 445
of lung, 156–163
of meninges, 830, 898
headache associated with, 830
of mouth, 752, 753, 754, 756, 757
of pancreas, 465
of penis, 656–657
of pituitary gland, and acromegaly, 548–550
and amenorrhea, 997
and Cushing's disease, 554, 555, 556, 557
and hyperprolactinemia, 575–577
of prostate, 653–656
of rectum, 476–479
of salivary glands, 754
of scrotum, 658
of skin, 377–382, 709–711, 731–733
premalignant, 733–736
recognition of malignant transformation of, mnemonic for, 732, 735
sun exposure and, 786
of stomach, 472–475
of testis, 657–658
of thymus, 856, 861
of thyroid, 584–587
thyroiditis in area of, 594
of tongue, 756
of upper urinary tract, 652
of urethra, 653
of urinary bladder, 652–653
of urogenital tract, 648–658
of uterine cervix, 1018–1021
of uterus, 1014–1018
of vulva, 1021–1026, 1022(t), 1024(t)
papillomavirus infection and, 727, 1023
pemphigus associated with, 768
polycythemia treatment and, 388
prolactin-secreting, 575–577
radiation therapy for. See *Radiation therapy*.
surgery for. See *Surgery, for tumors*.
Tumor lysis syndrome, 368, 372
Twenty-nail dystrophy, 723–724
Twins, delivery of, 950
Two-rescuer cardiopulmonary resuscitation, 224(t)
Type I diabetes mellitus, 487, 489–490, 493–499
hereditary hemochromatosis and, 346
Type II diabetes mellitus, 487, 490–492
Typhoidal tularemia, 135, 136
Typhoid fever, 140–142, 141(t)
Typhus fevers, 142–143, 143(t)

Ulcer(s). See also *Ulcerative* entries.
aphthous, 752–753
cutaneous, 758(t), 758–762
leishmaniasis and, 86
sickle cell disease and, 324
tularemia and, 135
decubitus, 759–762
duodenal, 469–472
Helicobacter pylori infection and, 469, 471–472
NSAID-induced, 469, 472
gastric, 469–472
Helicobacter pylori infection and, 469, 472
malignant, 474
NSAID-induced, 469, 472
genital, 666
leg, 758(t), 758–759
sickle cell disease and, 324
oral, 752–753, 755, 756, 757
oropharyngeal, tularemia and, 135
peptic, 9, 469–472
Helicobacter pylori infection and, 469, 471–472
medications for, 9, 470–472
NSAID-induced, 469, 472
surgery for, 472
bile reflux gastritis following, 443
pressure, 759–762
venous (stasis), 758–759
Ulcerative colitis, 426–433, 429(t)
Ulcerative gingivitis, acute necrotizing, 757
Ulcerative jejunoileitis, idiopathic chronic, 456
Ulceroglandular tularemia, 135
Ulnar neuropathies, 880
Ultrafiltration, for renal failure, 640
Ultrasonography, fetal, 331, 936–937, 937(t)
Ultraviolet A therapy, with psoralen, for cutaneous T-cell lymphoma, 380, 381, 382
for psoriasis, 713, 723
for vitiligo, 781
Ultraviolet B therapy, for pruritus, 37
Uncorrected congenital heart disease, effects of, 248
Ungual lesions, 721–725, 750
Unna boot, for stasis ulcer, 759
Unstable angina pectoris, 218–219, 221
Upper extremity, deep venous thrombosis in, 296, 297
Upper respiratory tract, infections of, symptomatic treatment of, 28(t), 29–30
surgery of, prophylaxis against endocarditis in, 119(t), 263(t)
Upper urinary tract, tumors of, 652
Ureaplasma urealyticum infection, 669, 670
Uremia. See also *Renal failure*.
Escherichia coli infection and, 11, 344
neuropathy associated with, 884
pericarditis associated with, 291
Ureter(s), calculi in. See *Urolithiasis*.
resection of, for cancer of upper urinary tract, 652
trauma to, 624
Urethra, *659*
cancer of, 653
dilatation of, for prostatic hyperplasia, 631
for strictures, 659–661

Urethra *(Continued)*
dysfunction of, and incontinence, 607–608
inflammation/infection of, 608, 669(t), 669–670, 1011, 1012(t)
obstruction of, due to prostatic hyperplasia, 627, 628
stricture of, 658–661, *660*
trauma to, 625–626
tumors of, 653
Urethral sphincter deficiency, intrinsic, 607–608
Urethritis, 608, 669(t), 669–670, 1011, 1012(t)
Urethrotomy, for stricture, 661
Uric acid, elevated serum levels of, 503, 504, 505
in renal failure, 639
Uric acid stones, 664
Uricosuric agents, 505
Urinary bladder. See also *Urinary incontinence.*
cancer of, 652–653
dysfunction of, 605–607
in patients with multiple sclerosis, 852–853
infection of, in female patients, 596–598, 621
in male patients, 595, 596
irrigation of, in warming of hypothermic patients, 1075
trauma to, 624–625
tumors of, 652–653
Urinary catheter, indwelling, infection associated with, 596, 599
Urinary incontinence, 604–608
in children, 601–604
in patients with multiple sclerosis, 852–853
Urinary retention, in patients with multiple sclerosis, 853
Urinary tract, bacterial infection of, 595–601
and acute-on-chronic renal failure, 644
and bacteremia, 57(t)
in female patients, 596(t), 596–601, 621–622
in male patients, 595(t), 595–596, 621, 669–670
obstruction of, due to prostatic hyperplasia, 627, 628
in chronic renal failure, 644
postmenopausal atrophic changes in, 1004
upper, tumors of, 652
Urine, bacteria in. See *Bacteriuria.*
detection of drugs in, 1040, 1041(t)
elevated calcium levels in, 663(t)
hemoglobin in. See *Hemoglobinuria.*
laboratory reference values for, 1139(t)
Urogenital tract. See also *Genital lesions* (and sex-specific organ entries); *Urinary* entries.
cancer of, 648–658
disorders of, in sickle cell disease, 326
gonococcal infection of, 667–668
surgery of, prophylaxis against endocarditis in, 119(t), 263(t)
trauma to, 623–626
tumors of, 648–658
Urokinase, for acute arterial occlusion, 294
for deep venous thrombosis, 297, 1027, 1027(t), 1028
for pulmonary embolism, 195(t)
Urolithiasis, 661–665, 662(t), 663(t)
Urolithiasis *(Continued)*
sarcoidosis and, 199
Urticaria, 776–779
drug reaction and, 695–696
solar, 786
transfusion and, 399
treatment of, 37, 696, 696(t), 777–779
Urticarial vasculitis, 777, 778
Uterine cervical cap, 1033, 1034
Uterine cervix, cancer of, 1018–1021, 1019(t)
inflammation/infection of, 1011, 1012(t)
Papanicolaou smear of, in screening for cancer, 1018
tumors of, 1018–1021
Uterus, absence of, 996
atony of, 956
bleeding from, dysfunctional, 993–994
cancer of, 1015–1018, 1016(t)
leiomyoma and, 1014
dysfunction of, 998
infection of, bacteremia as complication of, 57(t)
chlamydial, 1011
leiomyomas (fibroids, myomas) of, 1014–1015
leiomyosarcoma of, 1014
resection of, for cervical cancer, 1019, 1020
for endometrial cancer, 1016
for endometriosis, 992
for leiomyoma, 1015
for premenstrual syndrome, 1003
rupture of, in pregnancy, 944
tetanic contractions of, 950
tumors of, 1014–1018

Vaccination. See *Immunization.*
VACOP-B chemotherapy regimen, for non-Hodgkin's lymphoma, 376(t)
VAD chemotherapy regimen, for multiple myeloma, 383, 384, 384(t)
Vagal enhancing maneuvers, effect of, on tachycardia, 238, 238(t), 239(t), 240(t)
Vaginal bleeding, abnormal, causes of, 993(t)
late in pregnancy, 941–944
postpartum, 956
Vaginal delivery, anesthesia for, 949
pain following, 953
Vaginal spermicides, 1034
Vaginitis, 1006–1008, 1007(t)
atrophic, 1004, 1008
Vaginosis, bacterial, 1007, 1007(t)
Valproic acid, 811(t), 1103(t)
adverse effects of, 1060(t)
for Cushing's syndrome, 557, 557(t)
for epilepsy, 808, 809, 810, 810(t), 811(t), 816–817
in pediatric patient, 822, 823
for mania, 1060(t)
for panic disorder, 1066
therapeutic vs. toxic levels of, 1138(t)
Valvular heart disease. See *Mitral* entries and *Infectious endocarditis.*
Vancomycin, allergic reaction to, 699
for bacteremia, 57(t)
for brain abscess, 789, 789(t)
for cellulitis, 740
for *Clostridium difficile*–associated diarrhea, 14(t)
for endocarditis, 259, 260(t), 261
for meningitis, 101(t), 102(t)
Vancomycin *(Continued)*
for neutropenia and infection, 328
in patient with leukemia, 362, 369
for osteomyelitis, 928(t)
for sepsis, in newborn, 970(t)
for toxic shock syndrome, 1010
therapeutic vs. toxic levels of, 1138(t)
Vancomycin prophylaxis, for endocarditis, 119(t), 263(t)
Variant angina pectoris, 219
Varicella-zoster immune globulin, 68, 69
Varicella-zoster virus infection, 66–69, 742–743
acyclovir for, 67, 68, 69
following radiation therapy, 359
in immunocompromised patient, 52, 69, 190, 369, 386
Varicelliform eruption, Kaposi's, 741, 764
Variegate porphyria, 390(t), 393
Varix (varices), esophageal, bleeding, 413–417, *414*, 415(t)
oral, 752
Vasa praevia, 942, 944
Vascular access devices, long-term, in parenteral nutrition, 535, 536, 537
Vascular disease, cerebral, ischemic. See *Stroke syndrome.*
leading to hemorrhage, 797
sickle cell syndromes and, 325
intestinal, portal hypertension and, 407
lower extremity. See entries under *Lower extremity.*
Vascular muscle-contraction headache, 831
Vasculitis, 719–721
cutaneous, 719–721
neuropathy associated with, 886
pericarditis associated with, 291
urticarial, 777, 778
Vasectomy, 1035
Vasoconstrictors, for supraventricular tachycardia, 239(t)
Vasodilators, for hypertension, 273(t), 274
Vasopressin (antidiuretic hormone), for colonic diverticular bleeding, 425
for diabetes insipidus, 560, 561(t), 562, 574–575
for esophageal variceal bleeding, 414
for hemorrhagic portal hypertensive gastropathy, 443
Vasopressinase syndromes, 559, 563
VBAP chemotherapy regimen, for multiple myeloma, 384(t)
VBMCP chemotherapy regimen, for multiple myeloma, 384(t)
VDS-P chemotherapy regimen, for lung cancer, 162(t)
Vecuronium, in management of head trauma, 893, 894(t)
in treatment of tetanus, 130
Vena caval filter, for thromboembolism, 194, 297, 1030
Venereal diseases, 666–674, 1010–1014
Venereal warts (condylomata acuminata), 727, 728, 729, 735, 1023
Venesection (phlebotomy), for iron overload, 347
for polycythemia, 388
for porphyria cutanea tarda, 393
Venlafaxine, adverse effects of, 1060(t)
for depression, 1060(t)
Venom immunotherapy, for insect sting allergy, 702
Venous insufficiency, chronic, 296
Venous thrombosis, deep, 192, 296–298
in female patient, 1026–1031

Venous thrombosis *(Continued)*
prophylaxis for, 195, 297(t)
risk factors for, 192(t), 195(t), 296(t)
treatment of, 297, 1027–1029, 1028(t)
in pregnant patient, 1030
disseminated intravascular coagulopathy and, 343
heparin-induced thrombocytopenia and, 193, 340
nephrotic syndrome and, 610, 612
pancreatitis and, 463
polycythemia and, 388
subclinical, central venous catheter placement and, 537
superficial, 1031
Venous (stasis) ulcers, 758–759
Venovenous hemodialysis, continuous, for renal failure, 640, 640(t)
Ventilation, alveolar, ineffective, 148
mechanical. See *Mechanical ventilation.*
methods of, in cardiopulmonary resuscitation, 224(t), 226
Ventilation-perfusion abnormalities, 147
Ventilatory pump failure (hypercapnic respiratory failure), 147, 148, 149
Ventricle, single, surgery for, 246
Ventricular aneurysm, myocardial infarction and, 283
Ventricular arrhythmias, 237, 240(t), 240–241. See also *Ventricular tachycardia.*
development of, during cardiac rehabilitation, 287, 288
heart failure and, 256
neonatal, 244
mitral valve prolapse syndrome and, 252
nonsustained, 232, 240–241
sustained, 241
Ventricular dysfunction, asymptomatic, management of, 255
heart failure due to, 253
sudden cardiac death due to, 222, 240
Ventricular ectopy, mitral valve prolapse and, 252
premature beats due to, 231–233, 240, 241
significance of, in cardiac rehabilitation patient, 287, 288
sudden cardiac death due to, 222, 227, 232, 252
Ventricular failure. See *Heart failure.*
Ventricular fibrillation, 241
cardiac arrest due to, 222, 223, 225
myocardial infarction and, 283
treatment of, 224(t), 225
in hypothermic patient, 1074
Ventricular filling pressures, raised, in heart failure, 254
Ventricular infarction, 284(t)
Ventricular septal defect, myocardial infarction and, 284(t)
timing of surgery for, 247, 248
Ventricular tachycardia, 241
cardiac arrest due to, 222, 223, 225
cardiac death due to, 232
diagnosis of, in newborn with heart failure, 244
myocardial infarction and, 283
nonsustained, 232, 241
pulseless, treatment of, 224(t), 225
treatment of, 224(t), 225, 241, 241(t)
in pediatric patient, 244(t)
Ventriculostomy, in lowering of intracranial pressure, 891, 893, 894(t)
Verapamil, 1107(t)
for angina pectoris, 221(t)
Verapamil *(Continued)*
for atrial fibrillation, 228(t)
for cluster headache, 836
for hypertension, 277(t)
for migraine, 835
for myocardial infarction, 283, 284
for panic disorder, 1066
for supraventricular tachycardia, 238
for tachycardia, in stimulant-abusing patient, 1042
poisoning by, 1107(t)
Verrucae. See *Warts (verrucae).*
Verrucous carcinoma, of oral cavity, 753–754
of vulva, 1025
Vertebra(e), deformities of, sickle cell disease and, 324
fracture of, ankylosing spondylitis and, 913
osteoporosis and, 522, 523, 524
lumbosacral, limiting stress in region of, 40
Vertebrobasilar insufficiency, and vestibulopathy, 840(t)
Vertigo, 837–841
treatment of, 837–841, 838(t)–840(t), *839*
Very-low-calorie diet, for obesity, 514–515
Very-low-density lipoprotein, 506, 506(t)
high serum levels of, 507
treatment of, in patient with concurrent elevation of LDL levels, 510
Vesicoureteral reflux, in girls with urinary tract infection, 601
Vestibular compensation, 840–841
Vestibulopathy, 837–838, 839(t), 840(t)
Vibrio(s), cholera. See *Vibrio cholerae infection.*
marine, antimicrobials effective against, 1083
Vibrio cholerae infection, 13, 69–72, 75
antimicrobials for, 13, 14(t), 71–72, 75
rehydration in management of, 70, 70(t), 71
stool in, 71(t)
Vidarabine, for varicella-zoster virus infection, 742
Vinblastine, for bladder cancer, 653
for cutaneous T-cell lymphoma, 381
for Hodgkin's disease, 351(t)
for kidney cancer, 651
for lung cancer, 162(t)
for lymphoma, 351(t), 381
for testicular cancer, 658
for urethral cancer, 653
Vincent's infection, 757
Vincristine, for brain cancer, 898
for cutaneous T-cell lymphoma, 381
for Hodgkin's disease, 351(t)
for leukemia, 366, 367
for lymphoma, 351(t), 375, 376(t), 381
for multiple myeloma, 383, 384(t)
for non-Hodgkin's lymphoma, 375, 376(t)
Vindesine, for lung cancer, 162(t)
Vinegar soaks, for lesions due to contact with hazardous marine animals, 1084
Viral conjunctivitis, 65–66, 66(t)
neonatal, 65
Viral croup, 190
Viral encephalitis, 68, 111, 127, 844(t), 844–845, 845(t)
Viral hepatitis, 443–450
cirrhosis due to, 406, 445
hepatocellular carcinoma risk in, 412, 445
immunization against, 447–448, 448(t)
Viral hepatitis *(Continued)*
interferon for, 406, 448–449, 449(t)
transfusion-transmitted, 401, 446
Viral infection, and aplastic anemia, 299
in patient with leukemia, 369
in patient with multiple myeloma, 386
non-HIV, in AIDS patient, 46(t), 51–52
transfusion-transmitted, 334, 401, 446
Viral meningitis, 843–844
differential diagnosis of, 843(t)
Viral nasal infection, 203
Viral neurolabyrinthitis, 839(t)
Viral pericarditis, 291
Viral pneumonia, 68, 80, 189–190
Viral respiratory tract infections, 68, 80, 187–190
and asthma, 679
Viral rhinosinusitis, 203
Viral skin infection, 66–69, 727–729, 735, 740–745. See also specific infections, e.g., *Varicella-zoster virus infection.*
Viruses, food sources of, 75(t)
Visceral leishmaniasis (kala-azar), 83–86, 747
Visual disturbances, migraine and, 833, *833*
Visual hallucinations, levodopa usage and, 876
Visual loss, optic neuritis and, 864, 865
Vitamin(s), deficiencies of. See under specific vitamins.
multiple supplemental, for preterm infant, 975
provision of, in parenteral nutrition, 535(t)
recommended daily allowances of, 518(t)
signs of excess of, in patient receiving parenteral nutrition, 538
signs of insufficient intake/absorption of, 451(t)
Vitamin A, for patient with measles, 128
Vitamin B_1 (thiamine), 518(t), 519
deficiency of, 517, 518(t), 519
for comatose poisoning victim, 1089
for patient with status epilepticus, 818(t)
Vitamin B_2 (riboflavin), 518(t), 519
deficiency of, 518(t), 519
Vitamin B_6 (pyridoxine), 518(t), 519
as antidote, 1097(t)
deficiency of, 518(t), 519
for isoniazid-induced neuropathy, 884
for mushroom poisoning, 77
for premenstrual syndrome, 1002
Vitamin B_{12} (cobalamin), deficiency of, 311, 312
malabsorption of, 311
tropical sprue and, 454–455
need for, in megaloblastic anemia, 312–313
in short bowel syndrome, 458
in tropical sprue, 454–455
repigmentation with, in vitiligo, 781
test for absorption of, 452, 452(t)
Vitamin B supplements, for alcoholic neuropathy, 884
Vitamin C (ascorbic acid), 517, 518(t)
deficiency of, 517, 518(t)
for patient with pressure ulcer, 760
for patient with scurvy, 517, 518(t)
repigmentation with, in vitiligo, 781
use of, with deferoxamine, 316, 347
Vitamin D, for breast-fed infant, 979
for hyper- or hypoparathyroid patient, 568
for patient receiving prednisone, 903

Vitamin D *(Continued)*
reduced synthesis of, in chronic renal failure, 647
Vitamin E (tocopherol), for premenstrual syndrome, 1002
for yellow nail syndrome, 724
Vitamin K, 520
as antidote, 1098(t)
deficiency of, 520–521
patients requiring, 521, 809
use of, in newborn, 521, 979
in patient receiving parenteral nutrition, 534
in patient with cirrhosis, 412
to reverse effects of warfarin, 1029
Vitiligo, 780–781
VMCP chemotherapy regimen, for multiple myeloma, 384(t)
Vocal folds, abnormal closure of, and aspiration, 419
nodules of, 30
paralysis of, 31–32
Vocal tics, in Tourette syndrome, 824
treatment of, 825–827
Vocal tract hygiene, 27–29
Voice care, 26(t), 27, 27(t)
Voice misuse/abuse, 30–31
avoidance of, 26(t), 27
Voiding, dysfunctional. See also *Incontinence.*
in girls, 601, 604
Volume-assist mode, of mechanical ventilation, 150
Volume depletion, in chronic renal failure, 643
Volume expanders, administration of, in newborn, 962, 971
Vomiting, 4–8
anticipatory, 7–8
cancer chemotherapy and, 7(t), 7–8
causes of, 5(t)
delayed, 7
drugs for, 5–8, 6(t), 7(t), 78, 116, 137, 289, 842, 874
induction of, in patient exhibiting allergic drug reaction, 695
in poisoning victim, 78, 1087
signs of, in bulimic patient, 1050(t)
pancreatitis and, 459
Von Willebrand's disease, 335, 336(t)
VP16 (etoposide), for cutaneous T-cell lymphoma, 381
for lung cancer, 162(t)
for multiple myeloma, 384, 384(t)
for non-Hodgkin's lymphoma, 376(t)
for testicular cancer, 658
VP chemotherapy regimen, for lung cancer, 162(t)
Vulvar pruritus, 775–776
Vulvar tumors, 1021–1026, 1022(t), 1024(t)
Vulvovaginitis, 1006–1008

Warfarin, anticholinergic properties of, 1054(t)
Warfarin *(Continued)*
for stroke, 229, 800(t)
for thromboembolism, 195, 296, 1029
hemorrhage risk with, factors potentiating, 194(t)
teratogenic effects of, 1030
use of, prior to cardioversion for atrial fibrillation, 229
Warfarin embryopathy syndrome, 1030
Warm antibody autoimmune hemolytic anemia, 305(t), 305–308
Warming, of frostbitten patient, 1076
of hypothermic patient, 1075–1076
of newborn, 958–959, 965
of patient with cryopathic hemolytic anemia, 308
Warts (verrucae), 727–729, 735
cutaneous, 727–729, 735
genital (venereal), 727, 728, 729, 735, 1023
ungual, 724
Washed red blood cells, 394
Washing instructions, for patient with atopic dermatitis, 763
for patient with impetigo, 737
for patient with pruritus, 36, 776
for patient with varicella, 67
Water exposure, and cercarial dermatitis, 748, 1085
and contact with hazardous marine animals, 1082–1084
and infection by marine vibrios, 1083
and otitis externa, 1084–1085
effects of, on foot, 1076
Water-soluble vitamins. See specific types, e.g., *Vitamin B_6 (pyridoxine)* and *Vitamin C (ascorbic acid).*
Weakness (muscle weakness), sites of, in myasthenia gravis, 856, 860
Weaning, timing of, in infant feeding, 979
Wearing-off phenomenon, with levodopa usage, 875
Web(s), esophageal, 421
Weeping and laughing, in multiple sclerosis, 855
Weight reduction, by hypertensive patient, 267
by obese patient, 512–515
Weight standards, 511, 512(t)
Wet-to-dry compression dressing, for stasis ulcer, 759
Wheelchair, for hemiplegic patient, 805
Whipple's disease, 455
Whipworm infestation, 482(t), 483, 486
White coat hypertension, 264
White matter cerebral lesions, 888
in AIDS, 52
White superficial onychomycosis, 750
Whole blood, 393–394
Whole-bowel hyperosmotic cleansing solutions, 18
in management of poisoning, 1088
Whooping cough, 144(t), 144–146, 145(t)
WHO recommendations, on leprosy treatment, 89
Wilson's disease, 406
Withdrawal (abstinence syndrome). See also *Drug abuse.*
alcohol, management of, 1040
barbiturate, 1104
delirium due to, 1054
narcotic, 1044, 1118–1119
sedative hypnotic, 1045
stimulant, 1043
Withdrawal (treatment termination), steroid regimen, and adrenal insufficiency, 553
Wolff-Parkinson-White syndrome, 229–230
Wood alcohol, poisoning by, 1101–1102
Working Formulation, for classification of lymphoma, 375, 375(t)
Work recommendations, for patient with low back pain, 41
Work-related asthma, allergens causing, 679(t)
Work-related dermatoses, 781–784
Work-related pulmonary disease, 199(t), 199–201
World Health Organization recommendations, on leprosy treatment, 89
Worm infestation, intestinal, 479, 481(t)–482(t), 483–486
Wound cleansing, in management of impetigo, 737
Wound infection, and bacteremia, 57(t)
Wrist injury, sports-related, 931

Xenograft, porcine, for burns, 1072
Xerostomia, 751
radiation-induced, 359
X-linked immunodeficiency, Epstein-Barr virus infection in, 104
Xylene, poisoning by, 1112
Xylometazoline, for common cold, 188

Yellow nail syndrome, 724
Yersinia enterocolitica infection, 16
Yersinia pestis infection, 107–108

Zenker's diverticulum, 418, 422
Zidovudine (azidothymidine, AZT), adverse effects of, 44
for acquired immunodeficiency syndrome, 43–44, 45(t)
Zinc deficiency, in patient receiving parenteral nutrition, 538
Zollinger-Ellison syndrome, 457
Zolpidem, for seizures, 1106(t)
Zoster (shingles). See *Varicella-zoster virus infection.*

ISBN 0-7216-4052-4

L. Arango
Jun '95